369 0246381

Hunter's Tropical Medicine and Emerging Infectious Diseases

The Editors of the ninth edition of Hunter's Tropical Medicine and Emerging Infectious Diseases gratefully and sincerely acknowledge Dr G Thomas Strickland, the past Editor of editions 6 through 8. Dr Strickland has worked tirelessly to create and update a clinically useful textbook of tropical medicine. He continues his contribution to Hunter's as an author of chapters on viral hepatitis and schistosomiasis for the 9th edition. We also extend a special thank you to all our contributors for the 9th edition, a highly talented and experienced group of clinicians assembled from around the world. We also sincerely thank the professional production and editing staff at Elsevier who worked equally as hard as everyone else to complete this 9th edition. Most of all we would like to thank our wives and families who patiently watched and waited as we spent many late nights and weekends working to complete this 9th edition.

Content Strategist: Sue Hodgson/Belinda Kuhn
Content Development Specialist: Nani Clansey
Content coordinator: Kristen Lowson, Sam Crowe, Trinity Hutton
Project Manager: Maggie Johnson/Cheryl Brant
Design: Kirsteen Wright
Illustration Manager: Bruce Hogarth
Illustrator: Antbits
Marketing Manager(s) (UK/USA): Helena Mutak

Hunter's Tropical Medicine and Emerging Infectious Diseases

NINTH EDITION

Alan J. Magill, MD, MACP, FIDSA, FASTMH
COL US Army (retired)
Emeritus, Walter Reed Army Institute of Research
Associate Professor of Preventive Medicine and Biometrics
Associate Professor of Medicine
Uniformed Services University of the Health Sciences
Bethesda, MD, USA

Edward T Ryan, MD, FACP, FIDSA, FASTMH
Professor of Medicine
Harvard University
Director, Tropical Medicine
Division of Infectious Diseases
Massachusetts General Hospital
Boston, MA, USA

David R Hill, MD, DTM&H, FRCP, FFTM (RCPS Glasg), FASTMH
Professor of Medical Sciences
Director of Global Public Health
Frank H. Netter MD, School of Medicine
Quinnipiac University
Hamden, CT, USA

Tom Solomon, BA, FRCP, DCH, DTMH, PhD
Professor of Neurological Science
Honorary Professor of Medical Microbiology
Director, Institute of Infection and Global Health
University of Liverpool
Director, Walton Neuro-Centre NHS Foundation Trust
Liverpool, UK

SAUNDERS

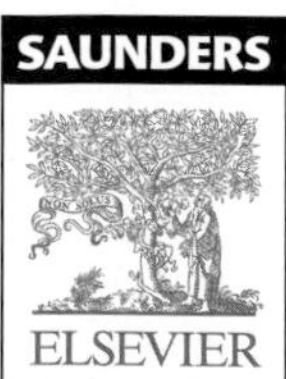

London • New York • Oxford • St Louis • Sydney • Toronto

SAUNDERS
ELSEVIER

An imprint of Elsevier Inc.

First edition 1945
Second edition 1954
Third edition 1960
Forth edition 1966
Fifth edition 1976
Sixth edition 1984
Seventh edition 1991
Eighth edition 2000

Notices

Knowledge and best practice in this field are constantly changing. As new research and experience broaden our understanding, changes in research methods, professional practices, or medical treatment may become necessary.

Practitioners and researchers must always rely on their own experience and knowledge in evaluating and using any information, methods, compounds, or experiments described herein. In using such information or methods they should be mindful of their own safety and the safety of others, including parties for whom they have a professional responsibility.

With respect to any drug or pharmaceutical products identified, readers are advised to check the most current information provided (i) on procedures featured or (ii) by the manufacturer of each product to be administered, to verify the recommended dose or formula, the method and duration of administration, and contraindications. It is the responsibility of practitioners, relying on their own experience and knowledge of their patients, to make diagnoses, to determine dosages and the best treatment for each individual patient, and to take all appropriate safety precautions.

To the fullest extent of the law, neither the Publisher nor the authors, contributors, or editors, assume any liability for any injury and/or damage to persons or property as a matter of products liability, negligence or otherwise, or from any use or operation of any methods, products, instructions, or ideas contained in the material herein.

ISBN: 978-1-4160-4390-4

Printed in China

Last digit is the print number: 9 8 7 6 5 4 3 2 1

Contents

PART 3 BACTERIAL INFECTIONS

Section A Infections of the Eye & Throat

Section B Respiratory Tract Infections

Section C Gastrointestinal Tract Infections

Section E Cestode Infections

PART 7 POISONOUS AND TOXIC PLANTS AND ANIMALS

PART 8 NUTRITIONAL PROBLEMS AND DEFICIENCY DISEASES

PART 9 VECTOR TRANSMISSION OF DISEASES AND ZOONOSES

PART 10 THE SICK RETURNING TRAVELER

PART 11 LABORATORY DIAGNOSIS OF PARASITIC DISEASES

PART 12 DRUGS USED IN TROPICAL MEDICINE

Preface

Hunter's Tropical Medicine grew out of the urgent need to provide training in tropical medicine to doctors preparing to support the massive American military expeditionary forces assembled during World War II. After America's official entry into the war in 1941, it was quickly apparent that millions of Allied military personnel would be deployed for years to tropical areas of the South Pacific, the China–Burma–India theatre, North Africa and, in smaller numbers, to South America and sub-Saharan Africa. The number of medical doctors who were knowledgeable and experienced in tropical infectious diseases to which they would be exposed was limited to a few specialized medical centers and the US military. It became necessary to educate a large cohort of military medical corps officers very quickly. Much of this training was done at the Army Medical School tropical and military medicine course taught at the Walter Reed Army Medical Center in Washington, DC.

The first edition of this book, entitled *A Manual of Tropical Medicine*, was published in 1945 by three of the course instructors, Colonel Thomas T Mackie, Major George W Hunter III, and Captain Brooke Worth. The focus of the original book was a single small volume of practical information that could be carried by each doctor to his new assignment where they would be taking care of patients often in relatively resource-poor environments. The same authors published a second edition in 1954. Colonel Hunter was joined by co-authors from Louisiana State University School of Medicine for the third, fourth and fifth editions were published in 1960, 1966, and 1976, respectively. George Hunter's contributions were acknowledged by adding his name to the book title in the sixth edition in 1984, edited By G Thomas Strickland, a retired US Navy Captain. Dr Strickland also edited the seventh and eighth editions published in 1991 and 2000, and remains as an important contributor to this edition.

Although much has changed in the more than 60 years since the first edition was published, the current ninth edition of Hunter's Tropical Medicine and Emerging Infectious Diseases (HTM9) retains its primary objective as a concise presentation of practical information on the essential clinical aspects of patient presentation, diagnosis, and treatment of medical conditions found in the tropics. To accomplish this ambitious goal, a highly experienced and dedicated new group of editors has assembled a team of over 250 contributors from around the world. Numerous authors are from the tropics, and most of the authors who are not from the tropics have spent years living and working in the endemic areas.

We have produced a single volume of information with the clinician in mind, focusing on the perspective of a physician taking care of an individual ill patient. Tropical medicine has a long history dating back to the late 1800s when the "germ theory" of disease was applied to the newly encountered diseases of the tropics as seen through the experience of European physicians sent out to new colonial destinations. For the purpose of HTM9, we use the term tropical disease as defined by the World Health Organization to specify a geographic area between the Tropic of Cancer (23.3 degrees latitude north) and Tropic of Capricorn (23.3 degrees latitude south). In practice, the term is often taken to refer to infectious diseases that thrive in hot, humid conditions, such as malaria, leishmaniasis, schistosomiasis, onchocerciasis, lymphatic filariasis, Chagas disease, African trypanosomiasis, and dengue, which are not endemic or are uncommon in temperate latitudes. Increasing human encroachment of tropical rainforests, deforestation, and rising migration, international air travel and tourism to and from tropical regions has led to an increased incidence and emergence of tropical diseases into temperate regions. Thus, we have added the title *Emerging Infectious Diseases* to the ninth edition of this series.

It is our sincere wish that all who use this book find it useful in the care of individual patients and that the knowledge gained leads to improved outcomes for our patients.

Alan J Magill, MD
Edward T Ryan, MD
David R Hill, MD
Tom Solomon, MD
September 2012

List of Contributors

Jose M Acuin, MD
Professor
Department of Otorhinolaryngology - Head and Neck Surgery
De La Salle Health Sciences Institute
Dasmariñas City, Philippines

Rodney D Adam, MD
Professor Emeritus
Infectious Disease Section
University of Arizona College of Medicine
Tucson, AZ, USA
Professor of Pathology,
Clinical Microbiology
Aga Khan University
Nairobi, Kenya

Tsiri Agbenyega, MBChB, PhD
Professor of Physiology
Principal Medical Officer in Child Health
Department of Physiology
School of Medical Science
Kwame Nkrumah University of Science and Technology
Kumasi, Ghana

AM Shamsir Ahmed, MBBS
Deputy Project Coordinator
Centre for Nutrition and Food Security
ICDDR,B
Dhaka, Bangladesh

Tahmeed Ahmed, MBBS, PhD
Director and Senior Scientist
Centre for Nutrition and Food Security
ICDDR,B
Dhaka, Bangladesh

S Asad Ali, MBBS, FAAP, MPH
Senior Instructor of Paediatrics and Child Health
Aga Khan University
Department of Paediatrics and Child Health
Karachi, Pakistan

Gregory M Anstead, MD, PhD
Associate Professor
Department of Medicine
Division of Infectious Diseases
University of Texas Health Science Center at San Antonio
Director
Immunosuppression and Infectious Diseases Clinics
South Texas Veterans Health Care System
San Antonio, TX, USA

George E Armah, BSc, MSc (Ghana), PhD (Osaka)
Senior Research Fellow
Electron Microscopy and Histopathology
Noguchi Memorial Institute for Medical Research
University of Ghana, Legon
Accra, Ghana

Stephen J Aston, BMedSc, MBChB, MRCP (UK), DTM&H
Specialist Registrar in Infectious Diseases
Tropical and Infectious Disease Unit
Royal Liverpool University Hospital
Liverpool, UK

Ronald C Ballard, MIBiol, PhD
Associate Director for Lab Science
Center for Global Health
Centers for Disease Control and Prevention
Atlanta, GA, USA

Elizabeth D Barnett, MD
Associate Professor of Pediatrics
Boston University School of Medicine
Boston, MA, USA

Imelda Bates, BSc, MBBS, FRCP, MD, DTM&H, FRCPath, MA (Education)
Senior Clinical Lecturer in Tropical Haematology
Liverpool School of Tropical Medicine
Liverpool, UK

Charles W Beadling, MD, FAAFP, IDHA, DMCC
Director
Center for Disaster and Humanitarian Assistance Medicine
Department of Military and Emergency Medicine
Uniformed Services University of the Health Sciences
Bethesda, MD, USA

Nicholas J Beeching, MA, BM, BCh, FRCP, FRACP, FFTM, RCPSG, DCH, DTM&H, Hon FCCP (SL)
Clinical Lead
Tropical and Infectious Disease Unit
Royal Liverpool University Hospital
Senior Lecturer (Clinical) in Infectious Diseases
Liverpool School of Tropical Medicine
Liverpool, UK

Michael L Bennish, MD
Senior Associate
Department of Population
Family and Reproductive Health
Bloomberg School of Public Health
Johns Hopkins University
Baltimore, MD, USA
Director
Mpilonhle
Mtubatuba, South Africa

Caryn Bern MD, MPH20
Medical Epidemiologist
Division of Parasitic Diseases and Malaria
Center for Global Health
Centers for Disease Control and Prevention
Atlanta, GA, USA

Frank J Bia, MD, MPH
Medical Director
AmeriCares Foundation
Stamford, CT
Professor (Emeritus)
Internal Medicine
Yale School of Medicine
New Haven, CT, USA

Brian H Bird, DVM, ScM, PhD
Veterinary Medical Officer
Centers for Disease Control and Prevention
Special Pathogens Branch
Atlanta, GA, USA

Allyson K Bloom, MD
Instructor
Massachusetts General Hospital
Department of Medicine
Division of Infectious Disease
Boston, MA, USA

Gerard Bodeker, EdD, EdM MPsych
Adjunct Professor of Epidemiology
Columbia University
Mailman School of Public Health
New York, NY, USA
Senior Clinical Lecturer Public Health
Green Templeton College University of Oxford
Oxford, UK

Robert W Bradsher Jr, MD, FACP, FIDSA
Ebert Professor of Medicine
Vice Chair
Department of Medicine
Director
Division of Infectious Diseases
University of Arkansas for Medical Sciences
Little Rock, AR, USA

Nynke van den Broek, FRCOG, PhD
Reader in Maternal and Newborn Health
Liverpool School of Tropical Medicine
Liverpool, UK

Simon Brooker, DPhil
Reader in Tropical Epidemiology and Disease Control
Department of Infectious and Tropical Disease
London School of Hygiene and Tropical Medicine
London, UK

John T Brooks, MD
Medical Epidemiologist
Centers for Disease Control and Prevention
Atlanta, GA, USA

W Abdullah Brooks, MD, MPH
Head
Unit of Infectious Diseases
Division of Health Systems & Infectious Diseases
International Centre for Diarrhoeal Disease Research
Associate Scientist
Bloomberg School of Health
Johns Hopkins University
Dhaka, Bangladesh

Philippe Brouqui, MD, PhD
Professor
Unité de Recherche sur les Maladies Infectieuses Emergentes et Tropicales
Faculty of Medicine
Marseille, France

Michael Brown, BM, BCh, MRCP, PhD, DTM&H
Senior Lecturer
London School of Hygiene and Tropical Medicine
Honorary Consultant Physician
Hospital for Tropical Diseases
London, UK

Fabrizio Bruschi, MD
Professor
Department of Experimental Pathology, M.B.I.E.
Università di Pisa School of Medicine
Pisa, Italy

Donald AP Bundy, PhD
Lead Health Specialist
Africa Health Program Leader
Human Development Network
The World Bank
Washington DC, USA

Danai Bunnag, FRCP, DTM&H
Emeritus Professor
Faculty of Tropical Medicine
Mahidol University
Bangkok, Thailand

Benjamin Caballero, MD, PhD
Professor
Department of International Health
Johns Hopkins Bloomberg School of Public Health
Baltimore, MD, USA

Michael V Callahan, MD
Division of Infectious Disease
Massachusetts General Hospital
Boston, MA, USA

Aulasa J Camerlin, MA, MPH
Research Assistant
Division of Epidemiology
The University of Texas Health Science Center at Houston School of Public Health
Brownsville, TX, USA

Grant L Campbell, MD, PhD, FACPM
Senior Consultant
Arboviral Diseases Branch
Centers for Disease Control and Prevention
Fort Collins, CO, USA

Jonathan R Carapetis, MBBS, Phd, FRACP, FAFPHM
Director
Menzies School of Health Research
Professor
Charles Darwin University
Casuarina, Darwin, Australia

Enitan D Carrol, MBChB, MRCPCH, MD, DTMH
Clinical Reader/Consultant in Paediatric Infectious Diseases
University of Liverpool Institute of Child Health
Alder Hey Children's NHS Foundation Trust
Liverpool, UK

Eric Caumes, MD
Professor of Infectious and Tropical Diseases
Consultant Dermatologist
Service des maladies infectieuses et tropicales
Groupe Hospitalier Pitié-Salpêtrière
Paris, French

Remi N Charrel, MD, PhD
Associate Professor
Department of Microbiology and Infectious Diseases
Unité des Virus Emergents
Aix-Marseille Université
Marseille, France

Anna M Checkley, MBChB, MRCP
Clinical Research Fellow
The Jenner Institute
Oxford University
Oxford, UK

Mala Chhabra, MBBS, MD
Joint Director
National Centre for Disease Control
Delhi, India

Tepirou Chher, DDS, MDSc
Dental Officer
The Oral Health Office
Preventive Medicine Department
Ministry of Health
Phnom Penh, Cambodia

Charlotte M Chiong, MD, FPCS, FPSO-HNS
Clinical and Research Associate Professor
Department of ORL
University of the Philippines
Manila, Philippines

M Jobayer Chisti, MBBS, MMed
Associate Scientist
Centre for Nutrition and Food Security
Consultant Physician
Intensive Care Unit
Dhaka Hospital
ICDDR,B
Dhaka, Bangladesh

David C Christiani, MD, MPH
Professor of Medicine
Professor of Occupational Medicine and Epidemiology
Harvard University
Boston, MA, USA

Bradley A Connor, MD
Clinical Associate Professor of Medicine
Weill Medical College of Cornell University
New York
New York, NY, USA

Edward S Cooper, MB, FRCP, FAAP
Retired Pediatrician and International
Health Consultant
London, UK

Philip J Cooper, PhD, FRCPath
Reader in Parasitology
Centre for Infection
St George's University of London
Tooting
London, UK

R Richard Coughlin, MD, MSc
Clinical Professor of Orthopaedic Surgery
University of California, San Francisco
School of Medicine
San Francisco, CA, USA

John H Cross, PhD (Deceased)
Professor
Tropical Public Health
Uniformed Services University of the Health
Sciences
Bethesda, MD, USA

Nigel N Cunliffe, BSc (Hons), MBChB, PhD, MRCP, FRCPath, DTM&H
Professor
Department of Clinical Infection,
Microbiology & Immunology
Institute of Infection and Global Health
Faculty of Health and Life Sciences
University of Liverpool
Liverpool, UK

Mark Danta, B Med, DTM&H, MPH, MD, FRACP
Hepatologist and Senior Lecturer in
Medicine
University of New South Wales
Sydney, Australia

Nicholas PJ Day, MA, BM BCh, DM, FRCP, FMedSci
Professor of Tropical Medicine
University of Oxford
Director
Wellcome Trust Mahidol University Oxford
Tropical Medicine Research Programme
Mahidol University Bangkok, Thailand

Paron Dekumyoy, BS (Biology), MSc (Trop. Med.), PhD (Trop. Med.)
Associate Professor
Head of Immunodiagnostic Unit for
Helminthic Infections
Mahidol University
Bangkok, Thailand

Nilanthi deSilva, MD
Professor of Parasitology
Faculty of Medicine
University of Kelaniya
Sri Lanka

Gregory Deye, MD
Investigator
Division of Experimental Therapeutics
Walter Reed Army Institute of Research
Silver Spring, MD, USA

Rebecca Dillingham, MD, MPH, FACP
Assistant Professor of Medicine
University of Virginia
Charlottesville, VA, USA

H Rogier van Doorn, MD, PhD
Consultant Clinical Microbiologist &
Virologist
Oxford University Clinical Research Unit
Hospital for Tropical Diseases
Ho Chi Minh City, Vietnam

Barbara Doudier, MD
Physician, Infectious Diseases Fellow
Assistant Professor
Department of Internal Medicine
Hopital Saint-Joseph
Marseille, France

Michel Drancourt, MD, PhD
Professor of Microbiology
Unité des Rickettsies
Faculté de Médecine
Marseille, France

Françoise Dromer, MD, PhD, F(AAM)
Head
Molecular Mycology Unit and National
Reference Center for Mycoses & Antifungals
Institut Pasteur
Paris, France

Michael Eddleston, MA, PhD, MRCP
Clinical Lecturer
Consultant in Clinical Pharmacology and
Toxicology
Clinical Pharmacology Unit
Queen's Medical Research Unit
University of Edinburgh
Edinburgh, UK

Samer S El-Kamary, MBChB, MSc, MPH, FAAP
Assistant Professor
Department of Epidemiology and Public
Health
Department of Pediatrics
Center for Vaccine Development
University of Maryland School of Medicine
Baltimore, MD, USA

Jeremy Farrar, FRCP, FMedAcSci, DPHil, OBE
Professor
Director of Oxford University
Clinical Research Unit
Hospital for Tropical Diseases
Ho Chi Minh City
Vietnam

Wafaie Fawzi, MBBS, MPH, MS, DrPH
Chair
Department of Global Health and
Population
Richard Saltonstall Professor of Population
Sciences
Professor of Nutrition
Epidemiology and Global Health
Boston, MA, USA

Nicholas A Feasey, BSc, MSc, MBBS, MRCP, FRCPath, DTM&H
Research Associate MLW Laboratory
Lecturer in Medicine
University of Malawi College of Medicine
Blantyre, Malawi

Vanessa Field, MBBS, MRCGP, DTM, DTMH, FFTM (RCPSG)
Associate Specialist in Travel Medicine
National Travel Health Network and Centre
Hospital for Tropical Diseases
University College London Hospitals NHS
Foundation Trust
London, UK

Marc Fischer, MD, MPH
Chief
Surveillance and Epidemiology Activity
Arboviral Diseases Branch
Centers for Disease Control and Prevention
Fort Collins, CO, USA

Susan Fisher-Hoch, MB, BS, MSc, MRCPath, MD
Professor
Division of Epidemiology
Genetic Diseases and Environmental Health
University of Texas School of Public Health
Brownsville, TX, USA

Kevin Forsyth, MD, PhD, FRACP
Professor of Paediatrics
Flinders University
Dean
Royal Australasian College of Physicians
Sydney, Australia

LeAnne M Fox, MD, MPH, DTM&H
Medical Officer
Deputy Team Leader for Disease Elimination
and Control
Parasitic Diseases Branch
Division of Parasitic Diseases and Malaria
Center for Global Health
Centers for Disease Control and Prevention
Atlanta, GA, USA

Arthur M Friedlander, MD
Adjunct Professor of Medicine
Uniformed Services University of the Health Sciences
Bethesda, MD
Senior Scientist
U.S. Army Medical Research Institute of Infectious Diseases
Frederick, MD, USA

Gerson Galdos-Cardenas, MD, MHS, PhD (c)
Research Associate
Global Disease Epidemiology and Control
International Health Department
Johns Hopkins School of Public Health
Baltimore, MD, USA

Hector H Garcia, MD, PhD
Professor
Department of Microbiology
Universidad Peruana Cayetano Heredia
Head
Cysticercosis Unit
Instituto Nacional de Ciencias Neurologias
Lima, Peru

Lynne S Garcia, MS, CLS, FAAM
Director
LSG & Associates
Santa Monica, CA, USA

Anna-Maria Geretti, MD, PhD, FRCPath
Professor of Infectious Diseases and Virology
Department of Clinical Infection, Microbiology and Immunology
Institute of Infection and Global Health
University of Liverpool
Liverpool, UK

Achilleas Gikas, MD, PhD
Associate Professor of Infectious Diseases
Department of Internal Medicine
University Hospital of Heraklion
Crete, Greece

Robert H Gilman, MD, DTMH (LOND)
Professor
Department of International Health
Johns Hopkins Bloomberg School of Public Health
Baltimore, MD, USA

Victor Javier Sanchez Gonzalez, MD, PhD
Medical Director
CJD Mexico
Guadalajara, Jalisco, Mexico

Melita A Gordon, BM MCh, MA, MRCP, DTM&H, MD
Senior Clinical Lecturer
Consultant in Gastroenterology
Gastroenterology Unit
Henry Wellcome Laboratories
University of Liverpool
Liverpool, UK

Richard A Gosselin, MD, MSc, MPH, FRCS(C)
Institute for Global Orthopaedics and Traumatology (IGOT)
University of California
San Fransisco, CA, USA

Stephen M Graham, FRACP, PhD
Associate Professor of International Child Health
Department of Paediatrics
University of Melbourne
Melbourne, Australia

Alison D Grant, MBBS, PhD, DTM&H
Reader in Epidemiology & Infectious Diseases
London School of Hygiene & Tropical Medicine
Honorary Consultant
Hospital for Tropical Diseases
London, UK

James J Gray, PhD, FIBMS, FRCPath
Head
Enteric Virus Unit
Centre for Infections
Health Protection Agency
London, UK

John R Graybill, MD
Professor Emeritus
Division of Infectious Diseases
University of Texas Health Science Center
San Antonio, TX, USA

Bertrand Graz, MD, MPH
Clinical Chief and Assistant Professor
Public Health and International Health
Geneva University
Geneva, Switzerland

Stephen Green, MD, BSc, FRCP(Lond & Glas), FFTM, DTM&H
Consultant Physician in Infectious Diseases & Tropical Medicine
Royal Hallamshire Hospital
Sheffield Teaching Hospitals NHS Trust
Honorary Professor of International Health
Sheffield Hallam University
Co-investigator
NIHR-funded Medical Tourism Project
York Management School
University of York
York, UK

Jeffrey K Griffiths, AB, MD, MPH&TM, FAAP
Director
Global Health
Department of Public Health and Community Medicine
Associate Professor of Public Health, Medicine, Nutrition, Veterinary Medicine, and Civil and Environmental Engineering
Tufts University
Boston, MA, USA

Bruno Gryseels, MD, DTMH, PhD
Director and Full Professor
Institute of Tropical Medicine
Antwerp, Belgium

Duane J Gubler, ScD, FAAAS, FIDSA
Professor and Program Director
Emerging Infectious Disease
Duke-NUS Graduate Medical School
Singapore

Rathi Guhadasan MBBS MRCPCH DTM&H MSc
University of Liverpool Institute of Child Health
Alder Hey Children's NHS Foundation Trust
Liverpool, UK

Aron J Hall, DVM, MSPH
Epidemiologist
Viral Gastroenteritis Team
Centers for Disease Control and Prevention
Atlanta, GA, USA

Davidson Hamer, MD
Associate Professor of International Health and Medicine
Boston University Schools of Public Health and Medicine
Adjunct Associate Professor of Nutrition
Tufts University Friedman School of Nutrition Science and Policy
Center for International Health and Development
Boston, MA, USA

David Harley, BSc, MBBS, PhD, FAFPHM, MMedSc (Clin Epid)
Associate Professor of Epidemiology
National Centre for Epidemiology and Population Health
The Australian National University
Canberra, Australia

Jason B Harris, MD, MPH
Assistant Professor of Pediatrics
Harvard Medical School
MassGeneral Hospital for Children
Boston, MA, USA

Amy L Hartman, PhD
Research Manager
University of Pittsburgh Regional Biocontainment Laboratory
Research Instructor
Department of Infectious Diseases and Microbiology
University of Pittsburgh Graduate School of Public Health
Pittsburgh, PA, USA

Oliver Hassall, MRCGP, MPH, DTM&H
Clinical Research Fellow
Department of Primary Health Care
University of Oxford
Devon, UK

Roderick J Hay DM, FRCP, FRCPath
Professor of Cutaneous Infection
Kings College London,
London, UK

Chris F Heyns, MB, ChB, MMed(Urol), PhD, FCSSA(Urol)
Professor of Urology
Department of Urology
Faculty of Health Sciences
University of Stellenbosch and Tygerberg Hospital
Tygerberg, South Africa

David R Hill, MD, DTM&H, FRCP, FFTM (RCPS Glasg), FASTMH
Professor of Medical Sciences
Director of Global Public Health
Frank H. Netter MD, School of Medicine
Quinnipiac University
Hamden, CT, USA

Martin H Hobdell, BDS, MA (j.o.), PhD
Visiting Professor
Department of Epidemiology and Public Health
University College London
London, UK

Caroline M den Hoed, PhD, MD
Drs, Erasmus MC
Erasmus University
Rotterdam, The Netherlands

Meredith L Holtz, MD
Medical Student,
Atlanta, GA, USA

M Iqbal Hossain, MBBS, DCH, PhD
Scientist
Centre for Nutrition and Food Security
Clinical Lead
Clinical Nutrition Unit
Dhaka Hospital
ICDDR,B
Dhaka, Bangladesh

Peter J Hotez, MD, PhD, FAAP
Professor of Pediatrics and Molecular Virology and Microbiology
Chief, Section of Pediatric Tropical Medicine
Baylor College of Medicine
Houston, TX, USA

Eric R Houpt, MD
Associate Professor
Division of Infectious Diseases and International Health
University of Virginia
Charlottesville, VA, USA

Cynthia R Howard, MD, MPHTM, FAAP
Assistant Professor of Pediatrics
University of Minnesota
Minneapolis, MN, USA

Chien-Ching Hung, MD, MSc
Assistant Professor of Medicine
Department of Internal Medicine
National Taiwan University Hospital
Taipei, Taiwan

Munirul Islam, MBBS, PhD
Associate Scientist
Centre for Nutrition and Food Security
Consultant Physician
Clinical Nutrition Unit
Dhaka Hospital
ICDDR,B
Dhaka, Bangladesh

Elizabeth Joekes, MD
Consultant Radiologist
The Royal Liverpool and Broadgreen University Hospitals NHS Trust
Liverpool, UK

Victoria Johnston, MB B.Chir, MRCP, DTM&H, MSc (epi)
Clinical Research Fellow
Department of Infectious and Tropical Diseases
London School of Hygiene and Tropical Medicine,
London, UK

Sam Kampondeni, MB, CHB, M.MED(RAD)
Associate Professor of Radiology
University of Malawi College of Medicine
Queen Elizabeth Central Hospital
Blantyre, Malawi

Gagandeep Kang, MD, PhD, FRCPath
Professor of Microbiology
The Wellcome Trust Research Laboratory
Department of Gastrointestinal Sciences
Christian Medical College
Vellore, India

Powel Kazanjian, MD
Professor and Chief of Infectious Disease
University of Michigan Health Center
Ann Arbor, MI, USA

Jay S Keystone, MD, MSc (CTM), FRCPC
Professor of Medicine
University of Toronto
Tropical Disease Unit
Toronto General Hospital
Toronto, Ontario, Canada

Wasif Ali Khan, MBBS, MHS
Associate Scientist
International Centre for Diarrhoeal Disease Research
Dhaka, Bangladesh

Arthur Y Kim, MD
Assistant Professor of Medicine
Harvard Medical School
Division of Infectious Diseases
Massachusetts General Hospital
Boston, MA, USA

Christopher L King, MD, PhD
Professor of International Health, Medicine and Pathology
Center for Global Health and Diseases
Case Western Reserve University
Veteran Affairs Medical Center
Cleveland, OH, USA

Amy D Klion, MD
Investigator
Eosinophil Pathology Unit
Laboratory of Parasitic Diseases
National Institutes of Health
Bethesda, MD, USA

Richard Knight, BA, BM, BCh, FRCP(E)
Professor of Clinical Neurology
National CJD Surveillance Unit
Western General Hospital
Edinburgh, UK

Peter James Krause, MD
Senior Research Scientist
Department of Epidemiology and Public Health
Yale School of Medicine
New Haven, CT, USA

Sanjeev Krishna, MA, BMBCh, FRCP, DPhil, ScD, FMedSci
Professor of Molecular Parasitology and Medicine
Division of Cellular and Molecular Medicine
Centre for Infection
St. George's University of London,
London, UK

Ernst J Kuipers, MD, PhD
Professor of Medicine
Chief
Department of Gastroenterology & Hepatology and Internal Medicine
Erasmus MC
Rotterdam, The Netherlands

Angelle D LaBeaud, MD, MS
Assistant Scientist
Associate Physician
Children's Hospital Oakland Research Institute
Oakland, CA, USA

David G Lalloo, MB, BS, MD, FRCP, FFTM, RCPSGlas
Professor of Tropical Medicine
Liverpool School of Tropical Medicine
Liverpool, UK

Xavier De Lamballerie, MD, PhD
Professor of Medicine
Faculté de Médecine
Universite de la Mediterranee (Aix-Marseille II) & IRD
Marseille, France

Saba Lambert, MBChB
Clinical Researcher
London School of Hygiene and Tropical Medicine
London, UK

Regina C LaRocque, MD, MPH
Assistant Professor of Medicine
Harvard Medical School
Massachusetts General Hospital
Boston, MA, USA

John Lawrenson, FCP(SA)
Consultant Cardiologist
Department of Paediatrics and Child Health
Stellenbosch University
Department of Paediatrics and Child Health
Stellenbosch University
Cape Town, South Africa

Myron M Levine, MD, DTPH
Professor of Medicine
University of Maryland School of Science
Baltimore, MD, USA

Daniel H Libraty, MD
Associate Professor of Medicine
Department of Medicine
University of Massachusetts Medical School
Worcester, MA, USA

Diana NJ Lockwood, BSc, MD, FRCP
Professor of Tropical Medicine
London School of Hygiene and Tropical Medicine
Consultant Physician & Leprologist
Hospital for Tropical Diseases
London, UK

Kinke M Lommerse, MD, MPhil
Department of Psychiatry
VU University Medical Centre and GGZ inGeest
Amsterdam, the Netherlands

Olivier Lortholary, MD, PhD
Service des Maladies Infectieuses et Tropicales
Hôpital Necker-Enfants maladies
Université Paris Descartes
Centre d'Infectiologie Necker-Pasteur, IHU Imagine
Paris, France

Rogelio López-Vélez, MD, DTM&H, CTropMed®, PhD
Head
Tropical Medicine & Clinical Parasitology
Infectious Diseases Department
Ramón y Cajal Hospital
Associate Professor of Medicine
Alcala University
Madrid, Spain

Benjamin A Lopman, PhD
Epidemiologist
Division of Viral Diseases/National Center for Immunization and Respiratory Diseases
Centers for Disease Control and Prevention
Atlanta, GA, USA

David Mabey, DM, FRCP
Professor of Communicable Diseases
London School of Hygiene & Tropical Medicine
Honorary Consultant Physician
Hospital for Tropical Diseases
London, UK

Alan J. Magill, MD, MACP, FIDSA, FASTMH
COL US Army (retired)
Emeritus, Walter Reed Army Institute of Research
Associate Professor of Preventive Medicine and Biometrics
Associate Professor of Medicine
Uniformed Services University of the Health Sciences
Bethesda, MD, USA

Ciro Maguiña, MD
Full Professor of Medicine
Deputy Director
Instituto de enfermedades tropicales "Alexander Von Humboldt"
Universidad Peruana Cayetano Heredia
Lima, Peru

Syed Faisal Mahmood, DABIM, DABIM (ID)
Assistant Professor, Infectious Diseases
Department of Medicine
The Aga Khan University Hospital
Karachi, Pakistan

Kathryn Maitland, MD, MRCPaeds, PhD
Senior Lecturer in International Child Health
Kemri Wellcome Trust Programme
Kilifi, Kenya

Hadi Manji, MA, MD, FRCP
Consultant Neurologist and Honorary Senior Lecturer
National Hospital for Neurology
London, UK

Barbara J Marston, MD
Medical Officer
Global Aids Program
Atlanta, GA, USA

Anu Mathew, BHB, MBChB
Researcher
Population Health Unit
Centre for Eye Research Australia
Melbourne, Australia

Christine E Mathews, MPH
Doctoral Student
University of Texas School of Public Health
Brownsville Regional Campus
Brownsville, TX, USA

Max Maurin, MD, PhD
Professor of Clinical Microbiology
Centre Hospitalier Universitaire de Grenoble
Grenoble, France

Paola J Maurtua-Neumann, MD
Pediatric Infectious Diseases Fellow.
Tulane University Medical Center
New Orleans, LA, USA

Philippe Mayaud, MD, MSc
Reader in Infectious Diseases and Reproductive Health
London School of Hygiene & Tropical Medicine
London, UK

Bongani M Mayosi, DPhil, FCP(SA), FRCP, FACC, FESC
Professor of Medicine and Physician-in-Chief,
Groote Schuur Hospital and University of Cape Town,
Department of Medicine,
Groote Schuur Hospital,
Cape Town, South Africa

Joseph B McCormick, MD, MS
Regional Dean
James H. Steele Professor of Epidemiology
Brownsville Regional Campus
University of Texas School of Public Health
Brownsville, TX, USA

Stephen McKew, MBChB, MRCP, MRCPath
Clinical Research Fellow
Liverpool School of Tropical Medicine
Liverpool, UK

Susan LF McLellan, MD, MPH
Associate Professor of Clinical Medicine (SOM)
Clinical Associate Professor of Tropical Medicine (SPHTM)
Tulane University School of Medicine
New Orleans, LA, USA

Peter C McMinn, MB,BS, BMedSc (Hons), PhD, FRCPA FRCPath
Bosch Chair of Infectious Diseases
Sydney Medical School
The University of Sydney
Sydney, Australia

Joseph D Mega, MD, MPH
Resident Physician
Contra Costa Family Medicine Residency Program
Martinez, CA, USA

Donald E Meier, MD, FACS, FWACS, FAAP
Professor of Pediatric Surgery
Paul L. Foster School of Medicine
Texas Tech University. Health Sciences Center
Lubbock, TX, USA

Matthieu Million, MD, MSc
Assistant Doctor
Infectious Disease Department
Hôpital Nord
Marseilles, France

Veena Mittal, MBBS, MD
Additional Director
National Centre for Disease Control
Delhi, India

Elizabeth M Molyneux, FRCP, FRCPCH, FRCPCH (Hons), FCEM, OBE
Professor of Pediatrics
Department of Pediatrics
College of Medicine
University of Malawi
Blantyre, Malawi

Susan P Montgomery, DVM, MPH
Veterinary Medical Officer
Centers for Disease Control and Prevention
Atlanta, GA, USA

Pedro Morera, MQC
Full Professor of Medical Parasitology
School of Medicine and Institute of Health Research
University of Cost Rica
San José, Costa Rica

Pedro L Moro, MD, MPH
Logistic Health Incorporated
Meningitis and Vaccine-Preventable Diseases Branch
Division of Bacterial Diseases
National Center for Immunization and Respiratory Diseases
Centers for Disease Control and Prevention
Atlanta, GA, USA

William J Moss, MD, MPH
Associate Professor
Department of Epidemiology
Department of International Health
Department of Molecular Microbiology and Immunology
Johns Hopkins Bloomberg School of Public Health
Baltimore, MD, USA

K Darwin Murrell, MSPH, PhD
Adjunct Professor
Rockville, MD, USA

Osamu Nakagomi, MD, PhD
Professor
Department of Molecular Microbiology and Immunology
Graduate School of Biomedical Sciences, and Global Center of Excellence
Nagasaki University
Nagasaki, Japan

Toyoko Nakagomi, MD, PhD
Associate Professor
Department of Molecular Microbiology and Immunology
Graduate School of Biomedical Sciences, and Global Center of Excellence
Nagasaki University
Nagasaki, Japan

Neha Nanda, MD
Assistant Professor of Medicine
Section of Infectious Diseases
Yale University School of Medicine
New Haven, CT, USA

James P Nataro, MD, PhD
Professor of Pediatrics, Medicine, Microbiology & Immunology, and Biochemistry and Molecular Biology
Center for Vaccine Development
University of Maryland School of Medicine
Baltimore, MD, USA

Eileen E Navaro, MD
Fellow and Instructor
Division of Infectious Diseases
Department of Medicine
University of Maryland School of Medicine
Baltimore
Biotechnology Fellow
National Cancer Institute
Immunocompromised Host Laboratory
National Institutes of Health
Bethesda, MD, USA

Ronald C Neafie, BS, MS
Parasitologist
American International Pathology Laboratories
Silver Spring, MD, USA

Ricardo Negroni, MD
Professor of Microbiology and Parasitology
Consultant Medical Doctor of Muñiz Hospital
Buenos Aires, Argentina

Ann M Nelson, MD
Medical Officer
Infectious Disease and AIDS Pathology
Joint Pathology Center
Silver Spring, MD, USA

Paul N Newton, BM, BCh, D.Phil, MRCP, DTM&H
Reader in Tropical Medicine
University of Oxford
Director
Wellcome Trust
Mahosot Hospital
Oxford Tropical Medicine Research Collaboration
Vientiane, Laos

Robert Newton, MBBS, D.Phil, FFPH
Reader in Clinical Epidemiology
Epidemiology and Genetics Unit
Department of Health Sciences
University of York
York, UK

Stuart T Nichol, PhD
Chief
Viral Special Pathogens Branch
Centers for Disease Control and Prevention
Atlanta, GA, USA

Francesca F Norman, MBBS, BMedSci
Tropical Medicine & Clinical Parasitology
Infectious Diseases Department
Ramón y Cajal Hospital
Madrid, Spain

Marcio RT Nunes, PhD
Researcher
Department of Arbovirology and Hemorrhagic Fevers
Instituto Evandro Chagas,
Deputy Director
National Institute for Viral Hemorrhagic Fevers
Ministry of Health
Ananindeua, Brazil

Thomas B Nutman, MD
Head
Helminth Immunology Section
Head
Clinical Parasitology Unit
Laboratory of Parasitic Diseases
National Institutes of Health
Bethesda, MD, USA

Richard A Oberhelman, MD
Professor of Tropical Medicine and Pediatrics
Tulane University
New Orleans, LA, USA

Edward C Oldfield III, MD, FACP, FIDSA
Professor of Medicine
Professor of Microbiology & Molecular Cell Biology
Eastern Virginia Medical School
Norfolk, VA, USA

Eloy E Ordaya, MD
Research Fellow
Instituto de enfermedades tropicales "Alexander Von Humboldt"
Universidad Peruana Cayetano Heredia
Lima, Peru

Christopher D Paddock, MD, MPHTM
Staff Pathologist
Infectious Diseases Pathology Branch
Centers for Disease Control and Prevention
Atlanta, GA, USA

Slobodan Paessler, DVM/PhD
Associate Professor of Pathology
Galveston National Laboratory
University of Texas Medical Branch
Galveston, TX, USA

Ilias C Papanikolaou, MD
Fellow in Pulmonary Medicine,
Sismanoglio General Hospital,
Athens, Greece

Georgios Pappas, MD
Physician
Head
Institute of Continuing Medical Education of Ioannina (ICMEI)
Ioannina, Greece

Luc Paris, MD
Practicien Hospitalier
Biologiste des Hopitaux
Service de Parasitologie et Mycologie
Groupe Hospitalier Pitie-Salpetriere
Paris, France

Philippe Parola, MD, PhD
Associate Professor of Infectious Diseases and Tropical Medicine
Unité de Recherche en Maladies Infectieuses et Tropicales Emergentes
Marseille, France

Christopher M Parry, BA (Hons), MB, BCh, PhD, MRCP, FRCPath, DTMH
Senior Lecturer (Honorary Consultant)
Medical Microbiology
School of Infection and Host Defence
University of Liverpool
Liverpool, UK

Manish M Patel, MD, MSc
Medical Epidemiologist
Division of Viral Diseases
National Center for Immunizations and Respiratory Diseases
Centers for Disease Control and Prevention
Atlanta, GA, USA

Sharon J Peacock, BM, BA, MSc, DTMH, FRCP, FRCPath, PhD
Clinical Microbiologist
Mahidol-Oxford Tropical Medicine Research Unit
Faculty of Tropical Medicine
Mahidol University
Bangkok, Thailand

Rosanna Peeling, BSc, MSc, PhD
Professor of Diagnostics Research
Chair of Diagnostics Research
Department of Infectious and Tropical Diseases
London School of Hygiene and Tropical Medicine
London, UK

Hans Persson, MD
Senior Consultant in clinical Toxicology
The Swedish Poisons Information Centre
Nacka, Sweden

Philip J Peters, MD, DTM&H
Medical Officer
Division of HIV/AIDS Prevention
Centers for Disease Control and Prevention
Atlanta, GA, USA

Jonathan J Phillips, BA
University of California, San Francisco/San Francisco General Hospital
Institute for Global Orthopaedics and Traumatology (IGOT)
San Francisco, CA, USA

Richard O Phillips, MBChB, PhD, FWACP
Consultant Physician
Department of Medicine
Kwame Nkrumah University of Science and Technology
Kumasi, Ghana

Farah Naz Qamar, MBBS, DCH, FCPS
Infectious Diseases Fellow
Paediatrics and Child Health
Aga Khan University
Karachi, Pakistan

Atif Rahman, PhD, MRCPsych
Professor of Child Psychiatry
University of Liverpool
School of Population, Community and Behavioural Sciences
Child Mental Health Unit
Alder Hey Children's NHS Foundation Trust
Liverpool, UK

Jamilla Rajab, MBChB, Mmed (path),MPH
Lecturer and Consultant Haematologist,
University of Nairobi,
School of Medicine,
Department of Haematology,
Nairobi, Kenya

Didier Raoult, MD, PhD
Professor of Microbiology
Unité des Rickettsies
University of the Mediterranean
Faculty of Medicine
Marseille, France

Michael F Rein, MD, FACP, FIDSA
Professor Emeritus of Medicine
Division of Infectious Diseases and International Health
University of Virginia
Charlottesville, VA, USA

Aurélié Renvoisé
Resident
Unité des Rickettsies
University of the Mediterranean
Faculty of Medicine
Marseille, France

Jean-Marc Reynes, DVM, PhD
Head of Virology service
Centre Pasteur du Cameroun
Yaoundé, Cameroon

Frank O Richards Jr, MD
Director
River Blindness Program
The Carter Center
Atlanta, GA, USA

John Richens, MD
Clinical Specialist in STIs & HIV
Course Organizer for MSc in STIs & HIV
UCL Research Department of Infection and Population Health
University College London
London, UK

Anne W Rimoin, PhD, MPH
Assistant Professor
Department of Epidemiology
UCLA School of Public Health
Los Angeles, CA, USA

Robert Riviello, MD, MPH
Instructor of Surgery
Department of Surgery
Division of Trauma, Burns, and Surgical Critical Care
Brigham and Women's Hospital
Boston, MA, USA

Ema G Rodrigues, DSc, MPH
Postdoctoral Fellow
Harvard School of Public Health
Boston, MA, USA

Allan R Ronald, MD
Emeritus Professor Internal Medicine
University of Manitoba
Winnipeg, Canada

Benjamin M Rosenthal, SD
Research Zoologist
Agricultural Research Service
US Department of Agriculture
Beltsville, MD, USA

David Rosmarin, MD
Instructor in Dermatology,
Department of Dermatology,
Harvard Medical School,
Boston, MA, USA

Ernesto Ruiz-Tiben, MS, PhD
Director
Dracunculiasis Eradication
The Carter Center
Tucker, GA, USA

Edward T Ryan, MD, FACP, FIDSA, FASTMH
Professor of Medicine
Harvard University
Director, Tropical Medicine
Division of Infectious Diseases
Massachusetts General Hospital
Boston, MA, USA

Debasish Saha, MBBS,MS
Clinical Epidemiologist
Medical Research Council (UK) Laboratories
Banjul, The Gambia

Arturo Saavedra, MD, PhD
Instructor in Dermatology,
Department of Dermatology,
Harvard Medical School,
Boston, MA, USA

Peter M Schantz VMD, PhD
Department of Global Health
Rollins School of Public Health
Emory University
Atlanta, GA, USA

Tony Schountz, PhD
Associate Professor of Microbiology
University of Northern Colorado
Greeley, CO, USA

Sandra K Schumacher, MD, MPH
Pediatric Infectious Diseases Fellow
Maxwell Finland Laboratory for Infectious Diseases
Boston Medical Center
Boston, MA, USA

James J Sejvar, MD
Neuroepidemiologist
Division of High-Consequence Pathogens and Pathology
National Center for Emerging and Zoonotic Infectious Diseases
Centers for Disease Control and Prevention
Atlanta, GA, USA

Aisha Sethi, MD
Assistant Professor of Medicine
Associate Residency Program Director
Section of Dermatology
University of Chicago
Chicago, IL, USA

Kwonjune J Seung, MD
Associate Physician
Division of Global Health Equity
Brigham and Women's Hospital
Boston, MA, USA

Om Prakash Sharma, MD, FRCP, DTM&H
Professor of Medicine,
LAC and USC Medical Center,
Los Angeles, CA, USA

Trueman W Sharp, CAPT, MC, USN (MD, MPH)
Chair,
Department of Military and Emergency Medicine
Uniformed Services University of the Health Sciences,
Bethesda, MD, USA

Anuraj H Shankar, DSc
Senior Research Scientist
Harvard School of Public Health-Nutrition Department
Boston, MA, USA

Sonya S Shin, MD, MPH
Assistant Professor
Harvard University
Associate Physician
Division of Infectious Diseases
Division of Global Health Equity
Brigham and Women's Hospital
Boston, MA, USA

David R Shlim, MD
Medical Director
Jackson Hole Travel and Tropical Medicine
Jackson, WY, USA

Nicholas J van Sickels, MD
Fellow
Tulane University
Section of Infectious Diseases
New Orleans, LA, USA

Freddy Sitas, BSc, MSC(MED), MSc(Epidemiology), D. Phil
Director
Cancer Research Division
Cancer Council New South Wales
NSW, Australia

Thomas L Snelling, BMBS(Hons.), DTM&H GDipClinEpid FRACP
Research Scholar
Menzies School of Health Research
Research Scholar
Charles Darwin University
Casuarina, Australia

Cristina Socolovschi, MD, PhD
Graduated Medical Doctor
Infectious Diseases and Tropical Medicine,
Unité de Recherche en Maladies Infectieuses et Tropicales Emergentes
Marseille, France

Tom Solomon, BA, BM BCh, FRCP, DCH, DTMH, PhD
Professor of Neurological Science
Honorary Professor of Medical Microbiology
Institute of Infection and Global Health
University of Liverpool
Director
Walton Neuro-Centre NHS Foundation Trust
Liverpool, UK

J Erin Staples, MD, PhD
Medical Epidemiologist
Centers for Disease Control and Prevention
Fort Collins, CO, USA

Robert C Stewart, MRCPsych
Lecturer in Psychiatry
College of Medicine
Department of Community Health
University of Malawi
Blantyre, Malawi

August Stich, MD, MSc (Clin.Trop.Med.), DTM&H
Professor of Tropical Medicine
Head of Department
Medical Mission Hospital
Wuerzburg, Germany

G Thomas Strickland, MD, PhD, DCMT, FACP
Professor of Epidemiology and Preventive Medicine
Professor of Microbiology and Immunology
International Health Division
Department of Epidemiology and Preventive Medicine
University of Maryland School of Medicine
Baltimore, MD, USA

Kathryn N Suh, MD, FRCPC
Assistant Professor of Medicine
University of Ottawa
Ottawa, Canada

Andreas Suhrbier, BA, MA, PhD
Principal Research Fellow
Queensland Institute of Medical Research
Professor
Griffith Medical Research College
Griffith University
Queensland, Australia

Khuanchai Supparatpinyo, MD
Professor of Infectious Disease
Department of Medicine
Faculty of Medicine
Chiang Mai University
Chiang Mai, Thailand

Catherine G Sutcliffe, PhD, ScM
Research Associate
Johns Hopkins Bloomberg School of Public Health
Baltimore, MD, USA

Brett E Swierczewski, PhD
Microbiologist
Division of Tropical Public Health
Department of Preventive Medicine and Biometrics
Uniformed Services University of the Health Sciences
Bethesda, MD, USA

John L Tarpley, MD, FWACS, FACS
Professor of Surgery and Anesthesiology
Vanderbilt University
Nashville, TN, USA

Hugh R Taylor, MD, FRANZCO
Harold Mitchell Chair of Indigenous Eye Health,
Melbourne School of Population Health,
The University of Melbourne,
Melbourne, Australia

Terrie Taylor, DO
University Distinguished Professor
Dept of Internal Medicine
East Lansing, MI, USA
Harold Mitchell Chair of Indigenous Eye Health,
Melbourne School of Population Health,
The University of Melbourne,
Melbourne, Australia

Harry J Thomas, BM BCh, MSc, DLSHTM
Gastroenterology Unit
Massachusetts General Hospital
Harvard Medical School
Boston, MA, USA

C Louise Thwaites, MSc, MBBS, MRCP, MD, LCOM
Researcher
Oxford University Clinical Research Unit
Ho Chi Minh City, Vietnam

Guy E Thwaites, MA, MBBS, MRCP, FRCPath, PhD
Clinical Reader in Infectious Diseases
Kings College London
London, UK

Tejpratap SP Tiwari, MD
Medical Epidemiologist
Centers for Disease Control and Prevention
Atlanta, GA, USA

Phan Van Tu, MD
Virologist
Deputy Head of Microbiology and Immunology
Pasteur Institute of Ho Chi Minh City
Ho Chi Minh City, Vietnam

Angus W Turner, MBBS, FRANZCO
Associate Professor
Lions Eye Institute
University of Western Australia
Perth, Australia

Edouard Vannier, PhD
Assistant Professor of Medicine
Division of Geographic Medicine and Infectious Diseases
Tufts Medical Center
Boston, MA, USA

Pedro FC Vasconcelos, MD, PhD
Chief
Department of Arbovirology and Hemorrhagic Fevers
Instituto Evandro Chagas
Director
National Institute for Viral Hemorrhagic Fevers
Director
WHO Collaborating Centre for Arbovirus Reference and Research
Ministry of Health
Ananindeua, Brazil
Professor of Pathology
Pará State University
Belém, Brazil

Fransisco Vega-López, MD, MSc, PhD, MFTM, RCPSG, FRCP
Cosultant Dermatologist
University College London Hospitals
NHS Foundation Trust
Honorary Professor in Infectious & Tropical Diseases
London School of Hygiene & Tropical Medicine
London, UK

Jorge J Velarde, MD
Pediatrics
Division of Infectious Diseases
Children's Hospital Boston
Boston, MA, USA

Nicholas J Vietri, MD, FIDSA
Assistant Professor of Medicine
Department of Medicine
Uniformed Services University of the Health Sciences
Bethesda, MD, USA
Chief
Bacterial Vaccines Section
Bacteriology Division
U.S. Army Medical Research Institute of Infectious Diseases
Fort Detrick, MD, USA

Govinda S Visvesvara, PhD
Microbiologist
Waterborne Disease Prevention Branch
Division of Foodborne, Waterborne & Environmental Diseases
Centers for Disease Control and Prevention
Atlanta, Georgia, USA

Keyur S Vyas, MD
Assistant Professor of Medicine
University of Arkansas for Medical Sciences
College of Medicine
Little Rock, AR, USA

Katie Wakeham, MBBS
Research Fellow
Medical Research Council
Uganda Research Unit on AIDS
Entebbe, Uganda
University of York
York, UK

Thomas J Walsh, MD
Chief
Immunocompromised Host Section
Pediatric Oncology Branch
National Cancer Institute
Bethesda, MD, USA

Mark H Wansbrough-Jones MB, MSc, FRCP
Consultant Physician
Senior Lecturer in Infectious Diseases
St George's Hospital
London, UK

David A Warrell, DM, DSc, FRCP, FMedSci
Emeritus Professor of Tropical Medicine
University of Oxford
Oxford, UK

Mary J Warrell, MB BS, MRCP, FRCPE, FRCPath
Hon. Clinical Virologist
Oxford Vaccine Group
Centre for Clinical Vaccinology & Tropical Medicine
University of Oxford
Oxford, UK

Haider J Warraich, MBBS
Research Associate
Department of Paediatrics and Child Health
Aga Khan University
Karachi, Pakistan

George Watt, MD, DTM&H
Associate Professor of Medicine
University of Hawaii at Manoa
John A. Burns School of Medicine
Consultant
Faculty of Tropical Medicine
Mahidol University
Bangkok, Thailand

Yupaporn Wattanagoon, MB, BS, DTM&H, Dip. Thai Board Of Internal Medicine
Associate Professor of Clinical Tropical Medicine
Faculty of Tropical Medicine
Mahidol University
Bangkok, Thailand

Dorn Watthanakulpanich, MD, PhD
Medical Parasitologist of Hospital for Tropical Diseases
Faculty of Tropical Medicine
Mahidol University
Bangkok, Thailand

Scott C Weaver MS, PhD
Director
Institute for Human Infections and Immunity
University of Texas Medical Branch
Galveston, TX, USA

Rachel B Webman, MD
Resident
Department of Surgery
NYU School of Medicine
New York, NY, USA

Paul J Weidle, Pharm.D., MPH
Research Support Officer
Centers for Disease Control and Prevention
Atlanta, GA, USA

Louis M Weiss, MD, MPH
Professor of Pathology
Division of Parasitology and Tropical Medicine
Professor of Medicine
Division of Infectious Diseases
Albert Einstein College of Medicine
Bronx, NY, USA

Nicholas J White, DSc, MD, FRCP, F Med Sci, FRS
Professor of Tropical Medicine
Faculty of Tropical Medicine
Mahidol University
Bangkok, Thailand

Christopher JM Whitty, FRCP
Professor
Clinical Research Department
London School of Hygiene & Tropical Medicine
London, UK

Dana M Woodhall, MD
Epidemic Intelligence Service Officer
Parasitic Diseases Branch
Centers for Disease Control and Prevention
Atlanta, GA, USA

Stephen G Wright, MB, FRCP, DCMT
Honorary Senior Lecturer
Department of Infectious and Tropical Diseases
London School of Hygiene and Tropical Medicine
Consultant Physician
King Edward VII Hospital,
London, UK

Ramnik J Xavier, MD
Chief of Gastroenterology
Massachusetts General Hospital
Boston, MA, USA

Lihua Xiao, DVM, PhD
Chief
Molecular Epidemiology Laboratory
Division of Parasitic Diseases
Centers for Disease Control and Prevention
Atlanta, GA, USA

Hongjie Yu, MD, MPH
Medical Epidemiologist
Office for Disease Control and Emergency Response
Chinese Center for Disease Control and Prevention (China CDC)
Beijing, China

Anita KM Zaidi, MBBS, SM, FAAP
Professor of Pediatrics and Child Health
Professor of Microbiology
Aga Khan University
Karachi, Pakistan

PART

1

CLINICAL PRACTICE IN THE TROPICS

SECTION

A

ORGAN-BASED CHAPTERS

1 Tropical Lung Diseases

Ilias C Papanikolaou, Om P Sharma

Key features

- Bacterial pneumonias are major causes of death in the tropics
- Symptoms and physical examination remain crucial for diagnosis and management
- Parasitic infections can manifest as wheezing, eosinophilic pneumonia or a pleural effusion
- Analysis of pleural fluid can help in management decisions
- Common diseases like chronic obstructive pulmonary disease (COPD) can have a different epidemiology and etiology in the tropics than in the developed world

INTRODUCTION

The term "tropics" refers to the region of the earth lying between the Tropic of Cancer and the Tropic of Capricorn. In the tropics, warm climate, poverty, lack of education, and poor sanitation provide an ideal environment for pathogens, vectors and intermediate hosts to flourish [1]. In this vast landmass, respiratory infections are a major cause of morbidity and mortality in children and adults [2]. In a typical tropical clinic, 20–40% of outpatients have respiratory complaints, and 20–30% of inpatients have lung disease (Table 1-1) [2].

Many tropical patients suffer from lung diseases that are found worldwide, e.g. asthma, bronchiectasis, chronic obstructive lung disease, HIV infection-related lung disease, and lung cancer. Numerous dust diseases, e.g. silicosis, asbestosis, byssinosis, hypersensitivity pneumonitis, and diseases due to microbial contamination of agricultural products, remain under-recognized. Diseases associated with pulmonary symptoms and infection that are concentrated in the tropics include malaria, pulmonary schistosomiasis, melioidosis, paragonimiasis, echinococcal cysts, tropical eosinophilia, and diseases related to nutritional deficiencies [3]. In addition, individuals who come in contact with birds or animals may develop zoonoses such as tularemia, psittacosis, Q fever and leptospirosis [4]. In the tropics, indoor air pollution caused by biomass fuels used for cooking and heating of the homes and huts is an important cause of obstructive lung disease and chronic lung infections [5].

The following are the common tropical pulmonary conditions:

- pneumonia: typical and atypical
- eosinophilic pneumonias and tropical pulmonary eosinophilia
- bronchiectasis, asthma and chronic obstructive pulmonary disease (COPD)
- pleural effusion
- nontuberculous granulomatous lung disease
- occupational lung diseases.

A reasonable approach to the patient with lung disease in the tropic starts with age, occupational exposure, physical examination, HIV status, chest x-ray and blood tests. In children, bacterial pneumonia is the most common and life-threatening disorder. Known immunodeficiency suggests tuberculosis, fungi and opportunistic pathogens. Peripheral blood eosinophilia with either a pleural effusion or diffuse parenchymal consolidation may suggest a parasitic infection, or, when combined with wheezing, tropical pulmonary eosinophilia. Worldwide diseases like COPD may affect nonsmoking individuals due to indoor pollutants.

PNEUMONIA

Streptococcus pneumoniae is the most common bacterial cause of pneumonia. Upper respiratory involvement often precedes the onset of pneumococcal pneumonia, which is characterized by fever, chills, malaise and sweating. The patient is flushed and febrile with a rapid pulse and respiratory rate. Dyspnea is associated with a nonproductive cough, and sputum, if present, may be thick, tenacious or "rusty". Severe pleuritic chest pain causing tachypnea and grunting respiration is often present. Such symptoms are abrupt in young, immunocompetent patients (Fig.1.1) [6].

In elderly patients, symptoms may be few and can be dominated by confusion, delirium and prostration [7]. Physical examination of the affected lung, usually the lower lobe, reveals diminished lung expansion, impaired percussion note, decreased breath sounds, crepitations (crackles/rales) and bronchial breath sounds. Cyanosis is common and a herpes simplex eruption may be seen on the lips. With proper treatment, most patients with pneumococcal pneumonia improve clinically and radiographically within 1–2 weeks. When resolution occurs, fever subsides within a week as the temperature decreases following a crisis pattern (Fig. 1.2A). Delayed resolution is seen in smokers, the elderly, and in those with poor nutrition, diabetes or other comorbid illnesses.

Staphylococcal pneumonia (*Staphylococcus aureus*), accounts for 2–10% of acute community-acquired pneumonias. It is an important cause of pneumonia in children, the elderly, patients recovering from influenza, people with diabetes mellitus, and those who are immunocompromised. Methicillin-resistant *Staphylococcus aureus* (MRSA) causes illness in 1% of cases of upper or lower respiratory tract infection in the community and in 10% of patients who are hospitalized. Patients with staphylococcal pneumonia are usually ill with high fever, shaking chills, chest pain, cough and purulent sputum. Chest x-ray films show patchy consolidation and cavities.

INVESTIGATIONS AND MANAGEMENT

Sputum examination is an important aid in the diagnosis of pneumonia. Color, amount, consistency and odor are helpful: mucopurulent sputum is commonly found in bacterial pneumonia or bronchitis; scanty watery sputum is often noted in atypical pneumonia; "rusty" sputum is seen in pneumococcal pneumonia; and currant-jelly or dark-red sputum suggests *Klebsiella pneumoniae*. Foul-smelling expectoration is associated with anaerobic infections due to aspiration,

FIGURE 1.1 (A) World Health Organization algorithm for diagnosing pneumonia in children (*modified with permission from World Health Organization, Family and Community Health Cluster, Department of Child and Adolescent Health and Development. Consultative meeting to review evidence and research priorities in the management of acute respiratory infections (ARI). Meeting report. Geneva: WHO; 2003:1–30.*). **(B)** IMCI (Integrated Management of Childhood Illness) guidelines for treating pneumonia (*modified with permission from WHO/UNICEF. Integrated Management of Childhood Illness (IMCI) for high HIV settings. Geneva: WHO; 2009;11:2.*)

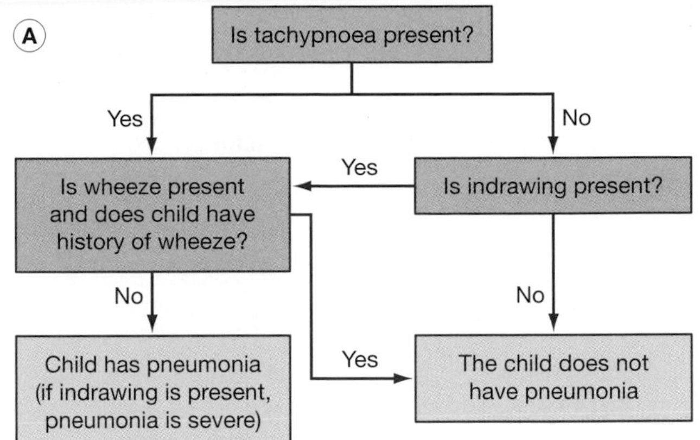

CHECK FOR GENERAL DANGER SIGNS

Ask:
- Is the child able to drink or breast feed?
- Does the child vomit everything?
- Has the child had convulsions?

Look:
- See if the child is lethargic or unconscious.
- Is the child convulsing now?

A child with any general danger sign needs urgent attention; complete the assessment and any permitted treatment immediately so that referral is not delayed.

CLASSIFY

THEN ASK ABOUT MAIN SYMPTOMS:
Does the child have a cough or difficult breathing?

If yes, ask:
- For how long?

Look, listen, feel:
- Count the breaths in one minute.
- Look for chest indrawing.
- Look and listen for stridor.
- Look and listen for wheezing.

} **Child must be calm**

If wheezing and either fast breathing or chest indrawing: *Give a trial of rapid-acting inhaled bronchodilator for up to three times 15–20 minutes apart. Count the breaths and look for chest indrawing again, and then classify.*

If the child is:	Fast breathing is:
2 months up to 12 months	**50** breaths per minute or more
12 months up to 5 years	**40** breaths per minute or more

Classify **cough** or **difficult breathing**

IDENTIFY TREATMENT

USE ALL BOXES THAT MATCH THE CHILD'S SYMPTOMS AND PROBLEMS TO CLASSIFY THE ILLNESS.

SIGNS	CLASSIFY AS	TREATMENT (Urgent pre-referral treatments are in bold print)
• Any general danger sign or • Chest indrawing or • Stridor in a calm child	**Severe pneumonia or very severe disease**	• **Give first dose of an appropriate antibiotic** • **Refer urgently to hospital**
• Fast breathing	**Pneumonia**	• **Give oral antibiotic for 5 days** • If wheezing (even if it disappeared after rapidly acting bronchodilator) give an inhaled bronchodilator for 5 days* • Soothe the throat and relieve the cough with a safe remedy • If coughing for more than 3 weeks or if having recurrent wheezing, refer for assessment for TB or asthma • Advise the mother when to return immediately • Follow-up in 2 days
• No signs of pneumonia or very severe disease	**Cough or cold**	• If wheezing (even if it disappeared after rapidly acting bronchodilator) give an inhaled bronchodilator for 5 days* • Soothe the throat and relieve the cough with a safe remedy • If coughing for more than 3 weeks or if having recurrent wheezing, refer for assessment for TB or asthma • Advise the mother when to return immediately • Follow-up in 5 days if not improving

*in settings where inhaled bronchodilator is not available, oral salbutamol may be the second choice

TABLE 1-1 Incidence of Pneumonia Cases and Pneumonia Deaths Among Children Under 5 Years of Age, by UNICEF Region, 2004*

UNICEF regions	Number of children under 5 years of age (in thousands)	Number of childhood pneumonia deaths (in thousands)	Incidence of pneumonia cases (episodes per child per year)	Total number of pneumonia episodes (in thousands)
South Asia	169,300	702	0.36	61,300
Sub-Saharan Africa	117,300	1,022	0.3	35,200
Middle East and North Africa	43,400	82	0.26	11,300
East Asia and Pacific	146,400	158	0.24	34,500
Latin America and Caribbean	56,500	50	0.22	12,200
CEE/CIS	26,400	29	0.09	2,400
Developing countries	533,000	2,039	0.29	154,500
Industrialized countries	54,200	1	0.03	1,600
World	613,600	2,044	0.26	158,500

*Modified from UNICEF/WHO. Pneumonia: the forgotten killer of children. Geneva: UNICEF/ WHO; 2006, p.13.

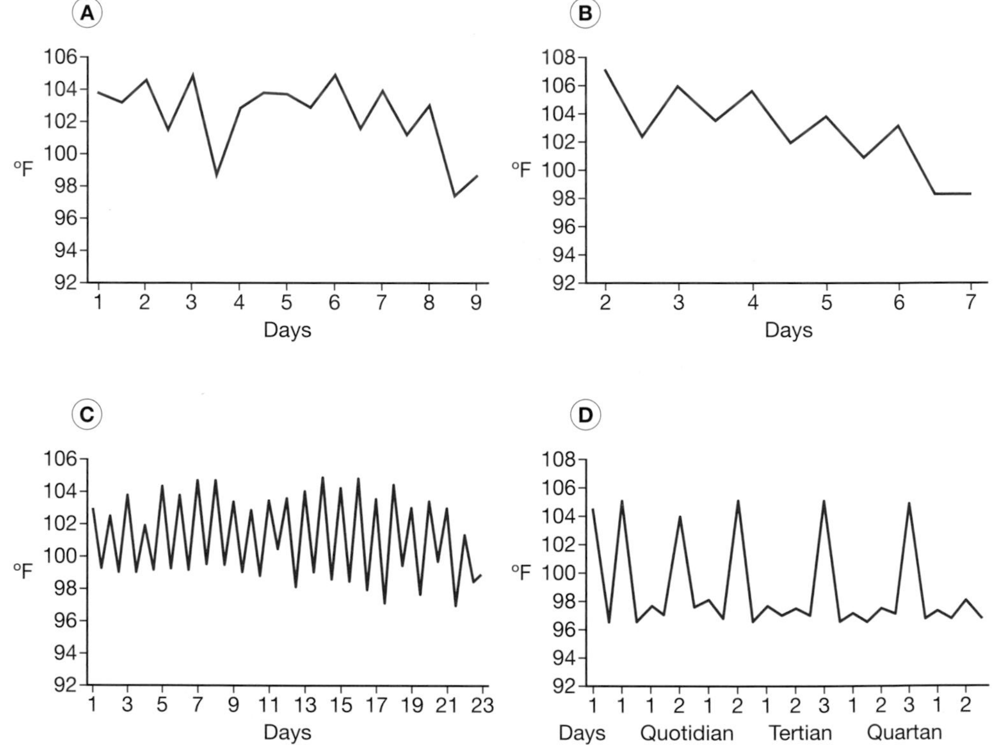

FIGURE 1.2 Various patterns of fever. **(A)** In lobar pneumonia, fever subsides by crisis within a week. **(B)** In bronchopneumonia, fever comes down slowly by lysis and takes longer. **(C)** In tuberculosis, fever is remittent. **(D)** In malaria, fever is typically intermittent.

lung abscess and necrotizing pneumonia. The presence of Gram-positive diplococci indicates pneumococcal pneumonia; small Gram-negative coccobacillary forms are typical of *H. influenzae*, and staphylococcal organisms appear in tetrads and grapelike clusters. In mycoplasma, viral and legionella pneumonia, typical bacterial organisms are not seen. If sputum is not available, a specimen can be obtained by tracheobronchial suction.

A blood count usually reveals leukocytosis in bacterial pneumonia, leukopenia in viral infection, and eosinophilia in parasitic infestation. When available, chest x-ray is extremely helpful (Table 1-2). Tuberculosis is omnipresent in the tropics; upper lobe lesions with or without cavities strongly suggest tuberculosis.

In children, the Integrated Management of Childhood Illness (IMCI) guidelines for treating pneumonia are recommended (see Fig. 1.1) [8]. Nevertheless, a patient's illness has to be assessed based on geography, prevalence of potential etiologies, virulence of the organism, and the drug sensitivity pattern (Box 1.1). In some areas, particularly Papua New Guinea, South Africa and Spain, resistance of the

TABLE 1-2 Clinical Features of Typical and Atypical Common Community-Acquired Pneumonias

	Pneumococcal	Mycoplasma	Viral
Causative agent	*Streptococcus pneumoniae*	*Mycoplasma pneumoniae*	Influenza virus A and B
Fever	Sustained 102–103°F	100–103°F	100–103°F unremitting
Chills	Abrupt onset	In 25%	Chilly sensation not rigors
Cough	Productive	Dry, nonproductive	Nonproductive to productive
Sputum	Purulent, blood-stained, rusty	Mucoid, if present	Scant to purulent, may be blood-stained
Gram stain	Diplococci, lance-shaped, often intracellular	No organisms, many alveolar macrophages	No organisms
Chest x-ray	Lobar consolidation	Diffuse perihilar, patchy infiltrates	Diffuse interstitial, perihilar infiltrates
Typical patient	All ages, high incidence in the elderly and alcoholics	Usually children and young adults	Severe illness in elderly
Complications	Meningitis, empyema	Anemia, Steven–Johnson syndrome, myringitis	Staphylococcal infection

BOX 1.1 Key Facts
Acute Respiratory Infections (ARIs) in Children

- 20% of all deaths in children under 5 years are due to ARIs
- 90% of all deaths due to ARIs are due to pneumonia
- *Streptococcus pneumoniae* and *Haemophilus influenzae* are two top causes of pneumonia
- Low-birthweight, malnourished and non-breastfed children are at high risk of having pneumonia
- High fever, rapid breathing, and retraction of the chest are indicators for hospitalization
- Children with malnutrition and edema should be admitted to hospital

pneumococcus to penicillin is common. For children with non-severe pneumonia, the World Health Organization (WHO) recommends oral trimethoprim–sulfamethoxazole (TMP-SMX) or oral amoxicillin for 5 days [9]. In severe pneumonia in hospitalized children, the policy in low-income countries is to first give benzylpenicillin injections, changing the therapy to oral amoxicillin when the child responds. In very severe pneumonia, in children in low-income settings, chloramphenicol may be given first with benzylpenicillin and gentamicin in combination as an alternative [10,11].

ATYPICAL PNEUMONIA

Atypical pneumonia is caused by *Mycoplasma pneumoniae, Chlamydia pneumoniae, Legionella* spp., viruses, tuberculosis, fungi and parasites. This syndrome is not extensively studied in the tropics because of the expense involved in culturing and isolating various organisms and obtaining serologic and immunologic tests.

Mycoplasma pneumoniae infections occur worldwide, affecting mostly school-aged children and young adults. A typical patient with mycoplasma pneumonia is an older child or young adult with an insidious onset of fever, malaise, tightness of the chest, and dry brassy cough. Constitutional symptoms are out of proportion to the respiratory symptoms. Hemoptysis, pleural pain and gastrointestinal symptoms are uncommon. The tropical physician should be aware of the non-respiratory manifestations of mycoplasma infection, including anemia, myringitis, Stevens–Johnson syndrome, hepatitis and neuritis [12] (see Table 1-2).

OTHER CONDITIONS ASSOCIATED WITH PULMONARY INFECTION

Leptospirosis is common in tropical areas where sanitation is poor and water supply primitive. Epidemics of leptospirosis occur after high rainfall in monsoon seasons when the water supply is contaminated by sewage or animal urine. About half of the patients with leptospirosis have fever, cough, hemoptysis and pneumonitis [13]. Other features are jaundice, conjunctivitis and impaired renal function.

Melioidosis, caused by *Burkholderia pseudomallei*, is endemic in Southeast Asia (Vietnam, Cambodia, Myanmar), northern Australia and West Africa. Melioidosis is hyperendemic in northern Australia, and in parts of northeastern Thailand it is an important cause of fatal community-acquired pneumonia [14]. Patients become infected while wading through fields, paddies, and flooded roads. Clinical presentation is protean and nonspecific. The radiologic picture of upper lobe infiltration and cavity formation can be indistinguishable from tuberculosis [15]. Diagnosis requires isolation of the organism. The mortality rate ranges from 20% to 50% but is higher in HIV-infected and immunocompromised hosts.

Respiratory symptoms of cough and chest pain in typhoid are present in up to 50% of cases at the onset of the disease. Pulmonary infiltrates may be associated with positive sputum cultures for *Salmonella typhi*. A fever chart showing continuous fever is highly suggestive of enteric fever. Diagnosis may be difficult without blood and stool culture facilities.

In brucellosis, the lungs are involved in about 5% to 10% of cases, usually following inhalation of organisms. Abnormalities include bronchopneumonia, solitary or multiple lung nodes, miliary interstitial lung disease, lung abscess and pleural effusion. Organisms can be identified on stains or sputum cultures.

Tularemia is a generalized infection caused by *Francisella tularensis* and occurs after skin or mucous membrane contact with infected mammals or through the bite of an arthropod, usually a tick or biting fly. Diagnosis should be considered in the presence of a skin ulcer associated with fever, generalized lymphadenopathy, cough and signs of pneumonia. Pneumonia, either primary from inhalation of an infected aerosol or secondary to systemic infection, occurs in about 20% of cases.

Pneumonic plague is less common than either bubonic or septicemic disease. Nevertheless, fatal bronchopneumonia can occur without lymphadenopathy and is characterized by watery, bloody sputum. A sputum Gram stain can show bipolar stunted rods. Pneumonic plague and tularemic pneumonia should be considered when a severe, rapidly progressive bronchopneumonia is reported in an endemic area, and "typical" bacterial pneumonias have been ruled out.

In slaughterhouses, meat-processing plants, and areas with sheep and goat husbandry, Q fever (*Coxiella burnetii*) can cause epidemics of atypical pneumonia. Inhalation of dried infected material is the chief source, and fever, headache and dry cough are the main symptoms. Occasionally, the sputum is blood-streaked.

Bornholm disease (caused by coxsackieviruses and occasionally other enteroviruses), also known as epidemic pleurodynia or Devil's grip, causes chest discomfort and cough. Widespread epidemics of Bornholm disease occur in the Pacific islands and South Africa.

In 2002–2003, an unusual coronavirus was responsible for more than 8000 cases of a severe acute respiratory syndrome (SARS) that spread via international travel across continents from its origin in Guandong Province, China. The SARS coronavirus was previously unknown in humans; a possible reservoir was identified in civet cats and raccoons. After droplet inhalation of the virus, there was an incubation period of 2–7 days, then fever, cough, malaise and headache occurred. Pulmonary inflammation was characterized by desquamation of pneumocytes, hyaline membrane formation and acute respiratory distress syndrome (ARDS). The chest x-ray showed diffuse opacities or consolidation, especially in the lower lung fields. Recovery could be slow and some patients developed fibrosis. Mortality was 10–20%, with the elderly and those with cardiovascular problems being especially at risk.

Kawasaki disease occurs in children under 5 years of age. This acute multisystem disease of unknown cause is characterized by fever of 5 days duration and four of five clinical features: non-purulent conjunctivitis; injected (or fissured) lips or pharynx or strawberry tongue; cervical adenopathy; a maculopapular rash; and changes in the extremities (erythema and edema of the palms and soles, associated with desquamation). Pneumonitis occurs in 10% of the children and coronary artery dilatation and aneurysms in 20–25% of untreated cases. In Brazil there has been a seasonal rise of the condition at the beginning and end of the monsoon season [16].

Cryptococcus neoformans and *C. gatti* are saprophytic fungi distributed worldwide and are particularly abundant in soil contaminated by pigeon droppings in the tropics as well as in temperate countries. Pulmonary infection results from inhalation of the organisms from environmental sources [17].

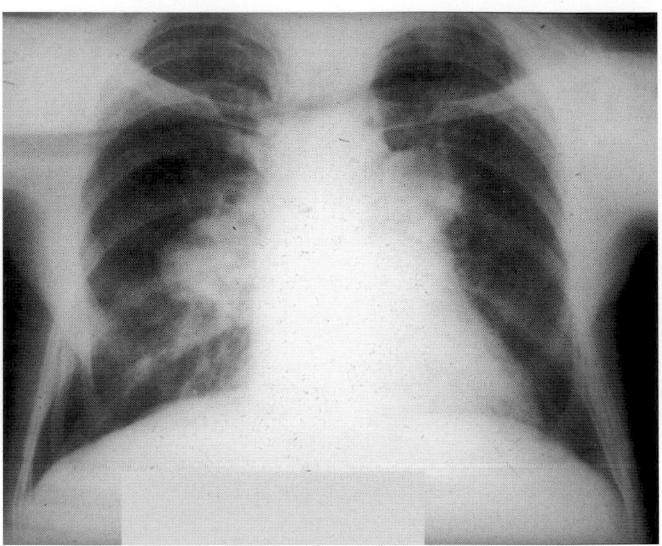

FIGURE 1.3 Bilateral pulmonary arteries dilatation in *schistosomiasis*.

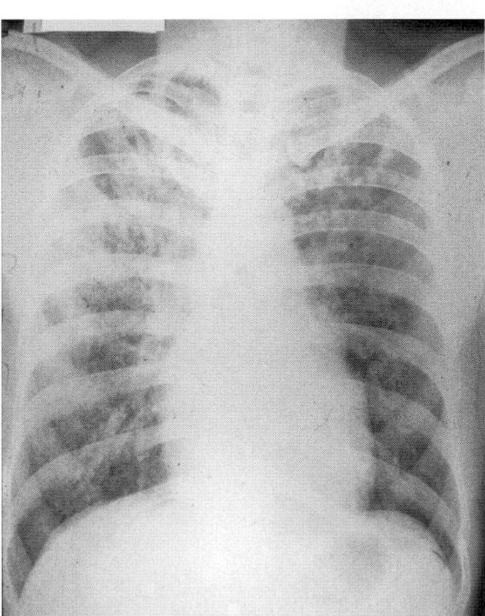

FIGURE 1.4 Predominant bilateral interstitial opacities affecting all lung fields, in a patient with *tropical pulmonary eosinophilia*.

EOSINOPHILIC PNEUMONIAS

Systemic helminth infection usually elicits eosinophilia and increased IgE. Although eosinophilia can be a clue to a pulmonary helminth infestation, the definitive diagnosis requires demonstration of ova or larvae in sputum, bronchial alveolar lavage fluid, pleural fluid or lung biopsy [18]. Loeffler's syndrome refers to "simple" pulmonary eosinophilia with no or minimal systemic and pulmonary symptoms. In many helminth infestations (ascaris, strongyloidiasis, hookworm), the larvae migrate through the lung and can cause fever, cough, dyspnea, wheezing, hemoptysis and lung infiltrate.

Schistosomes cause two clinical syndromes. In acute disease, immature schistosomula pass through the lung, and can lead to fever, eosinophilia and pulmonary infiltrate. In chronic schistosomiasis, especially when portal hypertension has led to venous shunts, eggs can bypass the liver and plug pulmonary capillaries and arterioles, producing granuloma and pulmonary hypertension. Radiographs may show dilated pulmonary arteries (Fig. 1.3).

In paragonimiasis, the lung is the predominantly involved organ. The diagnosis must be considered in a patient from Southeast Asia with cough, hemoptysis (which is recurrent in >80% of cases), a pulmonary cavity and pleural effusion.

Tropical pulmonary eosinophilia, typically in India and other South Asian countries, causes immunologic hyperresponsiveness to *Wuchereria bancrofti*, *Brugia malayi* or other microfilariae. Clinical presentation consists of nocturnal cough, wheezing, fever and weight loss. Chest radiographs show diffuse interstitial miliary infiltrates (Fig. 1.4); there is a high eosinophil count. In developed countries, serum IgE and antifilarial antibodies can be used to confirm the diagnosis (Table 1-3).

BRONCHIECTASIS, ASTHMA, CHRONIC OBSTRUCTIVE PULMONARY DISEASE

Bronchiectasis is a chronic, debilitating condition. Dilatation and distortion of the airways leads to impaired mucociliary clearance, which encourages bacterial colonization and bronchial inflammation. Patients have fever, chronic cough, mucopurulent sputum, hemoptysis (Table 1-4), wheezing, dyspnea and malaise (Box 1.2).

TABLE 1-3 Serum IgE Levels in Syndromes with Pulmonary Involvement and Eosinophilia

Normal <150 IU	Mildly high 150–500 IU	Moderately high 500–1000 IU	Extremely high >1000 IU
Tuberculosis	Coccidioidomycosis	Strongyloidiasis	Allergic bronchopulmonary aspergillosis
Brucellosis	Drug-induced	Schistosomiasis	Tropical pulmonary eosinophilia
Hydatid cyst	Loeffler's syndrome	Paragonimiasis	Churg–Strauss syndrome
Amebiasis	Sézary syndrome	Hydatid cyst, if it leaks	
Sarcoidosis	Polyarteritis nodosa		

TABLE 1-4 Causes of Hemoptysis

Worldwide	Tropical countries
Bronchiectasis	Tuberculosis
Bronchogenic carcinoma	Bronchiectasis
Chronic bronchitis	Paragonimiasis
Congestive heart failure	Melioidosis
Blood diseases	Leptospirosis
Tuberculosis	Hydatid disease
Endemic mycosis	Endemic mycosis

BOX 1.2 Key Facts
Bronchiectasis

- Dilatation and destruction of bronchi
- Cough, sputum, crackles, clubbing
- Chest x-ray: increased markings, honeycombing
- High-resolution CT scan: honeycombing, cysts, ring shadows
- Complications: hemoptysis, cor pulmonale, amyloidosis
- Treatment: antibiotics, surgery; prevention

The diagnosis of bronchiectasis in developed countries is confirmed by computed tomography of the chest (Fig. 1.5); whereas, in the tropics, the diagnosis is mainly clinical and depends upon a compatible history, presence of finger clubbing, sputum that settles into three layers (mucoid or frothy, mucopurulent, and purulent) and a chest x-ray, if available. Treatment includes regular chest percussion, broad-spectrum antibiotics for exacerbations, and influenza and pneumococcal vaccinations.

The incidence of asthma in the tropics is low for unclear reasons; however, the disease remains underdiagnosed and untreated. "All that wheezes is not asthma" is a dictum that is true in the tropics, as there are many entities that cause wheezing and difficulty in breathing, including tropical eosinophilia and mitral stenosis. Asthma monitoring in the tropics can be achieved by using an inexpensive peak flow meter. Treatment should fit the frequency and severity of attacks. Beta-agonists and cromolyn sodium (sodium cromoglycate) are usually available. Oral corticosteroids in short courses can be used to control severe episodes; however, long-term use of systemic corticosteroids, without adequate monitoring, is not safe. Aerosol inhalers are of great value but they are expensive, difficult to use, and require painstaking teaching.

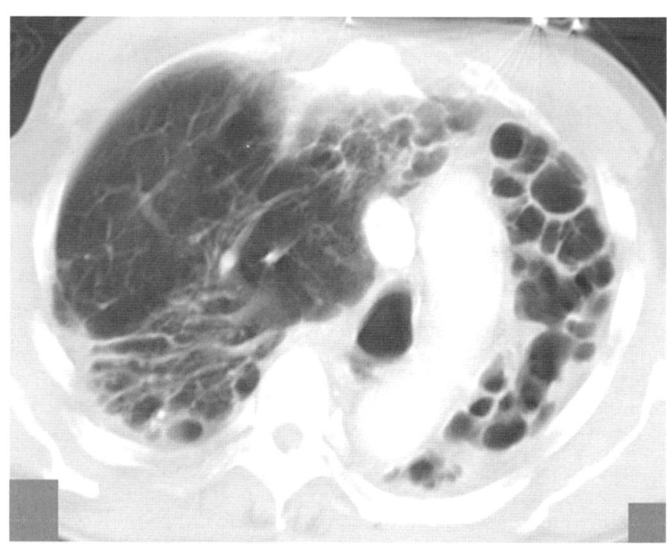

FIGURE 1.5 Computed tomography of the chest: cystic bronchiectasis.

BOX 1.3 Key Facts
COPD

- COPD is progressive obstructive lung disease
- An estimated 210 million people have COPD worldwide and more than 3 million people die each year of COPD
- 90% of COPD deaths are in low- and middle-income countries
- The primary cause of COPD is smoking
- COPD affects men and women equally
- COPD is not curable but can be prevented

Chronic obstructive lung disease is a progressive disease which is characterized by airway obstruction that is only partially reversible by bronchodilator therapy. The term COPD encompasses chronic bronchitis and emphysema. Once a common disease of men, COPD is now as frequent in women because of increased tobacco use and the widespread use of dung and biomass for indoor cooking and heating in low-income countries (Box 1.3). The most common symptoms are dyspnea and chronic cough. The onset of dyspnea is insidious; at first it is mild and occurs only on heavy exertion. With progression of airway obstruction, patients become more short of breath and eventually cannot breathe at rest. Physical examination in the early stage is normal, but in advanced disease, prolonged expiration and expiratory wheezes are audible. In severe cases, the thoracic cage becomes barrel-shaped with increased anterior–posterior diameter; percussion note is hyperresonant. When chest x-ray and pulmonary function testing are not available, a peak-flow meter is an inexpensive device to assess severity of airway obstruction and monitor the response to treatment.

Cessation of smoking is essential. Oral theophylline and beta-agonist drugs control symptoms. Antibiotics (ampicillin, tetracycline and sulfa drugs) are available to treat COPD exacerbations in the tropics.

PLEURAL EFFUSION

Pleural effusion is a frequent condition with variable clinical signs and symptoms. Small effusions can remain silent and are often detected only on chest radiography. Large effusions are associated with dyspnea and diminished chest movements on the affected side. Vocal fremitus is reduced; percussion note is stony dull; and auscultation reveals diminished breath sounds and decreased vocal resonance. Sometimes, bronchial breathing is heard at the upper level of dullness. In addition there may be a pleural friction sound.

If possible, all but the smallest effusions should be tapped. It should be established whether the fluid is serous, bloody, pus or chylous. The effusion can be further divided into transudative and exudative, according to pleural fluid characterization (Table 1-5). Laboratory tests that can guide the management of a pleural effusion are macroscopic appearance (Table 1-6), pleural fluid cell counts, biochemistry, pH and Gram stain. A simple test is centrifugation of the fluid. If an originally "milky" fluid clears with that process, it is presumably an empyema. If not, it is either a chylothorax (pleural fluid triglycerides >110 mg/dL, e.g. lymphoma, post thoracic surgery) or a cholesterol effusion (pleural fluid cholesterol >200 mg/dL).

Transudative pleural effusions occur in heart failure, liver disease, endomyocardial fibrosis, hypoproteinemia/malnutrition and hypothyroidism. The pleural fluid white blood cell count is typically <10,000 cells/mm^3, the pH >7.2, protein <3.0 g/L, the LDH <200 IU/L and the glucose ≥60 mg/dL. A bloody effusion is caused by hemothorax, trauma, malignancy and pulmonary embolism.

Exudative effusions typically have cell counts, protein and biochemical markers opposite to those of transudates. Exudates can be further classified into neutrophilic, lymphocytic and eosinophilic. Neutrophilic exudates may be due to bacterial infection, gastrointestinal diseases, pulmonary embolism, collagen-vascular diseases (CVD) and asbestos-related benign effusion. Pleural effusion occurs in about 50% cases of pneumonia, and can progress to a complicated effusion (pleural fluid pH<7.2, positive Gram stain) or to an empyema, both necessitating pleural fluid drainage with a chest tube thoracostomy in addition to antibiotic treatment. Empyema can occur in pneumococcal, staphylococcal (most often) and *Klebsiella* infections. A right-sided pleural effusion may be associated with amebic liver abscess.

The disease presenting with the highest pleural fluid lymphocytosis is tuberculous pleuritis; however, early in the course, there can be a neutrophilic exudate. A large volume of pleural fluid should be obtained for examination for acid-fast bacilli. In about one-third of cases, the tuberculin skin test is negative initially and converts to positive after 2–4 weeks. Knowledge of the HIV status of a patient with pleural effusion, if positive, significantly inclines to a tuberculosis.

An eosinophilic exudate is more common in the tropics. Endemic parasitic and fungal infections are major causes of such an effusion. Ascariasis, echinococcosis and paragonimiasis are some of the causative parasitic infections. Paragonimiasis is associated with low pleural fluid glucose and low pH. Fungal diseases responsible for such an effusion are histoplasmosis, cryptococcosis and coccidioidomycosis.

TABLE 1-5 Common Causes of Pleural Effusion

Worldwide	Tropical countries
Heart failure	Tuberculosis
Cancer	Paragonimiasis
Pulmonary embolism	Cryptococcosis
Hepatic cirrhosis	Histoplasmosis
Tuberculosis	Lung cancer

TABLE 1-6 Diagnostic Appearances of Pleural Fluid

Appearance	Disease
Pale, straw-colored	Tuberculosis, transudate
Blood-tinged/frank blood	Trauma, cancer, pulmonary infarct
Pus	Empyema
Anchovy sauce	Amebiasis
Milky/chylous/white	Filariasis, lymphoma, lymphatic abnormality, cholesterol effusion

NONTUBERCULOUS GRANULOMATOUS LUNG DISEASE

In the absence of chest x-ray or biopsy evidence, it is not possible to diagnose pulmonary involvement due to sarcoidosis and other granulomatous diseases. Consequently, in the tropics, these disorders remain undiagnosed. The possibility of sarcoidosis should be considered in a patient with dyspnea, uveitis, hepatosplenomegaly, peripheral lymphadenopathy, chronic skin lesions, and a chest x-ray film showing bilateral hilar adenopathy [18].

OCCUPATIONAL AND DUST LUNG DISEASES

The occupational disorders result from human social activity, and as such are preventable. The dusts that provoke occupational disorders can be classified into: those that induce granulomatous reaction (e.g. beryllium, talc and organic antigens); those that cause fibrosis (e.g. silica, asbestos and coal); and those that cause neither inflammation nor fibrosis, thus remaining inert (e.g. iron, barium and tin) (Table 1-7).

TABLE 1-7 Poorly Recognized Occupational Disorders in the Tropics

Disease	Antigen	Distribution
Silicosis	Silica	Widespread
Asbestosis, mesothelioma	Asbestos fibers	Widespread
Byssinosis	Cotton dust	Asia, Africa
Bagassosis	Sugar cane	Americas, Cuba, India
Hypersensitivity pneumonitis	Grain dust, vegetable matter	Widespread
COPD	Animal dung, biomass fuels	India, Africa, South America

Podoconiosis is an endemic nonfilarial elephantiasis occurring in individuals exposed to red clay soil derived from alkaline rock. A chronic and debilitating disease, it exerts a large economic burden. The silica particles are found in the skin, lymph nodes and lymphatics of affected and unaffected individuals. These individuals have reduced lung function as compared with adults living in areas of low silica concentration [19].

REFERENCES

1. Zumla A, James D. Immunological aspects of tropical lung disease. Clin Chest Med 2002;23:283–308.
2. UNICEF/WHO. Pneumonia: the forgotten killer of children. Geneva: UNICEF/WHO; 2006.
3. Vijayan V. Parasitic lung infections. Curr Opin Pulm Med 2009;15:274–82.
4. Charoenratanakul S. Tropical infections and the lung. Arch Chest Dis 1977;52:376–9.
5. Steinoff M. Pulmonary disease. In: Strickland GT, ed. Hunter's Tropical Medicine, 7th edn. Philadelphia: WB Saunders; 1991:1–7.
6. World Health Organization, Family and Community Health Cluster, Department of Child and Adolescent Health and Development. Consultative meeting to review evidence and research priorities in the management of acute respiratory infections (ARI). Meeting report. Geneva: WHO; 2003:1–30.
7. Metlay J, Schults R, Li Y, et al. Influence of age on symptoms and presentation in patients with community acquired pneumonia. Arch Intern Med 1997;157: 112–24
8. WHO/UNICEF. Integrated Management of Childhood Illness (IMCI) for high HIV settings. Geneva: WHO; 2009;11:2.
9. Catchup Study Group. Clinical efficacy of co-trimoxazole versus amoxicillin twice daily for treatment of pneumonia: a randomised controlled clinical trial in Pakistan. Arch Dis Child 2002;86:113–18.
10. Shann F, Barker J, Poore P. Chloramphenicol alone versus chloramphenicol plus penicillin for severe pneumonia in children. Lancet 1985;2:684–6.
11. Duke T, Poka H, Dale F, et al. Chloramphenicol versus benzylpenicillin and gentamicin for the treatment of severe pneumonia in children in Papua New Guinea: a randomised trial. Lancet 2002;359:474–80.
12. Martin G. Approach to the patient with tropical pulmonary disease. In: Guerrant RL, Walker DH, Weller PF, eds. Tropical Infectious Diseases: Principles, Pathogens and Practice. Philadelphia: Churchill Livingstone Elsevier; 2006: 1544–53.
13. Carvalho CRR, Bethlem EP. Pulmonary complications of leptospirosis. Clin Chest Med 2002;23:469–78.
14. Currie BJ, Fisher DA, Howard DM, et al. The epidemiology of melioidosis in Australia and Papua New Guinea. Acta Trop 2000;74:121–7.
15. Kronman K, Truett A, Hale B, Crum-Cianfione N. Melioidosis after brief exposure: a serological survey in US Marines. Am J Trop Med Hyg 2009; 80:182–4.
16. Magalhaes C, Vasconcelos P, Pereira M, et al. Kawasaki disease: a clinical and epidemiological study of 70 children in Brazil. Trop Doct 2009;39: 99–101.
17. Luna C, Faure C. Common tropical pneumonias. In: Sharma OP, ed. Lung Biology in Health and Disease: Tropical Lung Disease, 2nd edn. New York: Taylor & Francis; 2006:211:117–42.
18. Mihailovic-Vucinic V, Sharma O. Tropical granulomas: diagnosis. In: Sharma OP, ed. Lung Biology in Health and Disease: Tropical Lung Disease, 2nd edn. New York: Taylor & Francis; 2006:211:173–93.
19. Morrison C, Davey G. Assessment of respiratory function in patients with podoconiosis. Trans R Soc Trop Med Hyg 2009;103:315–17.

2 Cardiovascular Diseases

Bongani M Mayosi, John Lawrenson

Key features

- The pattern of cardiovascular disease is changing in tropical countries. Although infectious diseases still dominate, increasing urbanization is producing a new pattern of disease that includes hypertension, stroke, diabetes mellitus and ischemic heart disease
- While ischemic heart disease is increasing, it remains rare in rural areas of Africa, India and South America
- Rheumatic heart disease, tuberculous pericarditis, Chagas disease and cardiomyopathies are major contributors to cardiovascular disease in many lower-income countries
- Rheumatic heart disease still disables young patients and is the largest contributor to the cases of heart failure in children and young adults
- Peripartum cardiomyopathy is highly prevalent in parts of Africa; endomyocardial fibrosis is confined to the peri-equatorial tropical regions of Africa, America and Asia
- Chagas disease is a major cause of disability secondary to tropical diseases in young adults in Latin American countries
- HIV infection is associated with a shortening in life expectancy, a reduction in body mass index, and a fall in systolic blood pressure. There is also an increased incidence of inflammatory cardiovascular disorders, resulting in cardiomyopathy, tuberculous pericarditis, pulmonary hypertension, stroke and vasculopathy, in HIV-infected people. Antiretroviral treatments can be associated with insulin resistance, dyslipidemia and lipodystrophy
- Lack of access to resources leads to an excess of early deaths from congenital heart disease and the late presentation of survivors

COMMON SYNDROMES OF CARDIOVASCULAR DISEASE IN THE TROPICS

The principal syndromes of acquired cardiovascular disease are heart failure, stroke and vascular disorders. The causes of these clinical syndromes are summarized in Tables 2-1 to 2-3.

Congenital heart disease is discussed at the end of the chapter.

HEART FAILURE

Heart failure is a clinical syndrome of effort intolerance secondary to a cardiac abnormality with altered neurohumoral adaptation, leading to salt and water retention. Heart failure is the dominant form of cardiovascular disease in many tropical and subtropical regions of the world. The epidemiology of heart failure in the tropics differs from that in industrialized countries in several respects [1]. First, heart failure in the tropics is due largely to nonischemic causes. Second, the common causes of heart failure in the tropics (Table 2-1) present for the most part in children and young adults before middle-age. Finally, infections remain a significant cause of heart failure. Pulmonary hypertension due to lung disease and schistosomiasis, together with tuberculous pericarditis, accounts for at least 10% of cases of heart failure. The burden of tuberculous pericarditis and cardiomyopathy has increased in regions where HIV/AIDS has reached epidemic proportions. Chagasic heart disease due to *Trypanosoma cruzi* infection continues to exact a heavy toll on people living in Latin America [2].

In contrast to industrialized nations, where degenerative valvular heart disease predominates, valvular disease in the tropics is almost always the result of infection. Valvular disease in developed nations is an insidious disease of the elderly, who frequently have comorbidities. In developing countries, valvular disease (with a rapid course) is encountered in the young.

The epidemiology of nonrheumatic valvular disease in the tropics is poorly defined. Myxomatous mitral valve disease associated with mitral valve prolapse is an uncommon indication for mitral valve surgery compared with rheumatic valve disease. Congenital subvalvular aneurysms below the mitral and aortic valves are rare forms of valvular heart disease that were first described in Africa. These congenital subvalvular aneurysms can be associated with varying degrees of valve regurgitation, can rupture or compress the coronary arteries, or can predispose to infective endocarditis or thrombus with systemic embolization.

The major clinical aspects of infective endocarditis in the tropics are reminiscent of the experience in industrialized countries before the antibiotic era. Infective endocarditis is a disease of the young with high morbidity and mortality. Underlying rheumatic heart disease is the major predisposing factor [3].

STROKE

The World Health Organization (WHO) defines stroke as rapidly developing clinical signs of focal (or global) disturbance of cerebral function, with symptoms lasting 24 hours or longer or leading to death, with no apparent cause other than vascular origin. The age-standardized mortality, case fatality and prevalence of disabling stroke in the tropics are similar to or higher than those measured in most industrialized countries. In the tropics, stroke incidence is higher in people less than 65 years of age, and there is a greater proportion of hemorrhagic (30% vs 15%) compared to ischemic stroke than in industrialized countries. In the tropics, more than 90% of patients with hemorrhagic stroke and more than half with ischemic stroke are

TABLE 2-1 Causes of Heart Failure in the Tropics

Intracardiac causes		
Endocardial diseases	Valvular endocardium or annular defect	• Acute rheumatic fever • Rheumatic heart disease, infective endocarditis • Congenital submitral or subaortic aneurysm
	Mural endocardium	• Endomyocardial fibrosis
Myocardial diseases	Acute	• Acute rheumatic fever • Septic myocarditis • Diphtheria • Coxsackie B infection • Acute Chagas disease
	Chronic	• Dilated cardiomyopathy • Peripartum cardiomyopathy • HIV-associated cardiomyopathy • Chronic Chagas disease • Ischemic heart disease
	Nutritional	• Thiamine deficiency (beri-beri) • Selenium deficiency (Keshan disease)
Pericardial diseases	Acute	• Acute bacterial pericarditis with or without HIV infection • Acute rheumatic fever
	Chronic	• Tuberculous pericardial effusion or effusive constrictive pericarditis • Constrictive pericarditis
Extracardiac causes		
Increased peripheral resistance	• Hypertension	• Essential hypertension • Secondary to Takayasu arteritis, chronic glomerulonephritis
Increased pulmonary vascular resistance	• Cor pulmonale	• Destructive hypoxic lung disease • HIV-associated pulmonary hypertension • Schistosomal pulmonary arteriolitis
Conditions causing high cardiac output	• Anemia • Thiamine deficiency (beri-beri) • Thyrotoxicosis • Post-traumatic arteriovenous fistula	

hypertensive. While hypertension is the single most important factor for stroke, non-hypertensive causes explain nearly half of cases of ischemic stroke. These factors include structural heart disease, cardiac arrhythmia, HIV/AIDS and other infections (Table 2-2) [4].

Infection with HIV is associated with an increased risk of stroke. HIV-associated stroke occurs in younger patients and is due to an ischemic mechanism in the majority of cases. In tropical countries, treatable infections account for the majority of causes, with extracranial and intracranial vasculopathy contributing to 20% of cases [5].

VASCULAR DISORDERS

The range of arterial and venous syndromes includes diseases of the aorta, atherosclerotic diseases of medium-sized arteries, and unusual vascular disorders of the tropics (Table 2-3).

Atheroma and dissection of the aorta is present in communities with an accumulation of risk factors, including hypertension. Similarly, atheroma and aortic aneurysm is becoming more common in people living in tropical environments as their cardiovascular risk profile worsens. By contrast, aortitis resulting from syphilis is less common due to the early use of penicillin. Idiopathic tropical aortitis or Takayasu's disease is found in sub-Saharan Africa and Asia. The clinical manifestations depend on the stage and anatomy of the disease. The disease may present with angina, cerebral ischemic symptoms, absent pulses, and hypertension – a common presentation in children [6].

Atherosclerotic disease of the medium-sized vessels presents with a number of clinical syndromes including cardiac pain and coronary thrombosis, intermittent claudication and gangrene of the legs, and mesenteric artery occlusion. These ischemic syndromes are particularly common in people of Asian, Melanesian and Polynesian origin (who also have a high incidence of diabetes mellitus). Angina in the tropical environment may also be due to valvular heart disease, hypertrophic cardiomyopathy, dysrhythmias, syphilitic arteritis or anemia.

Hemoglobin disorders (such as sickle cell disease) contribute to the cardiovascular disease burden either by exacerbating existing cardiac disease with anemia, or by causing peripheral vascular occlusion or pulmonary hypertension.

Idiopathic gangrene of the extremities, gangrene associated with tropical phlebitis, and gangrene associated with acquired hemolytic anemia are unusual vascular disorders encountered in Africa. Idiopathic gangrene of the extremities presents mainly in infants and children with bilateral symmetrical gangrene. No cause is found, although infection with *Salmonella typhi*, *S. paratyphi* and *Neisseria meningitidis* has been incriminated. Predisposing factors are dehydration and malnutrition. The onset of the illness is acute, with fever,

TABLE 2-2 Causes of Stroke in the Tropics

Pathologic mechanism	Condition
Intracerebral hemorrhage	• Hypertension
Cerebral infarction due to embolism or thrombosis	• Valvular heart disease • Cardiomyopathy • Atrial fibrillation • HIV-associated vasculopathy or coagulopathy • Atherosclerosis of cerebral vessels
Subarachnoid haemorrhage	• Ruptured aneurysm at the base of the brain • Arteriovenous malformation • Trauma • Spontaneous
Cerebral venous thrombosis	• Dehydration • Sepsis • Pregnancy and puerperium
Infections	• In HIV-positive individuals, consider toxoplasma, CMV, lymphoma, meningitis, HIV-associated vasculopathy, and coagulopathy • Syphilis • Cerebral abscess • Cerebral cysticercosis • Tuberculoma • Echinococcus cysts
Malignancy	• Primary or secondary tumors
Trauma	• Subdural hematoma

TABLE 2-3 Vascular Disorders that are Encountered in the Tropics

Pathology	Clinical syndrome
Diseases of the aorta	• Aortic dissection • Aortic aneurysm • Syphilitic aortitis • Idiopathic tropical aortitis/ Takayasu aortitis
Atherosclerosis of medium-sized arteries (other than vertebrobasilar insufficiency and cerebral thrombosis resulting in stroke)	• Cardiac pain and coronary thrombosis • Intermittent claudication and gangrene of the leg • Mesenteric artery occlusion causing intestinal angina and infarction of the gut
Unusual vascular disorders of the tropics	• Idiopathic gangrene of the extremities • Gangrene associated with tropical phlebitis • Gangrene associated with acquired hemolytic anemia

malaise and petechial rash associated with symmetrical gangrene affecting the digits.

Gangrene of the limbs, associated with tropical phlebitis, is thought to be part of the same spectrum of disease as the peripheral gangrene syndrome. The veins are inflamed and later thrombosed and occluded. An adjoining artery may be affected. The cavernous sinus, internal jugular vein or limb veins may be affected [7].

AN APPROACH TO THE PATIENT WITH CARDIOVASCULAR DISEASE

Despite variable access to resources for investigation and treatment, the practitioner in a developing country may achieve a great deal with a thorough history and physical examination. The social and geographical context of the consultation should never be taken for granted.

The key syndromes of cardiovascular disease are recognized on clinical examination. Congestive heart failure is characterized by pedal edema, raised jugular venous pressure, and tender hepatomegaly, while stroke is recognized by the presence of a neurological deficit that is consistent with a vascular insult. Vascular disorders present with several clinical syndromes (see Table 2-3), depending on the type and location of the diseased vessel. Features of immunosuppression should be sought in patients with suspected HIV infection.

The essential tests in the evaluation of the patient with cardiovascular disease include urine analysis for protein, blood and glucose, electrocardiography (ECG), chest radiography and HIV serology. A full blood count and urea, creatinine, sodium and potassium levels are useful in excluding anemia, renal disease and electrolyte abnormalities as the reasons for presentation. In the evaluation of heart failure, echocardiography is required to define the nature of the cardiac abnormality. In stroke, the erythrocyte sedimentation rate (ESR) or C-reactive protein, syphilis serology and a computed tomographic (CT) scan of the brain are indicated. Other tests, such as carotid Doppler ultrasound, echocardiography, clotting screen, blood cultures, lumbar puncture and thrombophilia screen, may be conducted depending on the indication and available facilities. In vascular disease of the aorta and medium-sized vessels, angiography is essential for the delineation of the disease. Specific diagnostic tests, such as blood culture for infective endocarditis, will be required.

Magnetic resonance imaging (MRI) is playing an increasing role in the evaluation of patients with cardiovascular disorders but it is not widely available in tropical countries.

DIAGNOSIS AND DIFFERENTIAL DIAGNOSIS

Heart Failure

The differential diagnosis of heart failure is listed in Table 2-1. The diagnosis of cardiomyopathy is made by clinically excluding other causes of heart failure such as hypertension and valvular disease. Patients with hypertensive heart disease and severe systolic dysfunction may present initially with blood pressure in the normal range, with hypertension declaring itself after a period of treatment; their presenting blood pressure is low because of markedly reduced cardiac output. It may be difficult to distinguish hypertensive heart failure from idiopathic dilated cardiomyopathy, because the latter is accompanied by blood pressure readings in the hypertensive range in up to 8% of cases. This difficulty is compounded by the fact that the end-organ effects of hypertension, such as renal involvement and aortic dilatation, may not be apparent clinically.

It is essential to exclude reversible forms of nutritional heart muscle disease such as beriberi (thiamine deficiency). The diagnosis of beriberi should be considered when heart failure occurs in an alcoholic or in an impoverished person or child living in an area where polished rice forms the major part of the diet. In beriberi, neurologic symptoms such as paresthesiae and weakness of peripheral neuropathy and Wernicke's encephalopathy are occasionally present. The definitive diagnosis is made by demonstrating diminished erythrocyte transketolase activity, which increases after the addition of thiamine pyrophosphate. In areas where this testing is not available, a short course of thiamine supplementation in all patients with heart failure may be beneficial. A rapid response to therapy, with a decrease in cardiac size clinically and on x-ray seen within 2 weeks, will occur in the patient who is thiamine-deficient.

The forms of cardiomyopathy that are unique to people living in tropical environments include peripartum cardiomyopathy,

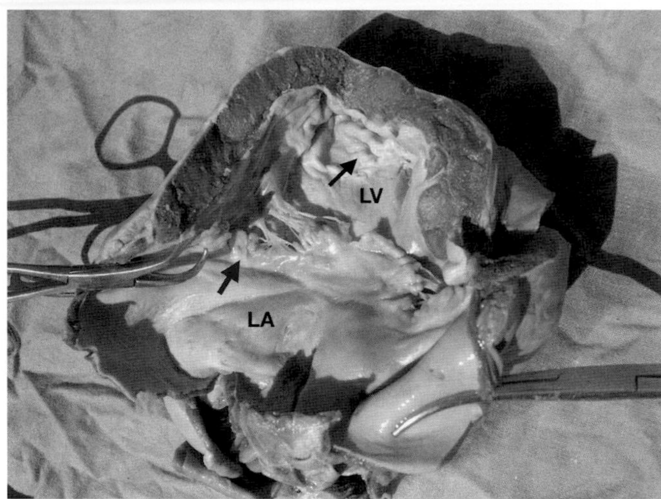

FIGURE 2.1 Postmortem heart specimen of a young boy who died as a result of severe mitral regurgitation caused by left-sided endomyocardial fibrosis. Black arrow indicates scar at the apex of the left ventricle. Note that the left ventricle is small and the left atrium is enlarged and the retracted posterior leaflet of the mitral valve is involved in the fibrotic process (blue arrow). *(With permission from Sliwa K, Damasceno A, Mayosi BM. Epidemiology and etiology of cardiomyopathy in Africa. Circulation 2005;112:3577–83.)*

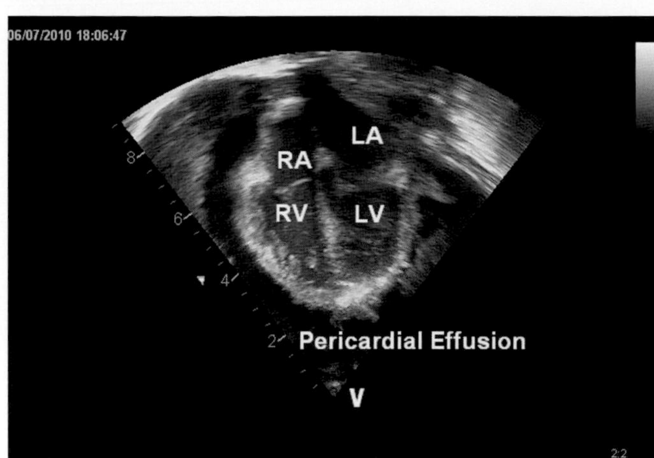

FIGURE 2.2 An echocardiogram of a patient with pericardial effusion, represented by the echo-free space around the heart, shows the "shaggy" surface of the heart that is typical of tuberculous pericarditis. RA, right atrium; LA, left atrium; RV, right ventricle; LV, left ventricle.

endomyocardial fibrosis and Chagas disease. The diagnosis of peripartum cardiomyopathy is confirmed by echocardiographic demonstration of left ventricular systolic dysfunction which is not explained by other forms of heart disease. The typical period of disease onset is in the last month of pregnancy and up to 5 months following delivery.

Tropical endomyocardial fibrosis (Fig. 2.1) affects children in very low socioeconomic groups in countries within 15 degrees latitude from the equator. Typically, symptoms are suggestive of congestive cardiomyopathy, but signs resemble constrictive pericarditis. Like congestive cardiomyopathy, patients present with dyspnea, orthopnea and peripheral edema. Like constrictive pericarditis, pulsus paradoxus, a raised jugular venous pressure (JVP) with rapid "x" and "y" descents, an early third heart sound, hepatomegaly and ascites are present. Unlike constrictive pericarditis, however, there is frequently a murmur of tricuspid and/or mitral regurgitation.

The diagnosis of endomyocardial fibrosis is made on the basis of clinical, echocardiographic and hemodynamic changes. Echocardiography shows increased ventricular wall thickness and cavity obliteration; and enlarged atria, with or without a small pericardial effusion. Cardiac catheterization is needed to demonstrate the combination of restricted filling and incompetence of the atrioventricular valves as well as to show excess fibrous tissue in endocardial biopsy specimens [8].

Chagas disease from *Trypanosoma cruzi* is acquired only in South and Central America; however, migrants from Latin America can present with chronic chagasic heart disease. Cardiac disease is characterized by anginal chest pain and symptomatic conduction system disease; severe, protracted, congestive cardiac failure, often predominantly right-sided, is the rule in advanced cases. Bifascicular block is present in more than 80% of cases and death from asystole and arrhythmia is common. Autonomic dysfunction is also common. Apical aneurysms and left ventricular dilatation increase the risk of thromboembolism and arrhythmias.

The chest x-ray demonstrates cardiomegaly. The ECG is abnormal as a rule in the late course of the disease. The echocardiographic features in advanced cases are those of dilated cardiomyopathy, including left ventricular posterior wall hypokinesia and preserved interventricular septum motion as well as an apical aneurysm. Chagas disease is diagnosed by demonstration of trypanosomes in the peripheral blood or amastigotes forms in a lymph node biopsy, or, in chronic disease, by a combination of serologic tests.

In tuberculous pericardial effusion, evidence of chronic cardiac compression mimicking heart failure is the most common presentation in parts of southern Africa. Tuberculous pericarditis as a cause of heart failure is less common than rheumatic heart disease, but more common than hypertensive heart disease and cardiomyopathy in parts of southern Africa. Although there is marked overlap between the physical signs of pericardial effusion and constrictive pericarditis, the presence of increased cardiac dullness extending to the right of the sternum favors a clinical diagnosis of pericardial effusion. It is easy to detect a pericardial effusion using echocardiography (Fig. 2.2). Unfortunately, it is not easy to determine etiology using ultrasound; nor is it readily possible to diagnose constrictive pericarditis.

Imaging by CT scanning or MRI (to diagnose constriction) can also be used but is seldom available in tropical areas. Signs and symptoms of tuberculous pericarditis are usually nonspecific and vague. A "definite" diagnosis of tuberculous pericarditis is based on the demonstration of tubercle bacilli in pericardial fluid or on a histologic section of the pericardium; "probable" tuberculous pericarditis is based on the proof of tuberculosis elsewhere in a patient with otherwise unexplained pericarditis, a lymphocytic pericardial exudate with elevated adenosine deaminase levels, and/or an appropriate response to a trial of antituberculosis chemotherapy [9].

The diagnosis of circulatory disease in patients living with HIV depends on the presenting symptoms. In patients presenting with symptoms of heart failure, three conditions should be considered: tuberculous pericarditis, HIV-associated cardiomyopathy, and primary pulmonary hypertension. The diagnosis of primary pulmonary hypertension is based on the presence of clinical, electrocardiographic, radiologic and hemodynamic changes of pulmonary hypertension in the absence of primary lung disease.

Stroke

The differential diagnosis of stroke in the tropics is similar to in other parts of the world, as outlined in Table 2-2. Radiologic evaluation by CT scan or MRI (which may be available only in tertiary referral hospitals) will establish the pathologic diagnosis (infarction or hemorrhage) and exclude other conditions that may mimic stroke, such as subarachnoid hemorrhage and brain tumor. A chest x-ray may reveal a primary source of malignancy. An echocardiogram is indicated if a cardiac source of embolism is suspected. In primary intracerebral hemorrhage, a clotting screen is indicated, and a thrombophilia screen in young patients with unexplained stroke. Lumbar puncture is indicated in suspected subarachnoid hemorrhage or meningitis as well as in those patients with an ischemic stroke who are HIV-positive.

Vascular Disorders

The clinical diagnosis of aortic and medium-sized vessel arterial disease should be confirmed using angiography if possible. In atherosclerotic disease of the aorta and medium-sized arteries, the etiology is related to cardiovascular risk factors which require specific testing and control. In aortitis, the etiologic diagnosis is between syphilis and idiopathic aortitis. When there is doubt about the diagnosis, a biopsy of the artery may be necessary.

MANAGEMENT AND OUTCOMES

The principles of management of patients with heart failure, stroke and vascular disease are the same in the tropics as elsewhere in the world. There is, however, a need for empiric treatment in certain instances before a definitive diagnosis is reached. For example, in patients presenting with a large pericardial effusion from a community where tuberculosis is endemic, it is appropriate to commence antituberculosis treatment if pericardiocentesis is not possible or before microbiology results become available.

In patients with valvular disease and heart failure due to rheumatic heart disease (Fig. 2.3), ongoing penicillin prophylaxis (past the age of 35 years) is recommended even if surgery is not undertaken [10].

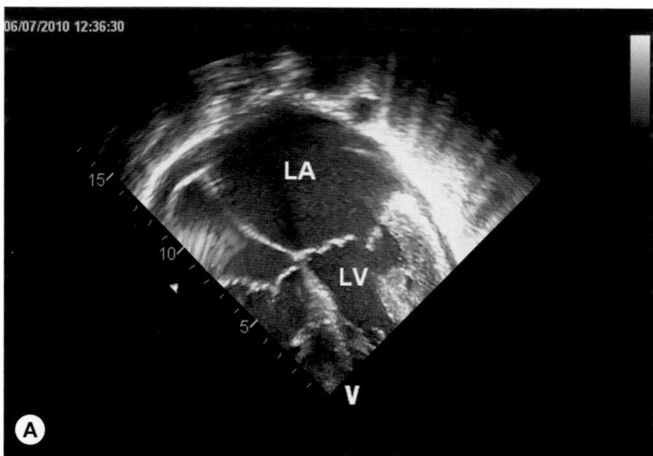

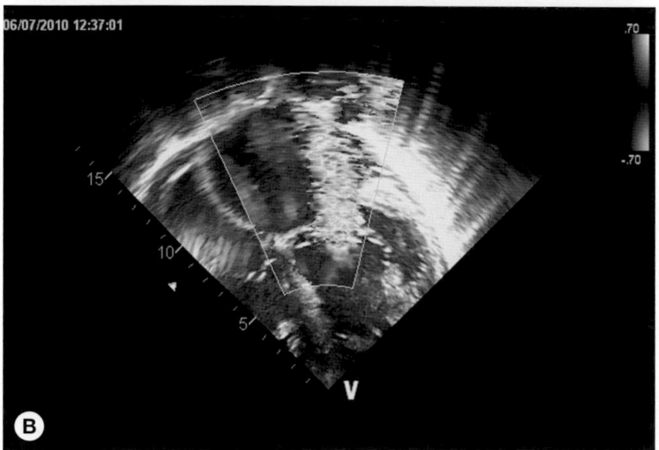

FIGURE 2.3 An echocardiogram of rheumatic mitral regurgitation showing a dilated left atrium, thickening and deformation of the anterior and posterior mitral valve leaflets **(A)**, and the mosaic pattern of severe mitral regurgitation extending to the back of the left atrium **(B)**.

There are few studies comparing the outcome of patients with heart failure and vascular disorders in the tropics versus nontropical regions. By contrast, a systematic analysis of stroke studies has shown several differences in relation to outcome in the tropics compared to the rest of the world. The available case fatality data from hospital-based prospective studies reveal a rate of about 30% at 1 month – a value much higher than the 20% reported for older populations in the rest of the world. The prevalence of disabling stroke in sub-Saharan Africa is at least as high as in high-income areas.

PEDIATRIC CONSIDERATION: CONGENITAL HEART DISEASE

Congenital heart disease refers to malformations of heart structure existing at birth (WHO). It is the most common congenital abnormality occurring in isolation or in combination with other genetic abnormalities. Whereas, as a result of access to surgery, survival into adulthood is the norm for more than 90% of patients born with congenital heart disease in industrialized nations, opportunities for surgical correction of defects are rare in developing nations. In many developing countries, the commencement and sustainability of surgical programs must be balanced against the need to control infectious disease and diseases related to poverty.

CLINICAL PRESENTATION

The cause of a congenital heart lesion in most cases is unknown. Exposure to teratogens and genetic syndromes account for a relatively small proportion of the total number of defects.

An approach to classification is shown in Figure 2.4.

Approximately 40% of all patients born with congenital heart disease will need surgery in the first years of life to survive. The introduction of a surgical program needs to coincide with major improvements in the under-5-year mortality in a country – a level of less than 30/1000 would appear to be the threshold value. Relatively few developing countries have established surgical programs which meet or partly meet the needs of the population in this regard.

The attrition of complex patients in early life therefore will mean that the practitioner is likely to encounter adults with moderate left-to-right shunts, uncomplicated valvular heart disease, and obstructive pulmonary vascular disease. In areas with a high prevalence of rheumatic heart disease, congenital heart disease is likely to be confused with valvular heart disease.

A heart lesion should be suspected in any patient with a recognizable genetic abnormality. The practitioner caring for the patient with Down syndrome or Marfan syndrome should be aware that cardiac disease is an integral part of the disorder.

As would be expected, the adult population with congenital heart disease is dominated by atrial septal defect, small ventricular septal defects, and mild to moderate aortic and pulmonary stenosis. The majority of patients seen are symptomatic, with dyspnea and palpitations being the commonest presenting complaints.

Table 2-4 compares the physical signs, ECG and chest x-ray findings in patients presenting in adulthood with the more common congenital heart lesions.

The final diagnosis will be confirmed by echocardiography; fortunately, the cost of quality echocardiographic machines has declined with time.

In patients with underlying congenital heart disease, comorbid conditions common in tropical climates can be present. For example, sickle cell disease is associated with significant risk of pulmonary hypertension.

Diuretics and digoxin are used to obtain symptomatic relief in patients with large left-to-right shunts. This practice is not based on evidence from controlled trials but is an extension from the practice in patients with heart failure.

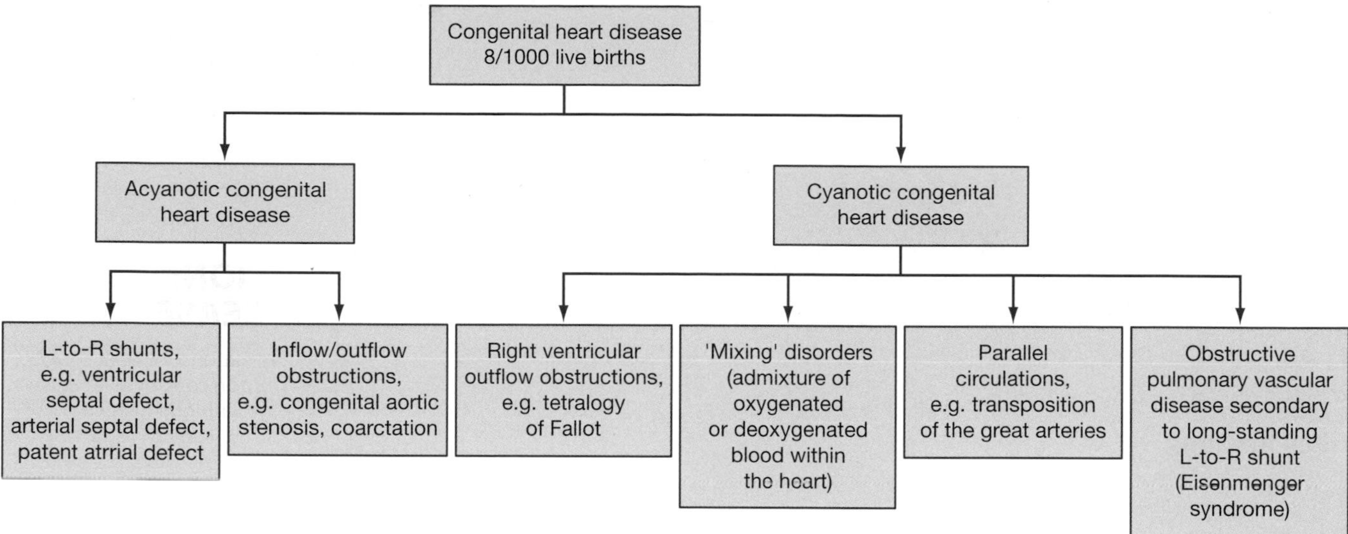

FIGURE 2.4 Classification of congenital heart disease.

TABLE 2-4 Comparison of Physical Signs and Investigative Findings in Patients Presenting in Adulthood with the More Common Congenital Heart Lesions

	ASD	VSD	PS	AS	Tetralogy of Fallot	Eisenmenger syndrome
Cyanosis	–	–	–	–	++	+
Cardiac size	RV lift	–	–	LVH (apex)	–	–
Murmur	ESM LSE MDM LSE	PSM LSE	ESM LSE	ESM LSE	ESM LSE	–
Heart sounds	Split S2	S2 normal	P2 soft, ejection click	A2 soft, additional ejection click	P2 soft	P2 loud/palpable Ejection click
ECG	RVH; atrial fibrillation	Normal	RVH	LVH	RVH	RVH
X-ray	Hilar enlargement plethora of vessels CTR increased				Boot-shaped heart, right arch; decreased peripheral vasculature	Small heart, large central PAs; pruning of peripheral vessels

Abbreviations: A2, aortic component of second sound; AS, aortic stenosis; ASD, atrial septal defect; CTR, cardiothoracic ratio; ESM, ejection systolic murmur; LSE, left sternal edge; LVH, left ventricular hypertrophy; MDM, mid-diastolic murmur; P2, pulmonary component of second sound; PAs, pulmonary arteries; PS, pulmonary stenosis; RV, right ventricle; S2, second sound; VSD, ventricular septal defect.

The relief of symptoms, however, will only be achieved with surgical repair. Access to surgery varies markedly. Many countries rely on charity; well-organized humanitarian missions (such as those offered by the Chain of Hope organization) to target countries can achieve improvements in health for individuals and are more effective than movement of patients to high-income countries. Some countries, such as Guatemala, have growing programs which aim to serve as training hubs for a region. Other countries, such as Brazil, have well-established programs offering high-quality and innovative surgery.

When surgery can be offered only to limited numbers of individuals, practitioners should select patients with straightforward conditions that need very limited long-term care.

REFERENCES

1. Ntusi NBA, Mayosi BM. Epidemiology of heart failure in sub-Saharan Africa. Exp Rev Cardiovasc Ther 2009;7:169–80.
2. Cubillos-Garzón LA, Casas JP, Morillo CA, Bautista LE. Congestive heart failure in Latin America: the next epidemic. Am Heart J 2004;147:412–17.
3. Nkomo VT. Epidemiology and prevention of valvular heart diseases and infective endocarditis in Africa. Heart 2007;93:1510–19.
4. Mensah GA. Epidemiology of stroke and high blood pressure in Africa. Heart 2008;94:697–705.
5. Tipping B, de Villiers L, Wainwright H, et al. Stroke in patients with human immunodeficiency virus infection. J Neurol Neurosurg Psychiatry 2007;78: 1320–4.
6. Chesler E. Chapter 19: Diseases of the aorta, pp. 389–98. In: Clinical Cardiology. New York: Springer-Verlag; 1992.
7. Parry E, Godfrey R, Mabey D, Geoffrey G. Chapter 76: The heart, pp. 837–86. In: Principles of Medicine in Africa, 3rd edn. Cambridge, UK: Cambridge University Press; 2004.
8. Sliwa K, Damasceno A, Mayosi BM. Epidemiology and etiology of cardiomyopathy in Africa. Circulation 2005;112:3577–83.
9. Mayosi BM. Contemporary trends in the epidemiology and management of cardiomyopathy and pericarditis in sub-Saharan Africa. Heart 2007;93: 1176–83.
10. World Health Organization (WHO). WHO Technical Report Series. Rheumatic fever and rheumatic heart disease: report of a WHO expert panel, Geneva 29 October–1 November 2001. Geneva: WHO; 2004.

3 Gastrointestinal Diseases

Ramnik J Xavier, Harry J Thomas

Key features

More common in the tropics

- Duodenal ulcer
- Gastrointestinal infections
- Tuberculosis of the abdomen and intestine
- Malabsorption due to
  - giardiasis, capillariasis, strongyloidiasis
  - tropical sprue
  - chronic calcific pancreatitis
  - malnutrition
  - alpha chain disease
  - hypolactasia
- Intestinal obstruction due to ascariasis
- Intestinal volvulus
- Intussusception

Less common in the tropics

- Gastric ulcer
- Celiac disease
- Mesenteric ischemia
- Diverticulosis
- Inflammatory bowel disease
- Ischemic colitis

PRESENTATIONS

Gastrointestinal diseases are among the most common problems encountered in the tropics. The principal syndromes are diarrhea, abdominal pain, abdominal distension, intestinal obstruction and gastrointestinal bleeding.

DIARRHEA

Diarrheal diseases are a major cause of morbidity and mortality in the tropics and subtropics [1]. Children are most often and most seriously affected, with 1.8 million children under the age of five dying each year due to diarrhea. Dehydration is the main cause of death, whereas malnutrition is the main cause of morbidity.

Etiology and Distribution

Rotavirus is the most common cause of severe diarrhea in infants and young children worldwide. The second most common cause of viral gastroenteritis is norovirus. Among the bacterial agents, enterotoxigenic *Escherichia coli* (ETEC) is the most common pathogen affecting both native residents of and visitors to developing countries. Salmonella is a common cause of food poisoning in developed countries; varying incidences have been reported from countries in the tropics. *Campylobacter* and *Shigella* spp. have a worldwide distribution and are relatively common causes of infectious diarrheal disease in all age groups. *E. coli* O157 causes a dysenteric illness very similar to shigellosis. Cholera remains endemic in many parts of Africa, Asia, and Central and South America.

Transmission and Epidemiology

Infection occurs by the ingestion of organisms in food and water contaminated by feces from a human or animal excreting the organism. This contamination is associated with inadequate public sanitation and low standards of personal hygiene. Defecation near pools and streams that are sources of water for domestic use is common, and simple sewage disposal systems often empty feces into the domestic water supply of the community. Person-to-person spread of infection also occurs. Seafoods such as shellfish, mussels and crabs transmit viruses causing gastroenteritis, *Vibrio cholerae* and *V. parahaemolyticus*. Flies carry bacteria from feces to food, on their mouthparts and legs. Low standards of kitchen hygiene in homes and public eating places also encourage transmission of intestinal infection. Precooked food kept warm for long periods may transmit a number of gut pathogens and contain enterotoxin formed by staphylococci growing in warmed food. Poultry and eggs are important sources of nontyphoidal salmonellae and campylobacter. An important and avoidable source of intestinal infection in infants results from bottle-feeding with powdered milk solution instead of breastfeeding. Unsterile bottles and nipples and contaminated water all contribute to the considerable risk of gut infection.

Pathogenesis

Diarrhea can be defined as an increase in the water content of stools. Physiologically, the cause may be that: (1) the small intestine secretes more fluid than it reabsorbs; (2) solute absorption in the small intestine is impaired so that the osmotic load retains fluid in the gut lumen; (3) the volume of fluid entering the colon exceeds its capacity for water absorption; (4) the water- and electrolyte-reabsorbing capacity of the colon is reduced as a result of enterotoxigenic infection such as cholera; or (5) the water-reabsorbing capacity and motility of the colon are altered by localized or generalized colonic inflammation and ulceration. Infectious agents produce diarrhea by causing one or more of these effects. Enterotoxin-producing bacteria include *V. cholerae*, enterotoxigenic *E. coli*, *Staphylococcus aureus*, and *Shigella* and *Salmonella* spp. Enteroinvasive bacteria include *Shigella*, *Salmonella* and *Campylobacter* spp.

Clinical Manifestations

The onset of symptoms can vary from a few hours after ingesting food containing preformed toxins, to several days after ingesting bacterial pathogens, to two or more weeks in parasitic infections. Acute infectious diarrhea can be classified into watery diarrhea and bloody diarrhea (dysentery) (Box 3.1). Noninfectious causes of acute diarrhea are less significant in the tropics, but causes that should be considered include toxin-induced (e.g. organophosphate poisoning), medication-related and ischemic colitis. The most important physical signs to be

BOX 3.1 Causes of Acute Infectious Diarrhea

- Intoxication
  - *Staphylococcus aureus*
  - *Clostridium perfringens*
  - *Bacillus cereus*
  - Botulism (uncommon)
- Infection
  - Viruses
    - Rotaviruses
    - Noroviruses
    - Enteric adenoviruses
    - Coronaviruses
  - Bacteria
    - *Escherichia coli* (enterotoxigenic, enteropathogenic, enteroadherent, enterohemorrhagic, enteroinvasive)
    - *Campylobacter* spp.
    - *Salmonella* spp.
    - *Shigella* spp.
    - *Vibrio cholerae, V. parahaemolyticus*
    - *Yersinia enterocolitica, Y. pseudotuberculosis*
    - *Clostridium difficile*
    - *Aeromonas* spp.
    - *Plesiomonas* spp.
  - Protozoa
    - *Cryptosporidium hominis/parvum*
    - *Giardia lamblia*
    - *Entamoeba histolytica*
    - *Cyclospora cayetanensis*

BOX 3.2 Dehydration Assessment

Mild dehydration

- Decreased urine output

Moderate dehydration (≥5% volume loss)

- Irritability
- Delayed capillary refill time
- Tachycardia
- Orthostatic hypotension
- Deep respirations
- Decreased skin turgor
- Dry mucous membranes
- Sunken eyes
- Sunken fontanelle (infants)

Severe dehydration (≥10% volume loss)

- Decreased consciousness
- Hypotension
- Deep respirations with an increase in respiratory rate
- Cool extremities
- Peripheral cyanosis

elicited concern the assessment of hydration (Box 3.2); the patient should be weighed at first presentation, as weight gain or loss can be a valuable guide to the effectiveness of rehydration.

The rapid onset of nausea, vomiting and diarrhea after food consumption is most often due to the ingestion of a preformed toxin produced by *Staphylococcus aureus, Bacillus cereus* or *Clostridium perfringens.*

Large-volume watery diarrhea indicates a small bowel etiology, e.g. due to *V. cholerae*, enterotoxigenic *E. coli* and rotavirus infections. Toxin-induced secretory diarrhea continues independent of food intake. Malabsorption of carbohydrate in the small intestine leads to fermentation of unabsorbed substrates by colonic bacteria; this may cause bloating, the passage of much rectal gas and frothy stools, which are all characteristic of giardiasis. Cryptosporidiosis can involve both small and large bowel, causing short-lived and self-limiting diarrhea; however, the infection can be prolonged in patients with impaired immune responses. *Cyclospora cayetanensis* can also cause acute and more chronic diarrhea with abnormalities of intestinal absorption.

Frequent bowel movements with small volumes of stool and the passage of blood and mucus suggest colonic infection. Causes of bloody diarrhea (dysentery) include invasive bacteria such as *Campylobacter* spp., enterohemorrhagic *E. coli*, and *Salmonella, Shigella* and *Yersinia* spp.; nonbacterial causes include *Entamoeba histolytica* (amebic dysentery) and *Balantidium coli*, which is spread by close contact with pigs. Colicky abdominal pain is common in many gut infections and is especially severe in campylobacteriosis and yersiniosis, mimicking acute appendicitis. Fever, chills and generalized myalgia are usually associated with infection by invasive organisms; these patients appear ill and have generalized abdominal tenderness.

Antibiotic-Associated Colitis

Antibiotics may cause diarrhea through a number of mechanisms, a common cause being pseudomembranous colitis due to infection with cytotoxigenic *Clostridium difficile*. Originally described in patients who had received clindamycin, *C. difficile* infection has since been found to complicate treatment with a number of antibiotic classes, especially fluoroquinolones. The burden of *C. difficile* infection in North America and Europe has greatly increased since the emergence of a hypervirulent strain in 2003; the incidence in other parts of the world is not yet fully known, but appears to be increasing. Patients develop fever, diarrhea and marked leukocytosis. Sigmoidoscopy reveals an inflamed mucosa with pseudomembranous plaques adhering to the mucosa. Management consists of discontinuing unnecessary antibiotics, treating with metronidazole or oral vancomycin, and, for life-threatening cases, colectomy.

Antibiotic-associated hemorrhagic colitis, a form of antibiotic-associated colitis in which *C. difficile* is absent, is associated with penicillin treatment and has been found to be caused by *Klebsiella oxytoca* [2].

Chronic Diarrhea

Most acute infections of the gut have resolved or are resolving within 2 weeks. The most common causes of chronic diarrhea are repeated infection and persistent infection. Persistent infection is commonly due to parasitic infections, including those caused by protozoa (*Giardia lamblia, Entamoeba histolytica, Isospora belli, Cyclospora cayetanensis, Cryptosporidium hominis/parvum*, microsporidia) and helminths (*Strongyloides stercoralis, Capillaria philippinensis*) (Box 3.3) [3]. Patients have frequent, pale, offensive stools, which are characteristic of malabsorption [4]. Noninfectious causes of mucosal malabsorption include celiac disease, tropical sprue, Crohn's disease, and neoplasms of the small bowel. Malabsorption may also be caused by intraluminal maldigestion, which occurs in pancreatic exocrine insufficiency and bacterial overgrowth of the small intestine. Other causes of chronic diarrhea include medication effects, endocrinopathies (particularly hyperthyroidism and diabetes mellitus) and hormone-producing neoplasms.

Complications

The leading cause of death in patients with acute diarrhea is dehydration, which requires prompt fluid and electrolyte replacement. The nutritional state of children often deteriorates because of anorexia, nutrient malabsorption, and the practice of not feeding children who have diarrhea. Hypolactasia is a sequela of many gut infections and may cause persistent diarrhea. Dysentery can be associated with severe local complications such as hemorrhage, toxic megacolon and bowel

BOX 3.3 Causes of Persistent/Chronic Diarrhea

- Infection
  - Parasitic
    - *Giardia lamblia*
    - *Entamoeba histolytica*
    - *Isospora belli*
    - *Cyclospora cayetanenis*
    - *Cryptosporidium hominis/parvum* (immunodeficient)
    - Microsporidia
    - *Strongyloides stercoralis*
    - *Capillaria philippinensis*
  - Mycobacterial
    - *Mycobacterium avium-intracellulare*
    - *Mycobacterium tuberculosis*
- Malabsorption
- AIDS enteropathy
- Inflammatory bowel disease

perforation. In addition, invasive organisms can result in systemic manifestations including hemolytic uremic syndrome (which can complicate *Shigella dysenteriae* and *E. coli* O157 infections), reactive arthritis (following shigellosis, salmonellosis, campylobacteriosis, yersiniosis, and *Clostridium difficile* infection) and Guillain–Barré syndrome (campylobacteriosis).

Diagnosis

The range of laboratory tests and expertise needed to make a specific microbiologic diagnosis in most patients with diarrhea requires facilities not often available in the tropics. Some simple tests can be useful in most circumstances. It is important to examine the stool sample for blood. A smear of fluid stools should always be examined by direct microscopy for trophozoites of *Entamoeba histolytica* and trophozoites and cysts of *Giardia lamblia*. The presence of any cellular exudate in the smear should also be noted: the presence of polymorphonuclear leukocytes suggests infection with enteroinvasive bacteria, whereas a predominance of red cells may suggest amebic dysentery. Culture of stool samples or rectal swabs gives the bacteriologic diagnosis. A proctosigmoidoscopy should be considered in patients with persistent dysentery: diffuse inflammation, ulceration and bleeding of the rectal mucosa are the usual appearances; ulcerated or bleeding areas of mucosa should be scraped and the material examined immediately for amebic trophozoites.

Treatment and Prognosis

The mortality from dehydrating diarrheal diseases will decline if measures to correct and maintain hydration are started as early as possible.

Treatment of Dehydration

After assessing the severity of dehydration, the first goal of therapy is to replace water and electrolyte deficits. If dehydration is severe, patients should receive an intravenous bolus of isotonic fluid (either saline or lactated Ringers) in order to prevent progression to hypovolemic shock. Oral rehydration therapy has markedly reduced mortality from dehydrating diarrheal diseases and is the treatment of choice in children with mild to moderate dehydration. Community health providers can distribute oral rehydration salts (ORS) and teach others how to make and give the solution. The formulation recommended by the World Health Organization (WHO) contains the following: a sugar such as glucose, which facilitates the absorption of sodium and water in the small intestine; sodium and potassium, to replace gastrointestinal losses of these electrolytes; and citrate or bicarbonate, which helps correct the acidosis that develops as a result of diarrhea. ORS solution is absorbed in the small bowel even in the presence of severe diarrhea. Use of a new reduced osmolarity formulation (containing 75 mEq/L of glucose and 75 mEq/L of sodium) is currently recommended.

Antimicrobial Agents

Antimicrobials usually have a limited or secondary role in the treatment of patients with secretory acute watery diarrhea. Empiric treatment, taking into account WHO protocols and local antimicrobial resistance patterns, should be given to patients who have symptoms and signs of infection with enteroinvasive organisms – fever, abdominal pain, toxicity, tenesmus, and frequent stools containing mucus and blood. Fluoroquinolones are effective against the enteroinvasive bacteria, including *Salmonella* and *Shigella* spp., though increasing resistance has been observed. Macrolides are the drug of choice for *Campylobacter* spp. infection. Giardiasis and amebiasis will require specific treatment with metronidazole or tinidazole.

Additional Therapy

Zinc supplementation reduces the duration and severity of diarrhea and mortality in children with intestinal infection [5]; a similar effect of vitamin A has not been shown. The adverse effects of diarrhea on nutrition can be lessened by continuing feeding and increasing breastfeeding in infants. Patients should be fed as soon as they want to eat, with energy-rich, low-osmolality foods given in frequent, small-volume meals, and there should be increased feeding after the diarrheal episode. Intestinal sedatives should be avoided, as the reduced frequency of bowel movements causes fluid stagnation in the gut lumen, encouraging proliferation of organisms and keeping organisms and their toxins in contact with the mucosa.

Prevention and Control

Providing clean drinking water and proper sewage disposal reduces the incidence of gut infections. Tube wells are one means of providing clean water. The construction of acceptable latrines will help to break the cycle of fecal–oral transmission of gut pathogens. Health education regarding the importance of good sanitary practices and breastfeeding should be given by trained members of the community. Although such measures will be effective in the long term, a short-term decrease in the incidence of diarrheal diseases requires more immediate measures such as vaccination. Rotavirus vaccination has been shown to be effective in children in both developed and developing countries. An oral cholera vaccine was effective in preventing cases during an outbreak in Mozambique in 2004 [6]. However, it has not been widely implemented, owing in part to its short duration of protection and issues of availability.

Control of epidemics of gastrointestinal infection includes finding the source(s) of infection, detection of cases, and treatment, as necessary, to prevent transmission of the disease. Handwashing prevents transmission of enteric infection, as does fly control.

Traveler's Diarrhea

People from developed countries who visit the tropics are at risk for developing traveler's diarrhea [7]. The risk appears to be increased in younger individuals, those taking proton pump inhibitors, and people who fail to adhere to personal hygiene precautions. The most common pathogens are enterotoxigenic *E. coli* and enteroaggregative *E. coli*; other identified bacteria include *Campylobacter, Shigella, Salmonella, Aeromonas, Plesiomonas* and *Vibrio* spp. [8,9]. Noroviruses and rotaviruses are the most common viral agents of traveler's diarrhea, and *Giardia lamblia, Entamoeba histolytica* and *Cryptosporidium hominis/parvum* the most common protozoan pathogens.

Typhoid and hepatitis A vaccines should be offered to people traveling to endemic areas. The risk of traveler's diarrhea may be lessened by the administration of bismuth subsalicylate or probiotics. Antibiotic prophylaxis has been shown to be effective in the prevention of traveler's diarrhea, but is not advised for the general population due to the potential adverse effects of antibiotics and the risk of antibiotic resistance.

In people who develop traveler's diarrhea, antibiotic therapy reduces the duration of symptoms, even in those in whom a pathogen cannot be identified. As the prevalence of fluoroquinolone-resistant *Campylobacter* spp. is increasing, azithromycin is emerging as an effective alternative in the treatment of traveler's diarrhea. Rifaximin is another option, though it is not recommended in patients with invasive disease. In addition to a short course of antibiotic therapy, patients should be advised regarding hydration and diet, and those without evidence of invasive disease may benefit from an antimotility agent.

ABDOMINAL PAIN

Upper abdominal pain is commonly due to peptic ulcer disease, and worsening of the symptoms may herald a complication such as perforation or penetration. The differential diagnosis of upper abdominal symptoms with ulceration in the stomach or duodenum includes infections (e.g. tuberculosis, *Mycobacterium avium intracellulare*, cytomegalovirus, herpes simplex virus), neoplasms (either primary tumor or metastatic disease) and infiltrative diseases. Acute pancreatitis is another cause of acute upper abdominal pain; gallstones and alcohol are the most common causes worldwide, though infectious etiologies are important in the immunocompromised. Chronic pancreatitis is characterized by abdominal pain, steatorrhea and diabetes mellitus. Alcohol abuse accounts for the majority of cases worldwide; however, in several parts of the tropics, the most common cause of chronic pancreatitis is tropical calcific pancreatitis, a condition of unknown etiology that commonly affects children. Pancreatic calcifications may be seen on plain film of the abdomen, and ductal dilatation may be evident on ultrasonography or computed tomography.

Right upper quadrant pain may be seen in biliary colic, acute cholecystitis, acute cholangitis, acute hepatitis, and liver abscess (see hepatobiliary chapter). Left upper quadrant pain may be caused by disorders of the spleen such as splenomegaly or splenic abscess or infarction. In evaluating the patient with upper abdominal pain, it is important to consider supradiaphragmatic causes such as pneumonia and myocardial infarction.

A number of parasitic worms may cause nonspecific gastrointestinal symptoms including epigastric pain. In addition, parasitic infections of the biliary tract may lead to acute pancreatitis, as exemplified by adult *Ascaris lumbricoides* worms, which can migrate from the jejunum and invade the papilla, obstructing the pancreatic and bile ducts.

Right lower quadrant pain is commonly due to acute appendicitis; not uncommonly, however, infection with *Yersinia* or *Campylobacter* can cause severe pain that is misdiagnosed as appendicitis. In females with acute lower abdominal pain, it is important to consider ectopic pregnancy, pelvic inflammatory disease, and adnexal pathologies.

Colicky abdominal pain is one of the cardinal features of bowel obstruction. It may also be seen in intussusception in children. Generalized abdominal pain and tenderness may be caused by peritonitis, which can occur as a result of perforated peptic ulcer, ileal perforation in typhoid fever, colonic perforation in amebic colitis, or rupture of a hydatid cyst. Severe abdominal pain with minimal or no tenderness is seen in acute mesenteric ischemia. In addition to considering such surgical emergencies, it is important to consider "medical" causes of abdominal pain. Patients with sickle cell disease may have acute painful episodes due to vaso-occlusion that is difficult to distinguish from other causes of an acute abdomen. Abdominal pain is a common symptom in several infectious diseases, most notably malaria.

ABDOMINAL DISTENSION

Patients with ascites may complain of abdominal pain, early satiety or dyspnea due to splinting of the diaphragm. Analysis of ascitic fluid is helpful in determining the cause of ascites: (1) to determine whether the fluid is infected (spontaneous bacterial peritonitis is defined as a polymorphonuclear leukocyte count over 250 cells/mL with a positive bacterial culture); and (2) to determine whether there is underlying portal hypertension (indicated by a serum–ascites albumin gradient of 1.1 g/dL or greater). Cirrhosis and tuberculous peritonitis are among the most common causes. Chronic hepatic schistosomiasis is a common cause of ascites in endemic areas. Malignancy can cause ascites through a number of mechanisms; while ascitic fluid cytology may be positive in peritoneal carcinomatosis, it will be negative if the ascites is due to portal hypertension from massive liver metastases. In chylous ascites, the ascitic fluid appears cloudy due to the high levels of triglycerides; the most common causes in developing countries are infections leading to lymphatic obstruction, such as tuberculosis and filariasis. Cardiac ascites may result from tricuspid regurgitation, constrictive pericarditis, or any cause of right-sided heart failure. Spontaneous bacterial peritonitis may complicate ascites due to cirrhosis; however, it is very rare in non-cirrhotic ascites, as these patients have a higher concentration of ascitic fluid opsonins. The classic presentation is with fever and abdominal pain and tenderness, but it may be asymptomatic or present with encephalopathy or renal failure.

A massive ovarian cyst can present with abdominal distension, but the central location of the swelling, presence of a fluid thrill, and absence of shifting dullness help to distinguish this from ascites.

Abdominal distension may be due to gas, either within or outside the bowel lumen. Extraluminal gas is seen in bowel perforation, which is a surgical emergency. Gaseous distension of the bowel may be due to mechanical obstruction or motility disorder. Bloating is a common symptom in lactose malabsorption, which is commonplace among Africans and Asians after childhood, and in irritable bowel syndrome.

INTESTINAL OBSTRUCTION

The cardinal features are colicky abdominal pain, vomiting, constipation and abdominal distension. A bolus of worms can cause intraluminal obstruction in children with heavy *Ascaris lumbricoides* infestation; it may also serve as a lead point for intussusception and volvulus. Colorectal carcinoma is increasingly recognized in the tropics, but may not be evident until presentation with obstruction of the large bowel. The differential diagnosis includes inflammatory masses that can lead to intramural obstruction, such as: ileocecal tuberculosis, histoplasmosis, actinomycosis, amebiasis, schistosomiasis and angiostrongyliasis. Extramural obstruction is most commonly due to incarcerated hernia. Umbilical hernias are more common in African children, but usually the defects close spontaneously. Symptoms and signs of small bowel obstruction may also be seen in paralytic ileus, in which there is bowel dilatation without mechanical obstruction. This is a common complication of abdominal surgery, but may also occur in peritonitis or after trauma. Plain film or computed tomography of the abdomen in paralytic ileus shows gas in the colon and rectum, helping to differentiate it from small bowel obstruction in which the colon is decompressed. Treatment is supportive, consisting of fluid resuscitation, correction of electrolyte abnormalities (especially hypokalemia) and discontinuation of antikinetic drugs. Another motility disorder that may be misdiagnosed as mechanical obstruction is chronic intestinal pseudo-obstruction, which may occur in Chagas disease [10]. Here, gross dilation of the colon (megacolon), most commonly involving the sigmoid colon, causes constipation; it may be complicated by toxic megacolon or volvulus.

GASTROINTESTINAL BLEEDING

Upper gastrointestinal bleeding, defined as bleeding emanating from a source proximal to the ligament of Treitz, presents with hematemesis and/or melena. It is most commonly due to bleeding peptic ulcer. In areas with a high prevalence of cirrhosis, bleeding from esophageal and gastric varices is common. Mallory–Weiss tears are mucosal lacerations at the gastroesophageal junction that are most commonly associated with repeated retching. Gastric and duodenal neoplasms can present with overt gastrointestinal bleeding, though occult blood loss is more common. Unusual causes of upper gastrointestinal bleeding include vascular abnormalities.

Hematochezia is most often due to colorectal sources but may be the first sign of a brisk upper gastrointestinal hemorrhage. Patients with infectious colitis present with bleeding in association with diarrhea, abdominal pain and systemic upset. Gastrointestinal bleeding is a common complication of typhoid fever. Many causes of lower gastrointestinal bleeding that are common in the West – colonic diverticular bleeding, ischemic colitis, colorectal cancer and hemorrhoids – are unusual in the tropics due to epidemiologic differences. Lymphoma and Kaposi sarcoma may affect any part of the gastrointestinal tract and are common causes of gastrointestinal bleeding in patients with AIDS.

The initial management of patients with acute gastrointestinal bleeding consists of fluid resuscitation and, if coagulopathy or thrombocytopenia is present, transfusion of blood products. Once patients are stabilized, endoscopy should be performed in order to diagnose and treat the source of bleeding. Cirrhotic patients with upper gastrointestinal bleeding are at risk for bacterial infections including spontaneous bacterial peritonitis; broad-spectrum antibiotics may reduce this risk.

ANATOMIC DIFFERENTIALS

MOUTH

Dental Caries

Dental caries is a chronic disease in which the composition of the oral flora is altered as a result of chronic consumption of high-sugar substances. This leads to demineralization of the enamel, eventually causing a dental cavity. Dental caries is a major oral health problem worldwide, and the incidence is increasing in developing countries as people engage in Western dietary practices [11]. Three factors are important in the prevention of caries: dietary counseling, oral hygiene, and fluoride supplementation.

Oral Cancer

Oral cancer should be suspected in any patient with a nonhealing ulcer or mass in the mouth. As with all squamous cell carcinomas of the head and neck, the major risk factors are tobacco and alcohol use. Additional risk factors include viral infection (Epstein-Barr virus, which is strongly associated with nasopharyngeal carcinoma, human papillomavirus and HIV) and betel-nut chewing, which is widespread in South and Southeast Asia.

Candidiasis

Oral infection with *Candida* ("thrush") is usually characterized by white plaques on the oral mucosa, though there is also an atrophic form that presents as erythema without plaques. It is a common finding in patients with HIV infection; other risk factors include treatment with antibiotics or steroids (both oral and inhaled). Treatment consists of a topical antifungal agent or, in patients with more severe disease, systemic therapy.

Herpes Simplex Virus Infection

Primary infection of the oral cavity with herpes simplex virus causes gingivostomatitis and pharyngitis. The lesions can be vesicular or ulcerative and may be associated with fever and cervical lymphadenopathy. Reactivation of the virus leads to vesicular lesions of the oral mucosa ("cold sores"). Treatment should be directed toward providing symptomatic relief; antiviral therapy may be helpful if primary infection is detected early or for patients with recurrent infection who can identify a characteristic precipitating factor or prodrome.

Cancrum Oris (Noma)

This is a gangrenous, polymicrobial infection affecting the orofacial tissues [12]. It starts as a gingival ulceration, which, if left untreated, spreads rapidly through the soft and hard tissues of the mouth and face, breaching normal anatomic barriers and resulting in gross deformity. It is thought to occur after fecal–oral transmission in young children who are at risk due to a complex interplay between infection, malnutrition and immunocompromise – a combination that is common in impoverished areas of Africa, Asia and Latin America. The acute stage may present with unilateral facial pain and swelling, halitosis, oral discharge and systemic upset; management consists of broad-spectrum antibiotics and local wound care together with treatment of associated diseases and nutritional deficiencies. However, most patients are not brought to medical attention until the infection is well established – characterized by a necrotic center with a well-demarcated perimeter – at which time reconstructive surgery is required.

ESOPHAGUS

Esophagitis

The main presenting features are odynophagia, dysphagia and retrosternal chest pain. While noninfectious conditions such as gastroesophageal reflux disease and pill esophagitis are the most common causes in immunocompetent hosts, infections of the esophagus are common in the immunocompromised. In patients with HIV infection, the most common cause is esophageal candidiasis. While the presence of oropharyngeal candidiasis can be a clue to esophageal infection, its absence does not rule it out. Diagnosis can be made by endoscopy, which reveals white plaques on the esophageal mucosa; biopsy reveals the presence of budding yeasts. An alternative strategy is to undertake a therapeutic trial of a systemic antifungal agent; if the symptoms do not resolve within days, then further investigation is warranted. Cytomegalovirus esophagitis causes similar symptoms, but endoscopy reveals ulcerative lesions. Ulcers are also seen in herpes simplex virus esophagitis, but they tend to have heaped-up borders as opposed to the more shallow lesions of cytomegalovirus; there may or may not be associated oropharyngeal lesions. It is important to note that a number of patients with HIV infection presenting with esophagitis may have simultaneous infection with more than one agent, whereas others will have no infection identified. The latter condition, named idiopathic esophageal ulcer, may respond to steroids.

Caustic Esophageal Injury

Caustic injuries to the esophagus may result from ingestion of acid or alkali. The main complaint is pain, and there may be signs of complications such as perforation, mediastinitis or peritonitis. Attempts at inducing emesis or neutralizing the ingested substance must be avoided, lest the injury be aggravated. Endoscopy may be helpful for risk stratification and guiding further management. Late complications include esophageal strictures, which cause dysphagia and necessitate dilation, and squamous cell carcinoma.

Esophageal Varices

Esophageal varices are relatively common in the tropics. The causes of portal hypertension can be classified as pre-hepatic, hepatic and post-hepatic. Pre-hepatic causes include the tropical splenomegaly syndrome and portal or splenic vein thrombosis. Hepatic causes may be classified as pre-sinusoidal, sinusoidal and post-sinusoidal, exemplified by schistosomiasis, cirrhosis and veno-occlusive disease, respectively. Budd–Chiari syndrome and cardiac causes (restrictive cardiomyopathy, congestive heart failure) are post-hepatic causes. Variceal bleeding carries a high mortality rate worldwide. Initial management consists of restoration of the circulating volume, with caution to avoid over-transfusion, the use of agents to reduce portal pressure (e.g. terlipressin or octreotide), and antibiotic prophylaxis. After stabilization, endoscopic variceal ligation is the ideal approach. For patients with refractory bleeding, balloon tamponade can be a temporizing measure while awaiting portosystemic shunting.

Megaesophagus

Marked dilation of the esophagus is the most common gastrointestinal manifestation of chronic Chagas disease and occurs due to a loss of neurons in the enteric nervous system. Dysphagia is the most prominent symptom, but patients may also complain of odynophagia and regurgitation; aspiration is a common complication. The condition cannot be reversed by antitrypanosomal agents, but symptomatic relief can be achieved through balloon dilations of the lower esophageal sphincter or through surgery.

Esophageal Cancer

Squamous cell carcinoma usually arises in the mid portion of the esophagus in patients with a history of tobacco and alcohol use or preexisting esophageal diseases. In contrast, adenocarcinoma affects the lower third of the esophagus in patients with Barrett's esophagus. Both types of cancer have a similar clinical presentation, with dysphagia and weight loss being the most common symptoms. Diagnosis is made at endoscopy with biopsy. Over half of patients present with incurable disease.

STOMACH

A variety of gastroduodenal pathologies are related to infection with *Helicobacter pylori*. This Gram-negative, spiral-shaped bacterium adheres to the gastric epithelium and is able to survive in the acidic environment of the stomach due to a urease that converts urea into ammonia, which increases the pH of the immediate vicinity. It is spread by person-to-person (likely fecal–oral) transmission and is usually acquired at an earlier age in developing countries than in developed countries. It is found worldwide, though the prevalence is decreasing with improved sanitation and hygiene. Infection causes acute gastritis, which leads to chronic gastritis. Peptic ulcer disease is a common complication, while a small minority of patients with *H. pylori* infection go on to develop gastric adenocarcinoma or MALT (mucosa-associated lymphoid tissue) lymphoma.

Gastritis

Both inflammation of the stomach (gastritis) and damage to the gastric epithelium with minimal or no inflammation (gastropathy) may cause epigastric pain and nausea and vomiting, but they may be asymptomatic. The most common infectious cause of gastritis is *H. pylori* infection. A number of agents cause gastropathy, the most common being nonsteroidal anti-inflammatory drugs (NSAIDs), alcohol, and bile reflux.

Peptic Ulcer Disease

Population-based endoscopy studies have shown that the prevalence of peptic ulcer disease is almost 10% in the East, twice as high as in Western countries [13]. Historically, duodenal ulcers were more common than gastric ulcers in the tropics – due to the higher prevalence of *H. pylori* and lower usage of NSAIDs – but this ratio is changing with time. While patients with peptic ulcer may be asymptomatic, the usual symptom is epigastric discomfort or pain, which may radiate to the back. The four major complications are hemorrhage, penetration, perforation, and gastric outlet obstruction. Bleeding peptic ulcer is a common cause of acute upper gastrointestinal hemorrhage; management consists of hemodynamic resuscitation, endoscopic therapy, and, for refractory cases, surgery. Treatment with a proton pump inhibitor reduces the risk of rebleeding after endoscopic hemostasis. Penetration of the ulcer through the bowel wall causes intense pain; further erosion results in bowel perforation, causing peritonitis and necessitating emergency laparotomy. Gastric outlet obstruction is usually a complication of a longstanding ulcer, due to chronic inflammation and fibrosis. A test for *H. pylori* should be performed in all patients with peptic ulceration; this may be performed either at endoscopy or noninvasively. If positive, eradication of *H. pylori* should be undertaken; this should consist of a proton pump inhibitor and two antibiotics, taking into account local resistance patterns. Unlike duodenal ulcers, which are very rarely neoplastic, gastric ulcers may be malignant in etiology, so follow-up endoscopy is necessary to ensure resolution.

Gastric Neoplasms

Gastric cancer is the second most common cause of death from cancer worldwide. Uncommon in developed countries, the incidence is highest in East Asia and parts of South America. Part of the geographic variation may be due to dietary factors and prevalence of *H. pylori*. The most common presenting symptoms are weight loss and abdominal pain; other features include dysphagia, early satiety, and iron deficiency anemia due to chronic blood loss. The majority of patients have metastatic disease at the time of presentation, precluding curative resection.

Over 90% of gastric cancers are adenocarcinomas; gastric MALT lymphomas make up a minority, but are important, as early lesions are curable with *H. pylori* eradication therapy alone. Nonresponsive or recurrent disease requires chemotherapy.

SMALL BOWEL

A wide variety of disease processes give rise to similar histologic abnormalities in the mucosa of the small intestine, resulting in predictable clinical manifestations. The first event is infiltration of lymphocytes into the epithelium, resulting in an intraepithelial lymphocytosis. Next, there is increased crypt cell proliferation, resulting in crypt hyperplasia. Then, loss of villous cells leads to increasing degrees of villous atrophy, eventually leading to a flat mucosa. As a consequence of mucosal malabsorption, patients present with diarrhea, steatorrhea and weight loss. Laboratory studies may be helpful in defining the extent of the malabsorption syndrome. Anemia may result from deficiencies of iron, folate and/or vitamin B12 – the latter implying that the mucosal damage extends to involve the terminal ileum. Prolongation of the prothrombin time may be due to a deficiency of vitamin K (one of the fat-soluble vitamins, along with A, D and E), which occurs in fat malabsorption. Hypophosphatemia, hypocalcemia and an elevated alkaline phosphatase are seen in vitamin D deficiency, which may cause osteomalacia or osteoporosis. Conditions that cause these histologic abnormalities and present with these clinical and laboratory features include parasitic infections, celiac disease, tropical sprue, bacterial overgrowth and Crohn's disease (Box 3.4). Similar clinical manifestations may be seen in other disorders with specific pathologic findings, such as intestinal lymphoma and amyloidosis. The general principles of treating disorders of the small intestinal mucosa include treating the underlying disease and correcting any nutrient deficiencies that may be present. In addition, a lactose-free, low-fat diet may be beneficial.

Tropical Sprue

Abnormalities of the small intestinal mucosa, resulting in increased intestinal permeability and decreased absorption, have been described in both residents of and visitors to certain tropical and subtropical

BOX 3.4 Causes of Malabsorption

- Infections
- Celiac disease
- Tropical sprue
- Bacterial overgrowth
- Crohn's disease
- Malignancies
  - Immunoproliferative small intestinal disease
  - Intestinal lymphoma
- Hypolactasia
- Pancreatitis
  - Alcoholic pancreatitis
  - Chronic calcific pancreatitis

countries. Variously referred to as tropical sprue or tropical enteropathy, the disorder is characterized by a chronic malabsorption syndrome, either following an episode of acute infectious diarrhea or developing more insidiously; it has even been reported to develop years after leaving an endemic area. Its incidence appears to be decreasing, mainly as a result of the increasing recognition of nontropical sprue, or celiac disease, and perhaps also due to the increasing use of antibiotics for patients with acute diarrheal diseases. It occurs in the Indian subcontinent, Southeast Asia and some parts of the Caribbean; however, it is not endemic in all tropical areas, being notably rare or absent in Africa and other parts of the Caribbean such as Jamaica. There is considerable heterogeneity in disease presentation among these areas, suggesting that tropical sprue may represent a spectrum of related disorders. The etiology is unknown, but infectious etiologies are considered likely given the epidemiology of the disease and its response to antibiotics; although a number of infectious agents have been implicated, there has been little consistency between studies. In addition, folate deficiency has been implicated in the etiology of tropical sprue, given the prevalence of folate deficiency in these patients and the histologic improvement observed upon folic acid repletion; this and other theories – for example, implicating malnutrition or excess T-cell activity – are flawed due to the inability to separate cause from effect. The clinical, laboratory and endoscopic features of tropical sprue are largely similar to those of celiac disease. While the mucosal lesion can be patchy in both conditions, the villous atrophy in tropical sprue tends to be less severe – with a flat mucosa being uncommon – but more diffuse throughout the small intestine. The key factors distinguishing tropical sprue from celiac disease are the absence of celiac disease-specific autoantibodies and the absence of clinical and histologic improvement on a gluten-free diet. Thus, tropical sprue is a diagnosis of exclusion, suggested by villous atrophy in a patient with malabsorption who is living or has lived in an endemic area. The disease can be cured with antibiotics, usually tetracycline for up to 6 months, in combination with folic acid.

Celiac Disease

Variously referred to as nontropical sprue or gluten-sensitive enteropathy, celiac disease is a chronic inflammatory disorder of the small bowel in which genetically susceptible individuals show an inappropriate immune response to wheat gluten and related proteins in barley and rye. Previously thought to be uncommon in the tropics, the discovery of specific and sensitive serologic tests has led to increased recognition of the condition, including among South Asians and Arabs of North Africa and the Middle East [14]. People from these areas with malabsorption and small intestinal villous atrophy, with no evidence of parasitic infection or bacterial overgrowth, were almost certainly misdiagnosed in the past as having tropical sprue. The prevalence of celiac disease in what was considered a low-risk group is evidenced by a study of 259 Indian children attending a pediatric gastroenterology clinic in New Delhi, in which over 40% were diagnosed with celiac disease. The condition classically presents after the introduction of gluten into the diet of infants, but adult-onset celiac disease is well recognized, and it can also present in the elderly; the prevalence is higher in females than males. Together with the increased recognition of celiac disease, there has been a greater appreciation of its protean manifestations: while classic disease presents with chronic diarrhea, abdominal distension, and failure to thrive or weight loss, a substantial proportion of patients present with atypical disease in which extraintestinal manifestations – for example, delayed menarche in girls, neuropsychiatric symptoms or osteomalacia – are more prominent; still others have silent or subclinical disease, with positive results on serologic testing and biopsy but no symptoms. Serologic tests are helpful in the diagnosis of celiac disease: the sensitivity and specificity of both of the currently used tests, IgA endomysial antibodies and IgA tissue transglutaminase antibodies, exceed 85% and 95%, respectively. However, small bowel biopsy remains the gold standard for the following reasons: in patients with positive serologic tests, biopsy helps to confirm the diagnosis and exclude complications such as lymphoma; and in patients with suggestive clinical features but negative serologic tests, it is important to continue the investigation, as approximately 10% of IgA-competent celiac disease patients are seronegative. Although the diagnosis was previously restricted to those individuals with villous atrophy on biopsy, it is now recognized that patients with lesser degrees of mucosal damage – that is, crypt hyperplasia or intraepithelial lymphocytosis alone – have a mortality rate that is at least as high as those with frank villous atrophy [15]. Thus, current diagnosis of celiac disease is based on a positive small bowel biopsy (defined as intraepithelial lymphocytosis with or without crypt hyperplasia and villous atrophy) with clinical and/or histologic improvement upon removal of gluten from the diet. Serologic tests, though not necessary for the diagnosis, are also helpful in the management of celiac disease – as a positive test will turn negative once the patient is on a strict gluten-free diet. Nonresponsive celiac disease is usually due to intentional or inadvertent ingestion of gluten; if these are ruled out, it may be due to coexistent diseases such as microscopic colitis (which is associated with celiac disease), refractory celiac disease, or enteropathy-associated T-cell lymphoma. Epidemiologic studies have shown that patients with celiac disease have an increased risk of both gastrointestinal and non-gastrointestinal malignancies.

Protein-Losing Enteropathy

Loss of protein into the gastrointestinal tract may occur as a result of: (1) erosive mucosal disease, in which protein leaks across damaged membranes; (2) non-erosive mucosal disease, in which protein loss is due to altered epithelial permeability; and/or (3) lymphatic disease, in which lymph leaks into the lumen. The most common cause of non-erosive mucosal disease is intestinal infection. Lymphatic dysfunction may be due to obstruction, as in mesenteric tuberculosis, or impaired drainage, as occurs in portal hypertension or right-sided heart failure. The diagnosis is suggested by the presence of hypoalbuminemia without protein malnutrition, proteinuria or liver disease. In addition to correcting the underlying disorder, treatment consists of providing medium-chain triglycerides for nutritional support.

Immunoproliferative Small Intestinal Disease

Also known as alpha heavy chain disease or Mediterranean lymphoma, immunoproliferative small intestinal disease (IPSID) is a form of MALT lymphoma, characterized by secretion of truncated immunoglobulin alpha heavy chains without an associated light chain by plasma cells infiltrating the bowel wall [16]. Owing to its unique epidemiology – only being found in the Mediterranean, the Middle East and Africa – the association with poor sanitation, and response to antibiotic therapy, it is thought that environmental factors, including one or more infectious agents, are critical in the etiology of IPSID. Given the association between *H. pylori* and gastric MALT lymphomas, investigators have sought to associate this pathogen with IPSID. Although one case report has been published of an association, a subsequent case series has failed to replicate this finding. Following the detection of *Campylobacter jejuni* in an index patient with IPSID, investigators examined six additional patients and found evidence of *C. jejuni* in four of them, suggesting that this bacterium might be responsible, at least in part, for driving the antigenic response in IPSID [17].

Pathology

The second, third and fourth parts of the duodenum and the proximal jejunum are areas of maximal involvement, although ileal or total small bowel involvement has been reported. Gastric and colonic involvement is even more rare. The mucosa is grossly thickened with infiltrations producing a cobblestone appearance, localized nodules or polypoid tumors. The normal villous pattern of the gut is totally effaced by the massive infiltration of plasma cells. Villi are shortened but crypts remain small and are rather buried in the infiltrate.

Clinical Manifestations and Diagnosis

The disease is characterized clinically by a severe malabsorption syndrome with diarrhea, abdominal pain and weight loss. An abdominal mass may be palpable, while hepatosplenomegaly is a sign of advanced disease. Laboratory findings are notable for hypoalbuminemia and hypogammaglobulinemia (from protein-losing enteropathy). The finding of alpha heavy chains in the serum is diagnostic, but this may be absent in a minority of patients; in the remainder, immunohistochemical staining of biopsy specimens is positive.

Treatment and Prognosis

Early-stage IPSID can be cured with antibiotic therapy, which historically has involved tetracycline with or without metronidazole (for associated parasitic infections) although newer agents may also be effective. In advanced disease, chemotherapy may be required. In unresponsive cases, surgery may be required for bulky abdominal disease causing obstruction.

Enteritis Necroticans (Pigbel)

This is a necrotizing infection affecting either the small or large intestine that occurs after ingestion of food containing the beta toxin of *Clostridium perfringens* type C. It classically affects chronically malnourished people who ingest a high-protein meal; it was first recognized in children and adults in Papua New Guinea after eating a pork feast, but has since been described in people from other parts of Asia and Africa. A cofactor for the infection is decreased trypsin activity, which is seen in protein malnutrition and in people ingesting foods with antitrypsin properties, such as sweet potatoes. The toxin causes tissue necrosis, usually affecting the small intestine but occasionally extending to involve the colon. Histologic examination reveals extensive inflammation and necrosis of the mucosa together with large numbers of bacteria on the affected surface. Patients present with abdominal pain and distension, bloody diarrhea, and shock. Surgical resection of the affected section of bowel may be curative, but the disease is often fatal.

Intussusception

Intussusception is defined as the telescoping of one part of the bowel into another. Ninety-five percent of cases occur in children, in whom the classic features are sudden onset of colicky abdominal pain and vomiting, a right-sided abdominal mass (as the ileocecal junction is the most common site), and currant-jelly stool (due to the mixture of blood and mucus). Most cases can be treated non-operatively using air, saline, or barium enemas. The majority of cases are idiopathic; in the remainder, a variety of lesions in the intestine can act as a lead point for intussusception – for example, Meckel's diverticulum, polyp or vascular malformation. The opposite is true in adults with intussusception, in whom an underlying disorder is almost always found; in addition to benign and malignant neoplasms, amebomas and schistosomal granulomas have been found to act as the lead point. Owing to the risk of underlying malignancies in adults with intussusception, surgical resection is favored over non-operative reduction.

COLON

Appendicitis

Acute appendicitis is one of the most common causes of the acute abdomen, occurring at all ages. Inflammation of the appendiceal wall leads to ischemia, necrosis, and eventually perforation, which may result in a localized abscess or generalized peritonitis. The inciting event is obstruction of the appendix, which is commonly due to fecaliths or calculi. However, the cause of the appendiceal obstruction varies by age, with lymphoid hyperplasia being common in children and tumors occasionally found in adults. In areas where schistosomiasis is endemic, schistosome ova have been found in the appendiceal wall in patients undergoing appendectomy, suggesting a potential causative role for certain parasitic infestations in the pathogenesis of acute appendicitis. Regardless of the etiology, the clinical features of acute appendicitis are similar: the classic symptoms include pain that migrates from the periumbilical area to the right iliac fossa, fever, anorexia and vomiting, though the diagnosis may be more challenging in children and the elderly who present with less specific features. Laboratory findings are nonspecific, though a leukocytosis is usually present. In areas with access to radiographic studies, ultrasonography or computed tomography may establish the diagnosis, though imaging should not delay surgical exploration in cases where the diagnosis of acute appendicitis is very likely based on the clinical assessment. For patients presenting soon after the onset of symptoms, the treatment of choice is immediate appendectomy, with the addition of broad-spectrum antibiotics in those with frank perforation; patients with a longer duration of symptoms may be managed non-operatively with antibiotics. The differential diagnosis of acute appendicitis includes acute gastroenteritis, in which diarrhea is usually a prominent symptom and abdominal pain is more diffuse. In contrast, gastroenteritis due to *Yersinia* infection may present with little diarrhea and right lower quadrant abdominal pain, causing it to be misdiagnosed as appendicitis.

Intestinal Tuberculosis

This can affect any part of the gastrointestinal tract, but the ileocecal region is an area of predilection. In addition to the classic constitutional symptoms of fever, night sweats and weight loss, abdominal involvement may be manifested by distension due to ascites, diarrhea due to malabsorption, obstruction due to stenosing disease, or the presence of an abdominal mass. Less than half of patients with intestinal tuberculosis have open pulmonary disease. Laboratory tests usually reveal anemia and raised inflammatory markers, though these are nonspecific. Tuberculin tests are usually strongly positive in patients who are adequately nourished but are frequently negative in those with malnutrition or HIV infection. Sputum and gastric washings should be examined for tubercle bacilli. Radiographic contrast studies of the gut show a range of changes, including mucosal ulceration, stricture formation, segmental narrowing, and fistula formation. Colonoscopy may establish the diagnosis when acid-fast bacilli or caseating granulomas are found on biopsy; however, these findings are not always present, and other endoscopic findings can be difficult to distinguish from other diseases of the colon, most notably Crohn's disease. Laparoscopy or laparotomy with microscopic examination and culture of biopsies may be the only means of establishing the diagnosis in some patients. If facilities for investigation are inadequate, it may be necessary to treat the patient with antituberculous drugs on the basis of a clinical diagnosis.

Inflammatory Bowel Disease

The inflammatory bowel diseases, Crohn's disease and ulcerative colitis, are chronic inflammatory disorders of the bowel that are thought to occur as a result of the interplay between genetic factors, environmental factors and the host immune response. Classically considered diseases of the West, it is now appreciated that the incidence is increasing in many developing countries. Although the hygiene hypothesis is almost certainly an oversimplification of the etiology of these diseases, the altered Th1/Th2 balance as a result of decreased exposure to helminths in childhood may be partly responsible for the increasing incidence in tropical countries that are undergoing demographic transition [18]. In addition, it is likely that a substantial proportion of true cases were misdiagnosed in the past as infectious colitis.

Crohn's disease can involve any part of the gastrointestinal tract, but has a predilection for the terminal ileum and cecum. Inflammatory lesions cause right lower quadrant abdominal pain, diarrhea and weight loss. The differential diagnosis of ileocecal inflammatory lesions includes: bacterial infections such as yersiniosis or actinomycosis; tuberculosis; histoplasmosis; parasitic infections such as amebiasis; and helminthic infections such as strongyloidiasis. Microscopic examination of biopsy specimens is notable for transmural inflammation, lymphoid aggregates, and noncaseating granulomas. It can be challenging to differentiate Crohn's disease from intestinal tuberculosis on the basis of clinical, endoscopic and histologic features; in areas where tuberculosis is endemic, an empiric trial of antituberculous drugs is undertaken [19]. Management of Crohn's disease involves both medical and surgical approaches: medical therapies include broad-spectrum antibiotics and immunosuppressive agents; surgical management is necessary if the disease is complicated by strictures, fistulizing disease or abscesses.

In ulcerative colitis, the inflammation starts at the rectum and spreads proximally; the mucosa appears red and raw on proctosigmoidoscopy. Histologic examination reveals that the inflammation is limited to the submucosa. In addition, there is an inflammatory cell infiltrate in the lamina propria, neutrophil accumulation in crypt abscesses, and depletion of goblet cells from the epithelium; granulomas are absent. Unlike Crohn's disease, in which lesions may occur throughout the bowel, ulcerative colitis is limited to the colon and rectum; thus, if the disease is not responsive to medical therapy, total colectomy is curative.

Megacolon

Patients with large bowel dilatation may be ill-appearing with abdominal pain, distension and tenderness. Toxic megacolon can complicate any of the infectious colitides, e.g. it is a relatively common complication of *C. difficile* infection; it is also seen in fulminant colitis from the inflammatory bowel diseases; rarely, it is due to drug-induced intestinal hypomotility. Abdominal examination is remarkable for a distended abdomen with absence of bowel sounds. Plain film of the abdomen shows a markedly distended colon. Stool should be sent for bacterial culture, *C. difficile* toxin, and examination for ova and parasites. However, regardless of the etiology, the treatment is colectomy; without surgical treatment, the risk of bowel perforation and peritonitis is unacceptably high.

In contrast, some patients may have large bowel dilatation without systemic toxicity. This results in constipation due to chronic intestinal pseudo-obstruction. It may be due to acquired absence of the ganglions in the enteric nervous plexus, as in Chagas disease.

Stenosing Lesions of the Colon and Rectum

Stenosing lesions of the bowel can be caused by amebiasis, schistosomiasis, tuberculosis and lymphogranuloma venereum, which involves the rectum. Strictures can also be inflammatory, occurring in Crohn's disease or after an episode of diverticulitis, or neoplastic.

The cecum is the most common site for ameboma formation, but any part of the colon may be affected. Occasionally, multiple amebomas occur in the same patient. Persisting diarrhea with blood in the stools and localized abdominal pain are the usual features, and one or more tender masses may be palpable in the abdomen. The lesion itself consists of granulation tissue with areas of necrosis and fibroblast proliferation. Amebas are often difficult to find, but serologic tests are positive in over 90% of cases. Rapid resolution follows specific treatment, and surgical excision is not required.

Granulomatous lesions of the colon due to schistosomiasis can cause narrowing of the bowel. Early lesions are reversible with antischistosomal treatment. The rare fibrotic strictures that form may require surgical removal.

RECTUM AND ANUS

Proctitis

Inflammation of the rectum causes rectal pain, tenesmus and a mucopurulent rectal discharge. While any of the infectious causes of colitis may involve the rectum, isolated proctitis is more commonly a sexually transmitted infection (STI), usually seen in men who have sex with men who engage in unprotected anal intercourse [20]. Common causes are gonorrhea, herpes simplex, lymphogranuloma venereum secondary to chlamydia (which is endemic in Africa, South and Southeast Asia, and Central and South America), and syphilis. Noninfectious causes of proctitis include the inflammatory bowel diseases, radiation, ischemia and neoplasia. Infectious workup should include rectal swab cultures for gonorrhea, lymphogranuloma venereum and herpes simplex virus, and blood for syphilis serologic testing. STI testing should be performed prior to rectal examination, as some lubricants are bacteriostatic. Anoscopy may not be possible due to pain; if performed, the mucosa is seen to be edematous, erythematous and friable with exudates or ulceration. If the proctitis is likely due to an STI but the causative agent is unknown, empiric antimicrobial therapy should be started; the combination of ceftriaxone, doxycycline and valacyclovir is effective against the four main causes. Sexual partners should be identified and treated; counseling regarding barrier protection is important, as proctitis increases the risk of HIV transmission.

Rectal Prolapse

Either the mucosa or all layers of the rectal wall may prolapse through the anus. This is almost always secondary to an underlying disorder. Common causes in children in the tropics are diarrheal diseases, especially shigellosis, parasitic infestations (e.g. with *Trichuris trichiura*), and malnutrition. Among adults, rectal prolapse is more common in elderly women due to pelvic floor weakness as a result of vaginal delivery. Treatment is focused on correcting the underlying disorder and, if repeated manual reductions are necessary, surgical repair.

Anal Lesions

Common benign lesions that occur around the anus include ulcers and warts. Both may cause pruritus, bleeding and pain. Ulcers are usually caused by herpes simplex virus, syphilis or chancroid; in addition, patients with HIV are susceptible to ulcers caused by cytomegalovirus, tuberculosis and fungal infection. A proportion of patients with HIV have ulcers without evidence of any of these infectious agents, so-called idiopathic anal ulcers. Condylomata acuminata (anal warts) are caused by human papillomavirus infection, which is related to sexual activity. These exophytic, flesh-colored lesions should be distinguished from the flat lesions of condyloma lata, seen in secondary syphilis.

Anal Cancer

Cancer of the anal canal, usually squamous cell carcinoma, makes up only a small proportion of gastrointestinal malignancies. However, the incidence is increasing worldwide, likely due to the widespread prevalence of human papillomavirus infection. The risk may be increased further in patients co-infected with HIV. Patients present with rectal bleeding or a mass at the anal verge. The treatment options are chemoradiotherapy or surgery.

GASTROINTESTINAL DISEASES IN PATIENTS WITH HIV/AIDS

Acute HIV-1 infection presents with a mononucleosis-like illness in which gastrointestinal symptoms are not usually prominent but may include nausea and vomiting and diarrhea. Rarely, patients may have pancreatitis or hepatitis. In contrast, advanced HIV infection commonly involves the gastrointestinal tract, with the main syndromes being esophageal disease and chronic diarrhea (Box 3.5). The causes of organ-specific disease in HIV-infected patients can usually be attributed to one of three causes: due to HIV infection itself; due to opportunistic infection; or due to the medications used to treat HIV or prevent its complications [21]. The etiologies vary depending on the degree of immunosuppression.

Chronic diarrhea is a common problem in patients with AIDS, causing significant morbidity and mortality. While the CD4 cell count is preserved, the causes are similar to those in patients without HIV. As the infection becomes more advanced, parasitic, fungal and viral infections become more prevalent. Many of these pathogens can also be identified in AIDS patients without diarrhea, showing that asymptomatic infection is common. Workup should include stool specimens for bacterial culture and ova and parasite examinations. If these

BOX 3.5 Gastrointestinal Involvement in AIDS

- Dysphagia
  - Candida esophagitis
  - CMV esophagitis
  - HSV esophagitis
  - Idiopathic esophageal ulcer
- Diarrhea
  - Opportunistic infections
    - CMV
    - Salmonellosis, campylobacteriosis
    - Tuberculosis, *Mycobacterium avium-intracellulare* infection
    - *Cryptosporidium hominis/parvum, Cyclospora cayetanensis, Isospora belli, Entamoeba histolytica, Giardia lamblia, Strongyloides stercoralis*
    - Microsporidiosis, cryptococcosis, coccidioidomycosis, histoplasmosis
  - AIDS enteropathy
  - Medications
  - Lymphoma
- Malignancy – any location, due to
  - Kaposi sarcoma
  - Non-Hodgkin lymphoma

are unrevealing, flexible sigmoidoscopy with biopsy may be helpful in the diagnosis, especially in the identification of cytomegalovirus infection. Treatment should be directed at the specific enteric pathogen identified and antiretroviral therapy, which is the only treatment for some infections such as cryptosporidiosis and microsporidiosis, should be initiated.

In a substantial proportion of AIDS patients with diarrhea, no enteric pathogens are isolated. Small intestinal biopsy specimens from these patients are notable for villous atrophy and lymphocytic infiltration into the lamina propria. This idiopathic condition is named AIDS enteropathy, and may represent the mucosal response to atypical pathogens, including HIV.

REFERENCES

1. Kosek M, Bern C, Guerrant RL. The global burden of diarrhoeal disease, as estimated from studies published between 1992 and 2000. Bull World Health Organ 2003;81:197–204.
2. Hogenauer C, Langner C, Beubler E, et al. *Klebsiella oxytoca* as a causative organism of antibiotic-associated hemorrhagic colitis. N Engl J Med 2006; 355:2418–26.
3. Pawlowski SW, Warren CA, Guerrant R. Diagnosis and treatment of acute or persistent diarrhea. Gastroenterology 2009;136:1874–86.
4. Ramakrishna BS, Venkataraman S, Mukhopadhya A. Tropical malabsorption. Postgrad Med J 2006;82:779–87.
5. Roy SK, Hossain MJ, Khatun W, et al. Zinc supplementation in children with cholera in Bangladesh: randomised controlled trial. BMJ 2008;336:266–8.
6. Lucas MES, Deen JL, von Seidlein L, et al. Effectiveness of mass oral cholera vaccination in Beira, Mozambique. N Engl J Med 2005;352:757–67.
7. Hill DR, Ryan ET. Management of travellers' diarrhoea. BMJ 2008;337:a1746.
8. Steffen R. Epidemiology of traveler's diarrhea. Clin Infect Dis 2005;41(Suppl 8):S536–40.
9. Shah N, DuPont HL, Ramsey DJ. Global etiology of travelers' diarrhea: systematic review from 1973 to the present. Am J Trop Med Hyg 2009;80:609–14.
10. Teixeira AR, Nitz N, Guimaro MC, et al. Chagas disease. Postgrad Med J 2006;82:788–98.
11. Section on Pediatric Dentistry and Oral Health. Preventive oral health intervention for pediatricians. Pediatrics 2008;122:1387–94.
12. Enwonwu CO, Falkler WA Jr, Phillips RS. Noma (cancrum oris). Lancet 2006;368:147–56.
13. Leong RW. Differences in peptic ulcer between the East and the West. Gastroenterol Clin North Am 2009;38:363–79.
14. Bhatnagar S, Gupta SD, Mathur M, et al. Celiac disease with mild to moderate histologic changes is a common cause of chronic diarrhea in Indian children. J Pediatr Gastroenterol Nutr 2005;41:204–9.
15. Ludvigsson JF, Montgomery SM, Ekbom A, et al. Small-intestinal histopathology and mortality risk in celiac disease. JAMA 2009;302:1171–8.
16. Al-Saleem T, Al-Mondhiry H. Immunoproliferative small intestinal disease (IPSID): a model for mature B-cell neoplasms. Blood 2005;105:2274–80.
17. Lecuit M, Abachin E, Martin A, et al. Immunoproliferative small intestinal disease associated with *Campylobacter jejuni*. N Engl J Med 2004;350: 239–48.
18. de Silva HJ, de Silva NR, de Silva AP, et al. Emergence of inflammatory bowel disease "beyond the West": do prosperity and improved hygiene have a role? Trans R Soc Trop Med Hyg 2008;102:857–60.
19. Almadi MA, Ghosh S, Aljebreen AM. Differentiating intestinal tuberculosis from Crohn's disease: a diagnostic challenge. Am J Gastroenterol 2009;104: 1003–12.
20. Davis TW, Goldstone SE. Sexually transmitted infections as a cause of proctitis in men who have sex with men. Dis Colon Rectum 2009;52:507–12.
21. Cello JP, Day LW. Idiopathic AIDS enteropathy and treatment of gastrointestinal opportunistic pathogens. Gastroenterology 2009;136:1952–65.

4 Hepatobiliary Diseases

Mark Danta, Arthur Y Kim

Key features

- Hepatobiliary abnormalities are common in resource limited and tropical settings
- Liver disease can be divided into: "pre-hepatic", involving the portal vein or hepatic artery; "hepatic", involving the parenchymal lobule, including hepatocytes, biliary and vascular sinusoids; and "post-hepatic", involving the hepatic vein or biliary systems
- Characterizing liver abnormalities involves a combination of clinical, biochemical, serologic, microbiologic, radiologic and histologic investigations
- Hepatitis is common, and most frequently due to viral infections and toxins
- Parasitic infection of the liver may be seen during echinococcosis, schistosomiasis and liver fluke infection, among other processes
- Many tropical diseases may result in cholestasis and jaundice, through varied mechanisms
- Focal liver diseases may be due to infection or neoplasia
- Hepatitis B and hepatitis C can lead to chronic liver disease, especially in setting of HIV co-infection
- Chronic liver disease can lead to cirrhosis, liver failure, and cancer

INTRODUCTION

Given the prevalence of hepatotropic infections and the exposure of the liver to gastrointestinal organisms and toxins, it is not surprising that many tropical diseases manifest primarily in the liver. Acute and chronic diseases of the hepatobiliary system pose major threats to the health of people living within, and travelers to, endemic regions. This chapter provides a framework to approach common presentations of liver diseases in the tropics. Each primary clinical presentation is discussed with emphasis on differential diagnosis; for individual conditions, the reader is referred to the specific chapter.

APPROACH TO LIVER DISEASE

The liver has a great capacity to regenerate; however, hepatic dysfunction and failure, which usually occurs in the context of cirrhosis, carries a poor prognosis. Specific etiologic agents cause a variety of liver injuries. The functional unit of the liver is the hepatic lobule. Blood enters from either the portal (70%) or systemic (30%) circulation, flowing across the liver sinusoids to the central vein and then back to the heart via the hepatic veins. The hepatocyte microvilli, which project basally into the perisinusoidal space and apically into the bile canaliculi, actively secrete and absorb fluids and solutes. The liver is integrally involved in the synthesis of proteins, metabolism of amino acids, fat and carbohydrate, and the detoxification of many compounds; receiving blood from the intestine, spleen and pancreas via the portal circulation. As a result, the liver is exposed to numerous potential infective and toxic pathogens from the gastrointestinal tract, particularly in the tropics and developing world. Hepatic infections most commonly spread to the liver hematogenously, but can also ascend via the biliary tract. Gastrointestinal organisms enter the liver via the portal circulation or biliary tract, and include pathogenic ameba, enteric bacteria, hydatids, liver flukes (Fasciola, Opisthorchis and Clonorchis) and schistosomes. Systemic infections seed the liver via the hepatic artery and include *Mycobacterium tuberculosis* (TB), *Burkholderia pseudomallei* (the cause of melioidosis), syphilis and fungal infections.

The spectrum of liver disease varies from asymptomatic liver lesions and abnormalities detected on routine blood tests to hepatic failure. Chronic inflammation and subsequent hepatic fibrosis can lead to cirrhosis, characterized by the formation of fibrous tissue and regenerative nodules in the liver that disrupt hepatocyte and biliary function, and obstruct flow through canaliculi and sinusoids. These histologic changes result in the clinical manifestations of liver disease. Acute and chronic liver failure are defined by the inability of the liver to maintain normal metabolic and synthetic function [1] with manifestations that include hyperbilirubinemia (leading to jaundice), coagulopathy (leading to bleeding), increased nitrogenous waste products (associated with encephalopathy), and hypoalbuminemia (contributing to edema and ascites). Vascular obstructions that affect sinusoidal blood flow can lead to portal hypertension, which itself then contributes to ascites and formation of varices [2].

The evaluation of the liver should determine the site of hepatic injury, the underlying etiology and the severity of the liver disease. Conceptually, liver disease can be divided into: "pre-hepatic", involving the portal vein or hepatic artery; "hepatic", involving the parenchymal lobule, including hepatocytes, biliary and vascular sinusoids; and "post-hepatic", involving the hepatic vein or biliary systems. Characterizing liver abnormalities may involve a combination of clinical, biochemical, serologic, microbiologic, radiologic and histologic investigations. These evaluations should be refined by knowledge of the geographic distribution of each condition, and understanding of risk factors for each disease. Evaluation should include a detailed history encompassing a review of symptoms (including right upper quadrant pain or discomfort, anorexia, jaundice, darkened urine, pruritus, fever), underlying conditions, past vaccination history and epidemiologic exposures (including exposures to water, food, blood and animals, and sexual practices). Examination should include assessment of signs and findings consistent with liver disease, including jaundice, occurrence of smooth-surfaced white spots or patches under the nails (leukonychia), palmar erythema, spider nevi and gynecomastia. Hepatomegaly can be associated with most causes of hepatitis and liver lesions, while splenomegaly in the context of liver disease represents either portal hypertension or an underlying cause, such as malaria.

The inaccurately termed "liver function tests" can be used to refine the site of liver disease (Fig. 4.1). Bilirubin is a breakdown product of

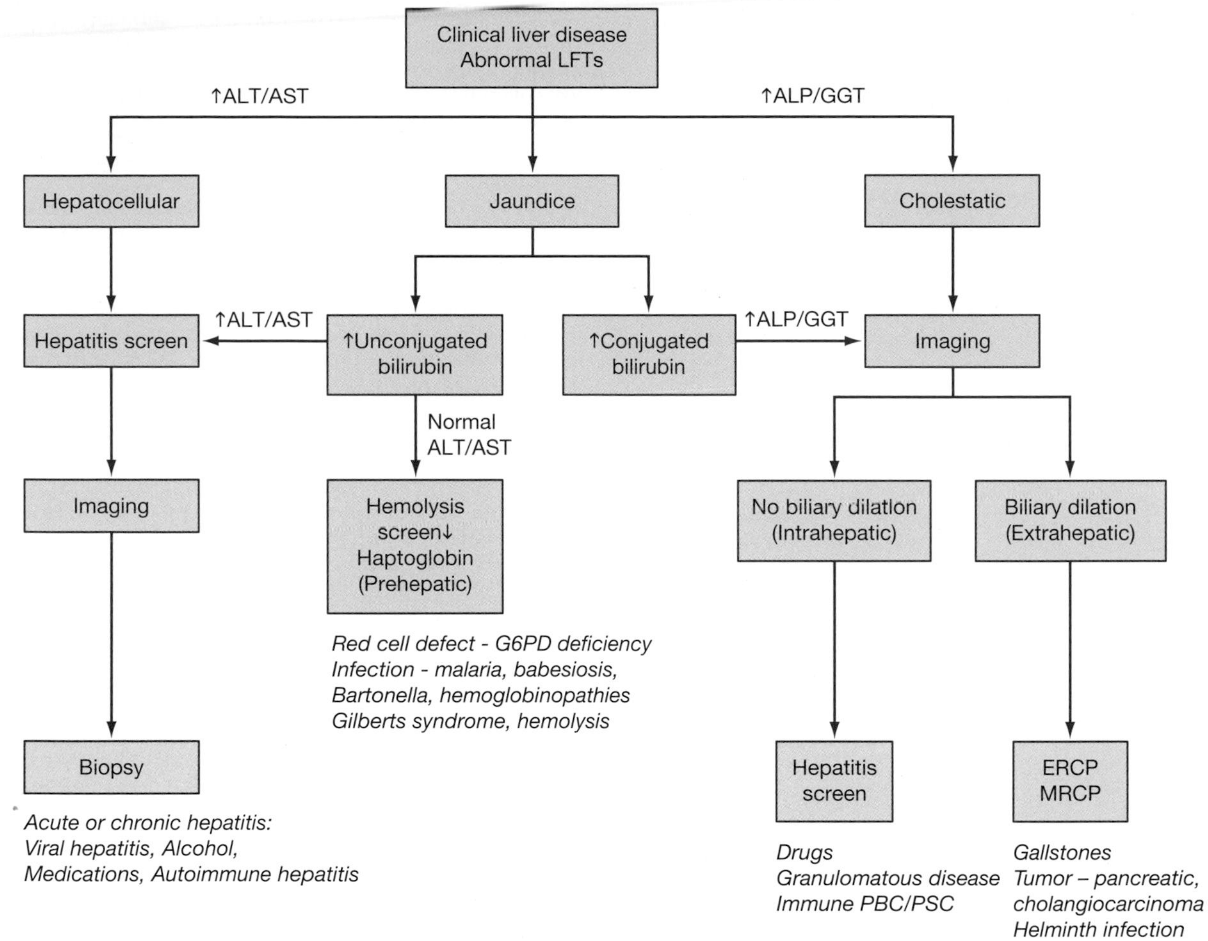

FIGURE 4.1 The initial screening tests for hepatic injury are "liver function tests", which are abnormal in a variety of tropical conditions. Abbreviations include: ALT, alanine aminotransferase (also termed SGPT or serum glutamic pyruvic transaminase); AST, aspartate aminotransferase (also termed SGOT or serum glutamic oxaloacetic transaminase); ALP, alkaline phosphatase; GGT, gamma-glutamyl transpeptidase. When jaundiced, the total bilirubin should be fractionated into unconjugated (also termed "indirect") and conjugated (also termed "direct"). Imaging is an important diagnostic tool to look for both biliary dilation and mass lesions (see Table 4-3) and to assess hepatic vasculature, with ultrasound more available in resource-limited settings than computed tomography. ERCP, or endoscopic retrograde cholangiopancreatography and MRCP, or magnetic resonance cholangiopancreatography, are useful for assessment of biliary disease.

hemoglobin which is conjugated by the liver. Elevation can result from an increased load (pre-hepatic), reduced hepatic conjugation or transport, or post-hepatic biliary obstruction. Elevation of hepatic cytosolic alanine aminotransferase (ALT) and mitochondrial aspartate aminotransferase (AST) indicates parenchymal inflammation and hepatocyte injury. In contrast, alkaline phosphatase (ALP), lining the hepatic canalicular membrane, and gamma-glutamyl transpeptidase (GGT), expressed on the epithelium of the bile ducts, are cholestatic enzymes that increase in biliary disease. However, alkaline phosphatase also increases in some parenchymal and granulomatous disease, while GGT can also be elevated following injury mediated by alcohol and drugs, such as phenytoin. Using these biochemical markers, however, patterns of liver injury can be characterized as hepatocellular (ALT/AST), cholestatic (ALP/GGT), or mixed. The true functional tests of hepatic function include assessing blood levels of albumin, bilirubin and coagulation factors. Thrombocytopenia in chronic liver disease is often secondary to portal hypertension. In the tropics, peripheral blood eosinophilia can be useful in suggesting certain parasitic infections. Based on clinical and blood parameters, two scoring systems exist that relate the severity of chronic liver disease and prognosis: the Childs Pugh classification and the Model for End-stage Liver Disease (MELD) score [3] (Table 4-1).

The primary approach to the differential diagnosis depends on the results of the initial examination and laboratory testing as outlined in Figure 4.1. Further investigations may include a hepatitis screen and imaging. A hepatitis screen usually includes viral serologies (hepatitis A, B and C), immune serologies (including antinuclear antibody [ANA], antimitochondrial antibody [AMA] and anti-smooth muscle antibody), and metabolic markers such as iron or copper studies. Applicability of tests will depend on local resources and prevalence of specific conditions. An ultrasound is a useful, usually accessible investigation that can identify parenchymal and biliary disease and cirrhosis. It may also detect evidence of portal hypertension, including reversal of portal vein flow and splenomegaly. More detailed investigations include computed tomography (CT) and magnetic resonance imaging (MRI) for parenchymal and vascular disease, and magnetic resonance cholangiopancreatography (MRCP) and endoscopic retrograde cholangiopancreatography (ERCP) for biliary disease. Finally, liver biopsy may be required for definitive diagnosis and staging of disease [4].

HEPATITIS AND JAUNDICE (Table 4-2 AND Fig. 4.1)

ACUTE HEPATITIS

Acute hepatitis can be defined as any syndrome that causes elevation of liver function tests (LFTs) for less than 6 months. This can be caused by a variety of infections, toxin/drug exposures, or metabolic

TABLE 4-1 Modified Childs-Pugh Classification

Parameter	Points assigned		
	1	*2*	*3*
Ascites	Absent	Slight	Moderate
Bilirrubin, mg/dL	</= 2	2–3	>3
Albumin, g/dL	>3.5	2.8–3.5	<2.8
Prothrombin time			
* Seconds over control	1–3	4–6	>6
* INR	<1.8	1.8–2.3	>2.3
Encephalopathy	None	Grade 1–2	Grade 3–4
Grade	**Points**	**One-year patient survival (%)**	**Two-year patient survival (%)**
A (total 5–6): well-compensated disease	5–6	100	85
B (total 7–9): significant functional compromise	7–9	80	60
C (total 10–15): decompensated disease	10–15	45	35

diseases, often with a typical hepatocellular, cholestatic, or mixed picture on LFTs. A variety of viruses, bacteria and other organisms can cause an acute elevation in liver enzymes, either due to direct infection (as in the viral hepatitides), or indirectly as a response to systemic infection (e.g. during sepsis, malaria, typhoid fever). These and other common toxins and drugs that commonly cause hepatitis are summarized in Table 4-2. Since distinguishing causality by clinical presentation alone is difficult, knowledge of the geographic distribution of infections and a history eliciting particular risk factors are critical in determining the likelihood of each entity and guiding evaluation and treatment.

Hepatitis A virus (HAV), a non-enveloped RNA virus in the picornavirus family, is the most common cause of viral hepatitis worldwide. HAV infection is transmitted by the fecal–oral route and in the developing world often occurs in the first years of life. HAV infection is usually asymptomatic when acquired in childhood and confers lifelong immunity. In adults, acute HAV is more likely to cause symptomatic illness, including prolonged jaundice with cholestasis and, rarely, fulminant hepatitis and liver failure, especially with older age. Tender hepatomegaly and splenomegaly may be present on physical examination. Overall, recovery and lack of sequelae are the outcomes in the vast majority of cases, especially among young children. Due to the unlikelihood of exposure that would generate natural immunity in many people in the developed world, HAV remains a significant risk to travelers from low-prevalence countries. Proper use of pooled immunoglobulin and inactivated hepatitis A vaccine can reduce the risk of acute infection significantly, and may be used for post-exposure prophylaxis [5]; restricting food preparation among infected individuals is also important to prevent further household transmission.

Hepatitis E virus (HEV), a calicivirus, is another virus that also has a fecal–oral route of transmission. HEV has a more localized distribution than HAV (Mexico, Asia, Africa and the Middle East), and should be considered in people living in areas with outbreaks or in travelers returning from those countries [6]. Most cases are self-limited, but fulminant hepatitis can occur, with overall mortality rates of about 0.5–4%. Pregnancy is a risk factor for severe HEV infection, with mortality as high as 20% if acquired during the third trimester. Diagnoses of both HAV and HEV rely on detection of specific IgM antibodies from sera (see Chapter 31).

In contrast, hepatitis B virus (HBV) and hepatitis C virus (HCV) are transmitted primarily through parenteral, sexual or perinatal exposure. In high-prevalence areas, HBV is primarily transmitted by vertical exposure from mother to child, and acute congenital infection is often asymptomatic with higher rates of chronicity (90%) than infections acquired later in life [7]. This course contrasts with the clinical outcome of HBV acquired during adulthood, generally through parenteral or sexual exposures. In this latter setting, symptomatic hepatitis is more prevalent along with spontaneous clearance of the virus (HBsAb positive with clearance of HBsAg). Thus, travelers or expatriates are at greater risk for acute HBV via occupational exposures (contact with blood), nosocomial exposures (contact with contaminated needles or medical equipment) or unprotected sexual contacts. Recombinant vaccines, immunoglobulin for neonates, universal precautions and safer sex are key to preventing HBV infection. Superinfection with hepatitis D virus (HDV) requires coexisting HBV infection and is generally transmitted by parenteral exposure. Diagnosis of acute HBV can be made by detection of surface antigen (HBsAg) and, more specifically for the acute stage, made by detection of IgM against the core protein (anti-HBc-IgM).

HCV is most efficiently transmitted via the parenteral route and in the majority (~75%) of infected people causes a lifelong chronic infection [8]. HCV is endemic throughout the world, but some countries and regions have a higher prevalence (e.g. Egypt has a prevalence of >10%), the epidemic amplified due to previous unsafe injection practices. Most acute infections are asymptomatic and thus do not come to medical attention, but acute symptomatic hepatitis with or without jaundice may occur. Fulminant hepatitis and mortality due to acute HCV is very rare; however, chronic liver disease that develops over decades is a major cause of morbidity and mortality. There is no approved prophylactic HCV vaccine. Diagnosis of acute HCV may be difficult, but ideally made by documentation of seroconversion and/or the presence of HCV RNA via molecular testing techniques in the presence of negative antibody.

Other tropical viral infections that affect the liver include vector-borne causes such as yellow fever, where hepatic necrosis may accompany up to 20% of cases (see Chapter 33.1) and dengue fever (see Chapter 32.1). A variety of viral hemorrhagic fevers may also involve the liver; some of these viruses (e.g. Lassa fever, Ebola virus; see Chapters 33.2 and 33.4) may require strict isolation precautions, if suspected. Herpesviruses not specific to the tropics (particularly cytomegalovirus and Epstein-Barr virus which can also cause splenomegaly) can also affect the liver.

Elevation of transaminases can occur during various systemic infections, including sepsis. Specific bacterial causes of acute hepatitis include spirochetal illness such as leptospirosis and relapsing fever, or syndromes caused by Gram-negative bacteria such as melioidosis, typhoid fever and tularemia, as well as scrub typhus and Q fever. Accompanying pulmonary symptoms may result from bacterial pneumonia, sepsis, Q fever or tuberculosis. Rarely, miliary tuberculosis may be associated with acute elevation in transaminases, but is more commonly associated with granulomatous hepatitis. Granulomatous hepatitis can be caused by several infectious and noninfectious etiologies, but primary diagnostic considerations should include tuberculosis (see Chapter 39), brucellosis (see Chapter 70) and Q fever (see Chapter 66). Eosinophilia may be caused by a variety of parasitic infections, but eosinophilia in the setting of symptomatic hepatitis or hepatomegaly may suggest schistosomiasis, trichinellosis, capillariasis or fascioliasis (see Chapters 122, 115, 107, or 124).

Noninfectious causes of liver enzyme abnormalities include acute hepatic injury from medications (Table 4-3) such as isoniazid or pyrazinamide, commonly used antimycobacterial drugs, acetaminophen, or toxins such as alcohol, mushrooms, carbon tetrachloride or aflatoxins.

TABLE 4-2 Etiology of Hepatitis

	Pre-hepatic	Hepatic (hepatocellular or intrahepatic cholestatic)	Post-hepatic
Infectious			
Fecal–oral		Hepatitis A virus Hepatitis E virus Typhoid Q fever Brucellosis	Microsporidiosis Cryptosporidiosis Ascariasis
Inhalation		Tuberculosis Adenovirus Psittacosis	
Water-borne	Schistosomiasis	Leptospirosis	Liver fluke: Fasciola Clonorchis Opisthorchis Ascariasis
Parenteral and permucosal		Hepatitis B virus Hepatitis D virus Hepatitis C virus Syphilis	
Vector-borne	Malaria Babesiosis Bartonellosis	Dengue Yellow fever Hemorrhagic fevers: Lassa, Ebola, Marburg, yellow fever, dengue	
Saliva		Epstein-Barr virus Cytomegalovirus	
Noninfectious	Hemolysis G6PD deficiency Hemoglobinopathy	Drug reaction Toxins – alcohol, aflatoxins, carbon tetrachloride Immune – primary biliary cirrhosis/primary sclerosing cholangitis Non-Hodgkin lymphoma	Cholangiocarcinoma Gallbladder cancer Pancreas: pancreatic tumor or pancreatitis Cholelithiasis
Vascular	Ischemic hepatitis Portal vein thrombosis	Sinusoidal obstruction syndrome (SOS) Nodular regenerative hyperplasia (NRH) Peliosis	Budd–Chiari Cardiac hepatopathy

TABLE 4-3 LFT Patterns with Drugs

Cholestatic	Hepatocellular
Amoxicillin/clavulanic acid Anabolic steroids Chlorambucil Chlorpromazine Chlorpropamide Erythromycin Estrogen (oral contraceptives) Tricyclics	Acetaminophen Antiretroviral therapy (ART) Allopurinol Amiodarone Aspirin and nonsteroidal anti-inflammatory drugs (NSAIDs) Carbamazepine Halothane Isoniazid Ketoconazole Nitrofurantoin Phenytoin Propylthiouracil Rifampin Statins Sulfonamides Tetracycline Valproic acid

CHRONIC LIVER DISEASE

Chronic hepatitis is arbitrarily defined as abnormal liver function tests for more than 6 months. The major consequence of chronic hepatitis is cirrhosis with its concomitant risk of liver failure and cancer. The most common cause of chronic hepatitis worldwide is hepatitis B virus, with an estimated 400 million people currently chronically infected worldwide. Untreated, about 20–25% of people with chronic HBV may die of complications of cirrhosis and/or hepatocellular carcinoma, and this course may be accelerated by coexisting HDV infection. Chronic HCV is also a cause of significant morbidity and mortality worldwide, with an estimated 190 million people chronically infected. While treatments have been developed for each of these viruses, their effectiveness is not universal, and their cost is often prohibitive.

Schistosomiasis (see Chapter 122) is another major cause of chronic liver disease [9]. Adult schistosome worms live in draining veins of the intestine or urinary tract. Eggs secreted by adult worms in mesenteric vessels can be flushed into the liver, and become trapped in presinusoidal portal venules, leading to intense inflammation, granulomas, and a "pipe-stem" fibrosis. This can result in portal hypertension out of proportion to the level of fibrosis and hepatic dysfunction. Given the prevalence and geographic overlap with chronic viral hepatitis, alternative causes of liver disease should be considered when true cirrhosis is found in the setting of chronic schistosomiasis. Moreover, given that each may be clinically silent for years to decades, a high index of suspicion is needed to diagnose these conditions. Early treatment with praziquantel can lead to regression of fibrosis due to schistosomiasis.

Other causes of chronic liver disease leading to hepatic failure include: granulomatous diseases, metabolic diseases and alcoholic liver disease. Systemic infections can be associated with granulomas in the liver. In addition to schistosomiasis, these include: mycobacteriosis, leishmaniasis, histoplasmosis, brucellosis and syphilis. Noninfectious causes include sarcoidosis, lymphoma, primary biliary cirrhosis, and drug reactions. High environmental copper ingestion in children can also lead to cirrhosis (copper-associated childhood cirrhosis or Indian childhood cirrhosis); recognition of how to prevent and treat this entity has decreased the incidence of this disease. African Bantu hemosiderosis is a disease of iron overload similar in manifestations to hemochromatosis; the presumed genetic basis of this disease is currently unknown. It is important to counsel those with chronic liver disease to avoid additional hepatic insults via prevention of exposures to infectious agents and toxins, as well as provision of vaccination against hepatitis A and hepatitis B viruses.

JAUNDICE AND BILIARY OBSTRUCTION

Many tropical diseases may result in cholestasis and jaundice, through varied mechanisms. Overload of unconjugated bilirubin can occur during acute hemolysis due to malaria, babesiosis, Oroya fever (caused by *Bartonella bacilliformis*), and hemolytic uremic syndrome caused by *E. coli* O157:H7 or *Shigella dysenteriae*, and sepsis related to *Clostridium perfringens*. Hemolytic crises can also complicate hemoglobinopathies and may be precipitated by infections. Jaundice may also be caused by processes that result in impaired conjugation and/or excretion of bilirubin by the liver. Some tropical diseases may be associated with both hemolysis and impaired excretion (i.e. leptospirosis). Non-obstructive causes include any causes of generalized liver dysfunction (i.e. during fulminant acute hepatitis or subsequent to chronic liver disease/cirrhosis). Obstructive causes include noninfectious causes (gallstones and tumors), helminthic infection (such as those caused by *Ascaris lumbricoides*. or *Clonorchis sinensis* and other liver flukes) and certain protozoa (such as *Cryptosporidium hominis/parvum*, particularly in those with HIV or other states of immunosuppression). Any biliary obstruction can be complicated by bacterial cholangitis. Some of these entities often cause obstruction by mass lesions (see below section) that may also involve blockage of the pancreatic duct; serum pancreatic enzymes and ultrasound and/or other imaging may be useful tests to help identify specific etiologies.

VASCULAR LIVER DISEASE (see Table 4-2)

Vascular diseases of the liver are uncommon and include: Budd–Chiari syndrome, which is obstruction of the intrahepatic portion of the inferior vena cava or hepatic veins; portal vein thrombosis; sinusoidal obstruction syndrome (previously termed veno-occlusive disease); nodular regenerative hyperplasia and peliosis [10]. Other causes include ischemic hepatitis and congestive hepatopathy as a result of cardiac failure, for example right heart failure related to mycobacterial constrictive pericarditis. Usually, these vascular lesions are associated with portal hypertension which precedes hepatic synthetic failure. Doppler ultrasound or contrast CT are useful imaging techniques for delineating the vessels of the liver.

FOCAL LIVER LESIONS (Table 4-4)

The evaluation of a focal liver lesion may include noninvasive tests, including serology, blood parameters, tumor markers and microbiologic assessment, as well as further imaging with ultrasound, CT or MRI. Biopsy may be required to differentiate lesions; however, in a large study of focal liver lesions, preoperative assessment was correct in 221 of the 225 cases (98.2%), suggesting that fine needle aspiration for diagnosis is not necessary in the majority of cases [11]. Determining the size and whether the lesion is solid or cystic are useful in stratifying the diagnostic approach (Table 4-4). As a rule, small lesions (<1 cm) are often benign, while larger lesions and those occurring in the context of chronic liver disease have higher potential for malignancy.

TABLE 4-4 Focal Liver Lesions

	Infection	Tumor
Cystic	Abscess Pyogenic Amebic Hydatid	Simple cyst Polycystic liver disease
Solid	Tuberculosis Syphilitic gumma Liver fluke: Fasciola Clonorchis Opisthorchis	Hepatocellular carcinoma (HCC) Adenoma Fibronodular hyperplasia (FNH) Hemangioma Regenerative nodule
		Metastatic disease Lymphoma
Biliary obstruction	Liver fluke: Fasciola Clonorchis Opisthorchis Microsporidiosis Cryptosporidiosis	Cholangiocarcinoma Gallbladder cancer Pancreas: pancreatic tumor or pancreatitis Gallstone

In an individual presenting with a cystic liver lesion associated with right upper quadrant pain and fever, consideration should be given to differentiating amebic from pyogenic abscesses. While both are associated with a significant mortality, treatment differs. The typical imaging appearance of a pyogenic abscess is a fluid-filled lesion with surrounding parenchymal edema. However, imaging could not satisfactorily differentiate pyogenic from amebic abscesses in a large series [12]. In this series, multivariate analysis identified pyogenic abscesses to be associated with older age (>50 years), pulmonary findings on examination, multiple lesions and negative amebic serology (<1:256 IU). The major route of seeding in both is the portal circulation. Pyogenic liver abscesses are commonly polymicrobial, usually caused by mixed enteric facultative and anaerobic species. *Klebsiella pneumoniae* and *Streptococcus milleri* are common pathogens [13]. Focal liver abscesses can also complicate melioidosis (caused by the Gram-negative bacillus *Burkholderia pseudomallei*). Melioidosis occurs in Southeast Asia, China and northern Australia populations, particularly in patients with diabetes, alcoholism or renal failure [14].

Pyogenic abscesses require early percutaneous drainage and broad-spectrum antibiotics. Studies do not support a difference between intermittent versus continuous drainage of these abscesses [15]. In contrast, amebic abscesses are usually treated medically. Liver abscess is the most common extraintestinal manifestation of *Entamoeba histolytica* infection (see Chapter 89), occurring in endemic areas such as Central and South America, West and South Africa, and India [16]. Amebic abscesses may be solitary or multiple, and often occur in the right hepatic lobe (75%). Diagnosis is usually based on detection of antibody in blood, or antigen in stool or hepatic aspirates, as well as response to empiric treatment [17] with metronidazole or its analogs, followed by a luminal amebicide such as paromomycin, iodoquinol or diloxanide furoate to eliminate infection [16]. Drainage, however, should be considered if there is impending rupture or involvement of the pleura or pericardium.

Other cystic lesions of the liver include simple hepatic cysts and cystic hydatid disease caused by *Echinococcus granulosus* (see Chapter 128) [18]. Hydatid cysts have a typical radiologic appearance which has led to a staging classification based on imaging appearance [19]. Generally, hydatid cysts have thick pericystic walls which may be calcified. The cysts usually have septa and may contain "daughter" cysts [20]. Unlike abscesses, surrounding liver tissue is normal. Anti- *E. granulosus* antibodies are positive in a majority of cases [19]. Current treatment usually involves albendazole with or without mechanical drainage or removal.

Primary malignant hepatobiliary tumors in the developing world often relate to underlying infectious etiologies. Hepatocellular carcinoma (HCC) leads to over 600,000 deaths annually worldwide, usually occurring in the context of chronic liver disease [21]. An estimated 85% of cases are associated with chronic viral hepatitis (HBV and HCV), which currently infects over 500 million people worldwide [22,23]. Levels of HBV viremia correlate with the risk of developing HCC [24], and successful anti-HBV vaccination programs lead to a significant reduction in the incidence of HCC [25]. Other risk factors for HCC include alcohol and aflatoxins, which may in part explain the higher incidence of HCC in West African and Chinese populations without underlying HBV-related cirrhosis [23]. Diagnosis usually involves a combination of consistent findings on imaging studies, and elevated alpha-fetoprotein (AFP) levels in the setting of chronic liver disease. Typically, HCCs appear as hypervascular lesions on imaging, a result of neovascularization from the hepatic artery. Approximately 70% of cases are associated with an elevated AFP. In the largest randomized study of ultrasound and AFP screening in over 18,000 Chinese patients, biannual screening reduced HCC mortality by 37% [26]. However, the benefit of screening in resource-limited settings is controversial [27].

To date, HCC treatment involves either locoregional therapies, including alcohol injection, radiofrequency ablation, or transarterial chemoembolization (TACE), or surgical resection in those with small tumors and sufficient hepatic reserve without portal hypertension. However, overall prognosis of HCC is usually poor. Newer targeted chemotherapies such as sorafenib are emerging, but their current cost precludes use in the resource-limited settings [28]. Benign parenchymal liver tumors include adenomas, fibronodular hyperplasia, and hemangiomas. Chronic biliary inflammation associated with persistent *Salmonella* infection of the biliary tract and Clonorchis/Opisthorchis liver flukes has also been associated with gallbladder cancer and cholangiocarcinoma, respectively [29]. Individuals with these entities may usually eventually present with biliary obstruction, with elevation of alkaline phosphatase and GGT with or without jaundice, and biliary dilation on ultrasound, CT or MRCP. ERCP or endoscopic ultrasound (EUS) with cytology can be diagnostic in biliary tract malignancies. Finally, in the context of systemic disease, metastatic malignancy and lymphoma should be considered.

HIV AND THE LIVER (Table 4-5)

The majority of people infected with HIV live in the lower-income world (see Chapter 27). HIV is associated with a number of specific diseases of the liver related to immunosuppression, immune reconstitution and drug effects. Broadly, the spectrum of liver disease relates to CD4 count and antiretroviral therapy (ART) exposure. In areas where ART is available, the burden of disease has shifted from opportunistic infection and malignancy to chronic diseases, with liver disease related to viral hepatitis becoming a leading cause of morbidity and mortality [30]. Chronic viral hepatitis and HIV co-infection is associated with reduced spontaneous clearance and accelerated progression of viral hepatitis to cirrhosis, hepatic decompensation and hepatocellular carcinoma [31]. However, in those who do not have access to ART, opportunistic infection and malignancy are still prevalent. Most conditions associated with liver disease are systemic and have spread hematogenously from other sites to involve the liver. These can be stratified by CD4 count, as most serious opportunistic infections (OIs) occur with severe immunodeficiency (CD4 <100 cells/μL). However, tuberculosis, non-Hodgkin lymphoma (NHL)

TABLE 4-5 HIV Infection and the Liver

	Infection	Tumor	Other
CD4 <100 cells/μL	*Mycobacterium avium* infection Cryptococcosis Cytomegalovirus	Non-Hodgkin lymphoma (NHL) Kaposi sarcoma (KS)	
CD4 >200 cells/μL	Tuberculosis	Non-Hodgkin lymphoma Kaposi sarcoma	
CD4 >500 cells/μL	Viral hepatitis (hepatitis B virus, hepatitis C virus)	Hepatocellular carcinoma	Drug-induced liver injury (DILI) Lipodystrophy Immune reconstitution

and Kaposi sarcoma (KS) can occur at moderate levels (CD4 >200 cells/μL) of immunodeficiency [32,33]. Of the OIs infecting the liver, *Mycobacterium avium* complex is the most common. Other infections include *Cryptococcus neoformans, Pneumocystis jiroveci,* cytomegalovirus and tuberculosis. In particular geographic areas, visceral or disseminated leishmaniasis is also prevalent. AIDS cholangiopathy is associated with cryptosporidial and microsporidial infection in patients with CD4 counts <100 cells/μL, and can lead to biliary obstruction [34]. While the presentation is variable, it is usually a variation of cholangitis with diarrhea, which is the result of the intestinal infection with these pathogens.

Following the initiation of ART in individuals with low CD4 T-cell counts (<100 cells/μL), approximately 10–30% of individuals present with a new opportunistic infection or worsening clinical symptoms of an already established infection, termed immune reconstitution syndrome [35]. This is of particular relevance for those co-infected with viral hepatitis with advanced hepatic fibrosis, as fatal hepatic flares have been reported [36]. Finally, drug-induced liver injury (DILI) is commonly associated with ART, and this entity is more likely when there is co-infection with viral hepatitis [37].

REFERENCES

1. O'Grady JG, Schalm SW, Williams R. Acute liver failure: redefining the syndromes. Lancet 1993,342:273–5.
2. Cardenas A, Gines P. Portal hypertension. Curr Opin Gastroenterol 2009, 25:195–201.
3. Kamath PS, Kim WR. The model for end-stage liver disease (MELD). Hepatology 2007,45:797–805.
4. Bravo AA, Sheth SG, Chopra S. Liver biopsy. N Engl J Med 2001,344: 495–500.
5. Betz TG. Hepatitis A vaccine versus immune globulin for postexposure prophylaxis. N Engl J Med 2008,358:531.
6. Aggarwal R, Naik S. Epidemiology of hepatitis E: current status. J Gastroenterol Hepatol 2009,24:1484–93.
7. Ganem D, Prince AM. Hepatitis B virus infection – natural history and clinical consequences. N Engl J Med 2004,350:1118–29.
8. Lauer GM, Walker BD. Hepatitis C virus infection. N Engl J Med 2001, 345:41–52.
9. Gryseels B, Polman K, Clerinx J, Kestens L. Human schistosomiasis. Lancet 2006,368:1106–118.
10. DeLeve LD. Vascular liver diseases. Curr Gastroenterol Rep 2003,5:63–70.
11. Torzilli G, Minagawa M, Takayama T, et al. Accurate preoperative evaluation of liver mass lesions without fine-needle biopsy. Hepatology 1999,30:889–93.
12. Lodhi S, Sarwari AR, Muzammil M, et al. Features distinguishing amoebic from pyogenic liver abscess: a review of 577 adult cases. Trop Med Int Health 2004,9:718–23.
13. Yang CC, Yen CH, Ho MW, Wang JH. Comparison of pyogenic liver abscess caused by non-*Klebsiella pneumoniae* and *Klebsiella pneumoniae*. J Microbiol Immunol Infect 2004,37:176–84.

14. Currie BJ, Fisher DA, Howard DM, et al. Endemic melioidosis in tropical northern Australia: a 10-year prospective study and review of the literature. Clin Infect Dis 2000,31:981–6.
15. Yu SC, Ho SS, Lau WY, et al. Treatment of pyogenic liver abscess: prospective randomized comparison of catheter drainage and needle aspiration. Hepatology 2004,39:932–8.
16. Stanley SL Jr. Amoebiasis. Lancet 2003,361:1025–34.
17. Haque R, Mollah NU, Ali IK, et al. Diagnosis of amebic liver abscess and intestinal infection with the TechLab Entamoeba histolytica II antigen detection and antibody tests. J Clin Microbiol 2000,38:3235–9.
18. Frider B, Larrieu E, Odriozola M. Long-term outcome of asymptomatic liver hydatidosis. J Hepatol 1999,30:228–31.
19. McManus DP, Zhang W, Li J, Bartley PB. Echinococcosis. Lancet 2003, 362:1295–304.
20. Doyle DJ, Hanbidge AE, O'Malley ME. Imaging of hepatic infections. Clin Radiol 2006,61:737–48.
21. Parkin DM, Bray F, Ferlay J, Pisani P. Global cancer statistics, 2002. CA Cancer J Clin 2005,55:74–108.
22. Wands JR. Prevention of hepatocellular carcinoma. N Engl J Med 2004, 351:1567–70.
23. Bosch FX, Ribes J, Borras J. Epidemiology of primary liver cancer. Semin Liver Dis 1999,19:271–85.
24. Chen CJ, Yang HI, Su J, et al. Risk of hepatocellular carcinoma across a biological gradient of serum hepatitis B virus DNA level. JAMA 2006,295: 65–73.
25. Chang MH, Chen CJ, Lai MS, et al. Universal hepatitis B vaccination in Taiwan and the incidence of hepatocellular carcinoma in children. Taiwan Childhood Hepatoma Study Group. N Engl J Med 1997,336:1855–9.
26. Zhang BH, Yang BH, Tang ZY. Randomized controlled trial of screening for hepatocellular carcinoma. J Cancer Res Clin Oncol 2004,130:417–22.
27. Danta M, Barnes E, Dusheiko G. The surveillance and diagnosis of hepatocellular carcinoma. Eur J Gastroenterol Hepatol 2005,17:491–6.
28. Llovet JM, Ricci S, Mazzaferro V, et al. Sorafenib in advanced hepatocellular carcinoma. N Engl J Med 2008,359:378–90.
29. Kumar S. Infection as a risk factor for gallbladder cancer. J Surg Oncol 2006,93:633–9.
30. Bica I, McGovern B, Dhar R, et al. Increasing mortality due to end-stage liver disease in patients with human immunodeficiency virus infection. Clin Infect Dis 2001,32:492–7.
31. Koziel MJ, Peters MG. Viral hepatitis in HIV infection. N Engl J Med 2007,356:1445–54.
32. Spano JP, Costagliola D, Katlama C, et al. AIDS-related malignancies: state of the art and therapeutic challenges. J Clin Oncol 2008,26:4834–42.
33. Engels EA, Pfeiffer RM, Goedert JJ, et al. Trends in cancer risk among people with AIDS in the United States 1980–2002. AIDS 2006,20:1645–54.
34. Margulis SJ, Honig CL, Soave R, et al. Biliary tract obstruction in the acquired immunodeficiency syndrome. Ann Intern Med 1986,105:207–10.
35. Crane M, Matthews G, Lewin SR. Hepatitis virus immune restoration disease of the liver. Curr Opin HIV AIDS 2008,3:446–52.
36. Crane M, Oliver B, Matthews G, et al. Immunopathogenesis of hepatic flare in HIV/hepatitis B virus (HBV)-coinfected individuals after the initiation of HBV-active antiretroviral therapy. J Infect Dis 2009,199:974–81.
37. Sulkowski MS, Thomas DL, Chaisson RE, Moore RD. Hepatotoxicity associated with antiretroviral therapy in adults infected with human immunodeficiency virus and the role of hepatitis C or B virus infection. JAMA 2000, 283:74–80.

Hematologic Diseases 5

Stephen McKew, Jamilla Rajab, Imelda Bates

ANEMIA

ETIOLOGY

Normal hemoglobin (Hb) varies with age, sex and pregnancy status but can also be influenced by genetic and environmental factors. Hb results must be interpreted with care. Individuals living in tropical regions who otherwise appear healthy commonly have a lower Hb than the reference levels indicated in Table 5-1. This is often as a result of environmental factors such as malaria and malnutrition, but also genetic factors such as higher frequencies of α+ thalassemia. Altitude has the effect of increasing Hb by approximately 0.25 g/dl per 1000 m above sea level.

Anemia can be caused by reduced production, excessive loss or destruction of red cells. In this chapter, only causes of anemia with particular relevance for low-income countries will be discussed.

EPIDEMIOLOGY

Anemia is a major global health problem that impacts on economic premature development, as well as health. Around 1.62 billion people are anemic worldwide; 24% of the global population (Table 5-2).

The greatest burden of anemia is in pregnant women and preschool children, with the highest prevalence in Africa and Southeast Asia (Table 5-3).

DIAGNOSIS

The accurate diagnosis of anemia in a resource-poor setting is challenging where there is often little, or no, laboratory support. Healthcare workers often rely on physical signs, but there are a number of portable diagnostic tools available to aid in the diagnosis of anemia.

Pallor is a commonly used physical sign in identifying anemia and there have been numerous studies looking at the diagnostic accuracy of conjunctival and palmar pallor. In patients with severe anemia, defined as a Hb <7 g/dl, conjunctival and palmar pallor can predict severe anemia with reasonable accuracy. These clinical signs, however, cannot be relied upon to diagnose mild and moderate anemia, and are frequently misleading.

The Hb color scale (HCS) is a rapid, cheap and simple method of estimating Hb levels using a blood spot obtained from a finger prick [1]. The test costs less than US$0.1, requires no laboratory support and can estimate the Hb concentration to within 1 g/dl [2]. Assessment of the HCS when used by professionals has indicated that it can be both sensitive and specific in assessing anemia, but further field testing is needed before its widespread use as a diagnostic tool can be recommended. The HemoCue method provides an accurate Hb measurement (to within 0.1 g/dl) from a finger-prick blood spot. The 301 model has been specifically designed for use in tropical environments. The main barrier to its widespread use is the recurrent cost associated with the disposable cuvettes.

CLINICAL FEATURES

Anemia results in a reduction in oxygen delivered to tissues. It is associated with increased perinatal mortality, poor growth, delayed development and poor cognitive development in children; in adults it results in reduced productivity.

Clinical manifestations depend on the rate of development of anemia, co-existent medical conditions and the age of the patient. If the onset of anemia is insidious and there is no cardiorespiratory disease ("compensated anemia"), the Hb can fall below 8 g/dl before symptoms become apparent, especially in children who can tolerate very severe anemia. In compensated anemia, there are few symptoms at rest, although there may be pallor and breathlessness on exertion. Cardiac output is increased and there is a rise in erythrocyte 2,3-diphosphoglycerate levels, which improves tissue oxygen delivery.

A severe reduction in Hb, particularly if this has occurred acutely, can be associated with breathlessness at rest, increased heart rate and

TABLE 5-1 Normal Red Cell Indices Expressed as Mean ±2SD (95% Range)[15]

	Hb (g/dl)	RBC ($\times10^{12}$)	PCV (l/l)	MCV (fl)	MCH (pg)	MCHC (g/dl)
Birth	18 ± 4	6.0 ± 1.0	0.6 ± 0.15	110 ± 10	34 ± 3	33 ± 3
1 month	14.0 ± 2.5	4.2 ± 2.5	0.43 ± 0.1	104 ± 12	33 ± 3	33 ± 4
1 year old	12.6 ± 1.5	4.5 ± 0.6	0.34 ± 0.04	78 ± 6	27 ± 2	34 ± 2
2–6 years	12.5 ± 1.5	4.6 ± 0.6	0.37 ± 0.03	81 ± 6	27 ± 3	34 ± 3
6–12 years	13.5 ± 2.0	4.6 ± 0.6	0.4 ± 0.05	86 ± 9	29 ± 4	34 ± 3
Men	15.0 ± 2.0	5.0 ± 0.5	0.45 ± 0.05	92 ± 9	29.5 ± 2.5	33 ± 1.5
Women	13.5 ± 1.5	4.3 ± 0.5	0.41 ± 0.05	92 ± 9	29.5 ± 2.5	33 ± 1.5

From Lewis SM, Bain BJ, Bates I. Dacie and Lewis. Practical Haematology, 10th edn. Philadelphia, PA: Churchill Livingstone; 2006.

cardiac output, and, eventually, heart failure ("decompensated anemia"). There may be severe breathlessness, angina and claudication with pulmonary edema, peripheral edema, and ascites and hypotension. Mortality is high once heart failure occurs.

MANAGEMENT PRINCIPLES

The cause of the anemia should be identified and treated. Blood transfusion rapidly corrects the anemia but may exacerbate cardiac failure and carries significant infection risks, especially in low-income countries, so it should only be used as a last resort. In low-resource settings, anemia is often caused by several factors acting simultaneously, for example malnutrition, hemoglobinopathies and infections [3, 4]. Some of these factors have a degree of interdependency, such as iron deficiency and infection, which may explain why the traditional single-treatment approaches have failed to make a significant impact on the huge public health burden of anemia. More than one of the factors causing anemia described in this section may, therefore, be present in an individual and anemia will not completely resolve unless all contributory causes are addressed.

ANEMIA CAUSED BY REDUCED RED CELL PRODUCTION

Underproduction anemia can be caused by a lack of hematinics (such as iron, folate, vitamin B12, vitamin A and riboflavin) and/or reduced bone marrow activity and is characterized by anemia with an inappropriately low reticulocyte count. Hematinic deficiencies are usually caused by poor nutrition and, because the deficiency develops gradually, quite severe degrees of anemia can be tolerated. Some of these deficiencies are associated with specific features described below.

TABLE 5-2 Global Anemia Prevalence in Different Populations[16]

Population Group	Prevalence of anemia (%)	Population affected (millions)
Pre-school children	47.4	293
School-age children	25.4	305
Pregnant women	41.8	56
Non-pregnant women	30.2	468
Men	12.7	260
Elderly	23.9	164
Total population	**24.8**	**1620**

From World Health Organization. Worldwide prevalence of anaemia 1993–2005. Geneva: World Health Organization; 2008.

Iron Deficiency (Table 5-4)

This may present with angular stomatitis, koilonychia, glossitis (Figs 5.1–5.2) and loss of melanin skin pigmentation.

The mean corpuscular volume (MCV) and mean corpuscular Hb (MCH) are reduced, the platelet count is often raised, and hypochromia, microcytosis and characteristic "pencil cells" are evident on the blood film (Fig. 5.2). Serum ferritin may be low but, as it is an acute phase protein, it has been suggested that the lower cut-off level

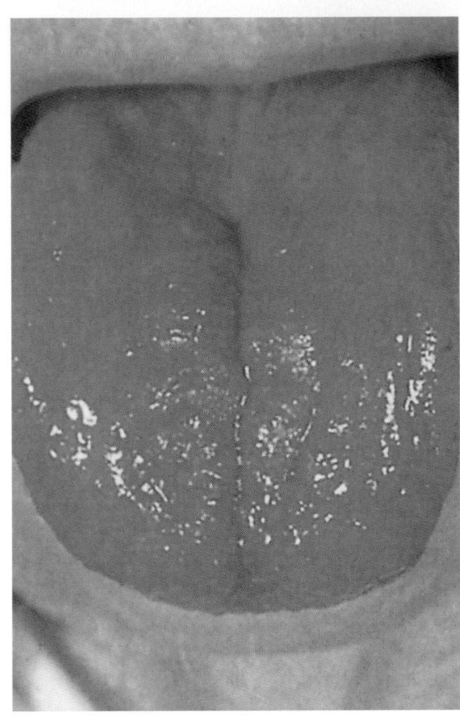

FIGURE 5.1 Tongue glossitis in iron deficiency *(reproduced with permission from Elsevier Inc. Atlas of Tropical Medicine and Parasitology, 6th edition, W. Peters and G. Pasvol, fig 1166).*

TABLE 5-3 Anemia Prevalence by WHO Region

WHO region	Pre-school age children		Pregnant women		Non-pregnant women	
	Prevalence (%)	*# affected (millions)*	*Prevalence (%)*	*# affected (millions)*	*Prevalence (%)*	*# affected (millions)*
Africa	67.6	83.5	57.1	17.2	47.5	69.9
Americas	29.3	23.1	24.1	3.9	17.8	39.0
South-east Asia	65.5	115.3	48.2	18.1	45.7	182.0
Europe	21.7	11.1	25.1	2.6	19.0	40.8
Eastern Mediterranean	46.7	0.8	44.2	7.1	32.4	39.8
Western Pacific	23.1	27.4	30.7	7.6	21.5	97.0
Global	**47.4**	**293.1**	**41.8**	**56.4**	**30.2**	**468.4**

Adapted from Iron Deficiency Anaemia: Assessment, Prevention and Control, World Health Organization, 2001.

TABLE 5-4 Common Causes of Iron Deficiency Anemia

Decreased iron intake	Inadequate diet Impaired absorption Coeliac disease Tannins, phytates (e.g. in grains and beans)
Increased loss	Gastrointestinal bleeding Hookworm Schistosomiasis Trichuriasis Gastroesophageal ulceration Malignancy NSAIDs use Menstrual loss Bladder neoplasm
Increased requirements	Infancy Pregnancy Lactation

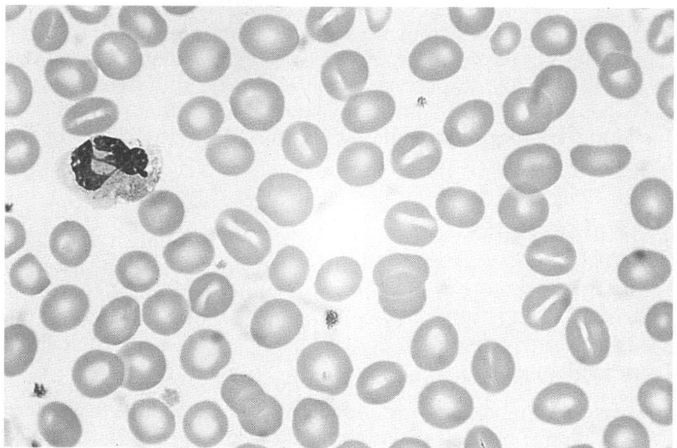

FIGURE 5.2 Photomicrograph of a blood film, Liver disease. Shows macrocytosis and stomatocytosis *(with permission from Elsevier, Dacie and Lewis: Practical Haematology, 11th edition, 2011, pp73, fig 5.11).*

should be raised in populations where infections are common [5]. Treatment is with ferrous sulfate (200 mg, three times a day) and absorption can be improved by combining it with vitamin C. Treatment should be continued for 6–12 weeks once a normal Hb is achieved to replenish body stores. If oral iron cannot be tolerated, parenteral iron should be used rather than blood transfusion. The underlying cause of the iron deficiency should also be addressed.

Folate Deficiency

Although folate is found in many foods (e.g. liver, green vegetables, tubers, bananas), deficiency is relatively common because it is destroyed by overcooking. Severe deficiency is associated with neutropenia and thrombocytopenia, and deficiency in pregnancy can cause neural tube defects and intrauterine growth retardation. Both folate deficiency and B12 deficiency cause hyperpigmentation of the skin, as well as an increase in MCV and neutrophil hypersegmentation on the blood film. A red cell folate assay and serum B12 level may be needed to differentiate between these two deficiencies. If these tests are not available, folate 5 mg/day can be tried; however, the patient should be closely monitored because if B12 deficiency is also present and untreated, the neurologic complications of B12 deficiency may become apparent (see below). Three weeks of treatment are usually adequate to replenish stores.

TABLE 5-5 Summary of the Relationship between Infections Causing Blood Loss and Anemia[17]

Infection	Relationship to anemia
Hookworm (heavy infections)	Very strong
Hookworm (light infections)	Strong
Trichuris (heavy infections)	Strong
Trichuris (light infections)	Moderate
Schistosomiasis	Strong/moderate
Ascaris	Weak/absent
Poly-infections	
≥3 soil-transmitted helminths (moderate/high-intensity infections) ± schistosomiasis	Very strong
≥3 soil-transmitted helminths (low-intensity infections) or <3 soil-transmitted helminths	Strong/moderate

Vitamin B12 Deficiency

Vitamin B12 is synthesized by microorganisms and is found in animal products, but not in vegetables. The daily requirement is extremely small and so deficiency generally develops over many years. The clinical and hematological picture of B12 deficiency is very similar to folate deficiency, but there are additional complications, such as peripheral neuropathy, optic atrophy, psychiatric abnormalities and subacute combined degeneration of the cord. Hyperpigmenatation of the skin may be more pronounced than in folate deficiency. Antibodies to intrinsic factor antibodies and gastric parietal cells may indicate pernicious anemia as the cause of B12 deficiency. The treatment of B12 deficiency is intramuscular hydroxocobalamin at a maintenance dose of 1 mg every 3 months.

ANEMIA CAUSED BY EXCESSIVE LOSS OF RED CELLS

Infections such as hookworm, trichuriasis and schistosomiasis occur predominantly in low-income countries and cause chronic blood loss from the bowel or urinary tract leading to iron-deficiency anemia (Table 5-5). They may also exacerbate anemia by interfering with intestinal absorption (e.g. strongyloides, ascaris) or by causing hypersplenism (e.g. intestinal schistosomiasis). Management consists of treating the underlying infection and replenishing iron stores. Blood transfusion should be avoided as it may precipitate cardiac failure in the presence of longstanding chronic anemia.

ANEMIA CAUSED BY REDUCED BONE MARROW ACTIVITY

Bone marrow activity can be reduced directly (e.g. by infiltration with malignant cells) or indirectly (e.g. infections, cytokines). Transient pancytopenia and myelodysplasia may occur in a variety of severe infections.

Anemia of Inflammation

Anemia of inflammation is associated with a wide range of infections, malignancies or chronic inflammatory conditions (Table 5-6). The anemia is related to cytokine production and is characterized by hypoferremia with ample reticuloendothelial iron stored in the bone marrow and other tissues, and reduced erythropoiesis in the bone marrow [6].

TABLE 5-6 Common Conditions Associated with Anemia of Inflammation

Chronic infections	Pulmonary infections (TB, abscesses, emphysema) HIV Osteomyelitis
Chronic diseases	Rheumatoid arthritis Rheumatic fever SLE Vasculitis
Malignancy	Any
Miscellaneous	Alcoholic liver disease Congestive cardiac failure Diabetes mellitus

The blood film is usually normal but may be microcytic and hypochromic in up to 25% of cases. Treatment should be targeted at the underlying condition.

Anemia and HIV

Anemia is the most common hematological consequence of infection with HIV and is an independent predictor of poor outcome. The cause of anemia is often multifactorial, including medication, poor nutrition, anemia of inflammation, opportunistic infections and malignancies. Management is by treating the HIV infection itself and addressing specific complications [7, 8].

Anemia and Parvovirus B19

In low-income countries, most children are exposed to parvovirus before the age of 2 years; protective antibodies are found in >90% of adults. The virus inhibits red cell production in the bone marrow and clinically significant anemia can occur in immunocompromised individuals or those with shortened red cell survival (e.g. sickle cell disease). Treatment is with blood transfusion, although intravenous immunoglobulin may be needed in those with immune deficiency.

ANEMIA CAUSED BY EXCESSIVE RED CELL DESTRUCTION (HEMOLYTIC ANEMIAS)

Red cells can be destroyed by abnormalities within the red cell (e.g. hemoglobinopathies, enzymopathies), abnormalities of the membrane (e.g. spherocytosis, elliptocytosis) or factors external to the red cell (e.g. drugs, antibodies, mechanical heart valves). Hemolytic anemias are characterized by anemia, jaundice, splenomegaly and gallstones, with increased reticulocyte count, unconjugated bilirubin and lactate dehydrogenase and reduced haptoglobin.

IMPORTANT TROPICAL INFECTIONS ASSOCIATED WITH ANEMIA

Malaria

Anemia can occur with all species of malaria but is especially common with *Plasmodium falciparum* infection. The cause of the anemia is multifactorial and includes intracellular parasites, hypersplenism and dyserythropoiesis caused by cytokine imbalance [9]. In malaria-endemic areas, anemia is most common in those with the highest prevalence of infection, such as young children and pregnant women. Anemia caused by malaria generally responds to antimalarial treatment but children need careful follow-up as anemia may recur or only improve slowly. Blood transfusion should be limited to those who have signs of life-threatening complications of anemia, such as cardiac failure and severe tissue under-perfusion, and are unresponsive to other resuscitation measures.

Hyper-reactive malarial splenomegaly occurs particularly in women in malaria-endemic areas and has a familial tendency. It is characterized by massive splenomegaly (≥10 cm) with hypersplenism, hepatomegaly and raised IgM levels [10]. Treatment is malarial prophylaxis (usually proguanil 100 mg/day) though other anti-malarials appropriate for long-term administration can be tried. The presence of a lymphocytosis may suggest an underlying lymphoma and should prompt referral to a specialist.

Visceral Leishmaniasis

Visceral leishmaniasis is associated with insidious onset of anemia and, eventually, pancytopenia primarily caused by hypersplenism. The diagnosis can be made by finding macrophages containing intracellular parasites (Leishman-Donovan bodies) in the bone marrow. The detection rate for parasites is higher in splenic aspirates (>95% positive compared with >85% for bone marrow) but these should only be performed if coagulation tests are normal. Treatment results in the splenomegaly and hematological abnormalities resolving after several months.

THALASSEMIAS

These are hereditary hemolytic anemias characterized by a genetic defect affecting the synthesis of one or more of the globin subunits of the Hb molecule, most commonly the α or β globin chains (α- and β- thalassemias). This leads to imbalanced globin chain production, ineffective erythropoiesis and anemia caused by destruction of the abnormal red cells.

β-Thalassemia

Approximately 3% of the world population (150 million people) carry a β-thalassemia gene mutation (Table 5-7). β-Thalassemia is most common (2–30% of the population) in the belt between the Mediterranean and Indonesia (Fig. 5.5a) but sporadic mutations occur in all populations.

β-thalassemia mutations can result in either a complete absence of the β globin chain (β^0thalassemia) or a variable reduction in production of the β globin chain (β^+thalassemia). β thalassemia is classified by the clinical severity of the disease. Thalassemia major is the most severe form and is characterized by transfusion-dependent anemia. In thalassemia intermedia, there is moderate anemia but regular transfusion is not required; thalassemia minor is generally asymptomatic.

β-Thalassemia Major

Pallor, failure to thrive, fever and splenomegaly become evident within the first 6 months of life. Without adequate blood transfusions, bone marrow hypertrophy leads to skeletal abnormalities, such as skull bossing (Fig. 5.3), prominent zygomatic bones and maxillary overgrowth with malocclusion. Ineffective erythropoiesis leads to progressive hepatosplenomegaly, gallstone formation and a hypermetabolic state with growth retardation and increased thrombosis risk.

Investigations

In non-transfused children, the Hb is 3–6 g/dl with a low MCV (50–60 fl) and MCH (12–18 pg). The peripheral blood film shows marked variation in red cell size with target cells, tear drop cells and red cell fragments. The red cells are extremely hypochromic with basophilic stippling and red cell inclusions (Pappenheimer bodies – precipitated α chains), and there are many nucleated red cells. Hb electrophoresis or high-performance liquid chromatography (HPLC) show increased levels of hemoglobin F (HbF) and hemoglobin α 2(HbA2) with absent (β^0thalassemia) or reduced normal hemoglobin α (HbA) Hb (β^+thalassemia).

TABLE 5-7 Estimated Prevalence of Carriers of Hemoglobin Gene Variants and Affected Conceptions[18]

WHO region	Demography 2003				% of the population carrying			Affected conceptions (per 1000)			Affected births (% of under-5 mortality)
	Population (millions)	*Crude birthrate*	*Annual births (1000s)*	*Under-5 mortality rate*	*Significant variant[a]*	*α^+Thalassemia[b]*	*Any variant[c]*	*Sickle-cell disorders[d]*	*Thalassemias[e]*	*Total*	
African	586	39.0	22895	168	18.2	41.2	44.4	10.68	0.07	10.74	6.4
American	853	19.5	16609	27	3.0	4.8	7.5	0.49	0.06	0.54	2.0
Eastern Mediterranean	573	29.3	16798	108	4.4	19.0	21.7	0.84	0.70	1.54	1.4
European	879	11.9	10459	25	1.1	2.3	3.3	0.07	0.13	0.20	0.8
South-east Asian	1 564	24.4	38139	83	6.6	44.6	45.5	0.68	0.66	1.34	1.6
Western Pacific	1 761	13.6	23914	38	3.2	10.3	13.2	0.00	0.76	0.76	2.0
World	6 217	20.7	128814	81	5.2	20.7	24.0	2.28	0.46	2.73	3.4

[a]Significant variants include Hb S, Hb C, Hb E, Hb D etc. β thalassemia, α^0thalassemia. [b]α^+thalassemia includes heterozygous and homozygous α^+thalassemia. [c]Allows for (1) coincidence of α and β variants, and (2) harmless combinations of β variants. [d]Sickle-cell disorders include SS, SC, S/β thalassemia. [e]Thalassemias include homozygous β thalassemia, hemoglobin E/β thalassemia, homozygous α^0thalassemia, α^0/ α^+thalassemia (hemoglobin H disease).

From Modell B, Darlison M. Global epidemiology of haemoglobin disorders and derived service indicators. Bull World Health Organ 2008;86:480–7.

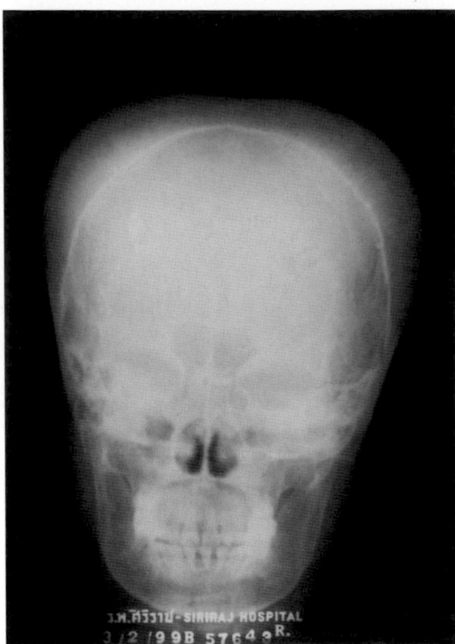

FIGURE 5.3 X-ray of skull in thalassemia.
Thalassemia disease produces this typical "hair-on-end" appearance of the skull in X-rays *(reproduced with permission from Elsevier Inc. Atlas of Tropical Medicine and Parasitology, 6th edition, W.Peter and G. Pasvol, fig 1212).*

Management and Outcome

The management of β-thalassemia major is complex and requires input from many specialities to deal with the complications and to provide psychological and social support for the patient and family. A red cell transfusion every 2–4 weeks is the mainstay of management, aiming for a Hb of 9.5–10 g/dl. Although blood transfusions can slow the development of complications, iron overload is an inevitable consequence causing endocrine failure, liver fibrosis, cardiac dysfunction and diabetes mellitus. Blood transfusions should therefore be utilized in conjunction with iron chelation (e.g. desferrioxamine, deferiprone), but this is not available in many low-income countries. Without transfusion, children may not survive beyond the age of 2 years, whereas those who receive intermittent transfusions may survive to early teenage years.

Splenectomy may be helpful in patients with hypersplenism and worsening anemia. Because of the risk of infection with encapsulated organisms, it is advisable to delay splenectomy until the child is 4–5 years old. They should be vaccinated against encapsulated organisms pre-operatively and started on lifelong penicillin prophylaxis in accordance with local guidelines for asplenic patients. Bone marrow transplantation from a well-matched sibling donor has a high success rate and, in the long-term, is probably cheaper than the transfusion-chelation regimen.

β-Thalassemia Intermedia

Thalassemia intermedia produces non-transfusion-dependent anemia with Hb levels of 5–9 g/dl. Patients present later than those with β-thalassemia major and have similar, but less severe, complications and hematological abnormalities. The need for regular blood transfusions is guided by the clinical condition of the patient, therefore growth, skeletal abnormalities and spleen size should be monitored. Transfusion may be required intermittently during periods of stress (e.g. infections, rapid growth, pregnancy) or during aplastic crises.

β-Thalassemia Trait

β-Thalassemia trait is usually asymptomatic with no, or only very mild, anemia. The MCV and MCH are markedly reduced and the blood film is hypochromic and microcytic (Fig. 5.4).

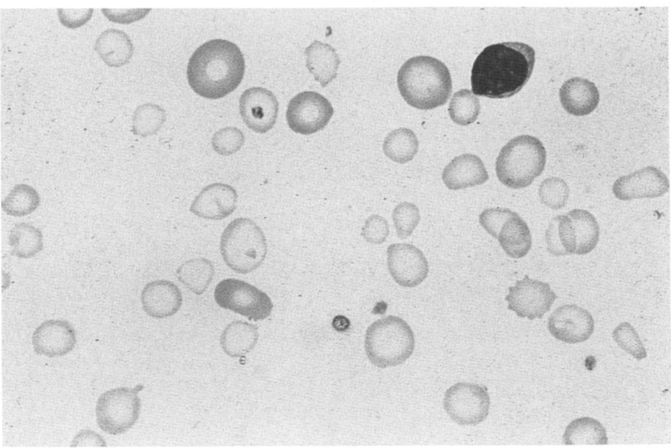

FIGURE 5.4 Photomicrograph of a blood film. Iron deficiency anemia. Shows a marked degree of hypochromia, microcytosis, marked anisocytosis and mild poikilocytosis: there are some normally hemoglobinized cells *(reproduced with permission from Elsevier, Dacie and Lewis: Practical Haematology, 11th edition, 2011, pp75, fig 5.15).*

α-Thalassemia

The α -thalassemias are common throughout the Mediterranean, sub-Saharan Africa, the Middle East, India, Southern China and Indonesia but sporadic mutations occur in all populations (Fig. 5.5).

As α genes are duplicated, there are four genes (αα/αα) responsible for production of the α chain. Deletion of one of the α genes (–α) results in α^+thalassemia, with reduced α chain production, while deletion of both genes (- -) results in α^0 thalassemia, with absent α chain production. The excess β and γ chains form tetramers: γ tetramers in fetal life (Hb Bart's) and β tetramers in adult life (HbH) which damage red cells leading to hemolysis and reduced erythropoiesis.

The α gene mutations result in four clinical conditions, increasing in severity: silent carrier, α-thalassemia trait, HbH disease and Hb Bart's hydrops fetalis.

Silent Carrier (-α/αα)

This is usually associated with a completely normal blood count and blood film or a trivial microcytic anemia.

α-Thalassaemia Trait (-α/-α or –/αα)

This is usually asymptomatic but there may be mild microcytic anemia.

Hemoglobin H Disease (HbH) (–/-α)

HbH is common in Southeast Asia and around the Mediterranean, but occurs rarely in those of African descent. Most patients have Hb 7–10 g/dl with few symptoms and mild hepatosplenomegaly. They may require occasional transfusions during pregnancy or episodes of infection. The blood film (Fig. 5.6) shows extreme variation in red cell size and shape, as well as hypochromia, microcytosis, polychromasia and basophilic stippling. Staining with brilliant cresyl blue demonstrates the characteristic "golf-ball" HbH inclusions in up to 90% of red cells. Hemoglobin electrophoresis and HPLC show increased HbH (<40%) with reduced HbA2.

Hemoglobin Bart's Hydrops Fetalis

There is complete failure of HbF and HbA production and the condition is not compatible with postnatal life. Newborns have marked hepatosplenomegaly and generalized edema and are stillborn or die shortly after birth. Globally, non-immune hydrops fetalis occurs in 1/1500–1/3800 births. It is a common reason for fetal loss in

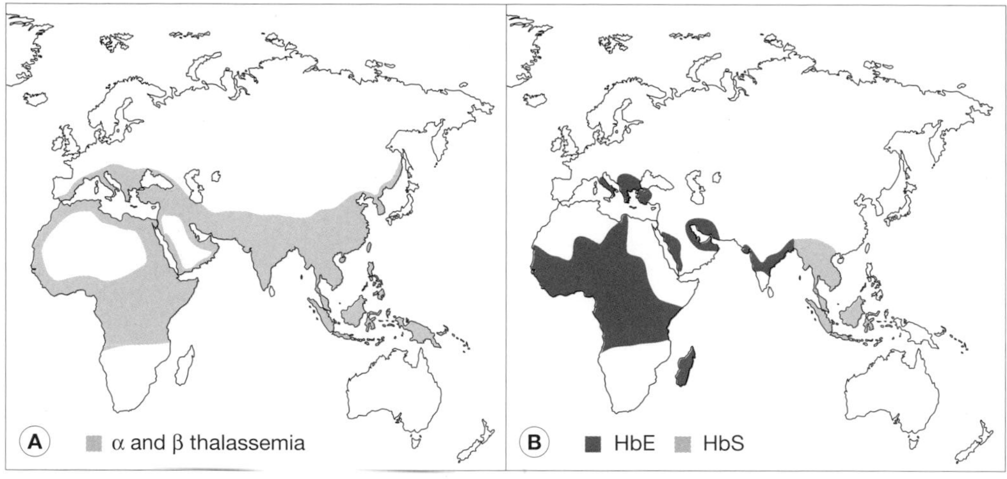

FIGURE 5.5 Global distribution of **(A)** α and β thalassemia and **(B)** haemoglobins S and E. *(Reproduced with permission from Weatherall DJ, Clegg JB. Inherited haemoglobin disorders: an increasing global health problems. Bulletin of the WHO 2001;79:704–11, Fig 2 and 3 p77).*

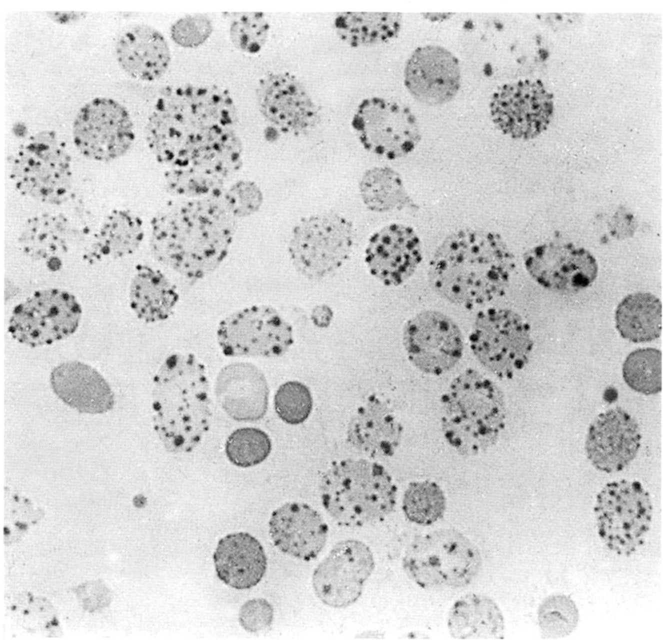

FIGURE 5.6 Hb H disease. Almost every erythrocyte is affected *(reproduced with permission from Elsevier, Dacie and Lewis: Practical Haematology, 11th edition, 2011, pp338, fig 15.7).*

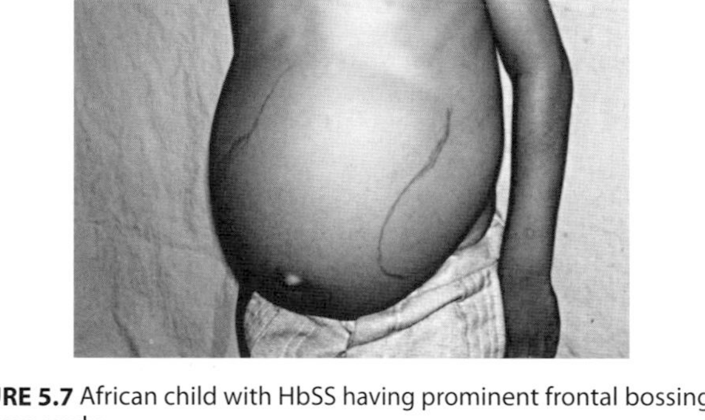

FIGURE 5.7 African child with HbSS having prominent frontal bossing and splenomegaly.

Southeast Asia, but is less common in the Mediterranean region and rare in infants of African descent.

SICKLE CELL HEMOGLOBINOPATHIES

Sickle hemoglobin (HbS) is caused by a mutation in the β globin gene which affects the stability and solubility of the β chain. When HbS is deoxygenated (e.g. during inflammation, infection, dehydration or hypoxia) it polymerizes and distorts the red cell, eventually resulting in the characteristic sickle shape. The red cell damage leads to hemolysis and vascular occlusion which is the basis for the clinical symptoms.

HbS is found in high frequency in Africa and also areas of the Middle East, where the prevalence can reach >30%. HbS occurs in parts of the world where *P. falciparum* malaria is endemic and it now has a global distribution contributed to initially by the transAtlantic slave trade and now by modern travel. Individuals with sickle cell trait (HbAS) have 10-fold protection against severe malaria compared with individuals with normal Hb. The mechanism of protection probably involves both innate and immune-mediated mechanisms.

SICKLE CELL DISEASE (HBSS) [11]

The high prevalence of HbS in sub-Saharan Africa leads to approximately 230,000 infants being born with sickle cell disease (HbSS) each year. These are mostly HbSS, but also Hb sickle cell (HbSC) and HbS/β+ thalassemia. In these infants, symptoms such as hemolytic anemia, splenomegaly and vaso-occlusive episodes become apparent after the first 6 months of life as the protective effect of HbF is lost. The age of onset of symptoms is variable, but most children will experience problems by the age of 6 years. Children with HbSS are stunted, with bossing of the bones of the skull similar to that seen in β-thalassemia (Fig. 5.7). Both conditions cause expansion of the bone marrow, which is the cause of the bossing and other abnormalities of

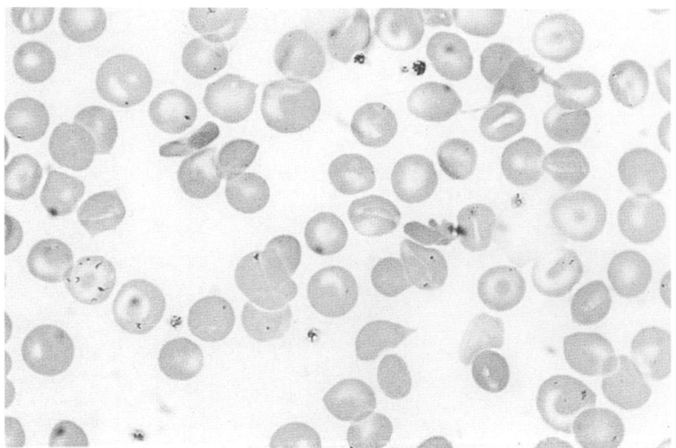

FIGURE 5.8 Photomicrograph of a blood film. Sickle cell anemia (homozygosity for hemoglobin S). Shows elliptical sickle cells, target cells and Pappenheimer bodies *(reproduced with permission from Elsevier, Dacie and Lewis: Practical Haematology, 11th edition, 2011, pp84, fig 5.55).*

development of the facial bones. HbS can be co-inherited with other Hb abnormalities (e.g. sickle cell/Hb C disease, sickle cell/β-thalassemia) when it produces a similar clinical picture to sickle cell disease. Cells containing HbSS form sickle-shaped cells in tissues where there is low oxygen tension. This triggers a complex process involving activation of adhesion, inflammation and coagulation which ultimately results in microthrombi and the pain crises so typical of sickle cell disease.

Investigations

The blood count is normal at birth but Hb falls during the first year of life. The adult Hb is 6–10 g/dl, but can drop to less than 2 g/dl during a crisis. Blood films (Fig. 5.8) show the typical sickle cells, as well as target cells, polychromasia and nucleated red cells. After the age of 3 years, features of hyposplenism (e.g. Howell-Jolly bodies) become apparent. Reticulocytes and the white cell count are often raised. Diagnosis can be confirmed by Hb electrophoresis or HPLC. A useful screening test for the presence of HbS is the sickle solubility test.

The sickle solubility test is based on the principle that HbS has reduced solubility at low oxygen tensions. A positive test indicates the presence of Hb S but does not differentiate between homozygotes (i.e. patients with sickle cell disease) and heterozygotes (i.e. sickle cell trait). A blood film is not a reliable way to differentiate sickle cell disease from sickle cell trait as in HbSS in steady state there may be very few sickled cells. False-negative sickle screening tests can occur if the patient is very anemic (ideally use packed cells to avoid this), if the reagents are out of date, if the infant is less than 6 months old or if the patient has had a recent transfusion. False-positives are associated with very high white cell counts and high protein results; this can also be minimized by the use of packed cells.

Management and Outcome

Sickle cell disease is a chronic condition requiring a multidisciplinary, long-term approach to the education and management of the patient and family. Early diagnosis is facilitated by antenatal screening; routine folic acid, penicillin prophylaxis and vaccinations to prevent infections are important. Sickle cell disease is characterized by both acute (Table 5-8) and chronic (Table 5-9) problems.

HbF has a protective effect in HbSS. Drugs such as hydroxycarbamide/hydroxyurea, which increase HbF levels, have been shown to reduce some of the complications of sickle cell disease, such as painful crises, acute chest syndrome and anemia.

Hydroxycarbamide is generally well-tolerated. It should be started at 500 mg per day (or 10–15 mg/kg in children) and increased to 1000 mg per day after 8 weeks. The dose can be increased further (2000 mg or 20–30 mg/kg) but the neutrophil count should be monitored regularly and the dose reduced if the neutrophil count falls. As in β-thalassemia major, a well-matched bone marrow transplant, even from a sibling with HbAS, may be the most cost-effective management strategy.

Life expectancy depends largely on the availability of healthcare. With high-quality health care, survival into middle age is common but, where health systems are weak, less than 2% of children born with HbSS will survive beyond 4 years.

TABLE 5-8 Acute Problems in Sickle Cell Disease

Dactylitis. Typically the bones of the hands and feet are affected with fever and leukocytosis. It is often the first event in young children and can occur multiple times until the age of 3 years

Painful crises. Typically occurs after the first few years in bones or occasionally abdominal viscera. Pain is due to ischemia and can be very severe. Crises are associated with low-grade fever and mild leukocytosis in comparison to osteomyelitis where fever and leukocytosis are more pronounced. Pain relief with paracetamol, non-steroidal anti-inflammatory drugs or opoids, as appropriate, should be instigated immediately. Supportive measures such as hydration, intravenously if necessary, and oxygen also help to reduce the duration of the pain crisis. Any precipitating cause such as infection, should be treated

Central nervous system events. Strokes occur in up to 17% of children and young adults. The pathogenesis is unclear but angiography often shows occlusions or stenosis. Recurrence is likely unless a long-term transfusion programme is initiated

Acute chest syndrome. This is a common cause of death presenting with fever, tachypnea chest pain, leukocytosis and chest pain often with a sudden drop in hemoglobin. It can be difficult to differentiate from infection, infarction and embolism. Common precipitating causes are pulmonary fat embolism and infections. Treatment is with transfusion (simple or exchange), antibiotics and aggressive treatment of hypoxia

Splenic sequestration. This occurs in children between 6 months and 2 years. It is caused by sudden trapping of red cells within the spleen producing a sudden drop in hemoglobin and rapidly enlarging spleen eventually leading to hypovolemic shock and death. Management includes early detection of the rapidly enlarging spleen and blood transfusion

Priapism. Engorgement of the penis can be short-lived and self-terminating or can last in excess of 24 hours and may lead to impotence. Initial management is with fluids and analgesia but persistent priapism (>12 hours) may need partial exchange transfusion and corporal aspiration

Infections. Overwhelming infection with *Streptococcus pneumonia* is the most common cause of death in children. Other common causes of infections in sickle cell disease include *H. influenzae* and *Salmonella*.[19] A significant reduction in the number of deaths from sepsis has resulted from the routine use of vaccinations against these organisms and antibiotic prophylaxis. Malaria prophylaxis should be considered in endemic areas

SICKLE CELL TRAIT

Individuals with sickle cell trait (HbAS) are generally asymptomatic with a normal Hb and normal life expectancy. Complications are extremely uncommon but can include poor perfusion of the renal papillae and increased bacteruria [12]. The blood film is either normal or shows a slight microcytosis. Diagnosis can be confirmed by Hb electrophoresis or HPLC. The sickle solubility test is positive.

TABLE 5-9 Chronic Problems in Sickle Cell Disease

Growth and development	Reduced height and weight Pubertal delay Cognitive impairment (recurrent small strokes)
Locomotor	Osteonecrosis of humeral and femoral heads Chronic leg ulcers
Cardiovascular	Myocardial infarction Left and right ventricular dilatation
Pulmonary	Pulmonary fibrosis Pulmonary hypertension Cor pulmonale
Genitourinary	Renal papillary necrosis – hematuria and tubular defects Chronic renal failure Frequent urinary tract infections in women Impotence (secondary to priapism)
Ocular	Proliferative retinopathy (30% of patients) Blindness (especially in SC disease) Retinal detachment

Hemoglobin Sickle Cell (SC) Disease

Hemoglobin sickle cell (SC) results from the inheritance of HbS from one parent and HbC from the other. The highest prevalence is in West Africa. The clinical features are similar to those in HbSS disease but slightly less severe. Splenic perfusion remains intact into adulthood and so splenomegaly, splenic infarcts and splenic sequestration can present in adulthood. Regular ophthalmic review should be undertaken as proliferative retinopathy may start in the second decade of life.

Anemia is less marked in HbSC than in HbSS (8–14 g/dl). The blood film in HbSC differs from that in HbSS as there are fewer sickle cells and more target cells, and rhomboid HbC crystals may be seen within ghost cells. The sickle solubility test is positive owing to the presence of HbS and diagnosis can be confirmed by Hb electrophoresis or HPLC.

Hemoglobin S (HbS) β-Thalassemia

Double heterozygous inheritance of HbS and β-thalassemia produces a variable clinical severity depending on the amount of β globin chain production. If there is no, or minimal, production ($S\beta^0$), the clinical picture is similar to HbSS.

ENZYMOPATHIES

The most common enzymopathy encountered in tropical practice is glucose-6-phosphate dehydrogenase (G6PD) deficiency, which has a prevalence of up to 25% and is associated with increased protection against malaria. G6PD is responsible for maintaining the integrity of the red cell by modulating the oxygen affinity of Hb. Cells deficient in G6PD undergo premature destruction and their half-life is directly related to the levels of G6PD in the red cells.

GLUCOSE-6-PHOSPHATE DEHYDROGENASE (G6PD) DEFICIENCY

G6PD deficiency is the most common metabolic disorder of red cells, affecting over 400 million people worldwide [13]. The gene is X-linked so deficiency is more common in boys, though it can also occur in girls. G6PD deficiency provides protection against malaria so tends to be more common in malaria-endemic areas. The clinical features vary according to the severity of the loss of enzyme activity [14]. Enzyme levels of >60% of normal are generally not associated with hemolysis. Lower levels cause varying degrees of intermittent hemolysis and if G6PD is virtually absent there may be persistent hemolysis. The African varieties of G6PD deficiency tend to be less severe than those found in other parts of the world, such as the Mediterranean region and Southeast Asia. The clinically important consequences of G6PD deficiency are neonatal jaundice and acute and, less commonly, chronic hemolysis.

NEONATAL JAUNDICE

G6PD deficiency is an important cause of neonatal jaundice. It is essential to treat high levels of unconjugated bilirubin with phototherapy and, in the most severe cases, with exchange transfusions in order to prevent kernicterus.

ACUTE HEMOLYSIS

Infections (e.g. *Salmonella, Escherichia coli*, β-hemolytic streptococci, malaria, pneumococcal pneumonia, viruses) are the most common trigger for hemolysis but it can also be caused by drugs (e.g. primaquine, sulfapyridine, nitrofurantoin) and certain foods (e.g. fava beans). In the African variety of G6PD deficiency, these triggers may result in a fall in Hb of 2–4 g/dl, resulting in mild jaundice. Usually, this does not require any specific treatment as the hemolysis will stop once the cells that are deficient in G6PD have hemolyzed. In contrast, in the more severe types of deficiencies, a life-threatening precipitous fall in Hb can occur, with the hemolysis occasionally causing acute renal failure. It is important to try to prevent further episodes of haemolysis by avoiding precipitating factors.

CHRONIC HEMOLYSIS

A small number of individuals have a very severe deficiency of G6PD with ongoing hemolysis in the absence of triggering factors. They have mild-to-moderate anemia (Hb 8–10 g/dl) and reticulocytosis of 10–15%.

INVESTIGATIONS

In the steady state, the Hb and blood film are normal in all except the most severe forms of G6PD deficiency. During a hemolytic episode, the blood film shows characteristic morphologic abnormalities with irregularly contracted cells, some with small inclusions caused by Heinz bodies, and "bite cells" where the Hb appears to have retracted within the cell. There are several simple screening tests for G6PD deficiency that depend on detecting nicotinamide adenine dinucleotide phosphate (NADPH) production. It is important to test individuals 6 weeks after the hemolytic episode, as a false-negative result can occur if testing is done during an acute attack because of the high numbers of young red cells. Quantitative G6PD assays are performed using spectrophotometry.

RED CELL MEMBRANE DEFECTS

The structure of the red cell membrane determines the shape, strength, flexibility and survival of the red cell. There are many hereditary and acquired defects of the red cell membrane which can alter these properties. These conditions often occur in malaria-endemic areas, as they may provide some protection against malaria. Examples include Southeast Asian ovalocytosis and elliptocytosis in Africa, both of which have autosomal dominant inheritance. Most of these hereditary red cell membrane defects are not associated with any clinical problems apart from occasional, mild hemolysis. The blood film is usually diagnostic.

WHITE CELL DISORDERS

Alterations in various components of the white cell count occur in many medical conditions and common causes of increased and

TABLE 5-10 Common Causes of Increased White Cells

Neutrophilia	Infection (bacterial, viral, fungal, parasitic) Inflammation (trauma, burns, infarction, autoimmune disease) Chemicals (e.g. drugs, steroids, hormones, venoms) Hematological malignancy (e.g. myeloproliferative disease, chronic myeloid leukemia) Other malignancies Hemorrhage Pregnancy and delivery Miscellaneous (e.g. cigarette smoking, post-splenectomy)
Lymphocytosis	Viral infections (e.g. measles, hepatitis, varicella, rubella) Protozoal infections (e.g malaria, *Toxoplasma gondii*) Childhood infection Leukemias and lymphomas Miscellaneous (e.g. stress, trauma, vigorous exercise, post-splenectomy)
Eosinophilia	Helminthic infections Allergic syndromes (e.g. asthma, eczema, urticaria) Many drugs Malignancy (e.g. Hodgkin's lymphoma, leukaemia) Miscellaneous (e.g. post-splenectomy, skin rashes, rheumatoid arthritis, sarcoidosis)
Monocytosis	Infection (e.g. malaria, trypanosomiasis, typhoid) Chronic infections (e.g. TB, brucellosis) Malignancy (e.g. myelodysplasia, Hodgkin's lymphoma)

TABLE 5-11 Common Causes of Reduced White Cells

Neutropenia	Viral infection (e.g. HIV, influenza) Overwhelming bacterial infection Parasitic infections Many drugs Hypersplenism Autoimmune disease Felty's syndrome Bone marrow failure (e.g. leukemia, lymphoma, aplastic anemia, malnutrition) Miscellaneous (e.g. familial, cyclical, idiopathic)
Lymphopenia	Infections (e.g. HIV, other viral infections) Autoimmune disease (e.g. SLE, rheumatoid) Bone marrow failure

decreased counts encountered in low-income countries are listed in Tables 5-10 and 5-11. Mild neutropenia is a normal finding in individuals of African descent.

Pancytopenia is a reduction in more than one type of blood cell and should raise the suspicion of leukemia, aplastic anemia or infections. Organisms associated with pancytopenia include intracellular pathogens such as *Leishmania, Mycobacteria, Histoplasma, Salmonella, Brucella* sp. , HIV, Epstein-Barr virus (EBV), hepatitis C and cytomegalovirus (CMV).

LEUKEMIA

The acute and chronic leukemias are a heterogeneous group of malignancies that arise from immature hematopoietic stem cells. They are classified as myeloid or lymphoid and further subclassified on the basis of morphology, cytochemistry, immunophenotype and genetics. Management varies with the subtype of leukemia but often the technology required to provide an accurate classification, and the full range of therapies, are not available in most hospitals in low-income countries. For this reason, and because the prognosis for patients with leukemia is better if they are managed in a specialist center, the sections below focus predominantly on features that may prompt referral to a specialist.

Acute Leukemias

Acute lymphoblastic leukemia (ALL) and acute myeloblastic leukemia (AML) have different epidemiologic patterns in low-income and industrialized countries. ALL occurs most commonly in childhood, with a peak at 2–4 years in industrialized countries and 5–14 years in less wealthy countries. This age difference is thought to be caused by delayed exposure to infection and possibly less breastfeeding in industrialized countries. The incidence of ALL in children in industrialized countries is fourfold higher than that of AML, whereas in low-income tropical countries, the incidence of childhood ALL and AML is similar. Risk factors for AML include smoking and exposure to chemicals and alkylating agents.

The clinical presentation of ALL and AML are similar because in both conditions the leukemic blast cells infiltrate the bone marrow causing pancytopenia. Patients therefore present with symptoms caused by bone marrow failure, such as anemia, fever, infection, bleeding and bony pains. Hepatosplenomegaly is commonly seen and some have infiltration of the skin and gums by leukemic cells. Chloromas, a solid mass of leukemic blasts, are more common in AML where they may occur in 10–20% of all patients and up to 30% of young boys.

Investigations

In both types of acute leukemia, the white cell count is usually raised because of the presence of blast cells, but occasionally it can be reduced, and the Hb and platelet count are often reduced. A blood film will usually show blast cells, but occasionally they may be absent or very infrequent. In children, the clinical features and blood film of acute viral infection may mimic those of ALL, and a leukemoid reaction mimicking AML may occur in severe tuberculosis. Suspicious blood films should therefore always be interpreted by a specialist. Cytochemical stains of peripheral blood with Sudan black, myeloperoxidase and nonspecific esterase can help to differentiate between ALL and myelomonocytic and monocytic AML. Flow cytometry and cytogenetic analysis undertaken at a specialist center can provide information to guide treatment strategies and to indicate prognosis.

Management and Outcome

Supportive care should be commenced while the diagnosis is being confirmed. Survival without definitive treatment is usually only a few months. Anemia, thrombocytopenia and any bleeding diathesis can be treated with appropriate blood products. Infections should be treated aggressively and allopurinol started for hyperuricemia. The treatment of ALL is complex, involving chemotherapy and radiotherapy, but can be extremely effective when delivered in specialist centers. In AML, blood transfusions and oral cytoreductive therapy, such as hydroxycarbamide/hydroxyurea, may achieve survival rates of 6–12 months. Curative treatment involves intensive regimens of cytotoxic drugs or bone marrow transplantation.

Chronic Myeloid Leukemia (CML)

Chronic myeloid leukemia (CML) is commonly associated with the Philadelphia chromosome t(9;22). This translocation results in the production of an abnormal tyrosine kinase-like protein which alters cell proliferation, differentiation and survival in several cell lines.

CML appears to occur uniformly throughout the world; incidence increases from late childhood. In low-income countries where populations are younger, CML is more commonly seen in those under 40. The clinical onset of symptoms is insidious with symptoms caused by anemia and hypercatabolic effects, such as progressive general fatigue and weight loss. Abdominal discomfort caused by splenomegaly and hepatomegaly is common.

Investigations

An increase in white cells, predominantly mature and immature neutrophils, of up to 500×10^9/l can occur, accompanied by anemia and, occasionally, increased platelets. A definitive diagnosis depends on a specialist laboratory demonstrating the 9;22 (Philadelphia) translocation by cytogenetics or *in situ* hybridization. Many inflammatory and infectious conditions can cause an increased neutrophil count with immature forms mimicking CML. These conditions tend to have lower basophil counts than in CML with toxic granulation of the neutrophils.

Management and Outcome

Once a diagnosis of CML has been made, supportive management and allopurinol should be started. Bone marrow transplantation may result in a cure but carries significant risks and is only appropriate for selected patients. In industrialized countries, first-line treatment in adults is Imatinib, a tyrosine kinase inhibitor. Currently, the manufacturer will provide Imatinib free-of-charge for low-income countries if the diagnosis can be confirmed and the patient meets certain criteria (program administered by The Max Foundation: www.themaxfoundation.org). Life expectancy with such treatment is not yet known but cure is unlikely. Cytoreductive therapy with drugs such as hydroxycarbamide/hydroxyurea or busulphan can produce some improvement in symptoms and blood count and may increase life expectancy to around 40–47 months. This may be extended by the addition of interferon α.

Chronic Lymphocytic Leukemia (CLL)

Chronic lymphocytic leukemia (CLL) usually originates from mature B lymphocytes. Incidence increases with age and there is a male predominance of 2:1. The onset of disease is gradual and it is often diagnosed incidentally. Symptoms include fever and weight loss with lymphadenopathy, splenomegaly and anemia, and an increased risk of infections.

Investigations

There is a lymphocytosis of $>5 \times 10^9$/l which occasionally can be as high as 400×10^9/l. Autoimmune anemia and thrombocytopenia can occur. The blood film shows excessive numbers of mature, but fragile, lymphocytes, so many of the cells appear "smeared". The diagnosis is confirmed by immunophenotyping, which differentiates CLL from other causes of lymphocytosis. "African CLL", which is associated with lymphocytosis and occurs predominantly in young women in Africa, is now thought to be a type of splenic lymphoma possibly related to chronic immune stimulation by malaria.

Management and Outcome

No treatment is necessary for asymptomatic CLL. Once symptoms develop, combinations of oral agents, such as chlorambucil or cyclophosphamide, are generally effective but are not curative and close monitoring is needed to avoid neutropenia. Median survival is approximately 8 years from diagnosis, but is less if the patient presents late in the course of the disease. Infection is a frequent complication and often the terminal event.

DISORDERS OF HEMOSTASIS

Disorders of haemostasis can be associated with an increased risk of either bleeding or clotting and can be acquired or congenital (Table 5-12).

TABLE 5-12 Common Bleeding Disorders

Acquired	Vitamin K deficiency Dietary deficiency or malabsorption Systemic illness (e.g. liver disease) Hemorrhagic disease of newborn Disseminated intravascular coagulation Viral and bacterial infections Obstetric disorders (e.g. septic abortion, placental abruption) Shock (e.g. trauma, surgical, burns) Envenomation Platelet disorders Infections (e.g. malaria, dengue) Hypersplenism DIC Immune (e.g. ITP, drugs, HIV) Others (e.g. cyclical, congenital, cytotoxic or non-steroidal drugs)
Congenital	Clotting factor deficiencies (e.g. FVIII – hemophilia A, FIX – hemophilia B) Von Willebrand's disease Platelet disorders (e.g. storage pool disorders, Bernard-Soulier)

ACQUIRED BLEEDING DISORDERS

Vitamin K Deficiency

Clotting factors (II, VII, IX and X) are dependent on vitamin K which is a fat-soluble vitamin. Vitamin K deficiency therefore causes prolongation of the prothrombin time (PT) and activated partial thromboplastin time (aPTT) and will respond to intravenous vitamin K (10 mg/day for 3 days orally or by intravenous injection). It should be noted that the PT and aPTT are not good predictors of the bleeding risk of a patient, as some clotting disorders associated with thrombosis (e.g. anti-phospholipid antibodies) will cause a prolongation of the aPTT.

Dietary and Absorption Deficiency

Deficiency of vitamin K because of poor diet, small bowel disease or bile flow obstruction can develop within a few weeks.

Hemorrhagic Disease of the Newborn (HDN)

In a newborn infant, vitamin K-dependent clotting factors may drop to around 5% of normal values at 48 hours. The risk of hemorrhage is highest in premature infants or those that have been exclusively breast-fed or exposed *in utero* to drugs for tuberculosis, convulsions or anti-coagulation. Newborns present in the first few days of life with bleeding into the skin and gut, bleeding from the umbilical stump or bleeding at circumcision. Prevention is with 1 mg of intramuscular vitamin K given at delivery. In some cases, hemorrhagic disease of the newborn (HDN) may present at 1–6 months with intracranial hemorrhage caused by cholestatic disease. In this case, rapid correction of the clotting abnormality can be achieved with fresh frozen plasma (FFP).

Disseminated Intravascular Coagulation (DIC)

This process is characterized by activation of hemostasis with widespread fibrin formation, activation of fibrinolysis and consumption of platelets and clotting factors. Disseminated intravascular coagulation (DIC) has many causes (e.g. tissue injury, obstetric complications, malignancies, infections) and is a life-threatening condition with a high mortality. Patients present with spontaneous bruising or excessive bleeding, for example from venepuncture sites or surgical incisions. Complications include renal failure, acute respiratory distress syndrome and microangiopathic hemolytic anemia.

The combination of depleted clotting factors (i.e. prolonged PT and aPTT) and a falling platelet count with red cell fragments on the blood film is strong evidence of DIC. Raised D-dimers or fibrin degradation products, and reduced fibrinogen levels are characteristic. Management involves treating or removing the underlying cause, correction of blood pressure and correcting the hemostatic abnormalities with combinations of platelets, cryoprecipitate and FFP.

Immune Thrombocytopenic Purpura (ITP)

Immune thrombocytopenic purpura (ITP) is caused by immune destruction of platelets. Although it is usually primary, it can be associated with underlying conditions, such as lymphomas and infections including HIV. It may present incidentally or with bruising. Bleeding from the nose or gums, or petichiae are more likely if the platelet count is <30 × 10^9/l. Spontaneous recovery occurs more often in children than in adults.

Increased numbers of platelet precursors in the bone marrow support a diagnosis of ITP. It is important to exclude other causes of thrombocytopenia, such as drugs, disseminated intravascular coagulation or sepsis. Treatment is usually only necessary if the platelet count is <30 × 10^9/l or if there is bleeding. Treatment is initially with prednisolone at doses of 0.25–0.5 mg/kg which should be tapered off over several weeks once the platelet count has improved. Second-line treatments include immunosuppressive agents and danazol. Splenectomy may result in a long-term improvement in platelet count but the benefits need to be balanced against the risks of splenectomy, particularly in low-income settings where infections are common. Platelet transfusions or intravenous gammaglobulin can be used to increase the platelet count in an emergency or prior to surgical procedures.

Congenital Bleeding Disorders

The congential bleeding disorders occur with the same frequency throughout the world. Hemophilia A has a prevalence of about 10/10,000, von Willebrand's deficiency is >10/10,000 and hemophilia B is <0.1/10,000. Although the diagnosis may be suspected from the patient's personal and family history, diagnosis should be confirmed by a specialist center. Treatment options include replacement of the missing coagulation factors and cryoprecipitate. Von Willebrand's disease may respond to desmopressin.

THROMBOPHILIA

Thrombophilia (hypercoagulability) may be inherited (e.g. deficiencies of thrombin, protein S or protein C) or acquired (e.g. antiphospholipids) and results in venous or arterial thromboembolism. The patient's personal and family history and the results of clinical and imagining examinations may suggest the diagnosis. Several laboratory tests are required to determine the cause and classify the type of thrombophilia. Interpretation of the results, understanding the limitations of the tests and explaining the implications to patients requires considerable expertise and should be done by specialists.

REFERENCES

1. Critchley J, Bates I. Haemoglobin colour scale for anaemia diagnosis where there is no laboratory: a systematic review. Int J Epidemiol 2005; 34:1425–34.
2. Medina Lara A, Mundy C, Kandulu J, et al. Evaluation and costs of different haemoglobin methods for use in district hospitals in Malawi. J Clin Pathol 2005;58:56–60.
3. Boele van Hensbroek M, Calis JC, Phiri KS, et al. Pathophysiological mechanisms of severe anaemia in Malawian children. PLoS ONE 2010;5:e12589.
4. Calis JC, Phiri KS, Vet RJ, et al. Erythropoiesis in HIV-infected and uninfected Malawian children with severe anemia. AIDS 2010;24:2883–7.
5. Phiri KS, Calis JC, Siyasiya A, et al. New cut-off values for ferritin and soluble transferrin receptor for the assessment of iron deficiency in children in a high infection pressure area. J Clin Pathol 2009;62:1103–6.
6. Deicher R, Horl WH. New insights into the regulation of iron homeostasis. Eur J Clin Invest 2006;36:301–9.
7. Volberding PA, Levine AM, Dieterich D, et al. Anemia in HIV infection: clinical impact and evidence-based management strategies. Clin Infect Dis 2004; 38:1454–63.
8. Calis JC, van Hensbroek MB, de Haan RJ, et al. HIV-associated anemia in children: a systematic review from a global perspective. AIDS 2008;22:1099–112.
9. Casals-Pascual C, Roberts DJ. Severe malarial anaemia. Curr Mol Med 2006; 6:155–68.
10. Bedu-Addo G, Bates I. Causes of massive tropical splenomegaly in Ghana. Lancet 2002;360:449–54.
11. Rees DC, Williams TN, Gladwin MT. Sickle-cell disease. Lancet 2010;376: 2018–31.
12. Tsaras G, Owusu-Ansah A, Boateng FO, Amoateng-Adjepong Y. Complications associated with sickle cell trait: a brief narrative review. Am J Med 2009; 122:507–12.
13. Nkhoma ET, Poole C, Vannappagari V, et al. The global prevalence of glucose-6-phosphate dehydrogenase deficiency: a systematic review and meta-analysis. Blood Cells Mol Dis 2009;42:267–78.
14. Cappellini MD, Fiorelli G. Glucose-6-phosphate dehydrogenase deficiency. Lancet 2008;371:64–74.
15. Lewis SM, Bain BJ, Bates I. Dacie and Lewis. Practical Haematology, 10th edn. Philadelphia, PA: Churchill Livingstone; 2006.
16. World Health Organization. Worldwide prevalence of anaemia 1993–2005. Geneva: World Health Organization; 2008.
17. Bates I, McKew S, Sarkinfada F. Anaemia: A useful indicator of neglected disease burden and control. PLoS Medicine 2007;4:e231.
18. Modell B, Darlison M. Global epidemiology of haemoglobin disorders and derived service indicators. Bull World Health Organ 2008;86:480–7.
19. Williams TN, Uyoga S, Macharia A, et al. Bacteraemia in Kenyan children with sickle-cell anaemia: a retrospective cohort and case-control study. Lancet 2009;374:1364–70.

Urinary Tract Diseases 6

Chris F Heyns

Key features

- Urinalysis (dipsticks and microscopy) remains an essential part of the clinical evaluation of any patient
- Ultrasonography is the best noninvasive imaging modality for evaluating patients with suspected urinary tract disease
- Causes of acute renal failure seen in tropical areas include malaria, infectious diarrhea, snakebites, insect stings, herbal medicines, and obstetric complications
- Causes of chronic renal failure include infection-related glomerulonephritis, schistosomiasis, tuberculosis, HIV infection, and sickle cell nephropathy
- Tropical parasites affecting the urinary tract include echinococcus (hydatid cysts) and filariasis (chyluria) and schistosomiasis (hematuria)
- Vesicovaginal fistulas in women and urethral strictures in men comprise a large burden of disease in some tropical countries

This chapter focuses on renal and urinary tract diseases that are more common in tropical countries; a wide spectrum of disease associated with renal and urinary tract pathology occurs in tropical regions (Table 6-1) [1].

INVESTIGATIONS

In addition to a complete history and physical examination, urinalysis, both dipstick (Fig. 6.1) and microscopy (Fig. 6.2), provides the most important clues to urinary tract disease. A midstream urine (MSU) specimen should be collected in a sterile container. In non-toilet-trained children, bag specimens can be used for obtaining a urine sample.

URINE DIPSTICK

Hematuria

Hematuria (blood in the urine) (Box 6.1) can be macroscopic (visibly red urine) or microscopic. A positive dipstick test for blood can be caused by either free hemoglobin or myoglobin, therefore microscopy is indicated to confirm the presence of red cells [2].

Leukocytes and Nitrites

Dipstick urinalysis that is positive for leukocytes as well as nitrites has a high specificity for UTI.[3]. Microscopy is more time-consuming and expensive than a dipstick, but is faster and less expensive than urine culture. If microscopy shows pyuria (white cells in the urine) and bacteriuria, it indicates UTI, and culture is not essential. If microscopy shows either pyuria or bacteriuria, but not both, confirmatory culture is necessary. Leukocyturia with negative urine culture (sterile pyuria) may be caused by several conditions (Box 6.2).

Proteinuria

Proteinuria (especially in the presence of edema, hypertension or elevated serum creatinine) indicates glomerular disease.

URINE MICROSCOPY

Red cell casts and dysmorphic red cells (acanthocytes) indicate glomerular disease (see Fig. 6.2). White cell casts indicate acute interstitial nephritis or severe pyelonephritis. Granular and epithelial casts indicate acute tubular necrosis (ATN), glomerulonephritis, or acute interstitial nephritis.

URINE CULTURE

Ideally, urine should be sent for culture before antibiotic treatment is started. However, this is not always feasible or affordable; therefore, empiric treatment is acceptable in the presence of symptoms, signs and urinalysis indicating UTI. Recurrent or persistent UTI is an indication for urine culture.

IMAGING

Ultrasonography is relatively inexpensive and avoids the risks associated with radiologic contrast and ionizing radiation (Fig. 6.3). It is especially valuable in the evaluation of patients with renal failure (Box 6.3).

Intravenous pyelography (IVP), or excretory urography (EUG), remains an excellent imaging study. The contraindications are iodine allergy, renal failure, pregnancy, hemorrhagic shock and dehydration.

Computed tomography (CT) is more accurate than ultrasonography or IVP for imaging all abdominal organs, but it is expensive and not readily available. Non-contrast-enhanced CT is becoming the modality of choice for imaging urinary tract stones.

In patients with renal failure, when ultrasound shows hydronephrosis, bladder catheterization may solve the problem if there is infravesical obstruction; if not, uni- or bilateral percutaneous nephrostomy can be life-saving.

KEY SYNDROMES

URINARY TRACT INFECTION (UTI)

UTI is most often caused by Gram-negative organisms. In women, further investigations are indicated only for recurrent, persistent or complicated UTI. However, in children and adult men, imaging is indicated to rule out underlying urinary tract abnormalities. UTI is

TABLE 6-1 Conditions Associated with Renal and Urinary Tract Disease

More common in tropical regions	Common in all regions of the world
Malaria	Congenital anomalies
Schistosomiasis	Hypertension
AIDS	Diabetes mellitus
Tuberculosis	Urinary tract infection
Sickle cell disease	Urolithiasis
Filariasis	Renal failure
Hydatid disease	Benign prostatic hyperplasia
Vesicovaginal fistula (females)	Cancer of the kidney,
Urethral stricture (males)	bladder and prostate

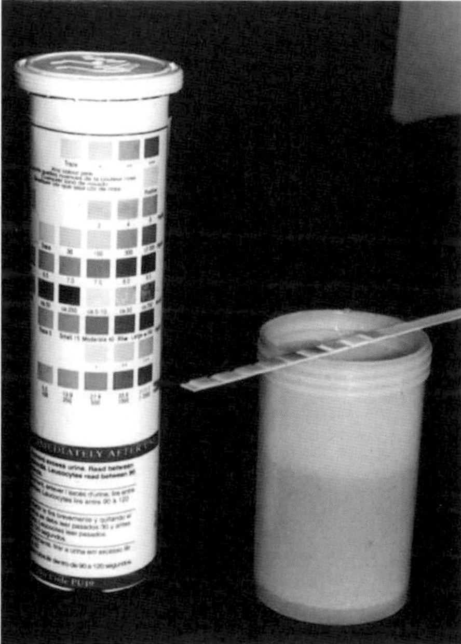

FIGURE 6.1 Urine dipstick – essential for the clinical evaluation of any patient.

BOX 6.1 Causes of Hematuria

- Contamination: red cells from balanitis or menstrual blood
- Trauma
- Infection: bacterial cystitis, schistosomiasis, tuberculosis
- Glomerulonephritis
- Interstitial nephritis
- Polycystic kidney disease
- Papillary necrosis (sickle cell disease, tuberculosis, diabetes mellitus)
- Urolithiasis
- Malignancy: renal, bladder or prostate cancer, Wilms tumor (children)
- Coagulopathy
- Miscellaneous: urethral caruncle, factitious

BOX 6.2 Causes of Sterile Pyuria

- Gram-negative UTI on antibiotic treatment
- Tuberculosis of the urinary tract
- Schistosomiasis
- Urolithiasis
- Papillary necrosis
- *Chlamydia trachomatis* infection
- Chemical or radiation cystitis
- Bladder cancer

BOX 6.3 Ultrasonography in Renal Failure

- Dilated renal calyces and pelvis ± thin cortex = obstructive uropathy
- Small, shrunken kidneys = chronic intrinsic renal disease
- Normal-sized, hyperechoic kidneys = acute glomerulonephritis or acute tubular necrosis
- Normal-sized kidneys with normal echogenicity = prerenal failure
- Enlarged kidneys = malignant infiltration, renal vein thrombosis, amyloidosis or HIV-associated nephropathy (HIVAN)

BOX 6.4 Treatment of UTI

Acute uncomplicated UTI:

- Oral trimethoprim ± sulfamethoxazole (TMP-SMX), fluoroquinolone (e.g. ciprofloxacin), cephalosporin (e.g. cefuroxime), nitrofurantoin, amoxicillin ± clavulanate

Complicated UTI:

- Parenteral ceftriaxone, fluoroquinolone, gentamicin (± ampicillin) – specific treatment according to urine culture

the cause of fever of unknown origin (FUO) in almost 10% of children <3 years of age in tropical countries, and UTI often coexists with gastroenteritis, protein energy malnutrition and acute respiratory infection [4]. Treatment of UTI is indicated in Box 6.4.

GLOMERULAR DISEASE

The clinical features of glomerular disease presentation in the tropics are shown in Box 6.5 and treatment in Boxes 6.6 and 6.7. The glomerulonephritides are more prevalent and severe in Africa than in Western countries, with nephrotic syndrome as the major presentation. The etiology is often undetermined, as is the histologic type, due to the infrequency of renal biopsies and absence of facilities for immunofluorescence and electron microscopy in many countries.

The incidence of post-streptococcal glomerulonephritis (PSGN) has decreased worldwide in the past two to three decades, but it remains common in developing countries [5]. It usually affects children, with a 2 : 1 predominance in boys.

Infections such as malaria, schistosomiasis, hepatitis B and HIV have been suggested as major causes of the nephrotic syndrome (NS) in African children, ascribed to an immune complex pathogenesis where parasitic antigens and host antibodies cause glomerular damage.

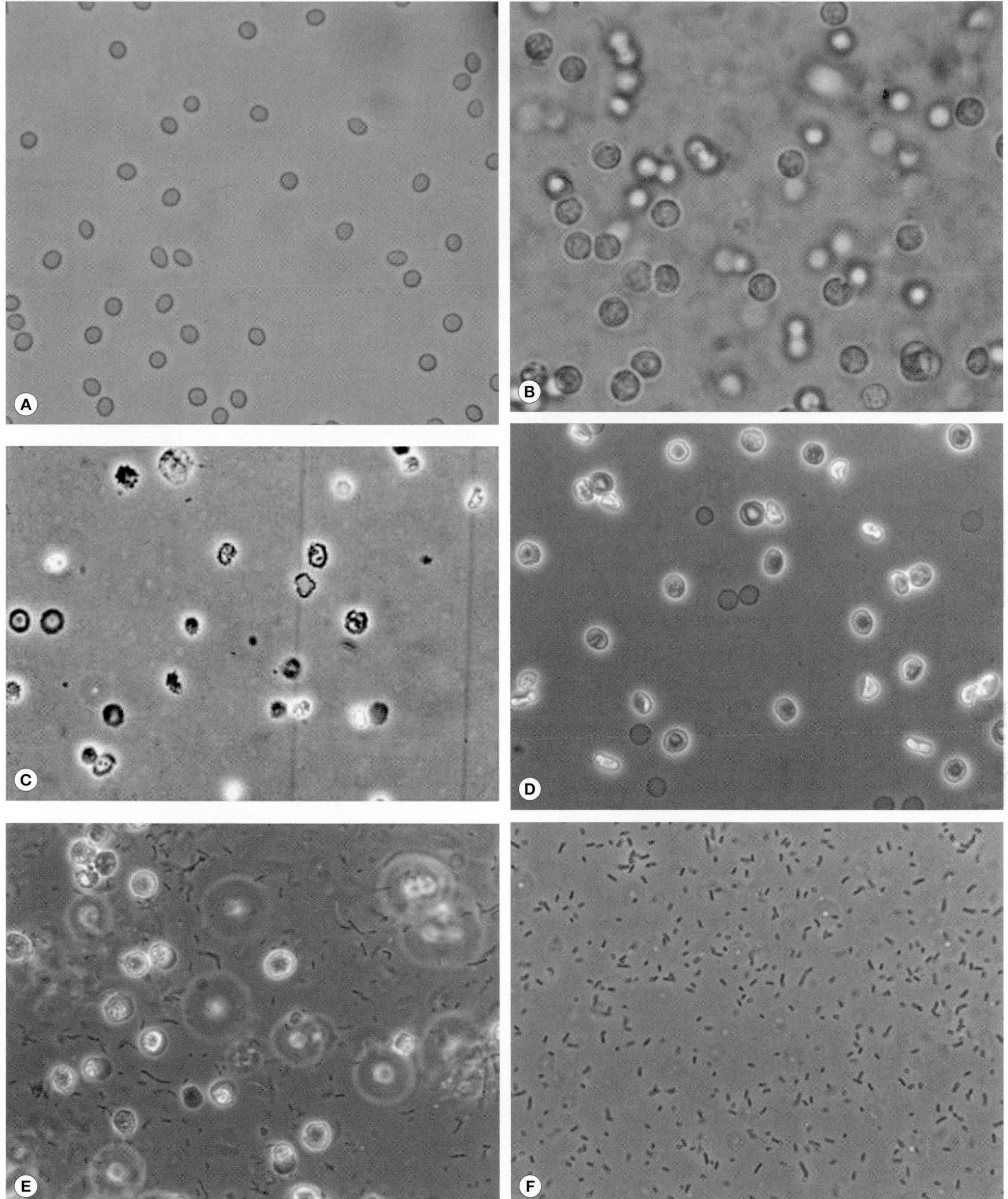

FIGURE 6.2 Urine sediment. Light microscopy of **(A)** normal red blood cells, **(B)** white blood cells, and **(C)** dysmorphic red cells; phase contrast microscopy of **(D)** red cells, **(E)** white cells, **(F)** bacteria (cocci);

Continued

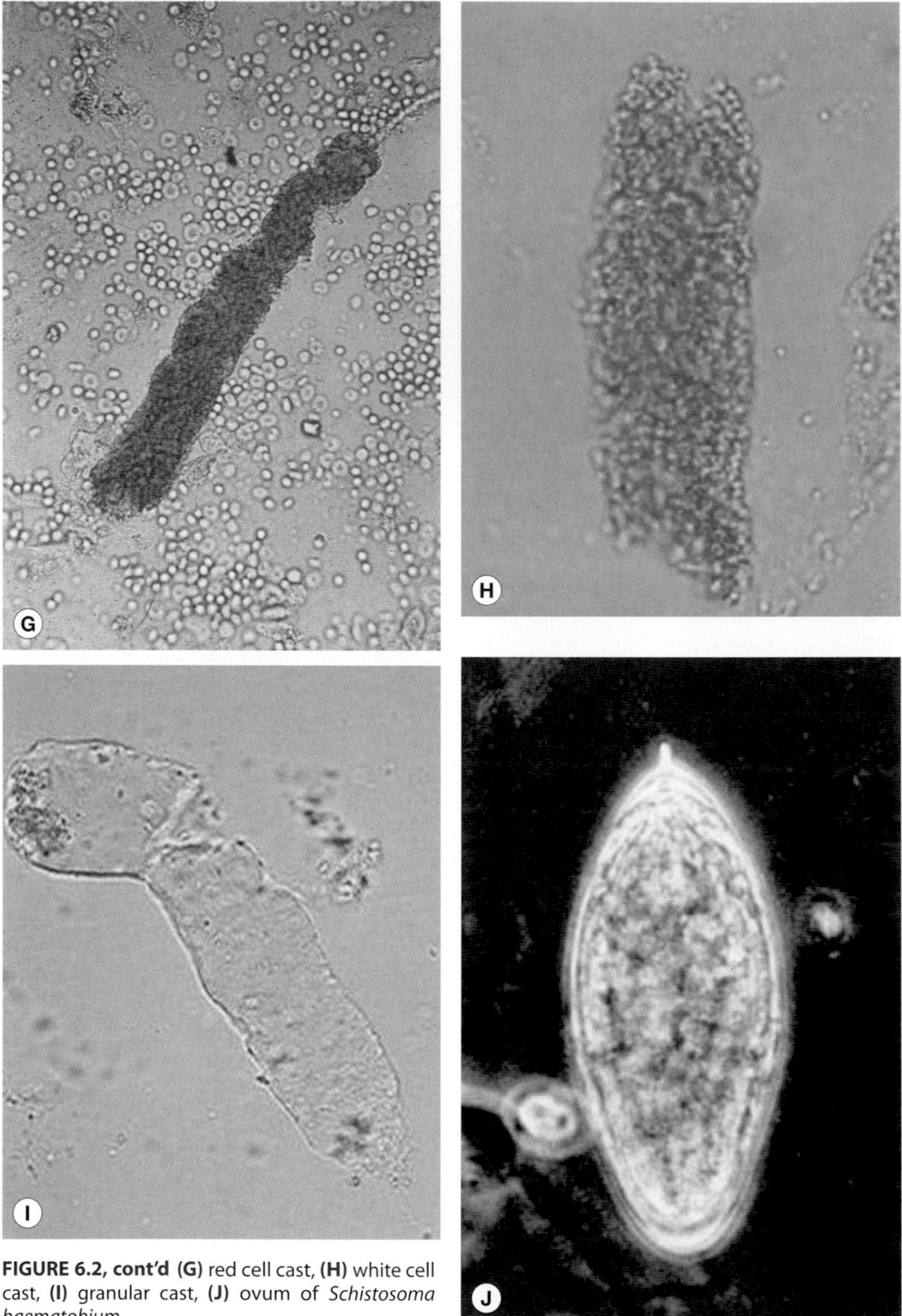

FIGURE 6.2, cont'd (G) red cell cast, **(H)** white cell cast, **(I)** granular cast, **(J)** ovum of *Schistosoma haematobium*.

However, recent reviews found little evidence for steroid-resistant "tropical glomerulopathies" in children with NS and suggested that the term "tropical nephrotic syndrome" should be discarded.

In Africa, focal segmental glomerulosclerosis (FSGS) is now becoming the most common cause of NS in renal biopsies instead of minimal change glomerulonephritis and amyloid, which were the most common causes prior to the AIDS pandemic.

RENAL FAILURE

Acute renal failure (ARF) in tropical regions may be caused by conditions not commonly seen in nontropical areas: infectious diarrheal disease, malaria, leptospirosis, snakebite, insect stings, herbal medicines and pregnancy-related conditions (septic abortion, eclampsia, peripartum hemorrhage and puerperal sepsis).

Chronic renal failure (CRF) in tropical countries is commonly caused by infection-related glomerulonephritis (possibly related to the high prevalence of soft tissue infections), diabetic nephropathy, hypertensive nephrosclerosis, malaria, schistosomiasis, tuberculosis, HIV infection and sickle cell nephropathy.

Facilities for hemodialysis are not readily available in many tropical countries. However, chronic ambulatory peritoneal dialysis (CAPD) is an effective and less expensive option, with the advantage that patients are less hospital-dependent. The risk of infective peritonitis is increased.

MALARIA

Malarial acute kidney injury (MAKI) predominantly affects adults and older children from areas of low intensity of malaria transmission,

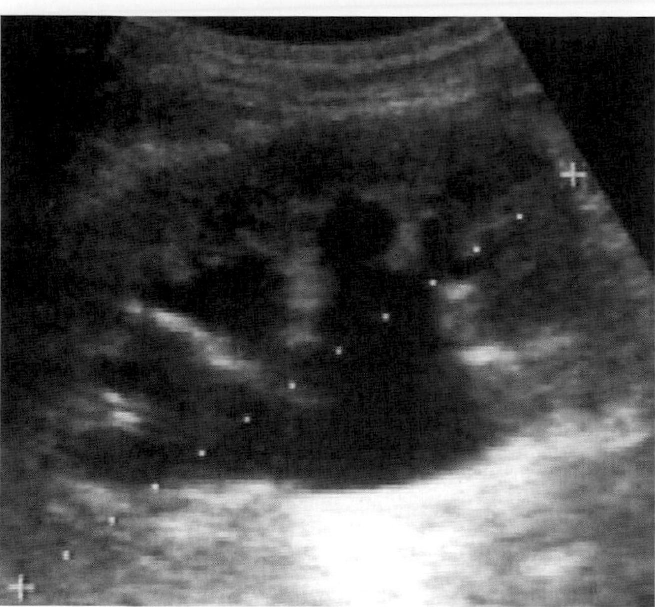

FIGURE 6.3 Ultrasound is the ideal imaging modality in patients with renal failure. This image shows hydronephrosis.

BOX 6.5 Clinical Presentations of Glomerular Disease

- Asymptomatic: proteinuria 150 mg to 3 g per day
- Hematuria:
  - microscopic: dysmorphic red cells
  - macroscopic: brown/red urine, painless
- Nephritic syndrome: abrupt onset, edema, hypertension, oliguria, hematuria (with red cell casts), proteinuria (<3 g/day)
- Nephrotic syndrome: edema, proteinuria (adult >3.5 g/day, child >40 mg/h per m^2), lipiduria, hypoalbuminemia (<3.5 g/dL), hypercholesterolemia
- Rapidly progressive glomerulonephritis: renal failure, proteinuria (<3 g/day), hematuria (with red cell casts), often normotensive
- Chronic glomerulonephritis: hypertension, renal insufficiency, proteinuria (>3 g/day)

BOX 6.6 Treatment of Acute Nephritic Syndrome

- Restricted sodium and water intake for 12–24 hours to establish the severity of oliguria and to achieve an early negative balance
- Patients with edema may benefit from IV furosemide
- For hypertension: oral nifedipine, IV hydralazine or diazoxide; hypertensive encephalopathy may require sodium nitroprusside
- Avoid: digitalis preparations (ineffective in this condition), spironolactone, angiotensin-converting enzyme inhibitors and propanolol (hyperkalemia), and alpha-methyldopa (ineffective, and risk of oversedation)
- Dialysis is indicated for uremia or hyperkalemia

BOX 6.7 Treatment of Nephrotic Syndrome

- Diuretics combined with moderate dietary sodium restriction, aiming at fluid removal of no more than 2 kg daily in adults
- If serum albumin is <2.5 g/dL, prophylactic low-dose anticoagulation is recommended if possible
- A high clinical suspicion for infection is vital
- Immunosuppressive therapy: corticosteroids, azathioprine or cyclophosphamide

BOX 6.8 Management of Malarial Acute Renal Failure

- Maintenance of fluid and electrolyte levels with central venous pressure monitoring
- If oliguria persists after fluid replacement, furosemide 40 mg or bumetanide 1 mg can be given
- The administration of albumin for volume expansion may reduce mortality rates
- Management of concomitant infection
- Nephrotoxic drugs should be avoided: angiotensin-converting enzyme inhibitors, nonsteroidal anti-inflammatory drugs, aminoglycosides
- Peritoneal or hemodialysis should be started early if there is a rapid increase of serum creatinine
- Indications for dialysis include uremic symptoms, pulmonary edema, congestive cardiac failure, pericardial rub, severe metabolic acidosis and hyperkalemia

and is invariably caused by *Plasmodium falciparum* malaria. It is characterized by oliguria and rapidly increasing serum creatinine. Risk factors for the development of MAKI are pregnancy, high parasitemia, severe jaundice, prolonged dehydration and NSAID therapy. The prognosis is worse in patients with jaundice, cerebral malaria (coma and convulsions), hypoglycemia and multi-organ dysfunction. The mortality is 15–50% [6].

Blackwater fever (BWF) is a clinical syndrome characterized by fever, anemia, jaundice, massive intravascular hemolysis, hemoglobinuria and ARF that is classically seen in European expatriates chronically exposed to *Plasmodium falciparum* and irregularly taking quinine [7]. Management is described in Box 6.8.

TROPICAL NEPHROTOXINS

Botanical nephrotoxins are encountered in common edible plants and medicinal herbs. Traditional medicines are a mix of herbs and unknown chemicals administered orally or as enemas. The prevalence of nephropathy caused by traditional medicines is related to poverty and lack of medical facilities [8].

Animal nephrotoxins (venoms of snakes and stinging insects) are complex mixtures of proteins, enzymes and chemicals. Acute kidney injury is attributed to decreased renal blood flow (anaphylactic shock, disseminated intravascular coagulation), intravascular hemolysis or rhabdomyolysis causing hemoglobinuria and myoglobinuria, or direct tubular toxicity.

Treatment consists of antihistamines, corticosteroids, hydration, diuretics, urine alkalinization and hemodialysis with hemofiltration.

HIV-ASSOCIATED NEPHROPATHY (HIVAN)

HIV/AIDS has a high prevalence in several tropical regions (especially sub-Saharan Africa) and HIVAN occurs in up to 10% of AIDS patients. It presents with proteinuria and renal failure, usually in patients with an AIDS-defining condition, CD4 counts <200 cells/μL, and normal to enlarged echogenic kidneys on ultrasonography. ESRD invariably develops, usually within 4–6 months. Some studies have demonstrated dramatic responses to ART.

HEMOLYTIC UREMIC SYNDROME (HUS)

HUS is a thrombotic microangiopathy that may present in (1) a classical form, associated with gastroenteritis, and (2) an idiopathic form, not associated with diarrhea. Classical HUS results from gastrointestinal infections with shiga toxin-producing *Escherichia coli* and *Shigella* spp. Most cases are in children 6 months to 4 years of age, but infants and adults can be affected. The mortality of HUS was reduced from nearly 50% to 2–4% with the use of peritoneal dialysis.

SCHISTOSOMIASIS (BILHARZIA)

The ova of *Schistosoma haematobium* are deposited in the wall of the bladder and ureters, where they evoke a granulomatous inflammatory reaction with eventual calcification of the bladder wall (Fig. 6.4) [9]. The typical presentation is painful terminal hematuria. Secondary bacterial infection may occur, particularly with *Pseudomonas*, *Proteus* or *Salmonella*, especially following instrumentation of the bladder.

Dipstick hematuria is valuable for screening children at risk of urinary schistosomiasis. Microscopic examination of a fresh urine sample usually shows *S. haematobium* ova (see Fig. 6.2). Serologic tests are useful in confirming the diagnosis in the absence of ova. Ultrasonography can assess bladder abnormalities and urinary tract obstruction. Cystoscopy and bladder biopsy should only be performed if the diagnosis can not be established noninvasively.

Treatment is usually with praziquantel. Praziquantel lacks efficacy against juvenile schistosomes, leading to lower cure rates in hyperendemic areas.

UROGENITAL TUBERCULOSIS (UGTB)

Most patients with UGTB are <50 years of age. The symptoms include LUTS, recurrent UTI, abdominal pain, epididymitis, macroscopic hematuria, hemospermia or infertility. On examination there may be hypertension, an abdominal mass secondary to hydronephrosis, or scrotal swelling.

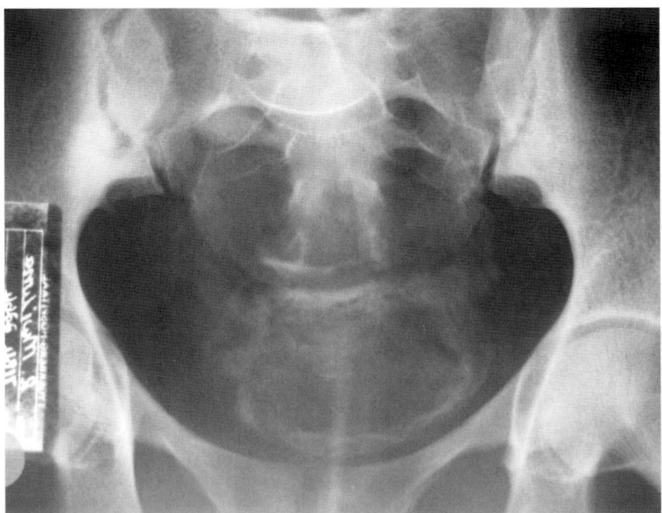

FIGURE 6.4 Plain x-ray of the pelvis showing calcification of *Schistosoma haematobium* granuloma in the bladder wall.

On urinalysis, acid sterile pyuria should raise the suspicion of TB, but in up to one-third of patients a Gram-negative organism is cultured. Micro- or macroscopic hematuria is often present. Ziehl–Neelsen (ZN) staining of urine has a high false-negative rate. At least three early morning urine specimens should be sent for TB culture.

IVP is the best imaging modality for suspected UGTB. Biopsy of the bladder wall, epididymis or prostate may confirm the diagnosis histologically.

Treatment of UGTB requires combination therapy to prevent bacterial resistance – usually four drugs for 2 months (isoniazid, rifampicin, pyrazinamide and ethambutol) and two drugs for the remaining 4 months (rifampicin and isoniazid). Drug-resistant TB can be treated with addition of streptomycin or ciprofloxacin.

SICKLE CELL DISEASE (SCD)

SCD is an autosomal recessive inherited disorder with a genetic prevalence of 25–50% in some West African areas. Relative hypoxia in the renal medulla leads to sickling, with obliteration of the vasa recta, papillary necrosis and macroscopic hematuria. Patients with SCD have an increased susceptibility to bacterial infections. Renal failure is the cause of death in about 14% of cases. A common problem in men with SCD is priapism (prolonged painful erection).

Microscopic examination of a blood smear may show sickle cells. Hemoglobin electrophoresis is required to establish the diagnosis. Treatment includes bed rest, IV fluids, diuretics, urine alkalinization with sodium bicarbonate, blood transfusion, bladder washout for removal of blood clots, and irrigation of the pelvicaliceal system with silver nitrate.

CHYLURIA

Chyluria is caused by microfilariae of a mosquito-borne nematode (*Wuchereria bancrofti*) causing rupture of lymphatic varices into the urinary tract [10]. It occurs in about 2% of filarial afflicted patients, mainly in South Asian countries. Chyluria may result in severe protein loss leading to hypoalbuminemia and anasarca. The urine is usually milky white, but may be pink if there is also hematuria. Spontaneous resolution occurs in >50% of cases. A low-fat diet and high fluid intake reduce the risk of urinary stasis and clot formation. Diethylcarbamazine (DEC) may result in long-term remission.

HYDATID DISEASE

The urinary tract is involved in 2–4% of cases of cystic hydatid disease caused by the tapeworm *Echinococcus granulosus*. Flank pain occurs in about 60% of cases. Hydaturia (scoleces in the urine) is rare (5%). Ultrasonography typically shows a complex cyst. The Casoni test or indirect hemagglutination test can be used to confirm the diagnosis. Percutaneous aspiration of the cyst carries the risk of anaphylaxis and hydatid seeding. Albendazole is the first-line treatment, because surgery carries the risk of dissemination if spillage occurs.

UROLITHIASIS

Risk factors for urolithiasis in the tropics include low urine volumes due to sweating or chronic diarrhea [11]. The incidence of upper urinary tract stones in adults is increasing in more affluent, urbanized populations. In children, bladder stones are more common in tropical countries, probably due to dietary factors or chronic diarrhea.

VESICOVAGINAL FISTULA (VVF)

Postpartum VVFs mostly occur in young women in remote areas where obstetric services are inadequate. Most are large, complex fistulas involving the continence mechanism. Vaginal repair can be performed under spinal anesthesia by adequately trained staff; however, currently, thousands of women remain untreated due to lack of facilities [12].

URETHRAL STRICTURES

In men, urethral strictures due to previous gonorrheal or chlamydial urethritis are relatively common in some tropical countries. It may present with UTI or urinary retention. Transurethral catheterization is impossible; therefore, a suprapubic catheter is required until dilatation, internal urethrotomy or urethroplasty can be performed.

REFERENCES

1. Hotez PJ, Kamath A. Neglected tropical diseases in sub-Saharan Africa: review of their prevalence, distribution, and disease burden. PLoS Negl Trop Dis 2009;3:e412.
2. Rodgers M, Nixon J, Hempel S, et al. Diagnostic tests and algorithms used in the investigation of haematuria: systematic reviews and economic evaluation. Health Technol Assess 2006;10:iii–iv, xi–259.
3. Whiting P, Westwood M, Bojke L, et al. Clinical effectiveness and cost-effectiveness of tests for the diagnosis and investigation of urinary tract infection in children: a systematic review and economic model. Health Technol Assess 2006;10:iii–iv, xi–xiii, 1–154.
4. Jeena PM, Coovadia HM, Adhikari M. Probable association between urinary tract infections (UTI) and common diseases of infancy and childhood: a hospital-based study of UTI in Durban, South Africa. J Trop Pediatr 1996;42:112–14.
5. Seedat YK. Glomerular disease in the tropics. Semin Nephrol 2003;23:12–20.
   Authoritative review of the etiology, histology, prevention, and management of glomerular diseases in the tropics.
6. Mishra SK, Das BS. Malaria and acute kidney injury. Semin Nephrol 2008;28:395–408.
   Clinically useful review of the management of acute renal dysfunction associated with malaria.
7. Bruneel F, Gachot B, Wolff M, et al. Corresponding Group. Resurgence of blackwater fever in long-term European expatriates in Africa: report of 21 cases and review. Clin Infect Dis 2001;32:1133–40.
8. Jha V, Chugh KS. Nephropathy associated with animal, plant, and chemical toxins in the tropics. Semin Nephrol 2003;23:49–65.
   Interesting review of the recently recognized entity of toxic nephropathy as an important segment of renal disease in tropical countries.
9. Jyding Vennervald B, Kahama AI, Reimert CM. Assessment of morbidity in Schistosoma haematobium infection: current methods and future tools. Acta Trop 2000;77:81–9.
10. Gulati S, Gupta N, Singh NP, et al. Chyluria with proteinuria or filarial nephropathy? An enigma. Parasitol Int 2007;56:251–4.
11. Robertson WG. Renal stones in the tropics. Semin Nephrol 2003;23:77–87.
12. Gutman RE, Dodson JL, Mostwin JL. Complications of treatment of obstetric fistula in the developing world: gynatresia, urinary incontinence, and urinary diversion. Int J Gynaecol Obstet 2007;99(Suppl 1):S57–64.
    Comprehensive review of existing literature and expert recommendations of the Gates Fistula Institute meeting on surgical repair of obstetric fistula, including its complications such as gynatresia and urinary incontinence.

7 Sexually Transmitted Infections

David Mabey, Philippe Mayaud

Key features

- The incidence and prevalence of sexually transmitted infections (STIs) are higher in developing than in developed countries
- STIs facilitate the sexual transmission of HIV and influence HIV replication and disease progression, and vice versa
- Syndromic management of STIs is recommended in resource-poor settings. It is less effective for the management of vaginal discharge than for other syndromes
- In regions with a high HIV prevalence, an increasing proportion of genital ulcers presenting to health facilities is due to herpes simplex virus
- Suppressive treatment for genital herpes has been shown to reduce the levels of HIV in the plasma and genital tract of dually infected individuals, but has not reduced the incidence of HIV in high-risk groups or transmission between HIV-serodiscordant couples
- Rapid, point-of-care tests for syphilis are now available which do not require electricity or laboratory equipment, and can be performed on blood samples obtained by finger prick
- Male circumcision has been shown to reduce HIV incidence by more than half in three trials in African men
- Effective vaccines against oncogenic strains of human papillomavirus (HPV) are now available and are being given to young women in developed countries

STIs IN DEVELOPING COUNTRIES

The impact of HIV/AIDS has been catastrophic in many developing countries; more than 20% of adults are infected in some parts of Africa. UNAIDS estimates that at least 60 million people have been infected with HIV, of whom more than 20 million have died; 2.7 million new HIV infections occurred in 2008, more than 90% of which were in developing countries; 33 million people are currently living with HIV, two-thirds of them in sub-Saharan Africa; and 2 million people died of HIV-related conditions in 2008 [1].

Few countries outside Western Europe and North America have accurate reporting systems for STIs other than HIV. Knowledge of STI epidemiology is based on the results of *ad hoc* prevalence surveys undertaken in convenient populations (e.g. STI or antenatal clinic attenders), but these are often unrepresentative of the population at large. STIs are more common in economically disadvantaged populations. Many rural villagers have migrated into cities in developing countries, and many more have been displaced by war or famine; poverty and lack of education drive many women into commercial sex; and poor people often lack access to effective treatment.

The worldwide incidence of curable STIs (syphilis, gonorrhea, trichomoniasis and chlamydial infection) has been estimated by WHO from prevalence data and the estimated duration of infection. This analysis suggests that, in 1999, there were over 340 million new cases of curable STIs; 174 million cases of trichomoniasis, 92 million cases of chlamydial infection, 62 million cases of gonorrhea, 12 million cases of syphilis, and 6 million cases of chancroid [2]. In view of the uncertainty surrounding the prevalence estimates, the duration of untreated STIs, and the mean duration before effective treatment is received, these figures cannot be considered definitive.

Large population-based surveys have confirmed the high prevalence of STIs in sub-Saharan Africa, even in asymptomatic rural populations; for example, syphilis (5–10% of adults infected), *Trichomonas vaginalis* (20–30% of women and 10% of men) and bacterial vaginosis (up to 50% of women) [3–5]. Syphilis is estimated to cause 490,000 stillbirths and neonatal deaths per year in Africa; this figure is almost twice the number of children dying of HIV/AIDS worldwide [6].

Genital herpes and human papillomavirus (HPV) infections are common among all sexually active populations, but cause a particularly heavy burden of disease in developing countries. Genital herpes, which is usually due to herpes simplex virus type 2 (HSV-2), is a lifelong infection, causing recurrent episodes of genital ulceration which are more frequent, more severe and longer-lasting in immunocompromised individuals. A very high prevalence of HSV-2 infection (30–50%) has been found in the general populations of several African countries [7]. The proportion of genital ulcers caused by HSV-2 has increased greatly in populations with a high HIV prevalence.

Cervical carcinoma is the most common malignancy in women in much of the developing world, reflecting the high incidence of sexually transmitted HPV infection.

The rate at which an STI spreads in a population depends on the average number of new cases generated by an infected individual – the basic reproductive number (R_0). This in turn depends on the mean rate of sexual partner change (c), the average duration of the infection (D), and its infectiousness (the likelihood of it being transmitted per sexual act, β). This relationship has been described by the simple formula: $R_0 = \beta * c * D$.

The duration of a curable infection depends on the time that elapses before effective treatment is given. A disease such as chancroid, which almost always causes painful symptoms, is likely to be treated rapidly in populations with access to effective treatment, and has almost disappeared from industrialized countries. It remains endemic in core groups in some developing countries, although its incidence has declined in the past decade, probably as a result of behavior change resulting from the HIV/AIDS epidemic. In contrast, chlamydial infection, which is often asymptomatic in both men and women, is likely to be of longer duration and therefore to persist even in affluent populations with good access to treatment. When R_0 declines below 1 in a given population, the infection will eventually disappear.

However, even when R_0 is less than 1, infections may be maintained in core groups with a high rate of sexual partner change (e.g. sex-workers and their clients), and may continue to occur in the general population as a result of sexual contact with members of high-risk groups.

INTERACTIONS BETWEEN HIV AND OTHER STIs

Ulcerative STIs such as chancroid, syphilis and herpes facilitate sexual transmission of HIV by increasing both infectivity and susceptibility. STIs causing genital discharge (e.g. gonorrhea) increase shedding of HIV in both seminal and cervicovaginal secretions [8].

A community-randomized trial conducted in Tanzania showed that improved services for the management of STIs, using the syndromic approach in rural health facilities, reduced the incidence of HIV infection by 40% over a 2-year period [3]. Trials of STI case management using either the syndromic approach or periodic mass treatment in Uganda failed to show any impact on HIV incidence [4,5]. Review of the data from these trials suggested that improved STI case management is more likely to reduce HIV incidence in the early stages of an HIV epidemic, when most HIV infections are concentrated in groups with high numbers of concurrent sexual partnerships who also have a high prevalence of other curable STIs [9].

HIV and HSV-2 each appears to facilitate the transmission of the other virus. Suppressive treatment for HSV-2 has been shown to reduce HIV shedding and plasma viral load in co-infected individuals but, disappointingly, two recent trials found no evidence that suppressive herpes treatment reduced the risk of HIV acquisition among high-risk groups, and one large trial found no impact of HSV suppressive therapy on HIV transmission among serodiscordant couples [10–13].

STIs represent important cofactors of HIV transmission, and STI control could significantly reduce the incidence of HIV infection worldwide, although the impact of interventions may vary according to the local epidemiologic context.

CLINICAL MANAGEMENT OF STIs

Prompt and effective treatment prevents sequelae and further transmission and should be the cornerstone of an STI control program. Yet STI treatment services are often accorded very low priority by health planners and ministries of health. If treatment for STIs is to be widely accessible in developing countries, it must be provided at the point of first contact with health services. It should be available at health centers and dispensaries in rural as well as urban areas. STI specialists and referral centers are best utilized to treat intractable cases, to train rural health workers, and to serve as a laboratory reference center to monitor antibiotic resistance.

Criteria for the selection of drugs used for STI treatment have been listed by the World Health Organization (WHO) (see Box 7.1). An important point is that drugs in all healthcare facilities that provide STI care should have an efficacy of at least 95%.

Since antimicrobial resistance of several sexually transmitted pathogens, in particular *Neisseria gonorrhoeae*, has been increasing in many parts of the world, special attention should be paid to the selection of drugs with high efficacy even if costly, since cheaper but inadequate drugs would result in increased treatment failures, referral, development of sequelae and further transmission.

History Taking and Examination

If clinical STI services are to be acceptable to populations at risk, certain criteria must be met: (1) privacy; an adequate sexual history and clinical examination can be taken only in private; (2) empathy; patients rarely attend clinics where staff treat them in a hostile or judgmental manner. Time is often short in health facilities in developing countries, but there are certain minimum requirements for the management of STI patients. The history should include details of the present complaint, including treatment already received, details of sexual partners since the onset of symptoms and in the preceding month; and past history of STIs.

BOX 7.1 Criteria for the Selection of STI Drugs

Drugs selected for treating STI should meet the following criteria:

- high efficacy (at least 95%)
- low cost
- acceptable toxicity and tolerance
- organism resistance unlikely to develop or likely to be delayed
- single dose
- oral administration
- not contraindicated for pregnant or lactating women

Appropriate drugs should be included in the national essential drugs list, and, in choosing drugs, consideration should be given to the capabilities and experience of health personnel.

Reproduced with permission from World Health Organization. Guidelines for the Management of Sexually Transmitted Infections; Revised version. Geneva: WHO; 2003.

Examination should include inspection of the mucous membranes, palms and anogenital region; palpation of the inguinal glands, penis and scrotum in men, with retraction of the foreskin, if present. In women, a speculum examination to visualize the cervix and a bimanual examination are required to assess possible lower abdominal tenderness (sign of pelvic inflammatory disease, PID, or for differential diagnosis with surgical conditions). The examination should be performed in private in a good light, and gloves should be worn.

Counseling

This is an essential component of clinical management. STI patients should be advised that they are placing themselves at risk of HIV infection and encouraged to reduce their number of sexual partners. They should be encouraged to avoid sex while symptomatic or to use condoms. Condoms should also be recommended for high-risk future contacts; use should be demonstrated and free samples provided. The importance of complying fully with treatment and of referring sexual contacts for treatment should be emphasized. Patients should be advised to return to the clinic promptly for treatment if they should develop symptoms of STI in the future.

KEY SYNDROMES

The Syndromic Approach

Most health centers and dispensaries in developing countries lack adequate laboratory facilities for the diagnosis of STIs. WHO recommends that STIs be treated syndromically, according to suggested treatment algorithms for the common STI syndromes: urethral discharge, genital ulcer, inguinal bubo, painful scrotal swelling, abnormal vaginal discharge, lower abdominal pain [14]. A more recent addition, which still requires validation, is the anorectal syndrome in men who have sex with men. The principle underlying syndromic management is that treatment for all likely causes of a syndrome at the first visit will prevent further transmission, and prevent sequelae in the patients.

WHO has developed simplified tools (flowchart or algorithms) to guide health workers in the implementation of syndromic management of STIs (Figs 7.1 to 7.9). It is strongly recommended that

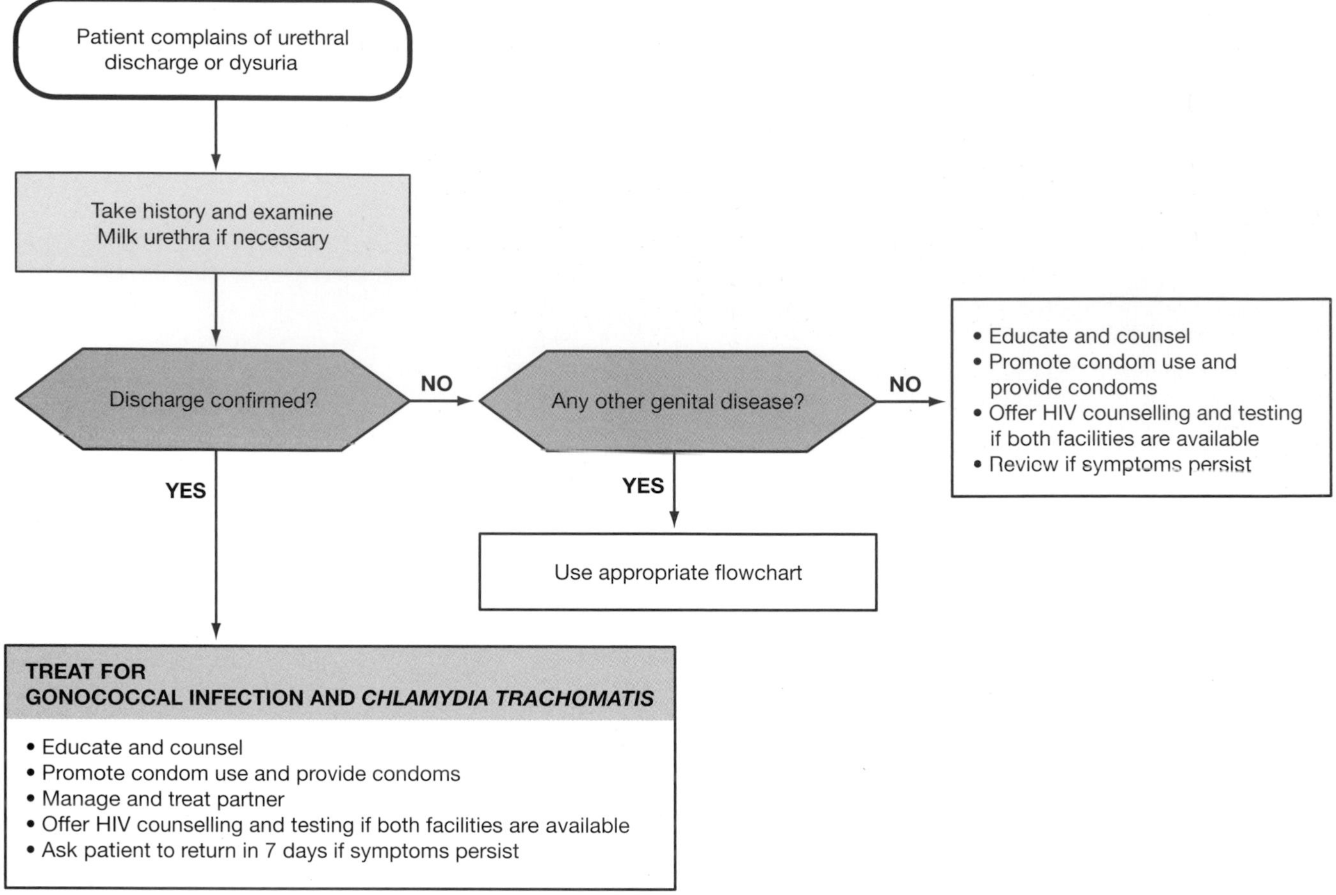

FIGURE 7.1 Urethral discharge. *Reproduced with permission from World Health Organization. Guidelines for the Management of Sexually Transmitted Infections; Revised version. Geneva: WHO; 2003.*

countries establish and use national standardized treatment protocols for STIs. These can help to ensure that all patients receive adequate treatment at all levels of healthcare services. The protocols can also facilitate the training and supervision of healthcare providers and can help to reduce the risk of development of resistance to antimicrobials. Finally, having a standardized list of antimicrobial agents can also facilitate drug procurement (see Table 7-1 for WHO-recommended drug regimens for the main STI pathogens and syndromes).

URETHRAL DISCHARGE (see Figs 7.1 & 7.2)

Most male patients presenting with urethral discharge or dysuria (when young) will have urethritis, defined as the presence of ≥5 polymorphonuclear leukocytes per high-power field on a Gram stain of a urethral swab, caused by one of four pathogens (see Table 7-1). In the syndromic management, treatment of a patient with urethral discharge (see Fig. 7.1) should adequately cover these most frequent organisms causing gonorrhea (*N. gonorrhoeae*) and non-gonococcal urethritis (*Chlamydia trachomatis*) which cannot always be distinguished by clinical presentation (presence of profuse purulent versus mucoid discharge) or incubation period (shorter usually for gonorrhea, 3 to 7 days, versus 5 to 21 days). Although variable by setting, dual infections are not uncommon, accounting for up to 10% of cases. If a microscope is available, the diagnosis of gonorrhea can be confirmed by the presence of intracellular diplococci on a Gram stain. Persistent or recurrent symptoms of urethritis may result from drug resistance, poor compliance or re-infection. Given the high prevalence of these once-neglected infections in some settings, *Trichomonas vaginalis* and *Mycoplasma genitalium* should be suspected in cases of persistent urethral discharge [15] (see Fig. 7.2).

SCROTAL SWELLING (EPIDIDYMO-ORCHITIS) (see Fig. 7.5)

Epididymitis is an important complication of gonococcal or chlamydial urethritis. It presents as a painful swelling of the scrotum, usually unilateral; the onset is usually more acute in gonococcal than in chlamydial disease. Torsion of the testis is an important differential diagnosis, requiring urgent surgical repair. Other differential diagnoses include trauma and tumor or other infectious causes such as mumps, tuberculosis or brucellosis. In men over 50 years of age, epididymo-orchitis is more likely to be secondary to a bacterial urinary tract infection than to urethritis, at least in developed countries.

GENITAL ULCER (see Fig. 7.3)

There are five common causes of genital ulceration (see Table 7-1). In most developing countries, in the 1980s and 1990s, the majority of genital ulcers were due to either syphilis or chancroid, and in some settings (e.g. Papua New Guinea, the Caribbean, South Africa), donovanosis (caused by *Klebsiella granulomatis*) or lymphogranuloma venereum (caused by L1–L3 strains of *C. trachomatis*). However, the pattern of genital ulcer disease (GUD) changes from locale to locale and over time. Since the advent of HIV/AIDS, genital herpes caused by HSV-2 has become the dominant etiology of GUD worldwide. Clinical differential diagnosis of genital ulcers is inaccurate, particularly in settings where several etiologies are common. Clinical manifestations and patterns of GUD may be further altered in the presence of HIV infection. Patients with ulcers should therefore be treated for syphilis and chancroid and all locally relevant bacterial etiologies.

TABLE 7-1 Major Curable and Incurable STIs and STI Syndromes and Their Treatment

Major curable STIs	Disease	Recommended treatment*
Neisseria gonorrhoeae	Gonorrhea	Ciprofloxacin, 500 mg orally, single dose OR Ceftriaxone, 125 mg by intramuscular injection, single dose OR Cefixime, 400 mg orally, single dose OR Spectinomycin, 2 g by intramuscular injection, single dose
Chlamydia trachomatis	Chlamydial infection, lymphogranuloma venereum (LGV 1–3 strains)	Doxycycline, 100 mg orally, twice daily for 7 days Azithromycin, 1 g orally, single dose Alternative regimen: Erythromycin, 500 mg orally, four times a day for 7 days For LGV: same treatment for 14 days
Treponema pallidum	Syphilis	Benzathine benzylpenicillin, 2.4 million IU, singe dose by intramuscular injection Alternative regimen, or if penicillin allergy: Doxycycline, 100 mg orally twice daily for 14 days
Haemophilus ducreyi	Chancroid	Ciprofloxacin, 500 mg orally, twice daily for 3 days OR Erythromycin, 500 mg orally, four times daily for 7 days OR Azithromycin, 1 g orally, single dose
Klebsiella granulomatis	Donovanosis (granuloma inguinale)	For at least 3 weeks/until lesions have completely epithelialized: Doxycycline, 100 mg orally, twice daily OR Azithromycin, 1g orally on first day, then 500 mg orally single dose
Trichomonas vaginalis	Trichomoniasis	Metronidazole, 2 g orally, single dose OR Metronidazole, 400 mg or 500 mg orally, twice daily for 7 days OR Tinidazole, 500 mg orally, twice daily for 5 days
Major incurable STIs	***Disease***	***Recommended treatment****
Herpes simplex virus (HSV)	Genital herpes	First episode: Acyclovir, 200 mg orally, five times daily for 7 days OR Acyclovir, 400 mg orally, three times daily for 7 days OR Valacyclovir, 1 g orally, twice daily for 7 days OR Famciclovir, 250 mg orally, three times daily for 7 days Recurrent episodes: Acyclovir: same dosages and duration as for primary infection OR Valacyclovir, 500 mg orally, twice daily for 7 days OR Valacyclovir, 1g orally, once daily for 7 days OR Famciclovir, 125 mg orally, twice daily for 7 days
Human papillomavirus (HPV)	Genital warts, cervical and other genital carcinomas	See Anogenital warts treatment
Human immunodeficiency virus (HIV)	HIV disease and AIDS	Antiretroviral therapy regimens are based on the combination of three classes: (1) nucleoside inhibitors, (2) non-nucleoside inhibitors, and (3) protease inhibitors, with new classes appearing (e.g. fusion inhibitors)

TABLE 7-1 Major Curable and Incurable STIs and STI Syndromes and Their Treatment—cont'd

Major curable STIs	Disease	Recommended treatment*
Major STI syndromes	***STI causes***	***Drug options***
Urethral discharge	*N. gonorrhoeae, C. trachomatis, T. vaginalis, Mycoplasma genitalium*	For gonorrhea: ciprofloxacin, ceftriaxone, spectinomycin or cefixime PLUS For chlamydia: doxycycline or azithromycin
Genital ulcer disease	*T. pallidum, H. ducreyi*, HSV, *Klebsiella granulomatis* (donovanosis), *C. trachomatis* LGV strains L1, L2 and L3	For syphilis: benzathine benzylpenicillin PLUS For chancroid: ciprofloxacin, erythromycin or azithromycin PLUS For HSV: acyclovir, valacyclovir or famciclovir PLUS Depending on local etiology, add drug options for LGV (doxycycline or erythromycin) and for donovanosis (doxycyline or azithromycin)
Inguinal bubo	*H. ducreyi* and *C. trachomatis* LGV strains L1, L2 and L3 (rule out limb infection or tuberculosis)	For chancroid: ciprofloxacin PLUS For LGV: doxycycline or erythromycin
Scrotal swelling	As urethral discharge, after ruling out other infections (mumps), trauma, torsion and cancers	For gonorrhoea: ciprofloxacin, ceftriaxone, spectinomycin or cefixime PLUS For chlamydia: doxycycline or azithromycin
Abnormal vaginal discharge	Cervical infections (*N. gonorrhoeae, C. trachomatis, Mycoplasma genitalium*) and vaginal infections (*T. vaginalis, Candida albicans*, bacterial vaginosis)	For gonorrhoea: ciprofloxacin, ceftriaxone, spectinomycin or cefixime PLUS For chlamydia: doxycycline or azithromycin PLUS For *T. vaginalis* or BV: metronidazole, tinidazole PLUS For vulvovaginal candidiasis: Miconazole or clotrimazole, 200 mg intravaginally, daily for 3 days OR Clotrimazole, 500 mg intravaginally, single dose OR Fluconazole, 150 mg orally, single dose
Lower abdominal pain/pelvic inflammatory disease (PID)	As vaginal discharge + anaerobic infections (*Bacteroides* spp. and Gram-positive cocci, *Mycoplasma hominis*)	Outpatient therapy: For uncomplicated gonorrhea: ciprofloxacin, ceftriaxone, cefixime or spectinomycin PLUS For chlamydia: doxycycline for 14 days PLUS For *T. vaginalis*, BV, anaerobic infections: metronidazole for 14 days
Neonatal conjunctivitis (ophthalmia neonatorum)	*N. gonorrhoeae, C. trachomatis*	Ceftriaxone, 50 mg/kg by intramuscular injection, single dose (max. 125 mg) OR Kanamycin, 25 mg/kg by intramuscular injection, single dose (max. 75 mg)
Anorectal syndrome	*N. gonorrhoeae, C. trachomatis, C. trachomatis* LGV strains L1, L2	For gononorrhoea: ciprofloxacin, ceftriaxone, cefixime or spectinomycin PLUS For chlamydia/LGV: doxycycline or azithromycin for up to 3 weeks
Anogenital warts	Human papillomavirus (HPV) types 6, 11	Removal of external warts by surgery, cryotherapy or podophyllin, podophyllotoxin or trichloroacetic acid solutions OR Patient-applied podophyllotoxin 0.5% or imiquimod gels

Reproduced with permission from World Health Organization. Guidelines for the Management of Sexually Transmitted Infections; Revised version. Geneva: WHO; 2003.

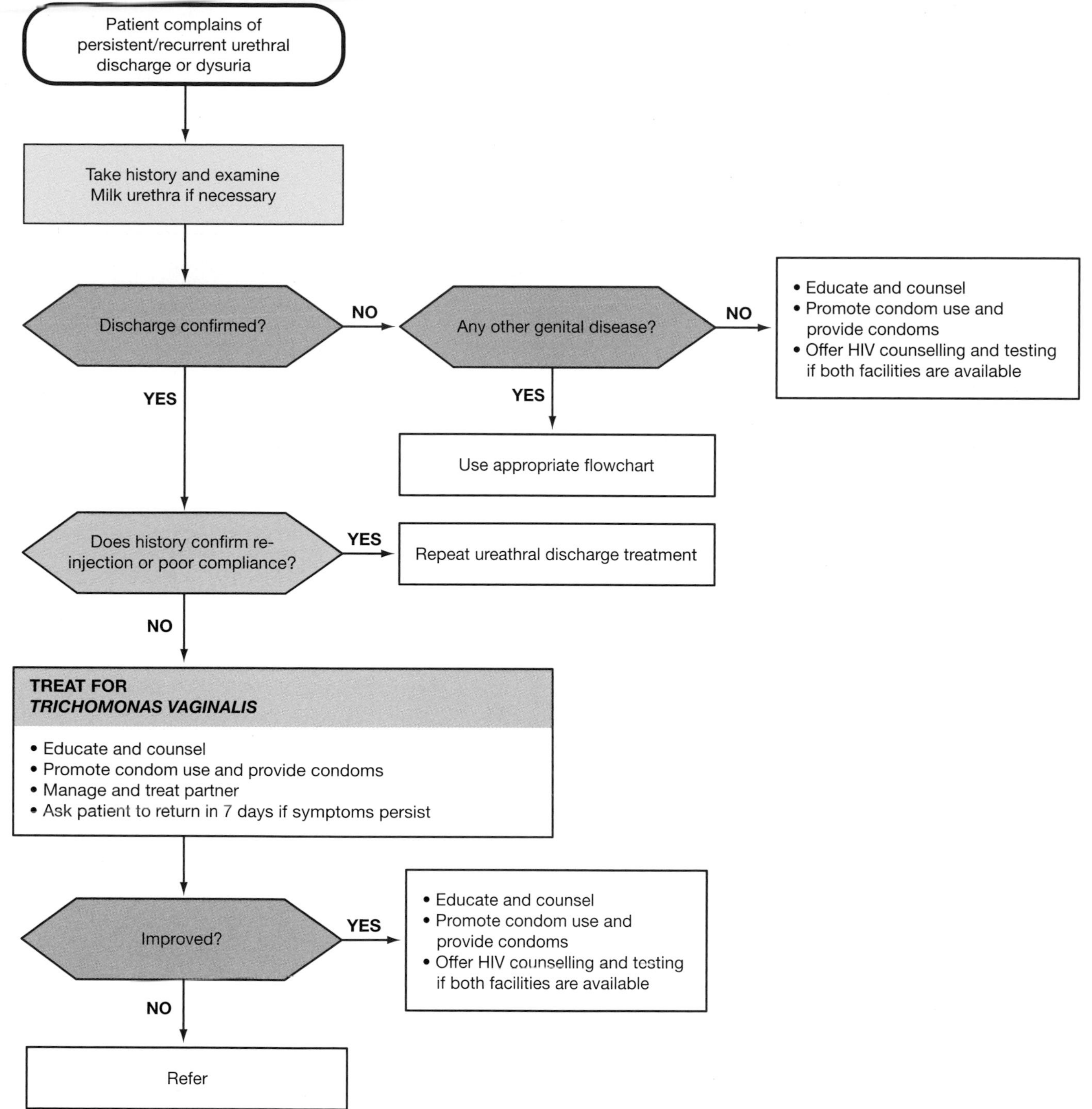

FIGURE 7.2 Persistent/recurrent urethral discharge in men. *Reproduced with permission from World Health Organization. Guidelines for the Management of Sexually Transmitted Infections; Revised version. Geneva: WHO; 2003.*

However, treatment of genital herpes with antivirals (e.g. acyclovir), even though it simply helps healing but does not cure the infection, is now recommended by WHO (see Fig. 7.3) in high HIV prevalence settings.

Laboratory-assisted differential diagnosis is rarely helpful for GUD, and mixed infections are common. Herpes simplex infection can be diagnosed by culture, antigen detection or PCR, but these are rarely available in resource-poor settings. Chancroid can be diagnosed by culture, but *Haemophilus ducreyi* is difficult to grow. PCR has been used in research settings, but there is no commercially available test. Dark-field microscopy for syphilis requires specialist expertise and lacks sensitivity. In areas of high syphilis prevalence, a reactive serologic test may be only a reflection of a previous infection, and a negative test does not necessarily exclude primary syphilis as seroreactivity may take 2–3 weeks to show.

INGUINAL BUBO (see Fig. 7.4)

Inguinal lymphadenopathy is a common feature of chancroid, lymphogranuloma venereum (LGV) and syphilis. Syphilitic adenopathy is usually painless and does not suppurate, in contrast to the buboes of chancroid and LGV. In males, a genital ulcer is usually visible when a bubo results from one of these conditions, although the primary lesion of LGV is often small, painless and transient. In women, the ulcer may be overlooked unless a careful speculum examination is

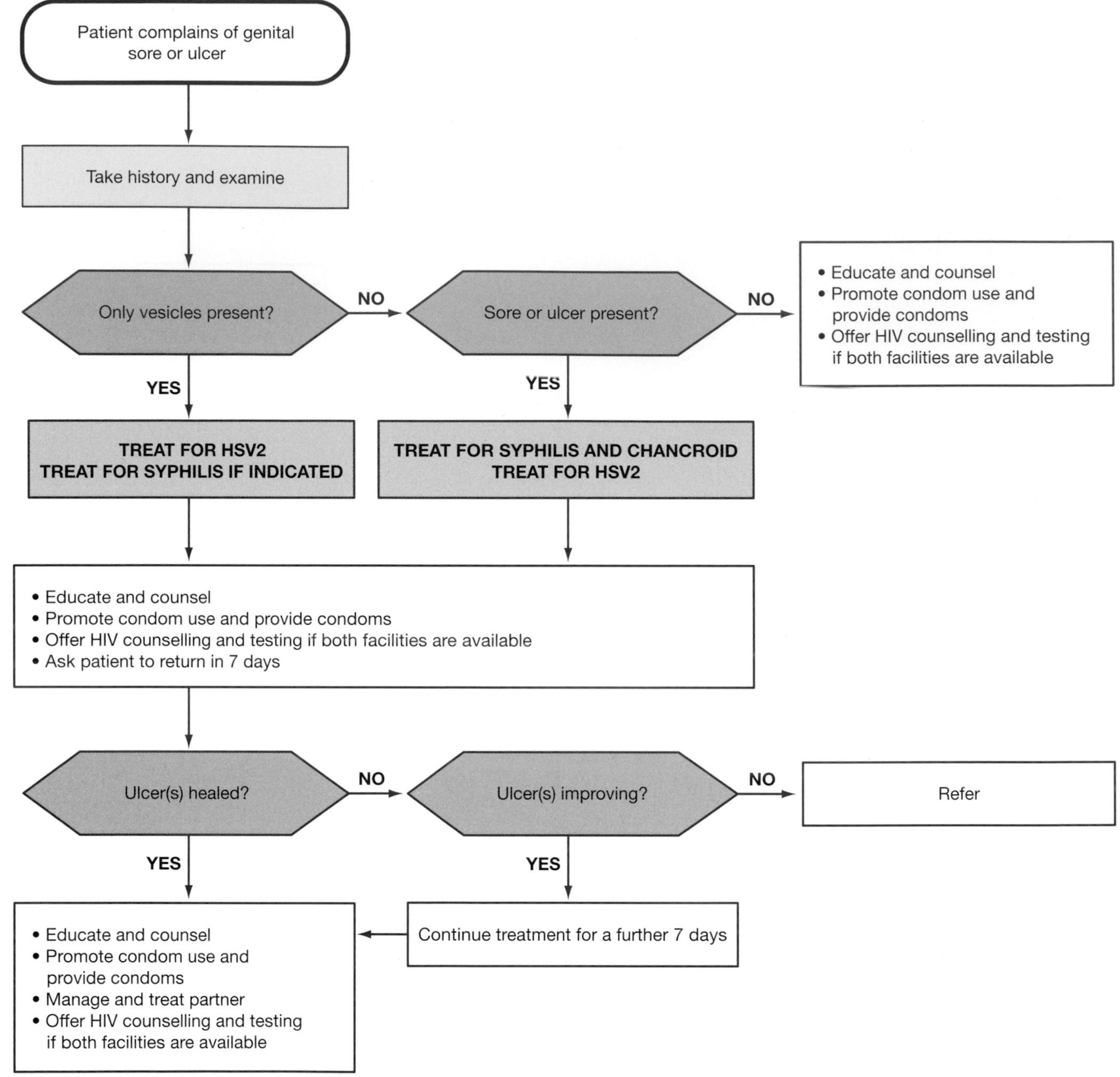

FIGURE 7.3 Genital ulcers. *Reproduced with permission from World Health Organization. Guidelines for the Management of Sexually Transmitted Infections; Revised version. Geneva: WHO; 2003.*

performed. The differential diagnosis includes inguinal hernia, septic lesion of the lower limb, HIV infection with generalized lymphadenopathy, filariasis, tuberculosis and plague. Laboratory investigation is rarely helpful, though elementary bodies of *C. trachomatis* may be detected by immunofluorescent staining in lymph node aspirates from cases of LGV.

VAGINAL DISCHARGE (see Figs 7.6–7.8)

The syndromic approach for the management of vaginal discharge syndrome aims to include treatment of cervicitis caused by *N. gonorrhoeae and C. trachomatis* alongside treatment of vaginitis caused by *T. vaginalis*, bacterial vaginosis (BV) and *Candida* spp. (see Fig. 7.6). The syndromic approach lacks both sensitivity and specificity, as most cervical infections are asymptomatic and only a minority of women presenting with vaginal discharge syndrome have cervical infections. To improve algorithm accuracy and to save costs linked to overtreatment, WHO has suggested the use of individual risk assessment scores, which are combinations of sociodemographic and behavioral risk factors and clinical signs found to be locally associated with cervical infections and/or the results of simple laboratory or bedside tests. Past evaluations of risk assessment scores have yielded mixed results, with sensitivities and specificities not usually exceeding 70%, and with higher positive predictive values and better cost-effectiveness profiles found in settings with higher *N. gonorrhoeae* or *C. trachomatis* prevalence [16]. Such findings imply that effectiveness may vary not just between countries, but also between settings within a country. The WHO STI guidelines have recommended that risk assessment scores incorporate background cervical infection prevalence levels in the target population.

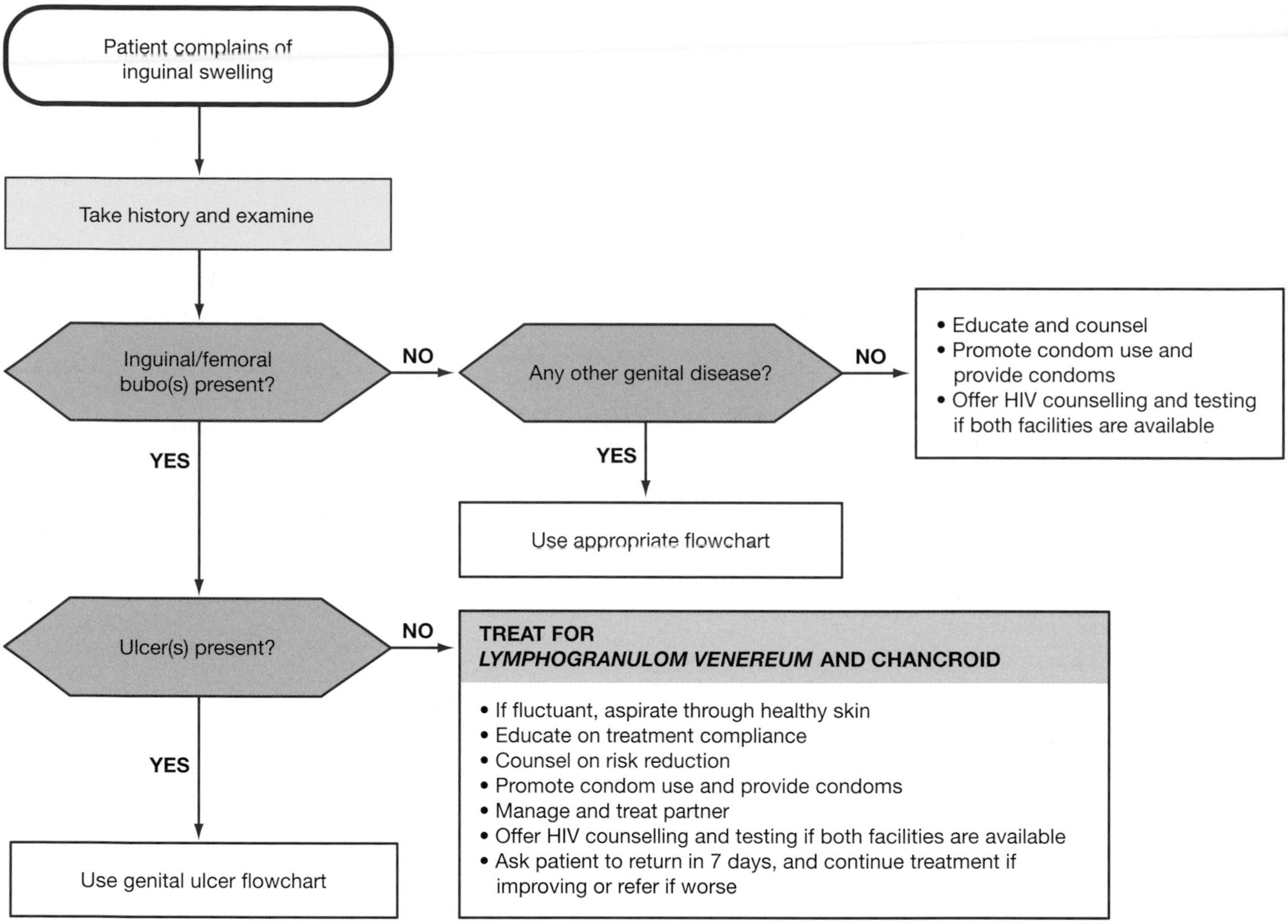

Patient complains of inguinal swelling

Take history and examine

Inguinal/femoral bubo(s) present?

NO

Any other genital disease?

NO

- Educate and counsel
- Promote condom use and provide condoms
- Offer HIV counselling and testing if both facilities are available

YES

Use appropriate flowchart

YES

Ulcer(s) present?

NO

TREAT FOR
***LYMPHOGRANULOM VENEREUM* AND CHANCROID**

- If fluctuant, aspirate through healthy skin
- Educate on treatment compliance
- Counsel on risk reduction
- Promote condom use and provide condoms
- Manage and treat partner
- Offer HIV counselling and testing if both facilities are available
- Ask patient to return in 7 days, and continue treatment if improving or refer if worse

YES

Use genital ulcer flowchart

FIGURE 7.4 Inguinal bubo. *Reproduced with permission from World Health Organization. Guidelines for the Management of Sexually Transmitted Infections; Revised version. Geneva: WHO; 2003.*

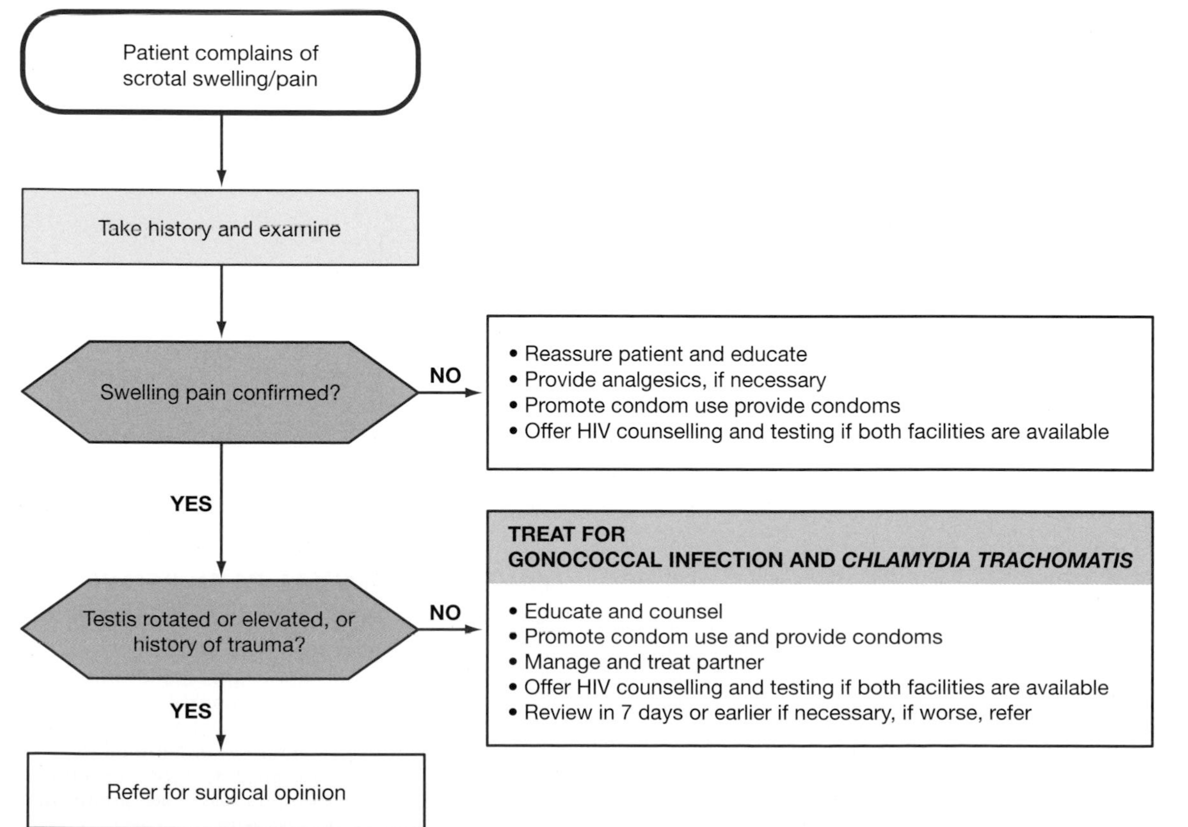

FIGURE 7.5 Scrotal swelling. *Reproduced with permission from World Health Organization. Guidelines for the Management of Sexually Transmitted Infections; Revised version. Geneva: WHO; 2003.*

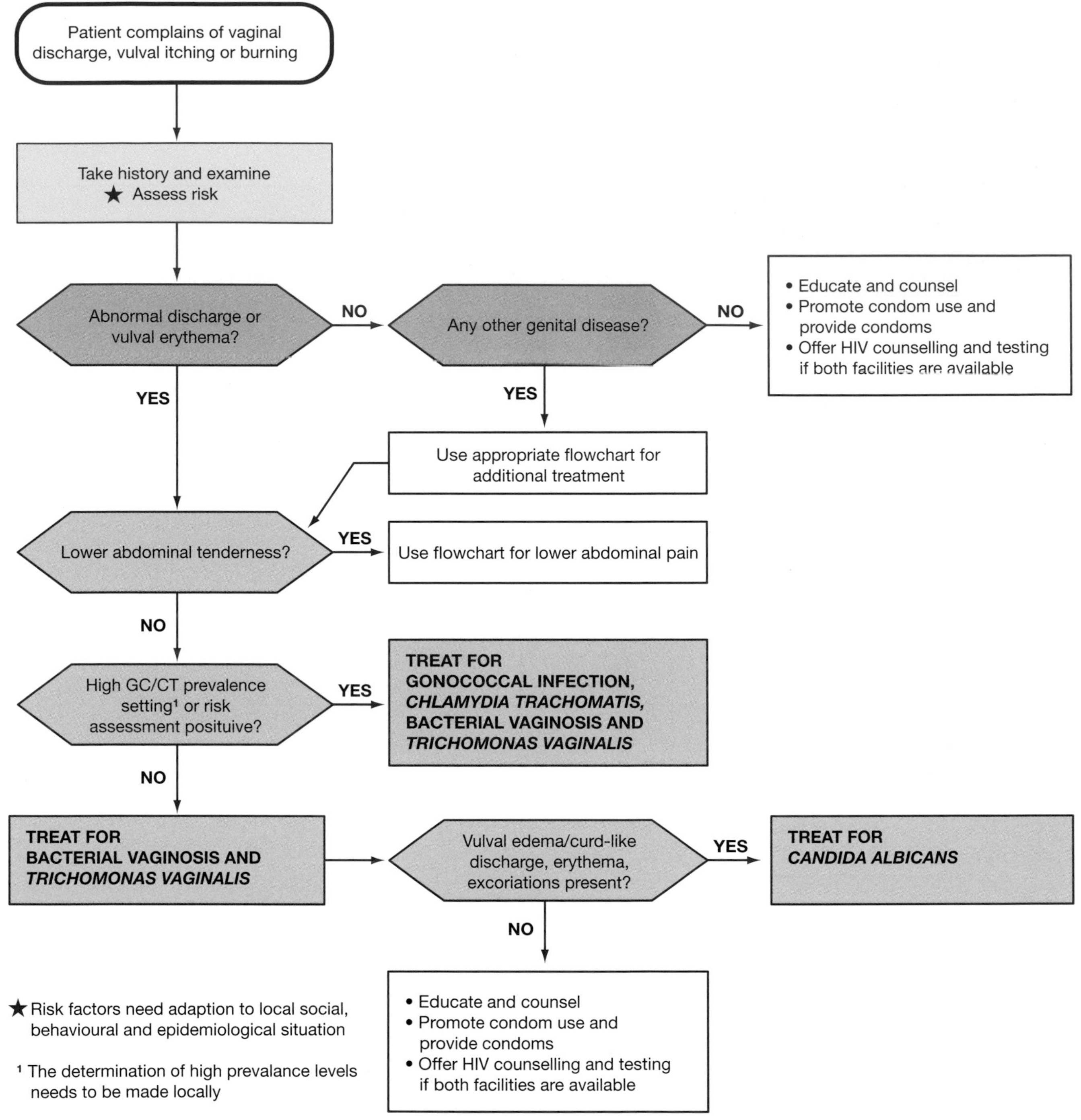

FIGURE 7.6 Vaginal discharge. *Reproduced with permission from World Health Organization. Guidelines for the Management of Sexually Transmitted Infections; Revised version. Geneva: WHO; 2003.*

Where speculum examination is possible, vulvovaginal candidiasis can often be diagnosed clinically (see Fig. 7.7). If a microscope is also available, the presence of motile trichomonads in a wet preparation confirms *T. vaginalis* infection, clue cells suggest bacterial vaginosis, and budding yeasts confirm the presence of *Candida* spp. (see Fig. 7.8). *C. trachomatis* and *N. gonorrhoeae* are usually diagnosed by nucleic acid amplification tests, which can be performed on self-administered vaginal swabs, in resource-rich settings, but these are expensive. There is an urgent need for simple, cheap diagnostic tests (e.g. dipsticks) to guide the management of vaginal discharge syndrome in resource-poor settings.

LOWER ABDOMINAL PAIN (PELVIC INFLAMMATORY DISEASE, PID) (see Fig. 7.9)

Infection of the female upper genital tract is commonly due to *N. gonorrhoeae* or *C. trachomatis*, in combination with ascending infection from organisms found in the normal vagina flora, e.g. *Streptococcus* spp., anaerobes. PID often follows trauma to the cervix caused by termination of pregnancy, insertion of an intrauterine contraceptive device, cesarean section or vaginal delivery. Gonococcal PID usually has a more acute onset and more severe symptoms than chlamydial PID, but either may cause irreversible damage to the fallopian tubes,

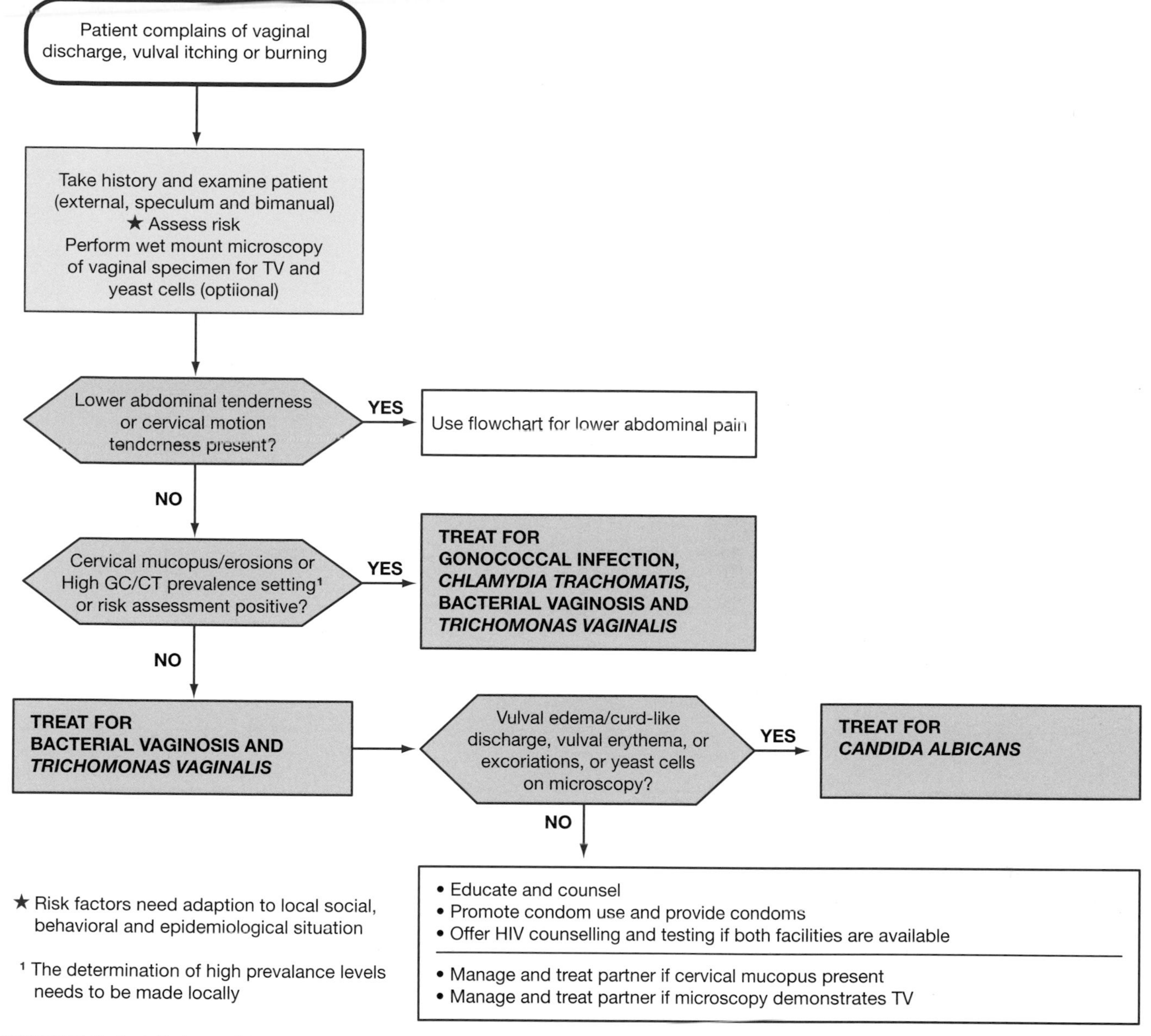

FIGURE 7.7 Vaginal discharge: bimanual and speculum, with or without microscope. *Reproduced with permission from World Health Organization. Guidelines for the Management of Sexually Transmitted Infections; Revised version. Geneva: WHO; 2003.*

leading to infertility or ectopic pregnancy. In developing countries, the diagnosis of PID is usually clinical (lower abdominal and cervical motion tenderness) (see Fig. 7.9). Laparoscopy is helpful when it is available. Important differential diagnoses include ectopic pregnancy, appendicitis and endometriosis. Treatment should cover *N. gonorrhoeae, C. trachomatis* and anaerobic bacteria.

ANORECTAL SYNDROME

In recent years, outbreaks of lymphogranuloma venereum (LGV) have been reported in Europe and North America, usually among HIV-positive men who have sex with men (MSM). Most patients presented with proctitis, and symptoms included severe rectal pain, mucoid and/or hemorrhagic rectal discharge, tenesmus, constipation and other signs of lower gastrointestinal inflammation, sometimes severe, whilst genital ulcers and inguinal adenopathy were rare. The resurgence of LGV in settings where only a few imported cases had been seen each year, with its unusual clinical presentation, highlighted the need to have more accurate diagnostic, management and control tools. Studies conducted among men and women in Asia and Latin America have shown a high prevalence of anorectal infections in MSM and in female sex-workers, yet no approach for case management was included in the WHO guidelines. It is likely that a substantial number of anorectal infections go unrecognized and untreated, especially when low levels of clinical suspicion are combined with stigmatization of anal intercourse. Thus, there have been calls to introduce a new algorithm for management of the anorectal syndrome, which will soon be published by WHO, but which will require further validation.

The likely infectious causes of anorectal syndrome in both men and women are *N. gonorrhoeae* and *C. trachomatis*, both non-LGV and LGV (L1–L3) strains, but can also include syphilis, HSV and HPV (involving the stratified squamous epithelium) as well as infections of the rectum and colon, e.g. shigella, campylobacter, cytomegalovirus, amebiasis. Differential diagnosis includes neoplastic lesions, perineal abscesses, and chronic conditions such as ulcerative colitis or Crohn's disease. Investigations sometimes performed in resource-rich settings include DNA amplification tests for *N. gonorrhoeae* and *C. trachomatis*, though these have not been approved by the Food and Drug Administration (FDA) for rectal specimens. Serology for syphilis and HIV are recommended.

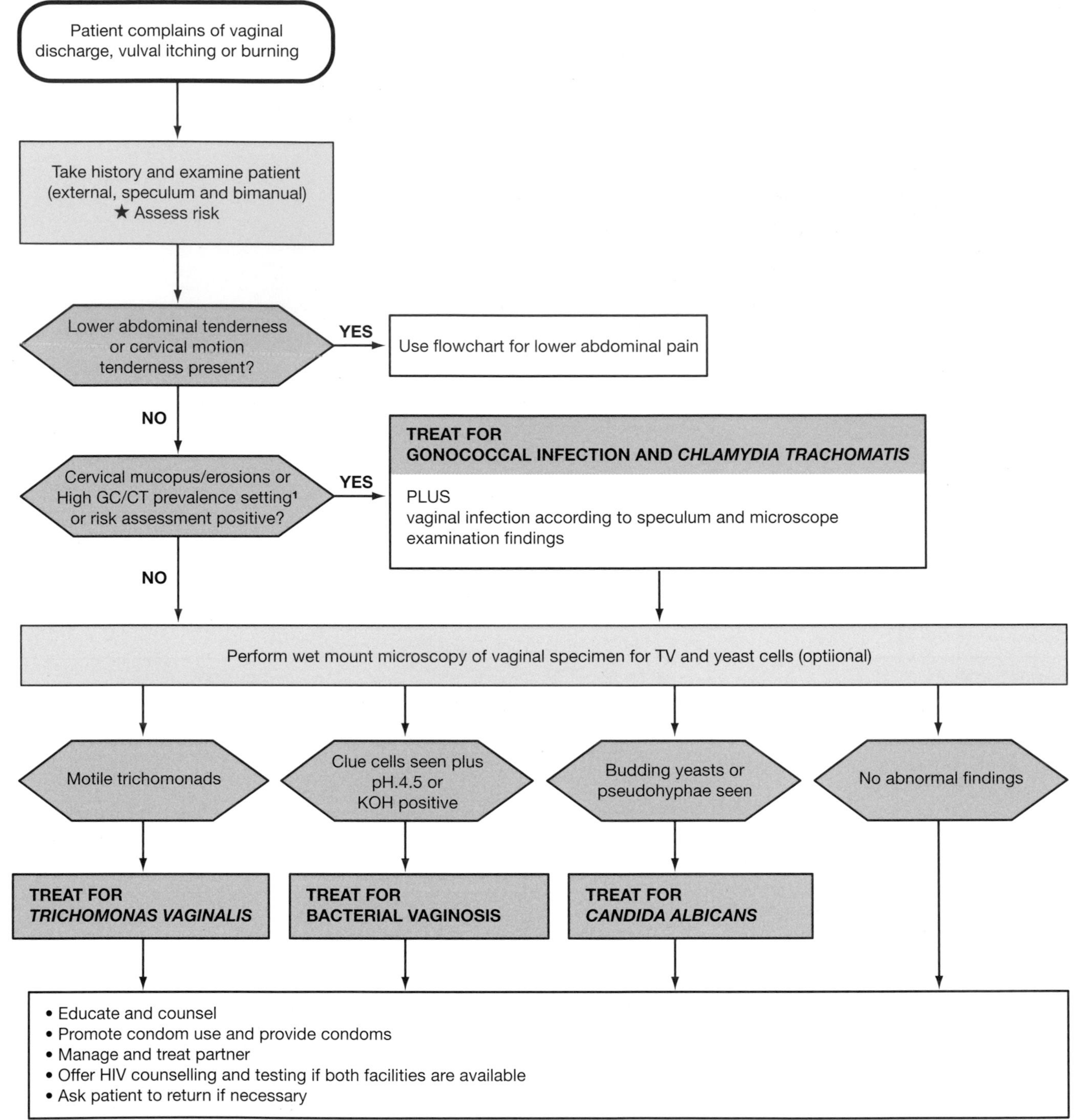

FIGURE 7.8 Vaginal discharge: bimanual, speculum and microscope. *Reproduced with permission from World Health Organization. Guidelines for the Management of Sexually Transmitted Infections; Revised version. Geneva: WHO; 2003.*

CONTROL OF STIs

Given sufficient resources, it is possible to control curable STIs through the provision of accessible, acceptable and affordable clinical services, combined with partner notification and screening programs in high-risk groups. In most developing countries, case management of STIs must be syndromic, because facilities for laboratory diagnosis are unavailable outside a few specialist centers.

Partner Notification

Even in the case of easily treatable STIs, control is difficult because of the high prevalence of asymptomatic infection in both men and women. Partner identification and treatment is an important approach to a frequently asymptomatic, high-risk population. In developing countries, resources are not usually available for the notification of partners by the healthcare provider. Patients must be relied on to refer their contacts(s). It is important that the clinician spend time

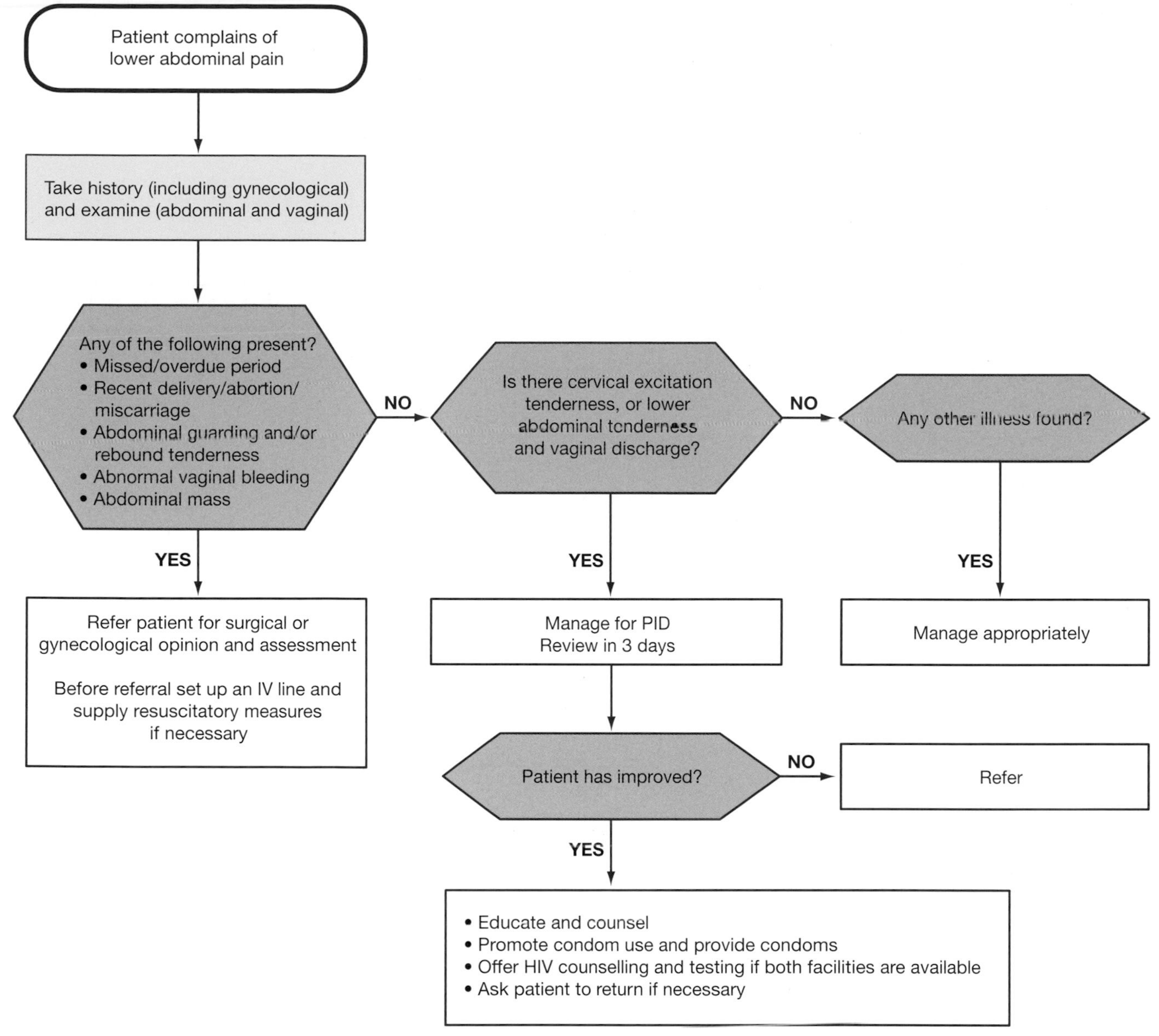

FIGURE 7.9 Lower abdominal pain. *Reproduced with permission from World Health Organization. Guidelines for the Management of Sexually Transmitted Infections; Revised version. Geneva: WHO; 2003.*

explaining the importance of treating partners, both to avoid re-infection and to prevent sequelae in the partner and any future children. Many clinics give contact notes to index cases to pass on to their sexual partners. Unfortunately, partner notification rarely results in the treatment of more than a small number of individuals. Alternative strategies, e.g. providing treatment to the index partner to provide to his or her partner(s), have been piloted in trials in developing countries, but it is difficult to ascertain their impact. Moreover, there are risks associated with partner notification in the context of syndromic management, since women with vaginal discharge syndrome frequently do not have an STI but an endogenous infection (VVC, BV). Requesting them to refer their partner(s) for STI treatment may be a waste of resources and may expose them to domestic violence.

Screening

In view of the serious consequences of syphilis in pregnancy, serologic screening for active syphilis is recommended for all women attending antenatal clinics [17,18]. Universal screening of pregnant women for syphilis, and treatment with single-dose benzathine penicillin before 28 weeks' gestation, could prevent more than 500,000 perinatal deaths per year [6]. This is one of the cheapest and most cost-effective health interventions available. New simple, rapid, cheap point-of-care serologic tests for syphilis, which can be performed on whole blood obtained from a finger prick, are now available [19]. Since they can be stored at room temperature, and require no laboratory equipment, they could greatly increase the coverage of prenatal syphilis screening at the primary healthcare level in developing countries.

Male circumcision

This has been shown to reduce HIV incidence by about 60% in three randomized controlled trials in African men, and also reduces the risk of acquiring some other STIs such as herpes and HPV [20,21].

Vaccination

There are no vaccines against bacterial STIs. However, safe and effective vaccination can be provided to prevent the sexual acquisition of hepatitis B virus (HBV), particularly in high-risk populations (e.g. homosexual men, injecting drug users, or prisoners). In addition, two effective vaccines against oncogenic HPV strains 16 and 18, which

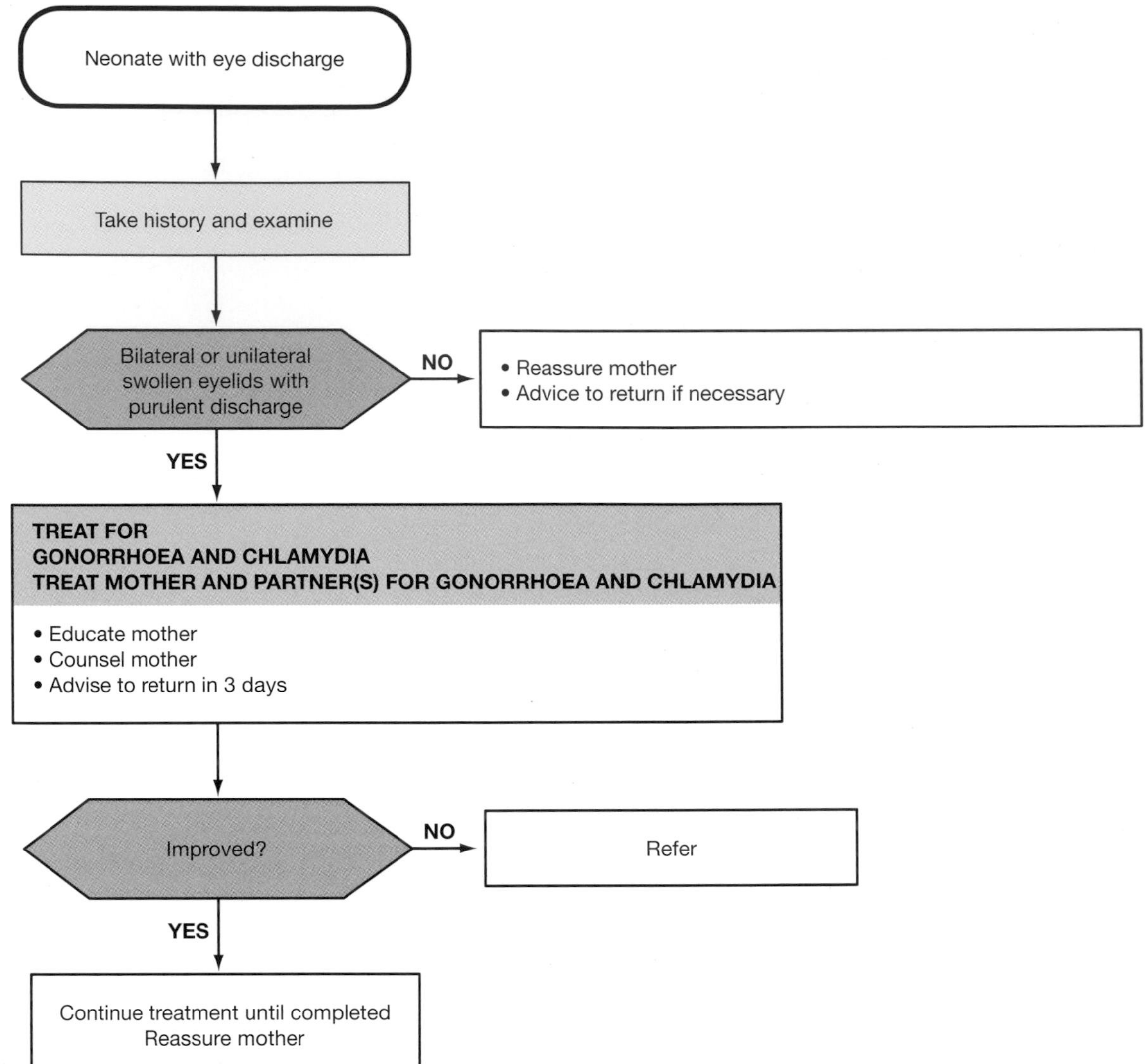

FIGURE 7.10 Neonatal conjunctivitis. *Reproduced with permission from World Health Organization. Guidelines for the Management of Sexually Transmitted Infections; Revised version. Geneva: WHO; 2003.*

cause around 70% of cervical cancers worldwide, are now available and are being given to young women in industrialized countries, but they are expensive and are not yet available in most developing countries [22]. WHO has produced useful guidelines for the introduction of HPV vaccines [23].

Ocular Prophylaxis

The prevention of neonatal conjunctivitis (also called ophthalmia neonatorum) due to *N. gonorrhoeae* or *C. trachomatis* should be a simple matter. More than 100 years ago, Crede prevented the disease by the instillation of 1% silver nitrate drops into the eyes of infants at delivery. More recently, 1% tetracycline ointment, which is cheap, widely available and easy to store, was shown to be equally effective [24]. Due to the spread of tetracycline-resistant gonococcal strains, erythromycin 0.5% eye ointment may be more effective. Given the high incidence of neonatal conjunctivitis and its devastating consequences (Fig. 7.10), this simple measure is one of the most cost-effective health interventions available. Yet there are very few developing countries in which prophylaxis of neonatal conjunctivitis is systematically carried out. Moreover, a quadrivalent vaccine has additional high effectiveness in preventing anogenital warts caused by HPV genotypes 6 and 11.

Ultimately, control of STIs depends on tackling social, cultural, gender and economic disparities in health and in accessing healthcare, and in improving living conditions for the poor, particularly women, in both the developed and the developing world.

REFERENCES

1. Joint United Nations Programme on AIDS (UNAIDS). http://data.unaids.org/pub/Report/2009/2009_epidemic_update_en.pdf
2. WHO. Global estimates of the prevalence and incidence of selected sexually transmitted infections: overview and estimates, 1999. Geneva: WHO; 2001. http://www.who.int/hiv/pub/sti/who_hiv_aids_2001.02.pdf
3. Grosskurth H, Mosha F, Todd J, et al. Impact of improved treatment of sexually transmitted diseases on HIV infection in rural Tanzania: randomised controlled trial. Lancet 1995;346:530–6.
   This community randomized trial showed that improved syndromic management of STIs in rural health centers in Tanzania reduced the incidence of HIV infection by 38%.
4. Wawer MJ, Sewankambo NK, Serwadda D, et al. Control of sexually transmitted diseases for AIDS prevention in Uganda: a randomised community trial. Rakai Project Study Group. Lancet 1999;353:525–35.
5. Kamali A, Quigley M, Nakiyingi J, et al. Syndromic management of sexually-transmitted infections and behaviour change interventions on transmission of HIV-1 in rural Uganda: a community randomised trial. Lancet 2003;361: 645–52.
6. Schmid G. Economic and programmatic aspects of congenital syphilis prevention. Bull World Health Organ 2004;82:402–9.

7. Weiss HA, Buvé A, Robinson NJ, et al. The epidemiology of HSV-2 infection and its association with HIV infection in four urban African populations AIDS 2001;15(Suppl 4):S97–108.
8. Fleming DT, Wasserheit JN. From epidemiological synergy to public health policy and practice: the contribution of other sexually transmitted diseases to sexual transmission of HIV infection. Sex Transm Infect 1999; 75:3–17.
This excellent review assesses the evidence that other STIs enhance the sexual transmission of HIV, and considers the public health implications of interactions between HIV and other STIs.
9. Korenromp EL, White RG, Orroth KK, et al. Determinants of the impact of sexually transmitted infection treatment on prevention of HIV infection: a synthesis of evidence from the Mwanza, Rakai, and Masaka intervention trials. J Infect Dis 2005;191(Suppl 1):S168–78.
10. Nagot N, Ouedraogo A, Foulongne V, et al. Reduction of HIV-1 RNA levels with therapy to suppress herpes simplex virus. N Engl J Med 2007;356: 790–9.
11. Watson-Jones D, Weiss HA, Rusizoka M, et al. Effect of herpes simplex suppression on incidence of HIV among women in Tanzania. N Engl J Med 2008; 358:1560–71.
12. Celum C, Wald A, Lingappa JR, et al. Acyclovir and transmission of HIV-1 from persons infected with HIV-1 and HSV-2. N Engl J Med 2010;362: 427–39.
This study among HIV-discordant couples in whom the HIV-positive partner was HSV-2 seropositive showed that suppressive treatment of the HIV-positive partner with acyclovir did not reduce transmission to the HIV-seronegative partner
13. Celum C, Wald A, Hughes J, et al. Effect of aciclovir on HIV-1 acquisition in herpes simplex virus 2 seropositive women and men who have sex with men: a randomised, double-blind, placebo-controlled trial. Lancet 2008;371: 2109–19.
This study, and reference 11, showed that suppressive treatment with acyclovir did not reduce the incidence of HIV infection among high-risk individuals who were seropositive for HSV-2.
14. World Health Organization. Guidelines for the Management of Sexually Transmitted Infections; Revised version. Geneva: WHO; 2003.
15. Pépin J, Sobéla F, Deslandes S, et al. Etiology of urethral discharge in West Africa: the role of *Mycoplasma genitalium* and *Trichomonas vaginalis*. Bull World Health Organ 2001;79:118–26.
16. Mayaud P, Ka-Gina G, Cornelissen J, et al. Validation of a WHO algorithm with risk assessment for the clinical management of vaginal discharge in Mwanza, Tanzania. Sex Transm Infect 1998;74(suppl 1):77–84.
17. Watson-Jones D, Changalucha J, Gumodoka B, et al. Syphilis and pregnancy outcomes in Tanzania. 1. Impact of maternal syphilis on outcome of pregnancy in Mwanza Region, Tanzania. J Infect Dis 2002;186:940–7.
18. Watson-Jones D, Gumodoka B, Changalucha J, et al. Syphilis in pregnancy in Tanzania II. The effectiveness of antenatal syphilis screening and single dose benzathine penicillin treatment for the prevention of adverse pregnancy outcomes. J Infect Dis 2002;186:948–57.
This study, conducted in antenatal clinics in Tanzania, showed that a single dose of benzathine penicillin, given before 28 weeks' gestation, prevents adverse pregnancy outcomes due to syphilis.
19. Mabey D, Peeling RW, Ballard R, et al. Prospective, multi-centre clinic-based evaluation of four rapid diagnostic tests for syphilis. Sex Transm Infect 2006;82(suppl v):v13–16.
20. Siegfried N, Muller M, Deeks JJ, Volmink J. Male circumcision for prevention of heterosexual acquisition of HIV in men. Cochrane Database Syst Rev 2009;(2):CD003362.
21. Tobian AA, Serwadda D, Quinn TC, et al. Male circumcision for the prevention of HSV-2 and HPV infections and syphilis. N Engl J Med 2009; 360:1298–309.
22. Louie KS, de Sanjose S, Mayaud P. Epidemiology and prevention of human papillomavirus and cervical cancer in sub-Saharan Africa: a comprehensive review. Trop Med Int Health. 2009;14:1287–302.
23. World Health Organization. Preparing for the introduction of HPV vaccines. Policy and programme guidance for countries. Geneva: WHO; 2006. http://www.who.int/reproductivehealth/publications/cancers/RHR_06.11/en/index.html
24. Laga M, Plummer FA, Piot P, et al. Prophylaxis of gonococcal and chlamydial ophthalmia neonatorum. A comparison of silver nitrate and tetracycline. N Engl J Med 1988;318:653–7.

8 Tropical Dermatology

Arturo Saavedra, David Rosmarin

Key features

- Though the most common culprits of acute dermatoses in the tropics are infectious agents, important inflammatory dermatoses should be considered, which often mimic infectious diseases
- When considering the differential diagnosis of an acute eruption, the primary morphology of the lesion is the most important factor to identify during the physical examination
- Due to significant interactions between systemic medications as well as poor excretion of drugs through the skin, topical regimens are often first-line agents that suffice in the therapy of most cutaneous disorders. However, exceptions do exist, particularly in the case of cutaneous manifestations of systemic infections as well as inflammatory autoimmune bullous disorders such as pemphigus
- Whenever the primary morphology of the lesion and/or its distribution are not sufficient for diagnosis, skin biopsy may be indicated, particularly to evaluate the primary effector cell in the infiltrate (i.e. lymphocyte, neutrophil or eosinophil)

In this chapter, we will highlight those dermatologic disorders and presentations that are either more commonly found in tropical or resource-limited regions, or that most frequently enter the differential diagnosis in such areas. Emphasis is placed on the physical examination. For ease of creating a differential diagnosis, diseases are discussed based on the predominant primary lesion and symptoms they cause. Special mention is made of those diseases that have multiple morphologies or transition to different appearance as the disease evolves. For detailed discussion on the epidemiology, pathophysiology, diagnosis and treatment for individual disorders, please refer to the corresponding disease-specific chapter.

VESICLES/BULLAE

Vesicles and bullae are fluid-filled lesions. Herpetic involvement of the skin classically includes a vesicular phase, and is among the most common dermatoses encountered by the clinician. Herpetic vesicles lay on an erythematous base, and the lesions ulcerate and eventually heal with crusting. Traditionally, herpetic ulcers show a scalloped border with serosanguineous drainage, pain at the site, and, occasionally, ipsilateral lymphadenopathy. Chronic disease may lead to scarring. The patient experiences early dysesthesias at the site of a future eruption in recurrent disease. Most importantly, the diagnosis should be suspected in those with chronic ulcers, particularly if they are immunosuppressed. Though HSV-1 is more common in orofacial disease and HSV-2 in genital lesions, both strains can be seen in either location. Often a fixed location in the body is noted; however, primary disease can affect any area of the body.

Zoster infection is caused by reactivation of varicella (chickenpox) virus that has laid dormant in basal root ganglia. Zoster usually presents with crop-like vesicles along a dermatome. Zoster can disseminate, especially in immunocompromised patients. Greater than 20 lesions outside a dermatome should raise suspicion for dissemination. Ulcerations may be chronic, especially in immunocompromised patients. It is important to remember this diagnosis, particularly when steroid-responsive diagnoses such as pseudo-vesicular Sweet's syndrome (or idiopathic neutrophilic dermatosis) are considered, as oral steroid use in patients with disseminated zoster can be lethal. The occasionally necrotic center of evolving lesions may easily be confused for a primary vasculitis. It is important to note, however, that vasculitis seen in the setting of zoster is usually reactive and not a primary disease requiring steroids or cytotoxic medication, even when it is clearly present on skin biopsy.

Pemphigus foliaceous is an autoimmune blistering disease overrepresented in the tropics. It is caused when pathogenic immunoglobulins against intraepidermal desmoglein 1 destroy intercellular connections, leading to single cell detachment. As little to no desmoglein 1 is expressed in mucosal skin, pemphigus foliaceous is primarily a disease of cutaneous surfaces, sparing the eyes and mouth. The blisters in pemphigus foliaceous are not tense, but flaccid (Fig. 8.1). They are readily expanded when side pressure is exerted, and further separation is created between the superficial layers of skin, the so-called Nikolsky's sign. It is important to highlight, however, that vesicles may only be seen in the acute, early phases of disease. Because these blisters are so fragile, by the time the patient presents for care, the physical examination is notable for crusted and scaly papules, erosions, or even psoriatic-like disease. The disease is strikingly photosensitive, so that the scalp and upper extremities and shawl distribution may be disproportionately affected.

Fogo selvagem refers to a prominent intensely inflammatory response with vesicles and bullae that can follow a fly bite in areas of South America. It is usually treated with steroids.

VASCULAR PAPULES AND NODULES (ANGIOMATOUS LESIONS)

Angiomatous lesions are reddish papules or nodules due to vascular proliferation and dilatation. Kaposi sarcoma, verruga peruana, pyogenic granulomas, cherry angiomas and pseudo-Kaposi can all present with these vascular lesions. If they are more nodular and deeper in the skin, the angiomata may appear violaceous.

Carrion disease is caused by *Bartonella bacilliformis* in focal areas of South America, and has two phases: Oroya fever and verruga peruana. In Oroya fever, soon after initial infection, fever, hemolysis, malaise, headaches and musculoskeletal pain develop. If the patient survives, the acute illness is followed by the chronic phase, verruga peruana, in

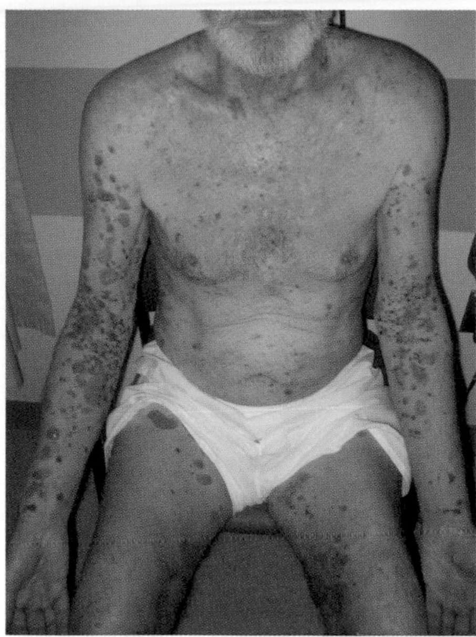

FIGURE 8.1 Pemphigus foliaceous. Note the presence of flaccid blisters on a mildly inflammatory border. Unlike herpetic bullae or erosions, the lesions of pemphigus foliaceous are usually photodistributed, can be larger, and are often fragile, so the patient rarely presents with intact blisters.

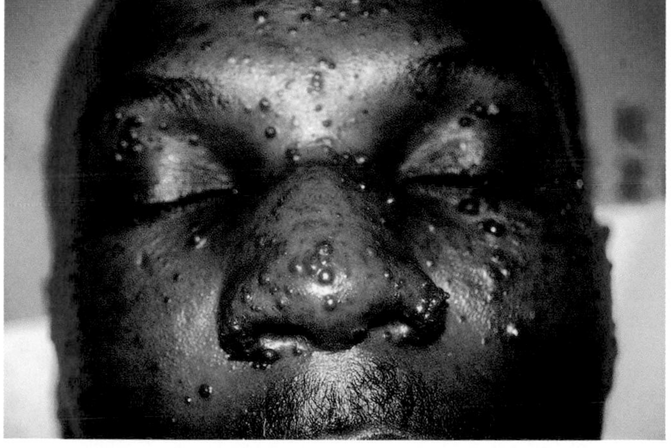

FIGURE 8.2 Bacillary angiomatosis. Lesions are often dome-shaped erythematous papules, resembling angiomas. This striking disseminated pattern raises suspicion for HIV infection, if not previously diagnosed.

which the patient develops multiple angiomatous lesions on the skin. These reddish papules or nodules sometimes have a collarette and may be eroded. They are very similar to the lesions seen in bacillary angiomatosis.

Bacillary angiomatosis caused by *Bartonella henselae* and *Bartonella quintana* most commonly affects immunosuppressed patients. Red angiomatous papules or nodules are very characteristic (Fig. 8.2). There is a great variation in the number of lesions that may develop. The lesions may bleed and erode and cause regional lymphadenopathy, as well as peliosis, blood-filled cystic spaces in the liver and spleen.

Kaposi sarcoma due to human herpesvirus-8 (HHV-8) is in the differential diagnosis of angiomatous lesions, and it is necessary to biopsy the lesion to ascertain the diagnosis. Lesions begin as macules, but develop into papules and then nodules, with symmetric, widespread reddish, violaceous or blue-black lesions. Edema can be an accompanying sign. There are five different types, with the AIDS-associated type commonly being the presenting manifestation that leads to a diagnosis of HIV. Gastrointestinal and pulmonary involvement by Kaposi sarcoma can lead to death from hemorrhage, hemoptysis or bowel obstruction.

PETECHIAE AND PURPURA

Purpura is blood that has leaked out of the vasculature into the skin but remains visible. If it occurs as small spots, it is referred to as petechiae; if it occurs in larger areas and in deeper structures, it is called ecchymoses. Characteristically, purpura will not blanch under pressure since the erythrocytes have escaped in the tissue and are no longer within compressible vessels. Common causes include coagulopathies, trauma, nutritional deficiencies, vasculitides, medicines such as aspirin and warfarin (Coumadin), and infections.

Rickettsial diseases have a predilection for the microvasculature, often causing petechiae. During louse-borne epidemic typhus caused by *Rickettsia prowazekii* and flea-borne endemic typhus caused by *Rickettsia typhi*, an erythematous macular eruption occurs on the trunk and spreads centrifugally, sparing the face, palms and soles. Patients are febrile and appear toxic. During Rocky Mountain spotted fever (RMSF), the eruption begins in the extremities, often involving the wrists, and spreads centripetally. In severe typhus and RMSF, the eruption may become hemorrhagic with gangrene of the distal structures – nose, fingertips, toes and earlobes.

Mite-borne scrub typhus is caused by *Rickettsia tsutsugamushi*, and the primary skin lesion is an erythematous papule at the site of inoculation by the mite, which is commonly in the genital area or legs. The original papule may form a vesicle and ultimately evolve into an ulcer with a necrotic eschar and surrounding indurated erythema with locoregional lymphadenopathy. A pink macular eruption may develop on the trunk and extend peripherally. Tinnitus and deafness can occur in untreated cases.

Patients with rickettsial spotted fevers such as RMSF, Mediterranean spotted fever, North Asian tick typhus, and others most frequently present with fever, headache, and an initially pink macular eruption on the extremities that spreads centripetally, and may develop into an erythematous papular eruption which becomes hemorrhagic and petechial. Though the face is often spared, the palms and soles are frequently involved, which should raise the suspicion of rickettsial illness.

Patients with bacterial meningitis due to *Neisseria meningitides* often present with fever and rash, the latter classically including petechiae. A useful clue is finding lesions on areas of skin pressure such as at the waist, where belts are worn, or shoulders, where a strap may have been resting. A patient may lack the hemorrhagic signs, and only have a morbilliform exanthem, even in the setting of photophobia and nuchal rigidity.

Patients with leptospirosis, caused by spirochetes of the genus *Leptospira*, can present with fever, hepatic and renal dysfunction, conjunctival suffusion, jaundice and a petechial eruption.

Patients with dengue fever may present with petechial lesions. Fever and myalgia in a patient from the Caribbean or Southeast Asia should prompt consideration of the diagnosis. The rash in dengue may extend to the trunk, and does not resemble dependent vasculitis as is seen in leukocytoclastic vasculitis. Hyperemia and a diffuse macular rash with central islands of sparing may be seen.

ULCERS/VERRUCOUS PLAQUES

Many diseases begin as an ulcer and later develop into a verrucous or warty plaque. Tuberculosis primarily affects the lung, although it can occasionally primarily involve the skin. Following direct inoculation into skin, a firm, red-brown papule may develop which ultimately ulcerates into a chancre and is covered by a dark, adherent crust. Sometimes the bacteria-rich ulcer is associated with erythema nodosum and may eventually spontaneously heal.

Tuberculosis verrucosa cutis occurs by direct contact. A papule forming a verrucous plaque with centrifugal progression and central scarring is typical.

Scrofula and scrofuloderma result when there is contiguous spread from underlying necrotic tuberculoid lymph nodes. The neck is the most common site of involvement. A firm, deep, adherent, purple-red nodule may become fluctuant, suppurate or ulcerate, and form a fistula. Less commonly, self-inoculation near natural orifices can lead to tuberculosis cutis orificialis that appears as yellow-red nodules in or near the mucosa. These lesions frequently ulcerate and are tender.

Lupus vulgaris is a destructive process that usually involves the face, leaving central atrophy. Lupus vulgaris needs to be differentiated from leishmaniasis, sarcoidosis, discoid lupus erythematosus, cutaneous T-cell lymphoma, tuberculoid leprosy, pyodermatitis vegetans and paracoccidioidomycosis. Dermatologic manifestations of disseminated miliary tuberculosis include papules and pustules that are diffusely distributed throughout the body. Papulonecrotic tuberculids are firm, pustulonecrotic, symmetric papules on the extensor surfaces that resolve over several weeks. Lichen scrofulosorum consists of tiny, flat-topped, keratotic papules on the trunk which grow in groups. Erythema induratum appears as symmetric, erythematous subcutaneous nodules on the posterior calves with overlying atrophy and slight scale, commonly in middle-aged women. It is thought to be a hypersensitivity reaction during tuberculosis. Erythema nodosum may appear similar, but is more often on the shins, is more painful, and does not ulcerate.

Skin lesions can also be due to nontuberculous mycobacteria. Rapidly growing *M. fortuitum* and *M. chelonae/abscessus* can cause subcutaneous abscesses or cellulitides. *M. marinum* can lead to erosions, verrucous papules or plaques, and is commonly acquired from aquariums or lakes. *M. marinum, M. kansasii* and other nontuberculous mycobacteria can cause lesions in a sporotrichoid (lymphangitic) pattern (Fig. 8.3). *M. ulcerans* is the cause of Buruli ulcer, a chronic process that first manifests as a solitary, indurated, painless nodule that ulcerates and develops undermined borders. Buruli ulcers most often affect children living in Australia and Africa, and less frequently in Latin America.

Rickettsialpox is caused by *Rickettsia akari* and transmitted by the bite of rodent-associated mites. At the site of inoculation, an erythematous papule first occurs, which then develops into a vesicle that then ruptures and ulcerates. An eschar can occur. There is often an accompanying papulovesicular eruption, as well as regional lymphadenopathy, and patients are febrile and report headache and myalgia.

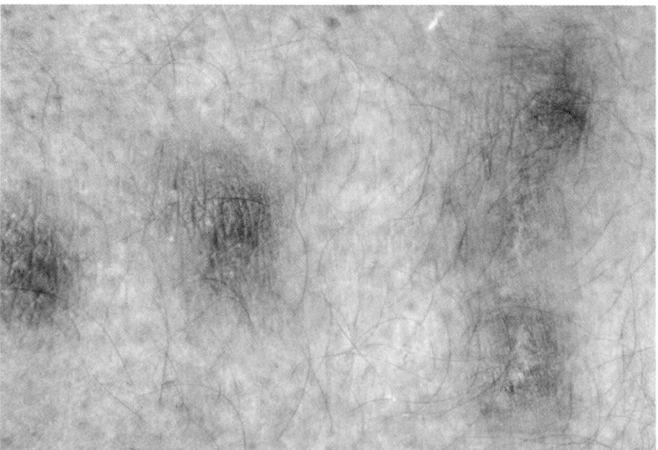

FIGURE 8.3 Atypical mycobacteria. These papulonodular lesions assemble almost in a linear distribution, suggestive of lymphangitic spread. Note the lack of scale or ulceration that could otherwise resemble papulonecrotic tuberculid.

Cutaneous anthrax, caused by *Bacillus anthracis*, is usually due to contact with livestock, animal products or soil. Initially, there is pruritus at the site of inoculation, followed by the development of a papule. Vesicles may surround the papule and coalesce until there is rupture and formation of a 4–6-cm ulcer. There is significant perilesional edema. The ulcer develops a thick black, depressed, painless eschar that is characteristic of the disease. Cutaneous infection can cause systemic illness. The differential diagnosis includes orf, bullous impetigo, plague, a burn, rickettsial eschar, ecthyma gangrenosum and cutaneous diphtheria, although perilesional edema surrounding an eschar strongly suggests cutaneous anthrax. In addition to the cutaneous form of anthrax, which represents 95% of cases, there are also gastrointestinal and pulmonary anthrax that follow ingestion and inhalation of spores, respectively.

Plague is caused by *Yersinia pestis* carried by fleas and is maintained in a number of rodent reservoirs. At the site of a flea bite, a papule, pustule, vesicle, ulcer or eschar may develop, and patients have high fever and appear systemically ill. Regional lymph nodes may become swollen, warm and very tender (buboes). If the bacteria enter into the blood, disseminated intravascular coagulopathy, sepsis, petechiae, purpura fulminans and acral gangrene can occur.

Cutaneous diphtheria, caused by *Corynebacterium diphtheriae*, presents in a variety of ways, including an anesthetic ulcer called ecthyma diphthericum which begins as a vesicle. A membrane may be adherent. Infection of the respiratory tract causes a low-grade fever, sore throat, and purulent nasal discharge which may become erosive. An adherent grayish pseudomembrane may develop on the tonsils, with significant "bull neck" cervical edema and lymphadenopathy.

Cancrum oris or noma pudenda is a progressive polymicrobial infection of the face that leads to destruction and ulceration, most commonly in severely malnourished children.

In Old World cutaneous leishmaniasis, a papule first forms at the site of a sandfly bite. Next, a well-defined ulcer with surrounding erythema, crusting and variable pyoderma is usually noted. The "oriental sore" may also exhibit undermined ulcer edges that have been confused for smaller lesions of pyoderma gangrenosum. Most lesions heal with minimal scarring, atrophy or depigmentation in a self-limited fashion over 6–24 months. The lesions may vary wildly in size and depth, as smaller satellite lesions may coalesce with the primary ulcer. Ulcers may be "wet" or "dry." Leishmanial lesions are not painful. Hyperkeratotic variants occur. In diffuse cutaneous leishmaniasis (DCL), the initial papule rarely ulcerates, but rather, several other papules appear with minimal erythema or pigmentation outwardly spreading from the initial site. As lesions evolve, they may become deeper and nodular. A chronic form of cutaneous disease called leishmania recidivans causes sarcoidal-appearing lesions, with outwardly enlarging dermal induration and central clearance. If pressed against a glass slide, the erythematous to violaceous coloration and dusky nature of the lesion may blanche into an "apple-green" appearance, reflecting the presence of histiocytes and other chronic inflammatory cells in tissue. Post-kala-azar dermal leishmaniasis (PKDL) refers to diffuse nodular involvement that occurs following resolution of visceral leishmaniasis (kala-azar). Multiple primary morphologies may be noted, including diffuse macules, papules and nodules.

Cutaneous New World leishmaniasis appears similar to the Old World variant. A specific New World mucocutaneous manifestation of *L. braziliensis* is termed espundia. Following resolution of a primary skin lesion, leishmania infection can relapse, specifically involving oro-naso-mucosal membranes, including the nasal septum, pharynx, larynx and buccal mucosa. Untreated, mucocutaneous leishmaniasis can be disfiguring and can lead to central destruction of the face.

Rhinosporidiosis may rarely be confused with mucosal leishmania. The physical examination is notable for pedunculated polyps, often arising from nasal mucosa and conjunctiva, but also may be found in the genitals. Rarely, cutaneous, non-mucosal disease is documented.

SUBCUTANEOUS MYCOSES

Direct inoculation of a fungus into the skin, often by a splinter or other trauma, may result in a subcutaneous mycosis. Clinically, subcutaneous mycoses result in an ulcer or verrucous plaque. The most common types are sporotrichosis, mycetoma, chromoblastomycosis, phaeohyphomycosis and lobomycosis. Treatment can be difficult and may require long courses of oral antifungals, cryotherapy or surgical excision, alone or in combination.

Sporotrichosis is caused by *Sporothrix schenckii* and follows direct inoculation, classically involving thorns or cats' claws. Lymphangitic spread is common. This type of sporotrichoid spread is also seen in atypical mycobacteriosis, leishmaniasis and nocardiosis, and differs from regional lymphadenopathy.

Chromoblastomycosis usually manifests as a classic verrucous plaque. Central atrophy with scarring may also be seen. Chromoblastomycosis is due to dematiaceous (melanin-producing) fungi, often *Fonsecaea pedrosoi*, and most commonly involves the lower extremities of individuals involved in soil-related occupations.

Phaeohyphomycosis can manifest in a number of ways, most commonly as black eschars with scalloped, erythematous borders. Subcutaneous abscesses should be excised.

Lobomycosis due to *Lacazia loboi* is reported in areas of Latin America, and manifests as asymptomatic, smooth-surfaced, keloidal lesions, often on the ear.

Mycetoma, or Madura foot, is caused by bacteria (actinomycetoma) or fungi (eumycetoma). The clinical presentation is one of an asymptomatic, subcutaneous swelling with sinus tracts that discharge "granules" or "grains." Granules from bacteria tend to be lighter in color, whereas granules from fungi tend to be dark. Radiologic imaging should be performed as bone involvement is common.

Zygomycoses are divided into two types – the opportunistic type typified by mucormycosis that affects hosts immunosuppressed by diseases other than AIDS, such as diabetes, and entomophthoromycosis that affects immunocompetent hosts living in the tropics. Mucormycosis commonly presents around the nose, forming black necrotic tissue and involving the orbit and brain, while entomophthoromycosis forms a solitary, painless nodule or slowly expansile mass, most commonly on an extremity.

DEEP MYCOSES

Aside from subcutaneous mycoses, deep cutaneous fungal infections often result from systemic infection. The cutaneous presentations are protean. Sometimes, cutaneous infection causes erythema nodosum, sterile, tender erythematous nodules on the shin which have a favorable prognosis. Other times, there is a nonspecific presentation such as a morbilliform eruption. Accompanying signs and symptoms of fever, gastrointestinal upset and emaciation aid in the diagnosis of a systemic infection.

Histoplasmosis may present with mucocutaneous ulcerations and granulomas. Care must be taken not to misdiagnose as sarcoidosis. Children sometimes present with purpura, fever, fatigue and gastrointestinal symptoms. Blastomycosis is endemic in North America and often affects the bone, particularly ribs and vertebrae along with the skin. The cutaneous lesions are multiple, growing slowly, forming verrucous and granulomatous lesions with thick crust overlying granulation tissue and sometimes central white scars. Paracoccidioidomycosis is endemic in Latin America. It may present with mucocutaneous disease, most commonly of the gingiva, with small papules and ulcerations. The disease is fifteen times more common in men than in women. Penicilliosis is endemic in Southeast Asia, sometimes causing umbilicated papules or oral lesions. Cryptococcus has a particular affinity for the central nervous system and skin.

In patients with AIDS, coccidioidomycosis, histoplasmosis, penicilliosis and molluscum contagiosum may all appear as umbilicated vesicles, and be indistinguishable on clinical examination. Primary cutaneous lesions may present with verrucous papules or ulcers similar to subcutaneous mycoses.

PAINLESS PAPULES

Molluscum contagiosum manifests as umbilicated papules that can coalesce into plaques. Clinicians may confuse the diagnosis with herpetic disease, but relatively simple bedside maneuvers can assist in diagnosis. Lancing lesions of molluscum leads to extravasation of a "white cheesy material" which can be stained with hematoxylin and eosin, revealing eosinophilic globules. In the patient with unknown HIV status, confluent facial molluscum contagiosum is a reason to test for HIV. Therapy is often via destruction with curettage or cryotherapy, or with reconstitution of the immune system in those with deficiencies.

PAINFUL PAPULES/URTICARIA

Infestation of skin with fly larvae is called myiasis. A large, tender, cyst-like structure or papule may be noted with surrounding erythema, a central punctum and occasional suppuration. Patients usually report movement within the lesions. Lesions may be multiple. New World myiasis is caused by the botfly; Old World disease is most commonly caused by the tumbu fly. Treatment involves asphyxiating the larvae, usually via application of an occlusive dressing or substance, followed by larval extrusion. Surgical excision may sometimes be required. Bacterial suprainfection can occur.

Tungiasis (also called jiggers) is caused by *Tunga penetrans*, the sand flea. The female flea burrows into skin, usually on the feet, but can involve any exposed skin area, creating a callus-like papule, often with some hyperpigmentation. The terminus of the flea is often visible in the center of the lesion. Pain is usually present. Treatment involves mechanical removal.

Many insect bites and plant dermatitides occur in the tropics. The physical examination is often helpful at suggesting the diagnosis. Insect bites may result in erythematous papules of variable size and distribution. Urticarial-like erythema is seen around lesions, at times enlarging far over 10 cm in diameter. A number of beetles, millipedes and centipedes can cause a severe contact dermatitis. Plant dermatitides may manifest in both acute and chronic forms, depending on the repetitive nature of contact. Whereas contact dermatitis is the most common presentation, characterized by vesicles on an erythematous base in a linear or geographic distribution, chronic disease may present as eczematous dermatitis. Occupational disease, as seen in florists or gardeners, can present as atopic dermatitis of the hands, with severe dryness, scaling, cracking, erythema, and even fibrotic-like constriction in palmar function.

PRURITUS AND PAPULES

Schistosomal cercarial dermatitis can occur at the site of skin penetration with the infectious form of *Schistosoma* spp. following water exposure. Nonhuman *Schistosome* spp., especially avian species, can cause prominent dermatitis that may manifest as multiple, highly pruritic, erythematous papules. Distribution is of skin exposed to infectious water. Seabather's eruption can cause similar lesions but is caused by larval forms of coelenterates (jelly fish), but distribution usually reflects a "bathing suit" distribution, since the larvae become entrapped by clothing. Pediculosis (or lice) is caused by louse infestation. Different lice are responsible for each form of human involvement: corporis (body), capitis (head) and pubis (genitals). Louse infestation can result in pruritus and excoriations. The body louse (*Pediculus humanus corporis*) takes a daily blood meal, but lives in clothing. It is transmitted from person to person, usually in overcrowded and impoverished conditions, and during periods of war and social unrest. The head louse (*Pediculus humanus capitis*) is also transmitted from person to person. It is particularly common in school-aged children. Pubic lice (*Phthirus pubis*) are spread by sexual contact, creating intense pruritus in the groin, commonly known as "crabs".

Lice can be seen adherent to pubic hair. Symptoms are regional, although lice and nits may occasionally be seen on eyelashes.

Scabies is an important infestation caused by *Sarcoptes scabei* mites; it is often misdiagnosed. The organism burrows superficially, just underneath the stratum corneum. It does not penetrate the skin, and as such it is not a true infection. Contrary to common belief, dermatitis does not occur immediately following infestation. Dermatitis occurs as a hypersensitivity reaction created by the mite, its eggs or its excrement, termed scybala. Clinical findings vary according to the immune status of the host. Immunocompetent patients suffer from extreme pruritus. Close inspection reveals erythematous papules or nodules, with superficial crusting and excoriation, and there is a particular predilection for involvement of genital, intertriginous and acral skin (Fig. 8.4). In immunosuppressed hosts, the infirm, or institutionalized patients, a functionally debilitating pruritic dermatosis can occur. There is a specific association of severe scabies and infection with HTLV-1. In these severe cases, patients present with disseminated eczematous dermatitis, nodules and, occasionally, generalized urticaria. Late findings include hyperpigmentation, lichenification and psoriatic-like lesions. Also denoted Norwegian or crusted scabies, this diffuse involvement may progress to wart-like lesions. In the elderly, lesions may appear bullous, often mimicking bullous pemphigoid. In the newborn, lesions may be vesicular, and the disease may present as failure to thrive. Pustular diseases of the newborn, including acropustulosis and neonatal acne, may be considered, but the disseminated nature of the disease, examination of the vesicular fluid, as well as a diagnostic examination of a scraping following application of mineral oil to identify mites or their products, can quickly aid in making the correct diagnosis. Topical treatments for limited disease include permethrin 5% cream, lindane, crotamiton 10% cream, sulfur, malathion and ivermectin lotion. Crusted or nodular scabies and disease in the immunosuppressed often require systemic ivermectin at 200 mcg/kg. The entire family, including pets, should be treated, and clothes, bedding, and frequently used fomites should be immediately washed in warm water. A second treatment a week after is usually recommended. Oral antipruritics may be needed.

Prurigo nodularis manifests as hyperkeratotic nodules, linear excoriations and lichenification, particularly over areas that the patient can reach. In this condition, patients may experience diffuse or focal pruritus. Rather than scratching, patients tend to "pick", creating "picker nodules". Therapy is with topical or injectable steroids or phototherapy. Nodules may also raise concern for scabies, particularly in the patient with severe pruritus. It is important to consider the diagnosis of papular eruption of HIV, where patients develop erythematous papules with urticarial-type erythema. Chronic cases may resemble prurigo nodularis. Recent reports have shown that the pathology of these lesions may mimic insect bites. Interestingly, symptoms as well as response to therapy may correspond with the CD4 count in HIV-infected individuals. Finally, when these papules show a necrotic center, the patient is less pruritic, and the diagnosis of papulonecrotic tuberculosis needs to be considered. Acne-like nodules and papules in a sun-exposed distribution should raise suspicion for eosinophilic folliculitis which may manifest during the immune reconstitution syndrome, but may also suggest viral resistance, worsening CD4 counts, or untreated infection altogether.

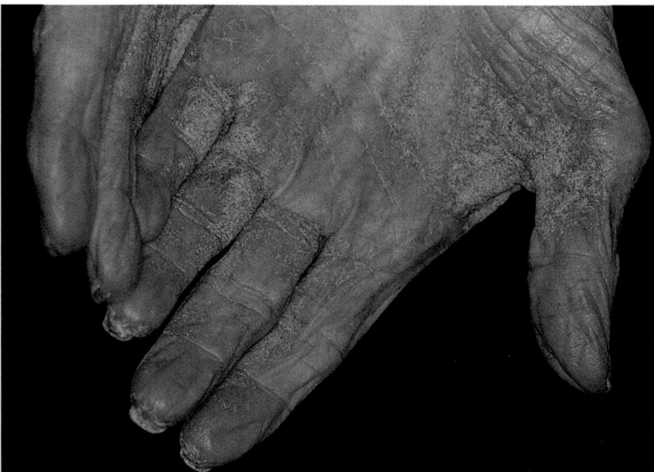

FIGURE 8.4 Scabies. Scabies incognito in which an elderly patient with a neuropathy had a nonspecific, asymptomatic hand "rash" that proved to be due to crusted scabies.

PRURITUS WITHOUT PRIMARY SKIN LESIONS

In patients who have severe pruritus and minimal primary skin manifestations, it is important to evaluate for underlying causes. The differential diagnosis includes obstructive liver disease, chronic hepatitis, uremia, hypo- and hyperthyroidism, hematopoietic diseases, polycythemia vera, lymphoma, leukemia, myeloma, internal malignancies, intestinal parasites, carcinoid, multiple sclerosis, AIDS, medications and neuropsychiatric diseases, especially anorexia nervosa. In a patient presenting with idiopathic pruritus, a thorough physical examination is warranted, along with the following laboratory tests: complete blood count with differential, thyroid-stimulating hormone, liver function tests, renal panel, hepatitis serologies, HIV antibody, urinalysis, stool guaiac, chest x-ray, stool for ova and parasites, and possibly serum protein electrophoresis. While topical steroids can often provide relief for patients who itch due to pruritic skin disorders, if there is an internal cause, the pruritus is often recalcitrant to topical treatments, and a search for correcting the underlying cause becomes even more essential.

HYPOPIGMENTATION/ DEPIGMENTATION

Vitiligo is a common autoimmune disease in the tropics. Caused by selective melanocyte destruction, patients present with depigmented patches that can involve all cutaneous surfaces and hair. Wood's light examination may be useful in distinguishing complete depigmentation from hypopigmented skin, particularly if post-inflammatory hypopigmentation resulting from prior dermatologic disease is suspected. Seborrheic dermatitis, pityriasis alba, early tinea infections and secondary syphilis may cause such hypopigmentation in skin. It is important to highlight that hypopigmentation may also be seen in so-called "trichrome" vitiligo, where a transition from normal skin to hypopigmented and then depigmented skin is noted. Unfortunately, the disease is often colloquially confused for leprosy, particularly in Southeast Asia, and affected patients can be subject to discrimination. Attention must also be paid to other systemic autoimmune diseases that may include anemia and thyroid disease.

MORBILLIFORM EXANTHEMS

Individuals with measles develop a morbilliform exanthem, usually in the setting of fever and coryza. For the purpose of this discussion, such an exanthem describes erythematous, blanchable macules, patches, papules, and occasionally even plaques, on a hyperemic background. Koplik spots are almost pathognomonic, and manifest in the mouth as white papules with surrounding erythema of sand-grain-like texture. They often precede the rash by 1–2 days. The exanthem starts in the forehead and neck, and then generalizes to the trunk and extremities. Clinical symptoms such as fever, malaise and coryza are often present. Cases may be difficult to correctly diagnose in those who have previously been vaccinated and present with atypical measles. Unlike its common form, patients with atypical measles lack coryza and Koplik spots, but may present with high fever, pneumonia, hepatitis, edema and paresthesias. In this case, skin lesions may be vesicular, hemorrhagic and urticarial. Clinical prodromes in addition to a morbilliform exanthem may indicate the presence of other viral infections.

Human monocytotropic ehrlichiosis (HME), caused by *Ehrlichia chaffeensis*, human granulocytotropic anaplasmosis (HGA), caused by *Anaplasma phagocytophilium*, and *Ehrlichiosis ewingii* infection lead to nonspecific symptoms such as fever, chills, headaches and leukopenia. A macular and papular skin eruption on the trunk and extremities is more common in pediatric patients with these infections than in adults. The cutaneous manifestations often occur after other systemic symptoms arise.

Trench fever, caused by *Bartonella quintana*, gives rise to a nonspecific morbilliform eruption of the trunk, along with systemic symptoms.

PAPULOSQUAMOUS AND ECZEMATOID LESIONS

Papulosquamous lesions are rashes that are both raised and have scale, such as psoriasis and tinea corporis (Table 8-1). In tineasis, the dermatophytes *Microsporum*, *Trichophyton* and *Epidermophyton* infect keratinized tissue. Characteristically, they appear as erythematous, annular plaques, with serpiginous borders, with scale at the leading edge, and are named based on the location of involvement: tinea capitis – scalp; tinea corporis – body; tinea faciei – face; tinea cruris – groin; tinea pedis – feet; tinea manuum – hand; tinea barbae – beard; tinea unguium – nails. Diagnosis can be confirmed by performing a scraping of the scale and applying one or two drops of potassium hydroxide (KOH) and visualizing the hyphal structures under 10× magnification. The differential diagnosis includes other papulosquamous or scaly raised lesions (see Table 8-1). For limited disease, topical antifungals are usually effective, except for tinea capitis and onychomycosis, which often require oral antifungal medications. As recurrence is common, multiple courses of therapy are often required.

Tinea capitis causes circular, scaly patches on the scalp with alopecia and black dots caused by breakage of the hair shaft. Some causative species such as *Microsporum audouinii* fluoresce on Wood's lamp examination. Favus is a particular type of tinea capitis which causes yellow, concave cup-shaped crusts on the scalp around loose hairs and is caused by *T. schoenleinii*. There is a characteristic mousy odor which aids in the diagnosis. KOH staining of an affected hair shows air bubbles in the shaft.

Tinea imbricata is a rare form of tinea corporis due to *Trichophyton concentricum* that causes concentric, polycyclic, scaly rings over the body. This can sometimes be confused with erythema gyratum repens which is associated with an underlying malignancy. However, a KOH stain will help differentiate these two diseases.

TABLE 8-1 Differential Diagnosis of Papulosquamous Lesions

Uniform scale	Annular scale
Psoriasis	Tinea types
Pityriasis rubra pilaris	Pityriasis rosea
Mycosis fungoides	Porokeratosis
Subacute lupus	Secondary syphilis
Drug eruption	Psoriasis
Pityriasis lichenoides chronica	Erythema annulare centrifugum
Seborrheic dermatitis	Subacute lupus
Lichen planus	
Secondary syphilis	
Tinea versicolor	
Confluent and reticulated papillomatosis	

Nondermatophyte superficial mycosis includes tinea versicolor, a chronic mildly pruritic scaly discoloration of the upper trunk, arms and neck caused by *Malassezia* spp. On KOH scraping, a characteristic "spaghetti and meatball" pattern is seen, corresponding to the short thick hyphae and spores. Even after treatment and cure, the hypopigmentation may persist for months.

Tinea nigra, caused by *Hortaea werneckii* or *Stenella araguat*, is found primarily in Africa, Asia, the Caribbean and Latin America. Clinically, it causes a solitary, asymptomatic, light brown macule, often on the palm, that darkens and grows. Though confused with melanoma, this lesion will scrape off, and can be confirmed with KOH staining. Topical azoles or keratolytics can be used for treatment.

Black piedra, caused by the astromycete *Piedraia hortae*, is found primarily in Africa, Asia and Latin America. It causes black, hard, fixed nodules attached to the hair. White piedra is most commonly caused by *Trichosporon beigelii*, and manifests as yellow or beige soft sheaths coating hair shafts. Treatment for black and white piedra consists of a short haircut, although antifungals can also be used.

Candida is a commensal inhabitant of the gastrointestinal and genitourinary tracts, but is also a pathogen which grows during conditions of warmth, moisture and increased pH. Thrush, or oral candidiasis, manifests as grayish-white plaques in the mouth that scrape off. Perlèche is candida-associated erythematous scaling at the angles of the oral commissure that can mimic some nutritional deficiencies. Candidiasis often affects the perianal region, inguinal folds and inframammary areas, and manifests as beefy red erythema with satellite lesions and occasional pustules. Antibiotics and immunosuppression predispose to candidiasis.

M. leprae usually affects skin on the extremities, which is cooler in temperature, while sparing warmer areas of the body, including the axilla and scalp. There is a wide range of disease, from the limited tuberculoid type to the diffuse lepromatous type of leprosy (Hansen's disease). In tuberculoid leprosy, there are well-demarcated solitary, hypopigmented plaques with raised borders and slight scale. The hypoesthesia, absence of hair and lack of sweating within the lesions is very characteristic. In lepromatous leprosy, owing to an absence of cell-mediated immunity, there are numerous small hypopigmented or erythematous macules that are ill-defined. Loss of the lateral eyebrow, leonine facies, madarosis, glove-and-stocking neuropathy, claw-finger and toe deformities are late manifestations. Borderline lesions exist between the continuum of tuberculoid and lepromatous leprosy.

Other diseases that cause hypopigmentation include pityriasis alba, post-inflammatory hypopigmentation and tinea versicolor. Tinea versicolor also causes a hypopigmented scaly thin plaque (Fig. 8.5). A Wood's lamp can be helpful in demonstrating that the lesions in leprosy and tinea are hypopigmented and not depigmented as in vitiligo. The differential diagnosis also includes papulosquamous disorders such as cutaneous T-cell lymphoma, pityriasis rosea, para-psoriasis, lupus erythematosus, sarcoidosis and secondary syphilis.

Lyme disease is caused by *Borrelia burgdorferi*, transmitted by *Ixodes* hard ticks. Erythema chronicum migrans (ECM) manifests as a bull's-eye lesion of a gradually expanding, non-scaly redness around the initial tick bite. Headache, stiff neck, myalgia and arthralgias may accompany the characteristic rash. Acrodermatitis chronica atrophicans, lymphocytoma and lichen sclerosus have all been associated with chronic Lyme disease.

Syphilis, caused by *Treponema pallidum*, can be divided into three main stages. During primary syphilis, a painless round, indurated chancre forms, which may form on extragenital sites, such as within the oral cavity, in addition to the genitalia. Secondary syphilis may manifest as a nonspecific maculopapular or, less commonly, a papulosquamous eruption, classically with involvement of the palms and soles.

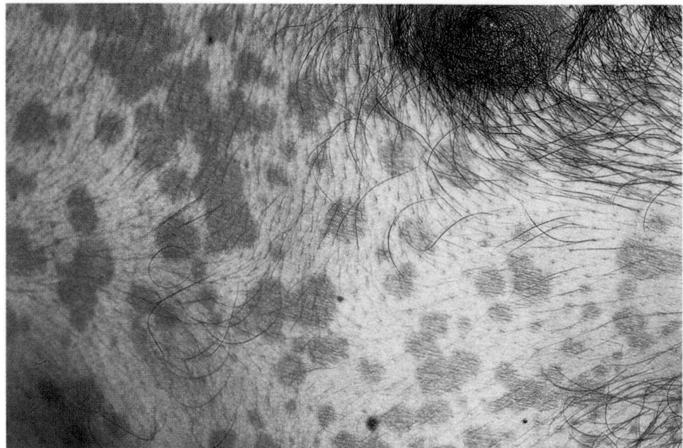

FIGURE 8.5 Tinea versicolor. This chronic disease is characterized by macules and thin patches and plaques with subtle scale. The term versicolor refers to the changing coloration of lesions, often appearing lighter than surrounding tan skin in the summer, but darker than sun-protected skin during colder months.

Tertiary, late-stage syphilis may manifest as noduloulcerative lesions consisting of reddish-brown firm nodules.

HTLV-1 infection may be associated with a number of dermatologic conditions. HTLV-1 infection is most frequently recognized in the Caribbean, and areas of Asia and Latin America, and in the latter is most frequently reported among Amerindian populations. Patients may present with recalcitrant eczematoid dermatitis, seborrheic dermatitis and blepharitis. The diagnosis is usually made after several attempts at controlling the eruption with topical steroids or immunomodulators. In adults, dermatologic disease may be a presenting manifestation of adult T-cell leukemia. Affected patients present with disseminated papules that coalesce into plaques and nodules, with striking infiltrative morphology. Patients also have systemic symptoms and the systemic evidence of acute T-cell leukemia, including hepatosplenomegaly, systemic lymphadenopathy and central nervous system involvement. Affected patients will exhibit circulating leukemic cells, termed "flower cells" or "ATL cells". The disease is often fatal, but smoldering forms, chronic disease and lymphoma-type disease have also been reported.

ERYTHRODERMA

Correctly diagnosing the cause of diffuse erythroderma or whole-body erythema presents a unique challenge to the physician. These patients may present with marked systemic symptoms, and can suffer severe morbidity from lack of epidermal barrier function, including dehydration, infection and severe pain. Ectropion may be seen. Diffuse erythema can lead to severe imbalances of electrolytes and minerals, and hypocalcemic tetany can occur. As the eruption improves, generalized exfoliation is the norm. The evaluation of patients with erythroderma often requires histopathologic evaluation, to exclude full-thickness epidermal necrosis, including toxic epidermal necrolysis (TEN). TEN is commonly caused by a drug, but infectious etiologies have also been implicated, particularly mycoplasma and herpetic infections.

Erythroderma may be caused by severe drug reactions. The presence of small, superficial pustules may indicate exanthematous generalized pustular dermatosis (AGEP), most commonly caused by β-lactam and cephalosporin antibiotics. Patients present with fever and can have peripheral blood leukocytosis, commonly prompting evaluation for an infectious disease. A similar finding may be noted in pustular psoriasis, which may occur in patients with no prior history of psoriasis. Though nail findings may be helpful in those with prior history, such findings may not be seen in those with an acute, first episode. Patients appear ill and are often hospitalized. Cultures of the pustules

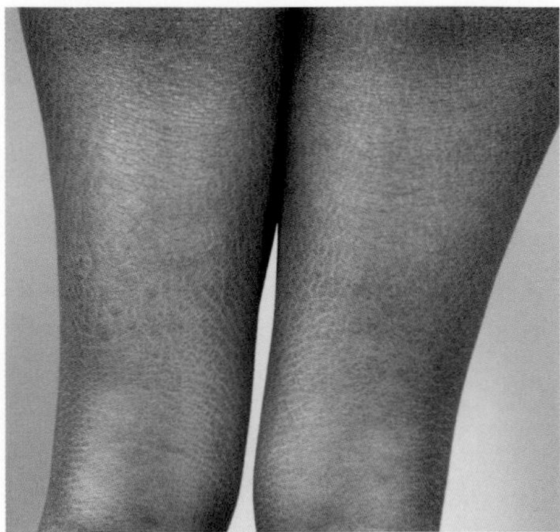

FIGURE 8.6 Ichthyosis. Note the fine white scales in the lower extremities.

fail to indicate a superficial cutaneous infection, though ectopic infection such as streptococcal pharyngitis may precipitate an attack. Though oral steroids may improve symptoms, upon withdrawal, disease can re-flare.

Pityriasis rubra pilaris, a close relative of psoriasis, may also be the cause of erythroderma. Patients often have conspicuous "islands of sparing", where seemingly normal skin is noted among erythrodermic skin. Hyperlinearity may be seen in palms and soles, in addition to a salmon-colored, sand-papered type of scale with sharp demarcation along transgrediens lines (the line boundary between cutaneous skin and the sole of the foot, for instance).

Other important diagnoses to consider include atopic dermatitis, viral exanthems, cutaneous T-cell lymphoma, which in the leukemic phase is termed Sézary syndrome, the staphylococcal skin scalded syndrome, as well as toxic shock syndrome. In HIV-positive individuals or those with other immunosuppressing disorders, seborrheic dermatitis may lead to erythroderma. Uncommonly, systemic malignancies such as colon and lung carcinoma, as well as lymphoma and leukemia, can also be culprits. In those who have had a bone marrow transplant, erythroderma may be a result of graft-versus-host disease. Red man syndrome indicates a state of erythroderma where no clear culprit can be ascertained.

ICTHYOSIS

Fish-like scaling on cutaneous surfaces (ichthyosis) may be seen in a variety of conditions, both congenital and acquired. Disease may range from limited and asymptomatic, to disseminated and life-threatening. Most commonly, ichthyosis vulgaris is inherited in an autosomal dominant fashion, and develops as scaling over relatively uninflamed skin. Usually, antecubital fossae are spared. Scales may become hyperpigmented and feel tightly adherent to underlying skin (Fig. 8.6). It may be coincident with atopic dermatitis or its associated findings, such as the follicularly based, spiny, hyperkeratotic papules of keratosis pilaris over the upper extremities and thighs. Though ichthyosis may be the presenting sign of a lymphoma, it is found most commonly in the general population and may go unnoticed. Congenital ichthyoses include lamellar disease, which is inherited in an autosomal recessive pattern. Ectropion and alopecia may be a distinguishing feature. The scale is often likened to "reptile skin". Though it can be seen in adults, patients readily exhibit disease in their early years, even at birth. X-linked ichthyosis presents as adherent fish-like scaling, usually hyperpigmented and giving an impression of "dirty skin".

SERPIGINOUS LESIONS

Cutaneous larva migrans is caused by zoonotic hookworms. Also referred to as "creeping eruption", the primary lesion is a serpiginous, slightly swollen, erythematous lesion that may induce local urticaria

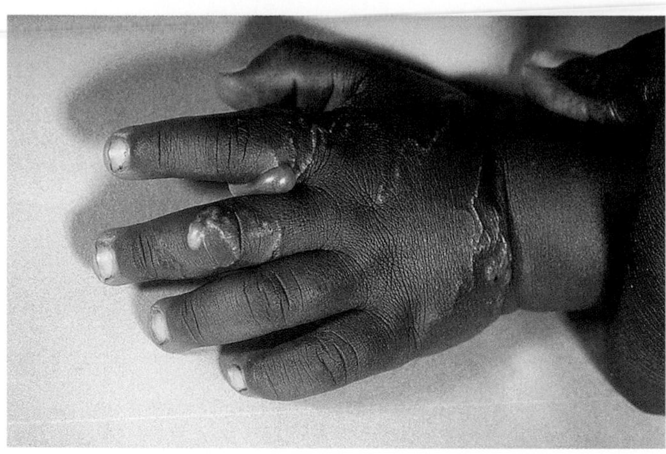

FIGURE 8.7 Cutaneous larva migrans. The key to the diagnosis is to identify a serpiginous lesion that is not static. The patient will report intense pruritus and a changing lesion, both in shape and location.

(Fig. 8.7). Infection is acquired cutaneously, most often from dog or cat hookworms (*Ancylostoma braziliense*). Interestingly, the advancing edge of the lesion does not accurately represent the body of the hookworm, bur rather the inflammatory reaction that trails it. Usually, the hookworm has advanced beyond the visible serpiginous border, so destructive therapies such as cryotherapy applied to the advancing edge may miss the hookworm altogether. If such treatments are performed, therapy should aim about 1 cm ahead of the advancing edge. Notably, the hookworms causing cutaneous larva migrans lack collagenase and are therefore restricted to the squamous epithelium in skin and are only rarely found in the dermis due to the presence of collagen IV in the basement membrane separating dermis from epidermis. This is in contrast to larva currens, which represents cutaneous transit of infective strongyloides larvae before entering the systemic circulation. Disseminated or hyperinfectious strongyloidiasis may be associated with sepsis, petechiae and purpura fulminans.

TABLE 8-2 Nutritional Deficiencies: Symptoms and Physical Examination Findings

Marasmus	<60% of ideal body weight, "monkey" facies, emaciation, no edema
Kwashiorkor	Protein deficiency, normal caloric intake, edema, "flag" sign of hair, potbelly, scaly skin, abnormal pigmentation
Essential fatty acids	Periorificial dermatosis, lighter hair, alopecia
Vitamin A	Phrynoderma "toad" skin, keratomalacia, Bitot's spots, xerophthalmia
Thiamin (B1)	Beriberi, polyneuropathy, Wernicke–Korsakoff encephalopathy
Riboflavin (B2)	Perlèche, genital dermatitis, photophobia
Niacin (B3)	Pellagra: dermatitis, Casal's necklace, seborrheic dermatitis, gastrointestinal symptoms, dementia
Pyridoxine (B6)	Seborrheic dermatitis, glossitis, atrophic glossitis
Cyanocobalamin (B12)	Glossitis, symmetric hyperpigmentation, atrophic glossitis
Vitamin C	"Scurvy," perifollicular petechiae, keratotic plugs, corkscrew hairs, gingivitis
Vitamin K	Purpura, hemorrhage
Iron	Koilonychia, glossitis, cheilitis, telogen effluvium, dysphagia
Biotin	Alopecia, brittle nails, periorificial dermatitis
Zinc	Acrodermatitis enteropathica, hypopigmentation, alopecia

EDEMA

Lymphatic filariasis is associated with lymphangitis, and recurrent and worsening episodes of lymphedema. Lymphedema is due to impedance in lymphatic flow, or outright lymphatic channel destruction. Lichenification, fissuring and scaling can be seen in longstanding infections. End-stage disease can be mistaken for elephantiasis verrucosa nostra from chronic stasis dermatitis, as well as podoconiosis, the latter caused by lymphatic obstruction secondary to silica-laden volcanic ash. Unilateral chronic extremity edema should prompt consideration of filariasis or a unilateral obstructing mass in the draining lymph nodes. Other important clues to the diagnosis of lymphatic filariasis include testicular hydrocele and lymphadenopathy.

Loiasis is a filarial infection in which the adult *Loa loa* worm migrates in subcutaneous tissue and across the conjunctiva ("eye worm"). Localized edema from a hypersensitivity reaction can occur over joints and bony prominences as the worm passes, so-called Calabar swellings. Peripheral eosinophilia is prominent. Compared to lymphatic filariasis, loaiasis-associated edema is transient and migratory.

Onchocerca volvulus, the causative organism of onchocerciasis (river blindness), is another filarial infection that often first manifests in the skin. Microfilariae are produced by adult worms that reside in subcutaneous nodules, so-called onchocermata. Microfilariae migrate freely through subcutaneous and ocular structures. Dying microfilariae provoke an intense inflammatory response, leading to pruritus and excoriations, and a diffuse papular dermatitis. Papules and plaques can be seen with overlying lichenified streaks indicating chronic scratching and rubbing by afflicted patients. Scabetic infection may enter the differential diagnosis, but linear burrows along interdigital web spaces, genital involvement, and evidence of the causative mite on a mineral oil preparation can usually readily diagnose the latter condition. Of note, hyperpigmentation is not a distinguishing feature in differentiating among these diseases, as chronic infection in both may lead to atopic dermatitis-like disease and patchy hypo/hyperpigmentation. Plate-like ichthyosis over leathery skin with hypo/hyperpigmentation, commonly referred to as leopard skin, would point to the diagnosis of chronic onchocerciasis. Loss of elasticity of skin can lead to "hanging groin".

Trichinosis can also be the cause of edema, though in this case, periorbital, nondependent edema is most commonly noted. Other dermatologic findings may include a hypersensitivity-like petechial rash, xerosis and subconjunctival hemorrhage.

American trypanosomiasis can be difficult to diagnose acutely given its nonspecific systemic and dermatologic manifestations. Distinguishing features of acute disease include the so-called "chagoma", where the protozoal inoculum causes subcutaneous swelling, induration and erythema accompanied by local lymphadenopathy. When the eye is the portal of entry, Romaña's sign may develop, comprised of unilateral, painless, periorbital edema and conjunctival swelling. African trypanosomiasis also includes skin manifestations. A chancre can develop at the site of a bite from an infecting tsetse fly. The lesion can rapidly enlarge and ulcerate, and can be associated with local lymphadenopathy. In East African trypanosomiasis, caused by *T. rhodesiense*, high fever and toxemia are common, and patients often present for clinical attention. A diffuse macular rash may also be present. In West African trypanosomiasis, caused by *T. gambiense*, initial skin involvement may be mild, and patients often only come to clinical attention in the late stages of the disease when the central nervous system is involved. Dracunculiasis can also be associated with swelling and pain in an extremity, often the legs. An acral nodule will progress to a blister on the affected limb, and upon immersion in water, part of the female worm will extrude through the ruptured blister.

CACHEXIA – NUTRITIONAL DEFICIENCIES

Signs to alert the physician that a patient may have a nutritional disorder include: cachexia, abnormal fat distribution, edema, glossitis of the tongue, seborrheic dermatitis, abnormalities in hair/nails, cheilitis and periorificial dermatitis. For specific clinical manifestations of nutritional deficiencies, see Table 8-2 and corresponding chapters.

REFERENCES

Ameen M. Chromoblastomycosis: clinical presentation and management. Clin Exp Dermatol 2009 Dec;34(8):849–54. Epub 2009 Jul 2.

Bonifaz A, Gómez-Daza F, Paredes V, Ponce RM. Tinea versicolor, tinea nigra, white piedra, and black piedra. Clin Dermatol 2010 Mar 4;28(2):140–5.

Cestari TF, Pessato S, Ramos-e-Silva M. Tungiasis and myiasis. Clin Dermatol 2007 Mar–Apr;25(2):158–64.

Haddad V Jr, Lupi O, Lonza JP, Tyring SK. Tropical dermatology: marine and aquatic dermatology. J Am Acad Dermatol 2009 Nov;61(5):733–50.

Handog EB, Gabriel TG, Pineda RT. Management of cutaneous tuberculosis. Dermatol Ther 2008 May–Jun;21(3):154–61.

Lupi O, Tyring SK. Tropical dermatology: viral tropical diseases. J Am Acad Dermatol 2003 Dec;49(6):979–1000.

Lupi O, Tyring SK, McGinnis MR. Tropical dermatology: fungal tropical diseases. J Am Acad Dermatol 2005 Dec;53(6):931–51.

Lupi O, Madkan V, Tyring SK. Tropical dermatology: bacterial tropical diseases. J Am Acad Dermatol 2006 Apr;54(4):559–78.

Naafs B, Padovese V. Rural dermatology in the tropics. Clin Dermatol 2009 May–Jun;27(3):252–70.

Ramos-e-Silva M, Rebello PF. Leprosy. Recognition and treatment. Am J Clin Dermatol 2001;2(4):203–11.

Sampaio SA, Rivitti EA, Aoki V, Diaz LA. Brazilian pemphigus foliaceus, endemic pemphigus foliaceus, or fogo selvagem (wild fire). Dermatol Clin 1994 Oct;12(4):765–76.

Welsh O, Vera-Cabrera L, Salinas-Carmona MC. Mycetoma. Clin Dermatol 2007 Mar–Apr;25(2):195–202.

Zeegelaar JE, Faber WR. Imported tropical infectious ulcers in travelers. Am J Clin Dermatol 2008;9(4):219–32.

Ophthalmological Diseases 9

Hugh R Taylor, Angus W Turner

Key features

- Disease burden:
  - Worldwide, 161 million people are blind or visually impaired
  - An additional 153 million have uncorrected refractive error
- Unique features in tropics – increased prevalence of:
  - Blinding infections, e.g. filariasis and corneal ulcers secondary to fungal infections
  - Ocular trauma
  - Acute glaucoma (Asian countries)
- Resource-poor countries:
  - Ocular sequelae of malnutrition, e.g. vitamin deficiency
  - Late presentation of disease, e.g. diabetic eye disease and glaucoma
- Industrialized countries:
  - Baseline of unavoidable blindness
  - Chronic conditions affecting elderly
  - Screening programs to detect asymptomatic disease
  - Expensive treatments for glaucoma and macular degeneration

INTRODUCTION

Globally, blindness remains one of the main causes of disability affecting humans. More than 161 million people are blind or vision-impaired due to eye diseases such as cataract, diabetic retinopathy, glaucoma, trachoma and macular degeneration (Fig. 9.1) [1]. An extra 153 million people are vision-impaired from uncorrected refractive error (Table 9-1) [2].

Many of the ocular conditions affecting people in tropical countries are preventable or treatable (see "Key features" box). Trained field workers are crucial for the control of blinding infections, malnutrition and filariasis; for primary care of simple ocular trauma and acute glaucoma; and for the recognition and referral of cases of chronic glaucoma, cataract and the more complicated diseases that require surgery.

The most important steps in assessing a patient's problem involve taking a careful and appropriate history and performing a proper examination. It is important to elicit a history of the onset, duration and characteristics of the presenting complaint, together with a review of the patient's general health and individual and family history. Specific information concerning vision – such as blurring, flashes or floaters, double vision, visual field loss and night blindness – should be sought, and questions about ocular discharge, pain and discomfort should be asked.

A basic part of the ophthalmic examination is the assessment of visual acuity, which is traditionally measured with a letter test chart, placed 6 meters away from the patient. The acuity of small children can be assessed by determining their ability to fixate upon and follow a target, such as a light, evaluating one eye at a time while the other eye is covered. Children will also often object to covering of the normal eye but not a poorly seeing eye. Picture charts are sometimes used for pre-literate children. An E chart is also used for illiterate adults, where the direction of the "tumbling E" of diminishing sizes is identified.

Simple observation of the eye will often give much information, especially in terms of the presence and site of infection or trauma (Fig. 9.2 – demonstrates ocular anatomy), the alignment and movement of the eyes, or their possible displacement. Careful examination of the front of the eye with a hand light will reveal gross corneal or conjunctival disease, including xerophthalmia, trachoma, foreign bodies and corneal ulcers. It also reveals much about the anterior chamber and lens, the presence of blood or pus in the eye, acute glaucoma and significant lens opacities (cataract). Whenever possible, the front of the eye should be examined with some magnification, e.g. 2.5× magnification loupe, or a direct ophthalmoscope using a +10 diopter lens.

The diagnosis of mild trachoma requires examination of the conjunctiva on the undersurface of the upper lid, which is accomplished by everting the eyelid (Fig. 9.3). The pupils can also be examined with a hand light, taking note of their size, shape and response to light. It is usually easier to examine the pupils in a somewhat darkened room. A direct ophthalmoscope is essential for examining the back of the interior eye, to search for abnormalities of the optic disc, macular region, blood vessels and other areas.

DIFFERENTIAL DIAGNOSIS OF THE PAINFUL, RED EYE – KEY SYNDROMES

The painful, red eye is one of the most common ocular problems. Many such patients have conjunctivitis, but all should be examined carefully, because a number of serious eye conditions can present with a similar picture. In almost every case, the correct diagnosis can be made from the history and a simple ocular examination (Fig. 9.4).

The most important conditions that present as a painful, red eye are conjunctivitis, keratitis (including keratoconjunctivitis), corneal trauma and foreign bodies, anterior uveitis and acute angle-closure glaucoma (Table 9-2).

CONJUNCTIVITIS

Conjunctivitis is the most common cause of red eye bilaterally. It is usually infective, although conjunctivitis may be allergic or traumatic. It is commonly bilateral; a unilateral red eye increases the likelihood of other diagnoses. Infectious conjunctivitis usually has an acute onset, which is accompanied by ocular discharge. In viral and chlamydial conjunctivitis, the discharge is usually thin and watery. With bacterial conjunctivitis or secondary bacterial infection, the discharge

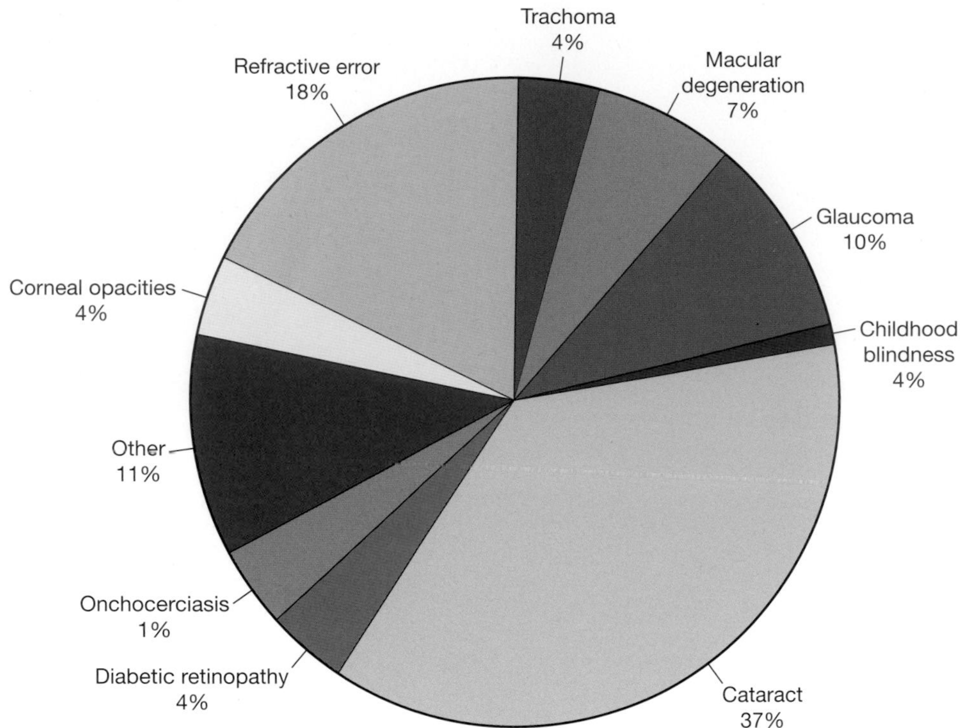

FIGURE 9.1 Global blindness causes.

TABLE 9-1 Global Loss of Vision Table with Blind and Low Vision

Presenting vision	Eye disease	Refractive error	Total
Blindness	37 million	8 million	45 million
Low vision	124 million	145 million	269 million
Total	161 million	153 million	314 million

Presbyopia: Difficulty 410 million; uncorrected 517 million – Total: 1.04 billion.

From Resnikoff S, Pascolini D, Mariotti SP, Pokharel GP. Global magnitude of visual impairment caused by uncorrected refractive errors in 2004. Bull World Health Organ 2008;86:63–70.

is mucopurulent or purulent. A frankly purulent discharge is especially common in gonococcal infections. Mucopurulent and purulent discharges frequently accumulate on the eyelashes and lid margins, causing the lids to stick together.

The most consistent sign of conjunctivitis is conjunctival injection. The superficial and tortuous vessels of the conjunctiva appear dilated and bright red or pink, giving rise to the common term "pink eye". In severe inflammation, pseudomembranes, or even true membranes, may be present. These are seen as dirty gray sloughs on the tarsal conjunctiva. In viral and chlamydial conjunctivitis, follicles are frequently present. Giant, fleshy papillae may occur in allergic conjunctivitis. A detailed description of trachoma and inclusion conjunctivitis is provided in Chapter 35.

Visual acuity is usually not affected in conjunctivitis. The cornea is clear and bright; the pupil is circular and reacts normally; and the anterior chamber is clear and of normal depth.

Bacterial conjunctivitis usually requires specific antibiotic treatment. Antibiotics such as chloramphenicol may be given topically as 0.5% drops (four times per day) and as 1.0% ointment at night. Alternatively, and especially in children, antibiotic ointment, such as 1.0% tetracycline (four times per day) may be used for 1 week. Other ophthalmic solutions may also be used, such as those containing fluoroquinolone antibiotics, although expense may be prohibitive in many regions of the world. Patients should be cautioned to keep their eyes clean by washing away accumulated discharge. They should wash their hands carefully and not share towels or clothes with others, to avoid spreading infection.

Neonatal gonococcal conjunctivitis is a medical emergency. The infant should be hospitalized to confirm response to therapy and a single dose of either ceftriaxone 25–50 mg/kg (not to exceed 125 mg) or cefotaxime 50 mg/kg should be administered intravenously or intramuscularly. The neonate should also receive treatment for presumptive chlamydial conjunctivitis with a 1–3-day course of oral azithromycin 20 mg/kg/day to maximal dose of 1 g or erythromycin syrup (50 mg/kg/day divided into four doses per day for 14 days). Saline irrigation of the eyes should be performed immediately and then at hourly intervals for as long as necessary to eliminate the purulent discharge [3].

Chlamydial conjunctivitis and trachoma in adults and non-neonatal children should be treated with systemic azithromycin with a 1 g single oral dose. In children, a dose of 20 mg/kg is given [4].

Viral conjunctivitis does not respond to antibiotics. Significant symptomatic relief can be obtained with the use of cold compresses and local vasoconstrictors, which also can be used for patients with allergic conjunctivitis. Topical steroids should never be used without the direct supervision of an ophthalmologist.

KERATITIS AND CORNEAL ULCERATION

Keratitis and corneal ulceration are common causes of painful, red eyes and are usually uni-ocular. Severe photophobia is often the main symptom, and the vision is usually blurred. Secondary uveitis may develop and cause ciliary injection. Ciliary injection shows a ring of redness, which is most intense around the limbus, and is a sign of inflammation of the ciliary body and iris. A history of trauma can often be elicited. At other times, a corneal ulcer and, more especially,

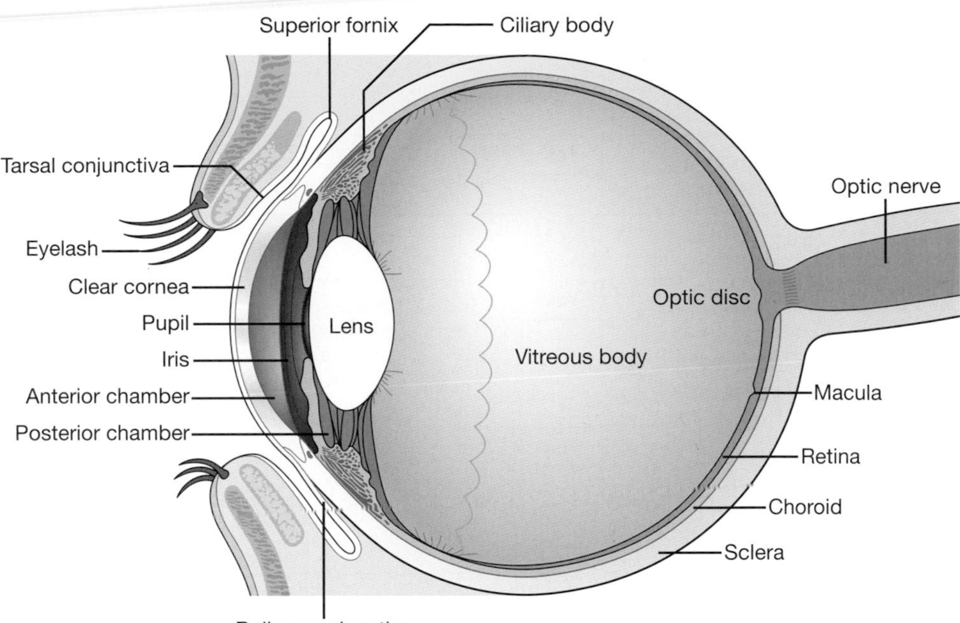

FIGURE 9.2 A diagram of the front of eye and a cross-sectional diagram of the eye.

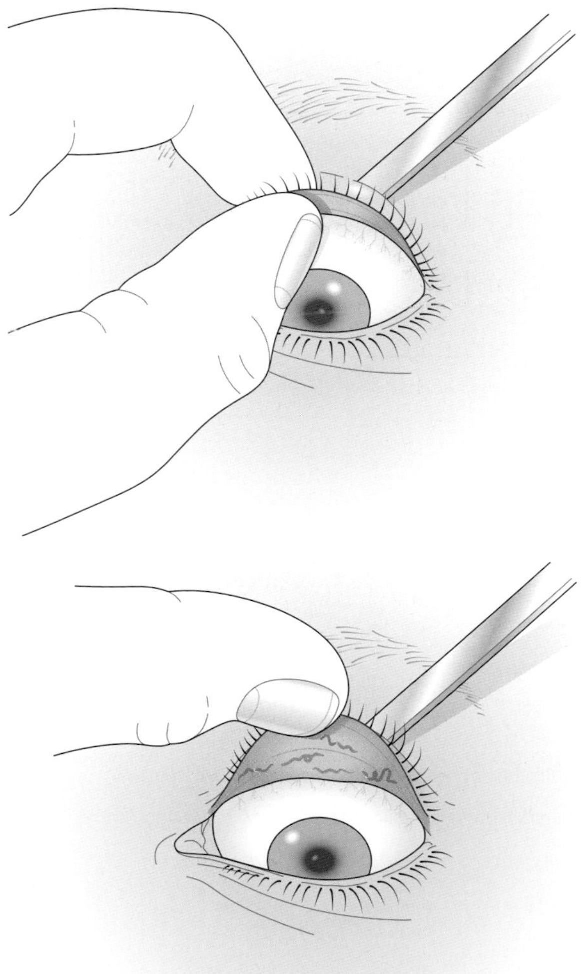

FIGURE 9.3 Eversion of the upper eye lid.

keratitis may occur as a result of viral or severe bacterial conjunctivitis, in which case the signs of conjunctivitis may coexist. Sometimes, corneal ulcers develop spontaneously, especially with herpetic keratitis and are particularly common following measles.

The most important diagnostic sign is the appearance of a corneal defect – either an opacity, which will obscure underlying iris details, or a surface defect, which will distort the surface light reflex. If an ulcer penetrates the cornea, the globe may collapse and the intraocular contents may be expelled. The hole in the cornea may be plugged with a knuckle of iris which then shows as dark tissue in the base of the ulcer. A small ulcer, such as a dendritic ulcer caused by herpes simplex, is best seen if fluorescein is instilled and the eye is observed with a blue light. Large infective ulcers frequently are filled with white sloughed material and other debris. At times, pus may accumulate in the anterior chamber as a hypopyon.

Most corneal ulcers are medical emergencies and these patients should be under the care of an ophthalmologist. Proper management frequently requires a microbiologic diagnosis of the infectious agent, using isolation cultures. Intensive topical antibiotics are used. For bacterial keratitis, commercially available antibiotics drops, e.g. chloramphenicol, ofloxacin or ciprofloxacin, can be used every hour.

Fungal keratitis is a major cause of infectious keratitis in tropical areas of the world. It represents a diagnostic and therapeutic challenge and clinicians need a high index of suspicion if keratitis was presumed to be bacterial but does not respond well to empirical antibiotic treatment. The corneal infiltrate typically has fluffy margins. Treatment is usually either topical natamycin or amphotericin drops (hourly initially, then tapering over more than 2 weeks or until infection has resolved).

If a characteristic dendritic lesion (Fig. 9.5) can be seen on the cornea and if the cornea has decreased sensation, a presumptive diagnosis of herpetic keratitis can be made. Dendritic ulcers are most appropriately treated with topical antiviral agents, e.g. trifluridine drops (eight times per day) or acyclovir ointment (five times per day) for 1 week [5]. Oral acyclovir is often also administered. A mydriatic, such as 2% homatropine (three times per day) may be used until the ulcer has healed.

Parasitic infections represent a rare but severe cause of infectious keratitis. Acanthamoeba is the most common. Treatment is polyhexamethylene biguanide (PHMB) 0.02% drops and Brolene drops administered hourly.

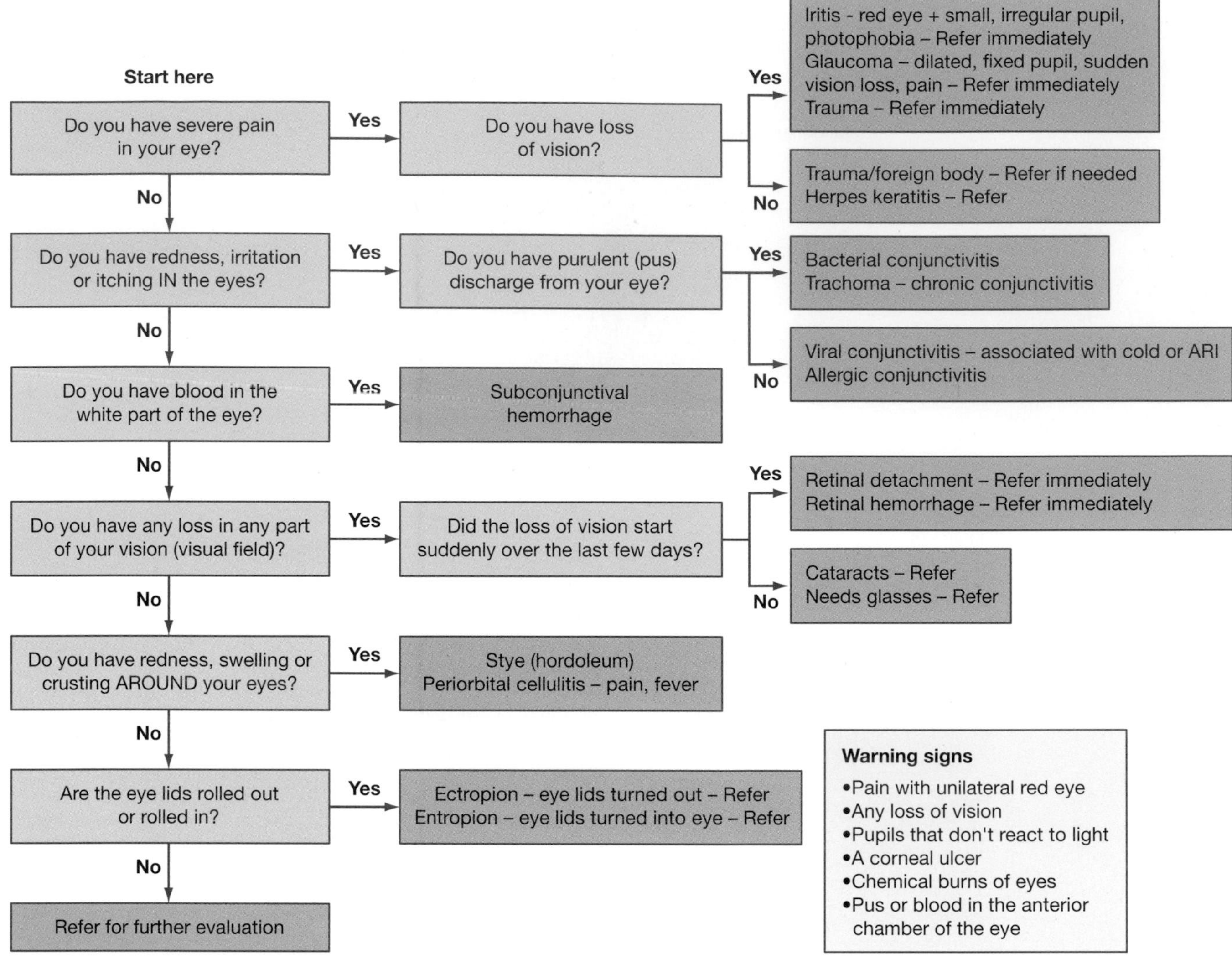

FIGURE 9.4 Algorithm for diagnosis and referral of common eye pathology. *Courtesy of the Nick Simons Institute, Nepal, 2009.*

TABLE 9-2 Differential Diagnosis of the Painful, Red Eye

	Acute conjunctivitis	Keratitis	Anterior uveitis	Acute angle-closure glaucoma
Occurrence	Very common	Common	Uncommon	Uncommon
Age	All ages, especially the young	All ages	Adolescents and adults	Elderly
Onset	Gradual	Sudden (trauma) or gradual	Gradual	Sudden
Pain	Itching, irritation	Moderate to severe	Headache, moderate	Severe, with nausea
Vision	Normal	Blurred	Blurred, sensitivity to light	Marked reduction, with halos
Injection	Conjunctiva, bright red	Ciliary or diffuse	Ciliary	Ciliary, purple
Discharge	Moderate to marked, watery to purulent	Variable, mild to marked	None	None
Cornea	Clear and bright	Abrasion, opacity, foreign body	Clear; keratic precipitates	Steamy, hazy
Pupil	Normal	Variable	Small, irregular, sluggish	Large, oval, unresponsive
Intraocular pressure	Normal	Normal	Usually normal	Markedly elevated

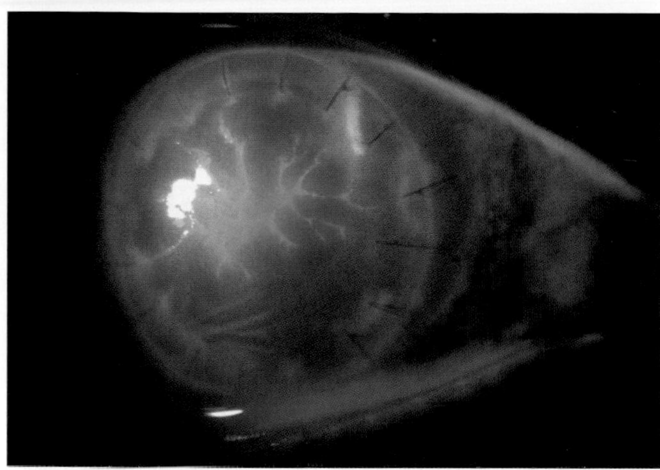

FIGURE 9.5 A dendritic ulcer due to herpetic keratitis in a patient with previous corneal graft.

TABLE 9-3 Proposed Clinical Classification of Uveitis (IUSG 2005)

Infectious	• Bacterial, e.g. syphilis, tuberculosis, brucellosis • Viral, e.g. herpetic, HIV • Parasitic, e.g. toxoplasmosis, cysticercosis • Fungal
Noninfectious	• Known systemic association, e.g. sarcoidosis, arthropathies • No known systemic association
Masquerade	• Neoplastic • Non-neoplastic

From Jabs DA, Nussenblatt RB, Rosenbaum JT, Standardization of Uveitis nomenclature (SUN) Working Group. Standardization of uveitis nomenclature for reporting clinical data. Results of the First International Workshop. Am J Ophthalmol 2005;140:509–16.

For both fungal and acanthamoeba corneal infections, a microbiologic diagnosis should be obtained before treatment is commenced. As with conjunctivitis, steroids should not be used in patients with corneal ulcers and keratitis unless under close supervision by an ophthalmologist.

CORNEAL NECROSIS

A number of systemic conditions are associated with corneal ulceration and necrosis, including collagen vascular diseases, leukemia and granulomatoses. In developing countries, nutritional keratopathy relating to vitamin A deficiency (xerophthalmia, keratomalacia) is a common cause of childhood blindness (Chapter 139). In many poorer Asian countries, measles is an important precipitating event for xerophthalmia (Chapter 28.1). Even in well-nourished Western children, measles may cause a mild, superficial, self-limiting keratitis that does not require therapy. In much of Africa, however, measles itself is considered an important blinding condition. The mechanism is not entirely clear. In many instances, it represents precipitation of acute xerophthalmia, as in Asia. In others, it appears to represent secondary herpetic infection, which also accounts for the accompanying stomatitis and skin ulcers. In still others, corneal damage is a chemical keratitis or bacterial infection secondary to the common practice of placing herbal and other traditional medicines in the eyes of measles patients.

CORNEAL TRAUMA

With trauma, ocular signs and symptoms are usually unilateral and the onset is sudden. A history of trauma or foreign bodies is usually present. Conjunctival foreign bodies cause pain and a feeling of having "something in the eye". Conjunctival vascular injection and some watering of the eye are usually present. A foreign body may be seen with a simple external examination. At other times, however, conjunctival foreign bodies lodge behind the upper eyelid and are not seen until the lid is everted, at which time they can be easily removed.

A corneal foreign body usually produces more severe pain and photophobia. After some time, it will often cause a secondary inflammation with ciliary-limbal injection. Most corneal foreign bodies can be removed fairly easily with a cotton-tipped swab, but if this is not possible, the case should be referred to an ophthalmologist. A single application of antibiotic ointment may be used prophylactically, if available.

In tropical environments in particular, corneal abrasions from plant matter, whether or not they leave a foreign body behind, carry a high risk of subsequent fungal infection. These can be notoriously difficult to treat and should be watched for closely.

Chemical burns to the eyes are best treated with immediate, thorough and copious irrigation. Ideally, sterile saline solution should be used, but rather than delay irrigation, tap water should be used if saline is not available. The damage caused by an acid burn can usually be determined immediately. Because alkali continues to penetrate the eye, alkaline burns are frequently much more severe than initially realized. All chemical burns should be assessed by an ophthalmologist.

Conjunctival hemorrhages, which may be traumatic or spontaneous, require no treatment and will resolve in 1 to 2 weeks. Minor conjunctival lacerations do not require suturing and will heal in a few days. Topical antibiotics are usually given until the eye has healed.

All cases of penetrating trauma to the eye and laceration to the globe, including corneal lacerations and intraocular foreign bodies, are medical emergencies that require prompt referral to and careful assessment by an ophthalmologist.

UVEITIS

The classification of uveitis may be anatomical, clinical, pathological or etiological. All systems may be useful for management purposes.

Anterior uveitis is a relatively uncommon cause of a sore, red eye. The term is used to describe inflammation of the anterior uveal structures – the iris and the ciliary body. The less common posterior uveitis refers to inflammation of the retina and choroid.

Uveitis may occur as a primary event, either in isolation or in association with some underlying systemic disease. Causes are considered to be infective, noninfective or masquerades (Table 9-3) [6]. Secondary anterior uveitis is commonly seen with corneal trauma and ulceration.

Primary anterior uveitis has a gradual onset, with moderate to severe pain and some blurring of vision. It may be unilateral or bilateral, and the patient may have a history of similar episodes. Ciliary injection is the most important feature. This injection decreases with distance from the limbus, and the conjunctiva of the fornices and lids is not inflamed. There is usually no discharge.

The other important sign in anterior uveitis is a pupillary change. The pupil is usually small and reacts poorly to light. Frequently, the pupil is irregular because of adhesions, called posterior synechiae, between the pupillary margin and the lens. On examination with a slit lamp, keratic precipitates or inflammatory cells may be seen on the back of the cornea and also inflammatory cells and an aqueous "flare" in the anterior chamber. In severe cases, these changes may be recognized during the examination of the front of the eye with an ophthalmoscope, using the +10 diopter lens. Posterior uveitis may be asymptomatic or involve severe vision loss if inflammation involves the macula.

Due to possible secondary causes, patients with recurrent episodes of anterior uveitis or other systemic symptoms should be examined in detail to exclude the possibility of such an underlying condition. All patients with posterior uveitis warrant further investigation.

Treatment for anterior uveitis involves cycloplegia and mydriasis obtained with topical drops, such as atropine 1% (three times per day). A systemic analgesic, such as aspirin, will often give symptomatic relief. Topical steroids are frequently indicated, but they should be given only at the direction of an ophthalmologist. If an underlying disease such as syphilis, tuberculosis or brucellosis is present, targeted systemic treatment should also be initiated. In severe uveitis and in chronic uveitis, secondary cataracts and secondary glaucoma may develop. These conditions require specific treatment.

Posterior uveitis is difficult to manage and requires referral to an ophthalmologist to manage the ocular inflammation and to investigate further. Treatment may involve topical, intraocular and systemic steroids or antimicrobials.

Endophthalmitis

Endophthalmitis refers to diffuse inflammation of the eye including uveitis and vitritis. Patients usually present with loss of vision. Involvement of the eye can be "exogenous" following eye surgery or trauma, or "endogenous" representing hematogenous seeding of the eye during bacteremia or fungemia. Patients often do not have fever unless there is an ongoing systemic infection. Examination of the eye may disclose a hypopyon and haziness of the vitreous. Treatment involves intraocular antibiotics, and all patients with endophthalmitis should be referred to an ophthalmologist. Endogenous infections should also be systemically treated.

ACUTE ANGLE-CLOSURE GLAUCOMA

Acute angle-closure glaucoma is a relatively uncommon cause of a painful, red eye, although its diagnosis is of great importance because irreversible blindness can result without prompt treatment. Acute angle-closure glaucoma is characterized by a sudden increase in intraocular pressure when the drainage channels for the intraocular fluid (aqueous humor) are obstructed. The persistence of elevated intraocular pressure can cause permanent and total loss of vision within 1 to 2 days. The condition is most frequent in Asian populations due to the anatomically short eye. A mature cataractous lens causes further crowding of the anterior segment and predisposes to angle-closure.

Acute angle-closure glaucoma usually starts with sudden and severe ocular pain, often severe enough to cause nausea and vomiting. Vision is markedly reduced, and the patient often complains of seeing halos or colored rings around lights. On examination, there may be ciliary injection, but the most striking features are the "steamy" or hazy cornea and the greatly increased intraocular pressure. The corneal changes are due to corneal edema. Intraocular pressure can be assessed by gently palpating the globe through the closed upper lid and comparing the degree of resilience of the affected eye with that of the other eye, or with that of the eye of a person with normal vision. Increased intraocular pressure causes the eye to feel firmer or hard.

The anterior chamber is usually very shallow in angle-closure glaucoma, and the iris appears to be almost touching the cornea. The pupil is frequently found to be semi-dilated and unreactive, and it may have an irregular or vertically oval shape.

Medical attempts to reduce intraocular pressure in such patients should be started without delay. Diuretics such as acetazolamide, 500 mg orally or intravenously, should be given up to four times daily. Any available anti-glaucoma pressure-lowering topical drops should also be given frequently. These patients require referral to an ophthalmologist. An iridectomy or laser iridotomy is generally indicated to prevent further episodes. Pilocarpine 1–2% should be initiated twice daily in the fellow eye to reduce the risk of an acute attack until definitive surgical prophylaxis [7].

CHRONIC DISEASES

Refractive error, cataracts, glaucoma and macular degeneration are major causes of blindness in aged populations of both developed and developing countries.

REFRACTIVE ERROR

Refractive errors include short-sightedness (myopia) and long-sightedness (hyperopia) with or without astigmatism (when an eye can only sharply focus a line in one meridian). These conditions can be rectified with appropriate optical correction. This is a cost-effective intervention and has an important impact on development and quality of life. Presbyopia is the progressive loss of near-vision ability that occurs in everyone over about 40 years of age. This may be easily corrected with ready-made magnifiers. Cost and access barriers to appropriate refractive correction are a problem in many developing areas, but much work is being carried out to rectify this situation.

CATARACT

Opacification of the lens interferes with transmission of clear images to the retina by both decreasing and scattering the light rays as they pass through. To the examiner, the pupillary area may look opaque and whitish or dark brown on hand-light illumination, and fundus details will be obscured when viewed with the direct ophthalmoscope. Aside from cataracts of rare congenital origin and those that result from chronic inflammation, most cataracts are lumped together under the heading "senile". These are undoubtedly of multifactorial origin. Because the precise causes of such cataracts are as yet unknown, preventive measures do not currently exist. Cataracts can be surgically removed with a high degree of technical success and likelihood of return of useful vision.

In general, cataracts are the leading cause of blindness in developing countries. Visually disabling cataracts appear to occur earlier in life in some cultures than in others. More importantly, surgical therapy is commonly unavailable to large segments of the population. Some countries are overcoming the paucity and maldistribution of ophthalmologists by conducting intensive rural "cataract camps"; others are doing so by training properly supervised paramedical personnel to remove cataracts. Because the potential for intraoperative complications and postoperative infections is high under these circumstances, these approaches require careful consideration and detailed organization. However, as no other recourse often exists, these methods require further development and extension.

Merely removing an advanced cataract can improve vision, but removal alone will not restore reading acuity. Some form of aphakic correction, most commonly intraocular lenses or spectacles, is also required.

GLAUCOMA

There are two major forms of glaucoma – acute and chronic. As already discussed, the acute form, with its red, injected, painful eyes, is the more dramatic. Chronic open-angle glaucoma, however, is much more common and is the more important cause of blindness.

Chronic elevation of intraocular pressure, at levels below those reached in acute angle-closure glaucoma, results in progressive destruction of the optic nerve. After many years (usually 10 to 20), this painless, asymptomatic destruction of the optic nerve results in loss of visual field, detectable by careful visual field examination. Antiglaucoma therapy may delay or prevent further damage, but it cannot replace the vision that has already been lost. Unfortunately, patients are usually unaware of the problem until late in the course of the disease, when central acuity is finally involved and little vision or optic nerve remains to be saved.

Glaucoma is the classic disease in which screening methods have played an important role. Unfortunately, the simplest technique, that of demonstrating by tonometry that the intraocular pressure is greater than 21 mmHg, is far from infallible. Half of those with established glaucomatous field loss will have a normal pressure on a single casual screening test, and only 1 in 20 or 30 people with an elevated pressure will already have field loss. The higher the pressure, however, the greater the likelihood of having, or soon developing, field loss. Screening is improved by combining tonometry with examination of the optic disc (by direct ophthalmoscopy or, preferably, with a slit lamp and contact lens). Deep, large, asymmetric optic disc cupping, equal to or greater than 0.6 disc diameter, suggests glaucomatous damage.

Ultimately, diagnosis requires demonstration of classic changes in the visual fields.

Treatment consists of lowering the intraocular pressure below 21 mmHg or to whatever level prevents further damage. A variety of topical medications may accomplish this: prostaglandin analogues are generally used first-line in developed countries. Beta-blockers such as timolol are less expensive and equally effective at lowering intraocular pressure. Alpha-agonists, e.g. brimonidine, and topical carbonic anhydrase inhibitors are also used. If one agent proves inadequate, others may be added to the regimen.

Glaucoma management requires careful monitoring of pressure and visual field and frequent adjustment of dosage and regimen, while compliance of patients with the treatment plan is generally poor.

Laser trabeculoplasty is effective at lowering intraocular pressure for 5–10 years and has far less complications than surgery. Improved compliance is a significant advantage over the topical medications. The treatment is also cost-effective as initial treatment.

When visual field loss continues, even on "maximum" medical therapy, the patient requires filtering surgery. A small channel is produced through the tough outer coats of the eye, so that some of the aqueous may percolate out of the eye into the subconjunctival space, where it is absorbed. Such artificial channels are at least temporarily successful, after one or more operations, in 85% of Caucasian patients. African patients do not fare so well because of their greater tendency for scarring, which closes the new channel. Concomitant local use of antimetabolites increases success.

Despite the potential for preventative measures, glaucoma is an especially difficult clinical problem in tropical countries; screening and diagnostic procedures are time-consuming and complex, and medical therapy is expensive, requires careful monitoring, and usually is attended by poor compliance.

AGE-RELATED MACULAR DEGENERATION

In temperate climates, age-related macular degeneration (AMD) is the first or second leading cause of blindness. AMD has received little attention in the tropics because it is difficult to diagnose without a dilated pupil fundus examination, occurs mainly in the elderly, and does not have easily available treatment options.

AMD has a strong genetic basis and is also associated with cigarette smoking [8]. Early in the disease, scattered, white, deep-retinal dots, known as drusen, can be seen concentrated in the macular area. Some, but not all, people with these signs eventually develop progressive degeneration of their retinal pigment epithelium and the underlying choroid. Loss of vision is gradual, unpredictable, and is usually confined to loss of fine reading acuity. Patients rarely develop "black blindness" (total loss of vision) and can usually care for themselves. In some, a net of new blood vessels grows from the choroid, and these vessels may leak or bleed. Such vascular networks may be treated with injections in the eye of anti-VEGF agents. However, these are very expensive, seldom available, and require repeated administration. Laser treatment may also be effective for certain subtypes.

DIABETIC RETINOPATHY

Diabetic retinopathy includes a wide, complex spectrum of changes. Because few long-time diabetics survive in the poor, rural communities of developing countries, diabetic retinopathy is less common than in developed countries and in increasingly affluent urban communities elsewhere. The major treatable component of the disease is the growth of neovascular membranes which extend into the vitreous from the surface of the optic nerve or retina. Timely laser therapy provides substantial benefit and dramatically reduces the risk of blindness. Laser treatment also benefits patients with fluid accumulation in the macula (macular edema) if they are treated early. Diabetics should have their eyes examined annually if possible to ensure that suitable laser treatment is applied prior to the development of sight-threatening complications.

PROPTOSIS

Abnormal protrusion of the eye is uncommon but usually signifies serious orbital pathology. Although included in this chronic section, there are a number of acute causes. Causes include: inflammatory disease, e.g. thyroid eye disease; infection, e.g. orbital cellulitis (bacterial, parasitic, fungal); tumors; and vascular anomalies, e.g. carotid–cavernous fistula (perhaps after trauma).

REFERENCES

1. Resnikoff S, Pascolini D, Etya'ale D, et al. Global data on visual impairment in the year 2002. Bull World Health Organ 2004;82:844–51.
2. Resnikoff S, Pascolini D, Mariotti SP, Pokharel GP. Global magnitude of visual impairment caused by uncorrected refractive errors in 2004. Bull World Health Organ 2008;86:63–70.
3. O'Hara MA. Ophthalmia neonatorum. Pediatr Clin North Am 1993;40: 715–25.
4. Taylor HR. Trachoma. Melbourne, Australia: Haddington Press; 2008:204.
5. Wilhelmus KR. Therapeutic interventions for herpes simplex virus epithelial keratitis. Cochrane Database Syst Rev 2008;(1):CD002898.
6. Jabs DA, Nussenblatt RB, Rosenbaum JT, Standardization of Uveitis Nomenclature (SUN) Working Group. Standardization of uveitis nomenclature for reporting clinical data. Results of the First International Workshop. Am J Ophthalmol 2005;140:509–16.
7. Salmon JF, Kanski JJ. Glaucoma, 3rd edn. Oxford, UK: Butterworth Heinemann; 2004:69.
8. Kanski JJ. Clinical Ophthalmology, 6th edn. Edinburgh, UK: Butterworth Heinemann; 2003:629.

10 Neurologic Diseases

Tom Solomon, Hadi Manji

Key features

Neurologic diseases present different challenges in the tropics:

- Increased incidence from infectious causes, particularly those that relate to sanitation (e.g. typhoid) or arthropods (e.g. cerebral malaria)
- Toxic and nutritional causes, e.g. peripheral neuropathies
- Rapid adoption of Western lifestyles and the associated chronic diseases (hypertension, obesity, diabetes) without the necessary public health campaigns and measures to limit them
- Increased incidence of vaccine-preventable diseases (polio, diphtheria, tetanus)
- Greater role of non-conventional medical practices—traditional medicines, and healers and psychiatric diagnoses as witch-craft
- Greater incidence of HIV and poorer access to drugs

The number of infectious and non-infectious causes of neurologic presentation is large (Table 10-1). In this chapter, for each of the key presenting neurologic syndromes, the clinical approach, investigation, diagnosis and management is considered.

MENINGISM AND MENINGITIS

KEY SYNDROMES AND CLINICAL APPROACH

Meningism is the clinical syndrome of headache, neck stiffness and photophobia, often with nausea and vomiting. It is most often caused by inflammation of the meninges (see below), but other causes include raised intracranial pressure. Kernig's sign is present if, with the patient supine and the hip and knee flexed, extension of the knee causes pain in the back and neck.

Brudzinski's sign is positive if passive flexion of the neck causes knee and hip flexion. Both signs have low sensitivity but high specificity for meningitis.

Meningitis is inflammation of the meninges. Bacterial, viral, and fungal infections are the most common causes, but meningitis can also be caused by carcinoma and drugs. Fever, neck stiffness and altered consciousness are described as the "classic triad", but they are only found in about half of adults with acute bacterial meningitis [1]. The term "meningoencephalitis" is used by some clinicians to describe patients with meningitis and altered consciousness, but by other clinicians to describe patients with meningitis or encephalitis. Therefore, it is probably best avoided!

In the history and examination pay particular attention to the presence of rash (meningococcus), macules or vesicles on the hands and feet and mouth ulcers (enterovirus causing hand, foot and mouth disease), buccal lesions (enterovirus) and otitis (pneumococcal

TABLE 10-1 Causes of Neurologic Disease (VIMTO)

Vascular			
	Ischemia/infarct		
	Subarachnoid/subdural/extradural/intracerebral hemorrhage		
	Hypertension/hypotension		
Infectious			
		Bacteria	
	Direct effect		*Meningococcus, Streptococcus, Haemophylus influenzae*, tuberculous
	on CNS		
		Viruses	
			Arboviruses, herpes viruses, enteroviruses, rabies

TABLE 10-1 Causes of Neurologic Disease (VIMTO)—cont'd

		Parasites			
			Protozoans		
				Malaria *(Plasmodium falcipaurm)*	African trypanosomiasis (*Trypanosoma brucei* gambiense and rhodesiense)
				Toxoplasmosis (*Toxoplasma gondii*)	Amoebiasis (*Entaboema histolytica*)
			Trematodes (Flukes)		
				Paragonimiasis, schistosomiasis (esp. *Schistosoma japonicum*)	
			Cestodes (tapeworms)		
				Cysticercosis (*Taenia solium*), hydatidosis (*Echinococcus granulosa*)	
			Nemotodes (round worms)		
				Ascariasis (*Ascaris lumbricoides*)	Parastronglyliasis (*Parastrongylus cantonensis*)
				Gnathostomiasis	Trichinosis (*Trichonella spiralis*)
		Spirochetes			
				Neurosyphilis (Treponema pallidum)	Lyme disease (*Borrelia burgdorferi*)
				Leptospirosis (Leptospira species)	Louse-borne/epidemic relapsing fever (*B. recurrentis*)
				Tick-borne/endemic- relapsing fever (*B. duttoni*)	
		Rickettsiae			
				Epidemic/louse-borne typhus (*Rickettsia prowazekii*)	Endemic/murine/flea-borne typhus (*R. typhi/ mooseri*)
				Scrub typhus (*R. tsutsugamushi*)	Rocky Mountain spotted fever (*R. rickettsii*)
		Fungi			
				Cryptococcosis	Histoplasmosis
				Aspergillosis	Coccidiomycosis
				Candidiasis	Paracoccidiomycosis
				Blastomycosis	Nocardia*
	Indirect effect	Toxin-mediated infectious diseases (tetanus, diphtheria, shigella)			
	of infection	Immune-mediated, post-infectious inflammatory (GBS, acute disseminated encephalomyelitis)			
Metabolic					
		Hypoglycemia, diabetic ketoacidosis, hepatic encephalopathy, uremia, hyponatremia, hypo-/hyperthyroidism, Addison's disease			
Tumors/trauma/ toxins					
		Alcohol, drugs (medical, recreational, traditional), pesticides, poisons			
Other		Hydrocephalus			
		Epilepsy			
		Psychiatric disease—hysteria			

*Nocardia is an actinomycetes bacteria that is grouped with fungi because of its morphology and behavior.
CNS, central nervous system; GBS, Guillain-Barré syndrome.

meningitis). Ask about possible contact with tuberculosis, or whether there is an outbreak of mumps in the community, for example. Is there a history of eating raw snails in Asia (*Angiostrongyloides*) or ingestion of unpasteurized milk or dairy products (*Brucella, Listeria*)? Look for needle injection marks and pointers to HIV infection (see Box 10.1).

APPROACHES TO INVESTIGATION, DIAGNOSIS AND MANAGEMENT

The cardinal investigation in diagnosing meningitis and determining its underlying cause is the lumbar puncture (LP). Although there is some controversy about which patients should receive LP (see Box

BOX 10.1 Pointers to HIV Infection

History

Risk factors for HIV—multiple sexual partners, male sex with males, sex workers, intravenous drug abuse, blood products

For children, death of mother and father

Weight loss; unexplained pyrexi

Persistent diarrhea

Clinical Signs

Wasting

Lymphadenopathy

Hairy leukoplaqia, oral candida on oral examination

Seborrhoebic dermatitis, Kaposi's sarcoma, molluscan contageosum, zoster, herpes simplex

Intravenous drug injection sites

Retinitis (cytomegalovirus, toxoplasma, syphilis), papilloedema, uveitis, iritis on ocular examination

Investigations

Low platelet count and white cell count

High erythrocyte sedimentation rate (ESR)

BOX 10.2 Lumbar Puncture Guidelines

All patients with a suspected CNS infection should have a lumbar puncture (LP) as soon as possible, unless there are contraindications. In Western industrialized settings, LP use declined somewhat in the 1990s, following concerns that it might precipitate brain shift and herniation syndromes in patients with incipient herniation. In the West, a CT scan is therefore recommended before LP in patients with clinical features suggestive of incipient herniation; whilst this is performed, appropriate antimicrobial therapy is started and a LP is performed as soon as it is deemed safe.

In the tropics, where CT is less readily available and infections are more common, the benefits of accurate diagnosis and appropriate treatment are often felt to outweigh the theoretical risk of herniation, and even patients with a relative contraindication often undergo a LP with no apparent harm.

Imaging preferred before lumbar puncture, if possible to exclude brain shift, swelling, or space-occupying lesion.

Antimicrobial treatment should be started whilst awaiting imaging.

If imaging shows no significant brain shift, lumbar puncture should be performed.

- Focal neurologic signs, other than cranial neuropathies
- Papilloedema
- Recent-onset seizures
- Moderate-to-severe impairment of consciousness, or rapidly falling level of consciousness
- Hypertension with bradycardia
- Immunocompromise (some patients)

Other contraindications to immediate LP:

- Bleeding disorder
- Anticoagulant treatment
- Sepsis over the spine

Notes

- In settings where CT is not readily available, the benefits of rapid accurate diagnosis from LP and appropriate treatment are often felt to outweigh the theoretical risk of herniation, and even patients with a relative contraindication often undergo a lumbar puncture with no apparent harm.
- There is no agreement on the depth of coma that necessitates imaging before LP; some argue Glasgow Coma Score <12, others say <10 or <8.
- Imaging is preferable in patients with known severe immunocompromise (e.g. advanced AIDS).

Modified from Solomon T. Meningitis. Brain's Diseases of the Nervous System. Oxford: Oxford University Press; 2009:1327–54.

10.2) and whether computed tomography (CT) scanning is indicated, LP is used more readily in the tropics than in Western industrialized nations. If all the equipment is not available, it can be fashioned out of readily available items (Box 10.3).

After LP, most patients will be classified as having normal cerebrospinal fluid (CSF), consistent with viral meningitis, bacterial meningitis or tuberculous meningitis (Box 10.4); in some patients a microorganism will have been seen on CSF microscopy, thus guiding treatment. If CSF is consistent with acute bacterial meningitis, empirical antibiotics (usually a third-generation cephalosporin) are started. If the initial CSF findings suggest tuberculosis meningitis (TBM), microbiologic confirmation requires large volumes of CSF (e.g. 6–10 ml). Therefore, unless the patient is very unwell, it is worth waiting 24 hours to repeat LP removing large CSF volumes. It is important to remember that the differential diagnosis of aseptic meningitis is broad (see Table 10-2).

There has, for many years, been controversy over the role of corticosteroids in treating acute bacterial meningitis. A recent meta-analysis of data from five studies, including two from Malawi and one from Vietnam, showed that dexamethasone did not reduce deaths or neurologic sequelae; a sub-group analysis showed it did reduce death and the composite analysis of death, neurologic sequelae and severe hearing loss in patients over 55 years old [2]. This is in contrast to TBM, where corticosteroids are thought to be of benefit [3].

The investigation and management of the common diagnoses are covered in individual chapters:

Bacterial Meningitis (Chapter 54).
Tuberculous Meningitis (Chapter 39).
Angiostrongyloides (Chapter 118).
Cryptococcus (Chapter 84).

ENCEPHALOPATHY AND ENCEPHALITIS

KEY SYNDROMES AND CLINICAL APPROACH

Encephalopathy is the syndrome of reduced or altered level of consciousness, ranging from the obvious (coma), to the subtle (changed

BOX 10.3 Lumbar Puncture Technique

- Time spent positioning the patient is time well spent. Insist on good lighting and help from nursing colleagues to keep the patient still.
- Use pillows (or equivalent) under the patient's head and between their legs to ensure the entire cranio-spinal axis is parallel to the bed.
- Take blood for plasma glucose just before performing the lumbar puncture (LP).
- Although a proper lumbar puncture needle with a stylet is preferred, in the tropics, standard 20 or 22 gauge needles are sometimes used if nothing else is available, especially in children.
- Measure the cerebrospinal fluid (CSF) opening pressure; an improvised manometer can be made by connecting any sterile tubing (e.g. from a drip) to a LP needle (using a three-way tap) and measuring CSF height against a ruler.
- If unable to obtain CSF, sit the patient on a chair facing the wrong way, and ask them to lean over the back of it; this opens up the inter-vertebral space and makes LP easier (however, do not measure the CSF opening pressure with the patient upright—it will be falsely elevated).
- If there is no formal biochemistry laboratory to measure CSF protein and glucose, and approximation can be made using a urine dipstick [8].

behavior or personality, which can be mistaken for psychiatric illness or witch-craft). The differential is very broad, including metabolic, toxic and infectious causes.

Encephalitis is inflammation of the brain parenchyma, often owing to infection; strictly speaking, this can only be diagnosed pathologically, with biopsy or autopsy. Because of the practical limitations of this, surrogate markers are used, such as CSF, pleocytosis or inflammatory change on imaging. Infectious causes of encephalitis include viruses and some bacteria, particularly small, intracellular bacteria. Acute disseminated encephalomyelitis (ADEM) is often a post- or para-infectious inflammation. Rarer causes include limbic encephalitis associated with systemic neoplasms. Clinically, encephalitis usually presents with a history of flu-like illness followed by altered consciousness and severe headache; in children there are often seizures and depending on the type and cause of encephalitis, there may be focal signs. Japanese encephalitis is often associated with tremors and other signs of Parkinsonism. Herpes simplex encephalitis may be associated with olfactory hallucinations.

The term "Acute Encephalitis Syndrome" is used in World Health Organization (WHO) surveillance guidelines in Asia to describe patients with a febrile illness and altered consciousness or seizures in whom encephalitis is suspected. Acute encephalopathy syndrome may be a more accurate term, as many of these patients turn out to have an encephalopathy rather than encephalitis.

The Patient in Coma

Before the history and detailed examination can be considered, patients in coma require emergency assessment, stabilization and treatment of any **immediately life-threatening conditions** (Box 10.5).

TABLE 10-2 Causes of Aseptic Meningitis

	Viruses	Bacteria	Other infections	Non-infectious causes
Common	Enteroviruses	Partially treated bacterial meningitis	*Cryptococcus* spp.	Drugs (non-steroidal anti-inflammatory drugs, antibiotics, others)
	Herpes simplex virus type 2	Parameningeal bacterial infections	*Toxoplasma gondii*	
	Arboviruses*	*Listeria monocytogenes*		
	HIV (seroconversion illness)	Tuberculous meningitis		
	Mumps	*Treponema pallidum* (syphillis)		
Less common	Other human herpes viruses (HSV 1, VZV, EBV, CMV, HHV-6, HHV-7)	*Mycoplasma pneumoniae*	Other fungi, (e.g. *Candida* spp., *Aspergillus* spp.)	Autoimmune disorders, vasculitis
	Other viruses (influenza A & B, measles, parvovoris B19, LVMC, rotavirus)	*Borrelia burgdorferi* (Lyme disease)	Parasites (e.g. *Angiostrongylus cantonensis, Naegleria fowleri, Acanthamoeba* spp.)	Sarcoid
		Leptospira spp.		Malignancy
		Brucella spp.		Behçets disease
		Rickettsia rickettsii		
		Erlichia spp.		
Other		*Nocardia* spp.		

*Varies greatly depending on geographical location
CMV, cytomegalovirus; EBV, Epstein-Barr virus; HHV-6, human herpes virus 6; HHV-7, human herpes virus 7; HSV 1, herpes simplex virus 1; VZV, varicella zoster virus.
Modified from From Solomon T. Meningitis. Brain's Diseases of the Nervous System. Oxford: Oxford University Press; 2009:1327–54.

BOX 10.4 Cerebrospinal Fluid (CSF) Interpretation—Typical CSF Findings in Central Nervous System Infections (CNS)

	Viral meningitis or encephalitis	Acute bacterial meningitis	Tuberculous meningitis	Fungal meningitis	Normal*
Opening pressure	Normal/high	High	High	High–very high	10–20 cm
Color	'Gin' clear	Cloudy	Cloudy/yellow	Clear/cloudy	Clear
Cells/mm^3	Normal–high	High–very high	Sl. increased	Normal–high	
	0–1000	1000–50,000	25–500	0–1000	<5
Differential	Lymphocytes	Neutrophils	Lymphocytes	Lymphocytes	Lymphocytes
CSF/plasma	Normal	Low	Low–very low	Normal–low	66%
Glucose ratio			(e.g.<30%)		
Protein (g/L)	Normal–high	High	High–very high	Normal–high	<0.5
	0.5–1	>1	1–5	0.2–5.0	

*Normal values:
Normal CSF opening pressure is <20 cm for adults, <10 cm for children below the age of eight years old.
Although 66% is quoted as the normal glucose ratio, only values below 50% are taken as being significant in many settings.
A bloody tap will falsely elevate the CSF white cell count and protein. To correct for a bloody tap, subtract 1 white cell for every 700 red blood cells/mm^3 in the CSF and 0.1 g/dL of protein for every 1000 red blood cells.
Some important exceptions:
In viral CNS infections, an early lumbar puncture (LP) may give predominantly neutrophils, or there may be no cells in early or late LPs.
In patients with acute bacterial meningitis that has been partially pretreated with antibiotics (or patients younger than one year old), the CSF cell count may not be very high and may be mostly lymphocytes.
Tuberculous meningitis (TBM) may have predominant CSF polymorphs early on.
Listeria can give a similar CSF picture to TBM, but the history is shorter.
CSF findings in bacterial abscesses range from near normal to purulent, depending on location of the abscess and whether there is associated meningitis or rupture.
A cryptococcal antigen test (CRAG) and India ink stain should be performed on the CSF of all patients in whom *Cryptococcus* is possible.

For assessing depth of coma in adults and children over the age of five, the Glasgow Coma score is used (Box 10.6); in children under the age of five, a range of scores are used, including the Alert, Voice, Pain, Unresponsive (AVPU) score (see Box 10.5) and the Blantyre Coma score (Box 10.7).

A careful history and examination greatly assist the classification of patients presenting with altered consciousness. Consider evidence for HIV infection or other immunocompromise (Box 10.1).

In the history pay attention to:

- Duration of onset of coma:
  - rapid (minutes–hours) suggests vascular cause, especially brainstem cerebrovascular accidents or subarachnoid hemorrhage; if preceded by hemispheric signs, then intracerebral hemorrhage;
  - coma caused by some infections (e.g. malaria, encephalitis) can also develop rapidly, especially when precipitated by convulsions;
  - intermediate (hours–days) suggests diffuse encephalopathy (metabolic or, if febrile, infectious);
  - prolonged (days–weeks) suggests tumors, abscess, chronic subdural hematoma.
- Any drugs?
- Any trauma?
- Important past medical history (e.g. hypertension)?
- Family history (e.g. tuberculosis)?
- Known epidemic area (e.g. viral encephalitis)?
- Exposure to insects—mosquitoes (malaria, flaviviruses), ticks (flaviviruses, borrelia).
- Exposure to sick animals—dogs, cats (rabies).
- Ingestion of contaminated food—snails (Angiostrongylus), unpasteurized milk/dairy products (brucella, listeria), fresh produce/water (cysticercosis, typhoid).
- Exposure to contaminated water (leptospirosis, schistosomiasis).
- Illness in the community (measles, mumps).
- Generalized illness (infectious mononucleosis).
- Time of year.
- Geographical location in the tropics.

The **general medical examination** can provide essential clues:

- Examine for signs of trauma (check ears and nose for blood or CSF leak).
- Smell breath for alcohol and ketoacidosis.
- Examine skin for:
  - rash (meningococcal rash, dengue or other hemorrhagic fever, typhus, relapsing fever);
  - needle marks of drug abuse;
  - recent tick-bite or eschar (tick-borne encephalitis, tick paralysis, tick-borne typhus or relapsing fever);
  - chancre, with or without circinate rash (trypanosomiasis, especially rhodesiense);
  - healed dog-bite (rabies);
  - snake bite.
- Check the fundi for papilloedema (longstanding raised intracranial pressure) or signs of hypertension.
- Lymphadenopathy (HIV, tuberculosis), hepatosplenomegaly.

A focused neurologic examination includes assessment of level of consciousness (**Boxes 10.6 and 10.7**), then examination of pupils, eye movements, breathing patterns and response to pain to help determine whether a patient has:

- a diffuse encephalopathy (usually metabolic or infectious);
- supratentorial focal damage (i.e. above the cerebellar tentorium), which usually manifests as hemispheric signs;
- damage in the diencephalon or brainstem (midbrain, pons or medulla), which may indicate a syndrome of cerebral herniation

BOX 10.5 Rapid Assessment of Patient with Coma in the Tropics

- Airways
- Breathing—give oxygen; intubate if breathing is inadequate or gag reflex impaired
- Circulation—establish venous access
  - obtain blood for immediate bedside blood glucose test (hypoglycemia)
  - malaria film (look for parasites and pigment of partially treated malaria)
  - full blood count, electrolytes, blood cultures, arterial blood gases
- Disability
  - Start IV: 10% dextrose (50 ml in adults, 5 ml/kg in children) irrespective of blood glucose
  - Give adults 100 mg thiamine intravenously (especially if alcohol abuse suspected)
  - Immobilize cervical spinal cord if neck trauma suspected
- Determine whether Alert, responds to Voice, to Pain, or Unresponsive (the AVPU scale)
  - If responds to pain or is unresponsive, examine the pupils, eye movements, respiratory pattern, tone and posture for signs of brain shift (herniation—see below)
  - If herniation suspected, start treatment for this
- If purpuric rash present, give cefotaxime for presumed meningococcal meningitis (after blood cultures)
- Look for, and treat, generalized seizures, focal seizures and subtle motor seizures (mouth or finger twitching, or tonic eye deviation)

BOX 10.6 Modified Glasgow Coma Scale for Adults and Children >5 Years Old

Best motor response
6 Obeys command
5 Localizes supraorbital pain
4 Withdraws from pain on nail bed
3 Abnormal flexion response
2 Abnormal extension response
1 None

Best verbal response
5 Oriented
4 Confused
3 Inappropriate words
2 Incomprehensible sounds
1 None

Eye opening
4 Spontaneous
3 To Voice
2 Pain
1 None

Total score ranges from 15 to 3; the term "unrousable coma" is sometimes used to reflect a score <9

BOX 10.7 Blantyre Coma Scale for Children <5 Years Old

Best motor response
2 Localizes painful stimulus
1 Withdraws limb from pain
0 Nonspecific or absent response

Best verbal response
2 Appropriate cry
1 Moan or inappropriate cry
0 None

Eye movements
1 Directed (e.g. follows mother's face)
0 Not directed

Total score ranges from 5 to 0; the term "unrousable coma" is sometimes used to reflect a score <2

through the tentorial hiatus or the foramen magnum (Box 10.8, Fig. 10.1).

Determining whether there are brainstem signs can be helpful prognostically.

Based on the history, general examination and neurological examination, patients will usually fall into one of the following categories, with differentials as shown.

Classification into Syndromes

Encephalopathy only (no brainstem or hemispheric signs; if moderate encephalopathy—just behavioral changes/confusion; if more severe—coma).

- If patient is febrile*, suspect central nervous system (CNS) infection, e.g. cerebral malaria, typhoid, dengue, or
- metabolic cause with secondary aspiration pneumonia.
- If no history of fever, coma is likely to be:
  - metabolic, (hypoglycemia, drugs, alcohol, diabetic ketoacidosis, toxins);
  - psychogenic;
  - subarachnoid hemorrhage (or other cerebrovascular accident).

Coma with focal signs (+/- meningism).

Decide if the signs are "hemispheric signs", "brainstem signs" or both.

- Hemispheric signs only:
  - if febrile, consider CNS infection, especially encephalitis, bacterial meningitis with empyema, abscess (tuberculoma);
  - if afebrile, consider space-occupying lesion, cerebrovascular accident, trauma.
- Brainstem signs only may be caused by either:
  - focal pathology within the brainstem, e.g. encephalitis (especially if markedly asymmetrical signs);
  - herniation of the brainstem (through the foramen magnum), secondary to a diffuse process (e.g. diabetic ketoacidosis or late bacterial meningitis) causing raised intracranial pressure.

*Note: patients with a history of fever are classified "febrile" even if not febrile when first examined.

BOX 10.8 Examination for Brainstem Signs (Figure 10.1)

Examine pupil size, and reaction to light

- Normal reaction (i.e. constriction)—diffuse encephalopathy.
- Unilateral large pupil—herniation of the temporal lobe uncus.
- Small or mid-sized but reactive pupil—diencephalic syndrome.
- Unreactive midsized pupils—midbrain or pontine lesions.
- Unreactive large pupils in medullary lesions.

Note: pinpoint pupils occur following opiate or organophosphate overdose, or in isolated pontine lesion; other drugs can cause large unreactive pupils.

Assess eye movements (holding eyelids open if necessary)

- Spontaneous eye movements (brainstem is intact).
- Oculocephalic (doll's eye) reflex (rotate the head, the eyes normally deviate away from the direction of rotation):
  - Normal indicates brainstem is intact (i.e. diffuse encephalopathy);
  - Reduced or absent responses occur in uncal herniation and in brainstem damage (or, rarely, in deep metabolic coma).

Assess breathing pattern

A normal pattern occurs in a diffuse encephalopathy.

Cheyne-Stokes breathing and hyperventilation occur in reversible herniation syndromes.

Shallow, ataxic or apneic respiration occurs in more severe brainstem syndromes (Figure 10.1).

Other causes of hyperventilation include:

- acidosis;
- aspiration pneumonia;
- flaccid paralysis of respiratory musculature.

Assess response to pain (to supraorbital ridge and nailbed of each limb)

- Hemiparesis most often indicates supratentorial hemispheric focal pathology (other signs include asymmetry of tone and focal seizures), but also occurs in uncal herniation.
- Flexor "decorticate" posturing (flexion of arms with extension of legs) damage in the diencephalon.
- Extensor "decerebrate" posturing (extension of arms and legs—midbrain/upper pontine damage) is prognostically worse.
- No response, or leg flexion only, is more severe.

Metabolic encephalopathies: symmetrical posturing (decorticate or decerebrate) and hemiparetic focal signs are also occasionally seen in metabolic encephalopathies (e.g. hypoglycemia; hepatic, uremic, or anoxic coma; sedative drugs), cerebal malaria and intra- or post-ictally. Other pointers to metabolic disease include asterixis, tremor and myoclonus preceding the onset of coma.

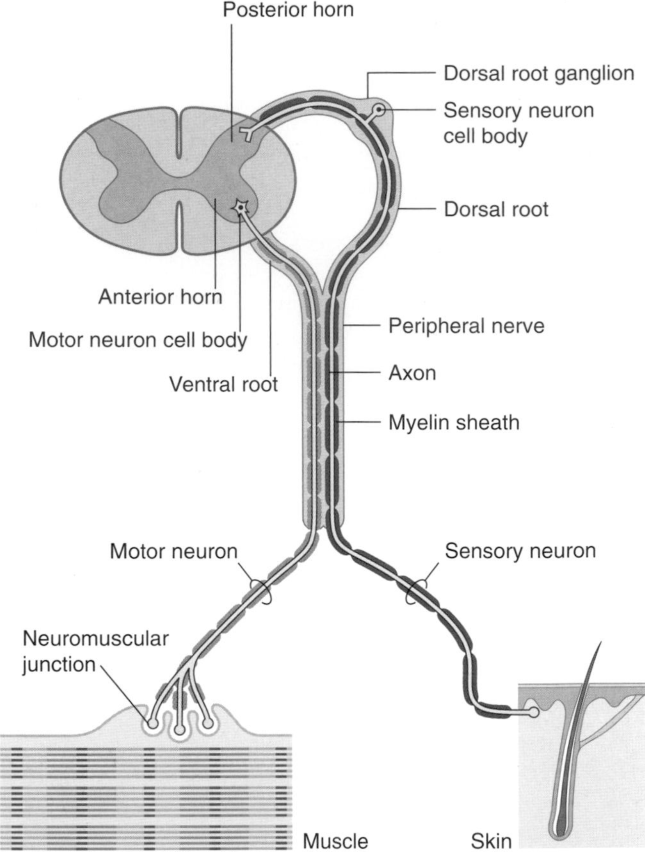

FIGURE 10.1 Peripheral nervous system (PNS). The PNS consists of all of the neural elements outside of the central nervous system (CNS; brain and spinal cord) and provides the connections between the CNS and all other body organ systems. The PNS consists of somatic and autonomic components. The somatic component innervates skeletal muscle and skin and is shown here (see Figure 2.15 for the autonomic nervous system). The somatic component of the peripheral nerves contains both motor and sensory axons. Cell bodies of the motor neurons are found in the anterior horn gray matter, whereas the cell bodies of sensory neurons are located in the dorsal root ganglia.

- Hemispheric and brainstem signs may be caused by either:
  - supratentorial lesion causing hemispheric signs and sufficient swelling to precipitate brainstem herniation (e.g. cerebral bleed, abscess);
  - patchy focal pathology in hemispheres and brainstem (e.g. toxoplasma, viral encephalitis).

APPROACHES TO INVESTIGATION, DIAGNOSIS AND MANAGEMENT OF ENCEPHALOPATHY

Essential blood tests in encephalopathic patients include blood sugar (hypoglycemia), a peripheral blood smear (*Plasmodium falciparum*), full blood count (leukocytosis in bacterial infection, leukopenia in some viral infections).

CSF examination is extremely helpful. If patients are mildly encephalopathic with only a moderate reduction in coma score, LP can proceed without imaging (see Box 10.2). If patients have brainstem signs, hemispheric signs or deep coma, imaging before LP is preferred where possible. A CT scan may reveal the cause in patients with supratentorial or hemispheric signs; it is less helpful in those with posterior fossa (cerebellar) or brainstem signs, in whom magnetic resonance imaging (MRI) is more useful.

In viral encephalitis, the CSF is usually lymphocytic, with some important exceptions (Box 10.4).

If enterovirus infection is suspected, swabs should be taken from the throat and any skin vesicles for enterovirus PCR and culture. In addition, rectal swabs or stool samples should be sent.

Neurophysiologic Investigations

An electroencephalogram (EEG) can be useful in helping determine whether a patient with abnormal behavior has an encephalopathy (with slow waves on the EEG) or has psychiatric illness (EEG normal). Its other role is in determining whether a patient with abnormal movements is in subtle motor status epilepticus. EEGs can also help characterize the nature of a patient's epilepsy. In many tropical settings, the equipment is found in psychiatric, rather than neurologic, departments.

Management of Patients with Encephalopathy and Encephalitis

Management of specific causes of encephalopathy and encephalitis is covered in the relevant chapters:

Bacterial Meningitis Causing Encephalopathy (Chapter 54);
Viral Encephalitis (Chapter 34);
TB Meningitis (Chapter 39);
Cryptococcus (Chapter 84).

Here, management of some of the common complications is considered. Regardless of the underlying etiology, common problems include seizures (Box 10.9) and raised intracranial pressure (Box 10.10).

Fluid management is also an issue in many patients with altered consciousness. Ask about how much fluid a patient has had in recent days and look for reduced skin turgor and sunken eyes indicative of dehydration. Although, in theory, one wants to avoid fluid overload in patients that may have cerebral edema, in practice most patients are dehydrated by the time they get admitted to hospital and fluid restriction may make things worse. Such patients need careful rehydration; the ability to measure central venous pressure can be helpful. If there is papilloedema or clinical signs of raised intracranial pressure and brain shift, mannitol or hypertonic saline are often given. Although there is little evidence for or against many conditions, data from children with cerebral malaria suggest that mannitol gives a transient reduction in pressure, but overuse can ultimately result in raised pressure [4]. A recent, multi-center study in Africa showed that bolus administration of fluid in children with a febrile illness and impaired perfusion (including those with coma) increased mortality [5].

EPILEPSY

Epilepsy is a major cause of neurodiability in the tropics. The incidence is increased as a result of infectious causes, such as cysticercosis, and head trauma and cerebral palsy. Common syndromes include:

- in adults: complex partial seizures with secondary generalizations;
- in children: primary, generalized epilepsies associated with cerebral palsy or developmental delay.

With a targeted history, resources such as brain imaging and EEG can be focused on those who will really benefit from them. In many settings, the only drugs available are phenytoin, phenobarbitone, sodium valproate and carbamazepine. Management is often complicated by local superstition about what causes epilepsy (curses, witchcraft, etc.), and poor access to health care. Severe burns, secondary to falling into an open fire, are a common complication of epilepsy in many parts of the tropics.

The management of status epilepticus is covered above (Box 10.11A) [6].

DEMENTIA AND COGNITIVE IMPAIRMENT

In the tropics, cognitive impairment secondary to chronic infection is more common than in the West.

Infectious disease causes of dementia include: bacteria, such as tuberculosis and syphilis; viruses, such as HIV and subacute sclerosing panencephalitis (SSPE) secondary to measles; cryptococcus and other fungi; and sleeping sickness.

Examination should include looking for posterior cervical lymphadenopathy (Winterbottom's sign in African trypanosomiasis), clues to HIV (Box 10.11A). In SSPE, there is a characteristic myoclonic jerking of the limbs with associated EEG abnormality; CSF protein is usually elevated and the diagnosis is confirmed by high titers of anti-measles antibodies in the serum and CSF.

HEMIPARESIS

As the populations in tropical countries rapidly adopt the unhealthy lifestyle of Western industrialized nations, including smoking and a diet high in saturated fats, they are developing the associated diseases, including hypertension and diabetes, leading to an increased risk of stroke. In addition, stroke in younger people is especially common, possibly because of the increased incidence of HIV.

Infectious space-occupying lesions may cause hemiparesis, altered consciousness, dementia or meningism depending on their etiology, location, speed of onset and the host response (Box 10.11B). They are especially important in the immunocompromised. Brain imaging is an essential investigation in such patients.

PERIPHERAL NERVE AND MUSCLE SYNDROMES

KEY SYNDROMES AND CLINICAL APPROACH

Peripheral nerve syndromes are the most frequent of the neuromuscular disorders encountered. The most common causes are diabetes, HIV, leprosy, drugs, toxins and nutritional deficiencies [although the complete list is much longer (Box 10.12)]. Identifying drug, toxin and nutritional causes rapidly is important as it will obviate the need for extensive investigations, and removal of the offending drug or toxin will stop progression and result in recovery if identified early enough. Similarly, treatment with the appropriate vitamins and nutrients will stop progression and help with recovery, although this may not be complete. Nowadays, and especially in the tropics, HIV, which can affect all areas of the neuro-axis, including nerve and muscle, features high on every list of differential diagnosis. Furthermore, as much of the developing world has a growing middle class who are rapidly adopting Western lifestyles and diets with fast foods and less exercise, diabetes and obesity are an increasing problem with the well-known consequences.

The prevalence of relatively common neuromuscular conditions such as Guillain-Barré syndrome (GBS), chronic inflammatory demyelinating polyneuropathy (CIDP), polymyositis and myasthenia gravis (MG) is unknown in the "tropics". For the most part, there is no reason why they should be more or less prevalent; however, the acute motor axonal neuropathy (AMAN) form of GBS, which is often associated with *Campylobacter jejuni* infection, was, at one time, especially common in China, probably because of the way domestic chickens were housed.

Neuro-anatomically, lesions may involve anterior horn cell (causing a motor neuronopathy), nerve root (radiculopathy), dorsal root ganglion (sensory neuronopathy), brachial or lumbo-sacral plexus, sensory and motor nerve, motor nerve only, sensory nerve only (large and/or small fibers), neuromuscular junction and muscle (Fig. 10.2).

BOX 10.9 Recognition and Management of Acute Symptomatic Seizures in Patients with Central Nervous System (CNS) Infection

- In some severe brain infections (cerebral malaria, viral encephalitis), children in status epilepticus may have subtle motor seizures, rather than generalized tonic clonic seizures. Usually, this is in children who had multiple tonic clonic seizures before hospitalization. Clinical manifestations include twitching of digit, mouth or eyelid, tonic deviation of the eyes, excess salivation and an abnormal respiratory pattern.
- A World Health Organization (WHO) algorithm for management of status epilepticus in children is shown below (taken from [6]). In many settings, facilities for intubation and ventilation are very limited and difficult decisions have to be made about which patients are likely to benefit. Bag and mask ventilation by family members is often employed for hours, and even days, through lack of facilities.

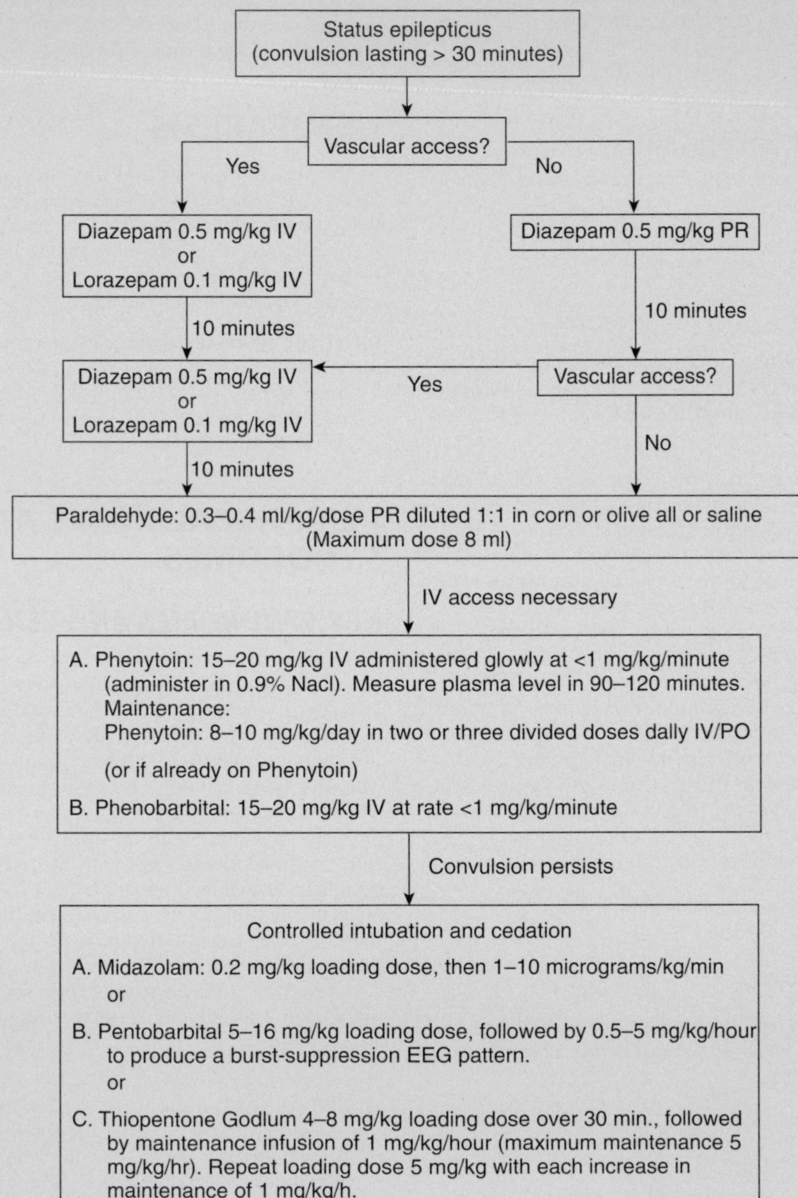

Reproduced with permission from Solomon (Chair), T. and Japanese Encephalitis Working Group. World Health Organization: Japanese encephalitis Clinical Care Guidelines. Geneva: World Health Organization; 2005.

BOX 10.10 Management of Raised Intracranial Pressure in Central Nervous System (CNS) Infections

- Manage the patient with the bed raised at 30°, use pillows to keep the head in the midline position (a bent neck can impair jugular venous outflow thus increasing intracranial pressure).
- Mannitol is often given, but recent studies in cerebral malaria show that after an initial reduction in pressure, repeated mannitol ultimately leads to increased pressure.
- Steroids are often given; their benefit has been shown in tuberculous meningitis (TBM), but the evidence suggests they are probably not beneficial in acute bacterial meningitis or in Japanese encephalitis.
- Raised pressure caused by over-production/impaired absorption of cerebrospinal fluid (CSF; as in cryptococcal meningitis) is treated by shunt insertion and ventriculo-peritoneal shunt.

BOX 10.11A Causes of Chronic Neurological Presentations in the Tropics

Infectious
Sleeping sickness (esp. *Trypanosoma brucei* gambiense)
Tuberculous meningitis
HIV encephalopathy
Toxoplasma gondii and other parasitic space-occupying lesions
Bacterial abscesses
Partially-treated bacterial meningitis
Neurosyphilis
Cryptococcal meningitis and other fungi
Subacute sclerosing pan-encephalitis
Progressive multifocal leukoencephalopathy

Other
Tumors
Chronic subdural hemorrhages
Lead and other heavy metal poisoning
Dementia
Vitamin deficiencies
Drugs
Toxins

PERIPHERAL NEUROPATHIC SYNDROMES

Sensory symptoms include positive symptoms, such as pins and needles (paraesthesiae), burning, sharp shooting or stabbing pains, or a band-like, tight sensation. These co-exist with negative symptoms of numbness (lack of feeling). Patients may also complain of allodynia (pain resulting from non-painful stimulus, such as light touch). Unsteadiness when walking and falling over in the dark or with the eyes closed (rhombergism) suggests significant large fiber or dorsal column involvement. Severe pain and localized edema may suggest a vasculitis process.

BOX 10.11B Infectious and Non-infectious Causes of Central Nervous System (CNS) Space-Occupying Lesions in the Tropics

Infectious
Bacterial abscesses
Tuberculomas
Parasites:
  Protozoa—toxoplasmosis, amoebiasis
  Tremotodes—paragonimiasis, schistosomiasis
  Cestodes—cysticercosis, hydatidosis
  Nemotodes—Ascariasis
Fungi:
  Aspergillosis, blastomycosis, nocardia

Non-Infectious
Tumors and metastases
Hemorrhage

BOX 10.12 Etiology of Peripheral Nerve Disorders

Metabolic: diabetes
Infectious:
  Viral—HIV, polio, HTLV-1, Hepatitis B and C
  Bacterial—*Mycobacterium leprae, Corynebacterium diptheriae, Clostridium botulinum* (strictly causes neuromuscular blockade), Borrelia and brucellosis (cause a radiculopathy)
  Parasitic: *Trypanosoma cruzi* (mainly autonomic dysfunction)
Post-infectious [typically Guillain-Barré syndrome (GBS)]: *Campylobacter jejuni*, Epstein-Barr virus, cytomegalovirus, HIV, malaria
Toxic:
  Drugs—anti-retrovirals (ddI, ddC, D4T), isoniazid, metronidazole, nitrofurantoin, chemotherapy (vinca alkaloids, cis-platin, thalidomide)
  Pesticides—organophosphates
  Heavy metals—arsenic, mercury, thallium, lead
  Organic solvents—acrylamide, carbon disulfide, n-hexane
  Alcohol—direct toxicity + thiamine deficiency
  Biological toxins—ciguatera toxin, brevetoxin B, tetrodoxtoxin
Nutritional:
  Strachan's syndrome (optic + peripheral neuropathy due to multifactorial deficiencies)
  Deficiencies—B1 (thiamine), beri-beri, B3 (niacin), pellagra, B6(pyridoxine), B12 (cyanocobalamin), subacute combined degeneration of the cord, folate, hypophosphatemia, vitamin E, copper
  Note: Excess B6 causes a dorsal root ganglionopathy
Neoplastic: (infiltration of root, plexus, nerve), paraneoplastic (anti-hu antibody)
Genetic: Charcot-Marie-Tooth (CMT1 = demyelinating, CMT2 = axonal)

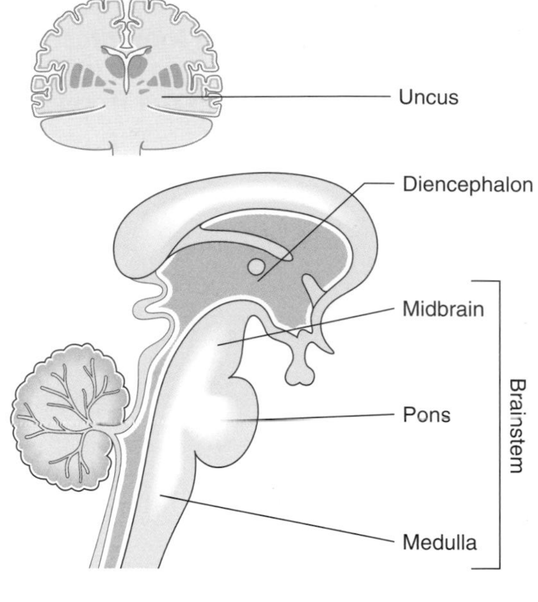

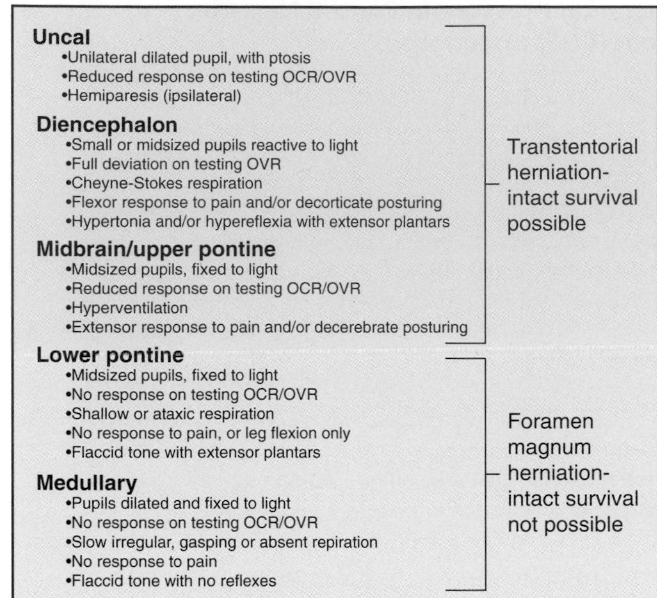

FIGURE 10.2 Sagittal section of brain showing anatomy and key abnormal findings of midline herniation syndromes, and (above) coronal section showing herniation of the uncus of the temporal lobe—this compresses the ipsilateral third nerve (to cause a palsy of CNIII) and the contralateral cerebral peduncle (to cause an ipsilateral hemiparesis). OCR, occulocephalic (doll's eye reflex); OVR, oculovestibular (caloric) reflex.

BOX 10.13 Patterns of Peripheral Nerve Syndromes

1. Symmetrical proximal and distal weakness and sensory loss, e.g. Guillain-Barré syndrome (GBS), chronic inflammatory demyelinating polyneuropathy (CIDP), vasculitis.
2. Symmetrical distal weakness and sensory loss, e.g. diabetes, leprosy, toxic neuropathies (arsenic), nutritional deficiency (thiamine).
3. Asymmetric distal weakness with sensory loss:
   multiple nerve involvement (mononeuritis multiplex), e.g. vasculitis, leprosy, HIV, infiltration (lymphoma, carcinoma, sarcoidosis);
   single nerve involvement, e.g. compression, but may be initial presentation of mononeuritis.
4. Asymmetic distal or proximal weakness without sensory loss, e.g. motor neuron disease (MND), polio, lead toxicity, post-infectious neuralgic amyotrophy, multifocal motor neuropathy with block (MMN).
5. Asymmetric proximal and distal weakness with sensory loss, e.g. GBS, CIDP, plexopathy due to diabetes or malignant infiltration, radiculopathies (e.g. tuberculosis, brucellosis).
6. Symmetric sensory loss without weakness—mainly small fiber involvement (pain and temperature loss), e.g. diabetes, HIV, nutritional deficiencies (thiamine, pyridoxine), toxins (ciguatera).
7. Symmetric sensory loss without weakness—large fiber (joint position and vibration sensory loss) and small fiber, e.g. diabetes, HIV, drugs, nutritional deficiencies, toxins (mercury, thallium).
8. Marked proprioceptive sensory loss, e.g. sensory ganglionopathies owing to Sjogrens, paraneoplastic, B6 toxicity, HIV.
9. Neuropathy with autonomic neuropathy, e.g. diabetes, GBS, *Trypanosoma cruzi* (Chagas'disease), amyloidosis.
10. Neuropathy with cranial nerve involvement, e.g. GBS, diphtheria, Lyme disease, HIV, malignant infiltration, sarcoidosis. (Note: Miller Fisher variant of GBS—ophthalmoplegia, ataxia, areflexia.)

Common motor symptoms include tripping because of weakness of ankle dorsiflexors (foot drop), unable to turn keys or open jars because of weakness of small hand muscles. Note: in GBS, bulbar and respiratory muscle weakness may be life-threatening.

Examination of patients with peripheral nerve disorders or radiculopathies may reveal evidence of a "lower motor neuron syndrome" with wasting ± fasciculation ± weakness in the distribution of a root(s), peripheral nerve(s) or plexus(i) ± depressed or absent reflexes ± sensory loss in the appropriate dermatomes. Note: in small fiber neuropathies, e.g. diabetes, HIV, and sometimes leprosy in the early stages, reflexes may remain present.

In order to reach a diagnosis for peripheral nerve syndromes, the following questions need to answered after the history and examination:

1. Temporal evolution?
   - acute (days up to 4 weeks), e.g. GBS, vasculitis, toxic (drugs such as anti-retrovirals), nutritional deficiency;

- subacute (4–8 weeks), e.g. subacute inflammatory demyelinating polyneuropathy (SIDP), vasculitis, toxins, nutritional deficiency;
- chronic (longer than 8 weeks), e.g. CIDP, toxins, infections (HIV, leprosy), nutritional deficiency.

2. Which parts or combinations of the peripheral nerve system are involved?
   - motor nerves;
   - sensory nerves;
   - autonomic nerves;
   - cranial nerves.

   The pattern of nerve involvement (Box 10.13) gives a clue to the etiology.
3. Clues to genetic neuropathy—family history, onset in childhood with delayed motor milestones. Examination for pes cavus (high arched feet), pes planus (flat feet), clawed toes, scoliosis. Commonest: Charcot-Marie-Tooth (CMT).

MYOPATHIC SYNDROMES

There are a more limited number of myopathic syndromes. The important ones to consider in the tropics include HIV and drugs used to treat it, such as azidothymidine (AZT) (Box 10.14).

BOX 10.14 Etiology of Myopathic Syndromes

Inflammatory: polymyositis, dermatomyositis, inclusion body myositis.
Infectious: HIV, HTLV1, coxsackie, influenza.
Drug-induced: azidothymidine (AZT), statins, corticosteroids, colchicines, chloroquine.
Endocrine: hypothyroidism, Cushing's syndrome.
Genetic: muscular dystrophies, myotonic dystrophy, mitochondrial myopathies.
Toxic: mushrooms (*Tricholoma equestre*), red yeast (*Monascus purpureus*), alcohol, snake venoms (e.g. taipan), spider venom (e.g. redback spider), toluene, organophosphates.

BOX 10.15 Investigations in Neuromuscular Syndromes

Peripheral nerve disorders

Basic facilities:
- full blood count, erythrocyte sedimentation rate;
- renal and liver function;
- fasting glucose;
- HIV;
- venereal disease research laboratory (VDRL) test, *Treponema pallidum* hemagglutination test (TPHA).

High-level facilities:
- $HbA1_c$;
- glucose tolerance test (GTT);
- B12, folate, B1, B6;
- immunoglobulins and protein electrophoresis;
- ANA (antinuclear antibody), dsDNA, ENA (extractable nuclear antibody), ANCA (antineutrophil cytoplasmic antibody);
- anti-neuronal antibodies (paraneoplastic syndromes);
- cryoglobulins;
- CSF examination [in Guillain-Barré syndrome (GBS), elevated protein level with normal cell count (< 5 cells)]; elevated CSF cell count—consider infections such as HIV seroconversion, Borrelia, lymphoma;
- Chest x-ray;
- Nerve conduction studies (NCT) and electromyography (EMG) —useful for categorizing demyelinating [GBS, chronic inflammatory demyelinating polyneuropathy (CIDP), diphtheria] and axonal neuropathies;
- Nerve biopsy—only sensory nerve (sural nerve, superficial peroneal nerve or dorsal ulnar nerve)—looking for vasculitis, demyelinating neuropathy (CIDP), amyloid, malignant infiltration or possible genetic neuropathy if no family history (note: diagnostic yield for biopsy is low in chronic axonal neuropathy and if nerve is normal on neurophysiologic tests);
- genetic tests—PMP 22 duplication for CMT 1a;
- Specific antibody tests—GQ1b (Miller Fisher variant of GBS) anti-MAG (myelin-associated glycoprotein) antibody;
- MRI brachial and lumbosacral plexus—thickened in inflammation and infiltration.

Muscle disorders

Basic facilities:
- creatinine phosphokinase (CPK);
- HIV.

High-level facilities:
- NCT and EMG;
- muscle biopsy;
- MRI muscles—defines affected muscles and helps localize best muscle for biopsy;
- genetic tests, e.g. Duchenne muscular dystrophy, myotonic dystrophy.

Myasthenic disorders

Basic facilities:
- CXR [malignancy in Lambert-Eaton myasthenic syndrome (LEMS)].

High-level facilities:
- acetylcholine receptor antibodies (present in 85% generalized MG, 50% ocular MG). If negative, muscle-specific kinase (MuSK) antibodies;
- voltage-gated calcium channels for LEMS (paraneoplastic or autoimmune);
- NCT and EMG—repetitive nerve stimulation and single fiber studies will discriminate between MG and LEMS;
- tensilon (edrophonium test)—rapid-onset, short-acting cholinesterase inhibitor drug given intravenously. Potential cardiac side effects (bradycardia). Require physical sign such as ptosis or ocular paresis or limb weakness that can be objectively tested before and after (note: botulism may give a false-positive result);
- CT chest (thymoma) in patients with MG;
- positron emission tomography (PET) scan in patients with LES (Lambert Eaton syndrome) (malignancy usually small cell lung cancer).

Symptoms: muscle pain (myalgia) and tenderness, dysphagia, dark urine (myoglobinuria). Weakness suggestive of proximal weakness (difficulty rising from the floor or chair, climbing stairs, reaching above the head). Exercise-induced muscle pains and cramps.

Examination: weakness of neck flexion (sternomastoid muscles), muscles around the shoulder girdle [shoulder abductors (deltoid muscle)], pelvic girdle [hip flexors and extensors (iliopsoas and glutei muscles)]. Reflexes are usually intact except in profoundly weak and wasted muscles, such as quadriceps (knee jerk, L3, L4).

Note: in inclusion body myositis (IBM, the commonest cause of inflammatory myopathy in patients over the age of 50 years), the forearm flexors and quadriceps muscles are selectively affected.

MYASTHENIC SYNDROMES

Symptoms: Painless, fluctuating weakness may affect ocular muscles [with drooping eyelids (ptosis) and double vision (diploplia)], bulbar and respiratory muscles (maybe life-threatening), as well as limb muscles.

Examination: in MG, fatiguability (increasing weakness with exertion, e.g. test shoulder abduction before and after 20 repetitive abduction, adduction movements at the shoulders) is pathognomonic, but in Lambert-Eaton syndrome (LEMS), the opposite occurs. In botulism, there is progressive weakness, starting with ocular muscles with pupillary involvement (fixed pupils), followed by bulbar and limb muscle weakness with autonomic dysfunction as the toxin binds irreversibly with post-synaptic receptors at the cholinergic neuromuscular junction.

Drugs such as penicillamine can rarely cause a myasthenic syndrome. Rare congenital syndromes are also described. Organophosphates, used as pesticides and in chemical warfare, may also be ingested with suicidal intent. This causes an acute cholinergic crisis as a result of acetylcholinesterase inhibition with ocular, bulbar, limb and respiratory weakness.

BOX 10.16 Management of Peripheral Nerve Syndromes

1. Guillain-Barré syndrome (GBS):
   - intravenous immunoglobulin (i.v. IG) (0.4g/kg/day) is the treatment of choice, but has similar efficacy to plasma exchange. Applies to HIV-associated GBS;
   - corticosteroids have no benefit;
   - general supportive measures essential. In the best centers, mortality is 5%. At one year, 15% unable to walk unaided. Poor outcome associated with older age, preceeding diarrheal illness, severity and rapid rate of decline to ventilation, and severe muscle wasting;
   - respiratory failure: inabilty to recognize this insidious complication is a common cause of mortality. Regular monitoring of vital capacity (VC), not peak flow (PEF), is essential. If ≤ 20 ml/kg (1.5 L for average adult), consider ITU (intensive treatment/care unit) transfer and ventilation. Decreased O_2 saturation is a very late sign;
   - swallowing: requires speech and language therapy assessment (SALT). If compromised, consider nasogastric tube;
   - cardiac: brady and tachy arrhythmias and labile blood pressure owing to autonomic involvement. ECG monitoring necessary;
   - thromboembolic: deep vein thrombosis (DVT) prophylaxis;
   - neuropathic pain is common: gabapentin. Avoid amitryptyline in early stages because of autonomic complications;
   - bowel function needs regulation with laxatives;
   - mood: depression common;
   - physiotherapy.
2. Chronic inflammatory demyelinating polyneuropathy (CIDP):
   - Corticosteroids, IV IG, plama exchange all efficacious with 80% response rate.
     - Corticosteroids start with 60 mg/day for 2 weeks, gradually tailing off. If steroid responsive add azathioprine (2 mg/kg) or methotrexate initially 7.5 mg/week + folic acid up to 15 mg/week as steroid-sparing agents.
     - After initial course of IV IG (2 g/kg), subsequent doses and timing depends on patient response.
3. Vasculitic neuropathy:
   - In nerve-specific vasculitis, i.e. no evidence of other organ involvement corticosteroids starting at 60 mg/day gradually tapering dose. If part of a generalized vasculitis add cyclophosphamide. Treat associated infectious etiology such as HIV appropriately. In hepatitis C, high-dose steroids can cause liver decompensation. Liaise with hepatologists.
4. Neuropathic pain:
   - Common problem in diabetes and HIV neuropathies.
     - Drugs to consider:
       - Amitryptyline or nortriptyline. Start dose 10 mg nocte, up to 100–150 mg nocte.
       - Gabapentin. Start dose 100 mg tds, up to 900 TDS.
       - Pregabilin. Start dose 25 mg bd, up to 300 mg bd.

BOX 10.17 Management of Inflammatory Myopathic Syndromes

1. Polymyositis and dermatomyositis
   - Unless indolent: methylprednisolone 500 mg IV for 5 days.
   - Followed by oral prednisolone 1 mg/kg/day (up to 100 mg) single oral dose until creatinine phosphokinase (CPK) reverts to normal and patient improving. Gradual taper with clinical and CPK monitoring. Prescribe treatment for steroid induced osteoporosis.
   - Usually also start immunosuppressants (azathioprine 25 mg/day up to 2.5 mg/kg/day over 6–8 weeks or methotrexate initially 7.5 mg per week with folic acid, as these may take months to become effective).
2. Inclusion body myositis
   - Unless biopsy shows a marked inflammatory infiltrate when a trial of steroids is indicated, at present no treatment of proven significant benefit.

BOX 10.18 Management of Myasthenic Syndromes

1. Myasthenia gravis
   - pyridostigmine:
     - 30mg bd, gradually up to 60 mg x5 daily. Doses > 300 mg rarely required and could cause a cholinergic crisis. Side effects of muscarinic smooth muscle abdominal pain and diarrea respond to propantheline 15–30 mg PRN.
   - corticosteroids:
     - initial starting dose 10 mg alternate days. Note risk of deterioration on starting steroids. Warn patient or, if possible, admit to hospital initially. Aim for 120 mg on alternate days. When in remission, gradually tail off. Prescribe treatment for steroid-induced osteoporosis.
   - steroid-sparing drugs:
     - Azathioprine. Therapeutic effect may not be apparent for 6–12 months. Check thiopurine methyltransferase (TPMT) levels as indicator of risk of hematological side effects. Azathioprine starting at 25 mg/day, increase weekly to 2.5 mg/day. Regular blood tests required every week for 2 months then 3-monthly.
   - Plasma exchange and IV Ig:
     - Used in myasthenic crises or if significant bulbar and respiratory symptoms before starting pyridostigmine and steroids.
   - thymectomy
     - indicated if thymoma present as it is locally invasive. Consensus of benefit in those <45 years age but is controversial in those older than 45 years.

BOX 10.19 Some Clinical Pearls in Approaching Patients with Peripheral Nerve and Muscle Syndromes

- Palpate nerves (ulnar, superficial radial, dorsal ulnar, common peroneal). Causes of thickened nerves: leprosy, chronic inflammatory demyelinating polyneuropathy (CIDP), Charcot-Marie-Tooth (CMT), malignant infiltration.
- Neck flexion weakness is a useful sign. Causes: myopathies, myasthenia gravis, motor neuron disease, myotonic dystrophy, Guillain-Barré syndrome (GBS).
- Demyelinating neuropathy clues: postural tremor, weakness but no wasting, thickened nerves, generalized areflexia.
- Coasting—drug and toxic neuropathies may continue deteriorating for a period despite stopping the offending drug.
- HIV causes a spectrum of neuropathies: distal sensory peripheral neuropathy (DSPN), demyelinating neuropathy (GBS, especially at seroconversion and CIDP), vasculitic neuropathy, dorsal root ganglionopathy and motor neuron syndrome. It is also associated with polymyositis. Drugs used in HIV may cause neuropathy (ddI, ddC, D4T) and myopathy [azidothymidine (AZT)].
- Always enquire about homeopathic, traditional medications and over-the-counter supplements, such as vitamins as these may contain lead, mercury and/or arsenic.

APPROACHES TO INVESTIGATION, DIAGNOSIS AND MANAGEMENT

The approach to investigation and diagnosis of peripheral nerve, muscle and myasthenic disorders depends on whether only basic or more advanced facilities are available (Box 10.15).

The management of peripheral nerve syndromes depends on the diagnosis. Approaches to managing GBS, CIDP, vasculitis and neuropathic pain are shown in Box 10.16. The approach to managing myopathic syndromes is given in Box 10.17, whilst in Box 10.18 an overview of the approach to MG is shown. Some clinical pearls in approaching patients with peripheral nerve and muscle syndromes are given in Box 10.19.

REFERENCES

1. van de Beek D, de Gans, J, Spanjaard L, et al. Clinical features and prognostic factors in adults with bacterial meningitis. N Engl J Med 2004;351:1849–59.
2. van de Beek D, Farrar JJ, de Gans J, et al. Adjunctive dexamethasone in bacterial meningitis: a meta-analysis of individual patient data. Lancet Neurol 2010;9:254–63.
3. Thwaites GE, Nguyen DB, Dung NH, et al. Dexamethasone for the treatment of tuberculous meningitis in adolescents and adults. N Engl J Med 2004; 351:1741–51.
4. Newton CRJC, Crawley J, Sowumni A, et al. Intracranial hypertension in Africans with cerebral malaria. Arch Dis Child 1997;76:219–26.
5. Maitland K, Kiguli S, Opoka RO, et al. for the FEAST Trial Group. Mortality after fluid bolus in African children with severe infection. N Engl J Med 2011;364:2483–95.
6. Solomon (Chair), T. and Japanese Encephalitis Working Group. World Health Organization: Japanese encephalitis Clinical Care Guidelines. Geneva: World Health Organization; 2005.
7. Solomon T. Meningitis. Brain's Diseases of the Nervous System. Oxford: Oxford University Press; 2009:1327–54.
8. Molyneux EM, Walsh AL, Phiri D, et al. Does the use of urinary reagent strip tests improve the bedside diagnosis of meningitis? Trans R Soc Trop Med Hyg 1999;93:409–10.

11 Psychiatric Diseases

Robert C Stewart, Kinke M Lommerse, Atif Rahman

Key features

- **High burden:** Neuropsychiatric conditions account for four of the top ten causes of years lived with disability (YLD) in low- and middle-income countries (LAMIC): unipolar depressive disorder (10.4% of total YLD), alcohol use disorders (3.5%), schizophrenia (2.8%), bipolar disorder (2.4%) [1]
- **Significant mortality:** >800,000 people commit suicide annually, 86% in LAMIC [2,3]
- **Socioeconomic risk factors for mental disorder are highly prevalent:** e.g. poverty, unemployment, low status of women, violence, rapid urbanization, poor education
- **Low priority is given to mental health:** Many LAMIC allocate less than 1% of health expenditure to mental health [2]
- **Human rights abuse:** Stigma may lead to structural discrimination and social exclusion. Low resources and outdated legislation increase risk of human rights abuses
- **Task shifting:** Extreme shortages of trained staff necessitate a Primary Health Care (PHC) approach, with a focus on training and task shifting to lower cadres
- **Cultural factors:** These influence conceptualization and manifestation of mental illness, and provision of care
- **Mental and physical ill-health are strongly interrelated**

GETTING ORGANIZED

For the general clinician:

- Identify staff responsible for psychiatric care and their activities.
- Make a list of local referral options, community support organizations, etc.
- Be familiar with commonly available medications, existing treatment protocols, and the basics of local mental health legislation.

If you are in charge of developing psychiatric services:

- Build relationships with medical colleagues, pharmacies, community organizations and NGOs.
- Provide training to as wide a range of healthcare workers as possible.
- Try to establish basic primary care for mental health using simple protocols for nonpsychiatric healthcare staff and community personnel.

CULTURE AND MENTAL HEALTH

Many aspects of the etiology, presentation, and treatment response of mental disorders are universal. However, it is important to appreciate cultural differences, as failure to do so can lead to misdiagnosis or misunderstanding.

- **Differences in norms of social interaction and nonverbal communication:** e.g. in some cultures, it may not be appropriate for patients to make eye contact with the doctor. This could be misinterpreted as evidence of depression or suspiciousness.
- **Beliefs about the influence of supernatural causes on daily life and disease:** e.g. people may attribute their difficulties to the action of witchcraft, spirits or "ancestors". It is important to differentiate these from psychotic experiences.
- **Cultural sanctioning of certain abnormal states of mind:** e.g. trance/possession states forming part of religious activities, use of psychoactive substances, and sometimes even true psychotic symptoms, may be experienced as beneficial.
- **Differing patterns of help-seeking behavior when emotionally distressed:** It may not be seen as either appropriate or beneficial to seek help for emotional or spiritual issues at "Western" medical facilities. Many people instead seek help from traditional or religious healers. These consultations often provide important social or spiritual meaning lacking in the Western biomedical model, but can also lead to late presentation or poor compliance with medication.
- **"Culturally related syndromes":** Syndromes that are predominantly restricted to localized cultures or populations. These are often anxious or dissociative states precipitated by interpersonal or societal stressors. They may overlap with "Western" diagnostic categories. Management requires understanding of social context and meaning [4]. Examples:
  - **Semen-loss syndrome** (also known as Dhat, sukra prameha, Indian subcontinent): fatigue and other somatic complaints, anxiety and dysphoria, associated with belief that semen has been "lost" in urine.
  - **Genital shrinking syndrome** (Koro, suo-yang, Chinese and Malay populations): belief that penis is retracting into body, associated fear of impotence or death. Epidemics have been reported.
  - **Brain Fag** (West Africa): pain and burning sensations around head and neck; impaired memory and concentration, blurred vision, sleep disturbance. Attributed to overwork or excessive studying.

ASSESSMENT

Basic Principles

- Ensure safety (see management of aggression below).
- Attempt to ensure confidentiality and explain the purpose of the interview.
- If using an interpreter:
  - Speak directly to the patient, with the interpreter repeating your questions.
  - Ask the interpreter to translate exactly what the patient says and not to tell you what he/she thinks was meant.
  - The interpreter may be a useful source of information on cultural issues.

History

- Personal details.
- Who referred and why?
- History of presenting complaint: Establishing accurate timelines for events may prove difficult. Refer to significant dates to help with this.
- Past psychiatric history including self-harm: Be wary of previous diagnoses as these may not be accurate.
- Past medical history: e.g. epilepsy, HIV status, pregnancy.
- Medication history: Note any medications known to have neuropsychiatric side effects (e.g. mefloquine (antimalarial), Efavirenz (antiretroviral)).
- Drugs and alcohol.
- Family psychiatric history.
- Personal history and current social circumstances.
- Forensic history.
- Premorbid personality: Is this new behavior or has the person always acted like this?

Mental State Examination

- Appearance and behavior: Note general physical condition.
- Speech.
- Mood: Subjective and objective.
- Thought: Delusions, e.g. persecutory, grandiose; cognitions typical of depression (guilt, worthlessness, hopelessness); suicidal ideas, thoughts of harm to others.
- Perception: Hallucinations: visual, auditory, other.
- Cognition: Level of consciousness, attention and concentration, orientation, memory.
- Insight.

Informant History and Previous Case Notes

- Informant history is particularly important in psychiatric illness (loss of insight) and high-risk situations.
- Take care not to breach confidentiality.

Physical Examination

- Any suspicion of delirium or organic cause should prompt investigation for infective and metabolic causes, head injury, substance misuse, poisoning, etc.
- People with chronic mental illness are at high risk for physical disorders (e.g. tuberculosis) but tend to be neglected by medical services.
- Improving general health by treating comorbid conditions (e.g. anemia, parasitic infections) can promote recovery.

Investigations

- Conduct focused and appropriate investigations as resources allow.
- If suspicion of delirium or organic cause: blood glucose, full blood count, urea and electrolytes, urinalysis, blood film for malaria, syphilis test, chest x-ray, lumbar puncture, brain CT scan.
- HIV (and CD4) testing with counseling and consent procedures, but can be done without if patient lacks capacity and outcome of test would change management.

BOX 11.1 Common Syndromes

- The acutely disturbed or stuporose patient
- The patient who is sad, worried or has unexplained somatic complaints
- The patient who is misusing alcohol or other substances
- Common psychiatric emergencies (see Boxes 11.2 & 11.3):
  - The aggressive patient
  - The suicidal patient
- The chronically confused patient (see Box 11.5).
- The disturbed child (see Box 11.6)

ASSESSMENT AND DIFFERENTIAL DIAGNOSIS OF COMMON SYNDROMES (Box 11.1)

THE ACUTELY DISTURBED OR STUPOROSE PATIENT

Patients may present with a mixture of symptoms and often an unclear history. Precise diagnosis may be difficult.

Delirium

Altered level of consciousness, impaired attention, disorientation and visual hallucinations. Cause indicated by history and examination, e.g. infective, traumatic, intoxication/poisoning, alcohol withdrawal (**delirium tremens**).

Acute Psychosis

Delusions, hallucinations, muddled thinking and loss of insight. Hostile and suspicious, restless and disinhibited, or withdrawn and stuporose. Many conditions can cause acute psychosis. Characteristic features will guide diagnosis:

- Recent substance misuse (e.g. cannabis, stimulants), some "organic" features (confusion, visual hallucinations) and short duration indicate **drug-induced psychosis** or **withdrawal**.
- Subtle confusion, physical signs or a history suggestive of a temporal relationship between psychiatric and physical symptoms, indicate **organic psychosis.**
- Epilepsy-associated psychiatric syndromes, e.g. **postictal confusion** (minutes/hours), **postictal psychosis** (days/weeks), and **interictal psychosis** (months/years).
- Acute onset in response to a clear stressor (e.g. bereavement, job loss) with no previous episodes suggests a **brief reactive psychosis** (likely to resolve quickly with good prognosis).
- Delusions that one's thoughts or actions are being controlled, auditory hallucinations in the third person, disjointed and "off-the-point" speech (formal thought disorder) and a history of gradual decline in work and social functioning (negative symptoms) suggest **schizophrenia.**
- Onset of psychosis soon after childbirth (mood symptoms or confusion may be prominent) indicates **puerperal psychosis.** Be sure to exclude delirium.

Mood Disorder

- Elated or irritable mood, disinhibition and recklessness (social, sexual, financial), pressured speech, flight of ideas (rapidly jumping between tenuously related topics), grandiose delusions

BOX 11.2 Psychiatric Emergencies – The Aggressive Patient

1. If patient is armed, immediately contact police/security.
2. Reduce external stimulation for the patient but do not become isolated from help. Talk in a calm, reassuring and confident manner. Ensure that you can move away from the patient if needed.
3. Attempt to assess mental and physical state. Ascertain if patient has already been given sedation, and any history of adverse drug reactions or cardiorespiratory problems.
4. Offer oral medication, e.g. diazepam 10–20 mg or lorazepam 1–4 mg and/or chlorpromazine 100–200mg or haloperidol 5–10 mg.
5. If the patient refuses oral medication, it should be given parenterally. Physical restraint may be needed. Gather adequate staff. Hold the patient lying on his/her back, avoid applying force to chest or head. Reassure and give explanation to the patient throughout. End restraint as soon as it is safe.
6. Local practice for parenteral sedation will vary. An acceptable regimen is benzodiazepine (e.g. lorazepam 1–4 mg IM or diazepam 5–20 mg IV) and/or typical antipsychotic (e.g. haloperidol 5–10 mg IM or chlorpromazine 50–200 mg IM). Choose lower dose in physical illness, the elderly, wasted, dehydrated, or treatment-naïve. In case of insufficient response, repeat the dose. Wait at least 10 minutes after IV and 30 minutes after IM dose. In case of drug intoxication/withdrawal, give benzodiazepine only. Monitor for side effects, e.g. respiratory depression, hypotension, acute dystonia.

BOX 11.3 Psychiatric Emergencies – The Suicidal Patient

1. If patient presents having attempted suicide (e.g. hanging, organophosphate poisoning), resuscitate and provide appropriate medical management.
2. Assess the severity of the attempt and risk of repetition. High intent is indicated by perceived lethality of method, extent of preparation and efforts to avoid detection. Risk of repeat also increased if: ongoing suicidal intent, thoughts of hopelessness for the future, mental illness (e.g. depression, schizophrenia), lack of social support, alcohol/substance misuse.
3. Assess stressors (e.g. life events, family or relationship problems) and support structures.
4. Monitor the patient and assess suicide risk regularly.
5. Initiate treatment for underlying mental illness. Problem-solving and engagement of community support can be helpful in life-difficulties. Organize early follow-up.
6. Legal consideration: In some countries, attempting suicide is an offence. The patient's wellbeing should always be the first concern for health workers. If police interference may harm a patient's wellbeing, you may decide not to inform the police.

and mood-congruent auditory hallucinations indicate an **acute manic episode**.

- A history typical of depressive illness (e.g. low mood, loss of pleasure and participation in activities), psychomotor retardation (although may be anxious and agitated), prominent negative content to delusions/hallucinations, and suicidal ideation suggest a **depressive psychosis.** Emaciation and dehydration are signs of the need for urgent treatment.
- Remember that depressive and manic presentations may also have an **organic cause** (e.g. HIV, syphilis, medications).

Other

- Prolonged abnormal posturing and/or alternating immobility and restlessness are features of **catatonia.** Causes include organic (e.g. intracerebral infection) and schizophrenia (in tropical settings, catatonia appears to be a more common presentation of schizophrenia than in Western settings). In severe form, it may be indistinguishable from **neuroleptic malignant syndrome** (a life-threatening side effect of typical antipsychotics).
- Nonpsychotic **acute stress reactions** (e.g. in response to family crisis, exam pressure) may be difficult to distinguish from acute psychosis but are likely to settle with reassurance and removal of the stressor. Such presentations appear to be common in cultures where verbal expression of psychologic distress may be difficult.

THE PATIENT WHO IS SAD, WORRIED OR HAS UNEXPLAINED SOMATIC COMPLAINTS

- Depression and anxiety are common in LAMIC, in part because of the high prevalence of socioeconomic risk factors.
- Even mild–moderate depression/anxiety is associated with significant disability.
- Severe depression can be life-threatening.
- Depression/anxiety often presents with somatic complaints rather than psychologic symptoms. However, questioning usually reveals anxious and depressive symptoms [5].
- Somatic complaints associated with psychologic distress vary across populations, e.g. "all over pain", headache, "heart pain", or tiredness.
- If somatization is suspected, conduct an appropriate medical workup but avoid over-investigation or unnecessary treatment.
- Explore the patient's beliefs about the symptoms and enquire about likely stressors.

  Depressive symptoms: low mood, loss of pleasure in activities, impaired energy and concentration, thoughts of worthlessness, guilt and hopelessness, suicidal ideas and acts, sleep and appetite disturbance.

  Anxiety symptoms: muscle tension, restlessness, dyspnea/hyperventilation, paresthesia, catastrophic thinking, avoidance and escape from triggers of anxiety.

Differential Diagnosis

- Mixed anxiety/depression (most common)
- Major depressive episode
- Bipolar affective disorder (BPAD) (if manic episodes too)
- Panic disorder
- Obsessive compulsive disorder (OCD)
- Post-traumatic stress disorder. People who have experienced severe traumatic events (e.g. war, torture, rape) may present with hypervigilance, re-living experiences ("flashbacks"), emotional "numbing", and avoidance of situations that trigger memories of the trauma
- Conversion symptoms (e.g. pseudoseizures, non-organic paralysis)
- Dissociative state (acute florid behavioral disturbance)
- Symptoms can be secondary to a general medical condition (e.g. chronic infection, thyroid disease, dysrhythmia, diabetes mellitus, etc.).

THE PATIENT WHO IS MISUSING ALCOHOL OR OTHER SUBSTANCES

Alcohol is widely used all over the world and is associated with major health and social harm. The pattern of other drug use (e.g. cannabis, opiates, cocaine, khat) varies between countries, depending on socio-economic, cultural and availability factors. Patients may present with intoxication, withdrawal syndrome, or the psychological, social and physical consequences of excessive use or dependence.

MANAGEMENT OF PATIENTS WITH PSYCHIATRIC ILLNESS

Basic Principles

- Teamwork is essential. Liaise with other specialities and facilities.
- Provide psychoeducation. Encourage hope.
- Follow local mental health legislation. Emergency management of delirium/psychosis should be carried out "in the patient's best interests" on the basis that the patient lacks capacity and is at immediate risk of harm. Longer-term enforced inpatient treatment of mental disorder will require use of the local mental health legislation. Ask for guidance on local policy.
- High risk of harm to self or others may require hospitalization and sometimes specialist services. If lower risk and supportive home environment, outpatient treatment may be preferable.

THE ACUTELY DISTURBED OR STUPOROSE PATIENT

Acute Psychosis

"Typical" antipsychotics are cheap, effective and widely available, e.g. chlorpromazine 100 mg nocte–200 mg three times daily (sedative, risk of photosensitivity), haloperidol 1–5 mg twice a day (increased risk of extrapyramidal side effects [EPSE]). Start on a low dose and review after 1–2 weeks if possible. If acute agitation, consider adjunctive *short-term* benzodiazepine.

If available, consider first-line use of **"atypical" antipsychotics** (less EPSE, may be more effective for negative schizophrenic syndrome, but more expensive), e.g. risperidone 1–3 mg twice daily, olanzapine 10–20 mg once daily.

Typical antipsychotics cause **extrapyramidal side effects** (EPSE). Treat **acute dystonia** with IV/IM anticholinergic, e.g. benzhexol 5 mg. Manage **parkinsonism** or **akathisia** by reducing dose, switching antipsychotic, and prescribing regular oral anticholinergic (e.g. benzhexol 5 mg up to three times daily). **Tardive dyskinesia** is caused by long-term typical antipsychotic use and may be irreversible.

Continued antipsychotic prescription reduces relapse risk. If possible, continue the dose that was effective in treating the acute episode, but tolerability may necessitate a lower dose. Ask whether the patient can access and afford an ongoing supply. Suggested continuation periods are:

- First episode psychosis – continue for 1–2 years.
- Schizophrenia with recurrent episodes – long-term treatment recommended.
- Brief stress-related psychosis – continue for 1 month after recovery.

If poor compliance or patient preference, consider **IM depot antipsychotic,** e.g. fluphenazine decanoate 25–100 mg 4-weekly. Give a small test dose initially. Steady state is achieved after two or three doses, so continue oral medication over this period before tapering down.

Management of chronic psychosis such as schizophrenia must also always include **psychosocial interventions,** e.g. family support and education, occupational therapy, rehabilitation.

Drug-Induced Psychosis

Toxic psychosis will resolve over hours/days with only containment and sedation. If symptoms persist, continue antipsychotic for several months post-recovery and longer if recurrent episodes.

Epilepsy-Associated Psychosis

Optimize seizure control. For psychosis, use haloperidol in preference to chlorpromazine, which lowers seizure threshold.

Catatonia

Investigate organic causes. If associated reduced level of consciousness and autonomic instability, treat on medical ICU if available. Stop antipsychotics and treat with benzodiazepines only. Consider referral for electroconvulsive therapy (ECT).

Acute Manic Episode

Use antipsychotic ± short-term benzodiazepine (as acute psychosis). Gradually reduce dose as patient recovers. If high risk of exhaustion or harm to others, and medication is ineffective, consider referral for ECT.

Bipolar Affective Disorder

If recurrent manic (± depressive) episodes, consider long-term treatment for relapse prevention ("mood stabilizers"). Consider carbamazepine, lithium (requires monitoring), sodium valproate (avoid in women of childbearing age) or atypical antipsychotics. Typical antipsychotics are also widely used in LAMIC although research evidence is lacking [6]. Choose the medication that is accessible and affordable over the long term.

Depressive Psychosis

Ensure adequate hydration and nutrition (IV fluids if needed). Close observation if high suicidal risk. Commence antidepressant ± antipsychotic. Consider referral for ECT.

DEPRESSION, ANXIETY AND SOMATIZATION

Use a "stepped-care approach" [7]:

1. For mild/moderate symptoms, use a psychosocial intervention such as problem solving (see Box 11.4).
2. If somatization is prominent, do not dismiss symptoms but educate the patient about how sadness and worry can cause physical complaints.
3. If psychosocial treatment is ineffective or the symptoms are severe/chronic, consider addition of medication. Advise the patient that antidepressants may take 3 weeks to act and should be continued for at least 6 months after recovery. Tricyclic antidepressants, e.g. amitriptyline 50–150 mg nocte (sedating, dangerous in overdose). Selective serotonin reuptake inhibitors (SSRIs), e.g. fluoxetine 20 mg mane (warn about initial agitation and nausea). Antidepressants are also effective in treating anxiety. SSRIs may worsen anxiety symptoms initially, so start at a low dose and gradually increase.
4. If available, refer for specific psychologic treatment, e.g. cognitive behavioral therapy.

SUBSTANCE DEPENDENCE

1. Engage the person in a non-judgmental manner.
2. Treat any comorbid mental and physical disorder.
3. Encourage recognition of the problem by helping him/her list all the reasons for reducing or stopping the substance use.
4. Decide with the person if he/she wishes to control his/her substance use or to be abstinent. If the substance use has caused severe health or social harm, abstinence is preferred.

BOX 11.4 A Brief Problem-Solving Intervention

1. Explain how difficulties in life can cause emotional problems that, in turn, make it hard to try to solve those difficulties.
2. Together with the patient, define the specific problems (e.g. work, relationships, physical health).
3. Summarize the problems to show you have understood.
4. Choose a problem that seems solvable.
5. With the patient, generate possible solutions and identify consequences of carrying these out. Agree on the best solution. Set specific achievable targets. The patient should lead in generating solutions but assist by helping him/her identify social supports and individual strengths. Ask colleagues for advice on local agencies that might help (e.g. govt., NGO).
6. At subsequent sessions, ask specifically what the person has achieved. If successful, reflect on how this affected the patient's mood. If unsuccessful, assess what the barriers were and consider another solution.
7. Repeat 5 and 6 for another problem.

(Adapted from Patel V, Where There Is No Psychiatrist – A Mental Health Care Manual. London: RCPsych Publications; 2003)

BOX 11.5 The Chronically Confused Patient

- There are rapidly growing numbers of elderly people in LAMIC, with a consequent increase in the prevalence of dementia [8].
- Dementia describes a syndrome of progressive global impairment of cognitive functions, including orientation, memory, language and personality. Associated depression and psychotic symptoms are common.
- The most common causes in the elderly are Alzheimer's type and vascular dementia.
- Particularly if there are atypical features or early onset, consider other causes, some of which may be treatable, e.g.
  - Infective: HIV, neurosyphillis, tuberculosis
  - Chronic subdural hematoma
  - Alcohol-related
  - Vitamin B12 deficiency
  - Hypothyroidism
  - Depression can present with complaints of cognitive impairment ("pseudo-dementia").
- Principles of management:
  - Optimize physical health.
  - Educate family/carers on nature of disorder and discuss how they can keep their relative safe but also active and involved in family life. Be vigilant for signs of carer fatigue.
  - Only if psychosis is present or the person is severely aggressive, consider low-dose typical antipsychotic (e.g. haloperidol). Review for side effects and stop if not beneficial. Avoid sedating medications.

BOX 11.6 The Disturbed Child

1. See the child with the parents/carers, but you may also wish to see child alone (particularly if older). Engage the child in an age-appropriate, non-judgemental manner. Get information from as many sources as possible.
2. History should include: home environment, friends, schooling; recent life changes (e.g. bereavement, orphaning); recent and past physical illness (including epilepsy, birth trauma); developmental history.
3. Observe for neurological or other physical signs. Observe the interaction between child and carers.
4. Differential diagnosis of disturbed behavior includes:
   - New-onset **organic cause** (e.g. meningitis/encephalitis, drug ingestion).
   - **Learning disability** (mental retardation). New troublesome behaviors may indicate comorbid physical disorder (e.g. infection, constipation) or psychiatric condition (e.g. psychosis, depression, reaction to abuse). Alternatively, carers may have sought help because of fatigue.
   - Poorly controlled **epilepsy** or side effects of antiepileptics.
   - Behavioral **reaction to stress** at home or school (e.g. exams, being sent to live with relatives, abuse). Look for symptoms of **depression**.
   - **Psychosis** (rare in children).
   - **Attention deficit hyperactivity disorder (ADHD)** presents with persistent restlessness and inattention at school and home. Onset may follow neurological insult, e.g. cerebral malaria.
   - **Conduct disorder** (repeated rule breaking, criminality, substance misuse) may be associated with poor home circumstances, family breakdown, and suboptimal parenting.
5. Management:
   - Investigate and treat organic causes. If epileptic, review antiepileptic treatment.
   - In learning disability, you may be asked to prescribe "calming" medication. Do not do so unless firm suspicion of comorbid psychosis or dangerously severe aggression (consider low-dose antipsychotic or carbamazepine). Always try non-pharmacological interventions first and regularly review need for medication.
   - If the problems followed an identifiable stressor (e.g. exam stress), educate carers about how children may express distress through their behavior. Encourage family communication and use problem-solving techniques.
   - Help parents and carers identify and access community support.
   - If there is evidence of abuse and/or the child is at immediate risk, involve colleagues and police to help devise a plan that best protects the child.
   - Seek expert review if available.
   - Always offer follow-up.

5. Using the problem-solving approach or other psychologic intervention, help the person avoid relapse by identifying and avoiding triggers (e.g. stress, particular social groups). If available, refer to a community support organization.
6. If someone is alcohol- or drug-dependent, he/she should not abruptly stop use, but taper down gradually to avoid withdrawal symptoms.
7. Treat **alcohol withdrawal/delirium tremens** with a reducing regimen of benzodiazepine, e.g. diazepam 10–20 mg three to four times a day, reducing to stop over 5 days. Give parenteral B vitamins if available, otherwise oral thiamine 100 mg three times a day for 4 weeks.

REFERENCES

1. World Health Organisation. ICD-10: The ICD-10 Classification of Mental and Behavioural Disorders: Clinical Descriptions and Diagnostic Guidelines. Geneva: WHO; 1992.
2. Prince M, Patel V, Saxena S, et al. No health without mental health. Lancet 2007;370:859–77.
3. Lancet Series on Global Mental Health, 2007.
4. Jilek WG. Culturally related syndromes. In: Gelder MG, Lopez-Ibor JJ, Andreasen N, eds. New Oxford Textbook of Psychiatry, Vol. 1. Oxford, UK: Oxford University Press; 2000:1061–6.
5. Patel V, Pereira J, Mann AH. Somatic and psychological models of common mental disorder in primary care in India. Psychol Med 1998;28:135–43.
6. Taylor D, Paton C. The Maudsley Prescribing Guidelines, 10th edn. London: Informa Healthcare; 2009.
7. Patel V, Simon G, Chowdhary N, et al. (2009) Packages of care for depression in low- and middle-income countries. PLoS Med 2009;6:e1000159.
8. Prince MJ, Acosta D, Castro-Costa E, et al. (2009) Packages of care for dementia in low- and middle-income countries. PLoS Med 2009;6:e1000176.

FURTHER READING

Patel V. Where There Is No Psychiatrist – A Mental Health Care Manual. London: RCPsych Publications; 2003.

Patel V, Thornicroft G. Packages of care for mental, neurological, and substance use disorders in low- and middle-income countries: PLoS Medicine Series. PLoS Med 2009;6:e1000160.

Semple D, Smyth R. Oxford Handbook of Psychiatry, 2nd edn. Oxford, UK: Oxford University Press; 2009.

Ungvari G, Kau LS, Wai-Kwong T, Shing NF. The pharmacological treatment of catatonia: an overview. Eur Arch Psychiatry Clin Neurosci 2001;251(Suppl 1);I31–4.

World Health Organisation. mhGAP intervention guide for mental, neurological and substance use disorders in non-specialised health settings: mental health Gap Action Programme (mhGAP), 2010.

12 ENT

Charlotte M Chiong, Jose M Acuin

Key features

- Hearing impairment is the most common cause of ear, nose and throat (ENT) disability worldwide
- Chronic otitis media is the most common cause of preventable hearing loss in the world
- Cancers of the head and neck also account for significant global morbidity and mortality
- Cleft lip and palate often go unrepaired in many resource-limited areas
- Over 70% of patients with acute rhinosinusitis improve after 7 days, with or without antimicrobial therapy
- The deep fascial spaces of the head and neck are potential cavities and can be involved in infections that extend from adjacent structures such as the teeth, tonsils, lymph nodes, salivary glands and soft tissues

GLOBAL BURDEN OF ENT DISEASES

The burden of ear, nose and throat (ENT) disorders is high in resource-limited countries due to the scarcity of otolaryngologists (ENT specialists), a high prevalence and severity of many infections of the head and neck, and the impact of immunocompromising disorders (HIV, malnutrition) and regional behavioral influences (betel nut chewing, cigarette smoking). Hearing impairment is the most common cause of ENT disability worldwide. Approximately 80% of the almost 300 million with disabling hearing impairment live in low- and middle-income countries [1]. According to Alberti [2], 50% of all disabling hearing losses are preventable by vaccination programs or better hearing protection from noise exposure. Cancers of the head and neck also account for significant morbidity and mortality. In Southeast Asia, 13% of all cancers involve the mouth or oropharynx [3]. Oropharyngeal cancer is more common in developing than developed countries, and the prevalence of oral cancer is particularly high among men. Cleft lip and palate often go unrepaired in many resource-limited areas.

DEAFNESS AND HEARING IMPAIRMENT

Disabling hearing impairment is defined by the World Health Organization (WHO) as hearing thresholds that fall above 30 db in the better ear in children, and thresholds that fall above 40 db in the better-hearing ear in adults. Hearing loss can be either congenital or acquired. The most common acquired conditions include chronic otitis media, ototoxicity, noise-induced hearing loss, presbycusis, and sudden hearing loss from trauma or specific infections such as scrub typhus (Box 12.1).

Basic ear evaluation includes first the inspection of the pinna and postauricular areas to look for swelling or fistulae, followed by examination with adequate illumination through a head mirror, head light, otoscope or otomicroscope. A 512-Hz tuning fork can detect the presence of either a conductive hearing loss (Weber's test lateralizes to worse ear with Rinne test negative or air conduction [AC] < bone conduction [BC]) or a sensorineural hearing loss (Weber's lateralizes to the good ear and Rinne test is positive or AC>BC).

Audiologic evaluation is performed when equipment is available and will usually include:

- OAE (otoacoustic emissions) – A pass or refer result is detected by clicks from an ear probe causing outer hair cell vibration-induced "echoes" to be detected by a sensitive microphone and mostly used for newborn hearing screening.
- PTA (pure tone audiometry) – From age 3 years, sound stimulation given through a headphone or an earphone is used to detect the threshold (minimum level at which sound is detected) in the frequencies 1 kHz, 2 kHz, 4 kHz, 8 kHz, 500 Hz and 250 Hz for both bone-conducted and air-conducted sounds.
- Speech audiometry – monosyllables and two-syllable words in a standardized word list are used to check for ability to understand speech.
- Tympanometry – measures pressure in the middle ear and checks the compliance of the tympanic membrane. Maximal compliance at atmospheric pressure is type A and found in normal ears; decreased compliance at atmospheric pressure from ossicular chain fixation is type As; increased compliance at atmospheric pressure in ossicular chain dislocation is type Ad; flat type B is when there is middle ear fluid or when there is a tympanic membrane perforation and type C is produced by peak compliance at negative pressure with Eustachian tube dysfunction.
- Auditory brainstem response (ABR) testing shows tiny brainstem waves (I–V) from more central auditory centers produced in response to sounds like tone bursts or clicks, allowing detection of hearing loss in both adults and children. It is also valuable as a screening tool for retrocochlear lesions or tumors in the cerebellopontine angle.
- Auditory steady state response (ASSR) testing – see Box 12.2.
- Genetic testing for hearing loss is now offered in more developed countries, followed by genetic counseling. This testing is not readily available in most developing countries.
- Radiologic imaging may include mastoid x-rays (Towne's view, Law's and Stenger's views) that can detect mastoiditis and the presence of cholesteatoma (Fig. 12.1) which is still common in the tropics. Complicated chronic suppurative otitis media is ideally investigated with computed tomography (CT) of the temporal bone to assess for labyrinthine fistula or facial canal erosions in cases of facial paralysis and tegmental erosion that might suggest intracranial involvement (Fig. 12.2); gadolinium-enhanced magnetic resonance imaging (MRI) gives soft tissue details in the internal auditory canals and cerebellopontine angles, and in cases of asymmetric hearing loss can rule out a vestibular schwannoma or other rare lesions such as hydatid cyst (Fig. 12.3). A three-dimensional CISS MRI of the inner ear may

BOX 12.1 Common Causes of Acquired Deafness

- Conductive hearing loss
  - Acute otitis media, otitis media with effusion, chronic otitis media
- Sensorineural hearing loss
  - Severe hypoxia
  - Lassa fever
  - Sepsis neonatorum
  - Bacterial meningitis
  - Viral infections, e.g. mumps
  - Hyperbilirubinemia
  - Noise-induced damage
  - Autoimmune sensorineural hearing loss
  - Presbycusis
  - Head trauma
  - Meniere's disease
  - Scrub typhus
  - Sudden idiopathic sensorineural hearing loss
  - HIV/AIDS, tuberculosis
  - Ototoxicity
  - Tumors, hydatid cyst in the cerebellopontine angle

BOX 12.2 Pediatric Note

Auditory steady state response (ASSR) testing uses pure tones modulated in amplitude and frequency so that stimulation at 120 db may produce responses in the majority of those without response to brainstem auditory evoked response (BAER) testing, and provides frequency-specific information for objective audiometric threshold estimation helpful in fitting infants and very young children with appropriate hearing aids.

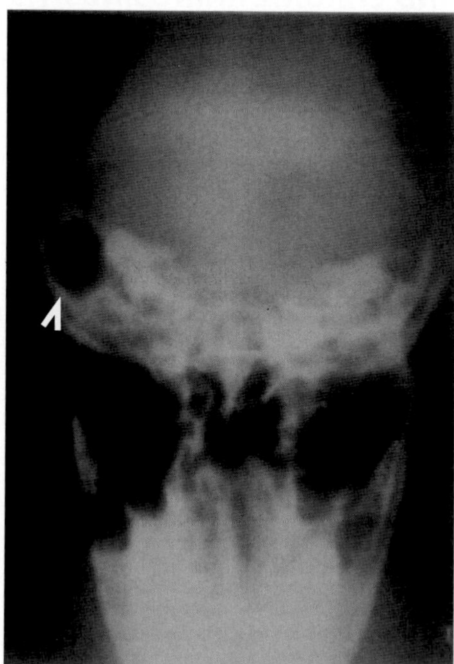

FIGURE 12.1 Towne's view x-ray of mastoiditis with radiolucent appearance of right mastoid cholesteatoma (arrowhead).

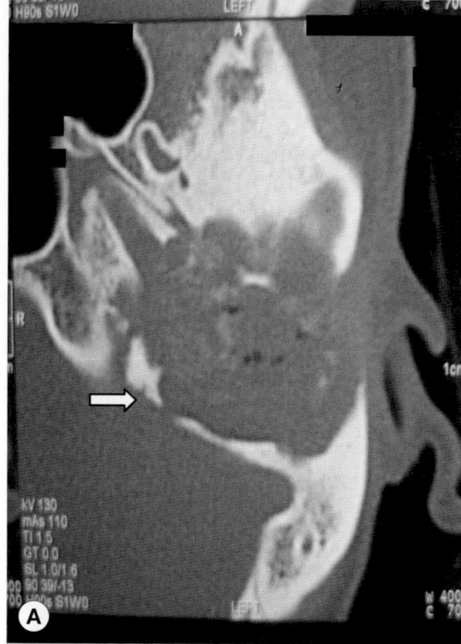

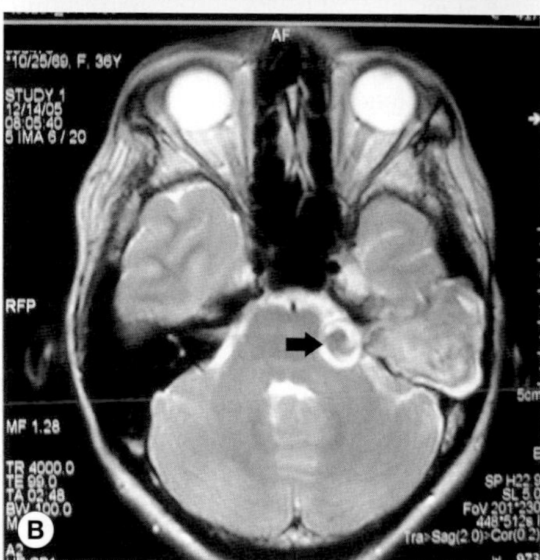

FIGURE 12.2 Extensive cholesteatoma with erosion in the left temporal bone seen on CT scan (**A**) suggesting intracranial extension (white arrow) and on MRI (**B**) shows a cerebellar extension (black arrow).

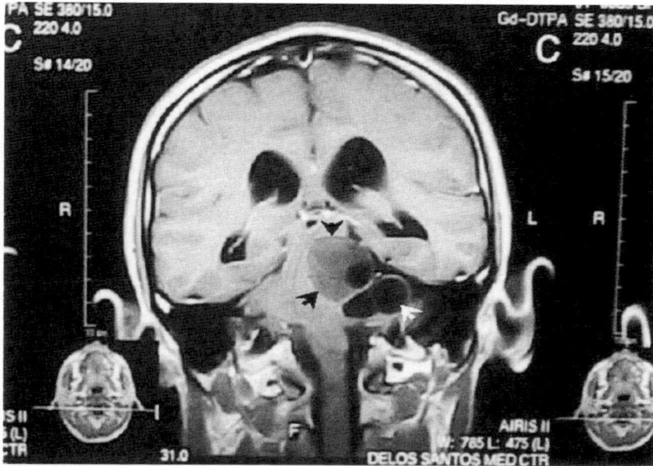

FIGURE 12.3 MRI showing a complex cerebellopontine angle hydatid cyst in a 30-year-old Filipino male with unilateral progressive hearing loss (black arrow).

demonstrate cochlear obliteration (following meningitis) or inner ear malformations such as cochlear absence or cochlear nerve aplasia in cases of congenital hearing loss.

Chronic otitis media is the most common cause of preventable hearing loss in the world [4]. Extracranial complications include subperiosteal abscess and labyrinthine fistula, facial weakness, foul ear discharge, postauricular swelling and abscess formation. Sequelae may include facial paralysis, profound deafness, and intracranial complications, including meningitis.

Patients with chronic suppurative otitis media should be treated with antibiotics. Topical antibiotics can have some benefit in the setting of an open communication to the middle ear, but ototoxic drugs (for example, topical aminoglycosides) should be avoided in this setting. A topical fluoroquinolone such as ciprofloxacin, or oral amoxicillin–clavulanic acid are commonly administered agents [4–7]. If intractable to medical treatment or when there is evidence of cholesteatoma, surgery is indicated. For non-cholesteatomatous ears, a Cochrane review revealed low-quality and scanty literature comparing tympanoplasty versus tympanoplasty with mastoidectomy in discharging ears [8]. In the setting of a cholesteatoma, a canal-wall-down mastoidectomy or open cavity technique may be indicated. There is level 3 evidence of improved or equivalent hearing outcomes with unstaged rather than staged tympanoplasty [9,10].

Given the tremendous surgical backlog in resource-limited countries because of the lack of ear surgeons, some countries hold "surgical ear camps" like the BRINOS (British Nepal Otological Surgery) and Rural Ear Foundation in Thailand.

Other Causes of Deafness

Ototoxicity: Many ototoxic drugs are routinely used in resource-limited settings, including streptomycin (used for tuberculosis treatment), neomycin, kanamycin and gentamicin.

Platinum-containing chemotherapy with cisplatin or carboplatin and radiotherapy for neck tumors may also cause hearing loss [11,12].

Noise-induced hearing loss can be caused by exposure to intense sounds, and if caused by a broadband noise such as in industrial settings, a characteristic 4-kHz notch or dip is noted on audiometric testing. Prevention by hearing conservation programs should include education on the risks of hearing loss with noise exposure, the effective use of hearing protection devices, monitoring hearing and noise levels at the workplace, and minimizing the duration of exposure.

Presbycusis is characterized as decreased high-frequency hearing sensitivity usually beyond the age of 50 years, typically involving both ears. Central auditory deficits also increase with age [13].

Sudden hearing loss should be considered an emergency since early treatment may reverse the loss. Sudden hearing loss is defined as a hearing loss of >30 db over 72 hours and affected patients may present with aural fullness although otoscopic findings are normal. Ideally, an MRI with gadolinium should be performed to evaluate for a retrocochlear lesion. An empiric trial of prednisone at 1 mg/kg/day for 2 weeks followed by a taper, or its methylprednisolone equivalent, has shown benefit in some patients. A study showed the group given steroids improved significantly, with 5 : 1 relative odds of >50% recovery [14]. A steroid-effective zone of 40–90 db (moderate to severe) loss was defined, with best results if treated within 10–14 days of onset. Empiric addition of acyclovir or valacyclovir did not improve results [15,16] Intratympanic steroids are now being tried in some centers, and initial results report this to be promising as a salvage treatment for patients who fail to respond to initial systemic steroids administration [17]. There are reports of acute hearing loss and otalgia following scrub typhus infection [18]. Scrub typhus is an acute febrile disease secondary to infection by an obligate intracellular bacterium, *Orientia tsutsugamushi*, transmitted via *Leptotrombidium* chigger mite bites. Symptoms include myalgia, diffuse lymphadenopathy, fever, eschars, and erythematous maculopapular rashes. Complications include pneumonia, myocarditis, meningitis, hepatitis, acute renal failure and hearing loss. Hearing loss can affect up to a third of those with scrub typhus. Severe otalgia, initially paroxysmal and intermittent, becomes persistent for several hours. Hearing loss and tinnitus tend to appear 2 weeks after the onset of scrub typhus. Otalgia appears during the first week. Hearing loss can be permanent.

AUDITORY REHABILITATION

Aural rehabilitation requires identification of the presence, type and degree of hearing loss. For hearing loss between 40 db and 85 db, conventional hearing aids provide the greatest benefit. However, the cost of hearing aids is prohibitive in most resource-limited settings, although low-cost solar battery options are being developed. For severe to profound sensorineural hearing loss, vibrotactile devices or cochlear implants may be helpful, but are usually not feasible or available.

CLEFT LIP AND PALATE

The global incidence of oral clefts has been variably reported as 1 per 500 to 1000 live births, making it one of the most common congenital anomalies [19]. Gender and race differences have been reported, and Asians in particular are at high risk. A 1997 study showed the incidence of oral clefts in the Philippines to be about 2 per 1000 live births [20]. Etiologic risk factors include micronutrient deficiency, maternal exposure to tobacco smoke, alcohol, corticosteroids, exogenous estrogen, organic pollutants and occupational chemicals. History and physical examination include a search for other possible abnormalities, as 300 syndromes (Stickler syndrome: Pierre Robin sequence plus myopia or retinal problems, velocardiofacial, Treacher–Collins, fetal alcohol, oro-facial-digital type) have been associated with cleft lip and palate. Evaluation and treatment is best done by a multidisciplinary team composed of an oral surgeon, otologist, speech pathologist, psychologist and education specialist. Genetic counseling of high-risk families is important. The timing of surgical repair should be emphasized: repair cleft lips at 3 months (with myringotomy and ventilation tube placement), palatoplasty at 18 months, speech intervention at 3–4 years, velopharyngeal surgery at 4–6 years, alveolar bone grafting at 9–11 years, nasal reconstruction at 12–18 years, and orthognathic surgery, when needed, after 16 years of age.

NOSE AND THROAT INFECTIONS

ACUTE AND CHRONIC RHINOSINUSITIS

Infections of the paranasal sinuses (ethmoid, maxillary, frontal and sphenoid sinuses) may occur as a result of contiguous infections (e.g. rhinitis, dental abscesses). Acute sinusitis is produced by inflammatory thickening of the mucoperiosteal lining of the sinus cavities and increased mucus secretions. Mucosal congestion and edema, occurring in the areas surrounding the sinus openings, result in blocked sinus drainage and accumulation and stasis of sinus secretions. Pressure on the nerve endings in the sinus mucosa produces facial pain and fullness. Suppurative complications, including meningitis and orbital cellulitis, can occur. Acute sinusitis may evolve into chronic sinusitis. In the latter condition, mechanical obstruction of sinus drainage occurs from persistently swollen mucosa, polyp formation, bony protuberances, nasal septal deviations or spurs. Longstanding infection can lead to squamous metaplasia of the normally cuboidal and columnar epithelia of the paranasal sinuses, leading to loss of functional mucociliary transport and thickening of sinus mucus.

Fungal sinusitis may manifest along a spectrum ranging from localized, largely asymptomatic colonization of the nasal and paranasal sinus mucosa, to chronic invasive rhinosinusitis with granuloma formation. Severe acute invasive rhinosinusitis is usually seen among immunocompromised patients, and is characterized by a fulminant, necrotizing process.

It is difficult to distinguish bacterial from viral rhinosinusitis. Anterior rhinoscopy, using a nasal speculum and sufficiently bright and focused illumination, may demonstrate purulent discharge from the middle meatus (next to the middle turbinate) in either condition. Transillumination in a darkened room, using a penlight held against the skin overlying the frontal or maxillary sinuses, may suggest acute sinusitis if there is unequal transillumination due to fluid accumulation. Sinus x-rays, CT and nasal endoscopy are recommended when the condition fails to respond to therapy, when the diagnosis or the extent of disease is in question, or when surgery is being planned. Paranasal sinus x-rays (Waters', Caldwell's and lateral views) or ultrasound may demonstrate fluid accumulation inside the maxillary sinus (x-rays must be taken with the patient upright) or varying degrees of sinus opacification or thickening of the sinus mucoperiosteum. In patients with chronic rhinosinusitis, nasal endoscopy using a 0 degree Hopkins rod telescope may be performed to more closely inspect the mucosa of the middle turbinate and middle meatus and visualize small polyps. This is an office procedure that requires minimal-to-no topical anesthesia. CT of the sinuses can better demonstrate the extent of sinus disease, bony and soft tissue abnormalities that obstruct critical nasal and sinus passageways, and soft tissue masses, such as sinus mucoceles, polyps and cysts. Bacterial culture, taken either by an endoscopically guided swab of the middle meatus or by a puncture of the maxillary sinus antrum, is considered the reference standard in diagnosing acute bacterial rhinosinusitis, but is only used when medical treatment fails. *Streptococcus pneumoniae* and *Haemophilus influenza* are the most commonly isolated organisms, although anaerobes may also be present [21].

Over 70% of patients with acute rhinosinusitis improve after 7 days, with or without antimicrobial therapy. Thus, patients with mild fever and facial pain should be given analgesics and observed regularly. About seven patients must be treated with antibiotics to achieve one more clinical cure beyond spontaneous resolution [22]. Ampicillin, amoxicillin, trimethoprim–sulfamethoxazole, macrolides and cefaclor, given for 7 to 14 days, have all been shown to be effective treatment for most cases of acute bacterial rhinosinusitis [23]. The final choice should be guided by local bacterial prevalence and antibiotic resistance patterns. Diarrhea and adverse events are 80% more common in patients who receive antimicrobials. If symptoms fail to resolve with antibiotics, the diagnosis should be reconfirmed, other illnesses should be excluded, risk factors should be addressed, and antibiotic treatment extended. For patients with chronic rhinosinusitis, antibiotics are often given for 4 weeks or more. If inhalant allergies are known or suspected, intranasal steroids may be prescribed to decrease mucosal inflammation associated with acute and chronic rhinosinusitis [24]. Surgery is indicated for extranasal spread of infection, evidence of mucocele or pyocele, fungal sinusitis or obstructive nasal polyposis, and is often performed in patients with recurrent or persistent infection not improved by drug therapy [25]. Surgical treatment of chronic rhinosinusitis is performed with fine surgical instruments under endoscopic control and is aimed at removing abnormal bone and mucosa in the natural sinus ostia and other critical sinus passageways to improve ventilation and preserve mucociliary function. The success of this procedure in resolving sinusitis is supported by evidence of variable quality [25] and depends on specific sinus conditions, the surgeon's expertise, and the patient's compliance with postoperative care.

Granulomatous Involvement of the Head and Neck

Granulomas of the head and neck can occur as single or multiple lesions in virtually any area. Mycobacterial pathogens are the leading cause. Although becoming increasingly rare, leprosy produces characteristic nodules and/or leonine deformities of the soft tissues of the face. Tuberculosis of the head and neck can result in granulomas of the face, salivary glands, oral, pharyngeal and laryngeal cavities, ear and temporal bone, nose and paranasal sinuses. Tuberculous infection of the lymph nodes of the neck (scrofula) can present as a slow-growing mass that then can rapidly enlarge, leading to tenderness and suppuration. Chronic recurrent breakdown of the overlying skin can results in multiple draining sinuses and scarring. Syphilitic involvement of the head and neck can be expressed as necrotizing chancres of the mouth, nose and paranasal sinuses, granulomas of the oropharynx, nose and nasopharynx, draining buboes of the neck, intracranial gummas, and cranial and peripheral neuropathies. Vertigo precipitated by loud sounds can be caused by syphilitic fixation of the stapes footplate to the oval window.

SALIVARY GLAND INFECTIONS

Bacterial infections of the parotid, submandibular and sublingual salivary glands may result from oral or dental infections. Acute enlargement of intraparotid nodes may be due to many viruses and can lead to swelling and secondary suppuration of the parotid gland. (Primary viral infections of the parotid gland are discussed elsewhere.) Intraductal and parenchymal edema and congestion can lead to stasis and accumulation of secretions and blockade of salivary drainage. The resulting swelling, pain and tenderness can produce trismus and dysphagia. Infections of the salivary glands are usually treated empirically. For fluctuant, painful swellings or for patients who do not respond to empiric antimicrobial therapy, aspiration or open drainage with culture and sensitivity testing of the purulent discharge may be required. The most common organisms involving salivary glands include *Staphylococcus aureus* and *Streptococcus pyogenes*. Treatment should include antibiotic therapy directed against these bacteria, anti-inflammatory agents and adequate hydration.

DEEP FASCIAL SPACE INFECTIONS

The deep fascial spaces of the head and neck are potential cavities and can be involved in infections that extend from adjacent structures such as the teeth, tonsils, lymph nodes, salivary glands and soft tissues. Involvement and abscess formation and edema can result in obstruction (swallowing and breathing), pain, tenderness, trismus and neck stiffness. Visible soft tissue swelling can result from infections of the peritonsillar, parapharyngeal, parotid, submandibular, suprahyoid, periauricular and masseteric spaces. Peritonsillar abscess formation, also known as Quinsy, presents with unilateral swelling of the soft palate above the tonsil. Abscess formation beneath the floor of the mouth, called Ludwig's angina, produces tense and tender swelling behind the chin and between the angles of the jaw. Vincent's angina, or trench mouth, presents with localized or multiple necrotic mucosal ulcerations and foul breath. Retropharyngeal and retroesophageal abscesses produce dysphagia and neck rigidity. Mediastinal spread is a potential complication that can lead to sepsis; rupture may lead to respiratory obstruction. Erosion of the great vessels of the neck can lead to catastrophic hemorrhage. Soft tissue lateral views of the head and neck may aid in diagnosing retropharyngeal and retroesophageal abscesses. Purulent material that is drained or aspirated from deep neck abscesses should be submitted for culture and sensitivity studies and the results used to adjust the selection of antibiotics. Treatment should include aggressive antibiotic therapy against both Gram-positive and Gram-negative organisms (including anaerobes), prompt incision and drainage of abscesses, and adequate nutrition and fluid therapy. Respiratory obstruction should be proactively addressed with consideration of artificial airways.

CYSTICERCOSIS

Cysticercosis can present as nontender, solitary or multiple subcutaneous or submucosal nodules in the face, eyes, neck, nose, mouth, tongue and pharynx [26,27].

ORAL ULCERS

Lesions of the mucosa of the lips, gums, tongue, floor of mouth, buccal cavity, palate and pharynx can be secondary to inflammatory, traumatic, neoplastic, metabolic, immunologic, hematologic and idiopathic causes. Different etiologies can be expressed in similar ways. For instance, infections, malignancies, autoimmune disorders and blood dyscrasias can all produce painful mouth ulcers. Oral disease caused by fungal, bacterial or viral infections can also be commonly found in immunocompromised hosts. For instance, oral lesions are strongly associated with HIV infection such as pseudomembranous oral candidiasis, oral hairy leukoplakia, HIV gingivitis and periodontitis, Kaposi sarcoma and non-Hodgkin lymphoma. All mucosal ulcers of the oral cavity that do not heal or do not show signs of healing within 2 weeks warrant further investigation. Microscopic examination of scrapings from the ulcer bed may demonstrate fungi such as *Candida albicans*. Tissue biopsies are required to assess for malignant involvement. Treatment is directed against the etiology of the ulcer, or symptomatically if a cause is not identified.

CANCRUM ORIS

Noma (cancrum oris, stomatitis gangrenosa) is a serious and often fatal condition characterized by a quickly spreading orofacial gangrene in children, caused by a combination of malnutrition, debilitation because of concomitant diseases (measles), and intraoral infections. Cancrum starts as a stomatitis followed by ulceration, spreads rapidly through orofacial tissues, and often has a blackened necrotic center. Management entails antisepsis, wound debridement, antibiotics (intravenous penicillin and metronidazole) and nutrition. Reconstructive plastic surgery is often required in survivors.

LEISHMANIASIS

Mucocutaneous leishmaniasis (MCL) or **espundia** is an occasional complication of New World cutaneous leishmaniasis caused by *L. (viannia) braziliensis* (New World CL). Naso-oropharyngeal symptoms may appear several years after resolution of the primary cutaneous lesion(s). Manifestations include chronic nasal symptoms, especially of the anterior nasal septum (leading to development of the characteristic "tapir nose") and progressing to extensive naso-oropharyngeal destruction. Secondary bacterial (or fungal) infections and associated problems are common [28].

MYIASIS

Human myiasis is caused by infestation of human tissue by dipteran larvae and can involve the head and neck (e.g. New World botfly, *Dermatobia hominis*), or eyes, nose, ears and pharynx (*Oestrus ovis*, the sheep nasal botfly). Pseudo-furuncles in dermal myiasis may be present. Treatment involves mechanical removal.

HALZOUN

Halzoun is due to infection of the nasopharyngeal tract by the pentastomid *Linguatula serrata*. The worm attaches to the back of the throat, causing pain and swelling. It is acquired by eating raw liver. Swallowed leeches and the pentastomid *L. serrata* can also cause this condition. Pentastomiasis due *to Armillifer armillatus* was very common in the snake-eating aboriginal forest dwellers of Malaysia [29].Similar infections in human due to *Prosthodendrium* and *Phaneropsulus* in Thailand may be due to the regional habit of eating intermediate host dragonfly nymphs.

HEAD AND NECK NEOPLASMS

Neoplasms of the head and neck may arise from skin, mucosa, soft tissues and salivary glands. Table 12-1 lists the most commonly encountered benign and malignant tumors in the different regions of the head and neck.

TABLE 12-1 The Most Commonly Encountered Benign and Malignant Tumors in Different Regions of the Head and Neck

	Benign	Malignant
Nose and paranasal sinuses	Nasal polyp, hemangioma, inverting papilloma, mucocele, dermoid, meningioma	Squamous cell carcinoma; esthesioneuroblastoma; sarcomas
Face	Nevus, epidermal inclusion cyst; sebaceous cyst	Squamous cell carcinoma; basal cell carcinoma; malignant melanoma
Oral cavity	Squamous papilloma; mucocele; torus mandibularis/palatinus; ameloblastoma, odontogenic cyst	Squamous cell carcinoma; sarcoma
Pharynx	Nasopharyngeal angiofibroma	Nasopharyngeal carcinoma; lymphoma
Larynx	Vocal fold nodules, polyps and cysts; laryngeal papilloma	Squamous cell carcinoma
Ears	Aural polyp; osteoma; acoustic neuroma	Squamous cell carcinoma
Neck	Dermoid, branchial cleft cyst, thyroglossal duct cyst; cystic hygroma; lymphangioma; goiter	Lymphoma; metastatic carcinoma; thyroid carcinoma
Salivary glands	Pleomorphic adenoma; Warthin's tumor	Adenoid cystic carcinoma; mucoepidermoid carcinoma

BENIGN NEOPLASMS

By far the most common nasal neoplasm is a mucosal polyp that develops in a patient with chronic rhinosinusitis. Polyps are edematous outpouchings of nasal mucosa covered by squamous epithelium and originate from the ethmoids and other sinuses. Untreated, they can fill the nasal vault up to the vestibule, widen the nasal dorsum, and result in severe obstruction to breathing and smelling. By obstructing the natural ostia of the sinuses and destroying bone, they often perpetuate the infectious process. Hemangiomatous polyps and hemangiomas often present with epistaxis or nosebleed. An inverting papilloma may present like a nasal polyp but aggressively proliferates, invades bony partitions, and may harbor carcinoma.

Benign neoplasms of the face and oral cavity are usually slow growing, well circumscribed, and produce few symptoms. An ameloblastoma is a tumor of the enamel organ of the tooth and presents as a uni- or multicystic mandibular mass. It can grow to enormous size and destroy significant portions of the lower jaw. Odontogenic cysts, such as dentigerous cysts and radicular cysts, are derived from dental tissue and occur in either the upper or lower jaw as solitary small or medium-sized masses.

Nasopharyngeal angiofibromas are highly vascular tumors that arise from the superolateral wall of the nasopharynx. They are found exclusively in adolescent males and present with recurrent, at times massive, epistaxis. They can spread to the adjacent nasal vault, ethmoid sinuses, pterygomaxillary fossa and infratemporal fossa, sphenoid and base of the skull. Branches of the internal maxillary artery may give rise to feeding vessels.

Benign neoplasms of the larynx include nodules, polyps and cysts that arise from the true vocal folds or adjacent tissues. These are single, circumscribed masses that may lead to hoarseness and subtle voice changes. They are associated with longstanding voice misuse or abuse. Laryngeal papilloma, either juvenile or the adult type, are usually multiple pedunculated masses arising from any area of the larynx, with a propensity to spread to the tracheobronchial tree. They are associated with human papillomavirus infection acquired either while passing through the birth canal of an infected mother or through intimate contact later in life.

Cervical lymph node enlargement associated with infections of the upper respiratory tract, oral cavity, scalp and face occurs frequently in children. Cystic hygroma and lymphangioma are both malformations of the lymphatic channels of the neck that present as solitary, soft, painless, poorly demarcated masses in young children. The malignant counterpart is lymphoma, either Hodgkin or non-Hodgkin, characterized by massive multiple enlargement of lymph nodes on the posterior triangle of the neck.

Benign neoplasms constitute 75% of salivary gland tumors, of which pleomorphic adenoma of the parotid gland is the most common. Other benign salivary gland tumors include Warthin's tumor, which occurs mostly in males at the fourth to fifth decade of life.

MALIGNANT NEOPLASMS

Squamous cell carcinoma is the most common malignancy of the head and neck. Depending on the stage at diagnosis, degree of differentiation, and the site of origin, it can present early or late, destroy overlying bone, invade adjacent soft tissues, extend intracranially or spread to the submandibular and deep jugular chain of neck nodes. The mass is usually fungating and bleeds easily to touch. Tobacco smoking and chewing, alcohol intake, infection by Epstein-Barr virus or human papillomavirus types 16, 18 and 31, and exposure to betel quid, heavy metals, leather tanning and woodworking products are risk factors. Symptoms include local pain, ulceration, bleeding and swallowing difficulty. Laryngeal cancer presents with hoarseness, hemoptysis, throat pain, cough and breathing difficulty. In the oral cavity, submucosal spread of the tumor should be determined by palpation. A second primary cancer should always be considered. Squamous cell carcinoma of the ear presents with ear mass, bleeding and pain, and may arise on a background of a chronic otitis media. Late symptoms include facial paralysis, sensorineural hearing loss, vertigo and severe ear pain.

Malignancies of the head and neck spread to the draining submental, submandibular, and deep jugular chain of lymph nodes in one or both sides of the neck. Distant metastasis to the lungs, liver and brain occur in late stages.

Verrucous carcinoma is a special type of well-differentiated squamous cell carcinoma which is wart-like, indolent and frequently recurs after excision. It arises from the skin of the lips and gums.

Nasopharyngeal carcinoma occurs as an undifferentiated lymphoepithelioma, or a poorly differentiated or a well-differentiated squamous cell carcinoma. It arises from the posterolateral nasopharyngeal walls and may initially present with hearing loss (from blockade of the Eustachian tube), diplopia (from impingement of the abducens nerve and consequent lateral rectus palsy) or epistaxis. It is not uncommon for patients to present with an enlarged lymph node just behind the angle of the jaw. It is common among people of Chinese descent and is associated with eating spicy preserved fish. This malignancy has a great potential for early spread to the deep jugular lymph nodes of the neck and the base of the skull. Lymphoma, either Hodgkin or non-Hodgkin type, can arise from the chain of lymphoid tissues encircling the oropharyngeal opening (i.e. the Waldeyer's ring consisting of the pharyngeal, palatine, tubal and lingual tonsils).

The malignant neoplasms of the skin include squamous cell carcinoma, basal cell carcinoma and malignant melanoma, the latter two being associated with sunlight exposure. While squamous cell carcinomas are expansile, aggressive and spreading, basal cell carcinomas are ulcerative, more indolent and localized. The areas around the lips, nose and cheeks are especially prone to this cancer. Malignant melanoma is a locally destructive superficial malignancy with a high tendency to postoperative and systemic spread.

Sarcomas, such as rhabdomyosarcoma, leiomyosarcoma, osteosarcoma, hemangiosarcoma and neurosarcoma, are solid and rapidly enlarging masses seen in younger patients. They quickly spread via the bloodstream into distant organs.

In the salivary glands, the malignant variants are adenoid cystic carcinoma and mucoepidermoid carcinoma. These are also commonly seen in the parotid gland. As a rule, however, minor salivary gland tumors tend to be malignant more often than parotid gland tumors.

Papillary carcinoma is by far the most common thyroid malignancy, followed by follicular cancer. Other rarer varieties include medullary cancer and undifferentiated (anaplastic) cancer.

INVESTIGATIONS

Neoplasms should usually be biopsied to establish a diagnosis. Fine needle (gauge 22) aspiration biopsy of soft tissue masses with intact surfaces is often the most feasible procedure to perform. Once the needle has penetrated the substance of the mass, the plunger of the syringe is pulled to maintain negative pressure while the needle is carefully and repeatedly plunged to sample several areas. The plunger is then released and the needle momentarily disconnected from the syringe to release any negative pressure and preserve the aspirated specimen within the bore of the needle. A bloody aspirate must be avoided as this obscures cellular detail. The specimen must be expressed from the needle on to several glass slides, smeared and soaked in 95% ethyl alcohol for 2 minutes. Training and experience are necessary to ensure correct diagnosis (86% and 96% for malignant and benign head and neck tumors, respectively [30]) and to minimize missed diagnoses to as low as 2% [31]. An accuracy level of 89% has been reported for solitary thyroid nodules [32]. Polyps, papillomas and similar pedunculated masses may be gently avulsed so that a representative portion can be submitted for histopathologic examination after immersing the entire specimen in 10% formaldehyde. Cysts of the soft tissues and bones of the face may be excised both for diagnosis and for definitive management. Tonsillectomy may be done when tonsillar lymphoma is suspected. Neck nodes are usually not biopsied unless the primary lesion has been identified by histopathology. This may require rigid or flexible endoscopic examination of the nose, pharynx, oral cavity, pharynx, larynx and esophagus. If endoscopic results are negative or equivocal for malignancy, a fine needle aspiration biopsy of the neck nodes may be performed. An open biopsy should be considered as the last resort. Biopsy should not be done for vascular tumors such as hemangiomas and nasopharyngeal angiofibromas. These often present with massive bleeding, so they are usually diagnosed on clinical grounds and appearance. Angiography may be required to visualize feeding blood vessels and to plan for arterial ligation or embolization prior to definitive excision.

DIAGNOSIS AND DIFFERENTIAL DIAGNOSIS

Benign and malignant neoplasms of the face, salivary glands, neck and external parts of the ears, mouth and nose present with lumps or masses. These may be present at birth, such as dermoid and cystic hygroma, at early childhood, such as branchial cleft cyst and thyroglossal duct cyst, at adolescence, such as nasopharyngeal angiofibroma, at adulthood. Their location may be determined by their embryologic origin; thus, dermoids occur in the midline and other fusion lines, and branchial cleft cysts are found along the paths of the branchial clefts present in early fetal life. Benign masses are usually circumscribed, mobile masses that exhibit little or slow change in size, consistency or number over time. Malignant masses exhibit more dynamic and rapid changes, and tend to involve adjacent tissues. Neoplasms that occur in cavities, such as the nose, paranasal sinuses, mouth, pharynx, larynx and ears, are less clinically apparent, and may initially present with subtle signs such as nosebleeds, mucosal discolorations, voice changes, and mild hearing impairment. As the tumor enlarges, it can obstruct preformed cavities, such as the larynx and the nasal cavity, or press on bony walls, such as the paranasal sinuses. Owing to the proximity of the base of the skull, neoplasms of the nose, paranasal sinuses, nasopharynx and ear can present with neurologic signs and symptoms such as facial paralysis, headache, seizures and diplopia. Destruction of bony walls and invasion of adjacent soft tissues suggest aggressive behavior, although they do not necessarily mean malignancy. Destruction of anatomic boundaries, marked enlargement of draining lymph nodes of the neck, and spread to distant sites are more typical of carcinomas and sarcomas.

MANAGEMENT AND OUTCOMES

Benign neoplasms that are small, circumscribed and solitary can be managed with simple excision. However, if they occur in the face or neck, careful placement of incisions, atraumatic handling of tissues, and meticulous skin and soft tissue closure must be observed to ensure good cosmetic results. With malignant lesions and extensive benign neoplasms, management must be planned according to the nature of the tumor, the preferences and circumstances of the patient, and the available medical and surgical expertise.

Simple excision is often curative of benign neoplasms of the head and neck. Several tumors, however, are particularly challenging to manage and are best referred to an ENT specialist or a head and neck surgeon. In general, polyps and other masses within the nose are best excised with special nasal forceps under endoscopic or headlight visualization. Inverting papillomas require excision of underlying bone to prevent recurrence, and these may require external approaches through the maxilla or nose. Nasopharyngeal angiofibroma is removed via a transpalatal or a transnasomaxillary approach. Since bleeding can be massive, preoperative embolization of feeding arterial vessels is preferred, and the ability to transfuse should be available. Laryngeal papillomatosis must be carefully excised with either cold knife or laser with endoscopic visualization under general anesthesia. Since these tumors are highly recurrent, ENT surgeons must balance disease control with organ preservation. Pleomorphic adenomas of the parotid gland should be removed by superficial parotidectomy with careful preservation of the facial nerve. Deeper tumors require removal of the deep lobe. Branches of the facial nerve may be sacrificed only if complete curative removal of parotid cancers requires it. Ameloblastomas of the maxilla and mandible are best treated with complete excision since enucleation carries with it a high recurrence rate. If a significant portion of the mandible is lost, then reconstruction with bone grafts and biocompatible materials may be needed. Large and deeply spreading branchial cleft cysts and cystic hygromas may be challenging to remove completely since their cyst walls blend with adjacent structures. Margins of excision must be sacrificed in order to preserve as much normal tissue as possible.

The main goals of therapy for head and neck squamous cell cancers are complete removal of the neoplasm while minimizing morbidity, preserving normal function and appearance, and maintaining reasonable quality of life. In 2003, the Radiation Therapy Oncology Group (RTOG) trial, which randomized patients with locally advanced, resectable laryngeal cancer to radiation therapy alone, induction chemotherapy followed by radiation therapy, or concurrent chemoradiation, showed that tumor control and larynx preservation were significantly better in the concurrent chemoradiation arm than in the other two arms. Overall survival rates among the three groups were similar, at approximately 55%. Thus, concurrent chemoradiation has become the standard of care for patients with locally advanced laryngeal cancer, with the goal of organ preservation [33]. If chemoradiation is not available, early-stage head and neck cancers (see Table 12-2 for common staging) may be managed with either surgery or chemoradiation. The results are comparable. In a 7-year review of cases, 5-year survival rates for laryngeal cancer patients (n=451) were 85% for stage I, 77% for stage II, 51% for stage III, and 35% for stage IV disease, and survival for patients with stage I–III disease was similar for patients treated operatively or nonoperatively (P=0.4). Patients with stage IV disease had significantly better survival with surgery (49%) than with chemoradiation (21%) or radiation alone (14%) (P<0.0001) [34]. As a rule, any treatment must be directed toward the primary tumor and its draining lymph nodes of the neck. Frank neck node metastasis may occur in 42% of oral cavity cancers [35] and this requires comprehensive dissection, but when the risk for positive neck lymph nodes exceeds 15–20%, elective neck dissection is indicated [36].

Studies have found significantly worse survival for stage IV, T4, N2 or N3 disease [37]. In 356 patients with oral cavity cancer, pathologic T stage (P<0.001) and tumor thickness cut-off of 5 mm (P=0.03) were independent predictors of disease-specific survival. With a median follow-up of 41 months, overall survival at 5 years was 59% and disease-specific survival was 73% [38].

Advanced tumors (stages III and IV) are usually managed with multimodality therapy. Patients with advanced head and neck cancer, despite aggressive treatment, generally have a 35% to 55% chance of remaining alive and disease-free 3 years after standard curative treatment. Locoregional recurrences develop in 30% to 40% of patients, distant metastases in 20% to 30%. Patients with recurrent small tumors, particularly of the larynx and nasopharynx, can be treated for cure with surgery or repeat irradiation. Patients who present with unresectable large recurrent tumors or those with recurrent tumors in previously irradiated areas, and patients with distant metastases, are usually approached with the intent of palliation [39].

TABLE 12-2 Common TNM Staging for Head and Neck Squamous Cell Carcinomas (Except Nasopharyngeal Carcinoma)*

Classification	Characteristic
T1	Tumor ≤2 cm in greatest dimension
T2	Tumor >2 cm but <4 cm in greatest dimension
T3	Tumor >4 cm in greatest dimension
T4	Tumor invades adjacent structure
N0	No regional LNs
N1	Single ipsilateral LN, ≤3 cm
N2a	Single ipsilateral LN, 3–6 cm
N2b	Multiple ipsilateral LNs, none >6 cm
N2c	Bilateral or contralateral LN, none >6 cm
N3	Any LN >6 cm
M0	No distant metastasis
M1	Distant metastasis

*LN, lymph node.

From Marur S, Forastiere AA. Head and neck cancer: changing epidemiology, diagnosis, and treatment. Mayo Clin Proc 2008;83:489–501.

REFERENCES

1. World Health Organization (WHO). WHO Fact Sheet No 300, March 2006. http://www.who.int/mediacentre/factsheets/fs300/en/index.html last accessed December 2009.
2. Alberti PW. The prevention of hearing loss worldwide. Scand Audiol Suppl 1996;42:15–19.
3. World Health Organization. Global Burden of Disease. 2004 Update. Geneva: World Health Organization; 2008.
4. Acuin J. Chronic Suppurative Otitis Media: Burden of Illness and Management Options. Child and Adolescent Health and Development Prevention of Blindness and Deafness. Geneva: World Health Organization; 2004.
5. Browning GG, Gatehouse S, Calder IT. Medical management of active chronic otitis media: a controlled study. L Laryngol Otol 1988;102:491–5.
6. Van Hasselt P, van Kregten A. Treatment of chronic suppurative otitis media with ofloxacin in hydroxypropyl methylcellulose ear drops: a clinical/ bacteriological study in a rural area of Malawi. Int J Pediatr Otorhinolaryngol 2002;63:49–56.
7. Shin J, Neely J. Chronic otitis media. In: Shin JJ, Hartnick CJ, Randolph GW, eds. Evidence-Based Otolaryngology. New York: Springer Science and Business Media, LLC; 2008:239–71.
8. Acuin JM, Chiong C, Yang N. Surgery for chronically discharging ears with underlying eardrum perforations (Protocol). Cochrane Database Syst Rev 2008;(1):CD006984.
9. Charachon R, Grtacap B, Elbaze D. Anatomical and functional reconstruction of old mastoidectomy cavities by obliteration tympanoplasty. Clin Otolaryngol 1989;14:121–6.
10. Minatogawa T, Jumoi T, Inamori T, et al. Hyogo ear bank experience with allograft tympanoplasty: review of tympanoplasty on 68 ears. Am J Otol 1990;11157–63.

11. Smits C, Swen S, Theo Goverts S, et al. Assessment of hearing in very young children receiving carboplatin for retinoblastoma. Eur J Cancer 2006; 42:492–500.
12. Jereczek-Fossa BA, Zarowski A, Milani F, Orecchia R. Radiotherapy-induced ear toxicity. Cancer Treat Rev 2003;29:417–30.
13. Bess F, Humes L. Audiology: The Fundamentals. Baltimore, MD: Lippincot Williams and Wilkins; 2009:198.
14. Wilson WR, Byl FM, Laird N. The efficacy of steroids in the treatment of idiopathic sudden hearing loss. Arch Otolaryngol Head Neck Surg 1980;106: 772–6.
15. Westerlaken BO, Stokroos RJ, Dhooge I, et al. Treatment of idiopathic sudden sensorineural hearing loss with antiviral therapy: a prospective randomized double blind clinical trial. Ann Otol Rhinol Laryngol 2003;112:993–1000.
16. Tucci DL, Farmer J, Kitch R, Witsell D. Treatment of sudden sensorineural hearing loss with systemic steroids and valacyclovir. Otol Neurol 2002;23: 301–8.
17. Gianoli GJ, Li JC. Transtympanic steroids for treatment of sudden hearing loss. Otolaryngol Head Neck Surg 2001;125:142–6.
18. Kang JI, Kim DM, Lee J. Acute sensorineural hearing loss and severe otalgia due to scrub typhus. BMC Infect Dis 2009;9:173.
19. Petersen PE, Bourgeois D, Ogawa H, et al. The global burden of oral diseases and risks to oral health. Bull World Health Organ 2005;83:661–9.
20. Murray JC, Daack-Hirsch S, Buetow KH, et al. Clinical and epidemiologic studies of cleft lip and palate in the Philippines. Cleft Palate Craniofac J 1997; 34:7–10.
21. Gwaltney JM Jr, Sydnor A Jr, Sande MA. Etiology and antimicrobial treatment of acute sinusitis. Ann Otol Rhinol Laryngol Suppl 1981;90:68–71.
22. Rosenfeld RM, Andes D, Bhattacharyya N, et al. Clinical practice guideline adult sinusitis. Otolaryngol Head Neck Surg 2007;137(3 Suppl):S1–31.
23. Lund V. Therapeutic targets in rhinosinusitis: infection or inflammation? Medscape J Med 2008;10:105.
24. Osguthorpe JD. Adult rhinosinusitis: diagnosis and management. Am Fam Physician 2001;63:69–76.
25. Chester AC, Antisdel JL, Sindwani R. Symptom-specific outcomes of endoscopic sinus surgery: a systematic review. Otolaryngol Head Neck Surg 2009; 140:633–9.
26. Kinnman J, Chi CH, Park JH. Cysticercosis in otolaryngology. Arch Otolaryngol 1976;102:144–7.
27. Del Brutto OH, Roos KL, Coffey CS, Garcia HH. Meta-analysis: cysticidal drugs for neurocysticercosis: albendazole and praziquantel. Ann Intern Med 2006;145:43–51.
28. Gill G, Beeching N. Lecture Notes: Tropical Medicine. Oxford, UK: Wiley-Blackwell; 2009:81.
29. Tappe D, Büttner DW. Diagnosis of human visceral pentastomiasis. PLoS Negl Trop Dis 2009;3(2):e320.
30. Fulciniti F, Califano L, Zupi A, Vetrani A. Accuracy of fine needle aspiration biopsy in head and neck tumors. J Oral Maxillofac Surg 1887;55:1094–7.
31. Ljung BM, Drejet A, Chiampi N, et al. Diagnostic accuracy of fine-needle aspiration biopsy is determined by physician training in sampling technique. Cancer 2001;93:263–8.
32. Pai BS, Anand VN, Shenoy KR. Diagnostic accuracy of fine-needle aspiration cytology versus frozen section in solitary thyroid nodules. The Internet Journal of Surgery 2007;12, Number 2.
33. Forastiere AA, Goepfert H, Maor M, et al. Concurrent chemotherapy and radiotherapy for organ preservation in advanced laryngeal cancer. N Engl J Med 2003;349:2091–8.
34. Gourin CG, Conger BT, Sheils WC, et al. The effect of treatment on survival in patients with advanced laryngeal carcinoma. Laryngoscope 2009; 119:1312–17.
35. Patel RS, Clark JR, Dirven R, et al. Prognostic factors in the surgical treatment of patients with oral carcinoma. ANZ J Surg 2009;79:19–22.
36. Gil Z, Fliss DM. Contemporary management of head and neck cancers. Isr Med Assoc J 2009;11:296–300.
37. Gourin CG, Conger BT, Sheils WC, et al. The effect of treatment on survival in patients with advanced laryngeal carcinoma. Laryngoscope 2009;119: 1312–17.
38. Patel RS, Clark JR, Dirven R, et al. Prognostic factors in the surgical treatment of patients with oral carcinoma. ANZ J Surg 2009;79:19–22.
39. Marur S, Forastiere AA. Head and neck cancer: changing epidemiology, diagnosis, and treatment. Mayo Clin Proc 2008;83:489–501.

13 Diseases of the Musculoskeletal System

Richard A Gosselin, Jonathan J Phillips, R Richard Coughlin

Key features

- Approximately 1.2 million people are killed in road traffic crashes each year and an estimated 50 million are injured worldwide. Many road traffic injuries result in significant musculoskeletal (MS) morbidity
- Advances in control have reduced the impact of some historically devastating infectious conditions that affect the MS system
- Timely recognition of infections of the bone and joints is especially important to prevent loss of mobility and MS integrity
- With increased life expectancy in most countries, age-related conditions account for an increasing percentage of the MS disease burden

INTRODUCTION

The toll of infectious diseases has drawn appropriate global attention; however, musculoskeletal diseases and injuries are becoming the "neglected burden" in low- and middle-income countries (LMIC). Beginning with the landmark Global Burden of Disease study in 1996 and subsequent update publications, the importance and significance of musculoskeletal diseases and injuries have been detailed (Fig. 13.1). Emergence of non-communicable and degenerative diseases such as diabetes and osteoarthritis increase the impact of musculoskeletal conditions. Further, despite the preponderance of a pediatric population in most developing countries, improving healthcare, vaccines and antibiotics have increased longevity and contribute to age-related conditions.

This chapter is divided into four sections; trauma and injury, orthopedic infections, pediatric conditions, and emerging age-related conditions. Each section will address key aspects of epidemiology, pathophysiology, clinical investigation, diagnosis, management and outcomes.

TRAUMA AND INJURY

Acute injuries are a leading cause of mortality and morbidity [1]. In 2001, injuries accounted for more than 11% of all disability-adjusted life-years (DALY) in LMIC, but only 7.5% in high-income countries (HIC) [2]. Road traffic injuries (RTI) alone are responsible for over a quarter of all injury-related DALYs. In LMIC, a significant amount of musculoskeletal care is provided by traditional healers, because of easier access and lower costs. Thus, many patients are seen late, with sequelae of neglected trauma such as non-unions or malunions, or even sequelae of treatment such as post-compartment syndrome contractures.

The numbers of drivers, passengers, motorized vehicles, and kilometers of paved road are steadily increasing in the developing world, and so are the numbers of high-energy injuries, seen more acutely at the district or referral hospitals (Table 13-1). Poor countries are often ill-prepared to manage this growing epidemic: lack of pre-hospital care systems, deficiencies in infrastructure, human, technologic and material capacities and resources, and absent or inadequate physical and social rehabilitation services [3]. Most countries have to focus their scarce resources on curative approaches, not on prevention strategies [4]. A recent country-wide survey in Sierra Leone, using a WHO situational assessment tool, has documented widespread deficiencies in basic parameters, such as availability of water and electricity, number of care providers (including surgeons, anesthesiologists, nurses and therapists), availability of oxygen, and capacity to insert a thoracic drain or even wash out an open fracture [5].

The WHO has recently estimated that over 25% of all hospital beds in LMIC are occupied by injured patients. Injuries are costly: RTIs alone can cost more than 2% of a developing country's GDP, over $100 billion per year worldwide, which is more than twice the total amount of dollars spent on development aid. Significant costs are also imposed on the victims: direct and indirect costs for care, and prolonged absence from gainful work can be ruinous for many poor families, reliant on subsistence farming. Selling of vital assets, severe indebtment and pulling children out of school all contribute to the vicious cycle of poverty.

The management of injuries depends on type, site and duration; if there was any prior treatment; the availability of local care providers, including surgeons and anesthesiologists; the presence of a safe surgical environment; and the availability of appropriate materials and supplies. As a general rule, most fractures will heal with conservative management, albeit not always in the optimal position. Wounds frequently present beyond the time when it is safe for closure.

Debridement and delayed closure, either primarily or by graft, are the norm. This is also true of open fractures, which are commonly treated with debridement and either external fixation, or a Plaster-of-Paris (POP) cast that is windowed for wound management. POP casting after reduction remains the cornerstone of management of most closed fractures, including humerus, forearm, hand, tibia, ankle and foot. Pins can be inserted percutaneously, particularly if fluoroscopic imaging is available, to improve and stabilize reduction, and then be incorporated in the cast. Skin traction in the pediatric group and skeletal traction in adults are still commonly used for femur fractures. In most LMIC, there is little pressure to minimize length of hospital stay, so conservative treatment involving weeks or even months of bed rest is not unusual. This is also the case for fractures of the spine or the pelvic ring.

Open reduction and internal fixation (ORIF) of long bone fractures has many advantages: earlier mobilization of the limb and of the patient, earlier return to home and to work, better functional results with less complications such as non-unions or malunions. The biggest drawback is the risk of deep infection, which in orthopedics can be catastrophic, sometimes salvageable only with a life-saving

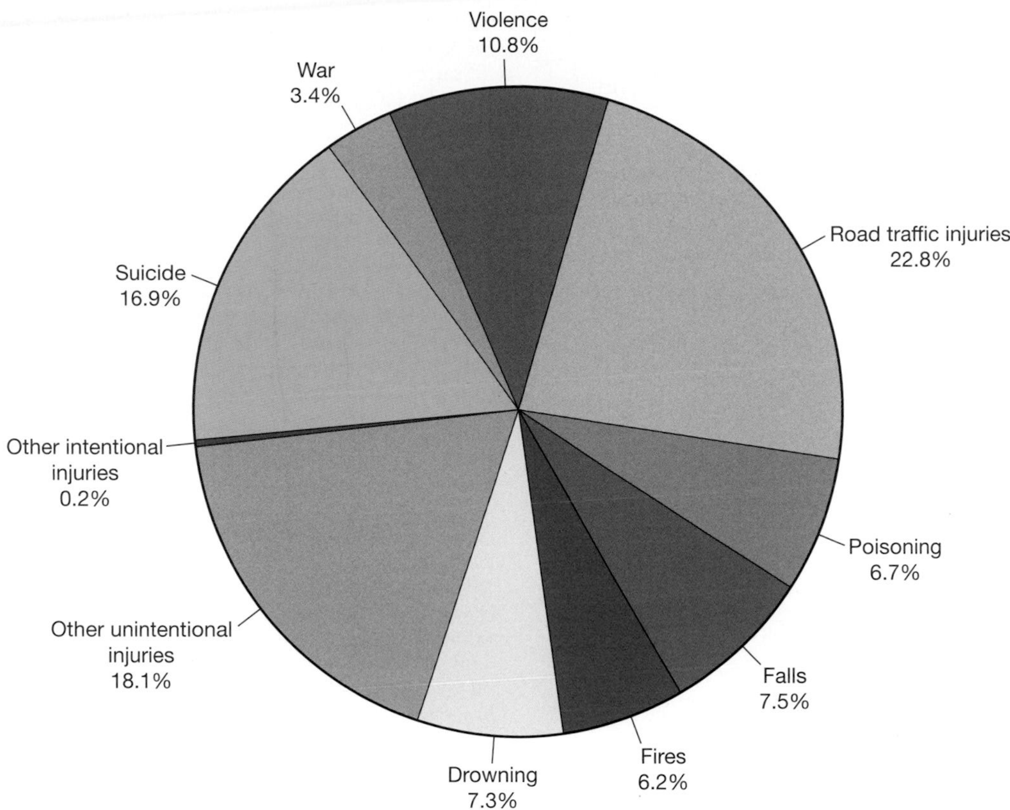

FIGURE 13.1 Distribution of global injury mortality by cause. *Redrawn from WHO Global Burden of Disease Project 2002, Version 1.*

amputation. A clean operating environment, skilled surgeon, trained personnel, adequate instrumentation and safe anesthesia are all absolute prerequisites to perform safe internal fixation of fractures. The surgeon should be well aware of the environment and be able to weigh potential risks and benefits of surgical versus conservative management. Even technically successful procedures, such as repair of lacerated finger flexor tendons, can have disappointing results, as the outcome is largely dependent on availability of good postoperative rehabilitation programs.

INTENTIONAL INJURIES

Rapid urbanization and crowding, combined with high unemployment and easier access to small arms and light weapons, can lead to an increase in interpersonal violence. In poorer countries, lacerations or stab wounds by knife or machete are more common than gun shot wounds (GSW). However, this trend is reversing in most middle-income countries. Furthermore, countries or regions afflicted by conflict, war, or chronic emergencies usually see a heavy toll of collateral damage in the civilian non-combatant population. Urban hospitals see more acute injuries, but late presentation is still common. Most wounds should be treated with a thorough debridement (sometimes called wound excision), and delayed closure or coverage.

Economic development goes hand in hand with rapid industrialization, and work-related injuries become more common. Safety laws may be absent or unenforced, and there is often no social safety net to help patients who cannot return to gainful employment after their recovery from injury. Injuries to the spine, mostly from falls or crush accidents, and to the fingers and hands are particularly common and can be quite disabling.

Economic development can also lead to more leisure time and an increase in sports-related injuries. Most soft tissue injuries, no matter how severe, are treated conservatively, and since rehabilitation services are often lacking, the results can be less than optimal. Appropriate bracing is a luxury out of reach for most LMIC.

ORTHOPEDIC INFECTIONS

Acute and chronic infections of bones, joints and soft tissues are a scourge in LMIC. The provider must be aware of the local prevalence and distribution of infections to facilitate diagnosis and orient treatment. Treatment is often empiric, based on the most likely pathogens, and adjusted according to clinical response. Poor sanitation, overcrowding, and chronic conditions that depress the immune response such as anemia, malnutrition or HIV infection, all contribute to the high prevalence of musculoskeletal infections in developing countries.

OSTEOMYELITIS (OSM)

There are three ways in which bones can become infected: hematogenous dissemination of pathogens, a contiguous focus of infection (e.g. discitis), or direct contact with the "outside world" from an open fracture or a surgical procedure. Acute OSM occurs more commonly in children, usually through hematogenous seeding. Any bone can be affected, but the femur and tibia account for around 50% of cases [6]. In the adult, infection usually follows an open fracture or as a complication from an orthopedic procedure. Chronic OSM is the result of untreated or poorly treated acute OSM, with residual foci of avascular bone and soft tissue debris leading to recurrent episodes of infections, with or without chronic sinus formation.

Acute hematogenous OSM starts in the metaphysis of long bones, where the microcirculation is sluggish (Fig. 13.2). As pressure builds up in the purulent material, the endosteal circulation is destroyed. If pus finds its way through the cortical bone, the periosteum is separated from the cortex, which then becomes completely avascular. The periosteum remains viable and attempts to wall-off the infectious process. This becomes visible on plain x-rays as a periosteal reaction within 10 to 20 days. The pus itself may perforate the periosteum and follow planes of least resistance to create soft tissue abscesses, and can even break through the skin to create a sinus or fistula. Eventually,

TABLE 13-1 The 20 Leading Non-fatal Injuries* Sustained as a Result of Road Traffic Collisions, World, 2002

Type of injury sustained	Rate per 100,000 population	Proportion of all traffic injuries
Intracranial injury† (short-term‡)	85.3	24.6
Open wound	35.6	10.3
Fractured patella, tibia or fibula	26.9	7.8
Fractured femur (short-term‡)	26.1	7.5
Internal injuries	21.9	6.3
Fractured ulna or radius	19.2	5.5
Fractured clavicle, scapula or humerus	16.7	4.8
Fractured facial bones	11.4	3.3
Fractured rib or sternum	11.1	3.2
Fractured ankle	10.8	3.1
Fractured vertebral column	9.4	2.7
Fractured pelvis	8.8	2.6
Sprains	8.3	2.4
Fractured skull (short-term‡)	7.9	2.3
Fractured foot bones	7.2	2.1
Fractured hand bones	6.8	2.0
Spinal cord injury (long-term§)	4.9	1.4
Fractured femur (long-term§)	4.3	1.3
Intracranial injury† (long-term§)	4.3	1.2
Other dislocation	3.4	1.0

*Requiring admission to a health facility.
†Traumatic brain injury.
‡Short-term = lasts only a matter of weeks.
§Long-term = lasts until death, with some complications resulting in reduced life expectancy.
Source: WHO Global Burden of Disease Project, 2002, Version 1.

the host response will attempt to reabsorb all the necrotic material, including the dead cortical bone, or sequestrum. The periosteum will lay down new living bone, called involucrum (Fig. 13.3). If the resorption process is incomplete, some of the sequestrum may be incorporated within the involucrum. This piece of dead bone acts as a foreign body that harbors bacteria, and cannot be sterilized by antibiotics alone. This is the stage of chronic OSM, with recurrent intermittent episodes of acute OSM-like symptoms that are relieved by antibiotics and/or spontaneous drainage from a re-opened fistula. Chronic drainage from permanently patent sinuses prevent pressure build-up within the bone and patients are less likely to have acute symptoms of pain and fever, but these longstanding fistulas are at increased risk of sarcomatous degeneration. Joints where the metaphyses are intra-articular (shoulder, elbow, hip and ankle) very often also have septic arthritis.

Acute OSM should always be suspected in a sick child complaining of limb pain, even if x-rays are normal. Fever, local swelling and tenderness, and guarding are common physical findings. Leukocytosis with a left shift, a very elevated erythrocyte sedimentation rate (ESR) and a negative malaria test are usual laboratory findings. Because malaria is a common cause of fever, patients with acute OSM often present late. Another reason for late presentation, as demonstrated in a study from Uganda, is that more than half of patients have first seen a traditional healer [7]. Thus, abnormal x-ray findings are common even at initial assessment.

Treatment involves antibiotics and often surgery. If culture results are available, appropriate antibiotics should be given according to sensitivity. However, this is rarely the case. *Staphylococcus aureus* is the most common pathogen globally and should always be covered when treating empirically [8]. As in developed countries, methicillin-resistant *S. aureus* (MRSA) is now seen in LMIC. The antibiotic regimen should also cover pathogens that are locally endemic. There is agreement that 6 weeks of total antibiotics is sufficient, at least 7 to 10 days of which should be given intravenously [8,9]. Surgery is indicated when clinical and radiographic findings are both found, where multiple drill holes in the metaphysis will help decompress the intraosseous pus, and hopefully before irreversible vascular damage has occurred. It is essential to disturb the periosteum as little as possible.

In chronic OSM, the clinical diagnosis is easier. Treatment will depend on the severity of the symptoms. The occasional painful flare-up can often be successfully managed by palliative antibiotics. Curative treatment is surgical, but recurrences are common.

SEPTIC ARTHRITIS

Bacterial septic arthritis can affect any joint, but hip, knee and shoulder are the most common, either as an isolated pathology or in conjunction with an intra-articular metaphyseal osteomyelitis. Late presentation is common. Parents often give a history of trauma: the patient fell a few days ago and has refused to bear weight ever since on the involved extremity. Examination usually reveals a septic child, with localized swelling over the involved joint, which is painful on palpation or passive mobilization. Basic laboratory findings are non-specific: elevated white blood cell count (WBC) and ESR. Plain x-rays can appear normal early on, or show only soft tissue swelling, but there will eventually be a widening of the joint space when compared to the contralateral side, which can lead to complete dislocation.

The differential diagnosis should include tuberculosis, inflammatory arthropathies, transient synovitis, post-traumatic hemarthrosis, and avascular necrosis. Joint aspiration can be very useful. *S. aureus* is the most common pathogen, but other bacteria can be involved, such as gonococcus in adolescents, *Haemophilus influenzae* in newborns and very young infants, and *Salmonella enterica* in patients with sickle cell disease. Surgical drainage should be considered whenever there is a clinical suspicion, and performed as early as possible. The downsides of a negative arthrotomy are far outweighed by the dire consequences of a neglected septic arthritis, particularly in a weight-bearing joint.

Other nonbacterial pathogens can involve the musculoskeletal system: fungi (histoplasmosis, actinomycosis, blastomycosis, aspergillosis), treponema (yaws, syphilis) or parasites (dracunculiasis or guinea worm, onchocerciasis). Their diagnosis and treatment are discussed in other sections of this text.

SOFT TISSUE INFECTIONS

Lacerations and penetrating injuries are seen in manual laborers, often with foreign bodies such as splinters, thorns, pieces of rock or metal, and shards of glass. They can lead to cellulitis, or superficial and deep abscesses. Some deep infections, such as hand flexor tendon

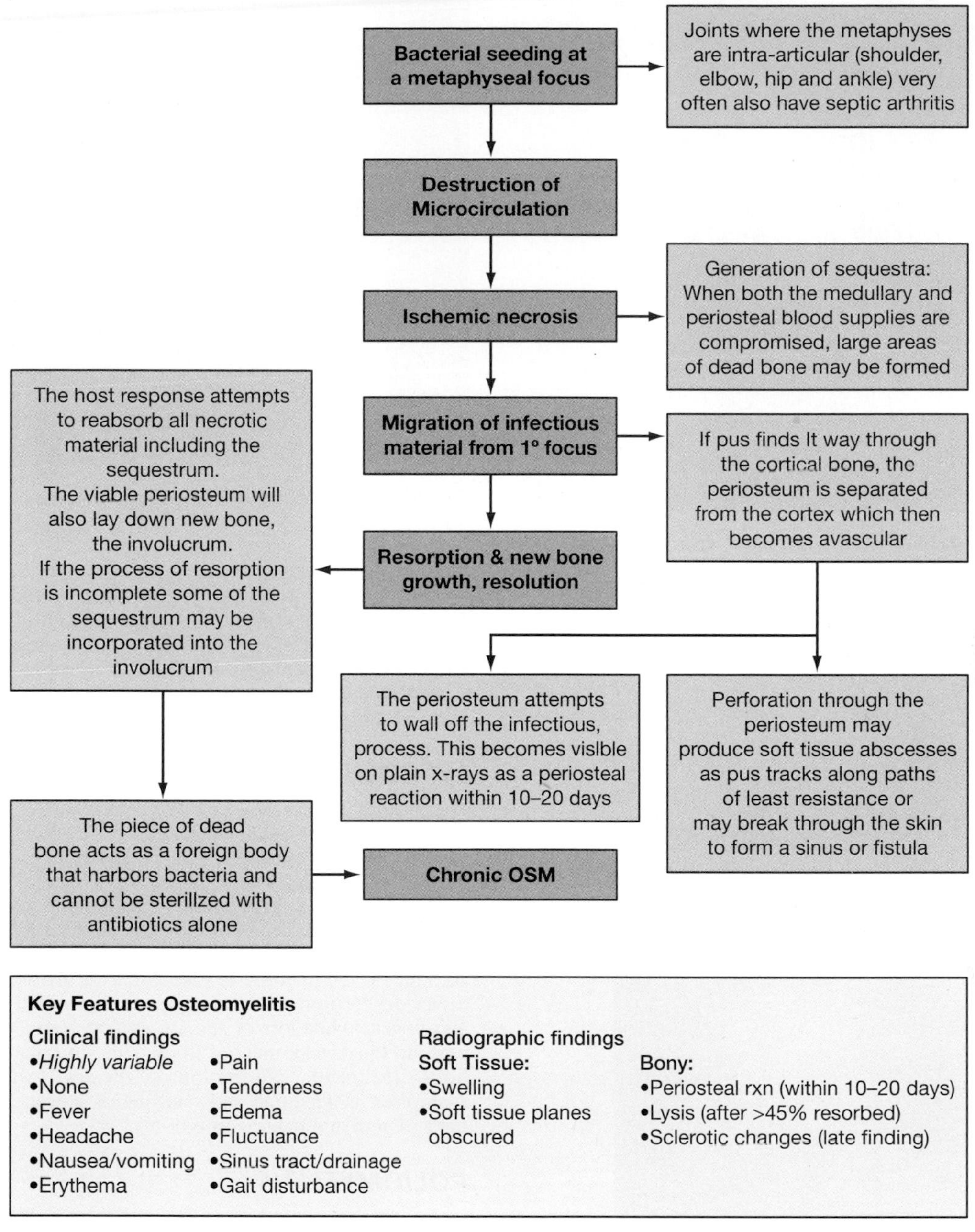

FIGURE 13.2 Osteomyelitis pathway.

sheaths, require early surgical debridement, or significant functional impairment can result.

Other soft tissue infections that can be seen in tropical environments are: atypical bacteria (tularemia, brucellosis), fungi (aspergillosis, cryptococcosis), and parasites (echinococosis, trichinosis).

Tropical pyomyositis was first described in Uganda in 1968 and presents with single to multiple suppurative lesions within skeletal muscle. It is more common in HIV-positive patients. Large muscles of the lower extremities and pelvic girdle are common sites of infection. Studies suggest up to 50% of patients report a previous injury. Examination usually reveals fever, diffuse fusiform swelling, and significant tenderness on palpation or passive stretching of the involved muscle, but usually no palpable fluid collection or fluctuation. The abscess is subfascial, within the muscle tissue itself, and poorly contained. *S. aureus* accounts for near 90% of cases. Multiple attempts at aspiration with a large-bore needle are often necessary to retrieve purulent material, and should be done when the diagnosis is suspected. Orthopedic management is incision and drainage of abscesses or debridement of necrotic tissue if involvement is extensive. Antibiotics are necessary.

TUBERCULOSIS

Approximately 5% of HIV-negative tuberculosis (TB) patients have involvement of their musculoskeletal system. This increases in HIV-positive TB patients. Thus, there could be at least one million people worldwide with TB of their bones and joints. Around half of skeletal TB involves the spine, 40% have articular disease, mostly hip and knee, and the remaining 10% have either isolated soft tissue or extra-articular osseous involvement (Figs 13.4 & 13.5).

Routine laboratory testing is nonspecific, with usually a mild to moderately elevated ESR and a normal to slightly elevated WBC. Aspiration can be nonspecific, with fluid ranging from mildly inflammatory

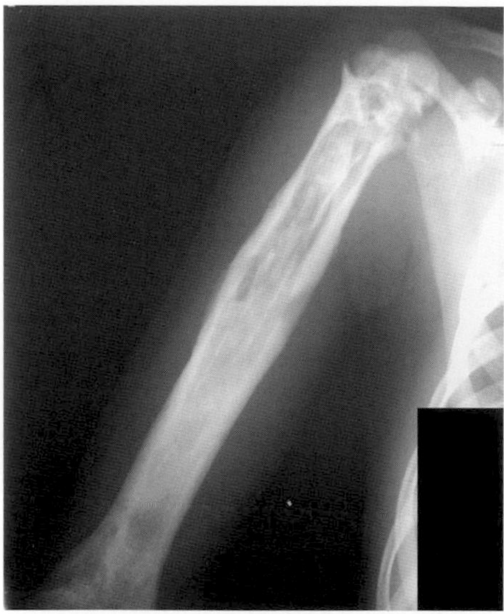

FIGURE 13.3 Osteomyelitis of the humerus with the formation of sequestrum and involucrum.

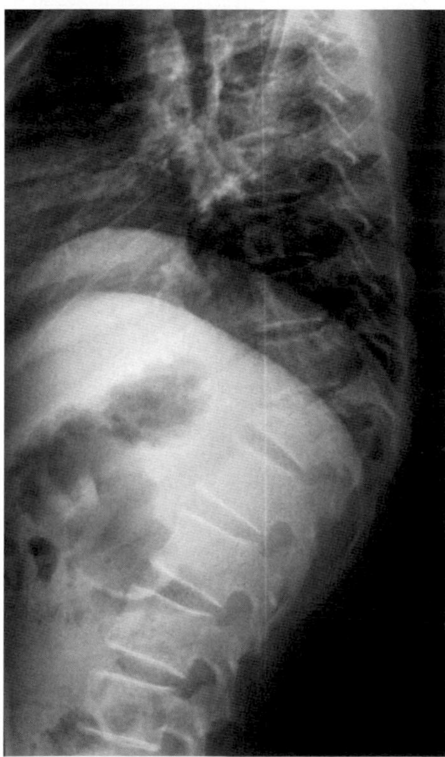

FIGURE 13.4 Characteristic spinal involvement of tuberculosis with contiguous disc involvement and kyphotic deformity.

to bloody to frankly caseous in appearance. Plain x-rays can be useful in identifying a primary pulmonary focus. The diagnosis rests on a high level of clinical suspicion, and chemotherapy is most often initiated on the basis of a combination of nonspecific findings.

The cornerstone of TB treatment is combination chemotherapy. Surgery may be indicated for diagnostic purposes if appropriate laboratory facilities are available. For spinal TB, surgery is indicated to decompress an epidural abscess compressing the cord and causing paraparesis, particularly with no improvement or continuous deterioration after initiation of the chemotherapeutic regimen (MRC). For osteoarticular TB, surgery is indicated as palliation in late-stage disease [6]. Some destroyed stiff and painful joints can be treated by resection

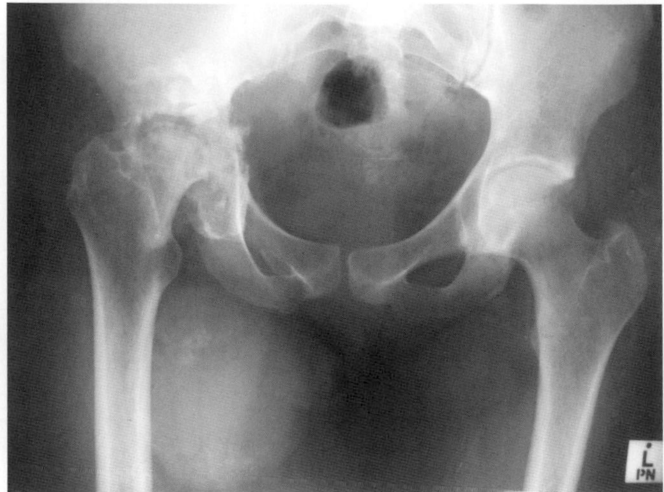

FIGURE 13.5 Disseminated tuberculosis with destructive infiltration of the hip joint.

arthroplasty, such as the hip (Girdlestone procedure) or the elbow. The trade-off is some degree of weakness and limb shortening. Other joints have a tendency to become unstable, and since in most poor countries access to quality orthotics is impossible, fusion becomes the surgical treatment of choice. This applies to wrist, knee and ankle joints in particular.

LEPROSY

The incidence of leprosy saw a 4% decrease in global cases in the period of 2007–2008; new cases detected in 2008 across 121 countries totaled 249,000. Leprosy is now largely limited to high prevalence pockets, including areas of India, Nepal, central Africa, and Brazil. Leprosy results in disabling limb deformities that have social implications and disrupt the ability of those afflicted to seek employment, or contribute to subsistence farming. Secondary changes to bone account for the majority of cases seen for orthopedic management. Motor denervation and fixed contractures result in clawing of the toes and fingers, while loss of afferent sensory nerve conduction predisposes to the development of trophic ulceration and secondary infections. Treatment with multidrug therapy (MDT) consisting of rifampicin, clofazimine and dapsone, is efficacious in interrupting transmission and treating infection.

POLIOMYELITIS

Four countries remain endemic for polio: India, Pakistan, Afghanistan and Nigeria. Several other countries in Africa, South Asia, and central Europe have reintroduced polio. New-onset disease is usually seen in the under-5 age group, however, much of what is encountered today may be residual disease. The seminal work of Huckstep remains the classic reference on the topic [10].

PEDIATRIC CONDITIONS

Early identification of pediatric conditions is important, as timely intervention can dramatically alter the course of a child's life. Pediatric orthopedic conditions include scoliosis, congenital hip dysplasia, limb length discrepancies, Legg–Calve–Perthes disease, genus varum, and osteogenesis imperfecta. This chapter describes congenital talipes equinovarus and cerebral palsy.

CONGENITAL TALIPES EQUINOVARUS

In the tropics, an important condition presenting at birth is that of congenital talipes equinovarus (CTE) or "clubfoot". Childbearing at home, in rural areas, outside the reach of an equipped medical facility, translates into higher rates of late-presentation clubfoot, requiring surgical correction. The late Dr Ignacio Ponseti revolutionized club foot management in the 1950s. He introduced a conservative non-operative technique to treat the deformity when it is recognized in infants and this is the gold standard across much of the world [11].

Management following the Ponseti technique involves gradual manipulation utilizing serial casting methods, with or without a simple percutaneous tenotomy, and has a near 95% success rate. Given the serial nature of the casting intervention, gradual reduction of the deformity takes place over a period of about 6 weeks, with subsequent bracing for an extended time.

CEREBRAL PALSY

Poor maternal–fetal and neonatal health services during the prenatal and postpartum periods are commonly cited as reasons for an increased incidence of cerebral palsy (CP). The neuromuscular disorder affects mobility, postural stability, and the ability to maintain balance, through variable effects on muscle tone. Orthopedic surgery is often required when deformities or contractures limit performance of daily activities, or decrease function.

AGE-RELATED CONDITIONS

Age-related musculoskeletal disease accounts for an increasing share of the musculoskeletal burden. Degenerative conditions can occur everywhere, but disability is greatest when weight-bearing joints are involved. Degenerative disease of joints can be primary (idiopathic) or secondary to a vast array of conditions: congenital (developmental dysplasia of the hip, talipes equinovarus), hereditary (osteogenesis imperfecta, achondroplasia), infectious (sequelae of septic arthritis), angular deformities (Blount's disease) or avascular necrosis (sickle cell disease, Legg–Perthes disease). They can also be the result of trauma, particularly of intra-articular fractures that have been unrecognized or neglected.

The rise of adult diabetes is associated with an increased incidence of neuropathic joints, particularly around the foot and ankle. Chronic low back pain (LBP) and significant osteoporosis are becoming more widespread (Fig. 13.6). Metastases to the bone secondary to neoplasms are also likely to increase. Clinical, radiographic, and basic laboratory parameters can be used for diagnosis. Inflammatory arthropathies are also increasingly recognized. Symptomatic treatment is with aspirin, analgesics, early generations of nonsteroidal anti-inflammatory drugs (NSAIDs), and corticosteroids.

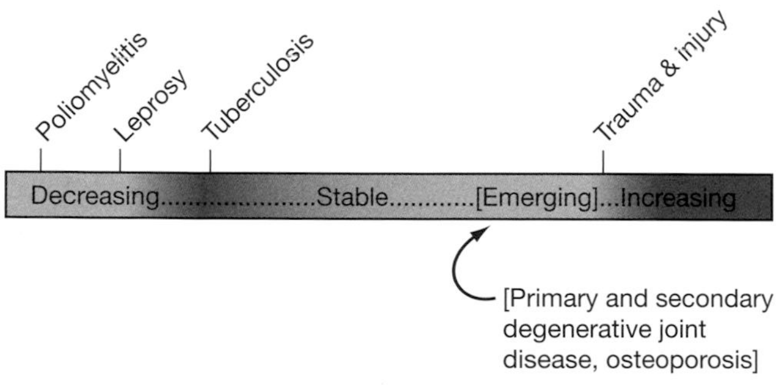

FIGURE 13.6 Thermal graph of emerging conditions.

Back pain is common worldwide. With greater than 80–90% of the workforce in the developing world undertaking strenuous physical labor, one might suspect that the prevalence of low back pain would be increased over that seen in industrialized nations. Osteoarthritis, spinal stenosis, disc degeneration, and osteoporosis all increase in aging populations.

The morbidity associated with osteoporosis is secondary to fractures that occur in fragile low-density bone. Common fracture sites are the spine, hip and upper extremity. Spine and hip fractures are particularly debilitating. Vertebral compression fractures lead to deforming scoliosis and painful nerve root compressions, while hip fractures necessitate long periods of hospitalization and may be fatal in up to 20% of cases. Where there is dependence upon subsistence farming, a debilitating spine or hip fracture can be of severe detriment.

Increasing age is a risk factor for the development of prostate, breast and lung cancers, each of which has a high propensity to metastasize to bone. It is likely that there will be an increase in the burden of secondary bone cancer. Slow development of many primary cancers, combined with lack of education and lack of access to chemotherapeutics and radiotherapy, result in the neglect of many primary cancers. Disruption of the structural integrity of bone by cancerous lesions reduces the load-bearing capacity. Pathologic fractures may result, and should be suspected in patients with nonspecific symptomatology who develop a fracture with a mechanism of injury inconsistent with fracture severity.

REFERENCES

1. Mock C, Cherian MN. The global burden of musculoskeletal injuries. Clin Orthop Relat Res 2008;466:2306–16.
2. Lopez AD, Mathers CD, Ezzati M, et al, eds. Global Burden of Disease and Risk Factors. Washington, DC: Oxford University Press; 2006.
3. Atijosan O, Rischewski D, Simms V, et al. A national survey of musculoskeletal impairment in Rwanda: prevalence, causes and service implications. PLoS One 2008;3:e2851.
4. Woolf A, Brooks P, Mody GM. Prevention of musculoskeletal conditions in the developing world. Best Pract Res Clin Rheumatol 2008;22:759–72.
5. Kingham TP, Kamara TB, Cherian MN, et al. Quantifying surgical capacity in Sierra Leone: a guide for improving surgical care. Arch Surg 2009;144: 122–7.
6. Spiegel DA, Penny JN. Chronic osteomyelitis in children. Techniques in Orthopaedics 2005;20:142–52.
7. Ibingira CB. Chronic osteomyelitis in a Ugandan rural setting. East Afr Med J 2003;80:242–7.
8. Akakpo-Numado GK, Gnassingbe K, Boume MA, et al. Current bacterial causes of osteomyelitis in children with sickle cell disease [French]. Sante 2008;18:67–70.
9. Mader JT, Shirtliff M, Calhoun JH. Staging and staging application in osteomyelitis. Clin Infect Dis 1997;25:1303–9.
10. Huckstep RL. Poliomyelitis: A Guide for Developing Countries, Including Appliances and Rehabilitation of the Disabled. Edinburgh, UK: Churchill Livingstone; 1975.
11. Siapkara A, Duncan R. Congenital talipes equinovarus: a review of current management. J Bone Joint Surg 2007;89:995–1000.

SECTION

B

SKILLS-BASED CHAPTERS

14 General Surgery in the Tropics

Donald E Meier, John L Tarpley, Robert Riviello

Key features

- Resource-poor areas (RPAs), particularly sub-Saharan Africa, have the highest surgical disease burden with the lowest concentration of surgical and anesthesia providers in the world
- Many operations in RPAs are performed by general practitioners with minimal formal surgical training
- In RPAs, surgeons are, by default, "general" surgeons, since they are expected to be local experts in all surgical disciplines, including obstetrics and gynecology
- Delayed patient presentation and gross deficiencies in basic infrastructure lead to the necessity of treating a large volume of patients with advanced disease using minimal equipment and supplies
- Improvisation, maintenance, and reuse of "disposable" items are essential RPA strategies
- Prudent patient selection and safe anesthesia are the keys to successful operations

INTRODUCTION

General surgery in more developed areas of the tropics parallels general surgery in advanced areas outside the tropics, and surgeons in these areas are well served by standard textbooks of surgery. Many tropical locations, however, are resource-poor. Surgery has been labeled "the neglected stepchild of global public health" [1]. Sub-Saharan Africa has the most concentrated surgical disease burden with the lowest concentration of surgical and anesthesia providers in the world (1 surgeon per 200,000 people in West Africa) [2]. Contrary to previously held beliefs, provision of essential surgical services in this setting is a cost-effective intervention [3,4]. The purpose of this chapter is to assist physicians practicing surgery, either full time or as short-term volunteers, in these resource-poor areas (RPAs).

PRACTICAL ASPECTS OF SURGERY IN RPAs

Many operations in RPAs are not performed by formally trained, board-certified surgeons, but by general practitioners with minimal formal surgical training. The term "surgeon" in this chapter will subsequently refer to any practitioner performing operations, regardless of training. Surgeons in RPAs, by default, are "general" surgeons expected to be local experts in all areas of surgery, including orthopedic, urologic, plastic, pediatric, otorhinolaryngologic, oral, neurologic, obstetric and gynecologic surgery. All surgeons in RPAs face a common set of problems: inadequate funding of health, hospitals, equipment and supplies, and poor infrastructure for the provision of water and electricity. Many resource-poor countries spend less than $10 per capita per annum on healthcare [5]. Professional isolation is the norm.

Operative complications are common in RPA hospitals but can be minimized using a surgical safety checklist [6]. Surgeons who try to render quality healthcare may be overcome by the volume of patients and lack of resources and can burn out. Many then secure positions elsewhere with better work hours and compensation, creating a vicious cycle where people with the greatest needs are served by the fewest surgeons.

Water and Electricity

Public water utilities, if available, may not be reliable, and water sources such as cisterns, wells, bore holes, and/or pumps for rivers or ponds must be incorporated as supplementary water sources. Electrical supply is often intermittent with wildly erratic voltage, requiring in-line stabilizers and circuit breakers to protect electrical equipment. Back-up generators are essential (although fuel scarcities may limit their usefulness) unless one plans to perform all operative procedures in the hours of daylight with the operating table next to a window in order to use the sun as an operating light.

Equipment and Supplies

Improvisation, maintenance, and reuse of "disposable" items are essential strategies. Decisions are based on the surgeon's needs and the hospital's capacity to acquire and maintain technologically appropriate materials. Operating room essentials include a pulse oximeter, an adjustable table, a lighting system, suction, and basic operative instruments. Nonessential but extremely useful items are an electrocautery, a bronchoscope/esophagoscope (particularly for pediatric foreign bodies), a fiberoptic headlight, and a table-mounted self-retaining retractor for upper abdominal procedures. Physicians, hospitals and organizations in more developed countries are sometimes willing to donate and ship used equipment to RPA hospitals; however, there may be exorbitant clearing and customs fees. Vetting donations to ensure that all equipment is functional, useful, and serviceable by the recipient institution is critical.

Cordless electric drills/bits for home use work well as bone drills when gas-sterilized and used on a low setting to minimize burn damage to the bone. An LED headlamp can substitute for an expensive fiberoptic headlight. Anal muscle stimulators for operations in children with anorectal malformations cost $3000 in more developed countries, but a substitute can be improvised using an anesthesia nerve stimulator ($50) and a piece of insulated, double-strand wire ($3) [7]. No improvisation is as good as the original, but all work surprisingly well and are better than having nothing.

Conditions in the tropics vary between hospitals, but expense, erratic availability, pilferage, deterioration, and lack of domestic production complicate the maintenance of an adequate central store. The tropical surgeon must decide which supplies and drugs are essential and then obtain them locally when possible, import them, or improvise from local materials. Nylon fishing line can substitute for monofilament suture, and carpet/sewing thread for multifilament suture. If disposable dressing gloves are not available, plastic bread bags can serve as inexpensive barrier-protection gloves when handling dressings, examining wounds, and performing digital rectal examinations. Worn sheets can be converted into rolled bandages, and towels cut to serve as laparotomy sponges. Non-chemically treated mosquito netting can substitute for medical-grade mesh for tension-free hernia repairs [8].

Sterilization

Reaching Western sterilization standards may not be possible. Sterilization techniques used in RPAs include steam autoclaving, soaking in antiseptic solution, boiling and gassing. Steam autoclaving can use electricity, gas, wood, coal or kerosene as an energy source and is preferred for instrument sets and cloth packs. Soaking solutions such as methyl alcohol (readily available in RPAs) is helpful in sterilizing scissors and blades that tend to dull or rust when steam-autoclaved. Boiling does not kill spores, but it can serve as a "flash" technique for dropped instruments. Gas sterilization is helpful in re-sterilizing rubber and plastic tubes, catheters, drains, electrical cords, and instruments such as diathermy pencils and power drills. Ethylene oxide ampoule systems are ideal, but relatively expensive for RPAs and cannot be transported by air or even on many container ships. An improvised gas sterilization system utilizes formaldehyde inside a discarded refrigerator with intact rubber seals. Inexpensive solar autoclaves made from locally available materials are currently being tested.

Wound infections in RPAs can be decreased by providing patients a place to bathe with water and soap before entering the operating room. For elective operations, on-the-table skin preparation with commercially available soap and methyl alcohol has been shown to be as effective as the more expensive Betadine technique [9].

Anesthesia

Safe anesthesia is the key component to successful operations in RPAs. Few formally trained physician anesthesia providers exist in RPAs outside of university hospitals. In most RPA hospitals, the anesthesia "department" usually consists of the surgeon and a personally trained nurse or technician. The surgeon must pay close attention to all activities on both sides of the ether screen. A functioning pulse oximeter is arguably the most important piece of equipment in an RPA operating room. Anesthetic options include vocal and hypnotic techniques, acupuncture, local and regional techniques, and dissociative and general techniques. The choice of technique depends on the patient, the procedure, the availability of drugs and trained personnel, and the preference of the patient and surgeon. Airway management is of prime importance in all techniques. The Eleven Golden Rules of Anesthesia [10] should be followed regardless of the level of medical sophistication (Box 14.1). General anesthesia capability necessitates additional equipment and personnel. Inhalational anesthetic systems that are technologically appropriate for RPAs have been developed. Drawover units, exemplified by the EMO (Epstein Macintosh Oxford) ether vaporizer, do not require compressed gases or electricity and have been modified for use with halothane. Because halothane has a cardiodepressant action, it should be given with oxygen enrichment. Portable oxygen concentrators can supply up to 6 L oxygen/minute to supplement these drawover systems (Fig. 14.1). Air compressors employed in combination with Boyle's type units can provide freshly compressed air as the carrier gas, thus eliminating the need for expensive and hard-to-find nitrous oxide.

Ketamine, a neuroleptic agent providing dissociative anesthesia, is used extensively in RPAs because of its effectiveness, availability, relatively low cost, and safety [11]. It rarely causes hypotension or respiratory depression, but airway monitoring, as with all anesthetic techniques, is mandatory. It may serve as the sole anesthetic agent (particularly in children), as an induction agent, or as one part of a balanced technique. It does not provide muscle relaxation, but intramuscular or intravenous ketamine safely anesthetizes children for abscess drainage, wound dressings, cast changes, burn debridement, herniorrhaphy, and, with repeated injections, for long procedures such as orthopedic and plastic procedures of the extremities. In adults, intravenous ketamine is especially useful as a short-duration anesthetic for dressing or cast changes and abscess drainage. Concomitant glycopyrrolate or atropine administration helps reduce hypersalivation. Benzodiazepine co-medication decreases emergence phenomena in adults but is not routinely needed in children since the incidence of emergence phenomena is quite low in children [11].

Emergency intra-abdominal procedures present an anesthetic challenge. Gastric decompression to minimize the risk of aspiration is obligatory before delivery of any anesthetic. Spinal anesthesia can be

BOX 14.1 The Eleven Golden Rules of Anesthesia

1. Perform an adequate history and physical examination
2. Perform operations on fasting patients. For abdominal emergencies, empty the stomach with a nasogastric tube and use a crash induction
3. Place the patient on a tilt-top table
4. Check the anesthetic equipment BEFORE you begin
5. Always have suction capability available
6. Keep the airway clear and open
7. Be prepared to control the patient's ventilation (have an ambu-type bag available)
8. Have a good IV line (optional in some instances of local anesthesia or IM ketamine)
9. Monitor the patient frequently
10. Have someone around to help
11. Be ready with equipment and agents to manage resuscitation from a cardiopulmonary arrest

After King M, ed. Primary Anesthesia. Oxford, UK: Oxford University Press; 1986.

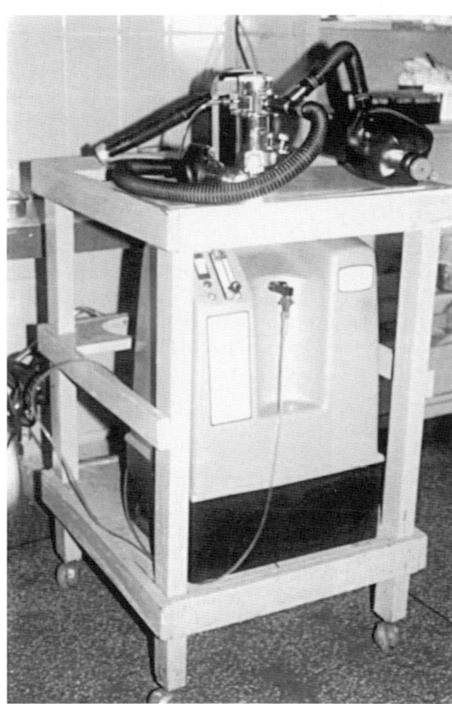

FIGURE 14.1 Drawover vaporizer and oxygen concentrator: inhalational general anesthesia without commercial gas cylinders.

used for emergency procedures below the diaphragm, but hypovolemia must be corrected before anesthesia delivery, because the spinal technique abolishes the sympathetic tone of the lower extremities, increases the capacitance, and produces hypotension. General anesthesia with a controlled airway is safer in emergency situations if appropriate equipment, agents and personnel are available.

Laboratory

The only consistently available tests in most RPA hospitals are: hematocrit, leukocyte count and urinalysis. Other tests, in order of decreasing availability, are: Gram stain, blood urea nitrogen, creatinine, liver enzymes, electrolytes, coagulation studies and blood cultures. Arterial blood gases are rarely available. HIV testing is available in most locations, but reagents and test kits may be in short supply.

Imaging and Endoscopy

Outside of teaching hospitals and certain urban medical centers, the tropical surgeon rarely encounters radiologists, functioning fluoroscopic units, or interventional technique capability. Ultrasound (US) is relatively inexpensive, noninvasive and portable, but is operator-dependent. US, especially useful in assessing the pelvis for obstetrics, can also provide the surgeon with important anatomic information about the biliary tract, liver, pancreas and kidneys. US can detect ascites, distinguish solid from cystic masses, and localize intra-abdominal abscesses. It is having an increasing role in the diagnosis and follow-up of parasitic diseases, e.g., schistosomiasis, hydatid cysts, amebic liver abscess and lymphatic filariasis.

Endoscopy has become more widespread, and flexible fiberoptic esophagogastroduodenoscopy is sometimes found even in peripheral areas. Initial cost and equipment maintenance, however, limit the availability of this valuable diagnostic tool.

Histopathology

Frozen-section capability is usually unavailable. The turnaround time for histopathologic reports can be months, and decisions relating to diagnosis, adequacy of margins, and institution of chemotherapy (e.g., antitubercular or antineoplastic) must often be made on clinical grounds alone or deferred for unacceptably long periods.

Transfusion Service

The transfusion service is largely a blood typing and collecting station and not a blood storage facility. Transfusions usually involve on-the-spot donor recruitment and immediate transfusion. Local customs and beliefs can inhibit blood donation, and consequently, establishing and maintaining a blood bank is difficult. "Walking" blood banks, whereby volunteers in an institution, organization or community are typed, can provide a measure of emergency supply.

AN OVERVIEW OF SURGICAL PRACTICE IN THE TROPICS

The tropical surgeon encounters few disease processes that the temperate surgeon does not encounter, but those common to both surgeons are usually far advanced on presentation in the tropics (Fig. 14.2). RPA surgeons therefore must treat patients with advanced problems often using minimal equipment and supplies. Patients in RPAs tend to be younger and more undernourished and to have less comorbid disease (atherosclerotic vascular disease and smoking-related pulmonary disease). Elective operating schedules are frequently difficult to achieve, since trauma, infection, and obstetric emergencies crowd out elective cases and consume most of the surgeon's time. Operating rooms in RPAs can have poor illumination and climate control, with dust and flying insects part of the operating room environment. Operative cases should be made as simple as possible. Distance, inconvenience, expense, and lack of perceived need limit patient follow-up, and the physician's knowledge of treatment outcomes is severely limited. Information sharing by surgeons is usually anecdotal.

GENERAL SURGERY

Trauma, infections, neoplasms, and abdominal problems including groin hernias constitute the four major areas of general surgery. Endocrine procedures are generally limited to the thyroid.

Trauma

Half of tropical surgery beds are filled by trauma victims. Mortality is high, and survivor morbidity and disability pose great socioeconomic costs for families and society. Some of the world's highest traffic fatality rates are reported from tropical countries. Crash scene and transport care is generally rendered by untrained "good Samaritans" without regard for spinal injuries. Emergency rooms are seldom equipped or staffed adequately for normal activities, much less for 50 mass casualty victims in various stages of dying, being delivered simultaneously. The RPA trauma surgeon must be a "general" surgeon with a functional knowledge of orthopedics, neurosurgery, urology, and plastic surgery in addition to general and thoracic surgery (Fig. 14.3). In the face of economic adversity, the proliferation of well-made, inexpensive motorcycles has led over the past decade to a threefold increase in motorcycle crashes with subsequent head and/or spine injuries and long-bone fractures. Motorcycle "taxis" are a ubiquitous scourge in many RPAs.

Infections, Bites and Stings

Stings from scorpions and bites from humans, dogs, cats, wild animals, snakes, spiders and insects cause local and systemic problems. A bite near a hand joint must be examined closely, opened if there is suspicion of violation, irrigated, and left unsutured with the patient admitted for antibiotic administration and extremity elevation. Rabies is a major concern, primarily from dog bites. Poisonous snakebites vary in incidence and type by topography and locale. Systemic antivenom may be indicated, and local care with wound excision and fasciotomy may be required to treat local and vascular compartment problems. Procaine infiltration, ice and analgesics can relieve the pain of scorpion envenomation. Black widow spider bites produce generalized muscle spasms while brown recluse spider bites produce a local ulcer with ischemic necrosis.

Abscesses of the skin, subcutaneous tissue, muscles (pyomyositis), bones (osteomyelitis), joints (pyarthrosis), thorax (empyema), and pericardial sac occur frequently and require drainage. *Staphylococcus aureus* is the most frequent etiologic agent. Multiple abscesses are common and may occur synchronously or metachronously. Early and wide drainage with antibiotic administration minimizes hematogenous spread of infection. Hand infections pose a special difficulty because most patients delay seeking medical care; and even after drainage, antibiotics, elevation and physiotherapy, residual hand deformity is frequently the outcome.

Clinically important mycoses include mycetoma, aspergillus granuloma, phycomycosis, histoplasmosis and chromoblastomycosis. Mycetoma (Madura foot) is a clinically defined lesion with swelling (chronic inflammation), multiple sinuses, and discharge of granules. Surgical treatment options include observation, local excision to healthy tissue, and amputation.

Cancer

The mortality rate from cancer in RPAs is higher than the rate in high-income areas [12]. Accurate statistics are not widely available, but cancers of the cervix, esophagus, stomach, liver, breast and prostate predominate. Primary hepatocellular carcinoma is more frequent in high hepatitis B and C virus areas. Most malignancies present at an advanced stage (see Fig. 14.2), and operations are usually palliative. Increased tobacco production and use in RPAs has been accompanied by an increase in tobacco-related illnesses, including lung cancer.

Abdominal Surgery

Tropical gastrointestinal surgeons have noted changing disease patterns. Appendicitis is increasing in incidence, and intestinal

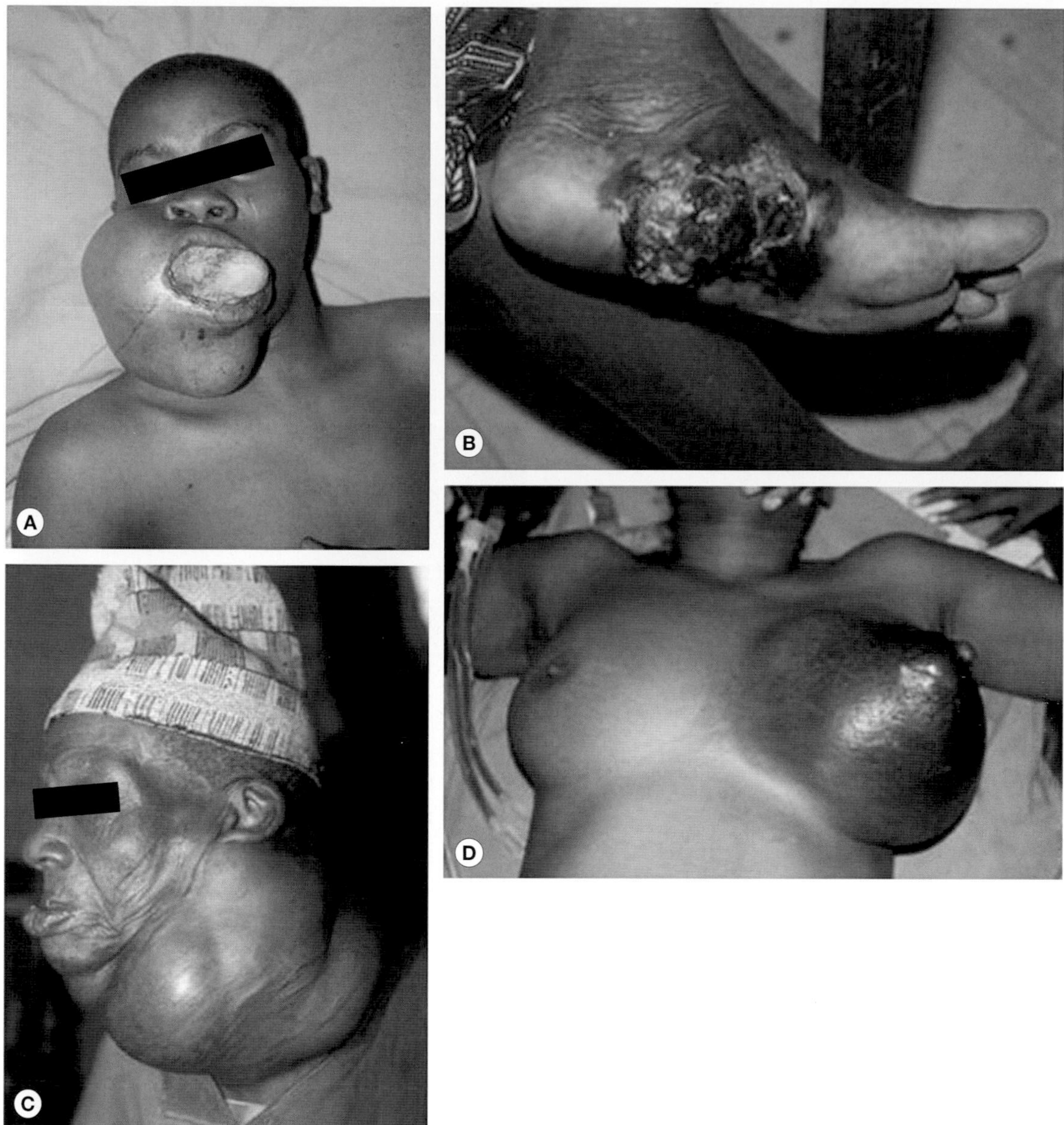

FIGURE 14.2 Typical stage at presentation: **A** 18-year-old male with ameloblastoma of the right mandible; **B** 55-year-old female with locally advanced and metastatic malignant melanoma; **C** 62-year-old male with thyroid carcinoma; **D** 43-year-old female with locally advanced and metastatic breast cancer.

obstruction is assuming a more Western pattern, with adhesions and neoplasms joining hernias as common causes. Appendiceal perforation, strangulated bowel (intestinal obstruction, hernia, volvulus), ileal typhoid perforations, and perforated duodenal ulcers are leading causes of secondary bacterial peritonitis and carry a high mortality rate because of advanced sepsis due to delays in seeking medical care. Since people rarely present until after a hernia is complicated (Fig. 14.4), obstruction, strangulation and peritonitis occur and sometimes cause fatalities.

Laparoscopy

The role of laparoscopy in RPAs is yet to be defined. To compensate for the lack of computed tomography (CT) and magnetic resonance imaging (MRI), diagnostic laparoscopy using non-disposable equipment and locally crafted dissectors can reduce the need for diagnostic laparotomy, especially in sexually active females when pelvic pathology is difficult to differentiate from appendicitis. Surgeons in India have decreased costs to $1.20 per patient [13]. However, initial equipment cost and subsequent maintenance remain obstacles to broader acceptance. It is also difficult to perform therapeutic laparoscopic procedures in RPA hospitals with a sporadic electrical supply. An ethical consideration in laparoscopy is the training of RPA surgeons. The teaching of open procedures should not be neglected when laparoscopy is added to a training curriculum, since surgical trainees who primarily learn laparoscopic procedures in teaching hospitals will find it difficult to function in situations where the only option is an open procedure.

Volvulus

Sigmoid volvulus is a leading cause of intestinal obstruction. Previously healthy patients will present with marked abdominal distention and tympany to percussion but without peritonitis unless strangulation or perforation has occurred. Although sigmoidoscopic deflation can be attempted, operation is the usual treatment since the colon is often strangulated. If at laparotomy the bowel is viable, a rectal tube can be passed under guidance, the loop deflated, and the volvulus manually reduced. After bowel preparation, an interval sigmoid resection can be performed to avoid the recurrence that is likely after

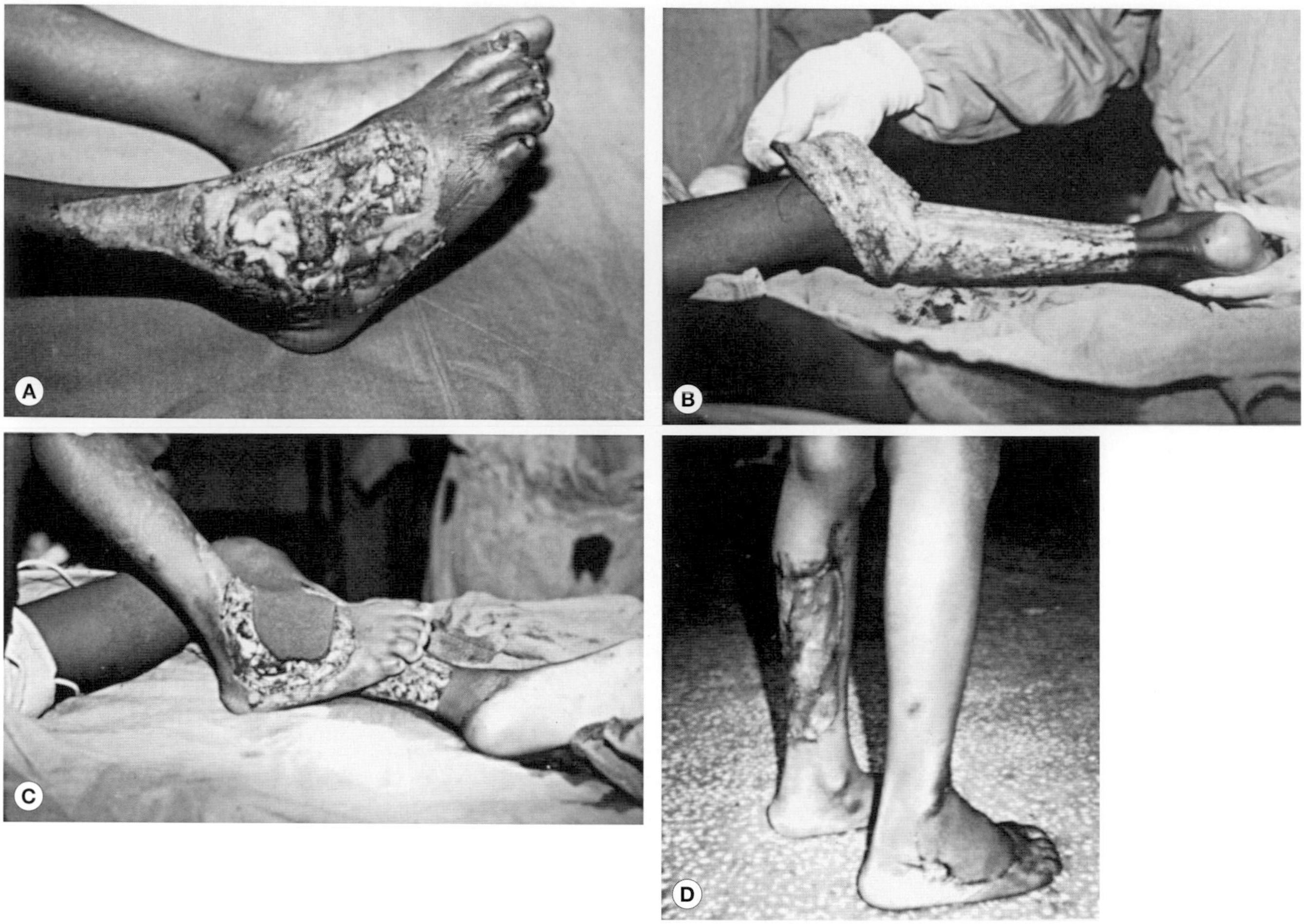

FIGURE 14.3 A 5-year-old boy's right foot traumatized by a taxi. **A** Preoperative view with exposed ankle joint, tarsal joints and soft tissue defect. **B** Fasciocutaneous flap elevated from the left calf. **C** Cross-leg flap placed to cover right foot defect. **D** Postoperative result: full coverage and function.

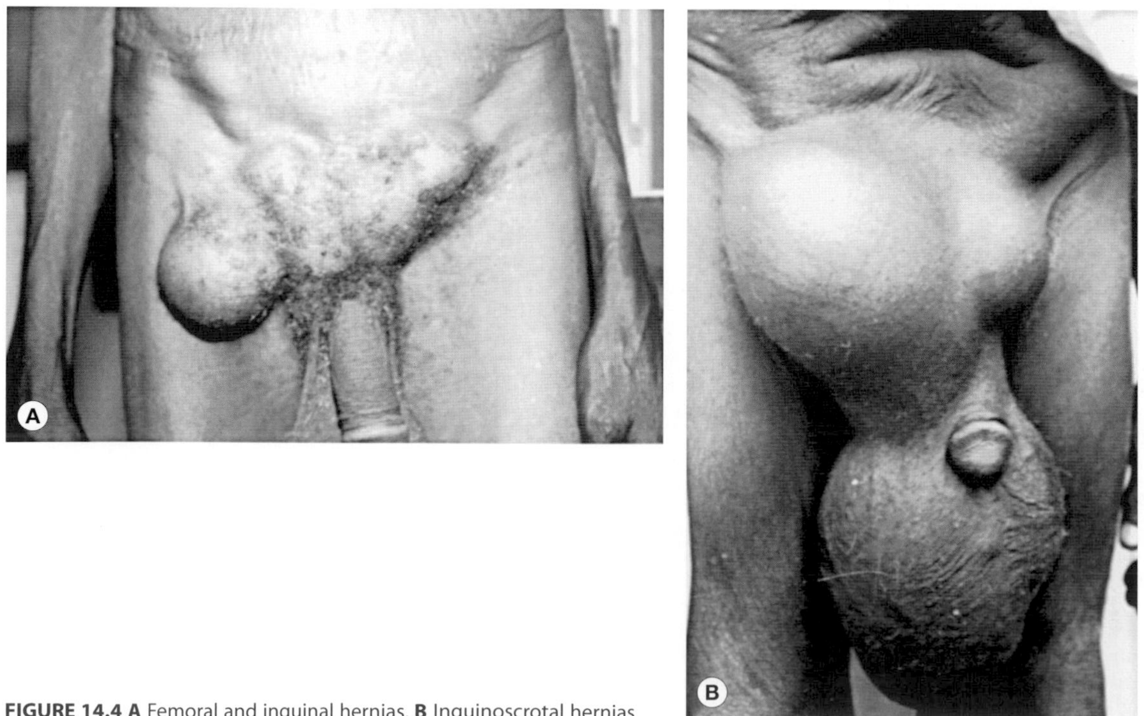

FIGURE 14.4 A Femoral and inguinal hernias. **B** Inguinoscrotal hernias

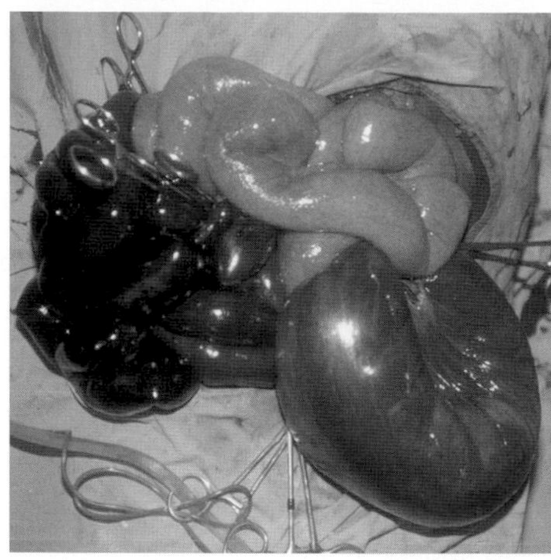

FIGURE 14.5 Ileosigmoid knotting with ischemic colon and frankly nonviable small bowel.

simple reduction. Alternatively, with viable bowel, an on-table lavage can be performed, the sigmoid resected, and alimentary continuity re-established by a primary anastomosis. When the sigmoid is strangulated, resection of the dead bowel with the creation of an end colostomy and mucus fistula or Hartmann pouch is recommended. Not infrequently, a loop of small bowel is caught in a twist of the sigmoid colon mesentery, producing a concomitant closed-loop obstruction and strangulation of the small bowel, the so-called compound volvulus or ileosigmoid knotting (Fig. 14.5). A small bowel resection and anastomosis must be performed in addition to correction of the colonic volvulus.

Gastrointestinal Obstruction and Inflammation

The leading operative indication for peptic ulcer disease in RPAs is gastric outlet obstruction. *Helicobacter pylori* may be the most common bacterial infection in Africa. *H. pylori* seropositivity was noted in 91% of Nigerian children under 20 years of age [14]. Mesenteric vascular diseases are not common. Inflammatory-type bowel diseases that can mimic regional enteritis or ulcerative colitis now occur in patients with HIV infections but are usually infectious, not idiopathic. Enteritis necroticans (pig-bel), a particular problem in the highlands of New Guinea, is a necrotizing enteritis produced by *Clostridium perfringens* toxin, and operative resection may be required to remove necrotic bowel.

Biliary Disease

Operative hepatobiliary and pancreatic diseases are not as frequent in sub-Saharan Africa as in Asia, where many are secondary to ascaris and liver flukes obstructing the biliary or pancreatic ducts. Cholecystitis is increasing in Saudi Arabia, probably secondary to changes in diet [15]. Gallbladder stones develop in patients with hemoglobinopathies; with increasing life expectancy in sub-Saharan Africa, sickle cell patients will more frequently present with complicated cholelithiasis.

OBSTETRICS AND GYNECOLOGY

These entities are covered in Chapter 6.

ORTHOPEDICS

Musculoskeletal problems in the tropics are covered in Chapter 13.

UROLOGY

Urologic problems can be congenital, infectious, obstructive or neoplastic. Undescended testes, hypospadias, posterior urethral valves, and torsion of the testis are congenital anatomic problems. Orchiopexy by 12 months maximizes the chances for spermatogenesis in cases of undescended testis. Children with hypospadias should not be circumcised at birth because the foreskin can be utilized later as a flap for hypospadia repair. Posterior urethral valves in males are diagnosed prenatally or shortly after birth in more developed areas, but in RPAs the diagnosis may not be made until several months of life, when the child presents with a chronic history of difficulty in initiating urination and a very weak urinary stream. A voiding cystourethrogram is the definitive test. Vesicostomy provides temporary treatment until definitive valve destruction can be performed endoscopically or through a perineal approach.

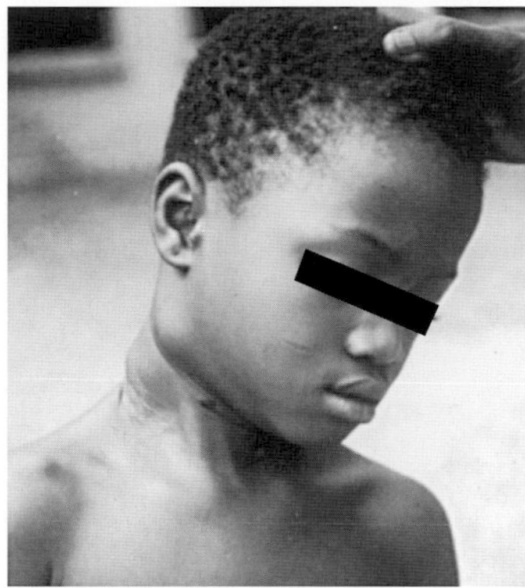

FIGURE 14.6 Tuberculosis cervical lymphadenitis (scrofula) in an 8-year-old Yoruba boy.

In the absence of ultrasound and flow Doppler examination, testicular torsion can be excluded only by direct visualization. In societies in which procreation is nearly mandatory, all males without progeny who present with a swollen, tender scrotum–testis should undergo scrotal exploration for diagnosis. Although the ipsilateral testis with torsion often is unsalvageable, orchiopexy of the contralateral testis can prevent future loss and resultant sterility.

Renal and ureteric stones are not prevalent in blacks, but Mediterranean Arabs have frequent stone problems. Since endoscopic and ultrasound techniques are generally not available, lithotomy is indicated for obstruction complicated by pain, progressive renal damage, or persistent infection. Lower urinary tract obstruction in older men generally results from benign prostatic hypertrophy, prostatic carcinoma, or urethral stricture secondary to prior gonococcal urethritis. Benign prostatic hypertrophy is treated by prostatectomy, usually open rather than transurethral. Urethral stricture is managed by repeated bougienage, suprapubic tube cystostomy, direct vision internal urethrotomy, or urethroplasty.

Cancers of the kidney, bladder, prostate, and penis (squamous cell carcinoma) are often seen at an advanced, non-operative stage. Urinary tuberculosis should be considered in patients with sterile pyuria. Infection by *Schistosoma haematobium* may produce granulomas of the ureters and bladder and result in bleeding, obstructive uropathy, pyelonephritis, or carcinoma of the bladder. Fournier's gangrene is a spontaneous gangrene of the skin of the scrotum and penis. Multiple organisms have been cultured, including *C. perfringens*. The onset is sudden and painful and is accompanied by fever and toxemia. Partial- or full-thickness scrotal slough can occur, exposing the testes. Treatment consists of antibiotics and aggressive debridement, and, on occasion, skin grafting.

EAR–NOSE–THROAT AND DENTAL SURGERY

Foreign bodies, neoplasia, infections, allergic conditions, maxillofacial trauma, and congenital anomalies are all seen in a tropical surgical practice. Tuberculous cervical adenitis (Fig. 14.6), Ludwig's angina,

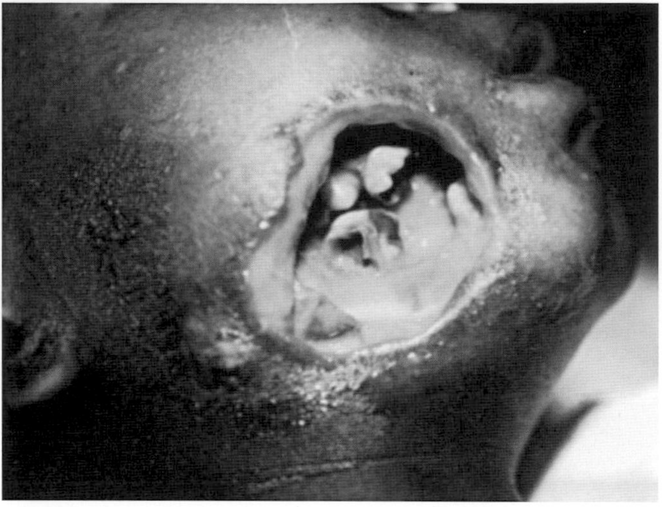

FIGURE 14.7 Cancrum oris (noma). Gangrenous stomatitis with soft tissue and bone defect producing an orocutaneous fistula in a 5-year-old malnourished boy.

dental abscesses, and otitis media with or without mastoiditis are common infections of the head and neck. Croup and laryngotracheobronchitis, especially as a complication of measles, may so compromise a child's airway that tracheostomy is mandatory. If nursing care, suctioning and humidification are deficient, serious complications may accompany tracheostomy. Cancrum oris (noma), usually seen in malnourished children, is a destructive, necrotic process (Fig. 14.7) that can produce oro-naso-cutaneous fistulas and ankylosis of the temporomandibular joint. Once infarction, infection and inflammation respond to debridement, penicillin and diet, the resultant fibrosis and tissue defects present a formidable reconstructive challenge. Myocutaneous flaps such as the pectoralis major island flap can be used to repair these complex problems. Dental care in RPAs is often extractive rather than preventative and preservative in nature and is not available in many rural areas.

PLASTIC SURGERY

Caring for large, infected, neglected wounds using a minimum of equipment and supplies occupies a large percent of the tropical surgeon's time. Simplified negative pressure wound therapy ("wound vacuuming") can often speed the rate of wound closure.

Thermal burns may receive inadequate initial treatment with resultant high mortality from renal failure and burn wound sepsis. In acute burn survivors, residual contractures and hypertrophic scarring are crippling. Skin-grafting capability for burn wound care is essential, with grafts taken freehand or with a drum or electric dermatome. The Tanner meshing technique allows expansion of the graft and improves graft "take". Early tangential excision and skin grafting should be considered except for extensive burns.

Burns of the hands are especially debilitating, but improved functional results can be obtained with early tangential excision and grafting, proper splinting, and conscientious physiotherapy. Infections and non-thermal hand injuries are very common and require prompt treatment to avoid fibrosis and contractures. Techniques of groin- and abdominal-flap coverage are particularly helpful in treating hand injuries.

A common congenital abnormality is cleft lip with or without a palatal defect. Access to corrective procedures and rehabilitation is often poor. Parents, disturbed by the neonate's deformity, want immediate repair. Counseling is indicated because lip repairs traditionally should not be undertaken until "10 weeks of age, 10 pounds of weight, and a hemoglobin level of at least 10 g/dL". Palatal repair is delayed until 1 year of age but should be performed before speech develops in order to prevent a nasalized speech pattern.

NEUROSURGERY

Imaging techniques, equipment and personnel to detect and treat tumors, arteriovenous malformations and various congenital abnormalities are rarely available. CT scanners are available at a few teaching hospitals and private clinics in the tropics, but scanner maintenance and expense limit availability and access.

Tropical neurosurgery focuses on trauma. Without benefit of sophisticated diagnostic equipment, head injury victims who have deterioration in their level of consciousness or who develop lateralizing neurologic signs should undergo exploration through burr holes with drainage if an epidural or subdural hematoma is found. Patients with open, depressed skull fractures require operation for debridement, hemostasis, elevation, and closure and coverage of the dura. Pond fractures (circular depressed fractures) in children can be observed or elevated using an obstetric vacuum extractor.

Spinal injuries from vehicular crashes or falls from trees are a major cause of morbidity and mortality. Spinal cord injury rehabilitation programs are rarely existent in RPAs; and if the para- or quadriplegic patient survives the in-hospital period of stabilization by traction, he or she often succumbs to urinary or decubitus ulcer-related sepsis after discharge. Spinal tuberculosis also causes paralysis. If deterioration of neurologic function in a patient with Pott's disease is recent or if it continues while the patient is receiving adequate antituberculous chemotherapy, drainage of the paraspinal abscess with spine stabilization should be considered.

PEDIATRIC SURGERY

Special concerns in tropical pediatric surgery include congenital anomalies of imperforate anus, bowel atresia, esophageal atresia, abdominal wall defects, and neural tube defects. These anomalies are apparent at birth before the child has been named and officially recognized as a family member, and parents may not seek treatment for such neonates and may refuse operative intervention if it is offered. Hirschsprung's disease, urinary tract abnormalities, and pediatric tumors, on the other hand, are usually detected after familial acceptance, and surgical help is sought, although stomas are often refused. Intussusception is a leading cause of intestinal obstruction in children 3 months to 2 years of age. Hydrostatic reduction is not routinely employed because of the uncertainty of adequate reduction as well as the scarcity of barium, film and fluoroscopy units. Operative reduction is the usual management for intussusception, and a nonviable intussusceptum is common. The mortality rate can be high [16].

CARDIOTHORACIC SURGERY

Pump oxygenators and the technological and financial support they require are rarely found in RPAs. Rheumatic fever with resultant valvular problems, congestive failure, congenital heart diseases, endomyocardial fibrosis and other cardiomyopathies, e.g., Chagas heart disease, and the pericardial problems of constriction (tuberculosis) and effusion (pyopericardium) are the major problems facing cardiologists and cardiac surgeons. Non-cardiac thoracic surgeons deal primarily with tuberculosis, thoracic empyema (commonly after measles), hemoptysis from destroyed lung, bronchiectasis, hydatid cyst, lung abscess, and trauma. Lung cancer is not widespread in RPAs but is increasing as tobacco use increases.

OPHTHALMOLOGY

Eighty percent of the world's preventable blindness occurs in patients living in the developing world. Causes of blindness include trauma, trachoma, onchocerciasis, corneal scarring, xerophthalmia (dryness and vitamin A deficiency) and cataracts. Cataracts blind 18 million people in the developing world, with the number doubling every 20–25 years. A nation may have major eye treatment centers, but only a select population has access to such care. Most people with treatable eye diseases never see an ophthalmic surgeon.

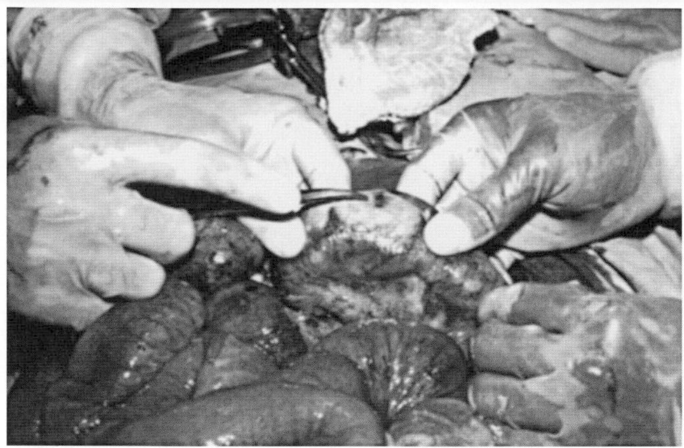

FIGURE 14.8 Perforation of the ileum in typhoid fever with secondary bacterial suppurative peritonitis.

TOPICS OF INTEREST TO SURGEONS AND NON-SURGEONS

TETANUS

See Chapter 55.

TYPHOID

Hemorrhage from and perforation of ileal ulcers are potentially fatal complications of typhoid. After prolonged periods of fever, catabolism and undernutrition, the patient can develop secondary bacterial peritonitis (Fig. 14.8). The best treatment is resuscitation followed by operative intervention to limit further contamination and to cleanse the peritoneal cavity. Simple two-layer closure in a transverse axis is adequate for one or two perforations. Multiple perforations require segmental resection with retention of the ileocecal valve if possible. Copious irrigation of the entire peritoneal cavity with saline is recommended. Operative mortality, although as low as 3–5% in some centers, is often in the 30% range.

LEPROSY (HANSEN'S DISEASE)

Patients with Hansen's disease may need surgical intervention to prevent or treat complications of the feet, hands and eyes. Foot ulcers, with or without accompanying osteomyelitis of the underlying bones, need bed rest, debridement, antibiotics, adequate footwear, and a change of lifestyle. Occasionally, ulcers require transtibial amputation. Tendon transfers can improve the pinch or intrinsic muscle function of a hand or counter a drop-foot gait, thus enhancing limb function and rehabilitation.

TUBERCULOSIS

The surgeon's role in tuberculosis is to obtain material for diagnosis (e.g., bronchoscopy, lymph node biopsy) and to treat complications. Tube thoracostomy is employed to treat pneumothorax, empyema and pyopneumothorax. Elective resections are used for bronchostenosis, bronchiectasis, destroyed lung, giant emphysematous bulla, resistant organisms, and recalcitrant patients with sputum-positive, localized open cavities. Elective pericardiectomy may be required in patients with constrictive pericarditis. Life-threatening hemoptysis may require emergency thoracotomy with lobectomy or pneumonectomy.

SCHISTOSOMIASIS

Schistosomiasis causes granuloma formation with bleeding, fibrosis and stricture in the lower gastrointestinal and genitourinary tracts. Schistosomiasis is a leading cause of portal hypertension. Treatment options for life-threatening variceal bleeding include medical management (vasopressin), balloon tamponade, injection sclerotherapy, variceal ligation, esophageal transection and portal decompression. Because of better liver function, patients with schistosomiasis do better following shunt procedures than do those who bleed from alcoholic or postviral cirrhosis. Urinary schistosomiasis can lead to an obstructive uropathy with progressive renal failure. Intraluminal obstruction of the distal ureter and damage to the ureteric muscle with loss of peristalsis produce hydronephrosis. Operative options for an abnormal distal ureter include ureteroneocystostomy and ureteric reconstruction. Cystoplasty using sigmoid, cecal or ileal bowel segments may be indicated in patients with a contracted bladder and can be combined with ureteric replacement. Urinary schistosomiasis can also contribute to the development of carcinoma of the bladder. Because such patients usually present with advanced disease, obstruction and renal failure, few are candidates for total cystectomy. Urinary diversion, with an ureterocolostomy to avoid a stoma and appliance, may provide palliation.

HYDATID CYST

Open surgical resection remains an important option for many patients with cystic hydatid disease, although excellent results following ultrasound-guided percutaneous aspiration, injection of scolicidal agents, and re-aspiration (PAIR) of hydatid cysts in the liver have been reported. Hypertonic saline solution or 0.1% cetrimide is recommended as the operative scolicide in preference to formalin. The operative goal is removal of the cyst without: (1) fluid leakage, which may cause toxic or anaphylactic reaction; (2) spillage of scolices or germinal epithelium, which may produce new cysts; or (3) bleeding and secondary infection. Alveolar hydatid disease of the liver requires a partial hepatectomy for treatment, and surgical resection, when possible, is recommended for polycystic hydatid disease.

AMERICAN TRYPANOSOMIASIS

The "megasyndromes" cause either dysphagia from megaesophagus or constipation from megacolon. Surgical treatment for megaesophagus includes partial or total resection of the esophagus, cardioplasty and myotomy. However, a report from Brazil noted a 62% incidence of complications in patients undergoing operation for chagasic megaesophagus, with one-third requiring reoperation and 88% having either a complication or postoperative dysphagia. Sigmoid resection is the operative treatment for megasigmoid. Toxic megacolon from Chagas disease warrants total colectomy.

FILARIAL ELEPHANTIASIS

Bancroftian, Malayan and Timorian filariasis can produce secondary lymphedema and the chronic obstructive signs of elephantiasis involving subcutaneous tissues of the scrotum and the lower extremities. Scrotal elephantiasis can be treated with excision of redundant tissue and placement of the testes in upper thigh adductor pockets or in a newly constructed scrotum. More than 20 operative procedures for the relief of chronic lower extremity lymphedema exist, indicating that none is superior. Operations for edematous extremities should be recommended only after careful consideration. The procedure most commonly employed is that of Charles (1912), in which the involved skin and lymphedematous subcutaneous tissue are excised down to deep fascia and the fascia then skin-grafted.

CONCLUSION

Developing and advancing a surgical practice in RPAs is challenging and frustrating, but can be quite rewarding. One must be vigilant not to let standards drop. Time-outs and an intentional focus on creating a culture of "safe surgery" can improve outcomes and job satisfaction. It helps to have local colleagues, to train interested nationals, to take care of one's own health, to take a long view, and to have a sense of humor. Two final aphorisms: Variability is the norm. Adversity is inevitable, but misery is optional.

REFERENCES

1. Farmer P, Kim J. Surgery and global health: a view from beyond the OR. World J Surg 2008;32:533–6.
2. MacGowan WAL. Surgical manpower worldwide. ACS Bulletin 1987;72:5–7.
3. Ozgediz D, Riviello R. The "other" neglected diseases in global public health: surgical conditions in sub-Saharan Africa. PLoS Med 2008;5:e121.
4. Gosselin RA, Thind A, Bellardinelli A. Cost/DALY averted in a small hospital in Sierra Leone: what is the relative contribution of different services? World J Surg 2006;30:505–11.
5. WHO Western Pacific Region – Fact sheets – Health, poverty and MDG. http://www.wpro.who.int/media_centre/fact_sheets/fs_20050621.htm.
6. Haynes AB, Wiser TG, Berry WR, et al. A surgical safety list to reduce morbidity and mortality in a global population. N Engl J Med 2009;360:491–9.
7. Meier DE. Opportunities and improvisations: a pediatric surgeon's suggestions for successful short-term surgical volunteer work in resource-poor areas. World J Surg 2010;34:941–6.
8. Freudenberg S, Sano D, Ouangré E, et al. Commercial mesh versus nylon mosquito net for hernia repair. A randomized double-blind study in Burkina Faso. World J Surg 2006;30:1784–90.
9. Meier DE, Nkor SK, Aasa D, et al. Prospective randomized comparison of two preoperative skin preparation techniques in a developing world country. World J Surg 2001;25:441–3.
10. King M, ed. Primary Anesthesia. Oxford, UK: Oxford University Press; 1986.
11. Meier DE, OlaOlorun DA, Nkor SK, et al. Ketamine – a safe and effective anesthetic agent for children in the developing world. Pediatr Surg Int 1996;11:370–3.
12. Parkin DM, Pisani P, Ferlay J. Global cancer statistics. CA Cancer J Clin 1999;49:33–64.
13. Udwadia TE, Udwadia RT, Menon K, et al. Laparoscopic surgery in the developing world. An overview of the Indian scene. Int Surg 1995;80:371–5.
14. Halcombe C, Tsimiri S, Eldridge J, et al. Prevalence of antibody to helicobacter pylori in children in northern Nigeria. Trans R Soc Trop Med Hyg 1993;87:19–21.
15. Tamini TM, Wosornu L, Abdul-Ghani A, et al. Increased cholecystectomy rates in Saudi Arabia. Lancet 1990;336:1235–7.
16. Meier DE, Coln CD, Rescorla FJ, et al. Intussusception in children – an international perspective. World J Surg 1996;20:1035–40.

Oral Health and Disease in the Tropics 15

Martin H Hobdell, Tepirou Chher

Key features

- Dental caries is the most prevalent non communicable disease worldwide and the most widespread childhood disease
- Late presentation of oral carcinoma, often the result of tobacco use (particularly chewing tobacco) and alcohol, is frequently lethal because of late presentation
- The highest prevalences of oral diseases are found in resource-poor tropical communities
- The majority of oral disease in resource-poor tropical countries remains untreated or is treated after a long delay, when treatment is more complex and resource-demanding, with poorer outcomes

INTRODUCTION

The most prevalent oral diseases in poor tropical communities are the result of poverty and institutional neglect combined with a lack of education. Dental caries (= dental decay) particularly of the primary (or baby) teeth is the most common childhood disease and the most frequent non-communicable disease worldwide. Most of the decay remains untreated and leads to infection of dental origin (= odontogenic) with serious impacts on child health and development [1].

The oral conditions with the most serious consequences are: oral cancer, the oral manifestations of HIV/AIDS, noma (or cancrum oris; = gangrene of the facial tissues), and trauma to the face and oral tissues (Boxes 15.1 & 15.2).

Providing dental care for patients in resource-poor communities poses the same problems as for other medical disciplines – limited equipment, materials and adequately trained personnel. This chapter presents simple frontline emergency care that can be provided using simple, but effective methods.

It is not exhaustive either in the provision of extensive clinical management details or in its presentation of detailed pathologic information on all oral diseases. It provides the basics necessary for a field officer to deal with the most commonly presenting oral conditions. Details of technical procedures can be found online at: http://www.hesperian.org/publications_download.php: look for *"Where there is no dentist"* by Murray Dickson.

BACKGROUND INFORMATION

The World Health Organization, since the 1960s, has been gathering data on the prevalence and severity of oral diseases, which are available online at: http://www.whocollab.od.mah.se/ and in more pictorial form at: http://www.oralhealthatlas.org/uniflip/index.html.

EXAMINING THE ORO-MAXILLO-FACIAL COMPLEX

A thorough oral examination begins outside the mouth because often there are signs of intraoral disease displayed outside the mouth, such as swelling, redness, trauma to the face, or sinus openings. Careful visual examination is essential together with palpation of the facial skeleton and of any swellings, which can reveal the nature of the swelling (hard, soft, fixed to underlying structures or free etc.). Like all clinical examinations it is best to develop a scheme that follows the same routine each time.

The intraoral examination likewise should always follow a fixed routine (Box 15.3). Begin by examining the lips and corners of the mouth for cuts, abrasions and/or ulcerations. In elderly edentulous patients, it is not uncommon to find signs of candida infection (cracks that are red and inflamed that may sometimes bleed when the patient stretches their mouth wide open).

Next, pull back the lips and examine their lining mucosa; then the cheeks, as far back as is possible, for ulceration or localized changes in color and/or texture. Ask the patient to open their mouth so that you can examine the hard and soft palate. Take a soft gauze and get the patient to protrude their tongue; grasp it gently with the gauze and examine the dorsal and ventral surfaces – again looking for ulceration or localized changes in color (be careful not to cut the soft ventral surface of the tongue on the incisal edges of the lower anterior teeth). Then examine the teeth for cavities (see section on dental caries) and how the teeth meet together. Check how the patient opens their mouth; is it smooth, without clicking, do the midlines of the jaws move parallel with each other?

DENTAL CARIES

DESCRIPTION

Dental caries most commonly presents as pain on eating or drinking, particularly of hot or cold foods. In its later stages, when pulpal infection has passed to the periapical tissues surrounding the root tip(s), there may be swelling, redness and heat of the infected area, and, if the infection has spread to the deeper tissues, trismus (= in ability to open the mouth). Other systemic symptoms are those of an acute infection: fever, malaise.

ETIOLOGY

The resting saliva of the mouth normally has a neutral or alkaline pH. This changes when the microorganisms attached to the surfaces of the teeth (or dental plaque) metabolize dietary sugars to produce acids. These acids, through chemical action, release calcium and phosphate ions from the hydroxyapatite crystallites that form the enamel

BOX 15.1 The Key Oral Diseases

- Dental caries
- Oral cancer, and other oral mucosal diseases including the oral manifestations of HIV/AIDS
- Noma
- Oro-facial trauma

BOX 15.2 Pediatric Considerations of Oral Conditions and Diseases

- Noma occurs largely in children 3–7 years of age, is a life-threatening and life-changing disease for which, if the initial infection is survived and halted, many reconstructive surgeries are necessary. Prevention is paramount
- Dental caries of the primary dentition, stunting and underweight are very common in resource-poor tropical countries
- There is some evidence that treatment of odontogenic infection in young undernourished stunted children increases their rate of growth and weight
- Oro-facial trauma in children is common in resource-poor tropical countries

BOX 15.3 Basic Instrumentation for Dental Examination and Simple Dental Treatment

Basic instrumentation for dental examination

- Mouth mirror
- Dental explorer (= probe)
- Gauze squares

Basic instrumentation for simple dental treatment

As above plus:

- Dental forceps for the extraction of upper and lower *primary* and *permanent* molars, bicuspids (= premolars), cuspids (= canines) and incisors
- Scalpel (for incisions needed for certain extractions and to achieve drainage of pus)
- Sutures (to close wounds – both surgical and traumatic)
- Needle holders
- Dental excavators (for preparing dental cavities for restoration)
- Dental plastic instruments (for manipulating restorative materials into prepared cavities)
- Spatula (for mixing the glass ionomer cement)

covering of the crowns of the teeth. The calcium and phosphate ions remain in the saliva.

The drop in the pH of the saliva around the teeth is relatively rapid – some few minutes. The resting neutral pH takes much longer to be re-established – around 40 minutes to 1 hour, depending, among other things, on the amount and stickiness of the sugary food eaten.

The very small, decalcified areas on the enamel surface are the initial lesions of the carious process. However, they are reversible lesions; if the salivary pH returns to neutral for a long enough time period, then the calcium and phosphate ions that have leeched out will re-mineralize back into the crystallite lattice. This information is important when preparing dietary and feeding information for young mothers and also in developing sound evidence-based preventive strategies.

If sugar is eaten frequently, then the pH of the saliva remains low and more enamel is dissolved; ultimately, a physical break in the integrity of the enamel surface results. This minute cavity is then colonized by microorganisms, which, in turn, produce acid from sugar, and so the process continues until a visible cavity results. Once the dentine of the tooth is infected, the process continues with other types of microorganisms becoming involved until the pulp cavity of the tooth is reached and infected – ultimately resulting in a dental abscess at the root(s) tip with the infection spreading to the surrounding periodontal ligament, bone. If this is neglected for long enough or infected with virulent organisms, infection spreads beyond into other soft tissues and tissue spaces. The visible sign when this has occurred is what are commonly called "gum boils" in young children. Sometimes the spread of infection to the surrounding tissues may be life-threatening if, for example, the infection spreads from the upper anterior region to the cavernous sinus or from a lower posterior tooth to the pharyngeal spaces.

SYMPTOMS/SIGNS AND DIFFERENTIAL DIAGNOSIS (Table 15-1)

CLINICAL DIAGNOSIS AND TREATMENT

- **Initial white spot lesions**: re-mineralize by coating the area with fluoridated toothpaste, varnish or gel repeatedly.
- **Initial cavitation**: small visible break in the surface enamel, in the enamel only, cover with fissure sealant.
- **More extensive cavitation, but small**: clean and fill with glass ionomer cement, coat with fissure sealant.
- **Cavitation involving outer layer of dentine**: use hand instruments to remove undermined enamel; remove soft and decayed dentine; restore with glass ionomer cement.
- **Cavitation with more extensive dentine involvement extending to more than one surface of the tooth, but not entering the pulp cavity**: refer for traditional restoration.
- **Cavitation with pulpal involvement**: treatment of choice in resource-poor tropical countries is tooth extraction under local anesthesia.
- **Management of infections associated with pulpal infections that have spread to surrounding tissues**: spreading infections from periapical abscesses can become life-threatening. Drain frank pus; prescribe wide-spectrum antibiotics. Once the infection is under control, extract the tooth under local anesthesia.

PREVENTION – INDIVIDUAL PROGRAMS

- **Dietary advice**: limit dietary use of sugars, particularly by reducing sugared and high-energy drinks, sweets and snacks, between-meal eating. There is little evidence that this alone is sufficient. It needs to be linked with one of the programs listed below. For details of the effectiveness and efficiency of the preventive measures listed below, go to: http://www.ohg.cochrane.org/reviews.html.
- **Toothbrushing with fluoridated toothpaste**: check that the toothpaste has fluoride – if possible, find one that has been approved by a dental organization like the American Dental Association or FDI World Dental Federation as not all toothpaste that states it contains fluoride has fluoride in it in many resource-poor tropical countries.
- **Fluoride mouth rinsing.**

- Fluoride varnish programs.
- Topically applied fluoride gels.

ORAL MUCOSAL LESIONS INCLUDING ORAL CANCER, OTHER TUMORS AND NOMA

DESCRIPTION

This section includes a brief summary of common oral mucosal conditions and a summary of their treatment (Table 15-2).

GENERAL ETIOLOGY

In general, the known causes for oral mucosal problems and tumors range from infectious agents – bacterial, viral and fungal infections – to trauma sustained over a long period as occurs in tobacco users either from smoke inhalation, heat from burning tobacco, or from specific components of the tobacco and any other substances with which it has been mixed. The effects of tobacco use appear to be exacerbated when combined with alcohol use. The cause of a number of invasive tumors, such as ameloblastomas, is not understood at the present time. Systemic diseases may also play a part in oral mucosal diseases.

TABLE 15-1 Toothache

Stimulus	Symptoms	Possible diagnosis	Actions
Cold or sweet substances	Intermittent pain that may be prolonged for a short while after stimulus ends	Exposed dentine: possibly dental caries, but if persistent for a short while could be exposed root surface, with reversible pulpitis	Examine tooth involved for either a cavity (dental caries) and/or exposed root surface not covered by enamel. If cavity, place temporary filling. If exposed root surface, apply fluoride toothpaste with patient's finger
Hot or cold substances	Intermittent pain that passes soon after stimulus ends	Dental caries	Examine tooth involved carefully for a cavity (dental caries). Place filling
Hot or cold substances	Intermittent pain that is prolonged after stimulus ends	Dental caries with reversible pulpitis	Examine tooth involved for a cavity (dental caries). Place temporary filling
Hot substances	Continuous dull aching pain	Dental caries with a pulpal abscess	Tap tooth gently with the handle of a mouth mirror. If painful, then root canal treatment or dental extraction
Hot substances	Strong continuous pain and tooth feels too high	Dental abscess or possibly a periodontal abscess	Examine gingiva and gum tissue around tooth for swelling near to gingival (gum) margin. If no swelling, then dental abscess. Root canal treatment or dental extraction
Going up or down stairs, or bending head down	A number of upper teeth hurt on one or both sides	Maxillary sinusitis	Treat maxillary sinusitis with decongestants

TABLE 15-2 Oral Mucosal Lesions – Ulcerations

Symptoms	Appearance	Possible diagnosis	Actions
Rapid onset and punched-out appearance; persists for normally around 2 weeks but may vary. Recurrent in nearly all age groups from 6 years upwards. Reportedly more common in patients with "tropical sprue"	Punched-out appearance; vary in size from very small pinhead to large penetrating lesions	Recurrent aphthous ulcers	Reassurance, 0.2% w/v chlorhexidine gluconate mouthwash may reduce oral bacteria load and aid healing
Usually in very young children (1–10 years) but can occur in adults. General malaise, fever and difficulty in eating and swallowing, profuse salivation	Bright red oral mucosa including the gingival tissues around the necks of the primary teeth	Primary herpes simplex infections (herpes simplex virus)	Elixir of erythromycin 250 mg four times a day rinsed around the mouth or on a cotton bud for very small children, mild antipyretics to reduce fever
Painful, usually small, watery papules around the mouth and on the lips	Watery vesicles with marked red halo	Secondary herpes simplex infections (herpes simplex virus): "cold sores"	Liberally apply 5% w/w acyclovir cream to the site at the first indication of an impeding vesicular eruption
Small erythematous areas on hands and feet, then oral ulceration soon after, with little systemic upset except in infants	Mild cases, only oral lesions present: small vesicles with erythematous base, very like aphthous ulcers. Skin lesions rarely ulcerate	Hand, foot and mouth disease (coxsackievirus)	Lesions heal after about 10 days. If the ulcers are large, keeping them clean with 0.2% w/v chlorhexidine gluconate mouthwash may help

Continued

TABLE 15-2 Oral Mucosal Lesions – Ulcerations—cont'd

Symptoms	Appearance	Possible diagnosis	Actions
Difficulty in opening mouth, which can be complete, with pain in last molar region, but usually no other symptoms. Unlike tetanus where there is also facial spasm on trying to smile and spasm of other muscles. No history of recent wound	Inflamed oral mucosa around partially erupted third molar (usually in the lower jaw). In the worst cases there may be extension of infection into pharyngeal spaces with fever and general malaise	Pericoronitis – inflammation of gum flap and surrounding tissues over third molar tooth	If systemic spread, high doses of broad-spectrum antibiotic in accordance with local protocol. In more mild cases, irrigation beneath gum flap with normal saline or 0.2% w/v chlorhexidine gluconate mouthwash. If upper third molar is biting hard on the gum flap, it should be extracted under local anesthesia
Apparent abscess formation some weeks after the extraction usually of a lower molar tooth, usually not very painful with or without spontaneous drainage	Abscess pointing on cheek at or near the corner of the mandible. Pus contains yellow (sulfur) granules	Actinomycosis	High and prolonged doses of amoxicillin 500 mg four times a day for 1–2 months
Foul-smelling rotten halitosis with gingival (gum margin) bleeding, general malaise and sometimes fever with lymphadenopathy of submandibular lymph nodes	"Punched-out" ulcerated interdental papillae (gum tips between adjacent teeth). Often a bloody yellow exudate	Fusospirochetal infection: acute necrotizing ulcerative gingivitis (ANUG)	Gentle cleaning around necks of teeth with a scaler to remove calculus (tartar) or toothbrush. Metronidazole 250 mg four times a day for 5–7 days
Sore mouth; difficulty in eating, swallowing and speaking. Cracking and sores at angles of mouth	White patches on the oral mucosa that wipe away easily leaving a raw bleeding surface. But may also be bright red patches (often under dentures) or red and hypertrophic. Not to be confused with oral leukoplakia, which will not wipe away and is a precancerous lesion. Seen frequently in sexually active, HIV-positive patients	Oral candida infections	Rinsing three times a day with 0.2% w/v chlorhexidine gluconate mouthwash and topical treatment with lozenges, ointments or creams. The drugs of choice include amphotericin B (lozenge, 10,000 IU slowly dissolved in the mouth 3–4 times per day after meals for 2 weeks minimum). You can cut a 100 mg clotrimazole vaginal insert into two pieces. In the morning, use one piece. Put in the mouth, let it slowly melt. Use the second at night. Package may say "do not take by mouth". This means do not swallow it. It is safe to let it melt in the mouth, then spit it out. Or use nystatin – cream, oral suspension or pastille – but do not use with chlorhexidine mouthwash
Largely painless, longstanding, red oral granulomatous ulceration of the oral mucosa. Could also present as a cold dental abscess	Patients with other symptoms/signs of tuberculosis, but initial diagnosis sometimes made in dental clinic from biopsy. Tuberculous abscess diagnosed from pus specimen and "collar stud" radiographic appearance	Tuberculosis	Treatment should follow the local protocol for the treatment of tuberculosis. The ulceration heals rapidly once treatment is commenced
Oral ulcer with relatively short duration on lips or hard palate; misshapen lower permanent incisors and/or first permanent molars; longstanding hard palate ulceration, which may perforate the palate into the nasal cavity	Primary lesion: painless brown ulcerated lump with a clear base (chancre) with submandibular lymphadenopathy on lips, tongue or elsewhere in the mouth. Congenital lesions: oral ulceration; and/or Hutchinson's chisel-shaped upper and/or lower incisors and/or "mulberry" nodular first molars. Tertiary lesions: chronic hard palate ulceration, which may perforate the hard palate into the nasal cavity	Syphilis	Treat according to the local protocol for the treatment of syphilis
Massive oral and facial ulceration, with or without bone necrosis in young children or sexually active adults	Usually seen in young children following an active infectious disease such as measles. In adults, increasingly seen in HIV-positive patients. Patients are usually severely malnourished and living in extreme poverty	Noma (cancrum oris)	Give IV fluids, whole blood and broad-spectrum antibiotics at high doses depending on body weight to control the spread of infection. Make sure the patient's mouth is cleaned regularly (at least once a day). Remove dead bony sequestra as required. Maintain liquid nutrition until patient has recovered sufficiently to eat

SIGNS/SYMPTOMS AND DIFFERENTIAL DIAGNOSIS (Table 15-2)

Differential Diagnosis (Table 15-3)

ORO-MAXILLO-FACIAL TRAUMA

DESCRIPTION

Oro-maxillo-facial trauma is particularly common in resource-poor tropical countries. It ranges from superficial flesh wounds to hard tissue damage and may have life-threatening implications if not dealt with appropriately. It can lead to permanent disfigurement and impaired function. Cut lips and bruised skin are frequent. Fractured teeth, alveolar bone fractures, maxillary and mandibular fractures are common. Oro-maxillo-facial trauma often occurs with other trauma to the patient's body.

AETIOLOGY

In many communities located in peri-urban, low-income, self-built, poor-housing areas, intentional violence is common. It involves beatings, knife and gun shot wounds. Industrial accidents are common in

TABLE 15-3 Swellings in the Mouth

Symptoms	Appearance	Possible diagnosis	Actions
Epithelial mass of granulation tissue at the gingival (gum) margin, but can occur elsewhere; more common in pregnant women	Darkish red mass on gingival margin that bleeds easily on touch	Pyogenic granuloma	Excision under local anesthesia and scaling away any calculus (tartar)
Smooth, painless, pale pink swelling on gingiva, or lining of cheek and elsewhere in the mouth	Can be pedunculated or not. Blanches on pressing but does not bleed	Fibroepithelial polyp or fibroma	Excision under local anesthesia
Usually painless hard swelling adjacent to the tip of a tooth root in the buccal sulcus (cheek pouch)	Swelling adjacent to a heavily filled or broken-down tooth, or one that has been traumatized in the past. Appears in a periapical radiograph as a dark area surrounding the root tip. The tooth is insensitive to hot or cold stimuli as it is dead. Radiolucency at tip of tooth root on x-ray. Usually much smaller than an odontogenic cyst	Radicular cysts	Root canal treatment or tooth extraction under local anesthesia, depending on size
Hard painless swelling anywhere in the jaws, but is sometimes masked in the maxilla as the cyst expands into the maxillary sinus. Can be very large	Associated with the crown of an unerupted tooth. On radiographs the tooth can usually be seen to be displaced by the growing cyst	Odontogenic cyst	If small, excision with unerupted tooth if it cannot be brought into position orthodontically, or if larger, marsupialization of the cyst, which later fills in from behind
Painless soft tissue swelling beneath the anterior part of the tongue, which may make swallowing difficult	Painless sessile rubbery swelling beneath the tongue arising from behind a sublingual salivary gland duct that has become blocked. Radiographic appearance may show calculus in gland duct in a view of the floor of the mouth	Ranula	Excision or marsupialization under local anesthesia
Painless swelling of the tooth-bearing part of the mandible or maxilla	Untreated, this tumor may become quite large. When small and within the cortical plates, it is hard, but as these are thinned by tumor growth, you may find "eggshell" crackling from minute fractures in the plates as you press them. It is a solid tumor with some cystic cavities. It is locally invasive, but rarely metastasizes. Radiographically, the roots of adjacent teeth may show resorption	Ameloblastoma	Excision of the tumor and a good margin of bone. Usually requires replacement with a bone graft
Relatively painless oral ulceration that has persisted for more than 3 weeks with or without treatment, with no obvious cause like a denture rubbing. It may appear anywhere on the oral mucosa	Any oral ulceration that has persisted for more than 3 weeks with or without treatment should be inspected carefully and biopsied if there is any doubt about the cause. Confirmation by biopsy	Oral carcinoma and precancerous lesions	Resection with a wide margin and application of the local protocol for the treatment of cancer
A painless, red-brown or purple-colored patch rather like a swollen bruise anywhere in the mouth	Nowadays, most commonly seen in sexually active HIV-positive patients. Rarely ulcerates	Kaposi sarcoma	Advice from an experienced clinician should be obtained as it can be treated with strong anticancer drugs or sometimes drugs used in the treatment of varicose veins
A rubbery swelling of the jaws; usually distorts the face in young children	The history – possible other swellings elsewhere in the body of a similar consistency should raise suspicions. Confirmation of the diagnosis is from biopsy findings	Burkitt's lymphoma	This is usually treated with cytotoxic drugs such as cyclophosphamide, but it should be treated using the recommended local protocol

TABLE 15-4 Oro-maxillo-facial Trauma

Symptoms	Appearance	Possible diagnosis	Actions
Broken tooth/teeth, sharp jagged tooth crown, mobile tooth	incomplete tooth crown, vertical or horizontal crack/split in tooth, with or without opening of the pulp chamber	Direct or indirect trauma to tooth, crown damage by dental caries (= decay) or large filling and tooth broken during chewing	In most cases, unless good restorative dental services available, tooth extraction under local anesthesia. This may be complicated by the fracture making it difficult to extract the complete root. Careful planning of extraction is necessary. If restorable and dental pulp is involved, root canal treatment is needed
Pain from lower jaw, inability to close teeth together normally, difficulty in opening and closing the mouth, blood in mouth. History of trauma	Occlusal plane (= line formed by tops of teeth) is disturbed, independent movement of one part of mandible. Blood seeping from the gum at the side of a tooth. Confirmed by lateral oblique radiograph of mandible on the side believed to be broken. To be differentiated from a dislocated mandible where the patient cannot close their mouth normally there is no obvious break in the bone and the heads of the mandibular condyles are anterior to their normal resting position – your fingers fit into a deep dimple on each side of the patient's face when you try to palpate the mandibular condyles	Mandibular fracture Mandibular dislocation	Urgent care. Position the patient comfortably – seated and leaning forward slightly and place a figure-of-eight bandage to hold the two fractured parts in a stable position. To reposition a recently dislocated mandible: stand in front of the seated patient. Place a thumb on the last molar, with your fingers under the tip of the chin. Press down hard on your thumbs, at the same time rotate the chin upwards and push the mandible backwards into the articular fossae. Instruct the patient to gently move their jaws but not to yawn or open widely for the next few days
Broken, displaced and mobile upper anterior teeth with broken alveolar bone	This is usually the result of being hit in the face or a fall. A mobile section of bone containing a number of upper anterior teeth	Simple dento-alveolar fracture of the maxilla	Managed by placing a splint attached to adjacent undamaged teeth either with eyelet wires and an arch bow or by splinting using composite resin
Major trauma involving the middle third of the face, from a hard direct impact often in a road traffic accident. Bleeding from the mouth, nose and possibly ears	Patient may have difficulty on breathing or swallowing and be bleeding from the nose and mouth. The orbits may be involved and consciousness impaired. Confirmation from posterior–anterior radiographs and other views, depending on the site of the major injuries	Simple or compound fractures of the maxilla. They may range from a fracture of the zygomatic arch to a complex fracture involving the base of the skull	An urgent assessment should be made of the extent of the injuries and if there is a concomitant brain injury. If brain injury suspected, attention to this takes precedence over the maxillary injuries. These cases require referral to specialist care

situations where health and safety issues are not strong components of industrial regulations/laws. To these have to be added motor vehicle accidents that occur in poor countries, caused by poor vehicle maintenance, poor driving and poor road conditions.

Less often seen are physical and chemical burns both to the face and inside the mouth. The flammable nature of housing and the use of kerosene lamps, heaters and cooking stoves make fire a frequent event in poor areas. Burns to the face and upper body occur often.

Chemical burns may occur because patients with untreated dental caries and toothache often resort to using aspirin or other substances. Believing their pain is associated with a particular tooth, they may place an aspirin in the buccal sulcus next to the painful tooth, not realizing of course that aspirin works systemically and not locally. If the aspirin remains in place for long, it will cause ulceration of the oral mucosa; a chemical burn. This ulcer is then painful itself and will take time to heal.

All serious trauma cases must receive emergency care promptly to maintain the airway, stop hemorrhage and maintain the heart rate and then be referred to those capable of making a full assessment and providing treatment.

SYMPTOMS/SIGNS AND DIFFERENTIAL DIAGNOSIS AND EMERGENCY ACTIONS (Table 15-4)

REFERENCE

1. Petersen PE, Bourgeois D, Ogawa H, et al. The global burden of oral diseases and risks to oral health. Bull World Health Organ 2005;83:661–9.

Maternal and Newborn Health 16

Nynke R van den Broek

Key features

- The difference in maternal mortality rates between developing and developed countries shows the greatest disparity of all health indicators
- An estimated 358,000 women die each year as a result of complications of pregnancy and childbirth. This is the leading cause of death in women aged 15–49 years
- There are an estimated 3.0 million stillbirths annually and 2.8 million early neonatal deaths
- Provision of Skilled Birth Attendance and availability of Essential (or Emergency) Obstetric Care coupled with Newborn Care are key strategies that, if implemented, will reduce maternal and neonatal mortality and morbidity
- The five main direct causes of maternal mortality are hemorrhage, eclampsia, sepsis, and complications of obstructed labour and abortion
- The main causes of neonatal death are prematurity, asphyxia and infection
- Women (and their babies) need access to, and availability of, a continuum of care that includes antenatal, intrapartum and postnatal care, newborn care and family planning services
- In order for care to be effective it must be evidence-based and of good quality

GENERAL INTRODUCTION

Each year, at least 358,000 women worldwide die from complications of pregnancy and childbirth [1]. Many more survive but suffer ill health and disability as a result of these complications. Ninety-nine percent of all maternal deaths occur in South Asia and sub-Saharan Africa. In addition, an estimated 4 million neonatal deaths occur each year, accounting for almost 40% of all deaths under the age of 5 years [2]. The health of the neonate is closely related to that of the mother and the majority of deaths in the first month of life could be prevented if interventions were in place to ensure good maternal health.

There have been significant global efforts to reduce maternal and newborn mortality and morbidity in the last few decades. The "Safe Motherhood Initiative" was launched in Nairobi in 1987. One of its stated aims was to reduce maternal mortality by 50% by the year 2000. However, figures at the turn of the millennium remained disappointingly unchanged from the start of the initiative. This was partly because of better data collection and documentation of the problems, and also because reducing maternal and newborn health requires a coordinated and multifaceted approach. In 2000, nearly 190 countries signed up to the Millennium Development Goals (MDGs) with two goals specifically targeted towards maternal and child health (Table 16-1). Very clearly defined and pertinent indicators to monitor progress towards these goals were also agreed. For MDG 5, the monitoring framework was revised during the 2005 World Summit to include one new target (5b) and four new indicators (5.3–5.6) (Table 16-2).

Politically, there is increased attention directed towards maternal health and many countries now see the status of maternal and newborn health as a signal or "litmus test" of the degree of functionality of their health system as a whole. But has progress been made and can MDG 5 be achieved? Medically speaking, the answer is yes—we know what is needed and we know what to do in case of complications of pregnancy and childbirth [3]. An agreed "continuum of care" that includes antenatal care, delivery care and postnatal care needs to be available and accessible to women [4]. The availability of Skilled Birth Attendance and Emergency (Essential) Obstetric Care for all women all over the world are seen as key [5]. This is in addition to basic neonatal care and family planning.

TABLE 16-1 The Millennium Development Goals (MDGs)

- To eradicate extreme poverty and hunger
- To achieve universal primary education
- To promote gender equality and empower women
- **To reduce child mortality**
- **To improve maternal health**
- To combat HIV/AIDS, malaria and other diseases
- To develop a global partnership for development

TABLE 16-2 Indicators for Progress Millennium Development Goal 5

Target 5a

To reduce maternal mortality by three quarters between 1990 and 2015:
- reduce the maternal mortality ratio
- increase the number of births attended by skilled health personnel

Target 5b

To achieve universal access to reproductive health by 2015:
- increase the contraceptive prevalence rate
- reduce adolescent birth rate
- increase antenatal care coverage
- reduce unmet need for family planning

TABLE 16-3 Estimates of maternal mortality ratio and number of maternal deaths by United Nations Regions for 2005 and 2008

Region	Maternal mortality ratio 2005	Annual number of estimated maternal deaths in 2005	Maternal mortality ratio 2008	Annual number of estimated maternal deaths in 2008
Africa	820	276,000	590	207,000
Asia	330	241,000	190	139,000
Latin America and the Caribbean	130	15,000	85	9200
Oceania	430	890	230	550
Developed Regions	9	960	14	1700
World Total	400	536, 000	260	358,000

From World Health Organization. Trends in Maternal Mortality:1990–2008. 2010, WHO, Geneva.

MATERNAL MORTALITY

The number of maternal deaths in a population is related both to the risk of mortality associated with each pregnancy or birth (reflected in the maternal mortality ratio, which is the number of maternal deaths per number live births, ×100,000) and the number of pregnancies experienced by women of reproductive age [reflected in the maternal mortality rate, which is the number of maternal deaths per number of women of reproductive age (taken as 15–49), ×100,000].

There is still a lack of accurate data, especially from developing countries where maternal mortality is high. In the absence of complete and accurate civil registration systems, which are almost non-existent in resource-poor settings, maternal mortality ratios and rates are estimated based on a variety of methods, including household surveys, "sisterhood" methods, reproductive age mortality studies, censuses and modeling. Since 1990, using all available data and/or statistical modeling, estimates have been developed by the United Nations (UN) agencies which allow for international comparison and analysis of progress. The latest estimates from 2008 show that of the 358,000 maternal deaths that are estimated to occur annually, the vast majority occur in developing countries. Almost two-thirds are in sub-Saharan Africa (207,000) followed by South Asia (139,000) (Table 16-3).

Analysis of trend shows that at the global level, the decrease in maternal mortality between 1990 and 2008 was estimated to be 2.3% overall, which is well below the estimated 5.5% decrease needed annually to achieve MDG 5 by 2015 [6].

CAUSES OF MATERNAL MORTALITY—WHY DO WOMEN DIE?

A seminal review by Thaddeus and Maine in 1994 introduced the "Three Delay Model" [7]. They acknowledged that there are numerous factors that contribute to maternal mortality and that when obstetric complications occur, with prompt adequate treatment, the outcome is usually satisfactory. They therefore examined the factors that affect the interval between the onset of an obstetric complication and its outcome. The three delays described and examined are: (i) delay in deciding to seek care; (ii) delay in reaching the healthcare facility; and, (iii) delay in receiving care after getting to the healthcare facility. This framework is now widely used to examine and address factors contributing to maternal deaths in many countries (Box 16.1).

BOX 16.1 The 3-Delay Model

Delay 1: Are women aware of the need for care and the danger signs of pregnancy?

Delay 2: Are services inaccessible because they are not available, because of distance and/or cost of services, or do socio-cultural barriers prevent women from accessing services?

Delay 3: Is the care received at the facility, timely and effective?

Medically, the main direct causes of maternal deaths are obstetric hemorrhage, hypertensive disorders (eclampsia and pre-eclampsia), sepsis or infection, and complications of obstructed labour and abortion. There is some variation both across and within geographical regions (Figs 16.1 and 16.2) [8]. Based on the need for much better identification and understanding of the causes of maternal deaths, a World Health Organization (WHO) Technical Working Group examined and reached a consensus on a new classification system for cause of maternal death in 2009. This new classification is aligned with International Classification of Diseases (ICD) 10 and will feed into the new ICD 11 system of classification [9].

HEMORRHAGE

Obstetric haemorrhage is the most commonly documented cause of maternal death. This can take the form of antepartum bleeding (e.g. as a result of placenta praevia or placental abruption), intrapartum bleeding (e.g. as a result of rupture of the uterus) or post-partum hemorrhage (e.g. as a result of atony of the uterus, associated with disseminated vascular coagulopathy, or trauma to the genital tract). Any bleeding during pregnancy and delivery should be considered a "danger" or warning sign and requires urgent attention.

Placental abruption can occur suddenly and unexpectedly. In many resource-poor settings, in the absence of ultrasonography, the warning signs of bleeding, coupled with the clinical sign of a "uterus en bois" (woody hard uterus which feels contracted), will alert the healthcare provider to this emergency. In the case of placenta previa, a cesarean section is needed.

Post-partum hemorrhage is commonly defined as blood loss of more than 500 ml and severe post-partum hemorrhage as a loss of more than 1000 ml. Most cases are unpredictable and it is vital that there is early recognition of excess blood loss and immediate action. The majority of cases are the result of uterine atony post-delivery, either after vaginal delivery or cesarean section. The recommended treatment is uterotonics (drugs to stimulate uterine contraction) and prompt replacement of volume lost to avoid hypovolemic shock.

There are a number of uterotonics available, including oxytocin and ergometrine (the traditional and well-proven first-line approach), as well as more recent prostaglandins, such as carboprost and misoprostol. Blood transfusion is frequently needed and many women in

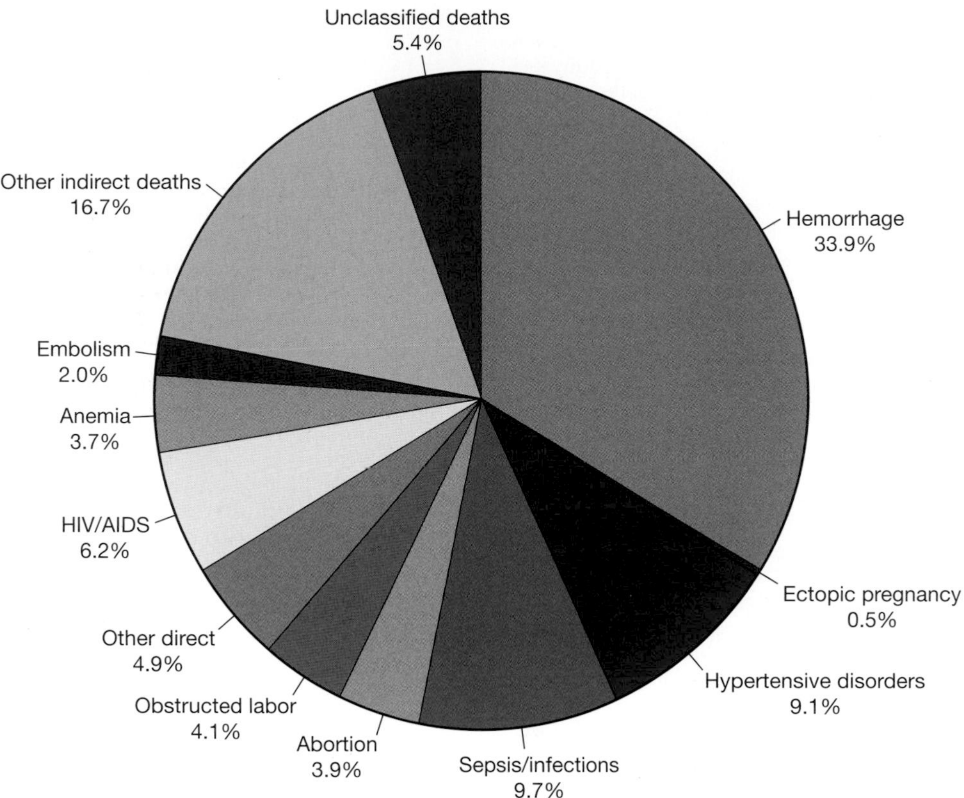

FIGURE 16.1 Causes of maternal deaths in Africa.

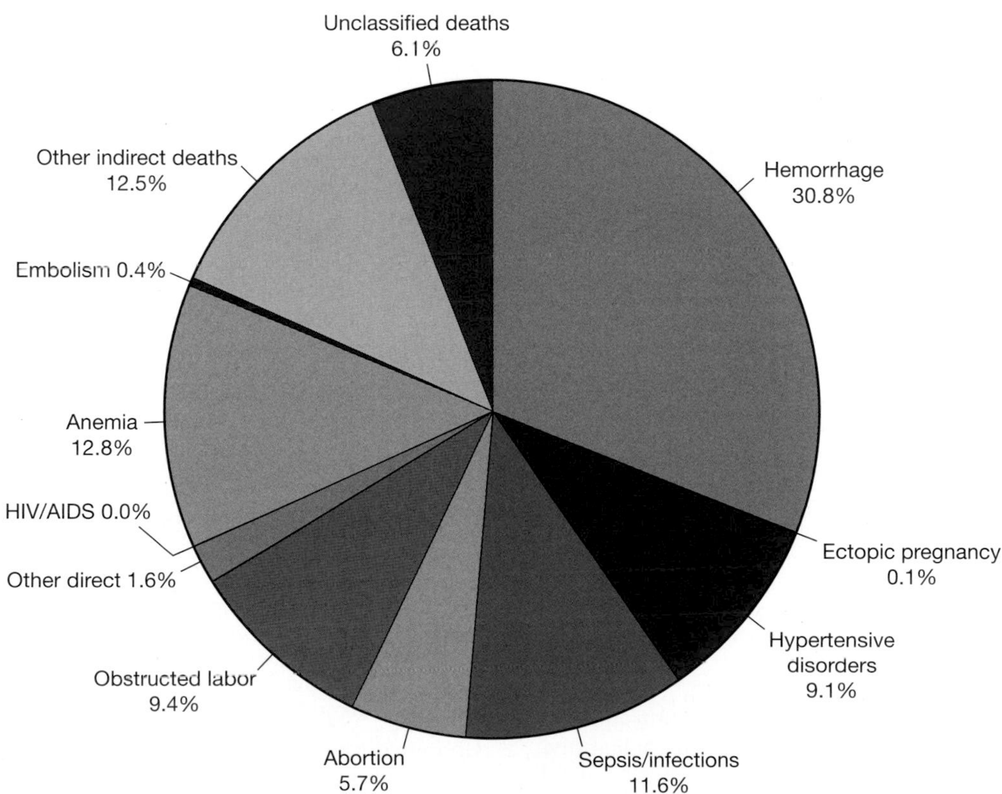

FIGURE 16.2 Causes of maternal deaths in Asia.

resource-poor areas do not survive hemorrhage because blood transfusion services are not available at all or insufficient blood is given. In addition, in cases of hemorrhage as a result of coagulopathy, such as is associated with abruption placenta and eclampsia, the availability of blood is crucial.

It may be necessary to explore the uterus for retained placental tissue. Retained placenta is a common problem leading to post-partum hemorrhage and all skilled birth attendants need to be able to carry out a manual removal of placenta under suitable analgesia (or anesthesia) and/or refer a woman with this condition to a higher level facility in good time. Retained placental tissue and/or membranes can lead to prolonged bleeding and high risk of infection. This requires careful exploration of the uterus under anesthesia and curettage. For hemorrhage occurring after a cesarean section, re-laparotomy may be necessary to check that this is not the result of unrecognized tears in the uterus and/or faulty surgical technique. In some cases with unstoppable hemorrhage, the only solution may be to perform a (subtotal) hysterectomy.

Post-partum hemorrhage can be prevented—it is recommended that all women have active management of the third stage of labor. This consists of administering a uterotonic (preferably oxytocin intramuscularly) at the time of delivery, together with clamping and cutting the cord and controlled cord traction (gentle cord traction with manual support of the uterus) to deliver the placenta. The oxytocin is given at the time of birth of the anterior shoulder; if it is not known whether this could be a multiple pregnancy, it should be given at the time of the birth of the baby, after checking there is no second baby. In some cases, this is combined with uterine massage or fundal pressure after delivery of the placenta. The routine administration of oxytocin reduces the risk of hemorrhage by more than half when compared with "physiologic" or expectant management (i.e. no oxytocic, no controlled cord traction, with the cord being clamped and cut after the placenta has been delivered by maternal effort only).

PRE-ECLAMPSIA AND ECLAMPSIA

Pre-eclampsia (hypertension with proteinuria) is specific to pregnancy and will progress to eclampsia (convulsions) if unrecognized. There is some evidence that eclampsia may be more common in certain developing countries, but good epidemiologic data are scarce. Pre-eclampsia is a multi-organ disease with unknown etiology. Early detection of hypertension and proteinuria is important and measurement of blood pressure with examination of urine must be done regularly during pregnancy, delivery and the postnatal period. Severe pre-eclampsia is associated with clinical signs and symptoms such as headache, visual disturbances, upper epigastric pain and hyperreflexia. An eclamptic convulsion is essentially the same as an epileptic fit with tonic and clonic seizures. Recurrent seizures can lead to maternal death but, most commonly, death is probably the result of intracerebral hemorrhage following untreated hypertension.

Delivery of the fetus and placenta is the "cure" for pre eclampsia and eclampsia, and, in many instances, a careful balance of risks needs to be made, especially if the fetus is premature. In addition to planning a timely delivery, magnesium sulfate has been consistently shown to be the drug of choice for pre-eclampsia in a number of important trials that included developing country populations. Magnesium sulfate can be given either intramuscularly or intravenously in cases of severe pre-eclampsia (to prevent eclampsia) and in eclampsia (to prevent seizures). Dosage can be monitored by checking the deep tendon reflexes and monitoring respiratory rate; absence of reflexes and respiratory depression indicate over-dosage.

Anti-hypertensive treatment must be given in pre-eclampsia and eclampsia. There are a variety of drugs available—all with proven benefit—including hydralazine (commonly preferred first-line drug), nifedipine and labetalol. Drugs often need to be given intravenously and may be combined with oxytocin, for example, to induce labor. Fluid input and output must be carefully monitored in the patient with pre-eclampsia and eclampsia. Cardiopulmonary overload is a frequent complication, especially when oxytocin (antidiuretic effect) is needed to induce labor. In addition, pre-eclampsia (a multi-organ disease) may be associated with kidney failure with reduced urine output.

SEPSIS

Most maternal deaths from infection occur in the postnatal period as a result of puerperal sepsis defined as "a temperature rise above 38.5 degrees Celsius maintained over 24 hours or recurring during the period from the end of the first to the end of the tenth day after childbirth or after abortion". Clinical signs and symptoms include fever, lower abdominal pain and uterine tenderness, subinvolution of the uterus with foul smelling, sometimes purulent, discharge with or without vaginal bleeding. Failure to recognize and manage puerperal sepsis early on will lead to septic shock and coagulopathy.

The clinical diagnosis of sepsis is relatively simple and does not require laboratory tests. In practice, fever in the post-partum period is often attributed solely to malaria, especially in malaria-endemic areas. Full clinical examination and a thick film slide will help with the differential diagnosis, as will the realization that, in many post-partum women, such fever is more likely to be associated with puerperal sepsis than malaria. Parenteral antibiotics are needed and generally given for 24–48 hours. There are various recommended regimens but in the absence of availability of blood-culture testing (as in most resource-poor areas), the best combination is ampicillin, gentamycin and metronidazol. The presence of retained placental fragments and/or fetal tissue in the case of abortion must be considered. Poor hygiene during delivery, during obstetric surgery, such as cesarean section or evacuation of the uterus (for termination of pregnancy or removal of retained products after an incomplete abortion), can all lead to puerperal sepsis. Good hand-washing practice and adequate sterilization of equipment used during surgical procedures are crucial preventive measures. Prophylactic antibiotics should be given in all cases of cesarean section. Infection with HIV is associated with reduced immunity, an increased risk of opportunistic infections and reported increased difficulty in treating post-partum sepsis, either after delivery or cesarean section.

COMPLICATIONS OF OBSTRUCTED LABOR

Obstructed labor is a condition contributing to maternal death in a number of ways, for example via haemorrhage as a result of rupture of the uterus or via sepsis. Morbidity associated with obstructed labor includes obstetric fistulae (vesico-vaginal and/or rectal). Obstructed labor is said to occur when there are good uterine contractions but there is no descent of the fetus through the pelvis. This may be because the fetus is too large for the pelvis (fetopelvic disproportion) and/or there are pelvic abnormalities (e.g. associated with rickets). Malposition of the fetus or congenital fetal abnormalities (e.g. hydrocephalus) can also be associated with obstructed labor. Clinical signs of rupture of the uterus include vaginal bleeding, hypovolemic shock, tender abdomen, an abnormal uterine contour, absent fetal heart and easily palpable fetal parts. A "Bandl's" ring can often be seen prior to rupture of the uterus and is a visible horizontal depression in the lower abdominal contour near the umbilicus which indicates the marcation between the thick muscular upper uterine segment and a very thin, stretched out lower uterine segment.

In cases of obstructed labor, in order to save both the mother and baby's lives, a timely cesarean section is needed. For this, the woman will need to be delivered in a health facility providing all the nine signal functions of Comprehensive Essential Obstetric Care (see Box 16.2) and referral may be needed if she is laboring at a lower-level facility. Such referral must be well organized and requires transport and communication systems to be in place.

Obstructed labor can be detected by using a partograph. This is a simple structured graphical one-page representation of the progress of a woman's labor and is recommended as a tool to monitor progress in all women during labor, as well as a documentation of the fetal condition. It consists of a graph depicting cervical dilatation in relation to time—in most cases also the degree of descent of the fetal presenting part—the strength and frequency of contractions and the

> **BOX 16.2 Levels of Essential Obstetric Care and their signal functions**
>
> **Basic**
> - Parenteral antibiotics
> - Parenteral oxytocics
> - Parenteral anticonvulsants
> - Manual removal of a retained placenta
> - Removal of retained products of conception (e.g. by manual vacuum aspiration)
> - Assisted vaginal delivery (e.g. vacuum extraction)
> - Basic neonatal resuscitation (e.g. with bag and mask)
>
> **Comprehensive:**
> - All seven basic functions, plus:
>   - obstetric surgery (e.g. cesarean section)
>   - blood transfusion

fetal heart rate. Other observations, such as maternal blood pressure, temperature, urine output, medication given, etc. are also recorded. Failure to progress in labor can be easily recognized using a partograph.

ABORTION

Each year many women die as a result of unsafe abortions [10]. The WHO defines unsafe abortion as "a procedure for terminating an unintended pregnancy either by individuals without the necessary skills or in an environment that does not conform to minimal medical standards, or both". Important causes of death include hemorrhage, infection and self-poisoning. Legalization of abortion and the availability of good-quality abortion services and post-abortion care have reduced the mortality in a number of countries.

The development of simple techniques and equipment, such as needed for manual vacuum aspiration to remove retained products of conception in the case of incomplete abortion (miscarriage) or to carry out termination of pregnancy where this is possible, have helped increase the availability of such services.

Many unwanted and unplanned pregnancies could be avoided with improved availability and access to effective contraceptives. Statistical models show that higher contraceptive prevalence and greater use of effective contraceptive methods will result in a reduced incidence of abortion. Where these are not available, women will seek to terminate their unintended pregnancies, despite a lack of safe abortion services and restrictive legislation. Restrictive legislation is associated with a high incidence of unsafe abortions, reluctance of women to access facilities when there are complications of abortion and of staff to extend services needed to manage complications of an unsafe abortion. Ensuring family planning services are accessible and available is part of the "continuum of care" that needs to be in place to improve women's health.

NEONATAL MORTALITY

Global estimates obtained from limited data and statistical modeling indicate that there are approximately 5.8 million perinatal deaths, 3 million stillbirths, 2.8 million early neonatal deaths and 3.7 million neonatal deaths (early and late) annually. Neonatal deaths account for up to 40% of mortality of those under the age of five years. Probably, around 75% of all neonatal deaths occur in the first week of life [11]. Although good data are scarce, the main causes of neonatal deaths in developing countries are thought to be prematurity (28%), infection (26%) and asphyxia (23%). These are all directly related to maternal health. Many of these deaths could be prevented with skilled birth attendance and access to essential obstetric and newborn care.

The majority of data available report on outcomes related to birth weight. The most important predictor of birth weight is, however, likely to be gestational age at time of birth. Recent articles report that the incidence of preterm birth (delivery before 37 weeks gestation) in many resource-poor populations is higher than in richer countries, with current estimates varying between 17% and 25%. It is difficult to prevent preterm labor occurring, but the administration of corticosteroids to the mother to enhance fetal lung maturity, as well as provision of Kangaroo Mother Care (See Chapter 17) are evidence-based interventions that will improve outcome.

Where infection is considered the cause of neonatal death, this has been documented as sepsis or septicemia, meningitis, pneumonia or acute respiratory tract infection, or simply as "neonatal infection". The causative organisms are rarely known and there is substantial uncertainty about the relative contribution and/or exact cause of death of the neonates in this category. Neonatal death owing to asphyxia can be the result of inability to resuscitate a baby with low apgar scores and neonatal encephalopathy with fits or coma. Many of these deaths include fresh stillbirths which could have been prevented with better monitoring of the fetal condition during labour (e.g. using the partograph) and expedited delivery where necessary. Neonatal tetanus accounts for around 7% of deaths. With vaccination of women in the antenatal period and clean cord care this can be prevented.

STRATEGIES TO REDUCE MATERNAL AND NEWBORN MORTALITY AND MORBIDITY

SKILLED BIRTH ATTENDANCE

A Skilled Birth Attendant is defined as:

"...an accredited health professional – such as a midwife, doctor or nurse with midwifery skills, who has been educated and trained to proficiency in the skills needed to manage normal (uncomplicated) pregnancies, childbirth and the immediate postnatal period, and in the identification, management and referral of complications in women and newborns" .

The term "Skilled Birth Attendance" includes the person (a skilled attendant) and an "enabling environment". This enabling environment is less well-defined but refers to a functioning health system within which the skilled birth attendant can work effectively and includes infrastructure, equipment, drugs and a functioning referral system. Global progress towards the availability and use of skilled birth attendants is being made, with an increase between 1990 and 2000 in births attended by a skilled worker (from 45% to 54%) in developing countries, with the exception of South Asia and sub-Saharan Africa [12]. In 2008, globally, an average of 65.7% of births were attended by a skilled health worker. Developed countries had over 99% coverage, while East Africa had the least coverage (33.7%), with 41.2% coverage in Western Africa, and 46.9% in South Central Asia.

With a heavy reliance on the proportion of births attended by a skilled attendant as the key indicator for measuring progress towards reducing maternal mortality, there is also need for an agreed monitoring and evaluation framework to inform policy makers on progress and impact of this strategy. Available evidence from around the world has shown that improving the recruitment, education, training and supervision of skilled attendants, as well as the provision of an enabling environment are all positive and crucial steps.

ESSENTIAL OBSTETRIC AND NEWBORN CARE

For an estimated 10–15% of all women, a potentially life-threatening complication develops during pregnancy, childbirth or the postpartum period. In most cases, this complication will be unexpected and unpredictable. Therefore, it is crucial that all women have access to good-quality essential (or emergency) obstetric care.

At least 80% of all maternal deaths result from five complications that are well understood and can be readily treated: hemorrhage, sepsis, eclampsia, ruptured uterus as a result of obstructed labor and complications of abortion; there are existing effective medical and surgical interventions that are relatively inexpensive. In 1997, the key interventions needed were bundled into a package now known as "Essential (or Emergency) Obstetric Care" (Box 16.2). There is unified agreement and criteria for what constitutes Essential Obstetric Care, as well as on what constitutes the minimum coverage levels needed at population level and on what constitutes good-quality evidence based practice [13–15].

Two levels of Essential (Emergency) Obstetric Care can be distinguished: Basic Essential Obstetric Care and Comprehensive Essential Obstetric Care. In addition to agreement on the components (signal functions), there are agreed specifications for levels of coverage needed. Thus, the UN agencies recommend that, for a population of 500,000, there should be at least one health facility that is able to provide the nine signal functions of comprehensive care and at least four that provide the seven signal functions of basic care. It is important that these facilities are equitably distributed geographically with regard to distance and time needed to travel to the health facility. In addition, the signal functions must be available 24 hours a day and 7 days a week for the facility to be considered fully functional.

A number of surveys have assessed the availability, accessibility and quality of essential obstetric care in countries with high maternal mortality. These surveys consistently find that coverage with facilities able to provide care is inadequate and minimum UN agreed standards are not yet in place. In many settings, there are relatively large numbers of health facilities but these are often not providing the full complement of signal functions for either basic or comprehensive essential obstetric care. In addition, the geographical distribution of facilities is such that these tend to be clustered in urban areas with poor coverage particularly in more rural areas [16].

QUALITY OF CARE

There is accumulating evidence that poor-quality care (or the third delay, as defined by the "three delay model") contributes significantly to adverse maternal and newborn outcomes in resource poor areas. Quality of Care should include the concept of effective care and timely access, and of reproductive health rights.

The quality of the provision of care and the quality of care as experienced by users are both essential components (Box 16.3). The use of services and outcomes are the result not only of the provision of care but also of women's experience of that care. Provision of care may be deemed of high quality against recognized standards of care but unacceptable to the woman and her family (the community). Conversely, some aspects of care may be popular with women but may be ineffective or harmful to health.

For maternal and newborn health in particular, there are well established tools for assessing and improving quality of care. These include maternal and perinatal death audit, "near miss" audit and standards (or criterion-) based audit. These tools have been successfully used in a variety of settings and such audit is recommended as part of everyday good clinical practice. All types of audit essentially ask the questions: what was done well, what was not done well and how can care be improved in future [17, 18]?

BOX 16.3 Quality of Care

"Quality of care is the degree to which maternal health services for individuals and populations increase the likelihood of timely and appropriate treatment for the purpose of achieving desired outcomes that are both consistent with current professional knowledge and uphold basic reproductive rights." (Hulton, 2010)

"The question should not be why do women not accept the service that we offer, but why do we not offer a service that women will accept." (Fathalla, 1998).

An absolutely fundamental principle is the importance of a non-threatening environment and a "no shame, no blame" approach. Wherever possible, confidentiality and anonymity must be maintained. Death reviews—conducted in this way—should result in recommendations for change. Such recommendations need to be (and in practice usually are) simple, affordable, effective and in line with evidence-based care.

Confidential enquiries are a systematic, usually multidisciplinary, anonymous review of all or a representative sample of maternal deaths occurring in an area, for example national or sub-national. Through aggregation of data, a confidential enquiry can make recommendations of a more general nature, inform wider health policy and practice, and can be used for advocacy to improve maternal and newborn health.

REFERENCES

1. Hogan MC, Foreman KJ, Naghavi M, et al. Maternal mortality for 181 countries, 1980–2008: a systematic analysis of progress towards Millennium Development Goal 5. Lancet 2010;375:1609–23.
2. World Health Organization. Neonatal and Perinatal mortality–Country, regional and global estimates 2004. Geneva: World Health Organization; 2007.
3. Enkin M, Keirse MJNC, Neilson J, et al. A guide to Effective Care in Pregnancy and Childbirth, 3rd edn. Oxford, UK: Oxford University Press; 2000 (reprinted 2004). Available at: www.childbirthconnection.org (last accessed 30/7/2012).
4. Kerber KJ, de Graft-Johnson JE, Bhutta ZE, et al. Continuum of care for maternal, newborn and child health: from slogan to service delivery. Lancet 2007; 370:1358–69.
5. World Health Organization. Making Pregnancy Safer: the critical role of the skilled attendant. A joint statement by WHO, ICM and FIGO. Making Pregnancy Safer, Department of Reproductive Health and Research. Geneva: World Health Organization; 2004.
6. World Health Organization. Trends in Maternal Mortality:1990–2008. Geneva: World Health Organization; 2010.
7. Thaddeus S, Maine D. Too far to walk: maternal mortality in context. Soc Sci Med 1994;38:1091–110.
8. Khan KS, Wojdyla D, Say L, et al. WHO analysis of causes of maternal death: a systematic review. Lancet 2006;367:1066–74.
9. Pattinson R, Say L, Souza JP, et al. on behalf of the WHO Working Group on Maternal Mortality and Morbidity Classifications. WHO maternal death and near-miss classifications. Bull World Health Organ 2009;87:734.
10. World Health Organization. Unsafe Abortion—global and regional estimates of the incidence of unsafe abortion and associated mortality in 2000, 4th ed. Geneva: World Health Organization; 2004.
11. Lawn JE, Cousens S, Bhutta ZA, et al. Why are 4 million newborn babies dying each year? Lancet 2004;364:399–401.
12. Adegoke A, van den Broek N. Skilled Birth Attendance—lessons learnt. BJOG 2009;116:33–40.
13. World Health Organization, United Nations Children's Fund, Averting Maternal Death and Disability. Monitoring emergency obstetric care: a handbook. Geneva: World Health Organization; 2009.
14. Fauveau V, de Bernis L. 'Good obstetrics' revisited—too many evidence-based practices and devices are not used. Int J Gynaecol Obstet 2006;94:179–84.
15. van den Broek N. Life Saving Skills Manual—Essential Obstetric and Newborn Care, revised edn. London: RCOG Press; 2007.
16. van den Broek NR, Hofman JJ, Increasing the capacity for essential obstetric and newborn care. In: Kehoe S, Neilson JP, Norman JE, eds. Maternal and Infant Deaths—Chasing Millennium Development Goals 4 and 5. London: RCOG Press; 2010.
17. Kongnyuy E, van den Broek N. Audit for maternal and newborn health services in resource poor countries. BJOG 2009;116:7–10.
18. Pattinson RC, Say L, Makin JD, Bastos MH. Critical Incident audit and feedback to improve perinatal and maternal mortality and morbidity. Cochrane Database Syst Rev 2005;CD002961.
19. Hulton L, Murray S, Thomas D. The evidence towards MDG5: a working paper. London: Options Consulting Services; 2010.
20. Fathalla M. Preface. Paediatric and Perinatal Epideiology 1988;12(suppl. 2): vii–viii.

Pediatrics in a Resource-constrained Setting 17

Elizabeth M Molyneux

Pediatrics in the tropics is challenging. It is not only the management of children with tropical diseases; it is caring for children in a health system that may be under-resourced, under-staffed and frequently overwhelmed by numbers. It is adapting to do the best with limited resources and few staff. It is the sharing of ideas and practice with a team that may have very different levels of medical education, but a common goal. It is to use clinical acumen for diagnosis and to be creative in finding solutions for what may seem, on first encounter, to be insuperable. It can be demanding, sometimes overwhelming, always interesting and very rewarding.

Most children in the world have their medical care provided by health workers with little access to diagnostic aids and with limited therapies. The first-line health worker may have received only minimal training. The World Health Organization (WHO) has provided guidelines for the diagnosis and management of common clinical problems based on pattern recognition of a collection of signs and symptoms, and syndromic treatment designed to treat the common causes of identified clinical problems. In the past, the management of individual illnesses was taught separately but these have been drawn together in the Integrated Management of Childhood Illnesses (IMCI) [1]. In this scheme, a child is assessed for danger signs, treated appropriately, referred when necessary and the family is counseled about immunizations, nutrition and follow-up (Fig. 17.1).

Syndromic management leads to over-treatment but simplifies looking after large numbers of patients with few staff. National policy should make appropriate drugs available for every level of healthcare.

IMCI strategy has three main components:

- To improve the case-management skills of health carers using locally adapted clinical guidelines that do not focus on a single diagnosis, but rather on selected signs and symptoms to guide rational treatment.
- This needs support through the provision of appropriate therapies and referral chains.
- The child is seen in the context of the family and the clinic visit because of an acute event which is used to provide, not only immediate curative treatment, but also attention to nutrition, immunization, counseling and other holistic health needs.

In Tanzania, this led to a 13% reduction in the cost of care and better outcomes [2]. A re analysis of these data to include the quality of care given showed that the cost of using IMCI was $4.02/person per annum compared with $25.70 without IMCI [3]. To reach these improvements requires all the ingredients of IMCI to be available—training, drugs, staff, immunizations and time; training alone will not suffice.

Although the ICMI works well in many settings, local and national constraints include low healthcare worker compliance, the perceived length and expense of training, inadequate counseling of child caregivers, the weakness of health systems to support ICMI policy and lack of institutional or governmental budget allocations for implementation. The need for support from national health policy, financial commitment and health system strengthening is emphasized [4].

Additional challenges have included the need to adapt it to take account of diseases that are important in particular settings, for example dengue is a much more important cause of illness in Asia than Africa. Because of its WHO endorsement, there may be a tendency for its implementation in inappropriate settings, for example in countries where healthcare workers are already trained to a high standard.

A seven-country audit of inpatient pediatric care was undertaken by the WHO in 1997. It showed that there were many gaps in health care delivery and there was a universal need for triage, emergency care and patient monitoring [5]. In response to these findings, the WHO produced the "Pocket Book of Hospital Care for Children: Guidelines for the Management of Common Illness with Limited Resources", also known as the The Hospital Pocket Book or Blue Book [6]. The book of guidelines is for use by doctors, senior nurses and other senior healthcare workers responsible for the inpatient and outpatient care of young children at the first referral level in developing countries (Fig. 17.2). The guidelines cover the most common diagnoses and problems in resource-constrained countries and assume that only basic laboratory support, essential drugs and inexpensive medicines are available, with no specialist care on site. It focuses on the major causes of childhood mortality, such as pneumonia, diarrhea, severe malnutrition, malaria, meningitis, measles, HIV infection and related conditions. It also covers neonatal problems and surgical conditions of children which can be managed in small hospitals. The Pocket Book can be purchased in a hardcopy or downloaded free from the WHO website [6]. A three-and-a-half-day course on Emergency Triage Assessment and Treatment (ETAT) is available on the WHO Child and Adolescent Health Division website [7].

PREVENTIVE SCHEMES

It is important to provide protection to vulnerable children in the form of immunizations, supplementary food, intermittent prophylactic drug therapy against malaria, bed nets, etc. All these tasks of testing and treating mothers and children, giving advice, giving medications or immunizations fall to the health assistant or the nurse. These community workers have gradually acquired a multitude of duties towards the child and their family. Each duty is small and important, but together they make for a heavy workload. Extended Programmes for Immunizations (EPI) days and antenatal visits are times when mothers and babies encounter the health service and these visits have acquired a lot of "add on" activities; all good but a lot for a worker to convey or a mother to recall (Table 17-1).

EXPANDED PROGRAMME FOR IMMUNISATION (EPI)

The EPI was established in 1974 through a World Health Assembly resolution to build on the success of the global smallpox eradication

ASSESS AND CLASSIFY THE SICK CHILD AGED 2 MONTHS UP TO 5 YEARS

ASSESS

Ask the mother what the child's problems are
- Determine whether this is an initial or follow-up visit for this problem.
- if follow-up visit, use the follow-up instructions on **Treat the child** chart
- if initial visit, assess the child as follows:

CHECK FOR GENERAL DANGER SIGNS

Ask:
- Is the child able to drink or breast feed?
- Does the child vomit everything?
- Has the child had convulsions?

Look:
- See if the child is lethargic or unconscious.
- Is the child convulsing now?

A child with any general danger sign needs urgent attention; complete the assessment and any permitted treatment immediately so that referral is not delayed.

CLASSIFY

THEN ASK ABOUT MAIN SYMPTOMS:
Does the child have a cough or difficult breathing?

If yes, ask:
- For how long?

Look, listen, feel:
- Count the breaths in one minute.
- Look for chest indrawing.
- Look and listen for stridor.
- Look and listen for wheezing.

} **Child must be calm**

If wheezing and either fast breathing or chest indrawing: *Give a trial of rapid acting inhaled bronchodilator for up to three times 15-20 minutes apart. Count the breaths and look for chest indrawing again, and then classify.*

If the child is:	Fast breathing is:
2 months up to 12 months	**50** breaths per minute or more
12 months up to 5 years	**40** breaths per minute or more

Classify **cough** or **difficult breathing**

IDENTIFY TREATMENT

USE ALL BOXES THAT MATCH THE CHILD'S SYMPTOMS AND PROBLEMS TO CLASSIFY THE ILLNESS.

SIGNS	CLASSIFY AS	TREATMENT
• Any general danger sign or • Chest indrawing or • Stridor in a calm child	**Severe pneumonia or very severe disease**	• **Give first dose of an appropriate antibiotic** • **Refer urgently to hospital**
• Fast breathing	**Pneumonia**	• **Give oral antibiotic for 3 days** • If wheezing (even if it disappeared after rapidly acting bronchodilator) give an inhaled bronchodilator for 5 days • Soothe the throat and relieve the cough with a safe remedy • If coughing for more than 3 weeks or if having recurrent wheezing, refer for assessment for TB or asthma • Advise the mother when to return immediately • Follow-up in 2 days
• No signs of pneumonia or very severe disease	**Cough or cold**	• If wheezing (even if it disappeared after rapidly acting bronchodilator) give an inhaled bronchodilator for 5 days • Soothe the throat and relieve the cough with a safe remedy • If coughing for more than 3 weeks or if having recurrent wheezing, refer for assessment for TB or asthma • Advise the mother when to return immediately • Follow-up in 5 days if not improving

FIGURE 17.1 The first page of the Integrated Management of Childhood Illness Chart Booklet, showing initial assessment for danger signs *(http://whqlibdoc.who.int/publications/2008/9789241597289_eng.pdf).*

programme and to ensure that all children in all countries benefited from life-saving vaccines. The first diseases targeted by the EPI were diphtheria, whooping cough, tetanus, measles, poliomyelitis and tuberculosis. In 2009, an estimated 82% of children globally had received at least three doses of diphtheria, pertussis, tetanus (DPT) vaccine (DPT3). Additional vaccines have now been added to the original six recommended in 1974. Most countries, including the majority of low-income countries, have added hepatitis B and *Haemophilus influenzae* type b (Hib) to their routine infant immunization schedules and an increasing number are in the process of adding pneumococcal conjugate vaccine and rotavirus vaccines to their schedules.

How to manage the airway in a child with obstructed breathing (or who has just stopped breathing) where neck trauma or possible cervical spine injury is suspected

1. Stabilise the neck
2. Inspect mouth and remove foreign body if present
3. Clear secretions from throat
4. Check the airway by looking for chest movements, listening for breath sounds and feeling for breath

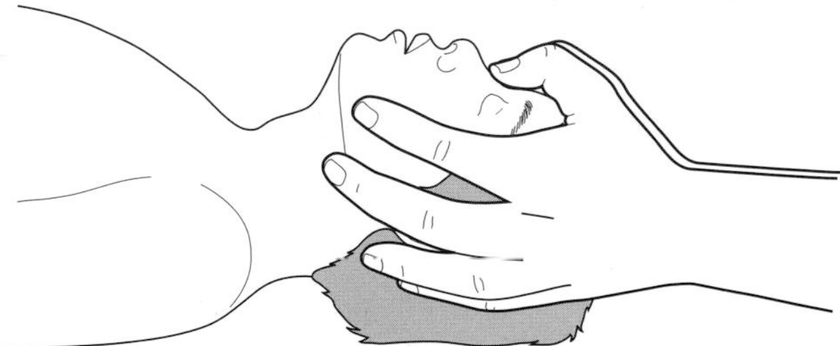

Use jaw thrust without head tilt. Place the 4th and 5th finger behind the angle of the jaw and move it upwards so that the bottom of the jaw is thrust forwards, at 90º to the body

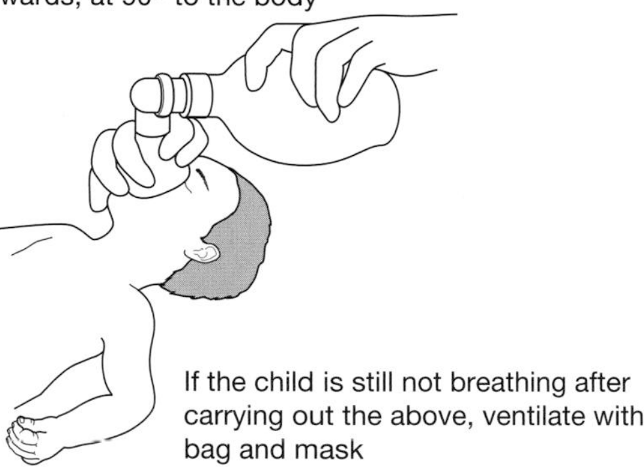

FIGURE 17.2 Page from the WHO Pocket Book showing how to manage the airway.

Table 17-1 Preventive care required from pregnancy through childhood

Antenatal care	Delivery	Postnatal	Childhood <5 yrs
Tetanus immunization	PMTCT	PMTCT	Cotrimoxazole prophylaxis
Maternal Hb level	Skilled care	Cord care	Pentavalent vaccine + polio
VDRL/RPR	Blood if needed	BCG/Polio	Supplementary feeds
IPDT*		KMC	Vitamin A
Breast feeding advice	Breast feeding advice	Breast feeding advice	Breast feeding advice
Bed net	Bed net	Bed net	Bed net
HIV test		HIV tests/PCR	HIV test / PCR[1]
BP			Measles immunisation
Weight		Weight	Weight/height/ MUAC[2]
Urine protein			iPDT*
Threats to good health and growth	MALNUTRITION AND HIV INFECTION		
	POVERTY, INACCESSIBILITY TO HEALTH CARE, PARENTAL SICKNESS, SOCIAL UNREST, ORPHANHOOD, WOODSMOKE		

BCG, Bacillus-Calmette-Guérin; BP, blood pressure; Hb, hemoglobin; IPDT, intermittent preventive drug therapy for malaria; KMC, Kangaroo Mother Care; MUAC, mid upper arm circumference; PMTCT, preventing mother to child transmission of HIV; RPR, rapid plasma reagin; VDRL, Venereal Disease Research Laboratory test.
*Intermittent preventive drug therapy for malaria.
[1]Polymerase chain reaction.
[2]Mid Upper Arm Circumference.

The overall coverage for childhood immunizations varies from country to country. In some countries (e.g. Malawi), the uptake is good, with 82% coverage for all three doses of the pentavalent vaccine [diphtheria, tetanus, whooping cough, hepatitis B and *H. influenza* type b (DPTHibHepB)] and 64% for measles. In other countries, the uptake is poor and the difference in urban/rural uptake is great [8]. EPI programs include the periodic distribution of vitamin A supplements to children. Not all countries have the pentavalent vaccine—many are still using DPT. The pentavalent vaccine raises the cost of vaccination 10-fold and can only be sustained with external funding, such as from the Global Alliance for Vaccines and Immunisation (GAVI).

Measles remains a cause of significant morbidity and mortality despite the availability of an effective vaccine (see Chapter 28.1). The WHO estimates that there are about 350,000 measles deaths a year [9]. Many of the deaths are not from acute measles, but from post-measles diarrhea and pneumonia. In countries where measles is common, it tends to occur in young children (<12 months of age). Therefore, children need to be immunized earlier than their counterparts in well-resourced countries. The measles vaccine is given at 9 months of age and is not repeated. Given at this age, it provides 80–90% protection [10].

Pneumococcal conjugate vaccine is not widely available in resource-constrained countries because of cost, but its introduction into the EPI service would be enormously beneficial. In HIV-infected infants, immunization is not as effective or as long-lasting compared with uninfected children, but a study from the Gambia showed an overall five-year protection measured by antibody levels to the nine serotypes of the study conjugate vaccine of 77% [confidence interval (CI) 95% 51.90] [11, 12].

The Pneumococcal Accelerated Development and Introduction Plan (pneumoADIP) is striving to make the seven-valent pneumococcal conjugate vaccine (PCV-7) available for young infants in resource-poor countries and Rwanda was the first country in Africa to introduce it into its infant EPI program. In 2010, the Rwandan Ministry of Health, with the help of international partners, made pneumococcal conjugate vaccine available through the EPI program to all infants. Through GAVI, it is anticipated that the cost of funded PCV-7 will be brought down to about US $1 for a three-dose course [13].

HIV/AIDS

Countries with a high HIV/AIDS burden are struggling to care for all the people who are living with AIDS (PLWA).

Prophylactic cotrimoxazole, recommended for all children (and adults) with HIV infection and HIV-exposed infants [14], and fixed combination drugs (FDC) are available and provided through the global fund. Local national programs provide registration procedures, protocols, training, stock control, prescribing controls and monitoring; the human resources required and logistical implications are huge. Children are expected to form about 10% of the total number of people on antiretroviral therapies (ARTs), but their access to therapy has been slower than that of adults. Reasons for this include difficulty in deciding how to provide suitable doses for children with a limited variety of FDC tablets available (and none of them child-friendly tablets), although pediatric combination tablets are now available. The need to confirm a diagnosis below the age of 15 months with PCR testing is a challenge. Studies have shown that infants started on ARTs before they develop opportunistic infections have a much better survival [15]. It is not easy to advise about infant feeding. What is best for babies whose chances of acquiring HIV infection from breast feeding are about 14–42% but whose chance of dying of gastroenteritis or malnutrition in a poor family if bottle fed is much greater? Recent studies from Zambia and Malawi both showed increased mortality with abrupt cessation of breast feeding of all infants and, in Malawi, there was no reduction in HIV transmission [16, 17]. The WHO recommends considering the ability of the mother to maintain artificial feeding under the headings Acceptability, Feasibility, Affordability, Sustainability and Safety (AFASS) before giving any advice [18], i.e. will replacement feeding be acceptable, feasible, affordable, sustainable and safe? Considerations include analyzing the family's access to clean water, electricity, hygienic latrines or toilets, their financial situation, and other social and economic factors necessary to support replacement feeding. A breast-feeding mother on ART that reduces her viral load to negligible amounts could breast feed her baby without fear of HIV transmission: this would seem the way forward in preventing vertical transmission of the disease, but not at the cost of infections and malnutrition that could be prevented by breast feeding.

NEWBORNS

Infant mortality has decreased in several countries, but this fall in the case fatality rate has been mainly in children over 2 months of age (Fig. 17.3). The United Nations Millennium Eight Development Goals were established following the Millennium Summit in 2000 [19]; they comprise eight international development goals that all 192 United Nations member states, and at least 23 international organizations, have agreed to achieve by the year 2015. To achieve the fourth Millennium Development Goal of halving child mortality by 2015, neonatal mortality must be tackled [20]. About 40% of all child deaths (4 million per year) occur in the neonatal period. Almost 75% of neonatal deaths occur in the first week of life, of which 85% are caused by prematurity, infection and birth asphyxia (Fig. 17.4). Skilled attendance at delivery, simple care of the premature—such as Kangaroo Mother Care (KMC)—and good hygiene would prevent many of these deaths. Tetanus can be prevented by maternal immunization. In Kenya, Opiyo et al. showed that a one-day training course in neonatal resuscitation led to a significant improvement in resuscitation steps and techniques (66% v 27% p=0.001) [21].The training was based on the one-day UK Resuscitation Council training [22] (Fig. 17.5) adapted to the Kenyan setting and included an A (Airway), B (Breathing) and C (Circulation) approach to resuscitation, laying down a clear, step-by-step strategy for the first minutes of resuscitation at birth with practical scenarios using infant manikins.

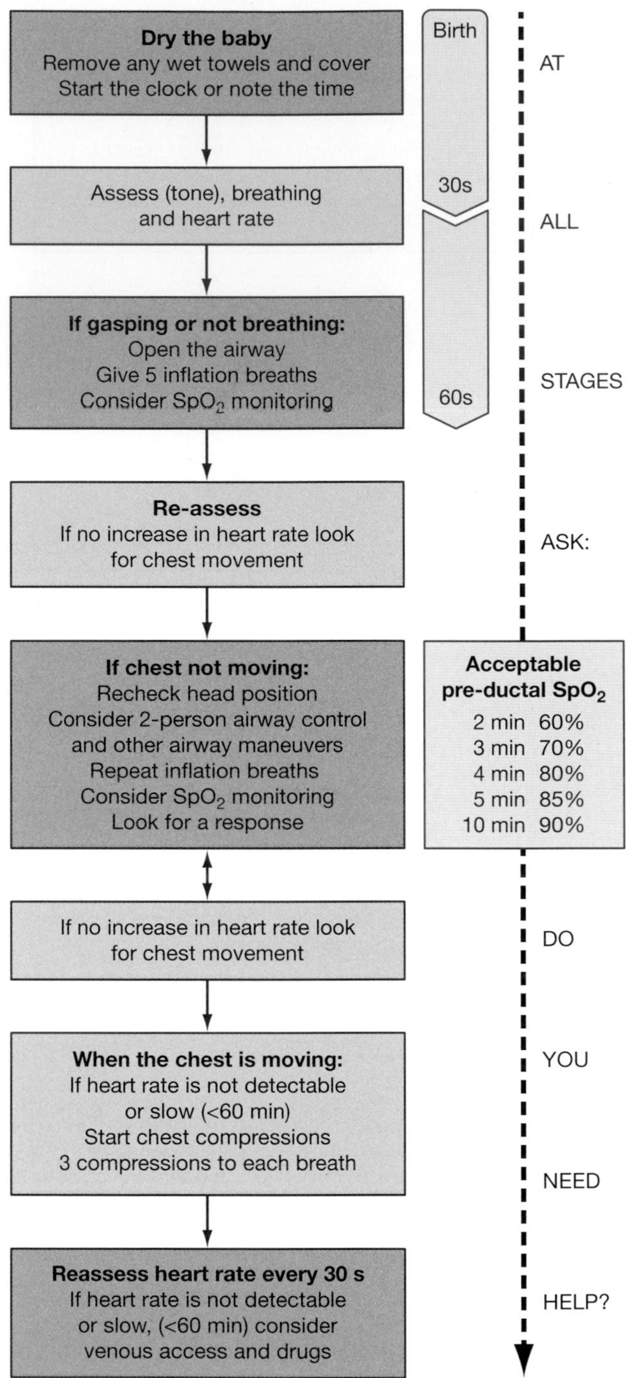

FIGURE 17.3 Steps to infant resuscitation from the UK Resuscitation Council Training Manual *[http://www.resus.org.uk/pages/nls.pdf (p. 121)].*

KMC is when a mother gives warmth, nutrition and love to her baby who is placed, skin-to-skin, between her breasts, and nursed there. The baby is kept in this position most of the day and night, providing a constant, even body temperature. KMC babies grow more quickly than those nursed in incubators. It is ideal care for premature and small-for-dates infants, and mothers can continue KMC at home until the baby's body weight is 2.5 kg. In hospital, this releases nurses to care for the very sick infants, as mothers provide most of the KMC for their infants [23].

PNEUMONIA

Pneumonia causes most deaths in childhood and the majority of these deaths occur in resource-constrained parts of the world. Qazi et al. showed that simple, standardized training in acute respiratory infection management, based on WHO recommendations, will reduce mortality and decrease the use of antibiotics [24]. The recommendations include assessment of the following:

- clinical signs in children presenting with a cough or difficult breathing;
- fast breathing;
- in-drawing of the lower chest wall;
- other specified danger signs.

Antibiotics are recommended for treatment of pneumonia, acute streptococcal pharyngitis, acute otitis media and mastoiditis, but not for treatment of acute upper respiratory infections, such as coughs and colds. Commercial cough remedies containing ineffective or harmful ingredients are discouraged.

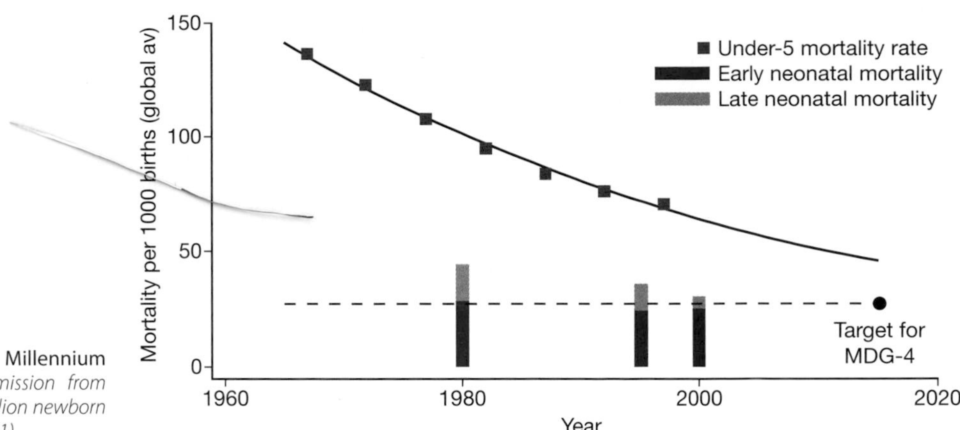

FIGURE 17.4 Neonatal deaths and the Millennium Development Goals *(Reproduced with permission from Lawn J, Cousens S, Bhutta Z, et al. Why are 4 million newborn babies dying each year? Lancet 2004;364:399–401).*

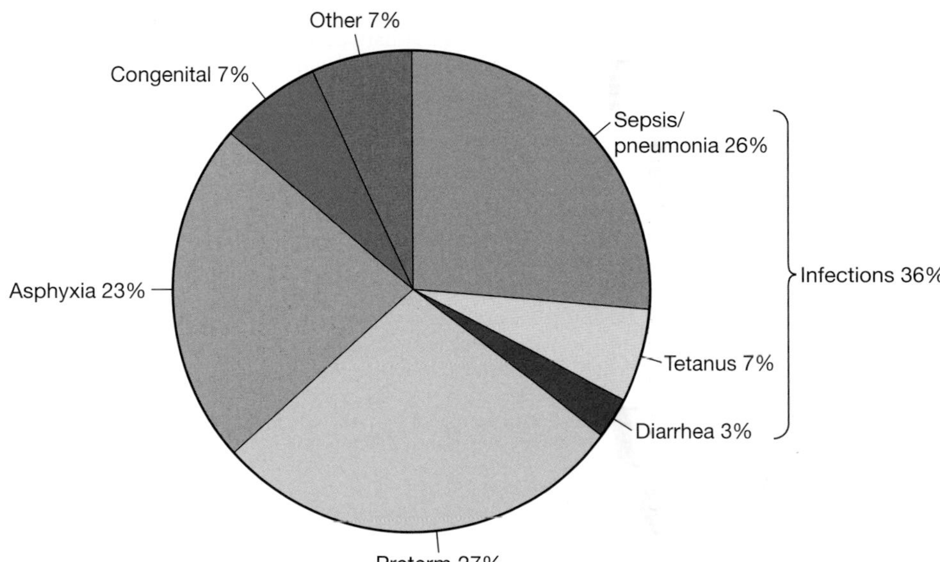

FIGURE 17.5 Common causes of infant deaths worldwide *(source: WHO).*

Despite the size of the problem, in Kenya and Papua New Guinea oxygen was unavailable in several health facilities and even fewer had oxygen saturation monitors [25]. In HIV-endemic areas, both the diagnosis and management of pneumonia have become increasingly difficult. HIV-infected children are prone to bacterial pneumonia (often caused by *Streptococcus pneumoniae)* but after repeated infections that cause structural damage and radiologic changes, it can be difficult to decide what is new, what is old and what is the best treatment for the present problem. Staphylococcal infections and carriage are more common in HIV-infected children. Bacterial pneumonia may occur on a background of lymphocytic interstitial pneumonitis (LIP) and/or tuberculosis (TB).

Pneumocystis jiroveccii pneumonitis (PCP) may be the presenting illness of HIV-infected infants aged 3–8 months. Despite treatment with high-dose cotrimoxazole and steroids, the prognosis is poor and it is hoped that by giving all HIV PCR-positive infants ART, the number and severity of all infections will be reduced. PCP has a distinctive clinical presentation—air hunger with hyperinflation of the lungs which are clear on auscultation. Body temperature is only minimally raised and even high flow oxygen often only marginally improves oxygenation.

On the other hand, TB can be difficult to diagnose. A contact history of TB is one of the most helpful findings in making the diagnosis. The purified protein derivative (PPD) skin tests are usually negative in HIV-infected children, but when strongly positive it can be very helpful. Sputum samples cannot be easily obtained and chest x-ray is seldom diagnostic. Gastric aspirates must be collected from an empty stomach and immediately placed in a buffered solution. In our hands, the results have been unrewarding. The mortality in HIV-infected children is higher than in HIV-negative children and is related to the CD4 count [26]. LIP has a characteristic lacy radiologic appearance and, clinically, there is generalized lymphadenopathy; fever is uncommon. LIP may be complicated by the presence of bronchiectasis and TB, making the diagnosis more complicated.

MALARIA

One million children die of malaria every year. Deaths are almost all caused by *Plasmodium falciparum* infections. Malaria comes in several forms and is most commonly asymptomatic or causes mild fever. Complicated malaria—accompanied by anemia or altered consciousness (cerebral malaria) and respiratory distress—carries a significant mortality [27]; urgent treatment is needed. Most countries with endemic *P. falciparum* malaria are using an artemisinin-based first-line combination therapy to overcome resistance to drugs such as chloroquine and sulfamethoxazole (SP). Combination drugs are used to slow down the development of resistance to artemisinins, which should not be prescribed on their own.

Several studies have identified malaria, particularly associated with convulsions, as a major cause of long-term neurologic sequelae, including epilepsy and behavioral disorders. It was always known that about 15–20% of children with severe or cerebral malaria developed gross neurologic sequelae, such as hemiplegia, blindness or cerebral palsy, but, more recently, subtle forms of sequelae have been studied and identified [28].

Bed nets, intermittent prophylactic therapeutic medication (iPTpd) and indoor residual spraying will help reduce the prevalence and severity of malaria; some malaria vaccines also look promising [29].

Malaria and malnutrition both lead to anemia and there is a known association between this anemia and non-typhoidal salmonellosis (NTS). NTS is the most common cause of bacteremia in malarial areas [30]. It is important to know the resistance pattern to antibiotics of the common pathogens in the region so that antibiotic guidelines can reflect the local findings.

GASTROENTERITIS

The use of oral rehydration solution (ORS) has greatly reduced the mortality from gastroenteritis but 1.4–6 million children still die every year from dehydration. ORS is a sodium and glucose solution prepared by diluting one sachet of ORS in 1 liter of safe water. In most countries, ORS packets are available from health centers, pharmacies, markets and shops. When a child has three or more loose stools in a day, begin to give ORS and encourage the child to drink as much as possible. A child under the age of 2 years needs at least a quarter to a half of a large (250-ml) cup of the ORS drink after each watery stool and a child aged 2 years or older needs at least a half to a whole large (250-ml) cup of the ORS drink after each watery stool. It is important to administer the solution in small amounts at regular intervals on a continuous basis. In case ORS packets are not available, caregivers at home may use homemade solutions consisting of half a teaspoon of salt and six level teaspoons of sugar dissolved in one liter of safe water [31]. Alternatively, lightly salted rice water, or even plain water, may be given. To avoid dehydration, increased fluids should be given as soon as possible after illness onset. All oral fluids, including ORS solution, should be prepared with the best available drinking water and stored safely. Continuous provision of nutritious food is essential and breastfeeding of infants and young children should continue [32].

Current guidelines for the acute management of severe sepsis in children place prime importance on early, rapid and substantial infusion of intravenous fluids; the immediate aim is to correct a possible fluid responsive hypodynamic circulation—the assumption being that, beyond this, an expansion of the circulating volume will attenuate hypotension, ameliorate the perceived impaired peripheral and end-organ perfusion, and correct abnormalities of base deficit and lactate. However, a recently published, multicenter, randomized, placebo-controlled trial of more than 3000 children in Uganda, Kenya and Tanzania found that fluid boluses significantly increased 48-hour mortality in critically ill children with impaired perfusion [33]. This unexpected finding is prompting some re-evaluation of the initial management of children with severe sepsis in resource-poor settings [33].

Rotavirus causes about 50–75% of cases of acute diarrhea and vomiting. Oral rotavirus vaccines have been approved by the WHO and it is anticipated that these vaccines, once introduced into national EPI programs, will have a huge impact on the number of gastroenteritis cases that occur [34]. Good hygiene, clean water and breast feeding all help prevent gastroenteritis and such simple methods of prevention must not be forgotten. If diarrhea does occur, oral zinc has been shown to be effective in reducing the frequency and volume of stools and length of the diarrheal episode [35].

REFERENCES

1. Integrated Management of Childhood Illnesses. UNICEF and CAH (WHO). Geneva: World Health Organization. Available at: http://www.who.int/child_adolescent_health/topics/prevention_care/child/imci/en/.
2. Adam T, Manzi F, Schellenberg JA, et al. Does the Integrated Management of Childhood Illness cost more than routine care? Results from the United Republic of Tanzania. Bull WHO 2005;83:369–77.
3. Bryce J, Cesar V, Habicht J-P, et al. The multicountry evaluation of the IMCI strategy: lessons for the evaluation of public health interventions. Am J Public Health 2004;94:406–15.
4. Ahmed HM, Mitchell M, Hedt B. National implementation of Integrated Management of Childhood Illness (IMCI): policy constraints and strategies. Health Policy 2010;96:128–33.
5. Nolan T, Angos P, Cunha AJ, et al. Quality of hospital care for seriously ill children in developing countries. Lancet 2001;357:86–7, 106–10.
6. WHO Pocket book for hospital care for children. Guidelines for the management of common illnesses with limited resources. Geneva: World Health Organization; 2005. Available at: http://www.who.int/child_adolescent_health/documents/9241546700/en/index.html.
7. WHO Emergency Triage Assessment and Treatment (ETAT). Manual for participants. Geneva: World Health Organization. Available at: http://www.who.int/child_adolescent_health/documents/.
8. Otten M, Kezaala R, Fall A, et al. Public-health impact of accelerated measles control in the WHO Africa region 2000–2003. Lancet 2005;366:832–9.
9. Centers for Disease Control and Prevention (CDC). Progress in global measles control and mortality reduction 2000–2006. MMWR 2007;56:1237–41.
10. Akramuzzaman SM, Cutts FT, Hossain MDJ, et al. Measles vaccination effectiveness and risk factors for measles in Dhaka, Bangladesh. Bull World Health Organ 2002;80:776–82.
11. Mahdi SA, Klugman KP, Kuwanda L, et al. Quantitative and qualitative anamnestic immune responses to pneumococcal conjugate vaccine in HIV-infected and HIV-uninfected children 5 years after vaccination. J Infect Dis 2009; 99;1168–76.
12. Saka M, Okoko BJ, Kohberger RC, et al. Immunogenicity and serotype-specific efficacy of 9- valent pneumococcal conjugate vaccine (PCV-9) determined during an efficacy trial in The Gambia. Vaccine 2008;26:3719–26.
13. Meehan A, Mackenzie D, Booy R. Protecting children with HIV against pneumococcal disease. Lancet Infect Dis 2009;9:394–5.
14. Chintu C, Bhat GJ, Walker AS, et al. Cotrimoxazole as prophylaxis against opportunistic infection in HIV-infected Zambian children (CHAP): a double blind randomised placebo-controlled trial. Lancet 2004;364:1865–71.
15. Violari A, Cotton MF, Gibb DM, et al; for the CHER Study Team. Early antiretroviral therapy and mortality among HIV-infeted infants. N Eng J Med 2008; 359:2233–44.
16. Kuhn L, Aldrovandi GM, Sinkala M, et al; for the Zambia Exclusive Breast Feeding Study. Effects of early, abrupt weaning on HIV-free survival of children in Zambia. N Eng J Med 2008;359:130–41.
17. Kumwenda NI, Hoover DR, Mofenson LM, et al. Extended antiretroviral prophylaxis to reduce breast-milk-HIV transmission. N Eng J Med 2008; 359:119–29.
18. Guidelines on HIV and infant feeding 2010. Principles and recommendations for infant feeding in the context of HIV and a summary of evidence. Geneva: World Health Organization; 2010.
19. http://www.un.org/millenniumgoals/.
20. Lawn J, Cousens S, Bhutta Z, et al. Why are 4 million newborn babies dying each year? Lancet 2004;364:399–401.
21. Opiyo N, Were F, Govedi F, et al. Effect of newborn resuscitation training of Health Worker practices in Pumwani Hospital Kenya. PLoS one 2008;3: e1999.
22. http://www.resus.org.uk/pages/glalgos.htm (Newborn Life Support Algorithm).
23. Blencowe H, Kerac M, Molyneux EM. Safety, effectiveness and barriers to follow up using an "Early Discharge" Kangaroo Care Policy in a resource poor setting. J Trop Paeds 2009; 55:244–8.
24. Qazi SA, Rehman GN, Khan MA. Standard management of acute respiratory infections in a children's hospital in Pakistan: impact on antibiotic use and case fatality. Bull World Health Organ 1996;74:501–7.
25. Graham SM, English M, Hazir T, et al. Challenges to improving case management of children with pneumonia at health facilities in resource constrained settings. Bull World Health Organ 2008;86:349–55.
26. Harries AD, Hargreaves NJ, Graham SM et al. Childhood tuberculosis in Malawi: nationwide case-finding and treatment outcomes. Int J Tuberc lung Dis 2002;6:424–31.
27. Crawley J, English M, Wariuru C, et al. Abnormal breathing patterns in childhood cerebral malaria. Trans R Soc Trop Med Hyg 1998;92:305–8.
28. Idro R, Ndiritu M, Ogutu B, et al. Burden, features, and outcome of neurological involvement in acute falciparum malaria in Kenyan children. JAMA 2007;297:2232–40.
29. Chattopadhyay R, Kumar S. Malaria vaccine: latest update and challenges ahead. Indian J Exp Biol 2009;47:527–36.
30. Gordon MA, Graham SM, Walsh AL, et al. Epidemic invasive non-typhoidal Salmonella infections among adults and children associated with multidrug resistance in Malawi. Clin Infect Dis 2008;146:963–9.

31. http://www.who.int/cholera/technical/en/.
32. Fischer Walker CL, Friberg IK, Binkin N, et al. Scaling up diarrhea prevention and treatment interventions: a Lives Saved Tool analysis. Plos Med 2001; 8(3):e10000428.
33. Maitland K, Kiguli S, Opoka RO, et al; FEAST Trial group. Mortality after fluid bolus in African children with severe infection. NEJM 2011;364(26): 2483–95.
34. Rotavirus vaccine: an update WHO. Weekly epidemiological record. No 51-52. 2009;84:533–40 http://www.who.int/wer/.
35. Zinc supplementation in the management of diarrhoea. http:/www.who.int/entity/elena/titles/zinc_diarrhoea/en/.

18 Disasters, Complex Emergencies, and Population Displacement

Trueman W Sharp, Charles W Beadling

Key features

- Disasters, either natural or man-made, disrupt the baseline functioning of a community, including food, water, sanitation and health. The resiliency of a community to recover from a disaster depends on existing economic and social structures. Poverty and inadequate economic and social systems are prevalent in tropical regions, making them extremely vulnerable to disasters
- Complex emergencies are the result of the near-total breakdown of authority and extreme violence due to conflict. Complex emergencies have increased dramatically in frequency since 1980 and are the leading cause of displaced populations
- Displaced populations are at increased risk of increased morbidity and mortality. Other vulnerable groups in the population include women, children, the elderly, and anyone with a physical or mental disability
- Leading causes of morbidity and mortality in displaced populations consistently include diarrhea, measles, malaria, acute respiratory infection and malnutrition

Disasters can strike anywhere, anytime. When one occurs in a resource-poor region already affected by economic or political strife, the extent of health needs and the challenges of providing effective relief can be greatly multiplied. This chapter will focus primarily on the most challenging and serious type of disaster, the complex emergency (CE), and one of its main consequences, population displacement, which is usually what causes the most morbidity and mortality after disasters. This chapter seeks to inform the medical care provider deploying to a relief effort, and to address many of the common myths regarding emergency disaster response [1]. Focusing on the CE is a way to explore the health impact of disasters in resource-poor settings and the fundamentals of emergency health response.

A disaster is an event of environmental disruption or destruction of sudden or gradual onset that is severe enough to overwhelm the resources of the affected community and necessitate outside assistance [2] (Box 18.1). Disasters often cause sufficient harm to a community's economic and social structures that its ability to survive is seriously undermined. The many types of disasters that can occur are often classified by etiology, and generally as natural or man-made disasters. Natural disasters include climatologic events such as typhoons or floods and geologic incidents such as earthquakes and tsunamis. The meltdown of the nuclear power plant in Chernobyl, Ukraine, in 1986, and the accidental release of methyl isocyanate in Bhopal, India, in 1979, are classic examples of sudden-onset man-made disasters. Intentional man-made disasters can also include large acts of terrorism, such as bombings, and some would argue famines and wars [3,4].

Even though the precipitating event of a disaster may be obvious and lend itself to simple classification, such as a typhoon or a hurricane, the consequences of even such natural disasters are usually the result of a complex mix of local circumstances, including the type and quality of building construction, local response capability, the specific location of the local population, cultural beliefs, current political systems, existing standards of medical care, and other factors. Natural disasters are often interwoven in the dynamic of conflict and complex emergencies. For example, the 1971 India–Pakistan war and subsequent refugee crisis was triggered by a cyclone. The disruption caused by this natural event greatly exacerbated already underlying social and political unrest. A severe drought was the principal catalyst for the civil war and humanitarian crisis in Somalia from 1991 to 1992 [5]. Thus, while the term "disaster" may invoke connotations of the unpredictable forces of nature, the hand of man is found in almost all disasters. What is identified as the disaster, even when it is a natural event, is often better understood as a trigger event that exposes underlying societal problems. Virtually every famine since 1977 has been the result of underdevelopment, armed conflict, inadequate economic and social systems, failed governments, and other man-made factors, even though they are sometimes believed to be caused by drought alone [6].

Since the 1980s, there has been a dramatic increase in a type of disaster often termed complex emergencies (CEs; also called complex humanitarian emergency or conflict-related complex emergency) (Fig. 18.1) which are humanitarian crises in a country, region or society where there is a breakdown of authority resulting from internal or external conflict and which requires an international response that goes beyond the mandate or capacity of any single agency and/or the ongoing United Nations (UN) country program [6,7]. These disasters involve an intricate interaction of political, military, economic and natural factors and have armed conflict as a central feature. CEs have been increasingly common since the end of the Cold War. Victims are usually large populations or specific ethnic or cultural groups, and violence against these groups is almost always a critical factor. Other high-risk groups in CEs include the elderly, very young, anyone with a disability, and females, especially if they are pregnant or lactating. Somalia in 1992 is an example of a CE in which civil violence was the most visible, proximate cause of the disaster, but years of underdevelopment, governmental failures, superpower intervention, ethnic conflict, drought, and famine all contributed substantially to the situation.

One of the hallmarks of CEs is displaced people; indeed, CEs are by far the leading cause of displaced people in the world today. CEs and displaced populations have been all too common in the resource-poor regions. In 2009, there were an estimated 42 million refugees and displaced people, more than 80% of whom were in the developing world [8] (Box 18.2).

THE HEALTH EFFECTS OF COMPLEX EMERGENCIES

Over the last two decades there has been an explosion in our understanding of the health effects of disasters and displaced populations and how to respond effectively to them. It is fair to say that disaster relief overall has become an important niche of medicine with a substantial body of scientific literature, standards of care, proven approaches, and ever more formal training programs [10]. While the reader is cautioned that all disasters are different, it is clear that most of the morbidity and mortality in disasters of all types results from population displacement. Displaced populations almost always have significantly higher morbidity and mortality than when they are in their baseline state.

Consistently, in resource-poor environments, while the relative order of importance may change, the five leading causes of death in the emergency phase of a crisis involving displaced people have been remarkably similar. The main causes of serious morbidity and mortality are almost invariably diarrheal illnesses, measles, malaria, acute respiratory infections and malnutrition [11] (Fig. 18.2). One of the most important principles for the health responder to keep in mind, though, is that while there are certainly common diseases, every disaster has a unique epidemiology and must be dealt with somewhat differently [12]. Whereas an earthquake often causes many immediate trauma deaths and usually does not result in food shortages, a flood typically causes few immediate deaths and disrupts food production and distribution networks. An earthquake in Haiti has a markedly different impact than an earthquake in southern California, because the extent of the development, the local building codes, population density, and local response capabilities are very different. One refugee population may be devastated by measles, while in another, in which vaccination coverage has been high, diarrhea may be the most important cause of morbidity and mortality. In the CEs of the 1970s, which were mainly in sub-Saharan Africa and Southeast Asia, infectious diseases in displaced populations were the predominant issue. This led to the recognition of the importance of interventions such as measles vaccine programs and diarrheal disease control programs [13]. In some of the CEs of the 1990s, in places such as the former

BOX 18.1 Definitions

Disaster – an event of environmental disruption or destruction that is severe enough to overwhelm the resources of the affected community and necessitates outside assistance.

Natural disaster – a humanitarian crisis caused by either climatologic or geologic events.

Man-made disaster (also called Technological) – a humanitarian crisis caused by either accidental (e.g. nuclear, chemical release) or intentional (e.g. terrorism, war) factors.

Complex emergency (also complex humanitarian emergency) – a humanitarian crisis in a country, region or society where there is a breakdown of authority resulting from internal or external conflict, usually characterized by extreme violence, and requires an international response that goes beyond the mandate of a single agency or the existing United Nations country program.

BOX 18.2 Refugees and Internally Displaced People

A ***refugee*** is a person outside of his or her country of nationality who is unable or unwilling to return because of persecution or a well-founded fear of persecution on account of race, religion, nationality, membership in a particular social group, or political opinions.

An ***internally displaced person*** (IDP) is a person who has been forced or obliged to flee or to leave their homes or places of habitual residence, in particular as a result of or in order to avoid the effects of armed conflict, situations of generalized violence, violations of human rights or natural or human-made disasters, and who has not crossed an internationally recognized State border.

Comment: Both refugees and IDPs have similar health needs; however, they have very different status and rights under international law. This distinction may seem artificial but can have major consequences with respect to their rights, protections, and access to relief. The region with the largest IDP population is Africa with some 11.8 million IDPs in 21 countries [9].

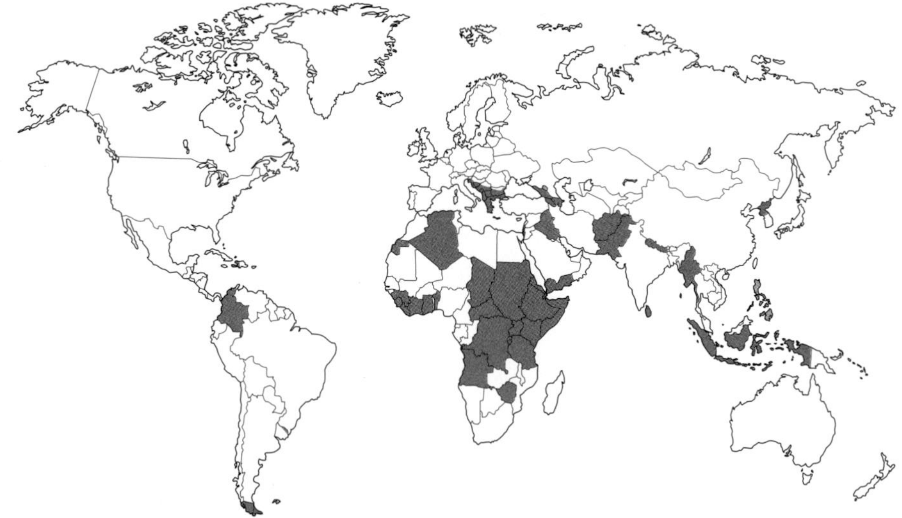

FIGURE 18.1 Complex emergencies. *From United Nations High Commissioner for Refugees. 2009 Global Trends: Refugees, Asylum-seekers, Returnees, Internally Displaced and Stateless Persons. Geneva, Switzerland; c 2010; cited 2010 July 4. Available from: http://www.unhcr.org/4c11f0be9.html Centre for Research on the Epidemiology of Disasters (CRED), Universite Catholique de Louvain. Complex Emergency Database. Brussels, Belgium: c2010; cited 2010 December 3. Available from: http://www.cedat.be.*

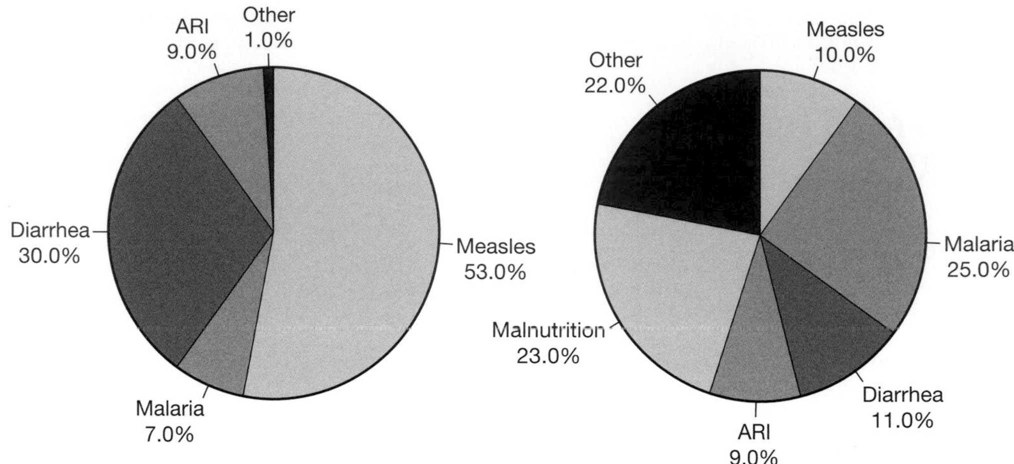

FIGURE 18.2 Leading causes of death in emergency phase of displaced people crisis in Sudan, 1985 (left) and Malawi, 1990 (right). *Adapted with permission from Toole MJ. Communicable diseases and disease control. In: Noji EK, ed. The Public Health Consequences of Disasters. New York: Oxford University Press; 1997:80–100.*

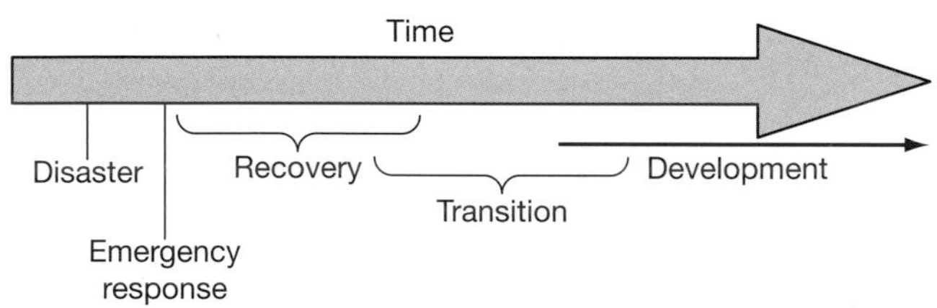

FIGURE 18.3 Hypothetical timeline of disaster response. *Adapted with permission from Burkholder BT, Toole MJ. Evolution of complex disasters. Lancet 1995;346:1012–15.*

Yugoslavia, trauma and chronic health conditions were more important causes of morbidity and mortality, requiring different types of interventions [14].

Furthermore, it is important to consider that within any given disaster, relief needs can evolve considerably over time. Some authors have described the phases of natural disasters, such as an impact phase, post-impact phase, and recovery phase, to discuss the importance of understanding how relief needs change markedly over time [15]. In the impact phase after earthquakes, for example, there may be an urgent need for trauma services in the first few days but then health needs shift to other conditions. Thus, deploying trauma hospitals that will arrive 4 or 5 days after the earthquake can be fruitless and wasteful.

It can sometimes be difficult to delineate clear phases of a CE. Because these disasters are usually the result of many years of complicated and deeply rooted problems, events may not unfold in a clear, linear fashion. Nevertheless, relief needs in complex emergencies can change substantially over time as well. For example, health needs for displaced people who have just arrived in a location – usually shelter, food, water, and basic medical care – will be quite different from what this population needs a few months after a camp has been established and matured. Dealing with infectious diseases such as leishmaniasis or tuberculosis often becomes much more important, and health needs such as family planning and medical care for chronic conditions and rehabilitation becomes more important (Fig. 18.3).

A critical concept for healthcare providers is that within a particular disaster, certain subpopulations may be more vulnerable, have fewer biological or social reserves to fall back on, and have less access to help (Box 18.3). Women and children, particularly small children, typically experience substantially increased morbidity and mortality. In Rwanda in 1999, for example, it was shown that refugee-camp children living in households headed by single women had a significantly higher risk of malnutrition because they had less access to food and other relief services [16]. Certain ethnic, religious, or cultural groups may be especially vulnerable. In Somalia, certain unarmed agriculturally based clans who were not participants in the fighting were particularly devastated by the civil conflict and had extremely limited access to emergency relief services. Even adults and adolescents, who are the most capable segments of the population, require special attention in some circumstances.

BOX 18.3 Displaced and Vulnerable Populations

Displaced populations in general are at increased risk of disease and injury due to degradation of sanitation and limited safe water, food, shelter and security. This is evidenced by a consistent, marked increase in crude mortality rates. However, some subgroups of the displaced population are at greater increased risks and considered especially vulnerable.

Vulnerable populations include, but are not limited to, women, especially pregnant or breastfeeding mothers, young children, the elderly, and anyone with a physical or mental disability. However, in some circumstances, certain ethnic groups and even young healthy males can be vulnerable as well.

THE HEALTH RESPONSE

Effectively addressing the health needs of a disaster-affected population requires gathering and monitoring appropriate information about the situation and the population, identifying vulnerable populations, providing appropriate clinical and nutritional services, and addressing the major public health issues. This must be done in the context of what is often a complex response network, and sometimes major political and security challenges. The rest of the chapter addresses the fundamental emergency health-related measures that should be pursued in the emergency phase of a disaster (Fig. 18.4).

Rapidly Assess the Health Status of the Affected Population and Establish a Health Information System

Effective relief depends on characterizing the situation with timely and sound clinical and public health data. Rapid assessment is essential as the first step in an emergency response to identify urgent needs and relief priorities for that particular situation (Box 18.4). The importance of rapid assessments has been increasingly recognized,

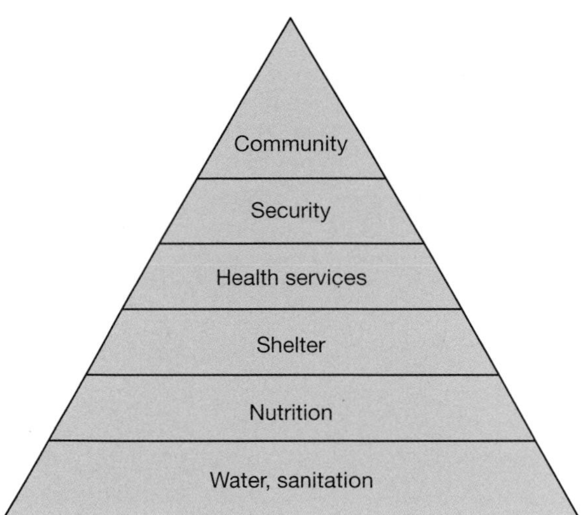

FIGURE 18.4 Pyramid of population needs in disasters.

and the science of conducting these assessments has developed considerably. It is now widely appreciated that in the absence of sound early assessments, relief efforts can easily be misguided and inappropriate no matter how well intentioned. After initial assessments, targeted surveys and specific investigations can be of great value in answering more focused questions, such as immunization coverage or the extent of malnutrition in a high-risk group. Then, standardized surveillance and health information systems need to be established (or re-established) after disasters to continually assess and monitor the needs of the affected population. Relief efforts should be modified accordingly as critical data become available. In the absence of mechanisms to constantly re-evaluate the health of the target population, priorities may become skewed and resources may be inappropriately directed or even wasted. The ongoing monitoring of important diseases and the use of this information is critical in designing and running effective relief efforts. There are innumerable examples in the disaster medicine literature of how early information collection and subsequent surveillance has been critical for successful disaster response and how failure to collect this information has at times even exacerbated the situation [17,18].

Immunize Against Measles and Provide Vitamin A

Measles in children has been shown repeatedly to be a major, and often the most important, cause of death in refugees and displaced people [19,20]. Measles outbreaks can be explosive after disasters and have

BOX 18.4 Tips for Rapid Assessment

It is imperative to base emergency relief efforts on a rapid assessment of the true situation and needs. Many relief efforts have gone awry because of a mismatch between real relief priorities and relief efforts based on presumed needs. The assessment ideally is done as soon as possible after the disaster and must balance the need for immediate information to guide relief activities with a certain degree of epidemiological rigor in collecting the data. Over the past decades, the methodology of rapid assessment has developed considerably. Rapid health assessments can be quite sophisticated or "quick and dirty". While many general templates and checklists are available, they must be adapted to the specific circumstances of the disaster and the organization conducting the assessment. Rapid assessments should always be followed by additional assessments and surveys or by establishment of surveillance and an ongoing health information system. The following is a sample outline of critical information that would be collected in a rapid health assessment after a sudden population displacement.

Key Characteristics of Affected Population

Population demographics
- Population size
- Percent male and female
- Percent less than age 5
- Nature and size of high-risk subgroups
- Average household or family size and degree of intact family structures
- Social and religious organization

Background health information
- Predominant health problems before displacement
- Normal crude mortality rates and other baseline health indicators
- Immunization status
- Usual sources and availability of healthcare
- Health beliefs and traditions
- Normal sanitary and excreta practices
- Burial practices

Availability of medical care and supplies
- Existing hospitals and clinics
- Availability of medical equipment and supplies
- Number and type of indigenous healthcare providers and community health workers

Nutrition and food
- Normal food types, diet, and sources
- Current availability and types of food
- Evidence of food shortages and malnutrition
- Availability of basic cooking supplies, utensils, and fuel

Emergency health indicators
- Overall crude mortality rate
- Age, sex, and cause-specific mortality rates
- Numbers, rates, and causes of morbidity

Water and sanitation
- Water sources, availability, and quality
- Availability of water transport capabilities
- Sanitation situation – availability of water treatment, soap, latrines
- Presence of disease-carrying and nuisance vectors

Material possessions and reserves
- Availability of blankets, shelter, building materials
- Availability of necessary clothing
- Presence of livestock and domestic animals
- Availability of transportation
- Money and other reserves

Physical location and security
- Current and potential locations of population(s)
- Topography, drainage, and access (roads, airfields)
- Current and anticipated climate and weather
- Security situation and threats

caused thousands of deaths in just a few weeks. Studies among refugees show that large measles outbreaks can occur even if vaccine coverage rates exceed 80%. Therefore, measles immunization campaigns must be given the highest priority. They should not be delayed until measles cases are reported or until other vaccines become available. Measles deaths occur primarily in young children, but children as old as 14 to 15 years have been affected. The most common nutritional deficiency in refugee and displaced populations is lack of vitamin A. Deficiency of this vitamin has been shown to be an important cause of mortality particularly in measles cases but also in mortality from all causes. Vitamin A supplementation is cheap and easy. Thus, mass administration of vitamin A at the same time as measles vaccination can be an important adjunct intervention to reduce the consequences of measles infection, particularly in malnourished populations (Boxes 18.5 & 18.6). In selected situations, vaccination against diphtheria, pertussis, tetanus, polio, tuberculosis, meningococcal meningitis, or

BOX 18.5 Top Ten Emergency Relief Measures

The following are ten priority emergency relief measures:

1. Rapid assessment of the emergency situation and the affected population
   - Magnitude of the emergency
   - Environmental conditions
   - Major health and nutritional needs of the population
   - Local response capacity
2. Provide adequate shelter and clothing
   - Exposure to elements can lead directly to death and increase caloric requirements
3. Provide adequate food
   - Minimum of 2000 kcal/person/day
   - Must consider mechanism for equitable distribution
   - Targeted supplemental and therapeutic feeding programs for vulnerable and severely malnourished individuals when resources are available
4. Provide elementary sanitation and clean water
   - Absolute minimum requirement 3 to 5 liters/person/day of reasonably clean water
   - Goal per Sphere standards are 15 liters/person/day
5. Institute communicable disease control programs
   - Community outreach for case prevention
   - Appropriate case management of severe diarrhea and dehydration
   - Improve sanitation and water source
6. Immunize against measles and provide vitamin A supplements
   - High priority in any displaced populations living in crowded conditions
   - Vitamin A deficiency is common in malnourished populations and contributes significantly to measles case fatality
7. Establish primary care medical treatment
   - Develop appropriate treatment algorithms for prevalent diseases based on treatment standards among the local population and use standard supplies
8. Establish disease surveillance and a health information system
   - Necessary to monitor effectiveness of health interventions and realign priorities
9. Organize human resources
   - Disaster victims are not helpless; most want to help themselves but need means
   - Identify leaders to organize food and water distribution and sanitation programs
   - Identify community health workers with pre-disaster experience
   - Identify interpreters
   - Identify surrogate families for unaccompanied minors
10. Coordinate activities
   - Local authorities, international relief organizations, governmental agencies, military

BOX 18.6 Pediatric Considerations

Dehydration

Often exacerbated by acute diarrhea, dehydration is a contributing factor to morbidity and mortality, especially in young children. Treatment is primarily by oral rehydration using Oral Rehydration Solution (ORS) (see Box 18.7).

Measles

Institute a vaccination program immediately, before cases present – target 6–23-month-old children for single dose, 0.5 mL of vaccine.

Supplement diet with vitamin A capsules, 100,000 IU or 200,000 IU.

6–11 months old	100,000 IU at vaccination
12–59 months old	200,000 IU at vaccination and every 6 months
Postpartum mothers	200,000 IU within 45 days of delivery to increase Vitamin A in breast milk

Note: Vitamin A should not be given to pregnant women or women of reproductive age due to risk of teratogenicity to the fetus.

Malnutrition

Kwashiorkor: severe protein insufficiency; edema of hands, feet and round "moon face"

Marasmus: total caloric insufficiency; gross muscle loss and wasting with "skin and bone" appearance

Moderate: minus 2–3 standard deviations (–2–3 Z-score), or 70–80% below median weight-for-height in population

Severe: minus >3 standard deviations (<–3 Z-score), or < 70% weight-for-height in the population, or edema; kwashiorkor malnutrition is always severe

Supplemental feeding program: to correct moderate malnutrition – weekly supplemental food distribution (preferred), 1000–1200 kcal/day, or daily on-site feeding, 500–700 kcal/day

Therapeutic feeding program: inpatient nutritional and medical care to correct severe malnutrition and concurrent illness – only milk-based supplements acutely, 70 kcal/100 mL, 10–12/day

cholera may be appropriate. But rarely, if ever, will these interventions be as important as immunization against measles. These other immunizations usually become considerations after the emergency phase has passed.

Institute Diarrhea Control Programs

Diarrheal diseases are often a principal cause of morbidity and mortality in complex emergencies [21]. Common pathogens such as rotavirus and *E. coli* are often important causes of diarrhea outbreaks, but *Vibrio cholera* and drug-resistant *Shigella* spp. have also caused devastating outbreaks. Prevention of all types of diarrhea involves providing good sanitation, clean water, and adequate personal hygiene. Simple emergency measures to prevent diarrhea include organizing chlorination brigades, isolating defecation fields, and providing soap. Simple measures such as providing soap are inexpensive and can substantially reduce person-to-person disease transmission. In some situations, though, and particularly in the emergency phases of a relief effort, preventive measures may not be feasible or effective. The critical intervention in coping with diarrheal disease then becomes preventing mortality through effective case management. Sound case management of diarrheal disease, even in cholera epidemics, can reduce case fatality rates to less than 1%. Effective case management of diarrhea is based primarily on providing fluid replacement through aggressive oral rehydration therapy (Box 18.7). Intravenous fluid replacement and antibiotics are used selectively and according to protocols relevant to the situation. While these concepts are easy to understand, experience has shown that effective diarrhea treatment programs require substantial organization and numerous personnel with experience and training. In northern Iraq in 1991, for example, the abundance of rehydration salts and enthusiastic medical providers was not enough in the absence of effectively run rehydration centers [22]. An important component of diarrhea control programs is developing community outreach programs to seek out cases that may not present to treatment facilities. Education of the community, particularly mothers, on the use of oral rehydration therapy, the importance of continuing breastfeeding, and the importance of personal hygiene is also a priority. Active case finding, surveillance, and outbreak investigation are essential in determining the causes of the outbreak. Care providers must appreciate that the approach to diarrhea management in a CE is different from the approach that would be followed in the developed world.

Provide Elementary Sanitation and Clean Water

Many of the diseases that occur in disasters, particularly in the setting of a CE, are to a great extent the consequence of poor environmental conditions [23]. Water is often in short supply and of poor quality. There are limited means to dispose of waste. Vectors of communicable diseases may be prevalent. The means for basic personal hygiene may be lacking. Addressing these environmental health issues, particularly providing potable water, usually is a very high priority. Water needs are frequently underestimated. Only 3 to 5 liters of potable water per day must be consumed for short-term survival, but adults need at least 15 to 20 liters per day for cooking, cleaning, medical care, and, sometimes, important ritual purposes. In some situations, such as when people are active in a hot environment, water needs are even greater. Medical facilities require much more water, usually at least 100 liters per patient per day. Environmental issues are often very difficult to resolve because they require considerable resources and technical expertise. Providing potable water to a group of refugees, for example, may require experienced engineers who can locate the best sources of water, whether from the ground, the surface, or a spring. Expertise, such as how to construct a proper well and select the appropriate pump, is needed to access the source. The characteristics of a water distribution system are important because they can greatly influence the way water is accessed and therefore used; if people have a difficult time obtaining water, they will use it sparingly. Assessing and maintaining water quality is a critical aspect of a water program. Local water may be a limited resource and local political considerations may be critical in its access and use. Cultural considerations can also be important factors in how water is accessed and used by the local population. The technical skills and other considerations in waste disposal, vector control, and personal hygiene can be equally complex. Some relief organizations attempt to focus on environmental health issues but most do not. The technical challenges and lack of donor appeal of environmental issues remain major problems.

Provide Adequate Shelter, Clothes and Blankets

Shelter is a basic human need. The provision of the basic means to be protected from the elements – sun, rain and cold – is a high priority. In populations with nutritional deficits, substantial energy can be expended simply in trying to keep warm. Consequently, some have argued that, in certain situations, distributing shelter, clothes and blankets may be more effective in preventing morbidity and mortality than is distributing food. As with environmental interventions, there is a substantial body of knowledge that deals with the technical considerations of emergency housing [24]. The selection of the specific sites for shelter, the layout of camps, and the type of materials used in construction are all important issues. Camps constructed in poor locations and with inadequate design can accelerate communicable disease transmission. Other factors to consider are the local availability of materials, the economic level of development of the population, the social habits, the local customs, and the political context. The decision to provide shelter can have significant long-term consequences. Simple shelters provided on an emergency basis may unintentionally evolve into a permanent camp and end up attracting more refugees to the site. Many of these issues may become a *fait accompli* before reasoned decisions can be made by relief officials. Refugees are often forced by circumstances into poor locations that would never have been chosen by relief workers who had been given the opportunity to make decisions based on health and safety.

Ensure Food Supplies are Adequate and Reach Intended Recipients

One of the hallmarks of complex emergencies is a shortage of food. Thus, providing at least 2000 kcal per day per person is an essential priority in emergency situations [25]. While it is often uncertain how many people actually die of starvation during complex emergencies, acute malnutrition has been shown to be a critical underlying cause of much morbidity and mortality [26]. There are many ways of providing emergency food relief. General food rations can be distributed widely to the population, perhaps in exchange for work or school attendance. General food rations consist of nutritionally balanced basic commodities that are appropriate to the situation and culture. Selective or supplemental feeding programs target food for certain high-risk people, such as malnourished children, tuberculosis patients, or lactating mothers. This food may be distributed as rations to take home or can be provided at feeding centers, such as "soup kitchens". Therapeutic or rehabilitative feeding can be provided for significantly malnourished people as a medical intervention and is usually given on an inpatient basis through assisted eating, nasogastric tube, or intravenous line. The mechanics of managing food distribution and feeding programs are often complex. For example, an intensive rehabilitative program for severely malnourished children must have mechanisms to identify patients in the affected population. To some extent, patients may be self-referred, but often they must be proactively sought through clinic referrals and community outreach workers. Protocols and procedures must be developed to screen patients and determine who is eligible. Refeeding is labor-intensive and requires care providers with training and experience. Patients typically have other aggravating illnesses and infections, such as malaria, that can complicate refeeding efforts. After discharge, follow-up programs must exist to prevent relapse. Sometimes family interventions are needed to counteract the social context that was a factor in the malnutrition. For example, in some cultures one child may be singled out to be deprived so that the other children may survive. The management of other food distribution programs can be

BOX 18.7 Additional Clinical Pearls

Vitamin A Deficiency

This is common in emergency affected areas. Vitamin A deficiency leads to blindness, lowered immunity, and increased morbidity and mortality, especially from diarrhea and measles. Vitamin A is a fat-soluble vitamin and supplementation can be dietary or capsule dosing. Target populations are children 6–59 months and lactating mothers.

Dietary sources: breast milk, whole milk, fish, meat, eggs, orange and yellow fruits and vegetables, green leafy vegetables.

Capsules: Vitamin A capsules are available from UNICEF in either 100,000 IU or 200,000 IU. Capsules are not swallowed. Administration is by cutting the nipple off one end of the capsule and squeezing drops into patient's mouth. Assistant should wash hands afterward.

Deworming

Intestinal parasite infection is a common problem in emergency affected areas due to inadequate sanitation and hygiene.

What: *Ascaris lumbricoides* (roundworm)
Ancylostoma duodenale and *Necator americanus* (hookworms)
Trichuris trichiura (whipworm)

Why: Improves nutritional status, immune response, growth and learning, as well as improved trust in community health workers
Decreases vitamin A deficiency and childhood morbidity and mortality.

Who: Target population is children 1–5 years old

How:

Drug	1–2 years old	2–5 years old	
Albendazole, 400 mg tablet	½ tablet	1 tablet	Single dose
Mebendazole, 500 mg tablet	½ tablet	1 tablet	Single dose

Oral Rehydration Salts (ORS)

Oral rehydration therapy (ORT) with ORS is the primary means of treating dehydration due to diarrhea. ORS is a balanced mixture of electrolyte salts and glucose recommended by the WHO and UNICEF. It is available as a pharmaceutical product, ORS sachets, containing sodium chloride, potassium chloride, trisodium citrate and glucose. Homemade ORS solutions can be used if prepared products are not available, or to begin treatment by parents or caregivers at the onset of diarrhea.

ORS sachets	One sachet per liter of safe drinking water
Homemade ORS	½ teaspoon salt + 6 teaspoons sugar per liter of safe drinking water

Administration:

<2 years old	50–100 mL at a time, up to ½ liter per day
2–9 years old	100–200 mL at a time, up to 1 liter per day
≥10 years old	As tolerated, up to 2 liters per day

Supplemental references:

- WHO position paper on oral rehydration salts to reduce mortality from cholera, www.who.int/cholera/technical/en
- First steps for managing an outbreak of acute diarrhea, www.searo.who.int/en/Section 1257/Section2263/info-kit/WHO-Managing_Diarrhea_outbreak.pdf
- WHO/UNICEF Joint Statement clinical management of acute diarrhea, www.whqlibdoc.who.int/hq/2004/WHO_FCH_CAH_04.7.pdf
- Oral rehydration salts production of the new ORS, www.whqlibdoc.who.int/hq/2006/WHO_FCH_CAH_06.1.pdf

complicated also and requires technical skills and experience. Food programs have not always been successful, due in part to formidable problems of logistics, security, and distribution. Food aid can be highly politicized and food relief misused. Food supplies must be nutritionally balanced and culturally appropriate, and there has been much debate about the appropriate number of calories and the best content of food rations. Remarkably, micronutrient deficiencies have occurred in populations relying on donated food [27]. The causes of food shortages are complex and may involve disruption of harvests, collapse of markets, lack of distribution systems, manipulation of food supplies by warring factions, and many other factors. Thus, an emergency feeding campaign must not only provide food urgently and effectively, but also begin to address the root problems of the crisis. Supplying seeds and agricultural implements may, in the long run, be as important as supplying emergency food. There are a number of agencies that specialize in managing the "food pipeline" to emergency situations: the procurement, processing, shipping, and storing of bulk food. The World Food Program is the principal international agency. In the US, some of the principal agencies include Care, Catholic Relief Services, World Vision, and Feed the Children. On the scene of an emergency, other agencies, such as the ICRC and private volunteer organizations, often assume responsibility for actually distributing food and for administering feeding programs.

Establish Appropriate Curative Services

Probably most importantly for direct care providers, establishing curative medical services that follow standard treatment protocols, are based on essential drug lists, and provide basic coverage to the community as a whole are a high priority in CEs. Providing acute medical care is one of the most visible and understandable aspects of a relief operation, and experience has shown that many external medical providers are willing to volunteer in an emergency. One of the hallmarks of emergency relief is the dispatch of medical teams from developed countries to treat sick victims. However, what medical care is actually needed should be carefully considered before providing curative services; noble intentions may not necessarily translate into effective patient management. As indicated above, much of effective relief has to do with public health programs. With regard to clinical care, substantial experience shows that medical care in emergency situations should be based on simple standardized protocols. There are basic, easily adaptable, field-tested protocols for managing diarrheal disease, respiratory infection, febrile illness, and other common problems [28]. Underlying these basic protocols are basic essential drug and supply lists [29]. Using standard protocols and basic supplies assures that the care provided will be appropriate and allows the most efficient use of limited resources. Following basic protocols enables physician assistants, nurses, and community health workers to provide effective medical care without time-consuming and unnecessary technical interventions. This allows care to be delivered that is appropriate for the population and the same level of care to be sustained after outside relief workers depart. The management of relief supplies has been a very difficult problem in many disaster efforts; using essential drug and supply lists helps assure that logistic resources are devoted to needed items. Medical providers must be prepared to treat the conditions they will face. Volunteer providers from sophisticated hospitals in developed nations may not be well trained in dealing with the common problems of displaced persons or in using basic protocols and techniques appropriate to the situation. They may be called on to use drugs and techniques that are no longer used in their countries. In many emergencies, field hospitals or specialty teams have been deployed when basic primary care that reaches a large number of the population was what was needed.

Organize Human Resources and Utilize Local Assets

Local preparedness and utilizing indigenous community health workers are essential in assuring that medical care in an emergency is truly community-based and oriented toward primary care [30]. While it is easy to focus on imported clinics and hospitals, community health workers are also the means by which health services actually reach much of the affected population. An effort should be made to ensure there is one community health worker for every 1000 individuals in the target population. Relief will only be effective if it is based on the needs and idiosyncrasies of the local cultures. Outside relief personnel may know little about local food preferences, sanitary mores, social customs, indigenous medical practices, and other such issues. A food program, for example, that provides culturally inappropriate commodities will not succeed. Community health workers will have insights into these matters that can profoundly affect the delivery of health services. The access that community health workers have to the community can be critical. They are essential in communicating with local leaders, who play a central role in the success or failure of relief programs. If local leaders do not support an urgent measles vaccination program, for example, few people will participate. There can be many barriers to seeking medical care in an emergency, some practical and some cultural. Community health workers are often able to locate those in need. In northern Iraq, severely malnourished and dehydrated children were sometimes kept in a dark corner of their shelter and were not brought into the clinic unless the community health worker actively sought them out [22]. Those from outside the affected population who are providing relief may tend to see aid recipients as helpless victims, but disaster-affected populations have a wealth of human resources. In fact, those affected by disasters are usually very anxious to help themselves and typically only lack the means. Community health workers are the key to mobilizing indigenous resources into relief efforts. In addition, utilizing community health workers and local health resources facilitates the often difficult transition from the emergency to long-term sustainable recovery [31].

Coordinate Activities of Local Authorities and Relief Agencies

A hallmark of a complex emergency is the complex response. In some respects, the response is every bit as complex as the disaster. A plethora of agencies and organizations – governmental and private, civilian and military, indigenous and external – become involved [32,33]. Relief workers must understand the other participants in the response and work collaboratively. Without effective cooperation and coordination, time, energy, money, supplies, and, most importantly, lives may be lost. Recently, the cluster approach, in which different agencies are assigned the lead for different aspects of the response, has been shown to be effective in allowing different and disparate groups to work more effectively together [34]. When appropriate communication and collaboration occur, the results can be dramatic [35,36] (Box 18.8).

BOX 18.8 Additional Help for the Practitioner who is Deploying to an Emergency Relief Effort

One of the best resources for the health professional leaving imminently to help in a disaster response is the **SPHERE handbook**. SPHERE is an initiative launched in 1997 by a group of humanitarian non-governmental organizations and the Red Cross and Red Crescent movement to bring consensus to critical areas of emergency health response. The participants framed a Humanitarian Charter and identified Minimum Standards to be attained in disaster assistance in each of five key sectors: water supply and sanitation, nutrition, food aid, shelter and health services. This resource provides practical information and guidance for the health practitioner in the field [24].

Another is **ReliefWeb**. ReliefWeb is an excellent source for timely, reliable and relevant humanitarian information and analysis. ReliefWeb was launched in October 1996, and is administered by the United Nations Office for the Coordination of Humanitarian Affairs (OCHA). The project was initiated by the US Department of State, Bureau of International Organization Affairs, which had noticed during the Rwanda crisis how poorly critical operational information was shared between NGOs, UN agencies and governments. To help those engaged in humanitarian action make sense of humanitarian crises worldwide, this organization constantly scans thousands of sources and ensures the most relevant content is readily available on their website, ReliefWeb, or through RSS, e-mail, mobile phone, Twitter and Facebook [33].

SUMMARY

Responding to any disaster is a daunting challenge, particularly the most difficult of all disaster situations, the CE. Understanding the needs of the specific situation and then working to assure that the response is appropriate and feasible will greatly increase the probability of a successful response. This also includes awareness of unique cultural issues and capabilities of the other responders and beneficiary population. The ideal is to contribute to a rebuilding of capacity and ultimately the return of stability and self-reliance.

REFERENCES

1. World Health Organization (WHO). Myths and Realities in Disaster Situations. Geneva: WHO; c2010; cited 2010 July 4. Available from: http://www.who.int/hac/techguidance/ems/myths/en/index.html
2. Lechat MF. The epidemiology of disasters. Proc R Soc Med 1976;69:421–6.
3. Toole MJ, Galson S, Brady W. Are war and public health compatible? Lancet 1993;341:1193–6.
4. Levy BS, Sidel VW, eds. War and Public Health. New York: Oxford University Press; 2008.
5. Chen LC, Rietveld A. Human security during complex emergencies: rapid assessment and institutional capabilities. Med Global Survival 1994;1:156–63.

6. Macrai J, Zwi AB. Food as an instrument of war in contemporary African famines: a review of the evidence. Disasters 1992;16:299–321.
7. Burkle FM. Complex, humanitarian emergencies, I: concepts and participants. Prehosp Disaster Med 1995;10:36–42.
8. Salama P, Spiegel P, Talley L, Waldman R. Lessons learned from complex emergencies over the past decade. Lancet 2004;364:1801–13.
9. United Nations High Commissioner for Refugees. 2009 Global Trends: Refugees, Asylum-seekers, Returnees, Internally Displaced and Stateless Persons. Geneva; c2010; cited 2010 July 4. Available from: http://www.unhcr.org/4c11f0be9.html
10. Noji, EK, ed. The Public Health Consequences of Disasters. New York: Oxford University Press; 1997.
11. Centers for Disease Control and Prevention. Famine-affected, refugee, and displaced populations: recommendations for public health issues. MMWR Recomm Rep 1992;41:1–76..
12. Noji EK. Disaster epidemiology. Emerg Med Clin North Am 1996;14: 289–300.
13. Toole MJ, Waldman RJ. Prevention of excess mortality in refugee and displaced populations in developing countries. JAMA 1990;263:3296–302.
14. Acheson D. Health, humanitarian relief, and survival in former Yugoslavia. BMJ 1993;307:44–8
15. Burkholder BT, Toole MJ. Evolution of complex disasters. Lancet 1995;346:1012–15.
16. Goma Epidemiology Group. Public health impact of Rwandan refugee crisis: what happened in Goma, Zaire, in July, 1994? Lancet 1995;345:339–44.
17. Bradt DA, Drummond CM. Rapid epidemiologic assessment of health status in displaced populations – an evolution toward standardized minimum data sets. Prehosp Disaster Med 2003;18:178–85.
18. Lillibridge SR, Noji EK, Burkle FM Jr. Disaster assessment: the emergency health evaluation of a population affected by a disaster. Ann Emerg Med 1993;22:1715–20.
19. Toole MJ, Steketee RW, Waldman RJ, Nieburg PI. Measles prevention and control in emergency settings. Bull World Health Organ 1989;67:381–6.
20. Nieburg P, Waldman RJ, Leavell R, et al. Vitamin A supplementation for refugees and famine victims. Bull World Health Organ 1988;66:689–97.
21. Toole MJ. Communicable diseases and disease control. In: Noji EK, ed. The Public Health Consequences of Disasters. New York: Oxford University Press; 1997:80–100.
22. Yip R, Sharp TW. Acute malnutrition and high childhood mortality related to diarrhea. JAMA 1993;270:587–90.
23. Landesman LY, ed. Public Health Management of Disasters: The Practice Guide, 2nd edn. Washington, DC: American Public Health Association; 2005.
24. The Sphere Project. Minimum Standards in Shelter, Settlement and Non-Food Items. Geneva: The Sphere Project; c2004; cited 2010 July 4. Available from: http://www.sphereproject.org/content/view/100/84/lang,english/
25. The Sphere Project. Minimum Standards in Food Security, Nutrition and Food Aid. Geneva: The Sphere Project; c2004. Available from: http://www.sphereproject.org/content/view/62/84/lang,english/
26. Yip R. Famine. In: Noji EK, ed. The Public Health Consequences of Disasters. New York: Oxford University Press; 1997:305–35.
27. Toole MJ. Micronutrient deficiencies in refugees. Lancet 1992;339:1214–16.
28. The Sphere Project. Minimum Standards in Health Services. Geneva: The Sphere Project; c2004; cited 2010 July 4. Available from: http://www.sphereproject.org/content/view/114/84/lang,english/
29. World Health Organization (WHO). The New Emergency Health Kit: Lists of Drugs and Medical Supplies for a Population of 10,000 Persons for Approximately 3 Months. Geneva: WHO; 1993. (Updated version available at: http://www.who.int/hac/techguidance/ems/new_health_kit_content/en/index3.html)
30. Musani A, Shaikh I. Preparedness for humanitarian crises needs to be improved. BMJ 2006;333:843–5.
31. Cuny F. From Disasters to Development. New York: Simon and Schuster; 1979.
32. Natsios AS. The international humanitarian response system. Parameters 1995;(Spring):68–81.
33. ReliefWeb. Serving the Needs of the Humanitarian Community. Geneva: United Nations Office for the Coordination of Humanitarian Affairs; c2010; cited 2010 July 4. Available from: http://www.reliefweb.int
34. ReliefWeb. The Cluster Approach. Geneva: United Nations Office for the Coordination of Humanitarian Affairs; c2010; cited 2010 July 4. Available from: http://www.reliefweb.int/humanitarianreform/
35. Auerbach PS, Norris RL, Menon AS, et al. Civil-military cooperation in the initial medical response to the earthquake in Haiti. N Engl J Med 2010; 362:e32.
36. Centre for Research on the Epidemiology of Disasters (CRED), Universite Catholique de Louvain. Complex Emergency Database. Belgium: Brussels; c2010; cited 2010 December 3. Available from: http://www.cedat.be/

SECTION

C

SERVICE-BASED CHAPTERS

19 Diagnostic Imaging in the Tropics

Elizabeth Joekes, Sam Kampondeni

Key features

Key differences in imaging in resource-poor countries, compared to industrialized countries:

- Ultrasound and plain radiography cover the majority of imaging indications
- Image acquisition and interpretation are frequently performed by non-specialists
- Lack of maintenance, quality assurance and radiation protection programs is widespread
- Very little evidence of the impact of imaging on patient management, outcome and cost is available

Key features unique to the tropics:

- Diagnostic imaging should be used within the framework of WHO-algorithm
- High prevalence of chronic and asymptomatic infections confounds image interpretation
- Imaging appearances of diseases vary with geographic location and endemic background

INTRODUCTION

Although the industrialized world has made great strides in diagnostic imaging, low-resource countries have remained at a disadvantage. This is related to a lack of basic equipment, accessories, maintenance and trained staff. Computed tomography (CT) and magnetic resonance imaging (MRI), which are standard in industrialized countries, are rare. Little evidence is available related to the impact and cost-effectiveness of imaging in the management of diseases in a low-resource setting.

EQUIPMENT AND SERVICE DEVELOPMENT

WHO guidance is available on the appropriate choice of equipment for each level of care [1,2]. A district hospital will ideally require a basic x-ray system and ultrasound. More advanced techniques such as fluoroscopy require contrast media and specialist knowledge. In the setting of a regional hospital with several specialists, this is an appropriate imaging modality. Specialist ultrasound applications, such as echocardiography, complex obstetric scanning and ultrasound-guided interventions, may also be available. At the tertiary teaching hospital level, services are generally supported by radiologists. More advanced techniques such as Doppler ultrasound, CT and MRI may be appropriate, depending on the clinical specialties and treatment options available.

Imaging equipment is extremely expensive to install and run and is very susceptible to break down: in particular in a setting of irregular power supply and in the absence of regular maintenance. It is essential that implementation is part of a wider national program of healthcare provision with appropriate imaging facilities chosen for the level of overall healthcare available [3]. Consideration of location, case mix and volume of patients is important, as high-cost equipment which is used sporadically will not be cost-effective. Choosing x-ray equipment requires specialist input and discussion with regional healthcare providers, national imaging societies and atomic energy commissions. Support is also available from international imaging societies [4,5] and WHO. No equipment should be donated or purchased without prior needs assessment, a long-term maintenance contract and appropriate training. Well-intended, but uncoordinated, second-hand equipment donations by hospitals in wealthy countries should be discouraged (Fig. 19.1). They have all too often resulted in the equipment standing idle or in misdirection of scarce local resources to run this equipment. Pooling resources for regional equipment servicing will reduce equipment breakdown and cost. Radiation protection and a quality assurance (QA) program should be in place. Poor image quality has been shown to be a major source of unnecessary radiation to patients in developing countries [6]. At a minimum, quality control should include regular equipment checks, radiation dose monitoring, and reporting incidents of inadvertent overexposure. However, other elements of QA which are helpful in improving imaging services are regular analysis of rejected films, review of referrals, and follow-up of the impact of the investigation on patient outcome and management. Ensuring staff have appropriate qualifications and access to continuing professional development are no less important. WHO has developed specifications for a basic, screen film-based x-ray system, the WHO Imaging System-Radiology, (WHIS-RAD), suited to the needs of district hospitals in low-resource settings. More recently, digital systems have been developed, solving the problems of film processing and the unreliable supply of film and dark room chemicals [7]. Digital systems reduce running costs and the need for retakes of poor-quality films [8]. The images are also suitable for tele-radiology purposes. WHO has published several manuals on maintenance, quality assurance and radiographic technique, available in print and online [9].

Ultrasound equipment is much cheaper and easier to install. It does not use radiation and is available in portable format. The downside is the need for intensive user training [10]. Without appropriate training there is a significant risk of misdiagnosis and harm to the patient. The choice of system will largely depend on the application required. Advice can be sought from national imaging societies or the World Federation for Ultrasound [11]. Maintenance is less complex than for x-ray equipment, but a regional engineer should be available.

If resources do not permit installation of both x-ray and ultrasound, traditional WHO guidance advocates implementation of x-ray before ultrasound, except in hospitals dedicated to obstetrics [2]. However, ultrasound in combination with appropriate training is cheaper and more versatile than x-ray installation and maintenance. Applications and impact of these two modalities differ and currently no evidence

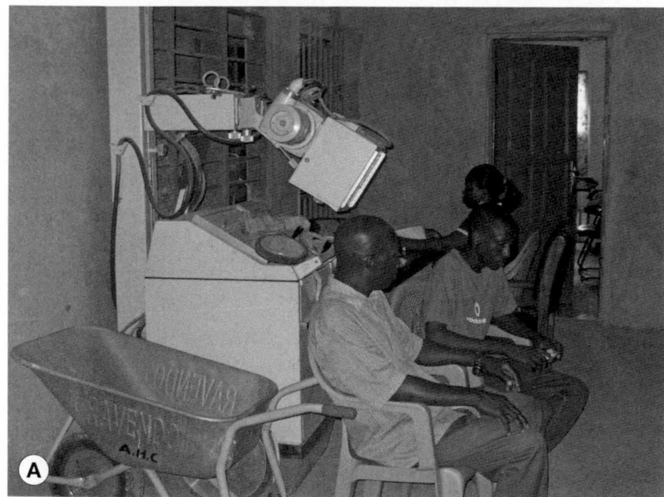

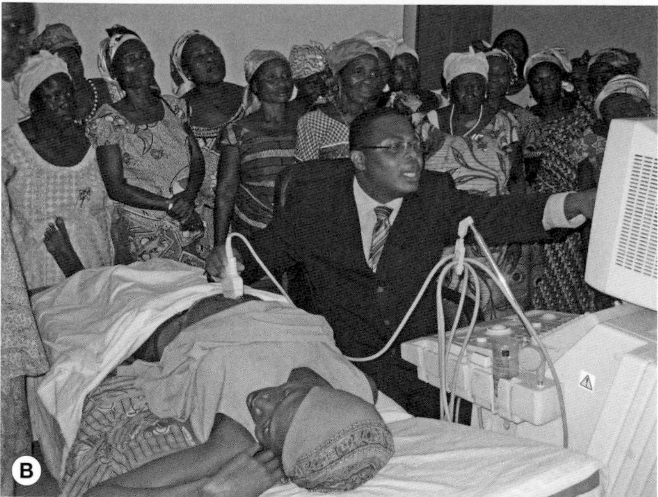

FIGURE 19.1 This x-ray machine **(A)** was donated to a district hospital without prior needs assessment or provisions for an x-ray room, consumables, staffing or maintenance. It was never used. Years later, in the same hospital, the ultrasound machine **(B)** was provided at the request of the hospital. A trained obstetrician has taken charge of the machine and a training program for midwives and general physicians was provided along with the machine.

is available on their relative merits and overall cost to the healthcare system.

PERSONNEL

Brain drain and a shortage of training programs in radiology, radiography and sonography are major issues in the tropics [12,13]. Equipment is frequently operated by untrained staff and images are interpreted by general physicians or non-medical health workers. Many studies have shown that interpretation errors may occur in up to half of all films when they are reported by non-radiologists [14,15]. If film quality is poor, the error rate increases even further [6]. The diagnostic value of an examination may be reduced significantly in these circumstances. In the absence of trained staff to interpret the images, the benefit of the test is unlikely to outweigh the considerable costs.

To improve matters, capacity building through hybrid programs between local countries and major regional centers is becoming increasingly popular. Ultrasound training programs, tailored to local needs, have been developed in the last decade [16]. Evidence of the impact of these programmes is scanty, but a few encouraging studies have been published recently [17,18]. Short intensive courses, followed by documentation of independently performed scans and regular review by trainers, ensure continuous learning and sustainability and allow evaluation of the impact of scans on patient outcome. Increasingly, teleradiology is being used to connect remote hospitals to large regional centers for expert second opinion [19,20]. Industrial image transfer systems come at a large cost, but simple images of films taken with a standard digital camera from a light box are sufficient for remote interpretation in most cases. Compression of these digital files on a home computer and sending them via e-mail provides a low-cost teleradiology option [21]. The rapid increase in internet connectivity in low-resource countries brings hope that this will be a great tool for supporting imaging in future.

> **BOX 19.1 Pediatric Considerations**
>
> - Radiographic exposures should be adjusted to age to avoid unnecessary radiation
> - Nutritional disorders such as rickets and scurvy can be diagnosed from skeletal x-rays
> - In neonates and infants, ultrasound can aid in the diagnosis of intracranial abnormalities, osteomyelitis and intussusception

THE IMAGING OF TROPICAL DISEASES

Most tropical diseases have established WHO algorithms for diagnosis and treatment. Imaging should be used in accordance with these algorithms, bearing in mind that there may be limited evidence to support the use of imaging in some. Where none exist, imaging should only be used when the test result is likely to have a significant impact on patient management. Plain radiographs and ultrasound should be the investigations of first choice whenever possible, even in the presence of fluoroscopy, CT or MRI.

PLAIN RADIOGRAPHS

A good-quality frontal chest x-ray is adequate in most situations. Routine lateral films are not necessary. Occasionally, they may be helpful to localize a retrosternal or retrocardiac lesion on a frontal film and to detect hilar adenopathy in children. Fluoroscopy is a real-time, dynamic x-ray investigation which is useful to assess the gastrointestinal tract for example. However, the resolution is relatively poor in order to keep radiation dose to a minimum and it cannot be used to replace a proper chest x-ray. In children, exposures should be adjusted to their age group to avoid unnecessary radiation (Box 19.1). Common indications for chest radiographs include the diagnosis of smear-negative tuberculosis (TB) in symptomatic patients [22] and the detection of complications such as pneumothorax. Screening of high-risk populations such as asymptomatic HIV-infected patients eligible for TB prevention therapy is a subject of ongoing debate [23,24]. TB in symptomatic HIV-infected patients with reduced CD4 counts commonly presents with a lobar pneumonia or an effusion on chest films, instead of the classical appearance of bilateral upper lobe cavitating bronchopneumonia. The x-ray may even be entirely normal in about 15% of cases [25]. In general, chest x-rays are not necessary in uncomplicated pneumonias, effusions or for follow-up during treatment.

Abdominal x-rays are helpful in diagnosing intestinal obstruction, perforation and renal calculi. Although a calcified bladder wall in schistosomiasis or a calcified hydatid cyst may be identified as an incidental finding, these films are not suitable to diagnose new, active infection and the appropriate laboratory tests or ultrasound should be performed.

Skeletal x-rays will mainly be used in the setting of trauma. Other indications in the tropics include acute or chronic osteomyelitis, hemoglobinopathies, and nutritional diseases such as rickets and scurvy. The widespread use of skull x-rays in head trauma should be strongly discouraged even in the absence of CT. Management will depend on the neurologic symptoms rather than on the presence or absence of a skull fracture on x-ray. Similarly, the use of lumbar spine x-rays in chronic back pain, in the absence of trauma or a suspicion of malignancy or TB, is not indicated as it will not significantly alter management.

As the imaging appearances of many tropical infections overlap, it is important to correlate all findings with the clinical presentation and laboratory test results. Even then it may be difficult to make a definitive diagnosis with the available imaging results. In addition, asymptomatic or previous infection with a wide variety of organisms is very common. They are often not the cause of the presenting symptoms, but may show abnormalities on imaging. For example, a fibrotic lung following successful TB treatment in the past may be mistaken for active infection. Assuming all these findings are active disease will lead to multiple diagnoses and overburdening of medical services. Similarly, differences in endemic background and comorbidities may change the way diseases present: HIV co-infection alters the presenting appearances of TB on chest x-rays [25], and primary infection patterns that are classically seen in children in endemic areas can be present in adults in non-endemic areas. Knowledge of local disease patterns is essential for accurate interpretation of imaging studies. Other pitfalls in the interpretation of imaging studies are the geographic variation in the appearances of both infectious and noninfectious diseases, as well as the variation in baseline standards between different populations. For example, Asian fetal biometric tables on low-cost Chinese ultrasound equipment cannot be applied in African countries, as the average birth weight of the Asian population is lower, leading to overestimation of fetal size in African countries.

ULTRASOUND

As in the industrialized world, antenatal care and emergency obstetrics are the most common indications for ultrasound in the tropics. Its application is now recognized as a valuable tool in low-resource settings [26]. Increasingly, ultrasound has also been implemented in general medical, surgical and tropical diseases. It is currently used extensively in the diagnosis of liver diseases, including abscesses, hydatid disease, and schistosomiasis-related peri-portal fibrosis [27–29]. In areas with a high incidence of cirrhosis and hepatocellular carcinoma (HCC), ultrasound can often reliably confirm the diagnosis (Box 19.2). Biliary pathology such as ascaris, flukes and HIV-related cholangiopathy are all readily diagnosed in the appropriate clinical setting. Ultrasound should be the first modality in investigation of the renal tract, where it will identify hydronephrosis, tumors, TB, and schistosomiasis-related abnormalities, in addition to simple calculi. This applies to all levels of care, including those with access to intravenous urography (IVU). If ultrasound is available, IVU should no longer be used as the primary investigation for hydronephrosis or hematuria. Ascites, effusions and soft tissue abscesses can be diagnosed with relative ease. In more experienced hands, ultrasound can pick up intra-abdominal adenopathy, TB peritonitis, psoas abscesses and bowel masses. It can guide biopsies and percutaneous treatment of abscesses and hydronephrosis. Pediatric applications include many of the above, as well as the diagnosis and treatment of intussusception and subperiosteal abscess [30]. In neonates and young infants, the large fontanelle can be used as a window to assess the brain for hydrocephalus, congenital malformations, hemorrhage and infections.

BOX 19.2 Summary

- Procurement of x-ray equipment should include a maintenance contract and QA programme
- Safe and effective use of ultrasound requires intensive user-training
- The relative merits of x-ray and ultrasound in different low-resource settings are unknown
- Errors in x-ray interpretation by non-radiologists can occur in up to half of all films
- Images taken off a light box with a digital camera can be sent via e-mail for remote second opinion
- Many different infections and diseases show similar appearances on chest x-rays
- Chest x-rays are normal in approximately 15% of HIV-infected patients with active pulmonary TB
- Ultrasound can diagnose many infectious diseases of the liver as well as cirrhosis and HCC
- IVU should be replaced by ultrasound in the initial assessment of suspected kidney disease

Although not specifically related to tropical diseases, assessment of the acute abdomen with ultrasound can reduce the need for exploratory laparotomy and thus avoid unnecessary morbidity and cost to the patient.

Overall, ultrasound is a very powerful diagnostic tool which is currently greatly underutilized in low-resource settings. However, as stated previously, to benefit from its full potential and to avoid unnecessary harm, further development of high-quality training programs and regulation of misuse are essential.

ADVANCED IMAGING TECHNIQUES

Fluoroscopy, CT, MRI and nuclear medicine are complex imaging techniques which fall outside the scope of this chapter. The main indications for fluoroscopy are related to the gastrointestinal tract and include esophageal strictures, stomach ulcers and ileocolitis.

In the current setting of soaring numbers of road traffic accidents, the greatest benefit of CT scanning probably lies in the assessment of head injuries rather than tropical diseases. Detection of neuro-infections such as TB, toxoplasmosis and cysticercosis is possible, but unlikely to be cost-effective in low-resource settings.

REFERENCES

1. [Anonymous]. Effective choices for diagnostic imaging in clinical practice. Report of a WHO Scientific Group. World Health Organ Tech Rep Ser 1990;795:1–131.
2. Palmer P. Imaging equipment for small hospitals. Trop Geogr Med 1990;45: 98–102.
3. Garner P, Kiani A, Supachutikul A. Diagnostics in developing countries. BMJ 1997;315:760–1.
4. International Society of Radiology http://www.isradiology.org/ (accessed 9 October 2009).
5. International Society of Radiographers and Radiological Technologists. http://www.isrrt.org/isrrt/default_EN.asp?SnID=330535879 (accessed 9 October 2009).
6. Muhogora WE, Ahmed NA, Almosabihi A, et al. Patient doses in radiographic examinations in 12 countries in Asia, Africa, and eastern Europe: Initial results from IAEA projects. AJR Am J Roentgenol 2008;190:1453–61.
7. World Health Imaging, Telemedicine and Informatics Alliance. http://www.worldhealthimaging.org/ (accessed 9 October 2009).
8. Akhtar W, Aslam M, Ali A, et al. Film retakes in digital and conventional radiography. J Coll Physicians Surg Pak 2008;18:151–3.
9. World Health Organization Diagnostic Imaging Documentation Centre. http://www.who.int/diagnostic_imaging/publications/en/index.html (accessed 9 October 2009).
10. [Anonymous]. Training in diagnostic ultrasound: essentials, principles and standards. Report of a WHO study group. World Health Organ Tech Rep Ser 1998;875:i–46; back cover.
11. World Federation for Ultrasound in Medicine and Biology. http://www.wfumb.org/ (accessed 9 October 2009).
12. Pearson B. The brain drain: a force for good? Mera 2004;Jan:10–11.
13. Broadhead R, Muula A. The challenges facing post-graduate medical training in Malawi. Mera 2004;Jan:13–15.
14. Mehrotra P, Bosemani V, Cox J. Do radiologists still need to report chest x-rays? Postgrad Med J 2009;85:339–41.

15. Eisen LA, Berger JS, Hegde A, Schneider RF. Competency in chest radiography: a comparison of medical students, residents, and fellows. J Gen Intern Med 2006;21:46–65.
16. Jefferson Ultrasound Research and Education Institute. Global affiliate network. http://www.jefferson.edu/jurei/affiliate/ (accessed 9 October 2009).
17. Shah S, Noble VE, Umulisa I, et al. Development of an ultrasound training curriculum in a limited resource international setting: successes and challenges of ultrasound training in rural Rwanda. Int J Emerg Med 2008;1:193–6.
18. Baltarowich OH, Goldberg BB, Wilkes AN, et al. Effectiveness of "teaching the teachers" initiative for ultrasound training in Africa. Acad Radiol 2009;166:758–62.
19. Corr P. Digital imaging and telemedicine. In: Pattern Recognition in Diagnostic Imaging. Geneva: WHO; 2001.
20. Fraser H. Information technology and telemedicine in sub-Saharan Africa. BMJ 2000;321:465–66.
21. Szot A, Jacobson FL, Munn S, et al. Diagnostic accuracy of chest X-rays acquired using a digital camera for low-cost teleradiology. Int J Med Inform 2004;73:65–73.
22. Tuberculosis Coalition for Technical Assistance. International Standards for Tuberculosis Care (ISTC). The Hague: Tuberculosis Coalition for Technical Assistance, 2006.
23. Havlir DV, Getahun H, Sanne I, Nunn P. Opportunities and challenges for HIV care in overlapping HIV and TB epidemics. JAMA 2008;300: 423–30.
24. Mosimaneotsile B, Talbot EA, Moeti TL, et al. Value of chest radiography in a tuberculosis prevention programme for HIV infected people, Botswana. Lancet 2003;362:1551–2.
25. Greenberg S, Frager D, Suster B, et al. Active pulmonary tuberculosis in patients with AIDS: spectrum of radiographic findings (including a normal appearance). Radiology 1994;193:115–19.
26. Kongnyuy E, van den Broek N. The use of ultrasonography in obstetrics in developing countries. Trop Doct 2007;37:70–2.
27. Benedetti NJ, Desser TS, Jeffrey RB. Imaging of hepatic infections. Ultrasound Q 2008;24:267–78.
28. Richter J, Hatz C, Häussinger D. Ultrasound in tropical and parasitic diseases. Lancet 2003;362:900–2.
29. Berhe N, Geitung JT, Medhin G, Gundersen SG. Large scale evaluation of WHO's ultrasonographic staging system of schistosomal periportal fibrosis in Ethiopia. Trop Med Int Health 2006;11:1286–94.
30. Justice FA, de Campo M, Liem NT, et al. Accuracy of ultrasonography for the diagnosis of intussusceptions in infants in Vietnam. Pediatr Radiol 2007; 37:195–9.

20 Blood Transfusion in Resource-limited Settings

Oliver Hassall, Imelda Bates, Kathryn Maitland

Key features

- The issues of blood safety, adequate supply, equitable access and rational use still remain major challenges throughout the world. The greatest concern is in resource-limited countries, the majority of which are in sub-Saharan Africa. This chapter focuses on the major challenges facing transfusion services in Africa, but these are relevant to other resource-limited countries
- Despite high demand, blood supply is inadequate to meet global needs. An average of only 2.3 units are donated per 1000 population in sub-Saharan Africa, compared with 8.1 and 36.7, respectively, in countries with a medium and high human developmental indices.
- Women and young children are the chief recipients of blood transfusions in sub-Saharan Africa, accounting for over three-quarters of the blood transfusion requirements
- Nearly half of the blood collected in sub-Saharan Africa is from family or paid donors, in whom infectious risks are higher than in voluntary and non-remunerated donors
- The risks of transfusion-transmitted infection (TTI) are often substantial in resource-limited settings because of the high background incidence of viral, bacterial and malarial infections, the frequent use of paid or replacement donors, and incomplete screening coverage
- The frequency of noninfectious adverse events related to blood transfusion is largely unknown as hemovigilance activities are very limited

INTRODUCTION

The transfusion of blood can be a life-saving intervention, and the provision of adequate supplies of safe blood for transfusion is an essential undertaking for any health system. In 1975, a World Health Organization (WHO) resolution recognized the importance of blood transfusion services and urged governments to "promote national blood transfusion services, based on voluntary non-remunerated donations, and to promulgate laws to govern their operation" [1]. More than 30 years later, the issues of blood safety, adequate supply, equitable access and rational use still remain major challenges throughout the world. The greatest concern is in resource-limited countries, many of which are in sub-Saharan Africa, which have struggled to achieve the four key goals of an integrated strategy of blood safety [2]:

- Establishment of a nationally coordinated blood transfusion service.
- Collection of blood only from voluntary non-remunerated blood donors from low-risk populations.
- Testing of all donated blood, including screening for transfusion-transmissible infections, blood grouping and compatibility testing.
- Reduction in unnecessary transfusions through the effective clinical use of blood, including the use of simple alternatives to transfusion (crystalloids and colloids), wherever possible.

With respect to these goals, this chapter focuses upon the major challenges facing transfusion services in countries in sub-Saharan Africa where the authors have immediate experience. The issues raised are likely to be relevant to other resource-limited countries.

BLOOD SUPPLY AND SAFETY

THE GLOBAL BLOOD SUPPLY (Fig. 20.1)

The Global Database on Blood Safety (GDBS) of the WHO reports that only 45% of all blood is donated in countries where 80% of the world's population live, and that the average blood donation rate in countries with a low human development index (HDI) is 2.3 per 1000 population, compared with 8.1 in countries with a medium HDI, and 36.7 in countries with a high HDI [3]. Although there is currently no model that takes into account disease burden and health service sophistication to define what constitutes an adequate national blood requirement, these figures undoubtedly indicate a serious inequity in the availability of blood globally and inadequate blood supplies in resource-limited countries.

BLOOD SUPPLY IN AFRICA

Published data with regard to blood supply in the WHO Africa Region are limited to the GDBS survey of 2004 [4], and are constrained by underreporting. Eight of 48 countries, including Africa's most populous, Nigeria, did not respond. Furthermore, within countries, there is bias in favor of data from national blood transfusion services, which may not give a true picture of the situation outside these organizations. In the 38 African countries for which data were provided, 2.2 million units of blood were reported to have been donated in 2004 for an estimated population of 431 million (72% of the total population of the region). This represents an average of 5.1 units donated per 1000 population per year. Of the 2.2 million units donated, 850,000 (39%) were donated in South Africa, which has a highly sophisticated blood transfusion service and an estimated population of 39 million (9% of the total). If South Africa is removed from the analysis, an average of 3.4 units of blood are donated per 1000 population for the rest of sub-Saharan Africa.

WHO estimates the blood requirement for countries in the region may be 10 to 20 units per 1000 population per year [4]. In resource-limited areas of Africa, demand is high predominantly because of

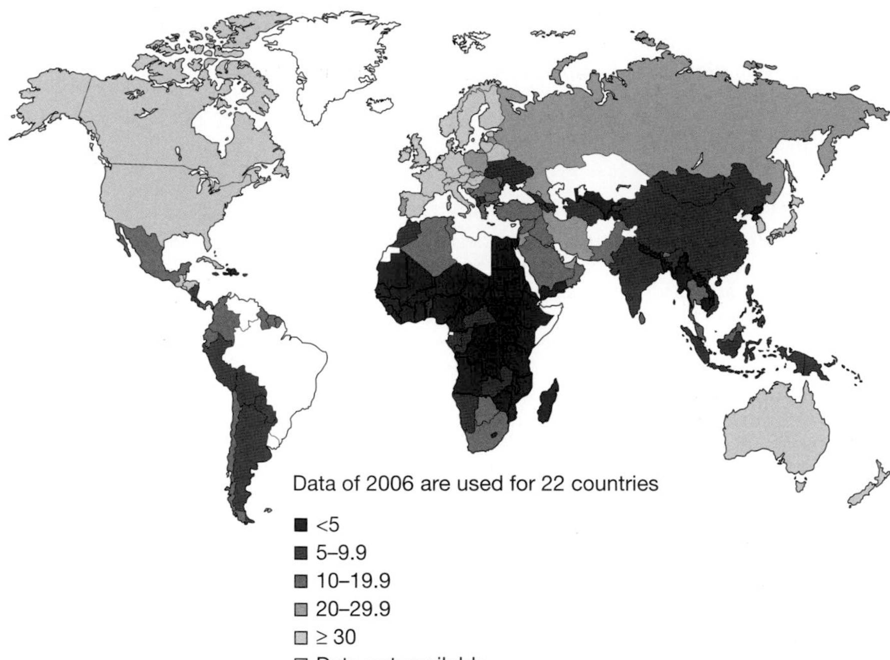

FIGURE 20.1 Global estimates for blood donations per 1000 population (2007).

severe anemia, infectious diseases, and bleeding in pregnancy. Based on the limited supply of data and using the lowest WHO estimate of demand (10 donations per 1000 population), the shortfall in blood donations for those countries responding to the survey and excluding South Africa is about 2.6 million units.

Although the magnitude of the shortage of blood for transfusion in sub-Saharan Africa is not certain, the patient groups who suffer the greatest impact are easier to identify. Young children have a high demand for blood, with the prevalence of severe anemia (defined as hemoglobin <5 g/dL) in hospitalized children ranging from 8% to 29% [5]. In malaria-endemic areas, *Plasmodium falciparum* malaria as well as other infections and nutritional deficiencies have also been associated with severe anemia in children [6–8]. In some hospitals, 50% of all children admitted are transfused, and children may account for up to 70% of all transfusions prescribed in malaria-endemic Africa [9–11].

Women of reproductive age are also major users of blood transfusions in resource-limited countries. Of the 20 countries worldwide with the highest maternal death rates, 19 are in sub-Saharan Africa, where the risk of maternal death is 1 in 16, compared with 1 in 2800 in industrialized countries. The most common cause of maternal death is severe bleeding, contributing to over 40% of maternal deaths, and it has been estimated that a quarter of these women die because of blood shortages [12].

BLOOD SAFETY

Infectious Risk of Blood Transfusions

Blood is a biologic tissue and when transferred from one individual to another it can transmit infection with potentially devastating consequences for the recipient. Viruses (e.g. HIV, hepatitis), bacteria (e.g. *Treponema pallidum*), parasites (e.g. malaria, trypanosomes) and prions (e.g. vCJD) may all be transmitted by blood transfusion. Reducing the risk of such an event is an important responsibility of providers of blood for transfusion.

The transfusion-transmissible infections (TTI) for which all blood for transfusion should be screened are HIV, hepatitis B, hepatitis C, and syphilis [13]. For any TTI, the risk of an infectious unit entering the donor pool is related to the prevalence and incidence of the infection within the donor population. The higher the prevalence, the more often a laboratory screening test will incorrectly identify an infected donation as uninfected, either because of imperfect test sensitivity or human error. The higher the incidence of new infection in the donor population, the greater the likelihood that blood will be donated during the window period before a serologic screening test is capable of detecting the infection.

Reducing the risk of TTI, therefore, has three main components: the identification of population groups with a low prevalence and incidence of TTI from which to recruit blood donors; health screening of potential donors to allow exclusion/self-exclusion of those with risk factors for TTI; and the screening of all blood donations for TTIs with sensitive and quality-assured tests in good laboratories.

HIV is readily transmitted by whole blood transfusion with a seroconversion rate of 96% [14] and, historically, blood transfusion was thought to account for 10% of all new HIV infections in sub-Saharan Africa [15]. In the mid-1990s, the risk of HIV infection from a blood transfusion in Kenya was 2% [16]. In a recent analysis, Jayaraman and colleagues constructed a mathematical model to quantify the transfusion risks of three viruses (HIV, hepatitis B and hepatitis C) in 45 sub-Saharan African countries [17]. Although the authors recognized methodologic bias in the epidemiologic sample base, they estimated that if projected annual transfusion requirements were met, transfusions alone would be responsible for 28,595 HBV infections, 16,625 HCV infections and 6650 HIV infections every year [17].

Another infectious risk of blood transfusion, for which laboratory screening is not routinely performed, is bacterial contamination. In wealthy countries, the risk of bacterial contamination of red cell products is low. In the Netherlands, a study of whole blood units cultured within 24 hours of donation reported a contamination rate of 0.34% [18], and the frequency of bacterial contamination of red blood cell concentrates is thought to be approximately 1 in 30,000 [19]. Clinically significant episodes resulting from bacterial contamination of blood products in wealthy countries are even rarer, with reported rates of 5.8 per million units (France) and 0.21 per million units (USA) [20,21].

Recent data from sub-Saharan Africa suggest that the risk of bacterial contamination in whole blood units may be much higher than in wealthy countries. Bacterial contamination, with predominantly environmental organisms, was found in 9% of pediatric transfusions issued in a Kenyan hospital [22]. Pediatric transfusions are particularly vulnerable to contamination in resource-limited countries, since, in the absence of pediatric transfusion packs, small volumes have to be drawn from adult (500 mL) packs. A recent study from northern Ghana on whole blood packs identified a contamination rate of 17.5%; the majority of contaminants in this case were thought to originate from the skin of the donor [23]. Another recent study from southern Ghana demonstrated a 13% bacterial contamination rate of whole blood [24].

Other Risks of Transfusion

Systems for the routine detection of adverse consequences of blood transfusions (hemovigilance) only exist where transfusion safety has been identified as a health priority by the government [25]. In low-income countries, the frequency of noninfectious adverse events related to blood transfusion is largely unknown as hemovigilance activities are very limited. The transfusion of the incorrect unit with the possibility of ABO incompatibility and a life-threatening hemolytic transfusion reaction remains the most common hazard of transfusion in the developed world [26,27]. Clerical and other human errors are frequently to blame, even in health systems that are sophisticated and well resourced.

In low-income countries, most blood is transfused as whole blood. Febrile nonhemolytic transfusion reactions (FNHTR) are therefore likely to be common because they are caused by biologically active substances associated with donor leukocytes, such as cytokines, complement fragments, antibodies and adhesion molecules [26,27]. Detection of these reactions in low-income countries is difficult because many transfusion recipients may already be febrile as a result of their underlying condition. In the only published study of its type, 40% of transfusions (26,973 units) in Yaounde, Cameroon were associated with fever [28]. In most resource-rich countries, leukocyte reduction of transfusion products has decreased the risk of immunogenicity and cytokine release, and significantly reduced the number of FNHTR [29,30], post-transfusion purpura, and transfusion-associated graft-versus-host disease [31].

The transfusion of whole blood may have other adverse consequences, such as activation of adhesion molecules that are thought to be important in the generation of transfusion-related acute lung injury resulting in noncardiogenic pulmonary edema [27,32]. Transfusion-associated immunomodulation is associated with accelerated disease progression and mortality in patients with HIV infection, due to transfusion-related immunosuppression [33].

Blood Donor Selection

One of the key goals of the WHO strategy is to ensure all donors are voluntary and non-remunerated, but many of the world's poorest countries are still struggling to achieve this goal (Fig. 20.2). For example, in 15 countries in Africa, accounting for 45% of the regions' population, only 25–50% of blood was collected from voluntary donors. Overall, 1.2 million units, nearly half of the 2.8 million units of blood collected in sub-Saharan Africa, were from family or paid donors [4]. Recent data indicate that the difference in HIV prevalence between voluntary and replacement donors may be related to their different age structures rather than whether they are voluntary or replacement donors [34]. Furthermore, the voluntary donors may have higher incidence rates of HIV infection because of their younger age profile [35]. In fact, the safest type of donor is one who is unpaid and donates regularly, irrespective of whether they were originally a voluntary or replacement donor.

PROGRESS IN IMPROVING BLOOD SUPPLY AND SAFETY IN SUB-SAHARAN AFRICA

Over the past decade, several countries in sub-Saharan Africa have made progress in achieving the goals defined by the WHO to improve blood safety, financed largely by international donors. For example, the US President's Emergency Plan For AIDS Relief (PEPFAR) provides direct support to 14 countries to strengthen blood transfusion services. Between 2003 and 2007, this resulted in an increase in the number of total blood donations and the proportion from voluntary donors, and a decrease in the percentage of donations reactive for HIV [36]. These improvements have been achieved by establishing regional centers, which make up a national blood transfusion service, to replace hospital-based systems. Although the increase in voluntary donors has reduced the number of replacement blood donors, many of the voluntary donors are secondary school students, so there is a risk of blood shortages during the school holidays, which may also coincide with periods of peak demand.

National blood transfusion services are more expensive than hospital-based facilities because they need to establish efficient donor recruitment and selection programs, maintain distribution and communication networks, and support quality-assured laboratory services. Most of the donors attending hospital-based facilities are recruited by families of patients (i.e. replacement donors), so the

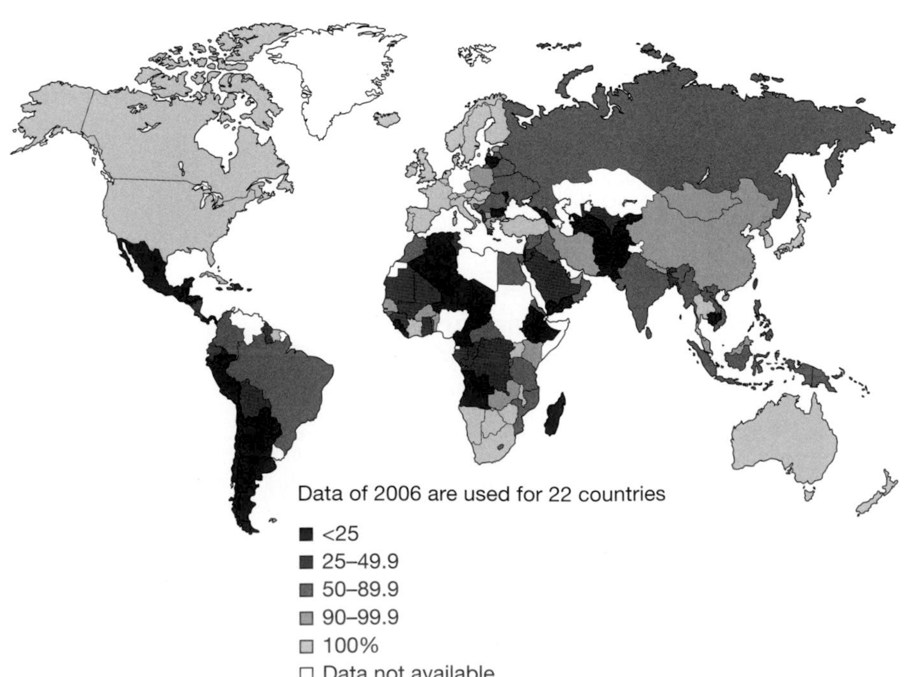

FIGURE 20.2 Global estimates for percentage of voluntary unpaid blood donations (2007).

hospitals do not bear the cost of donor recruitment [37]. There are, therefore, concerns about the sustainability of systems requiring a high level of financial support in low-income countries where cost recovery is unlikely.

CLINICAL USE OF BLOOD TRANSFUSION

WHO NEEDS BLOOD?

In wealthy countries, the use of blood is strictly monitored through specialist transfusion practitioners, hospital transfusion committees, and national reporting systems. In resource-limited countries, appropriate use of blood and blood products and monitoring of transfusions are poorly taught and rarely monitored. Evidence underpinning guidelines for the clinical use of blood in low-income countries is often weak or inappropriate for settings with few resources. The pattern of usage of blood in low-income countries, with most transfusions given predominantly as an emergency treatment to children and pregnant women, is very different from that in more wealthy countries (see Fig. 20.3A,B). The high percentage of blood used for pediatric transfusions (19–67%) and pregnancy-related complications in women (15–40%) contrasts markedly with equivalent figures of 1% and 4% from a district hospital in the UK. The majority of pediatric transfusions are for young children; in the studies for which data are available, children under the age of 5 years receive 43% to 62% of all blood transfusions.

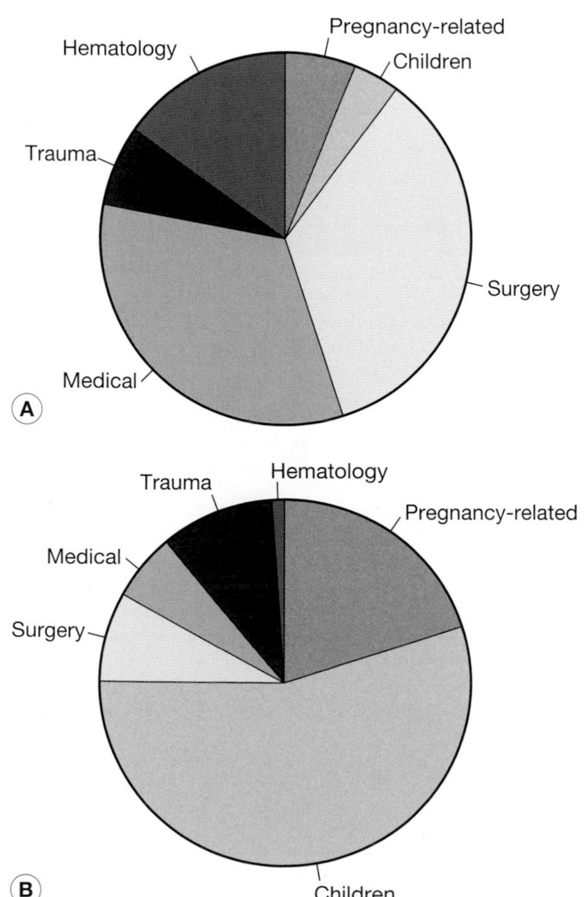

FIGURE 20.3 Estimates for the proportionate use of blood in the United Kingdom **(A)** and resource-limited countries in Africa **(B)**.

TRANSFUSION GUIDELINES

The decision whether or not to prescribe a blood transfusion should be based on an assessment of the clinical condition of the patient, taking into account their hemoglobin level. Trials based in wealthy countries have found that 30-day mortality was the same in two groups of critically ill patients irrespective of whether hemoglobin levels of 7 g/dL or 9 g/dL were used to trigger the transfusion [38]. In less acutely ill or younger patients, 30-day mortality was lower in the group with the trigger of 7g/dL [38]. One of the largest pediatric trials ever conducted also concluded that a hemoglobin transfusion threshold of 7 g/dL decreased transfusion requirements without increasing adverse outcomes [39]. Similar trials are needed in Africa, where, due to a shortage of blood, transfusion triggers tend to be much lower (4 g/dL or under 5 g/dL in symptomatic patients) [40].

Pediatric guidelines in low-income countries where malaria is prevalent often indicate that profound anemia (hemoglobin < 4 g/dL) should be treated with a transfusion [40]. Most transfusions received are whole blood and not packed red cells. This is supported by evidence suggesting that children with hemoglobin concentration less than 3.9 g/dL who were transfused had a lower mortality than those with similar hemoglobin concentrations who were not transfused [7]. Transfusions may be needed at higher hemoglobin levels if dehydration, shock, impaired consciousness, heart failure, or labored breathing are present.

MISUSE OF BLOOD TRANSFUSIONS

Even in wealthy countries with good supplies of blood, there can be significant overuse of blood transfusions [37]. In resource-limited countries, there is also often poor adherence to transfusion guidelines, and despite the lack of blood, 50–75% of blood transfusions may be given inappropriately [41,42]. This has led some to observe that "no other pharmaceutical preparation of comparable cost and toxicity is prescribed with [such] a cavalier attitude towards risk" [43]. Other studies have shown that over a third of transfused children did not have their hemoglobin measured prior to transfusion, and of those in whom the pre-transfusion hemoglobin was checked, 18% had levels above the recommended transfusion trigger of 6 g/dL without any additional indications for transfusion [42].

The decision to transfuse in resource-limited settings is often based on a clinical diagnosis of anemia using signs of severe pallor of the palms and/or the conjunctiva [44]. However, clinical assessment of pallor may over-diagnose anemia [41,42] or miss a large proportion of patients with severe anemia [45]. Clinical assessment of anemia is therefore not precise enough to inform the decision to prescribe a scarce and potentially dangerous therapy such as a blood transfusion. An accurate hemoglobin measurement is essential to avoid putting transfusion recipients at unnecessary risk, and to prevent inappropriate use and wastage of blood.

Manual measurement of hemoglobin requiring dilution techniques, as performed in laboratories in many resource-limited countries, is often inaccurate. Reasons include poorly maintained equipment, lack of supplies and quality standards, and inadequate training and supervision [46,47]. A photometric method (HemoCue® AB–Hb Photometer, Quest Diagnostics Ltd) does provide a direct hemoglobin reading on a small volume of blood, but uses disposable cuvettes which may be too expensive for resource-constrained laboratories with heavy workloads [48]. The packed cell volume is often used as a substitute for hemoglobin in pediatric practice [49], but this too does not give an accurate estimation of anemia [50,51]. The Hemoglobin Colour Scale (HCS) [52] is a simple, rapid and cheap method for assessing anemia, but its usefulness for guiding decisions about blood transfusions has not been evaluated in appropriate field trials in low-income countries [53].

OUTCOMES OF BLOOD TRANSFUSIONS

In-hospital case-fatality rates following blood transfusions in low-income African countries range from 6% to 20% [7,54–56]. In children, prostration, respiratory distress and profound anemia (hemoglobin <4 g/dL) are all associated with an increased risk of death. Around a third of these deaths occur within 6 hours of admission to hospital, so appropriate emergency management is crucial [9]. Recent studies have indicated that the respiratory distress and cardiovascular changes associated with acute severe anemia in children are due to hypovolemia rather than heart failure [57–59], and studies are underway to determine the optimal emergency management procedures for these children. In some children in malaria-endemic regions, anemia may fail to resolve or severe anemia may recur within a few weeks after discharge from hospital, possibly due to persistence of low-level malaria parasitemia [60,61].

ALTERNATIVES TO TRANSFUSION

Blood transfusions are a costly and risky therapy, especially in low-income countries, and should not be used if there are alternative therapies. Studies in healthy adult volunteers did not show evidence of poor oxygen delivery during isovolemic reduction of hemoglobin concentrations to 5 g/dL [62]. Healthy young adults are able to tolerate hemorrhage of up to 40% of their blood volume and can therefore be managed with crystalloid without the need for red cell transfusion. A study in the Gambia showed better recovery in children with hemoglobin levels of 4–5 g/dL who received iron treatment than in those who received a blood transfusion [54], and in Kenyan children, blood transfusion did not influence faster hemoglobin recovery at 1-month follow-up [60]. In obstetric bleeding, misoprostol (oxytocin) can stop hemorrhage and may be more cost-effective than blood products [63]. Transfusion should not be used as a source of blood volume [64], or to treat shock unless hypovolemia is associated with active hemorrhage. In such cases, volume expanders such as crystalloid solutions are cheaper and safer than blood. In children with severe malarial anemia with acidosis and shock, restoration of the circulating volume with saline or colloid while waiting for a blood transfusion did not cause pulmonary edema or a critical reduction in hemoglobin [65].

REDUCING TRANSFUSIONS BY PREVENTING ANEMIA

Anemia is a risk factor for poor outcome in pregnancy. Estimates for all-cause anemia-attributable direct and indirect mortality have been calculated as 6.4%, 7.3% and 3.0% for Africa, Asia and Latin America, respectively [66]. The prevalence of anemia in pregnant women and children in low-income countries commonly exceeds 50%, and the risk of needing a blood transfusion as a result of severe anemia or hemorrhage would be significantly reduced if early detection and management of anemia were improved. Therefore the best way to reduce the number of blood transfusions in low-income countries is to reduce the prevalence of anemia in the populations most at risk, such as children and pregnant women, through early detection and better management. Standard anemia treatment guidelines in low-income malarious areas focus on malaria, folate deficiency, and iron deficiency, but there is evidence that other factors such as bacteremia (especially nontyphoidal *Salmonella*), hookworm, HIV infection, vitamin A deficiency, and vitamin B12 deficiency may also be important [8].

REFERENCES

1. World Health Organization (WHO). Utilization and supply of human blood and blood products in Twenty-eighth World Health Assembly. Geneva: WHO; 1975.
2. WHO Department of Blood Safety. Aide-Memoire for National Blood Programmes: Blood Safety. Geneva: WHO; 2002:1–2.
3. World Health Organization (WHO). Global Database on Blood Safety: Report 2004–5. Geneva: WHO; 2008.
4. Tapko JB, Sam O, Diarra-Nama AJ. Status of blood safety in the WHO African Region: report of the 2004 survey. Brazzaville: WHO Regional Office for Africa; 2007:1–25.
5. World Health Organization (WHO). The prevention and management of severe anaemia in children in malaria-endemic regions of Africa: a review of research. Geneva: WHO; 2001.
6. Newton CR, Marsh K, Peshu N, Mwangi I. Blood transfusions for severe anaemia in African children. Lancet 1992;340:917–18.
7. Lackritz EM, Campbell CC, Ruebush TK 2nd, et al. Effect of blood transfusion on survival among children in a Kenyan hospital. Lancet 1992;340:524–8.
8. Calis JC, Phiri KS, Faragher EB, et al. Severe anemia in Malawian children. N Engl J Med 2008;358:888–99.
9. English M, Ahmed M, Ngando C, et al. Blood transfusion for severe anaemia in children in a Kenyan hospital. Lancet 2002;359:494–5.
10. Greenberg AE, Nguyen-Dinh P, Mann JM, et al. The association between malaria, blood transfusions, and HIV seropositivity in a pediatric population in Kinshasa, Zaire. JAMA 1988;259:545–9.
11. Jager H, N'Galy B, Perriens J, et al. Prevention of transfusion-associated HIV transmission in Kinshasa, Zaire: HIV screening is not enough. AIDS 1990;4: 571–4.
12. Bates I, Chapotera GK, McKew S, van den Broek N. Maternal mortality in sub-Saharan Africa: the contribution of ineffective blood transfusion services. BJOG 2008;115:1331–9.
13. World Health Organization (WHO). Screening Donated Blood for Transfusion-Transmissible Infections: Recommendations. Geneva: WHO; 2010:1–73.
14. Colebunders R, Ryder R, Francis H, et al. Seroconversion rate, mortality, and clinical manifestations associated with the receipt of a human immunodeficiency virus-infected blood transfusion in Kinshasa, Zaire. J Infect Dis 1991;164:450–6.
15. McFarland W, Mvere D, Katzenstein D. Risk factors for prevalent and incident HIV infection in a cohort of volunteer blood donors in Harare, Zimbabwe: implications for blood safety. AIDS 1997;11(Suppl 1):S97–102.
16. Moore A, Herrera G, Nyamongo J, et al. Estimated risk of HIV transmission by blood transfusion in Kenya. Lancet 2001;358:657–60.
17. Jayaraman S, Chalabi Z, Perel P, et al. The risk of transfusion-transmitted infections in sub-Saharan Africa. Transfusion 2010;50:433–42.
18. de Korte D, Marcelis JH, Soeterboek AM. Determination of the degree of bacterial contamination of whole-blood collections using an automated microbe-detection system. Transfusion 2001;41:815–18.
19. Hillyer CD, Josephson CD, Blajchman MA, et al. Bacterial contamination of blood components: risks, strategies, and regulation: joint ASH and AABB educational session in transfusion medicine. Hematology Am Soc Hematol Educ Program 2003:575–89.
20. Perez P, Salmi LR, Follea G, et al. Determinants of transfusion-associated bacterial contamination: results of the French BACTHEM case-control study. Transfusion 2001;41: 862–72.
21. Kuehnert MJ, Roth VR, Haley NR, et al. Transfusion-transmitted bacterial infection in the United States, 1998 through 2000. Transfusion 2001;41: 1493–9.
22. Hassall O, Maitland K, Pole L, et al. Bacterial contamination of pediatric whole blood transfusions in a Kenyan hospital. Transfusion 2009;49:2594–8.
23. Opoku-Okrah C. Bacterial contamination of donor blood at the Tamale Teaching Hospital, Ghana. Afr Health Sci 2009;9:13–18.
24. Adjei AA, Kuma GK, Tettey Y, et al. Bacterial contamination of blood and blood components in three major blood transfusion centers, Accra, Ghana. Jpn J Infect Dis 2009;62:265–9.
25. Faber JC. Worldwide overview of existing haemovigilance systems. Transfus Apher Sci 2004;31:99–110.
26. Williamson LM, Lowe S, Love EM, et al. Serious hazards of transfusion (SHOT) initiative: analysis of the first two annual reports. BMJ 1999;319: 16–19.
27. Snyder EL. The role of cytokines and adhesive molecules in febrile non-hemolytic transfusion reactions. Immunol Invest 1995;24:333–9.
28. Mbanya D, Binam F, Kaptue L. Transfusion outcome in a resource-limited setting of Cameroon: a five-year evaluation. Int J Infect Dis 2001;5:70–3.
29. Shanwell A, Kristiansson M, Remberger M, Ringden O. Generation of cytokines in red cell concentrates during storage is prevented by prestorage white cell reduction. Transfusion 1997;37:678–84.
30. Karam O, Tucci M, Toledano BJ, et al. Length of storage and in vitro immunomodulation induced by prestorage leukoreduced red blood cells. Transfusion 2009;49:2326–34.
31. Williamson LM, Stainsby D, Jones H, et al. The impact of universal leukodepletion of the blood supply on hemovigilance reports of posttransfusion purpura and transfusion-associated graft-versus-host disease. Transfusion 2007;47:1455–67.
32. Nishimura M, Hashimoto S, Takanashi M, et al. Role of anti-human leucocyte antigen class II alloantibody and monocytes in development of transfusion-related acute lung injury. Transfus Med 2007;17:129–34.
33. Sullivan P. Associations of anemia, treatments for anemia, and survival in patients with human immunodeficiency virus infection. J Infect Dis 2002;185 (Suppl 2):S138–42.

34. Allain JP, Sarkodie F, Asenso-Mensah K, Owusu-Ofori S. Relative safety of first-time volunteer and replacement donors in West Africa. Transfusion 2010;50:340–3.
35. Mumo J, Vansover A, Jehuda-Cohen T. Detecting seronegative-early HIV infections among adult versus student Kenyan blood donors, by using Stimmunology. Exp Biol Med (Maywood) 2009;234:931–9.
36. CDC. Progress toward strengthening blood transfusion services – 14 countries, 2003–2007. MMWR Morb Mortal Wkly Rep 2008;57:1273–7.
37. So-Osman C, Cicilia J, Brand A, et al. Triggers and appropriateness of red blood cell transfusions in the postpartum patient – a retrospective audit. Vox Sang 2010;98:65–9.
38. Hebert PC, Wells G, Blajchman MA, et al. A multicenter, randomized, controlled clinical trial of transfusion requirements in critical care. Transfusion Requirements in Critical Care Investigators, Canadian Critical Care Trials Group. N Engl J Med 1999;340:409–17.
39. Lacroix J, Hebert PC, Hutchison JS, et al. Transfusion strategies for patients in pediatric intensive care units. N Engl J Med 2007;356:1609–19.
40. Health Organization (WHO). Management of the Child with a Serious Infection or Severe Malnutrition: Guidelines for Care at the First-Referral Level in Developing Countries. Geneva: WHO; 2000.
41. Lackritz EM, Ruebush TK 2nd, Zucker JR, et al. Blood transfusion practices and blood-banking services in a Kenyan hospital. AIDS 1993;7:995–9.
42. Mosha D, Poulsen A, Reyburn H, et al. Quality of paediatric blood transfusions in two district hospitals in Tanzania: a cross-sectional hospital based study. BMC Pediatr 2009;9:51.
43. Fleming AF. HIV and blood transfusion in sub-Saharan Africa. Transfus Sci 1997;18:167–79.
44. World Health Organization (WHO). Hospital Care for Children: Guidelines for the Management of Common Illnesses with Limited Resources. Geneva: WHO; 2005.
45. Muhe L, Oljira B, Degefu H, et al. Evaluation of clinical pallor in the identification and treatment of children with moderate and severe anaemia. Trop Med Int Health 2000;5:805–10.
46. Critchley J, Bates I. Haemoglobin colour scale for anaemia diagnosis where there is no laboratory: a systematic review. Int J Epidemiol 2005;34: 1425–34.
47. Lara AM, Kandulu J, Chisuwo L, et al. Laboratory costs of a hospital-based blood transfusion service in Malawi. J Clin Pathol 2007;60:1117–20.
48. Neufeld L, Garcia-Guerra A, Sanchez-Francia D, et al. Hemoglobin measured by Hemocue and a reference method in venous and capillary blood: a validation study. Salud Publica Mex 2002;44:219–27.
49. Lee SJ, Stepniewska K, Anstey N, et al. The relationship between the haemoglobin concentration and the haematocrit in *Plasmodium falciparum* malaria. Malar J 2008;7:149.
50. Quinto L, Aponte JJ, Menendez C, et al. Relationship between haemoglobin and haematocrit in the definition of anaemia. Trop Med Int Health 2006;11:1295–302.
51. Carneiro IA, Drakeley CJ, Owusu-Agyei S, et al. Haemoglobin and haematocrit: is the threefold conversion valid for assessing anaemia in malaria-endemic settings? Malar J 2007;6:67.
52. Stott GJ, Lewis SM. A simple and reliable method for estimating haemoglobin. Bull World Health Organ 1995;73:369–73.
53. Paddle JJ. How objective are the supporters of the Haemoglobin Colour Scale? Bull World Health Organ 2002;80:987.
54. Bojang KA, Palmer A, Boele van Hensbroek M, et al. Management of severe malarial anaemia in Gambian children. Trans R Soc Trop Med Hyg 1997; 91:557–61.
55. Commey JO, Dekyem P. Childhood deaths from anaemia in Accra, Ghana. West Afr J Med 1995;14:101–4.
56. English M. Life-threatening severe malarial anaemia. Trans R Soc Trop Med Hyg 2000;94:585–8.
57. English M, Waruiru C, Marsh K. Transfusion for respiratory distress in life-threatening childhood malaria. Am J Trop Med Hyg 1996;55:525–30.
58. Maitland K, Pamba A, Newton CR, Levin M. Response to volume resuscitation in children with severe malaria. Pediatr Crit Care Med 2003;4:426–31.
59. English M, Muambi B, Mithwani S, Marsh K. Lactic acidosis and oxygen debt in African children with severe anaemia. QJM 1997;90:563–9.
60. Akech SO, Hassall O, Pamba A, et al. Survival and haematological recovery of children with severe malaria transfused in accordance to WHO guidelines in Kilifi, Kenya. Malar J 2008;7:256.
61. Lackritz EM, Hightower AW, Zucker JR, et al. Longitudinal evaluation of severely anemic children in Kenya: the effect of transfusion on mortality and hematologic recovery. AIDS 1997;11:1487–94.
62. Weiskopf RB, Viele MK, Feiner J, et al. Human cardiovascular and metabolic response to acute, severe isovolemic anemia. JAMA 1998;279:217–21.
63. Leduc D, Senikas V, Lalonde AB, et al. Active management of the third stage of labour: prevention and treatment of postpartum hemorrhage. J Obstet Gynaecol Can 2009;31:980–93.
64. World Health Organization (WHO). The Clinical Use of Blood Handbook. Geneva: WHO; 2002:1–221.
65. Maitland K, Pamba A, English M, et al. Pre-transfusion management of children with severe malarial anaemia: a randomised controlled trial of intravascular volume expansion. Br J Haematol 2005;128:393–400.
66. Brabin BJ, Premji Z, Verhoeff F. An analysis of anemia and child mortality. J Nutr 2001;131(2S-2):636S–645S; discussion 646S–8S.

21 Infection Control in the Tropics

Haider J Warraich, Syed Faisal Mahmood, Anita KM Zaidi

Key features

- Patients in developing countries suffer high rates of healthcare-associated infections
- Unique challenges of infection control in the tropics include:
    - Lack of resources and trained personnel
    - Low accessibility to clean water
    - Inappropriate use of invasive devices
    - Easy availability of over-the-counter antibiotics
    - Overcrowding and understaffing
    - Poor vector control
- Standard Infection Control Precautions (hand hygiene, patient isolation, aseptic technique, use of personal protective barriers, appropriate sterilization and disinfection of reused equipment, and safe injection practices) form the cornerstone of infection control in hospitals
- Adequate attention to hand hygiene compliance is the most important component of basic infection control
- Effective, low-cost, practical solutions addressing behavior modification to improve adherence to infection control practices, coupled with surveillance, and provision of essential resources can decrease the rate of healthcare-associated infections in developing countries
- Establishment of an effective infection control program in a health facility requires an infection control committee and strong institutional commitment to the program

Infection control policies and procedures are designed to prevent acquisition of healthcare-associated infections (HAIs) among patients as well as healthcare workers and visitors. The complexities of infection control in hospital environments have challenged medical systems throughout the world, and are constantly evolving with advances in medical technology and care of increasingly vulnerable patients. In this chapter, we have considered the tropics to be synonymous with developing countries, since most developing countries are located in tropical regions of the world. The term nosocomial infection has traditionally been used to refer to hospital-acquired infections among patients presenting 72 hours after hospitalization. We prefer the term healthcare-associated infections (HAIs) because many infections associated with the delivery of healthcare occur in outpatient settings and hospital-acquired infections may present sooner than 72 hours after admission. This chapter includes a review of the burden of HAIs in developing countries, selected problems unique to the tropics that have a great impact on the people and the health system, and a discussion of basic infection control measures.

BURDEN OF HEALTHCARE-ASSOCIATED INFECTIONS IN DEVELOPING COUNTRIES

HAIs are a serious problem in industrialized countries, with 1.7 million cases, and an estimated 100,000 deaths, per annum reported in the US alone [1]. However, with scant attention to infection control and poor quality of hospital care in most developing countries, HAIs are now recognized as a huge health burden in developing countries, too, responsible for both increased morbidity and mortality, and waste of precious resources. In addition, HAIs subvert patient expectations of quality medical care and increase negativity towards the formal health system in favor of other options, especially since the costs of HAIs are borne by the patients themselves in many developing countries. The World Health Organization (WHO) estimates that 1.4 million people suffer from HAIs worldwide. Furthermore, the risk of acquiring HAIs in developing countries is 2 to 20 times higher than in developed countries. Reducing the risk of HAIs faced by populations in developing countries is a major priority of the WHO [2].

RISK FACTORS FOR HEALTHCARE-ASSOCIATED INFECTIONS IN DEVELOPING COUNTRIES

Risk factors universally associated with an increased risk of HAIs are severity of underlying disease, length of hospital stay, inter-hospital transfers, use of invasive medical devices (intravascular devices, urinary catheters, intubation and mechanical ventilation), surgery, and prolonged and/or broad-spectrum antimicrobial therapy. An interplay of multiple complex factors lies at the heart of HAIs in developing countries (Table 21-1). These include lack of robust surveillance systems to control infections and outbreaks, indiscriminate antibiotic use, nonadherence to basic infection control practices such as hand washing, inadequate sterilization of medical equipment, reuse of single-use devices, and presence of reservoirs of infection such as contaminated food and water inside the hospital. Some of these are easier to address – for example, by staff training, adequate sterilization of equipment, and improving compliance with hand hygiene – than are others, such as overcrowding and understaffing.

MODES OF TRANSMISSION

In healthcare settings, most infections are transmitted through direct or indirect contact. In developing countries, lack of hand hygiene results in transmission of infectious agents from one infected patient to another. Table 21-2 provides a summary of different modes of transmission of infectious organisms, all of which necessitate specific transmission-based precautions.

SPECIAL PROBLEMS OF THE TROPICS

ANTIMICROBIAL RESISTANCE

Antimicrobial resistance is a major challenge [3]. HAIs in developing countries are dominated by Gram-negative organisms [4]. The proportion of resistant organisms, such as methicillin-resistant *Staphylococcus aureus*, extended-spectrum β-lactamase-producing *Enterobacteriaceae*, multidrug-resistant *Pseudomonas aeruginosa* and

TABLE 21-1 Factors Underlying Healthcare-Associated Infections in Developing Countries

Programmatic factors	Lack of resources (financial, programmatic, institutional) Low priority of infection control Lack of integration of infection control practices in routine medical care Over-the-counter availability and indiscriminate use of antibiotics Lack of infection surveillance systems Lack of microbiological laboratory facilities for reliable identification of infecting pathogens and antimicrobial susceptibility
Healthcare staff factors	Lack of infection control training Poor compliance with standard infection control practices, especially hand washing Carriage of organisms (hands, clothing, linen) Understaffing Inadequate sterilization and disinfection of equipment Use of devices (ventilators, central lines, urinary catheters) without aseptic precautions
Facility-related factors	Inadequate vector control (pests, rodents, arthropods) Overcrowding Lack of ventilation, climate control and effective isolation areas Lack of sinks and running water, soap, alcohol rubs, gloves, and other supplies Reservoirs of community infections in hospitals Re-use of single-use invasive devices (syringes, catheters, tubings) because of supply shortages Inadequate facilities for sterilization and disinfection
Host factors	Severity of underlying disease Length of hospital stay High burden of infectious diseases in the patient population
Pathogen factors	High prevalence of multidrug-resistant organisms

Acinetobacter spp., is also substantially higher in developing countries. Factors that predispose to infections with resistant organisms are poor hospital hygiene, high, and often irrational broad-spectrum antimicrobial use, overcrowding, lack of resources for infection control, unavailability of reliable microbiologic culture and antimicrobial susceptibility results, and a lack of personnel trained in controlling infections.

Control of antibiotic resistance requires strict adherence to infection control measures and restricted use of antibiotics. Hospitals can rationalize antibiotic use through antibiotic stewardship programs. However, antibiotic policies only have limited impact in countries where antimicrobials such as third-generation cephalosporin and fluoroquinolones are freely available over-the-counter and are widely and inappropriately used [5]. Misuse of antibiotics (inappropriate prescription, suboptimal dosing and duration) as well as low-potency formulations are widespread and a major factor associated with the emergence of resistant organisms. Although antibiotic stewardship programs can reduce and rationalize use of antibiotics, such programs are seldom implemented in developing countries. A review of antimicrobial use has shown that countries that adhere to WHO's essential drug policies provide greater access to essential drugs for vulnerable populations with less indiscriminate prescription of antimicrobials and injections [6].

TABLE 21-2 Modes of Transmission in Health Care Settings

Mode	Features
Contact transmission	Most common route. Divided into two sub-groups:
Direct contact	Organisms are transferred from one infected person to another without a contaminated intermediate, e.g. body fluid of patient directly enters healthcare worker's body through mucous membrane or cut in skin
Indirect contact	Transfer of organism through a contaminated intermediate object or person. Important intermediates include hands of healthcare workers, patient care devices and instruments, and clothing
Droplet transmission	Respiratory droplets (>5 μm) carry organisms directly from the respiratory tract of the patient, over short distances (usually ≤3 feet), necessitating facial protection such as with masks: e.g. *Bordetella pertussis, Mycoplasma pneumoniae*, respiratory syncytial virus and influenza virus
Airborne transmission	Transmission of droplet nuclei (≤5 μm) or small particles containing infectious agents that remain infective over time and distance, e.g., *Mycobacterium tuberculosis*, measles virus, varicella-zoster virus. These necessitate use of special air handling and ventilation systems

Access to reliable microbiologic data with information on etiology and antimicrobial susceptibility patterns of pathogens is also essential. Microbiology facilities are usually inadequate in resource-poor settings, contributing to high rates of empiric antimicrobial use, impeding surveillance, epidemiologic study of resistance patterns, and infection control.

DEVICE-ASSOCIATED INFECTIONS

Device-associated infections (DAIs) include central-line-associated bloodstream infections, catheter-associated urinary tract infections, and ventilator-associated pneumonia. The use of invasive devices in hospitals in developing countries has rapidly increased without equal attention given to instituting infection control, resulting in rates of device-associated infections that are much higher than in industrialized countries. Surveillance by the International Nosocomial Infection Control Consortium (INICC) in 98 ICUs in resource-poor settings in Latin America, Asia, Africa and Europe, using Centers for Disease Control and Prevention (CDC) definitions for HAIs, showed that among 43,114 patients over an aggregate of 272,279 days from 2002 through 2007, the pooled mean rates of DAIs were much higher compared to industrialized countries [7]. Catheter-associated bloodstream infection rates were 8.9 per 1000 central line (CL)-days compared to 2.4 per 1000 CL-days in comparable medical-surgical ICUs in the US, ventilator-associated pneumonia was 19.8 versus 3.6

per 1000 ventilator-days, and catheter-associated urinary tract infections rates were 6.6 versus 3.4 per 1000 catheter-days. Implementation of guidelines designed by the consortium for decreasing rates of infections from ventilators, catheters and central lines by using positive feedback programs for hand hygiene and central line, ventilator and urinary catheter care [8].

SURGICAL SITE INFECTIONS

Surgical procedures are associated with higher postoperative wound infection rates in developing countries due to inadequate attention to aseptic precautions. While most data are anecdotal, surgical wound infections are reported to be as high as 12.5% in Vietnam and 19.6% in Kenya. A surgical checklist developed by WHO has reduced surgical mortality and morbidity by encouraging use of simple measures by surgery, anesthesia and nursing staff. Ensuring delivery of antibiotic prophylaxis in the operating room using verbal confirmation alone improved antibiotic prophylaxis compliance from 56% to 83%. Chlorhexidine-alcohol is the antiseptic of choice for preoperative surgical site skin cleansing, and is superior to povidone-iodine in preventing postoperative wound infections [9]. Evidence also suggests that chlorhexidine-gluconate-based scrubs are more effective than povidone-iodine-based aqueous scrubs in reducing bacterial contamination on staff hands prior to operative procedures. A recent study showed that *S. aureus*-associated postoperative wound infections can be decreased by treating nasal carriers of *S. aureus* with preoperative mupirocin nasal-ointment and chlorhexidine soap. However, application in developing countries may be limited by the need to identify *S. aureus* carriers using rapid DNA detection methods such as real-time PCR.

UNSAFE INJECTIONS AND NEEDLE-STICK INJURIES

Unsafe injections are one of the most important sources of blood-borne pathogens such as hepatitis B and C, and HIV [10], and have been linked to nosocomial transmission of Ebola virus, Lassa fever and malaria. It is estimated that 16 billion syringes are sold worldwide each year, the vast majority in developing countries; injection rates vary from 1.7 to 11.3 per person per year depending on the geographic region. Up to 75% of these may be non-sterilized. Injections are mostly prescribed for nonspecific symptoms, gastroenteritis, fever or upper respiratory symptoms, and reuse of syringes is common.

Needle-stick injuries to healthcare workers are another source of infection with blood-borne pathogens. These injuries result from lack of adequate training, improper disposal and destruction of needles, attempts to recap needles, and other unsafe practices. Trainee staff and nurses are most at risk when drawing blood.

Improving injection safety requires programmatic reform on a national level. Although expensive, the availability of needle-disposal kits, and disposable "auto-destruct" syringes should be increased. Healthcare workers, medical and allied health students, and the public should be educated about the dangers of unsafe injections and the indications for injection medications. Healthcare workers should be trained in safe practices. Surveillance of needle-stick injuries and post-exposure prophylaxis for healthcare workers should be part of hospital infection control programs.

CROSSOVER OF COMMUNITY INFECTIONS INTO HOSPITALS

Outbreaks of several diseases such as cholera, measles, nontyphoidal *Salmonella* and other fecal–oral transmitted organisms have been reported [11]. Overcrowding, improper isolation of patients harboring these infections, and presence of visitors and outsiders are frequently implicated. Other sources of infection include contaminated food products brought in from the outside, and hospital food handlers who are infected [12].

Vector-borne illnesses such as malaria, dengue fever, leishmaniasis and filariasis are of concern in tropical environments [13]. Hospitals with inadequate vector control procedures serve as amplifiers of vector-borne illnesses because of the presence of infected patients in an overcrowded environment. Rodents such as mice and rats have been implicated in spread of infectious diseases. Attention to waste disposal, screened doors and windows, and traps are of use in vector control. New and more cost-effective LED insect traps have been shown to be effective in tropical climates, with minimal trap failures.

TUBERCULOSIS

Individuals co-infected with HIV and TB have rapidly progressive disease, and those with pulmonary disease are highly infectious, via aerosolized droplets, posing great challenges for infection control in resource-limited settings.

Healthcare workers, including laboratory workers, are at risk of acquiring TB. US CDC guidelines recommend rapid diagnosis and treatment, isolation in negative pressure rooms and special masks to prevent nosocomial transmission, which are rarely feasible in resource-poor settings. However, simple measures such as early diagnosis and treatment of patients with short-course chemotherapy, outpatient evaluation of suspected TB patients, a separate TB ward with adequate ventilation using exhaust fans and large open windows allowing UV rays from sunlight, early collection of samples, disinfecting sputum containers and treating the sputum with household bleach can be applied in resource-poor settings [14]. WHO has published guidelines to control transmission of TB in healthcare settings [15]. However, there is little evidence regarding efficacy and cost-effectiveness.

VIRAL HEMORRHAGIC FEVERS

Viral hemorrhagic fevers (VHF) present unique challenges for tropical countries and infection control measures taken are dependent on the specific VHF pathogens predominant in that area.

Spread of VHF viruses such as Lassa, Ebola, Marburg, and Crimean-Congo Hemorrhagic Fever has occurred in hospital environments, where healthcare providers are at risk. Transmission can occur directly from the patient, at time of transfer of the dead body, through contact with infectious fluids, contaminated equipment, or by needle-stick injuries. Standard precautions (see below) are necessary to prevent nosocomial transmission of VHF viruses. In areas where VHF viruses are known to circulate, suspected cases should be immediately isolated and placed in strict barrier precautions. Information from previous outbreaks can help define case definitions for sporadic cases. In cases of outbreaks, patients should be cohorted in a designated area. If a designated area cannot be set aside, patients can be housed in a portion of a larger ward, in an uncrowded corner of a large hall, in rooms designated for TB, or in private rooms. Healthcare workers and household members caring for these patients should be identified and other personnel should be restricted. Ideally, personal protective equipment (PPE) should include a scrub suit, thin gloves, and rubber boots (if the floor is soiled), upon which a disposable gown, plastic apron, thick gloves, HEPA filters and eyewear should be worn. In resource-limited settings, local alternatives may be used, such as old shirts for scrubs, washable cotton gowns for disposable gowns, plastic bags for boots and thick gloves, plastic sheets or plastic cloth for plastic aprons, commercially available eyeglasses for eye protection, and plastic bottles modified for sharps disposal. In regions prone to VHF outbreaks, a VHF coordinator should be appointed to oversee preparations and response, including serving as a focal point to coordinate activity and mobilize communities for rapid control [16].

BASICS OF INFECTION CONTROL

The fundamental concept of infectious disease control is that all patients admitted to the hospital are potentially infectious. An adequate body of knowledge about the basics of infection control exists which can be translated into action. However, the gap between knowledge and practice needs to be bridged with interventions feasible for developing-country settings.

BOX 21.1 Basic Infection Control Measures for Health Facilities

- Surveillance, either hospital-wide or targeted
- Hand hygiene
- Outbreak investigations
- Cleaning, disinfection, and sterilization of equipment and disposal of infectious waste
- Hospital employee health, specifically after exposure to either blood-borne or respiratory pathogens
- Review of antibiotic utilization, its relationship to local antibiotic resistance patterns, and antibiotic stewardship programs
- Prevention of infections due to surgical procedures and invasive devices (e.g. central venous catheters, urinary catheters and ventilators)
- Development of infection control policies and procedures
- Transmission risk-based patient isolation
- Oversight on the use of new products that directly or indirectly relate to the risk of healthcare-associated infections

Basic infection control measures deal with every aspect of the healthcare delivery system, since infection can spread at any point during the course of the patient's interaction with the system (Box 21.1).

STANDARD INFECTION CONTROL PRACTICES

Standard infection control precautions ("Standard Precautions") are measures that apply to all patients regardless of their reason for admission (Table 21-3) [17], and form the foundation of infection control. These precautions evolved from "Universal Precautions" that were developed by the CDC in the 1980s, specifically for blood-borne pathogens such as HIV and hepatitis B and C, and applied to blood and other body fluids containing visible blood, semen and vaginal secretions. "Standard Precautions" combined the principles of "Universal Precautions" and "Body Substance Isolation", and is now applicable to all patients, regardless of suspected or confirmed infection status.

The single most important aspect of Standard Precautions (Table 21-3) is hand hygiene, which can be hand washing with soap and water, or the use of alcohol-based gels or foams that do not use water. Guidelines published by the HICPAC/SHEA/APIC/IDSA Hand Hygiene Task Force provide specific recommendations to promote improved hand hygiene [18,19].

An "infection control committee" should be established to oversee compliance, efficacy and adequacy of infection control measures as well as develop institution-specific guidelines. Infection control committees are composed of representatives from the medical and surgical services as well as microbiology, infectious diseases, nursing, occupational health and various ancillary services. However, to be truly effective, strong administrative support and provision of resources are essential, as is an organizational commitment to a safety culture and strengthening of systems to convert knowledge into action. Unfortunately, infection control committees are often not present in most healthcare facilities in resource-limited countries, and when present, do not function efficiently. There may be a number of reasons for this, including lack of administrative commitment, no infrastructure within the institution, or a lack of expertise.

EVIDENCE FOR HAND HYGIENE

Hand hygiene remains the cornerstone of infection control. Simple, low-cost programmatic measures promoting hand hygiene, such as increased surveillance, increased sensitization of healthcare staff,

TABLE 21-3 Components of Standard Infection Control Precautions

Component	Recommendation
Hand hygiene	After touching blood, body fluids, secretions, contaminated items; immediately after removing gloves; between patient contacts
Personal protective equipment (PPE)	
- Gloves	For touching blood, body fluids, secretions, contaminated items; for touching mucous membranes and non-intact skin
- Gowns	During procedures and patient-care activities when contact of clothing/ exposed skin with blood/body fluids, secretions is anticipated
- Mask, eye protection	During procedures and patient-care activities when contact of clothing/ exposed skin with blood/body fluids, secretions is anticipated
Soiled patient-care equipment	Handle in a manner that prevents transfer of microorganisms to others and to the environment; wear gloves if visibly contaminated; perform hand hygiene
Environmental control	Develop procedures for routine care, cleaning, and disinfection of environmental surfaces, especially frequently touched surfaces in patient-care areas
Textiles and laundry	Handle in a manner that prevents transfer of microorganisms to others and to the environment
Needles and other sharps	Do not recap, bend, break, or hand-manipulate used needles; if recapping is required, use a one-handed scoop technique only; use safety features when available; place used sharps in puncture-resistant container
Patient resuscitation	Use mouthpiece, resuscitation bag, other ventilation devices to prevent contact with mouth and oral secretions
Patient placement	Prioritize for single-patient room if patient is at increased risk of transmission, is likely to contaminate the environment, does not maintain appropriate hygiene, or is at increased risk of acquiring infection or developing adverse outcome following infection
Respiratory hygiene/cough etiquette	Instruct symptomatic persons to cover mouth/nose when sneezing/coughing; use tissues and dispose in no-touch receptacle; observe hand hygiene after soiling of hands with respiratory secretions; wear surgical mask if tolerated or maintain spatial separation, >3 feet if possible

Adapted from Siegel JD, Rhinehart E, Jackson M, et al. Healthcare Infection Control Practices Advisory Committee 2007 Guideline for Isolation Precautions: Preventing Transmission of Infectious Agents in Healthcare Settings, June 2007. http:// www.cdc.gov/ncidod/dhqp/gl_isolation.html (accessed 4 November 2009).

positive feedback programs and appropriate attention to device care, have resulted in substantially lowering infection rates in ICUs in developing countries. Efforts to increase motivation and awareness of staff are crucial since lapses in hygiene practices are frequent unless continuously reinforced. Alcohol-based hand rubs are useful where access to running water is limited. They have better acceptability, less skin irritation compared to soap and water, and quicker application, resulting in improved compliance. Commercially prepared products are available, but an effective low-cost gel can be prepared by hospital pharmacies using 20 mL of glycerin, propylene glycol or sorbitol, mixed with 980 mL of >70% isopropanol. Gels combining chlorhexidine and alcohol may be more effective than alcohol alone because of chlorhexidine's prolonged bactericidal effect, but are expensive for routine hand hygiene. Their use is best limited to situations when a high degree of hand antisepsis is necessary, such as before surgical procedures and placement of invasive devices.

For optimal effectiveness, alcohol-based hand rubs should be combined with a multimodal intervention package that includes feedback and awareness messages, and other basic infection control practices.

EVIDENCE FOR OTHER INFECTION CONTROL INTERVENTIONS

Routine gowning is another intervention thought to be useful in controlling hospital-acquired infections. However, a Cochrane review assessing the role of routine gowning of visitors and attendants to prevent nosocomial infections in newborn nurseries showed no significant benefit in reducing mortality, systemic infection rates, bacterial colonization, length of hospital stay or hand-washing frequency [20]. Similarly, Cochrane reviews have found no benefit of preoperative "bathing or washing" with chlorhexidine over other wash products such as bar soap, and no benefit in reducing infection rates by preoperative shaving.

SURVEILLANCE FOR HEALTHCARE-ASSOCIATED INFECTIONS

Surveillance of resistant organisms and device- and procedure-related infections are well-recognized markers of effectiveness of infection control programs and interventions while providing an early alert for outbreaks. Using standardized definitions, rates of targeted HAIs can be calculated over time and compared across institutions as well as before and after interventions. Surveillance of resistant organisms is more problematic. While passive surveillance (based on clinically obtained samples) is less costly and labor-intensive, it tends to miss the reservoir of asymptomatic, colonized patients. Active surveillance, on the other hand, involves screening asymptomatic patients for resistant organisms and can be more effective in rapidly isolating colonized patients. However, cost considerations are major limiting factors. Which patient populations should be targeted for screening, what the optimal method of screening is, and under what circumstances is screening most effective remain unresolved. Hospitals should assess what can be done well in their setting and implement what is feasible. To overcome surveillance shortcomings, WHO has developed a low-cost computer-based antimicrobial resistance surveillance program (WHONET), which has been used successfully to monitor trends and generate locally applicable guidelines on antimicrobial use [21]. An additional impediment to surveillance of resistant organisms is the lack of reliable antimicrobial culture and susceptibility data. Standardization and quality assurance of clinical microbiology laboratories is not enforced in most developing countries and therefore assessing the true burden of antimicrobial resistance is challenging.

STRENGTHENING HEALTH SYSTEMS IN THE TROPICS

One of the major limitations that hospitals face is the lack of resources directed towards infection control. However, while many problems are attributed to this, there are means to achieve infection control if strong institutional commitment exists. Despite the enormity of the challenge, studies reviewing cost-effectiveness of infection control measures are universally optimistic. Even minimally effective hospital infection control programs are cost-effective, lowering the costs incurred from HAIs due to longer hospital stays, greater disease morbidity and mortality, and antimicrobial agents. Measures of the effectiveness of infection control can be used as an indicator of the quality of hospital care [22,23]. Any intervention program should comprise a holistic approach that includes basic infection control measures. WHO and CDC have issued guidelines to control spread of infections. However, the most effective solutions will be those that are indigenously developed and implemented, and improved through active learning cycles and feedback. Local research will be necessary to identify critical points in infection transmission and solutions to address these.

REFERENCES

1. Lynch P, Rosenthal VD, Borg MA, Eremin SR. Infection control: a global view. In: Jarvis WR, ed. Bennett and Brachman's Hospital Infections, 5th edn. San Francisco, CA: Lippincott Williams & Wilkins; 2008:255–71.
2. Pittet D, Allegranzi B, Storr J, et al. Infection control as a major World Health Organization priority for developing countries. J Hosp Infect 2008;68: 285–92.
3. Mir F, Zaidi AKM. Hospital infections by anti-microbial resistant organisms in developing countries. In: Sosa AJ, Byarugaba DK, Amabile-Cuemas CF, et al., eds. Antimicrobial Resistance in Developing Countries. New York: Springer; 2009.
4. Zaidi AK, Huskins WC, Thaver D, et al. Hospital-acquired neonatal infections in developing countries. Lancet 2005;365:1175–88.
5. Shears P. Poverty and infection in the developing world: healthcare-related infections and infection control in the tropics. J Hosp Infect 2007;67: 217–24.
6. Hogerzeil HV, Bimo, Ross-Degnan D, et al. Field tests for rational drug use in twelve developing countries. Lancet 1993;342:1408–10.
7. Rosenthal VD. Device-associated nosocomial infections in limited-resources countries: findings of the International Nosocomial Infection Control Consortium (INICC). Am J Infect Control 2008;36:S171.e7–12.
8. Rosenthal VD. Central line–associated bloodstream infections in limited-resource countries: a review of the literature. Clin Infect Dis 2009;49: 1899–907.
9. Darouiche RO, Wall MJ Jr, Itani KM, et al. Chlorhexidine-alcohol versus povidone-iodine for surgical-site antisepsis. N Engl J Med 2010;362:18–26.
10. Hutin YJ, Hauri AM, Armstrong GL. Use of injections in healthcare settings worldwide, 2000: literature review and regional estimates. BMJ 2003;327: 1075.
11. Mhalu FS, Mtango FD, Msengi AE. Hospital outbreaks of cholera transmitted through close person-to-person contact. Lancet 1984;2:82–4.
12. Nyarango RM, Aloo PA, Kabiru EW, Nyanchongi BO. The risk of pathogenic intestinal parasite infections in Kisii Municipality, Kenya. BMC Public Health 2008;8:237.
13. Schierhorn C. Bug out! Using an integrated management approach to pest problems. Health Facil Manage 2002;15:40–2, 44.
14. Harries AD, Maher D, Nunn P. Practical and affordable measures for the protection of health care workers from tuberculosis in low-income countries. Bull World Health Organ 1997;75:477–89.
15. WHO. Guidelines for the prevention of tuberculosis in health care facilities in resource-limited settings. http://www.who.int/entity/tb/publications/who_tb_99_269/en/index.html
16. Centers for Disease Control and Prevention and World Health Organization. Infection Control for Viral Haemorrhagic Fevers in the African Health Care Setting. Atlanta, GA: Centers for Disease Control and Prevention; 1998: 1e198.
17. Siegel JD, Rhinehart E, Jackson M, et al. Healthcare Infection Control Practices Advisory Committee 2007 Guideline for Isolation Precautions: Preventing Transmission of Infectious Agents in Healthcare Settings, June 2007. http://www.cdc.gov/ncidod/dhqp/gl_isolation.html (accessed 4 November 2009).
18. Boyce JM, Pittet D. Guideline for Hand Hygiene in Health-Care Settings. Recommendations of the Healthcare Infection Control Practices Advisory Committee and the HICPAC/SHEA/APIC/IDSA Hand Hygiene Task Force. Society for Healthcare Epidemiology of America/Association for Professionals in Infection Control/Infectious Diseases Society of America. MMWR Recomm Rep 2002;51:1–45.

19. Muto CA, Jernigan JA, Ostrowsky BE, et al. SHEA guideline for preventing nosocomial transmission of multidrug-resistant strains of Staphylococcus aureus and enterococcus. Infect Control Hosp Epidemiol 2003;24:362–86.
20. Webster J, Pritchard MA. Gowning by attendants and visitors in newborn nurseries for prevention of neonatal morbidity and mortality. Cochrane Database Syst Rev 2003;(3):CD003670.
21. Stelling JM, O'Brien TF. Surveillance of antimicrobial resistance: the WHONET program. Clin Infect Dis 1997;24 Suppl 1:S157–68.
22. Damani N. Simple measures save lives: an approach to infection control in countries with limited resources. J Hosp Infect 2007;65 Suppl 2:151–4.
23. Travis P, Bennett S, Haines A, et al. Overcoming health-systems constraints to achieve the Millennium Development Goals. Lancet 2004;364:900–6.

22.1 Microbiology

Christopher M Parry, Sharon J Peacock

Key Features

- Accurate diagnosis in resource-restricted settings is severely limited by the absence of good diagnostic laboratory services
- Laboratories in resource-restricted settings struggle with poor facilities, lack of reliable water and electricity, inadequate equipment and consumables, insufficient staff, poor training and low morale, absence of standard operating procedures and quality assurance programmes, and inadequate levels of biosafety
- A country plan for the development of a laboratory network requires consideration of the needs at primary, district, provincial/regional and national levels
- At District Hospital level, a quality-assured repertoire of essential laboratory tests can contribute to improved healthcare
- Surveillance by microbiology laboratories provides an understanding of the causes of infection in the local population and informs public health policy on appropriate antimicrobial therapy and preventive strategies
- There is increasing recognition of the need to support the development of a quality-assured laboratory service in resource-restricted settings and develop simple and robust point-of-care diagnostics
- Point-of-care rapid diagnostic tests are changing our approach to the diagnosis of some infectious diseases, but care needs to be taken about their usage and interpretation of results

INTRODUCTION

The effective management and containment of many treatable and preventable infectious diseases in resource-restricted countries is limited by the failure to make an accurate diagnosis. Access to accurate, affordable, easy to use, quality-assured, reliable and accessible diagnostic tests is severely lacking for most of the world's population and misdiagnosis of infectious diseases is common. Disease identification, appropriate treatment choice, and implementing public health measures for the prevention and control of endemic and epidemic infections all require laboratory support. This lack of reliable diagnostics compromises patient care. Laboratory diagnosis also highlights the increasing levels of resistance to antimicrobials in many infections and the need for newer, possibly unaffordable, antimicrobials such as broad-spectrum antimicrobials in bacterial sepsis, or second-line combination therapy for AIDS, malaria and tuberculosis. This issue is now being increasingly recognized and addressed in many regions.

THE NEED FOR LABORATORY SERVICES

In most resource-restricted settings, individual patient diagnosis is based on clinical signs and symptoms with little or no laboratory support. Diagnostic algorithms have been developed for situations with no laboratory backup, an approach adopted for example in the Integrated Management of Childhood Illness (IMCI). Unfortunately, for many infections, clinical features lack sufficient specificity to allow them to be used to differentiate the possible diagnoses, and overtreatment to cover the various possibilities is common.

In the assessment of the febrile child in the tropics, for example, malaria and systemic bacterial infections often have an indistinguishable clinical picture. Malaria may be diagnosed by smear microscopy but bloodstream infections require a blood culture service. It has become clear in recent years that bloodstream infections represent an underappreciated burden of disease and mortality. This was clearly demonstrated by a study conducted in Kenya in which bacterial bloodstream infections diagnosed by blood culture were responsible for 26% of deaths among children admitted to a rural district hospital [1]. Without an accurate diagnosis and specific treatment, bloodstream infections such as those due to *Salmonella enterica*, *Staphylococcus aureus*, *Streptococcus pneumoniae* or *Burkholderia pseudomallei* can carry a high mortality. Distinguishing cerebral malaria, bacterial meningitis and encephalopathic typhoid may be similarly difficult without laboratory support. Children in sub-Saharan Africa with clinical symptoms of pneumonia may have pneumococcal pneumonia, but can equally have malaria or invasive salmonellosis. A child with dysentery may be suffering from amebic colitis, *Shigella* infection or enterohemorrhagic *E. coli*. In adults, syndromic management of sexually transmitted infections is widespread but needs to be informed by periodic surveillance of antimicrobial susceptibility patterns. Emerging and potentially epidemic viral infections such as SARS and influenza (H5N1 and H1N1) require relatively sophisticated tests to confirm the diagnosis.

Infections by pathogens that are resistant to multiple antimicrobials are common in many tropical countries where there is widespread availability of over-the-counter antimicrobials. Appropriate therapy of these infections requires isolation of the causative organism and antimicrobial susceptibility testing.

Laboratories also have an important public health role within the healthcare system. The ability to investigate outbreaks of disease as part of epidemic preparedness is a key function. These might include outbreaks of watery or bloody diarrhea, epidemics of meningitis, or clusters of patients with fever of unknown etiology. In addition, laboratories are a critical component of disease control programs such as the national programs for the control of tuberculosis, HIV and malaria. The lack of laboratory capacity to support the expansion of diagnostic testing and antiretroviral therapy in HIV programs has made many international organizations appreciate the desperate plight of the laboratory service for the first time. Tuberculosis can be diagnosed in many patients with a Ziehl–Neelsen-stained smear of sputum, but to extend the diagnosis in those who are acid-fast bacilli negative or have multidrug-resistant disease requires more developed laboratory support. Furthermore, laboratories have an increasing role in infection control in healthcare settings and congregate facilities and in the prevention of healthcare-associated infections.

Accurate disease surveillance requires a laboratory network and is vital to inform public health policy concerning allocation of resources and disease prevention. Laboratories can help to define clinical problems by sampling surveys. For example, determining the antimicrobial susceptibilities of bacterial pathogens such *S. aureus*, *S. pneumoniae* or *S. enterica* for a selection of isolates can inform the appropriate empiric therapy in a particular area. An understanding of the burden of disease in an area – drug-resistant typhoid in an urban slum, for example – could lead to public health measures such as a vaccination program. Laboratory surveillance programs may produce the clue to the possibility of new organisms emerging – including both bacteria and viruses, most commonly at the animal–human interface.

At an international level, under revised International Health Regulations, countries are now committed to reporting events that could have health implications beyond their borders. Many countries do not have the capacity to do this. The World Health Organization (WHO), with other partners, have been working to address this issue by creating an international network of laboratories known as the Emerging and Dangerous Pathogens Laboratory Network for Response and Readiness. International organizations such as the American Society of Microbiology, the Centers for Disease Control and global academic institutions are actively contributing to training and mentoring of developing-country laboratory networks.

WHAT ARE THE PROBLEMS FOR LABORATORY SERVICES?

For many healthcare staff working in resource-restricted areas, the major problem is simply a lack of laboratory services. Hospital laboratories may be absent, or, if they are available, only offer a limited repertoire of tests. In other areas, particularly in Asia, there is a wide range of alternative services offered by private diagnostic laboratories, typically outside the front gate of the hospital but with uncertain quality. Even when the tests are available, they may not be used or the results ignored. Lack of use may stem from a poor perception of the laboratory, and tests may not be available because the costs are prohibitive.

Even when laboratories are present, they face the many challenges that are familiar to all areas of the healthcare sector. Inadequate facilities are common, with laboratories that lack space and a secure supply of electricity and water. Appropriate equipment may be unavailable or poorly maintained. Even basic equipment required for a functioning laboratory can be in disrepair because of the absence of regular care and servicing. A functioning microscope is a key piece of equipment for a basic microbiology laboratory but is frequently found in poor condition. In a survey of 90 microscopes in laboratories in nine districts in Malawi, only 50% were in good condition [2]. There were 1.1 functioning microscopes per 100,000 population and even microscopes in need of full servicing were still in daily use. The 90 microscopes were from 16 different manufacturers, illustrating the lack of standardization of laboratory equipment so frequently seen. The provision of biological safety cabinets is another area where equipment from multiple manufacturers, and lack of spare parts and maintenance is common, and in this case may lead to unsafe and hazardous conditions for laboratory workers. Standardization of equipment and consumables with central ordering, maintenance contracts and supplies of spare parts would seem a sensible response to this issue but is rarely seen. Tests may also be unavailable because of an inadequate supply route for consumables. This is another area where standardization of tests, central ordering and supply can lead not only to more reliable supply of quality-assured consumables but also to potential cost savings for the country.

The laboratory can generate results but the quality may be poor. Standard operating procedures may be absent and quality control of routine procedures non-existent. The absence of national or regional laboratory guidelines or programs of external quality assurance by the laboratory network is common. Communications between different levels within the laboratory network may be rudimentary so that specimens referred to the next level are not transported in a timely manner and results do not return in a time period that will influence clinical management. It is standard practice in tuberculosis programs that patients who fail treatment should have a sample cultured for tuberculosis so that susceptibility tests can be performed. In a study of the transport of such specimens to the central reference laboratory in Malawi, only 40% of specimens arrived in the reference laboratory and only 36% of those samples received were successfully cultured for susceptibility testing [3].

The shortage of staff with appropriate education and training is a further problem. Many laboratory workers have no formal training and are simply trained at the bench. At the peripheral level, there may be only one laboratory assistant, with no more than secondary school education. At district level, there may be assistants and technicians (formally educated in laboratory medicine for 3 years). At central level, technicians may work alongside technologists (with 2 years specialist post-technician training) and scientists (university science graduates). Regardless of qualifications, laboratory workers often have a lowly status within the health sector and the attrition of healthcare personnel out of government service results in low morale among those who remain. Private or research laboratories may attract the best technicians from the government sector. Diagnostic laboratories frequently have no representation at the local, provincial or national level, or, if they do, it is only as part of the support services. In many countries, the voice of the laboratory is rarely heard.

These many problems contribute to a poor biosafety situation in laboratories. The lack of equipment, knowledge and training mean that laboratory workers are processing samples with hazardous pathogens in an unsafe manner. In a study of tuberculosis laboratories in Korea, before safety conditions had been upgraded, the relative risk of being diagnosed with tuberculosis for the technicians performing drug susceptibility tests was 21.5 (95% CI 4.5–102.5) compared to non-laboratory workers [4]. The true magnitude of this problem in laboratory workers is difficult to gauge because surveillance of infection in laboratory workers is rarely performed or reported.

WHAT CAN BE DONE TO IMPROVE LABORATORY SERVICES?

At a national level, the important contribution of laboratories needs to be appreciated within the Ministry of Health, by national and local healthcare managers and by funding organizations. A representative of the laboratory services should be present in the key decision-making committees. Support is also needed from clinicians, who often have disproportionate influence within the system. A plan for the laboratory network should become part of the overall healthcare development plan. There needs to be a priority list of core and essential services provided in a quality-assured manner. The laboratory plan should include the provision for a tiered laboratory network at the primary, district, regional/provincial and national levels. The plans should be realistic, affordable and sustainable.

At the Level I or primary level, perhaps in a health post or health center serving outpatients, microscopy for malaria and tuberculosis and testing for HIV with a same-day service would be essential. These laboratories can serve as a collection point for samples that need referral to the next level. The Level II facility in the local District Hospital would have a dedicated laboratory space and a broader repertoire of tests serving inpatients and outpatients. The tests offered would depend on the spectrum of local diseases and resources available, and may be limited to microscopy, simple biochemistry and serology and blood transfusion, or may include bacterial culture facilities. Laboratories can act as a hub for the primary level laboratories, providing them with support, supplies of reagents, and quality assurance activities. At the Level III, provincial or regional level, laboratories will be located in larger referral hospitals. Laboratories at this level should be performing a more sophisticated range of tests with higher throughput. For example, facilities for tuberculosis culture might be available, together with molecular techniques for specific diseases and the ability to investigate disease outbreaks. Support for the Level II laboratories would be an important function, including periodic visits and laboratory assessment as part of a quality assurance program.

National reference laboratories at Level IV are likely to be located in the capital and serve specialized public health functions that may be linked to specific disease control programs such as the central reference laboratory for the National Tuberculosis Programme. It is important that laboratories at the national level should have links to regional supranational reference laboratories for advice and quality assurance. Level III and IV laboratories would conduct surveillance and monitoring of infections using laboratory data collected throughout the network, establish standard operating procedures and protocols, conduct training and quality improvement, and plan for equipment needs and maintenance throughout the network.

THE IMPORTANCE OF BIOSAFETY

Biosafety is an essential consideration at all levels of the laboratory network and depends on three principles [5]. Good laboratory practice and technique is fundamental and this requires established standard operating procedures and appropriate induction and training of staff. Safety equipment provides a primary barrier and this includes appropriate, properly maintained and used equipment (e.g. centrifuges, biological safety cabinets) and personal protective equipment (e.g. gloves, respirators). Finally, facility design and construction is a secondary barrier providing, for example, appropriate workflows (from clean to dirty areas) and directional airflows and containment if required.

Microorganisms are categorized into four hazard groups according to their risk to individuals and society and the availability of treatment and preventive measures (Table 22.1-1). Diagnostic laboratories are further categorized into biosafety levels (BSL) so that the facilities available are matched to the pathogens handled. A standard diagnostic laboratory would be at BSL2 and the basic requirements for such a laboratory are outlined in Table 22.1-2 and Box 22.1.1. More specialized laboratories such as tuberculosis reference laboratories where culture and susceptibility testing are performed require BSL3 facilities. BSL3 laboratories have particular design features to reduce the hazard of airborne transmission and incorporate directional airflows and the use of Biological Safety Cabinets. They are particularly appropriate for laboratories handling pathogens such as tuberculosis and influenza. However, BSL3 facilities are very expensive and difficult to build and maintain. WHO has recently indicated that in some circumstances, slightly less rigorous guidelines, so-called BSL2+ as outlined in Table 22.1-2, may be appropriate for selected laboratories, for example, processing samples for tuberculosis culture [6].

WHAT TESTS SHOULD BE AVAILABLE?

Healthcare staff working at the District Hospital level may be asked to advise on what would constitute an appropriate laboratory service for the hospital and district. The provision of an extensive range of tests is likely to be unaffordable and impractical. In a study evaluating the role of the laboratory in a District Hospital in Malawi, the services considered essential were blood transfusion (including blood grouping and compatibility testing and screening for HIV, hepatitis B and syphilis), hemoglobin estimation, and the microscopic diagnosis of malaria and tuberculosis [7]. This list will vary in different areas and the services of the laboratory should be orientated to the requirements of the district and the available resources. Other tests that

TABLE 22.1-1 Classification of Microorganisms on the Basis of Hazard

Class	Description of microorganism	Biosafety level	Laboratory type
1	Unlikely to cause human disease	Level 1	Basic teaching or research laboratory
2	May cause human disease; might be a hazard to laboratory workers; unlikely to spread in the community; laboratory exposure rarely causes infection; effective prophylaxis and therapy	Level 2	Routine diagnostic laboratory
3	May cause serious human disease; may be serious hazard to laboratory workers; may spread in the community; effective prophylaxis and therapy	Level 3	Special diagnostic laboratory (e.g. tuberculosis reference laboratory)
4	Causes serious human disease; serious threat to laboratory workers; high risk of spread in the community; no effective prophylaxis or therapy	Level 4	Supranational dangerous pathogen laboratories

Modified from World Health Organization (WHO). Laboratory Biosafety Manual, 3rd edn. Geneva: WHO, 2004.

BOX 22.1.1 Basic Requirements for a BSL2 Laboratory

- Access should be restricted to essential personnel, not including the general public – biohazard signs should be on the entry door
- A laboratory coat should be worn in laboratory area. Laboratory coats should be side or back fastening and made of strong material
- Gloves should be worn for contact or potential contact with infectious material
- All work should be performed using good microbiological technique
- Hands should be washed after handling infectious material before leaving laboratory area
- Eating, drinking, smoking, applying make-up not allowed
- No materials should be placed in mouth, including no pipetting by mouth
- The laboratory bench surfaces should be easy to clean
- There should be clear protocols for cleaning, decontamination and for dealing with spillages of potentially infected materials
- Potentially infected material should be decontaminated (by autoclaving, incineration or disinfection) before disposal

TABLE 22.1-2 Summary of Biosafety Level Requirements

	Biosafety level			
	1	**2**	**2+**	**3**
Isolation of laboratory	No	No	Yes	Yes
Room sealable for decontamination	No	No	No	Yes
Ventilation:				
Inward airflow	No	Desirable	Yes	Yes
Controlled ventilation system	No	Desirable	Yes	Yes
HEPA-filtered air exhaust	No	No	Desirable	Desirable
Double-door entry	No	No	Desirable	Yes
Anteroom	No	No	Desirable	Yes
Anteroom with shower	No	No	No	Desirable
Effluent treatment	No	No	No	Desirable
Autoclave:				
On site	No	Desirable	Yes	Yes
In laboratory room	No	No	Desirable	Desirable
Double ended	No	No	No	Desirable
Biological safety cabinets	No	Desirable	Yes	Yes
Safety monitoring capability	No	No	No	Desirable

Modified from World Health Organization (WHO). Laboratory Biosafety Manual, 3rd edn. Geneva: WHO, 2004; and World Health Organization (WHO). Guidance on bio-safety related to TB laboratory diagnostic procedures, 8–9 April 2009, Geneva, Switzerland. Online. Available: http://www.stoptb.org/wg/gli/assets/documents/Summary April 09.pdf.

require relatively little investment and can be done where there are limited resources include microscopy of urine and stool samples for ova, cysts and parasites, Gram stain and cell count in CSF and other sterile fluids, and Gram stains of pus samples. The microscopic appearance of some typical bacterial pathogens is shown in Figure 22.1.1 (available online). Guidelines for standard laboratory methods appropriate for resource-restricted areas are available [8]. A checklist of issues that should be considered when evaluating a diagnostic laboratory is in Box 22.1.2.

The diagnosis of infection depends on detection of the pathogen or the host response to the pathogen. Direct pathogen detection is traditionally performed by light microscopy, although antigen detection and nucleic acid amplification tests (such as PCR) are increasingly used. Pathogen detection may also be carried out by isolation of the microorganism by culture of relevant clinical samples and this allows susceptibility testing to be performed. Methods based on detecting the immune response mainly rely on detecting pathogen-specific IgM or IgG antibodies. Technologic advances in the design of testing methods have simplified antigen and antibody detection to the point that simple point-of-care test kits are now widely available. The rapid kits for HIV antibody detection have an established place in the voluntary counseling and testing framework being established in many countries. Rapid malaria detection tests have been recommended as a replacement for malaria microscopy in some guidelines and needs to be positive before antimalarial treatment is given.

In recent years, organizations such as the UNICEF/United Nations Development Programme/World Bank/WHO Special Programme for Research and Training in Tropical Diseases (TDR) and the Foundation for Innovative New Diagnostics (FIND) have played an important role in developing and evaluating new diagnostic tests for many tropical diseases. The WHO Sexually Transmitted Diagnostics Initiative has developed an approach to the characteristics of an ideal diagnostic test in the developing-country context. "ASSURED" tests should be affordable by those at risk of infection, sensitive and specific, user-friendly (simple to perform and requiring minimal training), rapid (to enable treatment at the first visit), robust (does not require refrigerated storage), equipment-free and able to be delivered to those who need it.

There have been considerable advances in the format and ease of use of molecular tests. This is exemplified by the increasing use in tuberculosis laboratories of nucleic acid amplification tests directly from acid-fast bacilli (AFB) smear-positive sputum, or from culture isolates. Line probe assays (LPAs) use a multiplex PCR amplification followed by reverse hybridization to identify *M. tuberculosis* complex and mutations in the genes associated with rifampicin and isoniazid resistance. LPA can be performed with results in 1 to 2 days, which is considerably quicker than the weeks required for traditional culture methods, and the overall agreement for the diagnosis of multidrug resistance between these tests and conventional methods is 99%. The format of these tests is being simplified so that the feasibility of their routine use in tuberculosis reference laboratories in developing countries is becoming a reality. These methods are an important component of the roll-out of the programmatic management of MDR tuberculosis globally.

Quality assurance (QA) is defined as "planned and systematic activities to provide adequate confidence that requirements for quality will be met". The QA system is the basis for a guaranteed result. If this system is not followed, patients may get the wrong results, with important consequences for their health – such as receiving inadequate treatment. A program of quality assurance in diagnostic laboratories involves not only internal quality control and external quality assurance but also attention to appropriate staffing, training and supervision, maintenance of equipment and facilities. International guidelines are now available and increasingly implemented for quality assurance in many areas of laboratory practice such as AFB smear microscopy and HIV testing.

BOX 22.1.2 A Laboratory Checklist

1. Management
   a. Clear management structure with representation in hospital management
2. Infrastructure
   a. A safe and suitable physical environment
   b. Sufficient space, power, climate control, water and transport access
   c. Uninterruptible power supply (UPS) supporting laboratory equipment in case of power surges
   d. Sufficient light, bench space, mains or bore hole water, and distilled water
3. Equipment
   a. Appropriate for the test repertoire
   b. Laboratory environment should have enough space to perform day-to-day operations safely
4. Testing repertoire
   a. Appropriate for local disease burden
   b. Standard operating procedures (SOPs) must be available, understood and implemented
5. Staffing
   a. Appropriate number of competent staff with adequate training
   b. Induction, performance appraisals, in-service training in place and implemented
6. Biosafety
   a. Appropriate standard operating procedures, personal protective equipment, and laboratory structure for pathogens being handled (BSL2, BSL2+ or BSL3)
   b. Staff health surveillance in place
7. Supplies
   a. Supply chain management system to provide adequate supplies of reagents, consumables and quality control (QC) materials
8. Quality assurance
   a. Routine performance of QC testing according to the established standards
   b. Participation in the EQA/proficiency testing (PT) programs available (e.g. acid-fast bacilli microscopy, HIV testing)

CONCLUSION

Accurate clinical diagnosis in resource-restricted settings relies strongly on the laboratory service. The increasing recognition of the need to support the development of a quality-assured laboratory service in such settings is therefore welcome. In many regions, international organizations are actively working with local providers to improve laboratory services. The development of laboratory services will contribute to improved health for the local population and ensure better use of scarce healthcare resources.

REFERENCES

1. Berkeley JA, Lowe BS, Mwangi I, et al. Bacteremia among children admitted to a rural hospital in Kenya. New Engl J Med 2005;352:39–47.
2. Mundy C, Ngwira M, Kadewele G, et al. Evaluation of microscope condition in Malawi. Trans R Soc Trop Med Hyg 2000;94:583–4.
3. Harries AD, Michongwe J, Nyirenda TE, et al. Using a bus service for transporting sputum specimens to the Central Reference Laboratory: effect on the routine TB culture service in Malawi. Int J Tuberc Lung Dis 2004;8:204–10.
4. Kim SJ, Lee SH, Kim IS, et al. Risk of occupational tuberculosis in National Tuberculosis Programme laboratories in Korea. Int J Tuberc Lung Dis 2007; 11:138.
5. World Health Organization (WHO). Laboratory Biosafety Manual, 3rd edn. Geneva: WHO, 2004.
6. World Health Organization (WHO). Guidance on bio-safety related to TB laboratory diagnostic procedures, 8–9 April 2009, Geneva, Switzerland. Online. Available: http://www.stoptb.org/wg/gli/assets/documents/Summary April 09.pdf
7. Mundy CJ, Bates I, Nkhoma W, et al. The operation, quality and costs of a district hospital laboratory service in Malawi. Trans R Soc Trop Med Hyg 2003;97:403–8.
8. Cheesbrough M. Medical Laboratory Manual for Tropical Countries. Vol II: Microbiology. London: Tropical Health Technology; 1998.

Approach to the Patient with Diarrhea 22.2

Regina C LaRocque, Jason B Harris

Key features

- Acute diarrheal disease is a major cause of global morbidity and mortality
- Diarrheal illness is classified as acute watery diarrhea, invasive diarrhea or persistent diarrhea
- In resource-limited settings, it is not usually necessary to make a specific etiologic diagnosis in order to provide appropriate management of diarrheal illness
- Rehydration is a critical component of the treatment of diarrhea. Oral rehydration therapy (ORT) is the preferred mode of fluid therapy in most cases
- Treatment of diarrheal illness includes the use of antibiotics in selected instances and dietary interventions and micronutrient supplementation in children to prevent and/or treat malnutrition
- Recognition and management of common comorbid conditions is an important part of the approach to the patient presenting with diarrheal illness

KEY SYNDROMES

Diarrheal disease is an important cause of morbidity globally, with an estimated 4.6 billion episodes worldwide per year [1]. Furthermore, diarrheal disease is the second most common infectious cause of death worldwide. In children under five years of age, diarrheal disease is a particularly important cause of death. Nearly two million children under the age of five years die from diarrheal disease every year; the majority of these deaths are in young children in resource-poor areas [2]. Diarrheal disease is also associated with malnutrition, which may cause irreversible deficits in physical and cognitive development and is the cause of millions of deaths annually [3].

Diarrhea is defined as the passage of loose or watery stools at least three times in a 24-hour period. Diarrheal illness is classified as acute watery diarrhea, invasive diarrhea or persistent diarrhea. This classification scheme reflects differences in the etiology, pathogenesis and management of each type of diarrheal illness.

ACUTE WATERY DIARRHEA

Infectious agents are the most common cause of acute watery diarrhea. In most cases of acute watery diarrhea it is not necessary to identify a specific microbiologic diagnosis and antibiotics are not indicated. An exception to this is *Vibrio cholerae* infection (Chapter 43), which often occurs in epidemics. It is useful to distinguish cholera from other causes of acute watery diarrhea as patients with severe cholera have more rapid fluid losses and benefit from antibiotic therapy. The diagnosis of cholera is suggested by vomiting and by the passage of voluminous watery diarrhea, which may have a characteristic rice-water appearance. Cholera should be suspected when otherwise healthy older children and adults die of watery diarrhea. Although numerous other pathogens also cause acute watery diarrhea, the most common etiologies are rotavirus in infants, and enterotoxigenic *Escherichia coli* (ETEC) in older children and adults. There is increasing recognition of the role of norovirus as a major cause of epidemic, and sporadic, acute watery diarrhea in adults and children.

Although acute watery diarrhea is most often caused by infection of the gastrointestinal tract, other systemic illnesses common in developing countries are also associated with acute watery diarrhea. Systemic viral infections associated with diarrhea include influenza, measles and dengue fever. Bacterial infections associated with diarrhea include urinary tract infection, pneumonia, and meningitis. Patients with malaria can present with diarrhea. Surgical emergencies, such as intussusception or appendicitis, may also present with diarrhea. For these reasons, the presence of acute watery diarrhea is not sufficient clinical evidence to exclude other potentially life-threatening infections, and a history and complete physical examination should be performed on all patients presenting with diarrhea (see "Differential Diagnosis" below).

INVASIVE DIARRHEA

Invasive diarrhea, or dysentery, is suggested by the presence of blood in stool. Invasive diarrhea is most often the result of inflammation of the small bowel or colon in response to invasive bacterial infection or amebiasis. In invasive diarrhea, the stool also typically contains visible mucus. Fecal leukocytes are usually detectable by direct microscopy. Fever usually accompanies invasive diarrhea, also resulting from the pronounced mucosal inflammatory response.

Worldwide, *Shigella* species are the most important bacterial pathogens causing invasive diarrhea. *Shigella flexneri* is the predominant species causing invasive diarrhea in children in resource-limited settings. *Shigella dysenteriae* serotype 1 (Sd1) is responsible for epidemic dysentery and is the most virulent of the four *Shigella* species. In addition to the frequent passage of small liquid stools that contain visible blood, abdominal cramps and tenesmus are common in shigellosis. Shigellosis cannot be distinguished reliably from other causes of bloody diarrhea on the basis of clinical features alone. Other etiologies of invasive diarrhea include *Salmonella enterica, Campylobacter* spp, enterohemorrhagic *E. coli*, enteroinvasive *E. coli* and the protozoan parasite *Entamoeba histolytica*. Enterohemorrhagic *E. coli* may cause epidemics of bloody diarrhea, similar to Sd1. Patients with enterohemorrhagic *E. coli* infection often have low, or absent, fever, while patients with shigellosis are usually febrile. The distinction is important as administration of antibiotics to patients with shigellosis is beneficial, while administration of antibiotics to patients with enterohemorrhagic *E. coli* infections markedly increases the risk of complications and renal failure.

PERSISTENT DIARRHEA

Diarrhea lasting longer than 2–4 weeks is classified as persistent, or chronic, diarrhea. In some cases, persistent diarrhea is associated with infection with enteroaggrative *E. coli* or *Cryptosporidium hominis/parvum*. However, the majority of cases of persistent diarrhea are thought to be triggered by an episode of acute gastroenteritis. In such cases, diarrhea is perpetuated by an inability to restore normal resorptive capacity after intestinal injury. Persistent diarrhea is associated with malnutrition and chronic enteropathy, and should also raise suspicion for underlying HIV infection; in HIV-infected persons, unexplained persistent diarrhea constitutes an AIDS-defining illness [4].

CLINICAL EVALUATION

The evaluation of individuals with acute diarrheal disease should include a careful history and physical exam, as well as classification of the diarrheal illness as acute watery diarrhea, invasive diarrhea or persistent diarrhea. The determination of hydration status provides essential information about the severity of the diarrheal illness and the need for rapid therapy and can be performed based on clinical features. In children, an assessment of nutritional status and evaluation for concomitant illness are also essential.

ASSESSMENT OF DEHYDRATION

Dehydration is the most important cause of mortality in patients with acute watery diarrhea, but may also contribute to mortality in patients with invasive and persistent diarrhea. Therefore, an initial assessment of the degree of dehydration, as well as a rapid estimate of ongoing fluid losses, is essential in the evaluation of any patient presenting with diarrhea. To estimate the initial hydration status, it is always necessary to use a combination of clinical signs and symptoms, because no single sign or symptom is sufficiently predictive of hydration status. The World Health Organization (WHO) recommends assessment of four clinical signs to estimate the degree of dehydration in children and adults (Fig. 22.2.1) [5].

ASSESSMENT OF NUTRITIONAL STATUS

Identification of malnutrition is important in the management of diarrheal illness. In patients with diarrhea and severe malnutrition, rehydration therapy can lead to the development of fluid overload and heart failure. There is also a high risk of occult, serious bacterial infection in malnourished children. Because of this, patients with diarrhea and severe malnutrition require a different approach to rehydration, antibiotic use and nutritional care. Diarrhea is also associated with vitamin A deficiency. For these reasons, children presenting with diarrhea in developing countries should be assessed for clinical signs of protein-energy malnutrition and vitamin A deficiency according to WHO standards.

EVALUATION FOR CONCOMITANT ILLNESS

Children with acute diarrhea, particularly those with malnutrition, should also be assessed for evidence of co-existing infections. Fever is a common presenting feature in patients with invasive diarrhea, but

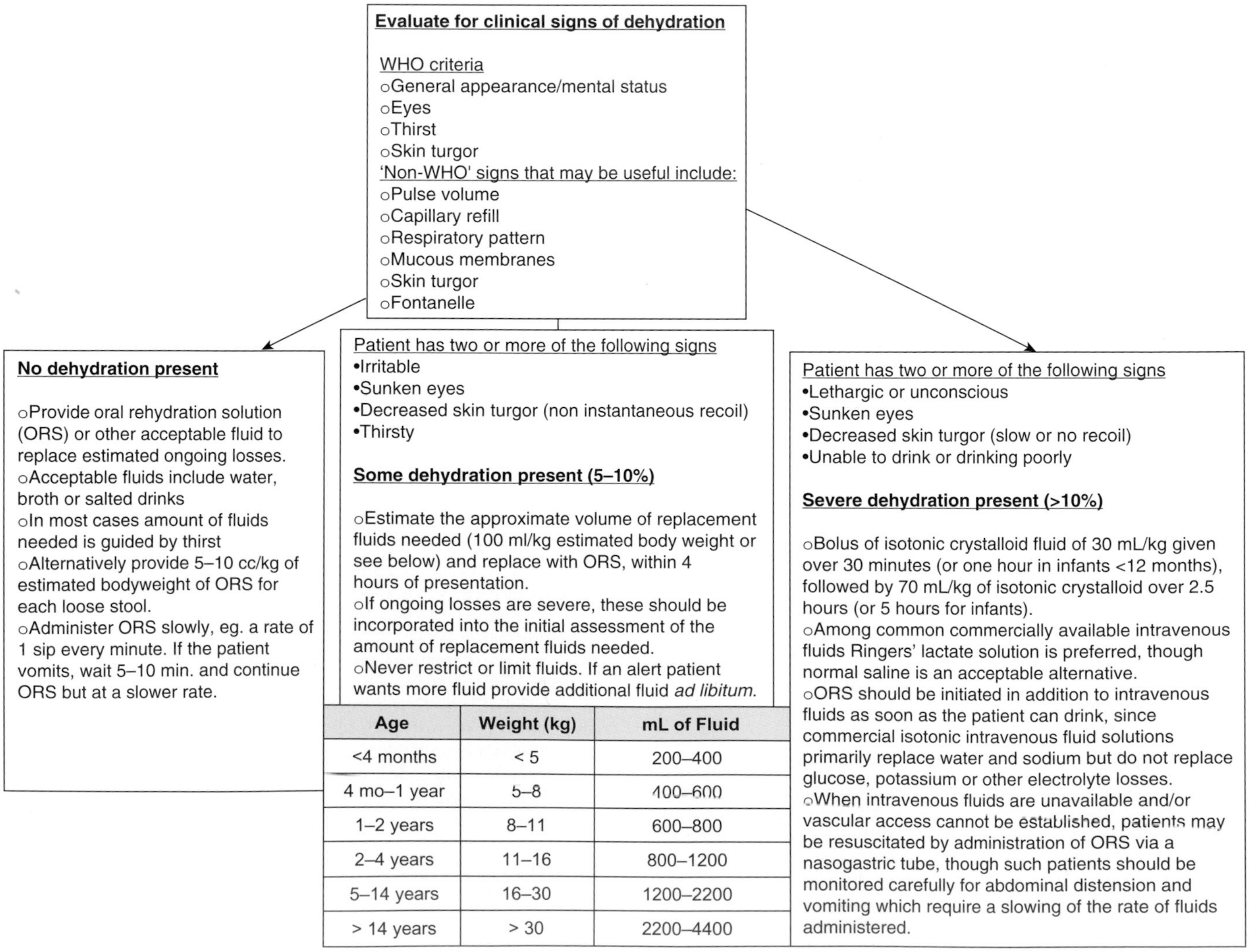

Evaluate for clinical signs of dehydration

WHO criteria
- General appearance/mental status
- Eyes
- Thirst
- Skin turgor

'Non-WHO' signs that may be useful include:
- Pulse volume
- Capillary refill
- Respiratory pattern
- Mucous membranes
- Skin turgor
- Fontanelle

No dehydration present

- Provide oral rehydration solution (ORS) or other acceptable fluid to replace estimated ongoing losses.
- Acceptable fluids include water, broth or salted drinks
- In most cases amount of fluids needed is guided by thirst
- Alternatively provide 5–10 cc/kg of estimated bodyweight of ORS for each loose stool.
- Administer ORS slowly, eg. a rate of 1 sip every minute. If the patient vomits, wait 5–10 min. and continue ORS but at a slower rate.

Patient has two or more of the following signs
- Irritable
- Sunken eyes
- Decreased skin turgor (non instantaneous recoil)
- Thirsty

Some dehydration present (5–10%)

- Estimate the approximate volume of replacement fluids needed (100 ml/kg estimated body weight or see below) and replace with ORS, within 4 hours of presentation.
- If ongoing losses are severe, these should be incorporated into the initial assessment of the amount of replacement fluids needed.
- Never restrict or limit fluids. If an alert patient wants more fluid provide additional fluid *ad libitum.*

Age	Weight (kg)	mL of Fluid
<4 months	< 5	200–400
4 mo–1 year	5–8	400–600
1–2 years	8–11	600–800
2–4 years	11–16	800–1200
5–14 years	16–30	1200–2200
> 14 years	> 30	2200–4400

Patient has two or more of the following signs
- Lethargic or unconscious
- Sunken eyes
- Decreased skin turgor (slow or no recoil)
- Unable to drink or drinking poorly

Severe dehydration present (>10%)

- Bolus of isotonic crystalloid fluid of 30 mL/kg given over 30 minutes (or one hour in infants <12 months), followed by 70 mL/kg of isotonic crystalloid over 2.5 hours (or 5 hours for infants).
- Among common commercially available intravenous fluids Ringers' lactate solution is preferred, though normal saline is an acceptable alternative.
- ORS should be initiated in addition to intravenous fluids as soon as the patient can drink, since commercial isotonic intravenous fluid solutions primarily replace water and sodium but do not replace glucose, potassium or other electrolyte losses.
- When intravenous fluids are unavailable and/or vascular access cannot be established, patients may be resuscitated by administration of ORS via a nasogastric tube, though such patients should be monitored carefully for abdominal distension and vomiting which require a slowing of the rate of fluids administered.

FIGURE 22.2.1 WHO-based approaches to the assessment and management of dehydration.

the presence of fever in a patient with acute watery diarrhea should increase suspicion for a co-existing infection. In particular, malaria should be considered in endemic areas.

Concomitant pneumonia is an important cause of mortality in patients presenting with diarrheal illness. Tachypnea is a common finding in patients with some (5–9%) dehydration, but the presence of cough, fever, crackles on chest auscultation, or persistent tachypnea after rehydration therapy should raise suspicion for pneumonia. Therefore, patients presenting with dehydration should be re-evaluated for the presence of pneumonia after rehydration.

Irritability is a common finding in moderate dehydration, while lethargy and coma are seen in severe dehydration. Encephalopathy is an important complication of shigellosis and may also be seen in systemic *Salmonella* infections. The differential diagnosis of seizures in a child with diarrhea includes hypoglycemia, hypo- or hypernatremia, encephalopathy, central nervous system (CNS) infection and febrile seizures. Consideration of a diagnosis of meningitis in children, especially infants, in whom typical meningeal signs are often absent, is warranted if there are seizures or abnormal CNS findings on exam.

LABORATORY INVESTIGATIONS

For most patients with diarrheal illness, laboratory studies and other investigations are not necessary. However, in complex cases, additional studies may be useful. In settings where microbiology laboratory resources are available, but limited, they can be utilized judiciously for surveillance to detect changing patterns in the etiology of diarrheal illness. Bacterial cultures and antibiotic susceptibility testing in cases of severe invasive diarrhea and in cases that do not respond to empiric antibiotic therapy are also an appropriate use of limited microbiology laboratory resources.

INVESTIGATIONS IN ACUTE WATERY DIARRHEA

Acute watery diarrhea is most often managed without any laboratory investigations. Assessing the degree of dehydration is a critical component of the evaluation of patients with diarrhea and can be performed using clinical parameters (see below). Serum and urine indices of dehydration do not provide additional predictive value beyond the clinical examination [6]. Similarly, determining the microbiologic etiology agent of acute watery diarrhea is usually unnecessary. *Vibrio cholerae* infection is an exception because patients with cholera may benefit from antibiotic therapy and because the diagnosis of cholera has public health implications. Cholera is definitively diagnosed based on bacterial culture using selective media; however, in countries where the disease is endemic, it can be diagnosed primarily on clinical grounds (see Chapter 43). A presumptive diagnosis of cholera can also be made using a rapid test (Crystal VC®, Span Diagnostics) or by the presence of motile *Vibrios*, which appear as "shooting stars" on dark field microscopic evaluation of stool.

When concomitant illnesses or life-threatening complications are suspected, the laboratory provides a useful adjunct to clinical evaluation and empiric therapy. Patients with seizures or altered consciousness should have a bedside glucose test and assessment for electrolyte disturbances. Appropriate laboratory investigations are warranted for children with suspected systemic infections such as pneumonia, sepsis, meningitis, urinary tract infection or malaria (see differential diagnosis).

INVESTIGATIONS IN INVASIVE DIARRHEA

The diagnosis of invasive diarrhea is made by the presence of blood and/or leukocytes in the stool. Direct microscopic examination of the stool, where available, is inexpensive and should support the clinical diagnosis by demonstrating abundant erythrocytes and polymorphonuclear cells in the stool. Most cases of invasive diarrhea in developing countries are caused by *Shigella* spp., and empiric antibiotics targeting *Shigella* spp. are warranted for invasive diarrhea. However, failure to improve within 48 hours should prompt consideration of performing a microbiologic analysis of stool including susceptibility profiles. Direct microscopy is also appropriate in such circumstances to evaluate for trophozoites of *E. histolytica* (Chapter 89), which warrants specific treatment for amebic dysentery.

INVESTIGATIONS IN PERSISTENT DIARRHEA

As with other categories of diarrheal illness, the identification of specific etiologic agents is not essential for the management of persistent diarrhea, as most cases will respond to empiric management. However, because of the associations between persistent diarrhea, malnutrition, HIV infection, and bacterial infections, patients presenting with persistent diarrhea should be evaluated for pneumonia, sepsis and other nonintestinal infections. Patients with unexplained persistent diarrhea should be tested for HIV.

MANAGEMENT AND OUTCOMES

Treatment of diarrheal illness involves rehydration, the use of antibiotics in selected instances, and nutritional interventions, including micronutrient supplementation in children. The WHO provides guidelines for the management of diarrheal illness in developing countries in "*The Treatment of Diarrhoea: A Manual for Physicians and Other Senior Health Workers*" [5].

REHYDRATION

The goal of rehydration therapy is to replace water and electrolytes lost in stool and vomitus (Fig. 22.2.1 and Table 22.2-1). Oral Rehydration Solution (ORS) – a mixture of water, salts and glucose administered by mouth – is the preferred mode of replacing these losses. Because fluid loss in acute watery diarrhea can be isonatremic, hyponatremic or hypernatremic, an advantage of correcting sodium imbalances with ORS is that the correction occurs relatively gradually, reducing the risk of neurologic complications that can occur with rapid shifts in osmolarity. Stool potassium losses commonly lead to hypokalemia, an important proximate cause of death among patients who die after rehydration therapy. Standard ORS contains more potassium than standard isotonic intravenous fluids, which is another advantage of oral rehydration. Hypo-osmolar ORS is inexpensive and widely available in developing countries. In rare cases, where ORS packets are not available, an acceptable solution can be prepared with six level teaspoons of sugar and one-half level teaspoon of table salt dissolved in one liter of safe water. Of note, patients with severe malnutrition require a distinct approach to rehydration (Box 22.2.1).

Rehydration is divided into replacement and maintenance phases.

Replacement Phase

The goal of the replacement phase is to rapidly correct the initial estimated fluid and electrolyte deficit. Patients without signs of dehydration do not require a specific replacement phase. In patients with signs of some (5–10%) dehydration, the patient should be kept under observation and fluid replacement should be continued until all signs of dehydration have resolved and the patient urinates. Optimally, this is achieved within four hours of initiation of therapy with ORS. However, 2–5% of patients presenting with some dehydration do not improve with ORS and have persistent signs of dehydration or progress to more severe (>10%) dehydration [7]. Failure of oral rehydration may be secondary to profound vomiting (more than twice an hour) or massive ongoing stool losses (more than 10 mL/kg/hour), such as seen in severe cholera.

Patients with severe dehydration should be treated emergently with isotonic intravenous fluids whenever possible. Ringer's lactate is the preferred fluid in most instances, but normal saline is an acceptable alternative. Blood products, colloids and hyptonic fluids should never be used for rehydration therapy. In addition, ORS should be initiated in addition to intravenous fluids as soon as the patient can drink, as isotonic intravenous fluid solutions primarily replace water and

TABLE 22.2-1 Composition of Diarrheal Stool and Rehydration Solutions (mmol/L)

Route	Solution	Na+	K+	Cl–	Base		Glucose/ Carbohydrate
					HCO^{3-}	Citrate	
Losses in Stool	Cholera stool – Adult	135	15	100	45	–	–
	Cholera stool – Child	105	25	30	30	–	–
	Non-cholera stool – Child	52	25	14	14	–	–
Oral Rehydration Solutions	Standard ORS	90	20	80	–	10	111
	Hypo-osmolar ORS*	75	20	65	–	10	75
	ReSoMal**	45	40	76	–	7	125
Intravenous Fluids	Ringer's Lactate	130	4	111	28	–	–
	Normal Saline	154	–	154	–	–	–

*Appropriate for rehydration of infants, children and adults with diarrhea.
**See Box 22.2.1.

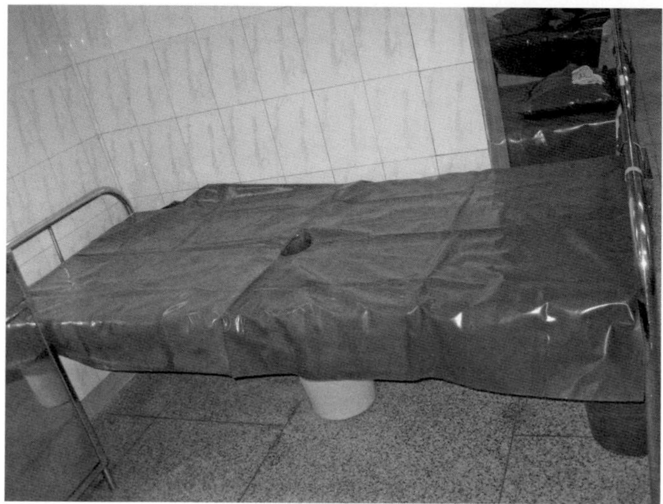

FIGURE 22.2.2 Cholera cot.

sodium, but do not replace glucose, potassium or other electrolyte losses.

Maintenance Phase

Maintenance phase begins once all signs of dehydration are absent. The goal of the maintenance phase is to counter ongoing losses of fluid and electrolytes in the stool and vomitus. Consumption of ORS or other suitable fluids *ad libitum* is appropriate in most cases. Although ORS is preferable, other suitable fluids include water, salted drinks and broths. Medicinal teas, coffee, carbonated beverages, and sweetened juices are not recommended and may exacerbate fluid losses.

In cases of massive ongoing losses, a cholera cot (Fig. 22.2.2) may facilitate recording of stool output in patients with severe diarrhea. Alternatively, stool losses can be estimated as 10–20 mL/kg per stool. The maintenance phase of rehydration is continued until all symptoms of diarrhea resolve.

ANTIBIOTICS

Antibiotics are not indicated for most individuals with acute watery diarrhea. Suspected cholera, particularly in outbreak settings, is an important exception in which antibiotic therapy can be useful in shortening the duration of illness and decreasing the amount of fluid resuscitation that is needed. Resistance is increasing in isolates of *V. cholerae*, hence data on local susceptibility should be used to guide treatment in suspected cholera cases (see Chapter 43).

Adults and children in resource-limited settings with invasive diarrhea should be treated promptly with an antimicrobial that is effective against *Shigella* (Chapter 44). This is of particular importance in those with higher risks of complications, including children younger than 5 years old, individuals with AIDS and the elderly. The choice of antimicrobial should be based on recent susceptibility data from *Shigella* strains isolated in the area, if available. In general, this will be sufficient to cover other common bacterial causes of invasive diarrhea. If clinical improvement does not occur within 48 hours after the initiation of antibiotic therapy, additional diagnostic testing for amebic dysentery (which will not respond to therapy directed at shigellosis) and culture for antibiotic resistant *Shigella* spp. is warranted. Alternatively, an empiric course of metronidazole or other agents directed at *E. histolytica* (Chapter 89) can be considered in patients with invasive diarrhea who do not respond to an appropriate trial of empiric treatment for shigellosis.

Antibiotics and the Risk of Hemolytic Uremic Syndrome

Sd1 produces shiga toxin, which is associated with hemolytic uremic syndrome. In patients with shigellosis treated with appropriate antibiotics, there does not appear to be an increase in toxin production or risk of hemolytic uremic syndrome [8]. This is in contrast to shiga toxin-producing strains of enterohemorrhagic *E. coli*, for which there is an increased risk of hemolytic uremic syndrome when antibiotics are administered. Fortunately, at this time, shiga toxin-producing *E. coli* remains a relatively rare cause of invasive diarrhea among children in resource-limited settings.

NUTRITION

The goals of nutritional intervention in patients with diarrhea are to identify and treat patients with severe nutritional deficiencies, and to prevent chronic enteropathy and malnutrition in otherwise apparently well-nourished children who are at risk of developing these sequelae after diarrheal illness.

Malnourished Children

The mortality among children with severe malnutrition and diarrhea may exceed 50%, but can be reduced to less than 10% using a standardized approach that incorporates the management of dehydration, nutrition, hypoglycemia and treatment of common concomitant infections [9]. Because of the increased risks of fluid overload and other complications of rehydration therapy, an alternative approach to assessing and treating dehydration is needed in severely malnourished patients (see Box 22.2.1). In addition, patients with severe malnutrition and diarrhea should be started on empiric broad-spectrum antibiotics immediately and on appropriate macro- and micronutrient therapy.

Apparently Well-Nourished Children

The continuous provision of nutritious food is important for all patients with diarrhea. Small meals should be provided frequently and should be initiated as soon as the patient is able to tolerate oral intake. Breastfeeding should always be continued in infants. Whenever possible, energy-rich food should be provided, including an extra meal (one meal more than usual) for at least two weeks after diarrheal symptoms resolve. In particular, children with persistent diarrhea require a calorie-rich diet; in some cases limitation of lactose intake may also be required.

Micronutrient Supplementation

In children, zinc supplementation reduces the severity and duration of diarrheal illness, as well as the incidence of subsequent episodes. The WHO recommends zinc supplementation for all children less than 5 years of age with diarrhea (10 mg/day for 10 days for children under 6 months and 20 mg/day for 10 days for children ages 6 months–5 years). Children with diarrhea are also at increased risk of vitamin A deficiency and should receive supplementation with vitamin A (administer a single dose; dosage is 50,000 IU for infants < 6 months, 100,000 IU for infants 6–12 months, and 200,000 IU for children >12 months). Children with xerophthalmia, severe malnutrition or measles should receive a series of three doses (administer a single dose, a second dose the following day, and a third at 2–4 weeks; dosage is as above).

OTHER THERAPIES

Antimotility agents, including loperamide, diphenoxylate-atropine and tincture of opium may cause paralytic ileus in children, while anti-emetics, including chlorpromazine, prochlorperazine, promethazine and metoclopramide have sedating effects that can interfere with rehydration and may cause extrapyramidal reactions. Therefore, these agents should be particularly avoided in children.

PREVENTION

Most cases of diarrhea are associated with contaminated food and water sources. Epidemics of diarrhea may affect individuals in refugee camps and unplanned urban settlements, with limited access to water and sanitation facilities. Direct contact with an infected individual may also contribute to the spread of epidemic dysentery caused by *Shigella* spp. Acute diarrheal diseases can be prevented with measures such as exclusive breastfeeding through to 6 months of age and continued breastfeeding with complementary foods through to 2 years of age, hand-washing, provision of safe drinking water, appropriate disposal of human waste, safe handling of food and control of flies. The WHO Strategic Advisory Group of Experts recommends that rotavirus vaccine be included in national immunization programs, particularly in countries where diarrheal deaths account for ≥10 percent of mortality among children aged <5 years.

BOX 22.2.1 Approach to Rehydration in the Severely Malnourished Child

- The ability to accurately predict the degree of dehydration based on the standard WHO clinical criteria is altered. For example, the lack of subcutanous fat, the presence of edema, and the presence of baseline apathy interfere with assessment of skin turgor and mental status as indicators of dehydration and intravascular volume.
- Cool or clammy extremities, diminished pulses and diminished urine output are all signs that suggest poor perfusion and indicate that additional fluids are needed to replace intravascular volume losses secondary to dehydration and/or sepsis.
- In general, rehydration in patients with severe malnutrition is approached cautiously because of the risks of fluid overload, hypernatremia, and hypokalemia.
- For these reasons, oral rehydration requires a specialized composition (ReSoMal – see Table 22.2-1) and should be given slowly as 70–100 ml/kg over 12 hours.
- Intravenous fluids should only be used in severely malnourished patients in the setting of overt shock.

REFERENCES

1. World Health Organization. The Global Burden of Disease: 2004 Update. Geneva: World Health Organization; 2008.
2. Boschi-Pinto C, Velebit L, Shibuya K. Estimating child mortality due to diarrhoea in developing countries. Bull World Health Organ 2008;86:710–17.
3. Bryce J, Boschi-Pinto C, Shibuya K, Black RE, WHO Child Health Epidemiology Reference Group. WHO estimates of the causes of death in children. Lancet 2005;365:1147–52.
4. World Health Organization. WHO case definitions of HIV for surveillance and revised clinical staging and immunologic classification of HIV-related disease in adults and children. Geneva: World Health Organization; 2007.
5. World Health Organization. The treatment of diarrhoea, a manual for physicians and other senior health workers. 4th revision. WHO/FCH/CAH/05.1. Geneva: World Health Organization; 2005 (last accessed on 8 January 2010 at: http://whqlibdoc.who.int/publications/2005/9241593180.pdf).
6. Steiner MJ, DeWalt DA, Byerley JS. Is this child dehydrated? JAMA 2004;29:2746–54.
7. Hartling L, Bellemare S, Wiebe N, et al. Oral versus intravenous rehydration for treating dehydration due to gastroenteritis in children. Cochrane Database Syst Rev 2006;3:CD004390.
8. Bennish ML, Khan WA, Begum M, et al. Low risk of hemolytic uremic syndrome after early effective antimicrobial therapy for shigella dysenteriae type 1 infection in Bangladesh. Clin Infect Dis 2006;42:356–62.
9. Ahmed T, Ali M, Ullah MM, et al. Mortality in severely malnourished children with diarrhoea and use of a standardised management protocol. Lancet 1999;353:1919–22.

SECTION

D

TOPIC-BASED CHAPTERS

23 Cancer in the Tropics

Katie Wakeham, Robert Newton, Freddy Sitas

Key features

- Cancer incidence and mortality are not well measured in many parts of the developing world and so understanding of the burden of disease is based on estimates
- Cancer incidence and mortality are increasing in the developing world
- Infections represent the most important cause of cancer in developing countries, although the impact of tobacco and other lifestyle factors normally associated with more affluent countries is increasing
- Many cancers can be prevented with modification of lifestyle, screening, or vaccination against oncogenic infections
- Methods for adequate diagnosis and management of cancer are not widely available in many developing countries

INTRODUCTION

In this chapter we describe patterns of cancer in developing countries, outline some of the most important causes, and briefly examine issues relating to screening and prevention. We then go on to discuss treatment and palliation in resource-poor settings. Clinical signs and symptoms of different cancer types are addressed in many other textbooks and are not discussed further here. Some of the content is updated from a chapter in the previous edition of this volume by Parkin and Ziegler.

Before going further, it is important to note that estimation of the burden of cancer (or any other disease) in developing countries is problematic and so data should be interpreted with appropriate caution. Overall, about 4–5% of the population of developing countries is covered by routine registration of mortality statistics. Cancer registries are another important source of data on cancer occurrence, but again, they cover only limited geographic areas – about 3% of the population of developing countries – although they can provide information on the current cancer profile and its evolution over time. Based on these limited data, it is possible to obtain working estimates of the burden of cancer in tropical countries and elsewhere (both incidence – usually expressed as the number of new cases per 100,000 people per year – and mortality), albeit with a number of important methodologic caveats.

In the year 2008, it is estimated that about 12.7 million people worldwide were diagnosed with cancer and about 7.6 million people died from the disease, an increase of about 25% since 1990 [1,2]. Overall, cancer causes about 10% of all deaths worldwide – 27% of deaths in developed countries, 15% in middle-income countries and about 6% in low-income countries – and is second only to cardiovascular disease as a cause of death globally [3]. Much of the disparity between developed and developing countries is the result of differences in the age structure of populations and the greater burden of infectious disease and perinatal mortality in the developing world. Over 80% of the population is aged less than 45 years in the developing world, compared to about 65% in the developed world (Fig. 23.1) and cancer is predominantly a disease of older people [1]. Despite this, although cancer is usually regarded as a problem of the developed world, about two-thirds of all cancers occur in the three-quarters of the world's population who live in developing countries, where comprehensive cancer control programs are limited or absent. There are more than 20 million people living with cancer at any time – the majority will not have access to appropriate diagnostic technology, curative treatment, or palliative care. Furthermore, the number of cases of cancer worldwide is likely to increase by about 50% by 2020 [2], primarily because of increasing longevity of many populations and because of trends in the prevalence of smoking and other important risk factors.

In the developed world, cancers of the lung, breast, prostate, colon and rectum and hematologic malignancies predominate, whereas in the developing world the pattern differs. Whilst cancers of the lung and breast remain frequent, cancers of the cervix, liver, stomach and esophagus are also relatively common, reflecting differences in the prevalence of underlying causal factors. These estimates are available from the GLOBOCAN database at http://www.iarc.fr [1]. Indeed, even for those cancers for which the cause is unknown, the large differences in the pattern of cancer incidence between populations and over time suggest that cancer might be largely avoided if the responsible environmental factors could be identified and moderated.

CANCER CAUSES AND CONTROL

TOBACCO

It is estimated that tobacco causes about 5 million deaths per year, corresponding to about a third of deaths in men aged 35–69 in North America and Europe and between 12% and 20% in the rest of the world [4]. It causes many diseases, of which the most important are cardiovascular disease, chronic obstructive lung disease, and various cancers, including a large proportion of those of the lung, pancreas, bladder, kidney, larynx, mouth, pharynx and esophagus. It is also associated with other types of cancer, such as stomach, liver, cervix, nasal cavities, colorectum and myeloid leukemia [5]. In parts of Southeast Asia in particular, the combination of tobacco use and chewing of betel quid is an important risk factor for cancers of the mouth and pharynx.

Stopping smoking at any age has a rapid beneficial effect on cancer risk. Indeed, in some developed countries, reductions in tobacco consumption have been associated with declining incidence of certain cancers, such as lung cancer. However, cigarette consumption is increasing markedly in developing countries. Because of this rising prevalence of smoking in developing countries, the incidence of many cancers and other tobacco-related diseases is rising, emphasizing the

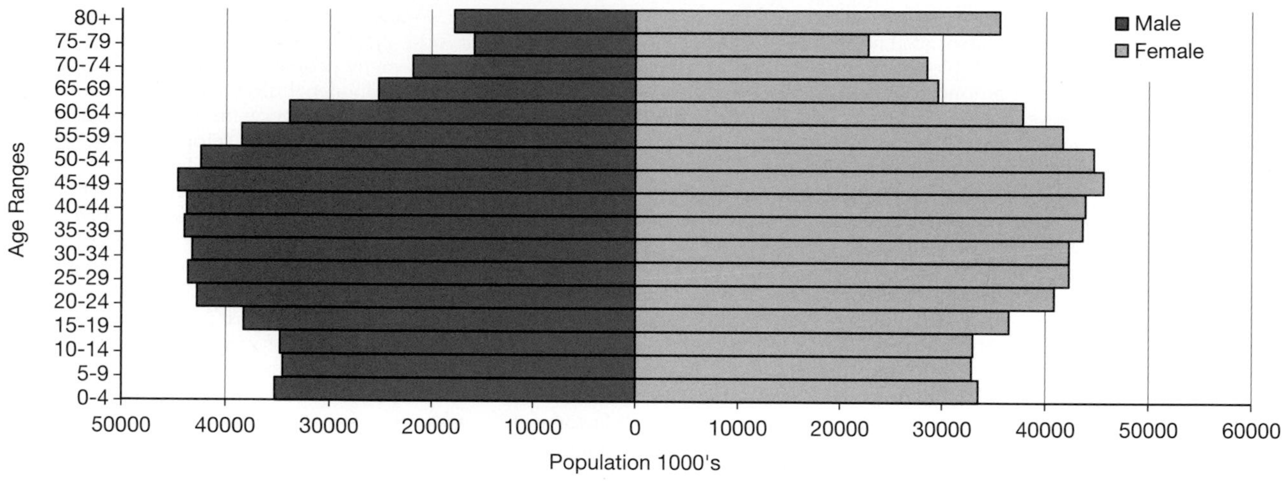

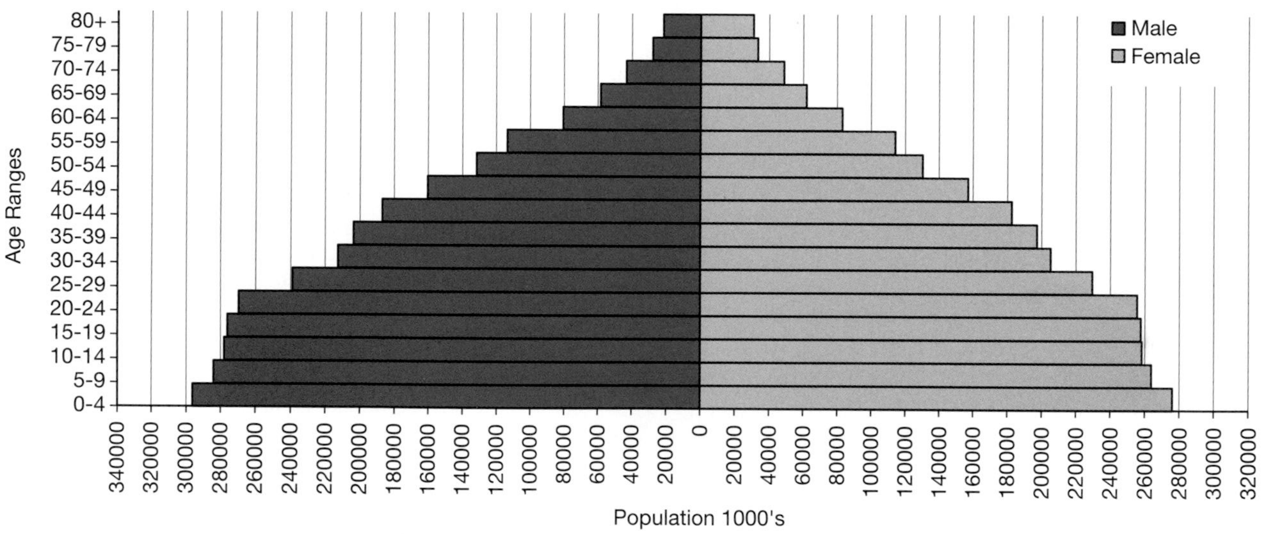

FIGURE 23.1 Age structure of developing (bottom) and developed (top) country populations.

importance of tobacco control programs. For example, in some Asian countries, lung cancer mortality rates have more than doubled in the last 30 years. Indeed, it has been estimated that if smoking rates could be halved, between 20 and 30 million premature deaths from all causes would be avoided by 2025 and about 150 million deaths by 2050 [4]. Efforts to reduce tobacco consumption are therefore central to preventing deaths from cancer and other diseases.

INFECTIONS

Collectively, infectious agents are the most important established cause of cancer after tobacco. Approximately 18% of cancers worldwide (about 1.6 million cases per year) are attributable to viral (13%), bacterial (5%), and helminth (0.1%) infections, the majority of which occur in the developing world [4]. In theory, if these infectious diseases were controlled, up to one in four cancers in developing countries, and one in ten cancers in developed countries, could be prevented.

More cancer cases are attributable to human papillomavirus (HPV) infection than to any other transmissible agent. It is well established that certain HPVs are the major causative agent for invasive cervical cancer. The most common HPV subtypes identified in tumors are HPV16, 18, 31, 33 and 45, although in some Asian countries the subtypes HPV52 and 58 are more common. The same subtypes also account for up to 80% of cancers of the anus and approximately one-third of cancers of the penis, vagina and vulva. HPV infection may also cause some cancers of the head and neck (particularly cancers of the oral cavity) [6]. In developed countries, cervical cancer screening programs that rely on the detection, by exfoliative cervical cytology, of treatable precancerous lesions, are established and are effective at reducing both the incidence and mortality of invasive cervical cancer. However, in many developing countries, screening procedures do not yet exist and incidence and mortality rates are still very high. Vaccination against the main HPV subtypes at an early age holds the most promise to substantially reduce the incidence of this cancer, although the cost remains prohibitively high. However, cheaper HPV DNA screening technology has emerged and this is proving to be much more cost-effective than vaccination at current costs [7].

Chronic infection with the hepatitis B virus is responsible for causing more than 300,000 liver cancers (specifically hepatocellular carcinoma) each year, which corresponds to about 60% of all primary liver cancers across the world [6]. Approximately 10% of the population in parts of sub-Saharan Africa, China, and Southeast Asia are infected with the hepatitis B virus. Transmission can occur from a mother to her child, from person to person during childhood, and via sexual or parenteral transmission during adulthood. About two-thirds of these people will develop chronic hepatitis, and a quarter of these will eventually die from primary liver cancer or cirrhosis, making liver cancer one of the most common cancers in these areas. Prospects for the prevention of hepatitis B virus-associated liver cancer are good. In developed countries, screening of blood and organ donors has reduced the spread of infection among adults. In areas where infection is most prevalent, however, the best hope for prevention lies with mass vaccination against the hepatitis B virus. Although it will be many years before an effect on the incidence of liver cancer is demonstrated in adults, the introduction of mass vaccination in Taiwan has already been associated with a sharp decline in the incidence of liver cancer in children and young adults [4].

The unrelated hepatitis C virus is also involved in the etiology of hepatocellular carcinoma and may cause about 25% of all liver cancers, with particularly high proportions in Africa (41%), Japan (36%) and Oceania (33%). The prevalence of hepatitis C virus infection is estimated to be about 1–1.5% in Europe and North America, about 3% in Japan and Oceania (excluding Australia and New Zealand), and up to 3.6% in Africa. Transmission is commonly via the parenteral route, although sexual and perinatal transmission can also occur. However, almost half of all hepatitis C-infected individuals have no identifiable risk factors [8]. Although a vaccine is not currently available, screening programs have greatly reduced transmission of hepatitis C via blood transfusions.

Infection with the Epstein-Barr virus (EBV) is involved in the etiology of several types of lymphoma (including Burkitt's lymphoma, Hodgkin disease, and immunosuppression-related lymphomas) and nasopharyngeal carcinoma, and may contribute up to 100,000 cancers per year worldwide [6]. Indeed, Burkitt lymphoma (associated with both EBV and malaria) is the commonest childhood cancer in many tropical areas. EBV infects more than 90% of the world's population and is usually acquired during childhood. It is transmitted orally in saliva and establishes a latent infection with lifelong persistence in the infected host. The overgrowth of virally transformed B cells is controlled by specific cytotoxic T-cell responses, the absence of which (in HIV-infected people for example) can result in lymphoma.

Kaposi's sarcoma-associated herpesvirus (KSHV) is related to the Epstein-Barr virus and is the principal cause of Kaposi's sarcoma [6]. It also causes a rare type of lymphoma (primary effusion lymphoma) and a lymphoproliferative B-cell disorder (Castleman's disease). KSHV is most prevalent in populations at highest risk of developing Kaposi sarcoma, such as homosexual men infected with HIV in Western countries and in African populations where the tumor has long been endemic.

Human T-cell leukemia virus type 1 (HTLV-1) is a causal agent of adult T-cell leukemia/lymphoma. It is estimated that there are about 15–20 million individuals infected with HTLV-1 worldwide, predominantly in Japan, the Caribbean, South America, and Central Africa. Adult T-cell leukemia/lymphoma develops in about 2–5% of HTLV-1-infected individuals and is especially frequent among those infected early in life. Perinatal transmission has been greatly reduced in Japan by avoidance of prolonged breastfeeding (i.e. more than 6 months), although this is not an option for many developing countries, where the risk of death from diarrheal disease rises markedly if breastfeeding is curtailed. Several countries have introduced universal screening of blood donors [6,8].

There is little evidence that the human immunodeficiency virus (HIV) has a direct oncogenic effect. Instead, its immunosuppressive effect appears to facilitate the development of Kaposi sarcoma, non-Hodgkin and Hodgkin lymphoma, and cancers of the cervix, anus and conjunctiva [6]. In areas of sub-Saharan Africa where HIV infection is highly prevalent, the incidence of Kaposi sarcoma has increased about 20-fold with the spread of HIV, such that in Uganda and Zimbabwe it is now the most common cancer in males and among the most common in females. There is evidence of a reduction in the increase in risk of both Kaposi's sarcoma and non-Hodgkin lymphoma among those on antiretroviral therapy for HIV [9]. However, in the developing world, the incidence of HIV-associated cancers is increasing as the epidemic spreads.

About half of the world's population is chronically infected with the bacterium *Helicobacter pylori*. This bacterium colonizes the stomach lining, and, although many people remain asymptomatic, some go on to develop gastric or duodenal ulcers. In a very small proportion of infected individuals, gastric adenocarcinoma and, to a lesser extent, gastric non-Hodgkin lymphoma may develop [6]. Although it is clear that *H. pylori* infection plays a role in the development of stomach cancer, other factors, such as diet, are also involved. The prevalence of infection is highest in developing countries and increases rapidly during the first two decades of life, such that 80–90% of the population may be infected by early adulthood; in most developed countries, the prevalence of infection is now substantially lower. Rates of infection with *H. pylori* have fallen over the last few decades, and this could explain much of the parallel decline in stomach cancer rates seen in most countries. This may be due to improvements in living conditions and trends towards a smaller family size, both of which are risk factors for *H. pylori* infection. Although antibiotics are effective in eradicating *H. pylori* in about 80% of cases, this has proved to be difficult to implement on a large scale and re-infection is common.

Infestation with the water-borne trematode *Schistosoma haematobium*, which causes schistosomiasis (bilharzia), is associated with an increased risk of squamous cell carcinoma of the bladder, and is the predominant cause of this cancer in tropical and subtropical areas. Schistosomiasis affects approximately 200 million people worldwide and is endemic in Northern Africa and the Middle East; in these areas, over half of the population is at risk of infection from contaminated water supplies (lakes, rivers, swamps) that contain the larvae. There is also some evidence that *S. japonicum* and, to a lesser extent, *S. mansoni* are related to the development of cancers of the liver and colorectum in China. Although treatable, preventative measures focusing on reducing contact with contaminated water supplies are currently the best method of reducing infection. Food-borne trematodes (liver flukes), such as *Opisthorchis viverrini*, *Opisthorchis felineus* and *Clonorchis sinensis*, are an established cause of cancer of the bile ducts (cholangiocarcinoma) in parts of Southeast Asia, due to consumption of raw or undercooked freshwater fish that contain the infective stage of the fluke. Control of infection has been achieved in some areas by a combination of chemotherapy, health education, and improved sanitation. However, eradication programs have, as yet, had little effect on the incidence of cholangiocarcinoma in these areas and a vaccine is not yet available.

OTHER FACTORS

Hormonal and reproductive factors play an important role in the etiology of a number of cancers in women, especially breast cancer. Established risk factors include early age at menarche, older age at first birth, low parity, and late age at menopause. The combination of these factors may explain much of the geographic variation in the incidence of breast cancer. Many of these reproductive factors suggest that cumulative exposure to estrogens during a woman's lifetime increases the risk of breast cancer. It is now known that high circulating levels of estrogens are directly associated with breast cancer risk, at least in postmenopausal women [10]. Further evidence for a role of hormones comes from consistent observations that current users of exogenous hormones, either in the form of oral and injectable contraceptives or hormone replacement therapy (HRT), have a 25–35% higher risk of developing breast cancer than never-users [10]. However, this risk appears to be transient and has largely disappeared after 10 years since stopping. Reproductive factors are also strongly related to ovarian cancer and, as for endometrial cancer, the most established protective factors are parity and use of hormonal contraceptives. In general, a first-term pregnancy is associated with about a 40% reduction in risk, with a smaller reduction in risk with each term pregnancy thereafter.

Several dietary factors, such as fat and meat, have been suggested to increase cancer risk, while other factors, such as fruit, vegetables and fibre, have been hypothesized to decrease risk. However, despite extensive research over the last two decades, few specific dietary determinants of cancer risk have been established, even for cancers such as colorectal cancer where dietary factors are the most obvious candidate risk factors. This is due to various reasons, the most important being the difficulty in accurately measuring dietary intake in epidemiologic studies. Other problems with epidemiologic studies of diet and cancer include the relatively narrow range of dietary exposures within one population, and the changes in dietary patterns over time, so that it is very difficult to determine whether dietary habits at a young age may affect cancer risk later in life. A high intake of alcoholic beverages increases the risk of cancers of the upper respiratory and digestive tracts (oral cavity, tongue, pharynx, larynx, esophagus). These cancers are also caused by smoking, and the increase in risk is particularly great for people who both smoke and drink heavily [5]. Heavy and prolonged alcohol consumption is also associated with liver cancer via the development of cirrhosis and alcoholic hepatitis. Cancers of the upper gastrointestinal tract are particularly associated with excessive alcohol consumption, although a moderate intake of 10 g of alcohol per day (approximately one drink) has been shown to increase the risk of breast cancer by around 7%.

Aflatoxins are mycotoxins produced by many species of the fungus *Aspergillus* and are among the most carcinogenic substances known. The fungi live in soil, particularly in warm and damp conditions, such as in the tropics, and are a common contaminant of cereals, oilseeds, nuts and spices. The toxin can also be found in milk from humans and livestock if the food supply is contaminated [11]. Consequences of exposure can include growth retardation and hepatic necrosis leading to cirrhosis and carcinoma of the liver. Concurrent infection with hepatitis B virus increases the risk of cancer further, since it interferes with the metabolism of aflatoxins.

Overweight and obesity are usually measured in terms of an individual's body mass index (BMI) (weight in kilograms divided by height in meters squared), where a BMI of greater than 25 kg/m^2 is considered overweight and a BMI of greater than 30 kg/m^2 is considered obese. Overweight and obesity increase the risk of colon cancer by about a third and increase the risk of breast cancer in postmenopausal (but not premenopausal) women by about a half. Overweight and obesity are associated with an approximate threefold increased risk of endometrial cancer in both pre- and postmenopausal women, and may account for up to 40% of endometrial cancer worldwide. Overweight and obesity also increase the risk of cancers of the kidney and gallbladder and of adenocarcinoma (but not squamous cell carcinoma) of the esophagus. It has been estimated that overweight and obesity account for about 5% of all cancers in Europe, most of which are cancers of the colon, endometrium and breast. Thus, up to 36,000 cases of cancer could be prevented each year if the prevalence of overweight and obesity in Europe was halved [12]. In countries such as the US, where the prevalence of obesity is higher than in Europe, an even higher proportion of cancers may be attributable to being overweight. Furthermore, the prevalence of obesity is increasing in both developed and developing countries, and is therefore expected to lead to a greater burden of cancers in the future.

MANAGEMENT OF CANCER

Cancer management requires multidisciplinary services and is often a complex and expensive process. In Western countries, the pathway starts with access to cancer services, often through screening or a primary care physician. Decisions surrounding the most appropriate treatment for an individual with cancer require: 1) an accurate pathologic diagnosis which may involve sophisticated immunohistologic and genetic profiling; 2) imaging, for stage, planning treatment, and monitoring; 3) biochemical markers, for example prostate-specific antigen (PSA), for monitoring, diagnosis, prognosis, response and relapse; and 4) laboratory work-up including hematology and renal and liver function tests. There are four general modalities of treatment for cancer: 1) surgery; 2) drugs, including hormones and chemotherapies; 3) radiotherapy; and 4) symptom control or palliative care. Outcome for treatment of malignant disease, in general, depends on the clinical and pathologic stage (tumor, size, nodal involvement, metastasis [local or distant], histologic features [spectrum from benign to aggressive]) and patient comorbidities or performance status.

Cure or long-term survival from cancer is largely dependent on cancer stage. All treatment modalities work best on small localized tumors with nonaggressive histologic features. In low-income settings, presentation with cancer (like other illnesses) is very often late with widespread neoplastic disease and a high burden of symptoms. Factors impacting on access to medical care are multifactorial, involving patient awareness of cancer and symptoms, fear of stigmatization, preference for traditional healers [13], cultural barriers that cancer is induced by supernatural forces and /or incurable [14], health worker knowledge, health infrastructure, and cost to patients. Once accessed, the availability of diagnostic and treatment modalities is often limited, resulting in generally poor survival in these settings. Adherence to treatment regimens is often low [15]. For countries already overstretched and grappling with infectious disease including HIV, TB and malaria, cancer is not a priority for healthcare. Cancer survival in resource-poor settings is currently very poor, particularly in sub-Saharan Africa [16,17], and is directly associated with per capita annual government healthcare expenditure and number of physicians [16]. Government expenditure on health in 2006 (US$), was $8 for low-income countries compared to $3076 in the USA, with only four physicians per 10,000 population in low-income countries compared to 27 per 10,000 in high-income countries [18].

Surgery is an essential part of treatment for solid neoplastic disease and the modality most likely to cure. Again, the probability of cure is increased when the cancer is small and localized, but surgery also plays a role in the management of metastasis and in palliation, for example of bowel obstruction, fistulas and gastrointestinal bleeds. There is a paucity of data from resource-poor settings on surgical oncology provision, but unmet surgical need it likely to be very high [19].

Cancer chemotherapies kill cancer cells by preventing cell division, disrupting DNA or RNA or nucleic acids. It is effective against systemic disease and can be used with both palliative and curative intent before and after surgery and/or radiotherapy. Other forms of drug treatments include hormones (for example, the anti-estrogen tamoxifen for estrogen receptor-positive breast cancer, and LHRH antagonists for prostate cancer) and immunotherapy (for example, interferon-alpha, used for some hematologic malignancies, and monoclonal antibodies, including trastuzumab and rituximab). Drugs with different mechanisms of action are often given in combination to increase efficacy. In resource-limited settings, low availability of cancer drugs – together with the drugs required to control side effects, including antiemetics and antibiotics is problematic. Cytotoxic agents, tamoxifen and steroids are listed in the WHO essential medicines complementary list, which presents essential medicines for priority diseases which need specialist care and/or high costs [20]. Chemotherapies ideally require specialist pharmacy rooms for preparation, a high degree of sterility, dedicated and highly trained staff and high levels of support to manage iatrogenic toxicities.

Radiotherapy is a common component of cancer treatment for cure or palliation and can be used alone or as an adjuvant to surgery to destroy cancer cells remaining in the tumor bed or with chemotherapy. Radiation acts by damaging cellular DNA by forming free radicals. Cancer cells have less ability to repair DNA damage than healthy cells and lose reproductive capacity or die by apoptosis. Radiotherapy can be broadly divided into external beam or local, where the radiation source is placed in the body, within or close to the cancer. External beam megavoltage radiation can be derived from a radioactive source such as cobalt-60 or by accelerating electrons at high energy to produce photons (linear accelerator). Resource-limited settings are more likely to use a radioactive source over a linear accelerator as it is comparatively cheaper, robust, requires only limited electricity and is much easier to maintain. Safe provision requires specifically designed buildings, monitoring, and an extensive team of trained medical, engineering and scientific staff.

Programme of Action for Cancer Therapy (PACT) is part of the International Atomic Energy Authority (IAEA). It was established

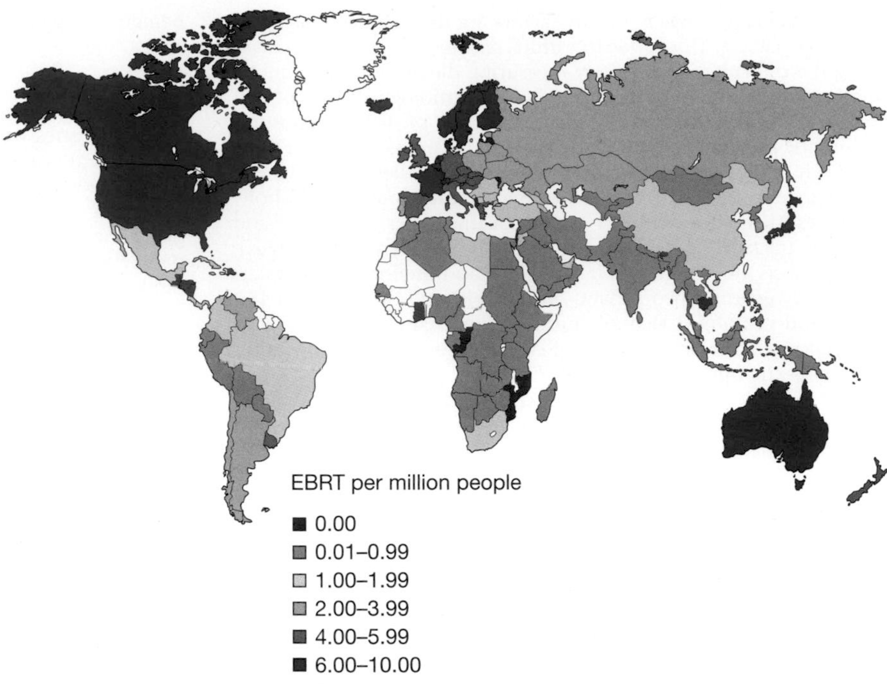

FIGURE 23.2 Worldwide distribution of external beam radiotherapy machines (EBRT machines). *(Source: Directory of Radiotherapy Centres [DIRAC], International Atomic Energy Agency, last accessed 4th November 2011 and Population Division of the Department of Economic and Social Affairs of the United Nations Secretariat (2009). World Population Prospects: The 2008 Revision. Highlights. New York: United Nations).*

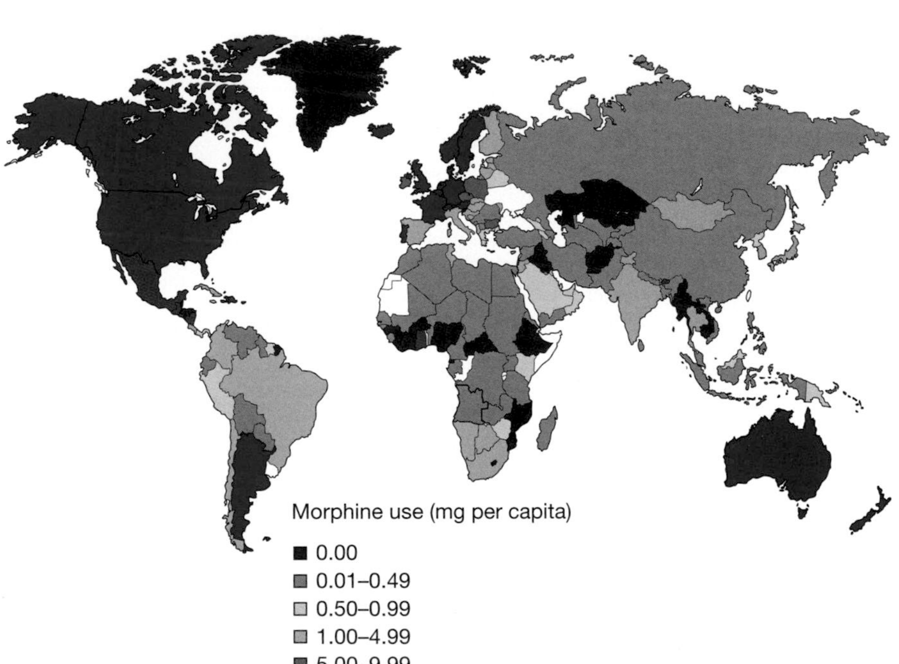

FIGURE 23.3 Countries that registered use of a strong opioid between 2003 and 2007 with the International Narcotics Control Board (INCB), with "low levels of opioid consumption indicating inadequate medical availability" (INCB Annual Reports 2003 to 2007, most recently available data taken for each country).

in 2004 to support and monitor radiotherapy in developing countries. A survey of Africa in 2002 reported that the provision of megavoltage radiotherapy machines was only 18% of the estimated need [21] (Fig. 23.2). Most low-income countries have less than one machine per million population and many have no machine at all.

The WHO state that "inadequate management of pain due to cancer is a serious public health problem in the world" [22]. Opioid analgesics are essential for pain relief. Morphine is highly effective for moderate and severe cancer pain. It is relatively cheap, the oral formulations are easy to administer, and it appears on the WHO three-step analgesic ladder and list of essential medicines. But few of those in need in a resource-limited setting have access to it or indeed to any opioid. Barriers to opioid access include: 1) cost, 2) lack of trained medical workforce to administer, 3) international regulations on manufacture and distribution of opioids, and 4) health worker and public attitude and knowledge due to concerns over addiction (Fig. 23.3). Advocacy groups, including Hospice Africa, have made great progress in improving access to symptom control by lobbying governments, training, increasing awareness and developing feasible models of care for resource-limited settings.

REFERENCES

1. www.iarc.fr
2. Ferlay J, Shin HR, Bray F, et al. Estimates of worldwide burden of cancer 2008: GLOBOCAN 2008. Int J Cancer 2010;127:2893–917.
3. www.who.int/healthinfo/global_burden_disease
4. Stewart BW, Kleihues P, eds. World Health Organization, World Cancer Report. Lyon: IARC Press; 2003.
5. Secretan B, Straif K, Baan R, et al. on behalf of the WHO International Agency for Research on Cancer Monograph Working Group. A review of human carcinogens – Part E: tobacco, areca nut, alcohol, coal smoke and salted fish. Lancet Oncol 2009;10:1033–4.
6. Bouvard V, Baan R, Straif K, et al. on behalf of the WHO International Agency for Research on Cancer Monograph Working Group. A review of human carcinogens – Part B: biological agents. Lancet Oncol 2009;10:321–2.
7. Canfell K, Shi JF, Lew JB, et al. Prevention of cervical cancer in rural China: evaluation of HPV vaccination and primary HPV screening strategies. Vaccine 2011;13:2487–94.
8. Newton R. Infections and cancer. In: Alison MR, ed. Cancer Handbook. London: Macmillan; 2002.
9. International Collaboration on HIV and Cancer. The impact of highly active anti-retroviral therapy on the incidence of cancer in people infected with the human immunodeficiency virus. J Natl Cancer Inst 2000;92:1823–30.
10. Allen N, Newton R, Banks E, et al. The causes of cancer. In: Franks L, ed. Introduction to the Cellular and Molecular Biology of Cancer, 4th edn. Oxford, UK: Oxford University Press; 2005:25–44.
11. IARC Working Group on the Evaluation of Carcinogenic Risks to Humans. Some traditional herbal medicines, some mycotoxins, naphthalene and styrene. IARC Monogr Eval Carcinog Risks Hum 2002;82:1–556.
12. Bergstrom A, Pisani P, Tenet V, et al. Overweight as an avoidable cause of cancer in Europe. Int J Cancer 2001;91:421–30.
13. Kazaura MR, Kombe D, Yuma S, et al. Health seeking behavior among cancer patients attending Ocean Road Cancer Institute, Tanzania. East Afr J Public Health. 2007;4:19–22.
14. Newton R, Ngilimana PJ, Grulich A, et al. Cancer in Rwanda. Int J Cancer 1996;66:75–81.
15. Anyanwu SN, Egwuonwu OA, Ihekwoaba EC. Acceptance and adherence to treatment among breast cancer patients in Eastern Nigeria. Breast 2011;20 Suppl 2:S51–3.
16. Ribeiro RC, Steliarova-Foucher E, Magrath I, et al. Baseline status of paediatric oncology care in ten low-income or mid-income countries receiving My Child Matters support: a descriptive study. Lancet Oncol 2008;9:721–9.
17. Sankaranarayanan R, Swaminathan R, Brenner H, et al. Cancer survival in Africa, Asia, and Central America: a population-based study. Lancet Oncol 2010;11:165–73.
18. World Health Organization (WHO). World Health Statistics 2009. Geneva: WHO; 2009.
19. Ozgediz D, Jamison D, Cherian M, McQueen K. The burden of surgical conditions and access to surgical care in low- and middle-income countries. Bull World Health Organ 2008;86:646–7
20. World Health Organization (WHO). The Selection and Use of Essential Medicines: Report of the WHO Expert Committee, 2009 (including the 16th WHO Model List of Essential Medicines and the 2nd WHO Model List of Essential Medicines for Children). WHO Technical Report Series 958. Geneva: WHO; 2009.
21. Barton MB, Frommer M, Shafiq J. Role of radiotherapy in cancer control in low-income and middle-income countries. Lancet Oncol 2006;7:584–95. Erratum in: Lancet Oncol 2006;7:797.
22. World Health Organization Department of Essential Drugs and Medicines Policy. Narcotic and Psychotropic Drugs: Achieving Balance in National Opioids Control Policy: Guidelines for Assessment. Geneva: World Health Organization; 2000.

24 Heat-associated Illness

Michael V Callahan

Key features

- Heat-associated illnesses are a spectrum of clinical syndromes ranging from minor heat exhaustion to life-threatening conditions characterized by rhabdomyolysis, renal failure and encephalopathy
- In the tropics, loss of shade trees, droughts, intense solar exposure and high humidity increase the incidence and severity of heat illness
- Hydration status, extremes of age, comorbidities and the use of certain traditional remedies, pharmaceuticals and alcohol can all impair physiologic cooling mechanisms, leading to heat illness
- Heat waves, or the combined effects of high heat, high humidity and lack of potable water and cool havens, may cause mass-casualty incidents that may overwhelm local medical resources
- Treatment of heat illness in the tropics requires an understanding of the physiology of heat load and heat loss, heightened clinical vigilance and prompt, effective use of cooling therapies

DEFINITION

Heat illnesses result from an imbalance of metabolic heat production or environmental heat loading and inadequate heat dissipation [1]. In healthy adults, thermoregulation dissipates metabolic and exogenous heat to maintain core body temperatures between 36 °C and 37.8 °C. Extreme heat loads can overwhelm thermoregulatory responses, resulting in heat illness. Heat illness syndromes should not be confused with fever, which is a physiologic increase in the temperature set point of the body, or with malignant hyperthermia – a hereditary metabolic hyperthermic response to certain pharmaceuticals or anesthetic gases. If overheating continues and the patient is left untreated, milder forms of heat illness, such as heat edema, may progress to more severe manifestations of heat illness, such as heat stroke, which, if untreated, can have a case fatality rate of 63%. The key syndromes associated with different heat illnesses are listed in Table 24-1.

EPIDEMIOLOGY

Heat illness is common among athletes, soldiers, foundry workers and in the general population during mass gatherings in hot environments such as the annual Hajj pilgrimage [2, 3]. Among young athletes, the most severe form of heat illness – heat stroke – is the second leading cause of death [4]. In tropical regions, heat casualties are common and may be increasing in developing economies as more workers are required to work under sweltering conditions. In many settings, inadequate access to cool havens or to cold, potable water increase the risk of heat illness. Epidemiologic studies on heat illness conducted in the USA and Europe [5, 6]indicate the groups at highest risk of heat illness are children under four years of age, the elderly, those with renal and endocrine disorders, and institutionalized and hospitalized patients [7, 8]. In particular, the importance of sweat-based evaporative cooling is demonstrated by the higher incidence of heat illness in the elderly and in patients being treated with anticholinergic medication [9, 10]. At this time, there are no convincing studies demonstrating differences in risk of heat illness between genders. Acclimatization to heat can reduce the risk of heat illness. Acclimatization involves near- and long-term physiologic adaptation; key findings include: rapid correction of water loss and improved sodium preservation and gradual normalization of plasma electrolytes, altered blood perfusion to the skin, and reduced sodium concentrations in sweat and urine. New arrivals to tropical climes undergo limited acclimatization over a 2–4–week period; subsequent advances in acclimatization are both limited and not definitively proven by the current literature.

PATHOPHYSIOLOGY

Heat illnesses are the result of excessive heat loads from the environment, the body's inability to dissipate heat or a combination of the two. In healthy individuals, the body compensates for heat stress by thermoregulatory processes and, less effectively, through adaptive processes. As total body heat load rises, a sensitive thermoregulatory system responds by stimulating the pre-optic nucleus of the anterior hypothalamus, which causes the dilation of cutaneous blood vessels and an increase in sweat production [11]. Familiarity with the mechanisms of heat loss allows the clinician to diagnose impaired thermoregulation and select the optimum cooling strategy for different patients and different treatment settings. There are four primary strategies that humans use to dissipate heat to the surrounding environment: evaporation, radiation, convection and conduction. Care providers who understand these mechanisms of heat loss are well positioned to exploit these mechanisms to greater effect using focal cold therapy. The major form of heat loss in hot, dry climates is evaporation of sweat or surface water from the skin or pulmonary system. Each of the four physical methods of heat loss is enhanced by compensatory physiologic processes such as increased sweat production, respiration and cardiac output, alterations in cutaneous and splanchnic blood flow, and reduction in physical activity. The physical mechanisms of heat loss are summarized in Table 24-2.

Physiologic thermoregulation expands upon physical mechanisms of heat loss through a combination of cutaneous vasodilation, increased sweat-based and respiratory evaporative cooling, and increased cardiac output. Environmental conditions greatly influence the efficiency of thermoregulation. For example, large temperature gradients between the body and surrounding air, convective loss from increased air movement, and low humidity all favor efficient cooling. Evaporative heat loss is limited by humidity greater than 75% and by impaired physiologic responses such as anhidrosis, perfusion abnormalities, low cardiac output and the effect of certain medications or ingested

TABLE 24-1 Clinical Spectrum of Heat Illness

Syndromes	Clinical features
Heat Edema	Self-limiting swelling of hands and feet resulting from cutaneous vasodilation and dependent pooling of interstitial fluid; resolves with early acclimatization.
Heat Rash (miliaria)	Pruritic, red vesicles found on skin covered by non-breathable clothing or sleeping pads. Occlusion of eccrine sweat ducts by keratinocytes leads to dilation and rupture. Secondary infection with bacteria including (in recent years) methicillin-resistant *Staphylococcus aureus* is common. Repeated occlusion of sweat ducts results in progression of inflammation and if untreated, chronic dermatitis.
Heat Cramps	Cramping of large muscle groups following exercise; common in un-acclimatized individuals and those unaccustomed to physical exercise in hot conditions. The syndrome is attributed to inefficient sodium recovery and hypernatremic sweat; resolves with acclimatization.
Heat Tetany	Hyperthermia-associated hyperventilation causes a primary respiratory alkalosis which in turn can cause perioral paresthesia, carpopedal or laryngeal spasm and Chvostek's sign.
Heat Exhaustion	Danger: symptoms include nausea, vomiting, fatigue, weakness and occasionally, diarrhea; clinical findings include orthostatic hypotension, tachycardia, syncope, hyperthermia (core temperature <40 °C; 104 °F) and minor mental status changes such as poor attention span. Caution: Heat exhaustion and heat stroke have overlapping symptoms; the primary differentiating criterion is that heat stroke is associated with more severe CNS disturbances and core body temperatures above 40 °C.
Heat Stroke	Life-threatening: heat stroke is a medical emergency characterized by core temperature >40 °C (105 °F) and CNS disturbances in patients with a history of heat exposure. Anhidrosis (absence of sweating) is often present but is no longer a criteria for diagnosis. Heat stroke occurs when thermoregulation fails completely leading to organ dysfunction and death. Caution: heat stroke is often missed in patients who may not have been physically active.

Adapted from Bouchama, A, Knochel, JP. Heat stroke. N Engl J Med 2002; 346: 1978 and Tek. D. Olshaker, JS. Heat Illness. Emerg Med Clin of North Amer; 1992;10;299.

toxins. Other major methods of heat loss, such as radiation of infrared energy from the skin, conduction of heat through contact with surrounding materials and convective heat loss, are less efficient when environmental temperatures are higher than skin temperatures. The body also has a limited ability to acclimatize to heat stress through increased shunting of blood to the skin, improved water preservation and increased aldosterone production to retain sodium. Unacclimatized individuals exposed to heat stress initially have high urine and sweat sodium content which reduces circulating plasma volume. Reduced renal blood flow from sodium and water loss stimulates aldosterone secretion which increases plasma sodium levels which,

TABLE 24-2 Physical Heat Loss

Evaporation	Evaporative cooling aids the efficiency of cutaneous heat transfer to the environment and is the primary mechanism of heat loss in healthy individuals. Evaporative cooling through respiration is critical for dogs upon which many classic heat stroke studies are based, but appear to be much less significant in humans compared to evaporation from the skin.
Conduction	Conduction is heat transfer through contact with a cooler material; the efficiency of conductive heat transfer varies with the properties of the conductive material, the temperature differential between surfaces and surface area. Conductive heat loss is improved when contact surfaces are of dense composition, contiguous or wet.
Radiation	Radiation is the loss of heat energy as electromagnetic waves, and accounts for up to 65% of total heat loss for temperatures <37 °C. When environmental temperatures are higher than body temperatures, the direction of heat exchange is reversed, resulting in a net heat gain
Convection	Convection is the loss of heat to surrounding air; as with radiation, the direction of heat transfer reverses when the air temperature is higher than the skin temperature.

in turn, increases intravascular fluid volume [12]. Under extreme physiologic conditions and high heat stress, vasodilation can be significant, leading to peripheral venous pooling, extravasation of fluids and reduced cardiac output. At temperatures above 42 °C (~108 °F), mitochondrial enzymes are inactivated, oxidative phosphorylation becomes uncoupled and ischemia of hepatocytes and renal parenchymal cells occurs. Heat damage to hepatorenal vascular beds results in microthrombi formation and prolonged prothrombin time (PT) and partial thromboplastin time (PTT); if cooling is not instituted, disseminated intravascular coagulation can occur, leading to multi-organ system failure and death [1, 13].

ASSESSMENT AND INVESTIGATIONS

The first priority in patient assessment is to confirm airway, breathing and circulation. Care providers should ensure that the patient is protected from further heat exposure. While assessment is underway, equipment and personnel should be recruited to assist with cooling. Appropriate initial steps include removal of clothing and preparation of cold water baths, water mist-convection systems and venous cooling dressings. Critically overheated patients may require more aggressive procedures, such as peritoneal lavage. If initial assessment suggests either heat exhaustion or heat stroke, peripheral intravenous access should be established and normal saline or lactated Ringers should be initiated at 200 ml/h. If available, unhumidified oxygen should be delivered by nasal cannula.

Initial work-up starts with a detailed history and thorough physical exam. If the patient is critically overheated, baseline vital signs should be obtained and re-assessed at 15-minute intervals; sphygmomanometer sites should be marked with indelible ink to ensure accurate measurements are obtained between care providers. Baseline body temperature needs to be established using a quality non-glass medical thermometer. Temperature measurements from axillary and inguinal sites are unreliable; however, they can be used to monitor trends in body temperature if rectal measurements are unsafe. If prolonged resuscitation is anticipated, a medical thermo-resistor probe should be placed in the rectum or esophagus. If none is available and the situation is dire, an inexpensive outdoor thermometer can be adapted for invasive monitoring by covering the probe with a prophylactic condom or glove and inserting the lead immediately beyond the anal verge. Continuous core temperature monitoring offers advantages in austere environments as monitoring will dictate triage priority and can be maintained during all phases of prehospital and hospital management. Mental status and the presence of focal neurologic problems should be assessed next. The cerebellum is highly sensitive to heat stroke and therefore finger–nose–finger or other exam to assess dysdiadochokinesia and cerebellar function should be performed. The oral cavity should be examined for evidence of gingival bleeding and the stool assessed for hemoglobin-positive results which may herald early coagulopathy. Pulmonary exam should assess for rales. Skin exam will help determine the patient's hydration status and the presence of miliaria. Muscle exams should include active and passive flexion of shoulders, thighs and calves; the presence of localized pain may indicate muscle breakdown. Urine should be collected by a Foley if necessary and inspected for evidence of myoglobin, hemoglobin and sediment. Disposable urine analysis "dip-sticks" are useful in the field as results guide rehydration and may aid detection of hemoglobinuria or myoglobinuria. In recent years, the proliferation of cartridge-based handheld blood chemistry units in field clinics increases the probability that basic blood chemistry may be obtained. The current-generation cartridges for these hand-held units require refrigeration; if test results are inconsistent with the clinical picture, the provider should suspect that the cartridges are outdated. If conventional coagulation studies are not possible, a whole-blood clotting assay can be used to assess for coagulopathy and a Weintraub sedimentation tube can be used to assess for hemoconcentration. The improvised coagulopathy and hemoconcentration tests discussed are most accurate when conducted with "controls" provided by a healthy bystander. Table 24-3 summarizes laboratory tests that are helpful in assessing heat illness casualties.

DIAGNOSIS

The differential diagnosis of heat illness requires a history of heat exposure, a detailed physical exam and bedside studies. Infectious etiologies and rare causes of hyperthermia need to be ruled out. The differential diagnosis should include malignant hyperthermia, neuroleptic malignant syndrome, endocrine and hypothalamic disorders, and fictitious hyperthermia. Heat edema and heat syncope are suggested by advanced patient age, deconditioning, low cardiac reserve and recent arrival in the tropics from cooler regions. Miliaria, a distinct heat dermatosis, is differentiated from other tropical skin maladies by the timing, distribution and physical appearance of skin vesicles. Miliaria responds promptly to antihistamines or dilute topical chlorhexidine. Heat cramps are a second common malady in unacclimatized individuals; diagnosis is suggested by resolution of cramps with rest and cool treatment, stretching and fluids, and electrolyte repletion. The two most dangerous heat illnesses – heat exhaustion and heat stroke – have overlapping clinical features and are discussed in greater detail below.

TABLE 24-3 Laboratory Assessment of Heat Illness

Mild cases: Obtain urine analysis; test for pH, specific gravity, urine sediment and hemoglobinuria and myoglobinuria
Moderate cases: Add basic blood chemistries; test for sodium, potassium, chloride, bicarbonate, blood urea nitrogen and creatinine.
Severe cases (e.g. CNS disturbances): Add aspartate transaminase (AST), alanine aminiotransferase (ALT), lactate dehydrogenase (LDH), uric acid, calcium, phosphate, coagulation studies (PT and PTT, fibrinogen); consider arterial blood gas for accurate determination of physiologic pH.

Heat exhaustion is an imprecise clinical syndrome characterized by nonspecific findings unified under a history of heat exposure. Core body temperature for heat exhaustion is <40°C. Common symptoms include nausea and vomiting, headache and weakness. Respiratory rate may be elevated. The cardiac and pulmonary exam may be normal; however, tachycardia may be present from concomitant dehydration. The presence of sweating in heat exhaustion patients is an important finding as it is frequently absent in heat stroke patients. The patient's mental status may suggest mild confusion and complaints may include dizziness. Symptoms of heat exhaustion tend to resolve with any modest interventions that lower body temperature.

Heat stroke is a life-threatening condition defined by a core body temperature >40°C and mental status or neurologic symptoms that do not respond to initial therapy (rest, cold treatment and hydration) [13]. Patients may be combative, with delirium, seizure, obtundation or coma. Clues to differentiate early heat stroke from heat exhaustion include significant mental status changes, diarrhea and dry skin in heat stroke. A minority of heat stroke casualties may present with sweating; however, this usually stops as thermoregulation continues to fail. Complications of heat stroke include acute renal failure from rhabdomyolysis, liver failure, disseminated intravascular coagulation (DIC), acute respiratory distress syndrome (ARDS), seizure, coma and death [1]. Select differential diagnostic features of heat stroke and heat exhaustion are listed in Table 24-4A, below. The differential diagnosis of hyperthermia is listed in Table 24-4B.

TABLE 24-4A Differential Diagnosis of Heat Exhaustion and Heat Stroke

Factor	Heat exhaustion	Heat stroke
Patient age	All ages	Often young/healthy
Symptoms	Nausea +/– vomiting	Nausea +/– diarrhea
Body temperature	<40C	>40C
CNS status	Normal: mild confusion	Delirium, ataxia, dysarthria, seizures, coma
Vital signs	+/– tachypneic	Tachypneic, tachycardia, hypotensive
Dermatologic findings	Sweating; +/– miliaria	Little or no sweat
Laboratory results	Normal	Elevated transaminases (AST > ALT); DIC, urine: muddy brown casts; Cr elevated; CBC: WBC elevated

TABLE 24-4B Differential Diagnosis of Hyperthermia

Environmental exposure	Hypothalamic stroke
Sepsis	Status epilepticus
Encephalitis	Cerebral hemorrhage
Brain abscess	Neuroleptic malignant syndrome
Meningitis	Alcohol, sedative-hypnotic withdrawal
Tetanus	Salicylate, lithium toxicity
Typhoid fever	Sympathomimetic toxicity
Thyroid storm	Anticholinergic toxicity
Pheochromocytoma	Dystonic reactions
Catatonia	Serotonin syndrome
Malignant hyperthermia	

TABLE 24-5 Treatment of Heat Illness

Heat illness	Treatment strategies
All	Rest, hydration, electrolytes, access to cool haven: initiate rapid cooling for temperatures >40 °C and any patient with mental status changes
Heat Edema	Elevation of legs, cold compresses on arms and legs or cold baths
Heat Syncope	Move to cool location, rest, fluids
Heat Syncope & Dehydration	Electrolyte replacement, consider decontinue antihypertensive and anticholingergic medications
Heat Cramps	Rest, hydration, electrolytes
Heat Tetany with Hyperventilation	Move to cool environment, restore normal respiration rates; in severe cases, rebreathing carbon monoxide or use of benzodiazepines
Heat Exhaustion	As above. Provide oral or intravenous hydration, mist water convective cooling and focal use of ice packs on large superficial veins, axilla and inguinal regions (see Figure 24.1)
Heat Stroke	Rapid cooling is the priority; use cold water immersion with rectal temperature monitoring; patient should be removed when rectal temperature reaches 39 C. Patients with coronary artery disease may develop coronary spasm with ice water immersion; patients with coronary risk factors should be treated less aggressively with mist water and convective cooling

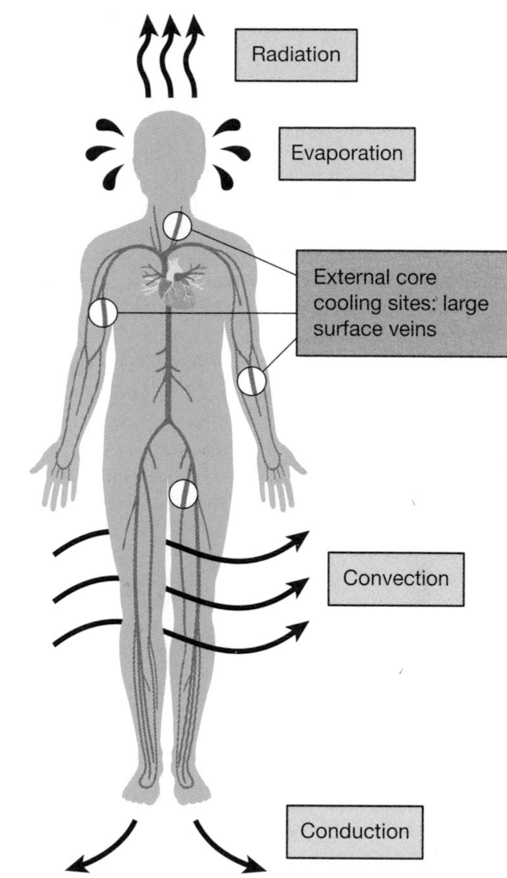

FIGURE 24.1 Thermoregulation and therapeutic cooling.

MANAGEMENT AND OUTCOMES

Treatment of heat illness is provided in Table 24-5. Management strategies exploit all four principal mechanisms of heat loss and cold therapy targeted to specific body locations (see Fig. 24.1). Minor heat illnesses are self-limiting if the patient is provided with fluids, rest and access to a cool environment. The majority of cases require only fluids and electrolytes for resolution of symptoms. Heat edema is prevented by exercise programs prior to travel to the tropics, optimization of diuretics and beta-blockers, and use of supportive compressive stockings.

Heat exhaustion is a more serious form of hyperthermia that requires close evaluation. Initial treatment of patients includes documentation of core temperature, assessment of blood chemistries, and treatment using hydration, moisture to the skin–preferably with convective cooling and oral electrolyte solutions. If symptoms are more severe or mental status changes are noted, the patient should be treated with intravenous normal saline. Both normal and abnormal serum chemistries should be rechecked after hydration and urine output is restored. Patients should be monitored until core body temperature has normalized. Heat exhaustion patients who have persistent or worsening mental status changes should have core temperature rechecked to confirm the diagnosis, and should receive more aggressive and prolonged cold treatment.

The treatment for heat stroke requires prompt, aggressive physical cooling. All measures for dissipating heat should be maximized: evaporation, radiation, convection and conductive cooling. Treatment of heat stroke in the tropics may be limited by inadequate water for cooling baths, unavailability of air-conditioning and unreliable electricity to power fans. Patient monitoring during treatment may be complicated by lack of quality thermometers or supportive laboratory tests. One frequently overlooked issue is that the conditions that caused one heat casualty are very likely to cause a large number of casualties. Initial assessment of a solitary heat illness casualty should therefore consider how local medical resources may efficiently scale to treat a large number of patients.

Of the available methods, evaporative cooling is the most available and scalable treatment for field management. Unlike water immersion and invasive techniques such as peritoneal lavage, evaporative cooling allows for constant patient monitoring, the use of additional cooling strategies and the scalability to treat multiple patients at one station. Evaporative cooling requires water to apply to the skin and an air movement source, such as an electric fan. The patient is undressed and placed supine close to the fan. The skin is moistened with water using a sponge or mist bottle. If local cultures, mores or religious beliefs prevent disrobing, the patient may be covered with a thin sheet that is kept wet; however, this dramatically reduces evaporative heat loss. Patients cooled with convective mist water systems need to be re-assessed regularly to ensure stable correction of body temperatures. Alcohol and other low vapor pressure fluids should not be applied to the skin as dilated cutaneous blood vessels may increase absorption, leading to intoxication. In many tropical clinics the only resources available for cooling the patient are ice packs: if supplies are limited, cold packs should be applied directly to large superficial veins on flexor surfaces such as the anticubital and popliteal fossa, axilla and inguinal region. If ice is used, it should be wrapped in a damp cloth and applied to superficial veins using non-compressive pressure (see Fig. 24.1). Current-generation chemical cold packs lack adequate cold capacity to treat heat casualties; however, they should be used if nothing else is available.

Cold (ice) water immersion is the most effective method for rapid cooling. Clinical experience indicates ice water immersion lowers body core temperature at twice the rate of convective mist-water cooling (mist water and electric fan). The advantage of cold water baths is that the rate of cooling can be controlled by changing the water temperature or the amount of body surface area in the water. In immersion cooling, the patient is undressed and placed in a tub of suitable depth to allow water to cover the extremities; cold immersion should only be used on alert patients. Heat stroke patients and those with comorbidities, such as underlying cardiac disease, should be monitored for arrhythmias or syncope and, if the situation is not critical, cooled using less aggressive methods. In developed regions, immersion cooling has fallen out of favor because of difficulties with patient telemetry. In refugee camps, however, a water bath is often constantly in use to treat heat illnesses.

Invasive cooling techniques are only to be used when cold water misting, evaporative cooling and cool water immersion are ineffective and the patient is critically overheated. Invasive cooling may correct temperature unevenly and result in unpredictable cooling rates, overcooling and possibly death. Current invasive cooling methods include gastric and peritoneal lavage with cold fluids, cooled intravenous fluids and cooled inhalational gas. The use of ice water gastric lavage is contraindicated in patients who have altered mental status or who are unable to protect their airway. Heat casualties with life-threatening elevated core temperatures and for whom gastric lavage is attempted should be intubated to protect the airway. Cold intravenous fluids require careful control, as proximal access and rapid infusion rates can induce cardiac arrhythmias. Cold peritoneal lavage is an invasive technique that requires sterile access and should not be used in patients suspected of having abdominal adhesions or who are pregnant. Cooled oxygen and oral hydration fluids lack the cold capacity necessary to justify use in emergency treatment. One new technology that has proven valuable to soldiers and athletes in hot climates is a small, portable vacuum cooling system known as "cooling gloves". This device consists of a negative pressure chamber for the hand and a small pump that circulates cold water to a handle. The hand is inserted into the chamber and grabs the handle. Air is then pumped out of the chamber, causing the vascular beds of the palm of the hand to be splinted open. Heat from the core is transmitted through the enlarged vascular bed to the cold conductive surface of the handle, resulting in rapid cooling of the body. A commercial vacuum cooling glove is illustrated in Figure 24.2.

Regardless of the cooling method used, care providers should continuously monitor core temperature to ensure cooling does not overshoot the desired temperature [16]. In cases involving rapid cooling of the core, treatment should be interrupted when core temperature drops below 40°C. The objective is to drop core temperature into a range where normal thermoregulation can again take control. Adjunct treatments that complement therapeutic cooling are limited. Dehydration is treated quickly with intravenous fluids or, in conscious patients, with water or sports drinks. Sports drinks should be diluted before use to prevent osmotic loading of the gastrointestinal (GI) tract, which, in turn, can cause GI distress. Antipyretic medications and drugs used to treat malignant hyperthermia have no value in the treatment of heat illnesses and should not be used [14]. One common complication of effective cooling with ice packs or immersion is shivering, which generates more body heat. In these situations, the careful use of short-acting benzodiazepines is reasonable. Although chlorpromazine is also used to treat shivering, the secondary alpha-1 blocking activity may make hypotension worse and therefore should not be used.

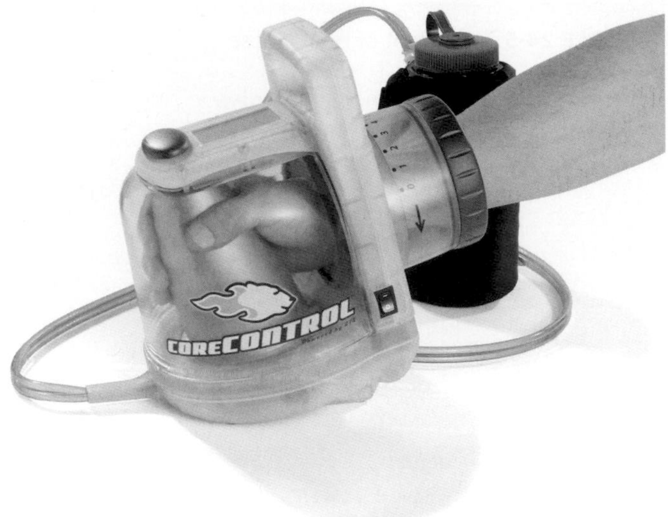

FIGURE 24.2 Commercial vacuum cooling glove.

Successful management of heat illness requires prompt recognition, triage, identification of exacerbating factors such as drug or alcohol ingestion, and efficient use of limited therapeutic cooling resources.

REFERENCES

1. Tek D, Olshaker JS. Heat illness. Emerg Med Clin North Am 1992;10: 299–310.
2. Centers for Disease Control and Prevention. Heat-related deaths – four states, July–August 2001, and United States, 1979–1999. MMWR Morb Mortal Wkly Rep 2002;51:567–70.
3. Al-Harthi SS, Nouh MS, Al-Arfaj H, et al. Non-invasive evaluation of cardiac abnormalities in heat stroke pilgrims. Int J Cardiol 1992;37:151–4.
4. Rav-Acha M, Hadad E, Epstein Y, et al. Fatal exertional heat stroke: a case series. Am J Med Sci 2004;328:84–7.
5. Heat-related deaths – Chicago, Illinois, 1996–2001, and United States, 1979–1999. MMWR Morb Mortal Wkly Rep 2003;52:610–13.
6. Misset B, De Jonghe B, Bastuji-Garin S, et al. Mortality of patients with heatstroke admitted to intensive care units during the 2003 heat wave in France: a national multiple-center risk-factor study. Crit Care Med 2006;34:1087.
7. Centers for Disease Control and Prevention. Heat-related deaths – four states, July–August 2001, and United States, 1979–1999. MMWR Morb Mortal Wkly Rep 2002;51:567–70.
8. Sierra Pajares Ortiz M, et al. Daily mortality in the Madrid community during 1986–1991 for the group between 45 and 64 years of age: its relationship to air temperature. Revista Española de Salud Pública, 1997,71:149–60.
9. Simon HB. Hyperthermia. N Engl J Med 1993;329:483–7.
10. Dann EJ, Berkman N. Chronic idiopathic anhydrosis – a rare cause of heat stroke. Postgrad Med 1992;68:750–2.
11. Khosla R, Guntapalli KK. Heat-related illness. Crit Care Clin 1999;15: 251–63.
12. Simon HB. Hyperthermia. N Engl J Med 1993;329:483–7.
13. Bouchama A, Knochel JP. Heat stroke. N Engl J Med 2002;346:1978–88.
14. Bouchama A, Cafege A, Devol EB, et al. Ineffectiveness of dantrolene sodium in the treatment of heatstroke. Crit Care Med 1991;19:176–80.

Traditional Medicine 25

Gerard Bodeker, Bertrand Graz

Key features

- Traditional medicines are used by many patients in all countries
- Although in part a profession, traditional medicine is often a home-based, familial practice
- Some traditional treatments are safe and some are unsafe or have adverse effects
- Some have been proven effective through controlled clinical trials; some have been shown ineffective
- An open-minded, critical and respectful perspective on traditional medicine is fundamental for a good professional partnership with the patients and the population
- In resource-poor areas, traditional medicines may not be a choice, but the only accessible form of healthcare. Such local resources may have a positive impact on the population health

DEFINITION

The local health traditions of developing countries and of indigenous communities are commonly referred to as "traditional medicine". As most have a theoretical basis, materia medica, a range of therapeutic modalities, an empirical approach to treatment and a tradition of training, a more appropriate term is "traditional health systems".

GENERAL PRINCIPLES

This chapter presents an overview of the question: how can a modern, Western-style health professional deal today with the major health traditions of regions in which tropical and traditional health systems interface? Survey chapters typically provide breadth of coverage at the expense of depth. However, the "References" contains publications that provide deeper coverage of the traditions, their treatment modalities and their efficacy.

WHY IS IT IMPORTANT FOR PHYSICIANS IN THE TROPICS TO KNOW ABOUT TRADITIONAL MEDICINE?

TRADITIONAL MEDICINE IS WIDELY USED

What has become clear since the publication of the World Health Organization (WHO) Global Atlas on Traditional, Complementary and Alternative Medicine in 2005 [1], is that the majority of the population in most developing countries rely on traditional medicine for their everyday health needs, often integrating it on an ad hoc basis with modern medicines [1].

Considerable use of traditional medicine exists in many developing countries: 40% in China and Colombia, 71% in Chile, while utilization in some African countries is estimated at 80% and above [2]. It can sometimes be difficult to differentiate what is traditional medicine and what is not, as in the example of the "kangaroo mother care" for preterm babies: although a "low-technology" method, it is actually a recent treatment modality [3].

TRADITIONAL MEDICINE IS OFTEN THE FIRST TREATMENT USED

There are many reasons why patients use traditional medicine. First, they may be in a remote location where modern medicine is simply not available when they need it. For cultural reasons, they may prefer traditional medicine, for example in an attempt to have fewer side effects. They may also have experienced a failure with a modern treatment and want to try a traditional one. Modern health facilities are sometimes avoided because they are perceived as expensive, dangerous, unfriendly or run with corruption. Patients may also fear the fact that many modern medicines sold on the market are counterfeit or "fake" drugs.

TRADITIONAL MEDICINE MAY INTERACT WITH MODERN TREATMENT

Some traditional treatments have known interactions with modern treatment. An example is St John's wort (*Hypericum perforatum*). It has become one of the most prescribed antidepressants, but must be used with caution by patients taking other drugs such as the contraceptive pill and some antiretroviral drugs, among others.

Therefore, it is prudent for physicians to discuss traditional medicine use with their patients. It is also useful to have some background in the safety, benefits and herb–drug interactions that may be involved, as well as familiarity with databases which provide such information.

TRADITIONAL MEDICINE MAY, IN SOME CASES, BE A VALUABLE OPTION

Most physicians are unaware that a considerable amount of clinical research has already been conducted and published on traditional medicine. It is therefore incorrect to state that there is "no evidence of effectiveness". As a matter of professional ethics, doctors need to know the present state of this knowledge through a regular check of the literature. If a treatment has a proven effectiveness and a good safety profile, this also must be known. In the same manner, if a treatment (e.g. a herbal tea) has potential secondary effects, doctors need to know this also (Box 25.1).

BOX 25.1 Databases on Complementary and Traditional Medicine

- Cochrane Complementary Medicine Group (http://cochrane.org/reviews/en/topics/22_reviews.html).
- University of Maryland School of Medicine Cochrane CAM Field offers summary of findings tables and plain language summaries of CAM-related Cochrane reviews (http://www.compmed.umm.edu/cochrane_about.asp).
- HerbMed: scientific data on the use of herbs for health (www.herbmed.org).
- MedicinesComplete: on interactions, clinical evidence, mechanisms of action (www.medicinescomplete.com).
- Natural Medicines Comprehensive Database (www.naturaldatabase.com). Contains "The Natural Product/Drug Interaction Checker" and "The Natural Products Effectiveness Checker".
- Globinmed (www.globinmed.com) has a section related to intellectual property rights and the development of traditional medicine.

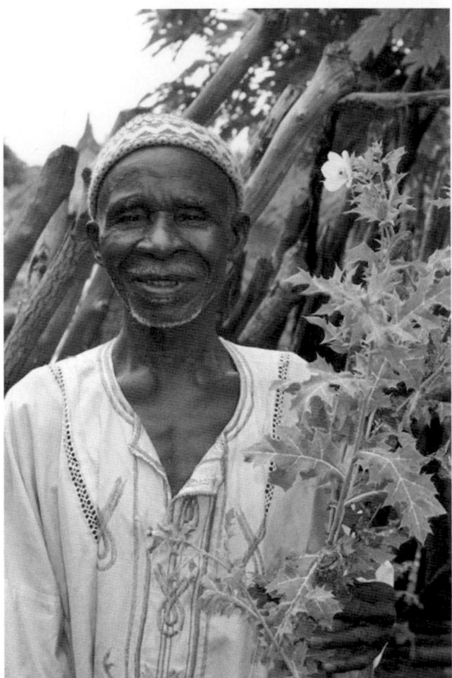

FIGURE 25.1 The traditional healer Thiemoko Bengaly and the plant *Argemone mexicana* used in his decoction against malaria (South Mali).

EFFECTIVENESS

CAN THE EFFECTIVENESS OF TRADITIONAL MEDICINE BE EVALUATED?

Traditional medicine can be evaluated as any other medicine. In most cases, it is possible to use a standard research method. For example, it is straightforward to organize a randomized, controlled trial (RCT) of a herbal treatment, provided one can make a placebo. For acupuncture trials, a "placebo acupuncture" (called "sham acupuncture") has been developed for control groups in clinical studies. Even very individualized treatments, such as complex mental techniques, can be evaluated through a prospective, randomized, controlled trial. Sometimes blinding (which makes it impossible to know whether the "real" treatment is given or the placebo) is impossible, just as for surgery research, but non-blinded studies can still be of high value.

Contrary to a commonly held myth, clinical studies (even RCTs) can be conducted at a relatively low cost if the researcher works with local/regional research institutes and with doctoral students, focusing on meaningful clinical measures rather than sophisticated laboratory analyses.

Recent studies on traditional medicine have begun to change perspectives on its effects and its role in the health of various populations. The safety and effectiveness of some traditional medicines have been studied, paving the way to better collaboration between modern and traditional systems. Traditional medicines still remain a largely untapped health resource: they are not only sources of new leads for drug discoveries, but can also provide novel approaches that may have direct public health and economic impacts [4].

SOME EXAMPLES OF EFFECTIVE TRADITIONAL TREATMENTS

The number of traditional treatments that have been scrutinized through clinical studies is high (>1500 clinical studies at the last count).

Malaria: from Local Practice to Global Solution

Cinchona and *Artemisia annua* have provided the basis for two of the three main classes of anti-malarials [5, 6], and many other plants contain antimalarial agents.

Case Study

It started with a "retrospective treatment-outcome" population survey in Mali that showed that all patients using a decoction of *Argemone mexicana* (Fig. 25.1) for uncomplicated malaria reported a complete cure with very few side-effects [7]. Subsequently, a dose-escalating prospective study showed a dose–response phenomenon [8]. A prospective, randomized, controlled trial was organized in a remote village: the "control" treatment was the artemisinin combination therapy (ACT) artesunate-amodiaquine. Deterioration to severe malaria was 1.9% in both groups in children aged ≤5 years (with 0% coma/convulsions), and there were no cases in patients aged >5 years.

The *A. mexicana* decoction could be proposed as a complement to standard modern drugs in high-transmission areas in order to reduce the drug pressure for development of resistance to ACT. It may also constitute a first-aid treatment when access to other anti-malarials is delayed [9]. A 3-month follow-up study confirmed that, even when all parasites were not eliminated, the rate of severe malaria and anemia remained low. Another plant of interest for malaria treatment is *Artemisia annua*. This plant provides the rough material for the production of ACT. It was reportedly used in China for a long time as a treatment for recurrent fevers. So, the question arose: why not cultivate the plant on the spot and use the plant itself [5, 6, 8]? The first consideration was that it does not grow everywhere. For example, it does not grow well in dry areas where *A. mexicana* grows—which could make these two plants complementary, geographically speaking. Another problem is that the content of artemisinine is quite low, even in selected species. It was, however, hypothesized that several active constituents might work in synergy. Clinical studies showed promising results, although with a relatively high recrudescence rate [10, 11].

Wounds

Herbal treatments are widely used for wounds in non-industrialized countries, as they are often more readily available and affordable, and may possibly be equally, or more, efficacious than the modern alternatives. Evidence indicates that a number of plant treatments are useful in a variety of dermatologic conditions, including wounds.

Centella asiatica extract is one of the most widely studied plant-based wound treatments. It is used in a number of tropical countries, including India, Malaysia, Madagascar and Sri Lanka. *In vivo* laboratory studies have shown its topical application to significantly accelerate wound healing and *in vitro* studies of treated granulating tissues have demonstrated a significant increase in fibroblast activity, total DNA and collagen content.

Research on *Aloe barbadensis* has shown it to be a powerful wound-healing agent. Extracts from *A. barbadensis*, or "*Aloe vera*" as it is commonly known, have been found to penetrate tissue, have anesthetic, antibacterial, antifungal and antiviral properties, serve as an anti-inflammatory agent, and dilate capillaries and increase blood flow [12, 13].

Chen et al. [14] studied the effects of "dragon's blood" (sap from the bark of *Croton lechleri* used as a wound-healing agent in South America). The researchers found that *C. lechleri* acts as a natural dressing which forms an occlusive layer with an antimicrobial environment and cell proliferative effects.

In Vietnam, research at the National Institute for Traditional Medicine in Hanoi has examined the mechanism by which *Cudrania cochinchinensis*, commonly used in Vietnam as a traditional wound-healing agent, produces a wound-healing effect. An extract of the plant was found to protect fibroblasts and endothelial cells against hydrogen peroxide-induced damage, leading to the suggestion that protection of cells against destruction by mediators of inflammatory processes may be mechanisms by which this plant contributes to wound healing [14, 15].

In studies at the Oxford Wound Healing Institute and Singapore General Hospital, Phan et al. studied the wound-healing properties of Eupolin, a topical agent produced from the leaves of *Chromolaena odorata*, and which is used widely for the treatment of burns and soft tissue wounds in Vietnam [16, 17]. Eupolin enhanced hemostasis, stimulated granulation tissue and re-epithelialization, and inhibited collagen contraction. These results suggest a mechanism for clinical reports on the effectiveness of Eupolin in reducing wound contraction and scarring, which are critical complications in post-burn trauma.

A comprehensive review of research by Burford et al. [18] on traditional medicine and wound healing presents information on utilization and research trends in this field.

Ophthalmic Conditions: a Range of Practices, from Harmful to Sight-Saving

Traditional eye treatment (TET) has been the cause of much concern becuase of serious eye infections and injury associated with some traditional treatments. Public health programmes have focused on training traditional practitioners to refer patients for eye treatment. Following an interactive training programme with traditional healers in Malawi, based on a collaborative approach to eye care, it was found that among the 175 pre-intervention and 97 post-intervention patients, delay in presentation improved slightly [19]. In a multicenter RCT at the All India Institute of Medical Sciences, an Ayurvedic herbal eye drop formulation was significantly more effective in treating trachoma and chronic conjunctivitis than placebo. Research by the same group has found that an Ayurvedic herbal eye drop significantly improved dry eye syndrome [20].

Trachoma is among the most frequent causes of preventable blindness in the world. At the trichiasis/entropion stage, there is only one officially advocated treatment: lid surgery. There are, however, numerous reports of its limitations (late attendance, poor uptake, imperfect outcome and common recurrence of the disease). A valuable complement to the "lid-surgery only" strategy would be a non-surgical, easy-to-apply, inexpensive and safe treatment.

A traditional treatment for trachomatous trichiasis was observed in the Sultanate of Oman: lashes contention. Based on the traditional treatment idea, a modern technique was devised (Fig. 25.2). Once the outside skin of the lid is clean and dry, malpositioned lashes are grasped with clean fingers and stuck on the outside skin with a small piece of sticking plaster. Check that eye opening and lid closure remain normal. The patient (or a friend or relative) is instructed to replace the sticking plaster when it falls off (this happens about once a week), for 3 months. This procedure was tested through a small, prospective, randomized clinical trial in China [21]. The results were that lashes contention with a sticking plaster was much more effective than epilation in relieving symptoms and correcting lashes—and similar to lid surgery.

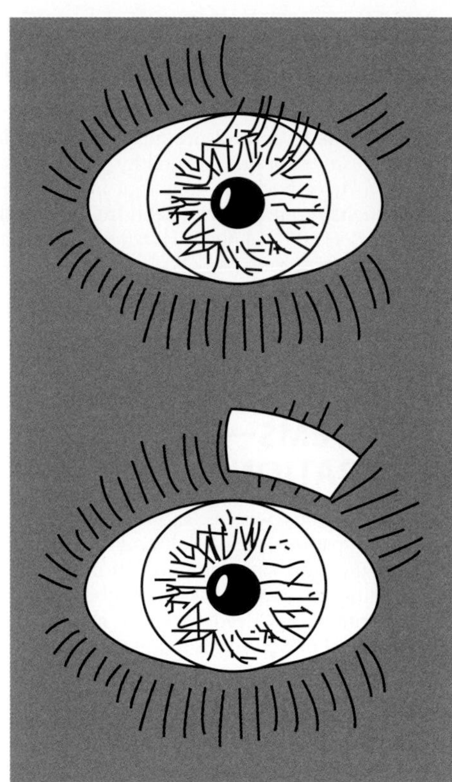

FIGURE 25.2 Based on a traditional method from the Arabic Peninsula, a non-surgical treatment of trachoma at the trichiasis stage was found safe and effective: lashes contention with a sticking plaster.

SAFETY OF TRADITIONAL MEDICINE

REGULATORY DEVELOPMENT

Regulatory requirements for herbal and traditional medicines vary from country to country, depending on their history. Countries such as China and Vietnam, with millennia of actual use and more than 50 years of official modern health sector incorporation of traditional medicine, safety and regulatory standards are highly developed. In other countries where traditions may be centuries old but official recognition is still absent or only recent, safety standards may not yet be fully developed.

Indonesia's Health Law Act, for example, classifies traditional medicines (*jamu*) into two groups: (1) traditional medicines produced by individual persons or by home industries, which do not require registration; (2) traditional medicines produced and packed on a commercial scale, which do require registration, including submission of data on safety, composition, dosage, efficacy, claimed indications and quality control.

COUNTERFEIT OR "FAKE" MEDICINES

The WHO has estimated that the annual earnings from the sales of counterfeit and substandard medicines are in excess of US$ 32 billion globally [22].

Traditional medicines do not escape the plague of counterfeit products. Irregularities have been detected in traditional preparations, including adulteration, substitution, contamination (e.g. with heavy metals or fungi), misidentification and incorrect preparation [23].

Attempts are being made to control products, with identification of constituents and assessment of product quality problems, be it intentional or not, and to trace back the source of inadequate products. Activities of drug quality control involve the International Criminal Police Organization (INTERPOL), the WHO, national authorities and non-governmental organizations (NGOs).

Improving the control of traditional preparations may, in turn, increase the level of public confidence in these products.

TRADITIONAL AND MODERN HEALTH SYSTEMS—THE NEED FOR COOPERATION

It is important for physicians, whether in private practice, working in a hospital, a research institute or in health administration to keep a close and lively relationship with the population that they are supposed to serve. Traditional medicine is one of the many community health factors that physicians need to know about and take into account. If a professional perspective is maintained along with a well-informed, constructive and non-judgemental attitude towards all health practices, community members will acknowledge this as a sign of respect and the outcome can be very rewarding in terms of relationship with the population.

EXAMPLES

In a Refugee Population

In a number of studies among refugees, it was found that Western physicians and treatments were not able to address cultural disease constructs or traditional practices, in some cases resulting in false diagnoses and inappropriate, or ineffective, care [24–26]. These lapses in understanding and care can (and have) compromise refugee health. Such oversight of cultural perceptions and practices has also deterred refugees from seeking timely, and often vital, Western health services for fear of misunderstandings or stigma attached to traditional practices.

When working in a refugee camp, it can be helpful to seek out those refugees interested in helping to set up and maintain the best possible interim health system, given the difficult situation that this population faces. There may be physicians and nurses who can readily work with the expatriate teams; there may be paramedics who will be ready to help in preventive interventions; and there may be traditional practitioners, who should be contacted for, at very the least, safety reasons. Because of their displacement, they may well be unfamiliar with local flora and could be at risk of providing unsafe preparations. Meetings between displaced and local traditional healers can be organized, if possible with a botanical outing, for refugees to learn to recognize local plants and avoid dangerous ones.

Many studies on psychosocial and primary health practices among refugees validate the effects of integrating traditional practices into refugee care. One of the first examples of such integration efforts was seen in the 1980s, when Dr J.P. Hiegel of the International Committee for the Red Cross (ICRC) helped Cambodian refugees in Thailand set up traditional medicine centers. Western clinicians and traditional practitioners cooperated to build a dual treatment system with effective, mutual referral procedures [27].

Another leading example is seen in Cambodia, where the Harvard Center for Refugee Trauma has shown that refugee trauma can be reduced by re-introducing traditional healing systems to dislocated communities [24]. Work with Karen refugees and internally displaced persons at the Thai–Burma border has included the training of refugee community health workers clinic staff in herbal medicine, research on refugee patients' use of, and belief in, traditional medicine and spiritual practices, and initial work on the development of networks of herbalists in the Thai–Burma border region [26, 28]. Training programs were found to have contributed to stimulating several grass-roots initiatives and to the development of herbal clinics along the border region.

These examples of integrating and supporting traditional health resources within refugee interventions highlight the need for increased international awareness regarding existing health resources within refugee populations.

In a Health District

Patients typically undertake their own self-referral, with few errors. They choose when they need to go to the modern medical system and when to turn to their traditional health practices. In the modern health center, the most frequent diagnoses (i.e. the 'case-mix') are typically infant and childhood diarrhea, pneumonia and malaria. In the traditional practitioner clinic, patients present with chronic and congenital disorders, mental problems, and functional and terminal diseases. These diagnoses represent a challenge for modern medicine which often has little to offer in resource-poor settings. Patients can be counselled and supported in making their choices in order to minimize mistakes.

DEVELOPMENT OF NEW DRUGS AND TREATMENTS; INTELLECTUAL PROPERTY RIGHTS

In the classical research process, many substances are selected through field studies (ethnobotany or ethnopharmacology), but very few are eventually found safe and effective in human studies. The selection process itself is questionable [29], as it is hard to find any treatment that has been found through this process in history. Conventional drug development is slow and expensive. The finished products are often unavailable and unaffordable to the poorest patients in remote areas, unless they are part of a heavily subsidized scheme.

In contrast, phytomedicines consisting of locally available products can, if proven safe and effective, become useful complements to imported drugs if they are cheaper and more readily available. The development of local phytomedicines of proven safety and effectiveness can be conducted through a relatively cheap and fast process called "reverse pharmacology" [30].

Exploitation of traditional medical knowledge for drug development without the consent of customary knowledge holders is not acceptable under international law {[United Nations (UN) Convention on Biological Diversity (CBD), [31]}. Under the CBD, state parties are required to "respect, preserve and maintain knowledge, innovations and practices of indigenous and local communities embodying traditional lifestyles ...and promote involvement of the holders of such knowledge and practices encourage the equitable sharing of the benefits arising from the utilisation of such knowledge, innovations and practices".

The International Society of Ethnobiology [32] has developed a comprehensive set of ethical guidelines for researchers working on traditional medicine, which can be accessed at: http://ethnobiology.net/code-of-ethics/.

The WHO's Global Strategy and Plan of Action on Public Health, Innovation and Intellectual Property [33] gives priority to research in this field and supports drug research and development in traditional medicine systems in developing countries (http://apps.who.int/gb/ebwha/pdf_files/A61/A61_R21-en.pdf).

CLINICAL SCENARIOS

The following anecdotal cases are not meant to recommend the particular intervention or strategy, but rather to illustrate that traditional medicine and practices are deeply established in many cultures and

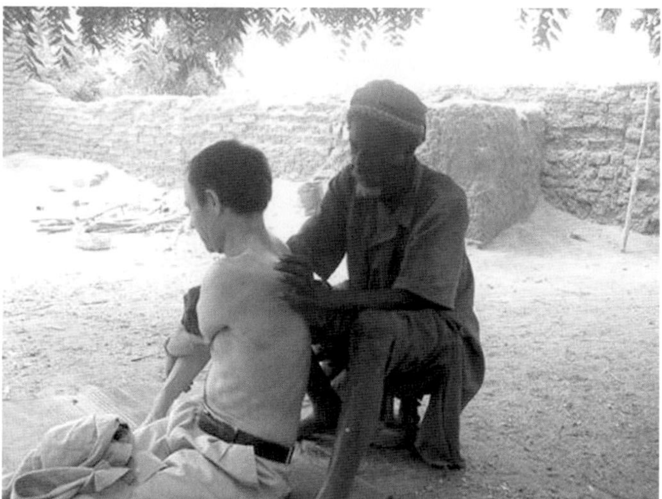

FIGURE 25.3 A traditional bone-setter in Mali taking care of a patient with acute low back pain.

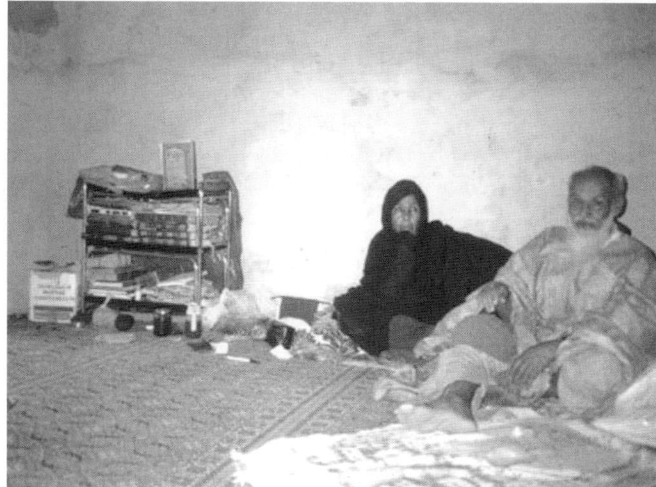

FIGURE 25.4 Traditional healers in the Sahara, practicing Greco-Arabic medicine (Mauritania).

often preferred by the local populations over accepted Western practices. In some cases, these traditional practices accomplish therapeutic goals as well as any Western intervention. In any case, the wise practitioner will seek to understand and work within the local traditional medicine culture.

A TRADITIONAL BONE-SETTER IN MALI

After 9 hours of travelling bumpy roads on the Dogon plateau in Mali, this visiting doctor was incapacitated for any further work, thanks to an attack of lower backache. His local colleague proposed visiting a well-known bone-setter. Once inside the courtyard, the patient (as the doctor was then) removed his shirt and was submitted to a series of energetic pulls and twists of trunk and limbs eliciting distinct cracking sounds. Five minutes later, he stretched, sprang up and found that he could walk again, the back pain almost gone. In such a case, there is no need for sophisticated clinical studies to conclude that we have observed a case of rapidly effective treatment for acute low back pain (Fig. 25.3).

LAST HOPE AFTER AN OPEN FRACTURE

In a clinic in the desert near Nouakchott, Mauritania, two traditional practitioners—a brother and sister—hold their consultations together on a carpet in a cool adobe house. Their practice is based on the Greco-Arabic tradition dating back to Avicenna and Hippocrates [34]. A boy of about 15 years of age is brought in by his parents. All three are in tears and despair: the boy, after an open fracture of the tibia, was taken to the National hospital where it was declared that his leg was deeply infected and must be amputated. The practitioner examines the leg and proposes a therapeutic trial. For several days, every morning he fills the purulent sinuses with powdered resin from a local tree (we learned later that this is a local variety of myrrh, *Commifora africana*). Three weeks later, we find the boy playing football in the courtyard. We took the resin to a microbiology lab for an antibiogram; the result was zero observed antibiotic properties. The effect—if there was any—remains of unknown nature. All we know is that, subsequently, we observed several other deep infections successfully treated with the same resin (Fig. 25.4).

TACKLING WATER-BORNE DISEASE THE TRADITIONAL WAY

The ancient texts of Ayurveda in India recommend the use of metals such as gold, silver and copper for water purification and, traditionally, Indian homes stored drinking water in copper and silver pots. In recent years, this practice has been replaced by the use of steel and plastic containers, as copper and silver have become expensive. Ayurvedic physicians, to the perplexity of the modern world, have argued that rising levels of childhood diarrhea and water-borne diseases are linked to this shift.

In a number of rural villages of India, water that contained *Escherichia coli*, *Salmonella typhi* and *Vibrio cholerae* was stored in copper pots or in glass containers along with a simple four-inch coil made of pure copper.

As expected by the Ayurvedic physicians, and to the considerable surprise of the modern medical research community, after 16 hours of storage, there was no growth of bacteria after overnight incubation with the copper pots or copper device, whereas control bottles without the device showed more than a 30-fold increase in *E. coli* counts and more than a fourfold increase in *S.* Typhi and *V. cholerae.* At the same time, the pH and levels of copper in the test containers were well within the permissible limits set by the WHO [35]. (This is part of ongoing evaluation of traditional health practices conducted by the Foundation for Revitalization of Local Health Traditions in Bangalore, India (www.frlht.org).)

CONCLUSION

The majority of the population of most tropical countries continue to use traditional medicine as a primary source of healthcare.

Accordingly, physicians in the tropics need to understand what traditional medicines and traditional therapeutic approaches their patients are using, in order to best advise on issues of herb–drug interactions, possible benefits and harms of traditional medicine and to work with local health practitioners on appropriate cross-referrals.

The tropical medicine practitioner may be faced with the negative effects of traditional medicine practice, but should not forget that only failures are seen (and the reverse is true: traditional healers only see the failures of modern medicine).

In view of the trust of local communities in traditional medicine and its practitioners, a policy of partnership with traditional health practitioners is warranted, based on mutually respectful exchange. In addition to enhancing a patient-centered approach to clinical practice, this will build a constructive relationship and credibility within the wider community.

ACKNOWLEDGMENTS

The Global Initiative for Traditional Systems (GIFTS) of Health, Oxford, UK (www.giftsofhealth.org) and the Research Initiative on Traditional

Antimalarial Methods (RITAM) (www.gifts-ritam.org); The Swiss Cooperation and the Organisation Antenna Technologies (Geneva) for their support; Merlin Willcox, Jacques Falquet and Jean-Claude François for their pictures; populations and authorities in the many tropical countries where the authors have gained experience: India, China, Vietnam, Thailand, Laos, Malaysia; Erytrea and Ethiopia; countries in East and Southern Africa, particularly Kenya, Tanzania, Uganda and South Africa; Madagascar; Mauritania, Mali, Oman, etc.

REFERENCES

1. Bodeker G, Ong C-K, Burford G, et al, eds. World Health Organization Global Atlas on Traditional and Complementary Medicine. Geneva: World Health Organization; 2005.
2. Kasilo OMJ, Alley ES, Wambebe C, Chatora R. Regional overview: African region. In: Bodeker G, Ong C-K, Burford G, et al, eds. World Health Organization Global Atlas on Traditional and Complementary Medicine. Geneva: World Health Organization; 2005.
3. Charpak N, Ruiz JG, Zupan J, Cattaneo A, et al. Kangaroo Mother Care: 25 years after. Acta Paediatr 2005;94:514–22.
4. Graz B, Kitua AY, Malebo HM. To what extent can traditional medicine contribute a complementary or alternative solution to malaria control programmes? Malar J 2011;10(suppl. 1:S6): http://www.malariajournal.com/supplements/10/S1 (accessed 12 March 2012).
5. Willcox M, Rasoanaivo P, Sharma VP, Bodeker G. Comment on: Randomized controlled trial of a traditional preparation of *Artemisia annua* L. (Annual Wormwood) in the treatment of malaria. Trans R Soc Trop Med Hyg 2004; 98:755–6.
6. Willcox M. Artemisia species: from traditional medicines to modern antimalarials-and back again. J Altern Complement Med 2009;15:101–9.
7. Diallo D, Graz B, Falquet J, et al. Malaria treatment in remote areas of Mali: use of modern and traditional medicines, patient outcome. Trans R Soc Trop Med Hyg 2006;100:515–20.
8. Willcox M, Graz B, Falquet J, et al. *Argemone mexicana* decoction for the treatment of uncomplicated falciparum malaria. Trans R Soc Trop Med Hyg 2007;101:1190–8.
9. Graz B, Willcox ML, Diakite C, et al. *Argemone mexicana* decoction versus artesunate-amodiaquine for the management of malaria in Mali: policy and public-health implications. Trans R Soc Trop Med Hyg 2010;104:33–41.
10. Mueller MS, Runyambo N, Wagner I, et al. Randomized controlled trial of a traditional preparation of *Artemisia annua* L. (Annual Wormwood) in the treatment of malaria. Trans R Soc Trop Med Hyg 2004;98:318–21.
11. Blanke CH, Naisabha GB, Balema MB, et al. Herba *Artemisiae annuae* tea preparation compared to sulfadoxine-pyrimethamine in the treatment of uncomplicated falciparum malaria in adults: a randomized double-blind clinical trial. Trop Doct 2008;38:113–16.
12. Grindlay D, Reynolds T. The aloe vera phenomenon; a review of the properties and modern uses. J Ethnopharmacol 1986;16:117–31.
13. Tian B, Hua YJ, Ma XQ, Wang GL. Relationship between antibacterial activity of aloe and its anthaquinone compounds. Zhongguo Zhong Yao Za Zhi 2003;28:1034–7 [in Chinese].
14. Chen ZP, Cai Y, Phillipson JD. Studies on the antitumor, antibacterial and wound healing properties of dragon's blood. Planta Medica 1994;60:541–5.
15. Van Hien T, Hughes MA, Cherry GWC. In vitro studies on the antioxidant and growth stimulatory activities of a polyphenolic extract from *Cudrania cochinchinensis* used in the treatment of wounds in Vietnam. Wound Repair Regen 1997;5:159–67.
16. Phan TT, Hughes MA, Cherry GW, et al. An aqueous extract of the leaves of *Chromolaena odorata* (formerly *Eupatorium odoratum*) inhibits hydrated collagen lattice contraction by normal human dermal fibroblasts. J Altern and Complement Med 1996;2:335–44.
17. Phan TT, Wang L, See P, et al. Phenolic compounds of *Chromolaena odorata* protect cultured skin cells from oxidative damage: implication for cutaneous wound healing. Biol Pharm Bull 2001;24:1373–9.
18. Burford G, Bodeker G, Ryan TJ. Skin disease. In: Bodeker G, Burford G, eds. Public Health and Policy Perspectives on Traditional, Complementary and Alternative Medicine. London: Imperial College Press; 2007.
19. Courtright P, Lewallen S, Kanjaloti S. Changing patterns of corneal disease and associated vision loss at a rural African hospital following a training programme for traditional healers. Br J Ophthalmol 1996;80:694–7.
20. Biswas NR, Beri S, Das GK, et al. Comparative double blind multicentric randomised placebo controlled clinical trial of a herbal preparation of eye drops in some ocular ailments. J Indian Med Assoc 1996;94:101–2.
21. Graz B, Xu JM, Yao, ZS, et al. Trachoma: can trichiasis be treated with a sticking-plaster? A randomised controlled trial in China. Trop Med Int Health 1999;4:222–8.
22. World Health Organization. Substandard and counterfeit medicines. Fact sheet N 275, November 2003: http://www.who.int/mediacentre/factsheets/2003/fs275/en/ (accessed 12 March 2012).
23. Yee SK, Chu SS, Xu YM, Choo PL. Regulatory control of Chinese proprietary medicines in Singapore. Health Policy 2005;71:133–49.
24. Mollica RF, Cui X, Mcinnes K, Massagli MP. Science-based policy for psychosocial interventions in refugee camps: a Cambodian example. J Nerv Men Dis 2002;190:158–66.
25. Dhooper SS. Health care needs of foreign-born Asian Americans: an overview. Health Soc Work 2003;28:63–73.
26. Bodeker G, Neumann C, Lall P, Oo ZM. Traditional medicine use and health worker training in a refugee setting at the Thai-Burma border. J Refugee Studies 2005;18:76–99.
27. Hiegel JP. Do Traditional Healers have a Role in Refugee Camps? Refugee Participation Network, 8: Oxford Refugee Studies Program; 1990.
28. Neumann C, Bodeker G. Humanitarian responses to traditional medicine for refugee care. In: Bodeker G, Burford G, eds. Public Health and Policy Perspectives on Traditional, Complementary & Alternative Medicine. London: Imperial College Press; 2007.
29. Heinrich M, Edwards S, Moerman DE, Leonti M. Ethnopharmacological field studies: A critical assessment of their conceptual basis and methods. J Ethnopharmacol 2009;124:1–17.
30. Willcox ML, Graz B, Falquet J, et al. A "reverse pharmacology" approach for developing an anti-malarial phytomedicine. Malar J 2011;10(suppl. 1): S8.
31. Convention on Biological Diversity (1993). Available at: http://www.biodiv.org/convention/articles.asp (accessed 12 March 2012).
32. International Society of Ethnobiology (2006). International Society of Ethnobiology Code of Ethics (with 2008 additions). Available at: http://ethnobiology.net/code-of-ethics/ (accessed 12 March 2012).
33. World Health Organization. World Health Organization's Global Strategy and Plan of Action on Public Health, Innovation and Intellectual Property; 2008. Available at: http://apps.who.int/gb/ebwha/pdf_files/A61/A61_R21-en.pdf (accessed 12 March 2012).
34. Graz B. Prognostic Ability of Practitioners of Traditional Arabic Medicine: Comparison with Western Methods Through a Relative Patient Progress Scale. Evidence Based Complementary and Alternative Medicine 2010;7:471–6.
35. Sudha VBP, Singh KO, Prasad SR, Venkatasubramanian P. Killing of enteric bacteria in drinking water by a copper device for use in the home: laboratory evidence. Trans R Soc Trop Med Hyg 2009;103:819–22.

Environmental Health Hazards in the Tropics 26

Ema G Rodrigues, David C Christiani

Key features

Features unique to the tropics and key differences in resource-poor areas

- Lack of alternative resources/options
- Less stringent or poorly enforced environmental and occupational regulations
- Burden of disease on families may be greater in developing countries
- Access to healthcare may be very limited

Pediatric considerations

- Children may be more likely to be exposed to some contaminants and toxins due to hand-to-mouth activity
- For a given exposure, children have greater exposures per unit of body weight
- Children less efficiently metabolize and excrete many toxic chemicals

INTRODUCTION

Diseases caused by environmental exposures are often not readily treatable, but are often preventable. Exposures to environmental hazards can be modified or controlled in many cases, thus reducing or preventing the risk of developing disease. Countries undergoing economic development may be especially vulnerable to environmental hazards since the introduction of new materials, processes, and industries into nascent or emerging economies often precedes the introduction of proper controls, regulation, and experience in those settings. The Environmental Kuznets Curve (EKC) hypothesizes that during the initial phase of a country's economic development, environmental emissions increase as per capita income increases, but that as the economy matures, pollutant levels may subsequently decrease. This inverted U-shaped curve was initially described by Simon Kuznets to represent the relationship between income and inequality, and represents the pattern of emissions of some pollutants quite well. The eventual decrease in pollution may result from the implementation of controls and environmental policies as the negative societal impact of pollution begins to outweigh the positive societal impact of production and economic growth.

The likelihood of exposure to environmental toxins is often affected by economic and regional factors. For instance, some pesticides that are banned in the USA and the EU (e.g. DDT) continue to be used in several countries worldwide, as these countries balance the low cost and high effectiveness of such agents against environmental health aspects. A more recent industry that has posed environmental health hazards to those in developing countries is the electronic waste (e-waste) recycling industry, with China being the largest importer of e-waste from developed countries [1]. While the majority of electronics are composed of iron, aluminum, plastic and glass, they also contain copper, platinum and lead which are often recycled for profit. The exportation of e-waste from the US and EU to less developed countries is often the result of more stringent environmental and occupational regulations in industrialized nations.

Access to training and healthcare are other important aspects that may affect a population's risk of developing environmental-related disease following exposure. This chapter will discuss methods used to control personal exposures to environmental hazards, but it is crucial that those who are required to work with hazardous substances be trained on ways to avoid or minimize toxicity. Similarly, individuals exposed to toxins should have access to healthcare to monitor exposure and to minimize and treat exposure-related disease. Unfortunately, this is not often the case in developing regions. For instance, workers in the industrialized world are typically exposed to chronic low-level exposures and preclinical effects can be detected with routine monitoring, while acute poisonings are more common in developing countries where exposures are typically higher and access to healthcare is often limited.

EXPOSURE CONCEPTS

Several considerations must be made when assessing the risk of exposure to environmental and occupational hazards. First, the source of the hazard must be identified. Is the source of the hazard in the workplace, home, or neighborhood? Typically, occupational exposures to substances are significantly higher than environmental exposures, but environmental contaminants usually affect a larger number of individuals. While workers are exposed to higher contaminant levels, they are typically healthier than the general population, which includes children, the elderly, and those who have chronic health conditions. In developing countries, this division between work and home may be less clear. For example, families may live on the agricultural lands where they work; all individuals may be exposed to occupational chemicals, such as pesticides and herbicides, throughout the day rather than only during certain work hours. Additionally, child labor remains common. Many children in developing countries contribute to both family and non-family work where exposures may be higher than those of the general population (Table 26-1).

Second, the route of exposure must be considered. Exposure to environmental contaminants occurs mainly through ingestion of contaminated food or water, inhalation of contaminated air, or dermal absorption of chemical or biological agents. The health effects associated with a hazard may vary depending on the route of exposure, since absorption differs by organ (lung, skin, or gastrointestinal tract). The absorbed dose, described as mass of chemical per mass of the individual's bodyweight, is an important consideration when determining how much exposure of a chemical is considered "safe". Because children have lower bodyweights than adults, equal exposures will result in higher doses for children. In addition to dose quantities, other considerations associated with the health effects of environmental hazards include duration and timing of exposure. In some cases, chronic exposures over a lengthy period of time may have cumulative effects leading to disease, whereas the effects of short-term or periodic exposures may be naturally repaired. For example, exposure to heavy metals may induce DNA damage, but DNA repair mechanisms may prevent the development of disease if exposures are short-term. Timing of exposure is also important since individuals are more susceptible to the health effects of environmental exposures during certain periods of life, such as during fetal development, childhood, and advanced age.

MAJOR ENVIRONMENTAL AND OCCUPATIONAL HAZARDS

AMBIENT AIR POLLUTION

Air pollution is a widespread environmental health hazard with sources ranging from anthropogenic sources (e.g. combustion of fossil fuels in power plants or motor vehicles) to natural sources (e.g. forest fires and dust storms). Air pollution is comprised of various contaminants, including particulate matter (PM), sulfur dioxide (SO_2), nitrogen dioxide (NO_2), carbon monoxide (CO), ozone (O_3) and polycyclic aromatic hydrocarbons (PAHs), among others. Rapid industrialization in several tropical countries has led to significantly higher concentrations of air pollutants compared to those in developed countries. Increase in some air pollutants, such as NO_2 and O_3, is often due to an increase in the use of motor vehicles, coupled with lack of environmental regulations to enforce controls [2].

TABLE 26-1 Child Labor, 5–14 Years (%), 1999–2007

Bangladesh	13
Belize	40
Brazil	6
Cambodia	45
Ghana	34
India	12
Mexico	16
Nicaragua	15

Data from: The State of the World's Children 2009, UNICEF.

Increased air pollution levels have been associated with cardiovascular disease, upper and lower respiratory tract infections, and lung cancer [3–5]. Additionally, individuals with chronic health conditions such as asthma, emphysema and cardiovascular disorders are more susceptible to the health effects associated with air pollution. Particulate matter, typically characterized by particle size defined by the aerodynamic diameter in microns (e.g. PM_{10}, $PM_{2.5}$, $PM_{1.0}$), has been shown to be especially harmful. While larger particles are typically trapped in the nose and throat, smaller particles are more likely to be inhaled into the deeper regions of the lung (i.e. alveoli), making smaller particles more likely to contribute to pulmonary and heart disease.

Weather conditions in many tropical zones may exacerbate the level of pollution. For instance, high temperatures in combination with high humidity and lack of rain lead to faster rates of the formation of smog, a term used to describe the interaction of nitrogen oxides, volatile organic compounds, and other pollutants, and there is some evidence that ambient PM_{10} concentrations have a greater effect on mortality and hospitalizations due to cardiovascular and respiratory causes during the warm periods and summer [6].

INDOOR AIR POLLUTION

The health effects associated with indoor air pollution (IAP) are of great concern in developing countries, where it has been estimated that more than 2.4 billion people use biomass fuels (BMF) such as wood, dung and coal for cooking and heating [7]. Figure 26.1 indicates that developing countries in tropical zones account for the majority of deaths attributed to exposure to indoor smoke from burning of solid fuels. BMF smoke is also associated with chronic obstructive pulmonary disease (COPD), tuberculosis, lung

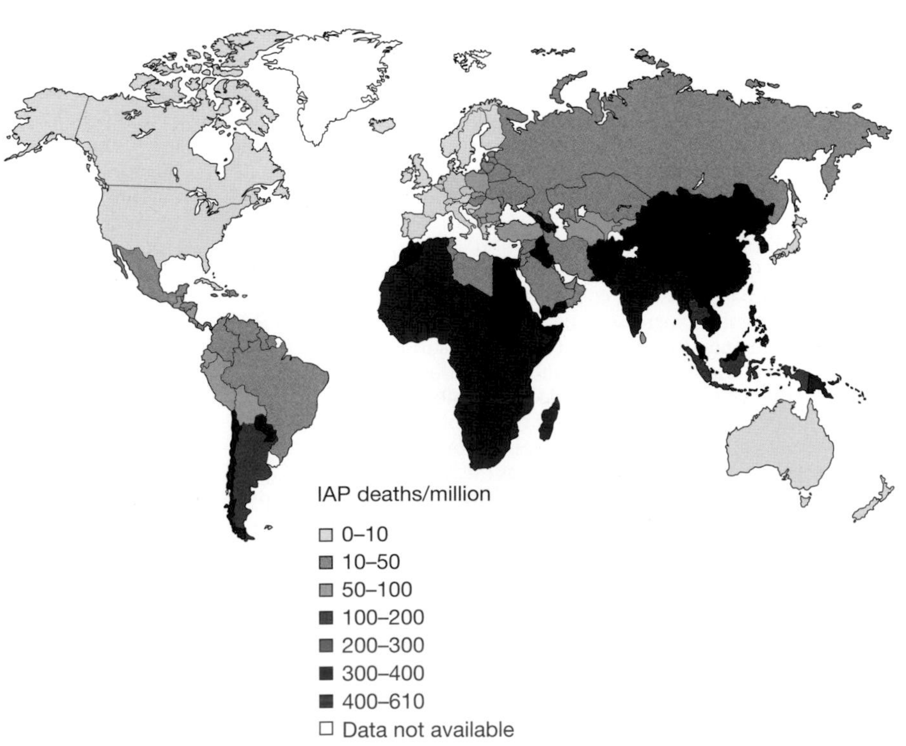

FIGURE 26.1 Deaths from indoor smoke from solid fuels. *Redrawn from WHO World Health Report, 2002.*

cancer, and an interstitial lung disease known as "hut lung". In developing countries, women are at highest risk of developing BMF smoke-related illness since they are exposed to the highest levels while cooking [8]. A recent study conducted in rural China reported a substantial decrease in the incidence of COPD among men and women after installation of household chimneys on previously un-vented stoves [9].

ARSENIC

Arsenic (As), a naturally occurring metal embedded in the earth's crust, is characterized as a known human carcinogen by the International Agency for Research on Cancer [10]. Exposure to arsenic occurs mainly through ingestion of contaminated water from deep wells (30–180 feet), but can also occur through food or inhalation of arsenic fumes from coal burning or smelting. Arsenic is leached into drinking water supplies from the bedrock surrounding the aquifers, and elevated arsenic levels in drinking water have been documented in several tropical countries such as India, Chile, Mexico, Bangladesh, Peru, Taiwan, Mongolia and Thailand, as well as in parts of the US. While inorganic arsenic occurs in several forms, the trivalent (As^{III}) and pentavalent (As^{V}) species are most toxic, whereas organic forms such as arsenobetaine occur in shellfish such as shrimp and are not toxic to humans.

In an effort to provide clean water free of microbial contamination, the United Nations Children's Fund (UNICEF) began to install tube wells in Bangladesh in the 1970s. While this effort was aimed at reducing the morbidity and mortality due to gastrointestinal disease, it also caused one of the largest arsenic poisonings in history. It has been estimated that more that 35–77 million people may be exposed to arsenic-contaminated drinking water across Bangladesh [11]. Also, large numbers of people in nearby West Bengal in India have been similarly affected. The clinical manifestations of chronic arsenic exposure are numerous, and include hyperpigmentation, keratoses, and skin, bladder and lung cancers (Fig. 26.2) [12–14]. There is no ideal treatment for chronic arsenic-related health effects, but affected individuals are usually told to avoid drinking additional arsenic-contaminated water and to consume a protein-rich diet. Additionally, higher selenium blood levels may reduce the risk of arsenic-related skin lesions [15]. In severe cases of arsenic poisoning, chelation with 2,3-dimercapto-1-propanesulfonate (DMPS) can increase the urinary excretion of arsenic and improve symptoms. Additionally, for arsenic-related cancers, surgical methods can be used to remove the cancer if it is detected early [16].

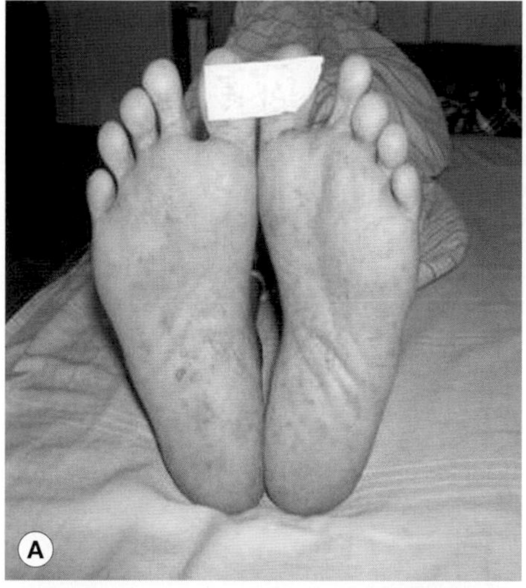

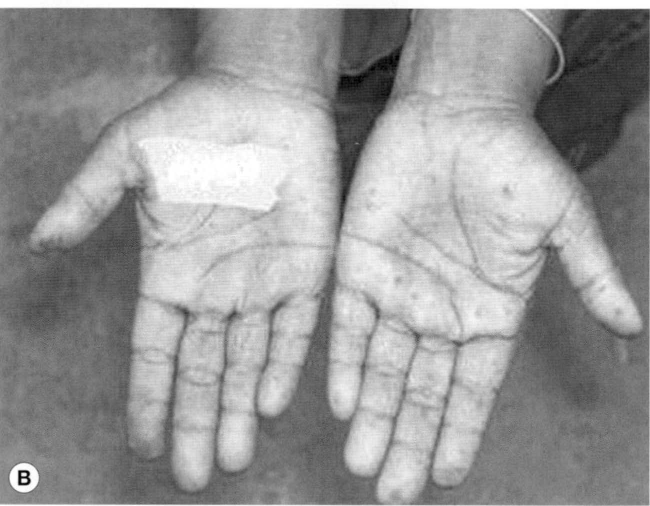

FIGURE 26.2 Hyperkeratotic rash of arsenic intoxication. Photos courtesy of Dr Molly Kile, Harvard School of Public Health

LEAD POISONING

Lead is a durable, malleable metal that is highly resistant to corrosion and is used worldwide for many applications. It has been used for the manufacture of water pipes, as an anti-knock agent in gasoline, as an anti-corrosive pigment in paint, additive in cosmetics, and in traditional medicines. Among the many uses, leaded gasoline is one of the major sources of airborne lead pollution and personal exposure. The phase-out of lead from gasoline has significantly reduced the air lead concentrations and blood lead levels in humans in many countries, including Austria, Brazil, Canada, Colombia, India [17], Japan, Pakistan [18], Slovakia, Sweden, Thailand and the US. Another source of lead, especially in developing countries, is lead glazes used in ceramics. When ceramic pottery is used for cooking or storing food, the lead contained in the glaze may leach into food [19]. Another source of lead exposure and poisonings in developing countries is the recycling of electronics containing lead and lead-acid batteries [20]. While lead exposures are very high in these workplaces, children and adults can also be exposed to dangerous levels of lead in air or soil while living near one of these facilities or living with an individual working with lead [21]. Cosmetics and traditional remedies containing lead are also commonly used in tropical countries.

Given its many uses, lead is a very common contaminant and is a leading cause of environmental-related illness among both children and adults worldwide. Lead is mainly absorbed into the bloodstream through ingestion and inhalation. Absorbed lead is redistributed and stored in bone and soft tissues until remobilized into the bloodstream. Because lead has a relatively long half-life for excretion ($T_{1/2}$ ~28 days), health effects associated with lead are chronic and long-lasting. Health effects related to increased blood lead levels in children include encephalopathy, and decreases in IQ, hemoglobin synthesis, growth, nerve conduction velocity and cognitive function (Box 26.1). Abdominal symptoms (called "lead colic") include abdominal pain, intermittent vomiting and constipation. High-level exposure can lead to interstitial nephritis. Research has shown that children in India under 3 years of age with blood lead levels ≥10 μg/dL are more likely to have moderate or severe anemia, but no lead level is considered safe [22]. Health effects in adults include anemia,

BOX 26.1 Pediatric Considerations – Lead

- Children absorb lead more efficiently than adults
- Children who are malnourished are particularly susceptible to lead due to lower intakes of iron and calcium which can reduce the absorption of lead
- Blood lead levels ≥10 μg/dL among children are considered elevated, but no level is considered safe

constipation, mental status changes, cardiovascular disease and hypertension, chronic renal dysfunction, decreased sperm count and increased abnormal sperm in men, and higher incidence of spontaneous abortions in women [23] (Table 26-2). Diagnosis usually rests on direct measurement of blood lead levels. Basophilic stippling of erythrocytes and gingival lead lines may be seen. Once internalized, lead enters bone, and boney tissues can act as long-term reservoirs. The most important feature of treatment is to minimize additional exposure. Chelation therapy can reduce immediate toxicity during acute exposures and severe intoxications, but may not appreciably alter long-term cognitive impairment.

PESTICIDES

In developing countries, acute pesticide poisonings are still a major health concern. Pesticides are widely available and widely used, and include insecticides, herbicides and rodenticides (Table 26-3). To maximize crop productivity, pesticides are in wide use in many areas of emerging economies. Health outcomes associated with pesticide exposures include death, and neurologic, reproductive, developmental, ophthalmic, genotoxic and carcinogenic effects. Many insecticides are organophosphates or carbamates, and are potent cholinesterase inhibitors. Signs and symptoms of intoxication relate to level, identity

TABLE 26-2 Health Effects Associated with Fibrogenic and Metal Dusts

Agent	Industry	Disease/health outcome	Clinical presentation/symptoms
Dusts			
Asbestos	Construction Fire proofing	Pleural plaques Malignant mesothelioma Pleural effusion	Chest pain Cough Shortness of breath Chest tightness
Silica	Ceramics Construction Cement manufacturing Glass manufacturing Semiconductors Metallurgy Sand blasting Stone cutting	Silicosis	Chronic cough Shortness of breath Fluid in lungs
Cotton dust	Textiles	Byssinosis	Chest tightness Cough Wheezing
Coal dust	Coal mining	Black lung disease	Breathlessness
Metals			
Lead	Battery recycling Construction/painting Electronics	Anemia Reproductive effects (male and female) Cardiovascular disease Encephalopathy Nephropathy Death	Fatigue Nausea Headaches Hypertension Constipation Increased blood lead levels Increased erythrocyte protoporphyrin
Manganese	Manganese processing Battery manufacturing Welding Steel production Mining Glass manufacturing Fungicides	Manganism Anemia	Neurological effects Slowed hand movements Behavioral changes Tremors Hypertension
Chromium	Steel production Chrome plating Leather industry Cement	Eczema Asthmatic bronchitis	Skin rashes/dermatitis Ulcers Kidney damage
Beryllium	Ceramics Nuclear weapons	Beryllium sensitization Chronic beryllium disease (CBD)	Shortness of breath
Mercury (inorganic)	Battery manufacturing Mercury recycling Auto manufacturing Thermometers Lighting	Minamata disease	Dermatitis Mood changes Memory loss Muscle weakness Tremors Kidney effects Respiratory failure Slurring of speech

TABLE 26-3 Adverse Health Effects Caused by Selected Classes of Pesticides*

Chemical/ chemical class	Examples of pesticides	Clinical presentation	Treatment	Route of exposure†
Arsenicals	Sodium arsenate	Abdominal pain, nausea, vomiting, garlic odor, metallic taste, bloody diarrhea, headache, dizziness, drowsiness, weakness, lethargy, delirium, shock, kidney insufficiency, neuropathy	Wash skin thoroughly and remove contaminated clothing Gastric lavage and/or activated charcoal (avoid cathartics as arsenicals can cause diarrhea) Intravenous fluid administration and monitoring of electrolytes Chelation: Agents include meso-2,3-dimercapto-succinic acid (succimer) or British Anti-Lewisite (BAL or dimercaprol); DMPS (sodium salt of 2,3-dimercapto-1-propane sulfonic acid) is also used but is not FDA-approved for use in the United States	O, R, D (rarely)
Borates (insecticide)	Borax	Upper airway irritation, abdominal pain, nausea, vomiting, diarrhea, headache, lethargy, tremor, kidney insufficiency	Wash skin thoroughly and remove contaminated clothing Gastric lavage (NOTE: activated charcoal has limited ability to absorb boric acid) Dialysis	O, R, D (broken skin)
Carbamates (insecticide)	Carbaryl thiram, aldicarb mecarbam	Malaise, weakness, dizziness, sweating, headache, salivation, nausea, vomiting, diarrhea, abdominal pain, confusion, dyspnea, dermatitis, pulmonary edema	Wash skin thoroughly and remove contaminated clothing Activated charcoal within first hour of ingestion Oxygen Endotracheal intubation often required for depressed mental status, bronchospasm, copious secretions, and respiratory depression Atropine Pralidoxime (must be given along with atropine)	O, D
Chloralose	Chloralose	Vomiting, vertigo, tremor, myoclonus, fasciculations, confusion, seizures, rhabdomyolysis	Gastric lavage and/or activated charcoal Benzodiazepines for seizures Intravenous fluids	O
Coumarins (rodenticide)	Brodifacoum warfarin	Ecchymoses, epistaxis, excessive bleeding, hematuria, prolonged prothrombin time, intracranial bleed, anemia, fatigue, dyspnea	Vitamin K Fresh frozen plasma +/– recombinant human factor VIIa for life-threatening bleeding GI decontamination if large ingestion	O, D (possible)
Diethyltoluamide (insect repellent)	DEET (N,N-diethyl-meta-toluamide	Dermatitis, ocular irritation, headache, restlessness, ataxia, confusion, seizures, urticaria	Gastric lavage within 1 hour and/or activated charcoal Benzodiazepines for seizures	O, D
Dipyridil (herbicide)	Paraquat, diquat	Mucous membrane and airway irritation, abdominal pain, diarrhea, vomiting, gastrointestinal bleeding, pulmonary edema, dermatitis, renal and hepatic damage, coma, seizures	Gastric lavage using diatomaceous earth clays (bentonite or Fuller's earth) Activated charcoal if diatomaceous earth clays not available Hemodialysis	O, D (via broken skin)
Phosphonates (herbicide)	Glyphosate	Airway, skin, and mucous membrane irritation, abdominal, pain, nausea, vomiting, shock, dyspnea, respiratory failure	Rinse mouth with milk or water Activated charcoal for later ingestions Monitor for acute lung injury and hypotension	O, R

Continued

TABLE 26-3 Adverse Health Effects Caused by Selected Classes of Pesticides—cont'd

Chemical/ chemical class	Examples of pesticides	Clinical presentation	Treatment	Route of exposure†
Fluoroacetate (rodenticide)	Sodium fluoroacetate	Vomiting, paresthesias, tremors, seizures, hallucinations, coma, confusion, arrhythmias, hypertension, cardiac failure	Gastric lavage within 1 hour and/or activated charcoal Monitor for and treat hypocalcemia (Administration of Monoacetin and ethanol have been used, but safety and efficacy have not been proven in humans)	O, D (possible)
Mercury, organic (fungicide)	Methyl mercury	Metallic taste, paresthesias, tremor, headache, weakness, delirium, ataxia, visual changes, dermatitis, renal dysfunction	Removal from source and gastric lavage and activated charcoal Chelation for acute neurologic symptoms or chronic toxicity: agents include penicillamine, BAL, DMPS, and dimercaptosuccinic acid (DMSA)	O, R, D
Metal phosphides (rodenticide, fumigant)	Zinc-, aluminum-, magnesium-phosphide	Abdominal pain, diarrhea, acidosis, shock, jaundice, paresthesias, ataxia, tremors, coma, pulmonary edema, tetany, dermal irritation	Wash skin thoroughly and remove contaminated clothing Be prepared to isolate vomited material as phosphine gas produced in stomach can off-gas into environment after vomiting	O, R, D
Halocarbons (fumigant)	Cellfume, methyl bromide	Skin/airway/mucous membrane irritant, cough, renal dysfunction, confusion, seizures, coma, pulmonary edema	Wash skin thoroughly and remove contaminated clothing Gastric lavage and/or activated charcoal if ingested	O, R, D
Organochlorines (insecticide)	Lindane, DDT	Cyanosis, excitability, dizziness, headache, restlessness, tremors, convulsions, coma, paresthesias, nausea, vomiting, confusion, tremor, cardiac arrhythmias, acidosis	Wash skin thoroughly and remove contaminated clothing Diazepam for convulsions Oxygenation Cholestyramine resin to enhance elimination	O, R, D
Organophosphates (insecticides)	Malathion, parathion dichlorvos chlorpyrifos	Headache, dizziness, bradycardia, weakness, anxiety, excessive sweating, fasciculations, vomiting, diarrhea, abdominal cramps, dyspnea, miosis, paralysis, salivation, tearing, ataxia, pulmonary edema, confusion, acetylcholinesterase inhibition	Same management as for carbamates	O, D
Organotin (fungicide)	Fentin acetate	Airway, skin and mucous membrane irritation, dermatitis, salivation, delirium, headache, vomiting, dizziness	Wash skin thoroughly and remove contaminated clothing Dilution with water or milk Activated charcoal	O, R, D
Phenol derivatives (fungicide, wood preservative)	Pentachlorophenol	Skin, airway and mucous membrane irritation, contact dermatitis, dyspnea, diaphoreses, urticaria, tachycardia, headache, abdominal pain, fever, tremor, hypotension, rhabdomyolysis	Gastric lavage and/or activated charcoal Intravenous fluids (NOTE: salicylates are contraindicated for fever)	O, R, D
Pyrethrins, pyrethroids	Allethrin cyfluthrin permethrin	Allergic reactions, anaphylaxis, dermatitis, paresthesias, wheezing, seizures, coma, pulmonary edema, diarrhea, abdominal pain	GI decontamination is usually not required For allergic or hypersensitivity reactions, antihistamines, inhaled beta-agonists, corticosteroids, or epinephrine may be used	R, D

TABLE 26-3 Adverse Health Effects Caused by Selected Classes of Pesticides—cont'd

Chemical/ chemical class	Examples of pesticides	Clinical presentation	Treatment	Route of exposure[†]
Strychnine (rodenticide)	Strychnine	Muscle rigidity, opisthotonus, rhabdomyolysis, hyperthermia, respiratory compromise	Endotracheal intubation is generally required High-dose benzodiazepines to control muscle activity Nondepolarizing neuromuscular blockade agents (e.g. vecuronium) may also be used in intubated patients Opioids (muscle contractions are extremely painful) Aggressive intravenous fluid administration	O
Thallium (rodenticide)	Thallium sulfate	Abdominal pain, nausea, vomiting, bloody diarrhea, headache, weakness, liver injury, hair loss, paresthesias, neuropathy, encephalopathy, cardiac failure	Gastric lavage and/or activated charcoal Insoluble Prussian blue to increase elimination rate Monitor for and treat hypocalcemia	O
Triazines (herbicide)	Atrazine, prometryn	Mucous membrane, ocular and dermal irritation	Gastric lavage and/or activated charcoal	O, R, D

Modified from Thundiyil JG, Stober J, Besbelli N, Pronczuk J: Acute pesticide poisoning: a proposed classification tool. Bull World Health Organ 2008;86:205–9.
*This list is an overview and is not meant to be a comprehensive list of all pesticides and pesticide classes. Gastric emptying is most effective when used within 1 hour of an acute and large dose ingestion, and should rarely be performed if more than 4 hours have elapsed since ingestion. Gastric emptying should in general not be performed following ingestion of corrosives and many hydrocarbons. Complications include aspiration and perforation.
[†]Route of exposure key: O, oral/ingestion; R, respiratory/inhalation; D, dermal or ocular.

BOX 26.2 Pediatric Considerations – Pesticides

- Approximately 70% of working children work in agriculture and may be exposed to pesticides at occupational levels worldwide
- Children are particularly vulnerable to the effects of pesticides because they have lower levels of enzymes involved in the metabolism and excretion of pesticides such as organophosphates

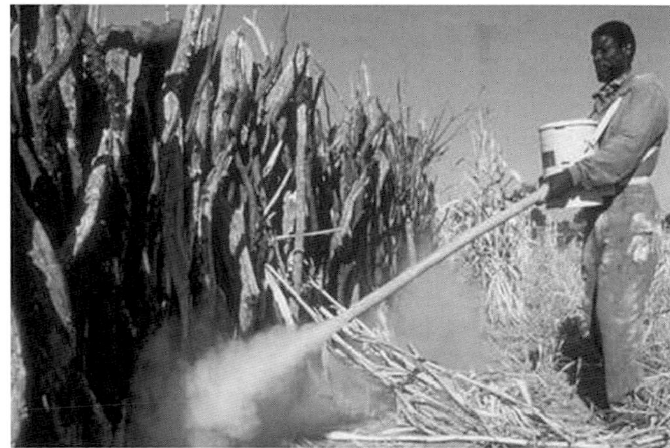

FIGURE 26.3 DDT spraying in Namibia. *Reprinted with permission from Peter Arnold, Inc.*

and fat solubility of the agent, and include: salivation, lacrimation, urination, defecation, gastric emesis, bronchorrhea, bronchospasm, bradycardia (SLUDGE/BBB), respiratory depression, cardiac arrhythmias, miosis, neuropathy and altered mental status. Death may result from respiratory and cardiovascular compromise. Diagnosis is usually one of clinical recognition. Treatment involves decontamination, supportive care, atropine, and oximes such as pralidoxime.

It has been estimated that 3 million cases of severe acute pesticide poisonings occur each year globally, resulting in 220,000 deaths annually, and that 99% of these deaths occur in the developing world. Globally, pesticides are also commonly used to commit suicide, since they are inexpensive, widely available, and effective. It is estimated that two-thirds of all pesticide-related deaths worldwide are the result of suicide [24].

Occupational exposure to pesticides can occur through inhalation, incidental ingestion, and dermal contact during job-related tasks such as mixing and spraying (Box 26.2). Pesticide containers should be clearly labeled in the local language with ample use of illustrations in low-literacy populations to communicate proper handling. Since many agricultural workers worldwide are illiterate, all workers should also be trained in proper handling and usage. While the use of personal protective equipment (PPE) such as respirators and impermeable gloves and clothing is effective in reducing exposures, PPE can be very costly and uncomfortable, and is less likely to be used in hot humid areas (Fig. 26.3). The lack of PPE use emphasizes the need to regulate the most toxic pesticides and replace them with less toxic alternatives. Additional interventions can include introducing crop rotation to minimize the need for pesticide use [25].

While pesticide use is essential in the developing world for agricultural purposes and the reduction of vector-borne diseases, actions can be taken to minimize the hazards of pesticide use, including self-poisonings. For the most part, highly toxic pesticides have been banned or are approved for restricted use by a certified applicator in developed countries (e.g. arsenic oxide, DDT, parathion), but these regulations are not normally extant or are not enforced in developing countries. In fact, DDT was banned in several African countries for several years before it was reintroduced for indoor use due to an increase in malaria deaths. Currently, a Global Environment Facility (GEF) initiative aims to phase-out the use of DDT by the early 2020s, while assuring that malaria infection rate reductions are met.

MOLD/FOOD IMPURITIES

The high heat, humidity, and long rainy seasons in tropical countries make infestation of mold a likely environmental problem, especially in agricultural communities. Aflatoxins, highly toxic metabolites produced by the fungi *Aspergillus flavus* and *Aspergillus parasiticus*, are contaminants found in animal feed and some crops such as corn, peanuts and cotton. Ingestion of aflatoxins can lead to liver necrosis, failure and cirrhosis. A recent outbreak of aflatoxin poisoning in eastern and central provinces in Kenya (2004) due to contaminated maize that had been stored in damp conditions lead to 317 cases of acute poisoning and 125 deaths. Levels of aflatoxin measured in maize from the households that were affected ranged from 20 ppb to 8000 ppb, up to 400 times the WHO recommended maximum limit [26]. Aflatoxin is also a major contributor to liver cancer [27,28] and is classified as a Group 1 human carcinogen by the International Agency for Research on Cancer (IARC) [29]. Diagnosis usually involves clinical recognition, especially of outbreaks from common ingestion, and measuring toxin or metabolites in blood or urine. Treatment is usually supportive.

Ergotism (also called St. Anthony's Fire), a disease caused by the ingestion of ergot alkaloids produced by ergot, is manifested in two forms: the gangrenous form and the convulsive form. The causative agent, alkaloid ergotamine, and derivatives affect vascular constriction and neurotransmission. The gangrenous form of ergotism is characterized by symptoms including edema of the legs, severe pain, and gangrene at the tendons, while the convulsive form is characterized by nausea and vomiting followed by drowsiness, twitching, uterine contractions and abortion, convulsions, blindness, hallucinations and paralysis. Chronic complications include cardiac valvular fibrosis. The main source of exposure to ergot alkaloids is contaminated grains (especially rye) that are stored in humid environments susceptible to contamination of fungi of the genus *Claviceps*. The clinical symptoms experienced by individuals who have ingested ergot alkaloids depend on the type of alkaloids produced by the various fungi. Ergotism can be prevented by thorough cleaning practices and by destroying the alkaloids by cooking and baking the flour products [30].

Farmer's lung disease (FLD) is a type of hypersensitivity pneumonitis resulting from an allergic reaction to inhaled microbial agents, including mold spores. Farmers may inhale fungal microorganisms typically found in hay stored in damp conditions with poor ventilation. The symptoms of this disease include shortness of breath, productive cough, bronchospasm, fever, and malaise. The chest x-ray shows bilateral, fleeting infiltrates. Additionally, patients with FLD have been shown to have higher precipitating immunoglobulin G (IgG) levels associated with various microbes, compared with farmers without the disease [31]. Chronic farmer's lung can lead to obliterating bronchiolitis and fibrosis. Treatment usually involves minimizing additional exposure and treatment with steroids (inhaled and systemic) and bronchodilators.

Melamine is another example of a toxic food impurity. Unlike mold contamination, food products containing melamine have been intentionally contaminated. Foods contaminated with melamine will appear to have higher protein content because melamine is rich in nitrogen, which is measured to determine protein levels. In an attempt to make some food items more marketable, a variety of products, such as infant formula and wheat flour used in pet food, originating in China have been contaminated with melamine. Tens of thousands of infants and young children in China have been hospitalized with kidney stones and obstructive renal failure after the consumption of melamine-contaminated formula. Some cases resulted in death [32]. Successful treatment of cases included dialysis to correct their electrolyte levels, hydration (orally or intravenously), alkalization, or surgical removal of the stones [33].

RECOGNITION OF ENVIRONMENTAL AND OCCUPATIONAL HAZARDS

Several methods can be used by physicians and public health professionals to identify diseases related to environmental conditions. Sentinel cases or unexpected cases of disease may give clues to causative agents. For example, in 1775, Percivall Pott was one of the first surgeons to observe a high incidence of scrotal cancers in young boys who worked as chimney sweeps. Pott suspected that this unexpected high incidence of cancer was a result of dermal contact with coal soot (that is now known to contain various polycyclic aromatic hydrocarbons and now known to be carcinogenic), and he noted that regular washing prevented the disease. Continuous surveillance and the maintenance of disease registries can also be valuable in the identification of an environmental or occupational health outcome. Registries allow for the methodical collection of demographic and occupational information from individuals who have developed specific illnesses (e.g. cancer, asthma, diabetes). Additionally, targeted registries can collect biological measurements on healthy people who may be at high risk for specific exposures (e.g. blood lead levels among construction workers).

Physicians play a crucial role in detecting and the critical role in treating individuals with disease relating to environmental exposure or poisoning. In many cases, the best treatment for an environmental disease is removal from exposure. Information about the patient's work environment as well as the home environment is crucial in the identification of disease. It is also important for physicians to consider previous jobs as well as current jobs. Some diseases have a long latency period and may have clinical impact years after the patient was exposed. Thorough exposure histories may identify a causative agent responsible for the patient's symptoms, and medical screening tests (e.g. beryllium sensitization test, pulmonary function) can be used to monitor exposed patients

CONTROL AND REDUCTION OF ENVIRONMENTAL AND OCCUPATIONAL HAZARDS

While several methods can be used to reduce the levels of personal exposure to environmental hazards, each method differs in terms of feasibility, expense and efficacy. The most efficient way to reduce the health effects associated with a hazard is to eliminate it from use or substitute it with a less hazardous substance. A common successful implementation of this is the elimination and substitution of lead in gasoline in several countries. Elimination of a hazard is the most desirable option, but it may not always be feasible. It is necessary to have a suitable less hazardous substitute that can be used for the purpose. When substitution is not an option, engineering controls, such as ventilation, or a redesigning of equipment can be used to minimize personal exposures to the hazard. While engineering controls are usually effective, they can be expensive to implement and maintain over time. The implementation of cooking stoves with enclosed wood-burning chambers with chimneys as opposed to open fires is an example of a redesign that reduced personal exposure to indoor air pollution and respiratory symptoms, specifically among women [34,35]. In the absence of feasible engineering controls, the use of administrative controls can reduce workplace exposures (not necessarily environmental exposures) to individuals by rotating jobs among workers or limiting the time a worker performs a specific task, such as spraying pesticides. Finally, workers can use personal protective equipment (PPE), such as respirators, and protective clothing (e.g. gloves, overalls, boots) to minimize the absorption of environmental hazards that cannot be controlled by any other means. The use of PPE may be effective, but it also poses additional challenges to workers. PPE requires routine cleaning and maintenance for efficacy and can be very cumbersome to wear, especially in hot and humid climates.

Other common control measures include regular hand washing to avoid exposure through hand-to-mouth contact while eating, drinking or smoking, and changing clothes after being exposed to dusts or chemicals to minimize further absorption and exposure to others.

REFERENCES

1. Ni HG, Zeng EY. Law enforcement and global collaboration are the keys to containing e-waste tsunami in China. Environ Sci Technol 2009;43:3991–4.
2. Chen B, Kan H. Air pollution and population health: a global challenge. Environ Health Prev Med 2008;13:94–101.
3. Zanobetti A, Schwartz J. The effect of fine and coarse particulate air pollution on mortality: a national analysis. Environ Health Perspect 2009;117:898–903.
4. Brunekreef B, Dockery DW, Krzyzanowski M. Epidemiologic studies on short-term effects of low levels of major ambient air pollution components. Environ Health Perspect 1995;103 Suppl 2:3–13.
5. Dockery DW. Epidemiologic evidence of cardiovascular effects of particulate air pollution. Environ Health Perspect 2001;109 Suppl 4:483–6.
6. Yi O, Hong YC, Kim H. Seasonal effect of PM(10) concentrations on mortality and morbidity in Seoul, Korea: a temperature-matched case-crossover analysis. Environ Res 2010;110:89–95.
7. International Energy Agency. World Energy Outlook 2004. Paris: Organization for Economic Co-operation and Development/International Energy Agency; 2004.
8. Fullerton DG, Bruce N, Gordon SB. Indoor air pollution from biomass fuel smoke is a major health concern in the developing world. Trans R Soc Trop Med Hyg 2008;102:843–51.
9. Chapman RS, He X, Blair AE, Lan Q. Improvement in household stoves and risk of chronic obstructive pulmonary disease in Xuanwei, China: retrospective cohort study. BMJ 2005;331:1050.
10. IARC. Arsenic and arsenic compounds. IARC Monogr Eval Carcinog Risk Chem Hum 1980;23:39–141.
11. Smith AH, Lingas EO, Rahman M. Contamination of drinking-water by arsenic in Bangladesh: a public health emergency. Bull World Health Organ 2000;78:1093–103.
12. McCarty KM, Ryan L, Houseman EA, et al. A case-control study of GST polymorphisms and arsenic related skin lesions. Environ Health 2007;6:5.
13. Smith AH, Hopenhayn-Rich C, Bates MN, et al. Cancer risks from arsenic in drinking water. Environ Health Perspect 1992;97:259–67.
14. Rahman MM, Ng JC, Naidu R. Chronic exposure of arsenic via drinking water and its adverse health impacts on humans. Environ Geochem Health 2009;31 Suppl 1:189–200.
15. Chen Y, Hall M, Graziano JH, et al. A prospective study of blood selenium levels and the risk of arsenic-related premalignant skin lesions. Cancer Epidemiol Biomarkers Prev 2007;16:207–13.
16. Guha Mazumder DN. Chronic arsenic toxicity: clinical features, epidemiology, and treatment: experience in West Bengal. J Environ Sci Health A Tox Hazard Subst Environ Eng 2003;38:141–63.
17. Nichani V, Li WI, Smith MA, et al. Blood lead levels in children after phase-out of leaded gasoline in Bombay, India. Sci Total Environ 2006;363:95–106.
18. Kadir MM, Janjua NZ, Kristensen S, et al. Status of children's blood lead levels in Pakistan: implications for research and policy. Public Health 2008;122:708–15.
19. Romieu I, Palazuelos E, Hernandez Avila M, et al. Sources of lead exposure in Mexico City. Environ Health Perspect 1994;102:384–9.
20. Haefliger P, Mathieu-Nolf M, Lociciro S, et al. Mass lead intoxication from informal used lead-acid battery recycling in Dakar, Senegal. Environ Health Perspect 2009;117:1535–40.
21. Zheng L, Wu K, Li Y, et al. Blood lead and cadmium levels and relevant factors among children from an e-waste recycling town in China. Environ Res 2008;108:15–20.
22. Jain NB, Laden F, Guller U, et al. Relation between blood lead levels and childhood anemia in India. Am J Epidemiol 2005;161:968–73.
23. Meyer PA, Brown MJ, Falk H. Global approach to reducing lead exposure and poisoning. Mutat Res 2008;659:166–75.
24. World Health Organization (WHO). Public Health Impact of Pesticides Used in Agriculture. Geneva: World Health Organization; 1990.
25. Eddleston M, Karalliedde L, Buckley N, et al. Pesticide poisoning in the developing world – a minimum pesticides list. Lancet 2002;360:1163–7.
26. Centers for Disease Control and Prevention (CDC). Outbreak of aflatoxin poisoning – eastern and central provinces, Kenya, January–July 2004. MMWR Morb Mortal Wkly Rep 2004;53:790–3.
27. Chuang SC, Vecchia CL, Boffetta P. Liver cancer: descriptive epidemiology and risk factors other than HBV and HCV infection. Cancer Lett 2009;286:9–14.
28. Wu HC, Wang Q, Yang HI, et al. Aflatoxin B1 exposure, hepatitis B virus infection, and hepatocellular carcinoma in Taiwan. Cancer Epidemiol Biomarkers Prev 2009;18:846–53.
29. IARC Working Group on the Evaluation of Carcinogenic Risks to Humans. Traditional herbal medicines, some mycotoxins, naphthalene and styrene. IARC Monogr Eval Carcinog Risk Chem Hum 2002;82:1–556.
30. Peraica M, Domijan AM. Contamination of food with mycotoxins and human health. Arh Hig Rada Toksikol 2001;52:23–35.
31. Erkinjuntti-Pekkanen R, Reiman M, Kokkarinen JI, et al. IgG antibodies, chronic bronchitis, and pulmonary function values in farmer's lung patients and matched controls. Allergy 1999;54:1181–7.
32. Kuehn BM. Melamine scandals highlight hazards of increasingly globalized food chain. JAMA 2009;301:473–5.
33. Sun Q, Shen Y, Sun N, et al. Diagnosis, treatment and follow-up of 25 patients with melamine-induced kidney stones complicated by acute obstructive renal failure in Beijing Children's Hospital. Eur J Pediatr 2010;169:483–9.
34. Granderson J, Sandhu J, Vasquez D, et al. Fuel use and design analysis of improved woodburning cookstoves in the Guatemalan Highlands. Biomass Bioenergy 2009;33:306–15.
35. Smith-Sivertsen T, Diaz E, Pope D, et al. Effect of reducing indoor air pollution on women's respiratory symptoms and lung function: the RESPIRE Randomized Trial, Guatemala. Am J Epidemiol 2009;170:211–20.

PART

2

VIRAL DISEASES

Introduction and General Principles

Tom Solomon, Anna-Maria Geretti

INTRODUCTION

Viruses represent the greatest infectious threat to human health, both in the tropics and globally!

Collectively, they are responsible for an enormous disease burden; the majority of the infectious diseases that have emerged or re-emerged in recent decades are viruses, particularly zoonotic ones, which have spread from animals to humans (Fig. P2.1) [1, 2].

One can consider viruses from a variety of viewpoints: their taxonomy, whether DNA or RNA (double-stranded or single-stranded, positive- or negative-sense), enveloped or not. From a clinical viewpoint, the most appropriate approach is to consider the disease syndromes with which they present and how to diagnose and manage them, and also to think about their epidemiology, how they are spread and how this might be prevented. In this section, viral diseases are grouped according to their clinical syndrome; the HIV chapters are followed by viruses that predominantly cause cutaneous, respiratory, then gastrointestinal disease; the hepatitis viruses are followed by arboviral causes of hemorrhagic fever and fever arthralgia rash syndromes; other hemorrhagic fever viruses come next, with central nervous system (CNS) infections coming last; prion diseases are included here as honorary viruses. Viruses that cause more than one clinical syndrome are primarily considered according to their most common or important manifestation.

EPIDEMIOLOGIC CONSIDERATIONS

Viruses are made up of small pieces of nucleic acid (DNA or RNA), surrounded by protein, whose sole purpose in life is to replicate. Because they do not have all the enzymes they need to do this, they have to muscle into "host" cells and borrow bits of their reproductive

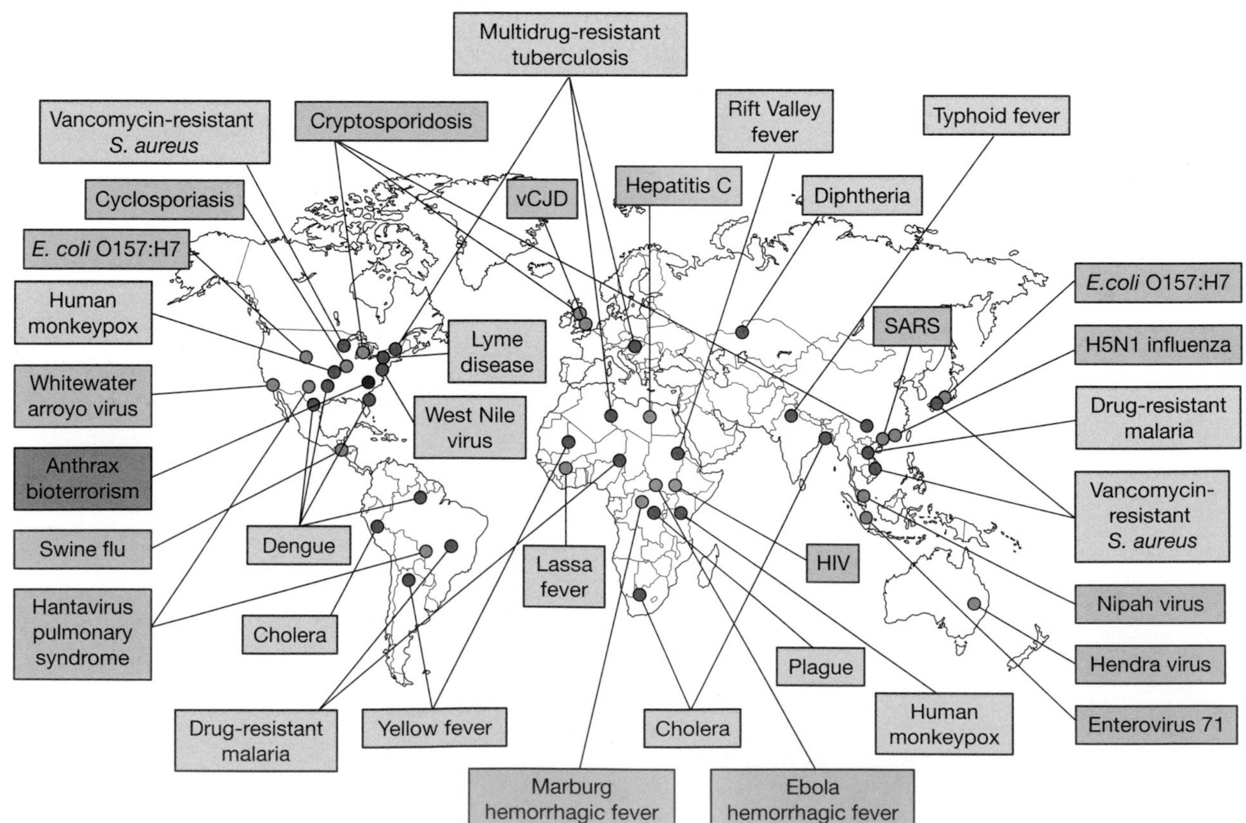

FIGURE P2.1 Global examples of emerging and re-emerging infectious diseases. Red represents newly emerging diseases; blue, re-emerging/resurging diseases; black, a "deliberately emerging" disease. Viruses are boxed. *Adapted, from [1].*

machinery. The host develops an immune response to fight off this unwanted invasion – sometimes successfully leading to short-lived infections, sometimes only partially leading to persistent infections – and the rest follows as a consequence of this eternal struggle.

Viruses have evolved a number of strategies to deal with the host response. Some, such as herpes viruses or HIV, hide deep within the host to form chronic infections, sometimes even integrating to become part of the host chromosome; HIV hides within the host and causes massive disruption of the host defenses – a very successful strategy. Other viruses put their effort into rapidly jumping to new immunologically naïve hosts; respiratory viruses do this in mucus and droplets of saliva; arthropod-borne viruses (arboviruses) get taken up and passed onto new hosts via blood-sucking insects or ticks [3]. The survival strategy adopted by viruses has a major impact on the clinical epidemiology of the diseases they produce; it is what distinguishes chronic infections, such as HIV, from acute epidemic diseases like influenza. Host defenses often deeply influence the outcome of the host/virus interactions, so that some people can clear infections, such as hepatitis B or hepatitis C spontaneously, while others become chronically infected.

CLINICAL SYNDROMES AND PATHOGENESIS

The clinical syndrome a virus produces is governed by a number of factors, particularly how the virus gets into the body, whether it has tropism for any particular tissues, whether other infections are present [4], and the pathogenesis and host response.

The epidermis of the skin is designed to keep pathogens, including viruses, out. Hence, many viral infections occur via soft warm moist mucosal surfaces, such as the respiratory, gastrointestinal, or genital tracts; in recent human history, some of those viruses which originally evolved to be transmitted sexually have also had a helping hand across the tough epidermis by way of needles – hepatitis B and HIV are probably the best examples. The arboviruses use nature's needles, such as mosquitoes, to get through the skin.

For many viruses, the site at which they enter the body is also the place where they cause most trouble; hence, respiratory syncytial virus causes coughs and colds, rotavirus causes diarrheal illness, etc. Others reach distant tissues, such as the liver or CNS. Although the term "tropism" is conventionally used, in reality viruses probably do not seek out particular organs; rather they infect, or attempt to infect, a whole range of cells, but different viruses have success in different tissues; thus encephalitic viruses manage to get across the blood–brain barrier and successfully replicate in the nervous system and the hepatitis viruses have a particular ability to replicate in the liver.

There are several common themes in disease mechanisms caused by viruses. First is the issue of how much damage at the cellular and tissue level is caused by viral replication itself, particularly its taking over of the host cell machinery, and how much is caused by the host innate and adaptive immune response trying to fight the infection [5, 6]. For most viral infections, there are elements of both. Some viruses leave cells by budding off the cell surface, others by causing lysis of the whole cell. The cell might respond by undergoing apoptosis, (programmed cell death) to try to shut down the production. Entry across the vascular endothelium into the tissue is a key event for many viruses that are in the blood stream; this in itself can disrupt the vascular endothelium, causing leakage and even necrotic damage; this is a key step for some of the hemorrhagic viruses. Inflammatory responses in viral-infected host tissues can themselves cause damage, particularly in physically restricted spaces, such as the skull. For acute viral infections there is resolution one way or the other: the host clears the virus and survives (though sometimes with severe damage), or, ultimately, the host succumbs to the infection. In chronic infections, this battle between virus and host rages on and is never won. Viruses, such as herpes simplex viruses, can become latent, lying low, hidden away from the immune response, but cropping up every now and again for sporadic attacks [7]; for others, such as cytomegalovirus (CMV) and HIV, there is ongoing warfare, waged especially by T cells [8, 9]. In the case of HIV, the virus usually ultimately wins, unless there is intervention in the form of drugs.

DIAGNOSTIC CHALLENGES

Broadly speaking, viral infections are diagnosed by showing that the virus (or some of its components) is there, or by showing that it has been there and the body has now developed a specific immune response to it. Some viruses can by visualized directly by electron microscopy if they occur in high enough titers, for example rotavirus in the stool or herpes simplex virus in skin lesions; however, the traditional method of viral detection is by culture in cell lines. Viral antigen detection has long been used for detecting the hepatitis B virus in the blood (surface antigen) and respiratory viruses in nasopharyngeal aspirates (various viral antigens); it has also proved useful for detecting HIV in the blood (p24 antigen) and, more recently, for dengue virus. The mainstay of viral diagnosis is now based on the detection of viral RNA or DNA by a variety of molecular techniques – most commonly PCR. These techniques, many would argue, have revolutionized clinical virology, particularly because they improve the sensitivity and speed of detection compared with virus isolation in cell culture [10]. Modern techniques, such as real-time PCR, also allow quantification of the amount of virus and are thus useful for disease monitoring, including planning and assessing responses to antiviral therapy. Over the years, there has been a large array of techniques for detecting antiviral antibody, with differing levels of technical complexity, sophistication, sensitivity, and specificity. Assays such as the complement fixation text and hemagglutination inhibition test are rather nonspecific and are no longer in routine use. Neutralization assays are useful because they show serum contains antibody which will actually neutralize viral function; however, because they involve live virus, they are technically demanding and require specialized laboratories. ELISAs for immunoglobulin are quite robust and those for IgM can be especially useful in showing acute infection. Antibody (and antigen) detection techniques have evolved through the years from the classic manual ELISA format to highly automated instrumentations. Some of these have now been modified to a card format, which gives a simple color change and can be used at the bedside [11, 12].

OPPORTUNITIES FOR TREATMENT

Our attempts at developing antiviral treatments for chronic infections have generally proven more successful than for acute viral infections. In part, this is probably because chronic diseases provide a larger disease burden and perhaps also because they are probably more amenable to investigation. The development of antiviral treatments for HIV has provided a spectacular showcase for the rational design of antimicrobial drugs [13–15]. There is now a specific anti-retroviral drug for almost every stage of the virus' replication cycle, from those that stop virus entry into the host cell (either by blocking binding of the viral envelope proteins to the CCR5 co-receptor or by preventing fusion of the virus envelope with the cell membrane), virus replication (with reverse transcriptase inhibitors which stop the viral RNA being transcribed into DNA and integrase inhibitors which inhibit virus integration in the host cell DNA) and virus maturation (protease inhibitors which interfere with the viral proteases needed for virus assembly, leading to the release of immature, non-infectious virus particles). In 1996, the understanding that it was possible to control HIV replication long-term through the combined used of drugs that target different stages of the virus cycle was a key milestone in the history of antiviral therapy.

The development of fixed-dose, co-formulated anti-retroviral drugs has rationalized the need for multiple tablets, and the discovery of human leukocyte antigen (HLA) associations with hypersensitivity to some anti-retroviral drugs has been a landmark in the development of personalized medicines [16]. Antivirals are also available for the herpes viruses, including herpes simplex, herpes zoster, and CMV, as well as for hepatitis B and C. In terms of acute infections, there are antivirals for influenza and respiratory syncytial virus, as well as Crimean-Congo hemorrhagic fever and Lassa fever [17–19].

Treatment with immune serum containing specific antibody has been used for a number of viral infections, including Ebola virus infection, where the outcome is unclear, and Argentine hemorrhagic fever, where it appears to be beneficial. Newer approaches with humanized monoclonal antibodies are being developed. One monoclonal antibody – Palivizumab – is available against respiratory syncytial virus [20].

One feature of antiviral therapy is the ease with which viruses can develop drug resistance. Antiviral drug resistance is a pressing worry whenever treating HIV, hepatitis B, hepatitis C, or influenza. Although more slow to emerge, antiviral resistance can also become a serious threat in the treatment of herpes virus infections in immunocompromised patients, including those with HIV or transplant recipients [21].

DISEASE CONTROL

Whereas development of drugs against viruses has, for many years, lagged behind those for bacteria, the vaccines developed against viruses have had a major impact on public health and the epidemiology of these diseases. The first, and most successful, vaccine was against smallpox – in this case the natural cowpox vaccine providing the source material [22]. Live vaccines against other diseases, including the Sabin vaccine for polio, 17D yellow fever vaccine and SA14-14-2 Japanese encephalitis vaccine were developed empirically by passing viruses through a range of substrates to come up with an attenuated strain that was immunogenic and safe. Other live-attenuated vaccines include measles, mumps, and rubella. Although live vaccines are highly efficacious, they may carry small risks of causing disease. The acceptability of such risks depends, to some extent, on the risks of the disease itself. Inactivated vaccines, whilst perhaps more attractive in terms of safety, tend to be more expensive, not least because larger doses are required with a killed rather than live virus; they include the Salk polio vaccine, and vaccines for rabies and hepatitis A. Subunit vaccines are made up of just part of the virion; the hepatitis B vaccine contains only the viral surface proteins, whilst influenza vaccines comprise hemagglutination and neuraminidase subunits [23]. Reverse genetics techniques are used to develop such vaccines. A recent major breakthrough in the control of viral disease through vaccination has been the development of non-infectious virus-like particles as vaccines for the prophylaxis of human papillomavirus (HPV) infection. These dramatically reduce the risk of cervical and other types of cancer associated with specific HPV types [24].

For other viruses, a range of different disease control efforts may be important. Clearly, for HIV, education and behavioral changes can limit spread. Other interventions that have been shown to be effective in limiting transmission of HIV include circumcision and the use of anti-retroviral therapy among infected people [25]. "Social distancing measures", for example closing schools and nurseries, are employed in Asia during large hand-foot-and-mouth disease outbreaks caused by enterovirus-71 (though their role is uncertain). For some of the arboviral diseases, such as dengue, vector control measures limit disease spread and safe hospital practices can certainly have a major impact on the spread of nosocomial infections, such as Ebola. Overall, though, the development of new vaccines probably offers the best means of controlling all the major viral infections, including HIV.

REFERENCES

1. Morens DM, Folkers GK, Fauci AS. The challenge of emerging and re-emerging infectious diseases. Nature 2004;430:242–9.
2. Tebit DM, Arts EJ.Tracking a century of global expansion and evolution of HIV to drive understanding and to combat disease. Lancet Infect Dis 2011;11: 45–56.
3. Solomon T, Whitley RJ. Arthropod-borne viral encephalitides. In: Scheld WM, Whitley RJ, Marra CM, eds. Infections of the Central Nervous System, 3rd edn. Philadelphia: Lippincott Williams & Wilkins; 2004:205–30.
4. da Silva SR, de Oliveira DE. HIV, EBV and KSHV: viral cooperation in the pathogenesis of human malignancies. Cancer Lett 2011;305:175–85.
5. Rothman AL. Immunity to dengue virus: a tale of original antigenic sin and tropical cytokine storms. Nat Rev Immunol 2011;11:532–43.
6. Bertoletti A, Maini MK, Ferrari C. The host-pathogen interaction during HBV infection: immunological controversies. Antivir Ther 2010;15(suppl. 3): 15–24.
7. Gupta R, Warren T, Wald A. Genital herpes. Lancet 2007;370:2127–37.
8. Brenchley JM, Paiardini M. Immunodeficiency lentiviral infections in natural and non-natural hosts. Blood 2011;118:847–54.
9. Derhovanessian E, Larbi A, Pawelec G. Biomarkers of human immunosenescence: impact of Cytomegalovirus infection. Curr Opin Immunol 2009;21: 440–5.
10. Ramaswamy M, McDonald C, Smith M, et al. Diagnosis of genital herpes by real time PCR in routine clinical practice. Sex Transm Infect 2004;80:406–10.
11. Campbell S, Fedoriw Y. HIV testing near the patient: changing the face of HIV testing. Clin Lab Med 2009;29:491–501.
12. Khanom AB, Velvin C, Hawrami K, et al. Performance of a nurse-led paediatric point of care service for respiratory syncytial virus testing in secondary care. J Infect 2011;62:52–8.
13. Siegfried N, Uthman OA, Rutherford GW. Optimal time for initiation of antiretroviral therapy in asymptomatic, HIV-infected, treatment-naive adults. Cochrane Database Syst Rev 2010;(3):CD008272.
14. Border S. The development of antiretroviral therapy and its impact on the HIV-1/AIDS pandemic. Antiviral Res 2010 Jan;85:1–18.
15. Siegfried N, van der Merwe L, Brocklehurst P, Stint TT. Antiretrovirals for reducing the risk of mother-to-child transmission of HIV infection. Cochrane Database Syst Rev 2011;(7):CD003510.
16. Phillips EJ, Mallal SA. Pharmacogenetics of drug hypersensitivity. Pharmacogenomics 2010;11:973–87.
17. Rosen HR. Clinical practice. Chronic hepatitis C infection. N Engl J Med 2011; 364:2429–38.
18. Ascioglu S, Leblebicioglu H, Vahaboglu H, Chan KA.Ribavirin for patients with Crimean-Congo haemorrhagic fever: a systematic review and meta-analysis. J Antimicrob Chemother. 2011;66:1215–22.
19. Charrel RN, Coutard B, Baronti C, et al. Arenaviruses and hantaviruses: from epidemiology and genomics to antivirals. Antiviral Res 2011;90:102–14.
20. Krilov LR. Respiratory syncytial virus disease: update on treatment and prevention. Expert Rev Anti Infect Ther 2011;9:27–32.
21. Soriano V, Vispo E, Poveda E, et al. Directly acting antivirals against hepatitis C virus. J Antimicrob Chemother 2011;66:1673–86.
22. Keegan R, Dabbagh A, Strebel PM, Cochi SL. Comparing measles with previous eradication programs: enabling and constraining factors. J Infect Dis. 2011;204(suppl. 1):S54–61.
23. Minor PD. Vaccines against seasonal and pandemic influenza and the implications of changes in substrates for virus production. Clin Infect Dis 2010;50: 560–5.
24. Kwak K, Yemelyanova A, Roden RB. Prevention of cancer by prophylactic human papillomavirus vaccines. Curr Opin Immunol. 2011;23:244–51.
25. Padian NS, McCoy SI, Karim SS, et al. HIV prevention transformed: the new prevention research agenda. Lancet 2011;378:269–78.

Human Immunodeficiency Virus Infection 27

Philip J Peters, Barbara J Marston, Paul J Weidle, John T Brooks

INTRODUCTION

As of the end of 2009, the World Health Organization (WHO) estimated that 33.3 million (31.4–35.3 million) persons were living with HIV infection [1]. During 2009, an estimated 2.6 million (2.3–2.8 million) new infections occurred worldwide. Sub-Saharan Africa has been most heavily affected by the HIV pandemic and bears the greatest burden of both prevalent (22.5 million or 68%) and new (1.8 million or 69%) infections. The majority (52%) of persons living with HIV worldwide are women. Since the late 1990s, the global annual number of new infections has steadily declined (Fig. 27.1). Likewise, with the significant scale up of antiretroviral therapy (ART), AIDS-related deaths have also decreased globally by 14% since 2004, when the availability of ART in the developing world dramatically expanded. As a result, prevalence has continued to increase (Fig. 27.2), although at a slower pace during the past decade.

The first cases of AIDS were recognized in the USA in 1981 [2]. Phylogenetic analysis of HIV sequences suggests that HIV originated in Central Africa and may have been transmitted to humans around 1930 [3]. By 1985, human HIV infection had been identified in every region of the world [4].

In some African countries, HIV has reduced life expectancy by more than 20 years, slowed economic growth and deepened household poverty [5]. Globally, AIDS is the leading cause of death among people aged 15–59 years old in low-income countries (especially sub-Saharan Africa) [6]. Despite the remarkably rapid scientific advances that have been made in epidemiology, basic science and treatment, in 2011, the HIV pandemic continues to represent one of the world's most urgent public health challenges.

HIV has also changed the practice of tropical medicine [7]. In many countries in eastern and southern Africa, 50–75% of adult medical inpatients at urban hospitals are HIV-infected [8–10]. As a result of the immunosuppression caused by HIV infection, susceptibility to, and severity of, other infectious diseases, especially opportunistic infections (e.g. tuberculosis, cryptococcal meningitis) is increased. HIV-infected patients can exhibit atypical clinical presentations of infections (e.g. fever as the only presenting symptom of cryptococcal meningitis) [11] and immunosuppressed HIV-infected patients can have multiple pathologic processes occurring simultaneously. The differential diagnoses for infectious diseases in HIV-infected persons can be broad, making empiric therapy difficult. Thus, rapid and accurate diagnostic testing—when available—is important.

The HIV pandemic has also heightened our global consciousness to health disparities, social justice and human rights, and mobilized unprecedented political, financial and human resources to scale-up

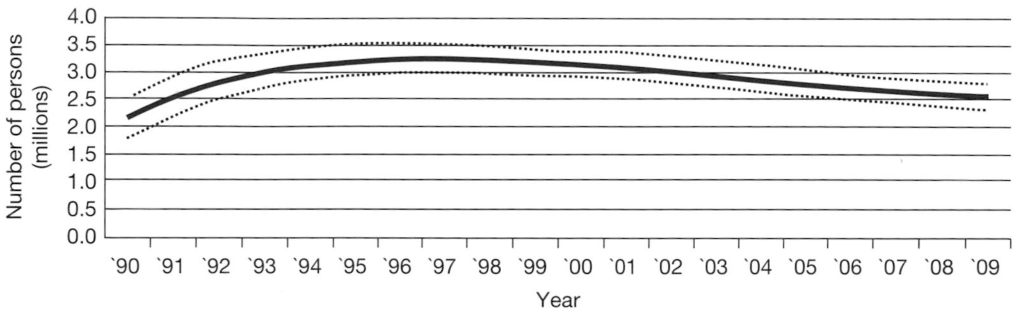

FIGURE 27.1 Annual number of people newly infected with HIV, worldwide 1990–2009. *Source: Joint United Nations Programmed on HIV/AIDS (UNAIDS). Global report: UNAIDS report on the global AIDS epidemic 2010. Available at: http://www.unaids.org/globalreport/Global_report.htm (accessed 5 May 2011).*

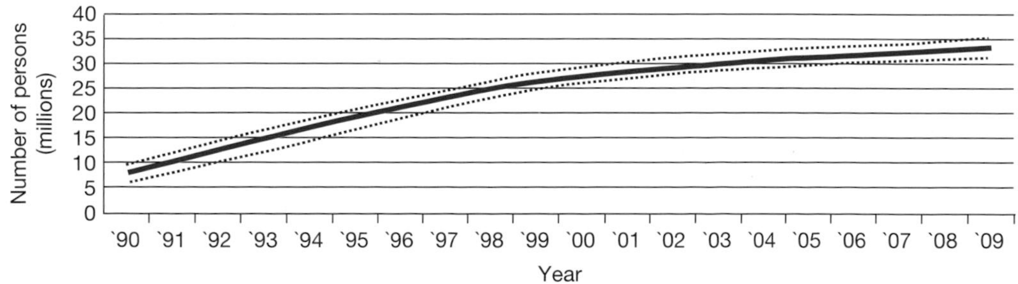

FIGURE 27.2 Number of people living with HIV, worldwide 1990–2009. *Source: Joint United Nations Programmed on HIV/AIDS (UNAIDS). Global report: UNAIDS report on the global AIDS epidemic 2010. Available at: http://www.unaids.org/globalreport/Global_report.htm (accessed 5 May 2011).*

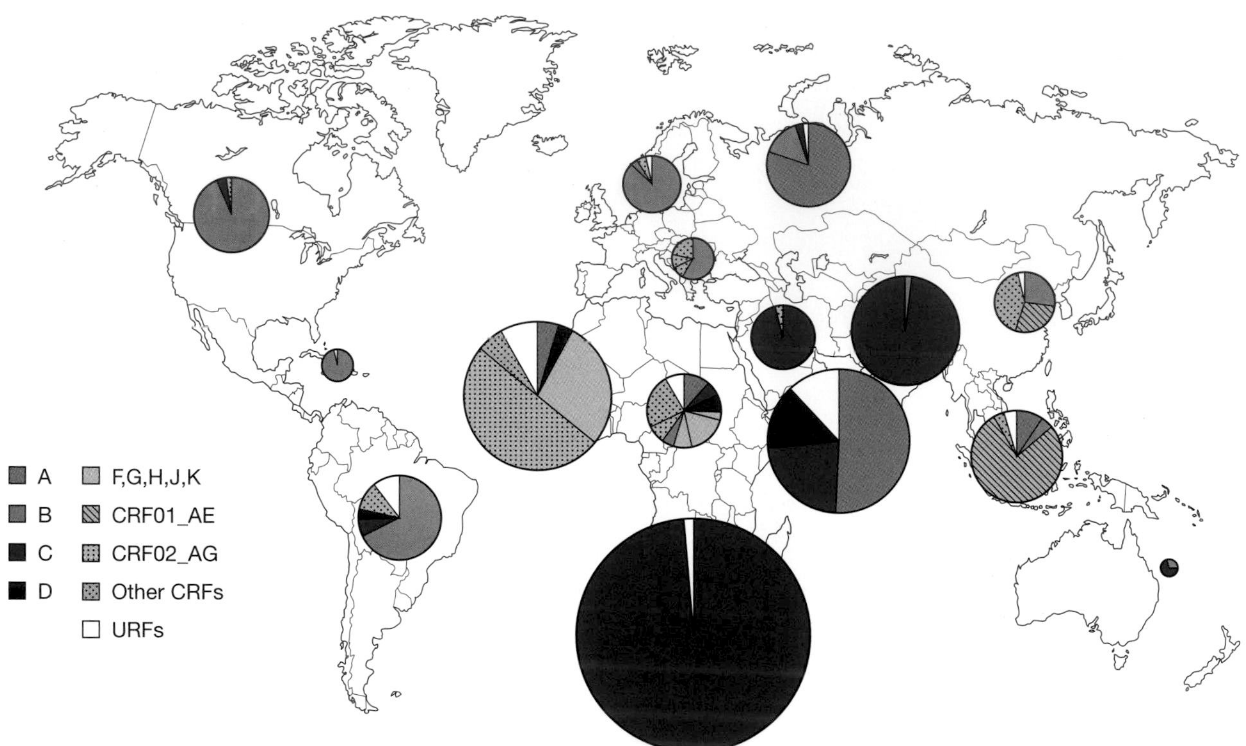

FIGURE 27.3 Global distribution of HIV-1 subtypes and recombinants, 2004–2007. *(Source: Hemelaar J, Gouws E, Ghys PD, Osmanov S. Global trends in molecular epidemiology of HIV-1 during 2000–2007. AIDS 2011;25:679–89).*

HIV prevention, care and treatment programs in the most affected countries [12–15].

EPIDEMIOLOGY

MOLECULAR EPIDEMIOLOGY

There are two main types of HIV (a lentivirus): HIV-1 and HIV-2. HIV-1 comprises three phylogenetically distinct groups, termed group M (main), group O (outlier), and group N (non-M, non-O) [16]. A fourth group (group P) has been proposed based on a single infection with a genetically unique HIV strain [17]. Each group has likely evolved from independent cross-species transmissions of chimpanzee simian immunodeficiency virus (SIVcpz) to humans [18–20]. HIV-1 group M has spread to every region of the world and is the virus responsible for the current global pandemic [21]. Group O infections are uncommon and limited to people living in, or epidemiologically linked to, Central Africa (especially Cameroon) [22]. Group N infections have been described rarely and only in Cameroon [23].

HIV-2 is a primate lentivirus related to HIV-1 that is less pathogenic and transmissible (see HIV-2 section) [24, 25]. HIV-2 evolved from the cross-species transmission of sooty mangabey SIV (SIVsm) to humans [19, 26]. Although HIV-2 infections have been reported throughout the world, they are most prevalent in Guinea-Bissau [27, 28] and in surrounding West African countries, as well as other nations with economic or cultural links to the region (e.g. Portugal, India, Angola, Mozambique, Cote d'Ivoire, Senegal, France) [24]. Recent data suggest the prevalence of HIV-2 in Guinea-Bissau has declined to less than 5% [27, 28]. Dual infection with HIV-1 and HIV-2 has been described but the viruses do not appear to recombine with each other [29].

High rates of viral replication coupled with continuous mutation and recombination events have resulted in the rapid genetic diversification of HIV-1 group M viruses into 9 distinct subtypes (or clades) and over 49 circulating recombinant forms (CRFs) [30]. The number of described CRFs is cataloged at the Los Alamos HIV sequence database [30]. There are also a variety of unique recombinant forms (URFs) that have only been identified in a single person or in an epidemiologically linked pair of persons. The effects of variation between HIV-1 subtypes on pathogenesis, transmission, drug resistance, and immune control are not well understood.

The initial genetic diversification of HIV-1 group M viruses likely occurred in Central Africa, where the greatest diversity and earliest cases of HIV-1 have been identified [31]. Subsequently, HIV-1 subtypes have spread with a geographically heterogeneous distribution (Fig. 27.3) [21]. Subtype C, the dominant subtype in Southern Africa, Ethiopia, and India, causes nearly half (48%) of HIV infections worldwide [21]. The predominance of subtype C, especially in countries with high-prevalence epidemics driven by heterosexual sexual contact, has led to speculation that subtype C might have an increased fitness for transmission [32, 33]. Subtype A accounts for 12% of infections worldwide and has a broad geographic distribution. CRF01_AE and CRF02_AG are two additional recombinant viruses involving subtype A that are epidemiologically important in Southeast Asia and West Africa respectively [21]. The emergence of these CRFs has raised concern that recombination may contribute to the selection of viruses with increased fitness, immune escape or transmissibility [34]. Subtype B predominates in the Americas, western and central Europe, and Australia. Finally, URFs are important components of the epidemics in East Africa, Central Africa, West Africa, and South America, and it is expected that some of these URFs will emerge as important CRFs in the future [21, 35–37].

Modes of Transmission

HIV can be transmitted by sexual contact; through contact with infected blood, blood products, or human tissues; and from mother to child (Table 27-1) [38, 39]. Although HIV has been isolated from a variety of body fluids, only blood, semen, genital fluids, and breast milk have been proven as sources of infection. HIV is not transmitted

TABLE 27.1 Estimated Per-Act Risk for Acquisition of HIV by Exposure Route*

Exposure Route	Risk per 100 exposures to an HIV-infected source
Blood transfusion	90.
Needle-sharing injection-drug use	0.67
Percutaneous needle stick	0.3
Receptive anal intercourse	0.5
Receptive penile–vaginal intercourse	0.1
Insertive anal intercourse	0.065
Insertive penile–vaginal intercourse	0.05
Receptive oral intercourse	0.01
Insertive oral intercourse	0.005
Mother-to-child transmission (without breastfeeding)	30.
Breastfeeding for 18 months	15.

*Estimates of risk for transmission from sexual exposure assume no condom use.

Sources: 1) Smith DK, Grohskopf LA, Black RJ, et al. Antiretroviral post exposure prohylaxis after sexual, injection-drug use, or other nonoccupational exposure to HIV in the United States: recommendations from the U.S. Department of Health and Human Services. MMWR Recomm Rep 2005 Jan 21;54(RR-2):1–20. and 2) KourtisAP, LeeFK, AbramsEJ, JamiesonDJ, BulterysM. Mother-to-child transmission of HIV-1: timing and implications for prevention. Lancet Infect Dis 2007;6(11):726–32.

TABLE 27.2 Select Host Factors Affecting Susceptibility to HIV Infection and Disease Progression

Select Host Factors	
Innate	Autoantibodies Chemokines Cytokines
Genetic	HLA haplotype CCR5 gene/promoter CCR2 gene/promoter CCL3L1 gene copy number
Acquired	Cytotoxic T-cell activity Helper T-cell function Neuralizing antibodies
Intrinsic	APOBEC3G/3F TRIM5α

HLA=Human leukocytic antigen; CCR=chemokine receptor; CCL3L1 = chemokine ligand like-1; APOBEC = apolipoprotein B mRNA editing complex

Source: Simon V, Ho DD, Abdool Karim Q. HIV/AIDS epidemiology, pathogenesis, prevention, and treatment. Lancet 2006;368:489–504.

though routine household contact or provision of medical care when universal precautions[1] are followed.

Unprotected sexual contact is the predominant mode of HIV transmission globally [1]. Despite a relatively low efficiency of transmission per sexual act [40], numerous factors increase transmission, including mucosal microtrauma, bleeding (e.g. menstruation), concurrent sexually transmitted infections (STIs; especially those that cause genital ulcerations), the stage of HIV infection and HIV viral load [41]. Concurrent sexual partners, and not simply the absolute number of partners, augment HIV's spread in a community [42]. Male circumcision reduces female-to-male transmission of HIV and may reduce male-to-female transmission to a lesser extent [43–45]. Certain genetic factors also decrease the probability of HIV transmission (Table 27-2) [46].

Among injection drug users (IDUs), HIV is transmitted by exposure to HIV-infected blood through shared contaminated needles and other injection equipment. People who have sex with an IDU are at risk through sexual transmission [1, 47]. Nosocomial transmission in hospitals from reuse of syringes and needles has been documented [48–50], and the risk of acquiring HIV from a transfusion with HIV-contaminated blood products approaches 100% [51].

Mother-to-child transmission can take place during pregnancy, labor and delivery, and during breastfeeding. In non-breastfeeding populations, the majority of transmissions occur during the short interval before delivery when the placenta separates from the uterine wall and labor occurs. An additional 30% of transmissions occur during late labor and the actual passage through the birth canal. In breastfeeding populations, approximately 40% of transmissions occur in the postnatal breastfeeding period. Overall rates of transmission are 25–40% (depending on breastfeeding practices) without prevention but can be reduced to 1% with antiretroviral prophylaxis to the infant and mother during pregnancy, labor and delivery, and during breastfeeding (see "*Prevention*" below) [39, 52]. Pre-chewing and feeding of food by an HIV-infected adult caregiver to an HIV-uninfected infant has been a potential cause of three HIV infections in North America [53]. No evidence suggests that saliva alone can transmit HIV.

GEOGRAPHIC EPIDEMIOLOGY

The prevalence of HIV infections varies dramatically with a disproportionate number of infections in sub-Saharan Africa (Fig. 27.4). New HIV infections appear to have peaked in some regions and, in 22 countries in sub-Saharan Africa, rates have declined by more than 25% between 2001 and 2009 [1]. In several high-prevalence countries, HIV prevalence among young women attending antenatal clinics (a sentinel population in generalized HIV epidemics) has declined in association with increases in condom usage and reductions in high-risk sexual behaviors (e.g. decreased number of partners, delayed sexual debut) among young people [1]. Improvements in surveillance, which include expanding surveillance sites to antenatal clinics in rural areas and conducting population-based surveys, can make trends difficult to interpret.

For the purposes of surveillance, UNAIDS and the WHO classify HIV epidemics as generalized, concentrated or low-level [54]. Generalized epidemics are defined by a HIV prevalence consistently over 1% in pregnant women, a sentinel population used to assess trends in HIV prevalence and to estimate the adult HIV prevalence[2], indicating that sexual networking in the general population is sufficient to sustain an epidemic independent of high-risk groups. Concentrated epidemics are defined by an HIV prevalence consistently over 5% in at least one defined high-risk group (i.e., men who have sex with men (MSM), IDU, commercial sex workers) and an HIV prevalence below 1% in pregnant women in urban areas indicating that HIV infection is not well established in the general population. Low-level epidemics are defined by an HIV prevalence that has not exceeded 5% in any defined high-risk group.

Sub-Saharan Africa

HIV is a generalized epidemic in many parts of sub-Saharan Africa, which contains 68% of all infections worldwide, but only 12.5% of

[1] "Universal precautions", as defined by the Centers for Disease Control and Prevention (CDC), are a set of precautions designed to prevent transmission of bloodborne pathogens, such as HIV, when providing first aid or health care. Information can be found at the Joint United Nations Programmed on HIV/AIDS (UNAIDS) website: http://www.unaids.org/en/KnowledgeCentre/Resources/PolicyGuidance/Techpolicies/Univ_pre_technical_policies.asp and the CDC website: http://www.cdc.gov/ncidod/dhqp/bp_universal_precautions.html.

[2] Adult prevalence—prevalence among the proportion of the population 15–49 years old (adults of reproductive age).

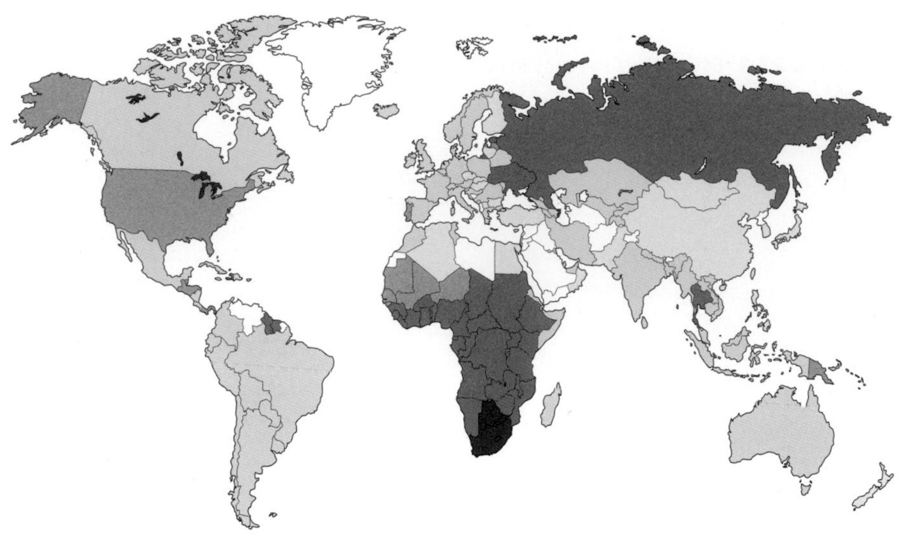

FIGURE 27.4 Global prevalence of HIV infection, 2009. *Source: Joint United Nations Programmed on HIV/AIDS (UNAIDS). Global report: UNAIDS report on the global AIDS epidemic 2010. Available at: http://www.unaids.org/globalreport/Global_report.htm (accessed 5 May 2011).*

the world's total population [1, 55]. Although considerable efforts have improved access to antiretrovirals, 1.3 million Africans died of AIDS in 2009 (72% of the AIDS deaths worldwide) [1]. Southern Africa now has the highest adult HIV prevalence in the world, followed by East Africa. Most countries in West and Central Africa have maintained a relatively low HIV prevalence (12 countries in West and Central Africa had an HIV prevalence of ≤2% in 2009). Geographic prevalence varies within countries. In Kenya, for example, HIV prevalence estimated in 2007 varied from 0.8% in the northeast to 14.9% in the western province of Nyanza [56].

HIV arrived late in southern Africa (South Africa had a HIV prevalence of less than 1% in 1988) but has spread rapidly (Fig. 27.5). Swaziland now has the most intense HIV epidemic in the world with an estimated one in four (26%) adults living with HIV infection in 2009 [1]. The nine countries with the highest adult HIV prevalence worldwide (with an HIV prevalence greater than 10%) are all located in southern Africa. Various social and biologic factors have played a role in the high prevalence rates. These include high rates of men migrating for work, concurrent sexual partnerships, genital herpes, low rates of male circumcision and gender-based inequalities [57].

Before the mid-2000s, new HIV infections in sub-Saharan Africa combined with AIDS-related deaths led to substantial decreases in life expectancy (Fig. 27.6) [58]. In Botswana, life expectancy fell from 65 years in 1985 to 34 years in 2006; however, with antiretroviral scale-up covering approximately 90% of eligible persons, AIDS-related deaths have been cut in half from an estimated 18,000 in 2002 to 9100 in 2009 [59]. In Malawi, provision of ART has been linked to a 10% drop in the adult death rate between 2004 and 2008 [60].

Efforts at preventing new infections are gaining traction. In Zambia, there is delayed sexual debut and increased condom usage among young adults age 15–19 years with coincident reductions in multiple sexual partnerships [1]. Throughout southern Africa, declining HIV prevalence among young adults, increased testing and counseling services, and provision of perinatal ART for prevention of mother-to-child transmission (PMTCT) have reduced new infections among children by 32% [1].

Denial of risk remains a barrier. In a 2005 South African survey, half of people who tested HIV-positive believed they were not at risk of acquiring infection [61]. In a 2007 Kenyan survey of adult men and women who reported not testing for HIV because they were low risk, the HIV prevalence was 4.9% and 5.9% respectively [56]. Only recently has the burden of HIV infections among MSM [62–66] and IDUs [67] in sub-Saharan Africa begun to be appreciated. The contribution of infections by MSM is estimated to be greater than that by IDU because many MSM also have sex with women, whereas injection drug use is a new, and smaller, phenomenon that provides fewer opportunities for bridging transmissions [67, 68].

Asia

Although the adult HIV prevalence is lower in Asia (Fig. 27.7) than sub-Saharan Africa, there were still an estimated 4.5–5.5 million people living with HIV in 2009, with over 360,000 new infections and more than 300,000 deaths in 2009 [1]. Prevalence is highest in Southeast Asia, where commercial sex work, sex between men and injection drug use are the primary modes of transmission. HIV in the region is concentrated in high-risk groups (there are no generalized epidemics) and in many countries there are significant regional variations in their HIV prevalence. In China, for example, five provinces account for over 50% of people living with HIV [69]. In India, unprotected sex accounts for the majority of new infections (90%); however, sharing contaminated injection equipment is the main mode of transmission in India's north-eastern states [70].

In Thailand and Cambodia, HIV spread rapidly in the late 1980s and early 1990s. Initial cases were reported among MSM and IDUs, and, later, among female sex workers. Extensive public education and prevention campaigns have had some success. In Thailand, increased knowledge of HIV and changes in sexual behavior (e.g. increased condom usage, fewer visits to sex workers) have correlated with reductions in HIV prevalence among new military conscripts [71]. Thailand's "100% Condom" campaign, which educated sex workers and promoted condom use, has also decreased HIV transmission from female commercial sex workers [72].

Latin America

Brazil, the most populous country in Latin America, had an estimated 460,000–810,000 people living with HIV in 2009 [1]. In the

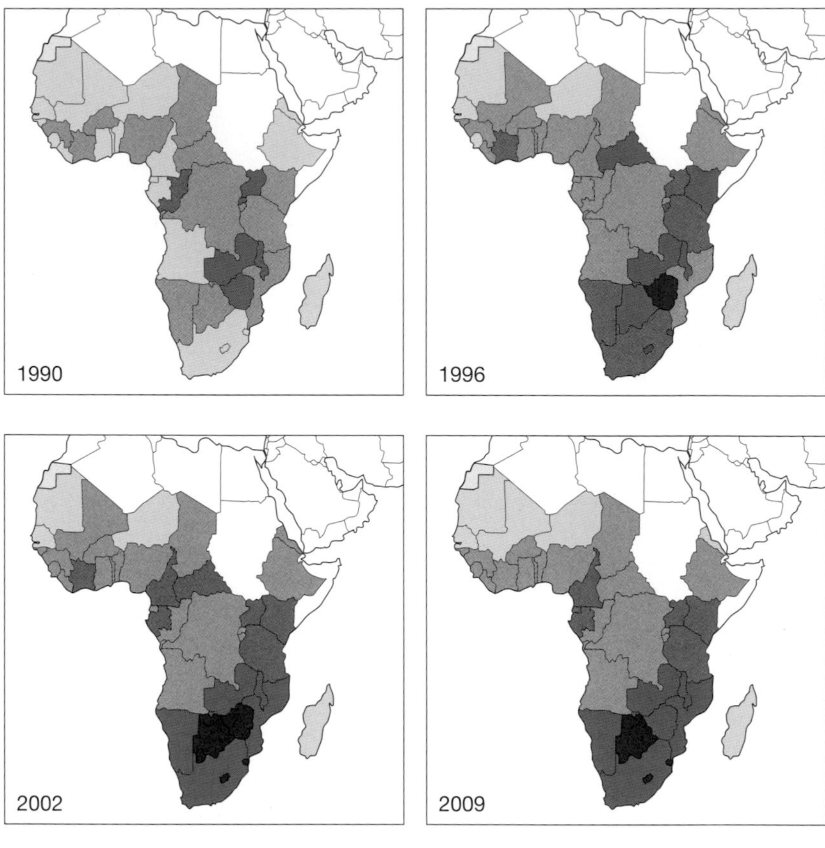

FIGURE 27.5 HIV prevalence among adults aged 15–49 years in sub-Saharan Africa, 1990–2009. *Source: Joint United Nations Programmed on HIV/AIDS (UNAIDS). Global report: UNAIDS report on the global AIDS epidemic 2010. Available at: http://www.unaids.org/globalreport/Global_report.htm (accessed 5 May 2011).*

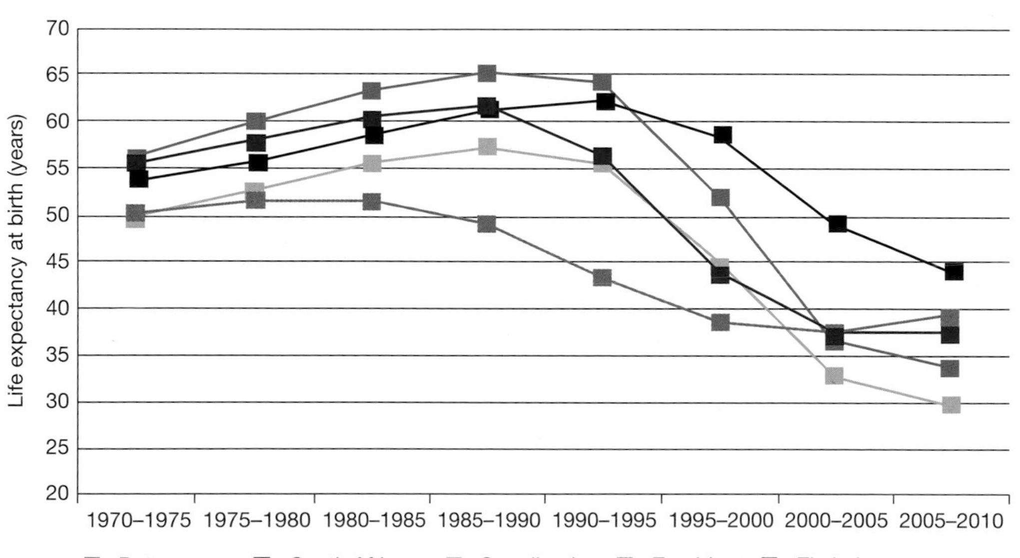

FIGURE 27.6 Impact of HIV on life expectancy in five African countries, 1970–2010. *Source: United Nations Population Division. World Population Prospects: The 2004 Revision, database. Available at: http://www.un.org/esa/population/publications/WPP2004/wpp2004.htm (accessed 5 May 2011).*

1990s, many experts predicted that Brazil's epidemic would rapidly accelerate. However, the country's sustained campaign to promote sex education, condom use, harm reduction and HIV testing, and to provide universal ART has held adult prevalence below 1% [1]. The majority of HIV infections in South America occur among MSM [73] and IDU [67]. Incarcerated men are at particularly high risk [74]. In addition, in Central America, a high proportion of MSM (22%) have reported having sex with at least one female partner in the previous 6 months, underscoring the potential for HIV to bridge to women in this region [75].

More detailed global and regional information is published annually by the WHO and UNAIDS (http://www.unaids.org; http://www.who.int/hiv/en/).

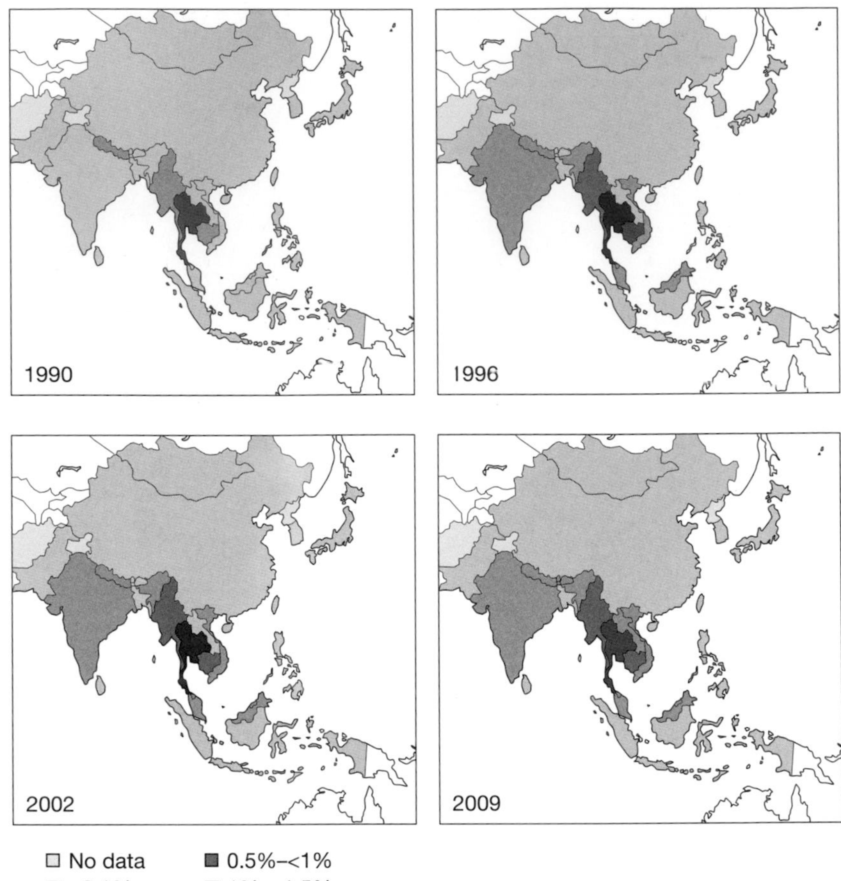

FIGURE 27.7 HIV prevalence among adults aged 15–49 years in Asia, 1990–2009. *Source: Joint United Nations Programmed on HIV/AIDS (UNAIDS). Global report: UNAIDS report on the global AIDS epidemic 2010. Available at: http://www.unaids.org/globalreport/Global_report.htm (accessed 5 May 2011).*

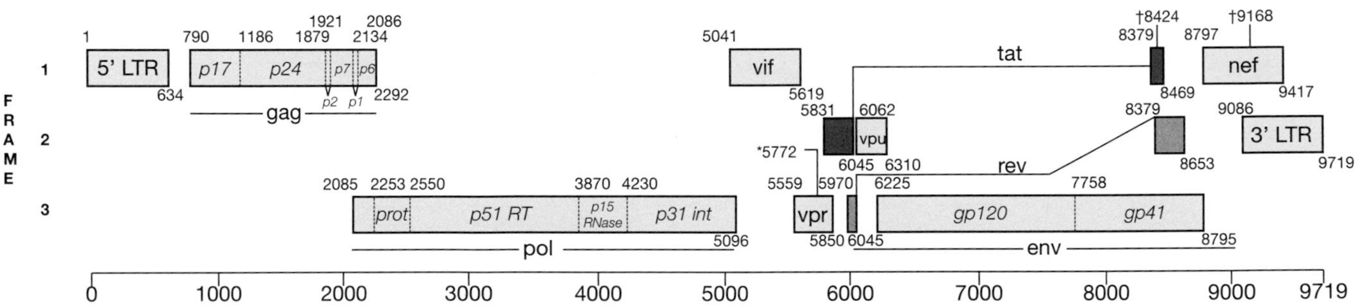

FIGURE 27.8 HIV-1 gene map. *Source: Los Alamos National Laboratory. The circulating recombinant forms(CRFs), HIV sequence database. Available at: http://www.hiv.lanl.gov/content/sequence/HIV/CRFs/CRFs.html (accessed 5 May 2011).*

NATURAL HISTORY, PATHOGENESIS AND PATHOLOGY

The HIV-1 genome is organized into three major regions: *gag*, encoding structural proteins, *pol*, encoding enzymes (e.g. reverse transcriptase, protease and integrase) necessary for viral replication, and *env*, encoding envelope proteins (Fig. 27.8) [76]. In addition, the HIV genome contains six regulatory genes (*tat, rev, nef, vpr, vpu*, and *vif*) that facilitate viral replication and host immune evasion. HIV is spherical with a diameter of 1/10,000 of a millimeter (Fig. 27.9) [77]. The outer coat, known as the viral envelope, is composed of two lipid layers taken from the membrane of a human cell when a newly formed virus particle buds. Within the inner viral protein core are two copies of positive, single-stranded RNA that are tightly bound to nucleocapsid proteins and viral enzymes necessary for replication.

HIV is able to avoid intracellular antiviral defenses (e.g. APOBEC3G/3F and TRIM5α), while activating and exploiting cellular machinery to replicate (Fig. 27.10). HIV infects and replicates in cells that express the CD4 receptor, in particular CD4$^+$ T lymphocytes. HIV's envelope protein (gp120) binds to the CD4 receptor and to additional co-receptors (i.e. CCR5 or CXCR4), leading to viral fusion with the cell and entry of HIV's inner viral core (steps 1 and 2 in Fig. 27.10) [77]. HIV's reverse transcriptase then converts the single-stranded HIV RNA genome into double-stranded DNA (step 3). Reverse transcriptase is error prone and it is at this step that mutations and strand recombinations generate genetically distinct viral variants. The viral DNA then complexes with HIV integrase, is transported into the host cell's nucleus and is integrated with the help of host DNA repair enzymes into a transcriptionally active location in the host's chromosomal DNA (step 4). This step irreversibly transforms the cell into a producer of virus. A certain proportion of cells infected by HIV are

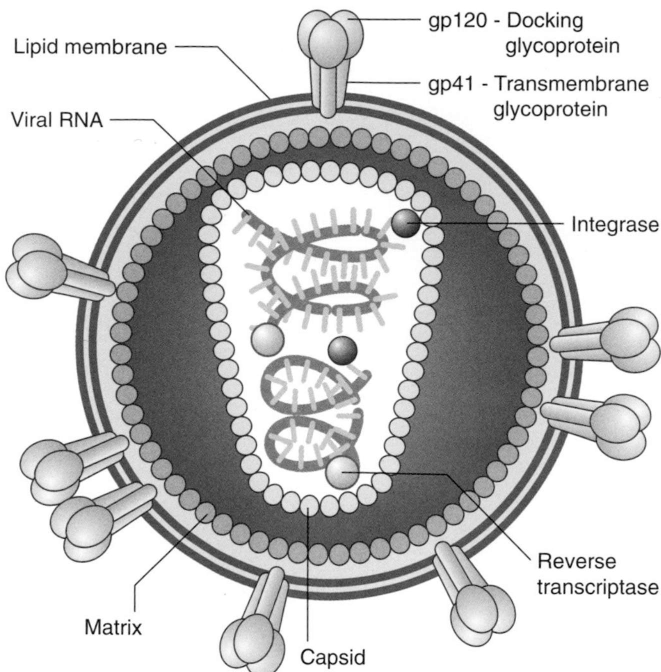

FIGURE 27.9 HIV-1 structure. *Source: National Institute of Allergy and Infectious Diseases. HIV Replication Cycle. Available at: http://www.niaid.nih.gov/topics/HIVAIDS/Understanding/Biology/Pages/hivReplicationCycle.aspx (accessed 26 April 2011).*

TABLE 27.3 Signs and Symptoms of Acute HIV Infection

Sign and Symptoms	Percent of patients with acute HIV infection
Any sign or symtom	84%
Fever	55%
Pharyngitis	43%
Myalgia	39%
Lymphadenopathy	36%
Headache	33%
Diarrhea	27%
Nausea	26%
Meningismus	20%
Photophobia	16%
Rash	16%
Vomiting	13%
Oropharyngeal sores	6%

Reprinted with permission from: Celum CL, Buchbinder SP, Donnell D, et al. Early human immunodeficiency virus (HIV) infection in the HIV Network for Prevention Trials Vaccine Preparedness Cohort: risk behaviours, symptoms, and early plasma and genital tract virus load. J Infect Dis 2001;183:23–35.

resting memory T lymphocytes, which provide the virus with a persistent, long-lived reservoir that currently available antivirals are unable to eliminate. Both host and viral factors stimulate transcription of viral RNA from the integrated DNA. This new viral RNA is translated into viral proteins (step 5) and these materials move to the cell membrane and new, immature HIV virions form and bud off from the cell with the help of host proteins (step 6). Once released, the HIV virion matures when HIV protease enzyme cleaves the gag-pol polyprotein into smaller functional proteins (step 7).

HIV transmission is inefficient (especially sexual transmission) and many HIV exposures do not result in HIV infection (Table 27-1). Successful HIV transmission occurs when HIV is able to cross the host's mucosal barrier and infect $CD4^+$ T lymphocytes, macrophages, and dendritic cells. At this early stage, HIV must avoid host defenses that could extinguish the infection while recruiting target cells, specifically $CD4^+$ T lymphocytes, to the site of infection. These initially infected cells return to regional lymph nodes where HIV is able to amplify by infecting other $CD4^+$ T lymphocytes. When these infected lymphocytes migrate into the bloodstream, HIV is dispersed throughout the body and causes massive infection of susceptible $CD4^+$ T lymphocytes in the gastrointestinal tract, lymph system, spleen, and bone marrow. Up to 60% of memory $CD4^+$ T lymphocytes in the gut-associated lymphoid tissue are infected and killed within weeks of infection [78–80]. This infection corresponds to a peak in HIV plasma viremia and the appearance of clinical symptoms of acute HIV infection (Fig. 27.11).

In response, the host generates both a humoral and cellular adaptive immune response and HIV viremia declines. This decline results primarily from the immune response (particularly the development of cytotoxic $CD8^+$ T lymphocytes against HIV) but also, to a lesser degree, from the depletion of available target cells. Within 6 months, an individual's viral load will reach a set-point; many individuals will be asymptomatic for years, although they remain infectious. The HIV viral load set-point varies greatly among individuals (in one study of 74 HIV-infected adults, the median HIV viral load set-point was 36,000 copies/mL (range: 200–717,000 copies/ml) at 120 days after HIV infection [81]) because of host and viral factors (Table 27-2), and a higher viral set-point predicts more rapid disease progression [82, 83]. Although clinically quiescent, this stage of HIV infection is characterized by on-going viral replication. The half-life of an individual HIV virion is short—the entire plasma viral population is replaced every 30 minutes [84]. To keep pace, T lymphocyte proliferation is greatly upregulated. However, over time, there is a gradual destruction of naïve and memory CD4 T lymphocytes. The rate of CD4 decline is variable [85, 86]. The median rate of CD4 decline has ranged from 37–74 cells/μl/year in studies from Africa [87, 88].

MANIFESTATIONS AND MANAGEMENT OF HIV INFECTION AND COMPLICATIONS OF HIV DISEASE

As the CD4 cell count declines, an HIV-infected person's susceptibility to infections and infection-related malignancies that are normally controlled by the cell-mediated immune system increases. This susceptibility is greatest when the CD4 cell count declines below 200 cells/μl. In high-income countries, the term "AIDS" describes the most advanced stage of HIV-infection characterized by severe immunodeficiency (e.g. CD4 cell count < 200 cells/μl in the USA) and development of opportunistic illnesses. In addition, HIV causes chronic inflammation and has direct effects on a variety of organs; many patients suffer from enteropathy, myopathy, neuropathy, or encephalopathy. Disease progression in the absence of ART varies with characteristics of the infecting virus, the host immune response and other factors. In general, disease progression is more rapid in children and older adults. Among infants, acquisition of HIV *in utero* predicts more rapid disease progression in the absence of treatment [89].

ACUTE HIV INFECTION

Acute HIV infection is the stage between HIV acquisition and development of detectable anti-HIV antibodies [90]. An estimated 40–90% of persons experience symptoms during acute HIV infection [91]. Acute HIV often presents as an infectious mononucleosis-like or influenza-like syndrome, but the clinical features can be highly variable. Symptoms typically begin a median of 10 days after HIV acquisition (Table 27-3), and include fever, maculopapular rash, arthralgia,

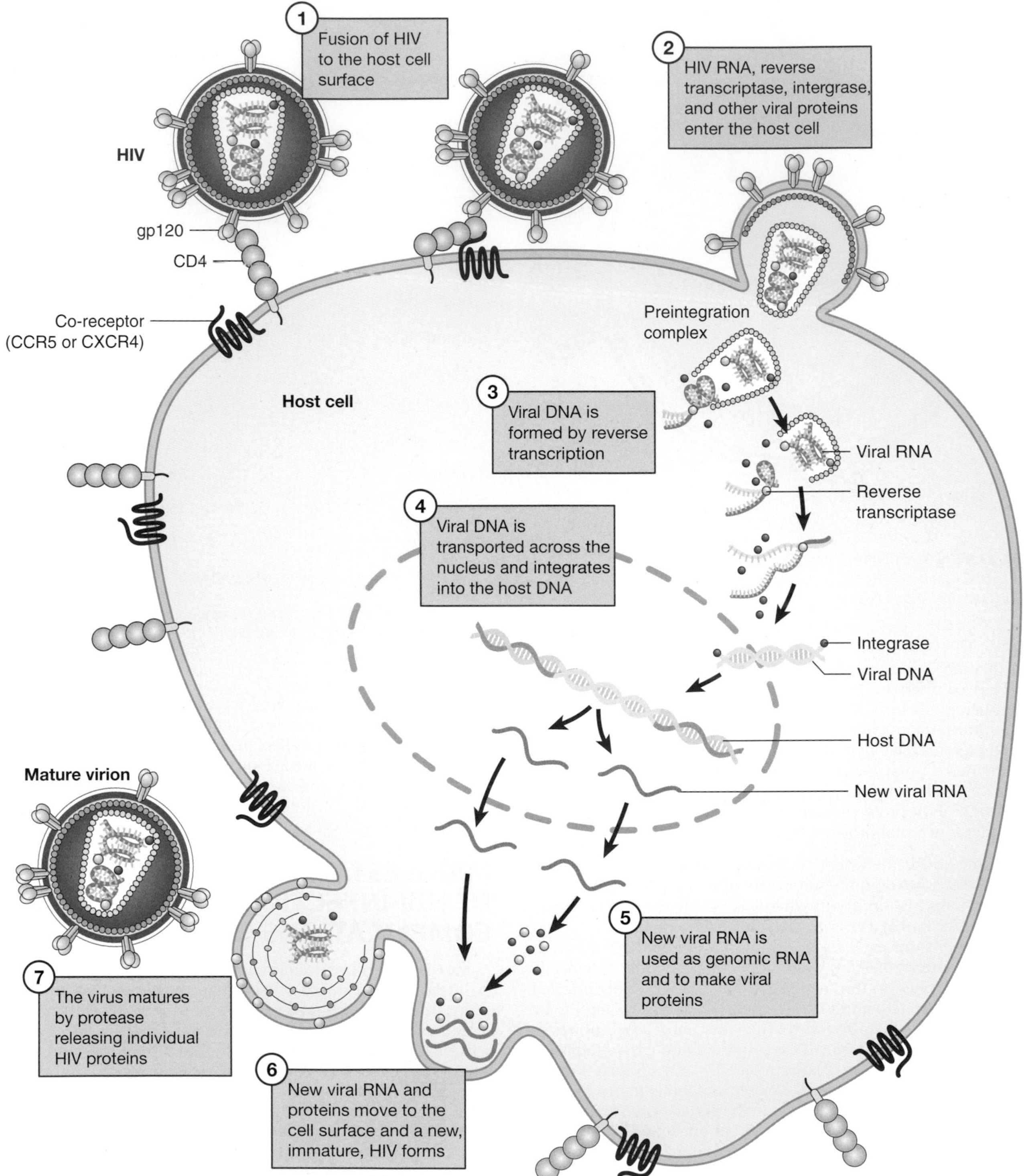

FIGURE 27.10 HIV life cycle. *Source: National Institute of Allergy and Infectious Diseases. HIV Replication Cycle. Available at: http://www.niaid.nih.gov/topics/HIVAIDS/Understanding/Biology/Pages/hivReplicationCycle.aspx (accessed 26 April 2011).*

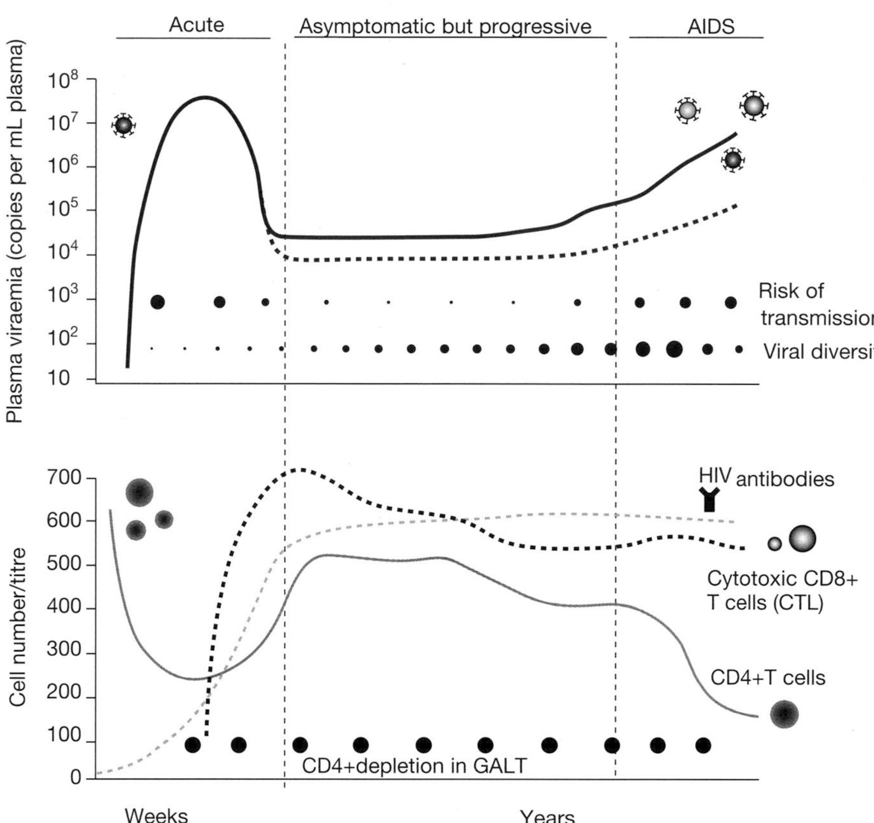

FIGURE 27.11 The course of HIV-1 infection. Plasma viremia (top) and dynamic changes in T lymphocyte compartments and HIV-specific antibodies (bottom). Primary infection characterized by high plasma viremia (solid dark blue line, top), low CD4 cells (solid light blue line, bottom) and absence of HIV-1 specific antibodies (light gray dashed line, bottom). Viremia drops as cytotoxic CD8$^+$ T lymphocytes (CTL) develop (black dashed line, bottom) and an individual viral-load set point is reached during chronic infection. Viral set points differ greatly among individuals (e.g. top) and predict disease progression. Viral diversity increases throughout the disease (closed circles, top). The risk of transmission is highest in the first weeks when viremia peaks (closed circles, top). GALT, gut-associated lymphoid tissues. *Source: Simon V, Ho DD, Abdool Karim Q. HIV/AIDS epidemiology, pathogenesis, prevention, and treatment. Lancet 2006;368:489–504.*

myalgia, malaise, lymphadenopathy, oral ulcers, pharyngitis, and weight loss [92]. The presence of fever and rash has the best positive predictive value [93]. Unfortunately, acute symptomatic HIV infection is rarely diagnosed by healthcare providers as its symptoms are often attributed to other viral infections or secondary syphilis [94].

Acute HIV infection is defined as having detectable HIV RNA[3] or HIV p24 antigen (a major core protein of HIV) in the presence of a negative or indeterminate serologic HIV antibody test [97]. Although a positive HIV RNA or HIV p24 antigen in the setting of a negative or indeterminate serologic HIV antibody test is diagnostically consistent with acute HIV infection, the diagnosis should be confirmed with an HIV antibody test performed over the next 3 months to document seroconversion [98, 99]. New advances in HIV testing technology [i.e. the increased use of fourth-generation enzyme immunoassay (EIA) tests that can detect both p24 antigen and anti-HIV antibodies] may improve its diagnosis [100, 101]. Identifying individuals during acute HIV is an important public health goal. During acute infection, HIV replicates extensively and can achieve a very high viral load, which increases the risk of further transmission (Fig. 27.11) [41, 46]. Pregnant women in high HIV prevalence settings may be particularly vulnerable to acute HIV infection and subsequent mother-to-child transmission of HIV [102]. Diagnosis should prompt preventive counseling to inform patients that they are highly infectious and to help reduce their risk of transmitting HIV. If testing for HIV RNA is not available but acute HIV is suspected, the patient should receive preventive counseling and repeat HIV antibody testing in 3–6 months.

[3]HIV RNA can be detected by qualitative and quantitative nucleic acid amplification tests (NAAT). The level of HIV viremia usually peaks with the onset of clinical symptoms of acute HIV infection [46]. Clinicians should suspect a false positive NAAT result if the HIV RNA level is less than 10,000 copies/ml in a patient with symptoms suggestive of acute HIV infection [95, 96]. In this setting, a repeat NAAT test should be performed as a rising HIV RNA level would suggest a true positive result.

STAGING OF HIV DISEASE

The two commonly used systems for the clinical staging of HIV disease are those developed by the WHO [103] and the USA Centers for Disease Control and Prevention (CDC) [104]. While these staging systems were defined primarily for surveillance purposes, they provide important prognostic and management information. The WHO clinical staging system classifies patients from Stage 1 (asymptomatic) to Stage 4 (life-threatening opportunistic infections or HIV-associated conditions) based on clinical and laboratory findings (Table 27-4). In resource-limited settings, inadequate laboratory capacity can limit the ability to measure CD4 cell counts or diagnose HIV-associated illnesses and accurately stage disease. The CDC surveillance case definitions are: Stage 1 (CD4$^+$ T-lymphocyte count ≥500 cells/μl); Stage 2 (CD4$^+$ T-lymphocyte count = 200–499 cells/μl); Stage 3 (CD4$^+$ T-lymphocyte count of <200 cells/μL or an AIDS-defining condition); or Stage unknown (Table 27-5).

In the absence of effective ART, HIV infection induces progressive immune suppression. Opportunistic illnesses closely relate to the degree of immune suppression. The risk for specific opportunistic illness can be anticipated based on the patient's CD4$^+$ count. Conversely, the occurrence of certain opportunistic illnesses can be a marker for the degree of HIV disease progression. Figure 27.12 illustrates the CD4$^+$ T lymphocyte counts at which opportunistic illnesses typically occur.

OPPORTUNISTIC ILLNESSES

Variation in risk by gender for some opportunistic illnesses has been reported (i.e. higher rates of tuberculosis among HIV-infected men [105]); however, observed differences have not been great enough to alter screening and prophylaxis recommendations for women compared with men. Disease in children mirrors that in adults with several important differences [106]. Cytomegalovirus (CMV) and disseminated herpes simplex (HSV) infections are more common in adults, whereas lymphoid interstitial pneumonia (also known as

TABLE 27.4 WHO Case Definitions of HIV for Surveillance and Revised Clinical Staging and Immunological Classification of HIV-Related Disease in Adults and Children

Primary HIV infection
Asymptomatic
Acute retroviral syndrome
Clinical stage 1
Asymptomatic
Persistent generalized lymphadenopathy (PGL)
Clinical stage 2
Moderate unexplained weight loss (<10% of presumed or measured body weight)
Recurrent respiratory tract infections (RTIs, sinusitis, bronchitis, otitis media, pharyngitis)
Herpes zoster
Angular cheilitis
Recurrent oral ulcerations
Papular pruritic eruptions
Seborrheic dermatitis
Fungal nail infections of fingers
Clinical stage 3
Conditions where a presumptive diagnosis can be made on the basis of clinical signs or simple investigations
Severe weight loss (>10% of presumed or measured body weight)
Unexplained chronic diarrhea for longer than one month
Unexplained persistent fever (intermittent or constant for longer than one month)
Oral candidiasis
Oral hairy leukoplakia
Pulmonary tuberculosis (TB) diagnosed in the last two years
Severe presumed bacterial infections (e.g. pneumonia, empyema, pyomyositis, bone or joint infection, meningitis, bacteremia)
Acute necrotizing ulcerative stomatitis, gingivitis, or periodontitis
Conditions where confirmatory diagnostic testing is necessary
Unexplained anemia (<8 g/dl), and/or neutropenia (<500/mm^3) and/or thrombocytopenia (<50000/mm^3)
Clinical stage 4
Conditions where a presumptive diagnosis can be made on the basis of clinical signs or simple investigations
HIV wasting syndrome
Pneumocystis pneumonia
Recurrent severe or radiological bacterial pneumonia
Chronic herpes simplex infection (orolabial, genital, or anorectal of > 1 month's duration)
Esophageal candidiasis
Extrapulmonary tuberculosis
Kaposi's sarcoma
Central nervous system toxoplasmosis
HIV encephalopathy

TABLE 27.4 WHO case definitions of HIV for surveillance and revised clinical staging and immunological classification of HIV-related disease in adults and children—cont'd

Conditions where confirmatory diagnostic testing is necessary:
Extrapulmonary cryptococcosis including meningitis
Disseminated non-tuberculous mycobacterial infection
Progressive multifocal leukocephalopathy (PML)
Candida of trachea, bronchi, or lungs
Cryptosporidiosis
Isosporiasis
Visceral herpes simplex infection
Cytomegalovirus (CMV) infections (retinitis or of an organ other than liver, spleen, or lymph nodes)
Any disseminated mycosis (e.g. histoplasmosis, coccidiomycosis, penicilliosis)
Recurrent non-typhoidal *Salmonella* septicaemia
Lymphoma (cerebral or B cell non-Hodgkin)
Invasive cervical carcinoma
Visceral leishmaniasis

Adapted from: WHO 2007. WHO case definition of HIV for surveillance and revised clinical staging and immunological classification of HIV-related disease in adults and children. http://www.who.int

TABLE 27.5 CDC Staging of HIV Infection* for Adults and Adolescents

Stage	**Laboratory evidence**[†]	**Clinical evidence**
Stage 1	CD4+ T-lymphocyte count of >500 cells/μL or CD4+ T-lymphocyte percentage of >29	and no AIDS-defining condition
Stage 2	CD4+ T-lymphocyte count 200-499 cells/μL or CD4+ T-lymphocyte percentage of 14-28	and no AIDS-defining condition
Stage 3 (AIDS)	CD4+ T-lymphocyte count <200 cells/μL or CD4+ T-lymphocyte percentage of <14[§]	or documentations of an AIDS-defining condition[§]
Stage unknown	no information on CD4+ T-lymphocyte count or percentage	and no AIDS-defining conditions

*Laboratory confirmed HIV infection

[†]The CD4+ T-lymphocyte percentage is the percentage of total lymphocytes. If the CD4+ T-lymphocyte count and percentage do not correspond to the same HIV infection stage, select the more severe stage.

§Documentation of an AIDS-defining condition supersedes a CD4+ T-lymphocyte count of >200 cells/μL and a CD4+ T-Lymphocyte percentage of total lymphocytes of >14. Definitive diagnostic methods for these conditions are available in the 1933 revised HIV classification system and the expanded AIDS case definition (CDC. 1933 Revised classification system for HIV infection and expanded surveillance case definition for AIDS among adolescents and adults. MMWR 1992;41[No. RR-17]) and from the National Notifiable Diseases Surveillance System (available at *http://www.cdc.gov/epo/dophsi/casedef/case_definitions.htm*).

Adapted from: CDC. Revised Surveillance Case Definitions for HIV Infection Among Adults, Adolescents, and Children Aged <18 Months and for HIV Infection and AIDS Among Children Aged 18 Months to <13 Years – United States, 2008. MMWR 2008;57(No. RR-10):[1–12].

Available at http://www.cdc.gov/mmwr/preview/mmwrhtml/rr5701a1.htm. Accessed May 12 2011.

pulmonary lymphoid hyperplasia) causes substantial illness among HIV-infected children [107]. For unclear reasons, the prevalence of *Pneumocystis jirovecii* pneumonia (PCP) among adults in most of sub-Saharan Africa is low compared with other parts of the world, but PCP is a substantial cause of morbidity and mortality among African children [108].

Visceral leishmaniasis occurs in parts of sub-Saharan Africa, around the Mediterranean Sea, on the Indian subcontinent and in South America. In Southeast Asia, most notably Thailand, systemic infection with the fungus *Penicillium marneffei* occurs with advanced immunosuppression (CD4 cell count <50 cells/μl) [109]. *Histoplasma capsulatum* occurs throughout central and southern USA, the tropics and subtropics, but is rare in Europe and Asia [110, 111]. Finally, there is substantial overlap between geographic areas affected by HIV, tuberculosis, and malaria (Fig. 27.13 and 27.14) [112].

Management of opportunistic illnesses is complex and must be tailored to the local spectrum of disease [108, 113]. The WHO and others have developed and updated international guidelines for the

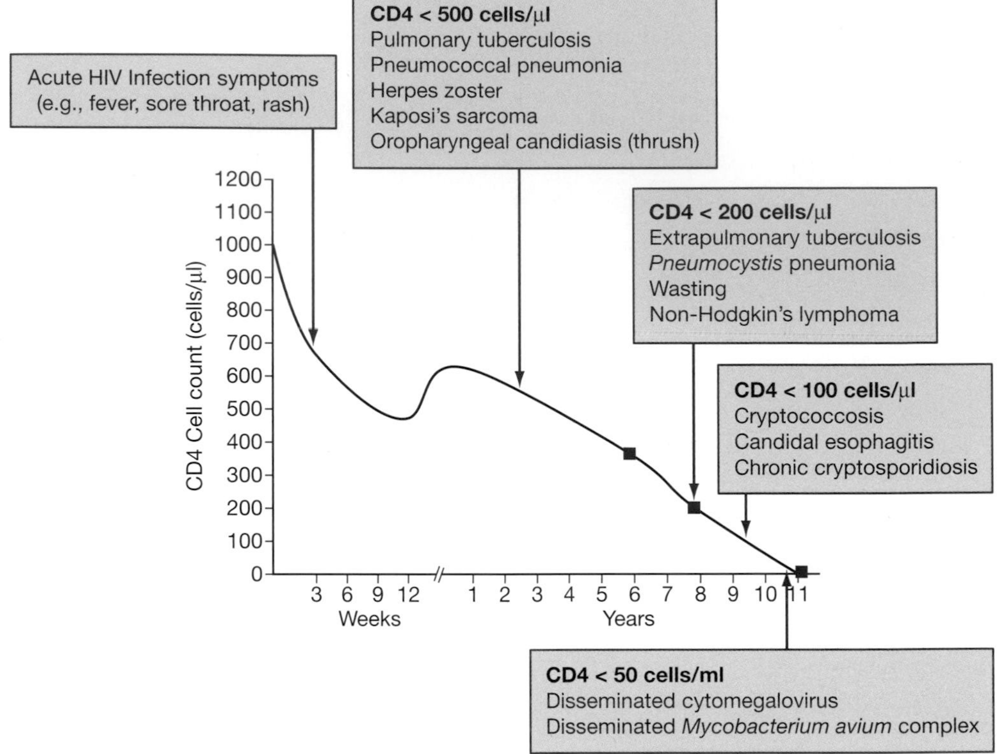

FIGURE 27.12 HIV disease progression and the occurrence of select complications. Natural history of untreated HIV infection and relationship of specific opportunistic infections to CD4 count. *(Reprinted with permission from Hanson DL, Chu SY, Farizo KM, et al. Distribution of CD4 + lymphocytes at diagnois of acquired immunodeficiency syndrome—defining and other human immunodeficiency viruse-related illnesses. Arch Intern Med 1995;155:1537–42) and (Reprinted with permission from Fauci AS, Pantaleo G, Stanley S, Weissman D. Immunopathogenic mechanismsof HIV infection. Ann Intern Med 1996;124:654–63)*

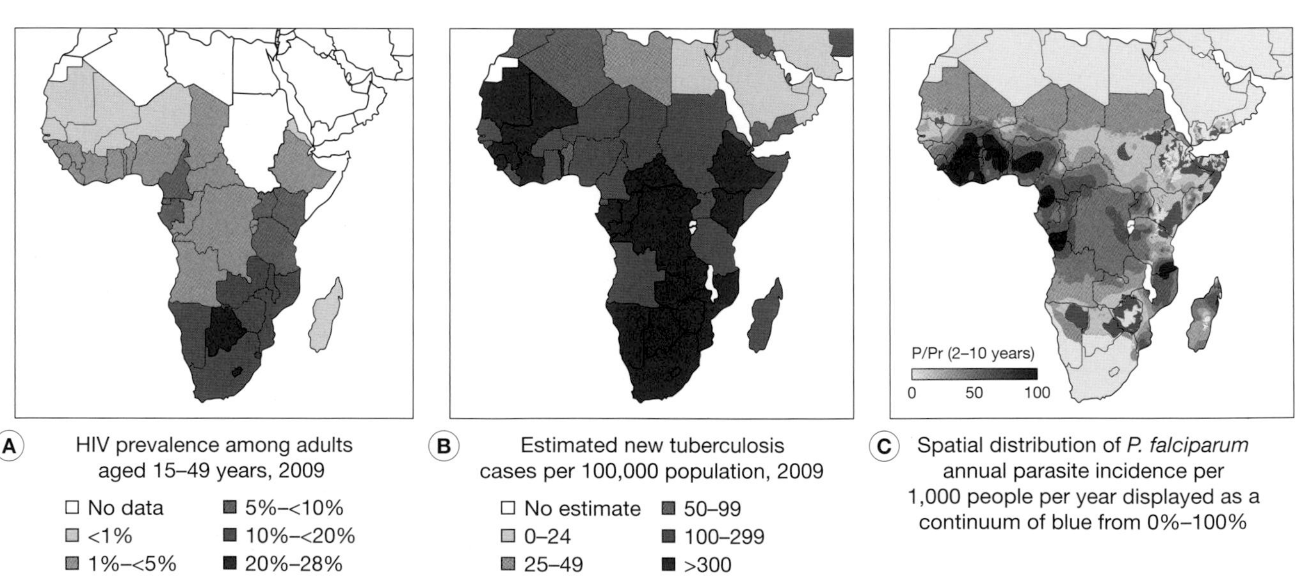

FIGURE 27.13 Prevalences of HIV infections, tuberculosis and *P. falciparum* malaria in sub-Saharan Africa, 2009. *(A) Joint United Nations Programmed on HIV/AIDS (UNAIDS). Global report: UNAIDS report on the global AIDS epidemic 2010. Available at: http://www.unaids.org/globalreport/Global_report.htm (accessed 5 May 2011). (B) World Health Organization. Global Control of Tuberculosis 2010. Geneva: World Health Organization; 2010. (C) Reprinted with permission from Hay SI, Guerra CA, Gething PW, et al. A world malaria map: Plasmodium falciparum endemicity in 2007. PLos Med 2009;6:1000048.*

management of opportunistic infections [114, 115]. High costs, drug availability, the need for a cold chain, intensive nursing support or specialized laboratory monitoring limits the ability to manage some infections. Selected opportunistic infections, HIV-associated malignancies and disease syndromes are described below.

SELECT MAJOR OPPORTUNISTIC INFECTIONS AND CO-INFECTIONS

[Note: issues regarding HIV and tuberculosis (see Chapter 27.1, "*Tuberculosis*") and malaria (see Chapter 96, "*Malaria*") are discussed in detail in dedicated chapters and are, therefore, not included here.]

FUNGAL INFECTIONS—FOCUS ON CRYPTOCOCCAL MENINGITIS AND PNEUMOCYSTIS PNEUMONIA

Cryptococcal Meningitis

Infection with *Cryptococcus neoformans* rivals tuberculosis as a cause of death in persons with HIV infection [116]. It usually manifests as meningitis but can also present as pneumonia. Cryptococcal meningitis is characterized by headache, fever, altered mental status, and cranial nerve palsies; notably, meningismus may not be prominent or completely absent.

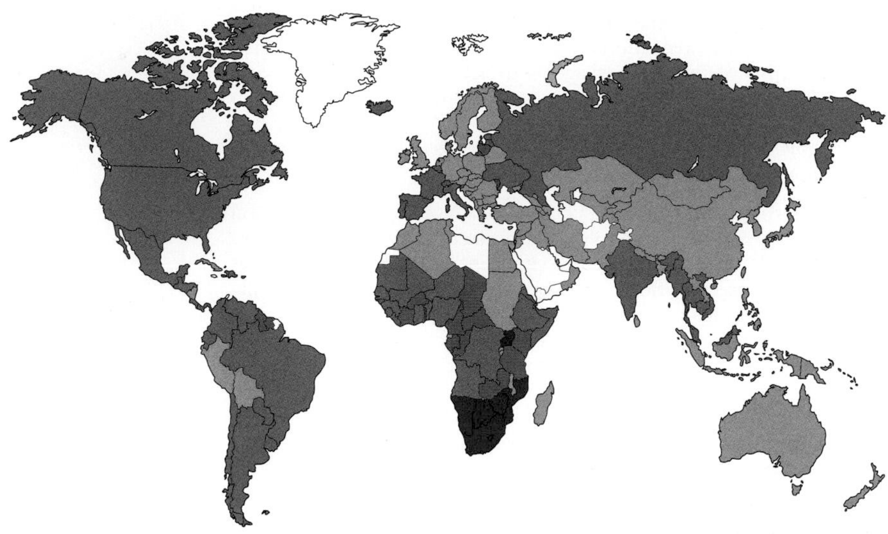

FIGURE 27.14 Estimated HIV prevalence in new tuberculosis cases, 2009. *Source: World Health Organization. Global Control of Tuberculosis 2010. Geneva: World Health Organization; 2010.*

Approximately 50% of HIV-infected patients with cryptococcal meningitis have elevated baseline intracranial pressures [i.e. >25 cm of cerebrospinal fluid (CSF)] and patients with a higher intracranial pressure tend to have a higher fungal burden [117]. The organism can be cultured from CSF in the majority of patients and from the blood in up to 75% of patients [115]. Testing for cryptococcal antigen (CrAg) in CSF or in serum is sensitive and specific [118–120]. Serum CrAg testing can be useful for screening or when lumbar puncture cannot be performed.

The most effective treatment for cryptococcal meningitis (see Chapter 84) is a combination of amphotericin B and flucytosine with management of increased intracranial pressure, such as by repeated lumbar punctures [121]. Fluconazole is an alternative when amphotericin cannot be given and should be combined with flucytosine if flucytosine and laboratory monitoring are available [122, 123]. Monotherapy with fluconazole is likely inferior [124] but, in some situations, may be the only option.

In persons with acute cryptococcal meningitis, there are conflicting data regarding the optimal timing of ART (e.g. concurrent with initiation of antifungal therapy or delayed) [125–128]. A randomized clinical trial in Zimbabwe evaluated the timing of ART in HIV-infected patients who were newly diagnosed with cryptococcal meningitis and treated with fluconazole monotherapy. In this trial, early initiation of ART (within 72 hours of the cryptococcal meningitis diagnosis) was associated with increased mortality [presumably as a result of immune reconstitution inflammatory syndrome (IRIS)] compared with delaying ART for 10 weeks [126]. Thus, it may be prudent to delay initiation for at least 2 weeks—possibly longer if fluconazole monotherapy is used. For persons who recover from an initial episode, secondary prophylaxis is recommended. While there are few data from resource-limited settings, it is assumed that discontinuation following immune recovery on ART is safe. Primary prophylaxis with fluconazole prevents cryptococcal disease, and may be cost effective in settings with high disease prevalence [129]. Alternate approaches to reducing the burden of cryptococcal disease are early initiation of ART or pre-emptive antifungal therapy to persons with asymptomatic cryptococcal infection [130].

Pneumocystis Pneumonia

PCP disease progression can be rapid, particularly in children, thus prevention by primary antimicrobial prophylaxis is a priority (see *"Prevention: Special Considerations for Antimicrobial Prophylaxis in Resource-Limited Settings"* below). PCP is most common in patients with CD4 cell counts <200 cells/μl. PCP typically presents with fever, a dry cough and progressive dyspnea. Hypoxia is common, serum lactate dehydrogenase is typically elevated and chest x-ray usually reveals diffuse interstitial infiltrates that are often perihilar.

BACTERIAL INFECTIONS

While identification of bacterial illness is unusual in resource-limited settings, epidemiologic studies have confirmed the importance of *Streptococcus pneumoniae* and non–typhoid *Salmonella* in adults and children with HIV [131, 132], and *Haemophilus influenzae* in children [133, 134]. Clinical manifestations of *S. pneumoniae* vary; pneumococcal infection presents most commonly as pneumonia or sinusitis, but meningitis also occurs and any presentation can be accompanied by pneumococcal bacteremia. WHO guidelines on the treatment of diarrhea and pneumonia in HIV-infected children and infants should be consulted for up-to-date recommendations: (http://whqlibdoc.who.int/publications/2010/9789241548083_eng.pdf) [135].

SEXUALLY TRANSMITTED INFECTIONS (STIs)

Many HIV-infected persons are at risk for STIs; these can also increase the risk of HIV transmission and acquisition [136]. Diagnosis and management of STIs in persons with HIV is similar to persons without HIV. However, clinical presentations of some STIs can be more severe with HIV, for example ulcerative lesions may be more extensive. Algorithms for syndromic management of STIs have not performed as well in persons with HIV and specific diagnoses should be confirmed where possible [137].

VIRAL HEPATITIS

Prevalence of hepatitis B (HBV) and hepatitis C (HCV) in HIV-infected persons can be higher than in HIV-uninfected persons because of shared routes of transmission [138]. Co-infection of HIV with HBV or HCV increases the mortality risk, but may have modest impact on the progression of HIV disease. However, co-infected patients are at increased risk of cirrhosis, liver failure, and hepatocellular carcinoma.

All persons with HIV and viral hepatitis should avoid alcohol consumption and use precautions to prevent transmission of viral hepatitis. A number of antiretroviral agents are active against both HIV and HBV. Therefore, guidelines now recommend that ART be started in any person diagnosed with active HBV or HCV [98, 139–141] (see *"Antiretroviral Therapy: What to Start—Special Considerations in Patients with Chronic Hepatitis B Infection"* below).

Baseline testing of HIV-infected persons for active hepatitis B infection can identify persons who should be prioritized to receive dually active antiretroviral regimens [142]. In settings where HBV prevalence is high, it may be cost-effective to consider empiric ART with dually active (i.e. active against both HIV and HBV) regimens. The objectives of treating HBV are normalization of alanine aminotransferase, hepatitis B e antigen seroconversion, suppression of hepatitis B viral load and improvement in liver histology. Withdrawal of dually active therapy in HBV-co-infected patients can lead to HBV reactivation [143, 144]. Therefore, HBV-infected patients on dually active regimens should be advised against self-discontinuation and closely monitored for hepatic injury if the regimen must be stopped.

Cure of HCV infection, defined as the sustained elimination of HCV RNA from the serum and liver, is possible. The existing standard of care—HCV protease inhibitors, pegylated interferon and ribavirin—is complex to manage because of the usual occurrence of adverse events that require clinical and laboratory monitoring. Directly-acting agents against HCV infection (e.g. HCV protease inhibitors) are in development [145–150].

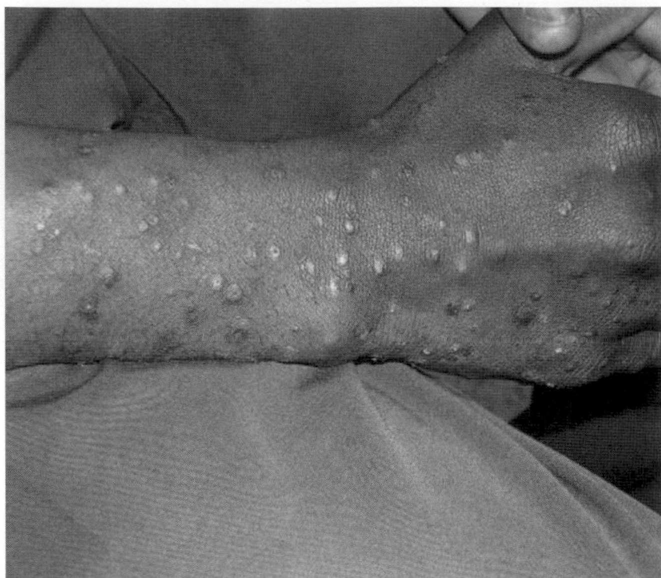

FIGURE 27.15 Pruritic papular eruption of HIV disease. Pruritic papular eruption occurring in individuals with human immunodeficiency virus infection. Detail from dorsal surface of hand showing excoriated papules. *(Reprinted with permission from Amerson EH, Maurer TA. Dermatologic manifestations of HIV in Africa. Top HIV Med 2010;18:16–22)*

SELECT MAJOR CLINICAL SYNDROMES

FEVER

Prolonged fever is common, especially among patients with low CD4 cell counts (e.g. <200 cells/ml) who are not receiving ART [151], and differential diagnosis is broad and varies geographically. Infectious etiologies are responsible for the majority of fevers.

Tuberculosis should be considered in all patients with fever especially if cough, shortness of breath, weight loss, night sweats, or lymphadenopathy are present (see Chapter 39, *"Tuberculosis"*) [131]. Other causes of fever are cryptococcal disease (e.g. *C. neoformans* bloodstream infection), bacteremia (e.g. *Salmonella*, *Rhodococcus*), pneumonia, both bacterial (e.g. *S. pneumoniae*) and fungal (e.g. PCP), malaria, CMV, and lymphoma. Multiple concurrent etiologies occur.

The diagnostic work-up for fever should be driven by the clinical presentation and availability of diagnostic tests. Blood cultures, blood smear for malaria, mycobacterial blood cultures and serum cryptococcal antigen testing can be helpful. Chest radiography, urine culture, bone marrow aspirate and biopsy, and other radiologic studies (e.g. brain imaging, abdominal imaging) may be necessary. Certain etiologies such as mycobacterial disease, *Pneumocystis*, *Bartonella*, lymphoma and certain fungal infections can be particularly difficult to diagnose and should be considered when fever persists despite a diagnostic work-up.

DERMATOLOGIC DISEASE

Dermatologic disease can have a broad differential diagnosis, especially in patients with advanced immunosuppression [152]. The International AIDS Society-USA (www.iasusa.org) has useful reference materials [152].

Pruritic papular eruption (PPE) is common in tropical environments. PPE may be caused by a hypersensitivity to insect bites and presents with extremely pruritic papules (<1 cm) predominately on the extremities that can be hyperpigmented and excoriated from scratching [153] (Fig. 27.15). PPE is diagnosed clinically and improves with ART; topical steroids and capsaicin can help. Bacterial folliculitis (e.g. staphylococcal folliculitis) can present with lesions similar to PPE. However, the lesions are follicular, fewer in number, variably pruritic and occur more commonly on the upper trunk and buttocks. Staphylococcal folliculitis can be treated with topical or oral anti-staphylococcal antibiotics. Eosinophilic folliculitis presents with pruritic papules on the face, neck, and upper trunk, and can mimic acne. It responds best to ART, but may paradoxically worsen. Topical steroids or oral itraconazole can improve symptoms.

Scabies can present with pruritic papular lesions similar to those seen with PPE; however, scabies lesions tend to be clustered in the finger webs, waist, ankles, axillae, breasts, and genital areas, and burrows can sometimes be seen. Severe scabies ('Norwegian' scabies) can present with a crusted thick grayish scale teeming with mites. Scratching of scabies lesions can lead to bacterial superinfection. Oral ivermectin or topical agents are effective. Prurigo nodularis—a condition that results from intense scratching—presents with larger (>1 cm) pruritic nodules that often start on the extremities with a symmetric distribution; management should identify the underlying cause of pruritis. Topical steroids, topical capsaicin, and oral antihistamines can ameliorate symptoms.

Seborrheic dermatitis presents with dandruff and indistinct plaques of yellowish scale involving the scalp, face, chest, back, and groin. Although it can typically be seen on the hair-bearing area of the head (e.g. eyebrows, outer ear canal), in the context of HIV infection, and especially in Africa, it occurs at skin folds (e.g. axillae, inner thighs). Mild cases respond to dandruff shampoo (e.g. selenium sulfide or zinc pyrithione). More severe cases require topical antifungals (e.g. ketoconazole) directed against *Pityrosporum* yeasts such as *Malassezia furfur* and steroids. Refractory cases may require oral ketoconazole.

Photodermatitis frequently occurs in Africa and presents with an itchy, scaly rash. It is differentiated from seborrheic dermatitis by its distribution on sun-exposed areas of skin. Although sulfonamides can be photosensitizing, their use in treating HIV infection is important and they should not be stopped, if possible, because of photodermatitis.

Human herpesvirus 8 infection (HHV-8), the cause of Kaposi's sarcoma (KS), is endemic to much of Africa. KS commonly occurs in patients with advanced HIV disease (see *"HIV-associated Malignancies"* below) [154]. It presents with reddish, violaceous or brown non-tender macules and papules that progress to nodules. KS often involves the head and neck but can involve several anatomical sites; oral lesions on the tongue, palate, and buccal mucosa may precede skin disease. Advanced KS causes widely disseminated skin disease with lymphatic obstruction and involvement of the lungs and gastrointestinal tract. KS can regress with ART, especially if detected at an early stage. Bacillary angiomatosis caused by infection with *Bartonella henselae* or *quintana* can cause similar lesions as KS but is treated effectively with antibiotics. Likewise, dermal non-Hodgkin lymphoma can have a similar presentation but occurs rarely.

Molluscum contagiosum is caused by a poxvirus and is common in HIV-infected children. It presents with dome-shaped umbilicated papules. Disseminated cryptococcosis can present with similar lesions that precede the development of systemic disease but the onset is usually abrupt.

Genital and non-genital warts caused by human papillomavirus are common in tropical environments and HIV-infected children may develop hundreds of flat warts. Syphilis should be considered in patients presenting with disseminated maculopapular skin disease or condylomata lata.

The possibility of drug eruptions should always be considered. Mucocutaneous eruptions, blisters or other erosive dermal lesions should prompt consideration of Stevens-Johnson syndrome or toxic epidermal necrolysis [155, 156]. Decisions on whether to stop treatment with the suspect agent or to "treat through" need to be made on a case-by-case basis.

OPHTHALMOLOGIC DISEASE

Eye disease is an important complication [157–159]. CMV retinitis is the most common cause of retinal disease and vision loss with advanced immunosuppression (i.e. CD4 cell count < 50 cells/μl) [158]. CMV retinitis can be diagnosed by retinal examination that demonstrates large white or creamy lesions with granular borders and associated hemorrhage (Fig. 27.16). Lesions often begin in the periphery and progress centrally; patients complain of unilateral floaters followed by progressively decreased visual acuity and eventual blindness. CMV retinitis should be treated with ART and CMV antiviral therapy (e.g. oral valganciclovir, intravenous ganciclovir, or intraocular ganciclovir). It can be confused with HIV retinopathy, which has characteristic "cotton-wool" spots on retinal examination. These lesions are not sight threatening and often resolve spontaneously [160]. Other causes of rapid vision loss are progressive outer retinal necrosis caused by varicella-zoster virus and, less commonly, by herpes simplex. Squamous cell carcinoma of the conjunctiva, corneal microsporidiosis, ocular tuberculosis, and syphilitic chorioretinitis and uveitis can cause ophthalmologic disease in low-income settings.

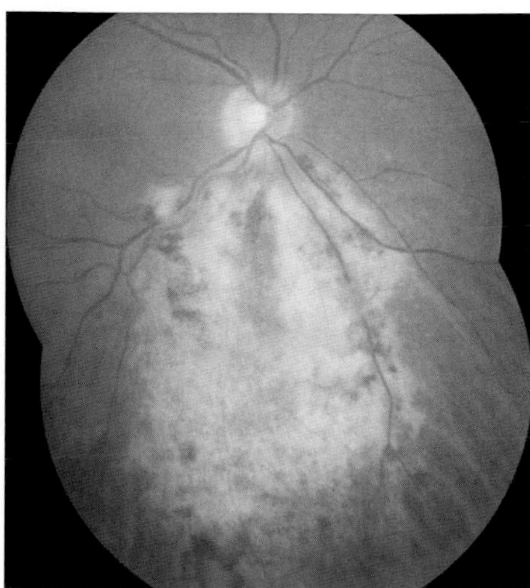

FIGURE 27.16 Retinal photograph of CMV retinitis. CMV retinitis is characterized by large white or creamy retinal lesions with granular borders and variable associated hemorrhage. *(Reprinted with permission from Heiden D, Ford N, Wilson D, et al. Cytomegalovirus retinitis: the neglected disease of the AIDS pandemic. PLoS Med 2007;4:e334.)*

PULMONARY DISEASE

In most clinical and autopsy case series of lung disease in HIV-infected patients, tuberculosis is among the most frequently identified pathogens and should be considered with any pulmonary infection (see Chapter 39, "*Tuberculosis*"). Community-acquired pneumonia, frequently caused by *S. pneumoniae*, is the next most common cause of lung disease [161, 162]. Tuberculosis and community-acquired pneumonia can occur at any time during HIV infection, but risk increases as the CD4 cell count declines. Cotrimoxazole prophylaxis and pneumococcal conjugate vaccination may be effective prevention strategies [163, 164]. PCP presents as a subacute process. KS, histoplasmosis, cryptococcosis, nocardiosis and, in children, lymphoid interstitial pneumonititis, are less common causes.

Pleural effusions are most often secondary to infection or malignancy [165]. Pleural tuberculosis can occur with or without parenchymal disease. Tuberculous pleural effusions are exudative, lymphocytic and not acidic or hypoglycemic. They typically demonstrate concentrations of adenosine deaminase (ADA) greater than 50 U/l [166]. A pleural fluid acid-fast smear is positive in less than 15% of cases, but a sputum smear may be positive. Pleural biopsies with examination for acid-fast bacilli and granulomas have the highest likelihood of confirming pleural infection. Bacterial pneumonia often causes parapneumonic effusions. KS, multicentric Castleman's disease, primary effusion lymphoma, B-cell non-Hodgkin lymphoma, and lung cancer are malignant causes of effusion.

ESOPHAGEAL DISEASE

Dysphagia (i.e. difficulty swallowing with a sensation of food sticking) and odynophagia (i.e. pain on swallowing) occur with advanced HIV infection and suggest esophagitis. Candidiasis is the most common cause [115, 167] and is usually associated with oropharyngeal candidiasis (thrush) (Fig. 27.17). Empiric treatment for candidal esophagitis with fluconazole is usually indicated, especially in patients with a CD4 count <200 cells/μL or if oral thrush is present. Patients who do not respond to fluconazole can be treated with a higher dose, and patients who still do not respond should be considered for upper endoscopy with biopsy. Other etiologies are CMV, herpes simplex virus, and aphthous ulcers, each of which tends to be associated with more prominent odynophagia (often without dysphagia).

GASTROENTERITIS/DIARRHEAL DISEASE

Acute diarrhea suggests a viral or bacterial pathogen although certain parasitic infections (*Isospora belli*, *Entamoeba histolytica*) can present

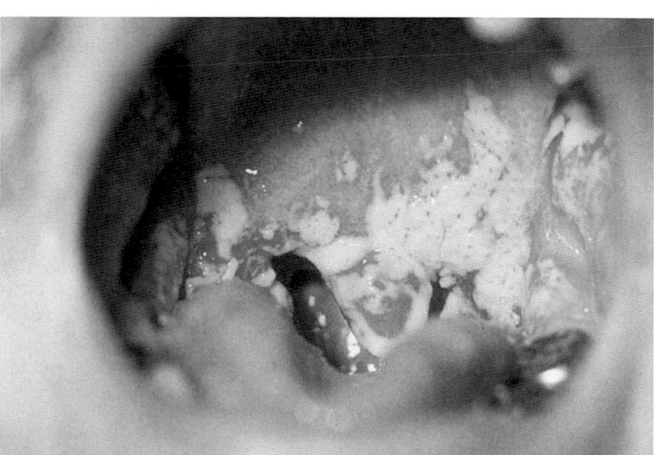

FIGURE 27.17 Oral candidiasis (thrush). Oral candidiasis is a fungal infection, also known as thrush, which presents as white or yellowish patches, sometimes with erythema. If wiped away, there will be redness or bleeding underneath. Lesions can appear anywhere in the mouth. *Source: Anon. Public Health Image Library. Available at: http://phil.cdc.gov/phil/quicksearch.asp (accessed 1 April 2011).*

acutely. Diarrhea and fever suggest *Salmonella, Shigella,* or *Campylobacter*, especially if mucus or blood are in the stool [168]. Bacterial diarrhea should be treated with antibiotics [115] guided by culture and antimicrobial sensitivity testing. Enteric viruses (e.g. norovirus, rotavirus, adenovirus) and pathogenic *Escherichia coli* (e.g. enteroaggregative, enterotoxigenic and enterohemorrhagic *E. coli*) can also cause acute diarrhea [169, 170]. *Clostridium difficile* occurs among HIV-infected patients in developed nations exposed to antibiotics or who have been hospitalized [171]. Non-infectious etiologies of acute diarrhea can be secondary to drugs, food poisoning (e.g. bacterial or marine toxins), lactose intolerance, inflammatory bowel disease, or infiltrative diseases (i.e. lymphoma or Kaposi's sarcoma). ART, especially protease inhibitors (e.g. nelfinavir), can also be associated with diarrhea and should be considered if other etiologies can be ruled out [172]. ART-associated diarrhea can often be managed symptomatically but in severe cases may require a single drug substitution to an alternative medication.

In patients with a low CD4 count (<200 cells/µl), cryptosporidiosis owing to infection with *Cryptosporidium parvum, C. hominis,* or *C. maleagridis* is a cause of chronic diarrhea [173–176]. Other causes are isosporiasis, microsporidiosis, *Mycobacterium avium* complex, cyclosporiasis, and CMV. Giardiasis, amoebiasis, and strongyloidiasis can occur at any stage of HIV infection. Even with access to diagnostic testing (e.g. stool leukocyte evaluation, stool culture, stool examination for ova and parasites with a modified acid-fast stain for *Cryptosporidium*) and endoscopy with biopsy, a significant proportion of chronic diarrhea has no pathogen identified and is attributed to HIV enteropathy [177]. While some causes of chronic diarrhea can be treated (i.e. trimethoprim-sulfamethoxazole for isosporiasis and cyclosporiasis), cryptosporidiosis and microsporidiosis are often refractory to antimicrobial therapy alone. For these patients, immune reconstitution with ART is necessary [178].

FOCAL CENTRAL NERVOUS SYSTEM (CNS) LESIONS

HIV-infected patients with advanced immunosuppression who present with focal neurologic symptoms or seizures often have a central nervous system (CNS) mass lesion caused by an opportunistic infection or HIV-associated malignancy. The evaluation and management of these lesions can be challenging if access to radiography [e.g. computed tomography (CT), magnetic resonance imaging (MRI)] and neurosurgery are limited [179, 180]. The most common etiology of focal CNS lesions in low-income settings has been tuberculosis (tuberculomas) [179], but neurocysticercosis, toxoplasma encephalitis, primary CNS lymphoma, non-Hodgkin lymphoma, bacterial brain abscess, cryptococcosis and, in South America, brain chagoma caused by *Trypanosoma cruzi*, are considerations. Tuberculosis should be strongly suspected if there is evidence of non-neurologic tuberculosis (e.g. lung disease), basal meningeal enhancement on CT scan or a CSF pleocytosis with a high protein.

Toxoplasma encephalitis presents with fever, headache, weakness, altered mental status or confusion, and possibly seizures; physical exam usually demonstrates focal neurologic abnormalities [181]. Most patients have a CD4 cell count <100 cells/µl and positive toxoplasma serology [182]. Empiric therapy with pyrimethamine, sulfadiazine, and leucovorin is indicated; clinical improvement should be seen within 1–2 weeks if the diagnosis is correct. In resource-limited settings, use of trimethoprim-sulfamethoxazole may be considered if the first-line drugs are not available [183, 184].

Progressive multifocal leukoencephalopathy (PML) is an insidious and progressive disorder caused by John Cunningham (JC) virus that usually presents with one or more rapidly progressive focal neurologic deficits without fever in advanced HIV infection [115]. The diagnosis can be made by identification of JC virus in CSF or demonstration of characteristic lesions by CNS imaging. No specific therapy exists; treatment is ART to restore immunity against the JC virus.

IMMUNE RECONSTITUTION INFLAMMATORY SYNDROME (IRIS)

Occasionally, and especially in persons with low CD4 cell counts, immune reconstitution following initiation of ART can unmask a clinically quiescent co-infection or lead to paradoxical worsening of an active previously diagnosed co-infection; in both cases the patient's clinical condition can worsen [185]. This ART-mediated IRIS occurs with mycobacterial infections, usually tuberculosis, as well as CMV retinitis, cryptococcal meningitis, and PML [185]. However, it has occurred with almost every AIDS-associated opportunistic infection and a variety of non-AIDS-associated infections and illnesses [186, 187]. In general, the benefits of early initiation of ART outweigh the risk of IRIS. IRIS can usually be managed without interrupting ART by treating the associated co-infection and providing supportive care, which can include non-steroidal anti-inflammatory drugs (NSAIDs) or corticosteroids. ART should be stopped with IRIS that is either life-threatening or that cannot be managed with supportive care.

HIV-ASSOCIATED MALIGNANCIES

Persons with HIV infection are at increased risk for three malignancies: KS, non-Hodgkin lymphomas, and cervical cancer [104, 188]. The incidence of KS and non-Hodgkin lymphomas has declined dramatically in high-income countries among persons receiving ART [189–191]. In regions where life expectancies of persons living with HIV infection have increased, the incidence of non-AIDS-associated malignancies has increased at rates in excess of rates for the same cancers in HIV-uninfected persons [192]. Whether similar trends are occurring in resource-limited settings is difficult to determine [193]. Many non-AIDS malignancies are associated with chronic oncogenic viral infections: human papillomavirus (HPV; anal and oropharyngeal cancer), Epstein-Barr virus (non-Hodgkin lymphoma), and viral hepatitis B and C (hepatoma) [194, 195]. Others are associated with lifestyle factors that are more prevalent among certain populations (e.g. tobacco use). Some data suggest that HIV infection independently increases risk for non-AIDS malignancies; however, it is not evident whether ART affects this risk [196–198].

Kaposi's Sarcoma (KS)

KS is caused by HHV-8 and the endemic prevalence (i.e. HIV-unassociated) generally correlates with regional HHV-8 seroprevalence; however, immunosuppression from HIV can increase the incidence and prevalence of KS [199–202]. KS is common in African countries of Zambia, Democratic Republic of Congo, Zimbabwe, Uganda, Rwanda, and Burundi [203–205]. Although endemic KS is uncommon in the Americas, Europe, and Asia, persons with HIV infection, and especially MSM, experience greater incidence of disease [206]. With ART, KS may regress [207] and protease inhibitors appear to have specific activity against HHV-8 [208]. Extensive visceral or rapidly progressive disease often requires cytotoxic chemotherapy and radiation therapy, which are generally palliative and not curative [201].

Non-Hodgkin Lymphoma

Non-Hodgkin lymphomas are the second most common malignancy associated with HIV infection and comprise a heterogeneous group of tumors that are almost all of B-cell origin [209]. Many of these tumors appear causally related to either Epstein-Barr virus or HHV-8 [210]. Incidence is increased substantially among patients with low CD4 cell counts. Diagnosis is based on clinical presentation (e.g. lymphadenopathy, fevers, night sweats, weight loss) and biopsy. Treatment and prognosis vary according to the type of tumor and available therapy.

Cervical Cancer

Cervical cancer is a leading cause of death among women worldwide and a common AIDS-related malignancy [211]. The vast majority of cervical cancers, including among HIV-infected women, are caused by infection with oncogenic types of HPV [212, 213]. HPV infections are more common and persistent in women with HIV. Risk for cervical cancer is not correlated with CD4 cell count. Incidence of cervical cancer has not declined significantly in high-income settings where ART use is widespread [193], although women who are adherent to ART demonstrate lower incidence and prevalence of oncogenic HPV types [214].

Screening and earlier intervention are key aspects of preventing cervical cancer. Traditional population-based cervical cancer prevention programs that rely upon examination of cervical cells face substantial barriers to sustainability in resource-limited settings. These include a lack of resources (e.g. cytopathology services, surgery and chemotherapy, infrastructure to support screening, and treatment) and trained healthcare workers (e.g. persons that collect specimens, cytotechnologists, clinicians for medical and surgical management of cervical disease), and the requirement that patients attend multiple medical visits [215]. Innovative "see-and-treat" programs, where women with cervical pathology during direct visual examination of the cervix after application of acetic acid are treated at the same visit with cryotherapy, show great promise [215]. National programs to vaccinate young women and men against HPV prior to sexual debut could substantially reduce the burden of cervical cancer and other HPV-associated malignancies (e.g. anal cancer, head and neck cancer). Studies of the effectiveness of HPV vaccination in HIV-infected women are ongoing (www.clinicaltrials.gov).

PATIENT EVALUATION, DIAGNOSIS AND DIFFERENTIAL DIAGNOSIS

HIV TESTING

Many persons with HIV infection do not get tested until late in their disease [216]. Not only is their access to ART delayed, but they remain unaware that they need to protect their sex or needle-sharing partners from becoming infected. Many HIV-infected persons will decrease risk behaviors when they are aware of their positive HIV status [217, 218]. Medical treatment that lowers plasma HIV viral load also reduces risk for transmission to others [219–221]. An international randomized clinical trial demonstrated that treating an HIV-infected individual with antiretrovirals can reduce the risk of sexual transmission of HIV to their HIV-uninfected partner by 96% [222].

In countries with generalized epidemics, the WHO recommends HIV testing all persons accessing health care. Testing should be considered a part of the standard of routine clinical care, and patients should be informed that they will be tested for HIV infection and that they can "opt-out". The highest priority for testing should be given to persons with syndromes that suggest HIV infection (Table 27-4) and to persons whose behaviors or exposures substantially increase their risk of acquiring HIV, such as persons with other STIs, commercial sex workers, IDUs, MSM, and children whose mothers have HIV infection.

All pregnant women should be tested at their initial antenatal visit. HIV testing can identify women who need their own treatment and who need to receive prenatal prophylaxis to PMTCT of HIV. In the absence of perinatal prophylaxis or interventions to prevent transmission at birth [223–226] and through breastfeeding [227, 228], approximately 15–40% of infants born to HIV-infected mothers will become infected. Timely perinatal prophylaxis for the mother and infant, and administration of ART to the mother or infant while breastfeeding, can reduce the rate to <1% [39, 52, 229–233].

Clinicians should also consider testing all women during their third trimester or at delivery, especially in regions where the HIV epidemic is generalized among women of reproductive age. Among women whose previous testing was negative, re-testing can identify women who have become HIV infected or who were seroconverting. A second HIV test during the third trimester is cost-effective [234, 235].

HIV-testing should be available and offered to persons in the general population. Effective models have used rapid test kits that allow for immediate delivery of test results and have employed trained lay counselors in settings with healthcare worker shortages. In populations with a high HIV prevalence, testing is feasible in rural settings and can be effectively offered by teams going door-to-door [236]. HIV testing results should be presented with counseling about HIV prevention and risk reduction. For persons who test positive, it is critical to provide psychosocial support and clinical services, and to ensure patients are referred to, and linked into, medical care [237] (see *"HIV counseling"* below).

HIV DIAGNOSIS

HIV infection should be diagnosed with a rapid or conventional serologic assay for antibodies against HIV (e.g. an EIA). Rapid HIV testing is faster (tests results are often available in less than 30 minutes), less costly and increases the number of clients who receive their results [238]. Most rapid tests do not require access to running water or electricity and some can be performed on oral fluids.

Results that are reactive by a serologic assay should be confirmed with another assay. Clinicians should follow local guidelines for confirmatory testing, which may involve repeat HIV testing with a different rapid EIA test, performing a Western blot for antibodies against specific HIV proteins or an assay that directly detects HIV RNA.

In low-income settings with a high HIV prevalence, there are algorithms using a series of rapid tests to confirm HIV infection (Fig. 27.18). Although HIV serology has sensitivities and specificities that approach 99.9%, false-positive and false-negative results occur. False-positive serology is more frequent among persons with autoimmune disease, multiple myeloma, chronic renal failure, in persons recently vaccinated, in women who have experienced multiple pregnancies and in persons who have been vaccinated with a candidate HIV vaccine in clinical trials. Importantly, in low-prevalence situations (e.g. <0.1% HIV prevalence), even tests with high specificity may yield a relatively high proportion of falsely positive results. False-negative results can occur during acute HIV infection when the person has not yet developed detectable anti-HIV antibodies (i.e. seroconversion), termed the "window period". Certain tests can detect HIV RNA and other HIV antigens (e.g. p24) early in infection during this "window period"; however, there still remains a period of time between infection and the ability to detect the virus, termed the "eclipse phase". During both the window period and eclipse phase, HIV-infected persons can transmit infection.

HIV infection in infants and children younger than 18 months cannot be reliably diagnosed with serology because of the persistence of transplacentally acquired maternal antibody [239]. Prompt diagnosis of HIV-infected infants with molecular testing is essential because a high proportion (15–20%) experience rapid disease progression within the first year of life [240]; HIV-infected infants require early initiation of ART and opportunistic infection prophylaxis to survive. Molecular HIV testing of newborns and infants can be performed by either quantifying HIV RNA or HIV proviral DNA (preferred if the mother is taking ART). The availability of these tests is limited in low-income settings.

HIV testing algorithms should use HIV diagnostic tests that have a high sensitivity for locally circulating HIV subtypes (clades). Most HIV EIA tests can detect the vast majority of emerging HIV-1 subtypes and CRFs; certain assays can also detect HIV-1 Group O and N [241–245]. Most current EIA tests also detect both HIV-1 and HIV-2, but only a few tests will distinguish between them. Patients whose EIA suggests dual infection should be confirmed with HIV-1 and HIV-2 specific RNA testing or other confirmatory tests. Many commercial molecular tests can detect and quantify most HIV subtypes; certain assays can quantify group O and N viruses [246, 247]. False-negative molecular tests, however, have been reported with URFs [248, 249].

HIV COUNSELING

Post-test counseling is necessary for all patients who test positive [237]. Emotional support should be provided to address issues of stigma and fear of disclosing one's HIV status. Risk reduction information and the value of male and female condoms should be provided

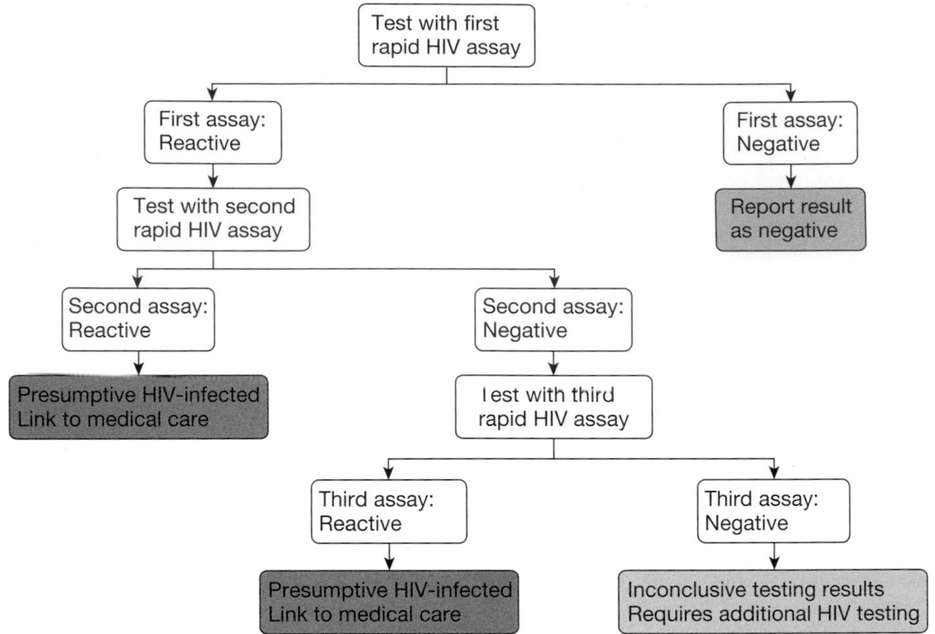

FIGURE 27.18 Example of a rapid HIV testing algorithm. *Reproduced with permission from Bennett BB, Delaney K, Owen M, et al. HIV Testing Algorithms: A Status Report. A publication of the Association of Public Health Laboratories and CDC. 2009, updated March 2010. Available at: http://www.aphl.org/aphlprograms/infectious/hiv/Pages/HIVStatusReport.aspx (accessed 24 June 2011).*

in non-judgmental language. Ideally, these devices should be made available to the client. Counseling should emphasize that HIV infection can be treated. Patients should be encouraged to disclose their status to trusted family members and friends. Any known sexual or needle-sharing contacts should seek HIV testing. Providers should also provide referrals to appropriate follow-up services.

INITIAL EVALUATION OF THE NEWLY DIAGNOSED PATIENT

Guidelines and recommendations for the evaluation of HIV-infected adults and children, and for treating and monitoring patients should be consulted (Table 27-5) [140, 250–254]. All patients diagnosed need a detailed history, examination and assessment of their social and economic circumstances. Patients in resource-limited settings often experience poor nutritional status, inadequate housing and limited access to clean water. Such factors increase the susceptibility to opportunistic infections. The medical history should screen for opportunistic infections and note any past HIV-related illnesses, other medical conditions or hospitalizations. A detailed sexual history should review sexual practices, past STIs, obstetric/gynecologic history (including plans for pregnancy), contraceptive use (including condoms), all sexual partners and recreational drug use (including cigarette and alcohol use). The physical exam should be performed with attention to the skin, lymphatic, oral and fundoscopic examination. Women should undergo pelvic examination with assessment for cervical disease by cytology (e.g. Papanicolaou smear) or acetic acid whitening. Baseline laboratory testing typically includes assessment for anemia and abnormalities in liver and kidney function.

Patients should be staged clinically and immunologically. The WHO staging system classifies patients from Stage 1 (asymptomatic) to Stage 4 (life-threatening opportunistic infections or other HIV-associated conditions) based on clinical and laboratory findings (Table 27-4) [103]. Where available, immunologic staging according to the patient's CD4 cell count provides the most accurate assessment of risk for opportunistic illnesses and death. Measurement of CD4 cell count is also used to guide initiation of ART and opportunistic infection prophylaxis and to monitor the response to treatment [98]. HIV infection among adults and adolescents aged ≥13 years can also be staged according to the 2008 revised CDC surveillance case definitions: Stage 1 (CD4+ T lymphocyte count ≥500 cells/μl), Stage 2 (CD4+ T lymphocyte count = 200–499 cells/μl), or Stage 3 (CD4+ T lymphocyte count of <200 cells/μl or an AIDS-defining condition), or Stage unknown (Table 27-5) [255]. HIV RNA viral load measurement and HIV genotypic resistance testing provide information useful for assessing prognosis and optimizing ART regimens. These tests are not widely available in resource-limited settings. In areas with a high burden of tuberculosis, active disease can be present in up to 20–30% of HIV-infected persons receiving clinical care [250].

INITIAL EVALUATION OF NEWLY DIAGNOSED WOMEN OF REPRODUCTIVE AGE

All newly diagnosed women of reproductive age should be assessed for pregnancy and, if pregnant, referred for ART and counseling to prevent perinatal HIV transmission to their infant [256]. Clinicians should query non-pregnant women regarding their intentions for future pregnancies and provide contraceptive counseling. Use of dual methods (i.e. hormonal contraception combined with male or female condoms) may be appropriate in some settings. HIV-infected women who are contemplating pregnancy should receive pre-conception counseling (e.g. eliminating alcohol and cigarette smoking, folic acid supplementation) and counseling regarding the risk for HIV transmission to their infant. HIV-infected women on ART who are contemplating pregnancy should not take potentially teratogenic drugs (i.e. efavirenz) and should attain a stable, suppressed maternal viral load prior to conception [257].

ANTIRETROVIRAL THERAPY (ART)

INTRODUCTION

Expert guidance on ART is available from the WHO, the United States Department of Health and Human Services, the International AIDS Society-USA, the British HIV Association, and the European AIDS Clinical Society (Table 27-6). Most resource-limited countries develop specific national guidance.

Combination ART became the standard of care in developed nations following its introduction in 1996. However, in resource-limited settings, few had access to these life-saving drugs. Starting in the early 2000s, governments, the private sector, human rights advocates and other stakeholders have reduced the cost of ART and initiated the

TABLE 27.6 Sources of Authoritative Information on HIV/AIDS

Source	Website
World Health Organization	http://www.who.int/hiv/
U.S. Department of Health and Human Services	http://aidsinfo.nih.gov/
European AIDS Clinical Society	http://europeanaidsclinicalsociety.org/
British HIV Association	http://www.bhiva.org/
International AIDS Society - USA	http://www.iasusa.org/
NAM - aidsmap	http://www.aidsmap.com/
HIV InSite	http://www.hivinsite.com/

infrastructure necessary to deliver ART and HIV care. By the end of 2009, more than 5.2 million of the estimated 15 million treatment-eligible people residing in low- and middle-income countries were receiving ART [1].

GOALS OF ART

The goal of ART is to maximally suppress HIV replication and improve the health of the individual. Improving the survival of young and middle-aged adults reduces the number of orphaned children and is associated with improved economic outcomes [258]. At the individual level, ART is associated with a reduction in sexual transmission of HIV from an HIV-infected individual to their HIV-uninfected partner [222]. At the population level, reduction of the viral load of the community of HIV-infected persons leads to decreases in new HIV infections [259, 260].

ART: WHEN TO START

ART should be initiated in persons who have developed an AIDS-related opportunistic infection or illness (WHO Stage 4 or CDC Stage 3 illness), who have symptoms of advanced HIV disease (WHO Stage 3 illness) or who have a CD4 cell count <200 cells/μl (CDC Stage 3 illness) (Tables 27-4 and 27-5). HIV-infected persons with CD4 cell counts <200 cells/μl can be asymptomatic for prolonged periods before developing a WHO clinical indication for treatment, thus, it is important to assess the CD4 cell count. The introduction of simplified formulations (e.g. once or twice daily combination pills), more tolerable and durable medications, and antiretrovirals that target new steps in HIV's lifecycle (e.g. integrase inhibitors, CCR5 inhibitors) have improved treatment options during earlier stages of disease (i.e. at higher CD4 cell counts). Observational cohort studies have also demonstrated that initiation of continuous ART at higher CD4 cell counts improves survival, increases AIDS-free survival, reduces non-AIDS associated outcomes (e.g. end-organ disease) [261–263] and may help control inflammatory responses related to chronic HIV infection [262–264]. A randomized trial in Haiti confirmed that initiation of ART and CD4 cell counts ≤350 cells/μL was associated with lower mortality and lower rates of tuberculosis than initiation at a CD4 cell count of 200 cells/μl [265]. Definitive randomized controlled trials of starting ART at even higher CD4 cell counts are underway [details can be found at: www.clinicaltrials.gov (Identifier: NCT00867048) or at http://insight.ccbr.umn.edu/start/].

As of 2011, the WHO recommends treating all patients with CD4 counts of ≤350 cells/μl, irrespective of their WHO clinical stage of disease [141]. Multiple guidelines from developed countries have moved the CD4 cell count threshold for ART initiation to 350–500 cells/μl and some recommend ART at any CD4 cell count as soon as HIV infection is diagnosed considering the harmful impact of ongoing HIV replication [98, 139, 140, 266]. The initiation of ART at CD4 cell count >350 cells/μL in resource-limited settings will be problematic until there is the availability of more options for second-line regimens when resistance to first-line ART develops.

ART: Initiating Therapy for Women of Reproductive Age

Most HIV-infected women and men remain sexually active, and many continue to have children or to not use any form of contraception [267–269]. Women of reproductive age presenting for care must be assessed for pregnancy before starting therapy and referred for contraceptive counseling if not pregnant (see "*Initial evaluation of newly diagnosed women of reproductive age*" above). ART should be offered to pregnant women with HIV infection who need it for their own health and started as early as possible in pregnancy for PMTCT.

ART: WHAT TO START

More than 20 antiretroviral drugs are commercially available. Antiretrovirals are characterized within five drug classes according to their mechanism of action (Table 27-7). The oldest, and most widely used, drugs against HIV are nucleoside/nucleotide analogues that inhibit HIV reverse transcriptase (NRTIs). Non-nucleoside reverse-transcriptase inhibitors (NNRTIs) target reverse-transcriptase but are structurally dissimilar to endogenous nucleosides, and to each other. Protease inhibitors inhibit the HIV protease and interrupt assembly of the mature virion. Protease inhibitors are typically co-administered with a low dose (e.g. 100 mg) of the protease inhibitor ritonavir that "boosts" the serum concentration of the other protease inhibitors by inhibiting their hepatic metabolism. Integrase inhibitors target HIV's integrase enzyme and block integration of HIV DNA into the host genome. Entry inhibitors block entry of HIV into the cell and include fusion inhibitors and agents that block the CCR5 co-receptor. As of 2011, this class is not available in most resource-limited settings.

Since 2002, the WHO has recommended use of standardized treatment regimens in resource-limited settings with reduced frequency of monitoring compared with high-income countries [141, 270]. Table 27-8 lists combinations of first-line antiretrovirals recommended by the WHO [141]. Standardization of treatment simplifies training of clinicians, medication dispensers (e.g. pharmacists, pharmacy technicians, and technologists), counselors, and community workers. There are also standards for treatment during pregnancy and co-infection with tuberculosis (for special considerations in patients with tuberculosis see Chapter 39, "*Tuberculosis*") or hepatitis B.

ART: What to Start—Special Considerations for Women Previously Given Antiretroviral Drugs as Prevention of Mother-to-Child Transmission (PMTCT) of HIV

Women who require PMTCT should be given highly active triple combination ART; this strategy reduces the risk of perinatal HIV transmission and minimizes development of resistance. In resource-limited settings, many programs have used only one or two drugs. Antiretroviral resistance can emerge under these circumstances [271], particularly resistance to lamivudine [272] and nevirapine [273, 274]. The resistance mutation to lamivudine confers increased susceptibility of HIV to other NRTIs. Thus, if this is the sole mutation present, then lamivudine can be used in combination with other NRTIs to treat mothers and their HIV-infected infants. Women who can wait at least one year after having received nevirapine prophylaxis for PMTCT respond as well to NNRTI-containing highly active antiretroviral therapy (HAART), as women who had not been exposed to nevirapine [275–282]. However, if less than a year has passed, a protease inhibitor-based regimen is preferred [283]. Antiretroviral resistance testing should be conducted for all women and HIV-infected infants

TABLE 27.7 Antiretroviral Drugs

Year Approved by US FDA	Generic Name	Trade Name(s)	Common Acronym
1. Nucleoside/Nucleotide Reverse Transcriptase Inhibitors			
1987	Zidovudine	Retrovir	AZT, ZDV
1991	Didanosine	Videx	ddl
1994	Stavudine	Zerit	d4T
1995	Lamivudine	Epivir	3TC
1998	Abacavir	Ziagen	ABC
2001	Tenofovir	Viread	TDF
2003	Emtricitabine	Emtriva	FTC
2. Non-nucleoside Reverse Transcriptase Inhibitors			
1996	Nevirapine	Viramune	NVP
1997	Delavirdine	Rescriptor	DLV
1998	Efavirenz	Sustiva, Stocrin	EFV
2008	Etravirine	Intelence	ETR
2011	Rilpivirine	Edurant	RPV
3. Protease Inhibitors			
1995	Saquinavir	Invirase	SQV
1996	Ritonavir	Norvir	RTV
1996	Indinavir	Crixivan	IDV
1997	Nelfinavir	Viracept	NFV
2000	Lopinavir/ ritonavir	Kaletra, Aluvia	LPV
2003	Atazanavir	Reyataz	ATV
2003	Fosamprenavir	Lexiva	FPV
2005	Tipranavir	Aptivus	TPV
2006	Darunavir	Prezista	DRV
4. Integrase Inhibitors			
2007	Raltegravir	Isentress	RGV
2012	Elvitegravir		EVG
5. Entry and Fusion Inhibitors			
2003	Enfuvirtide	Fuzeon	T-20
2007	Maraviroc	Selzentry, Celsentri	MVC

US FDA = United States, Food and Drug Administration
Sources: 1) Panel on Antiretroviral Guidelines for Adults and Adolescents. Guidelines for the use of antiretroviral agents in HIV-1-infected adults and adolescents. Department of Health and Human Services. January 10, 2011;1–166. Available at http://www.aidsinfo.nih.gov/ContentFiles/AudltandAdolescentGL.pdf Last accessed May 12, 2011. 2) Fact Sheet 402. Drup names and manufacturers. Revised November 3, 2010. Available at http://www.aidsinfonet.org. Last accessed November 3, 2010.

TABLE 27.8 Combinations of Antiretroviral Drugs Recommended by WHO as First-Line Therapy for Adults and Adolescents in 2010

Recommended Combinations
Zidovudine, lamivudine, efavirenz
Zidoudine, lamivudine, nevirapine
Tenofovir, lamivudine (or emtricitabine), efavirenz
Tenofovir, lamivudine (or emtricitabine), nevirapine

Source: WHO. Antiretroviral therapy for HIV infection in adults and adolescents: recommendations for a public health approach. – 2010 rev. http://www.who.int

exposed to PMTCT prior to initiation of their own ART. Such testing remains unavailable in many areas, in which case clinicians must consider the content and timing of prior ART and the likelihood of resistance.

ART: What to Start—Special Considerations for Pregnant Women

The NNRTIs nevirapine and efavirenz are both effective antiretroviral agents for pregnant women. Efavirenz has been associated with potential teratogenicity [284]; some guidelines recommend against its use during the first trimester of pregnancy [257.], though others consider the risk of teratogenicity to be small enough to allow for its use [266]. Rash and life-threatening hepatotoxicity have been associated with nevirapine in women with CD4 cell counts >250 cells/μl [285, 286]. However, clinical experience has been reassuring regarding the safety of nevirapine in women in resource-limited settings who have CD4 cell counts >250 cells/μl [287]. Nonetheless, pregnant women starting nevirapine should be counseled about the risk of rash and hepatotoxicity, and advised to seek immediate evaluation if problems occur.

ART: What to Start—Special Considerations in Patients with Chronic Hepatitis B Virus (HBV) Infection

Patients with HBV and HIV co-infection are at increased risk for chronic HBV and its complications [288]; earlier initiation of ART is associated with a reduction in liver disease (see *"Select Major Opportunistic Infections—Viral Hepatitis"* above). Several antiretroviral agents, including lamivudine, emtricitabine, and tenofovir, are active against both HIV and HBV. Selecting ART that contains two of these agents, such as tenofovir with emtricitabine or lamivudine, is recommended [98, 139–141]. Inclusion of a single agent with dual HIV and HBV activity is not recommended as it may not suppress HBV replication and can increase the risk of HBV drug resistance.

ART: ADHERENCE TO THERAPY

Adherence, including retention in care, is a cornerstone of effective ART [289–291]. Aspects of ART that make adherence difficult are: pill burden; complexity of regimens; side effects; patient knowledge and attitudes; distance from the clinic; transportation costs; user-friendliness of the services; competing priorities (e.g. employment, child care); mental illness (e.g. depression, addiction); and social instability. Systems issues, such as inadequate supplies and stockouts, can also lead to nonadherence. Suboptimal adherence is associated with treatment failure (e.g. viral breakthroughs, lower CD4 cell counts, increased mortality) and can lead to viral resistance.

All patients should receive adherence counseling at initiation of treatment. The WHO recommends client-centered counseling, pillboxes, and treatment supporters [141, 250]. As part of this counseling, the provider should assess readiness to commit to lifelong treatment, identify barriers to adherence and options to overcome them, and provide resources for assistance [292, 293].

Training healthcare personnel and community workers as treatment supporters can be facilitated if there is a set of essential messages. For advanced disease, improved health with ART (e.g. weight gain, increased strength, improved social functioning) can provide positive reinforcement. For those with less symptomatic disease, side effects are a challenge, especially if the patient experiences minimal improvements in their perceived wellbeing. Adherence can be improved if the health workers, and patient, understand what to expect after initiating ART and how to differentiate minor side effects from more severe events that require clinical evaluation.

Initiatives to maximize retention in care should identify persons who have lapsed (e.g. missed clinic visits, missed pharmacy refills) and reach out to those patients in the community [294]. Successful interventions have ranged from community workers making home visits to the use of cell phones and text messaging that enable staff at a central clinic to contact patients and community workers. Refilling antiretroviral medications more regularly (a proxy for adherence to medications and retention in care) has been associated with improved virologic response and survival [295–297]. It is important to retain persons who do not yet qualify for ART, but who need regular visits for CD4 count testing and other benefits such as cotrimoxazole prophylaxis [298].

ART: MONITORING THE EFFECTIVENESS OF ART

The WHO recommends a minimum standard for monitoring clinical response to ART [141, 299]. Immunologic (i.e. CD4 cell count) and virologic (i.e. HIV RNA viral load) monitoring are not emphasized, recognizing that access to laboratory capacity can be limited. Where laboratory testing is available, guidelines recommend measuring the CD4 cell count at initiation of ART and at least twice a year thereafter. Monitoring CD4 cell counts provides prognostic information and informs the use of opportunistic illness prophylaxis. Although adding CD4 cell counts to clinical monitoring improves outcomes [300, 301], discordant responses (e.g. viral load suppression without an accompanying increase in the CD4 cell count) can occur in 20% or more of patients [302].

Monitoring plasma HIV RNA viral load is controversial. Most authorities recommend HIV RNA viral load testing, although in resource-limited settings, adding this to routine patient monitoring does not improve outcomes [300, 303]. HIV RNA viral load provides the most direct measure of antiretroviral effectiveness and can indirectly assess adherence. Confirming virologic failure rather than poor adherence generally requires a repeat test. In developed countries, genotypic or phenotypic antiretroviral resistance testing is recommended prior to starting treatment and as needed during treatment to optimize ART in patients who are virologically failing [98, 304]. The WHO's standardized approach to second-line ART for resource-limited settings limits the need for HIV-resistance testing by making treatment recommendations based on the assumption that prior treatment could have induced resistance.

ART: MONITORING FOR TOLERABILITY

Antiretroviral drugs have early and late-onset side effects that can affect tolerance. Some side effects, such as headache and nausea, are common at treatment initiation but are usually transient and manageable. Table 27-9 lists some of the most common severe antiretroviral side effects.

TABLE 27.9 Severe and Life-Threatening Complications of Antiretroviral Drugs

Reaction	Drugs indicated	Onset	Common Manifestations
Early toxicities			
Severe rash (including Stevens-Johnson Syndrome)	Nevirapine (most common), efavirenz, etravirine Also reported with many protease inhibitors	First few days to weeks	Skin eruptions with mucosal alterations that may evolve to epidermal detachment or necrosis. May be accompanied by systemic symptoms (fever, malaise, myalgias, arthralgias)
Hypersensitivity reaction	Abacavir	Within first 1–6 weeks	Usually presents with multiple symptoms that may include: Fever, skin rash, malaise, nausea, headache, myalgias, chills, diarrhea, vomiting. Abdominal pain, dyspnea, arthralgias
Hepatotoxicity	Non-nucleoside reverse transcriptase inhibitors Protease inhibitors	Within first few weeks to months	May be asymptomatic or associated with non-specific symptoms such as anorexia, fatigue, weight loss, abdominal pain Elevated serum transaminases
Hypersensitivity with hepatic failure	Nevirapine	Within first 6–18 weeks	Abrupt onset of flu-like symptoms, abdominal pain, jaundice, or fever with or without skin rash. May present with drug rash with eosinophilia and systemic symptoms (DRESS) May progress to fulminant hepatic failure
Late toxicities			
Pancreatitis	Stavudine, didanosine, Tenofovir + didanosine may have increased risk	Usually weeks to months after starting	Abdominal pain, nausea, vomiting, diarrhea Increased serum amylase and lipase
Lactic acidosis/ hepatosteatosis (potentially with pancreatitis) (severe mitochondrial toxicities)	Stavudine, didanosine, zidovudine, other nucleoside reverse transcriptase inhibitors	After months or years	Nonspecific gastrointestinal symptoms that may rapidly progress with tachycardia, respiratory distress, jaundice, muscle weakness. Mortality up to 50% in severe cases Increase lactate, low arterial pH, low serum bicarbonate, increased anion gap, elevated serum transaminases

Source: Panel on Antiretroviral Guidelines for Adults and Adolescents. Guidelines for the use of antiretroviral agents in HIV-1 infected adults and adolescents. Department of Health and Human Services. January 10, 2011;1–166. Available at **http://www.aidsinfo.nih.gov/ContentFiles/AdultandAdolescentGL.pdf**

Directed assessments for adverse events (e.g. questionnaires that review specific signs and symptoms, monofilament testing for peripheral neuropathy) can help ensure that early side effects are identified when it is possible to change therapy to prevent their progression. As ART continues, the frequency of assessment can be decreased. It is not currently possible to identify which patients will develop side effects; however, the risk for ART-related events may be greater in patients with more advanced disease [305–307].

If available, routine laboratory monitoring is an important adjunct to care and can be used to monitor for ART-associated toxicities (e.g. liver enzymes to assess for nevirapine-associated hepatotoxicity, hemoglobin to assess for zidovudine-associated anemia). Laboratory monitoring, however, is not a prerequisite for the initiation of ART [141]. In high-income settings, guidelines typically recommend quarterly or semi-annual testing of complete blood counts, serum chemistries and urinalyses, as well as CD4 cell count and plasma HIV RNA viral load [98]. If resources are limited, laboratory testing should be directed by clinical signs and symptoms (see Table 27-9) [141]. The WHO also recommends testing that is tailored to the ART (e.g. creatinine clearance for tenofovir) [141].

Most patients with advanced HIV disease starting ART experience a return to health with improvements in functional status and laboratory parameters. However, high early mortality during the first 3–6 months of treatment has been observed among persons with advanced disease in resource-limited settings [308, 309]. Contributors to early mortality include undiagnosed or untreated opportunistic infection, IRIS, and severe malnutrition [310].

ART: METABOLIC COMPLICATIONS DURING TREATMENT

ART has been associated with the development of metabolic complications: abnormal changes in body fat distribution (lipoatrophy and lipoaccumulation), serum dyslipidemias, insulin resistance and glucose intolerance, and osteopenia [311]. Many metabolic complications increase the risk for chronic medical conditions (e.g. myocardial infarction, stroke, hepatic and renal failure, fragility bone fracture), and some, particularly lipodystrophy, can impair the quality of life. In industrialized nations, the care of HIV-infected persons is increasingly dominated by management of these complications.

ART: WHEN TO CHANGE ART

The goal of ART is to maintain maximal suppression of HIV replication for as long as possible and to change therapy when virologic failure occurs. Adherence should always be assessed. HIV RNA viral loads should be obtained at least every 6 months [98, 141]. However, where laboratory resources are limited, clinicians can limit HIV RNA viral load testing to confirm virologic failure when there is a declining CD4 cell count or clinical change in a person's health.

Clinicians should strive to maintain HIV RNA viral load below the limit of detection for the assay (usually <50 copies/ml) [98]. In resource-limited settings, a more lenient approach to virologic suppression has been advocated [141], with virologic failure defined as a plasma HIV RNA concentration >5000 copies/ml after at least 6 months of treatment. This allows programs with limited formularies to treat more patients and limit switching to costly second- or third-line regimens. Low-level viral replication in the presence of ART, however, increases the risk of developing ART resistance [312–314].

The occurrence of an AIDS-defining illness or a decline in CD4 count below a threshold (e.g. fall to baseline value or lower, 50% fall from on-treatment peak value, CD4 cell count persistently below 100 cells/μl) in a patient who had demonstrated clinical improvement after initiating ART suggests a need to change treatment. Some patients who initiate ART demonstrate no clinical improvement after a sufficient course of ART (e.g. 6 months). In this situation, the patient may have been infected with a strain with primary resistance.

ART: HOW TO CHANGE (SWITCH) ART

If genotypic or phenotypic antiretroviral resistance testing is available, clinicians should optimize regimens according to those results [312]. Resistance testing should be obtained while the patient is taking the failing antiretroviral regimen or shortly after treatment discontinuation. If the first-line regimen consisted of two NRTIs combined with an NNRTI, a reasonable second-line regimen would consist of a ritonavir-boosted protease inhibitor combined with two new NRTIs. Importantly, for HIV-infected patients who have chronic active hepatitis B infection, the second-line and subsequent regimens should maintain two antiretrovirals with activity against hepatitis B.

ART FOR CHILDREN

For perinatally infected children, ART should be started within the first few months of life as, without treatment, opportunistic illnesses and death can occur very early. ART may need to be initiated in infants with a presumptive diagnosis of severe HIV disease (criteria are published by the WHO at: http://www.who.int/hiv/pub/guidelines/art/en/), as access to infant diagnosis (i.e. HIV proviral DNA testing) may not be available (see "*HIV Diagnosis*" above) [239, 315]. These infants must be closely monitored and must have their HIV diagnosis confirmed as soon as possible (at the latest, with HIV antibody testing at 18 months of age) [316]. In all settings, pediatric ART has been complicated by the lack of approved drugs in child-friendly formulations (e.g. liquid products). As children grow, dosages must be adjusted. Some manufacturers have produced child-friendly tablets at pediatric dosages in fixed-dose combination tablets that are scored for easy splitting and are dispersible in water [317–320].

Perinatally infected children can be at greater risk of infection with strains of HIV that have primary resistance to antiretrovirals that the mother has taken for PMTCT. Treating all HIV-infected mothers with triple antiretroviral prophylaxis for PMTCT creates a barrier to transmitting drug-resistant infection [256]. Drug resistance can also emerge in HIV-infected children administered extended-prophylaxis with nevirapine (with or without concomitant zidovudine) during breastfeeding [321, 322] or if exposed to antiretroviral drugs through breastfeeding when their mothers are taking ART [323]. Lamivudine, nevirapine, efavirenz, but not zidovudine, are transmitted in biologically significant concentrations via breast milk [257].

PREVENTION

SPECIAL CONSIDERATIONS FOR ANTIMICROBIAL PROPHYLAXIS IN RESOURCE-LIMITED SETTINGS

[Note isoniazid prophylaxis is discussed in Chapter 39, "*Tuberculosis*".]

Trimethoprim-Sulfamethoxazole/ Cotrimoxazole

In resource-limited settings, daily prophylaxis with trimethoprim-sulfamethoxazole (cotrimoxazole) in adults and children reduces the incidence of pneumonia, diarrhea, malaria, and bacterial bloodstream infections [324–327], and reduces mortality in areas with high prevalences of malaria [326] and in persons with both HIV and active tuberculosis [325]. Cotrimoxazole prophylaxis is also beneficial for persons initiating ART [328–330]. The intervention has additional benefits in pregnant women and reduces the rate of low birth weight in newborns [331].

The WHO strongly recommends cotrimoxazole prophylaxis for HIV-infected persons, including children and pregnant women [332]. Countries may tailor its provision according to stage of disease (e.g. all HIV-infected persons vs. only persons with advanced disease). Cotrimoxazole prophylaxis increases pill burden and costs modestly, but is well-tolerated and is cost-effective [333–335]. It creates selection pressure leading to cotrimoxazole-resistant infections among a small number of individuals [336]; however, its use has been associated with decreases in overall rates of sulfa-resistant malaria [337]. Cotrimoxazole prophylaxis against *Pneumocystis* pneumonia can be safely discontinued in individuals who maintain CD4 cell counts >200 cells/μl for >3 months [115]. It is less clear whether cotrimoxazole in resource-limited settings should be discontinued; a marked increase in the risk of malaria and diarrheal disease following its discontinuation has been demonstrated [338].

Fluconazole and Itraconazole

Randomized clinical trials conducted in the USA, Uganda, and Thailand demonstrated that primary prophylaxis with fluconazole or itraconazole reduces the incidence of cryptococcal disease in adults with advanced HIV disease, particularly those with CD4 counts <50–100 cells/μl [129, 339–343], and, in one trial, improved survival [340]. Primary prophylaxis is not recommended in high-income countries with a low prevalence of cryptococcosis [115] but may be beneficial in countries with a high prevalence of azole-susceptible fungal opportunistic illness (e.g. cryptococcosis, penicilliosis) [250]. Fluconazole can also reduce the risk of recurrent candidal infections but the benefits are felt to be outweighed by cost and concerns about induction of fluconazole resistance [250]. Because of possible teratogenicity, women prescribed azoles should take effective birth control [344].

Non-Tuberculosis Anti-Mycobacterials [*Mycobacterium Avium* Complex (MAC)]

Prophylaxis against *Mycobacterium avium* complex (MAC) is recommended in developed countries for HIV-infected adults with CD4 cell counts <50 cell/μl [115]. The organism is ubiquitous in the environment worldwide [345–347]. However, MAC infections have not emerged as a substantial cause of disease in HIV-infected persons outside of North and South America and Europe. Primary prophylaxis against MAC is not addressed in WHO guidelines [141].

NON-PHARMACOLOGIC INTERVENTIONS

Insecticide-treated bed nets or indoor residual spraying for mosquitoes can prevent malaria, especially the associated risk for placental infection and its complications. Interventions to improve point-of-use water safety and hand hygiene (e.g. latrines, soap-and-water handwashing) can decrease the risk of diarrheal disease at both the family, clinic and community levels. Reducing the burden of tuberculosis in persons with HIV should also include infection control measures, such as early triage and separation of persons with suspected tuberculosis and efforts to optimize ventilation [348].

CHRONIC PRIMARY CARE CONSIDERATIONS

Smoking Cessation

Adult male prevalence estimates for daily cigarette smoking in 2006 ranged from 4–27% for countries in Africa, 18–57% for countries in Asia, and 2–39% for countries in the Americas [348]. In many countries, rates of tobacco smoking in HIV-infected adults are substantially higher than rates in the general population [196, 349–351]. HIV-infected adults are at increased risk of many diseases for which the burden is greater in tobacco smokers: cardiovascular disease (e.g. myocardial infarction), pulmonary disease (e.g. bacterial pneumonia, chronic obstructive pulmonary disease (COPD), tuberculosis [352]), and cancer (e.g. lung cancer) [348]. Smoking cessation is among the most cost-effective interventions for reducing long-term morbidity and mortality for HIV-infected persons [353].

Mental Health

Mental health conditions, such as depression and substance abuse, are common among people with HIV, reduce quality of life and present challenges to adherence and retention in care [354]. All patients should be screened for mood and thought disorders, and drug and alcohol dependency. Where feasible, supportive counseling, medication, and referral to specialists or specialized treatment programs should be provided [355].

Vaccinations

Vaccination guidelines for international travel and primary prophylaxis are available [342, 356–358]. Safety is a concern with some live virus vaccines and their use should be avoided when possible, especially in persons with CD4 cell counts <200 cells/μl. Generally, vaccinations are more immunogenic in persons with higher CD4 cell counts. For persons in whom immune reconstitution is anticipated and vaccine resources are limited, vaccination can be deferred until the CD4 cell count has improved (e.g. ≥200 cells/μl). Persons with low CD4 cell counts can be vaccinated at entry to care, and then reassessed once their CD4 cell count has improved and be revaccinated if warranted.

Nutrition

Food insecurity, inadequate energy intake, malnutrition, and specific micronutrient deficiencies are endemic in many areas with high HIV prevalence [359–362]. The diet and nutritional status of people living with HIV should be routinely assessed. In developed nations where patients have had long-standing access to ART, "return to health" has been associated with increased rates of obesity [363]. For patients whose expected lifespan has increased significantly, dietary counseling and exercise promotion are indicated.

PRIMARY HIV PREVENTION

Comprehensive, sustained prevention programs can reduce HIV transmission [364]; however, interventions do not reach most people at risk. Successful behavioral interventions engage high-risk populations and offer educational messages coupled with prevention skills, such as how to negotiate condom use and how to refuse sex.

HIV testing is an important component of primary HIV prevention as half of all persons living with HIV worldwide are unaware of their status [365]. Offering opt-out HIV testing in most clinical settings (e.g. antenatal clinics, pediatric and adult general medicine clinics, inpatients settings) has been widely recommended. Couples testing and counseling is acceptable in high-risk populations where transmission is predominately heterosexual [216]. Couples testing can be linked to ART of an HIV-infected partner, which can reduce transmission to the HIV-negative partner by as much as 96% through suppression of viral load [221, 222, 366].

A safe and effective HIV vaccine would be a major advance and is the subject of intense research efforts [367]. Male circumcision reduces a man's risk of acquiring HIV heterosexually by 50–60% [43–45]. In high prevalence areas where a large fraction of the regional population is uncircumcised, large-scale implementation of male circumcision has the potential to prevent many new infections.

Interventions that women can control, such as vaginal microbicides containing antiretrovirals, have shown early promise (39% reduction in HIV incidence) [368], and are the subject of intense investigation. Daily oral administration of antiretroviral drugs to high-risk, HIV-negative individuals, termed "pre-exposure prophylaxis", has been demonstrated in one trial to prevent HIV infection among MSM (44% reduction in HIV incidence) [369]. Trials among heterosexual men and women have also demonstrated an HIV prevention benefit from pre-exposure prophylaxis in Botswana (62% reduction in HIV incidence) and in Kenya and Uganda (67–75% reduction in HIV incidence) [370, 371]. Higher levels of protection were observed with more consistent use of pre-exposure prophylaxis in these trials. However, another trial conducted in Kenya, South Africa, and Tanzania among high-risk, HIV-negative women failed to demonstrate benefit; it is likely that low overall adherence contributed to the lack of efficacy, though other contributing factors may have made pre-exposure prophylaxis less effective [372].

PREVENTION WITH POSITIVES

Interventions that help patients maintain their health and reduce their risk of transmitting, often termed "prevention with positives", play a critical role in HIV prevention [216]. Maintaining a suppressed plasma HIV viral load reduces their infectiousness to others. Use of male and female condoms and clean needles for IDUs prevents exposure of uninfected persons to HIV and reduces the likelihood that an HIV-infected person could become infected with a resistant strain of HIV (termed "superinfection"). Encouraging patients to reduce their number of sexual partners, to disclose their HIV status, to encourage their partners to be tested and to use lubrication during intercourse can further reduce HIV transmission risk. Screening and treating for STIs may reduce their infectiousness to others [137].

PALLIATIVE CARE

Although there has been a 14% decline in the number of HIV-related deaths worldwide from 2004 to 2009, an estimated 1.8 million HIV-related deaths still occurred in 2009 [1]. Palliative care focuses on improving the quality of life of patients with life-threatening illnesses and helping patients live as actively as possible until death [373]. Palliative care can be offered throughout the course of HIV infection, not only at end-of-life situations. It can be provided in a healthcare setting or at home by family and community caregivers. Important goals are: (i) to provide relief from pain and other distressing symptoms (i.e. diarrhea, nausea, shortness of breath) which can be common with advanced HIV disease and opportunistic infections; and (ii) to provide support for the psychological, social, spiritual and cultural needs of the patient and family, including bereavement care. For pain relief, an analgesic ladder with three standard drugs is usually recommended and includes a non-opioid (e.g. aspirin or paracetamol), a weak opioid (e.g. codeine, dextropropoxyphene or methadone), and a strong opioid (e.g. morphine). Detailed guidelines on palliative care have been developed by the WHO [374].

REFERENCES

1. Joint United Nations Programmed on HIV/AIDS (UNAIDS). Global report: UNAIDS report on the global AIDS epidemic 2010. Available at: http://www.unaids.org/globalreport/Global_report.htm (accessed 5 May 2011).
2. Pneumocystis pneumonia—Los Angeles. MMWR Morb Mortal Wkly Rep 1981;30:250–2.
3. Korber B, Muldoon M, Theiler J, et al. Timing the ancestor of the HIV-1 pandemic strains. Science 2000;288:1789–96.
4. Joint United Nations Programmed on HIV/AIDS (UNAIDS). 2006 Report on the global AIDS epidemic. Available at: http://www.unaids.org/en/media/unaids/contentassets/dataimport/pub/globalreport/2006/2006_gr-executive summary_en.pdf (accessed 5 May 2011).
5. Joint United Nations Programmed on HIV/AIDS (UNAIDS). Report on the global HIV/AIDS epidemic 2008. Available at: http://www.unaids.org/en/dataanalysis/epidemiology/2008reportontheglobalaidsepidemic/ (accessed 5 May 2011).
6. World Health Organization. The global burden of disease: 2004 update. Available at: http://www.who.int/healthinfo/global_burden_disease/2004_report_update/en/index.html (accessed 5 May 2011).
7. Moore E. HIV is changing the face of tropical medicine. BMJ 2006;332:1280.
8. Colvin M, Dawood S, Kleinschmidt I, et al. Prevalence of HIV and HIV-related diseases in the adult medical wards of a tertiary hospital in Durban, South Africa. Int J STD AIDS 2001;12:386–9.
9. Nyirenda M, Beadsworth MB, Stephany P, et al. Prevalence of infection with hepatitis B and C virus and coinfection with HIV in medical inpatients in Malawi. J Infect 2008;57:72–7.
10. Wanyenze RK, Nawavvu C, Namale AS, et al. Acceptability of routine HIV counselling and testing, and HIV seroprevalence in Ugandan hospitals. Bull World Health Organ 2008;86:302–9.
11. French N, Gray K, Watera C, et al. Cryptococcal infection in a cohort of HIV-1-infected Ugandan adults. AIDS 2002;16:1031–8.
12. Samb B, Evans T, Dybul M, et al. An assessment of interactions between global health initiatives and country health systems. Lancet 2009;373:2137–69.
13. Biesma RG, Brugha R, Harmer A, et al. The effects of global health initiatives on country health systems: a review of the evidence from HIV/AIDS control. Health Policy Plan 2009;24:239–52.
14. Harries AD, Jensen PM, Zachariah R, et al. How health systems in sub-Saharan Africa can benefit from tuberculosis and other infectious disease programmes. Int J Tuberc Lung Dis 2009;13:1194–9.
15. Rabkin M, El-Sadr WM, De Cock KM. The impact of HIV scale-up on health systems: A priority research agenda. J Acquir Immune Defic Syndr 2009;52(suppl. 1):S6–11.
16. Robertson DL, Anderson JP, Bradac JA, et al. HIV-1 nomenclature proposal. Science 2000;288:55–6.
17. Plantier JC, Leoz M, Dickerson JE, et al. A new human immunodeficiency virus derived from gorillas. Nat Med 2009;15:871–2.
18. Gao F, Bailes E, Robertson DL, et al. Origin of HIV-1 in the chimpanzee Pan troglodytes troglodytes. Nature 1999;397:436–41.
19. Hahn BH, Shaw GM, De Cock KM, Sharp PM. AIDS as a zoonosis: scientific and public health implications. Science 2000;287:607–14.
20. Corbet S, Muller-Trutwin MC, Versmisse P, et al. env sequences of simian immunodeficiency viruses from chimpanzees in Cameroon are strongly related to those of human immunodeficiency virus group N from the same geographic area. J Virol 2000;74:529–34.
21. Hemelaar J, Gouws E, Ghys PD, Osmanov S. Global trends in molecular epidemiology of HIV-1 during 2000–2007. AIDS 2011;25:679–89.
22. Vessiere A, Rousset D, Kfutwah A, et al. Diagnosis and monitoring of HIV-1 group O-infected patients in Cameroun. J Acquir Immune Defic Syndr 2010;53:107–10.
23. Vallari A, Bodelle P, Ngansop C, et al. Four new HIV-1 group N isolates from Cameroon: Prevalence continues to be low. AIDS Res Hum Retroviruses 2010;26:109–15.
24. de Silva TI, Cotten M, Rowland-Jones SL. HIV-2: the forgotten AIDS virus. Trends Microbiol 2008;16:588–95.
25. Campbell-Yesufu OT, Gandhi RT. Update on Human Immunodeficiency Virus (HIV)-2 Infection. Clin Infect Dis 2011;52:780–7.
26. Hirsch VM, Olmsted RA, Murphey-Corb M, et al. An African primate lentivirus (SIVsm) closely related to HIV-2. Nature 1989;339:389–92.
27. Tienen C, van der Loeff MS, Zaman SM, et al. Two distinct epidemics: the rise of HIV-1 and decline of HIV-2 infection between 1990 and 2007 in rural Guinea-Bissau. J Acquir Immune Defic Syndr 2010;53:640–7.
28. da Silva ZJ, Oliveira I, Andersen A, et al. Changes in prevalence and incidence of HIV-1, HIV-2 and dual infections in urban areas of Bissau, Guinea-Bissau: is HIV-2 disappearing? AIDS 2008;22:1195–202.
29. Curlin ME, Gottlieb GS, Hawes SE, et al. No evidence for recombination between HIV type 1 and HIV type 2 within the envelope region in dually seropositive individuals from Senegal. AIDS Res Hum Retroviruses 2004;20:958–63.
30. Los Alamos National Laboratory. The circulating recombinant forms(CRFs), HIV sequence database. Available at: http://www.hiv.lanl.gov/content/sequence/HIV/CRFs/CRFs.html (accessed 5 May 2011).
31. Kalish ML, Robbins KE, Pieniazek D, et al. Recombinant viruses and early global HIV-1 epidemic. Emerg Infect Dis 2004;10:1227–34.
32. Walker PR, Pybus OG, Rambaut A, Holmes EC. Comparative population dynamics of HIV-1 subtypes B and C: subtype-specific differences in patterns of epidemic growth. Infect Genet Evol 2005;5:199–208.
33. Renjifo B, Gilbert P, Chaplin B, et al. Preferential in-utero transmission of HIV-1 subtype C as compared to HIV-1 subtype A or D. AIDS 2004;18:1629–36.
34. Njai HF, Gali Y, Vanham G, et al. The predominance of Human Immunodeficiency Virus type 1 (HIV-1) circulating recombinant form 02 (CRF02_AG) in West Central Africa may be related to its replicative fitness. Retrovirology 2006;3:40.
35. Brennan CA, Bodelle P, Coffey R, et al. The prevalence of diverse HIV-1 strains was stable in Cameroonian blood donors from 1996 to 2004. J Acquir Immune Defic Syndr 2008;49:432–9.
36. Delgado E, Ampofo WK, Sierra M, et al. High prevalence of unique recombinant forms of HIV-1 in Ghana: molecular epidemiology from an antiretroviral resistance study. J Acquir Immune Defic Syndr 2008;48:599–606.
37. Brennan CA, Brites C, Bodelle P, et al. HIV-1 strains identified in Brazilian blood donors: significant prevalence of B/F1 recombinants. AIDS Res Hum Retroviruses 2007;23:1434–41.
38. Smith DK, Grohskopf LA, Black RJ, et al. Antiretroviral postexposure prophylaxis after sexual, injection-drug use, or other nonoccupational exposure to HIV in the United States: recommendations from the U.S. Department of Health and Human Services. MMWR Recomm Rep 2005;54:1–20.
39. Kourtis AP, Lee FK, Abrams EJ, et al. Mother-to-child transmission of HIV-1: timing and implications for prevention. Lancet Infect Dis 2006;6:726–32.
40. Royce RA, Sena A, Cates W Jr, Cohen MS. Sexual transmission of HIV. N Engl J Med 1997;336:1072–8.
41. Cohen MS, Pilcher CD. Amplified HIV transmission and new approaches to HIV prevention. J Infect Dis 2005;191:1391–3.

42. Halperin DT, Epstein H. Concurrent sexual partnerships help to explain Africa's high HIV prevalence: implications for prevention. Lancet 2004;364: 4–6.
43. Auvert B, Taljaard D, Lagarde E, et al. Randomized, controlled intervention trial of male circumcision for reduction of HIV infection risk: the ANRS 1265 Trial. PLoS Med 2005;2:e298.
44. Gray RH, Kigozi G, Serwadda D, et al. Male circumcision for HIV prevention in men in Rakai, Uganda: a randomised trial. Lancet 2007;369: 657–66.
45. Bailey RC, Moses S, Parker CB, et al. Male circumcision for HIV prevention in young men in Kisumu, Kenya: a randomised controlled trial. Lancet 2007;369:643–56.
46. Simon V, Ho DD, Abdool Karim Q. HIV/AIDS epidemiology, pathogenesis, prevention, and treatment. Lancet 2006;368:489–504.
47. HIV infection among injection-drug users—34 states, 2004–2007. MMWR Morb Mortal Wkly Rep 2009;58:1291–5.
48. Yerly S, Quadri R, Negro F, et al. Nosocomial outbreak of multiple bloodborne viral infections. J Infect Dis 2001;184:369–72.
49. Hersh BS, Popovici F, Apetrei RC, et al. Acquired immunodeficiency syndrome in Romania. Lancet 1991;338:645–9.
50. Ahmad K. Kazakhstan health workers stand trial for HIV outbreak. Lancet Infect Dis 2007;7:311.
51. Donegan E, Stuart M, Niland JC, et al. Infection with human immunodeficiency virus type 1 (HIV-1) among recipients of antibody-positive blood donations. Ann Intern Med 1990;113:733–9.
52. Paintsil E, Andiman WA. Update on successes and challenges regarding mother-to-child transmission of HIV. Curr Opin Pediatr 2009;21: 94–101.
53. Gaur AH, Dominguez KL, Kalish ML, et al. Practice of feeding premasticated food to infants: a potential risk factor for HIV transmission. Pediatrics 2009;124:658–66.
54. Joint United Nations Programmed on HIV/AIDS (UNAIDS)/World Health Organization (WHO) Working Group on Global HIV/AIDS and STI Surveillance. Guidelines For Second Generation HIV Surveillance. 2000. Available at: http://data.unaids.org/publications/irc-pub01/jc370-2ndgeneration_en.pdf (accessed 20 May 2011).
55. Population Division of the Department of Economic and Social Affairs of the United Nations Secretariat. World Population Prospects: The 2008 Revision. Available at: http://esa.un.org/unpp (accessed 5 April 2011).
56. Kenya AIDS Indicator Survey 2007 (KAIS 2007) Final Report. 2009. Available at: http://www.aidskenya.org or: http://www.nacc.or.ke/index.php?option=com_booklibrary&task=view&id=9&catid=124&Itemid=122 (accessed 5 May 2011).
57. Beyrer C. HIV epidemiology update and transmission factors: risks and risk contexts–16th International AIDS Conference epidemiology plenary. Clin Infect Dis 2007;44:981–7.
58. United Nations Population Division. World Population Prospects: The 2004 Revision, database. Available at: http://www.un.org/esa/population/publications/WPP2004/wpp2004.htm (accessed 5 May 2011).
59. Stover J, Fidzani B, Molomo BC, et al. Estimated HIV trends and program effects in Botswana. PLoS One 2008;3:e3729.
60. Jahn A, Floyd S, Crampin AC, et al. Population-level effect of HIV on adult mortality and early evidence of reversal after introduction of antiretroviral therapy in Malawi. Lancet 2008;371:1603–11.
61. Shisana ORT, Simbayi L, Parker W, Zuma K, et al. South African National HIV Prevalence, HIV Incidence, Behaviour and Communication Survey, 2005.
62. Baral S, Trapence G, Motimedi F, et al. HIV prevalence, risks for HIV infection, and human rights among men who have sex with men (MSM) in Malawi, Namibia, and Botswana. PLoS One 2009;4:e4997.
63. Lane T, Raymond HF, Dladla S, et al. High HIV prevalence among men who have sex with men in Soweto, South Africa: Results from the Soweto Men's Study. AIDS Behav 2011;15:626–34.
64. Parry C, Petersen P, Dewing S, et al. Rapid assessment of drug-related HIV risk among men who have sex with men in three South African cities. Drug Alcohol Depend 2008;95:45–53.
65. Sanders EJ, Graham SM, Okuku HS, et al. HIV-1 infection in high risk men who have sex with men in Mombasa, Kenya. AIDS 2007;21:2513–20.
66. Wade AS, Kane CT, Diallo PA, et al. HIV infection and sexually transmitted infections among men who have sex with men in Senegal. AIDS 2005;19: 2133–40.
67. Mathers BM, Degenhardt L, Phillips B, et al. Global epidemiology of injecting drug use and HIV among people who inject drugs: a systematic review. Lancet 2008;372:1733–45.
68. Gelmon LKP, Oguya F, Cheluget B, Hailee G. Kenya: HIV Prevention Response and Modes of Transmission Analysis. 2009. UNAIDS. Available at: http://siteresources.worldbank.org/INTHIVAIDS/Resources/375798-1103037153392/KenyaMOT22March09Final.pdf (accessed 5 May 2011).
69. Wang L, Wang N, Li D, et al. The 2007 Estimates for people at risk for and living with HIV in China: Progress and challenges. J Acquir Immune Defic Syndr 2009;50:414–18.
70. National AIDS Control Organisation. UNGASS country progress report 2008: India. New Delhi, Ministry of Health and Family Welfare. 2008.
71. Nelson KE, Celentano DD, Eiumtrakol S, et al. Changes in sexual behavior and a decline in HIV infection among young men in Thailand. N Engl J Med 1996;335:297–303.
72. Rojanapithayakorn W. The 100% condom use programme in Asia. Reprod Health Matters 2006;14:41–52.
73. Baral S, Sifakis F, Cleghorn F, Beyrer C. Elevated risk for HIV infection among men who have sex with men in low- and middle-income countries 2000–2006: a systematic review. PLoS Med 2007;4:e339.
74. Coelho HC, Perdona GC, Neves FR, Passos AD. HIV prevalence and risk factors in a Brazilian penitentiary. Cad Saude Publica 2007;23:2197–204.
75. Soto RJ, Ghee AE, Nunez CA, et al. Sentinel surveillance of sexually transmitted infections/HIV and risk behaviors in vulnerable populations in 5 Central American countries. J Acquir Immune Defic Syndr 2007;46:101–11.
76. Kuiken C, Foley B, Leitner T, et al., eds. HIV Sequence Compendium 2010. Los Alamos National Laboratory: Theoretical Biology and Biophysics Group, LA-UR 10-03684.
77. National Institute of Allergy and Infectious Diseases. HIV Replication Cycle. Available at: http://www.niaid.nih.gov/topics/HIVAIDS/Understanding/Biology/Pages/hivReplicationCycle.aspx (accessed 26 April 2011).
78. Guadalupe M, Reay E, Sankaran S, et al. Severe CD4+ T-cell depletion in gut lymphoid tissue during primary human immunodeficiency virus type 1 infection and substantial delay in restoration following highly active antiretroviral therapy. J Virol 2003;77:11708–17.
79. Mehandru S, Poles MA, Tenner-Racz K, et al. Primary HIV-1 infection is associated with preferential depletion of CD4+ T lymphocytes from effector sites in the gastrointestinal tract. J Exp Med 2004;200:761–70.
80. Brenchley JM, Schacker TW, Ruff LE, et al. CD4+ T cell depletion during all stages of HIV disease occurs predominantly in the gastrointestinal tract. J Exp Med 2004;200:749–59.
81. Schacker TW, Hughes JP, Shea T, et al. Biological and virologic characteristics of primary HIV infection. Ann Intern Med 1998;128:613–20.
82. Mellors JW, Munoz A, Giorgi JV, et al. Plasma viral load and CD4+ lymphocytes as prognostic markers of HIV-1 infection. Ann Intern Med 1997; 126:946–54.
83. Mellors JW, Margolick JB, Phair JP, et al. Prognostic value of HIV-1 RNA, CD4 cell count, and CD4 Cell count slope for progression to AIDS and death in untreated HIV-1 infection. JAMA 2007;297:2349–50.
84. Ramratnam B, Bonhoeffer S, Binley J, et al. Rapid production and clearance of HIV-1 and hepatitis C virus assessed by large volume plasma apheresis. Lancet 1999;354:1782–5.
85. Wolbers M, Babiker A, Sabin C, et al. Pretreatment CD4 cell slope and progression to AIDS or death in HIV-infected patients initiating antiretroviral therapy—the CASCADE collaboration: a collaboration of 23 cohort studies. PLoS Med 2010;7:e1000239.
86. Rodriguez B, Sethi AK, Cheruvu VK, et al. Predictive value of plasma HIV RNA level on rate of CD4 T-cell decline in untreated HIV infection. JAMA 2006;296:1498–506.
87. Peters PJ, Karita E, Kayitenkore K, et al. HIV-infected Rwandan women have a high frequency of long-term survival. AIDS 2007;21(suppl. 6):S31–7.
88. Kiwanuka N, Robb M, Laeyendecker O, et al. HIV-1 viral subtype differences in the rate of CD4+ T-cell decline among HIV seroincident antiretroviral naive persons in Rakai district, Uganda. J Acquir Immune Defic Syndr 2010;54:180–4.
89. Little K, Thorne C, Luo C, et al. Disease progression in children with vertically-acquired HIV infection in sub-Saharan Africa: Reviewing the need for HIV treatment. Current Hiv Research 2007;5:139–53.
90. Quinn TC. Acute primary HIV infection. JAMA 1997;278:58–62.
91. Kahn JO, Walker BD. Acute human immunodeficiency virus type 1 infection. N Engl J Med 1998;339:33–9.
92. Celum CL, Buchbinder SP, Donnell D, et al. Early human immunodeficiency virus (HIV) infection in the HIV Network for Prevention Trials Vaccine Preparedness Cohort: risk behaviors, symptoms, and early plasma and genital tract virus load. J Infect Dis 2001;183:23–35.
93. Hecht FM, Busch MP, Rawal B, et al. Use of laboratory tests and clinical symptoms for identification of primary HIV infection. AIDS 2002;16: 1119–29.
94. Weintrob AC, Giner J, Menezes P, et al. Infrequent diagnosis of primary human immunodeficiency virus infection: missed opportunities in acute care settings. Arch Intern Med 2003;163:2097–100.

95. Rich JD, Merriman NA, Mylonakis E, et al. Misdiagnosis of HIV infection by HIV-1 plasma viral load testing: a case series. Ann Intern Med 1999;130:37–9.
96. Schwartz DH, Laeyendecker OB, Arango-Jaramillo S, et al. Extensive evaluation of a seronegative participant in an HIV-1 vaccine trial as a result of false-positive PCR. Lancet 1997;350:256–9.
97. Keele BF, Giorgi EE, Salazar-Gonzalez JF, et al. Identification and characterization of transmitted and early founder virus envelopes in primary HIV-1 infection. Proc Natl Acad Sci U S A 2008;105:7552–7.
98. Panel on Antiretroviral Guidelines for Adults and Adolescents. Guidelines for the Use of Antiretroviral Agents in HIV-1-Infected Adults and Adolescents. Department of Health and Human Services. March 27, 2012; 1–240. Available at: http://www.aidsinfo.nih.gov/ContentFiles/AdultandAdolescentGL.pdf (accessed 14 Aug 2012).
99. Bennett BB, Delaney K, Owen M, et al. HIV Testing Algorithms: A Status Report. A publication of the Association of Public Health Laboratories and CDC. 2009, updated March 2010. Available at: http://www.aphl.org/aphlprograms/infectious/hiv/Pages/HIVStatusReport.aspx (accessed 24 June 2011).
100. Cohen MS, Gay CL, Busch MP, Hecht FM. The detection of acute HIV infection. J Infect Dis 2010;202(suppl. 2):S270–7.
101. Branson BM. The future of HIV testing. J Acquir Immune Defic Syndr 2010;55(suppl. 2):S102–S105.
102. Kharsany ABM, Hancock N, Frohlich JA, et al. Screening for 'window-period' acute HIV infection among pregnant women in rural South Africa. HIV Med 2010;11:661–5.
103. World Health Organization. WHO Case Definitions of HIV for Surveillance and Revised Clinical Staging and Immunological Classification of HIV-Related Disease in Adults and Children. 2006. Available at: http://wwwwhoint/hiv/pub/vct/hivstaging/en/indexhtml (accessed 5 May 2011).
104. Centers for Disease Control. 1993 revised classification system for HIV infection and expanded surveillance case definition for AIDS among adolescents and adults. MMWR Recomm Rep 1992;41:1–19.
105. Holmes CB, Hausler H, Nunn P. A review of sex differences in the epidemiology of tuberculosis. Int J Tuberc Lung Dis 1998;2:96–104.
106. Nesheim SR, Kapogiannis BG, Soe MM, et al. Trends in opportunistic infections in the pre- and post-highly active antiretroviral therapy eras among HIV-infected children in the Perinatal AIDS Collaborative Transmission Study, 1986–2004. Pediatrics 2007;120:100–9.
107. Graham SM. Non-tuberculosis opportunistic infections and other lung diseases in HIV-infected infants and children. Int J Tuberc Lung Dis 2005;9:592–602.
108. Maartens G. Opportunistic infections associated with HIV infection in Africa. Oral Dis 2002;8(suppl. 2):76–9.
109. Sirisanthana T. Penicillium marneffei infection in patients with AIDS. Emerg Infect Dis 2001;7:561.
110. Sotgiu G, Mantovani A, Mazzoni A. Histoplasmosis in Europe. Mycopathologia 1970;41:53–74.
111. Randhawa HS. Occurrence of histoplasmosis in Asia. Mycopathologia 1970;41:75–89.
112. Slutsker L, Marston BJ. HIV and malaria: interactions and implications. Curr Opin Infect Dis 2007;20:3–10.
113. Grant AD, Kaplan JE, De Cock KM. Preventing opportunistic infections among human immunodeficiency virus-infected adults in African countries. Am J Trop Med Hyg 2001;65:810–21.
114. Joint United Nations Programmed on HIV/AIDS (UNAIDS). HIV-related opportunistic diseases: UNAIDS Technical Update. 1998. Available at: http://data.unaids.org/Publications/IRC-pub05/opportu_en.pdf (accessed 11 May 2011).
115. Kaplan JE, Benson C, Holmes KH, et al. Guidelines for prevention and treatment of opportunistic infections in HIV-infected adults and adolescents: recommendations from CDC, the National Institutes of Health, and the HIV Medicine Association of the Infectious Diseases Society of America. MMWR Recomm Rep 2009;58:1–207; quiz CE1–4.
116. Park BJ, Wannemuehler KA, Marston BJ, et al. Estimation of the current global burden of cryptococcal meningitis among persons living with HIV/AIDS. AIDS 2009;23:525–30.
117. Bicanic T, Brouwer AE, Meintjes G, et al. Relationship of cerebrospinal fluid pressure, fungal burden and outcome in patients with cryptococcal meningitis undergoing serial lumbar punctures. AIDS 2009;23:701–6.
118. Tanner DC, Weinstein MP, Fedorciw B, et al. Comparison of commercial kits for detection of cryptococcal antigen. J Clin Microbiol 1994;32:1680–4.
119. Asawavichienjinda T, Sitthi-Amorn C, Tanyanont V. Serum cyrptococcal antigen: diagnostic value in the diagnosis of AIDS-related cryptococcal meningitis. J Med Assoc Thai 1999;82:65–71.
120. Powderly WG, Cloud GA, Dismukes WE, Saag MS. Measurement of cryptococcal antigen in serum and cerebrospinal fluid: value in the management of AIDS-associated cryptococcal meningitis. Clin Infect Dis 1994;18:789–92.
121. Sloan DJ, Dedicoat MJ, Lalloo DG. Treatment of cryptococcal meningitis in resource limited settings. Curr Opin Infect Dis 2009;22:455–63.
122. Perfect JR, Dismukes WE, Dromer F, et al. Clinical practice guidelines for the management of cryptococcal disease: 2010 update by the infectious diseases society of america. Clin Infect Dis 2010;50:291–322.
123. Larsen RA, Bozzette SA, Jones BE, et al. Fluconazole combined with flucytosine for treatment of cryptococcal meningitis in patients with AIDS. Clin Infect Dis 1994;19:741–5.
124. Bicanic T, Meintjes G, Wood R, et al. Fungal burden, early fungicidal activity, and outcome in cryptococcal meningitis in antiretroviral-naive or antiretroviral-experienced patients treated with amphotericin B or fluconazole. Clin Infect Dis 2007;45:76–80.
125. Zolopa A, Andersen J, Powderly W, et al. Early antiretroviral therapy reduces AIDS progression/death in individuals with acute opportunistic infections: a multicenter randomized strategy trial. PLoS One 2009;4:e5575.
126. Makadzange AT, Ndhlovu CE, Takarinda K, et al. Early versus delayed initiation of antiretroviral therapy for concurrent HIV infection and cryptococcal meningitis in sub-saharan Africa. Clin Infect Dis 2010;50:1532–8.
127. Bicanic T, Jarvis JN, Muzoora C, Harrison TS. Should antiretroviral therapy be delayed for 10 weeks for patients treated with fluconazole for cryptococcal meningitis? Clin Infect Dis 2010;51:986–7; author reply 7–9.
128. Grant PM, Aberg JA, Zolopa AR. Concerns regarding a randomized study of the timing of antiretroviral therapy in zimbabweans with AIDS and acute cryptococcal meningitis. Clin Infect Dis 2010;51:984–5; author reply 7–9.
129. Chang LW, Phipps WT, Kennedy GE, Rutherford GW. Antifungal interventions for the primary prevention of cryptococcal disease in adults with HIV. Cochrane Database Syst Rev 2005:CD004773.
130. Meya DB, Manabe YC, Castelnuovo B, et al. Cost-effectiveness of serum cryptococcal antigen screening to prevent deaths among HIV-infected persons with a CD4+ cell count < or = 100 cells/microL who start HIV therapy in resource-limited settings. Clin Infect Dis 2010;51:448–55.
131. Crump JA, Ramadhani HO, Morrissey AB, et al. Invasive bacterial and fungal infections among hospitalized HIV-infected and HIV-uninfected adults and adolescents in northern Tanzania. Clin Infect Dis 2011;52:341–8.
132. Feikin DR, Jagero G, Aura B, et al. High rate of pneumococcal bacteremia in a prospective cohort of older children and adults in an area of high HIV prevalence in rural western Kenya. BMC Infect Dis 2010;10:186.
133. Mangtani P, Mulholland K, Madhi SA, et al. *Haemophilus influenzae* type b disease in HIV-infected children: a review of the disease epidemiology and effectiveness of Hib conjugate vaccines. Vaccine 2010;28:1677–83.
134. Berkley JA, Lowe BS, Mwangi I, et al. Bacteremia among children admitted to a rural hospital in Kenya. N Engl J Med 2005;352:39–47.
135. World Health Organization. WHO recommendations on the management of diarrhoea and pneumonia in HIV-infected infants and children: integrated management of childhood illness (IMCI). Geneva: World Health Organization; 2010.
136. Ward H, Ronn M. Contribution of sexually transmitted infections to the sexual transmission of HIV. Curr Opin HIV AIDS 2010;5:305–10.
137. Celum CL. Sexually transmitted infections and HIV: Epidemiology and interventions. Top HIV Med 2010;18:138–42.
138. Barth RE, Huijgen Q, Taljaard J, Hoepelman AIM. Hepatitis B/C and HIV in sub-Saharan Africa: an association between highly prevalent infectious diseases. A systematic review and meta-analysis. Int J Infect Dis 2010;14:E1024–31.
139. Thompson MA, Aberg JA, Hoy JF, et al. Antiretroviral treatment of adult HIV infection: 2012 recommendations of the International Antiviral Society-USA panel. JAMA 2012;308(4):387–402.
140. The European AIDS Clinical Society (EACS). Guidelines for the Clinical Management and Treatment of HIV-Infected Adults in Europe, version 6. Available at: http://europeanaidsclinicalsociety.org/guidelinespdf/EACSEuroGuidelines_FullVersion.pdf (accessed 14 Aug 2012).
141. World Health Organization. Antiretroviral Therapy for HIV Infection in Adults and Adolescents: Recommendations for a public health approach. 2010 revision. Available at: http://whqlibdoc.who.int/publications/2010/9789241599764_eng.pdf (accessed 3 May 2011).
142. Wiersma ST, McMahon B, Pawlotsky JM, et al. Treatment of chronic hepatitis B virus infection in resource-constrained settings: expert panel consensus. Liver Int 2011;31:755–61.
143. Bellini C, Keiser O, Chave JP, et al. Liver enzyme elevation after lamivudine withdrawal in HIV-hepatitis B virus co-infected patients: the Swiss HIV Cohort Study. HIV Med 2009;10:12–18.

144. Dore GJ, Soriano V, Rockstroh J, et al. Frequent hepatitis B virus rebound among HIV-hepatitis B virus-coinfected patients following antiretroviral therapy interruption. AIDS 2010;24:857–65.
145. McHutchison JG, Manns MP, Muir AJ, et al. Telaprevir for previously treated chronic HCV infection. N Engl J Med 2010;362:1292–303.
146. Hezode C, Forestier N, Dusheiko G, et al. Telaprevir and peginterferon with or without ribavirin for chronic HCV infection. N Engl J Med 2009;360: 1839–50.
147. McHutchison JG, Everson GT, Gordon SC, et al. Telaprevir with peginterferon and ribavirin for chronic HCV genotype 1 infection. N Engl J Med 2009; 360:1827–38.
148. McHutchison JG, Lawitz EJ, Shiffman ML, et al. Peginterferon alfa-2b or alfa-2a with ribavirin for treatment of hepatitis C infection. N Engl J Med 2009;361:580–93.
149. Poordad F, McCone J Jr, Bacon BR, et al. Boceprevir for untreated chronic HCV genotype 1 infection. N Engl J Med 2011;364:1195–206.
150. Bacon BR, Gordon SC, Lawitz E, et al. Boceprevir for previously treated chronic HCV genotype 1 infection. N Engl J Med 2011;364:1207–17.
151. Sepkowitz KA, Telzak EE, Carrow M, Armstrong D. Fever among outpatients with advanced human immunodeficiency virus infection. Arch Intern Med 1993;153:1909–12.
152. Amerson EH, Maurer TA. Dermatologic manifestations of HIV in Africa. Top HIV Med 2010;18:16–22.
153. Resneck JS Jr, Van Beek M, Furmanski L, et al. Etiology of pruritic papular eruption with HIV infection in Uganda. JAMA 2004;292:2614–21.
154. Parkin DM, Sitas F, Chirenje M, et al. Part I: Cancer in Indigenous Africans—burden, distribution, and trends. Lancet Oncol 2008;9:683–92.
155. Roujeau JC, Stern RS. Severe adverse cutaneous reactions to drugs. N Engl J Med 1994;331:1272–85.
156. Fagot JP, Mockenhaupt M, Bouwes-Bavinck JN, et al. Nevirapine and the risk of Stevens-Johnson syndrome or toxic epidermal necrolysis. AIDS 2001;15: 1843–8.
157. Cunningham ET Jr, Margolis TP. Ocular manifestations of HIV infection. N Engl J Med 1998;339:236–44.
158. Lewallen S, Courtright P. HIV and AIDS and the eye in developing countries: a review. Arch Ophthalmol 1997;115:1291–5.
159. Moraes HV Jr. Ocular manifestations of HIV/AIDS. Curr Opin Ophthalmol 2002;13:397–403.
160. Heiden D, Ford N, Wilson D, et al. Cytomegalovirus retinitis: the neglected disease of the AIDS pandemic. PLoS Med 2007;4:e334.
161. Hull MW, Phillips P, Montaner JS. Changing global epidemiology of pulmonary manifestations of HIV/AIDS. Chest 2008;134:1287–98.
162. Murray JF. Pulmonary complications of HIV-1 infection among adults living in Sub-Saharan Africa. Int J Tuberc Lung Dis 2005;9:826–35.
163. Zar HJ. Global paediatric pulmonology: out of Africa. Paediatr Respir Rev 2006;7(suppl. 1):S226–8.
164. Zar HJ, Madhi SA. Pneumococcal conjugate vaccine–a health priority. S Afr Med J 2008;98:463–7.
165. Afessa B. Pleural effusions and pneumothoraces in AIDS. Curr Opin Pulm Med 2001;7:202–9.
166. Gopi A, Madhavan SM, Sharma SK, Sahn SA. Diagnosis and treatment of tuberculous pleural effusion in 2006. Chest 2007;131:880–9.
167. Bonacini M, Young T, Laine L. The causes of esophageal symptoms in human immunodeficiency virus infection. A prospective study of 110 patients. Arch Intern Med 1991;151:1567–72.
168. Brooks JT, Ochieng JB, Kumar L, et al. Surveillance for bacterial diarrhea and antimicrobial resistance in rural western Kenya, 1997-2003. Clin Infect Dis 2006;43:393–401.
169. Giordano MO, Martinez LC, Rinaldi D, et al. Diarrhea and enteric emerging viruses in HIV-infected patients. AIDS Res Hum Retroviruses 1999;15: 1427–32.
170. Kelly P, Hicks S, Oloya J, et al. Escherichia coli enterovirulent phenotypes in Zambians with AIDS-related diarrhoea. Trans R Soc Trop Med Hyg 2003; 97:573–6.
171. Sanchez TH, Brooks JT, Sullivan PS, et al. Bacterial diarrhea in persons with HIV infection, United States, 1992–2002. Clin Infect Dis 2005;41:1621–7.
172. Guest JL, Ruffin C, Tschampa JM, et al. Differences in rates of diarrhea in patients with human immunodeficiency virus receiving lopinavir-ritonavir or nelfinavir. Pharmacotherapy 2004;24:727–35.
173. Nel ED, Rabie H, Goodway J, Cotton MF. A Retrospecive study of cryptosporidial diarrhea in a region with high HIV prevalence. J Trop Pediatr 2011;57:289–92.
174. Lule JR, Mermin J, Ekwaru JP, et al. Effect of home-based water chlorination and safe storage on diarrhea among persons with human immunodeficiency virus in Uganda. Am J Trop Med Hyg 2005;73:926–33.
175. Gumbo T, Sarbah S, Gangaidzo IT, et al. Intestinal parasites in patients with diarrhea and human immunodeficiency virus infection in Zimbabwe. AIDS 1999;13:819–21.
176. Wuhib T, Silva TM, Newman RD, et al. Cryptosporidial and microsporidial infections in human immunodeficiency virus-infected patients in northeastern Brazil. J Infect Dis 1994;170:494–7.
177. Weber R, Ledergerber B, Zbinden R, et al. Enteric infections and diarrhea in human immunodeficiency virus-infected persons: prospective community-based cohort study. Swiss HIV Cohort Study. Arch Intern Med 1999; 159:1473–80.
178. Carr A, Marriott D, Field A, et al. Treatment of HIV-1-associated microsporidiosis and cryptosporidiosis with combination antiretroviral therapy. Lancet 1998;351:256–61.
179. Modi M, Mochan A, Modi G. Management of HIV-associated focal brain lesions in developing countries. QJM 2004;97:413–21.
180. Smego RA Jr, Orlovic D, Wadula J. An algorithmic approach to intracranial mass lesions in HIV/AIDS. Int J STD AIDS 2006;17:271–6.
181. Porter SB, Sande MA. Toxoplasmosis of the central-nervous-system in the acquired-immunodeficiency-syndrome. N Engl J Med 1992;327:1643–8.
182. Luft BJ, Brooks RG, Conley FK, et al. Toxoplasmic encephalitis in patients with acquired immune-deficiency syndrome. JAMA 1984;252:913–17.
183. Torre D, Casari S, Speranza F, et al. Randomized trial of trimethoprim-sulfamethoxazole versus pyrimethamine-sulfadiazine for therapy of toxoplasmic encephalitis in patients with AIDS. Italian Collaborative Study Group. Antimicrob Agents Chemother 1998;42:1346–9.
184. Dedicoat M, Livesley N. Management of toxoplasmic encephalitis in HIV-infected adults (with an emphasis on resource-poor settings). Cochrane Database Syst Rev 2006;3:CD005420.
185. Muller M, Wandel S, Colebunders R, et al. Immune reconstitution inflammatory syndrome in patients starting antiretroviral therapy for HIV infection: a systematic review and meta-analysis. Lancet Infect Dis 2010;10: 251–61.
186. Lawn SD. Immune reconstitution disease associated with parasitic infections following initiation of antiretroviral therapy. Curr Opin Infect Dis 2007;20: 482–8.
187. Ratnam I, Chiu C, Kandala NB, Easterbrook PJ. Incidence and risk factors for immune reconstitution inflammatory syndrome in an ethnically diverse HIV type 1-infected cohort. Clin Infect Dis 2006;42:418–27.
188. Mbulaiteye SM, Katabira ET, Wabinga H, et al. Spectrum of cancers among HIV-infected persons in Africa: the Uganda AIDS-Cancer Registry Match Study. Int J Cancer 2006;118:985–90.
189. Buchacz K, Baker RK, Palella FJ Jr, et al. AIDS-defining opportunistic illnesses in US patients, 1994–2007: a cohort study. AIDS 2010;24:1549–59.
190. Simard EP, Pfeiffer RM, Engels EA. Cumulative incidence of cancer among individuals with acquired immunodeficiency syndrome in the United States. Cancer 2011;117:1089–96.
191. Shiels MS, Pfeiffer RM, Hall HI, et al. Proportions of Kaposi sarcoma, selected non-Hodgkin lymphomas, and cervical cancer in the United States occurring in persons with AIDS, 1980-2007. JAMA 2011;305:1450–9.
192. Patel P, Hanson DL, Sullivan PS, et al. Incidence of types of cancer among HIV-infected persons compared with the general population in the United States, 1992–2003. Ann Intern Med 2008;148:728–36.
193. Casper C. The increasing burden of HIV-associated malignancies in resource-limited regions. Annu Rev Med 2011;62:157–70.
194. Dienstag JL. Hepatitis B virus infection. N Engl J Med 2008;359:1486–500.
195. Castellsague X. Natural history and epidemiology of HPV infection and cervical cancer. Gynecol Oncol 2008;110:S4–7.
196. Clifford GM, Polesel J, Rickenbach M, et al. Cancer risk in the Swiss HIV Cohort Study: associations with immunodeficiency, smoking, and highly active antiretroviral therapy. J Natl Cancer Inst 2005;97:425–32.
197. Shiels MS, Cole SR, Kirk GD, Poole C. A meta-analysis of the incidence of non-AIDS cancers in HIV-infected individuals. J Acquir Immune Defic Syndr 2009;52:611–22.
198. Silverberg MJ, Neuhaus J, Bower M, et al. Risk of cancers during interrupted antiretroviral therapy in the SMART study. AIDS 2007;21:1957–63.
199. Cancer incidence in five continents. Volume VIII. IARC Sci Publ 2002:1–781.
200. Antman K, Chang Y. Kaposi's sarcoma. N Engl J Med 2000;342:1027–38.
201. Casper C, Wald A. The use of antiviral drugs in the prevention and treatment of Kaposi sarcoma, multicentric Castleman disease and primary effusion lymphoma. Curr Top Microbiol Immunol 2007;312:289–307.
202. Casper C. New approaches to the treatment of human herpesvirus 8-associated disease. Rev Med Virol 2008;18:321–9.
203. Parkin DM, Wabinga H, Nambooze S, Wabwire-Mangen F. AIDS-related cancers in Africa: maturation of the epidemic in Uganda. AIDS 1999;13: 2563–70.

204. Wabinga HR, Parkin DM, Wabwire-Mangen F, Nambooze S. Trends in cancer incidence in Kyadondo County, Uganda, 1960–1997. Br J Cancer 2000;82: 1585–92.
205. Chokunonga E, Levy LM, Bassett MT, et al. Cancer incidence in the African population of Harare, Zimbabwe: second results from the cancer registry 1993–1995. Int J Cancer 2000;85:54–9.
206. Martin JN. The epidemiology of KSHV and its association with malignant disease. In: Arvin A, Campadelli-Flume G, Mocarski E, et al., eds. Human Herpes viruses. Cambridge: Cambridge University Press; 2007.
207. Yoshioka MC, Alchorne MM, Porro AM, Tomimori-Yamashita J. Epidemiology of Kaposi's sarcoma in patients with acquired immunodeficiency syndrome in Sao Paulo, Brazil. Int J Dermatol 2004;43:643–7.
208. Gantt S, Carlsson J, Ikoma M, et al. The HIV protease inhibitor nelfinavir inhibits Kaposi sarcoma-associated herpesvirus replication in vitro. Antimicrob Agents Chemother 2011;55:2696–703.
209. Aboulafia DM, Pantanowitz L, Dezube BJ. AIDS-related non-Hodgkin lymphoma: still a problem in the era of HAART. AIDS Read 2004;14: 605–17.
210. Engels EA. Infectious agents as causes of non-Hodgkin lymphoma. Cancer Epidemiol Biomarkers Prev 2007;16:401–4.
211. Parkin DM, Bray F, Ferlay J, Pisani P. Global cancer statistics, 2002. CA Cancer J Clin 2005;55:74–108.
212. Schiffman M, Castle PE, Jeronimo J, et al. Human papillomavirus and cervical cancer. Lancet 2007;370:890–907.
213. Palefsky JM. Cervical human papillomavirus infection and cervical intraepithelial neoplasia in women positive for human immunodeficiency virus in the era of highly active antiretroviral therapy. Curr Opin Oncol 2003; 15:382–8.
214. Minkoff H, Zhong Y, Burk RD, et al. Influence of adherent and effective antiretroviral therapy use on human papillomavirus infection and squamous intraepithelial lesions in human immunodeficiency virus-positive women. J Infect Dis 2010;201:681–90.
215. Mwanahamuntu MH, Sahasrabuddhe VV, Pfaendler KS, et al. Implementation of 'see-and-treat' cervical cancer prevention services linked to HIV care in Zambia. AIDS 2009;23:N1–5.
216. Bunnell R, Mermin J, De Cock KM. HIV prevention for a threatened continent: implementing positive prevention in Africa. JAMA 2006;296: 855–8.
217. The Voluntary HIV-1 Counseling and Testing Efficacy Study Group. Efficacy of voluntary HIV-1 counselling and testing in individuals and couples in Kenya, Tanzania, and Trinidad: a randomised trial. Lancet 2000;356: 103–12.
218. Allen S, Meinzen-Derr J, Kautzman M, et al. Sexual behavior of HIV discordant couples after HIV counseling and testing. AIDS 2003;17:733–40.
219. Quinn TC, Wawer MJ, Sewankambo N, et al. Viral load and heterosexual transmission of human immunodeficiency virus type 1. Rakai Project Study Group. N Engl J Med 2000;342:921–9.
220. Donnell D, Baeten JM, Kiarie J, et al. Heterosexual HIV-1 transmission after initiation of antiretroviral therapy: a prospective cohort analysis. Lancet 2010;375:2092–8.
221. Baeten JM, Kahle E, Lingappa JR, et al. Genital HIV-1 RNA predicts risk of heterosexual HIV-1 transmission. Sci Transl Med 2011;3:77ra29.
222. Cohen MS, Chen YQ, McCauley M, et al. Prevention of HIV-1 infection with early antiretroviral therapy. N Engl J Med 2011;365:493–505.
223. Connor EM, Sperling RS, Gelber R, et al. Reduction of maternal-infant transmission of human immunodeficiency virus type 1 with zidovudine treatment. Pediatric AIDS Clinical Trials Group Protocol 076 Study Group. N Engl J Med 1994;331:1173–80.
224. Guay LA, Musoke P, Fleming T, et al. Intrapartum and neonatal single-dose nevirapine compared with zidovudine for prevention of mother-to-child transmission of HIV-1 in Kampala, Uganda: HIVNET 012 randomised trial. Lancet 1999;354:795–802.
225. Wiktor SZ, Ekpini E, Karon JM, et al. Short-course oral zidovudine for prevention of mother-to-child transmission of HIV-1 in Abidjan, Cote d'Ivoire: a randomised trial. Lancet 1999;353:781–5.
226. Lallemant M, Jourdain G, Le Coeur S, et al. Single-dose perinatal nevirapine plus standard zidovudine to prevent mother-to-child transmission of HIV-1 in Thailand. N Engl J Med 2004;351:217–28.
227. Nduati R, John G, Mbori-Ngacha D, et al. Effect of breastfeeding and formula feeding on transmission of HIV-1: a randomized clinical trial. JAMA 2000; 283:1167–74.
228. Moodley D, Moodley J, Coovadia H, et al. A multicenter randomized controlled trial of nevirapine versus a combination of zidovudine and lamivudine to reduce intrapartum and early postpartum mother-to-child transmission of human immunodeficiency virus type 1. J Infect Dis 2003; 187:725–35.
229. Cooper ER, Charurat M, Mofenson L, et al. Combination antiretroviral strategies for the treatment of pregnant HIV-1-infected women and prevention of perinatal HIV-1 transmission. J Acquir Immune Defic Syndr 2002;29: 484–94.
230. Thomas TK, Masaba R, Borkowf CB, et al. Triple-antiretroviral prophylaxis to prevent mother-to-child HIV transmission through breastfeeding—The Kisumu Breastfeeding Study, Kenya: A Clinical Trial. PLoS Med 2011;8: e1001015.
231. Taha TE, Li Q, Hoover DR, et al. Post-exposure prophylaxis of breastfeeding HIV-exposed infants with antiretroviral drugs to age 14 weeks: Updated efficacy results of the PEPI-Malawi trial. J Acquir Immune Defic Syndr 2011;57:319–25.
232. Kumwenda NI, Hoover DR, Mofenson LM, et al. Extended antiretroviral prophylaxis to reduce breast-milk HIV-1 transmission. N Engl J Med 2008; 359:119–29.
233. de Vincenzi I. Triple antiretroviral compared with zidovudine and single-dose nevirapine prophylaxis during pregnancy and breastfeeding for prevention of mother-to-child transmission of HIV-1 (Kesho Bora study): a randomised controlled trial. Lancet Infect Dis 2011;11:171–80.
234. Branson BM, Handsfield HH, Lampe MA, et al. Revised recommendations for HIV testing of adults, adolescents, and pregnant women in health-care settings. MMWR Recomm Rep 2006;55:1–17; quiz CE1–4.
235. Sansom SL, Jamieson DJ, Farnham PG, et al. Human immunodeficiency virus retesting during pregnancy: costs and effectiveness in preventing perinatal transmission. Obstet Gynecol 2003;102:782–90.
236. De Cock KM, Bunnell R, Mermin J. Unfinished business—expanding HIV testing in developing countries. N Engl J Med 2006;354:440–2.
237. World Health Organization. A Handbook for Improving HIV Testing and Counseling Services. Field-test version. Geneva: World Health Organization; 2010.
238. Ekwueme DU, Pinkerton SD, Holtgrave DR, Branson BM. Cost comparison of three HIV counseling and testing technologies. Am J Prev Med 2003; 25:112–21.
239. World Health Organization. Antiretroviral Therapy for HIV Infection in Infants and Children: Towards Universal Access. Recommendations for a public health approach. 2010 revision. Available at: http://wwwwhoint/hiv/pub/guidelines/art/en/ (accessed 26 April 2011).
240. Kourtis AP, Ibegbu C, Nahmias AJ, et al. Early progression of disease in HIV-infected infants with thymus dysfunction. N Engl J Med 1996;335:1431–6.
241. Lee S, Wood O, Tang S, et al. Detection of emerging HIV variants in blood donors from urban areas of Cameroon. AIDS Res Hum Retroviruses 2007; 23:1262–7.
242. Aghokeng AF, Mpoudi-Ngole E, Dimodi H, et al. Inaccurate diagnosis of HIV-1 group M and O is a key challenge for ongoing universal access to antiretroviral treatment and HIV prevention in Cameroon. PLoS One 2009; 4:e7702.
243. Owen SM, Yang C, Spira T, et al. Alternative algorithms for human immunodeficiency virus infection diagnosis using tests that are licensed in the United States. J ClinMicrobiol 2008;46:1588–95.
244. Pavie J, Rachline A, Loze B, et al. Sensitivity of five rapid HIV tests on oral fluid or finger-stick whole blood: a real-time comparison in a healthcare setting. PLoS One 2010;5:e11581.
245. Makuwa M, Souquiere S, Niangui MT, et al. Reliability of rapid diagnostic tests for HIV variant infection. J Virol Methods 2002;103:183–90.
246. de Mendoza C, Soriano V. Update on HIV viral-load assays: new technologies and testing in resource-limited settings. Future Virology 2009;4:423–30.
247. Ting PW, Schmid KL, Lam CS, Edwards MH. Objective real-time measurement of instrument myopia in microscopists under different viewing conditions. Vision Res 2006;46:2354v62.
248. Kim JE, Beckthold B, Chen Z, et al. Short communication: identification of a novel HIV type 1 subtype H/J recombinant in Canada with discordant HIV viral load (RNA) values in three different commercial assays. AIDS Res Hum Retroviruses 2007;23:1309–13.
249. Bruzzone B, Ventura A, Bisio F, et al. Impact of extensive HIV-1 variability on molecular diagnosis in the Congo basin. J Clin Virol 2010;47:372–5.
250. World Health Organization. Essential Prevention and Care Interventions for Adults and Adolescents Living with HIV in Resource-Limited Settings. 2008. Available at: http://wwwwhoint/hiv/pub/guidelines/EP/en/indexhtml (accessed 3 May 2011).
251. Mukherjee JS, ed. The PIH Guide to the Community-Based Treatment of HIV in Resource-Poor Settings, 2nd edn. Boston: Harvard Medical School Division of Social Medicine and Health Inequalities, Brigham and Women's Hospital François-Xavier Bagnoud Center for Health and Human Rights, Harvard School of Public Health; 2006.
252. Aberg JA, Kaplan JE, Libman H, et al. Primary care guidelines for the management of persons infected with human immunodeficiency virus: 2009 Update

by the HIV Medicine Association of the Infectious Diseases Society of America. Clin Infect Dis 2009;49:651–81.

253. Hammer SM. Clinical practice. Management of newly diagnosed HIV infection. N Engl J Med 2005;353:1702–10.
254. Bell SK, Little SJ, Rosenberg ES. Clinical management of acute HIV infection: best practice remains unknown. J Infect Dis 2010;202 (suppl. 2):S278–88.
255. Schneider E, Whitmore S, Glynn KM, et al. Revised surveillance case definitions for HIV infection among adults, adolescents, and children aged <18 months and for HIV infection and AIDS among children aged 18 months to <13 years—United States, 2008. MMWR Recomm Rep 2008;57:1–12.
256. World Health Organization. Antiretroviral Drugs for Treating Pregnant Women and Preventing HIV Infection in Infants. Recommendations for a public health approach. 2010 revision. Available at: http://www.who.int/hiv/pub/mtct/antiretroviral2010/en/index.html (accessed 24 May 2011).
257. Panel on Treatment of HIV-Infected Pregnant Women and Prevention of Perinatal Transmission. Recommendations for Use of Antiretroviral Drugs in Pregnant HIV-1-Infected Women for Maternal Health and Interventions to Reduce Perinatal HIV Transmission in the United States; 31 Jul 2012: pp. 1–235. Available at: http://aidsinfo.nih.gov/ContentFiles/PerinatalGL.pdf (accessed 14 Aug 2012).
258. Anema A, Au-Yeung CG, Joffres M, et al. Estimating the impact of expanded access to antiretroviral therapy on maternal, paternal and double orphans in sub-Saharan Africa, 2009–2020. AIDS Res Ther 2011;8:13.
259. Das M, Chu PL, Santos GM, et al. Decreases in community viral load are accompanied by reductions in new HIV infections in San Francisco. PLoS One 2010;5:e11068.
260. Montaner JS, Lima VD, Barrios R, et al. Association of highly active antiretroviral therapy coverage, population viral load, and yearly new HIV diagnoses in British Columbia, Canada: a population-based study. Lancet 2010; 376:532–9.
261. El-Sadr WM, Lundgren JD, Neaton JD, et al. CD4+ count-guided interruption of antiretroviral treatment. N Engl J Med 2006;355:2283–96.
262. Sterne JAC, May M, Costagliola D, et al. Timing of initiation of antiretroviral therapy in AIDS-free HIV-1-infected patients: a collaborative analysis of 18 HIV cohort studies. Lancet 2009;373:1352–63.
263. Kitahata MM, Gange SJ, Abraham AG, et al. Effect of early versus deferred antiretroviral therapy for HIV on survival. New Engl J Med 2009;360: 1815–26.
264. Collaboration TH-C. When to initiate combined antiretroviral therapy to reduce mortality and AIDS-defining illness in HIV-infected persons in developed countries. Ann Int Med 2011;154:509–15.
265. Severe P, Juste MA, Ambroise A, et al. Early versus standard antiretroviral therapy for HIV-infected adults in Haiti. N Engl J Med 2010;363:257–65.
266. British HIV Association Guidelines for the treatment of HIV-1 positive adults with antiretroviral therapy 2012. Available at: http://www.bhiva.org/documents/Guidelines/Treatment/2012/120430TreatmentGuidelines.pdf (accessed 14 Aug 2012).
267. Nakayiwa S, Abang B, Packel L, et al. Desire for children and pregnancy risk behavior among HIV-infected men and women in Uganda. AIDS Behav 2006;10:S95–104.
268. Yeatman SE. The impact of HIV status and perceived status on fertility desires in rural Malawi. AIDS Behav 2009;13(suppl. 1):12–19.
269. Cliffe S, Townsend CL, Cortina-Borja M, Newell ML. Fertility intentions of HIV-infected women in the United Kingdom. AIDS Care 2011:1–9.
270. World Health Organization. Scaling up Antiretroviral Therapy in Resource-Limited Settings. 2002. Available at: http://whqlibdoc.who.int/hq/2002/i9241545674.pdf (accessed 29 April 2011).
271. Weidle PJ, Nesheim S. HIV drug resistance and mother-to-child transmission of HIV. Clin Perinatol 2010;37:825–42, x.
272. Mandelbrot L, Landreau-Mascaro A, Rekacewicz C, et al. Lamivudine-zidovudine combination for prevention of maternal-infant transmission of HIV-1. JAMA 2001;285:2083–93.
273. Jackson JB, Becker-Pergola G, Guay LA, et al. Identification of the K103N resistance mutation in Ugandan women receiving nevirapine to prevent HIV-1 vertical transmission. AIDS 2000;14:F111–15.
274. Eshleman SH, Mracna M, Guay LA, et al. Selection and fading of resistance mutations in women and infants receiving nevirapine to prevent HIV-1 vertical transmission (HIVNET 012). AIDS 2001;15:1951–7.
275. Stringer JS, McConnell MS, Kiarie J, et al. Effectiveness of non-nucleoside reverse-transcriptase inhibitor-based antiretroviral therapy in women previously exposed to a single intrapartum dose of nevirapine: a multi-country, prospective cohort study. PLoS Med 2010;7:e1000233.
276. Jourdain G, Ngo-Giang-Huong N, Le Coeur S, et al. Intrapartum exposure to nevirapine and subsequent maternal responses to nevirapine-based antiretroviral therapy. N Engl J Med 2004;351:229–40.
277. Lockman S, Shapiro RL, Smeaton LM, et al. Response to antiretroviral therapy after a single, peripartum dose of nevirapine. N Engl J Med 2007; 356:135–47.
278. Zijenah LS, Kadzirange G, Rusakaniko S, et al. A pilot study to assess the immunologic and virologic efficacy of generic nevirapine, zidovudine and lamivudine in the treatment of HIV-1 infected women with pre-exposure to single dose nevirapine or short course zidovudine and their spouses in Chitungwiza, Zimbabwe. Cent Afr J Med 2006;52:1–8.
279. Coffie PA, Ekouevi DK, Chaix ML, et al. Maternal 12-month response to antiretroviral therapy following prevention of mother-to-child transmission of HIV type 1, Ivory Coast, 2003–2006. Clin Infect Dis 2008;46:611–21.
280. Chi BH, Sinkala M, Stringer EM, et al. Early clinical and immune response to NNRTI-based antiretroviral therapy among women with prior exposure to single-dose nevirapine. AIDS 2007;21:957–64.
281. Kuhn L, Semrau K, Ramachandran S, et al. Mortality and virologic outcomes after access to antiretroviral therapy among a cohort of HIV-infected women who received single-dose nevirapine in Lusaka, Zambia. J Acquir Immune Defic Syndr 2009;52:132–6.
282. Coovadia A, Hunt G, Abrams EJ, et al. Persistent minority K103N mutations among women exposed to single-dose nevirapine and virologic response to nonnucleoside reverse-transcriptase inhibitor-based therapy. Clin Infect Dis 2009;48:462–72.
283. Lockman S, Hughes MD, McIntyre J, et al. Antiretroviral therapies in women after single-dose nevirapine exposure. N Engl J Med 2010;363:1499–509.
284. Chersich MF, Urban MF, Venter FW, et al. Efavirenz use during pregnancy and for women of child-bearing potential. AIDS Res Ther 2006;3:11.
285. Food and Drugs Adminstration (FDA) advisory on nevirapine. AIDS Treat News 2005:7.
286. Dieterich DT, Robinson PA, Love J, Stern JO. Drug-induced liver injury associated with the use of nonnucleoside reverse-transcriptase inhibitors. Clin Infect Dis 2004;38(suppl. 2):S80–S89.
287. Peters PJ, Stringer J, McConnell MS, et al. Nevirapine-associated hepatotoxicity was not predicted by CD4 count >/=250 cells/muL among women in Zambia, Thailand and Kenya. HIV Med 2010;11:650–60.
288. Thio CL, Seaberg EC, Skolasky R Jr, et al. HIV-1, hepatitis B virus, and risk of liver-related mortality in the Multicenter Cohort Study (MACS). Lancet 2002;360:1921–6.
289. Mills EJ, Nachega JB, Bangsberg DR, et al. Adherence to HAART: a systematic review of developed and developing nation patient-reported barriers and facilitators. PLoS Med 2006;3:e438.
290. Smart T. Adherence and retention in HIV care in resource-limited settings. 2011. Available at: http://www.aidsmap.com/Adherence-and-retention-in-HIV-care-in-resource-limited-settings/page/1761429/ (accessed 29 April 2011).
291. Fox MP, Rosen S. Patient retention in antiretroviral therapy programs up to three years on treatment in sub-Saharan Africa, 2007-2009: systematic review. Trop Med Int Health 2010;15 (suppl. 1):1–15.
292. Weidle PJ, Wamai N, Solberg P, et al. Adherence to antiretroviral therapy in a home-based AIDS care programme in rural Uganda. Lancet 2006;368: 1587–94.
293. Coetzee D, Boulle A, Hildebrand K, et al. Promoting adherence to antiretroviral therapy: the experience from a primary care setting in Khayelitsha, South Africa. AIDS 2004;18 (suppl. 3):S27–31.
294. Rosen S, Fox MP, Gill CJ. Patient retention in antiretroviral therapy programs in sub-Saharan Africa: A systematic review. PloS Medicine 2007; 4:1691–701.
295. Nachega JB, Hislop M, Dowdy DW, et al. Adherence to highly active antiretroviral therapy assessed by pharmacy claims predicts survival in HIV-infected South African adults. J Acquir Immune Defic Syndr 2006;43:78–84.
296. Nachega JB, Hislop M, Dowdy DW, et al. Adherence to nonnucleoside reverse transcriptase inhibitor-based HIV therapy and virologic outcomes. Ann Intern Med 2007;146:564–73.
297. Bisson GP, Gross R, Bellamy S, et al. Pharmacy refill adherence compared with CD4 count changes for monitoring HIV-infected adults on antiretroviral therapy. PLoS Med 2008;5:e109.
298. Geng EH, Nash D, Kambugu A, et al. Retention in care among HIV-infected patients in resource-limited settings: emerging insights and new directions. Curr HIV/AIDS Rep 2010;7:234–44.
299. World Health Organization. Patient monitoring guidelines for HIV care and antiretroviral therapy. Geneva: World Health Organization; 2006.
300. Coutinho AMJ, Ekwaru J, Were W, et al. Utility of routine viral load, CD4 cell count, and clinical monitoring among HIV-infected adults in Uganda: A randomized trial. Abstract # 125 presented at the 15th Conference on Retroviruses and Opportunistic Infections (CROI), February 3–6, 2008 Boston, MA, USA Available at: http://wwwretroconferenceorg/2008/Abstracts/30881htm (accessed 26 April 2011).

301. Mugyenyi P, Walker AS, Hakim J, et al. Routine versus clinically driven laboratory monitoring of HIV antiretroviral therapy in Africa (DART): a randomised non-inferiority trial. Lancet 2010;375:123–31.
302. Moore DM, Hogg RS, Yip B, et al. Discordant immunologic and virologic responses to highly active antiretroviral therapy are associated with increased mortality and poor adherence to therapy. J Acquir Immune Defic Syndr 2005;40:288–93.
303. Sayana S, Javanbakht M, Weinstein M, Khanlou H. Clinical impact and cost of laboratory monitoring need review even in resource-rich setting. J Acquir Immune Defic Syndr 2011;56:e97–8.
304. European AIDS Clinical Society. Guidelines: Clinical Management and Treatment of HIV-Infected Adults in Europe. Version 5.4: April 2011. Available at: http://www.europeanaidsclinicalsociety.org/guidelines.asp (accessed on 21 April 2011).
305. Russell EC, Charalambous S, Pemba L, et al. Low haemoglobin predicts early mortality among adults starting antiretroviral therapy in an HIV care programme in South Africa: a cohort study. BMC Public Health 2010; 10:433.
306. Cesar C, Shepherd BE, Krolewiecki AJ, et al. Rates and reasons for early change of first HAART in HIV-1-infected patients in 7 sites throughout the Caribbean and Latin America. PLoS One 2010;5:e10490.
307. May M, Boulle A, Phiri S, et al. Prognosis of patients with HIV-1 infection starting antiretroviral therapy in sub-Saharan Africa: a collaborative analysis of scale-up programmes. Lancet 2010;376:449–57.
308. Lawn SD, Harries AD, Anglaret X, et al. Early mortality among adults accessing antiretroviral treatment programmes in sub-Saharan Africa. AIDS 2008; 22:1897–908.
309. Lawn SD, Harries AD, Wood R. Strategies to reduce early morbidity and mortality in adults receiving antiretroviral therapy in resource-limited settings. Curr Opin HIV AIDS 2010;5:18–26.
310. Dao CN, Peters PJ, Kiarie J, et al. Hyponatremia, Hypochloremia, and Hypoalbuminemia Predict an Increased Risk of Mortality during the First Year of Antiretroviral Therapy among HIV-infected Zambian and Kenyan Women. AIDS Res Hum Retroviruses 2011;Nov:1149–55.
311. Kotler DP. HIV and antiretroviral therapy: lipid abnormalities and associated cardiovascular risk in HIV-infected patients. J Acquir Immune Defic Syndr 2008;49(suppl. 2):S79–85.
312. Hirsch MS, Gunthard HF, Schapiro JM, et al. Antiretroviral drug resistance testing in adult HIV-1 infection: 2008 recommendations of an International AIDS Society-USA panel. Clin Infect Dis 2008;47:266–85.
313. Aleman S, Soderbarg K, Visco-Comandini U, et al. Drug resistance at low viraemia in HIV-1-infected patients with antiretroviral combination therapy. AIDS 2002;16:1039–44.
314. Karlsson AC, Younger SR, Martin JN, et al. Immunologic and virologic evolution during periods of intermittent and persistent low-level viremia. AIDS 2004;18:981–9.
315. Panel on Antiretroviral Therapy and Medical Management of HIV-Infected Children. Guidelines for the Use of Antiretroviral Agents in Pediatric HIV Infection. 16 August 2010; pp. 1–219. Available at: http://aidsinfo.nih.gov/ContentFiles/PediatricGuidelines.pdf. (accessed 21 April 2011).
316. World Health Organization. Antiretroviral Therapy for HIV Infection in Infants and Children: Towards Universal Access. Recommendations for a public health approach. 2006. Available at: http://wwwwhoint/hiv/pub/guidelines/art/en/ (accessed 26 April 2011).
317. L'Homme RF, Kabamba D, Ewings FM, et al. Nevirapine, stavudine and lamivudine pharmacokinetics in African children on paediatric fixed-dose combination tablets. AIDS 2008;22:557–65.
318. Mulenga V, Cook A, Walker AS, et al. Strategies for nevirapine initiation in HIV-infected children taking pediatric fixed-dose combination "baby pills" in Zambia: a randomized controlled trial. Clin Infect Dis 2010;51:1081–9.
319. Van der Linden D, Callens S, Brichard B, Colebunders R. Pediatric HIV: new opportunities to treat children. Expert Opin Pharmacother 2009;10: 1783–91.
320. Vanprapar N, Cressey TR, Chokephaibulkit K, et al. A chewable pediatric fixed-dose combination tablet of stavudine, lamivudine, and nevirapine: pharmacokinetics and safety compared with the individual liquid formulations in human immunodeficiency virus-infected children in Thailand. Pediatr Infect Dis J 2010;29:940–4.
321. Lidstrom J, Li Q, Hoover DR, et al. Addition of extended zidovudine to extended nevirapine prophylaxis reduces nevirapine resistance in infants who were HIV-infected in utero. AIDS 2010;24:381–6.
322. Fogel J, Hoover DR, Sun J, et al. Analysis of nevirapine resistance in HIV-infected infants who received extended nevirapine or nevirapine/zidovudine prophylaxis. AIDS 2011;25:911–17.
323. Zeh C, Weidle PJ, Nafisa L, et al. HIV-1 drug resistance emergence among breastfeeding infants born to HIV-infected mothers during a single-arm trial of triple-antiretroviral prophylaxis for prevention of mother-to-child transmission: A secondary analysis. PLoS Med 2011;8:e1000430.
324. Anglaret X, Chene G, Attia A, et al. Early chemoprophylaxis with trimethoprim-sulphamethoxazole for HIV-1-infected adults in Abidjan, Cote d'Ivoire: a randomised trial. Cotrimo-CI Study Group. Lancet 1999;353: 1463–8.
325. Wiktor SZ, Sassan-Morokro M, Grant AD, et al. Efficacy of trimethoprim-sulphamethoxazole prophylaxis to decrease morbidity and mortality in HIV-1-infected patients with tuberculosis in Abidjan, Cote d'Ivoire: a randomised controlled trial. Lancet 1999;353:1469–75.
326. Mermin J, Lule J, Ekwaru JP, et al. Effect of co-trimoxazole prophylaxis on morbidity, mortality, CD4-cell count, and viral load in HIV infection in rural Uganda. Lancet 2004;364:1428–34.
327. Chintu C, Bhat GJ, Walker AS, et al. Co-trimoxazole as prophylaxis against opportunistic infections in HIV-infected Zambian children (CHAP): a double-blind randomised placebo-controlled trial. Lancet 2004;364:1865–71.
328. Lowrance D, Makombe S, Harries A, et al. Lower early mortality rates among patients receiving antiretroviral treatment at clinics offering cotrimoxazole prophylaxis in Malawi. J Acquir Immune Defic Syndr 2007;46:56–61.
329. Walker AS, Ford D, Gilks CF, et al. Daily co-trimoxazole prophylaxis in severely immunosuppressed HIV-infected adults in Africa started on combination antiretroviral therapy: an observational analysis of the DART cohort. Lancet 2010;375:1278–86.
330. Hoffmann CJ, Fielding KL, Charalambous S, et al. Reducing mortality with cotrimoxazole preventive therapy at initiation of antiretroviral therapy in South Africa. AIDS 2010;24:1709–16.
331. Walter J, Mwiya M, Scott N, et al. Reduction in preterm delivery and neonatal mortality after the introduction of antenatal cotrimoxazole prophylaxis among HIV-infected women with low CD4 cell counts. J Infect Dis 2006; 194:1510–18.
332. World Health Organization. Guidelines on co-trimoxazole prophylaxis for HIV related infections among children adolescents and adults. Geneva: World Health Organization; 2006.
333. Yazdanpanah Y, Losina E, Anglaret X, et al. Clinical impact and cost-effectiveness of co-trimoxazole prophylaxis in patients with HIV/AIDS in Cote d'Ivoire: a trial-based analysis. AIDS 2005;19:1299–308.
334. Pitter C, Kahn JG, Marseille E, et al. Cost-effectiveness of cotrimoxazole prophylaxis among persons with HIV in Uganda. J Acquir Immune Defic Syndr 2007;44:336–43.
335. Ryan M, Griffin S, Chitah B, et al. The cost-effectiveness of cotrimoxazole prophylaxis in HIV-infected children in Zambia. AIDS 2008;22:749–57.
336. Chiller TM, Polyak CS, Brooks JT, et al. Daily trimethoprim-sulfamethoxazole prophylaxis rapidly induces corresponding resistance among intestinal *Escherichia coli* of HIV-infected adults in Kenya. J Int Assoc Physicians AIDS Care (Chic) 2009;8:165–9.
337. Hamel MJ, Greene C, Chiller T, et al. Does cotrimoxazole prophylaxis for the prevention of HIV-associated opportunistic infections select for resistant pathogens in Kenyan adults? Am J Trop Med Hyg 2008;79:320–30.
338. Campbell JD, Moore D, Degerman R, et al. HIV-infected ugandan adults taking antiretroviral therapy with CD4 counts >200 cells/μL who discontinue cotrimoxazole prophylaxis have increased risk of malaria and diarrhea. Clin Infect Dis 2012;54:1204–11.
339. Chariyalertsak S, Supparatpinyo K, Sirisanthana T, Nelson KE. A controlled trial of itraconazole as primary prophylaxis for systemic fungal infections in patients with advanced human immunodeficiency virus infection in Thailand. Clin Infect Dis 2002;34:277–84.
340. Chetchotisakd P, Sungkanuparph S, Thinkhamrop B, et al. A multicentre, randomized, double-blind, placebo-controlled trial of primary cryptococcal meningitis prophylaxis in HIV-infected patients with severe immune deficiency. HIV Med 2004;5:140–3.
341. Goldman M, Cloud GA, Wade KD, et al. A randomized study of the use of fluconazole in continuous versus episodic therapy in patients with advanced HIV infection and a history of oropharyngeal candidiasis: AIDS Clinical Trials Group Study 323/Mycoses Study Group Study 40. Clin Infect Dis 2005;41:1473–80.
342. McKinsey DS, Wheat LJ, Cloud GA, et al. Itraconazole prophylaxis for fungal infections in patients with advanced human immunodeficiency virus infection: randomized, placebo-controlled, double-blind study. National Institute of Allergy and Infectious Diseases Mycoses Study Group. Clin Infect Dis 1999;28:1049–56.
343. Smith DE, Bell J, Johnson M, et al. A randomized, double-blind, placebo-controlled study of itraconazole capsules for the prevention of deep fungal infections in immunodeficient patients with HIV infection. HIV Med 2001; 2:78–83.
344. Kremery V Jr, Huttova M, Masar O. Teratogenicity of fluconazole. Pediatr Infect Dis J 1996;15:841.

345. Fordham von Reyn C, Arbeit RD, Tosteson AN, et al. The international epidemiology of disseminated *Mycobacterium avium* complex infection in AIDS. International MAC Study Group. AIDS 1996;10:1025–32.
346. Falkinham JO 3rd. Epidemiology of infection by nontuberculous mycobacteria. Clin Microbiol Rev 1996;9:177–215.
347. von Gottberg A, Sacks L, Machala S, Blumberg L. Utility of blood cultures and incidence of mycobacteremia in patients with suspected tuberculosis in a South African infectious disease referral hospital. Int J Tuberc Lung Dis 2001;5:80–6.
348. World Health Organization. WHO Report on the Global Tobacco Epidemic. Implementing smoke-free environments. 2009. Available at: http://whqlibdoc.who.int/publications/2009/9789241563918_eng_full.pdf (accessed 29 April 2011).
349. Webb MS, Vanable PA, Carey MP, Blair DC. Cigarette smoking among HIV+ men and women: examining health, substance use, and psychosocial correlates across the smoking spectrum. J Behav Med 2007;30:371–83.
350. Burkhalter JE, Springer CM, Chhabra R, et al. Tobacco use and readiness to quit smoking in low-income HIV-infected persons. Nicotine Tob Res 2005; 7:511–22.
351. Benard A, Bonnet F, Tessier JF, et al. Tobacco addiction and HIV infection: toward the implementation of cessation programs. ANRS CO3 Aquitaine Cohort. AIDS Patient Care STDS 2007;21:458–68.
352. Lin HH, Ezzati M, Chang HY, Murray M. Association between tobacco smoking and active tuberculosis in Taiwan Prospective Cohort Study. American Journal of Respiratory and Critical Care Medicine 2009;180: 475–80.
353. Kwong J, Bouchard-Miller K. Smoking cessation for persons living with HIV: a review of currently available interventions. J Assoc Nurses AIDS Care 2010; 21:3–10.
354. Gordillo V, del Amo J, Soriano V, Gonzalez-Lahoz J. Sociodemographic and psychological variables influencing adherence to antiretroviral therapy. AIDS 1999;13:1763–9.
355. Baingana F, Thomas R, Comblain C. HIV/AIDS and Mental Health. 2005. Available at: http://www.worldbank.org/ (accessed 29 April 2011).
356. Geretti AM, Brook G, Cameron C, et al. British HIV Association guidelines for immunization of HIV-infected adults 2008. HIV Med 2008;9:795–848.
357. Recommended adult immunization schedule—United States, 2011. MMWR Morb Mortal Wkly Rep 2011;60:1–4.
358. Jong EC, Freedman DO. The immunocompromised traveler. In: Brunette GW, Kozarsky PE, Magill AJ, et al., eds. CDC Health Information for the International Traveler 2010. Altanta: US Department fo Health and Human Services, Public Health Service; 2009:457–65.
359. Ivers LC, Cullen KA, Freedberg KA, et al. HIV/AIDS, undernutrition, and food insecurity. Clin Infect Dis 2009;49:1096–102.
360. Au JT, Kayitenkore K, Shutes E, et al. Access to adequate nutrition is a major potential obstacle to antiretroviral adherence among HIV-infected individuals in Rwanda. AIDS 2006;20:2116–18.
361. World Bank. HIV/AIDS, nutrition and food security: what we can do. A synthesis of international guidance. 2007. Available at: http://www.worldbank.org/ (accessed 29 April 2011).
362. Oldewage-Theron WH, Dicks EG, Napier CE. Poverty, household food insecurity and nutrition: coping strategies in an informal settlement in the Vaal Triangle, South Africa. Public Health 2006;120:795–804.
363. Maia Leite LH, De Mattos Marinho Sampaio AB. Progression to overweight, obesity and associated factors after antiretroviral therapy initiation among Brazilian persons with HIV/AIDS. Nutr Hosp 2010;25:635–40.
364. Burns DN, Dieffenbach CW, Vermund SH. Rethinking prevention of HIV type 1 infection. Clin Infect Dis 2010;51:725–31.
365. World Health Organization. Towards universal access: scaling up priority HIV/AIDS interventions in the health sector: progress report 2009. 2009. Available at: http://wwwwhoint/hiv/pub/2009progressreport/en/indexhtml (accessed 26 April 2011).
366. Attia S, Egger M, Muller M, et al. Sexual transmission of HIV according to viral load and antiretroviral therapy: systematic review and meta-analysis. AIDS 2009;23:1397–404.
367. Johnston MI, Fauci AS. An HIV vaccine—evolving concepts. N Engl J Med 2007;356:2073–81.
368. Abdool Karim Q, Abdool Karim SS, Frohlich JA, et al. Effectiveness and safety of tenofovir gel, an antiretroviral microbicide, for the prevention of HIV infection in women. Science 2010;329:1168–74.
369. Grant RM, Lama JR, Anderson PL, et al. Preexposure chemoprophylaxis for HIV prevention in men who have sex with men. N Engl J Med 2010;363: 2587–99.
370. Baeten JM, Donnell D, Ndase P, et al. Antiretroviral Prophylaxis for HIV Prevention in Heterosexual Men and Women. N Engl J Med 2012;367:399–410.
371. Thigpen MC, Kebaabetswe PM, Paxton LA, et al. Antiretroviral Preexposure Prophylaxis for Heterosexual HIV Transmission in Botswana. N Engl J Med 2012;367:423–34.
372. Van Damme L, Corneli A, Ahmed K, et al. Preexposure prophylaxis for HIV infection among women. N Engl J Med 2012;367:411–22.
373. World Health Organization. Palliative Care. 2002. Available at: http://www.who.int/hiv/topics/palliative/PalliativeCare/en/ (accessed 24 May 2011).
374. World Health Organization. Palliative Care: Symptom Management and End-of-Life Care. 2004. Available at: http://www.who.int/3by5/publications/documents/en/genericpalliativecare082004.pdf (accessed 24 May 2011).
375. Hanson DL, Chu SY, Farizo KM, et al. Distribution of CD4+ lymphocytes at diagnois of acquired immunodeficiency syndrome—defining and other human immunodeficiency viruse-related illnesses. Arch Intern Med 1995; 155:1537–42.
376. Fauci AS, Pantaleo G, Stanley S, Weissman D. Immunopathogenic mechanisms of HIV infection. Ann Intern Med 1996;124:654–63.
377. Hay SI, Guerra CA, Gething PW, et al. A world malaria map: Plasmodium falciparum endemicity in 2007. PLos Med 2009;6:1000048.
378. World Health Organization. Global Control of Tuberculosis 2010. Available at http://www.who.int/tb/publications/global_report/en/ (accessed 1 April 2011).
379. Anon. Public Health Image Library. Available at: http://phil.cdc.gov/phil/quicksearch.asp (accessed 1 April 2011).

27.1 HIV, Tuberculosis, Malaria and *Streptococcus pneumoniae*

Alison D Grant

Key features

- HIV underlies the global resurgence of tuberculosis since the 1980s; the two epidemics overlap maximally in southern Africa, where more than half of patients with tuberculosis also have HIV infection
- All people with tuberculosis or pneumonia should know their HIV status
- In settings of high tuberculosis prevalence, people with HIV should be screened for tuberculosis at every clinical encounter
- Accumulating evidence supports starting antiretroviral therapy as soon as feasible after tuberculosis treatment for people with both diseases
- Care for people with HIV in resource-limited settings should include:
  - isoniazid preventive therapy to reduce the risk of tuberculosis
  - measures to prevent malaria in settings of stable malarial transmission
- Measures to minimize the risk of tuberculosis transmission are essential in healthcare facilities providing care for people with HIV

HIV AND TUBERCULOSIS

THE EFFECT OF HIV ON TUBERCULOSIS

The HIV epidemic is the main cause of the global resurgence of tuberculosis since the 1980s, with southern Africa most severely affected by the dual epidemic, such that more than half of people in this region who have active tuberculosis also have HIV infection. HIV infection increases the risk of active tuberculosis by about 20-fold [1]. People with HIV infection are more likely to progress to active tuberculosis following recent tuberculosis infection, and are more likely to reactivate latent tuberculosis. People with tuberculosis are more likely to die if they also have HIV infection, underlining the importance of coordinated management of both diseases.

HIV infection alters the clinical presentation of tuberculosis, making it harder to diagnose clinically because clinical manifestations may be atypical and more subtle. People with HIV and pulmonary tuberculosis, particularly the more immunosuppressed, are less likely to have upper lobe disease or to have cavitation. They can have atypical radiographic appearances of interstitial infiltrates or lymphadenopathy; they can also have normal chest x-rays, even in the presence of sputum culture-positive disease. People with HIV are more likely to have extrapulmonary (for example, pleural or pericardial) and disseminated tuberculosis.

HIV infection further complicates the management of tuberculosis by making laboratory diagnosis more difficult. People with HIV infection are less likely to have acid-fast bacilli visible on sputum smear microscopy. This presents problems in many resource-limited settings where smear microscopy is the only widely available diagnostic tool. Sputum culture, particularly using liquid culture media, is more sensitive and, where available, should be used in addition to microscopy. Newer, more sensitive diagnostic tools are in development. An automated PCR-based assay (Xpert MTB/RIF) can detect *Mycobacterium tuberculosis* and rifampin resistance in sputum (including smear-negative) within 2 hours with high specificity and sensitivity [2]. High cost is likely to limit its accessibility.

Tuberculosis is a common cause of immune reconstitution disease, which may be classified as paradoxical (worsening of tuberculosis manifestations among people who start antiretroviral therapy when already on anti-tuberculous treatment) or unmasking (tuberculosis with prominent inflammatory features that becomes clinically apparent after the start of antiretroviral therapy) [3].

The treatment of tuberculosis in people with HIV infection is, in principle, the same as for people without HIV infection. However, it is complicated by potential drug interactions, particularly between the key antituberculous agent, rifampin, and two of the main classes of antiretroviral agent: protease inhibitors and non-nucleoside reverse transcriptase inhibitors (see http://www.hiv-druginteractions.org/). The World Health Organization (WHO)-recommended approach in resource-limited settings is to use standard rifampin-based anti-tuberculosis treatment along with an efavirenz-based antiretroviral regimen [4]. Evidence is accumulating to support initiation of antiretroviral therapy as soon as possible after the start of anti-tuberculous treatment; earlier antiretroviral therapy is associated with reduced mortality, which outweighs concerns about overlapping drug toxicities and the risk of morbidity caused by immune reconstitution syndrome. A possible exception is when tuberculosis involves the central nervous system.

People with HIV infection are more likely to experience recurrence of tuberculosis after successful treatment. Where tuberculosis is common, studies using molecular epidemiology show that this is more often caused by re-infection than to relapse.

There is no clear evidence that HIV infection makes drug-resistant tuberculosis more common. However, since people with HIV are more likely to progress rapidly to active tuberculosis following new infection, in settings where drug-resistant tuberculosis is transmitted, HIV-infected persons are likely to be disproportionately affected. This problem was illustrated in an outbreak of extensively drug-resistant tuberculosis linked to an HIV clinic in KwaZulu Natal, South Africa [5].

THE EFFECT OF TUBERCULOSIS ON HIV DISEASE

Laboratory studies have been interpreted as suggesting that tuberculosis accelerates the progression of HIV disease. People with tuberculosis who also have HIV infection are at higher risk of death, particularly if antiretroviral treatment is delayed. However, epidemiologic studies indicate that, after controlling for confounders, mortality among people with HIV infection in settings of high and low prevalence of tuberculosis is similar, suggesting that tuberculosis is more likely to be a marker of HIV disease progression than a cause of it [6].

MANAGEMENT POINTS

- All people diagnosed with, or under investigation for, tuberculosis should know their HIV status.
- People diagnosed with HIV-associated tuberculosis should take cotrimoxazole preventive therapy.
- WHO guidelines recommend antiretroviral therapy for all people with HIV infection diagnosed with tuberculosis, starting as soon as possible after the start of anti-tuberculous therapy.
- People diagnosed with HIV infection should be screened for tuberculosis. In southern Africa, the prevalence of active tuberculosis among people presenting with HIV is so high that investigation (preferably with sputum culture) is justified for all. A symptom screen for tuberculosis (cough, fever, night sweats, weight loss) should be part of every clinical encounter.
- Sputum microscopy for acid-fast bacilli is less sensitive among people with HIV infection; more sensitive tests, such as culture or molecular testing, should be used, if available.
- Isoniazid preventive therapy reduces the risk of developing tuberculosis and should be part of the package of care for people with HIV infection.
- Measures to minimize the risk of tuberculosis transmission are essential in healthcare settings serving people with HIV infection.

HIV AND MALARIA

THE EFFECT OF HIV ON MALARIA

Mathematical modeling suggests that in southern Africa, HIV may have contributed to an increase in episodes of clinical malaria by up to 28%. In areas of stable malaria transmission, pregnant women with HIV infection are more likely to have clinical malaria, higher parasitemia, anemia and placental parasitemia leading to adverse birth outcomes than are their HIV-negative counterparts. In settings of stable malaria, HIV impairs acquired immunity to malaria among adults and older children such that they are more likely to have asymptomatic parasitemia and clinical malaria that is proportional to the degree of immunosuppression. In settings of unstable malaria, non-immune adults with HIV are more likely to experience severe malaria and death [7].

HIV infection has been associated with an increased risk of failure of malaria treatment, although most studies used suboptimal drug therapy and recurrence may be caused by reinfection rather than recrudescence.

In settings of stable malaria, the effect of co-trimoxazole preventive therapy in reducing HIV-associated morbidity is, in part, as a result of a reduction of symptomatic malaria. Co-trimoxazole preventive therapy has also been associated with an increased risk of failure of antimalarial treatment with sulfadoxine-pyrimethamine (which has a similar mechanism of action and of resistance). Some antiretroviral agents have antimalarial activity; however, to date, there is no clear evidence that this has clinical relevance. There are potential interactions between antimalarial and antiretroviral drugs, for example protease inhibitors can increase levels of quinine or lumefantrine.

THE EFFECT OF MALARIA ON HIV

HIV viral load has been noted to increase transiently after an episode of malaria in HIV-infected people not taking antiretroviral therapy; however, there is no clear evidence that this has clinical relevance. Malarial anemia, particularly among children, has indirectly contributed to HIV transmission via transfusion of unscreened, HIV-infected blood.

MANAGEMENT POINTS

- In malarial areas, antimalarial prevention measures, such as insecticide-treated bednets, should be part of the package of care for people with HIV infection.
- People with HIV infection who present with fever while taking co-trimoxazole preventive therapy are unlikely to have malaria and need further investigation; if malaria is diagnosed, sulfadoxine-pyrimethamine should not be used for treatment.
- Pregnant women with HIV infection in settings of stable malaria should receive three doses of intermittent presumptive malaria treatment during pregnancy (rather than two) if they are not taking co-trimoxazole preventive therapy. If they are taking co-trimoxazole, they should not receive sulfadoxine-pyrimethamine as presumptive treatment.
- There may be interactions between antimalarial drugs and antiretroviral therapy (see http://www.hiv-druginteractions.org/).

HIV AND *STREPTOCOCCUS PNEUMONIAE*

INTERACTIONS

People with HIV infection are at a greatly increased risk of pneumococcal disease [8]. Pneumococcal disease can occur at any CD4 count, but occurs more frequently among those whose CD4 is lower; pneumonia is more common among smokers. The clinical presentation of pneumococcal pneumonia with fever, chest pain, and cough, is similar among people with and without HIV; people with HIV are more likely to have pneumococcal bacteremia. HIV infection is also associated with pneumococcal meningitis; *Streptococcus pneumoniae* is the dominant cause of bacterial meningitis among people with HIV in southern Africa and has high mortality.

MANAGEMENT POINTS

- People with presumed/confirmed pneumococcal disease should be recommended to test for HIV.
- In people with HIV who have suspected bacterial pneumonia, the possibility of underlying tuberculosis should be considered. If possible, the empirical use of fluoroquinolones should be avoided in view of their anti-tuberculous activity, which may delay diagnosis and complicate treatment of tuberculosis.
- Although the evidence supporting the efficacy of 23-valent polysaccharide pneumococcal vaccination for adults with HIV is weak, many guidelines recommend it—particularly for people with CD4 counts above 200 cells/μL. Limited data suggest that newer, conjugate pneumococcal vaccines may be more efficacious, but there are fewer serotypes in the conjugate vaccine. Pneumococcal conjugate vaccine is efficacious in children with and without HIV, and there is evidence that vaccination of children under 5 years of age provides protection for adults with HIV in the same household.

REFERENCES

1. World Health Organization. Global Tuberculosis Control 2009: epidemiology, strategy, financing. Geneva: World Health Organization; 2009. Available at: http://www.who.int/tb/publications/global_report/2009/en/index.html.
2. Boehme CC, Nabeta P, Hillemann D, et al. Rapid molecular detection of tuberculosis and rifampin resistance. N Engl J Med 2010;363:1005–15.
3. Meintjes G, Lawn SD, Scano F, et al. Tuberculosis-associated immune reconstitution inflammatory syndrome: case definitions for use in resource-limited settings. Lancet Infect Dis 2008;8:516–23.
4. World Health Organization. Antiretroviral therapy for HIV infection in adults and adolescents: recommendations for a public health approach—2010 revision. Geneva: World Health Organization; 2010. Available at: http://www.who.int/hiv/pub/arv/adult2010/en/index.html.
5. Gandhi NR, Moll A, Sturm AW, et al. Extensively drug-resistant tuberculosis as a cause of death in patients co-infected with tuberculosis and HIV in a rural area of South Africa. Lancet 2006;368:1575–80.
6. Glynn JR, Murray J, Shearer S, Sonnenberg P. Tuberculosis and survival of HIV-infected individuals by time since seroconversion. AIDS 2010;24:1067–9.

7. Slutsker L, Marston BJ. HIV and malaria: interactions and implications. Curr Opin Infect Dis 2007;20:3–10.
8. Klugman KP, Madhi SA, Feldman C. HIV and pneumococcal disease. Curr Opin Infect Dis 2007;20:11–15.

FURTHER READING

World Health Organization. Essential prevention and care interventions for adults and adolescents living with HIV in resource-limited settings. Geneva: World Health Organization; 2008. Available at: www.who.int/hiv/pub/guidelines/EP/en/index.html.

World Health Organization. Guidelines for intensified tuberculosis case-finding and isoniazid preventive therapy for people living with HIV in resource-constrained settings. Geneva: World Health Organization; 2010. Available at: http://whqlibdoc.who.int/publications/2011/9789241500708_eng.pdf.

Viral Infections with Cutaneous Lesions 28

28.1 Measles

William J Moss

Key features

- Highly contagious mucocutaneous disease caused by measles virus
- One of the most important infectious diseases of humans, responsible for millions of deaths prior to the development of measles vaccines
- Prodromal illness characterized by fever, cough, coryza and conjunctivitis
- Koplik's spots, small white lesions on the buccal mucosa, appear before the rash
- Characteristic erythematous and maculopapular rash appears first on the face and behind the ears and then spreads to the trunk and extremities
- Widespread use of measles vaccines has resulted in dramatic declines in incidence and mortality

INTRODUCTION

Measles is a highly contagious disease caused by measles virus. Endemic areas are largely confined to the tropics, although outbreaks and deaths continue to occur in temperate zones among unvaccinated individuals (Fig. 28.1.1). Measles is one of the most important infectious diseases of humans and has caused millions of deaths since its emergence thousands of years ago. Measles virus (genus Morbillivirus, family Paramyxoviridae) most closely resembles rinderpest virus, a pathogen of cattle. It is thought to have evolved from an ancestral virus as a zoonotic infection in communities where cattle and humans lived in close proximity. Measles virus is believed to have become established in human populations about 5000–10,000 years ago when human populations achieved sufficient size in Middle-Eastern river valley civilizations to maintain virus transmission.

EPIDEMIOLOGY

Remarkable progress has been made in reducing the global measles incidence and mortality as a consequence of measles vaccination (Fig. 28.1.2) [1]. In the Americas, intensive vaccination and surveillance efforts have interrupted endemic transmission of the virus. More recently, progress has been made in sub-Saharan Africa as a consequence of increasing routine measles vaccine coverage and provision of a second opportunity for measles vaccination through mass measles vaccination campaigns [2].

Measles virus is one of the most highly contagious, directly transmitted pathogens and outbreaks can occur even in populations in which fewer than 10% of people are susceptible. There are no latent or persistent measles virus infections that result in prolonged contagiousness and no animal reservoirs for measles virus. Measles virus can only be maintained in human populations by an unbroken chain of acute infections.

Infants become susceptible to measles virus infection when the passively acquired maternal antibody is lost [3]. The average age of measles patients depends upon the rate of contact with infected persons, the rate of decline of protective maternal antibodies and the vaccine coverage rate. In densely populated urban settings with low vaccination coverage, measles is a disease of infants and young children. As measles vaccine coverage increases, or population density decreases, the age distribution shifts toward older children. As vaccination coverage increases further, the age distribution of cases may be shifted into adolescence and adulthood.

When endemic, measles incidence has a typical temporal pattern characterized by yearly seasonal epidemics superimposed upon longer epidemic cycles of 2–5 years or more. These cycles result from the accumulation of susceptible persons over successive birth cohorts and the subsequent decline in the number of susceptible people following an outbreak. In the tropics, measles outbreaks have variable relationships with rainy seasons. This seasonality, combined with high birth rates, can result in highly irregular, large outbreaks of measles [4].

NATURAL HISTORY, PATHOGENESIS AND PATHOLOGY

Measles virus is primarily transmitted by respiratory droplets over short distances and, less commonly, by small particle aerosols that remain suspended in the air for long periods of time. The time from infection to clinical disease is approximately 10 days to the onset of fever and 14 days to the onset of rash. Persons with measles are infectious for several days before and after the onset of rash, when levels of measles virus in blood and body fluids are highest and when the symptoms of cough, coryza and sneezing are most severe. The host immune response at sites of virus replication is responsible for the signs and symptoms of measles.

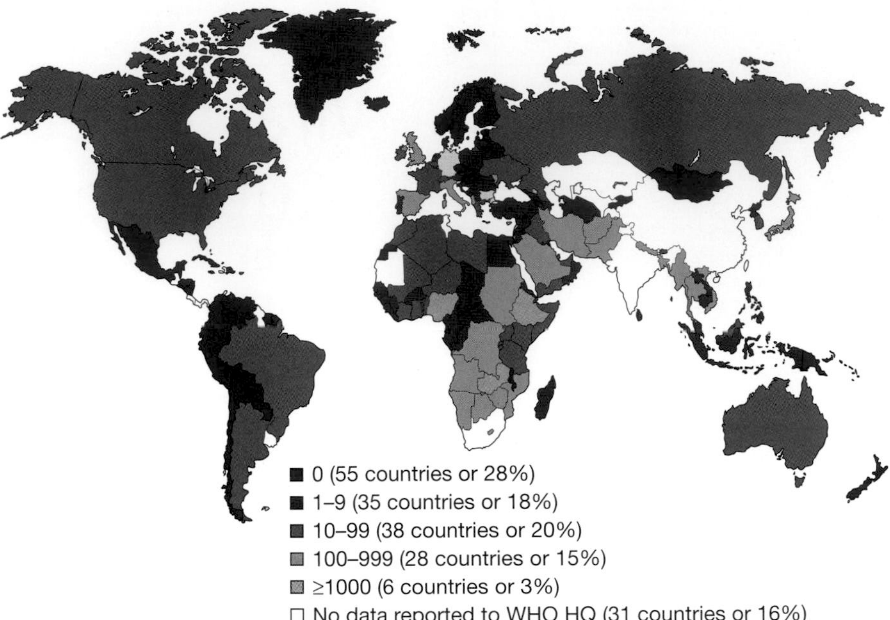

FIGURE 28.1.1 Reported measles cases with date of onset between July 2010 and January 2011 *(redrawn from World Health Organization. Measles Surveillance Data. Available at: http://www.who.int/immunization_monitoring/diseases/measles_monthlydata/en/index.html.) © 2011 Geneva, World Health Organization.*

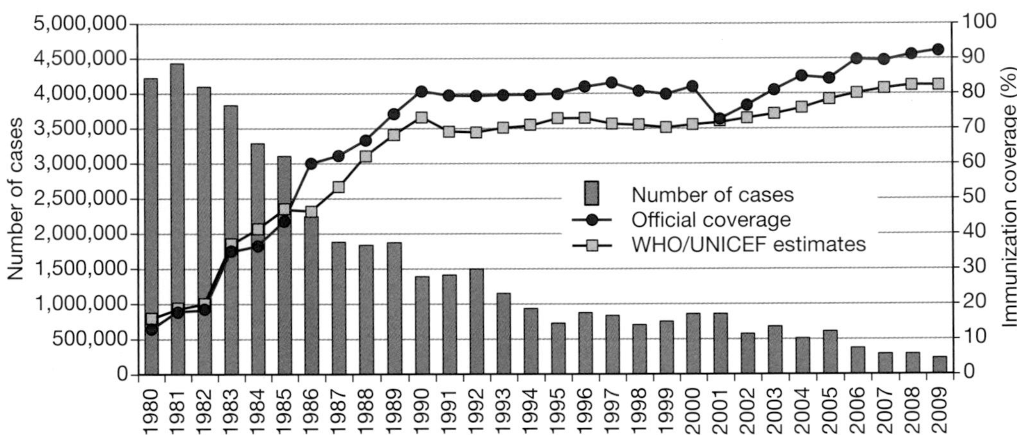

FIGURE 28.1.2 Global annual reported measles cases and measles vaccine coverage, 1980–2009 *(redrawn from World Health Organization, Department of Immunization, Vaccines and Biologicals. WHO vaccine-preventable diseases: monitoring system. 2010 global summary. Immunization, Vaccines and Biologicals. Available at: http://www.who.int/immunization/documents/who_ivb_2010/en/index.html. Geneva: World Health Organization; 2010.)*

Host immune responses to measles virus are essential for viral clearance, clinical recovery and the establishment of long-term immunity [5]. The protective efficacy of antibodies to measles virus is illustrated by the immunity conferred to infants from passively acquired maternal antibodies and the protection of exposed, susceptible individuals following administration of anti-measles virus immune globulin. The duration of protective immunity following wild-type measles virus infection is generally life-long [6]. The immune responses to measles virus infection are associated with depressed responses to unrelated (non-measles virus) antigens, lasting for several weeks to months. This state of immune suppression enhances susceptibility to secondary bacterial and viral infections causing pneumonia and diarrhea, and is likely responsible for much of measles-associated morbidity and mortality [7]. Vitamin A deficiency is a recognized risk factor for severe measles. The vitamin is essential for the maintenance of normal epithelial tissues throughout the body; measles virus itself infects and damages these tissues.

CLINICAL FEATURES

Clinically, features begin with a prodromal illness characterized by fever, cough, coryza and conjunctivitis (Fig. 28.1.3). Koplik's spots (small white lesions on the buccal mucosa) may be visible during the prodrome and allow the astute clinician to diagnose measles prior to the onset of rash (Fig. 28.1.4). The prodromal symptoms intensify several days before the onset of rash. A characteristic erythematous and maculopapular rash appears, first on the face and behind the ears, and then spreads, in a centrifugal fashion, to the trunk and extremities (Fig. 28.1.5). The rash lasts for 3–4 days and fades in the same manner as it appeared. Malnourished children may develop a deeply pigmented rash that desquamates or peels during recovery [8].

In uncomplicated measles, clinical recovery begins soon after appearance of the rash. Complications can occur in up to 40% of measles cases; the risk of complication is increased by extremes of age and malnutrition (Fig. 28.1.6). The respiratory tract is a frequent site of

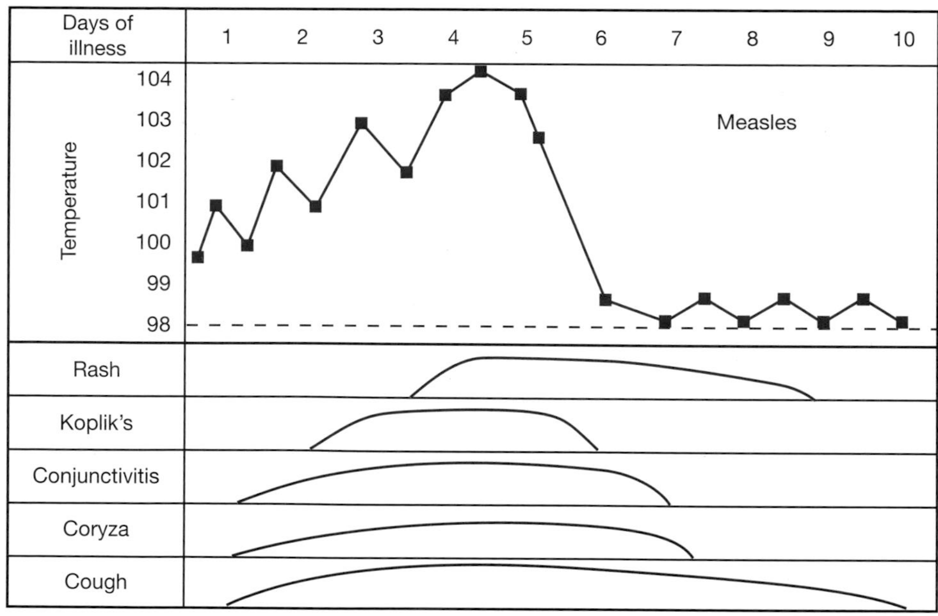

FIGURE 28.1.3 Clinical course of measles *(redrawn from Krugman S, Katz SL, Gershon AA, Wilfert CM, eds. Infectious Diseases of Children, 9th edn. St Louis: Mosby; 1992.)*

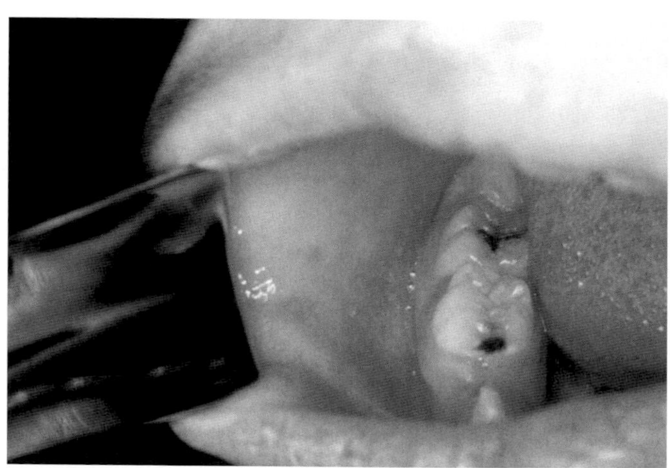

FIGURE 28.1.4 Koplik's spots of measles *(reprinted from Centers for Disease Control and Prevention http://phil.cdc.gov/phil/details.asp?pid=6111).*

complication, with pneumonia accounting for most measles-associated deaths [9]. Pneumonia is caused by secondary viral or bacterial infections, or by the measles virus itself. Other respiratory complications include laryngotracheobronchitis (croup) and otitis media. Mouth ulcers, or stomatitis, may hinder children from eating or drinking. Many children with measles develop diarrhea, which further contributes to malnutrition. Keratoconjunctivitis is common after measles, particularly in children with vitamin A deficiency, and is a frequent cause of blindness [10].

Because the measles rash is a consequence of the cellular immune response, persons with impaired cellular immunity, such as those with AIDS, may not develop the characteristic measles rash [11]. These persons have a high case fatality and may develop a giant cell pneumonitis caused by measles virus.

Measles virus causes three rare, but serious, central nervous system complications: post-measles encephalomyelitis, sub-acute measles encephalitis and subacute sclerosing panencephalitis (SSPE). Post-measles encephalomyelitis occurs in approximately 1 in 1000 cases, mainly in older children and adults. The syndrome develops within two weeks of the onset of rash and is characterized by fever, seizures and a variety of neurologic abnormalities. Around 15% of patients die and half are left with severe sequelae. The finding of periventricular demyelination, the induction of immune responses to myelin basic protein and the absence of measles virus in the brain suggest that it is an autoimmune disorder triggered by measles virus infection.

Subacute measles encephalitis (also known as measles inclusion body encephalitis) is a rare, but fatal, complication associated with progressive neurologic deterioration that affects individuals with defective cellular immunity and typically occurs 2–6 months after infection. There is lethargy, mental confusion, seizures, myoclonus and diffuse cerebral dysfunction which relentlessly progress to death in a few months. Pathologically, inflammatory changes are seen throughout the brain and there are eosinophilic inclusions in the nuclei of neurons.

SSPE is a slowly progressive disease that affects approximately one per million of those who have had measles, occurring 5–15 years after the initial infection. It is characterized by seizures and progressive deterioration of cognitive and motor functions, followed by death within two years [12]. SSPE most often occurs in persons infected with measles virus before the age of two years.

PATIENT EVALUATION, DIAGNOSIS AND DIFFERENTIAL DIAGNOSIS

Healthcare workers should consider measles in patients with fever and generalized rash, particularly when measles virus is known to be circulating, or in individuals with a history of travel to endemic areas. Physical examination should focus on the clinical features of measles, specifically Koplik's spots and rash, as well as potential sites of secondary infections, including pneumonia and otitis media. Appropriate precautions need to be taken to prevent transmission within health-care settings.

Measles is readily diagnosed on clinical grounds by clinicians familiar with the disease, particularly during outbreaks. Koplik's spots are especially helpful as they appear before the rash and are pathognomonic (Fig. 28.1.4). Clinical diagnosis is more difficult in regions where the incidence of measles is low, as other pathogens are

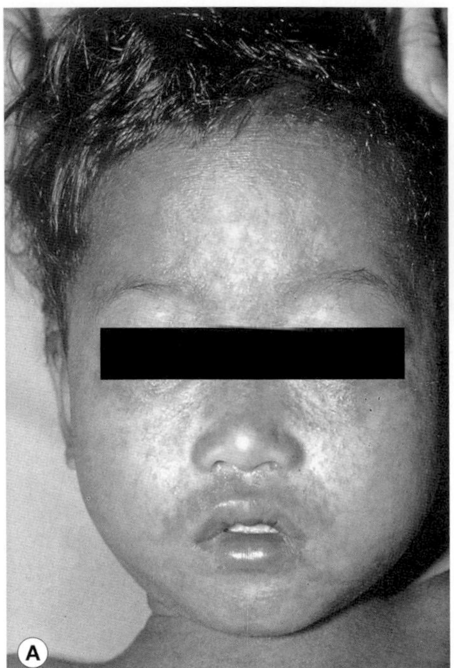

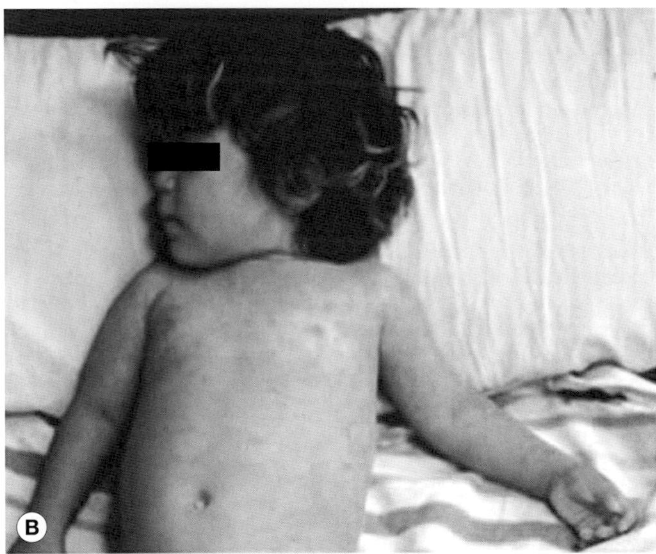

FIGURE 28.1.5 Measles rash. **(A)** *Courtesy Centers for Disease Control and Prevention.* **(B)** *Reprinted from Moss WJ, Griffin DE. Global measles elimination. Nat Rev Microbiol 2006;4:900–8.*

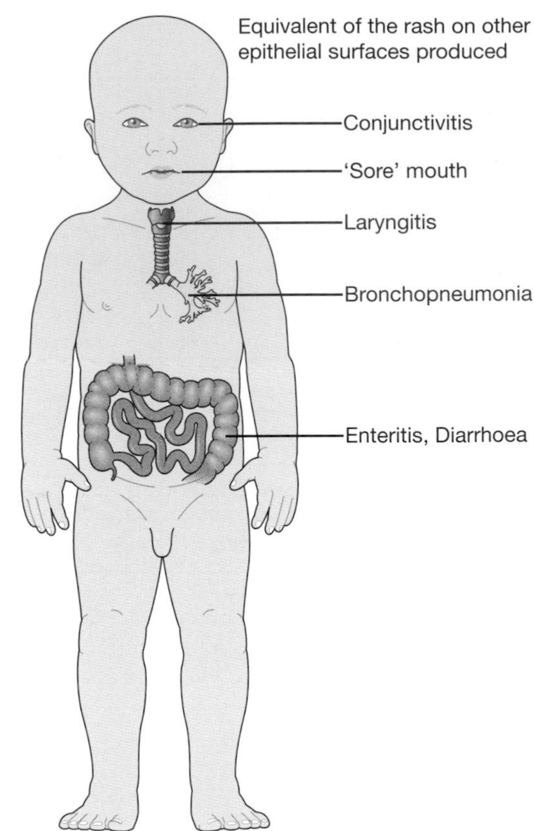

External rash
Normal rash develops
Rash darkens to a deep red and violet colour
Desquamation (the amount depends on the extent of darkening of the rash)

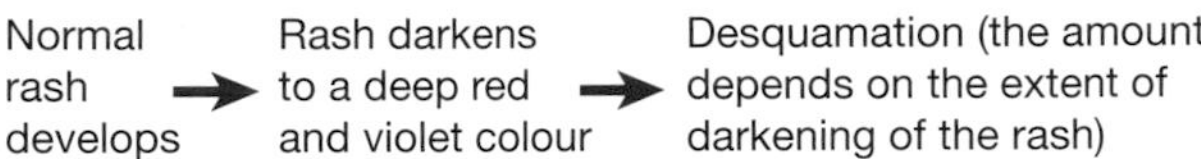

FIGURE 28.1.6 Complications of measles.

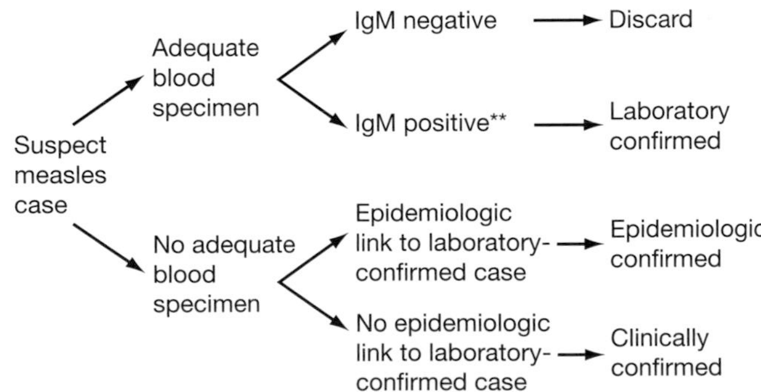

FIGURE 28.1.7 Classification of measles cases for measles surveillance *(redrawn from World Health Organization, Department of Vaccines and Biologicals. WHO recommended standards of surveillance of selected vaccine-preventable diseases. Geneva: World Health Organization; 2003.)*

responsible for the majority of illnesses with fever and rash (Table 28.1-1). The World Health Organization (WHO) clinical case definition for measles consists of any person with fever and maculopapular rash (i.e. non-vesicular), and cough, coryza or conjunctivitis [13]. Although this is not very specific, it is devised primarily for outbreak control and monitoring, rather than clinical use.

The detection of measles virus-specific IgM in a single specimen of serum or oral fluid is considered diagnostic of acute infection and is the most common method of laboratory confirmation (Fig. 28.1.7) [14]. IgM antibodies may not be detectable until four days or more after rash onset and usually fall to undetectable levels within 4–8 weeks of rash onset. Alternatively, acute infection can be confirmed with a fourfold, or greater, increase in measles virus-specific IgG antibody levels between acute and convalescent sera. The presence of IgG antibodies in a single serum specimen is evidence of prior infection or immunization, which cannot be distinguished serologically. Commercially available enzyme immunoassays (EIA) for detecting IgM or IgG antibodies are the most frequently used diagnostic assays.

Measles also can be diagnosed by isolating measles virus in cell culture from respiratory secretions, nasopharyngeal and conjunctival swabs, blood or urine. Detection of measles virus RNA by reverse transcriptase-PCR (RT-PCR) of clinical specimens can be accomplished using primers targeted to highly conserved regions of measles virus genes. When combined with nucleotide sequencing, these assays

TABLE 28.1-1 Differential Diagnosis of Measles

Diagnosis	Distinguishing characteristics
Rubella	Mild illness with distinctive lymphadenopathy involving the posterior cervical, suboccipital and posterior auricular nodes
Roseola	Rash appears after fever subsides
Dengue	Headache, myalgia and hemorrhagic lesions are not seen with measles
Scarlet fever	Often with evidence of streptococcal infection
Infectious mononucleosis	Atypical lymphocytosis, in contrast to the lymphopenia of acute measles
Enterovirus infection	Mild illness without the complications of measles
Adenovirus infection	Epidemics of keratoconjunctivitis usually not associated with rash
Rickettsial infection	Rash not as confluent as with measles and patient may have exposure history
Kawasaki disease	Prolonged illness that evolves in stages; a number of characteristics not found in measles
Drug sensitivity reaction	History of exposure to drugs, such as sulfonamides

permit the precise identification and characterization of virus genotypes for molecular epidemiologic studies, and can distinguish wild-type and vaccine measles virus strains.

The differential diagnosis of measles (Table 28.1-1) includes other causes of fever, rash and conjunctivitis, such as rubella, roseola, dengue, scarlet fever, infectious mononucleosis, and enterovirus or adenovirus infections. Less common causes include rickettsial infections (e.g. Rocky Mountain spotted fever), Kawasaki disease and drug reactions. Rubella, commonly mistaken for measles, is a milder illness without cough and with distinctive lymphadenopathy involving the posterior cervical, suboccipital and posterior auricular nodes. The rash of roseola (exanthema subitum) appears after the fever has subsided. The atypical lymphocytosis in infectious mononucleosis contrasts with the leukopenia commonly observed in children with measles.

PREVENTION AND TREATMENT

The best means of preventing measles is active immunization with measles vaccine [15]. Measles vaccines are live, attenuated viral vaccines that replicate within the host to induce protective immunity. The recommended age of first vaccination varies from 6–15 months and is a balance between the optimum age for seroconversion and the probability of acquiring measles before that age. The proportions of children who develop protective levels of antibody after measles vaccination are approximately 85% at 9 months of age and 95% at 12 months of age. As not all children develop protective immunity after vaccination, an opportunity for a second dose is needed to eliminate measles virus transmission. The second dose can be provided either through the primary healthcare system or mass vaccination campaigns (also called supplemental immunization activities).

TABLE 28.1-2 Vitamin A Treatment of Measles

Age	1st Day	2nd Day*
≥12 months	200,000 IU	200,000 IU
6–11 months	100,000 IU	100,000 IU
<6 months	50,000 IU	50,000 IU

*A third dose is recommended 2–4 weeks later in children with evidence of vitamin A deficiency.
Evidence: randomized controlled trials.

The duration of vaccine-induced immunity is at least several decades, if not longer [16]. Secondary vaccine failure rates have been estimated to be approximately 5% at 10–15 years after immunization, but are probably lower when vaccination is given after 12 months of age. Decreasing antibody titers do not necessarily imply a complete loss of protective immunity, as a secondary immune response usually develops after re-exposure to measles virus, with a rapid rise in antibody titers without overt clinical disease.

Standard doses of currently licensed measles vaccines are safe in immunocompetent children and adults. Fever to 39.4°C (103°F) occurs in approximately 5% of seronegative vaccine recipients and 2% of vaccine recipients develop a transient rash. Mild transient thrombocytopenia has been reported with an incidence of approximately 1 in 40,000 doses of the combined measles, mumps and rubella (MMR) vaccine.

Measles vaccines are well tolerated and immunogenic in HIV-infected children and adults, although antibody levels may be lower than uninfected children when vaccination occurs in later infancy and antibody levels may wane faster. Because of the potential severity of wild-type measles virus infection in HIV-infected children, measles vaccination is recommended for routine administration to these children at six and nine months of age, except those who are severely immunocompromised.

Other than general supportive measures, such as hydration and antipyretics, there is no specific antiviral therapy for persons with measles. Secondary bacterial infections are a major cause of morbidity and mortality following measles and effective case-management involves prompt treatment with antibiotics. Antibiotics are indicated for persons with measles who have clinical evidence of bacterial infection, including pneumonia and otitis media. *Streptococcus pneumoniae* and *Haemophilus influenza* type b are common causes of bacterial pneumonia following measles; vaccines against these pathogens likely lower the incidence of secondary bacterial infections following measles.

Vitamin A is effective for the treatment of measles and can result in marked reductions in morbidity and mortality (Table 28.1-2). The WHO recommends administration of once-daily doses of 200,000 IU of vitamin A for two consecutive days to all children aged 12 months or older with measles. Lower doses are recommended for younger children: 100,000 IU per day for children aged 6–12 months and 50,000 IU per day for children younger than 6 months old. A third dose is recommended 2–4 weeks later in children with evidence of vitamin A deficiency [17].

REFERENCES

1. World Health Organization. Global reductions in measles mortality 2000–2008 and the risk of measles resurgence. Weekly Epidemiol Rec 2009;84: 509–16.

2. Centers for Disease Control and Prevention. Progress toward measles control—African region, 2001–2008. MMWR Morb Mortal Wkly Rep 2009;58: 1036–41.
3. Caceres VM, Strebel PM, Sutter RW. Factors determining prevalence of maternal antibody to measles virus throughout infancy: a review. Clin Infect Dis 2000;31:110–19.
4. Ferrari MJ, Grais RF, Bharti N, et al. The dynamics of measles in sub-Saharan Africa. Nature 2008;7:679–84.
5. Moss WJ, Scott S. WHO Immunological Basis for Immunization Series: Measles. Geneva: World Health Organzation; 2009.
6. Amanna IJ, Carlson NE, Slifka MK. Duration of humoral immunity to common viral and vaccine antigens. N Engl J Med. 2007;357:1903–15.
7. Akramuzzaman SM, Cutts FT, Wheeler JG, Hossain MJ. Increased childhood morbidity after measles is short-term in urban Bangladesh. Am J Epidemiol 2000;151:723–35.
8. Morley D. Severe measles in the tropics. Brit Med J 1969;1:297–300.
9. Duke T, Mgone CS. Measles: not just another viral exanthem. Lancet 2003; 361:763–73.
10. Semba RD, Bloem MW. Measles blindness. Surv Ophthalmol 2004;49: 243–55.
11. Moss WJ, Cutts F, Griffin DE. Implications of the human immunodeficiency virus epidemic for control and eradication of measles. Clin Infect Dis 1999; 29:106–12.
12. Bellini WJ, Rota JS, Lowe LE, et al. Subacute sclerosing panencephalitis: more cases of this fatal disease are prevented by measles immunization than was previously recognized. J Infect Dis 2005;192:1686–93.
13. Department of Vaccines and Biologicals, World Health Organization. WHO-recommended standards of surveillance of selected vaccine-preventable diseases. Geneva: World Health Organization; 2003.
14. Bellini WJ, Helfand RF. The challenges and strategies for laboratory diagnosis of measles in an international setting. J Infect Dis 2003;187(suppl. 1):S283–90.
15. World Health Organization. Measles vaccines. Weekly Epidemiol Rec 2009; 84:349–60.
16. Dine MS, Hutchins SS, Thomas A, Williams I, et al. Persistence of vaccine-induced antibody to measles 26–33 years after vaccination. J Infect Dis 2004; 189(suppl. 1):S123–30.
17. D'Souza RM, D'Souza R. Vitamin A for the treatment of children with measles–a systematic review. J Trop Pediatr 2002;48:323–7.
18. World Health Organization. Measles Surveillance Data. Available at: http://www.who.int/immunization_monitoring/diseases/measles_monthlydata/en/index.html. Geneva: World Health Organization.
19. World Health Organization, Department of Immunization, Vaccines and Biologicals. WHO vaccine-preventable diseases: monitoring system. 2010 global summary. Immunization, Vaccines and Biologicals. Available at: http://www.who.int/immunization/documents/who_ivb_2010/en/index.html. Geneva: World Health Organization; 2010.
20. Krugman S, Katz SL, Gershon AA, Wilfert CM, eds. Infectious Diseases of Children, 9th edn. St Louis: Mosby; 1992.
21. Moss WJ, Griffin DE. Global measles elimination. Nat Rev Microbiol 2006; 4:900–8.
22. World Health Organization, Department of Vaccines and Biologicals. WHO-recommended standards of surveillance of selected vaccine-preventable diseases. Geneva: World Health Organization; 2003.

28.2 Poxviruses

Catherine G Sutcliffe, Anne W Rimoin, William J Moss

Key features

- Smallpox, caused by variola virus, historically the most important poxvirus of humans, was declared eradicated in 1980 following widespread vaccination with vaccinia virus
- Monkeypox:
  - zoonosis endemic in central and western Africa, clinically similar to smallpox although lymphadenopathy is more prominent and the mortality rate lower
  - transmitted by direct contact with infected animals or person to person via respiratory droplets
  - prior vaccination with vaccinia virus (smallpox vaccine) results in milder disease and significantly lower mortality
- Other important poxviruses diseases include:
  - Molluscum contagiousm – small umbilicated papules on the face, trunk or extremities of children worldwide
  - Orf – a zoonotic infection acquired from goats and sheep that manifests as papules, nodules and pustules at the site of inoculation

INTRODUCTION

Poxviruses belong to the family Poxviridae. Those which infect humans are found among four genera (*Orthopoxvirus, Parapoxvirus, Molluscipoxvirus* and *Yatapoxvirus*) within the Chordopoxvirinae subfamily (Table 28.2-1). The majority of poxvirus infections in humans are zoonoses, with only variola and molluscum contagiosum viruses being uniquely human pathogens. Poxviruses are large, generally brick-shaped virions containing double-stranded DNA that, in contrast to many other DNA viruses, replicate within the cytoplasm rather than in the nucleus [1].

Variola virus is the etiologic agent of smallpox and has been responsible for millions of deaths over thousands of years. The earliest archeological evidence dates to the Eighteenth Dynasty in ancient Egypt (1580–1350 BC). Large epidemics of smallpox have occurred in most civilizations, with 10–30% of cases resulting in death. Smallpox was eradicated through an intensive global campaign based on vaccination with vaccinia virus, a related *Orthopoxvirus* likely derived from cowpox virus. The last endemic case of smallpox occurred in Somalia in 1977; in 1980 the World Health Organization (WHO) officially declared smallpox eradicated [2].

More recently, concern has been raised about the use of variola virus as a biological weapon, resulting in increased interest in poxviruses. With more frequent global travel and the expansion of human populations into new habitats, the public health importance of zoonotic poxviruses and their potential to cause outbreaks have been

TABLE 28.2-1 Genera and Species of the Family Poxviridae, Subfamily Chordopoxvirinae that Affect Humans

Genus and species	Geographical distribution	Other infected animals	Reservoir
Orthopoxvirus			
Variola	Eradicated (formerly worldwide)	Humans	None
Monkeypox	Africa (USA)*	Humans, primates, zoo animals, prairie dogs	Squirrels, dormice, Gambian giant rat, hedgehog, Jerboa, opossum, woodchuck
Cowpox	Western Eurasia	Humans, cats, cows, elephants, gerbils, rats, okapi, zoo animals	Rodents (bank voles, long-tailed field mouse)
Vaccinia	Worldwide	Humans, cows, buffalo, rabbits, pigs	Most likely rodents
Parapoxvirus			
Bovine papular stomatitis	Worldwide	Humans, cows	Unknown (cows?)
Orf (contagious ectyma, contagious pustular dermatitis)	Worldwide	Humans, sheep, goat, artiodactyla, other ruminants	Unknown (sheep? goats?)
Pseudocowpox (paravaccinia, milker's nodule)	Worldwide	Humans, cows	Unknown (cows?)
Parapoxvirus of seals	Worldwide	Humans, seals	Unknown (seals?)
Parapoxvirus of reindeer	Finland	Humans, reindeer	Unknown
Molluscipoxvirus			
Molluscum contagiosum	Worldwide	Humans	Humans
Yatapoxvirus			
Tanapox	Africa	Humans, rodents	Mosquitoes(?), rodents(?)
Yabapox	Africa	Humans, primates	Unknown (primates?)
Yaba monkey tumor	Africa	Primates	Unknown

*Import of monkeypox to the USA with Gambian giant rats.
Adapted from Damon IK. Poxviruses. In: Knipe DM, Howley PM, eds. Field's Virology. Philadelphia: Lippincott Williams & Wilkins; 2007:2948–75, Essbauer S, Pfeffer M, Meyer H. Zoonotic poxviruses. Vet Microbiol 2009; 229–36, and Breman, JG. Poxviruses. In: Strickland GT, ed. Hunter's Tropical Medicine, 8th edn. Philadelphia: Saunders; 2000:207–10.

recognized. Monkeypox virus is a zoonotic poxvirus currently regarded as the most important *Orthopoxvirus* infection in humans since the global eradication of smallpox and is the focus of this chapter.

EPIDEMIOLOGY

Monkeypox virus was first identified in captive monkeys at the State Serum Institute in Copenhagen in 1958, although they are not the natural viral reservoir. Monkeypox virus is endemic to tropical rainforests of central and western Africa, with the majority of human cases occurring in the Democratic Republic of Congo (formerly Zaire) (Fig. 28.2.1). However, reports of monkeypox have increased in neighboring Republic of Congo and a cluster of cases were reported in 2006 in Sudan for the first time [3, 4]. In 2003, the first report of human monkeypox outside of the African continent occurred in the mid-western USA, and was associated with imported African rodents [5].

Outbreaks typically occur in small villages where inhabitants are engaged in hunting and gathering [2]. Humans contract monkeypox through direct contact with infected animals or humans. The majority of cases are contracted through direct contact with infected body fluids or lesions during hunting, skinning, killing or cooking animal carcasses. Such mammals include the great apes (chimpanzees and orangutans), many species of monkey, domestic pigs, African hedgehogs, opossums, many species of squirrel, dormice, African porcupines, rats, jerboa and shrews. The natural reservoir species is unknown; however, squirrels or other terrestrial rodents that inhabit the forests of central and western Africa are considered the most likely viral reservoirs [6, 7].

The first documented human case of monkeypox was a child in the Democratic Republic of Congo in 1970, two years after the last case of smallpox had occurred in the area [8]. After subsequent cases were recognized, the WHO began active surveillance in the Democratic Republic of Congo between 1981 and 1986, which identified a further 338 cases, with 28% attributed to secondary human-to-human transmission. The largest reported outbreak of monkeypox occurred in the Kasai Oriental region of the Democratic Republic of Congo during 1996 and 1997, although confusion with a concurrent varicella outbreak made precise estimates of the size of the outbreak difficult [9]. With increased global travel and interest in exotic pets, the geographic range of monkeypox has expanded. In 2003, the first outbreak of monkeypox outside of Africa occurred in the mid-western USA, with 71 cases, of which 35 were laboratory-confirmed [10]. Many cases had direct contact with infected pet prairie dogs. The outbreak was traced to imported giant Gambian rats from Ghana that were housed with prairie dogs. Despite this importation and the potential for monkeypox virus to infect a broad range of mammals, the virus does not appear to have established an endemic animal reservoir within the USA [6, 11].

Person-to-person transmission of monkeypox virus accounts for 10–30% of cases [9]. Transmission is through large respiratory droplets during prolonged face-to-face contact, although transmission through

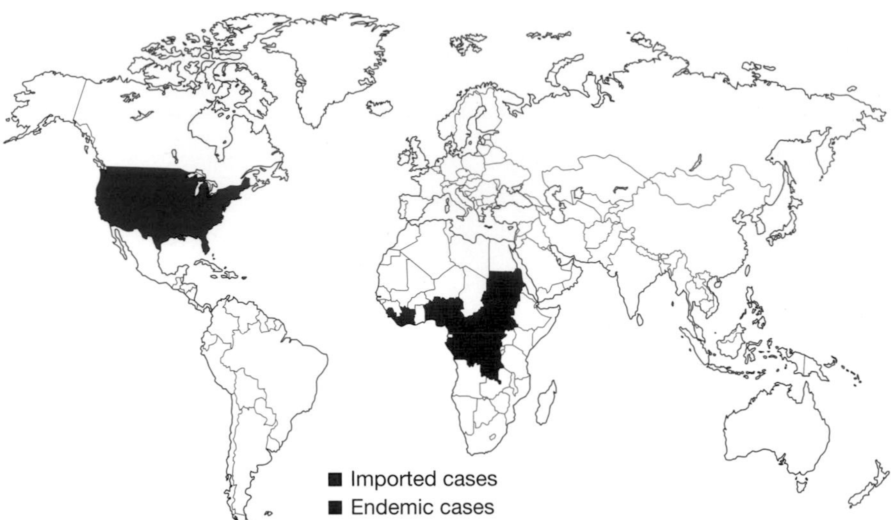

FIGURE 28.2.1 Map of endemic and imported Monkeypox cases since 1970.

contact with infected fomites or aerosols may occur [6]. Person-to-person transmission of monkeypox virus is less efficient than for variola virus and the longest recorded human chain of transmission is six generations [3]. Studies conducted in the 1980s suggested that household transmission from an index case occurred in 8–15% of contacts [12]. These data were used to create a stochastic model for the spread of monkeypox between humans, which indicated that monkeypox virus was highly unlikely to sustain itself in human populations and therefore did not constitute a major public health problem [13]. When these studies were conducted, the majority of household members were vaccinated against smallpox, which provided cross-protective immunity to monkeypox infection. Today, the majority of households are now vaccine-naïve, potentially increasing the risk for human-to-human transmission.

In endemic regions, transmission of human monkeypox has been reported throughout the year with no peak month or season. Incidence is highest in unvaccinated individuals under the age of 15 years and is slightly higher in males than females in this age group. In 1981, serologic surveys were carried out in four countries in central and western Africa to determine the prevalence of *Orthopoxvirus* infection and, in particular, monkeypox virus infection [14]. The prevalence of antibodies to orthopoxvirus was 15.4% among people without a history of smallpox vaccination. Only 0.7% of people tested were seropositive for monkeypox virus, with seroprevalence highest among children aged 5–9 years. More recently, a study conducted in the Republic of Congo after an outbreak of monkeypox in 2003 found a seroprevalence of 57% for orthopox viruses, with some seropositivity likely attributable to prior smallpox vaccination [15]. A 20-fold increase in the incidence of monkeypox was found in the Democratic Republic of Congo by active surveillance 30 years after cessation of smallpox and unvaccinated individuals were at a 5.2-fold increased risk of monkeypox [16].

The age distribution of cases and the secondary attack rate for monkeypox have changed, most likely as a result of cessation of smallpox vaccination and waning immunity among vaccinated persons. In the 1970s and 1980s, the majority of cases occurred among unvaccinated children younger than five years of age. Secondary cases tended to be older and were likely to be among mothers of infected children. As susceptibility to monkeypox increased, both the average age of infection and the proportion of secondary infections increased (Table 28.2-2). In the Democratic Republic of Congo, the mean age of cases of monkeypox increased from 4.4 years during the period 1981–1986 to 15.4 years during the period 2001–2004 [17].

Other poxviruses of humans include molluscum contagiosum, orf and tanapox viruses (Table 28.2-1). Molluscum contagiosum is the most common poxvirus infection of humans and causes umbilicated papules of 1–5-mm in size on the face, trunk or extremities of children worldwide. Orf, the most common *Parapoxvirus* infection of humans, is a zoonotic infection acquired from goats and sheep manifesting as papules, nodules and pustules at the site of inoculation. Tanapox virus, in the genus *Yatapoxvirus* and endemic in equatorial Africa, is transmitted by nonhuman primates via an arthropod vector or by direct contact, and results in a febrile illness with papulonodular skin lesions and lymphadenopathy.

NATURAL HISTORY AND PATHOGENESIS

Monkeypox begins with infection of either the dermis (after transmission from infected animals) or the respiratory epithelium (after transmission from an infected person). The virus disseminates through the lymphatic system resulting in primary viremia and systemic infection. A secondary viremia results in infection of epithelium, producing skin and mucosal lesions. As a consequence of replication in mucosal surfaces the virus can be transmitted through oropharyngeal secretions to close contacts. The risk of transmission likely depends on the density of oropharyngeal lesions, the proximity and duration of contact, and virus survival, despite host immune responses. Monkeypox virus, like other poxviruses, has evolved mechanisms to evade host immune responses. Monkeypox virus is likely to be stable on fomites and the number of virions required for infection is thought to be low, based on potential similarities with variola virus. Strain differences may exist—monkeypox strains circulating in western Africa appear to be more attenuated and less transmissible than those in the Congo basin [18].

The incubation period from exposure to the onset of clinical symptoms and signs is 10–14 days. Patients are infectious during the first week of rash and should be isolated [11]. Most people infected with monkeypox virus are symptomatic, but subclinical infection can occur. Serologic studies of household contacts of acutely infected cases in the Democratic Republic of Congo suggest that approximately 28% of all monkeypox infections are subclinical. More recently, immunologic evidence of exposure to monkeypox virus was identified in several asymptomatic contacts of infected people in the USA [19, 20].

HIV and other conditions that suppress cell mediated immunity may alter the natural history of disease. No data exist for monkeypox but other poxvirus infections, specifically vaccinia and molluscum contagiosum viruses, are more severe in those that are infected with HIV.

TABLE 28.2-2 Comparison of Epidemiologic Features of Human Monkeypox by Surveillance Period and Epidemiological Setting

Feature	1970–1979	1981–1986	1996–1997	2001–2004	2003
Location	Central and western Africa	Democratic Republic of Congo	Democratic Republic of Congo	Democratic Republic of Congo	Central USA
Epidemiologic setting	Passive surveillance	Active surveillance	Outbreak	Passive surveillance	Outbreak
Number of reported cases	47	338	419*	136	81
% laboratory confirmed	87	100	Unknown	37.5	40
Median age (yrs)	4	Unknown	Unknown	11	27
Suspected primary source	Unknown	Forest animals	Unknown	Squirrels, rodents, monkeys	Prairie dog, Gambian giant rat
Primary cases (%)	91	72	22	Unknown	100
Secondary cases (%)	9	28	78	Unknown	0
Secondary attack rate (%)	3.3	3.7†	8.0	Unknown	0
Case-fatality rate (%)	17	10	1.5	Unknown	0
Previous vaccinia vaccination	9% (with vaccine scar)	13%	6% (with vaccine scar)	Unknown	25%§

*Excludes 92 cases that were identified in an earlier investigation of the same outbreak but not included in the analysis of the subsequent cases.
†Among household contacts.
§Proportion of the confirmed cases for which information was available.
Sources: Di Giulio DB, Eckburg PB. Human monkeypox: an emerging zoonosis. Lancet Infect Dis 2004;4:15–25; Rimoin AW, Kisalu N, Kebela-Ilunga B, et al. Endemic human monkeypox, Democratic Republic of Congo, 2001–2004. Emerg Infect Dis 2007;13: 934–7.

CLINICAL FEATURES

The clinical features of monkeypox resemble those of smallpox (variola) (Table 28.2-3). Symptoms begin with a prodromal illness of fever and malaise lasting 1–3 days, followed by the characteristic rash. In contrast to smallpox, prominent submandibular, cervical, post-auricular, axillary or inguinal lymphadenopathy occurs in many infected persons 1–2 days before rash onset. Lymphadenopathy is not a typical feature of smallpox and can serve to clinically distinguish monkeypox from smallpox (Fig. 28.2.2; Table 28.2-3). As with smallpox, lesions develop concurrently and progress at a similar rate over 2–4 weeks, depending on the disease severity. The rash begins as small, 2–5-mm papules and progresses through vesicular, pustular and crusted stages over 2–3 weeks (Fig. 28.2.3). Like smallpox, it tends to be more severe on the head and extremities, including the palms and soles, and less intense on the trunk. The scabs slough off during recovery, leaving de-pigmented scars. Complications of monkeypox include secondary bacterial infection of the skin lesions, pneumonitis and eye involvement. Death occurs during the second week of illness in approximately 10% of cases. Prior vaccination with vaccinia virus (smallpox vaccine) results in milder disease with fewer skin lesions, less lymphadenopathy and significantly lower mortality [21].

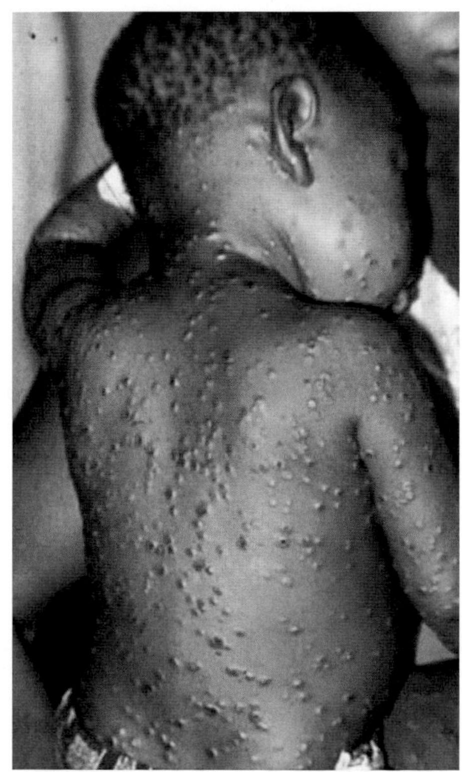

FIGURE 28.2.2 Posterior auricular lymphadenopathy in a child with monkeypox. *(Photo courtesy of Leo Lanoie, Prince Albert Parkland Health Region, Saskatchewan, Canada.)*

PATIENT EVALUATION, DIAGNOSIS, AND DIFFERENTIAL DIAGNOSIS

Poxvirus infection should be considered when evaluating a patient with a febrile illness and vesiculopustular rash, particularly when the patient resides in an area endemic for monkeypox virus (Fig. 28.2.1) or has contact with animals capable of transmitting poxviruses. A presumptive diagnosis of monkeypox can often be made clinically based on the characteristic rash and lymphadenopathy, although the skin lesions may be difficult to distinguish from chickenpox early in the course of illness (Table 28.2-3). Smallpox should be considered if bioterrorism is possible. Suspected cases of monkeypox should be reported to local health authorities.

TABLE 28.2-3 Differential Diagnosis of Monkeypox, Smallpox and Chickenpox

Variable	Monkeypox	Smallpox	Chickenpox
Incubation period, days	7–17	7–17	12–14
Prodrome period, days	1–4	2–4	0–2
Symptom			
Fever, severity	Moderate	Severe	Mild or none
Malaise, severity	Moderate	Moderate	Mild
Headache, severity	Moderate	Severe	Mild
Lymphadenopathy, severity	Moderate	None	None
Lesions			
Depth (diameter in mm)	Superficial to deep (4–6)	Deep (4–6)	Superficial (2–4)
Distribution	Centrifugal (mainly)	Centrifugal	Centripetal
Evaluation	Homogenous rash	Homogenous rash	Heterogeneous rash
Time to desquamation, days	14–21	14–21	6–14
Frequency of lesions on palms or soles of feet	Common	Common	Rare

From Nalca A, Rimoin AW, Bavari S, Whitehouse CA. Reemergence of monkeypox: prevalence, diagnostics, and countermeasures. Clin Infect Dis 2005;41: 1765–71.

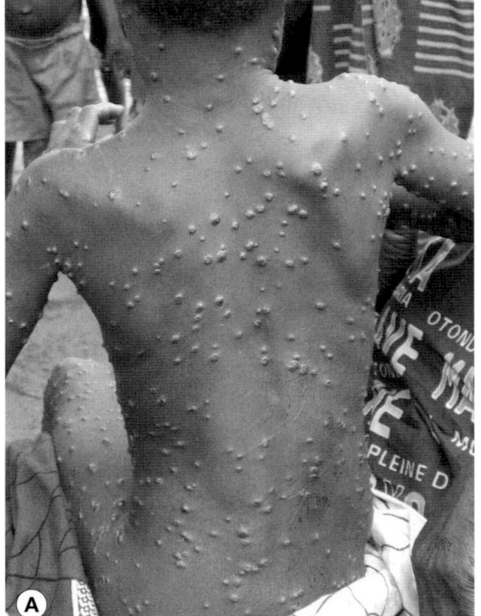

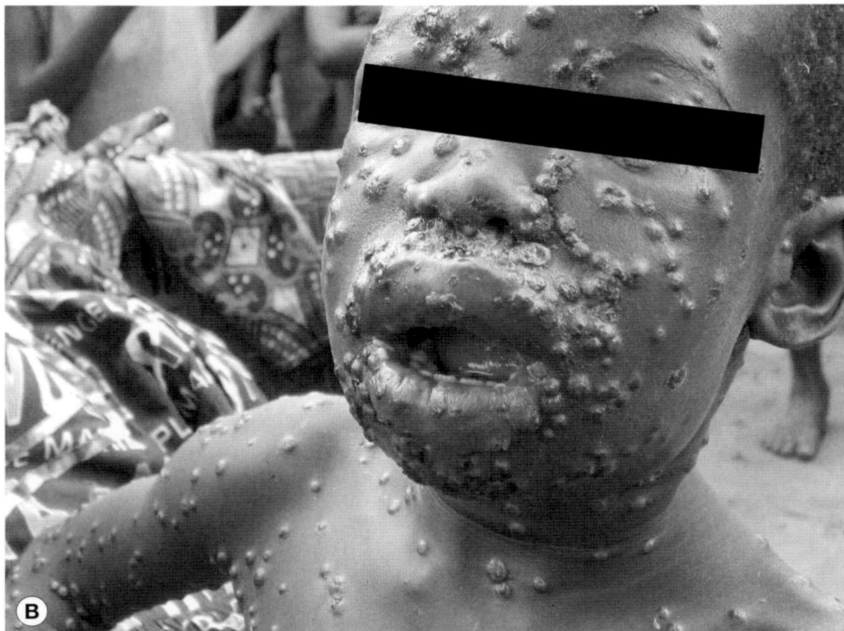

FIGURE 28.2.3 Human monkeypox in a 7-year-old girl, Tokondo, Kasai Oriental, Democratic Republic of Congo. *(Photos courtesy of Dr Anne W. Rimoin, UCLA-DRC Monkeypox Study. Tokondo, Democratic Republic of Congo.)*

Laboratory diagnosis is necessary to confirm the diagnosis of monkeypox and differentiate infection from other causes of vesiculopustular rash. The case definition developed by the Centers for Disease Control and Prevention (CDC) after the 2003 outbreak in the USA is shown in Table 28.2-4. Optimum clinical specimens for diagnostic testing include scabs or swabs of the base of vesicles applied to a microscope slide and air dried. Samples potentially infected with monkeypox virus should be handled in Biosafety Level 2 facilities. Monkeypox virus can be identified by cell culture or PCR-based assays. Serologic assays have insufficient sensitivity to reliably diagnose monkeypox infection.

With the exception of smallpox, monkeypox is most commonly confused clinically with varicella (chickenpox) (Table 28.2-3). Varicella can be distinguished from monkeypox because the skin lesions of chickenpox are pleomorphic (in different stages of development), concentrated on the trunk and rarely involve the palms and soles. Lymphadenopathy does not occur in uncomplicated varicella and the

TABLE 28.2-4 Centers for Disease Control and Prevention Case Definition for Monkeypox

Criteria for classification		
Clinical criteria	*Epidemiologic criteria*	*Laboratory criteria*

• Rash (macular, popular, vesicular, or pustular; generalized or localized; discrete or confluent)
• Fever (subjective or measured temperature of ≥99.3° F [≥ 37.4° C])
• Other signs and symptoms:
  ◦ Chills and/or sweats
  ◦ Headache
  ◦ Backache
  ◦ Lymphadenophathy
  ◦ Sore throat
  ◦ Cough
  ◦ Shortness of breath
	• Exposure* to an exotic wild mammalian pet† obtained on or after April 15, 2003, with clinical signs of illness (e.g. conjunctivitis, respiratory symptoms, and/or rash)
	• Exposure* to an exotic or wild mammalian pet† with or without clinical signs of illness that has been in contact with either a mammalian pet§ or a human with monkeypox
	• Exposure¶ to a suspect, probable, or confirmed human case of monkeypox
		• Isolation of monkeypox virus in culture
		• Demonstration of monkeypox virus DNA by polymerase chain reaction testing of a clinical specimen
		• Demonstration of virus morphologically consistent with an orthopoxvirus by electron microscopy in the absence of exposure to another orthopoxvirus
		• Demonstration of presence of orthopoxvirus in tissue using immunohistochemical testing methods in the absence of exposure to another orthopoxvirus

Case classification		
Suspect case	*Probable case*	*Confirmed case*

• Meets one of the epidemiologic criteria, AND
• Fever or unexplained rash, AND
• Two or more signs or symptoms with onset of first sign or symptoms <21 days after last exposure meeting epidemiologic criteria
	• Meets one of the epidemiologic criteria, AND
	• Fever, AND
	  ◦ Vesicular-pustular rash with onset of first sign or symptom <21 days after last exposure meeting epidemiologic criteria, OR
	  ◦ If rash is present but the type is not described, demonstrates elevated levels of IgM antibodies reactive with orthopox virus between at least days 7 to 56 after rash onset**
		• Meets one of the laboratory criteria

Exclusion criteria		
• An alternative diagnosis can fully explain the illness,†† OR • The case was reported on the basis of primary or secondary exposure to an exotic or wild mammalian pet or a human (see epidemiologic criteria) subsequently determined not to have monkeypox, provided other possible epidemiologic exposure criteria are not present, OR • A case without a rash does not develop a rash within 10 days of onset of clinical symptoms consistent with monkeypox.§§ • The case is determined to be negative for non-variola generic orthopoxvirus by polymerase chain reaction testing of a well samples rash lesion by the approved Laboratory Response Network (LRN) protocol, OR • The case is determined to have undetectable levels of IgM antibody during the period 7–56 days after rash onset.¶¶		

*Includes living in a household, petting or handling, or visiting a pet-holding facility (e.g. pet store, veterinary clinic, pet distributor).
†Includes prairie dogs, Gambian giant rats and rope squirrels.
§Includes living in a household or originating from the same pet-holding facility as another animal with monkeypox.
¶Includes skin-to-skin or face-to-face contact.
**Levels of circulating IgM antibody reactive with orthopoxvirus antigen are determined by ELISA and reported as optical density (OD) values. Values greater than three standard deviations above the mean OD of six independent negative controls are considered "elevated". IgM antibody levels may be elevated in persons who have been recently (within one year) vaccinated for smallpox.
††Factors that might be considered in assigning alternate diagnoses include the strength of the epidemiologic exposure criteria for monkeypox, the specificity of the diagnostic test, and the compatibility of the clinical presentation and course of illness for the alternative diagnosis.
§§If possible, obtain convalescent-phase serum specimen from these patients.
¶¶The optimal timing of specimen collection for determination of IgM levels is between days 7 and 56 post-rash onset. However, elevated levels of IgM antibodies may be detectable prior to day 7 or after day 56 post-rash onset; therefore, a negative result during this phase should not be interpreted to indicate an absence of monkeypox infection.
From Centers for Disease Control and Prevention. Updated Interim Case Definition for Human Monkeypox, Available at: http://www.cdc.gov/ncidod/monkeypox/ (last accessed: 6 March 2012). January 2004.

illness resolves in two weeks. Other causes of a vesiculopapular rash include drug eruptions, eczema herpeticum, dermatitis herpetiformis, rickettsialpox, and molluscum contagiosum [9].

PREVENTION AND TREATMENT

Access to basic health care in remote forested areas of western and central sub-Saharan Africa can be difficult, and the prevention and treatment of monkeypox is severely limited in the absence of external assistance. Data from the Democratic Republic of Congo in the early 1980s suggested that pre-exposure smallpox vaccination provided approximately 85% protection against monkeypox [22]. Prior smallpox vaccination, however, did not provide complete protection against monkeypox in the USA [19]. The CDC recommends pre-exposure smallpox vaccination for field investigators, veterinarians and healthcare workers investigating or caring for patients with suspected monkeypox. No information is available on the efficacy of post-exposure vaccination with vaccinia virus, although extrapolation from post-exposure vaccination for the prevention of smallpox suggests vaccination may prevent monkeypox disease or reduce severity. Hence, the CDC recommends post-exposure smallpox vaccination within four days of exposure to monkeypox and consideration of vaccination within two weeks of exposure.

Treatment of persons with monkeypox is supportive. Data are not available on the effectiveness of vaccinia immune globulin for the prevention or treatment of complications of monkeypox; however, the CDC recommends immune globulin be considered for prophylactic use in persons exposed to monkeypox virus with severe cellular immunodeficiency for whom smallpox vaccination is contraindicated [23]. Cidofovir has anti-monkeypox viral activity *in vitro* and in animal studies [24]. Whether humans may benefit is not known, but the CDC recommends that cidofovir therapy be considered in persons with severe monkeypox [23].

REFERENCES

1. Damon IK. Poxviruses. In: Knipe DM, Howley PM, eds. Field's Virology. Philadelphia: Lippincott Williams & Wilkins; 2007:2948–75.
2. Fenner F, Henderson DA, Arita I, et al. Smallpox and Its Eradication. Geneva: World Health Organization; 1988.
3. Learned LA, Reynolds MG, Wassa DW, et al. Extended interhuman transmission of monkeypox in a hospital community in the Republic of the Congo, 2003. Am J Trop Med Hyg 2005;73:428–34.
4. Damon IK, Roth CE, Chowdhary V. Discovery of monkeypox in Sudan. N Engl J Med 2006;355:962–3.
5. Reed KD, Melski JW, Graham MB, et al. The detection of monkeypox in humans in the Western Hemisphere. N Engl J Med 2004;350:342–50.
6. Parker S, Nuara A, Buller RM, Schultz DA. Human monkeypox: an emerging zoonotic disease. Future Microbiol 2007;2:17–34.
7. Essbauer S, Pfeffer M, Meyer H. Zoonotic poxviruses. Vet Microbiol 2009; 229–36.
8. Ladnyj ID, Ziegler P, Kima E. A human infection caused by monkeypox virus in Basankusu Territory, Democratic Republic of the Congo. Bull World Health Organ 1972;46:593–7.
9. Di Giulio DB, Eckburg PB. Human monkeypox: an emerging zoonosis. Lancet Infect Dis 2004;4:15–25.
10. Centers for Disease Control and Prevention. Update: multistate outbreak of monkeypox—Illinois, Indiana, Kansas, Missouri, Ohio, and Wisconsin, 2003. MMWR Morb Mortal Wkly Rep 2003;52:642–6.
11. Nalca A, Rimoin AW, Bavari S, Whitehouse CA. Reemergence of monkeypox: prevalence, diagnostics, and countermeasures. Clin Infect Dis 2005;41: 1765–71.
12. Jezek Z, Grab B, Szczeniowski MV, et al. Human monkeypox: secondary attack rates. Bull World Health Organ 1988;66:465–70.
13. Jezek Z, Grab B, Dixon H. Stochastic model for interhuman spread of monkeypox. Am J Epidemiol 1987;126:1082–92.
14. Jezek Z, Nakano JH, Arita I, et al. Serological survey for human monkeypox infections in a selected population in Zaire. J Trop Med Hyg 1987;90:31–8.
15. Lederman ER, Reynolds MG, Karem K, et al. Prevalence of antibodies against orthopoxviruses among residents of Likouala region, Republic of Congo: evidence for monkeypox virus exposure. Am J Trop Med Hyg 2007;77: 1150–6.
16. Rimoin AW, Mulembakani PM, Johnston SC, et al. Major increase in human monkeypox incidence 30 years after smallpox vaccination campaigns cease in the Democratic Republic of Congo. Proc Natl Acad Sci USA 2010;107: 16262–7.
17. Rimoin AW, Kisalu N, Kebela-Ilunga B, et al. Endemic human monkeypox, Democratic Republic of Congo, 2001–2004. Emerg Infect Dis 2007;13: 934–7.
18. Chen N, Li G, Liszewski MK, et al. Virulence differences between monkeypox virus isolates from West Africa and the Congo basin. Virology 2005;340: 46–63.
19. Karem KL, Reynolds M, Hughes C, et al. Monkeypox-induced immunity and failure of childhood smallpox vaccination to provide complete protection. Clin Vaccine Immunol 2007;14:1318–27.
20. Lewis MW, Graham MB, Hammarlund E, et al. Monkeypox without exanthem. N Engl J Med 2007;356:2112–14.
21. Hammarlund E, Lewis MW, Carter SV, et al. Multiple diagnostic techniques identify previously vaccinated individuals with protective immunity against monkeypox. Nat Med 2005;11:1005–11.
22. Fine PE, Jezek Z, Grab B, Dixon H. The transmission potential of monkeypox virus in human populations. Int J Epidemiol 1988;17:643–50.
23. Centers for Disease Control and Prevention. Updated Interim CDC Guidance for Use of Smallpox Vaccine, Cidofovir, and Vaccinia Immune Globulin (VIG) for Prevention and Treatment in the Setting of an Outbreak of Monkeypox Infections. 2003.
24. De Clercq E. Cidofovir in the treatment of poxvirus infections. Antiviral Res 2002;55:1–13.
25. Breman, JG. Poxviruses. In: Strickland GT, ed. Hunter's Tropical Medicine, 8th edn. Philadelphia: Saunders; 2000:207–10.
26. Centers for Disease Control and Prevention. Updated Interim Case Definition for Human Monkeypox, Available at: http://www.cdc.gov/ncidod/monkeypox/ (last accessed: 6 March 2012). January 2004.

28.3 Nonpolio Enterovirus Mucocutaneous Infections

Catherine G Sutcliffe, William J Moss

Key features

- Enteroviruses replicate within the gastrointestinal tract or other mucosal surfaces
- Acute hemorrhagic conjunctivitis is primarily caused by enterovirus 70 and a variant of coxsackievirus A24
- Epidemics of hemorrhagic conjunctivitis can be explosive, with up to 100% of household members and 15% of the population ultimately infected
- Hand-foot-and-mouth disease is most commonly caused by coxsackievirus A16 and enterovirus 71
- Rarely, hand-foot-and-mouth disease caused by enterovirus 71 may be associated with severe neurologic complications (see Chapter 34.2)

INTRODUCTION

Enteroviruses are members of the *Picornaviridae* family and are nonenveloped viruses with a single-stranded RNA genome that replicate within the gastrointestinal tract or other mucosal surfaces. More than 90 subtypes of enteroviruses have been identified. Human enteroviruses were formally divided into five subgroups: polioviruses; group A and B coxsackieviruses; echoviruses; and the numbered human enteroviruses. In 2000, the International Committee on Taxonomy of Viruses re-classified human enteroviruses into four species consisting of human enteroviruses A, B, C (containing the polioviruses) and D (Table 28.3-1) [1]. In addition to the four human enterovirus species A–D (shown in Table 28.3-1), other enteroviral species include: human rhinoviruses (A–C); and porcine, bovine and simian enteroviruses. Echoviruses 22 and 23 were reclassified as a new genus called parechoviruses (human parechoviruses 1 and 2).

Enteroviruses are ubiquitous and most infections are asymptomatic. Some enteroviruses, best known for mucocutaneous disease, are

TABLE 28.3-1 Enteroviral Species and Types Currently Recognized

Enterovirus species	Types
Human enterovirus A	Human coxsackievirus A2–8, 10, 12, 14, 16
	Human enterovirus 71, 76, 89–92
Human enterovirus B	Human coxsackievirus A9, B1–6
	Human echovirus 1–9, 11–21, 24–27, 29–33
	Human enterovirus 69, 73–75, 77–88, 93, 97, 98, 101, 106, 107
Human enterovirus C	Human poliovirus 1–3
	Human coxsackievirus A1, 11, 13, 15, 17–22, 24
	Human enterovirus 95, 96, 99, 102, 104, 105, 109
Human enterovirus D	Human enterovirus 68, 70, 94

Modified from Wong SS, Yip CC, Lau SK, Yuen KY. Human enterovirus 71 and hand, foot and mouth disease. Epidemiol Infect 2010;138:1071–89.

discussed in this chapter. Enteroviruses that are best known for causing neurologic disease, including polioviruses and enterovirus 71, are discussed in Chapter 34.2. Several new enteroviruses have emerged that have pandemic potential, including those causing acute hemorrhagic conjunctivitis and hand-foot-and-mouth disease (HFMD).

EPIDEMIOLOGY

Acute hemorrhagic conjunctivitis is primarily caused by enterovirus 70 and a variant of coxsackievirus A24; however, other enteroviruses, including echoviruses 7 and 11, coxsackieviruses B1 and B2, and several adenoviruses can also cause acute hemorrhagic conjunctivitis, sporadic conjunctivitis and keratoconjunctivitis. The first pandemic of hemorrhagic conjunctivitis was identified in Ghana in 1969 with subsequent spread to other countries in Africa and Southeast Asia, India, Japan and England between 1969 and 1971, affecting millions of people [2]. Enteroviruses capable of causing hemorrhagic conjunctivitis are highly transmissible, particularly in densely populated areas in the tropics, where good hygiene is not easy, and are spread either directly through ocular and respiratory secretions or indirectly through contaminated fomites (inanimate objects such as toys). Epidemics of hemorrhagic conjunctivitis can be explosive, with up to 100% of household members and 15% of the population ultimately infected. Outbreaks can be seasonal, particularly in the western hemisphere. Individuals of both sexes and all ages are susceptible, although adolescents and young adults are most commonly infected [3].

HFMD is most commonly caused by coxsackievirus A16 and enterovirus 71. Other enteroviruses associated with HFMD include: coxsackieviruses A4–A7, A9, A10, A24, and B2–B5; echoviruses 1, 4, 11 and 18; and enterovirus18. HFMD was first described during an outbreak in 1958 [1] and has been reported in North and South America, Europe and Asia. However, since the 1990s, enterovirus 71-associated outbreaks have occurred most frequently in Taiwan, Singapore, Malaysia, China, Vietnam and Australia [4] (see Chapter 34.2).

NATURAL HISTORY, PATHOGENESIS AND PATHOLOGY

Direct transmission of enterovirus 70 or coxsackievirus A24 from infected hands or fomites to the eye permits viral replication in the palpebral and bulbar conjunctivae and corneal epithelial cells. Both viruses bind to sialic acid on ocular epithelium but coxsackievirus A24 can also bind to cells expressing sialic acid in the respiratory tract— accounting for concurrent respiratory symptoms [5]. Viral replication in the conjunctivae and cornea leads to the destruction of cells and resulting hemorrhagic conjunctivitis. The incubation period from the time of exposure to conjunctivitis is typically 24–72 hours. Disease severity is variable and depends on the number of infected cells and extent of inflammation. Protective immune responses are elicited following enterovirus 70 and coxsackievirus A24 infections; however, immunity to enterovirus 70 wanes within seven years, leaving individuals susceptible to re-infection [6].

The pathogenesis of HFMD remains unclear but fecal–oral transmission likely leads to virus replication in the lower gastrointestinal tract, followed by viremia and further replication in the oropharynx (see Chapter 34.2).

CLINICAL FEATURES

Most enteroviral infections are asymptomatic or associated with a nonspecific febrile illness. Signs and symptoms of respiratory tract infection (coryza, pharyngitis and pneumonia) and herpangina (multiple oral ulcers at the back of the oral cavity) may occur, but it remains unclear if enteroviruses are a significant cause of vomiting, diarrhea or abdominal pain. Rare, serious clinical manifestations include neonatal sepsis, meningoencephalitis and myopericarditis. Infection with enterovirus 71 can result in pulmonary edema, pulmonary hemorrhage and cardiopulmonary failure. Chronic enterovirus infection can occur in persons with defective B-lymphocyte function, including those with X-linked agammaglobulinemia, severe combined immunodeficiency or common variable immunodeficiency.

Individuals with acute hemorrhagic conjunctivitis have abrupt onset of eye pain, photophobia and swelling of the eyelids. Fever, headache and pre-auricular lymphadenopathy may occur. Subconjunctival hemorrhage is the characteristic clinical manifestation and occurs in the majority of ocular infections caused by enterovirus 70 but is less common with coxsackievirus A24 ocular infection. Signs and symptoms typically peak on the first day of infection and resolve within several days without complications.

Children with HFMD usually present with fever, sore throat and refusal to eat. Physical examination reveals vesicles and ulcers on the buccal mucosa and tongue, and papules and vesicles with surrounding erythema on the hands, feet, wrists, ankles, buttocks and genitalia. HFMD caused by enterovirus 71 and coxsackievirus A16 is usually indistinguishable, although some observers state that the skin lesions associated with coxsackievirus A16 infection are larger and the lesions of enterovirus 71 infection are more commonly papular and petechial [7]. Rarely, HFMD caused by enterovirus 71 may be associated with severe neurologic complications, including aseptic meningitis, brainstem or cerebellar encephalitis, and acute flaccid paralysis (see Chapter 34.2). Permanent paralysis or death can result.

Other severe systemic manifestations of enterovirus infections include: acute respiratory disease, particularly with coxsackie A21 and A24 and echovirus 11; epidemic pleurodynia, characterized by chest pains, and caused by coxsackie B viruses; myocarditis and pericarditis, caused by coxsackie B viruses; and neonatal enterovirus infections, caused, in particular, by echovirus 11 and coxsackievirus B.

PATIENT EVALUATION, DIAGNOSIS AND DIFFERENTIAL DIAGNOSIS

Enterovirus infection should be suspected in persons with hemorrhagic conjunctivitis and those with vesicles and papules on the

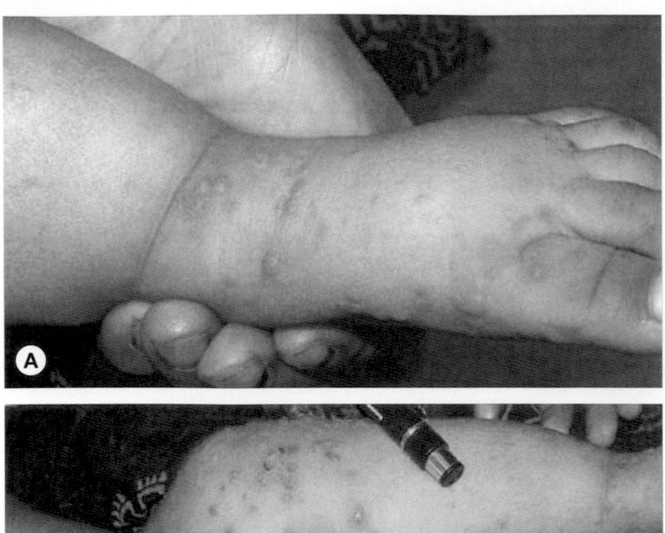

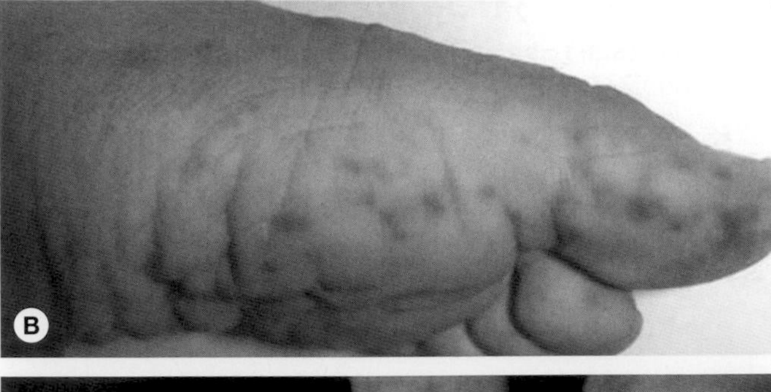

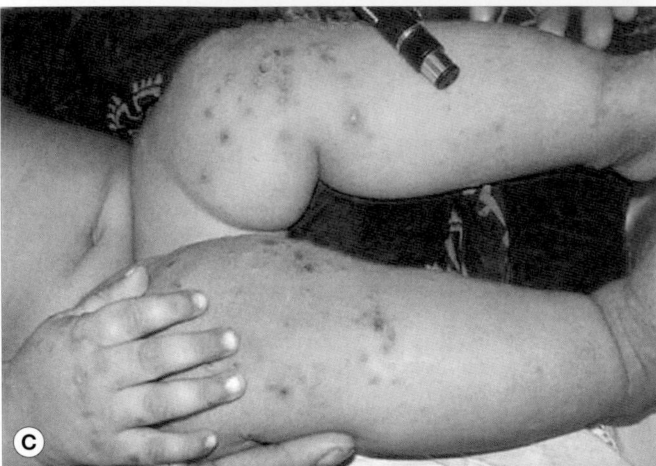

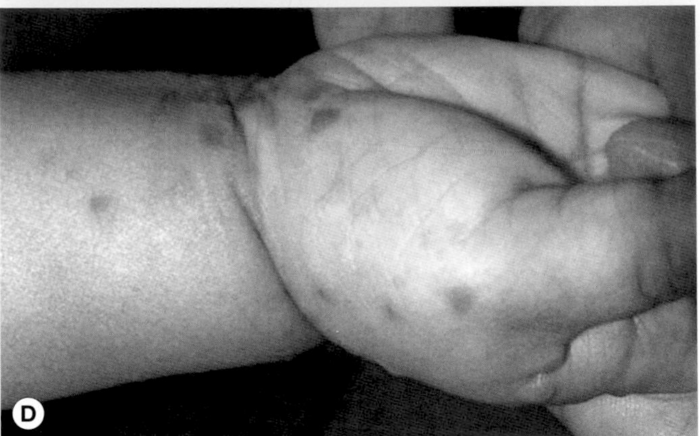

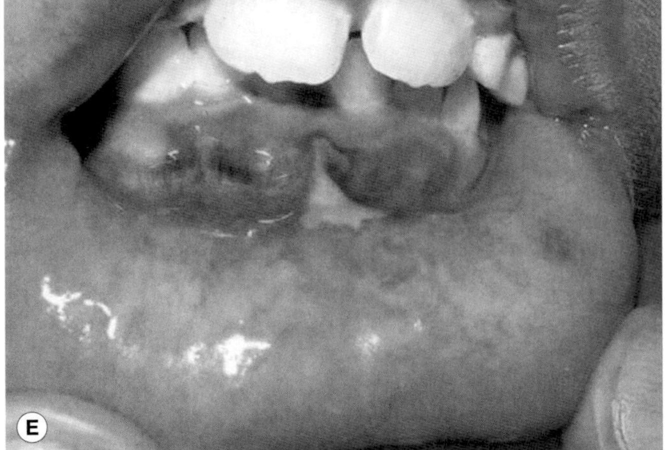

FIGURE 28.3.1 Clinical symptoms of hand-foot-and-mouth disease. **(A)** Severe involvement of the dorsum of the foot with multiple vesicles. **(B)** Erythematous papules without vesicles over the margin of the foot. **(C)** Multiple papulo-vesicular eruptions over the knee and the hand. **(D)** Erythematous papules with mild vesiculation over thenar eminence and margin of the hand. **(E)** Diffuse erythema over the lower gum along with erosion from a ruptured vesicle over the inner side of lip *(reproduced from Sarma N, Sarkar A, Mukherjee A, et al. Epidemic of hand, foot and mouth disease in West Bengal, India in August, 2007: a multicentric study. Indian J Dermatol. 2009;54:26–30.)*

hands, feet and in the oropharynx (Fig. 28.3.1). The diagnosis is usually first made on clinical grounds but enterovirus infection can be confirmed by cell culture or identification of viral RNA by reverse-transcriptase PCR. The generalized rash associated with enterovirus infection can resemble that of measles, rubella or roseola. Acute hemorrhagic conjunctivitis can be caused by enteroviruses other than enterovirus 70 and coxsackievirus A24, as well as adenoviruses (particularly type 11). However, these viral causes cannot be clinically distinguished. The skin lesions of HFMD may resemble those of herpes simplex virus or varicella-zoster virus infections (Table 28.3-2) [3], and the acute flaccid paralysis can be confused with paralytic poliomyelitis

PREVENTION AND TREATMENT

Good hygiene, particularly hand-washing, limits fecal–oral or ocular transmission and is the primary method of preventing enterovirus infection. Social distancing measures, such as closing schools, are also used [8]. Vaccines against enterovirus 71, including live-attenuated virus, inactivated whole virus, recombinant viral protein, virus-like particle and DNA vaccines are in development, but none are currently licensed for use [9]. No specific therapy for enterovirus infection is recommended. The antiviral agent pleconaril has activity against enteroviruses but evidence supporting clinical efficacy is lacking [10]. Intravenous immune globulin has been used to treat severe

TABLE 28.3-2 Comparison of Acute Hemorrhagic Conjunctivitis and Other Common Types of Conjunctivitis

Feature	Acute hemorrhagic conjunctivitis	Adenoviral conjunctivitis	Epidemic keratoconjunctivitis	Pharyngoconjunctival fever	Primary herpes simplex
Age group	All ages	All ages	All ages	Mostly children	Young children
Etiologic agent	Enterovirus 70, coxsackievirus A24	Adenovirus	Adenovirus types 8, 19	Adenovirus types 1, 2, 3	Herpes simplex virus
Duration	5–10 days	1–2 weeks	2–4 weeks	3 weeks	2–3 weeks
Physical findings					
Bilateral involvement	80%	Frequent	Usually	Often unilateral	Rare
Subconjunctival hemorrhage	Frequent	Rare	Occasional	Rare	Rare
Keratitis	Frequent	Occasional	Marked but rare early	Occasional	Occasional
Subepithelial opacities	Occasional	Occasional	Frequent	Occasional	Rare
Pseudomembrane	No	Occasional	Occasional	No	Occasional
Follicles	Slight	Marked	Marked	Marked	Moderate
Other symptoms	Upper respiratory tract infection common in coxsackievirus A24	Respiratory symptoms common	Upper respiratory tract infection, diarrhea common in children	Triad of fever, pharyngitis and conjunctivitis	Dendritic keratitis rare with primary conjunctivitis

Reproduced with permission from Wright PW, Strauss GH, Langford MP. Acute hemorrhagic conjunctivitis. Am Fam Physician 1992;45:173–8.

enteroviral infections, including overwhelming infection in neonates, myocarditis and meningoencephalitis, but data from controlled clinical trials are not available.

REFERENCES

1. Wong SS, Yip CC, Lau SK, Yuen KY. Human enterovirus 71 and hand, foot and mouth disease. Epidemiol Infect 2010;138:1071–89.
2. Mirkovic RR, Kono R, Yin-Murphy M, et al. Enterovirus type 70: the etiologic agent of pandemic acute haemorrhagic conjunctivitis. Bull World Health Organ 1973;49:341–6.
3. Wright PW, Strauss GH, Langford MP. Acute hemorrhagic conjunctivitis. Am Fam Physician 1992;45:173–8.
4. Ooi MH, Wong SC, Lewthwaite P, et al. Clinical features, diagnosis, and management of enterovirus 71. Lancet Neurol 2010;9:1097–105.
5. Nilsson EC, Jamshidi F, Johansson SM, et al. Sialic acid is a cellular receptor for coxsackievirus A24 variant, an emerging virus with pandemic potential. J Virol 2008;82:3061–8.
6. Aoki K, Sawada H. Long-term observation of neutralization antibody after enterovirus 70 infection. Jpn J Ophthalmol 1992;36:465–8.
7. Lee TC, Guo HR, Su HJ, et al. Diseases caused by enterovirus 71 infection. Pediatr Infect Dis J 2009;28:904–10.
8. Solomon T, Lewthwaite P, Perera D, et al. Virology, epidemiology, pathogenesis, and control of enterovirus 71. Lancet Infect Dis 2010;10.778–90.
9. Lee MS, Chang LY. Development of enterovirus 71 vaccines. Expert Rev Vaccines 2010;9:149–56.
10. Webster AD. Pleconaril—an advance in the treatment of enteroviral infection in immuno-compromised patients. J Clin Virol 2005;32:1–6.
11. Sarma N, Sarkar A, Mukherjee A, et al. Epidemic of hand, foot and mouth disease in West Bengal, India in August, 2007: a multicentric study. Indian J Dermatol. 2009;54:26–30.

28.4 Kaposi's Sarcoma-associated Herpesvirus

Catherine G Sutcliffe, William J Moss

Key features

- Kaposi's sarcoma-associated herpesvirus (KSHV) is associated with three lymphoproliferative disorders: Kaposi's sarcoma, which is a cutaneous malignancy; primary effusion lymphoma; and multi-centric Castleman's disease
- The epidemiology of KSHV transmission varies, with sexual transmission predominant in many regions and salivary transmission common among children in parts of sub-Saharan Africa

Key features—cont'd

- Kaposi's sarcoma occurs in four clinical and epidemiologic types: classic, endemic, immunosuppressed-associated and AIDS-associated
- Endemic Kaposi's sarcoma is found in central Africa where children are prone to a rapidly fatal, lymphadenopathic form
- Highly active anti-retroviral therapy can reduce the incidence of Kaposi's sarcoma and the severity of pre-existing lesions in persons co-infected with human immunodeficiency virus (HIV)

INTRODUCTION

Kaposi's sarcoma-associated herpesvirus (KSHV), also called human herpesvirus 8 (HHV-8), is a member of the lymphotropic gammaherpesviruses, which includes Epstein-Barr virus. As with other herpesviruses, KSHV likely evolved and migrated out of Africa with modern humans. Kaposi's sarcoma, a multifocal cutaneous neoplasm of vascular endothelium, was first described by the Hungarian dermatologist Moritz Kaposi in 1872 as an indolent neoplasm of older men residing in Eastern Europe and the Mediterranean. A more aggressive form of endemic Kaposi's sarcoma was subsequently identified in children and adults in Africa, particularly in the region surrounding Lake Kivu in the Democratic Republic of Congo and Rwanda, where it accounts for up to 10% of all malignancies in children. With the advent of immunosuppressive therapies for organ transplantation, Kaposi's sarcoma was recognized as a complication of immune suppression and the disease became widely known as a signal event of the AIDS epidemic [1]. These four variants correspond to the classic, endemic, immunosuppressed-associated and AIDS-associated forms. The etiology of Kaposi's sarcoma remained elusive until KSHV was identified in 1994 by representational difference analysis of viral DNA fragments from tissue samples [2].

EPIDEMIOLOGY

KSHV is only found in humans. There are four distinct subtypes of KSHV: subtypes A and C are predominantly found in Europe, the USA, Asia and the Middle East; subtype B is predominantly found in sub-Saharan Africa; and subtype D is predominantly found in south Asia, Australia and the Pacific Islands.

While infection with KSHV occurs worldwide, the prevalence of infection varies (Table 28.4-1) [3, 4]. In the USA, Asia, Europe, South America and the Caribbean, the overall prevalence of KSHV infection is less than 10%. In these regions, KSHV is primarily sexually transmitted. Pre-pubertal children are not usually infected and the prevalence of infection increases with age after the onset of sexual activity. In these epidemiologic settings, KSHV infections are more common among men than women. Homosexual transmission appears to be more efficient than heterosexual transmission, with seroprevalences ranging from 25–60% among male homosexuals and increasing with the number of sexual partners.

In the Mediterranean, the prevalence of KSHV infection ranges from 15–25%. In sub-Saharan Africa and American Indian populations in South America, however, KSHV is endemic, with the prevalence of infection 50–60% or higher (Fig. 28.4.1). In these regions, infection is equally prevalent among men and women and the majority of infections are acquired in childhood, suggesting transmission through non-sexual routes [4]. Salivary transmission, often through contact within the family, is the predominant mode of transmission. Following puberty, the prevalence of KSHV rises slowly as a result of less efficient heterosexual transmission. Mother-to-child transmission of KSHV can occur, but is infrequent [5], and the virus is not found in breast milk [6]. Studies in Africa have found different age-related patterns of KSHV infection, suggesting different patterns of transmission within endemic regions [7].

NATURAL HISTORY, PATHOGENESIS AND PATHOLOGY

The natural history of KSHV begins with infection of endothelial cells and B lymphocytes following contact with infected secretions. Viral latency is established in B lymphocytes, resulting in life-long infection. KSHV cycles between two phases: a latent phase during which the virus lies silent with limited gene expression, and a lytic phase with active replication in the oropharynx and viral shedding in saliva. Similar to other herpesviruses, KSHV evolved mechanisms to evade host immune responses, including modulation of immune surveillance and antiviral responses [8]. The viral genome also encodes oncogenic proteins capable of dysregulating cell growth that are likely

TABLE 28.4-1 Patterns of Kaposi's Sarcoma-Associated Herpesvirus (KSHV) Infection and Non-HIV Kaposi's Sarcoma (KS)

KS Incidence*	Regions	Population KSHV prevalence	Transmission	Risk groups
Low	North America, North Europe, Asia	<5%	Sexual	Homosexual men, STD clinic attendees, transplant recipients
Intermediate	Mediterranean, Middle Eastern countries, Caribbean	5–20%	Sexual, non-sexual?	Homosexual men, STD clinic attendees, transplant recipients, older adults
High	Africa, parts of Amazon basin	>50%	Non-sexual, sexual	Older adults, lower socioeconomic status

*AIDS-KS rates are highly dependent on local HIV infection rates and risk groups.
STD, sexually transmitted diseases.
Reproduced with permission from Ganem D. Kaposi's Sarcoma-associated Herpesvirus. In: Knipe DM, Howley PM, eds. Field's Virology. Philadelphia: Lippincott Williams & Wilkins; 2007:2847–88.

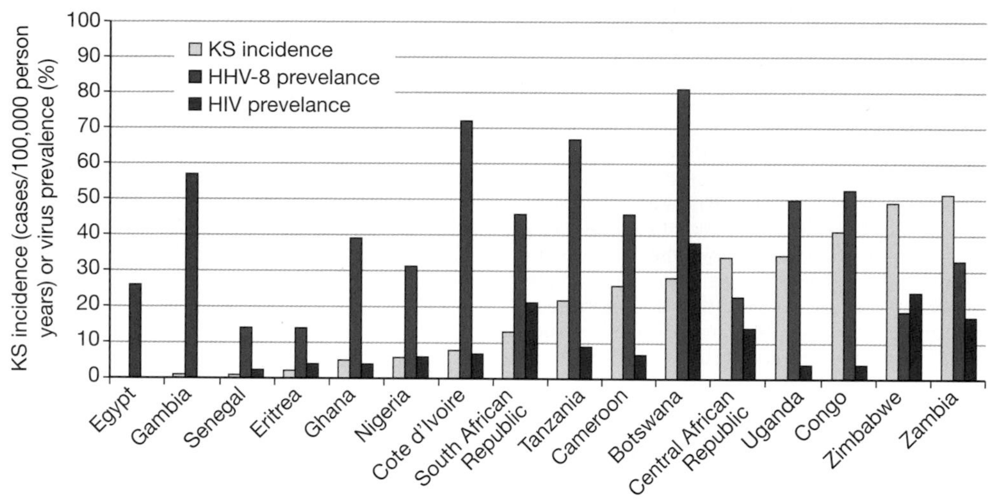

FIGURE 28.4.1 Prevalence of HHV-8 and HIV infection and incidence of Kaposi's sarcoma (KS) in select African countries, ranked according to incidence of KS *(reproduced with permission from Casper C. New approaches to the treatment of human herpesvirus 8-associated disease. Rev Med Virol 2008;18:321–9.)*

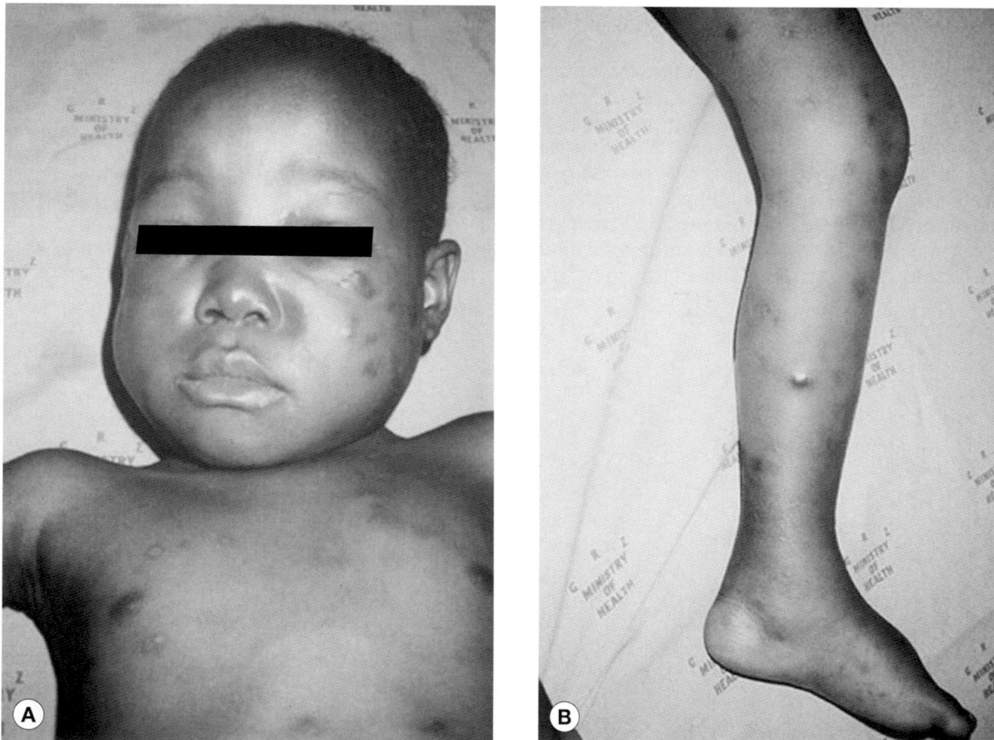

FIGURE 28.4.2 African child with lymphadenopathic Kaposi's sarcoma. The raised nodules with purple hue are evident on the face, trunk and leg. Lymphatic obstruction resul ted in facial edema *(courtesy of William Moss MD)*.

involved in the pathogenesis of the associated proliferative disorders [9]. Histologically, Kaposi's sarcoma is characterized by spindle cells with vascular spaces and extravasated red blood cells. The lesions of Kaposi's sarcoma are multicentric in origin and not the result of metastases.

CLINICAL FEATURES

Infection with KSHV is asymptomatic in most individuals, but some children with primary infection may have a nonspecific febrile illness [10]. More importantly, KSHV infection is associated with three lymphoproliferative disorders, primarily in immunocompromised hosts: Kaposi's sarcoma; primary effusion lymphoma; and multicentric Castleman's disease [8]. The lesions of Kaposi's sarcoma are commonly flat or raised nodules, 0.5–2.0 cm in diameter, with a purple hue as a consequence of numerous, poorly oxygenated red blood cells (Fig. 28.4.2). With more advanced disease, these nodules may coalesce. Lesions are common in the mouth and on the face, nose and extremities, but can also occur in the lung, biliary tract, and gastrointestinal tract. Children in endemic areas are more likely to have a rapidly fatal lymphadenopathic form that leads to edema (Fig. 28.4.2). Some lesions of Kaposi's sarcoma may spontaneously regress, confounding the evaluation of treatment strategies.

PATIENT EVALUATION, DIAGNOSIS AND DIFFERENTIAL DIAGNOSIS

Infection with KSHV is diagnosed serologically or by detection of viral DNA in saliva, tissue or blood samples. The diagnosis of Kaposi's sarcoma should be considered in patients with compatible skin or mucus membrane lesions and who reside in an endemic area or are HIV-infected or immunosuppressed. The diagnosis is made by careful physical examination of the skin and mucosal surfaces. Pathological examination of the biopsied lesions shows the characteristic highly vascular, spindle-shaped cells, although histologic variants with mixed cell or anaplastic types are not uncommon. Detection of gastrointestinal or pulmonary lesions requires imaging studies, such as a chest radiograph, although pulmonary findings are often non-specific. Clinical diagnosis is usually not problematic in persons with multiple lesions and with the appropriate clinical context. Isolated lesions, however, may be confused with hemangiomas, dermatofibromas or pyogenic granulomas. Kaposi's sarcoma may be clinically confused with bacillary angiomatosis caused by the Gram-negative bacteria *Rochalimaea,* with the two distinguished by histology.

PREVENTION AND TREATMENT

Methods to prevent sexually transmitted infections, such as the use of condoms, may prevent sexual transmission of KSHV. For persons co-infected with HIV, highly active anti-retroviral therapy is associated with a reduction in the incidence of Kaposi's sarcoma and regression in the size and number of existing lesions. Local therapy for palliation of symptomatic lesions or for cosmetically-unacceptable lesions can be achieved through a variety of means, including radiation therapy, surgical excision, cryotherapy, intralesional administration of anti-neoplastic agents and topical retinoids. Systemic therapy is reserved for rapidly progressive or severe disease and includes immune modulators (e.g. interferon-α) and chemotherapy. Antiviral therapy with ganciclovir, foscarnet or cidofovir has demonstrated some efficacy in small studies, but the virus is resistant to acyclovir.

REFERENCES

1. Durack DT. Opportunistic infections and Kaposi's sarcoma in homosexual men. N Engl J Med 1981;305:1465–7.
2. Chang Y, Cesarman E, Pessin MS, et al. Identification of herpesvirus-like DNA sequences in AIDS-associated Kaposi's sarcoma. Science 1994;266:1865–9.
3. Ablashi D, Chatlynne L, Cooper H, et al. Seroprevalence of human herpesvirus-8 (HHV-8) in countries of Southeast Asia compared to the USA, the Caribbean and Africa. Br J Cancer 1999;81:893–7.
4. de Sanjose S, Mbisa G, Perez-Alvarez S, et al. Geographic variation in the prevalence of Kaposi sarcoma-associated herpesvirus and risk factors for transmission. J Infect Dis 2009;199:1449–56.
5. Mantina H, Kankasa C, Klaskala W, et al. Vertical transmission of Kaposi's sarcoma-associated herpesvirus. Int J Cancer 2001;94:749–52.
6. Brayfield BP, Kankasa C, West JT, et al. Distribution of Kaposi sarcoma-associated herpesvirus/human herpesvirus 8 in maternal saliva and breast milk in Zambia: implications for transmission. J Infect Dis 2004;189: 2260–70.
7. Butler LM, Dorsey G, Hladik W, et al. Kaposi sarcoma-associated herpesvirus (KSHV) seroprevalence in population-based samples of African children: evidence for at least 2 patterns of KSHV transmission. J Infect Dis 2009;200: 430–8.
8. Sullivan RJ, Pantanowitz L, Casper C, et al. HIV/AIDS: epidemiology, pathophysiology, and treatment of Kaposi sarcoma-associated herpesvirus disease: Kaposi sarcoma, primary effusion lymphoma, and multicentric Castleman disease. Clin Infect Dis 2008;47:1209–15.
9. Wen KW, Damania B. Kaposi sarcoma-associated herpesvirus (KSHV): Molecular biology and oncogenesis. Cancer Lett 2010;28:140–50.
10. Andreoni M, Sarmati L, Nicastri E, et al. Primary human herpesvirus 8 infection in immunocompetent children. JAMA 2002;287:1295–300.
11. Ganem D. Kaposi's Sarcoma-associated Herpesvirus. In: Knipe DM, Howley PM, eds. Field's Virology. Philadelphia: Lippincott Williams & Wilkins; 2007:2847–88.
12. Casper C. New approaches to the treatment of human herpesvirus 8-associated disease. Rev Med Virol 2008;18:321–9.

Viral Respiratory Infections 29

H Rogier van Doorn, Hongjie Yu

Key features

- Global distribution of multiple pathogens causing similar diseases
- Varying burden geographically and seasonally
- Spectrum of pathogens from established, endemic human-adapted viruses to emerging, highly pathogenic viruses from animal reservoirs with pandemic threat
- Clinical disease from common cold to severe lower respiratory tract infection with systemic dissemination
- Severe disease can occur in all age groups but young children, the elderly and the immunocompromised are more at risk for severe disease (during the recent H1N1 influenza pandemic pregnant women and young adults were especially at risk)

INTRODUCTION

Globally, acute respiratory illnesses caused by viruses and bacteria are the most frequently occurring illnesses in all age groups. Disease is mostly limited to the upper airways and is self-limiting, but a small percentage can progress to lower respiratory tract infections as bronchiolitis and pneumonia. Children and elderly people are at increased risk, especially in developing countries. Childhood pneumonia is the leading single cause of mortality in children aged less than 5 years. The incidence in this age group is estimated to be 0.29 episodes per child-years in developing countries and 0.05 episodes per child-years in developed countries. This translates into about 156 million new episodes each year worldwide, of which 151 million episodes are in the developing world. Pneumonia is responsible for about 19% of all deaths in children aged less than 5 years, of which more than 70% take place in sub-Saharan Africa and Southeast Asia. On the other side of the age spectrum, pneumonia is also a major cause of morbidity and mortality in older people, with an annual incidence for non-institutionalized patients estimated at between 25 and 44 per 1000 population – up to four times that of patients younger than 65 years of age.

The most important etiologic agents of severe lower respiratory illness are bacteria such as *Streptococcus pneumoniae* and *Haemophilus influenzae*, and viruses such as respiratory syncytial virus (RSV) and influenza virus. Viruses are more important in mild upper and middle respiratory tract infections and in bronchiolitis in children, whereas bacteria are the main cause of pneumonia, especially in adults. Clinical syndromes considerably overlap and there is increasing evidence of bacterial-viral co-infections and of bacterial pneumonia being secondary to a viral respiratory tract infection [1–4].

A wide range of viruses from different families can cause respiratory infections; the most important are the ortho- and paramyxoviridae, picornaviridae, coronaviruses and adenoviruses. Recent etiological studies from tropical and subtropical regions are summarized in Table 29-1 [5–13].

EPIDEMIOLOGY

With some notable exceptions described below, most respiratory viruses are spread from person-to-person by the respiratory route – to a varying extent by large droplets, small-particle aerosols and by fomites with hand contamination and subsequent self-inoculation. Patients are most infectious early in disease: at symptom onset or even before. Secondary attack rates may be especially high in semi-closed populations, for example among schoolchildren, inpatients and nursing home residents. Children play a major role in respiratory virus outbreaks among families and communities. Frequent hand-washing and covering of the mouth when coughing or sneezing may partially prevent transmission.

Many of the viruses display significant seasonal variation, especially in temperate regions. Influenza virus and RSV epidemics occur in the winter months in temperate regions. In tropical areas, seasonal patterns are less clear: viruses may circulate throughout the year and peaks may coincide with either lower temperatures or increased rainfall. Parainfluenza virus 3 causes epidemics in the spring, while viruses 1 and 2 do so in autumn and early winter in temperate regions [14].

ORTHOMYXOVIRIDAE: INFLUENZA A, B AND C VIRUSES

Orthomyxoviridae are divided into three genera: A, B and C. Influenza A viruses are further subtyped based on the two major antigens: hemagglutinin (HA; H1–H16), responsible for host receptor binding/cell entry; and neuraminidase (NA; N1–N9), responsible for cleavage of the HA-receptor complex to release newly formed viruses. Key amino acids in these proteins, particularly in HA, are associated with host specificity and transmissibility in humans. Aquatic birds are the natural reservoir of influenza A viruses, harboring all possible subtypes. A selection of subtypes has established endemicity among a range of land and water mammals (e.g. humans, pigs, horses, seals; Fig. 29.1). Influenza B and C viruses are mainly human pathogens, with rare reports of influenza B virus infection in dogs, cats, swine and seals. Influenza C rarely causes human infections and will not be further discussed.

Yearly epidemics of influenza are caused by influenza A and B viruses with mutations in the regions of the HA and NA genes that encode antigenicity, allowing them to escape the hosts' immunity against parent strains (antigenic drift).

New lineages of influenza A virus emerge every few decades, resulting in global pandemics with varying severity owing to the absence of immunity in the human population. New human viruses have emerged through re-assortment of gene segments in animal hosts infected with two different viruses (antigenic shift – 1918 Spanish flu: H1N1; 40–100 million deaths, 1957 Asian flu: H2N2; 2 million deaths and 1968 Hong Kong flu: H3N2; 500,000 deaths) [19]. After

TABLE 29-1 Results of Recent Etiological Studies on Respiratory Viral Infections in Tropical and Subtropical Regions

Country	Years	Setting	Patients	Method	Disease	Number	RSV	hMPV	FluA	FluB	PIV1	PIV2	PIV3	PIV4	Adeno	Entero	Corona				Rhino	Boca	KI-WU
																	NL63	*HKU1*	*229E*	*OC43*			
Korea	2000–2005	H	Children	RT-PCR	LRTI	515	122	24	24	9	9	0	32	X	35	X	8	X	X	X	30	58	X
Bangladesh	2000–2001	O	Children	Serology	ARI	107	3	20	10	14	0	0	9	X	4	X	X	X	X	X	X	X	X
India	2002–2004	HO	Children	Antigen/ Culture	LRTI	385	101	X	21		8				4	X	X	X	X	X	X	X	X
Iran	2001–2002	H	Children	Antigen	ARI	202	26	X	16	7	13	13	32	X	12	X	X	X	X	X	X	X	X
Brazil	2001–2003	O	Adults	Antigen/ RT-PCR	ARI	420	10	24	52	37	1	1	2	X	17	9	X	X	6	12	103	X	X
Brazil	2003	H	Children	RT-PCR	LRTI	336	81	60	17	0	2	0	28	X	23	X	X	X	X	X	X	X	X
Brazil	2003–2005	H	Children	Antigen/ RT-PCR	CAP	184	28	X	17		31				5	9	X	X	X	X	39	X	X
Nepal	2004–2007	HO	Children	RT-PCR	CAP	2219	334	93	164	84	98	17	129	X	X	X	X	X	X	X	X	X	X
India	2005–2007	HO	Children	RT-PCR	LRTI	301	61	11	9	0	10	17	22	X	X	X	X	X	X	X	X	X	X
Brazil	2006–2007	HO	Children	RT-PCR	ARI	205	4	8	6	0	0	0	0	0	2	X	4	1	0	3	38	7	2
Hong Kong	2005–2006	H	Children	RT-PCR	ARI	475	40	7	34	16	19	6	14	3	23	2	X	X	16	2	17	X	X
Singapore	2005–2007	H	Children	Antigen/ RT-PCR	ARI	500	59	29	4	2	4	0	8	X	1	X	3		X	X	X	40	X
Singapore	2006–2007	O	Adults	RT-PCR	ARI	1354	0	9	326	159	1	0	4	0	5	X	X	X	0	1	15	X	X
Vietnam	2007–2008	H	Children	RT-PCR	ARI	958	217	43	146	2	7	5	36	X	49	X	X	X	X	X	270	19	X

Adeno, Adenovirus; ARI, Acute Respiratory Infection; CAP, Community Acquired Pneumonia; Entero, Enterovirus; FluA, influenza virus A; FluB, influenza virus B; H, Hospitalized; hMPV, human metapneumovirus; HO, Hospitalized and Outpatients; LRTI, Lower Respiratory Tract Infection; O, Outpatients, PIV, parainfluenza virus; RSV, respiratory syncytial virus; RT-PCR, Reverse Transcription-Polymerase Chain Reaction; Corona, Coronavirus; Rhino, Rhinovirus; Boca, Bocavirus, KI-WU, KI and WU polyomaviruses.

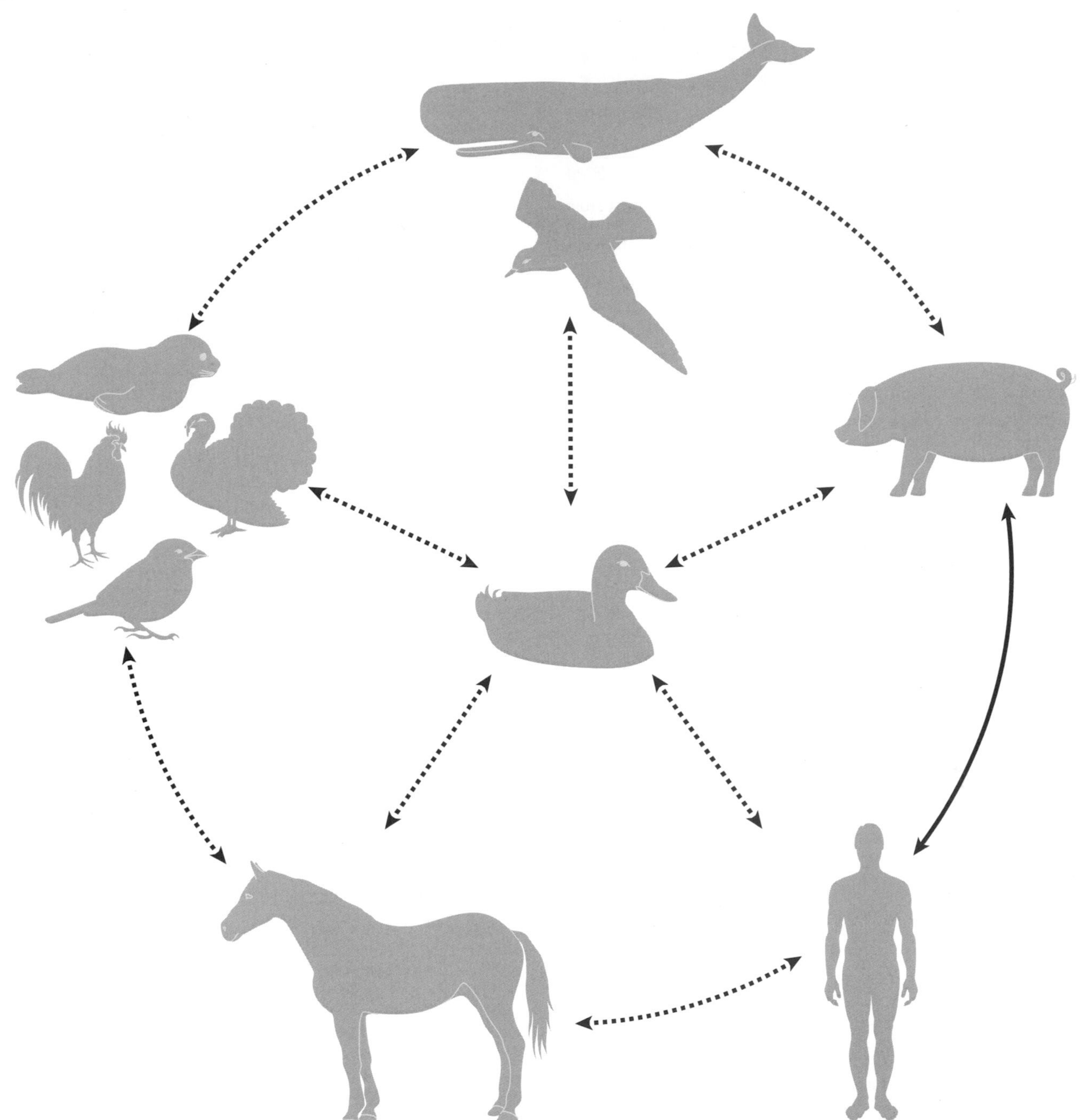

FIGURE 29.1 The reservoir of influenza A viruses. The working hypothesis is that wild aquatic birds are the primordial reservoir of all influenza viruses for avian and mammalian species. Transmission of influenza has been demonstrated between pigs and humans (solid lines). There is extensive evidence for transmission between aquatic birds and other species including pigs and horses and indirect transmission to humans through pigs and evidence for direct transmission to humans from chickens *(with permission from Elsevier Ltd, Encyclopedia of Virology 2nd edition; 1999; pp 824-829).*

such an introduction, the new virus becomes the dominant circulating lineage of influenza A. One exception was the re-introduction of H1N1 in the human population in 1977, which was possibly caused by an escape from a research laboratory. Since 1977, two lineages of H1N1 and H3N2 influenza A viruses have been co-circulating among humans, causing yearly seasonal epidemics worldwide (Fig. 29.2). Influenza B viruses co-circulate with influenza A viruses and also cause yearly epidemics but have not been associated with pandemics.

In 2009, a novel lineage of H1N1 influenza A virus emerged, most likely from pigs, in North America and caused a worldwide pandemic of relatively mild influenza. At the time of writing, the pandemic has passed and around 18,000 people died from infection during the pandemic phase. The virus has now become established as a seasonal virus, has largely replaced the former H1N1 virus and is co-circulating with H3N2.

Sporadic, dead-end human infections of animal viruses are known to occur and have caused concern about the pandemic potential of these viruses. H7N7, H7N3 and H9N2 viruses have caused conjunctivitis and mild, flu-like illness in patients who were in close contact with infected birds or seals. In contrast, H5N1 avian influenza viruses have caused severe human respiratory illness in Asia and North Africa, with a mortality of over 50%. Highly pathogenic H5N1 viruses were first detected in birds in 1996 in China. Transmission to 18 humans

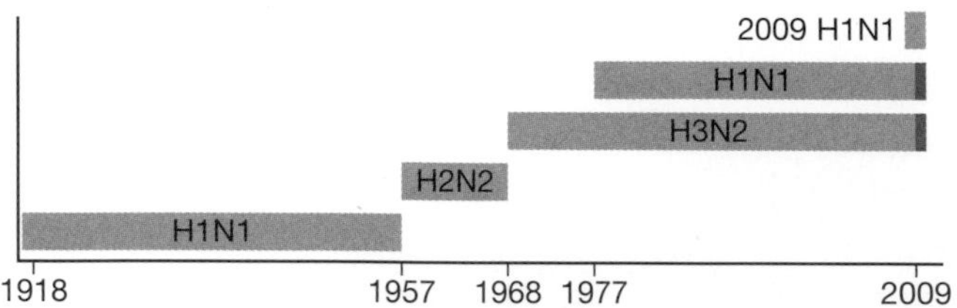

FIGURE 29.2 Timeline of circulating subtypes of influenza virus A from 1918 onwards. In 1977, H1N1 was reintroduced and has since then co-circulated with H3N2. In 2009 a new H1N1 lineage (pdm09) was introduced which has replaced the former H1N1 subtype.

occurred in Hong Kong, six of which were fatal. During the next 6 years, no human or animal cases were recorded. In 2003, the virus re-emerged in China. Since then, it has become panzootic among poultry and wild birds and, at the time of writing, has caused 584 sporadic infections (345 fatal) in humans, most of whom reported close contact with wild birds or domestic poultry. Despite their worldwide presence for many years, and the huge human–animal interface in Asia, no efficient human-to-human transmission episodes have been recorded. The possibility of mutations or re-assortment in these viruses remains a cause for concern and warrants continuous monitoring and surveillance of H5N1 viruses [15].

PARAMYXOVIRIDAE: RESPIRATORY SYNCYTIAL VIRUS (RSV), PARAINFLUENZA VIRUS 1–4 AND HUMAN METAPNEUMOVIRUS (HMPV)

These six human viruses are the most important causes of lower respiratory tract infections in children worldwide. RSV is the single most important cause of bronchiolitis and the leading cause of respiratory tract infections requiring hospitalization. Human metapneumovirus (hMPV) causes similar, but less frequent, disease, whereas the parainfluenza viruses are associated with croup.

Infections with these viruses are very common and virtually all children will have been infected with RSV by 2 years of age and by hMPV at 5 years of age. Immunity against all viruses is incomplete, although re-infections tend to be milder. Severe disease is common from RSV and hMPV in the first year of life. Re-infection with RSV or parainfluenza viruses is also a common cause of pneumonia in elderly and immunocompromised patients [6]. Other paramyxoviridae, such as rubeola virus (measles) or the zoonotic nipah virus may also be associated with respiratory disease as part of disseminated infection. These are discussed in separate chapters.

CORONAVIRUSES AND SEVERE ACUTE RESPIRATORY SYNDROME (SARS)-CORONAVIRUS

The four main human respiratory coronaviruses (229E, OC43, NL63 and HKU1) are associated with relatively mild upper respiratory infections and may cause 10–25% of episodes of common colds, but are less frequently implicated in severe infections requiring hospitalization.

In 2002–2003, a novel, severe form of pneumonia of unknown etiology emerged in Guangdong, China and was named Severe Acute Respiratory Syndrome (SARS). After smoldering for several months, the disease then spread rapidly across the world, facilitated by international air travel and a few so-called "super-spreaders", with the most notable outbreaks in Hong Kong and Toronto. Twenty-one percent of affected cases were healthcare workers. The rapidly identified culprit, SARS coronavirus, is thought to have jumped to humans from Civet cats (considered a delicacy in Asia) in live animal markets in Guangdong. Wild civet cats, however, do not carry these viruses but certain bat species have been implicated as the natural reservoir. The epidemic of SARS, with 8096 cases and 744 deaths in 29 countries across 5 continents, started in November 2002 and came to an end in July 2003. Few sporadic community- and laboratory-acquired infections, including limited person-to-person transmission, have been recorded since. SARS was characterized by fever and myalgia, rapidly progressing to a respiratory syndrome of cough and dyspnea followed by acute respiratory distress syndrome. Mortality was significantly lower in children.

SARS is primarily spread by the respiratory route, but oral–fecal transmission has also been implicated. Why the SARS epidemic did not continue to spread is subject to much speculation. Explanations may include the fact that SARS is most infectious in a later stage of infection, allowing for timely containment, and an extraordinary worldwide public health effort to control spread [16].

PICORNAVIRUSES: RHINOVIRUSES, ENTEROVIRUSES AND PARECHOVIRUSES

Rhinoviruses are the most important cause of the common cold and may be associated with exacerbations of asthma and chronic bronchitis. Enterovirus and parechoviruses typically present with aseptic meningitis but are also associated with (mild) respiratory illness.

ADENOVIRUSES

Adenoviruses are a frequent cause of epidemic infective conjunctivitis in developing countries and of respiratory tract infections in children and young adults worldwide. Outbreaks can occur in closed communities such as day care centers and boarding schools, and among military recruits. Most adenoviral infections remain subclinical.

NATURAL HISTORY AND PATHOGENESIS

Acute respiratory viral infections usually start in the upper respiratory tract as the port of entry is the nose, mouth or eyes. Spread to the lower parts of the airways occurs within two to four days. Syndromes overlap considerably, are usually accompanied by symptoms such as fever, cough and malaise, and can be caused by any of the pathogens described above.

In developing countries in particular, crowding of large families in small houses, low levels of sanitation and personal hygiene, indoor and outdoor smoke pollution, malnutrition, vitamin and mineral deficiencies, and a high frequency of respiratory infections may have detrimental effects on the integrity of the respiratory mucosa, respiratory function and the immune status, making the patient more prone to repeated, and more severe, viral infection and to secondary bacterial infection. Old and very young age, including prematurity are additional risk factors for a more severe course.

CLINICAL FEATURES

Common Cold

The common cold, or coryza, is the most frequent disease worldwide. Specific symptoms include a runny or stuffed nose, sneezing and sore throat. Picorna- and coronaviruses are often involved. Symptoms are caused by local infection of the ciliated nasal mucosal epithelium cells and surrounding increased vascular permeability. Disease is usually self-limiting.

Pharyngitis

Sore throat often accompanies the common cold but is typically not the result of inflammation of the throat, rather it is caused by excretion of chemical inflammation mediators that stimulate pain nerve endings. Bacteria are a common cause of true pharyngitis, as are coxsackieviruses, Epstein-Barr virus (EBV) and cytomegalovirus (CMV).

Acute Laryngotracheobronchitis (Croup)

Croup affects children under the age of 3 years; the hallmark symptoms are a barking cough and acute inspiratory stridor. Symptoms are caused by localized subglottic inflammation and edema leading to airflow impediment.

Tracheitis and Tracheobronchitis

These are most often caused by infection of the tracheal and bronchial epithelium by influenza A and B viruses and are characterized by tracheal tenderness, substernal discomfort on inhalation and nonproductive cough.

Bronchiolitis

This is a distinct syndrome of infants and young children. The major symptom is wheezing, accompanied by flaring of the nostrils, use of accessory respiratory muscles and cyanosis in more severe cases. Direct viral infection of the bronchiolar epithelial cells, followed by necrosis, infiltration of lymphocytes, submucosal swelling and increased mucus secretion results in the formation of dense plugs of debris that cause impediment of airflow, particularly expiratory. Children may experience repeated episodes of wheezing after recovery from bronchiolitis. Associations with later development of asthma and a causative role of the immune system in pathogenesis of bronchiolitis have been suggested.

Viral Pneumonia

Development of primary viral pneumonia, as described for influenza virus, is defined by dysfunctional gas exchange accompanying inflammation of the lung parenchyma, usually resulting in radiographic changes. There is acute generalized illness and a dry cough, rhinitis and conjunctivitis may be present. An increased respiratory rate is an early feature, with cyanosis developing in very severe disease. Viruses reach the small airways either through continuous spread or by inhalation of aerosols. Mucosal infection leads to destruction of epithelial cells, submucosal hyperemia, edema of the airways and hemorrhaging. Additional cellular infiltration and fibrin depositions may further compromise respiratory volume and gas exchange surface [17]. Viral pneumonia can be part of severe forms of measles and varicella, and may be secondary to generalized infections with EBV or CMV. In infections with New World hantaviruses, pulmonary symptoms are dominant but are, instead, caused by immune-mediated capillary leak.

Secondary bacterial pneumonia may follow any respiratory viral illness and presents as a recurrence or protracted fever and respiratory symptoms after initial recovery. *Streptococcus pneumoniae* and *Staphylococcus aureus* are common causes.

DIAGNOSIS

Epidemiologic characteristics, patient history, clinical features and accompanying signs and symptoms may give important clues in establishing the diagnosis of specific viral agents, but clinical syndromes overlap and are nonspecific. Diagnosis can only be reliably made by detection of virus, antigens or nucleic acids in respiratory or other specimens.

Rapid antigen tests exist for RSV and influenza virus, but these are, in general, not very sensitive (up to 70%). Viral culture is still considered the gold standard, but is complicated, cumbersome, slow and can also lack sensitivity. Instead, (reverse transcriptase)-PCR assays are rapid and sensitive and, when used in multiplex format, can detect most common respiratory viruses. Unfortunately, they are expensive by themselves and require even more expensive equipment, laboratory infrastructure and well-trained staff to be performed adequately, limiting their application in developing countries [17].

The identification of one viral agent does not rule out a double infection or mixed bacterial–viral infection. Recently, several novel viruses have been identified in the human respiratory tract (Bocavirus, WU and KI polyomaviruses, amongst several others). The exact significance of the role of these viruses as pathogens has yet to be established.

PREVENTION AND TREATMENT

Vaccines against influenza virus containing inactivated forms of the at-that-time predominant lineages of H3N2, H1N1 and B viruses are produced twice a year for the northern and southern hemispheres. Use in developing countries is limited because of the high cost and the need for annual re-vaccination. Vaccines for the other respiratory viruses are currently not available. Earlier attempts at the production of a formaldehyde-inactivated RSV vaccine were associated with more severe forms of disease in vaccinees.

Cidofovir is available for severe adenovirus infections but causes severe side effects and needs to be administered simultaneously with probenecid. Oral or aerosolized formulations of the broad-spectrum antiviral ribavirin inhibit replication of several respiratory viruses, including influenza virus and RSV; however, they are expensive, studies have not shown consistent benefit for patients with severe RSV infection and they should not be used routinely. Use of ribavirin in combination with other specific anti-influenza drugs for treatment of severe influenza infection has shown promising *in vitro* effects and is under investigation *in vivo*. Humanized anti-RSV immunoglobulins (palivizumab) are available for the prevention of RSV infection in high-risk groups (neonates and infants with congenital heart or lung disease), but are very expensive. Pleconaril was developed for the common cold and inhibits picornavirus replication, but the risks (reduction of efficacy of some hormonal contraceptives and drugs used to treat HIV) outweighed the benefits for its use in the prevention and treatment of uncomplicated infections.

The adamantanes (amantadine and rimantadine) and the neuraminidase inhibitors (oseltamivir and zanamivir) are specific antiviral drugs for influenza. The adamantanes and oseltamivir are available as oral preparations; zanamivir is administered through inhalation. Both have shown benefit in the prevention and treatment of uncomplicated influenza, especially when given early in the disease. For severe forms of influenza or H5N1 infection, treatment with oseltamivir is also of benefit when initiated in a later stage. The role of concomitant steroids for these infections is unclear. Oseltamivir was widely used in the developed world and, to a lesser extent, in the developing world to treat infection with 2009 H1N1. Development of resistance during treatment for both classes of drugs is a common phenomenon and is more frequently observed in children. In addition, the dominant lineages of H3N2 and H1N1 in the 2007–2008 season were resistant against adamantanes and oseltamivir, respectively. Resistance against zanamivir is rare, but its route of administration limits use in severe disease.

Parenteral formulations of oseltamivir and zanamivir, and two new neuraminidase inhibitors (peramivir and laninamivir) are under investigation for the treatment of severe influenza. Convalescent plasmatherapy, monoclonal antibodies and other forms of immunomodulation have shown promising results, warranting further evaluation in clinical trials. Supportive and, if needed, intensive care and various forms of oxygen supplementation for severe respiratory distress (tachypnea, retractions, cyanosis) are often the mainstay of treatment of respiratory viral infections. Extracorporeal membrane oxygenation (ECMO) is a last resort for maintaining oxygen saturation during severe viral pneumonia.

In some parts of the world (especially Southeast Asia), antibiotics are extensively used to treat any form of mild respiratory illness. Although there may be some benefit of the use of antibiotics in preventing secondary bacterial infection, over-the-counter availability of antibiotics, self-medication or medication by untrained pharmacy workers should be discouraged because of the selection and subsequent spread of resistance in commensal oral and gut flora.

REFERENCES

1. Brooks WA, Goswami D, Rahman M, et al. Influenza is a major contributor to childhood pneumonia in a tropical developing country. Pediatr Infect Dis J 2010;29:216–21.
2. Guerrant RL, Walker DH, Weller PF. Tropical Infectious Diseases: Principles, Pathogens, & Practice. Philadelphia, PA: Elsevier Churchill Livingstone; 2006.
3. Janssens JP, Krause KH. Pneumonia in the very old. Lancet Infect Dis 2004;4: 112–24.
4. Rudan I, Boschi-Pinto C, Biloglav Z, et al. Epidemiology and etiology of childhood pneumonia. Bull World Health Organ 2008;86:408–16.
5. Choi EH, Lee HJ, Kim SJ, et al. The association of newly identified respiratory viruses with lower respiratory tract infections in Korean children, 2000–2005. Clin Infect Dis 2006,43:585–92.
6. Abdullah Brooks W, Erdman D, Terebuh P, et al. Human metapneumovirus infection among children, Bangladesh. Emerg Infect Dis 2007;13:1611–13.
7. Yeolekar LR, Damle RG, Kamat AN, et al. Respiratory viruses in acute respiratory tract infections in Western India. Indian J Pediatr 2008;75:341–5.
8. Mathisen M, Strand TA, Sharma BN, et al. RNA viruses in community-acquired childhood pneumonia in semi-urban Nepal; a cross-sectional study. BMC Med 2009;7:35.
9. Bharaj P, Sullender WM, Kabra SK, et al. Respiratory viral infections detected by multiplex PCR among pediatric patients with lower respiratory tract infections seen at an urban hospital in Delhi from 2005 to 2007. Virol J 2009;6:89.
10. Albuquerque MC, Pena GP, Varella RB, et al. Novel respiratory virus infections in children, Brazil. Emerg Infect Dis 2009;15:806–8.
11. Sung RY, Chan PK, Tsen T, et al. Identification of viral and atypical bacterial pathogens in children hospitalized with acute respiratory infections in Hong Kong by multiplex PCR assays. J Med Virol 2009;81:153–9.
12. Tan BH, Lim EA, Seah SG, et al. The incidence of human bocavirus infection among children admitted to hospital in Singapore. J Med Virol 2009;81: 82–9.
13. Seah SG, Lim EA, Kok-Yong S, et al. Viral agents responsible for febrile respiratory illnesses among military recruits training in tropical Singapore. J Clin Virol 2010:47:289–92.
14. Brankston G, Gitterman L, Hirji Z, et al. Transmission of influenza A in human beings. Lancet Infect Dis 2007;7:257–65.
15. Abdel-Ghafar AN, Chotpitayasunondh T, Gao Z, et al. Update on avian influenza A (H5N1) virus infection in humans. N Engl J Med 2008;358:261–73.
16. Peiris JS, Yuen KY, Osterhaus AD, Stohr K. The severe acute respiratory syndrome. N Engl J Med 2003;349:2431–41.
17. Richman DD, Whitley RJ, Hayden FG. Clinical Virology, Washington: ASM Press; 2009.
18. Webster RG, Bean WJ, Gorman OT. Evolution and ecology of influenza A viruses. Microbiol Rev 1992;56:152–79.
19. Smith GJ, Bahl J, Vijaykrishnaa D, et al. Dating the emergence of pandemic influenza viruses. PNAS 2009;106:11709–12.

Viral Gastroenteritis 30

Osamu Nakagomi, Nigel A Cunliffe

Key features

- Viruses are the major etiologic agents of acute gastroenteritis, both in developing and developed countries, particularly in children younger than 5 years of age; in this age group diarrhea is the second most common cause of death
- All gastroenteritis viruses, also referred to as diarrhea viruses, cause acute-onset, watery, non-bloody diarrhea
- There are currently four genera and one species of viruses recognized as established causes of gastroenteritis in humans: *Rotavirus, Norovirus, Sapovirus, Astrovirus* and *Human adenovirus F* (also referred to as enteric adenoviruses)
- Diarrhea caused by these gastroenteritis viruses is indistinguishable by clinical features alone; etiologic diagnosis requires laboratory investigation
- The disease is self-limiting in otherwise healthy individuals, but oral or intravenous rehydration therapy is required for mildly or severely dehydrated patients
- Vaccines are available for rotavirus—one of the most important causes of viral diarrhea

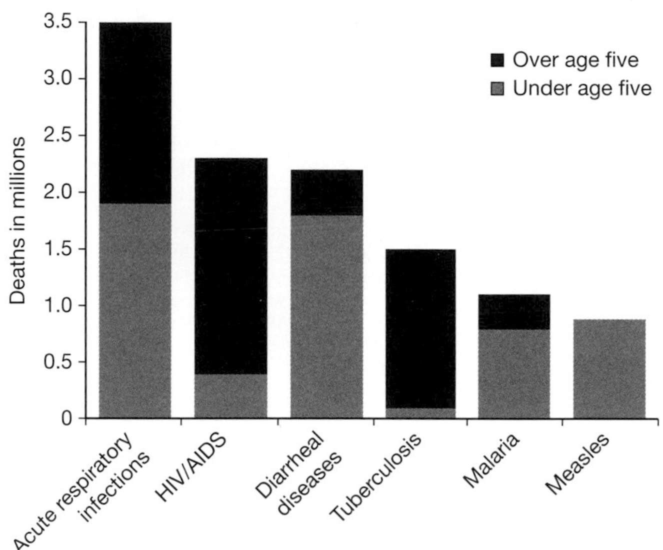

FIGURE 30.1 Leading causes of death in the world from infectious diseases in 2008 *(adapted with permission from http://www.who.int/infectious-disease-report/pages/graph5.html).*

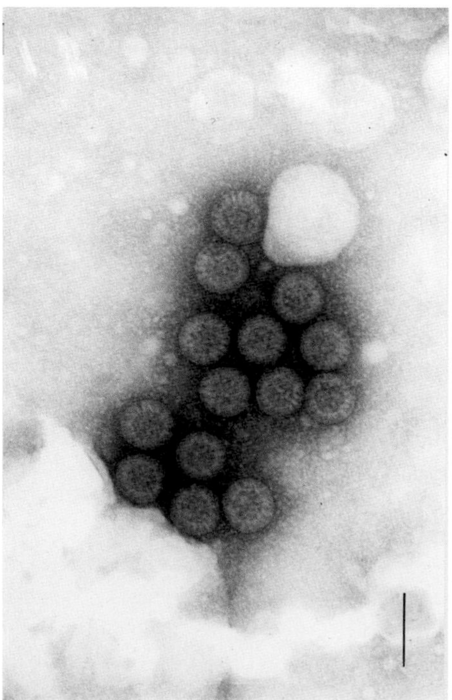

FIGURE 30.2 Negative-stain electron micrograph of rotavirus particles. The bar represents 100 nm *(courtesy of Brian Getty, University of Liverpool).*

INTRODUCTION

Acute diarrhea is the cardinal symptom of viral gastrointestinal infection and is defined as the passage of three or more watery or looser-than-usual stools within the preceding 24 hours for less than 2 weeks' duration. Globally, diarrhea is the second most common cause of death (18%, 10.8 million) in children younger than 5 years of age and it causes more deaths in this age group than HIV/AIDS, tuberculosis and malaria put altogether (Fig. 30.1). Viruses account for the major proportion of causative agents responsible for acute gastroenteritis both in developing and developed countries.

Viral gastroenteritis generally presents a similar clinical picture—whatever the virus—requiring laboratory investigation for establishing its etiology. Signs and symptoms of typical acute viral gastroenteritis include acute onset of diarrhea, often with preceding vomiting, and sometimes with fever and abdominal pain. The most important complication is dehydration and this requires oral or intravenous fluid replacement therapy depending on the degree of dehydration. The disease typically lasts 3–5 days and is self-limiting. The viruses are transmitted feco-orally and infect the epithelial cells of the small intestine. Damage to the villous epithelium of the small intestine affects the absorption of fluid and causes watery diarrhea. No inflammation occurs as the viruses only multiply within the enterocytes in the intestinal epithelium and do not spread into the submucosa.

TABLE 30-1 Characteristics of the Major Gastroenteritis Viruses

Virus	Morphology, size	Methods of detection	Detection proportion in AGE cases (%)	Epidemiologic features
Group A rotavirus (species *Rotavirus A*, genus *Rotavirus* family *Reoviridae*)	Characteristic wheel-like capsid, 70 nm in diameter, double-stranded RNA genome	EM, ELISA, PAGE, PCR	30–50	The most important cause of acute gastroenteritis in infants and young children. Vaccines are available
Group B rotavirus (species *Rotavirus B*, genus *Rotavirus* family *Reoviridae*)	Characteristic wheel-like capsid, 70 nm in diameter, double-stranded RNA genome	EM, PAGE, PCR	Rare	Reports from China, India, and Bangladesh. Affects both children and adults
Group C rotavirus (species *Rotavirus C*, genus *Rotavirus* family *Reoviridae*)	Characteristic wheel-like capsid, 70 nm in diameter, double-stranded RNA genome	EM, ELISA, PAGE, PCR	Rare	Sporadically reported. Affects more often school-age children
Norovirus (family *Caliciviridae*)	Indistinct substructure of virion surface, 27–32 nm in diameter, single-stranded (+) RNA	EM, ELISA, PCR	10–20	Causes gastroenteritis in all age groups. Major cause of food-borne gastroenteritis
Sapovirus (family *Caliciviridae*)	Characteristic cup-like depression on the surface, 27–32 nm in diameter, single-stranded (+) RNA	EM, PCR	<5	Similar age distribution of cases as group A rotavirus
Enteric adenovirus (family *Adenoviridae*)	Characteristic icosahedrons, 70 nm in diameter, double-stranded DNA	EM, ELISA, PCR	5–10	Serotypes 40/41 Causes sporadic cases of acute gastroenteritis
Astrovirus (family *Astroviridae*)	Characteristic star-like structure on the surface, 27–32 nm in diameter, single-stranded (+) RNA	EM, ELISA, PCR	<5	Causes sporadic cases of acute gastroenteritis

AGE, acute gastroenteritis; EM, electron microscopy; PAGE, polyacrylamide gel electrophoresis.

There are currently four genera and one species of viruses recognized as established causes of gastroenteritis in humans: *Rotavirus, Norovirus, Sapovirus, Astrovirus* and *Human adenovirus F* (to which serotypes 40 and 41 belong and which are also referred to as enteric adenoviruses). As these viruses are often shed in large numbers into stool, they can be identified by direct, negative-stain electron microscopy based on their characteristic morphology (Fig. 30.2). What were previously called small-round structured viruses (SRSV) roughly correspond to norovirus and morphologically identified human caliciviruses correspond to sapovirus; however, the distinction of both norovirus and sapovirus is to be made at the level of nucleotide sequence. The use of the term "human calicivirus" is discouraged because it is sometimes confusing whether human calicivirus refers to both norovirus and sapovirus (they are calicivirses causing disease in humans) or only morphologically identified human caliciviruses, in which case noroviruses are excluded.

The major features of these gastroenteritis viruses are summarized in Table 30-1.

30.1 Rotavirus

Osamu Nakagomi, Toyoko Nakagomi, Nigel A Cunliffe

Key features

- Group A rotaviruses are the single most important cause of acute gastroenteritis in infants and young children worldwide
- Protective immunity against rotavirus infection is mediated by rotavirus-specific secretory IgA antibodies on the intestinal mucosal surface
- The diagnosis of rotavirus gastroenteritis is usually made by demonstration of the characteristic wheel-shaped virus particles in stool by electron microscopy, or by the detection of viral antigen using a variety of immunologic methods

Key features—cont'd

- A distinct winter seasonality of rotavirus infection is evident in temperate countries, whereas year-round infection is common in tropical countries
- Five major combinations of G and P types (G1P[8], G2P[4], G3P[8], G4P[8], and G9P[8]) together comprise more than 75% of global rotavirus strains; however, in some developing countries other serotypes may predominate (e.g. G5, G8). In addition, G12 has emerged globally in recent years
- Rehydration and restoration of electrolyte balance are the primary aims of treatment of acute rotavirus gastroenteritis
- Two live, oral rotavirus vaccines are now licensed globally and have been incorporated into childhood immunization schedules in more than a dozen countries with a substantial reduction of rotavirus hospitalizations

INTRODUCTION

Among multiple etiological agents causing acute gastroenteritis accounting for approximately 17% of deaths occurring in children younger than 5 years of age [1], rotavirus has been recognized as the single most important agent [2]. The annual global burden of rotavirus diarrhea is estimated at more than 110 million episodes, 25 million physician visits, 2 million hospitalizations and more than half a million deaths [3]. Everywhere in the world a child will experience at least one rotavirus infection by 3–5 years of age. However, the consequence of infection is strikingly different between developing and developed countries: more than 90% of the rotavirus-associated deaths occur in developing countries. This uneven distribution of rotavirus mortality is staggering among the developing countries; more than 65% of the global deaths caused by rotavirus occur in 11 countries in Asia and Africa, where an estimated 345,000 children under the age of 5 years die each year [4] (Fig. 30.1.1).

The recognition of this huge burden of rotavirus disease led to the development of rotavirus vaccines soon after its discovery in 1973 on thin-section electron microscopy of duodenal biopsies from a child with acute gastroenteritis [5]. Rotavirus was also found in large numbers in stool specimens by negative-stain electron microscopy and significant antibody titer rises were shown between acute and convalescent sera from children with acute gastroenteritis by immune electron microscopy [6]. The name "rotavirus" was coined by its characteristic wheel-shaped (*rota* is Latin for wheel) morphology on electron microscopy. The virus is a double-stranded RNA virus: genus *Rotavirus*, family *Reoviridae*.

EPIDEMIOLOGY

Rotavirus infections occur worldwide. Globally, rotavirus accounts for a median of 39% (interquartile range: 29–45%) of hospitalizations caused by acute gastroenteritis [3]. Most symptomatic infections occur in children between 3 months and 2 years of age; the peak incidence tends to be shifted to a younger age in developing countries [2]. In temperate countries, rotavirus infections show winter seasonality, whereas infections occur year-round in most tropical countries.

Rotavirus spreads feco-orally, primarily through person-to-person transmission. Only a few virus particles are sufficient to infect the susceptible host.

Among group A rotaviruses, two independent serotypes, termed G and P serotypes, are distinguished on the basis of the antigen residing on the outer capsid VP7 and VP4 proteins respectively. These antigenic specificities are more often predicted by molecular assays than determined by traditional serologic assays. Thus, the term genotype is frequently, and virtually interchangeably, used. However, the numbering system for P serotype and P genotype is different, so the convention is adopted such that the number describing the P genotype is bracketed. While many G and P serotypes have been reported for human and animal rotaviruses, five G and P serotype (genotype) combinations account for more than 75% of rotaviruses detected in humans. They are: G1P[8], G2P[4], G3P[8], G4P[8] and G9P[8] [7, 8]. However, rotavirus serotypes that are uncommon in temperate regions (e.g. serotype G5 in Brazil and G8 in Malawi and other African countries) may be commonly seen in tropical regions [9].

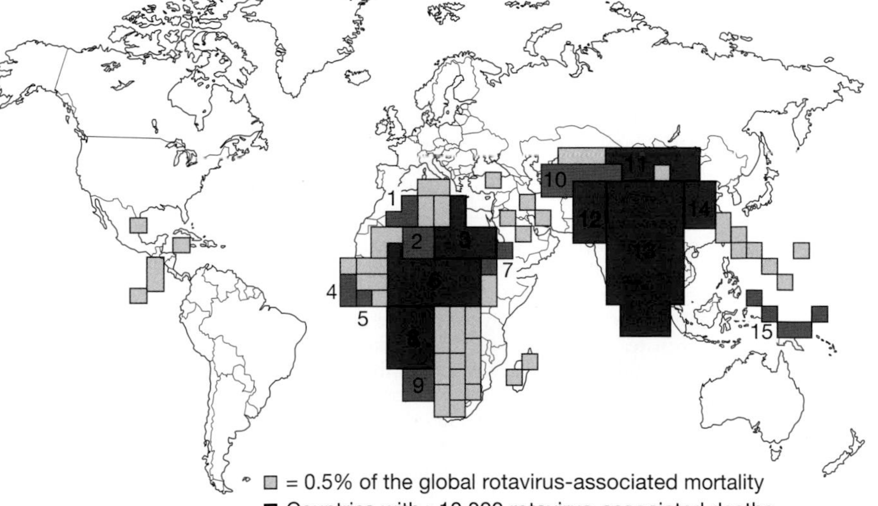

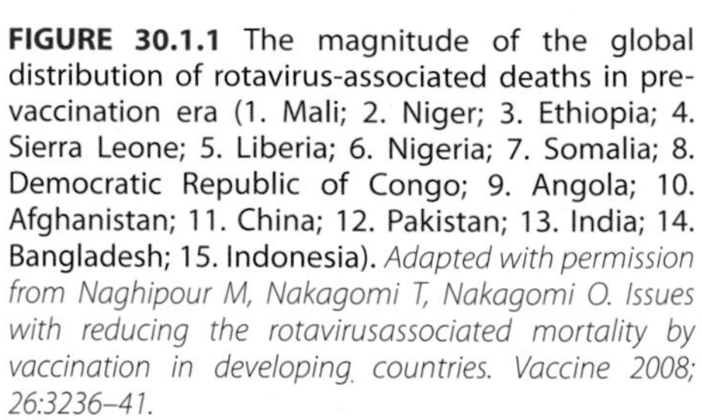

FIGURE 30.1.1 The magnitude of the global distribution of rotavirus-associated deaths in pre-vaccination era (1. Mali; 2. Niger; 3. Ethiopia; 4. Sierra Leone; 5. Liberia; 6. Nigeria; 7. Somalia; 8. Democratic Republic of Congo; 9. Angola; 10. Afghanistan; 11. China; 12. Pakistan; 13. India; 14. Bangladesh; 15. Indonesia). *Adapted with permission from Naghipour M, Nakagomi T, Nakagomi O. Issues with reducing the rotavirusassociated mortality by vaccination in developing countries. Vaccine 2008; 26:3236–41.*

NATURAL HISTORY, PATHOGENESIS AND PATHOLOGY

Rotavirus infection occurs throughout life. Multiple rotavirus infections commonly occur during infancy and early childhood. The first rotavirus infection typically results in the most severe disease outcome, although infection in the neonatal period often tends to be asymptomatic. Subsequent rotavirus infections, irrespective of infecting serotypes, are associated with milder disease or may even be asymptomatic [10, 11]. Although severe disease is less common, rotavirus infection may, nevertheless, cause gastroenteritis in older children and adults [12], and elderly people appear to become more susceptible as their immunity wanes [13].

Rotaviruses replicate exclusively in the epithelial cells of the small intestine and are released in large numbers into the intestinal lumen. The damage caused by multiplication in the epithelial cells causes impairment of the absorption of water and electrolytes from the lumen, leading to diarrhea which is followed by dehydration. However, other mechanisms have also been proposed, including viral nonstructural protein NSP4 acting as enterotoxin [14], secretion mediated by the enteric nervous system [15] and an increase in paracellular permeability [16].

The infection triggers a humoral and cell-mediated immune response at the mucosal level and the virus is normally cleared within a week. However, infection in the immunodeficient child may persist with severe chronic diarrhea associated with rotavirus excretion that can last many months [17]. Rotavirus-specific IgA antibodies on the enteric mucosal surface are thought to mediate protective immunity. Infection with one serotype provides serotype-specific (homotypic) protection and repeated infections lead to partial cross-serotype (heterotypic) protection. Thus, serotype does not appear to be the sole determinant in providing protective immunity [18].

CLINICAL FEATURES

The onset of symptoms is abrupt after a short incubation period of 1–2 days. Fever, vomiting and watery diarrhea are seen in the majority of infected children and last for 2–6 days. The stool is usually pale and watery or loose, and is rarely blood-stained. The major complication is dehydration that appears shortly after the onset of disease and varies in severity. The cause of death after rotavirus infection is dehydration, leading to metabolic disturbances and shock.

Extraintestinal manifestations during rotavirus gastroenteritis, such as encephalopathies, transaminase elevation and biliary atresia have been reported but causality is not established.

PATIENT EVALUATION, DIAGNOSIS AND DIFFERENTIAL DIAGNOSIS

The patient with acute gastroenteritis should first be evaluated regarding the presence and the degree of dehydration before seeking the etiology of the disease. It is not possible to distinguish rotavirus gastroenteritis from other viral or bacterial causes of non-inflammatory diarrhea solely on clinical grounds. To establish an etiological diagnosis, stool specimens from the patient in the acute phase of the disease can be examined by a variety of methods for the presence of rotavirus. Electron microscopy easily detects the characteristic virus particles. In the majority of cases, there are sufficient numbers of virions in the stool to allow the identification of characteristic RNA patterns (electropherotypes) upon polyacrylamide gel electrophoresis. Antigen detection tests include latex agglutination assays (latex particles are coated with rotavirus-specific antibody) and, more recently, immunochromatographic assays have been developed that can be used at the point of care. However, ELISAs offer the most sensitive diagnostic approach and are, therefore, the most commonly used method for rotavirus detection in routine clinical practice.

The diagnosis of rotavirus infection can also be made by demonstration of a fourfold, or greater, rise in antibody titers with serologic assays, including anti-rotavirus IgG and IgA ELISAs, complement-fixation tests and virus neutralization assays. However, these assays are predominantly applied in a research context.

TREATMENT AND PREVENTION

The mainstay of therapy for dehydration associated with rotavirus gastroenteritis consists of oral rehydration with fluids of specified electrolyte and glucose composition [19]. Intravenous rehydration therapy is indicated for the patient with severe dehydration, shock or reduced level of consciousness. Anti-motility agents are discouraged, particularly in infants and young children, as they are reported to be associated with rare, but severe, complications (Box 30.1.1).

Personal hygienic measures, such as hand-washing, safe disposal of feces and disinfection of contaminated surfaces, are important in reducing the risk of transmission.

Two, live-attenuated, oral rotavirus vaccines are licensed globally, and universal vaccination of infants is the most important preventive strategy to reduce the number of hospitalizations and deaths caused by rotavirus worldwide [20–22]. These two rotavirus vaccines were, to date, shown to be equally safe and efficacious in preventing severe rotavirus gastroenteritis in various settings. Attenuation of virulence has been achieved either by repeated passage in cell culture, or by substitution through genetic re-assortment of serotype-determining gene segments of a human rotavirus into the backbone of an animal rotavirus which is both naturally attenuated to humans and attenuated through repeated cell-culture passage (Table 30.1-1).

The first licensed rotavirus vaccine, a rhesus monkey rotavirus-based tetravalent human reassortant vaccine (RotaShield), enjoyed only a short lifespan in the market before being withdrawn after this vaccine was associated with the development of intestinal intussusception in approximately 1 : 10,000 vaccine recipients in the USA. Thus, rigorous safety clinical trials with respect to intussusception were successfully conducted for the currently licensed rotavirus vaccines [23, 24]. These vaccines include the monovalent G1P[8] human rotavirus vaccine, Rotarix [23], and the pentavalent human-bovine reassortant rotavirus vaccine, RotaTeq, which includes the most globally common human serotypes G1, G2, G3, G4 and P[8] on a bovine rotavirus background [24]. Both vaccines are highly (> 90%) effective in preventing severe diarrhea and hospitalization following rotavirus infection where the predominant circulating serotype is G1P[8] [23, 24]. While there was concern about to what extent the G1P[8] monovalent vaccine would be efficacious against strains fully heterotypic to the vaccine strain,

BOX 30.1.1 Treatment Considerations for Children with Acute Rotavirus Gastroenteritis

- The mainstay of treatment for uncomplicated rotavirus gastroenteritis comprises oral rehydration solutions providing essential electrolyte replacement plus sugar.
- For severe dehydration, shock and reduced level of consciousness, intravenous rehydration therapy is required.
- Anti-motility agents are discouraged, particularly in infants and young children, as they are reported to be associated with rare, but severe, complications.
- Either two doses of the monovalent rotavirus vaccine, Rotarix, or three doses of the pentavalent bovine-human reassortant vaccine, RotaTeq, are to be administered starting at SIX weeks of age and then according to the Expanded Programme on Immunization schedule to prevent severe rotavirus gastroenteritis and hospitalization.

TABLE 30.1-1 Characteristics of Globally Licensed Rotavirus Vaccines

	Monovalent vaccine (Rotarix)	Pentavalent vaccine (RotaTeq)
Manufacturer	GlaxoSmithKline	Merck and Co.
Parental strain	Human rotavirus strain RIX4414, G1P[8]	Bovine rotavirus strain WC3, G6P[5]
Formulation	Same as the original constellation of genomic RNA segments	5 reassortants G1×WC3, G2×WC3, G3×WC3, G4×WC3, P[8]×WC3
Vaccine titer	$\geq 10^{6.0}$ median cell culture infective dose per dose	$\geq 10^7$ infectious units per dose
Method of attenuation	Cell culture passage (43 times)	Naturally attenuated (animal strain); cell culture passage
Cell substrate	Vero cells	Vero cells
Volume per dose	1 mL	2 mL
Buffer	Calcium carbonate	Sodium citrate and phosphate
Dose regimen	2 oral doses	3 oral doses
Shedding	>50%	<10%

Adapted with modifications from Cunliffe NA, Nakagomi O. A critical time for rotavirus vaccines: a review. Expert Rev Vaccines 2005;4:521–32.

recent studies showed that it was reasonably effective in preventing severe rotavirus gastroenteritis and hospitalizations in a resource-poor setting in Latin America [25].

Another concern was related to the efficacy of both vaccines in high disease burden, impoverished countries in Africa and Asia, where infants commonly suffer with comorbidities (e.g. malnutrition, HIV, concomitant infections) and where a wide diversity of rotavirus strains typically circulate. However, recent data from a clinical trial undertaken in Malawi and South Africa demonstrated that, while vaccine efficacy against severe rotavirus gastroenteritis was lower than that observed in more developed countries (61% in Malawi and South Africa vs >90% in Europe), the impact of vaccination could be high because of a higher incidence of severe rotavirus disease [26].

From a technological perspective, it seems likely that we are equipped with safe and reasonably efficacious vaccines against rotavirus gastroenteritis for global use, although there is scope to improve vaccine efficacy. The most imminent hurdle to overcome from the perspective of substantial reduction of rotavirus mortality in the world's poorest countries may be to ensure vaccine delivery to those infants who most need them, and ensuring adequate cold chain facilities.

REFERENCES

1. Bryce J, Boschi-Pinto C, Shibuya K, et al. WHO estimates of the causes of death in children. Lancet 2005 365:1147–52.
2. Hart CA, Cunliffe NA, Nakagomi O. Diarrhoea caused by viruses. In: Cook GC, Zumla AI, eds. Manson's Tropical Diseases, 22nd edn. Philadelphia, PA: Saunders; 2009:815–24.
3. Parashar UD, Gibson CJ, Bresse JS, Glass RI. Rotavirus and severe childhood diarrhea. Emerg Infect Dis 2006;12:304–6.
4. Naghipour M, Nakagomi T, Nakagomi O. Issues with reducing the rotavirus-associated mortality by vaccination in developing countries. Vaccine 2008 26:3236–41.
5. Bishop RF, Davidson GP, Holmes IH, Ruck BJ. Virus particles in epithelial cells of duodenal mucosa from children with acute non-bacterial gastroenteritis. Lancet 1973;2:1281–3.
6. Kapikian AZ, Kim HW, Wyatt RG, et al. Reovirus like agent in stools: association with infantile diarrhea and development of serologic tests. Science 1974;185:1049–53.
7. Gentsch JR, Laird AR, Bielfelt B, et al. Serotype diversity and reassortment between human and animal rotavirus strains: implications for rotavirus vaccine programs. J Infect Dis 2005;192(suppl. 1):146–59.
8. Santos N, Hoshino Y. Global distribution of rotavirus serotypes/genotypes and its implication for the development and implementation of an effective rotavirus vaccine. Rev Med Virol 2005;15:29–56.
9. Cunliffe NA, Gentsch JR, Kirkwood CD, et al. Molecular and serologic characterization of novel serotype G8 human rotavirus strains detected in Blantyre, Malawi. Virology 2000;274:309–20.
10. Bishop RF, Barnes GL, Cipriani E, et al. Clinical immunity after neonatal rotavirus infection. A prospective longitudinal study in young children. N Engl J Med 1983;309:72–6.
11. Velazquez FR, Matson DO, Calva JJ, et al. Rotavirus infections in infants as protection against subsequent infections. N Engl J Med 1996; 335:1022–8.
12. Nakajima H, Nakagomi T, Kamisawa T, et al. Winter seasonality and rotavirus diarrhoea in adults. Lancet 2001; 357:1950.
13 Anderson EJ, Weber SG. Rotavirus infection in adults. Lancet Infect Dis 2004; 4:91–9
14. Ball JM, Tian P, Zeng CQ, et al. Age-dependent diarrhea induced by a rotaviral nonstructural glycoprotein. Science 1996;5:272:101–4.
15. Lundgren O, Svensson L. Pathogenesis of rotavirus diarrhea.Microbes Infect 2001;3:1145–56.
16. Stintzing G, Johansen K, Magnusson KE, et al. Intestinal permeability in small children during and after rotavirus diarrhoea assessed with different-size polyethyleneglycols (PEG 400 and PEG 1000). Acta Paediatr Scand 1986;75: 1005–9.
17. Saulsbury FT, Winkelstein JA, Yolken RH. Chronic rotavirus infection in immunodeficiency. J Pediatr 1980;97:61–5.
18. Ward RL. Rotavirus vaccines: how they work or don't work. Expert Rev Mol Med 2008;10:e5.
19. King CK, Glass R, Breese JS, et al. Managing acute gastroenteritis among children: oral rehydration, maintenance, and nutritional therapy. MMWR 2003;52:1–16
20. Cunliffe NA, Nakagomi O. A critical time for rotavirus vaccines: a review. Expert Rev Vaccines 2005;4:521–32.
21. Nakagomi O, Cunliffe NA. Rotavirus vaccines: entering a new stage of deployment. Curr Opin Infect Dis 2007;20:501–7.
22. Tate J, Patel M, Cortese M, et al. Global impact of rotavirus vaccines. Expert Rev Vaccines 2010;9:295–307.
23. Ruiz-Palacios GM, Pérez-Schael I, Velázquez FR, et al. Safety and efficacy of an attenuated vaccine against severe rotavirus gastroenteritis.N Engl J Med 2006;354:11–22.
24. Vesikari T, Matson DO, Dennehy P, et al. Safety and efficacy of a pentavalent human-bovine (WC3) reassortant rotavirus vaccine. N Engl J Med 2006; 354:23–33.
25. Correia JB, Patel MM, Nakagomi O, et al. Effectiveness of monovalent rotavirus vaccine (Rotarix) against severe diarrhea caused by serotypically unrelated G2P[4] strains in Brazil. J Infect Dis 2010;201:363–9.
26. Madhi SA, Cunliffe NA, Steele D, et al. Effect of human rotavirus vaccine on severe diarrhea in African infants. N Engl J Med 2010;362:289–98.

30.2 Norovirus

Aron J Hall, Manish M Patel, Benjamin A Lopman, George E Armah

Key features

- Also referred to as Norwalk virus, Norwalk-like virus, Calicivirus, small-round structured virus, viral gastroenteritis, "stomach flu" and "winter vomiting disease"
- Leading cause of epidemic gastroenteritis worldwide and a significant contributor to the diarrheal disease burden across all age groups
- Highly transmissible by the fecal-oral or vomitus-oral routes, including direct person-to-person contact, ingestion of contaminated food or water, and contact with contaminated fomites
- Disease characterized by acute-onset, watery, non-bloody diarrhea and/or vomiting lasting 1–3 days
- Generally self-limiting in otherwise healthy individuals, although medical attention may be necessary for dehydration caused by excessive fluid loss
- Treatment is primarily supportive consisting of either oral or intravenous fluid therapy, depending on the degree of dehydration

INTRODUCTION

Gastroenteritis is a leading cause of morbidity and mortality worldwide, accounting for over 1.8 million deaths annually in children aged <5 years, the vast majority of which occur in developing countries [1]. Although long recognized as common causes of epidemic gastroenteritis, noroviruses, which are positive-sense RNA viruses, have only recently been appreciated as important etiologies in the global gastroenteritis burden, significantly impacting both children and adults. Since the 1990s, the advent and widespread application of molecular diagnostic techniques have led to a vastly improved understanding of the epidemiology, natural history and clinical manifestations of norovirus infection. Nonetheless, lack of sensitive clinical assays and the inability to culture the virus *in vitro* continue to hamper further progress in characterization, prevention and control of norovirus.

EPIDEMIOLOGY

Noroviruses are the most common cause of gastroenteritis across all age groups and second only to rotavirus as a cause of severe gastroenteritis among children aged <5 years [2]. With the introduction of universal rotavirus immunization of infants and the consequent reduction of the burden of severe rotavirus diarrhea, the relative public health impact of noroviruses will continue to increase. This is evidenced by widespread acquisition of norovirus antibodies prior to adulthood—early exposure to norovirus occurs in both developed and developing countries [3]. Noroviruses frequently result in outbreaks and cause approximately 50% of all epidemic gastroenteritis worldwide [4]. Outbreaks have been reported in all age groups and commonly occur in nursing homes, hospital wards, daycare centers, schools, cruise ships and restaurants. The groups most vulnerable are the elderly, young children, travelers and the immunocompromised.

Noroviruses have a worldwide distribution with a prevalence of 5–36% among severe gastroenteritis cases in all age groups [5]. Studies in the USA have likewise shown norovirus to be responsible for 5–31% of gastroenteritis hospitalizations and 5–36% of clinic visits [6]. More than 90% of all nonbacterial gastroenteritis outbreaks in the USA have been attributed to noroviruses [7]. Although data are sparse from developing countries in Africa and Asia, where there is high morbidity and mortality from diarrhea in children <5 years of age, norovirus infection appears common [8, 9]. Each year, noroviruses cause approximately 64,000 episodes of diarrhea requiring hospitalization.

900,000 clinic visits among children in industrialized countries and up to 200,000 deaths of children younger than 5 years of age in developing countries [5].

There is substantial genetic diversity amongst circulating noroviruses. Based on sequencing of the viral genome, five distinct norovirus genogroups have been identified: GI–GV. Viruses from genogroups GI, GII and GIV infect humans, among which at least 25 genotypes have been identified thus far, whilst viruses from the GIII and GV genogroups have only been found in animals. Global norovirus surveillance studies show that GII strains, specifically those within the GII.4 genotype, predominate among human infections. Genetic drift, re-assortment and population immunity appear to drive the continued emergence of new viral strains, which have subsequently resulted in a pattern of successive global pandemics [10].

NATURAL HISTORY, PATHOGENESIS AND PATHOLOGY

Infection can be acquired by the fecal-oral or vomitus-oral routes, either directly by person-to-person transmission or indirectly through contaminated food, water or environmental surfaces (Fig. 30.2.1). Because there is no long-lasting acquired immunity to norovirus infection and there is little heterotypic protection to the diverse viral populations, infection can occur at any age and multiple times throughout a person's lifetime. Much of what is known about the natural history of norovirus infection and clinical disease comes from a collection of volunteer studies conducted since the 1970s. However, the amount of virus fed to volunteers in these classic studies considerably exceeded the minimum infectious dose (10^6 compared with 18 particles), so it remains unclear how the characterization of immunity and pathogenesis are representative of what occurs following natural exposure [15].

An intriguing observation made in these studies was that when volunteers were challenged with virus, some individuals developed infection and disease, while others (some with and some without pre-existing antibody) did not develop infection [16]. Recently, the innate resistance to infection in the latter group has been explained by genetic susceptibility. Noroviruses recognize histo-blood group antigens (HBGAs) that reside on the mucosal epithelia of the digestive tract. As determined by expression of the fucosyltransferase-2 (FUT2) gene, persons who are secretors (approximately 80% of Caucasian populations) are susceptible to infection, while those who are non-secretors are resistant [11]. However, binding is strain specific and there is a range of HBGAs in human populations; therefore, individuals resistant to one strain may be susceptible to others [17].

Following infection, histologic changes include broadening and blunting of the intestinal villi, crypt-cell hyperplasia, cytoplasmic

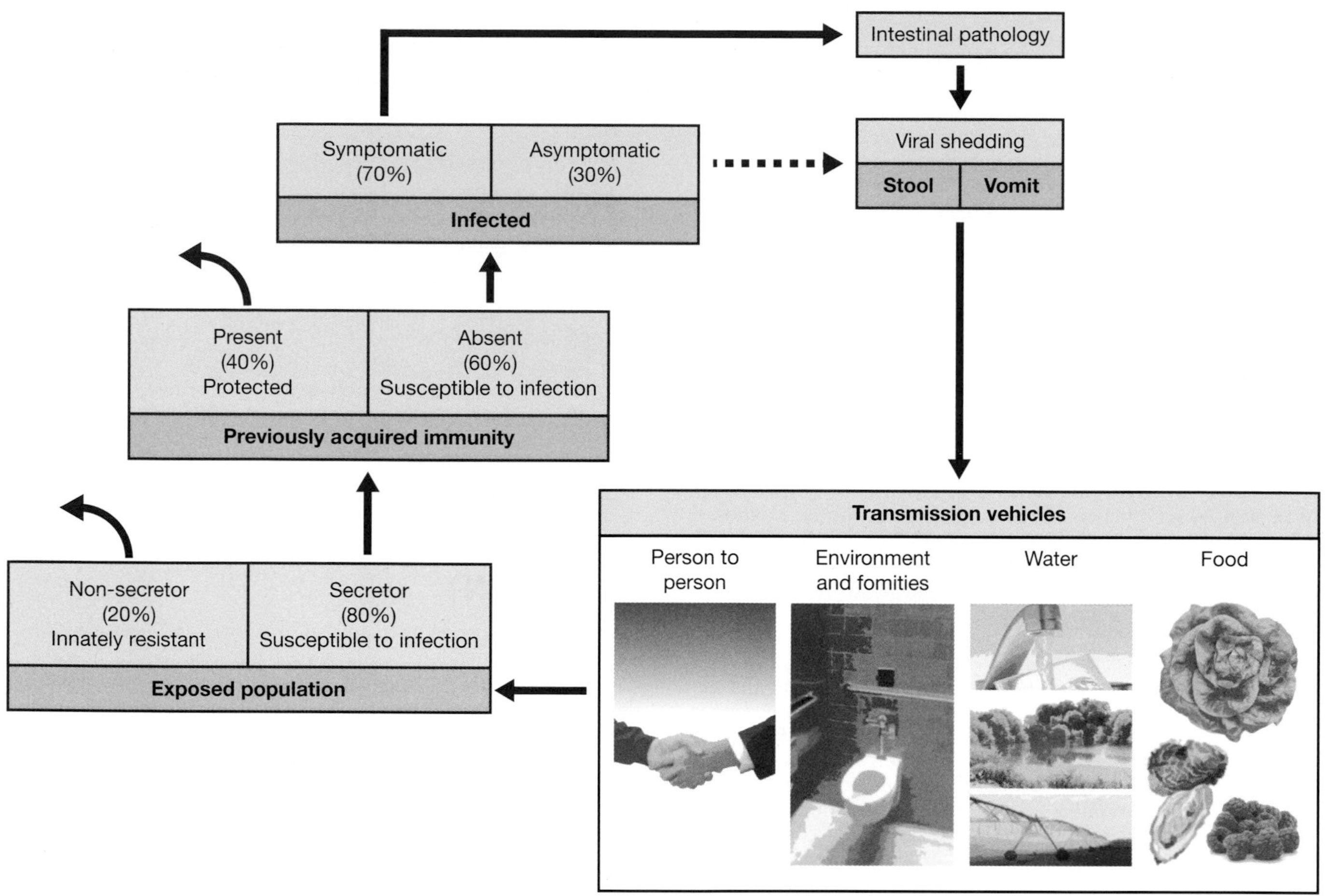

FIGURE 30.2.1 The cycle of norovirus transmission begins with infected individuals, including both symptomatic and asymptomatic infections. Symptomatic infection causes intestinal pathology, including blunting of villi, increased cytotoxicity and increased cell proliferation at the base of crypts. The virus is then shed in stool and vomit of symptomatic individuals, as well as the stool of asymptomatic individuals. Subsequent transmission vehicles may include raw or ready-to-eat foods, drinking or recreational water, contaminated fomites or environments, and direct person-to-person contact. Note that cross-contamination may occur among these vehicles, such as the contamination of fresh produce with irrigation water or shellfish with wastewater. The population exposed to these contaminated vehicles include both innately susceptible and resistant individuals, as denoted by secretor status. Among exposed secretors, a proportion will have previously acquired immunity and therefore be protected from infection. Those without innate or acquired immunity then become infected and the cycle begins anew. The specific proportions of individuals that are secretors, have previously acquired immunity, and develop symptomatic infections may vary depending on population, setting and strain [11–14].

vacuolization, and infiltration of polymorphonuclear and mononuclear cells into the lamina propria, while the mucosa itself remains intact. Enzymatic activity is decreased resulting in mild steatorrhea and transient carbohydrate malabsorption [18]. Recent work has demonstrated severe epithelial barrier dysfunction resulting in a leak flux mechanism whereby ions and water ''leak back'' from the subepithelial capillaries into the intestinal lumen as a result of the increased permeability of the tight junction, in addition to anion secretion in the norovirus-infected small intestine [12]. The physiologic and molecular mechanisms underlying the rapid onset of diarrhea, vomiting and other symptoms are not fully understood. Virus is shed in stool for an average of four weeks following infection, although peak shedding occurs 2–5 days after infection and at a magnitude of 95 billion viral particles per gram of feces [13]. Up to 30% of norovirus infections are asymptomatic although still capable of significant viral shedding, albeit less than that of symptomatic infections [14].

CLINICAL FEATURES

Norovirus typically causes disease after an incubation period of 12–48 hours and is characterized by acute-onset of diarrhea, vomiting, nausea and abdominal cramps. Some patients may experience only vomiting or diarrhea. Diarrheal stools tend to be watery without blood, mucus or leukocytes. Diarrhea is more prevalent in children aged <1 year, while persons aged >1 year more often develop vomiting [19]. Low-grade fever is present in approximately 40% of patients and typically resolves within 24 hours. Other constitutional symptoms, including myalgias, headache and chills are also commonly reported. Although symptoms may be severe, they typically resolve without treatment after 1–3 days in otherwise healthy individuals. However, more prolonged courses of illness lasting 4–6 days can occur, particularly among children, the elderly and hospitalized patients [19, 20]. While community-based studies suggest clinical disease associated with norovirus infection is generally milder than that of rotavirus, hospitalized children infected with either virus have similar severity scores. As such, severity alone does not readily distinguish norovirus disease from other causes of gastroenteritis.

In industrialized countries, up to 10% of patients with norovirus gastroenteritis seek medical attention, which may include hospitalization and treatment for dehydration [21]. Given the increased prevalence of malnutrition, co-infection with other enteric pathogens and other comorbidities, more severe disease manifestations and frequent hospitalizations may occur in tropical settings, although data are limited. Norovirus-associated deaths have been reported among the elderly and in the context of outbreaks in long-term care facilities [22, 23]. Although long-term sequelae do not appear to result following infection, secondary features that have been reported include necrotizing enterocolitis in neonates, chronic diarrhea (>1 year) in immunosuppressed patients and post-infectious irritable bowel syndrome resolving after 3 months [24–26]. Norovirus infections have also been implicated in causing neurologic manifestations, including benign seizures in infants and encephalopathy, as evidenced by detection of the virus in cerebrospinal fluid [27, 28]. Prospective, analytical studies are needed to better assess these anecdotal observations and determine the relative frequency of these complications among those infected with norovirus.

PATIENT EVALUATION, DIAGNOSIS AND DIFFERENTIAL DIAGNOSIS

A broad range of bacteria, viruses, preformed toxins and chemicals may cause symptoms of acute gastroenteritis mimicking norovirus infection. Norovirus gastroenteritis is typically characterized by short incubation, short duration, sudden onset (often with no prodrome) and high frequency of vomiting. The 12–48 hour incubation period following infection with norovirus can help in distinguishing it from organisms that produce a preformed bacterial toxin and typically have a shorter incubation period of 4–6 hours (e.g. *Staphylococcus aureus* or *Bacillus cereus*). In contrast, bacterial pathogens, such as *Campylobacter* spp., *Salmonella* spp., Shiga toxin-producing *Escherichia coli* and *Shigella* spp., tend to have a longer incubation period and more often cause bloody, mucoid stools compared with norovirus. Other viral etiologies are difficult to clinically differentiate from norovirus. In children, rotavirus is the most common virus to consider in the differential, which typically causes a pronounced dehydrating illness. Other, less common, viruses that clinically mimic norovirus include astrovirus, adenovirus 40/41 and sapovirus.

In general, no readily-available sensitive diagnostic assay exists for clinical diagnosis of norovirus infection. This shortcoming in the clinical setting is less problematic for norovirus compared with bacterial pathogens because, as yet, laboratory confirmation of a case rarely informs clinical management of norovirus gastroenteritis. Nonetheless, laboratory confirmation is crucial for surveillance and infection control purposes. Norovirus was discovered using electron microscopy, which remained the diagnostic method of choice until the 1990s. Reverse transcription (RT)-PCR is now the reference standard diagnostic for detecting virus in stool, as well as in water and food. With the advancement of molecular techniques, gel-based RT-PCR is being replaced by a real-time platform using a Taqman probe that allows simultaneous detection and quantification [29]. Immunoassays are commercially available in Europe and Japan, and are used aboard some cruise liners and other sea vessels in outbreak settings. These assays are specific for norovirus, but lack adequate sensitivity for routine clinical use.

A cocktail of primers for RT-PCR or a panel of cross-reactive antibodies for immunoassays is required to detect the diverse range of norovirus strains. Viral load in stool can peak as early as 48 hours after infection so fecal specimens should be collected as soon as possible after the onset of symptoms. However, molecular diagnostics may be sensitive enough to detect virus for a week or more after onset of symptoms. Therefore, for certain epidemiologic investigations (e.g. a suspected link between an ill food-handler and a cluster of cases), collection of specimens later in the course of illness may be warranted. Often, the goal of diagnosis is to determine the cause of an outbreak. In such situations, specimens should be collected from at least five cases, given that 2 or more positive specimens are usually recommended for definitive attribution [30]. Molecular diagnostics for norovirus are largely confined to reference or public health laboratories and are not routinely available to most clinical settings nor in developing countries. Epidemiologic characteristics (known as Kaplan criteria) have also been validated and used to attribute outbreaks to norovirus [31], although laboratory diagnostics are still required to confirm etiology.

BOX 30.2.1 Treatment Considerations for Pediatric Patients with Acute Norovirus Gastroenteritis

- For uncomplicated norovirus gastroenteritis, first-line therapy should be oral rehydration solutions providing essential electrolyte replacement plus sugar.
- Severe dehydration and shock may warrant intravenous fluid replenishment.
- As tolerated, initiating oral caloric intake early in the illness may enhance patient recovery.
- In developing countries, adjuvant therapy with zinc may reduce the duration and frequency of diarrhea.
- Antimotility agents should be avoided in children less than 3 years old as they can be associated with rare, severe, adverse complications, such as ileus, lethargy or death.

TREATMENT

No specific therapeutic interventions exist for acute norovirus gastroenteritis. Recommended therapy is similar to that for other causes of viral gastroenteritis which includes replenishment of intravascular depletion of volume and essential electrolytes. Oral rehydration solutions that provide electrolyte replacement plus glucose or sucrose are recommended as the first-line therapy for uncomplicated diarrheal illness [32]. A Cochrane Review failed to identify any important differences in outcome between oral and intravenous rehydration for acute diarrhea [33]. Thus, unless the patient is in shock or manifests signs and symptoms of severe dehydration or paralytic ileus, initial rehydration efforts with oral solutions should be attempted prior to intravenous rehydration (Box 30.2.1). When severe dehydration is present, more rapid fluid replacement may be necessary using intravenous fluids. As tolerated, patients should begin taking food early in the illness as adequate caloric intake has been found to enhance patient recovery [34, 35].

Few clinical trials have compared the effectiveness of anti-emetics in children with vomiting associated with acute gastroenteritis [36]. Although evidence is weak, the use of ondansetron and metoclopramide may reduce the number of episodes of vomiting related to gastroenteritis. Clinical investigations suggest that zinc replacement may shorten the duration of diarrheal episodes in children aged 6 months or older in developing countries with a high prevalence of micronutrient malnutrition [37]. Probiotics (e.g. *Lactobacillus spp*, yeast *Saccharomyces*) appear to reduce the duration of diarrhea when used as an adjunct to rehydration therapy; however, studies are insufficient to inform evidence-based treatment guidelines of specific probiotics in defined age groups [38]. Antimotility agents such as diphenoxylate or loperamide appear to reduce the duration and frequency of diarrhea, but should be avoided in children younger than 3 years old as they may be harmful in some cases [39]. Antibiotic therapy for the treatment of uncomplicated viral gastroenteritis is not recommended. Research efforts towards the development of antiviral agents against noroviruses have identified candidate drugs but clinical trials have not yet been conducted [40].

REFERENCES

1. Bryce J, Boschi-Pinto C, Shibuya K, Black RE. WHO estimates of the causes of death in children. Lancet 2005;365:1147–52.
2. Moreno-Espinosa S, Farkas T, Jiang X. Human caliciviruses and pediatric gastroenteritis. Semin Pediatr Infect Dis 2004;15:237–45.
3. Jiang X, Wilton N, Zhong WM, et al. Diagnosis of human caliciviruses by use of enzyme immunoassays. J Infect Dis 2000;181(suppl. 2):S349–59.
4. Patel MM, Hall AJ, Vinje J, Parashar UD. Noroviruses: a comprehensive review. J Clin Virol 2009;44:1–8.

5. Patel MM, Widdowson MA, Glass RI, et al. Systematic literature review of role of noroviruses in sporadic gastroenteritis. Emerg Infect Dis 2008;14: 1224–31.
6. Glass RI, Parashar UD, Estes MK. Norovirus gastroenteritis. N Engl J Med 2009;361:1776–85.
7. Fankhauser RL, Monroe SS, Noel JS, et al. Epidemiologic and molecular trends of "Norwalk-like viruses" associated with outbreaks of gastroenteritis in the United States. J Infect Dis 2002;186:1–7.
8. Monica B, Ramani S, Banerjee I, et al. Human caliciviruses in symptomatic and asymptomatic infections in children in Vellore, South India. J Med Virol 2007;79:544–51.
9. Sdiri-Loulizi K, Gharbi-Khelifi H, de Rougemont A, et al. Acute infantile gastroenteritis associated with human enteric viruses in Tunisia. J Clin Microbiol 2008;46:1349–55.
10. Koopmans M. Progress in understanding norovirus epidemiology. Curr Opin Infect Dis 2008;21:544–52 (annotated review).
11. Lindesmith L, Moe C, Marionneau S, et al. Human susceptibility and resistance to Norwalk virus infection. Nat Med 2003;9:548–53.
12. Troeger H, Loddenkemper C, Schneider T, et al. Structural and functional changes of the duodenum in human norovirus infection. Gut 2009;58: 1070–7.
13. Atmar RL, Opekun AR, Gilger MA, et al. Norwalk virus shedding after experimental human infection. Emerg Infect Dis 2008;14:1553–7.
14. Graham DY, Jiang X, Tanaka T, et al. Norwalk virus infection of volunteers: new insights based on improved assays. J Infect Dis 1994;170:34–43.
15. Teunis PF, Moe CL, Liu P, et al. Norwalk virus: how infectious is it? J Med Virol 2008;80:1468–76.
16. Parrino TA, Schreiber DS, Trier JS, et al. Clinical immunity in acute gastroenteritis caused by Norwalk agent. N Engl J Med 1977;297:86–9.
17. Tan M, Jin M, Xie H, et al. Outbreak studies of a GII-3 and a GII-4 norovirus revealed an association between HBGA phenotypes and viral infection. J Med Virol 2008;80:1296–301.
18. Agus SG, Dolin R, Wyatt RG, et al. Acute infectious nonbacterial gastroenteritis: intestinal histopathology. Histologic and enzymatic alterations during illness produced by the Norwalk agent in man. Ann Intern Med 1973;79: 18–25.
19. Rockx B, De Wit M, Vennema H, et al. Natural history of human calicivirus infection: a prospective cohort study. Clin Infect Dis 2002;35:246–53.
20. Lopman BA, Reacher MH, Vipond IB, et al. Clinical manifestation of norovirus gastroenteritis in health care settings. Clin Infect Dis 2004;39:318–24.
21. Widdowson MA, Sulka A, Bulens SN, et al. Norovirus and foodborne disease, United States, 1991–2000. Emerg Infect Dis 2005;11:95–102.
22. Harris JP, Edmunds WJ, Pebody R, et al. Deaths from norovirus among the elderly, England and Wales. Emerg Infect Dis 2008;14:1546–52.
23. Norovirus activity—United States, 2006–2007. MMWR Morb Mortal Wkly Rep 2007;56:842–6.
24. Turcios-Ruiz RM, Axelrod P, St John K, et al. Outbreak of necrotizing enterocolitis caused by norovirus in a neonatal intensive care unit. J Pediatr 2008;153:339–44.
25. Westhoff TH, Vergoulidou M, Loddenkemper C, et al. Chronic norovirus infection in renal transplant recipients. Nephrol Dial Transplant 2009;24: 1051–3.
26. Marshall JK, Thabane M, Borgaonkar MR, James C. Postinfectious irritable bowel syndrome after a food-borne outbreak of acute gastroenteritis attributed to a viral pathogen. Clin Gastroenterol Hepatol 2007;5:457–60.
27. Chen SY, Tsai CN, Lai MW, et al. Norovirus infection as a cause of diarrhea-associated benign infantile seizures. Clin Infect Dis 2009;48:849–55.
28. Ito S, Takeshita S, Nezu A, et al. Norovirus-associated encephalopathy. Pediatr Infect Dis J 2006;25:651–2.
29. Kageyama T, Kojima S, Shinohara M, et al. Broadly reactive and highly sensitive assay for Norwalk-like viruses based on real-time quantitative reverse transcription-PCR. J Clin Microbiol 2003;41:1548–57.
30. Hall AJ, Vinjé J, Lopman B, et al. Updated norovirus outbreak management and disease prevention guidelines. MMWR Recomm Rep 2011;60(RR-3): 1–20.
31. Kaplan JE, Feldman R, Campbell DS, et al. The frequency of a Norwalk-like pattern of illness in outbreaks of acute gastroenteritis. Am J Public Health 1982;72:1329–32 (defines epidemiologic criteria indicative of norovirus outbreaks, including: (1) vomiting in more than half of affected persons; (2) mean (or median) incubation period of 24–48 hours; (3) mean (or median) duration of illness of 12–60 hours; and (4) absence of bacterial pathogen in stool culture).
32. Practice parameter: the management of acute gastroenteritis in young children. American Academy of Pediatrics, Provisional Committee on Quality Improvement, Subcommittee on Acute Gastroenteritis. Pediatrics 1996;97: 424–35.
33. Hartling L, Bellemare S, Wiebe N, et al. Oral versus intravenous rehydration for treating dehydration due to gastroenteritis in children. Cochrane Database Syst Rev 2006;3:CD004390.
34. Brown KH, Gastanaduy AS, Saavedra JM, et al. Effect of continued oral feeding on clinical and nutritional outcomes of acute diarrhea in children. J Pediatr 1988;112:191–200.
35. King CK, Glass R, Bresee JS, Duggan C. Managing acute gastroenteritis among children: oral rehydration, maintenance, and nutritional therapy. MMWR Recomm Rep 2003;52:1–16.
36. Alhashimi D, Al-Hashimi H, Fedorowicz Z. Antiemetics for reducing vomiting related to acute gastroenteritis in children and adolescents. Cochrane Database Syst Rev 2009:CD005506.
37. Lazzerini M, Ronfani L. Oral zinc for treating diarrhoea in children. Cochrane Database Syst Rev 2008:CD005436.
38. Allen SJ, Okoko B, Martinez E, et al. Probiotics for treating infectious diarrhoea. Cochrane Database Syst Rev 2004:CD003048.
39. Li ST, Grossman DC, Cummings P. Loperamide therapy for acute diarrhea in children: systematic review and meta-analysis. PLoS Med 2007;4:e98.
40. Tan M, Jiang X. Norovirus gastroenteritis, increased understanding and future antiviral options. Curr Opin Investig Drugs 2008;9:146–51.

30.3 Enteric Adenoviruses

James J Gray, Gagandeep Kang

Key features

- Adenoviruses of species F, serotypes 40 and 41 are a common cause of gastroenteritis worldwide
- The main route of transmission is feco–oral
- Diarrhea, fever and vomiting are common and symptoms may last 3–11 days
- Adenoviruses have been isolated from as many as 40% of cases of intussusception
- Treatment is by oral rehydration with fluids containing electrolytes and sugar

INTRODUCTION

Adenoviruses are non-enveloped icosahedral viruses of 70–80 nm diameter, possessing a genome of linear dsDNA of approximately 35,000 bp. The virus capsid consists of 240 hexons and 12 pentons at the vertices which carry projecting fibers (Fig. 30.3.1). Their three-dimensional structure has been elucidated.

Human adenoviruses occur in 51 distinct serotypes ordered into six different species (A–F, previously designated groups or subgroups) within the genus *Mastadenovirus* of the *Adenoviridae* family. The classification is based on biologic, biochemical and immunologic differences. Within species, serotypes are differentiated by the reactivity of the two major capsid proteins, hexon and fiber. Within each species, DNA sequence homology is greater than 85%. Adenoviruses of

TABLE 30.3-1 Incidence of Enteric Adenovirus Gastroenteritis in Countries in Europe, South America, Africa, Asia and the Far East

Country	Age groups	Number of subjects	Adenovirus incidence	Method	Reference
Saudia Arabia	All	1000	1.4%	PCR	[9]
Thailand	All	262	1.5%	ELISA	[10]
South Korea	All	10,028	2.6%	ELISA	[11]
Brazil	All	415	3.6%	ELISA	[12]
The Netherlands	All	709	3.8%	ELISA	[13]
India	Children	439	7.7%	PCR	[14]
Tunisia	Children	632	2.7%	ELISA	[15]
Brazil	Children	470	6.4%	ELISA	[16]
Taiwan	Children	257	19.8%	PCR	[17]
Nigeria	Children	282	23.0%	ELISA	[18]
UK	Children	305	7.9%	PCR	[19]
Finland	Children	832	6.0%	PCR	[20]
Spain	Children	820	3.0%	ELISA	[21]

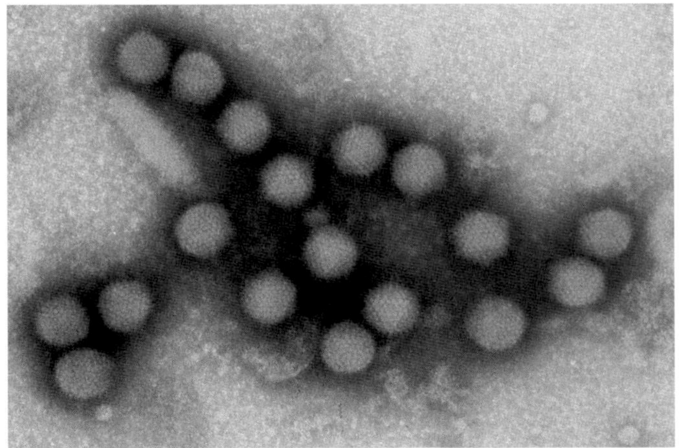

FIGURE 30.3.1 Electron micrograph of adenovirus particles showing characteristic icosahedral, non-enveloped particles of 80–110 nm in diameter.

species F, serotypes 40 and 41 are a common cause of gastroenteritis worldwide [1].

EPIDEMIOLOGY

Adenovirus cause epidemic, endemic or sporadic infections. The main route of transmission is feco-oral, but possibly also by droplet or close contact. Enteric adenoviruses are mainly endemic, but outbreaks in hospitals and boarding schools have been reported. Most infections are in infancy and early childhood, with the incidence of enteric adenovirus infections reported to be between 4 and 7 per 100 person years in small children [2], without a seasonal preference. The incidence of enteric adenovirus infections determined in burden of disease studies worldwide using ELISA and PCR methods ranged from 1.5–23.0% and 1.4–19.8%, respectively (Table 30.3-1). These differences cannot be solely associated with the sensitivity of the detection methods used, but may reflect the higher rates seen in children when compared with the whole population, or geographical differences associated with areas of poor sanitation or a lack of access to clean drinking water. By the age of 2 years, more than 40% of children possess neutralizing antibodies to adenoviruses types 40 and 41, suggesting that there are likely to be many unreported or unapparent infections [3]. In immunocompromised persons, adenoviruses can cause severe systemic disease.

NATURAL HISTORY, PATHOGENESIS AND PATHOLOGY

All adenoviruses grow well in human epithelial cells, with the exception of the fastidious or enteric adenoviruses types 40 and 41. Viral replication is initiated through cell attachment and is facilitated by the fiber protein, with uptake via receptor-mediated endocytosis. Members of the immunoglobulin superfamily have been implicated as receptors and integrins, possibly as co-receptors with CD46 identified as a receptor for species B and species D adenoviruses.

Adenoviruses replicate in the epithelia of the human respiratory and gastrointestinal tracts, as well as in the conjunctiva and in lymphocytes. Various viral factors contribute to the pathogenesis. Whilst the pentons are directly cytotoxic, early viral proteins counteract tumor necrosis factor (TNF) and apoptosis, and down-regulate the expression of major histocompatibility complex (MHC) Class I molecules, thus preventing recognition by cytotoxic T cells. Adenovirus infection may persist in lymphoid cells, but the mechanism is poorly understood. A serotype-specific humoral immune response provides homotypic protection.

CLINICAL FEATURES

Clinically, adenovirus-associated diarrhea does not differ from that caused by other viruses, although the duration of symptoms may be slightly longer (3–11 days). Fever and vomiting are common and stools are watery and non-bloody (in contrast to some bacterial diarrheas).

Intussusception is the most common cause of intestinal obstruction among young children aged 3 months to 3 years, occurring when one segment of the intestine invaginates (telescopes) an adjacent segment of the distal intestine. It causes severe colic, vomiting and the passage of blood and mucus rectally ("currant jelly" stool). This condition may result in arterial obstruction and subsequent bowel necrosis.

In the majority of childhood intussusception cases, no clear etiology is identified but reports indicate that adenovirus may by isolated from as many as 40% of cases. Interestingly, the majority of adenoviruses associated with intussusception belong to the non-enteric groups commonly associated with respiratory or conjunctival illness. This would suggest that intussusception is not associated with a particular adenovirus serotype or variant, but is likely to be host-related and driven by the immune response to adenovirus colonization.

PATIENT EVALUATION, DIAGNOSIS AND DIFFERENTIAL DIAGNOSIS

Detection of enteric adenoviruses in fecal specimens is mainly by ELISA using species F-specific monoclonal antibodies. Enteric adenoviruses grow very poorly in cell cultures and, therefore, virus isolation is not the diagnostic method of choice. In contrast, electron microscopy permits the detection of adenoviruses on the basis of their characteristic morphology. Enteric adenoviruses are shed in large numbers, approximately 10^8–10^9 particles per gram, and are readily detected. Adenoviruses are detected in 4–15% of stools from children with gastroenteritis in many hospitals, outpatients clinics and daycare centers [4]. Viral genome detection by means of PCR, which has much greater sensitivity (10–100 DNA molecules are detectable per reaction), is being increasingly used in adenovirus diagnosis [5]. However, of all the adenoviruses detected in feces, only 30–50% belong to species F, comprising types 40 and 41 [4, 6], the others being mainly members of species B and D, primarily infecting the respiratory tract.

PREVENTION AND TREATMENT

At present, there is no vaccine candidate for enteric adenoviruses. Public health measures to confine outbreaks include: cohort nursing of patients; use of gloves, gowns and goggles; disinfection with sodium hypochlorite; frequent hand-washing; removal of infected feces and contaminated food or water; and, exclusion of infected individuals from work. Outbreaks in clinical wards may require temporary closure to new admissions and restrictions on visiting and placements of staff.

Usually, adenovirus gastroenteritis is a mild disease and treatment is symptomatic and largely follows guidelines that have been established since 1985, mainly using oral rehydration fluids containing electrolytes and sugar [7]. Bismuth subsalicylate has been found to be beneficial in children with acute watery diarrhea [8]. Agents used against abdominal cramping such as diphenoxylate or loperamide should be avoided as they can have serious side effects. In severe cases of diarrhea, rapid fluid replacement by parenteral administration may be required. In developing countries where children are often malnourished, supplementary nutrition is an important component of the therapy. Cidofovir is active against adenovirus *in vitro* and has been used in the treatment of disseminated adenovirus infections in bone marrow transplant recipients. When it occurs, intussusception is usually reduced hydrostatically using a barium or air enema, but surgical intervention is sometimes required. An air enema is preferable to barium which occasionally enters the peritoneum through a clinically unsuspected perforation causing significant peritonitis.

REFERENCES

1. Wold WSM, Horwitz MS. Adenoviruses. In: Knipe DM, Howley PM, et al, eds. Fields Virology, 5th edn. Philadelphia: Wolters Kluwer Health/Lippincott Williams and Wilkins; 2007;2395–436.
2. Mistchenko AS, Huberman KH, Gómez JA, Grinstein S. Epidemiology of enteric adenovirus infections in prospectively monitored Argentine families. Epidemiol Infect 1992;109:539–46.
3. Shinozaki T, Araki K, Ushijima H, Fujii R. Antibody response to enteric adenovirus types 40 and 41 in sera from people in various age groups. J Clin Microbiol 1987;25;1679–82
4. Krajden M, Brown M, Petrasek A, et al. Clinical features of adenovirus enteritis: a review of 127 cases. Ped Infect Dis J 1990;9:636–41.
5. Avellón A, Pérez P, Aguilar JC, et al. Rapid and sensitive diagnosis of human adenovirus infections by a generic polymerase chain reaction. J Virol Methods 2001;92:113–20.
6. Lew JF, Moe CL, Monroe SS, et al. Astrovirus and adenovirus associated with diarrhoea in children in day care settings. J Infect Dis 1991;164:673–8.
7. Desselberger U. Rotavirus infections: guidelines for treatment and prevention. Drugs 1999;58:447-52.
8. Figueroa-Quintanilla D, Salazar-Lindo E, Sack RB, et al. A controlled trial of bismuth subsalicylate in infants with acute watery diarrheal disease. New Engl J Med 1993;328:1653–8.
9. Tayeb HT, Dela Cruz DM, Al-Qahtani A, et al. Enteric viruses in pediatric diarrhea in Saudi Arabia. J Med Virol 2008;80: 1919–29.
10. Kittigul L, Pombubpa K, Taweekate Y, et al. Molecular characterisation of rotaviruses, noroviruses, sapovirus, and adenoviruses in patients with acute gastroenteritis in Thailand. J Med Virol 2009;81:345–53.
11. Huh J-W, Kim W-H, Moon S-G, et al. Viral etiology and incidence associated with acute gastroenteritis in a 5-year survey in Gyeonggi province, South Korea. J Clin Virol 2009;44:152–6.
12. Andreasi MSA, Cardoso DD, Fernandes SM, et al. Adenovirus, calicivirus and astrovirus detection in fecal samples of hospitalised children with acute gastroenteritis from Campo Grande, MS, Brazil. Mem Inst Oswaldo Cruz (Rio de Janeiro) 2009;103:741–4.
13. De Wit MAS, Koopmans MPG, Kortbeek LM, et al. Sensor, a population-based cohort study on gastroenteritis in the Netherlands: Incidence and aetiology. Am J Epidemiolo 2001;154:666–74.
14. Verma H, Chitambar SD, Varanasi G. Identification and characterisation of enteric adenoviruses in infants and children hospitalised for acute gastroenteritis. J Med Virol 2009;81:60-4.
15. Sdiri-Loulizi K, Gharbi-Khelifi H, de Rougemont A, et al. Acute infantile gastroenteritis associated with human enteric viruses in Tunisia. J Clin Microbiol 2008;46:1349–55.
16. Magalhaes GF, Nogueira PA, Grava AF, et al. Mem Inst Oswaldo Cruz (Rio de Janeiro) 2007;102:555–7.
17. Chen S-Y, Chang Y-C, Lee Y-S, et al. Molecular epidemiology and clinical manifestations of viral gastroenteritis in hospitalised pediatric patients in northern Taiwan. J Clin Microbiol 2007;45:2054–7.
18. Aminu M, Ahmad AA, Umoh JU, et al. Adenovirus infection in children with diarrhoea in northwest Nigeria. Ann African Med 2007;6:168–73.
19. Simpson R, Aliyu S, Iturriza-Gomara M, et al. Infantile viral gastroenteritis: on the way to closing the diagnostic gap. J Med Virol 2003; 258–62.
20. Pang XL, Honma S, Nakata S, Vesikari T. Human caliciviruses in acute gastroenteritis of young children in the community. J Infect Dis 2000; 2(Suppl):S288–94.
21. Roman E, Wilhelmi I, Colomina J, et al. Acute viral gastroenteritis: proportion and clinical relevance of multiple infections in Spanish children. J MedMicrobiol 2003;52:435–40.

30.4 Astroviruses

Gagandeep Kang, James J Gray

Key features

- Important cause of viral gastroenteritis, particularly in children
- World-wide distribution, winter peaks in temperate climates
- Distinctive appearance of a star on electron microscopy
- Shedding may be prolonged in immunocompromised individuals
- Maintenance of hydration is the key to therapy

INTRODUCTION

Human astrovirus is the prototype of the *Astroviridae*, a family of non-enveloped positive-sense RNA viruses belonging to the genus ***Mamastrovirus***, measuring 38–41 nm with icosahedral symmetry. The genome of astrovirus consists of positive-sense, single-stranded RNA of 6.8–7.2 kb in length. These viruses were first described by Madeley and Cosgrove as 28-nm particles seen in infantile gastro-enteritis. By direct electron microscopy, astroviruses recovered from stool display a distinctive surface star-like appearance (Fig. 30.4.1), consisting of an electron-dense center surrounded by triangular electron lucent areas. Virus grown in cell culture shows spike-like projections.

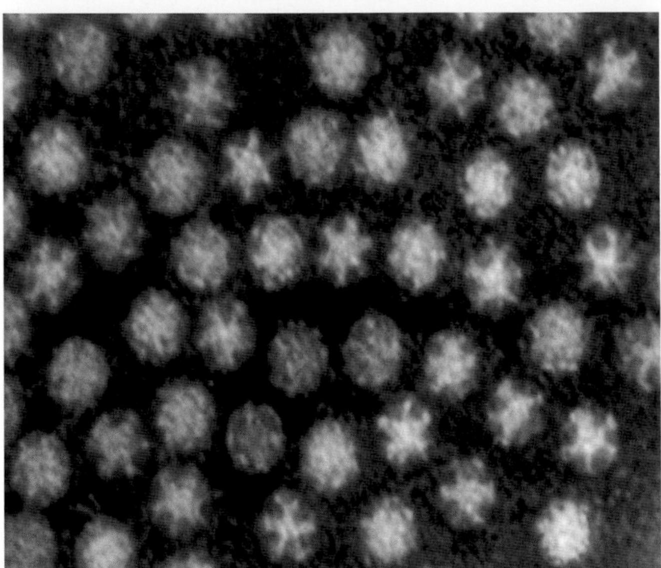

FIGURE 30.4.1 Astroviruses are spherical particles about 30 nm in diameter without an envelope. Nucleo-capsids have a regular surface structure and appear star-like with five or six points.

Astroviruses are classified into serotypes based on the reactivity of the capsid proteins with polyclonal sera and monoclonal antibodies. The number of viral structural proteins appears to vary with the serotype, with between one and three reported for the human viruses. Astroviruses can also be classified into genotypes on the basis of the nucleotide sequence of a 348-bp region of the genome; there is a good correlation with the serotypes. There are eight established genotypes designated human astroviruses 1–8 (HAstV1–HAstV8), which are considered "classical", as well as several newly described astroviruses [1].

EPIDEMIOLOGY

Person-to-person spread by the fecal–oral route is thought to be the most common route of transmission. Recent work with sensitive assay techniques has shown the prevalence of this virus to be much higher than previously thought and all eight HAstV serotypes or genotypes have been widely detected around the world, with HAstV-1 most commonly found using both serotyping and genotyping (Table 30.4-1).

Astroviruses are seen in stools of children with diarrhea, generally at rates lower than rotavirus and the noroviruses. Symptomatic infection occurs mainly in small children and the elderly, In hospital- and community-based studies in many countries, rates range up to 16%. In addition, outbreaks have been described in a range of settings, including schools, daycare centers and hospital wards. Generally, gastroenteritis is reported in young children, but outbreaks have been described in adults and in elderly populations.

Some studies have reported higher prevalence in winter in temperate climates, while infection does not appear to be seasonal closer to the equator. Seroprevalence studies show that infection is common, with children rapidly acquiring antibodies. Studies from the USA have shown that 94% of children have antibodies to HAstV1 and 42% to HAstV3 by the age of 9 years [2]; seroprevalence figures suggest that individuals can become infected by more than one serotype [3].

NATURAL HISTORY, PATHOGENESIS AND PATHOLOGY

The pathogenesis of the disease has not yet been fully elucidated. In volunteer studies, astrovirus infection by oral administration of stool filtrates has been shown to induce diarrhea and an immune response. Viral replication is thought to occur in intestinal tissue. In animal studies, there are inflammatory infiltrates in the lamina propria and atrophy of the intestinal villi; the osmotic diarrhea that follows is thought to be caused by decreased intestinal disaccharidase activity. Studies using model systems have shown intestinal permeability is increased following apical infection, modulated by the viral capsid protein. Increased permeability correlated with disruption of the tight-junction protein occludin and decreased actin stress fibers in the absence of cell death. Reactive oxygen species (e.g. nitric oxide) are thought to play a role in limiting infection.

Volunteers with no pre-existing antibodies were more likely to have severe symptoms and more likely to shed virus [4], indicating that neutralizing antibodies may be important in limiting infection. Studies of human intestinal biopsies have suggested that cellular immunity, specifically astrovirus-specific Th1-type CD4 cells in the gut mucosa, may also be involved in the anti-astrovirus response. Additionally, animal models have implicated innate immunity. The interactions between these various effector arms of the immune system which result in immunity and resistance to astrovirus infection are still unknown [5].

TABLE 30.4-1 Astrovirus Prevalence in Non-Outbreak Gastroenteritis Reported during the Period 2005–2010

Country	Age group	Number with diarrhea	Astrovirus prevalence (%)	Methods	Reference
Japan	Children	314	1.6	PCR	[11]
Czech Republic	Children	2606	0.8	ELISA	[12]
Italy	Children	215	7.0	ELISA	[13]
China	Children	335	9.9	PCR	[14]
Kenya	Children	476	6.3	ELISA	[15]
Vietnam	Children	1010	0.6	PCR	[16]
Brazil	Children	318	14	PCR	[17]
Brazil	Children	2534	6.1	PCR	[18]
Albania	Children	313	1.6	PCR	[19]
Vietnam	Children	502	13.9	PCR	[20]
Madagascar	Children	237	2.1	PCR	[21]
Bangladesh	Children	916	0.4	PCR	[22]
Nigeria	Children	134	5.0	ELISA	[23]
Taiwan	Children	415	2.9	ELISA	[24]
Saudi Arabia	Children	1000	1.9	ELISA	[25]
Brazil	Children	354	3.1	PCR	[26]
Thailand	Children	296	2.4	PCR	[27]
Egypt	Children	230	1.7	ELISA	[28]
Korea	All	10,028	3.4	ELISA	[29]
India	Children	416	7.5	PCR	[1]
USA	Children	466	2.8	PCR	[1]
Greece	Children	4604	2.4	ELISA	[30]
Japan	Children	877	4.6	PCR	[31]
Tunisia	Children	788	3.6	ELISA/PCR	[32]
Russia	All	4562	1.5	PCR	[33]
India	All	1340	3.1	PCR	[34]
China	Children	664	7.8	PCR	[35]

CLINICAL FEATURES

The majority of infections in adults are likely to be asymptomatic and, in children, rapid acquisition of antibodies indicates that exposure rates are high and infection does not always result in disease. When disease occurs, symptoms are mild and it is likely that many cases go unreported, resulting in an under-estimate of attributable illness. Astrovirus gastroenteritis consists of diarrhea associated with headache, nausea, low-grade fever and vomiting [6, 7]. The incubation period is estimated to be about 3 days and illness is short and self-limiting, typically 3–5 days. PCR assessment of virus shedding has shown that shedding may continue for over a month after the cessation of symptoms [6]. The disease does not appear to be more severe in children with HIV or those with other forms of immunocompromise, such as bone marrow transplantation or hematological malignancies. Recently, an association with necrotizing enterocolitis in neonates [8] and with intussusception has been reported [9].

PATIENT EVALUATION, DIAGNOSIS AND DIFFERENTIAL DIAGNOSIS

Astrovirus gastroenteritis is similar, but milder, to other viral gastroenteritis, resulting in an acute watery diarrhea that is, generally, self-limited. The techniques that have been used to diagnose astrovirus disease depend on virus visualization, virus culture antigen detection or genome amplification. Serology has been occasionally used to study outbreaks. Electron microscopy is generally an insensitive technique because a high concentration of viral particles is required for detection. Although astroviruses are shed in large numbers, the typical five- or six-pointed star morphology is seen in less than 10% of particles. Immune electron microscopy may increase diagnostic yield beyond basic electron microscopy. Enzyme immunoassays (EIA) have been developed, including streptavidin-biotin assays for increased sensitivity of detection, and are used in diagnostic laboratories. EIA is of comparable sensitivity (91%) and specificity (98%)

to immune electromicroscopy. For epidemiologic research, astrovirus-specific reverse transcription (RT)-PCR has recently been the screening method of choice. While some investigators have used highly sensitive primers targeted to conserved genomic regions coding for the nonstructural proteins and untranslated regions, others prefer to use primers from the capsid coding region which can be less sensitive but provides typing information. Recently, other approaches to nucleic acid amplification [1] and a DNA array for detecting astrovirus have been described that are increasing our understanding of virus diversity.

TREATMENT

Illness associated with astrovirus is generally self-limited and treatment, if required at all, is supportive and directed at replacing fluids and electrolytes, as directed by the estimated degree of dehydration. Oral rehydration is recommended for preventing and treating early dehydration and continued replacement therapy for continuing fluid losses. Severe dehydration may require intravenous therapy. Children should be fed a normal diet, if tolerated. Anti-emetics, antidiarrheal agents and antibiotics are not recommended. In developing countries, the World Health Organization recommends zinc supplementation for 2 weeks following an acute diarrheal episode.

Prevention of infection may be difficult to achieve, given the rapidity with which children are infected, but, as with all viral gastroenteritis, secondary transmission may be prevented by strict attention to hygiene, particularly hand-washing after contact with an infected person. Although immunity to astrovirus is not well understood, one report suggests that infection is associated with at least short-term protection against re-infection with the same serotype [10], raising the possibility of developing vaccines in the future.

REFERENCES

1. Finkbeiner SR, Holtz LR, Jiang Y, et al. Human stool contains a previously unrecognized diversity of novel astroviruses. Virol J 2009;6:161.
2. Mitchell DK, Matson DO, Cubitt WD, et al. Prevalence of antibodies to astrovirus types 1 and 3 in children and adolescents in Norfolk, Virginia. Pediatr Infect Dis J 1999;18:249–54.
3. Koopmans MP, Bijen MH, Monroe SS, Vinjé J. Age-stratified seroprevalence of neutralizing antibodies to astrovirus types 1 to 7 in humans in The Netherlands. Clin Diagn Lab Immunol 1998;5:33–7.
4. Kurtz JB, Lee TW, Craig JW, Reed SE. Astrovirus infection in volunteers. J Med Virol 1979;3:221–30.
5. Koci MD. Immunity and resistance to astrovirus infection. Viral Immunol 2005;18:11–16.
6. Mitchell DK, Monroe SS, Jiang X, et al. Virologic features of an astrovirus diarrhea outbreak in a day care center revealed by reverse transcriptase-polymerase chain reaction. J Infect Dis 1995;172:1437–44.
7. Dennehy PH, Nelson SM, Spangenberger S, et al. A prospective case-control study of the role of astrovirus in acute diarrhea among hospitalized young children. J Infect Dis 2001;184:10–15.
8. Bagci S, Eis-Hubinger AM, Franz AR, et al. Detection of astrovirus in premature infants with necrotizing enterocolitis. Pediatr Infect Dis J 2008;27:347–50.
9. Jakab F, Peterfai J, Verebely T, et al. Human astrovirus infection associated with childhood intussusception. Pediatr Int 2007;49:103–5.
10. Naficy AB, Rao MR, Holmes JL, et al. Astrovirus diarrhea in Egyptian children. J Infect Dis 2000;182:685–90.
11. Phan TG, Nguyen TA, Kuroiwa T, et al. Viral diarrhea in Japanese children: results from a one-year epidemiologic study. Clin Lab 2005;51:183–91.
12. Pazdiora P, Jelinkova H, Svecova M, Taborska J. First experience with diagnosing astroviral infections in children hospitalized in Pilsen (Czechia). Folia Microbiol (Praha) 2006;51:129–32.
13. Colomba C, De Grazia S, Giammanco GM, et al. Viral gastroenteritis in children hospitalised in Sicily, Italy. Eur J Clin Microbiol Infect Dis 2006; 25:570–5.
14. Liu MQ, Yang BF, Peng JS, et al. Molecular epidemiology of astrovirus infection in infants in Wuhan, China. J Clin Microbiol 2007;45:1308–9.
15. Kiulia NM, Mwenda JM, Nyachieo A, et al. Astrovirus infection in young Kenyan children with diarrhoea. J Trop Pediatr 2007;53:206–9.
16. Nguyen TA, Yagyu F, Okame M, et al. Diversity of viruses associated with acute gastroenteritis in children hospitalized with diarrhea in Ho Chi Minh City, Vietnam. J Med Virol 2007;79:582–90.
17. Victoria M, Carvalho-Costa FA, Heinemann MB, et al. Genotypes and molecular epidemiology of human astroviruses in hospitalized children with acute gastroenteritis in Rio de Janeiro, Brazil. J Med Virol 2007;79:939–44.
18. Gabbay YB, Leite JP, Oliveira DS, et al. Molecular epidemiology of astrovirus type 1 in Belem, Brazil, as an agent of infantile gastroenteritis, over a period of 18 years (1982-2000): identification of two possible new lineages. Virus Res 2007;129:166–74.
19. Fabiana A, Donia D, Gabrieli R, et al. Influence of enteric viruses on gastroenteritis in Albania: epidemiological and molecular analysis. J Med Virol 2007;79:1844–9.
20. Nguyen TA, Hoang L, Pham le D, et al. Identification of human astrovirus infections among children with acute gastroenteritis in the Southern Part of Vietnam during 2005–2006. J Med Virol 2008;80:298–305.
21. Papaventsis DC, Dove W, Cunliffe NA, et al. Human astrovirus gastroenteritis in children, Madagascar, 2004–2005. Emerg Infect Dis 2008;14:844–6.
22. Dey SK, Islam A, Mizuguchi M, et al. Epidemiological and molecular analysis of astrovirus gastroenteritis in Dhaka City, Bangladesh. J Trop Pediatr 2008;54: 423–5.
23. Aminu M, Esona MD, Geyer A, Steele AD. Epidemiology of rotavirus and astrovirus infections in children in northwestern Nigeria. Ann Afr Med 2008;7:168–74.
24. Lin HC, Kao CL, Chang LY, et al. Astrovirus gastroenteritis in children in Taipei. J Formos Med Assoc 2008;107:295–303.
25. Tayeb HT, Dela Cruz DM, Al-Qahtani A, et al. Enteric viruses in pediatric diarrhea in Saudi Arabia. J Med Virol 2008;80:1919–29.
26. Andreasi MS, Cardoso DD, Fernandes SM, et al. Adenovirus, calicivirus and astrovirus detection in fecal samples of hospitalized children with acute gastroenteritis from Campo Grande, MS, Brazil. Mem Inst Oswaldo Cruz 2008;103:741–4.
27. Malasao R, Maneekarn N, Khamrin P, et al. Genetic diversity of norovirus, sapovirus, and astrovirus isolated from children hospitalized with acute gastroenteritis in Chiang Mai, Thailand. J Med Virol 2008;80:1749–55.
28. Kamel AH, Ali MA, El-Nady HG, et al. Predominance and circulation of enteric viruses in the region of Greater Cairo, Egypt. J Clin Microbiol 2009;47: 1037–45.
29. Huh JW, Kim WH, Moon SG, et al. Viral etiology and incidence associated with acute gastroenteritis in a 5-year survey in Gyeonggi province, South Korea. J Clin Virol 2009;44:152–6.
30. Levidiotou S, Gartzonika C, Papaventsis D, et al. Viral agents of acute gastroenteritis in hospitalized children in Greece. Clin Microbiol Infect 2009;15: 596–8.
31. Nakanishi K, Tsugawa T, Honma S, et al. Detection of enteric viruses in rectal swabs from children with acute gastroenteritis attending the pediatric outpatient clinics in Sapporo, Japan. J Clin Virol 2009;46:94–7.
32. Sdiri-Loulizi K, Gharbi-Khelifi H, de Rougemont A, et al. Molecular epidemiology of human astrovirus and adenovirus serotypes 40/41 strains related to acute diarrhea in Tunisian children. J Med Virol 2009;81:1895–902.
33. Podkolzin AT, Fenske EB, Abramycheva NY, et al. Hospital-based surveillance of rotavirus and other viral agents of diarrhea in children and adults in Russia, 2005–2007. J Infect Dis 2009;200(suppl. 1):S228–33.
34. Verma H, Chitambar SD, Gopalkrishna V. Astrovirus associated acute gastroenteritis in western India: Predominance of dual serotype strains. Infect Genet Evol 2010;10:575–9.
35. Guo L, Xu X, Song J, et al. Molecular characterization of astrovirus infection in children with diarrhea in Beijing, 2005–2007. J Med Virol 2010;82: 415–23.

30.5 Sapovirus

Osamu Nakagomi, Toyoko Nakagomi, Nigel A Cunliffe

Key features

- Sapovirus is a non-enveloped RNA virus which, on electronic microscopy, has a characteristic cup-like depression, often described as the "Star of David"
- Sapovirus causes acute-onset, watery, non-bloody diarrhea in infants and young children and is typically less severe than rotavirus
- Sapovirus accounts for 3–5% of acute gastroenteritis in children less than 5 years of age in both developing and developed countries
- Sapovirus rarely causes food-borne gastroenteritis or sporadic cases of acute gastroenteritis in adults
- The disease is self-limiting and oral or intravenous rehydration therapy is adminstered as required

INTRODUCTION

Sapovirus is a non-enveloped, positive-sense, single-stranded RNA virus with characteristic cup-like depressions on the surface of the virion, often described as the "Star of David". While both sapovirus and norovirus belong to the *Caliciviridae* family, the distinction of sapovirus from norovirus is made by its genome coding strategy in which, unlike norovirus, sapovirus encodes the capsid protein contiguous to the large, nonstructural polyprotein (ORF1).

The type species, Sapporo virus, is named after the city of Sapporo, Japan, where the virus was first identified in association with gastroenteritis during an outbreak in an orphanage [1].

EPIDEMIOLOGY

Sapovirus generally accounts for less than 5% of cases of acute gastroenteritis in children and is distributed globally. A 3-year study in Kenya detected sapovirus in 2.2% of outpatients with acute diarrhea aged <6 years old, but 70–90% of infants and adults were positive for antibodies to sapovirus [2]. Another study in India showed that sapovirus was detected in 3.4% of acute gastroenteritis, of all severities, in a community cohort which followed children up to the age of 3 years old and in 5.1% of children less than 5 years of age hospitalized because of acute gastroenteritis [3]. Sapovirus gastroenteritis may occur year-round, although it seems to occur more frequently in winter in temperate countries. The virus rarely causes outbreaks of foodborne gastroenteritis and is spread by the fecal–oral route. To date, five genogroups (GI–GV) of sapovirus have been described, which appear to correlate with antigenic differences in the VP1 protein [4].

NATURAL HISTORY, PATHOGENESIS AND PATHOLOGY

Gastroenteritis caused by sapovirus predominates in infants and young children [2]; virtually all children appear to have experienced infection with sapovirus by the age of 5 years. Sapovirus rarely causes disease in adults. The lack of cases in adults, as well as a high prevalence of antibodies in adults, suggests immunity persists after symptomatic infection in childhood.

CLINICAL FEATURES

After an incubation period of 1–3 days, sapovirus infection typically begins with the abrupt onset of watery, non-bloody diarrhea associated with vomiting, fever and abdominal pain. When it occurs, dehydration tends to be less severe than that caused by rotavirus [5].

PATIENT EVALUATION, DIAGNOSIS AND DIFFERENTIAL DIAGNOSIS

Diagnosis of viral gastroenteritis requires laboratory investigation of stool specimens collected in the acute stage of disease. Typical calicivirus-like morphology observed under negative-stain electron microscopy is indicative of sapovirus infection; however, definite diagnosis relies on the identification of sapovirus genome by reverse transcription (RT)-PCR.

Differential diagnosis includes other forms of viral gastroenteritis and pathogenic *Escherichia coli*.

TREATMENT

If present, the point of treatment is in the management of dehydration and dependent on the severity. There is neither specific antiviral chemotherapy nor a vaccine available.

REFERENCES

1. Chiba S, Sakuma Y, Kogasaka R, et al. An outbreak of gastroenteritis associated with calicivirus in an infant home. J Med Virol 1979;4:249–54.
2. Nakata S, Honma S, Numata K, et al. Prevalence of human calicivirus infections in Kenya as determined by enzyme immunoassays for three genogroups of the virus. J Clin Microbiol 1998;36:3160–3.
3. Monica B, Raman S, Banerjee I, et al. Human calicivirus in symptomatic and asymptomatic infections in children in Vellore, South India. J Med Virol 2007;79:544–51.
4. Hansman GS, Oka T, Sakon N, Takeda N. Antigenic diversity of human sapoviruses. Emerg Infect Dis 2007;13:1519–25.
5. Sakai Y, Nakata S, Honma S, et al. Clinical severity of Norwalk virus and Sapporo virus gastroenteritis in children in Hokkaido, Japan. Pediatr Infect Dis J 2001;20:849–53.

31 Viral Hepatitis

G Thomas Strickland, Samer S El-Kamary

Key features

- Hepatitis caused by viruses is a huge cause of illness in less developed countries
- Two viruses (hepatitis A virus and hepatitis E virus) are transmitted feco-orally and cause acute viral hepatitis
- Two viruses (hepatitis B virus and hepatitis C virus) are transmitted parenterally and cause both acute and chronic hepatitis
- Hepatitis D virus sometimes occurs with hepatitis B virus infection
- Hepatitis B and C are the greatest cause of chronic liver disease (cirrhosis and hepatocellular carcinoma)
- There is no specific treatment for hepatitis A or E; therapy for hepatitis B and C is costly, toxic, prolonged and has limited efficacy
- Excellent vaccines exist for Hepatitis A, B and E viruses (this one currently unavailable), but none exist for hepatitis C

INTRODUCTION

At least five viruses belonging to five different families cause hepatitis in humans [1, 2]. Two, hepatitis A virus (HAV) and hepatitis E virus (HEV), are acquired chiefly through ingestion of fecally-contaminated food or water and cause a self-limited acute illness [3–5]. Hepatitis B virus (HBV), hepatitis C virus (HCV) and hepatitis D virus (HDV) are transmitted, in varying degrees, by blood, and by percutaneous, perinatal and sexual exposures [6–12]. These three frequently cause acute hepatitis and persistent infection (often occult) that can lead to chronic hepatitis and cirrhosis and its complications [13, 14]. Additional hepatotropic viruses (non-A–E) are suspected but none have been confirmed. Epstein-Barr virus (EBV) and cytomegalovirus (CMV) also cause human hepatitis, but it is not their principal clinical characteristic [15, 16].

Changes in human ecology and socioeconomic status have influenced the impact of hepatitis viruses. Improved sanitation has reduced the importance of HAV in developed countries, but it remains a serious public health problem in less developed countries and travelers to these areas are at risk for infection [1]. Improvements in screening blood products and the HBV vaccine have reduced transmission of HBV and HCV in developed countries, but these safeguards are not always available in less developed countries [17]. These five hepatitis viruses are a major worldwide public health problem because of the morbidity and occasional mortality during acute infections, and, more importantly, the long-term consequences of chronic infection with HBV and HCV, i.e. cirrhosis, chronic liver failure and hepatocellular carcinoma [13, 14, 18].

NATURAL HISTORY, PATHOGENESIS, AND PATHOLOGY

Site of viral entry can be oral or parenteral, with the virus spreading from the intestines, in the case of HAV and HEV, or in the blood in the case of HBV and HCV, to the liver. Common to all causes of acute viral hepatitis are focal hepatocyte necrosis and histocytic periportal inflammation. The reticulin framework of the liver is well preserved except in cases of massive necrosis. Hepatocyte necrosis is usually multifocal with the more severe changes occurring in centrilobular areas. A mononuclear cellular infiltration, which is particularly marked in the portal zones, is accompanied by some proliferation of the bile ducts. Kupffur cells and endothelial cells proliferate. Chlolestasis may occur and plugs of bile thrombi may be present in the bile canaliculi. Lesions in patients with anicteric hepatitis (i.e. without jaundice) are generally less severe, consisting of focal inflammation and necrosis. Either viral infection of hepatocytes and/or the host's immune response to the infection is the etiology of the pathologic lesions in viral hepatitis. One or both mechanisms may predominate [19, 20].

Repair occurs by regeneration of hepatocytes. There is a gradual disappearance of the mononuclear cell infiltrate from the portal tracts, but elongated histiocytes and fibroblasts may persist. The outcome of acute viral hepatitis may be complete resolution or fatal massive hepatic necrosis. In HBV and HCV infections, the virus may persist and chronic hepatitis, with lymphocytic inflammation and lymphoid aggregation in portal tracts, occurs (Fig. 31.1). There may also be microvesicular fatty changes and damage to the bile ducts and acidophilic changes in the hepatocytes. Cirrhosis and hepatocellular carcinoma may develop in 15–35 years in those having persistent active infections [21].

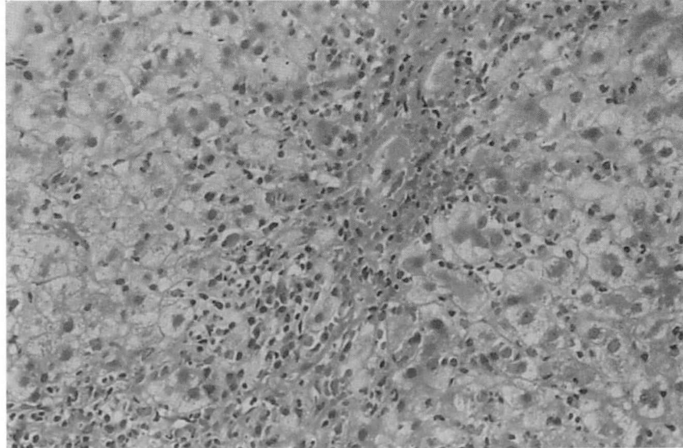

FIGURE 31.1 Histologic illustration of chronic hepatitis from a patient with chronic HCV infection. Note bridging fibrosis and piecemeal necrosis.

CLINICAL FEATURES

The particular virus causing hepatitis can rarely be clinically ascertained. However, hepatitis viruses have some tendency to manifest differently.

ACUTE HEPATITIS

Characteristically, there are four phases of viral hepatitis. After exposure, the virus *incubates* for from 2–6 weeks for HAV and HEV, and from 4–10 weeks for HBV and HCV [4, 22]. Then there may be a *prodromal illness*, characterized by fever, chills, headache, fatigue, malaise, rash, arthritis, right upper quadrant pain and a tender liver. Several days later and often coincident with an improvement in *systemic symptoms*, the patient will have more pronounced anorexia, nausea, vomiting, weight loss and right upper quadrant abdominal pain. Jaundice is usual and may persist for several weeks in association with dark urine, light (clay-colored) stools, and pruritus [2, 25, 26]. Often, the patient feels better following the onset of jaundice. Most symptoms of viral hepatitis abate within 1–3 weeks. Acute HCV infections are usually anicteric and are often not diagnosed. During outbreaks of HAV, and particularly HEV, there are many asymptomatic, mild and anicteric cases. As the acute hepatitis continues to *convalesce*, the patient may, or may not, remain icteric, but they almost always have anorexia, nausea, weight loss, and, if they smoke cigarettes, lose their taste for smoking. Patients infected with HAV or HEV are more likely to have intestinal symptoms, while those with HBV infections may have rash, arthralgias and arthritis [2].

CHRONIC HEPATITIS

While acute infections with hepatitis A and E resolve, HBV, HCV and HDV infections may persist. The frequency of persistence varies with the virus and the host and inversely correlates with the severity of acute infection suggesting that cell mediated immunity (CMI) is involved in resolving the infection. HBV infection persists in less than 5% of those infected as adults, but in greater than 80% of those infected as infants. Acute HCV infection is symptomatic less frequently than hepatitis B and is less likely to become chronic in children than in adults and in women than in men. Published prevalence of persistence of HCV infections range from 60–85%.

Patients with persistent hepatitis B and C often develop a smoldering chronic hepatitis that usually remains asymptomatic for 15–35 years before complications of cirrhosis and hepatocellular carcinoma occur. Bouts of mild acute hepatitis can occur intermittently in patients with occult chronic HCV infections [25]. They usually have mild flu-like symptoms and mild jaundice with alanine transaminase (ALT) levels 100–200 mg/dL. These abnormalities and symptoms often clear in of 2–3 weeks. There have been recent reports of persistent HEV infections which led to chronic hepatitis, but these are very rare.

COMPLICATIONS

Usually, the symptoms of acute hepatitis abate after 2–3 weeks, but malaise, fatigue, anorexia and weight loss may persist for up to 6–8 weeks.

Fulminating Hepatitis

Rarely, acute viral hepatitis may be fulminant, associated with altered mental status, coagulopathy and severe jaundice, leading to death. Fulminating hepatitis occurs more frequently during acute HEV infections, particularly in pregnant women in the Indian subcontinent, but this complication is less common in other areas. It has been reported in less than 1 in 200 cases of HAV, is very rare in acute HCV infections, but is more common in acute HBV, particularly when there is a concomitant HDV infection.

Cirrhosis

Chronic hepatitis B and C are the most common cause of cirrhosis of the liver. Several factors are associated with the fibrosis progression rate: duration of infection, age, male gender, alcohol consumption, HBV, HCV and HIV co-infections, and low CD4 count. Steatosis, being overweight and diabetes are cofactors of fibrogenesis. The viral genotype and viral load have no relationship with the development of cirrhosis.

PATIENT EVALUATION

The classical finding in acute viral hepatitis is jaundice, although patients with milder infections may have bilirubin levels below the 2.0–2.5 mg/dL in which jaundice is not detectable. Patients with chronic hepatitis usually do not have jaundice. In both conditions, the patient has other symptoms and signs listed in other sections. The classic laboratory abnormalities of acute hepatitis are elevated serum ALT and aspartate aminotransferase (AST) 10–20 times higher than normal. The serum bilirubin is usually elevated, often peaking 10–15-times normal. Clinical jaundice is noted when it exceeds 2.5–3.0 mg/dL. There may be elevations in alkaline phosphatase, and atypical lymphocytes can be noted in the peripheral blood film in the presence of a normal leukocyte count. Bilirubin is often also present in the urine. These laboratory abnormalities can help detect mild and asymptomatic cases [2, 25].

Diagnosis of anicteric cases of hepatitis are often based upon obtaining a history of potential exposures to patients with hepatitis or risk factors of infection. The severity of acute viral hepatitis is best measured by the clinical symptoms and serum levels of bilirubin, ALT or AST. The severity of chronic hepatitis is best measured by these same findings and may be supplemented by liver biopsy, ultrasonography and other noninvasive tests of hepatic fibrosis.

Each virus elicits a characteristic antibody response. Detection of virus-specific IgM class immunoglobulins generally represents acute infection, while IgG antibodies may be present years after resolution of disease. Recognition of viral antigens or nucleic acid represents ongoing infection and correlates with transmissibility.

TREATMENT AND PREVENTION

There is no specific treatment for acute HAV and HEV hepatitis. Supportive care, including rest, is important [26, 27]. Silymarin, a milk thistle extract, was reported to slightly accelerate recovery of some symptoms of acute clinical hepatitis; however, the most effective dose schedule has not been ascertained [28]. Secondary transmission should be prevented through active and passive immunization and careful sanitation and behavior modification.

See subchapters on HBV, HCV and HDV below on treatment of acute and chronic infection with these viruses.

Highly effective vaccines are available for preventing HAV and HBV infections [3, 17, 23, 30]. Phase III clinical trials for HEV vaccines were 95% effective, but they are not commercially available [111, 112]. Several preventive and/or therapeutic HCV vaccines are currently undergoing Phase II clinical trials [29]. HDV infections requiring HBV replication can be prevented by immunization for HBV.

31.1 Hepatitis A

Key features

- Enterically-transmitted virus with both sporadic cases and epidemic outbreaks (usually water-borne)
- More asymptomatic or mild infections than jaundiced patients following exposure
- Clinical illness rare in residents of endemic areas because of protection offered by early childhood exposures; major risk to travelers to these areas
- Classical findings are jaundice, anorexia, nausea, hepatic discomfort and elevated alanine transaminase (ALT) and aspartate aminotransferase (AST)
- Vaccine offers excellent protection to travelers and others with potential exposures

INTRODUCTION

HAV causes *short-incubation infectious hepatitis* that is transmitted by the fecal-oral route and has caused epidemics, particularly when it contaminates the water supply [3]. HAV is a small, non-enveloped, icosahedral, positive-sense RNA virus in the family *Picornaviridae*, genus *hepatovirus* [3] (Fig. 31.2) Although there are four HAV genotypes recognized in humans, there is only one HAV serotype such that neutralizing antibody to any HAV strain will protect against infection worldwide.

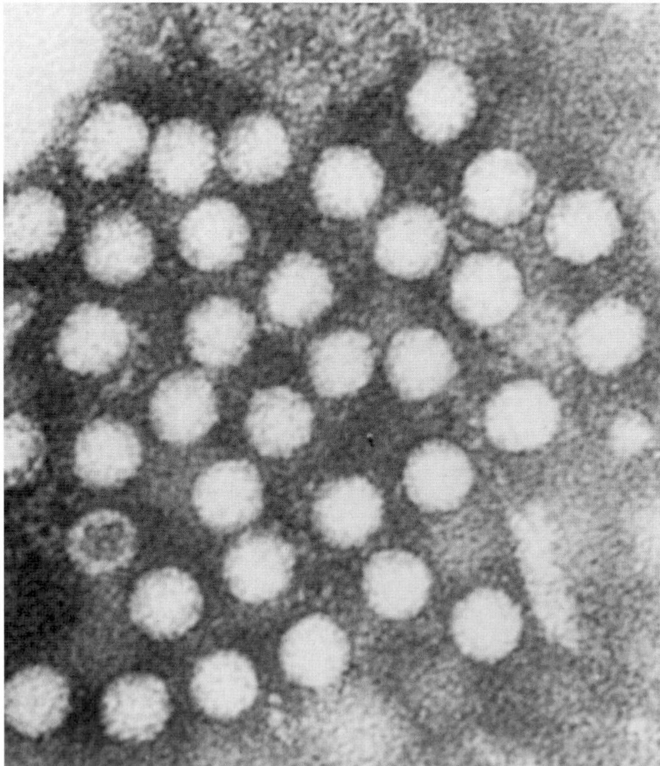

FIGURE 31.2 Hepatitis A virus particles in a fecal extract obtained from a patient during the late incubation period of the infection. The particles measure 25–27 nm in diameter and possess cubic symmetry (× 300,000).

Most infections in developing countries occur early in life and cause few, or no, symptoms, whereas infections in transitional or developed countries often lead to acute viral hepatitis in adolescents and adults. Unlike HBV and HCV, HAV never causes chronic infection [1].

Although *epidemic jaundice* has been recognized from epidemics of "campaign jaundice" that affected armies during the Middle Ages up until the Korean and Vietnam conflicts, HAV was not identified until about 50 years ago [26, 27]. Diagnostic serologic tests are commercially available and an effective vaccine is licensed [30].

EPIDEMIOLOGY

AGE AND PATTERN OF INFECTION

Although HAV infection occurs worldwide, the epidemiology differs according to sanitary conditions, for example water purification, sewage disposal and crowding. Nearly all inhabitants of some economically developing countries are infected with HAV during their first 2 or 3 years, when infection causes no or few symptoms. Low-income regions (sub-Saharan Africa and parts of South Asia) have high endemicity and almost no susceptible adolescents and adults, while middle-income regions in Asia, Latin America, Eastern Europe and the Middle East have an intermediate level of endemicity. In countries undergoing economic transformation, infection is often delayed to the second and third decades, and, thus, paradoxically, HAV becomes a greater public health problem [31]. Higher-income regions (Western Europe, Australia, New Zealand, Canada, USA, Japan, the Republic of Korea and Singapore) have very low HAV endemicity and a high proportion of illness-susceptible adults [32]. Large outbreaks of hepatitis A may occur in economically middle- and high-income nations, generally because of exposure to a common source of contaminated food or water; HAV infection is a particular threat to persons traveling from non-endemic to endemic areas (Fig. 31.3).

ROUTES OF TRANSMISSION

HAV-caused acute viral hepatitis is principally transmitted person-to-person by a fecal-oral route 2–6 weeks following exposure. It usually requires levels of exposures that occur within a family or between playmates. Asymptomatic transmission between children and then to a parent is especially characteristic, illustrating why daycare centers may be implicated in the spread of infection. Food- and water-borne HAV infection often involves a food handler with hepatitis A who failed to observe hand-washing protocol after defecation. Contamination of inadequately chlorinated water sources has led to both epidemic and sporadic HAV infections. Shellfish are particularly associated with HAV transmission, as they concentrate the virus by filtering large volumes of contaminated water. A massive epidemic of HAV occurred in Shanghai in 1988 following ingestion of undercooked shellfish. The short period of viremia before the onset of symptoms makes parenteral transmission possible, but this is rare.

Specific risk factors for HAV infection in developed countries include contact with another person with hepatitis or jaundice, homosexuality, travel to a less developed country, contact with children attending daycare centers and intravenous drug abuse. HAV infection is still endemic among Native Americans in the western states of the USA and Alaska.

CLINICAL FEATURES

After a susceptible person ingests HAV, viral replication occurs principally in the liver. Virions can be detected in stool and blood before the onset of symptoms. Serum transaminases increase several days after viral replication begins, indicating that hepatocellular damage

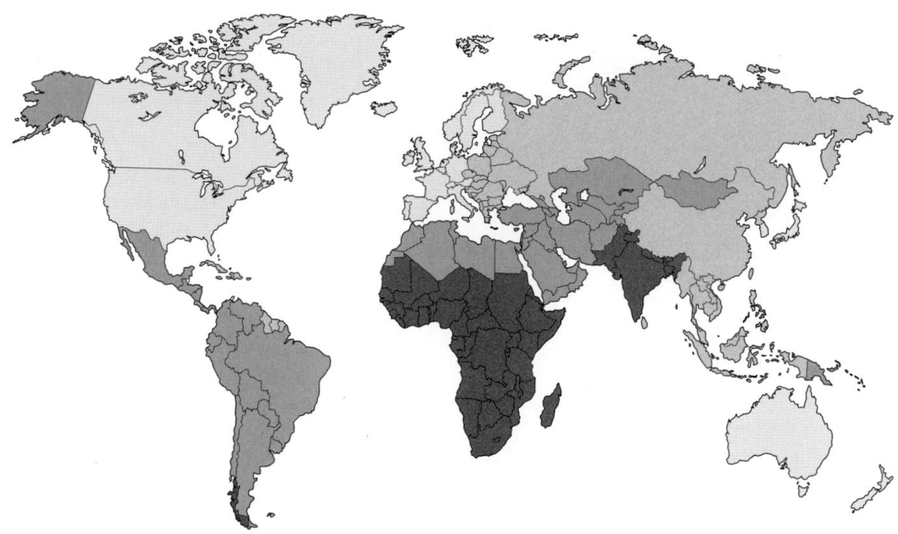

FIGURE 31.3 Geographic distribution of chronic hepatitis A virus infection as manifested by the prevalence of hepatitis A surface antigen (HBsAg) rates in the general population *(courtesy of the Centers for Disease Control and Prevention).*

may be immunologically mediated [3]. Up to 2 weeks after viral excretion and, on average, 25–30 days after exposure, prodromal symptoms may occur. The prodrome, which has an abrupt onset and consists of fever, fatigue, malaise, anorexia, nausea and vomiting, occurs in over 60% of adults but is uncommon among young children. After several days, flu-like symptoms give way to jaundice, which occurs in over 60% of adults and less than 25% of children. About 60% of symptomatic children have diarrhea, which occurs in 20% of adults with hepatitis A. Within two weeks of the onset of jaundice, HAV is generally not detected in stool. The serum bilirubin peaks after 7–10 days at a level usually greater than 10 mg/dL. Within 2–4 weeks of the onset of symptoms, jaundice resolves and transaminases return to normal. Post-hepatitis A convalescence symptoms of malaise, fatigue and anorexia may be prolonged for months. Hepatic failure occurs in 1 in 300 hepatitis A cases and generally does not result in death or the need for liver transplantation.

Relapsing hepatitis occurs in up to a fifth of adult patients within six months of resolution of the acute illness. This may include acute viral hepatitis symptoms along with viral excretion and elevated transaminases. Variations include asymptomatic resurgence in liver enzymes, which may persist for as long as a year, and more than one relapse. Prolonged cholestasis with fever, pruritus and diarrhea can last for months. Although the acute illness may be prolonged, there is no chronic liver disease after HAV infection [33].

DIAGNOSIS

HAV infection is generally diagnosed by detecting IgM antibodies to the virus (IgM anti-HAV) in the blood at the onset of symptoms. It peaks 4–6 weeks after exposure and persists for 3–12 months. IgG HAV antibodies, which can be detected one week after the IgM response, have neutralizing activity and may persist for life. Thus, IgG anti-HAV, when present without IgM anti-HAV, represents past HAV infection and means the individual is protected against recurrent infection. IgG anti-HAV may also be detected for 2–6 months after immunoglobulin (IG) administration or HAV vaccination. HAV virus can also be detected in stool by electron microscopy, but virus culture is not a practical technique.

TREATMENT

There is no specific treatment for Hepatitis A [26, 27].

PREVENTION AND CONTROL

SANITATION

The most important measures to reduce HAV infection involve improvements in sewage disposal, crowding and hygiene. Food handlers who are ill and persons with hepatitis A or unexplained jaundice should be restricted from work, and hand-washing should be strictly enforced. If hospitalization is necessary, enteric isolation is recommended for one week after the onset of jaundice which coincides with the highest quantities of viral excretion in stool. Additional precautions are needed only in incontinent or demented patients.

IMMUNIZATION

When exposure has occurred or is anticipated, HAV infection can be prevented through passive immunoprophylaxis using concentrated IG that contains at least 100 IU/mL of anti-HAV and vaccination with inactivated HAV. The two vaccines licensed in the USA are formalin-inactivated viral particles produced in infected human diploid fibroblasts. Protection is sustained for 10 or more years, an important feature for susceptible persons living in, or traveling frequently to, developing countries. Adverse events, for example mild soreness at the injection site and fever, are rare. Over 95% of healthy adults develop anti-HAV antibodies within a month of receiving a single dose of the vaccine. A booster dose, recommended six months after the first dose, raises the IgG anti-HAV titer. In clinical trials, a single 25 U dose of vaccine completely prevented symptomatic HAV hepatitis in heavily exposed children 18 days or more after immunization. Because immunization restricts hepatic viral replication, it reduces fecal viral shedding and interrupts transmission [23].

People who move or travel to regions where HAV is endemic should receive a first dose of vaccine at least one month before departure. The criteria for vaccine use in other situations are influenced by cost and exposure. It is recommended that all American children receive HAV vaccine at 1 year of age [34]. Early childhood asymptomatic infections usually protect the majority of inhabitants of lower and middle income countries from HAV-caused acute viral hepatitis. However, the more affluent people in these countries could miss having this early exposure and might benefit from immunization.

31.2 Hepatitis B

Key features

- Parenteral-transmitted hepatitis virus that causes both acute and chronic hepatitis in 400 million people
- Transmitted by infusion of blood products, inoculations, sexual intercourse and from mother to her fetus
- The incidence of HBV infections has been reduced since the application of diagnostic tests to screen blood and childhood immunization
- Chronic HBV remains a major cause of cirrhosis and hepatocellular carcinoma
- Treatment is expensive, toxic and not very efficacious
- Very effective vaccine is available

INTRODUCTION

Up until the late 1960s, the diagnosis of *long-incubation serum hepatitis* was made on the basis of jaundice occurring 60–120 days following injection of human blood or plasma or the use of inadequately sterilized syringes and needles. Serum hepatitis followed vaccination for smallpox in the 19th century and became more prevalent with the increasing use of syringes and needles to treat syphilis in the first half of the 20th century. During the 1940s, epidemics of hepatitis, later determined to be caused by HBV, followed the administration of yellow fever vaccines stabilized by adding human serum. In 1965, the Australia antigen was discovered by Blumberg and colleagues. Subsequently, this protein in the sera, hepatitis B surface antigen (HBsAg), was shown to be a marker of HBV infection and was used in a very effective vaccine. HBV is a small, enveloped, incompletely double-stranded DNA virus of the genus *Orthohepadnavirus*, family *Hepadnaviridae*, which has three distinct viral particles [7] (Fig. 31.4). Humans and higher-order primates are the only known hosts. It has three distinct viral particles (Fig. 31.4). HBV replication occurs by reverse transcription that predisposes to mutations. Mutation in the pre-core region of the genome interrupts translation of mRNA into HBeAg. Viral replication and synthesis of core polypeptide still occur, as indicated by HBV-DNA in plasma, but HBeAg is not detected. HBeAg is not required for viral replication but seems necessary for the establishment of chronic infection by acting as a tolerogen. Clinically, detection of HBeAg correlates with high-level viremia.

EPIDEMIOLOGY

It is estimated there are 400 million people living with chronic HBV infection (the majority in Asia, sub-Saharan Africa and other developing countries). Half a million deaths occur annually because of HBV-associated cirrhosis and hepatocellular carcinoma; an additional 40,000 die of acute HBV infection [24].

GEOGRAPHIC DISTRIBUTION

There are marked geographic differences in the prevalence of HBV infection (Fig. 31.5) and principal routes of transmission. The incidence of infection has been markedly reduced by wide-spread use of the HBV vaccines, serologic tests to screen blood transfusions and blood products, and by the availability and use of disposable syringes and needles. Despite a marked reduction in transmission in developed countries over the past 30–35 years, HBV remains a major cause of chronic liver disease. This is mostly because of the delay (15–35 years on average) between infection and severe medical complications. In most areas, higher HBV rates are found in persons of low socioeconomic status. Immigrants from countries with high HBV prevalence have a higher probability of being infected and developing chronic liver disease.

MODES OF TRANSMISSION [6]

HBV transmission is facilitated by the large human reservoir of HBV carriers. The virus can be transmitted by transfusions and injections of blood products, by needle-stick, by heterosexual or homosexual activities, and from mothers to their unborn or newborn infants. It is the most infectious of the major blood-borne viruses. In Asia, HBV transmission often occurs perinatally or during early childhood, whereas in sub-Saharan Africa and other developing countries, hepatitis B is generally acquired in the first decade of life through horizontal transmission within families and among playmates or, later, by heterosexual sex. In the USA, Europe and other developed nations, homosexual and heterosexual exposures and use of illicit drugs are the most important risk factors for HBV infection. Blood transfusions can still be an important mode of transmission where screening of blood prior to transfusion is inadequate or not carried out. HBV may also be transmitted to patients or healthcare workers by contaminated equipment or the environment during hemodialysis, by tattoos, acupuncture, surgery, barbers during shaving, male and female circumcisions or human bite.

The patterns of HBV transmission relate to the relative presence of infectious virions in body fluids, exposure to those fluids and the environmental stability of the fluids. The highest concentration of HBV is found in the blood of HBeAg-positive patients. HBsAg (infectious virions) has also been detected in saliva, semen, cerebrospinal fluid, tears, urine, feces, breast milk and other body fluids. Oral inoculation of high concentrations of virus from serum may cause mild infection. Thus, non-parenteral transmission requires high

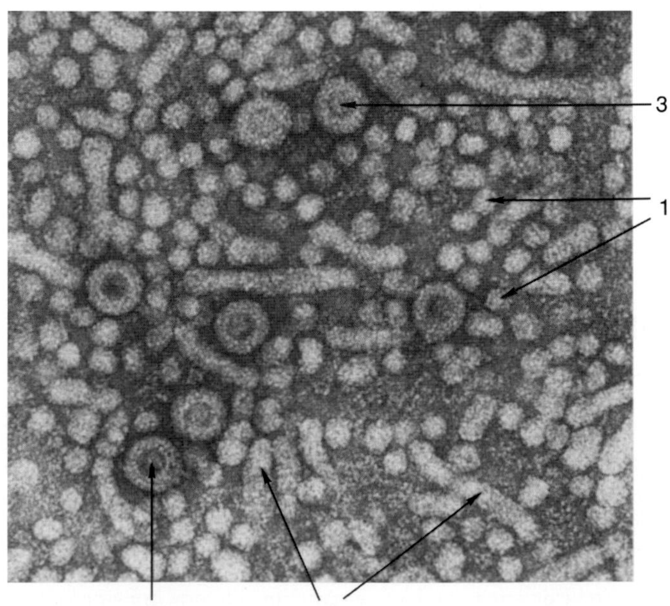

FIGURE 31.4 Electron micrograph showing the complex morphology of hepatitis B virus in serum: (1) small spherical particles of HBsAg; (2) tubular structures of the surface antigen; (3) large spheroidal particles and the complete virus particle, which may be solid or double-shelled (× 252,000).

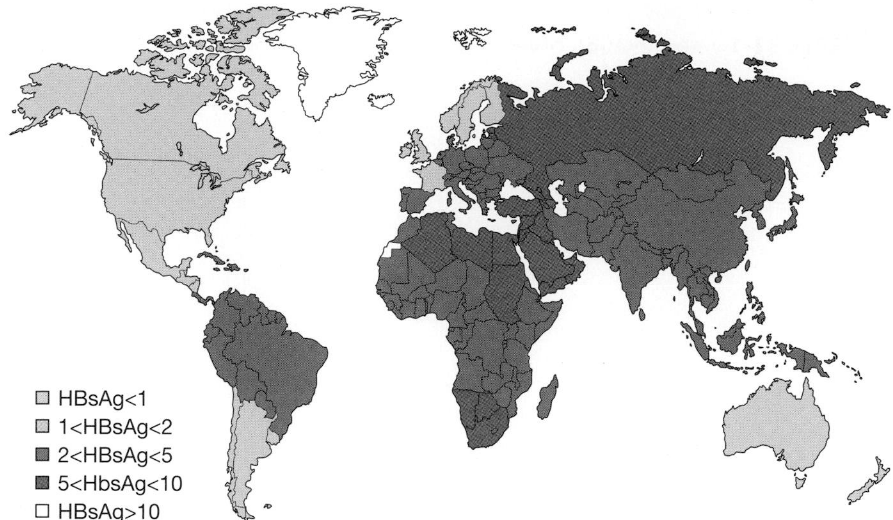

FIGURE 31.5 Geographic distribution of chronic hepatitis B virus infection as manifested by prevalence of hepatitis B surface antigen (HBsAg) rates in 2006 *(courtesy of the Centers for Disease Control and Prevention. Source:* http://wwwnc.cdc.gov/travel/yellowbook/2010/chapter-2/hepatitis-b.aspx*)*.

concentrations of virus or a break in mucosal barriers, for example as might occur with anal receptive intercourse, in someone with a genital ulcer, and between children with ulcerative skin lesions.

CLINICAL FEATURES

ACUTE INFECTIONS [7, 35]

From 2–4 months after exposure, prodromal symptoms occur in less than half of HBV infections. Approximately 15% of adult patients have a serum sickness-like illness characterized by fever, malaise, symmetric distal joint pain and urticaria; jaundice occurs in 25–35%. There may be right upper quadrant tenderness with an enlarged liver. Rarely, acute hepatitis B becomes fulminant, with a shrinking liver, increased abdominal pain, fever, vomiting and encephalopathy. This rare complication occurs more frequently in the elderly and in those with HDV, HCV or HIV co-infection.

CHRONIC INFECTIONS AND COMPLICATIONS [13]

Acute HBV infection is self-limited in 95% of adults who are not immunosuppressed but persists in almost all infants infected during the perinatal period and in 40–50% of children infected before the age of five [13]. Acute clinical illness is directly related to the immune response to the virus; those having no or minimal symptoms are more likely to become chronic carriers. This reverse relationship between symptoms and persistent infection is highly influenced by the age of when the infection occurs. Thus, young children are likely to have asymptomatic chronic HBV infections, while adults usually have acute viral hepatitis without a persisting infection.

Many with persistent HBV infection have waxing and waning of symptoms and serum levels of ALT and AST with eventual progression to cirrhosis and liver failure. The disease may also progress without apparent symptoms or remain indolent for 15–35 years.

Chronic Hepatitis and Cirrhosis [13, 19]

Most patients with persistent HBV infection are asymptomatic and have little histologic evidence of liver damage by biopsy (inactive carrier phase). These "healthy" carriers are HBsAg-positive but generally lose HBeAg, developing anti-HBe in association with transient clinical exacerbations. Others progressively develop liver disease, sometimes in association with systemic symptoms, for example fatigue and malaise. Long-term complications of this progression include cirrhosis, liver failure and hepatocellular carcinoma. Evidence of persistence can generally be detected histologically (immune active phase). In one study, the five-year survival was 86% in patients with chronic active hepatitis and 55% once cirrhosis was evident.

Hepatocellular Carcinoma [13, 19]

HBV infection increases the risk of hepatocellular carcinoma 100–200-fold and those with chronic infections develop hepatocellular carcinoma at a rate of 0.5–1.0% per year. Mechanisms include increasing malignant transformation of cells indirectly by increasing cell turnover and fibrogenesis and the induction of oncogenes or proto-oncogenes. The risk of hepatocellular carcinoma is much higher in those with cirrhosis, is greater in males, in those that consume large amounts of alcohol and in those with HCV co-infections. The tumors present with weight loss, right upper quadrant pain and, occasionally, fever or gastrointestinal bleeding. Hepatomegaly and ascites are common, but a discrete mass is often not palpable. Tumors are slow-growing and uncommonly metastasize.

Co-Infections with HIV [36]

Compared with HIV-negative patients, HIV-positive patients more often have HBeAg, HBV genotype A and co-infection with HCV or HDV. HIV positive patients were more often on HBV therapy leading to undetectable serum HBV DNA levels. In HIV positive patients, older age, lower initial HBV DNA levels, and longer time on HBV therapy significantly correlated with undetectable HBV DNA. HBsAg, but not HBe, loss was more often observed in HIV positive patients, sometimes followed by HBsAg re-appearance after withdrawal of HBV treatment. HIV infection did not have a negative impact on the likelihood of HBV therapeutic success.

DIAGNOSIS [37]

A guide to the interpretation of diagnostic tests is shown in Table 31-1.

DETECTION OF HBV ANTIGENS AND ANTIBODIES

During the 6–8 week incubation period, before biochemical evidence of liver dysfunction or the onset of jaundice, HBV-DNA, HBsAg and HBeAg can be detected in the plasma. The presence of HBeAg correlates with the number of virus particles and relative infectivity. Anti-HBc is present in the serum 2–4 weeks after the appearance of HBsAg. Core antibody of the IgM class becomes undetectable within six months of the onset of uncomplicated acute infection, but IgG core antibody persists for many years—possibly for life. Antibodies to the

TABLE 31-1 Interpretation of results of serologic tests for hepatitis B

HBsAg	HBeAg	Anti-HBe	Anti-HBc		Anti-HBs	Interpretation
			IgM	*IgG*		
+	+	–	–	–	–	Incubation period
+	+	–	+	+	–	Acute hepatitis B
+	+	–	–	+	–	Persistent carrier state
+	–	+	+/–	+	–	Persistent carrier state
–	–	+	+/–	+	+	Convalescence
–	–	–	–	+	+	Recovery
–	–	–	+	–	–	Infection with hepatitis B virus without detectable HBsAg
–	–	–	–	+	–	Recovery with loss of detectable anti-HBs
–	–	–	–	–	+	Immunization without infection. Repeated exposure to antigen without infection, or recovery from infection with loss of detectable anti-HBc

From [38].

surface (anti-HBs) and e (anti-HBe) antigens then appear, with anti-HBe indicating low infectivity and resolving infection [37].

DETECTION OF HBV-DNA

The presence of HBV-DNA represents viral replication and infectivity and is present early in acute cases of HBV and persistently in chronic infections. In addition, the loss of HBV-DNA has been used as a marker of successful therapy.

TREATMENT [39, 41]

HBV therapy is complicated and it is recommended that more detailed instructions be used for its management. Clearance of HBsAg naturally occurs in about 2% of chronic carriers each year. Seroclearance is greater in older individuals and those with lower viral loads; HBV-DNA levels almost always become undetectable before HBsAg clears [42]. Treatment is given for chronic hepatitis B to prevent the development of cirrhosis and hepatocellular carcinoma. Treatment criteria are based on HBV replication status and stage of liver disease, modulated by the patient's age and HBeAg status. Therapeutic end points are viral suppression, ALT normalization, HBeAg and HBsAg loss, and improvement in liver histology [41].

Two formulations of interferon and five orally-administered nucleos(t)ide analogs are approved for use in the USA. These therapies are effective in suppressing HBV replication and prevent disease progression. They have reduced the number of patients requiring liver transplants and age -elated HBV deaths. However, there is still uncertainty about when to start treatment: which medication should be used first, when can treatment be stopped?

Treatment is clearly indicated for patients with acute liver failure, decompensated cirrhosis, advanced fibrosis with high serum HBV DNA levels, and those who are HBsAg positive who will be receiving cancer or immunosuppressive chemotherapy. Therapy is also often recommended for patients with compensated cirrhosis who have high levels of HBV replication, i.e. HBeAg positive and/or high levels of serum HBV DNA. As chemotherapy reduces the incidence of hepatocellular carcinoma, these criteria may be broadened to treat all patients with compensated cirrhosis.

The decision to use nucleos(t)ide or interferon therapy is based on patient characteristics and preference. Interferon is not recommended for patients with hepatic decompensation, immunosuppression, or medical or psychiatric contraindications. The advantage of interferon is that it is administered for a finite duration and is associated with a higher rate of HBsAg and HBeAg clearance and sustained suppression of viral replication. The main disadvantages of interferon are the need for parenteral administration and its frequent side effects. Nucleos(t)ide analogs are administered orally and are well tolerated; however, viral relapse is common once treatment is discontinued, necessitating long durations of treatment with associated risks of antiviral drug resistance.

The nucleos(t)ide analogs in use for treating hepatitis B fall into three groups: L-nucleosides, including lamivudine and telbivudine; acyclic nucleoside phosphonates, including tenofovir and adefovir; and entecavir, a deoxyguanosine analog. Mutations associated with drugs in one group confer some resistance to other drugs within the same group and may reduce the sensitivity to drugs in other groups. The selection of the initial treatment should be based on antiviral activity and risk of antiviral resistance. Entecavir, telbivudine and tenofovir have more potent antiviral activity, while entecavir and tenofovir have a lower rate of resistance. Nucleos(t)ide analogs are most appropriate for patients with decompensated liver disease, or contraindications to interferon, and who will tolerate long durations of treatment. Entecavir and tenofovir have the best profile regarding efficacy, safety and drug resistance. Entecavir is preferred in patients with other medical conditions that are associated with increased risks of renal insufficiency, whereas tenofovir is preferred in young female patients contemplating pregnancy and patients who may have been exposed to lamivudine in the past. Lamivudine and telbivudine should not be used as first-line therapy because of high rates of drug resistance, whereas adefovir is largely superseded by tenofovir because of its weak antiviral activity.

Peginterferon-alpha-2a (40 kD; PEG INF) is used to treat adults with HBeAg-positive or HBeAg-negative chronic hepatitis B with compensated liver disease having viral replication and hepatic inflammation. It is given subcutaneously once a week; 48 weeks of therapy with PEG INF with, or without, lamivudine was more effective than lamivudine alone in achieving a sustained response in patients with HBeAg-positive or -negative chronic hepatitis B. A long-term follow-up study in patients with HBeAg-positive disease who received PEG INF monotherapy revealed an HBeAg seroconversion rate of 42% one year after the end of treatment. A five-year follow-up after the end of treatment of HBeAg-negative patients who received PEG INF with, or without, lamivudine reported HBsAg clearance in 12% of patients and inactive chronic hepatitis B in 17%.

A meta-analysis of 15 studies reported that 33% and 37% of interferon-treated patients had undetectable levels of HBeAg and HBV-DNA compared with 12% and 17% among those given placebo. The nucleos(t)ide analogues can reduce HBV replication and increase the rate of HBeAg clearance and decrease hepatic inflammation. However, in most patients the effect is not sustained when the drug is discontinued, which has lead to the recommendation that treatment be given for years. Clearance of HBeAg following treatment has been associated with improved biochemical, virologic and histologic outcomes in both HBeAg-positive and -negative patients. For a few patients this is associated with resolution of infection. For others it leads to remission and a reduced risk of progressing to cirrhosis, hepatocellular carcinoma, liver transplant and death. For others who do not respond, or who relapse, re-treatment with another agent can be considered.

PREVENTION AND CONTROL [6]

HBV infection can be prevented by reducing exposures, by passive immunoprophylaxis and by immunization. Dramatic reductions in post-transfusion HBV infection have been achieved by screening blood and blood products for HBsAg. Infection control policies to prevent transmission in hemodialysis units and healthcare centers also have reduced nosocomial transmission. Reductions in high-risk sexual and drug-related practices led to declining rates of HBV infection in some homosexual and drug-using populations.

HBV VACCINATION

Vaccination is the most important means of reducing HBV transmission. The heat-inactivated or chemically-inactivated subviral particles derived from chronic HBsAg carriers (plasma-derived vaccine) has largely been replaced by HBsAg particles expressed from recombinant DNA in the yeast *Saccharomyces cerevisiae* (recombinant vaccine). Combination vaccines that contain recombinant HBsAg coupled with HAV, *Haemophilus influenzae* and other childhood vaccines are also available, as are recombinant vaccines that include pre-S and S antigens.

Hepatitis B vaccines are among the safest and most immunogenetic products available. Mild injection-site reactions occur in about 20% of people, but fever and other systemic symptoms are uncommon. Protection occurs in more than 95% of healthy infants, children and adults. Although the recommended schedule includes three doses at 0, 1 and 6 months, minor alterations in the timing of vaccine administration does not reduce the immunogenicity. Protection is evident within a couple of weeks of the second dose correlates with anti-HBs titers above 10 mIU/mL. Generally, immunization schedules include a booster dose 4–6 months after primary immunization in order to obtain higher antibody titers and more durable protection.

A nationwide HBV vaccination program in Taiwan has markedly reduced the prevalence of HBsAg carriage [43]. This program, which was started in 1984, had already markedly reduced the incidence of hepatocellular carcinoma in Taiwanese children by 1994 [44]. Even in North America, Europe and other areas with low HBV incidence, the high risk of chronic disease resulting from HBV infection occurring in childhood, the difficulty reaching persons at risk later in life and other factors make universal vaccination of infants a rational strategy [45].

POST-EXPOSURE PROPHYLAXIS

HBV infection can also be prevented after exposure has occurred [46]. Common examples include perinatal or sexual exposures, and needle-stick accidents. Anti-HBsAg should be assessed in individuals who have been vaccinated or who are at high risk of infection. Those with anti-HBs titers greater than10 mIU/mL can be reassured. Previously vaccinated persons with anti-HBs titers less than10 mIU/mL should receive HBV-enriched immunoglobulin (HBIG) and a dose of vaccine. Individuals without prior HBV vaccination or infection should receive HBIG and three doses of vaccine. This regimen can markedly reduce the incidence of HBV infection in infants born to HBeAg-positive mothers and to those having occupational or sexual exposures [47, 48].

31.3 Hepatitis D [9]

Key features

- Hepatitis delta virus (HDV) infection occurs either with acute HBV (*co-infection*) or in a patient chronically infected with HBV (*superinfection*)
- Transmission by parenteral, sexual and household exposures
- Superinfection in person with chronic HBV is associated with more severe hepatitis and increased progression to cirrhosis
- Can be prevented by HBV immunization

INTRODUCTION

In 1981 an outbreak of severe hepatitis was investigated among Amerindians in Venezuela. The disease, having a high mortality, especially among young children and adolescents, was caused by the delta agent. The clinical and epidemiologic features of the outbreak were similar to those in previous reports of Labrea hepatitis (black fever) in the upper Amazon River basin along the Purus and Juruá Rivers in Brazil [49, 50].

HDV is an unclassified RNA virus that is dependent on HBV envelope proteins for replication [51]. HDV is distinct from antigenic determinants of HBV and is localized in the nuclei of liver cells of patients with HBV infection. HDV-RNA encodes for two forms of the nucleocapsid protein, the delta antigen (HDAg). The two HDAg products function differently, the short form being necessary for viral replication while the longer is required for packaging the genome and suppressing replication.

EPIDEMIOLOGY

The distribution and transmission of HDV infection has three patterns: (1) endemic and associated with non-parenteral spread in Italy, other Mediterranean countries and the Middle East; (2) endemic-epidemic in the Amazon area and other remote areas of South America; and, (3) sporadic and associated with parenteral transmission in almost all other geographic areas. Like HBV and HCV, HDV is parenterally transmitted [9]. HDV in developed countries is most prevalent in certain high-risk groups, for example illicit intravenous drug users. It can be transmitted both sexually and through non-sexual household contacts; the latter is the most common route of transmission in indigenous populations in South America, Africa and parts of Central and Southeast Asia.

CLINICAL FEATURES AND NATURAL HISTORY [9]

HDV infection can occur with acute HBV (*co-infection*) or in a patient chronically infected with HBV (*superinfection*). After an incubation of 4–8 weeks, there is a viral hepatitis syndrome that is generally more severe than with other hepatitis viruses and which may be fulminant. When HDV and HBV *co-infection* occurs, recovery is the rule. In contrast, HDV *superinfection* of chronic hepatitis B persists in more than 60% of patients and is associated with a threefold increased rate of progression to cirrhosis [9].

A retrospective study of 188 Italian patients studied the impact of viral and patient features on survival [52]. Eighty-two patients (43%) had chronic hepatitis at histology; the remaining 106 individuals had a clinical/histologic diagnosis of cirrhosis. Ninety-six patients received interferon or lamivudine therapy; 27 (30%) attained a sustained viral cure. During follow up, 21 of the treated patients with chronic hepatitis progressed to cirrhosis. Of the 127 cirrhotic patients, hepatic decompensation occurred in 33% and hepatocellular carcinoma in 13%. The 5- and 10-year survival free of events were 96.8% and 81.9%, respectively, for patients with chronic hepatitis, and 83.9% and 59.4% for cirrhotics. Lack of antiviral therapy, cirrhosis at presentation and male sex independently predicted a worse outcome. Half of HDV-infected patients who develop cirrhosis advanced to liver failure and interferon therapy was recommended to slow, or alter, the natural course of liver disease [52].

DIAGNOSIS

Acute HDV and HBV *co-infection* is recognized by transient detection of HDAg or, more often, antibody to HDAg (anti-HD) with the typical serologic profile for acute HBV infection. Within months of infection, there may be no serologic evidence of HDV *co-infection*. HDV *superinfection* occurs in a HBsAg-positive patient and is recognized by anti-HD (IgG or IgM) and/or HDV RNA or HDAg. Persistent detection of these HDV markers generally signifies chronic infection.

PREVENTION

There is no antiviral treatment for HDV. HDV infection is deterred by prevention of HBV infection using its vaccine.

31.4 Hepatitis C

Key features

- Parenterally-transmitted virus that infects 130 million people, most in lesser developed countries
- Most new infections in developed countries are caused by intravenous drug use, but multiple causes of transmission, including injections from healthcare providers and familial exposures in less developed countries
- Minority of those infected have acute hepatitis, but 15–20% of the 70–80% having chronic infections develop cirrhosis and hepatocellular carcinoma over decades
- Treatment of chronic hepatitis C virus (HCV) infection remains expensive, toxic, prolonged and is only effective in 40–80% of patients depending on the HCV genotype and therapeutic regimen given
- Serologic tests allow screening blood products but there is no preventive vaccine

INTRODUCTION

HCV was cloned and sequenced in 1989 [53, 54]. Shortly thereafter assays were developed to detect HCV-RNA and antibodies [55]. Huge epidemics of both HCV and HBV occurred following well-intended efforts to control endemic infectious diseases during the middle half of the 20th century [56, 57]. Impact from these exposures to parenteral therapy for schistosomiasis, sleeping sickness, malaria, etc. is much more important for HCV as persistent infection with this virus is much more common, other than in neonates, than it is for HBV.

The majority of initial infections are asymptomatic. Based upon observing children and adults with high exposure risks having HCV-specific cellular immunity in the absence of both HCV antibody and RNA, viremia sometimes spontaneously clears [58, 59]. Those who have persistent chronic infection usually have a smoldering asymptomatic chronic hepatitis that may progress over 15–35 years to cirrhosis and hepatocellular carcinoma [14]. HCV has become the leading cause of chronic liver disease in many countries. Unlike for HBV, there is no vaccine for HCV [29, 60]. Current therapy is expensive, toxic, complex, only partially effective, and many of those with HCV infections are co-infected with HIV [40]. New therapies under development offer challenges of their own, including increased side-effects, development of viral resistance and high cost [61]. The major biologic difficulty in controlling HCV is the diversity of the virus, both within patients and among populations which allows it to evade both the immune response and therapeutic regimens [62].

The virus is a single-stranded, positive-sense RNA virus from the genus *Flavivirus*, family *Flaviviridae* [63]. It has an RNA polymerase that lacks a proof reading ability and has a replication rate of an estimated 10^{12} virions per day, thereby making it potentially possible to generate a mutation in every single position of the genome in one infected host every day [64]. This astounding ability to produce immune-evading sequences is mainly attributed to a highly polymorphic region in E2, designated as the hypervariable region 1 (HVR 1). Within an individual, there are innumerable HCV variants that constitute a quasispecies, whose presence often confounds the immune response and complicates vaccine development [65]. In addition, HCV isolates from different people may have as little as 50–60% nucleic acid identity. Based upon this genetic heterogeneity, HCV strains can be divided into seven genotypes that share less than 80% sequence homogeny with each other [66]. Some genotypes of HCV are geographically restricted, others have worldwide distribution. Genotype 6 is in Southeast Asia and Types 1 and 2 predominate in the USA and Europe. Genotype 4 is found predominately in Egypt and other parts of Africa (Fig. 31.6).

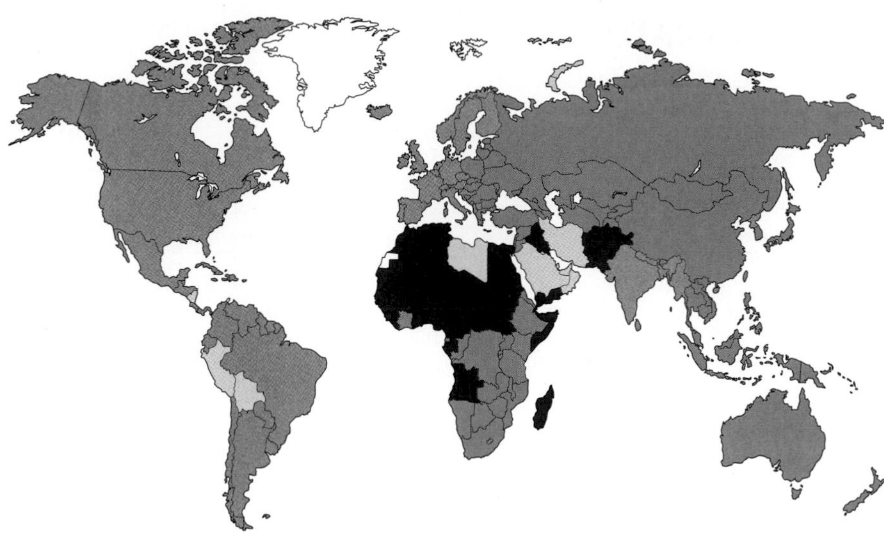

FIGURE 31.6 Worldwide prevalence of hepatitis C infection *(courtesy of the Centers for Disease Control and Prevention. Source: http://wwwnc.cdc.gov/travel/yellowbook/2010/chapter-5/hepatitis-c.aspx.).*

EPIDEMIOLOGY

DISTRIBUTION

Although the prevalence of HCV in the adult population of most countries is 1–2%, infection rates increase with age and are much higher in high-risk groups. The World Health Organization (WHO) estimates that 2.2% of the world's population has been infected with HCV and that 130 million persons are chronic carriers [67]. (Fig. 31.6) There may be 8 million carriers in Egypt alone; nearly 4 million Americans are infected with HCV, with an estimated 17,000 new infections each year, and it is believed to be responsible for the deaths of 10,000 Americans annually [57, 68–70, 70a]. In some villages in Egypt, sub-Saharan Africa and Japan, anti-HCV rates of 10–40% have been reported [70]. Travelers and immigrants from countries with high HCV prevalence have a higher probability of being infected and can develop chronic liver disease.

TRANSMISSION

Sharing of needles by injecting illicit drugs account for most hepatitis C cases in developed countries [14, 68]. Inhabitants of developing countries are usually infected from parenteral exposures from injections and other activities that penetrate the skin, inadequate screening of blood and blood products before transfusion, during renal dialysis, as well as from "interfamilial exposures" [10, 71–74].

In developed countries such as the USA, Europe and Japan, HCV infection as a result of blood transfusions has become rare. However, in some developing countries with high rates of HCV infections, transfusions remain risky because there is inadequate screening of blood or blood products for HCV. Two to six percent of infants born to HCV-infected mothers have persistent infections [11, 12]. In children, perinatal transmission, albeit rare, is the commonest route of transmission in developed countries and is more likely when the mother is dually infected with HIV-1 and when there are high quantities of maternal virus [75, 76]. Breastfeeding is not an important transmission route [12, 77]. Assessment of infant HCV infection should include HCV-RNA detection, as antibody-negative infection has been documented and maternal HCV antibodies are passively transferred to infants [11]. Sexual transmission of HCV also occurs, but with low frequency [78]. In over a third of HCV infections, no specific exposure is identified.

The high prevalence in Egypt and equatorial Africa is believed to be caused by various percutaneous exposures. For example, from the 1950s through the 1970s, the Egyptian government sponsored a national schistosomiasis control program that used intravenous tartar emetic in mass treatment campaigns. Healthcare providers in Central African Republic and Cameroon during the same period treated and controlled African trypanosomiasis, malaria and other endemic infectious diseases with intravenous medications [56, 71]. Exposure to blood by injections from conventional and traditional village health workers, dental procedures, cuts from barbers, male and female circumcisions and other activities are believed to continue HCV transmission in communities with a large HCV reservoir [10, 71–74, 79].

PATHOGENESIS AND PATHOLOGY

Individuals with chronic hepatitis C generally have lymphocytic inflammation with lymphoid aggregation in portal tracts (Fig. 31.1). There may also be microvesicular fatty changes and damage to bile ducts and acidophilic changes in hepatocytes—histologic findings that may also occur with HBV infection, but are more characteristic of hepatitis C. Cirrhosis may also be present, being associated with a long duration of infection [80].

HCV infections usually persist, owing, at least in part, to the rapid replication of the virus and its tendency to mutate, hence forming variants not contained by the immune response [81]. Some of the resulting population of viral strains, the HCV quasi-species, may be neutralized. However, other quasi-species may still transmit HCV infection. Chimpanzees can be experimentally re-infected with inoculates of HCV and natural re-infections have been reported in children with thalassemia who received multiple blood transfusions and in adult intravenous drug users [82].

CLINICAL FEATURES

ACUTE INFECTIONS [22]

The onset of HCV infection is usually unrecognized. Within 1–3 weeks of exposure, HCV RNA can be detected in blood. Transaminases may become elevated 3–9 weeks (average 50 days) later, but only 20–25% are jaundiced or are symptomatic. HCV is the cause of 20% of the cases of acute viral hepatitis in the USA and the Middle East [22]. When symptoms are experienced, there is a prodrome that tends to have a gradual onset and to be mild. The mean incubation period until the onset of symptoms is 7 weeks and clinical illness usually lasts from 2–12 weeks. ALT and AST return to normal and HCV RNA becomes undetectable within that time. Fulminating hepatitis from HCV infection is rare.

CHRONIC INFECTIONS [14]

HCV RNA can be persistent in 60–80% of patients who do not clear infections early after exposure. However, the viral titers may drop below the level of detection and, thus, detectable RNA may be intermittent. The chronic HCV-carrier often has intermittent elevations in transaminases and mild jaundice. These individuals are often diagnosed as mild cases of acute viral hepatitis [25]. Not all viremic patients have elevated ALT levels. Liver biopsies in HCV-positive patients with persistently normal ALT levels usually reveal evidence of inflammation. Nevertheless, their prognosis is better than if ALTs were elevated. Clinical symptoms or signs of liver disease tend to initially be nonspecific, mild and intermittent: fatigue described as lethargy, malaise, lack of energy, anorexia, nausea, arthralgia, myalgia, weakness and weight loss.

Many chronic HCV-carriers have no symptoms from their HCV infection and die of other conditions. The duration of infection and co-factors, for example the use of alcohol, concurrent HIV-1 infection or the HCV genotype causing the infection, may affect hepatitis C prognosis. However, although persistence and progression appear to be the rule, it remains difficult to predict the outcome for an individual patient [30].

Cirrhosis

Ten to twenty percent of HCV-infected patients develop cirrhosis over a period of 15–30 years. Once cirrhosis develops, marked fatigue, muscle weakness and wasting, fluid retention with edema and ascites, easy bruising, dark urine, jaundice, itching and upper gastrointestinal hemorrhage can occur. Hepatic failure is more likely in those who have additional causes of liver disease, for example schistosomiasis, concomitant HBV or HIV, and alcoholic liver disease. Staging of the fibrosis as detected on liver biopsy can predict clinical outcomes, the need for liver transplantation and liver-related death [83].

Hepatocellular Carcinoma [84, 85]

The annual incidence of hepatocellular carcinoma is 2–3% in those who have been HCV carriers for 30 years, particularly in the elderly, who can develop liver cancer sooner. There are geographic differences in the incidence of HCV-caused hepatocellular carcinoma; perhaps because of the length of time HCV has been transmitted in the local area or to differences in the prevalence of other hepatocellular carcinoma-causing cofactors. HCV-related hepatocellular carcinoma usually occurs in the context of cirrhosis. In the USA and many other areas, chronic HCV with cirrhosis is the most important risk factor for hepatocellular carcinoma.

EXTRAHEPATIC COMPLICATIONS

HCV infection has been associated with several extra-hepatitic syndromes, including essential mixed cryoglobulinemia (with or without vasculitis) and membranoproliferative glomerulonephritis. There are also reported correlations of HCV infection with arthritis, type 2 diabetes mellitus, keratoconjunctivitis sicca, lymphoma, Hashimoto's thyroiditis, lichen planus and porphyria cutanea tarda. This occurs in several types of chronic liver disease, often in association with iron overload.

Essential Mixed Cryoglobulinemia [86]

Hepatitis C appears to be the most common cause of this syndrome, which is marked by varying combinations of fatigue, myalgia, arthralgia and arthritis, hives, purpura or vasculitis, neuropathy and glomerulonephritis. Cryoglobulins, composed of immune complexes of HCV and anti-HCV, immunoglobulins, rheumatoid factor and complement, are present in the serum. Cryoglobulins are detectable in up to a third of patients with chronic hepatitis C, but the clinical syndrome of essential mixed cryoglobulinemia occurs in less than 2%; it sometimes improves with treatment of the HCV infection.

Non-Hodgkin Lymphoma (NHL) [87]

HCV is lymphotropic, as well as hepatotropic, and chronic HCV infection is a risk factor for Non-Hodgkin lymphoma. Case series have had a higher than expected prevalence of NHL in patients with essential mixed cryoglobulinemia (EMC) and chronic HCV infection, and a higher prevalence of HCV infections in case series of NHL.

DIAGNOSIS

HCV infections are diagnosed by detection of anti-HCV in plasma or serum. Reverse transcription (RT)-PCR assays are used to detect and quantitate the virus [88]. About 60–80% of those who are positive by the third-generation enzyme immunoassay (EIA) tests are also positive by RT-PCR and are considered to have active HCV infections. The remaining 20–40% of anti-HCV positive subjects who are RT-PCR negative have usually cleared their viremia. Differentiation of the IgM and IgG response to HCV has not been diagnostically useful.

Detection of HCV RNA indicates ongoing infection and transmissibility. Studies of perinatal hepatitis C have demonstrated that anti-HCV positive, HCV-RNA negative mothers do not transmit infection to their infants, whereas HCV-RNA positive mothers can [11]. HCV-RNA may rarely be detected in anti-HCV negative individuals. RT-PCR can be used to determine HCV genotypes; the response to antiviral therapy differs between HCV genotypes. Also, the quantity of HCV-RNA correlates with perinatal and sexual transmission; patients having sustained virologic response to interferon-based therapy generally have lower pretreatment levels of HCV than do non-responders. Thus, HCV-RNA assays can help to select HCV patients likely to benefit from treatment.

TREATMENT

JUSTIFICATION FOR TREATMENT

During natural history studies, 60–80% of individuals with acute hepatitis C progress to chronic infections [88]. Spontaneous resolution is more common among infected infants, children and young women [11, 73]. Spontaneous clearance of acute HCV infection and therapeutic response of patients with chronic hepatitis C is associated with a single nucleotide polymorphism (SNP) upstream of the interleukin (IL) 28B gene [89, 90]. Spontaneous clearance of infection was much more common in patients with the C/C genotype (64%) than in the C/T genotype (24%), and rare in those having the T/T genotype (6%). It is suggested that patients with the C/C genotype have a more favorable and efficient innate immune response, whereas HCV clearance in those with the C/T and T/T genotypes relates to an acquired cell-mediated immunity as jaundice is a positive risk factor for viral clearance in persons having these genotypes. There are racial differences in spontaneous clearance of acute HCV and sustained viral response following treatment with pegylated interferon alpha a or b (PEG) and ribavirin, with black patients having poorer responses than Caucasians. Chronic HCV infection increases the risk of infection among the infected person's contacts and for progression to cirrhosis and/or hepatocellular carcinoma among those who are infected. People with HCV-related cirrhosis are at 30% risk over 10 years of developing hepatic decompensation, as well as hepatocellular carcinoma (1–3% per year). A liver biopsy and/or noninvasive fibrosis marker can assist in selection of individuals who might benefit from antiviral therapy, as the level of fibrosis is a predictor for the development of cirrhosis.

THERAPEUTIC GOALS

Therapy is given to prevent complications, including renal disease in those having mixed cryoglobulinemia, and death [88, 91, 92]. However, interferon-based therapy is often toxic, prolonged, expensive, and has limited efficacy. More than 80% of persons with genotypes 2 and 3 HCV infection achieve a sustained viral response to standard-of-care treatment, whereas the response to treatment in persons infected with HCV genotypes 1 and 4 is only about 50%. Because of the slow evolution of the chronic HCV complications, surrogate responses, for example ALT normalization, histologic improvement in biopsy fibrosis score and clearance of HCV-RNA from the serum, are used to measure therapeutic success. The most important criteria for cure is the sustained viral response being HCV-RNA negative by a sensitive RT-PCR assay 24 weeks following the end of therapy. If the patient has a rapid virologic response, i.e. being aviremic after 4 weeks of therapy, or has an early virologic response, i.e. positive at 4 weeks, but negative or having a more than 2 log reduction by 12 weeks, then they are more likely to achieve a sustained viral response. Patients who fail to have a reduction in viral load by 12 weeks are unlikely to achieve sustained viral response.

THERAPEUTIC REGIMENS

HCV treatment is complicated and newer therapeutic regimens are being evaluated [93]. Up-to-date references should be consulted. Currently, a combination of PEGINF and ribavirin remains the standard of care. PEGINF is given once weekly, subcutaneously. Ribavirin, which is given daily by mouth, improves the response to PEGINF and reduces the relapse rate of monotherapy with PEGINF. The current optimal length of therapy for genotypes 1 and 4 is 48 weeks, while genotypes 2 and 3 should be treated for 24 weeks. If the HCV-RNA is negative at 36 weeks, that length of treatment may be sufficient for patients with genotype-4 HCV [94, 95]. There are insufficient data to recommend a PEGINF-ribavirin regimen for patients infected with genotype 5 or 6 HCV. The best predictors of a sustained viral response are a C/C IL28B genotype, infection with HCV genotypes 2 or 3 and a viral load of less than 600,000 IU/mL.

Other antiviral therapies are being evaluated [93]. To date, two protease products have completed Phase III clinical trials and have been approved by the Food and Drugs Adminstration (FDA). Telaprevir and bocepravir are both protease inhibitors that significantly increased the sustained virologic response when used in combination with PEGINF and ribavirin [96–98].

TREATMENT OF ACUTE HEPATITIS C

A minority of acute HCV infections is diagnosed, but up to half of patients with symptomatic acute hepatitis C spontaneously clear their infections, usually within 12 weeks. This compares with little evidence that asymptomatic initial infections spontaneously clear. The sustained viral response in patients with acute hepatitis C treated with standard PEGINF monotherapy is better than 90% [98a, 98b]. It is currently recommended that this be delayed by 8–12 weeks after infection to allow for spontaneously resolution [88].

PREVENTION AND CONTROL

Dramatic reductions in post-transfusion hepatitis C occurred after the institution of screening of blood donors for HCV antibodies. However, screening of blood products may be variable in some developing countries where the risk of infection is increased because of a high prevalence of chronic HCV infection. Activities in the communities, for example cuts from barbers, dental procedures and injections from traditional healers, as well as healthcare providers, may all transmit HCV and can be influenced by appropriate health education [71]. The relatively high percentage of cases that occur without identifiable exposures, other than HCV infections among family members, complicates preventive efforts [10].

There is no available vaccine to prevent HCV infection, and, owing to the extent of viral heterogeneity, a universally effective HCV vaccine will be difficult to develop, although several are undergoing clinical trials [29]. However, protective immunity to HCV has been demonstrated. Some HCV epitopes produce neutralizing antibodies in experimental animals; primates have been protected from challenge from homologous strains when immunized with recombinant antigens; and individuals at high risk of exposure have HCV-specific cell-mediated immunity (CMI) T-cell responses in the absence of HCV-antibody or RNA. Therapeutic vaccines that assist in clearance of chronic infections or that hinder development of chronic infections could prevent chronic complications of the infection.

31.5 Hepatitis E

Key features

- Enteric transmitted virus causing 20–30% of acute viral hepatitis in many developing countries and rarely in the USA and Europe
- It has a single serotype and six genotypes
- Some genotypes, for example genotype-1, cause acute viral hepatitis in humans while others, for example genotype-3, are zoonotic and primarily cause infection in animals—primarily pigs
- Water-borne outbreaks occur, primarily in the Indian subcontinent; it is also transmitted feco–orally and by viremic blood exposure and by eating undercooked pork
- Prevention is primarily related to improving sanitation; two effective vaccines have been developed but have not yet been marketed

INTRODUCTION

In 1983, hepatitis E virus (HEV) was visualized by immune electron microscopy (IEM) in stool from infected patients. It was then transmitted to a human volunteer and cynomolgus monkeys, thereby establishing its role in enterically transmitted non-A, non-B (NANB) hepatitis [99]. Development of specific diagnostic tests followed cloning of the HEV genome in 1990 and by recombinant DNA technology expressing viral antigens [100]. HEV was retrospectively recognized as a major cause of fecal-oral transmitted NANB hepatitis when clinical samples collected during epidemics of water-borne hepatitis in India in the 1950s and 1960s were serologically tested [101, 102]. HEV is a single-stranded, positive-sense RNA virus that has been placed in the genus, *Hepevirus*, but has not been assigned to a viral family. Although genomic and virulence variability occurs among geographically distinct isolates, HEV has at least one major cross-reactive epitope.

EPIDEMIOLOGY

HEV infections, transmitted by a fecal-oral route, are rarely detected in the USA or other developed countries. However, sporadic cases of HEV have been recognized in most developing countries, and major water-borne epidemics have been reported in India, Pakistan, Nepal and Africa [100]. HEV is also endemic to the remainder of Central and Southeast Asia, the Middle East, Africa and Central America (Fig. 31.7). In these areas, HEV is the etiologic cause of 20–30% of cases of acute viral hepatitis and, even more so, in the Indian subcontinent and during outbreaks. HEV is a risk to travelers to endemic areas, albeit less so than HAV [103].

Although sharing the same basic route of transmission as HAV, HEV infection in endemic countries occurs more often in the second and third decades of life, while HAV infection more commonly occurs in the first and second decades. Also, the secondary attack rate is lower for HEV than for HAV. Although not completely explaining the differences in transmission rates, lower quantities of HEV are excreted in the stool for shorter periods of time. Links to a common source of contaminated water are the rule during large outbreaks, and these often follow heavy rains. As with HAV, HEV infection can occur after exposure to contaminated blood products, owing to viremia that occurs during acute infection.

HEV is a zoonosis, having been isolated from pigs, rats, and other animals. The rare cases of HEV reported in North America, Europe or Japan are caused by human genotype-1 infections in travelers to endemic areas or because of porcine genotype-3 infections in people exposed to pigs, or who ate rare pig or boar in Japan [104]. Genotype-3 HEV has been isolated from pigs in Egypt (which are rare in the country) and genotype-1 has been isolated from a few cases of HEV-caused acute viral hepatitis in humans. HEV causes 20–25% of the cases of acute viral hepatitis in Egypt [31], but it is uncertain whether zoonotic transmission of genotype-3 is the cause of the 70–80% rate of HEV-antibodies in the country [105, 106].

CLINICAL FEATURES

The course of HEV infection is similar to that of hepatitis A. The incubation period averages 40 days (range 15–60 days). After oral inoculation, the virus principally replicates in the liver and produces cytopathic changes. HEV can be detected in stool and blood 3–4 weeks after ingestion, prior to the onset of symptoms, and for 1–2 weeks afterwards. Like hepatitis A, there are many more asymptomatic and anicteric infections with HEV than diagnosed cases of acute viral hepatitis. Children often have asymptomatic, anicteric infections, while the clinical attack rate is higher in the 15–40 year age group, and severity of illness increases with age.

Symptoms and signs are similar to those caused by other types of viral hepatitis: malaise, fatigue, anorexia, nausea and vomiting, jaundice and dark urine, abdominal pain, fever and hepatomegaly. The most common laboratory findings include elevated bilirubin, ALT, AST, and alkaline phosphatase. Histopathologic findings in biopsies from patients with HEV hepatitis have included both cholestatic hepatitis and classic acute viral hepatitis changes.

Clinical symptoms, hyperbilirubinemia and elevated aminotransferase levels generally resolve 1–6 weeks after onset of illness. Jaundice may be prolonged with HEV infection, which may also cause fulminant hepatitis; 10–20% of pregnant women in the third trimester who are hospitalized with acute HEV infection during outbreaks in India were reported to have fatal fulminant hepatitis [107, 108]. HEV very rarely causes chronic infection in immunosuppressed patients [109, 110].

DIAGNOSIS

Acute HEV infection can be diagnosed by detecting IgM HEV antibody, high titers of IgG anti-HEV or increasing titers of total HEV antibody by commercial enzyme immunoassays (EIAs) using recombinant-expressed proteins or synthetic peptides in patients with acute viral hepatitis [4]. The titer of IgM anti-HEV declines rapidly but can be detected in some patients for 5–6 months. IgG HEV-antibodies persist and have often been detected in persons from regions without

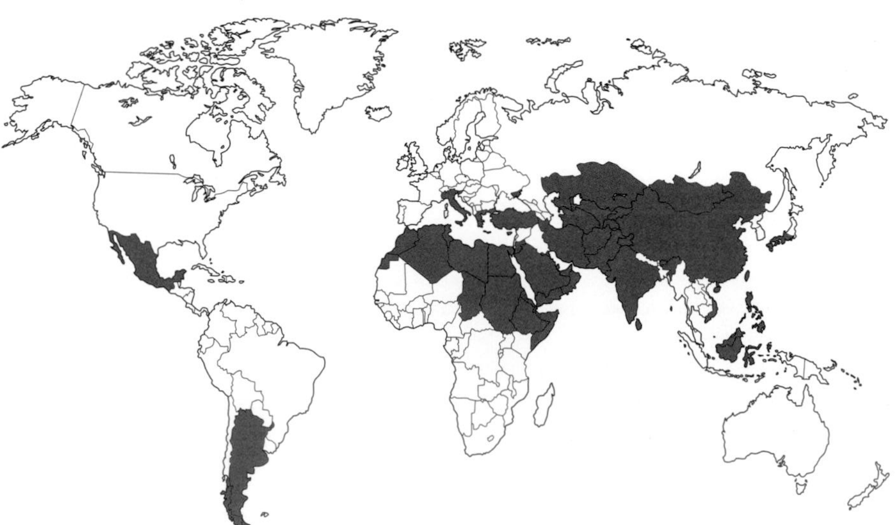

FIGURE 31.7 Geographic distribution of clinically significant hepatitis E among adults in selected regions *(modified from Purcell RH, Emerson SU. Hepatitis E: an emerging awareness of an old disease. J Hepatol 2008;48:494–503).*

recognized infection. Their presence must be coupled with the appropriate clinical and epidemiologic presentation. Acute HEV infection can also be diagnosed by detection of HEV in the stool or blood with PCR.

TREATMENT

Like other clinical cases of acute viral hepatitis, supportive care, including rest, is recommended [26, 27], and, if available, oral silymarin may be used to alleviate some symptoms [28].

PREVENTION AND CONTROL

HEV-caused acute viral hepatitis rarely occurs in developed countries. The primary means of control is through improvements in hygiene, especially by providing non-contaminated food and potable water. Immunization with recombinant HEV proteins can prevent HEV infection. Immunization with a vaccine based on the ORF-2 protein protected rhesus monkeys from intravenous challenge with both homologous and heterologous HEV. Protective vaccines have undergone successful phase III clinical trials in Nepal and China but are not yet commercially available [111, 112].

31.6 Non-A-to-E Hepatitis

Two to twenty percent of acute hepatitis cases are not caused by any of the well-described hepatitis viruses. Induction of hepatitis in primates with plasma from some non-A–E patients suggests that at least some are caused by an infectious disease [113]. A novel RNA virus has been recognized in the plasma of humans with acute non-A–E hepatitis, persons injecting illicit drugs, dialysis patients and blood donors. It has been provisionally named hepatitis G virus (HGV) or GB virus C [114]. This agent is a single-stranded, positive-sense RNA virus with approximately 25% nucleic acid identity with HCV. Its occurrence in humans can be demonstrated by detection of RNA and antibody to the viral envelope. HGV/GBV-C infection appears to persist with a frequency intermediate between those of HBV and HCV. Neither HGV/GBV-C or TT virus has not been associated with liver disease, and these viruses are probably not hepatropic. HGV has been detected in cases of fulminant hepatitis not caused by other recognized viruses. However, there are no data suggesting it causes either acute or chronic liver disease [115].

REFERENCES

1. Purcell RH. Hepatitis viruses: changing patterns of human disease. Proc Natl Acad Sci USA 1994;91:2401–6.
2. Ghabrah TM, Strickland GT, Tsarev S, et al. Acute viral hepatitis in Saudi Arabia: seroepidemiological analysis, risk factors, clinical manifestations, and evidence for a sixth hepatitis agent. Clin Infect Dis 1995; 21:621–7.
3. Martin A, Lemon SM. Hepatitis A virus: from discovery to vaccines. Hepatology 2006;43(suppl. 1):S164–S172.
4. Purcell RH, Emerson SU. Hepatitis E: an emerging awareness of an old disease. J Hepatol 2008;48:494–503.
5. Aggarwal R, Naik S. Epidemiology of hepatitis E: current status. J Gastroenterol Hepatol 2009;24:1484–93.
6. Alter MJ. Epidemiology of hepatitis B in Europe and worldwide. J Hepatol 2003;39(suppl. 1):S64–S69.
7. Liang TJ. Hepatitis B: the virus and disease. Hepatology 2009;49(suppl. 5):S13–S21.
8. Thomas DL. Hepatitis C epidemiology. Curr Top Microbiol Immunol 2000; 242:25–41.
9. Wedemeyer H, Manns MP. Epidemiology, pathogenesis and management of hepatitis D: update and challenges ahead. Nat Rev Gastroenterol Hepatol 2010;7:31–40.
10. Mohamed MK, Abdel-Hamid M, Mikhail NN, et al. Intrafamilial transmission of hepatitis C in Egypt. Hepatology 2005;42:683–7.
11. Shebl FM, El-Kamary SS, Saleh DA, et al. Prospective cohort study of mother-to-infant infection and clearance of hepatitis C in rural Egyptian villages. J Med Virol 2009;81:1024–31.
12. Arshad M, El-Kamary SS, Jhaveri R. Hepatitis C virus infection during pregnancy and the newborn period - are they opportunities for treatment? J Viral Hepat 2011;18:229–36.
13. McMahon BJ. The natural history of chronic hepatitis B virus infection. Hepatology 2009;49(suppl. 5):S45–S55.
14. Thomas DL, Seeff LB. Natural history of hepatitis C. Clin Liver Dis 2005; 9:383–98, vi.
15. Kofteridis DP, Koulentaki M, Valachis A, et al. Epstein Barr virus hepatitis. Eur J Intern Med 2011;22:73–6.
16. Varani S, Landini MP. Cytomegalovirus as a hepatotropic virus. Clin Lab 2002;48:39–44.
17. Zanetti AR, Van Damme P, Shouval D. The global impact of vaccination against hepatitis B: a historical overview. Vaccine 2008;26:6266–73.
18. Yang JD, Roberts LR. Hepatocellular carcinoma: A global view. Nat Rev Gastroenterol Hepatol 2010;7:448–58.
19. Chisari FV, Isogawa M, Wieland SF. Pathogenesis of hepatitis B virus infection. Pathol Biol 2010;58:258–66.
20. Guidotti LG, Chisari FV. Immunobiology and pathogenesis of viral hepatitis. Annu Rev Pathol 2006;1:23–61.
21. Alter HJ, Seeff LB. Recovery, persistence, and sequelae in hepatitis C virus infection: a perspective on long-term outcome. Semin Liver Dis 2000;20: 17–35.
22. Maheshwari A, Ray S, Thuluvath PJ. Acute hepatitis C. Lancet 2008;372: 321–32.
23. Nothdurft HD. Hepatitis A vaccines. Expert Rev Vaccines 2008;7:535–45.
24. Sorrell MF, Belongia EA, Costa J, et al. National Institutes of Health Consensus Development Conference Statement: management of hepatitis B. Ann Intern Med 2009;150:104–10.
25. Meky FA, Stoszek SK, Abdel-Hamid M, et al. Active surveillance for acute viral hepatitis in rural villages in the Nile Delta. Clin Infect Dis 2006;42: 628–33.
26. Chalmers TC, Eckhardt RD, Reynolds WE, et al. The treatment of acute infectious hepatitis. Controlled studies of the effects of diet, rest, and physical reconditioning on the acute course of the disease and on the incidence of relapses and residual abnormalities. J Clin Invest 1955;34:1163–235.
27. Chalmers TC, Reynolds WE, Eckhardt RD, et al. Treatment of acute infectious hepatitis in the Armed Forces; advantages of ad lib. bed rest and early reconditioning. J Am Med Assoc 1955;159:1431–4.
28. El-Kamary SS, Shardell MD, Abdel-Hamid M, et al. A randomized controlled trial to assess the safety and efficacy of silymarin on symptoms, signs and biomarkers of acute hepatitis. Phytomedicine 2009;16:391–400.
29. Strickland GT, El-Kamary SS, Klenerman P, Nicosia A. Hepatitis C vaccine: supply and demand. Lancet Infect Dis 2008;8:379–86.
30. Innis BL, Snitbhan R, Kunasol P, et al. Protection against hepatitis A by an inactivated vaccine. JAMA 1994;271:1328–34.
31. Zakaria S, Fouad R, Shaker O, et al. Changing patterns of acute viral hepatitis at a major urban referral center in Egypt. Clin Infect Dis 2007;44:e30–6.
32. Jacobsen KH, Wiersma ST. Hepatitis A virus seroprevalence by age and world region, 1990 and 2005. Vaccine 2010;28:6653–7.
33. Cuthbert JA. Hepatitis A: old and new. Clin Microbiol Rev 2001;14:38–58.
34. Fiore AE, Wasley A, Bell BP. Prevention of hepatitis A through active or passive immunization: recommendations of the Advisory Committee on Immunization Practices (ACIP). MMWR Recomm Rep 2006;55:1–23.
35. Shiffman ML. Management of acute hepatitis B. Clin Liver Dis 2010;14:75–91; viii–ix.
36. Piroth L, Pol S, Lacombe K, et al. Management and treatment of chronic hepatitis B virus infection in HIV positive and negative patients: the EPIB 2008 study. J Hepatol 2010;53:1006–12.

37. Bonino F, Piratvisuth T, Brunetto MR, Liaw YF. Diagnostic markers of chronic hepatitis B infection and disease. Antivir Ther 2010;15(suppl. 3):35–44.
38. Zuckerman AJ. Priorities for immunisation against hepatitis B. Br Med J (Clin Res Ed) 1982;284:686–8.
39. Wiegand J, van Bommel F, Berg T. Management of chronic hepatitis B: status and challenges beyond treatment guidelines. Semin Liver Dis 2010;30: 361–77.
40. Klenerman P, Fleming V, Barnes E. What are the prospects for controlling hepatitis C? PLoS Med 2009;6:e1000096.
41. Perrillo RP. Therapy of hepatitis B—viral suppression or eradication? Hepatology 2006;43(suppl. 1):S182–S193.
42. Liu J, Yang HI, Lee MH, et al. Incidence and determinants of spontaneous hepatitis B surface antigen seroclearance: a community-based follow-up study. Gastroenterology 2010;139:474–82.
43. Chen HL, Chang MH, Ni YH, et al. Seroepidemiology of hepatitis B virus infection in children: Ten years of mass vaccination in Taiwan. JAMA 1996; 276:906–8.
44. Chang MH, Chen CJ, Lai MS, et al. Universal hepatitis B vaccination in Taiwan and the incidence of hepatocellular carcinoma in children. Taiwan Childhood Hepatoma Study Group. N Engl J Med 1997;336:1855–9.
45. Kane M. Global programme for control of hepatitis B infection. Vaccine 1995;13(suppl. 1):S47–S49.
46. Iwarson S. Post-exposure prophylaxis for hepatitis B: active or passive? Lancet 1989;2:146–8.
47. Mast EE, Margolis HS, Fiore AE, et al. A comprehensive immunization strategy to eliminate transmission of hepatitis B virus infection in the United States: recommendations of the Advisory Committee on Immunization Practices (ACIP) Part I: immunization of infants, children, and adolescents. MMWR Recomm Rep 2005;54:1–31.
48. Mast EE, Weinbaum CM, Fiore AE, et al. A comprehensive immunization strategy to eliminate transmission of hepatitis B virus infection in the United States: recommendations of the Advisory Committee on Immunization Practices (ACIP) Part II: immunization of adults. MMWR Recomm Rep 2006; 55:1–33; quiz CE1–4.
49. Bensabath G, Hadler SC, Soares MC, et al. Hepatitis delta virus infection and Labrea hepatitis. Prevalence and role in fulminant hepatitis in the Amazon Basin. JAMA 1987;258:479–83.
50. Gomes-Gouvea MS, Soares MC, Bensabath G, et al. Hepatitis B virus and hepatitis delta virus genotypes in outbreaks of fulminant hepatitis (Labrea black fever) in the western Brazilian Amazon region. J Gen Virol 2009;90: 2638–43.
51. Casey JL. Hepatitis delta virus: molecular biology, pathogenesis and immunology. Antivir Ther 1998;3(suppl. 3):37–42.
52. Niro GA, Smedile A, Ippolito AM, et al. Outcome of chronic delta hepatitis in Italy: a long-term cohort study. J Hepatol 2010;53:834–40.
53. Choo QL, Kuo G, Weiner AJ, et al. Isolation of a cDNA clone derived from a blood-borne non-A, non-B viral hepatitis genome. Science 1989;244: 359–62.
54. Houghton M. The long and winding road leading to the identification of the hepatitis C virus. J Hepatol 2009;51:939–48.
55. Scott JD, Gretch DR. Molecular diagnostics of hepatitis C virus infection: a systematic review. JAMA 2007;297:724–32.
56. Frank C, Mohamed MK, Strickland GT, et al. The role of parenteral antischistosomal therapy in the spread of hepatitis C virus in Egypt. Lancet 2000; 355:887–91.
57. Strickland GT. Liver disease in Egypt: hepatitis C superseded schistosomiasis as a result of iatrogenic and biological factors. Hepatology 2006;43: 915–22.
58. Al-Sherbiny M, Osman A, Mohamed N, et al. Exposure to hepatitis C virus induces cellular immune responses without detectable viremia or seroconversion. Am J Trop Med Hyg 2005;73:44–9.
59. Hashem M, El-Karaksy H, Shata MT, et al. Strong hepatitis C virus (HCV)-specific cell-mediated immune responses in the absence of viremia or antibodies among uninfected siblings of HCV chronically infected children. J Infect Dis 2011;203:854–61.
60. Houghton M, Abrignani S. Prospects for a vaccine against the hepatitis C virus. Nature 2005;436:961–6.
61. De Francesco R, Migliaccio G. Challenges and successes in developing new therapies for hepatitis C. Nature 2005;436:953–60.
62. Simmonds P. Genetic diversity and evolution of hepatitis C virus—15 years on. J Gen Virol 2004;85:3173–88.
63. Lindenbach BD, Rice CM. Unravelling hepatitis C virus replication from genome to function. Nature 2005;436:933–8.
64. Neumann AU, Lam NP, Dahari H, et al. Hepatitis C viral dynamics in vivo and the antiviral efficacy of interferon-alpha therapy. Science 1998;282: 103–7.
65. Smith JA, Aberle JH, Fleming VM, et al. Dynamic coinfection with multiple viral subtypes in acute hepatitis C. J Infect Dis 2010;202:1770–9.
66. Kuiken C, Simmonds P. Nomenclature and numbering of the hepatitis C virus. Methods Mol Biol 2009;510:33–53.
67. Global burden of disease (GBD) for hepatitis C. J Clin Pharmacol 2004; 44:20–9.
68. Alter MJ, Kruszon-Moran D, Nainan OV, et al. The prevalence of hepatitis C virus infection in the United States, 1988 through 1994. N Engl J Med 1999; 341:556–62.
69. Armstrong GL, Wasley A, Simard EP, et al. The prevalence of hepatitis C virus infection in the United States, 1999 through 2002. Ann Intern Med 2006; 144:705–14.
70. El-Zanaty F, Way A. Egyptian Demographic and Health Survey 2008. Journal [serial on the Internet]. 2009. Available from: http://www.measuredhs.com/pubs/pdf/FR220/FR220.pdf (accessed 24 February 2012).
70a. El-Kamary SS, Jhaveri R, Shardell MD. All-cause, liver-related, and non-liver-related mortality among HCV-infected individuals in the general US population. Clin Infect Dis 2011;15;53(2):150–7.
71. Strickland GT. An epidemic of hepatitis C virus infection while treating endemic infectious diseases in Equatorial Africa more than a half century ago: did it also jump-start the AIDS pandemic? Clin Infect Dis 2010;51: 785–7.
72. Mohamed MK, Magder LS, Abdel-Hamid M, et al. Transmission of hepatitis C virus between parents and children. Am J Trop Med Hyg 2006;75: 16–20.
73. Saleh DA, Shebl F, Abdel-Hamid M, et al. Incidence and risk factors for hepatitis C infection in a cohort of women in rural Egypt. Trans R Soc Trop Med Hyg 2008;102:921–8.
74. Saleh DA, Shebl FM, El-Kamary SS, et al. Incidence and risk factors for community-acquired hepatitis C infection from birth to 5 years of age in rural Egyptian children. Trans R Soc Trop Med Hyg 2010;104:357–63.
75. Thomas DL, Villano SA, Riester KA, et al. Perinatal transmission of hepatitis C virus from human immunodeficiency virus type 1-infected mothers. Women and Infants Transmission Study. J Infect Dis 1998;177: 1480–8.
76. El-Kamary SS, Serwint JR, Joffe A, et al. Prevalence of hepatitis C virus infection in urban children. J Pediatr 2003;143:54–9.
77. Resti M, Azzari C, Mannelli F, et al. Mother to child transmission of hepatitis C virus: prospective study of risk factors and timing of infection in children born to women seronegative for HIV-1. Tuscany Study Group on Hepatitis C Virus Infection. BMJ 1998;317:437–41.
78. Tohme RA, Holmberg SD. Is sexual contact a major mode of hepatitis C virus transmission? Hepatology 2010;52:1497–505.
79. Habib M, Mohamed MK, Abdel-Aziz F, et al. Hepatitis C virus infection in a community in the Nile Delta: risk factors for seropositivity. Hepatology 2001;33:248–53.
80. Liang TJ, Rehermann B, Seeff LB, Hoofnagle JH. Pathogenesis, natural history, treatment, and prevention of hepatitis C. Ann Intern Med 2000; 132:296–305.
81. Bowen DG, Walker CM. Adaptive immune responses in acute and chronic hepatitis C virus infection. Nature 2005;436:946–52.
82. Lai ME, Mazzoleni AP, Argiolu F, et al. Hepatitis C virus in multiple episodes of acute hepatitis in polytransfused thalassaemic children. Lancet 1994;343: 388–90.
83. Castera L. Invasive and non-invasive methods for the assessment of fibrosis and disease progression in chronic liver disease. Best Pract Res Clin Gastroenterol 2011;25:291–303.
84. Thomas MB, Jaffe D, Choti MM, et al. Hepatocellular carcinoma: consensus recommendations of the National Cancer Institute Clinical Trials Planning Meeting. J Clin Oncol 2010;28:3994–4005.
85. Gebo KA, Chander G, Jenckes MW, et al. Screening tests for hepatocellular carcinoma in patients with chronic hepatitis C: a systematic review. Hepatology 2002;36(suppl. 1):S84–S92.
86. Dore MP, Fattovich G, Sepulveda AR, Realdi G. Cryoglobulinemia related to hepatitis C virus infection. Dig Dis Sci 2007;52:897–907.
87. Marcucci F, Mele A. Hepatitis viruses and non-Hodgkin lymphoma: epidemiology, mechanisms of tumorigenesis, and therapeutic opportunities. Blood 2011;117:1792–8.
88. Ghany MG, Strader DB, Thomas DL, Seeff LB. Diagnosis, management, and treatment of hepatitis C: an update. Hepatology 2009;49:1335–74.
89. Ge D, Fellay J, Thompson AJ, et al. Genetic variation in IL28B predicts hepatitis C treatment-induced viral clearance. Nature 2009;461:399–401.
90. Thomas DL, Thio CL, Martin MP, et al. Genetic variation in IL28B and spontaneous clearance of hepatitis C virus. Nature 2009;461:798–801.
91. Seeff LB, Ghany MG. Management of untreated and nonresponder patients with chronic hepatitis C. Semin Liver Dis 2010;30:348–60.

92. Gebo KA, Jenckes MW, Chander G, et al. Management of chronic hepatitis C. Evid Rep Technol Assess (Summ) 2002;60:1–7.
93. Vermehren J, Sarrazin C. New HCV therapies on the horizon. Clin Microbiol Infect 2011;17:122–34.
94. Kamal SM, El Kamary SS, Shardell MD, et al. Pegylated interferon alpha-2b plus ribavirin in patients with genotype 4 chronic hepatitis C: The role of rapid and early virologic response. Hepatology 2007;46:1732–40.
95. Khattab MA, Ferenci P, Hadziyannis SJ, et al. Management of hepatitis C virus genotype 4: Recommendations of An International Expert Panel. J Hepatol 2011;54:1250–62.
96. Bacon BR, Gordon SC, Lawitz E, et al. Boceprevir for previously treated chronic HCV genotype 1 infection. N Engl J Med 2011;364:1207–17.
97. Poordad F, McCone J, Jr, Bacon BR, et al. Boceprevir for untreated chronic HCV genotype 1 infection. N Engl J Med 2011;364:1195–206.
98. Pawlotsky JM. The results of Phase III clinical trials with telaprevir and boceprevir presented at the Liver Meeting 2010: a new standard of care for hepatitis C virus genotype 1 infection, but with issues still pending. Gastroenterology 2011;140:746–54.
98a. Jaeckel E, Cornberg M, Wedemeyer H, et al. Treatment of acute hepatitis C with interferon alfa-2b. N Engl J Med 2001;345(20):1452–7.
98b. Santantonio T, Fasano M, Sinisi E, et al. Efficacy of a 24-week course of PEG-interferon alpha-2b monotherapy in patients with acute hepatitis C after failure of spontaneous clearance. J Hepatol Mar 2005;42(3):329–33.
99. Kane MA, Bradley DW, Shrestha SM, et al. Epidemic non-A, non-B hepatitis in Nepal. Recovery of a possible etiologic agent and transmission studies in marmosets. JAMA 1984;252:3140–5.
100. Bryan JP, Tsarev SA, Iqbal M, et al. Epidemic hepatitis E in Pakistan: patterns of serologic response and evidence that antibody to hepatitis E virus protects against disease. J Infect Dis 1994;170:517–21.
101. Arankalle VA, Chadha MS, Tsarev SA, et al. Seroepidemiology of water-borne hepatitis in India and evidence for a third enterically-transmitted hepatitis agent. Proc Natl Acad Sci USA 1994;91:3428–32.
102. Khuroo MS, Rustgi VK, Dawson GJ, et al. Spectrum of hepatitis E virus infection in India. J Med Virol 1994;43:281–6.
103. Teshale EH, Hu DJ, Holmberg SD. The two faces of hepatitis E virus. Clin Infect Dis 2010;51:328–34.
104. Tamada Y, Yano K, Yatsuhashi H, et al. Consumption of wild boar linked to cases of hepatitis E. J Hepatol 2004;40:869–70.
105. Fix AD, Abdel-Hamid M, Purcell RH, et al. Prevalence of antibodies to hepatitis E in two rural Egyptian communities. Am J Trop Med Hyg 2000;62:519–23.
106. Stoszek SK, Engle RE, Abdel-Hamid M, et al. Hepatitis E antibody seroconversion without disease in highly endemic rural Egyptian communities. Trans R Soc Trop Med Hyg 2006;100:89–94.
107. Aggarwal R. Clinical presentation of hepatitis E. Virus Res 2011;161:15–22.
108. Arankalle VA, Jha J, Favorov MO, et al. Contribution of HEV and HCV in causing fulminant non-A, non-B hepatitis in western India. J Viral Hepat 1995;2:189–93.
109. Kamar N, Selves J, Mansuy JM, et al. Hepatitis E virus and chronic hepatitis in organ-transplant recipients. N Engl J Med 2008;358:811–17.
110. Dalton HR, Bendall RP, Keane FE, et al. Persistent carriage of hepatitis E virus in patients with HIV infection. N Engl J Med 2009;361:1025–7.
111. Shrestha MP, Scott RM, Joshi DM, et al. Safety and efficacy of a recombinant hepatitis E vaccine. N Engl J Med 2007;356:895–903.
112. Zhu FC, Zhang J, Zhang XF, et al. Efficacy and safety of a recombinant hepatitis E vaccine in healthy adults: a large-scale, randomised, double-blind placebo-controlled, phase 3 trial. Lancet 2010;376:895–902.
113. Chu CM, Lin DY, Yeh CT, et al. Epidemiological characteristics, risk factors, and clinical manifestations of acute non-A-E hepatitis. J Med Virol 2001;65:296–300.
114. Stapleton JT. GB virus type C/Hepatitis G virus. Semin Liver Dis 2003;23:137–48.
115. Reshetnyak VI, Karlovich TI, Ilchenko LU. Hepatitis G virus. World J Gastroenterol 2008;14:4725–34.

32 Viral Febrile Illnesses

32.1 Dengue and Dengue Hemorrhagic Fever

Daniel H Libraty

Key features

- Dengue is the most common and significant arboviral disease throughout the world. It is caused by infection with any one of the four dengue virus serotypes (DENV 1–4)
- The clinical manifestations of a DENV infection can range from an inapparent or mild febrile illness, to the more symptomatic and well-described dengue fever, to the most severe, and sometimes fatal, form of illness, dengue hemorrhagic fever
- The distinguishing characteristic of dengue hemorrhagic fever is a vascular leakage syndrome that develops around the time of defervescence. The relative risk for developing dengue hemorrhagic fever is increased with sequential heterologous DENV infections
- Patients with dengue, or suspected dengue, who manifest predefined "warning signs" require close monitoring and supportive care during the critical phase of illness
- The case-fatality rate for severe dengue is <1% with early recognition and appropriate supportive care and management

INTRODUCTION

Dengue is the most prevalent and widespread human arboviral disease in the 21st century. Dengue is caused by infection with any one of the four dengue viruses (DENV1–4), single-stranded RNA viruses that belong to the family *Flaviviridae*, genus *Flavivirus*. The DENVs are transmitted to humans through the bite of infected urban and peri-urban mosquitoes. The principal mosquito vector throughout the world is *Aedes aegypti*; the next most common mosquito vector is *Aedes albopictus*. Outbreaks of dengue-like illnesses were recognized and recorded in the 17th and 18th centuries, and perhaps even earlier [1]. There has been a dramatic increase in the incidence and global spread of dengue over the past 50 years [2, 3]. Today, dengue is poised as the vector-borne disease of globalization. The increased movement of people and goods across borders promotes the mix of DENVs, mosquitoes and people. Increased urbanization and growing economic power bring with them the discarded accessories of modern life and provide the breeding sites for *Aedes* mosquitoes.

EPIDEMIOLOGY

The global distribution of dengue essentially corresponds to the global distribution of the *A. aegypti* mosquito (Fig. 32.1.1). In the Asian tropics, all four DENV serotypes co-circulate continuously, creating a large region of hyperendemicity. Dengue outbreaks occur with predictable seasonality and periodicity. The majority of dengue cases are seen during the rainy season in a given year, when *Aedes* mosquito breeding and activity are at their highest levels. Through a complex interplay of population immunity, vector biology and environmental conditions, a shift in the dominant circulating DENV serotype typically occurs every 4–6 years. The shift in the dominant circulating DENV serotype often leads to waves of large-scale epidemic dengue activity [4]. Historically, the Americas were characterized by isolated and interspersed dengue outbreaks of a single infecting serotype. Over the past several decades, there has been introduction of "Asian genotype" DENV strains into the Americas, increased co-circulation of multiple DENV serotypes and geographic spread of dengue activity [5]. As such, the dengue disease and transmission patterns in the Americas are shifting towards the Asian hyperendemic patterns.

DENV infections produce clinical illness in tens of millions each year throughout the Asian and American tropics and subtropics. This is estimated to produce severe morbidity in approximately 2 million persons/year and approximately 20,000 deaths/year, predominantly in children [6]. Severe dengue is a major cause of hospitalization in children and often strains the healthcare systems of endemic countries during large outbreaks.

NATURAL HISTORY, PATHOGENESIS AND PATHOLOGY

The human dengue cycle is maintained by DENV transmission back and forth between mosquito vectors and viremic individuals. Following the bite of a DENV-infected mosquito, there is local viral replication in Langherhan's cells and cutaneous dendritic cells, and spread to regional lymph nodes. Thereafter, the virus rapidly disseminates throughout the reticuloendothelial system and skin leading to viremia. The primary target cells for viral replication appear to be

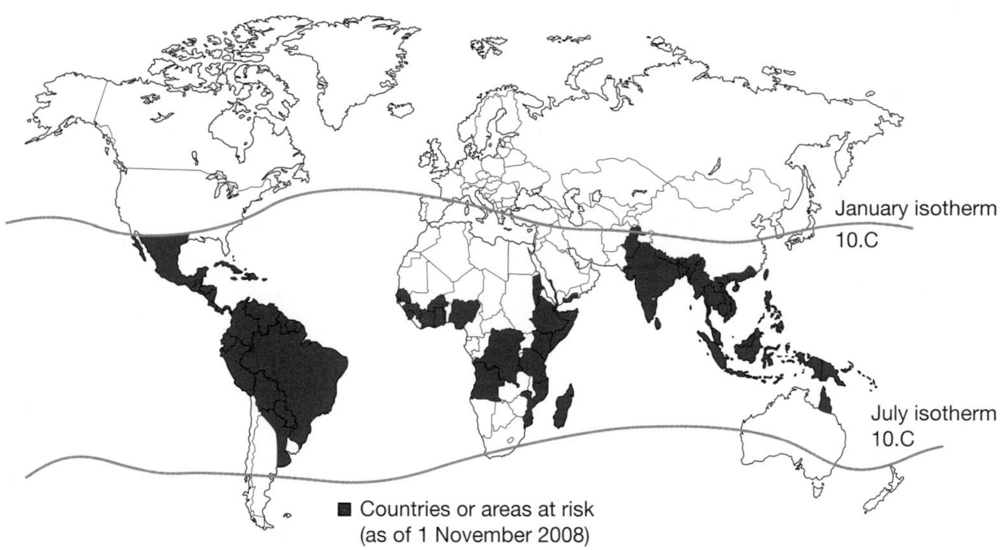

FIGURE 32.1.1 Global distribution of the *Aedes aegypti* mosquito as at 1 November 2008 *(redrawn with permission from WHO map. Public Health Information and Geographic Information Systems (GIS) WHO).*

those of myeloid lineage—dendritic cells, macrophages and monocytes. The incubation period between the mosquito bite and onset of symptoms varies from 3–10 days. Viremia generally lasts for 4–5 days and the disappearance of virus from the blood correlates with the resolution of fever [5, 7].

The most severe, and sometimes fatal, form of dengue is dengue hemorrhagic fever. The distinguishing pathophysiologic characteristic of dengue hemorrhagic fever is a transient and rapid increase in vascular permeability. The plasma leakage syndrome is most often characterized by hemoconcentration and transudate accumulation across serosal surfaces (i.e. pleural effusions and ascites). In its extreme form (dengue shock syndrome), hypovolemic shock ensues [8, 9]. The plasma leakage syndrome that distinguishes dengue hemorrhagic fever/dengue shock syndrome develops rapidly at the time of defervescence and clearance of viremia, and is transient (hours to days). Primary infection with a DENV serotype produces long-term protective immunity against re-infection with the homologous serotype (homotypic immunity), but only short-term protective immunity against heterologous serotypes (heterotypic immunity) [10, 11]. The relative risk of developing dengue hemorrhagic fever/dengue shock syndrome is increased 15- to 100-fold with sequential heterologous DENV infections compared with a primary DENV infection [12–14]. Primary DENV infections in infants <12 months old also appear more likely to lead to dengue hemorrhagic fever/dengue shock syndrome than primary DENV infections in children or adults [15]. The prevailing hypothesis to explain the apparent immunopathogenesis of dengue hemorrhagic fever has been antibody-dependent enhancement of DENV infection [3, 16, 17]. The antibody-dependent enhancement model for dengue hemorrhagic fever proposes that anti-DENV IgG, either actively acquired from a previous heterologous DENV infection or passively acquired in infants born to dengue-immune mothers, enhances DENV infection of Fc receptor-bearing cells and triggers a cytokine storm that leads to dengue hemorrhagic fever. The antibody-dependent enhancement hypothesis for dengue hemorrhagic fever/dengue shock syndrome immunopathogenesis remains controversial [18–20], and other contributing factors to dengue hemorrhagic fever immunopathogenesis are being investigated.

CLINICAL FEATURES

The most likely outcome of a primary or secondary DENV infection in all age groups is either asymptomatic infection or a mild, undifferentiated febrile illness of short duration. The mild febrile illness is often characterized by nonspecific constitutional and respiratory symptoms. This is particularly true in children, whereas DENV infections may be more likely to present as classic dengue fever in adults [5].

Classic dengue fever begins with the abrupt onset of fever, retro-orbital headache, backache and severe myalgias ("breakbone fever") [5, 21, 22]. The febrile illness typically lasts for 5–7 days and can be accompanied by anorexia, nausea/vomiting and prolonged asthenia. There is accompanying leukopenia, thrombocytopenia and often mild hepatic transaminase elevation. Petechiae may develop spontaneously, but, most commonly, can be elicited in a positive tourniquet test (>10 or 20 petechiae/square inch on the forearm after inflation of a blood pressure cuff) [23]. Clinically significant bleeding (e.g. epistaxis, gastrointestinal hemorrhage, menorrhagia/metrorrhagia) is much less common, but can occasionally be severe or life-threatening. Towards the end of the febrile period, the classic rash of dengue may appear (Herman's rash). It is a confluent erythematous macular rash over the extremities with scattered, well-circumscribed areas of sparing ("a sea of red with islands of normal skin"). The appearance of this rash is essentially pathognomonic for a DENV infection.

Dengue hemorrhagic fever is the dengue clinical syndrome whose distinguishing feature is abrupt plasma leakage from the intravascular to the extravascular space. When severe, the decrease in plasma volume leads to hypotension and shock (dengue shock syndrome). The World Health Organization (WHO) clinical case definition for dengue hemorrhagic fever incorporates three additional clinical criteria beyond dengue fever and established a grading scale of I–IV for dengue hemorrhagic fever severity (Table 32.1-1) [22]. Despite the moniker "hemorrhagic fever", most often the hemorrhagic manifestations may only be a positive tourniquet test, or spontaneous skin or mucosal petechiae. Severe coagulopathy is nearly always seen in the context of profound shock and multi-organ failure. Recently, WHO guidelines have moved away from the dengue hemorrhagic fever clinical case definition and, instead, proposed a case definition termed "severe dengue" (Table 32.1-1) [24]. Whether defined as dengue hemorrhagic fever or severe dengue, the overwhelming majority of serious morbidity and mortality caused by DENV infections is caused by a vascular leakage syndrome leading to hypotension and shock. Clinically significant hemorrhage can sometimes occur in the absence of vascular leakage, particularly in adults. Other uncommon, but serious, complications of DENV infections have also been recognized and include hepatic necrosis, encephalopathy or encephalitis, and chorioretinitis [8, 25].

TABLE 32.1-1 Case Definitions for Dengue Hemorrhagic Fever/Dengue Shock Syndrome, Severe Dengue and Warning Signs for Severe Dengue

Dengue hemorrhagic fever (DHF) case definition and severity classification	Case definition for "severe dengue"	Warning signs for severe dengue
Signs/symptoms of dengue fever and: 1. thrombocytopenia (platelet count < 100,000/mm^3), and 2. evidence of plasma leakage (hematocrit rise ≥ 20% from baseline, pleural effusion, or ascites), and 3. hemorrhagic manifestation (see below) • DHF Grade I = Criteria 1 + 2 + positive tourniquet test • DHF Grade II= Criteria 1 + 2 + spontaneous bleeding • DHF Grade III= DHF Grade I/II criteria + circulatory failure (hypotension, weak pulse) • DHF Grade IV = DHF Grade I/II criteria + profound shock	Probable or laboratory-confirmed dengue and: 1. severe plasma leakage (shock or fluid accumulation with respiratory distress), or 2. severe hemorrhage (as evaluated by clinician), or 3. severe organ impairment: a. liver: AST or ALT ≥ 1000 U/ml b. central nervous system: impaired consciousness c. heart and other organs	• Abdominal pain or tenderness • Persistent vomiting • Clinical fluid accumulation • Mucosal bleed • Lethargy, restlessness • Liver enlargement >2 cm • Increase in hematocrit concurrent with rapid decrease in platelet count

ALT, alanine aminotransferase; AST, aspartate transaminase.

PATIENT EVALUATION, DIAGNOSIS, AND DIFFERENTIAL DIAGNOSIS

Dengue should be considered in all individuals, particularly children, presenting with an abrupt-onset febrile illness in endemic regions. Dengue can be effectively excluded if the fever lasts more than 10–14 days. Otherwise, the initial clinical findings in DENV infections are fairly nonspecific and can be difficult to distinguish from other common febrile illnesses in the tropics. The differential diagnosis for dengue-like illnesses includes typhoid fever, leptospirosis, rickettsial infections or malaria. In the appropriate clinical setting, measles, influenza, other childhood viral illnesses and Chikungunya are also possibilities. Early in the febrile course, the suspicion for a DENV infection can be heightened by the presence of leukopenia, thrombocytopenia, mild aspartate aminotransferase elevation, and a positive tourniquet test or spontaneous petechiae. The positive predictive value for combinations of these early clinical findings has generally been good when dengue is highly prevalent (i.e. during the rainy season in DENV hyperendemic regions) [23, 26]. Their utility in distinguishing dengue from other acute febrile illnesses in other settings has not been well established. Among infants, an early macular rash and infantile febrile seizures should also raise suspicion for a DENV infection [27].

The critical phase of any DENV infection is the 24–48 hours surrounding defervescence—generally around days 5–7 of the febrile illness. This is the time period when plasma leakage will take place in patients developing dengue hemorrhagic fever. A challenge in patients with dengue, or suspected dengue, is to identify those at risk for severe disease before the critical phase is reached. A group of warning signs and symptoms have been identified in DENV-infected patients (mostly children) that often presage the deterioration to dengue hemorrhagic fever or severe dengue (Table 32.1-1) [24]. These patients always require close monitoring and supportive care during the critical phase of illness.

Laboratory diagnosis remains the most reliable way to identify a DENV infection. Reverse transcription (RT)-PCR can detect viral RNA in the blood for up to 5–7 days after the onset of fever in primary infections and 3–4 days after in secondary infections. However, DENV RT-PCR is not routinely available in most clinical settings. Viremia can also be detected by antigen-detection assays that measure circulating levels of a DENV nonstructural protein, NS1. The most widely used serologic assay for dengue is IgM/IgG ELISA. A single positive dengue IgM or high titer IgG can only provide a presumptive diagnosis of dengue. Definitive serologic diagnosis requires paired acute and convalescent sera. Anti-DENV IgM antibody levels do not generally become positive until the fifth or sixth day of illness and can be affected by other flavivirus infections (e.g. Japanese encephalitis virus). Therefore, the diagnostic sensitivity and specificity of anti-DENV IgM ELISA assays often depend on the timing of the blood sample, co-circulating flaviviruses in the region and the manufacturer [28]. Ideally, a laboratory approach to identifying DENV infections should incorporate more than method.

TREATMENT

There are no specific antiviral therapies available for dengue. The vast majority of uncomplicated dengue can be managed on an outpatient basis with rest, oral fluids and oral rehydration solution, and analgesia/antipyretics. The use of aspirin or nonsteroidal anti-inflammatory drugs (NSAIDs) should be avoided as they can exacerbate platelet dysfunction and mucosal bleeding. Patients and the parents of affected children should be notified of the warning signs and symptoms that should prompt an immediate return to medical attention.

The key to minimizing the morbidity and case-fatality rate of dengue is close monitoring, frequent re-assessment, and appropriate supportive care of patients with early suspicion of severe illness or impending deterioration. In-hospital management should be arranged for patients with the predefined warning signs, early evidence of plasma leakage (including narrow pulse pressure), bleeding or severe hematologic abnormalities, comorbid conditions, or those with unreliable access to outpatient follow-up care. For hospitalized patients without frank hypotension or shock, the key aspect of supportive therapy is judicious intravascular volume replacement as the critical phase is entered. This is accomplished by the careful administration of intravenous isotonic crystalloid solutions (e.g. 0.9% saline, Ringer's lactate, Hartmann's solution) with frequent re-assessment of intravascular volume status and urine output. The overly aggressive use of intravenous fluids or the failure to adequately monitor therapy can lead to serious complications of fluid overload during the critical phase of illness. For hospitalized patients with compensated or uncompensated hypotensive shock, more aggressive fluid resuscitation and monitoring are indicated. Treatment guidelines are shown in Figure 32.1.2.

Prophylactic platelet transfusions have not proven to be useful in dengue and should be avoided. Platelet transfusions can be considered in patients with thrombocytopenia and clinically significant hemorrhage. Similarly, packed red blood cell and whole blood transfusions should be used based on bleeding severity. Intramuscular injections, multiple large-bore intravenous lines and diagnostic or prophylactic placement of nasogastric tubes should be avoided, except as needed in the most severe cases. If possible, complicated, or unusual, severe dengue cases should be transferred to experienced referral centers in the area. The case-fatality rate for severe dengue is <1% with early recognition and appropriate supportive care and management.

PREVENTION

Dengue prevention can be approached by strategies to minimize human–vector contact and control mosquito vector populations (especially *A. aegypti*). Functioning window and door screens, and insecticide-treated bed nets for daytime sleeping (e.g. in infants) can reduce mosquito vector contact indoors. Personal measures that afford some protection against the daytime biting habits of female *A. aegypti* include wearing clothing that minimizes skin exposure and appropriate use of repellants on exposed skin or clothing. Effective repellants should contain N,N-diethyl-3-methylbenzamide (DEET), 3-(N-acetyl-N-butyl)-aminopropionic acid ethyl ester (IR3535) or 1-piperidinecarboxylic acid, 2-(2-hydroxyethyl)-1-methylpropylester (Icaridin) [24].

At the public health level, a sustained and integrated vector control strategy is generally needed to consistently reduce *A. aegypti* population densities. *Aedes aegypti* mosquitoes proliferate in many peridomestic water-containing habitats. These include purposely filled man-made containers (e.g. water storage barrels, flowerpots/vases), rain-filled solid waste containers (e.g. used tires, plastic bottles) and natural habitats (e.g. tree holes, rock holes). Successful vector control programs against *A. aegypti* have combined the identification and environmental management of productive breeding containers and the targeted application of larvicides (chemical and/or biological) and adulticides [24]. Novel strategies being explored for vector control and management include the release of genetically modified male *A. aegypti* that cannot produce viable offspring and the use of microbes to shorten the lifespan of adult female *A. aegypti*.

Dengue vaccine development has moved forward with encouraging advances. Given the potential for increased disease severity upon sequential infection with heterologous DENV serotypes, a general consensus has been that effective vaccination strategies will require simultaneous immunization to the four DENV serotypes (tetravalent vaccines). A chimeric, live-attenuated viral vaccine strategy, where the envelope proteins from DENVs1–4 have been engineered onto the yellow fever (YF)-17D vaccine backbone, has advanced to late-stage clinical trials. Other approaches in preclinical and early-stage clinical trials include chimeric, live-attenuated vaccines on a DENV backbone, inactivated virus vaccines and recombinant protein vaccines. In the future, the potential combination of effective dengue vaccination with

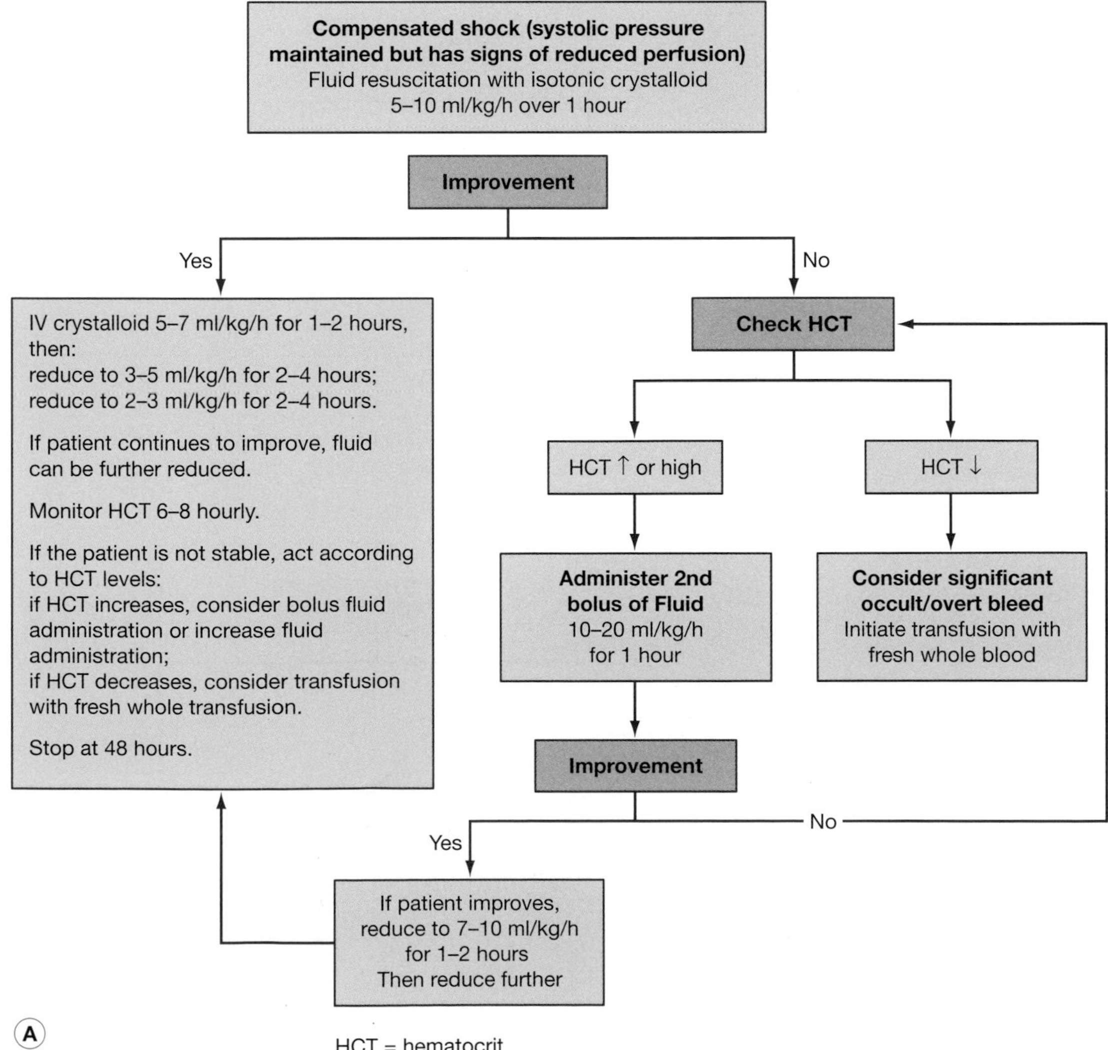

FIGURE 32.1.2 Treatment guidelines for dengue and dengue hemorrhagic fever.

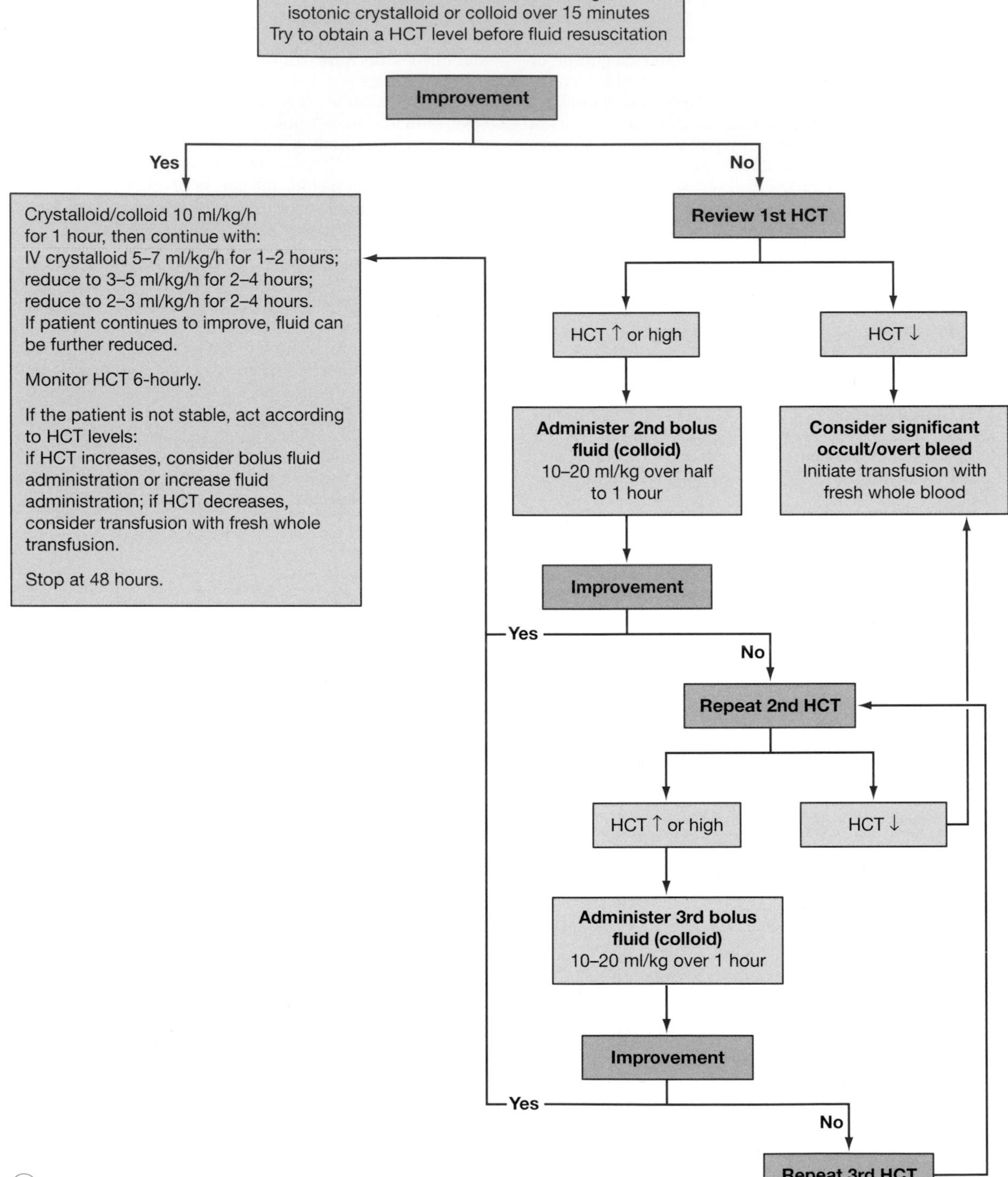

FIGURE 32.1.2, cont'd

vector control strategies will open up the possibility of severely halting, or even eradicating, DENV transmission in many endemic regions.

REFERENCES

1. Vasilakis N, Weaver SC. The history and evolution of human dengue emergence. Adv Virus Res 2008;72:1–76.
2. Kyle JL, Harris E. Global spread and persistence of dengue. Annu Rev Microbiol 2008; 62:71–92.
3. Halstead SB. Dengue. Lancet 2007;370:1644–52.
4. Cummings DA, Irizarry RA, Huang NE, et al. Travelling waves in the occurrence of dengue haemorrhagic fever in Thailand. Nature 2004;427: 34 -7.
5. Rigau-Perez JG, Clark GG, Gubler DJ, et al. Dengue and dengue haemorrhagic fever. Lancet 1998;352:971–7.
6. International Vaccine Institute. Global Burden of Dengue; 2009. Available at: http://www.pdvi.org/about_dengue/GBD.asp. (accessed 16 July 2009).
7. Halstead SB. Pathogenesis of dengue: challenges to molecular biology. Science 1998;239:476–81.
8. Nimmannitya S. Dengue hemorrhagic fever: diagnosis and management. In: Gubler DJ, Kuno G, eds. Dengue and Dengue Hemorrhagic Fever. New York: CAB International; 1997.
9. Wills BA, Oragui EE, Dung NM, et al. Size and charge characteristics of the protein leak in dengue shock syndrome. J Infect Dis 2004;190:810–18.
10. Sabin A. Research on dengue during World War II. Am J Trop Med Hyg 1952; 1:30–50.
11. Halstead SB. Pathogenesis of dengue: challenges to molecular biology. Science 1988;239:476–81.
12. Burke DS, Nisalak A, Johnson D, Scott RM. A prospective study of dengue infections in Bangkok. Am J Trop Med Hyg 1988;38:172–80.
13. Guzman MG, Kouri GP, Bravo J, et al. Dengue hemorrhagic fever in Cuba. Am J Trop Med Hyg 1990;42:179–84.
14. Halstead SB, Nimmannitya S, Cohen SN. Observations related to pathogenesis of dengue hemorrhagic fever. IV. Relation of disease severity to antibody response and virus recovered. Yale J Biol Med 1970;42;311–28.
15. Halstead SB, Lan NT, Myint TT, et al. Dengue hemorrhagic fever in infants: Research opportunities ignored. Emerg Infect Dis 2002;8:1474–79.
16. Halstead SB. Antibody, macrophages, dengue virus infection, shock, and hemorrhage: a pathogenetic cascade. Rev Infect Dis 1989;11(suppl. 4):S830–9.
17. Takada A, Kawaoka Y. Antibody-dependent enhancement of viral infection: molecular mechanisms and in vivo implications. Rev Med Virol 2003; 13:387–98.
18. Kliks SC, Nisalak A, Brandt WE, et al. Antibody-dependent enhancement of dengue virus growth in human monocytes as a risk factor for dengue hemorrhagic fever. Am J Trop Med Hyg 1989;40:444–51.
19. Laoprasopwattana K, Libraty DH, Endy TP, et al. Dengue Virus (DV) enhancing antibody activity in preillness plasma does not predict subsequent disease severity or viremia in secondary DV infection. J Infect Dis 2005;192: 510–19.
20. Libraty DH, Acosta LP, Tallo V, et al. A prospective nested case-control study of Dengue in infants: rethinking and refining the antibody-dependent enhancement dengue hemorrhagic fever model. PLoS Med 2009;6:e1000171.
21. Rothman AL, Ennis FA. Toga/Flaviviruses: Immunopathology. In: Cunningham M, Fujinami R, eds. Effects of Microbes on the Immune System. Philadelphia, PA: Lippincott Williams & Wilkins; 2000.
22. Anonymous. Dengue haemorrhagic fever: diagnosis, treatment, prevention and control, 2nd edn. Geneva: World Health Organization; 1997.
23. Kalayanarooj S, Vaughn DW, Nimmannitya S, et al. Early clinical and laboratory indicators of acute dengue illness. J Infect Dis 1997;176:313–21.
24. Dengue: guidelines for diagnosis, treatment, prevention and control—new edition. France: World Health Organization; 2009.
25. Nimmannitya S. Clinical spectrum and management of dengue haemorrhagic fever. Southeast Asian J Trop Med Public Health 1987;18:392–7.
26. Potts JA, Rothman AL. Clinical and laboratory features that distinguish dengue from other febrile illnesses in endemic populations. Trop Med Int Health 2008;13:1328–40.
27. Capeding RZ, Brion JD, Caponpon MM, et al. The incidence, characteristics, and presentation of dengue virus infections during infancy. Am J Trop Med Hyg 2010;82:330 6.
28. Hunsperger EA, Yoksan S, Buchy P, et al. Evaluation of commercially available anti-dengue virus immunoglobulin M tests. Emerg Infect Dis 2009;15: 436–40.

32.2 Chikungunya Fever

Mala Chhabra, Veena Mittal

Key features

- Chikungunya fever is a re-emerging arboviral disease characterized by the abrupt onset of fever with severe arthralgia followed by constitutional symptoms and rash lasting for 1–7 days
- It is transmitted by the bite of infected *Aedes aegypti* and, to some extent, by *Aedes albopictus* mosquitoes
- The disease is nearly always self-limited and rarely fatal. There is no specific treatment. Supportive care with rest is indicated during the acute symptoms
- As there is not yet an effective vaccine, preventive efforts focus on the avoidance of mosquito bites and mosquito vector control

INTRODUCTION

Chikungunya (CHIK) fever is an arboviral disease transmitted by *Aedes aegypti* and *Aedes albopictus* mosquitoes. Its name is derived from the Makonde (African language) word meaning "that which bends up" in reference to the stooped posture that develops as a result of the arthritic symptoms of the disease. The sudden onset of the febrile illness (fever, chills, headache, nausea, vomiting, low back pain and rash) accompanied by crippling arthralgias (Fig. 32.2.1) and frequent arthritis is clinically distinctive. The disease is nearly always self-limiting and rarely fatal [1]. CHIK virus (CHIKV) is a single-stranded positive-sense RNA virus belonging to the family *Togaviridae*, genus *Alphavirus*. Molecular characterization has demonstrated two distinct strain lineages that cause epidemics in Africa and Asia. A single point mutation in the viral envelope protein gene was associated with *A. albopictus* rather than *A. aegypti* transmission during an outbreak in La Reunion in 2005–6.

EPIDEMIOLOGY

A few centuries ago, CHIK virus was probably an infection of primates in the forests and savannahs of Africa. It continues to be maintained in a nonhuman primate cycle by sylvatic *Aedes* mosquitoes. Today, however, CHIK is also responsible for extensive *A. aegypti*-transmitted urban disease in the cities of Africa and has produced major epidemics in Asia.

The African and Asian genotypes of CHIKV exhibit differences in their transmission cycles. In Africa, the virus is predominantly maintained in a nonhuman primate sylvatic cycle, whereas in Asia, the predominant virus lifecycle is between humans and *A. aegypti* or *A. albopictus* mosquitoes.

CHIKV is known to cause epidemics after periods of quiescence. The first recorded epidemic occurred in Tanzania in 1952–53. In Asia, CHIKV was first isolated in Bangkok, Thailand, in 1958. Virus transmission continued until 1964. After a hiatus, virus activity re-appeared in the mid 1970s and declined by 1976. In India, well-documented outbreaks occurred in 1963 and 1964 in Calcutta and Southern India respectively. Thereafter, a small outbreak of CHIK was reported from the Sholapur district, Maharashtra in 1973. The virus emerged in the islands of the southwest Indian Ocean viz. French island of La Reunion, Mayotee, Mauritius and Seychelles, in February 2005. After three decades of quiescence, CHIKV then re-emerged in India in December 2005. The 2005–2006 outbreak in India involved approximately 1.35 million suspected cases in 12 states. The attack rate reached up to 45% owing to the lack of herd immunity and a large susceptible population [1].

Imported cases of CHIK infection have been reported from Europe and the USA in returning travelers from areas with high incidence rates. *Aedes albopictus*, a competent vector for CHIK virus, has been introduced into several European countries, Central America, Brazil and the USA through the trade in used tires and ornamental plants [2].

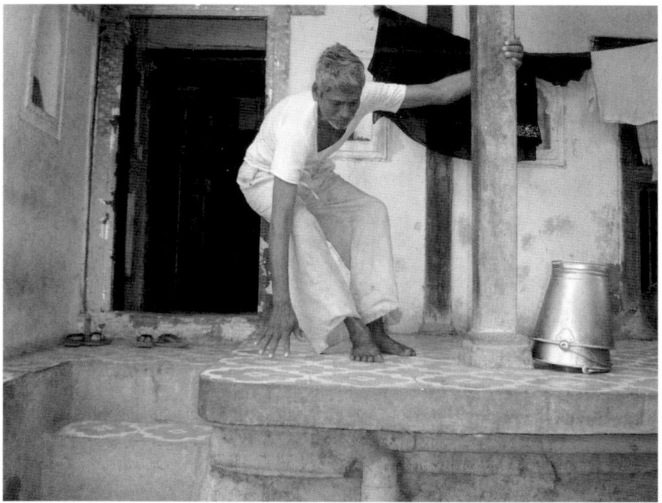

FIGURE 32.2.1 Inability to stand or walk without support due to involvement of joints in a chikungunya case (stooped posture).

NATURAL HISTORY, PATHOGENESIS AND PATHOLOGY

Following the bite of an infected mosquito, the virus replicates leading to a viremia that can be very high; the skin, joints and muscles are especially affected—the nervous system, heart and liver less frequently. Monocytes appear to be the main target of infection during the viremic phase. More severe symptoms relate to a higher viral titer, and stronger pro-inflammatory response. Chronic arthralgia is associated with high levels of interleukin-6 and granulocyte macrophage colony-stimulating factor (GM-CSF). There is little pathologic information available because the disease is rarely fatal.

CLINICAL FEATURES

Chikungunya is an acute infection of abrupt onset, heralded by fever and severe arthralgia, and followed by other constitutional symptoms and rash lasting for a period of 1–7 days. The incubation period is usually 2–3 days, with a range of 1–12 days. Fever rises abruptly, often reaching 39–40°C accompanied by intermittent shaking chills. This acute phase lasts 2–3 days. The temperature may remit for 1–2 days after a gap of 4–10 days, resulting in a "saddle back" fever curve that is characteristic of arthropod-borne virus infections.

The arthralgias are polyarticular, migratory and predominantly affect the small joints of the hands, wrists, ankles and feet (Fig. 32.2.2) with lesser involvement of larger joints. During the acute phase, patients complain bitterly of pain when asked to move. They characteristically lie still in the attitude of flexion. Pain on movement is worse in the morning, improved by mild exercise and exacerbated by strenuous exercise. Swelling may occur but fluid accumulation is uncommon. Patients with milder articular manifestation are usually symptom-free within a few weeks, but more severe cases require months to resolve entirely [1, 3]. A study indicated that over 12% of patients develop chronic joint symptoms. Generalized myalgias, as well as back and shoulder pain is common [4].

Cutaneous manifestations are typical with many patients. Initially, many present with facial and trunk flushing. This is usually followed by a maculopapular rash. The trunk and limbs are commonly involved (Fig. 32.2.3), but the face, palms and soles may also show lesions. The rash may simply fade or desquamate. Petechiae may occur alone or in association with the rash.

During the acute phase, most patients will have headache, but it is not usually severe. Photophobia and retro-orbital pain may also

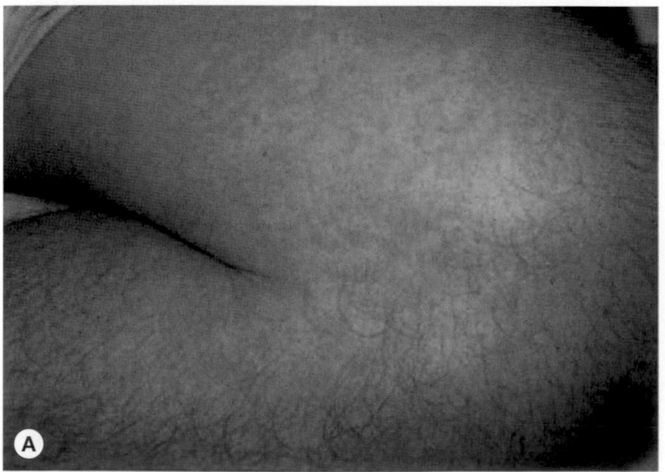

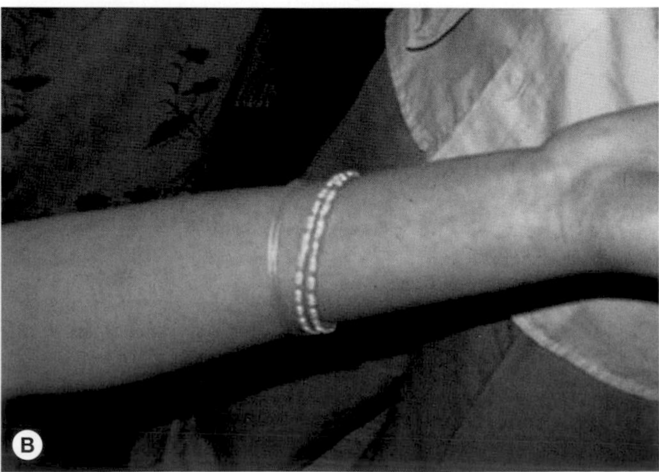

FIGURE 32.2.2 Maculopapular rash on lower extremities (A) and upper extremities (B) in cases of chikungunya fever.

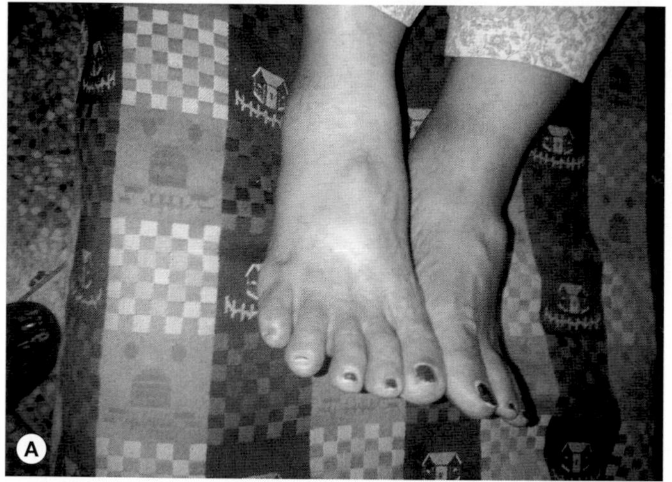

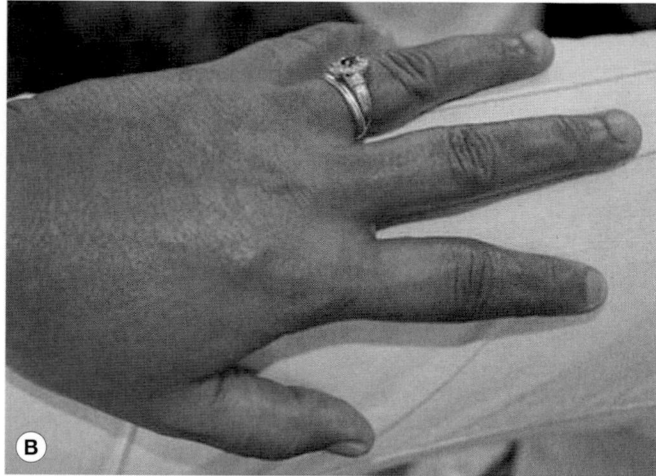

FIGURE 32.2.3 Swelling of ankle joints **(A)** and small joints of hands **(B)** in cases of chikungunya fever.

occur. Conjunctival redness is present in some cases. Some patients complain of a sore throat and have pharyngitis on examination [3]. CHIKV infection infrequently produces a meningoencephalitis, particularly in newborns [5, 6] and those with pre-existing medical conditions. Pregnant women can pass the virus to their infant. The Reunion South Hospital Group observed 84 pregnant women who had laboratory-confirmed CHIK infection. In 88% of these women (all involving infections relatively distant from delivery), the newborns appeared asymptomatic. Conversely, 10 newborns had severe attacks soon after birth (4 with meningoencephalitis and 3 with intravascular coagulation) and required intensive care support. No infant died; however, one suffered from intracerebral hemorrhage after severe thrombocytopenia [7]. Severe cases of CHIK can occur in the elderly, newborns and immunocompromised individuals. CHIK outbreaks typically result in several hundreds or thousands of cases, but deaths are rarely encountered.

PATIENT EVALUATION, DIAGNOSIS AND DIFFERENTIAL DIAGNOSIS

Symptoms of CHIKV infection can be clinically indistinguishable from dengue fever. Dual infection of CHIK and dengue fever has been reported [1, 2]. Other acute febrile illnesses in the differential diagnosis of CHIK include O'nyong-nyong virus infection and Sindbis virus infection [1–3].

The clinical laboratory findings in CHIK are not remarkable. A few patients may present with leukopenia with relative lymphocytosis; however, most patients will have normal blood counts. The platelet count may be moderately depressed. The erythrocyte sedimentation rate and C-reactive protein levels are elevated in acute cases [3]. A definitive diagnosis can only be made by laboratory means, but CHIK should be suspected when epidemic disease occurs with the characteristic triad of fever, rash and arthralgia.

Virus-specific IgM antibodies can be readily detected by 5–7 days of illness using capture ELISA in patients recovering from CHIK infection; they decline within 3–6 months. Diagnosis can be confirmed by virus isolation or reverse transcription (RT)-PCR by amplifying a fragment of the E-2 gene. Combined detection and genotyping of CHIKV targeting nsP1 and E1 genes has been developed [8]. Blood samples for virus isolation and RT-PCR should be collected within the first 5 days of illness when viremia is detectable.

TREATMENT

There is no specific treatment for CHIK. The illness is usually self-limiting and resolves with time. Supportive care with rest is indicated during the acute joint symptoms. Movement and mild exercise tend to improve stiffness and morning arthralgia, but heavy exercise may exacerbate rheumatic symptoms. Aspirin and other nonsteroidal anti-inflammatory drugs (NSAIDs) are recommended for chronic pain. In unresolved arthritis refractory to NSAIDs, Chloroquine 250 mg has proved to be useful [9].

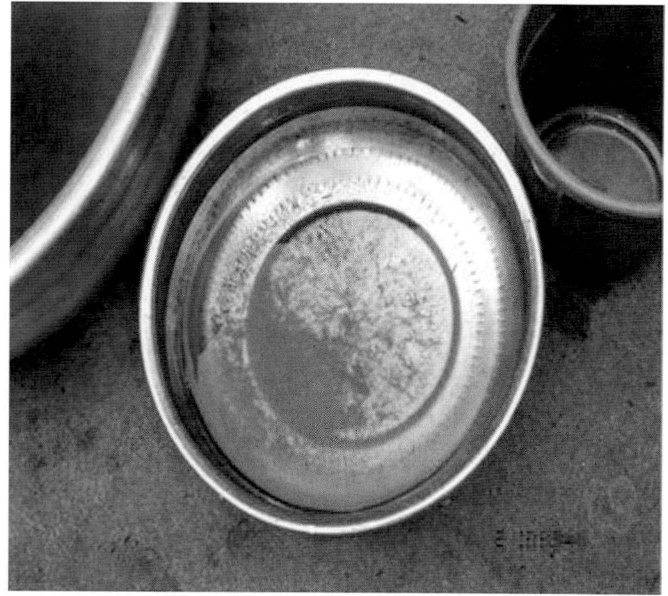

FIGURE 32.2.4 *Aedes* breeding in water storing containers at home.

A vaccine or specific medication is not yet available against CHIK infection. Thus, vector control is very important in controlling or preventing CHIKV transmission. Elimination of breeding sites or source reduction is an effective method of control. *Aedes aegypti* is typically a container-habitat species (Fig. 32.2.4) and breeds primarily in artificial containers and receptacles. Therefore, all water tanks, cisterns, barrels, trash containers, etc. need to be covered tightly with a lid. Old tires, tin cans, buckets, drums, bottles, etc. should be removed as mosquitoes may breed in these containers if they accumulate water. In ornamental garden water tanks, larvivorous fish (e.g. gambusia, guppy) can be introduced. Weeds and tall grass should be cut short—adult mosquitoes look for these shady places to rest during the hot daylight hours. In case water containers cannot be emptied on a daily or weekly basis, Temephos (1 ppm) should be applied.

Aedes mosquitoes are principally day-time biters. Thus, children should sleep under an insecticide-treated bed net during the daytime. Insecticide spraying should be done to kill mosquitoes. For knock-down, well-planned fogging operations are strongly recommended with 2% pyrethrum space spray in high-risk villages/wards and where clustering of cases has been reported. Insect repellant containing *N,N*-diethyl-m-toluamide (DEET) or another registered active ingredient should be applied on exposed skin. People should be advised to wear long sleeves and pants and have secure screens on windows and doors to keep mosquitoes out.

Infected persons should be protected from further mosquito exposure (staying indoors and/or under a mosquito net during the first few days of illness) so that they cannot contribute to the transmission cycle.

A vaccine or specific medication is not yet available against CHIK infection. Vector control is thus very important in controlling or preventing CHIKV transmission.

REFERENCES

1. Chhabra M, Mittal V, Bhhatacharya D, et al. Chikungunya Fever: A reemerging viral infection. Indian J Med Microbiol 2008;26:5–12
2. Pialoux G, Gaüzère B-A, Jauréguiberry S. Chikungunya, an epidemic arbovirosis. Michel Strobel. Lancet Infect Dis 2007;7:319–27
3. Fields BN, Knipe DM, Howley PM, eds. Alphaviruses. In: Fields Virology, 3rd edn, Vol. 1. Philadelphia: Lippincott-Raven Publishers; 1996:858–98.
4. Brighton SW. Chloroquine phosphate treatment of chronic Chikungunya arthritis: An open pilot study. S Afr Med J 1984;66:217–18.
5. Chatterjee SN, Chakravarti SK, Mitra AC, Sarkar JK. Virological investigation of cases with neurological complications during the outbreak of haemorrhagic fever in Calcutta. J Indian Med Assoc 1965;45:314–16.
6. Schuffenecker I, Iteman I, Michault A, et al. Genome microevolution of Chikungunya viruses causing the Indian Ocean outbreak. Plos Medicine. Available at: http://www.plosmedicine.org/article/info:doi/10.1371/journal.pmed.0030263.
7. Robillard PY, Boumahni B, Gerardin P, et al. Vertical maternal fetal transmission of the chikungunya virus. Presse Med 2006;35:785–8
8. Hasebe F, Parquet MC, Pandey BD, et al. Combined detection and genotyping of Chikungunya virus by a specific reverse transcription polymerase chain reaction. J Med Virol 2002;67:370–4.
9. Brighton SW. Chloroquine phosphate treatment of chronic Chikungunya arthritis: An open pilot study. S Afr Med J 1984;66:217–18

32.3 O'nyong Nyong Fever

Gregory Deye

Key features

- Alphavirus transmitted by anophiline mosquitoes in sub-Saharan Africa
- Typically occurs in large epidemics with high attack rates. Endemic or sporadic cases are rare with almost no disease activity between epidemics
- Fever and severe symmetrical arthralgias are nearly universal. Pruritic maculopapular rash is common
- Lymphadenitis (especially posterior cervical) is common but cannot help to differentiate it from other arboviral infections
- Diagnosis is by PCR in the first 3 days or by serology
- Treatment is supportive, with acute symptoms resolving in 5–7 days

INTRODUCTION

O'nyong nyong fever (ONN) is an arboviral disease caused by an alphavirus of the Semliki Forest complex and most closely related to chikungunya virus (CHIKV). Like other members of this complex, ONN causes a febrile arthalgic illness. It is unique among alphaviruses in its adaptation to anopheles mosquito vectors, which are primarily responsible for its transmission.

The disease was undescribed prior to 1959 when an epidemic began in the Acholi district in northwestern Uganda. By the end of the epidemic in 1962, it had involved 2 million people in a band-like distribution across Uganda, Kenya and Tanzania. Investigation of this epidemic led to the discovery of the novel virus, which was named after an Acholi term meaning "the joint breaker" [1].

EPIDEMIOLOGY

ONN has generally been described in epidemics occurring in sub-Saharan Africa. Sporadic cases outside of epidemic settings have occasionally been described. After the end of the initial epidemic in 1962, no clinical cases were recognized until a subsequent epidemic occurred in Uganda in 1996–97 resulting in several hundred cases. An illness with clinical features very similar to ONN had been described in 1967 in Nigeria. The causative agent was isolated and named Igbo Ora virus. Subsequent studies have shown that Igbo Ora is actually a strain of ONN [2]. The genetic similarities of Igbo Ora and the 1996–97 ONN virus to the 1959 ONN virus, together with serosurveys from Kenya, Cameroon and West Africa, indicate that unrecognized endemic transmission may occur during interepidemic periods. During epidemics, rates of infection of up to 68% have been seen in affected villages [3].

The virus is principally transmitted by *Anopheles funestus* and *Anopheles gambiae*, both of which also serve as important vectors of malaria. No vertebrate reservior has been identified. Risk factors for infection are likely to be related to risk of mosquito exposure and are likely to be similar to risk factors associated with malaria.

CLINICAL FEATURES

The ratio of symptomatic to inapparent infections is roughly 2:1 [3]. After an incubation period of about 8 days, clinical symptoms begin with sudden onset of fever and joint pains. Joint involvement is generally symmetrical, involving knees (90%), ankles (83%), elbows (75%), wrists (75%) or fingers (63%) [4]. Joint pain lasts for an average of 6 days, although durations as long as 90 days have been reported. Arthralgia was sufficiently severe to lead to immobilization in 78% of cases for an average of 4 days, although there was considerable variability in the reported durations, with immobility lasting as long as 28 days reported [4]. Additional symptoms include headache, a generalized pruritic maculopapular rash, cervical lymphadenopathy and conjunctival suffusion.

A mild neutropenia has been reported during the acute phase of the illness [5]. In both the 1959–62 epidemic and the 1996–97 epidemic, there were no reported fatalities, despite a total of more than 2 million cases.

PATIENT EVALUATION, DIAGNOSIS AND DIFFERENTIAL DIAGNOSIS

Although some clinical features, such as the presence of cervical lymphadenopathy may be suggestive, ONN cannot be differentiated from similar arboviruses, such as CHIKV and dengue on clinical grounds alone. Careful history and physical exam should be directed at excluding other illnesses, as well as finding supportive features such as rash. Virus can be detected in whole blood by molecular amplification (PCR) with greatest sensitivity during the first 3 days after the onset of illness. Serology can help to establish the diagnosis which can be made by the detection of specific IgM or by paired acute and convalescent sera showing development of specific IgG. IgM titers peak roughly 21 days after the onset of illness and remain elevated for over 60 days. IgG titers begin to rise by day 21 and are long-lasting [6]. Care must be taken in the interpretation of serologic results because of a well-known, one-way cross-reactivity with CHIKV (i.e. ONN patients will display antibodies to CHIK, but CHIK patients will not usually react to ONN) [7].

TREATMENT AND CONTROL

The illness is self-limited, but therapy with nonsteroidal antiinflamatory drugs (NSAIDs) may benefit joint symptoms. Preventive measures against exposure to malaria vectors, for example insecticide-treated bed nets and indoor residual insecticides, should also be effective in controlling epidemic ONN.

REFERENCES

1. O'nyong-nyong. Lancet 1962;279:363–4.
2. Powers AM, Brault AC, Tesh RB, Weaver SC. Re-emergence of Chikungunya and O'nyong-nyong viruses: evidence for distinct geographical lineages and distant evolutionary relationships. J Gen Virol 2000;81:471–9.
3. Sanders EJ, Rwaguma EB, Kawamata J, et al. O'nyong-nyong fever in south-central Uganda, 1996–1997: description of the epidemic and results of a household-based seroprevalence survey. J Infect Dis 1999;180:1436–43.
4. Kiwanuka N, Sanders EJ, Rwaguma EB, et al. O'nyong-nyong fever in south-central Uganda, 1996–1997: clinical features and validation of a clinical case definition for surveillance purposes. Clin Infect Dis 1999;29:1243–50.
5. Shore H. O'nyong-Nyong fever: an epidemic virus disease in East Africa; III. Some clinical and epidemiological observations in the Northern Province of Uganda. Trans R Soc Trop Med Hyg 1961;55:361–73.
6. Bessaud M, Peyrefitte CN, Pastorino BAM, et al. O'nyong-nyong Virus, Chad. Emerg Infect Dis 2006;12:1248–50.
7. Blackburn NK, Besselaar TG, Gibson G. Antigenic relationship between chikungunya virus strains and o'nyong nyong virus using monoclonal antibodies. Res Virol 1995;146:69–73.

32.4 Ross River Virus Disease

David Harley, Andreas Suhrbier

Key features

- Synonyms include epidemic polyarthritis and Ross River fever
- Endemic/epidemic transmission in Australia and Papua New Guinea, with a mean of ~4000 cases per annum in Australia
- Notable clinical features include peripheral symmetrical polyarthralgia/arthritis, predominantly involving small joints. Illness is self-limiting and usually progressively resolves over 3–6 months
- Diagnosis is made by specific IgM/IgG ELISA

INTRODUCTION

Ross River virus (RRV) is a mosquito-borne virus that, in Australia, causes several thousand cases per year with polyarthralgia or polyarthritis being the predominant clinical feature. This single-stranded, positive-sense RNA virus (~11.8 kb genome) belongs to the genus *Alphavirus* and the family *Togaviridae*. The virus was first isolated from *Aedes vigilax* mosquitoes trapped beside the Ross River in Queensland (Fig. 32.4.1) in 1959 [1]. Following a series of outbreaks, the disease was originally called "epidemic polyarthritis" [2, 3].

EPIDEMIOLOGY

RRV disease is notifiable to public health authorities in Australia. There has been a mean of ~4,000 (range 1454–5650) reported cases per year, equating to a yearly incidence of 7–26 per 100,000 between 2000–2009 [4]. Disease typically occurs in adults between 25 and 39 years old, with no clear predominance in males or females. Symptomatic infections are rare, or absent, in children [1].

RRV is endemic in Australia and Papua New Guinea. Most cases occur in northern Australia during the wet season (usually December–February) and individuals with high exposure to mosquitoes are at greatest risk [3]. In 1979–80, RRV also caused a large epidemic in the South Pacific (Fig. 32.4.1).

NATURAL HISTORY, PATHOGENESIS AND PATHOLOGY

RRV is transmitted in enzootic cycles with macropods (kangaroos and wallabies) as the natural vertebrate hosts. The virus is transmitted to humans from vertebrate hosts (and/or other humans during epidemics) by mosquitoes, principally *A. vigilax*, *Aedes camptorhynchus* and *Culex annulorostris* [1].

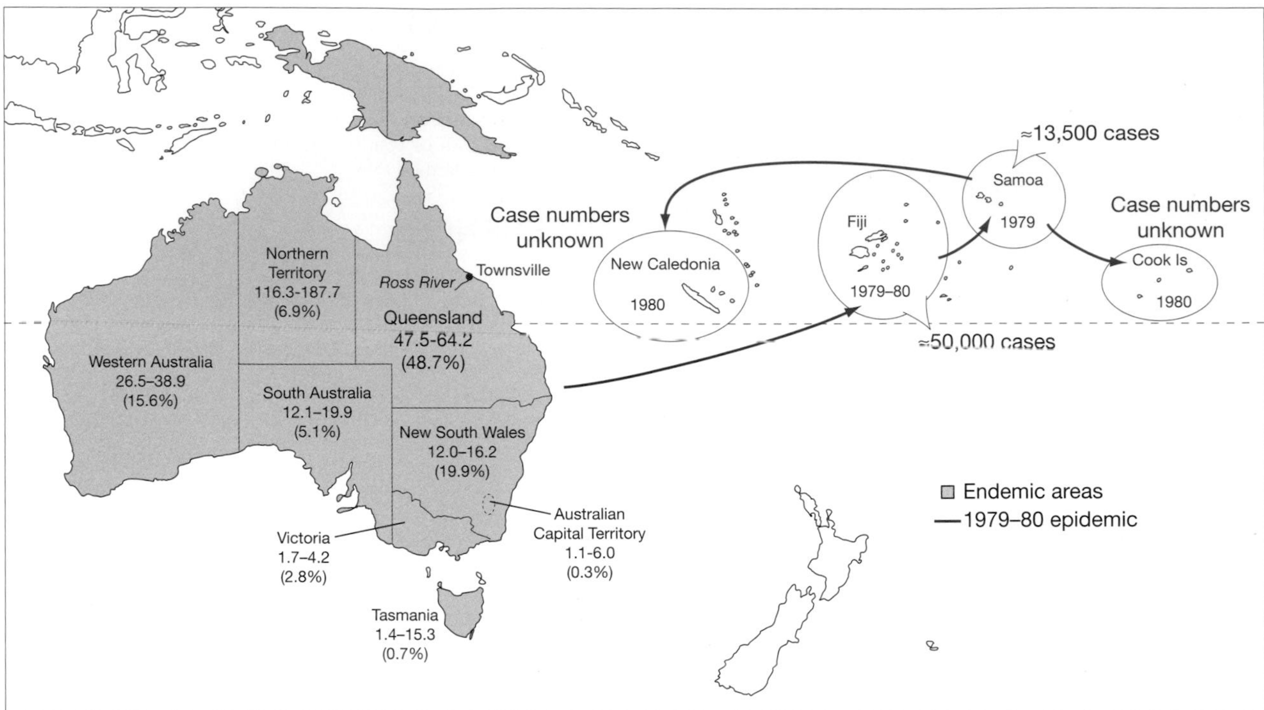

FIGURE 32.4.1 The figure shows the course of the 1979–80 epidemic in the Pacific islands (arrows); the blue shaded areas show where RRV is endemic. The range of incidence rates per 100,000 per annum and the mean percentage of total Australian cases (for 2007–9) are given for each state/territory of Australia. *Data was obtained from the Communicable Disease Network Australia Communicable Diseases Network Australia. Available at: http://www9.health.gov.au/cda/Source/Rpt_4_sel.cfm.*

Rheumatic disease is believed to arise from adaptive and/or innate immune responses directed at RRV antigens persisting in affected tissues. These responses produce classical arthrogenic pro-inflammatory mediators [5]. Joint effusions predominantly contain mononuclear cells and RRV has been detected in synovial fluids by PCR [6]. However, joint aspirations and PCR have limited value for diagnosis [3]. RRV infections can be subclinical, with the asymptomatic/symptomatic ratio estimated to be between 1.2 : 1 and 3 : 1 [1].

Virus-specific antibodies, probably neutralizing antibodies, are believed to be the principal protective adaptive immune response to RRV [7]. Immunity appears to be life-long, with no reports of re-infection.

CLINICAL FEATURES

The incubation period for RRV is usually 7–9 days, with a possible range of 3–21 days [1]. Acute disease typically presents as a triad of constitutional symptoms, joint involvement and rash [1, 3, 8]. Arthralgia/arthritis occurs in nearly all patients. The joints most commonly affected are multiple peripheral small joints and the knees, usually with a symmetrical pattern (Table 32.4-1). Effusions are often present but are usually small [8]. There may be tendonitis. Rash occurs in ~50% of patients, most commonly presenting as erythematous macules and papules (1–5 mm diameter). Fatigue, myalgia, fever and lymphadenopathy are common constitutional features. Fatigue typically affects over 50% of patients and is often protracted. Myalgia occurs in up to 58% of patients. Fever affects 33–50% of patients. Encephalitis or meningitis may occur, but is rare [1, 8].

There is a popular misconception that RRV disease, particularly rheumatic symptoms, last for years. However, prospective studies using validated questionnaires illustrated that, in patients with RRV disease (and no other diagnoses), rheumatic symptoms usually progressively resolve over 3–6 months with no long-term sequelae [9, 10].

TABLE 32.4-1 Joint Involvement in Ross River Virus Disease. The Percentage of Patients Who Have Arthritis/Arthralgia in the Indicated Joint(s) is Shown with the Range Reflecting the Data Obtained from Several Studies

Joint	Percent with involvement
Wrist	36–100
Knee	39–100
Ankle	50–97
Interphalangeal (fingers)	50–81
Elbow	17–71
Cervical spine	12–70
Shoulder	38–62
Interphalangeal (thumb)	53–58
Thoracolumbar spine	36–56
Tarsus	36–49
Interphalangeal (toes)	47
"Hand" including metacarpophalangeal joints	45
Hip	4–27
Temporomandibular joint	10–15

Data from Harley D, Sleigh A, Ritchie S. Ross River virus transmission, infection, and disease: a cross-disciplinary review. Clin Microbiol Rev 2001;14:909–32, and papers cited therein.

PATIENT EVALUATION, DIAGNOSIS AND DIFFERENTIAL DIAGNOSIS

A detailed history is helpful, especially with regard to geographical location, season and mosquito exposure. Rapid onset of arthritic symptoms is usual, with pain on movement, tenderness and slight swelling (that can be hard to detect) the most common signs. Tenderness, swelling, heat, redness and intolerance to movement or pressure can be extreme. Rash usually occurs within a few days after the onset of symptoms and resolves within 5–10 days, but can persist or recur. Rash distribution varies considerably, with the trunk and limbs most affected. The face is less affected and, rarely, the rash may be confined to palms, soles and/or digital webs. Lymphadenopathy is frequently present, if sought. Aside from fatigue, constitutional symptoms usually resolve within a week [1, 8].

Diagnosis is usually made by a primary-care physician aided by a commercial serodiagnostic ELISA-based test (widely available in Australia). Paired serologic testing at least 10–14 days apart is recommended. Peripheral blood counts are usually normal except for a possible slight neutrophilia. An elevated erythrocyte sedimentation rate can occur, but decreases within a few weeks. Serum C reactive protein levels are rarely elevated. Erosive changes in x-rays are generally not seen [8].

The differential diagnoses at initial disease presentation include related Old World alphaviruses (e.g. chikungunya, Barmah Forest or Sindbis virus. [6]), dengue and Epstein-Barr virus. Other viral arthritides may also be considered, for example rubella or parvovirus B19 [5, 8]. Drug reactions, autoimmune arthritides (e.g. rheumatoid arthritis and systemic lupus erythematosis) and other infectious arthritides may also be among the differential diagnoses. Persistent distinct monoarticular arthritis is not consistent with RRV disease [8].

In patients diagnosed with RRV disease, but in whom symptoms last longer than 3–6 months, other differential diagnoses should be actively sought. In a survey of RRV disease patients, about half the patients reported disease lasting longer than six months. However, in nearly all these patients, other rheumatic conditions (primarily autoimmune) or depression were subsequently diagnosed [9]. There is no evidence that RRV disease predisposes to other rheumatic diseases [9], but it may contribute to post-infective depression or fatigue [11].

TREATMENT

RRV disease is generally treated with nonsteroidal anti-inflammatory drugs (NSAIDs), with most patients being satisfied with this treatment [9, 10]. Anecdotal experience suggests different NSAIDs may need to be tried [8]. Risk factors and contraindications for NSAID use should also be considered [12]. Aspirin and/or paracetamol are also used by some patients [9, 10]. Steroids are not generally recommended [13]. There is some observational evidence for rest and physical therapies. There is currently no commercially available vaccine and preventative measures include avoiding mosquito bites in endemic areas [7].

REFERENCES

1. Harley D, Sleigh A, Ritchie S. Ross River virus transmission, infection, and disease: a cross-disciplinary review. Clin Microbiol Rev 2001;14:909–32.
2. Johnston RE, Peters CJ. Alphaviruses. In: Fields BN, Knipe DM, Howley PM, eds. Fields Virology, 3rd edn. Philadelphia, PA: Lippincot-Raven; 1996:843–98.
3. Barber B, Denholm JT, Spelman D. Ross River virus. Aust Fam Physician 2009;38:586–9.
4. Communicable Diseases Network Australia. Available at: (http://www9.health.gov.au/cda/Source/Rpt_4_sel.cfm).
5. Suhrbier A, Mahalingam S. The immunobiology of viral arthritides. Pharmacol Ther 2009;124:301–8.
6. Suhrbier A, La Linn M. Clinical and pathologic aspects of arthritis due to Ross River virus and other alphaviruses. Curr Opin Rheumatol 2004;16:374–9.
7. Kistner O, Barrett N, Bruhmann A, et al. The preclinical testing of a formaldehyde inactivated Ross River virus vaccine designed for use in humans. Vaccine 2007;25:4845–52.
8. Fraser J, Marshall I. Epidemic polyarthritis handbook. Canberra: Department of Community Services and Health; 1989.
9. Mylonas AD, Brown AM, Carthew TL, et al. Natural history of Ross River virus-induced epidemic polyarthritis. Med J Aust 2002;177:356–60.
10. Harley D, Bossingham D, Purdie DM, et al. Ross River virus disease in tropical Queensland: evolution of rheumatic manifestations in an inception cohort followed for six months. Med J Aust 2002;177:352–5.
11. Hickie I, Davenport T, Wakefield D, et al. Post-infective and chronic fatigue syndromes precipitated by viral and non-viral pathogens: prospective cohort study. BMJ 2006;333:575.
12. Tielemans MM, Eikendal T, Jansen JB, van Oijen MG. Identification of NSAID users at risk for gastrointestinal complications: a systematic review of current guidelines and consensus agreements. Drug Safety 2010;33:443–53.
13. Mylonas AD, Harley D, Purdie DM, et al. Corticosteroid therapy in an alphaviral arthritis. J Clin Rheumatol 2004;10:326–30.

32.5 Oropouche Virus

Marcio RT Nunes, Pedro FC Vasconcelos

Key features

- The most prevalent arboviral disease in South America, after dengue fever
- Over 30 epidemics reported in the last three decades in the Brazilian Amazon region, Peru, Panama and Trinidad and Tobago, with an estimated occurrence of over 500,000 infections
- Clinical picture caused by Oropouche fever virus is an acute febrile disease with headache, chills, myalgia, nausea/vomiting, retro-ocular pain and dizziness
- Some patients develop aseptic meningitis and virus can be recovered from blood but also from cerebrospinal fluid. Four genotypes of Oropouche fever virus (I, II, III and IV) are recognized
- Urban cycle is responsible for outbreaks' transmission and is transmitted by the midge *Culicoides paraensis*
- Diagnosing of Oropouche fever virus is by IgM-ELISA, virus isolation and molecular biology techniques [mainly reverse transcription (RT)-PCR] and nucleotide sequencing
- There is no vaccine available to prevent Oropouche fever virus and personal protection is recommended during epidemics

INTRODUCTION

Oropouche virus (OROV), a member of the *Orthobunyavirus* genus in the *Bunyaviridae* family, is the causative agent of Oropouche fever [1, 2]. The first case of Oropouche fever was described in 1955, when the virus was isolated from the blood sample of a febrile patient in the West Indies and from a pool of *Coquillettidia venezuelensis* mosquitoes. A large epidemic was recorded in the 1960s in Belém, Brazil involving an estimated 11,000 people [1]. Over the past five decades, it is estimated that more than half a million people have been infected by the virus in the tropical areas of South and Central America, mainly in the Amazon region [3, 4].

EPIDEMIOLOGY

OROV has been found in Brazil, Panamá, Peru and Trinidad, and is basically maintained by two different lifecycles. One occurs in urban areas of tropical cities in the Amazon region and involves humans as the vertebrate hosts with *Culicoides paraensis* midges as the major vector. The other described lifecycle is sylvatic, involving wild mammals and birds as the vertebrate hosts. The arthropod vector in the sylvatic life cycle is unknown, but may include *C. paraensis* [1, 2].

Many outbreaks of Oropouche fever have been characterized by epidemics spreading in numerous villages within one geographic area and over a short period of time. The spread of the virus is probably a consequence of the circulation of viremic people in localities where the transmitting vector can be found and where there is a large concentration of susceptible individuals [4].

NATURAL HISTORY, PATHOGENESIS AND PATHOLOGY

Oropouche is a self-limiting febrile illness with no fatalities recorded. Using molecular typing methods, four different OROV genotypes have been described in the Americas [3–5]. Little is known about the pathogenesis of the Oropouche fever in humans—most of the information on pathogenesis has been obtained in golden hamsters. As in humans, the viremic period in these animals is brief and reaches titers high enough to easily infect *C. paraensis* midges [2]. In lethal infections in hamsters, an intense encephalitis is observed with a prominent hepatitis [1].

CLINICAL FEATURES

Clinical Oropouche fever is characterized by the sudden onset of high fever, headache, myalgia, arthralgia, anorexia, dizziness, chills and photophobia. Some patients present with a morbilliform exanthem that resembles rubella. Nausea, vomiting, diarrhea, conjuntival congestion, epigastric and retro-ocular pain, and other constitutional symptoms are also common [1]. Some patients may display a picture of aseptic meningitis. A recrudescence of mild symptoms several days after waning of the initial febrile episode is commonly seen (biphasic illness). Recovery is complete in all individuals without apparent sequelae, even in the most severe cases. There are no reports of proven lethality caused by Oropouche fever [2].

PATIENT EVALUATION, DIAGNOSIS AND DIFFERENTIAL DIAGNOSIS

The differential includes other causes of febrile illness, particularly dengue fever and malaria. Blood samples collected during the acute phase of illness (up to 5 days after the onset of the symptoms) can be used for virus detection methods. The most commonly applied molecular method is reverse transcription (RT)-PCR [3–5]. Virus isolation can be attempted in newborn mice (1–3 days), or in Vero or C6/36 cell cultures. For viral identification, suspensions prepared from brains of mice or supernatants of infected Vero or C6/36 cells are used as antigens in complement fixation or immunofluorescence assays with OROV hyperimmune serum. For specific identification of OROV, neutralization and hemagglutination inhibition tests can be also performed [2].

TREATMENT

Treatment is supportive.

REFERENCES

1. Pinheiro FP, Travassos da Rosa APA, Travasssos da Rosa JFS, et al. Oropouche virus. I. A review of clinical, epidemiological and ecological findings. Am J Trop Med Hyg 1981;30:149–60.
2. Pinheiro FP, Travassos da Rosa APA, Vasconcelos PFC. Oropouche fever. In: Feigin RD, ed. Textbook of Pediatric Infectious Diseases, 5th edn. Philadelphia: Saunders; 2004:2418–23.
3. Nunes MRT, Vasconcelos HB, Medeiros DBA, et al. A Febre do Oropouche: Uma Revisão dos Aspectos Epidemiológicos e Moleculares na Amazônia Brasileira. Cad Saúde Colet 2007;15:303–18 [in Portuguese].
4. Vasconcelos HB, Azevedo RSS, Nunes MRT, et al. Oropouche fever epidemic in Northern Brazil: Epidemiology and molecular characterization of isolates. J Clin Virol 2008;44:129–33.
5. Saeed MF, Wang H, Nunes MRT, et al. Nucleotide sequences and phylogeny of the nucleocapsid gene of Oropouche virus. J Gen Virol 2000;81:743–8.

32.6 Mayaro Virus

Pedro FC Vasconcelos, Marcio RT Nunes

Key features

- Mayaro fever virus is an alphavirus responsible for sporadic cases and several outbreaks of illness with fever, arthralgia and rash in northern South America
- Some infected patients develop severe arthralgia during the defervescence period that can last up to a year
- Two Mayaro fever virus genotypes are recognized
- Mayaro fever virus is transmitted by *Haemagogus* mosquitoes, particularly *Haemagogus janthinomys*
- The vertebrate hosts are nonhuman primates
- In the Brazilian Amazon, the specific antibody rate ranges from 5–60%; it is higher among closed communities (South America Indians) in the forests

INTRODUCTION

Mayaro virus is a single-stranded, positive-sense, arthropod-borne RNA virus in the family *Togaviridae*, genus *Alphavirus*. Typically, it causes Mayaro fever, an acute fever, arthralgia and rash syndrome [1]. It typically causes sporadic cases or small outbreaks in forest workers, but has caused a few larger epidemics, particularly in Brazil and nearby South American countries. The first isolation of Mayaro virus occurred in Trinidad in 1954 from the blood of febrile patients. Two major epidemics were described in the Brazilian Amazon region [2]; smaller epidemics have been recognized since then in other parts of Brazil and in Santa Cruz, Bolivia [3, 4]. Mayaro virus is maintained in nature in a cycle involving mammals, birds and arhropods. New World nonhuman primates and marmosets have been implicated as natural hosts [5]. The virus has been isolated several times from *Haemagogus* spp. mosquitoes, mainly from *Haemagogus janthinomys* species, which is considered the primary potential vector. There are two distinct genotypes of virus. In addition, a unique strain of Mayaro virus has been recovered from *Coquillettidia venezuelensis* in Trinidad, two others from *Sabethes* spp. and one from *Culex* spp.

EPIDEMIOLOGY

Mayaro virus has been isolated from patient residents in tropical areas of Central and South America, mainly in Brazil, Trinidad, Bolivia and Surinam. The virus has also been isolated in French Guiana, Colombia, Panama and Peru. Detection of antibodies to the virus has been also demonstrated in certain populations of these countries, as well as in Guyana, Colombia and Peru [2]. Most cases occur in forest workers, who are typically adult males. In the Brazilian Amazon, the specific antibody rate ranges from 5–60%; it is higher among closed communities (South American Indians).

Only a few major Mayaro fever epidemics have been reported in the Americas: two in Brazil, one in Bolivia and one in Peru [2, 6]. Between 1955 and 1991, epidemics of Mayaro fever were restricted to Brazil, beginning in the municipality of Guamá, Pará state (1955), spreading toward to other localities in the São Miguel do Pará state, such as Belterra (1978), Conceição do Araguaia (1981), Itaruma in Goias state, Central region of Brazil (1981), Benevides, Pará state (1991) and Peixe, Tocantins state (1991). In the following years, the agent reached other Peruvian Amazon counties (Tumbes, Aucayacu and Huanuco in 1995) [6]. In 2008, the virus re-emerged in Pará state causing an outbreak in the Municipality of Santa Bárbara, Pará State, 50 km from Belém in northern Brazil [4].

NATURAL HISTORY, PATHOGENESIS AND PATHOLOGY

Little is known about the pathogenesis of Mayaro fever in humans, as the virus has not been associated with deaths. Thus, no material is available for histopathologic examination [1]. The data regarding its pathogenesis are a result of experimental *in vitro* studies using Vero cell cultures. These have indicated intense cytopathic effects and cell death with casein kinase 2 (CK2) having an important role during the Mayaro virus infection cycle [7].

CLINICAL FEATURES

Mayaro fever is clinically characterized as an acute febrile illness, generally accompanied by headache, myalgia, chills and photophobia. Dizziness, eye pain, nausea and vomiting are less frequently reported. Arthralgia, predominantly affecting the wrists, fingers, ankles and toes, as well as a cutaneous rash are also commonly observed [2, 3]. Occasionally, there may also be painful joint swelling that may persist. In some patients, arthralgia lasts up to a year.

PATIENT EVALUATION, DIAGNOSIS AND DIFFERENTIAL DIAGNOSIS

Leukopenia is a common finding in unspecific laboratory tests within the first week of illness, and a white cell count of about 2500/mm^3 is observed; platelet counts and liver function tests are usually normal. The differential diagnosis includes other causes of fever, arthralgia and rash, particularly dengue. The laboratory diagnosis of Mayaro fever either depends on virus isolation attempts and serologic diagnostic and molecular methods for genome detection. For virus isolation, biologic samples (serum or blood) obtained from viremic patients (up to 5 days after the onset of the symptoms) are used for inoculation in newborn mice or in Vero cells. Suspensions prepared from brains of mice or supernatants of infected cells are used as antigens in either complement fixation tests or an immunofluorescence assay against hyperimmune sera of different arboviruses circulating in the region. Specific identification of Mayaro virus is carried out using neutralization and hemagglutination inhibition tests [1] and by reverse transcription (RT)-PCR [3, 4].

TREATMENT AND PREVENTION

Treatment is supportive. Some patients require hospitalization but no deaths have been reported. In theory, personal protection against mosquito bites (insect repellent and long sleeves and trousers) should be protective, but this is not practical for most forest workers. Bed nets and window screens are of little benefit because *Haemagogus* mosquitoes are day-biters.

REFERENCES

1. Pinheiro FP, LeDuc JW. Mayaro vírus disease. In: Monath TP, ed. The Arboviruses—Epidemiology and Ecology, Vol. III. Boca Raton: CRC Press; 1986:137–50.
2. Pinheiro FP, Freitas RB, Travassos da Rosa JFS, et al. An outbreak of Mayaro virus disease in Belterra, Brazil. I. Clinical and virological findings. Am J Trop Med Hyg 1981;30:674–81.
3. Powers AM, Aguilar PV, Chandler LJ, et al. Genetic relationships among Mayaro and Una viruses suggest distinct patterns of transmission. Am J Trop Med Hyg 2006;75:461–9.
4. Azevedo RSS, Nunes MRT, Silva EPV, et al. Mayaro fever virus outbreak, Santa Barbara, Pará State, Brazilian Amazon. Emerg Infect Dis 2009;15:1830–2.
5. Watts DM, Ramirez G, Cabezas C, et al. Arthropod-borne viral diseases in Peru. In: Travassos da Rosa APA, Vasconcelos PFC, Travassos da Rosa JFS, eds. An overview of arbovirology in Brazil and neighbouring countries. Belem: Instituto Evandro Chagas; 1998:193–218.
6. Woodall JP. Virus research in Amzônia. In: Lent H, ed. Atas Simpósio Biota Amazônica, Vol. 6. Rio de Janeiro: Conselho Nacional de Pesquisas; 1967: 31–63.
7. Barroso MMS, Lima CS, Silva-Neto MAC, Da Poian AT. Mayaro virus infection cycle relies on casein kinase 2 activity. Biochem Biophys Res Comm 2002;5:1334–9.

32.7 Sandfly Fever

Remi N Charrel, Xavier de Lamballerie

Key features

- Phlebovirus infections are transmitted by sandflies
- Synonyms: pappataci fever, phlebotomus fever or 3-day fever
- High seroprevalence rates indicate that the majority of cases are unrecognized, possibly owing to asymptomatic or mild disease
- Clinical disease generally manifests as an undifferentiated systemic febrile illness
- One phlebovirus, Toscana virus, is neurotropic and may cause meningitis, encephalitis and peripheral neuropathy
- All countries where *Phlebotomus perniciosus*, *Phlebotomus perfiliewi* and *Phlebotomus papatasi* are present (Mediterranean basin and beyond) are at risk for sandfly-transmitted phlebovirus infections

INTRODUCTION

The viral etiology of the nonspecific febrile illness, sandfly fever, was recognized during World War II in Allied troops affected after landing in Southern Italy [1]. Within the group of sandfly-transmitted phleboviruses, three Old World viruses are recognized as etiologic agents of symptomatic human infections: Sicilian, Naples and Toscana viruses; the latter two belonging to sandfly fever Naples virus (SFNV), whilst the former belongs to the genetically and antigenically distinct sandfly fever Sicilian viruses (SFSV). Toscana virus is the only one of these viruses known to cause central nervous system (CNS) manifestations [2, 3] and data from Italy, France and Spain indicate that it is among the three leading causes of aseptic meningitis during periods of sandfly activity [4]. The other viruses are associated with systemic febrile illnesses but not CNS infections.

Chagres and Punta Toro viruses ("new world phleboviruses") have been isolated in Panama from the sandflies *Lutzomyia trapidoi* and *Lutzomyia ylephilator*. Candiru and Alenquer viruses have been isolated in Brazil. *Lutzomyia tarpidoi* is a highly anthropophilic species. The seroprevalence of antibodies to Chagres and Punta Toro viruses in residents of Panama has been reported to be as high as 17% and 35% respectively. However, only sporadic cases of illness have been recognized in this region.

EPIDEMIOLOGY

Phlebotomine flies are present in most of the countries surrounding the Mediterranean and extend towards the east (Fig. 32.7.1). For countries where clinical and epidemiologic studies were conducted, the imbalance between high seroprevalence rates and low numbers of clinical cases suggests that the majority of infections produce mild or asymptomatic disease, or are not diagnosed when they cause severe disease [5].

Phlebotomine flies are active during the warm season (April–October in the Mediterranean basin). Only the adult females bite: they are small (2–3 mm) and readily pass through bed nets and screens intended to protect from mosquitoes. Sandfly fever viruses are transmitted in transovarial and transstadial fashion in their vector species. In some endemic areas, high rates of virus-infected sandflies are common (1 : 100–1 : 200) with equal numbers of males and females. Traditionally, *Phlebotomus papatasi* is the principal vector of Naples and Sicilian virus, and *Phlebotomus perniciosus* and *Phlebotomus perfiliewi* are the chief vectors of Toscana virus. Most recently, Sicilian-like viruses were detected in sandflies other than *P. papatasi*, such as *P. perniciosus* and *Phlebotomus longicuspis*. Investigations to identify a vertebrate reservoir have so far failed but need to be pursued.

NATURAL HISTORY, PATHOGENESIS AND PATHOLOGY

There are currently less than 50 articles referenced in PubMed corresponding to clinical cases of Toscana virus infections and other sandfly transmitted phlebovirus infections. Therefore, clinicians are often unaware of sandfly-transmitted phleboviruses as a possible cause of febrile illness, with or without CNS symptoms—at least in the Old World. As cases are rarely fatal, there is little information about pathogenesis or pathology. The quality of clinical specimens and timing of sampling is of great importance for diagnosis as the duration of viremia is short (less than a week) and the viral load in cerebrospinal fluid (CSF) is modest.

CLINICAL FEATURES

Current clinical knowledge is based on the description of case reports or small series, and likely does not represent the entire spectrum of syndromes caused by these viruses.

Sandfly fever is a typical arboviral fever, presenting with high fever, headache, muscle and joint aches. This may be preceded by generalized fatigue, abdominal pain and chills. There may also be facial flushing and tachycardia. Rarely, bradycardia and hypotension may follow, but all patients make a complete recovery.

In Toscana virus infection, after an incubation period ranging from a few days to 2 weeks, disease onset is abrupt with headache, fever, nausea and vomiting in most patients; some also have myalgia [2, 3]. Physical examination may show Kernig's sign and neck rigidity in the majority, with depressed levels of consciousness in about 10% and, rarely, nystagmus, tremors and paresis. CSF analysis usually demonstrates a mild pleocytosis (>5–10 cells) with normal glucose and protein levels. Blood samples may show leukocytosis or, less commonly, leukopenia. The mean duration of the disease is 7 days and the outcome is usually favorable. However, a small number of severe cases have been reported in the literature. To date, there is no published data to suggest that Toscana virus causes other clinical manifestations.

PATIENT EVALUATION, DIAGNOSIS AND DIFFERENTIAL DIAGNOSIS

The lack of knowledge about infections caused by sandfly-transmitted phleboviruses is largely because of a lack of diagnostic means and laboratory detection.

Serodiagnosis is performed using either indirect immunofluorescence or ELISA assays looking for seroconversion and detection of IgG and IgM. There is almost no antigenic cross-reactivity between viruses within the SFNV group and those within the SFSV group. Ultimate serologic confirmation of specific virus infection relies on neutralizing antibody assays, but only a handful of laboratories perform these techniques. Virus isolation from either CSF or blood can be achieved

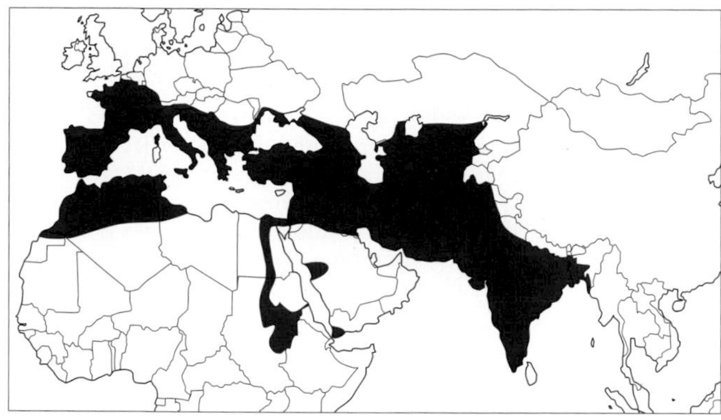

FIGURE 32.7.1 Distribution of sandflies in the Old World.

through inoculation onto mammalian Vero, BHK-21 or CV-1 cells. Molecular techniques, mostly real-time reverse transcription (RT)-PCR assays, are now the technique of choice for diagnostics [6, 7]. Interestingly, during the three last decades, no human case of Naples virus has been reported, suggesting that this virus may have become extinct for unknown reasons.

Recent years have witnessed the discovery of novel sandfly-transmitted phleboviruses through studies conducted in previously unexplored geographic areas, such as Algeria, Tunisia and Turkey [8–11]. Their role in human disease remains unknown.

TREATMENT

Treatment is largely supportive. There are no specific antiviral treatments or vaccines for these infections. There has been little research into prevention, but control of sandfly proliferation in areas where people are highly exposed has been suggested and personal protective measures against sandfly bites in areas known to be affected is advised.

REFERENCES

1. Hertig M, Sabin AB. Sand fly fever. In: Preventive Medicine in World War II, Vol. VII. Washington: Office of the Surgeon General, Department of the Army; 1964:109–74.
2. Braito A, Corbisiero R, Corradini S, et al. Toscana virus infections of the central nervous system in children: A report of 14 cases. J Pediatr 1998; 132:144–8.
3. Cusi MG, Savellini GG, Zanelli G. Toscana virus epidemiology: from Italy to beyond. Open Virol J 2010;4:22–8.
4. Charrel RN, Gallian P, Navarro-Mari JM, et al. Emergence of Toscana virus in Europe. Emerg Infect Dis 2005;11:1657–63.
5. De Lamballerie X, Tolou H, Durand JP, et al. Prevalence of Toscana virus antibodies in volunteer blood donors and patients with central nervous system infections in southeastern France. Vector Borne Zoonotic Dis 2007;7:275–7.
6. Pérez-Ruiz M, Collao X, Navarro-Marí JM, et al. Reverse transcription, real-time PCR assay for detection of Toscana virus. J Clin Virol 2007;39:276–81.
7. Weidmann M, Sanchez-Seco MP, Sall AA, et al. Rapid detection of important human pathogenic phleboviruses. J Clin Virol 2008;41:138–42.
8. Moureau G, Bichaud L, Salez N, et al. Molecular and serological evidence for the presence of novel phleboviruses in sandflies from northern Algeria. Open Virol J 2010;4:15–21.
9. Collao X, Palacios G, de Ory F, et al. Granada virus: a natural phlebovirus reassortant of the sandfly fever Naples serocomplex with low seroprevalence in humans. Am J Trop Med Hyg 2010;83:760–5.
10. Charrel RN, Moureau G, Temmam S, et al. Massilia virus, a novel Phlebovirus (Bunyaviridae) isolated from sandflies in the Mediterranean. Vector Borne Zoonotic Dis 2009;9:519–30.
11. Papa A, Velo E, Bino S. A novel phlebovirus in Albanian sandflies. Clin Microbiol Infect 2011;17:585–7.

32.8 Sindbis Fever

Gregory Deye

Key features

- Self-limited febrile illness with rash and polyarthropathy
- Arthritis may persist for longer than 12 months
- Broad geographic range

INTRODUCTION

Sindbis virus is an alphavirus within the Western Equine Encephalitis Virus complex. Like other alphaviruses, it has a single-stranded, positive-sense genome contained within a small, enveloped virion. The virus was first isolated in 1952 from *Culex univittatus* mosquitoes trapped in the Sindbis district of Egypt. Although seroprevalence surveys had previously suggested human infections occur, Sindbis virus was first identified as a human pathogen when it was isolated from febrile patients in Uganda in 1961. An epidemic in South Africa in 1974 caused hundreds of cases. During the 1980s, Ockelbo disease (Sweden), Karelian fever (Russia) and Pogosta disease (Finland), which have nearly identical clinical presentations were shown to be caused by Sindbis virus infection. Although Sindbis virus antigenic variations have been described in Australia, Europe and Africa, these have not been correlated with clinical differences.

EPIDEMIOLOGY

The virus is typically transmitted in an avian–mosquito cycle with the participation of various *Culex* species as the principal vector in different locations. *Aedes cinereus* and *Aedes communis* may function as bridging vectors from infected birds to humans. Numerous passerine avian species have been shown to be effective viral amplifiers.

Sindbis fever is principally recognized in Africa, the Middle East and Northern Europe, but sporadic cases and viral isolates have been reported from Australia and Asia. In South Africa and Europe, disease incidence tends to be clustered in discrete outbreaks occurring on a background of sporadic endemic cases. The seasonality of cases mirrors changes in local *Culex* mosquito populations. Cases in Scandanvia generally occur from July to September, whereas outbreaks in South Africa have occurred during the austral summer from December to April. Sindbis fever outbreaks occasionally occur in conjunction with outbreaks of West Nile Virus infection as they share the same *Culex* mosquito vectors.

Although Sindbis virus is the most widely distributed mosquito-borne virus collected in Australia and New Guinea, human cases in these areas are rarely recognized.

Seroprevelance rates vary dramatically within endemic areas, ranging from 9–17% in Finland [1] and up to 23% in endemic areas of South Africa. Age distribution has been reported in Sweden, with an incidence greatest between the fourth and seventh decades of life, and a similar incidence for males and females [2].

CLINICAL FEATURES

The incubation period is around 8–9 days. The majority of infections result in asymptomatic or subclinical infection, with approximately 6% of cases manifesting clinical symptoms [3]. Disease manifestations primarily consist of fever, rash and polyarthropathy, although malaise, headache, myalgia, conjunctivitis and pharyngitis have also been described. Fever is present in about half of cases and typically has a sudden onset and persists for less than 2 days [4].

A maculopapular rash occurs in the majority of cases, usually beginning within days after the onset of fever. The rash is occasionally pruritic and may vesiculate. The trunk and lower extremities are most frequently involved, although distribution can include all four extremities, including palms and soles; the face is usually spared. The rash may perisist for more than 5 days.

Symmetric oligoarthropathy is nearly universally present with or without joint effusions. The joints most commonly involved include ankles, knees, fingers and wrists, with less frequent involvement of hips, shoulders, neck and back. Joint symptoms are typically present during the acute illness and can persist often as long as 3 years, and may cause a significant degree of disability [5].

PATIENT EVALUATION, DIAGNOSIS AND DIFFERENTIAL DIAGNOSIS

Clinical presentation can be difficult to distinguish from infection with other arboviruses, particularly those that cause fever, arthralgia and rash, such as dengue, chikungunya and Ross River virus; however, the importance of these various viruses differs according to the geographical location. Reactive arthritis should also be considered.

Virus can be amplified by reverse transcription (RT)-PCR from whole blood or skin biopsy from only a minority of patients, even when samples are obtained within the acute illness. Diagnosis is typically based on serologic confirmation. Elevation of specific IgM is typically detectable within 1 week of symptom onset and persists for up to 6 months. IgG is generally elevated 8–9 days after symptom onset and is persistent.

TREATMENT

There are no specific therapies. Symptomatic therapy with nonsteroidal anti-inflammatory drugs (NSAIDs) and rest may provide some relief, although effectiveness may vary in individuals. Preventative measures include avoidance of the bites of *Culex* mosquitoes.

REFERENCES

1. Laine M, Vainionpää R, Oksi J, et al. The prevalence of antibodies against Sindbis-related (Pogosta) virus in different parts of Finland. Rheumatology (Oxford) 2003;42:632–6.
2. Lundstrom JO, Vene S, Espmark A, et al. Geographical and temporal distribution of Ockelbo disease in Sweden. Epidemiol Infect 1991;106:567–74.
3. Brummer-Korvenkontio M, Vapalahti O, Kuusisto P, et al. Epidemiology of Sindbis virus infections in Finland 1981–96: possible factors explaining a peculiar disease pattern. Epidemiol Infect 2002;129:335–45.
4. Kurkela S, Manni T, Myllynen J, et al. Clinical and laboratory manifestations of Sindbis virus infection: prospective study, Finland, 2002–2003. J Infect Dis 2005;191:1820–9.
5. Kurkela S, Helve T, Vaheri A, Vapalahti O. Arthritis and arthralgia three years after Sindbis virus infection: clinical follow-up of a cohort of 49 patients. Scand J Infect Dis 2008;40:167–73.

Viral Hemorrhagic Fevers 33

33.1 Yellow Fever

J Erin Staples, Marc Fischer

Key features

- Yellow fever is a mosquito-borne viral disease
- Yellow fever virus is endemic to sub-Saharan Africa and tropical South America and is estimated to cause 200,000 disease cases and 30,000 deaths annually
- Yellow fever can result in jaundice and hemorrhagic manifestations and is fatal in 20–50% of persons with severe disease
- Because no treatment exists for yellow fever, prevention through vaccination and the use of personal protective measures is critical to lower disease risk and mortality

INTRODUCTION

Yellow fever virus (YFV), a mosquito-borne flavivirus, is present in tropical areas of Africa and South America (Figure 33.1.1). In humans, the majority of YFV infections are asymptomatic. Clinical disease varies from a mild, undifferentiated febrile illness to severe disease with jaundice and hemorrhage. Because no specific antiviral treatment exists for yellow fever, prevention is critical to lower disease risk and mortality.

EPIDEMIOLOGY

The World Health Organization (WHO) estimates that YFV causes 200,000 cases of clinical disease and 30,000 deaths each year. However, the majority of cases and deaths are not recognized because of the predominantly rural nature of the disease and inadequate surveillance and reporting. Over the past few decades, hundreds of cases have been reported annually in South America, primarily among men with occupational exposures in forested areas. In Africa, the number of cases reported annually varies substantially (range: 1–5000 cases) and is likely attributable to variations in recognition and reporting. The natural occurrence of disease can also fluctuate, being absent in certain areas for years before re-appearing. Delineation of affected areas depends on surveillance for animal reservoirs and vectors, accurate diagnosis and prompt reporting of all human cases [1].

NATURAL HISTORY, PATHOGENESIS, AND PATHOLOGY

YFV is a positive-sense RNA virus that belongs to the genus *Flavivirus* (Family *Flaviviridae*). It is antigenically related to West Nile, St Louis encephalitis and Japanese encephalitis viruses. YFV has three transmission cycles: jungle, savannah and urban [2]. The jungle cycle involves transmission of the virus between nonhuman primates and tree-hole-breeding mosquito species (i.e. *Aedes* or *Haemagogus* spp.) found in the forest canopy. The virus is transmitted via mosquitoes from monkeys to humans when they encroach into the jungle during occupational or recreational activities. In Africa, a savannah cycle involves transmission of the virus from tree-hole-breeding *Aedes* spp. to humans living or working in jungle border areas. In this cycle, mosquitoes may also transmit the virus between humans. The urban cycle involves transmission of the virus between humans and urban mosquitoes, primarily *Aedes aegypti*. Humans infected with YFV experience the highest levels of viremia and are infectious to mosquitoes shortly before the onset of fever and for 3–5 days thereafter. Direct person-to-person transmission of YFV has not been documented, but might theoretically occur through blood transfusion, organ transplantation, intrauterine transmission or breastfeeding.

CLINICAL FEATURES

The majority of people infected with YFV remain asymptomatic. For those with clinical disease, the incubation period is usually 3–6 days. In its mildest form, yellow fever is a self-limited infection characterized by acute onset of fever and headache. A subset of patients experience other symptoms, including chills, myalgias, lumbosacral pain, anorexia, nausea, vomiting and dizziness [3]. Physical examination may demonstrate relative bradycardia in relation to elevated body temperature (Faget's sign). The patient is usually viremic during this period, which lasts for approximately 3 days. Most have an uneventful recovery but, in approximately 15% of cases, the illness recurs in a more severe form within 48 hours following the viremic period. Symptoms include fever, vomiting, epigastric pain, jaundice, renal insufficiency and cardiovascular instability. The virus is generally absent from the blood during this phase of symptom recrudescence. A bleeding diathesis with hematemesis, melena, metrorrhagia, hematuria, petechiae, ecchymoses and epistaxis. Physical findings include scleral and dermal icterus, hemorrhages and epigastric tenderness without hepatic enlargement.

PATIENT EVALUATION, DIAGNOSIS AND DIFFERENTIAL DIAGNOSIS

Laboratory findings in patients with yellow fever vary based on the severity and stage of illness. In the first week, leukopenia may occur; however, during the second week there may be leukocytosis. Hyperbilirubinemia may be present as early as the third day but usually peaks towards the end of the first week of illness. Elevations of serum transaminase levels occur in severe hepatorenal disease and may remain elevated for up to 2 months after onset. Patients with

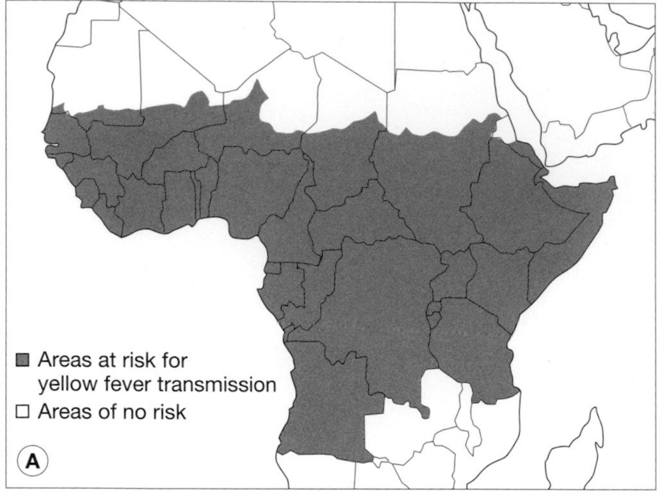

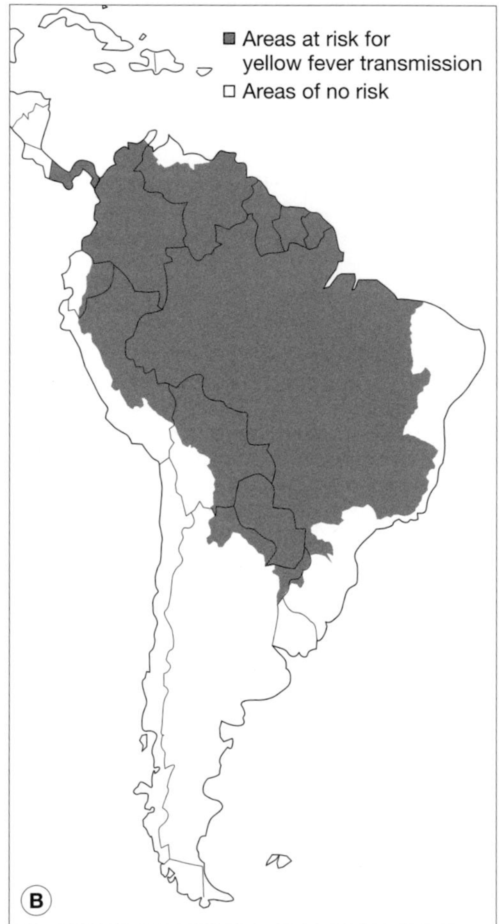

FIGURE 33.1.1 Areas at risk for yellow fever transmission—Africa **(A)** and South America **(B)**, 2009.

hemorrhagic manifestations often have elevated prothrombin and partial thromboplastin times, decreased platelet counts and fibrinogen, and presence of fibrin-split products.

Laboratory diagnosis is generally accomplished by testing serum for virus-specific IgM and IgG antibodies. Serologic cross-reactions occur with other flaviviruses (e.g. West Nile or dengue viruses), so positive results should be confirmed with a more specific test (e.g. plaque-reduction neutralization test). During the first 3–4 days of illness, the virus may be detectable in the serum by isolation or reverse transcription (RT)-PCR. However, by the time a diagnosis of yellow fever is considered, the virus or viral RNA usually is undetectable. Therefore, virus isolation and RT-PCR should not be used for excluding the diagnosis of yellow fever. Immunohistochemical staining of formalin-fixed material can detect YFV antigen in pathologic specimens. Healthcare providers should contact their state or local health department or national laboratories for assistance with diagnostic testing for YFV infections.

Preliminary diagnosis is based on the patient's clinical features, yellow fever vaccination status and travel history, including location, time of year and activities [1]. Mild yellow fever cannot be clinically distinguished from a range of other infections. Cases of yellow fever with jaundice must be differentiated from viral hepatitis, malaria, leptospirosis, Congo–Crimean hemorrhagic fever, Rift Valley fever, typhoid, Q fever and typhus, as well as drug-induced and toxic causes of jaundice. Other viral hemorrhagic fevers, which usually present without jaundice, include: dengue hemorrhagic fever; Lassa fever; Marburg and Ebola virus diseases; and Bolivian, Argentinean and Venezuelan hemorrhagic fevers.

TREATMENT AND PREVENTION

Although multiple drugs have been evaluated or empirically used for yellow fever, none has shown specific benefit [4]. Management is supportive and based on symptoms and the organ systems involved. Rest, fluids and nonsteroidal anti-inflammatory drugs (NSAIDs) or acetaminophen can relieve milder symptoms of fever and myalgias. Aspirin should be avoided because of the risk for hemorrhagic complications.

Because no treatment exists, prevention through use of personal protective measures and vaccination is critical to lower disease risk and mortality. Mosquito prevention measures that may lower the risk for yellow fever and other vector-borne infectious diseases include using insect repellent, wearing permethrin-impregnated clothing and staying in accommodation with screened or air-conditioned rooms.

A live-attenuated yellow fever vaccine is recommended for those ≥9 months of age who are traveling to, or living in, areas of South America and Africa with a risk of YFV transmission. International Health Regulations allow some countries to require proof of yellow fever vaccination (at least 10 days earlier) as a condition of entry for travelers arriving from certain countries to prevent importation and indigenous transmission of YFV. The yellow fever vaccination certificate for international travel is valid for 10 years.

The most common adverse events reported following vaccination include fever, headache, myalgias and injection site reactions [5]. Rare, but serious, adverse events following vaccine administration include immediate hypersensitivity or anaphylactic reactions, yellow fever vaccine-associated neurologic disease and yellow fever vaccine-associated viscerotropic disease [1]. To minimize the risk for serious adverse events, healthcare providers should vaccinate only persons who are at risk for exposure to YFV or who require proof of vaccination for country entry, and observe the contraindications and consider the precautions before administering yellow fever vaccine.

REFERENCES

1. Centers for Disease Control and Prevention. Yellow fever vaccine: Recommendations of the Advisory Committee on Immunization Practices (ACIP). MMWR 2010;59:1–27.
2. Barrett AD, Monath TP. Epidemiology and ecology of yellow fever virus. Adv Virus Res 2003;61:291–315.
3. Tuboi SH, Costa ZGA, Vasconcelos PFC, Hatch D. Clinical and epidemiological characteristics of yellow fever in Brazil: analysis of reported cases 1998–2002. Trans Roy Soc Trop Med Hyg 2007;101:169–75.
4. Monath TP. Treatment of yellow fever. Antiviral Res 2008;78:116–24.
5. Monath T, Cetron MS, Teuwen DE. Yellow fever vaccine. In: Plotkin SA, Orenstein WA, Offit PA, eds. Vaccines, 5th edn. Philadelphia: Saunders Elsevier; 2008:959–1055.

33.2 Lassa Fever

Aulasa J Camerlin, Joseph B McCormick

Key features

- Lassa virus causes Lassa fever, a hemorrhagic disease characterized by fever, generalized weakness, muscle pain, nausea and vomiting with mucosal bleeding
- Fatality occurs in about 15–30% of hospitalized patients; fatality is associated with endothelial dysfunction leading to intractable hypovolemic shock, gross edema of the head and neck with pulmonary edema, and respiratory distress
- Lassa fever is endemic to West Africa through persistent infection of *Mastomys natalensis*, a peridomestic rodent
- Transmission occurs via direct contact with infected rodents or their secretions, or by close person-to-person contact causing nosocomial spread
- An estimated 300,000–500,000 cases occur annually in West Africa with approximately 5000 deaths per year
- The disease can be successfully treated, particularly within the first week of illness, by the antiviral drug ribavirin
- Synonyms: Lassa virus, Lassa fever

INTRODUCTION

Lassa virus, a member of the genus *Arenavirus* (family *Arenaviridae*), is the etiologic agent of the hemorrhagic disease Lassa fever. The virus is naturally maintained by peridomestic rodent hosts in which persistent, lifelong infection is established. High titers of the virus are present in rodent urine and exposed humans may become infected as accidental hosts. The virus may be transmitted from person-to-person. Lassa fever is endemic to West Africa, but, occasionally, cases occur in non-endemic areas among returning travelers. An estimated 300,000–500,000 cases occur annually, resulting in approximately 5000 deaths per year. Although Lassa fever was first described in West Africa in the 1950s, the virus was not isolated until 1969 [1–4].

EPIDEMIOLOGY

Seroconversion to Lassa virus ranges from 5–22% annually among susceptible (seronegative) populations in endemic areas. Among seroconverters, 9–26% develop acute illness. Between 1 and 18 percent are re-infections. Estimates of prevalence of antibody to Lassa virus range from 4–52% among populations in endemic areas. Viruses from different geographic areas may vary in virulence. Case fatality rate among the general population can be as low as 1–2%; however, rates increase among hospitalized patients (15 to 30%). At least 20 imported cases of Lassa fever have been seen in the USA, the UK, Germany, the Netherlands, Israel, Japan and Canada [5].

Lassa virus affects people of all ages, races and gender. However, the only confirmed reservoir of Lassa virus is *Mastomys natalensis*; the disease is endemic to West Africa. Transmission is suspected to occur through direct contact with infected rodents or their secretions. Transmission is highly associated with indiscriminate food storage and catching of rodents. Person-to-person transmission occurs via direct contact with fluid or secretions from infected persons including blood, urine, sputum and seminal fluid on exposed cuts or abrasions, or mucous membranes. Nosocomial transmission is usually caused by injuries with needles and other sharp instruments, ill-advised surgery on infected patients or exposure to bodily fluids [1–4, 6, 7].

Symptoms of Lassa fever include: fever; sore throat; cough; vomiting; diarrhea; conjunctivitis; facial swelling; proteinuria; mucosal bleeding; and pain in the back, abdomen and chest. Neurologic symptoms include loss of hearing, tremors and encephalitis.

NATURAL HISTORY, PATHOGENESIS AND PATHOLOGY

Fatal Lassa fever is directly associated with uncontrolled viral replication and severe intravascular events, including leaky capillary syndrome, pulmonary edema and hypovolemic shock. In general, high titers of replicating virus in all organs are associated with fatality, whereas a rapid drop in viremia and viral clearance is correlated with survival. There is apparently suppressed cellular immune response in fatalities, whereas recovery from Lassa fever is associated with strong adaptive immune responses characterized by a high number of activated circulating monocytes and T cells, as well as Lassa virus-specific $CD4^+$ and $CD8^+$ T cells [1–4, 8, 9].

The critical events in fatal disease are: intractable hypovolemic shock; convulsions; bleeding; and gross edema of the head and neck with pulmonary edema and respiratory distress. Respiratory distress and/or convulsions with precipitous drop in body temperature and blood pressure indicate impeding death. Some of these manifestations are caused by disturbances in the intravascular compartment, particularly increased endothelial cell permeability. Disseminated intravascular coagulation is not a significant component of fatal Lassa fever. No clear evidence of virus replication and microscopic damage to endothelium has been demonstrated. An inhibitor of platelet function has been identified in the serum of patients and nonhuman primates with severe Lassa fever, suggesting that the underlying pathology in fatal infections is a disordered cytokine and chemokine response, as has been shown in Ebola and other fatal viral infections [1–4, 9, 10].

Lassa virus-specific IgM antibodies are detected 9–12 days post-infection; IgG antibodies are seen 12–16 days post-infection. However, antibody titers are not directly associated with viral clearance. Neutralizing antibodies are detected only after recovery and do not appear to be associated with immunity to reinfection [1–4].

CLINICAL FEATURES

Following an incubation period of 7–18 days, Lassa fever insidiously begins with fever, weakness and malaise. More than 50% of patients experience joint and lumbar pain, and 60% or more have a nonproductive cough. Most patients also have severe headache, usually frontal, and a painful sore throat. Many also develop severe retrosternal chest pain and about half have vomiting or diarrhea and abdominal pain. On physical examination, respiratory rate, temperature and pulse rate are elevated and blood pressure may be low. About a third have conjunctivitis and more than two thirds have pharyngitis, half of whom have exudates with diffusely inflamed and swollen posterior pharynx and tonsils but with few, if any, petechiae [1–4].

Up to a third of hospitalized patients progress to a prostrating illness 6–8 days after onset of fever. They are often dehydrated on admission, with elevated hematocrit. Bleeding occurs in only 15–20% of patients, limited primarily to the mucosal surfaces or, occasionally, conjunctival hemorrhages or gastrointestinal or vaginal bleeding. Edema of the face and neck occurs in severe disease and carries a poor prognosis—this may indicate capillary leakage, rather than cardiac dysfunction or impaired venous return. Approximately half of all patients have diffuse abdominal tenderness, but there are no localizing signs and bowel sounds are usually active. On more than one occasion, surgery has been performed which is contraindicated. Proteinuria occurs in two thirds of patients and blood urea nitrogen levels may be moderately elevated [1–4].

Crepitations in the lungs, and pleural and pericardial rubs usually develop in early convalescence in about 20% of patients, occasionally in association with congestive heart failure. Severe retrosternal or epigastric pain seen in many patients may be caused by pleural or pericardial involvement. Most patients have abnormal electrocardiographies (ECGs) and changes include nonspecific ST-segment and T-wave abnormalities, ST-segment elevation, generalized low-voltage complexes and changes reflecting electrolyte disturbance. None of these abnormalities correlate with clinical severity of disease, serum aminotransferase levels or eventual outcome. Neurologic signs are infrequent but also carry a poor prognosis, progressing from fine tremors and confusion to severe encephalopathy with, or without, generalized seizures but without focal signs. The cerebrospinal fluid (CSF) is usually normal, but there may be a few lymphocytes. Virus titers are lower in the CSF than in the serum. The most significant hematologic changes are in platelet function. Thrombocytopenia is moderate, even in severely ill patients, and function is markedly depressed, or even absent. This abnormality is usually maximal on admission to the hospital and is characteristically present, even when circulating platelet numbers remain normal. A circulating inhibitor of platelet function has been associated with severe disease. The mean white blood cell count in Lassa fever on admission to hospital is $6000/mm^3$ and there is characteristically early lymphopenia, relative thrombocytopenia and sometimes a relative, or absolute, neutrophilia. Neutrophil counts as high as $30{,}000/mm^3$ have been recorded in severe disease [1–4, 11, 12].

Serum aminotransferase levels >150 IU/L on admission are associated with a case-fatality rate of 50%. The level of viremia [blood virus level >1 X 10^3 mL, median tissue culture infective dose ($TCID_{50}$) per milliliter] is also associated with increased case fatality. The synergistic effect of both factors is a mortality risk of 80%. Other indicators of poor prognosis include: shock; bleeding; neurologic manifestations; thrombocytopenia; lymphopenia; and leukocytosis with neutrophilia [1–4].

Lassa fever is a common cause of maternal mortality in many areas of West Africa. In Sierra Leone, Lassa virus accounts for 25% of all maternal deaths. Case fatality rates in pregnancy are as high as 40%, with the worst prognosis occurring in the third trimester. This is true even for women who receive adequate obstetric care. Prognosis for the mother improves with uterine evacuation at any stage of gestation; the highest case fatality rates occur in women with a fetus *in utero*. Spontaneous abortion occurs in 80% of women who are infected with Lassa virus during the first or second trimesters of pregnancy. Stillbirth and neonatal death occur in 75% of maternal cases in the third trimester. Virus titers in the placenta are as high as 10^9 $TCID_{50}$/mL. Virus is also shed in milk from infected mothers and is believed to be transmitted through breastfeeding [13].

Up to 30% of patients with Lassa fever experience an acute loss of hearing in one or both ears; in two-thirds of these patients, the loss is permanent. Unlike other viral infections that are known to cause hearing loss during the acute stage of infection, hearing loss associated with Lassa virus often occurs during the convalescent stage of infection, or even after apparent recovery, and is thought to be immune-mediated; early administration of ribavirin has little effect on hearing outcomes [14].

PATIENT EVALUATION, DIAGNOSIS, DIFFERENTIAL DIAGNOSIS AND VACCINATION

All persons performing procedures must wear adequate personal protective equipment (e.g. gloves, mask, and gown). Additionally, freshly made disinfectant (e.g. 10% hypochlorite) must be on site for immediate disinfection of contaminated materials. Particular care must be taken with all sharp instruments. Specimens should be drawn into a vacuum tube system, if available, to minimize risk of spills. Blood should be allowed to clot at room temperature and serum should be separated and placed in a plastic vial with exterior screw cap for storage and/or transfer. Urine should be mixed with an equal amount of bovine serum albumin at pH 7.4 before freezing. Other fluids should be frozen undiluted. All of these specimens keep best if they are frozen at −70 °C or in liquid nitrogen as soon as possible [1–4].

Lassa fever is difficult to diagnose because its manifestations are not specific and easily confused with early manifestations of many common infections (e.g. malaria, arbovirus infections and typhoid fever). In young babies, marked edema has been reported. In older children, the disease may manifest as diarrhea, pneumonia or an unexplained prolonged fever. Among adults in an endemic area, fever with pharyngitis, proteinuria and retrosternal chest pain has a positive predictive value for Lassa fever of 81% and a specificity of 89%. However, this triad's diagnostic sensitivity is only 50%. Bleeding and sore throat have a sensitivity and specificity for fatal outcome of about 90% [1–4].

The standard field method for the laboratory over many years has been detection of virus-specific antibody by indirect fluorescent antibody (IFA). Slides of inactivated Lassa virus-infected tissue culture cells may be stored at −20 °C for 6 months or at −70 °C for several years. Generally, an IgG titer of at least 16 and an IgM titer of 4 are considered specific for Lassa infection. At least 50% of Lassa fever patients have measurable IgG or IgM IFA antibodies by day 5 of illness, and virtually all have antibodies by days 12–14. The IgG antibodies are directed against the glycoprotein and nucleocapsid of Lassa virus; they are often present simultaneously with high levels of viremia and during the most severe stage of illness. Alternatives to IFA include indirect ELISA to detect IgG and/or IgM antibodies using either recombinant antigens or tissue culture, or reverse ELISA where the amount of antibody can be measured using a directly labeled antigen or by a labeled monoclonal antibody. Reverse transcription (RT)-PCR techniques detecting fragments of the S gene of the virus coding for the glycoprotein have also been used successfully. This technique is rapid, accurate and sensitive. RNA extraction techniques effectively inactivate the virus, so the procedure carries minimal laboratory hazards [15, 16].

Lassa virus isolation requires laboratory Biosafety Level 4 (BSL-4) facilities and may easily be isolated in cell culture (the E6 clone of vero cells) or suckling mice. It has also been isolated from throat swabs during acute illness, breast milk, spinal fluid, pleural and pericardial transudate, and autopsy material. Virus may be recovered for 1–2 months in urine during convalescence, albeit at low titer [15].

TREATMENT

Ribavirin, a guanosine analog, is the only antiviral drug that has been successfully used in humans to treat acute Lassa fever. When administered within the first 6 days of illness, ribavirin decreases the case fatality rate from 55% to 5%. A smaller, but still significant, decrease in fatality has also been demonstrated in patients treated later in illness. Patients treated with ribavirin undergo a significant reduction in viremia, regardless of outcome. The drug is most successful when given intravenously as a 2-g loading dose, followed by 1 g every 6 hours for 4 days, and then 0.5 g every 8 hours for 6 more days. There is some evidence that oral ribavirin may also be effective, particularly when given early in milder cases. Alternatives to ribavirin are currently under investigation. Certain HIV antivirals have been effective in treating Lassa virus infection in cell culture or animal models. Tetherin, a membrane-associated protein that prevents HIV-1 release by retaining progeny virions on cell-surfaces, inhibits Lassa virus-like particle release *in vitro*. Zidampidine, an aryl phosphate derivative of azidothymidine (AZT), significantly improves the survival rates of mice challenged with Lassa virus. Stampidine, a nucleoside analog known for its strong antiviral activity against HIV-1 and HIV-2, has also proven effective against Lassa virus in mouse models. Other antiviral strategies include T-705, a pyrazine derivative currently under clinical development for treatment of influenza virus, as well as interferon-α and -γ therapies [17–24].

Fluid, electrolyte, respiratory and osmotic imbalances should be corrected to prevent clinical shock. However, even vigorous support of this kind may be insufficient to prevent fatal progression of advanced disease when antiviral treatment is started late in infection. Furthermore, the tendency of patients to develop pulmonary edema may be exacerbated by injudicious fluid replacement [1–4].

VACCINATION

Lassa vaccine strategies have evolved from killed to live vaccines. The early killed vaccines invoked good humoral response to Lassa virus proteins, but failed to protect Lassa virus-challenged nonhuman primates. Focus then shifted to activating cellular response. A comprehensive study involving 44 nonhuman primates evaluated the efficacy of recombinant vaccinia viruses expressing Lassa virus proteins. The vaccine was highly successful in protecting against lethal disease; however, the vaccinia platform was found unsuitable for human use as a result of potential side effects, particularly among immunosuppressed individuals. The safety profile of another recombinant vaccine, vesicular stomatitis virus expressing the complete Lassa virus GPC, has yet to be sufficiently explored. The most viable strategy appears to be a reassortment vaccine, ML29, which encodes the NP and GPC of Lassa virus and the Z and L proteins from the Mopeia virus (a non-pathogenic arenavirus). ML29 successfully protected mice, guinea pigs and small nonhuman primates challenged with Lassa virus. Further safety studies must be undertaken to examine the potential dangers of natural re-assortment in this vaccine [25–29].

REFERENCES

1. McCormick JB. Epidemiology and control of Lassa fever. Curr Top Microbiol Immunol 1987;134:69–78.
2. McCormick JB, Fisher-Hoch SP. Lassa fever. Curr Top Microbiol Immunol 2002;262:75–109.
3. McCormick JB, King IJ, Webb PA, et al. A case-control study of the clinical diagnosis and course of Lassa fever. J Infect Dis 1987;155:455.
4. McCormick JB, Webb PA, Krebs JW, et al. A prospective study of the epidemiology and ecology of Lassa fever. J Infect Dis 1987;155:437–44.
5. Macher AM, Wolfe MS. Historical Lassa fever reports and 30-year clinical update. Emerg Infect Dis 2006;12:835–7.
6. Fisher-Hoch SP, Price ME, Craven RB, et al. Safe intensive-care management of a severe case of Lassa fever with simple barrier nursing techniques. Lancet 1985;2:1227–9
7. Fisher-Hoch SP, Tomori O, Nasidi A, et al. Review of cases of nosocomial Lassa fever in Nigeria: The high price of poor medical practice. BMJ 1995; 311:857.
8. Baize S, Marianneau P, Loth P, et al. Early and strong immune responses are associated with control of viral replication and recovery in Lassa virus-infected cynomolgus monkeys. J Virol 2009;83:5890–903.
9. Khan SH, Goba A, Chu M, et al. New opportunities for field research on the pathogenesis and treatment of Lassa fever. Antiviral Research 2008;78: 103–15.
10. Fisher-Hoch SP, Mitchell SW, Sasso DR, et al. Physiologic and immunologic disturbances associated with shock in a primate model of Lassa fever. J Infect Dis 1987;155:465–74.
11. Cummins D, Bennett D, Fisher-Hoch SP, et al. Electrocardiographic abnormalities in patients with Lassa fever. J Trop Med Hyg 1989;92:350–5.
12. Cummins D, Fisher-Hoch SP, Walshe KJ, et al. A plasma inhibitor of platelet aggregation in patients with Lassa fever. Br J Haematol 1989;72:543–8.
13. Price ME, Fisher-Hoch SP, Craven RB, McCormick JB. A prospective study of maternal and fetal outcome in acute Lassa fever infection during pregnancy. Br Med J 1988;297:584–7.
14. Cummins D, McCormick JB, Bennett D, et al. Acute sensorineural deafness in Lassa fever. JAMA 1990;264:2093–6.
15. Bausch DG, Rollin PE, Demby AH, et al. Diagnosis and clinical virology of Lassa fever as evaluated by enzyme-linked immunosorbent assay, indirect fluorescent-antibody test, and virus isolation. J Clin Microbiol 2000;38: 2670–7.
16. Emmerich P, Thome-Bolduan C, Drosten C, et al. Reverse ELISA for IgG and IgM antibodies to detect Lassa virus infections in Africa. J Clin Virol 2008; 37:277–81.
17. Asper M, Sternsdorf T, Hass M, et al. Inhibition of different Lassa virus strains by alpha and gamma interferons and comparison with a less pathogenic arenavirus. J Virol 2004;78:3162–9.
18. Baize S, Kaplon J, Faure C, et al. Lassa virus infection of human dendritic cells and macrophages is productive but fails to activate cells. J Immunol 2004; 172:2861–9.
19. Baize S, Pannetier D, Faure C, et al. Role of interferons in the control of Lassa virus replication in human dendritic cells and macrophages. Microb Infect 2006;8:1194–202.
20. Gowen BB, Smee DF, Wong MH, et al. Treatment of late stage disease in a model of arenaviral hemorrhagic fever: T-705 efficacy and reduced toxicity suggests an alternative to ribavirin. PLoS One 2008;3:e3725
21. Gowen BB, Wong MH, Jung KH, et al. In vitro and in vivo activities of T-705 against arenavirus and bunyavirus infections. Antimicrob Agents Chemother 2007;51:3168–76.
22. McCormick JB, King IJ, Webb PA, et al. Lassa fever: effective therapy with ribavirin. N Engl J Med 1986;314:20–6.
23. Sakuma T, Noda T, Urata S, et al. Inhibition of Lassa and Marburg virus production by tetherin. J Virol 2008;83:2382–5.
24. Uckun FM, Venkatachalam TK, Erbeck D, et al. Zidampidine, an aryl phosphate derivative of AZT: in vivo pharmacokinetics, metabolism, toxicity, and anti-viral efficacy against hemorrhagic fever caused by Lassa virus. Bioorg Med Chem 2005;13:3279–88.
25. Carrion R, Patterson JL, Johnson C, et al. A ML29 reassortant virus protects guinea pigs against a distantly-related Nigerian strain of Lassa virus and can provide sterilizing immunity. Vaccine 2007;25:4093–102.
26. Fisher-Hoch SP, McCormick JB. Lassa fever vaccine: a review. Expert Rev Vaccines 2004;3:103–11.
27. Geisbert TW, Jones S, Fritz EA, et al. Development of a new vaccine for the prevention of Lassa fever. PLoS Med 2005;2:e183.
28. Lukashevich IS, Carrion R, Salvato MS, et al. Safety, immunogenicity, and efficacy of the ML29 reassortant vaccine for Lassa fever in small non-human primates. Vaccine 2008;26:5246–54.
29. Lukashevich IS, Patterson UJ, Carrion R, et al. A live attenuated vaccine for Lassa fever made by reassortment of Lassa and Mopeia viruses. J Virol 2005; 79:13934–42.

33.3 South American Hemorrhagic Fevers

Slobodan Paessler

Key features

- South American hemorrhagic fevers are a series of similar, geographically restricted hemorrhagic fever syndromes caused by several related "Old World" arenaviruses: Junin virus causes Argentine hemorrhagic fever; Machupo virus causes Bolivian hemorrhagic fever; Guanarito virus causes Venezuelan hemorrhagic fever; and Sabia virus causes Brazilian hemorrhagic fever

Key features—cont'd

- South American hemorrhagic fever has a 6–14-day prodromic phase and 8–12 days after onset about 20–30% of patients advance to the neurologic and hemorrhagic phase
- Symptoms include confusion, convulsions, coma and bleeding from body orifices
- Survivors have a long convalescence period of 1–3 months duration
- The causative agents of South American hemorrhagic fevers have a significant impact on public health within their endemic regions, with case fatality rates of 10–30%

INTRODUCTION

South American arenaviruses cause chronic infections of rodents and severe disease in humans. Junin virus (JUNV), for example, causes Argentine hemorrhagic fever, a disease mostly endemic to the pampas region of Argentina, with about five million people at risk. In addition, increased traveling to and from endemic regions may lead to the importation of hemorrhagic fever into non-endemic metropolitan areas of various countries. In addition to its impact on public health, some of the viruses such as JUNV, possess features that might make them potential biological weapons; JUNV is very stable, highly infectious and exhibits high morbidity and significant mortality at low doses.

Argentine hemorrhagic fever was first described in 1953 and the virus was isolated several years later. A similar disease was reported in Bolivia in 1959 and the causative agent, Machupo virus, was first isolated in 1965. In 1989, an outbreak of Venezuelan hemorrhagic fever occurred among a rural population; the isolated virus was named Gunarito virus. The most recent isolate of South American hemorrhagic fever viruses occurred in Brazil in 1990 where Sabia virus (a causative agent of Brazilian hemorrhagic fever) was isolated. All of these viruses belong to the family of *Arenaviridae.*

EPIDEMIOLOGY

South American hemorrhagic fever viruses cause chronic infections of rodents, with a wide regional distribution. Infected rodents move freely in their natural habitat and may invade human dwellings. Humans are infected through mucosal exposure to aerosols or by direct contact of abraded skin with infectious material. Person-to-person transmission is very rare and may occur via direct contact with infected body fluids (e.g. sexual transmission) of a viremic patient; nosocomial infections have also been reported. Nevertheless, agricultural workers (mostly male adults) have historically been at the highest risk for infection while working around potentially infected rodents in fields.

ARGENTINE HEMORRHAGIC FEVER

Epidemics predominantly occur during the major sugar cane harvesting season in Argentina, with a peak incidence in the month of May, at the end of the Argentine summer. The disease is four times as prevalent in males as in females, and is more prevalent among rural workers than in urban populations [1]. The annual incidence of Argentine hemorrhagic fever is positively correlated with local population densities of the reservoir. This epidemiologic pattern is being further modified through vaccination of high-risk populations.

BOLIVIAN HEMORRHAGIC FEVER

The reservoir for Machupo virus is a species of the genus Calomys. The host species resides in habitats where grassland intergrades into forest and, unlike *C. musculinus,* thrives in villages and near human habitations. Bolivian hemorrhagic fever tends to be a seasonal disease, with more cases occurring in the dry season, at the peak of agricultural activity. Epidemics in towns may occur during epizootic conditions when rodent densities reach unusually high levels and rodents invade towns or villages. In 1963–1964, a Bolivian hemorrhagic fever epidemic occurred in the village of San Joaquin resulting in 637 cases and 113 deaths among the town's 3000 residents [2]. Under these conditions, transmission to humans is likely from the inhalation of infectious aerosols; however, direct contact of broken skin or mucous membranes with rodent excreta or contaminated fomites, such as food, should also be considered. Person-to-person transmission, likely *via* direct contact with infectious body fluids, may occur in familial or nosocomial settings. Transmission by intimate contact during convalesence is also possible [3].

VENEZUELAN HEMORRHAGIC FEVER

In 1989, a severe hemorrhagic fever was recognized in the municipality of Guanarito, Guanarito State, Venezuela. The causative agent was soon isolated and shown to be an arenavirus (Guanarito). Guanarito virus is specifically associated with *Zygodontomys brevicauda,* while a second arenavirus, Pirital virus, is associated with co-occurring *Sigmodon alstoni.* While cases have been observed throughout the year, epidemics appear to have a seasonal peak from November to January, coinciding with maximum agricultural activity in the endemic region. As for Argentine hemorrhagic fever, the highest risk is among adult male agricultural workers. Thus, transmission to humans likely occurs outside the home and is potentially related to agricultural activities [4]. Person-to-person transmission or nosocomial infection has not been observed in Venezuelan hemorrhagic fever patients.

NATURAL HISTORY, PATHOGENESIS AND PATHOLOGY

Usually, hemorrhage is present in many organs and effusions can be found in serous cavities. There is widespread necrosis, which may be present in any organ system, varying from modest and focal to massive in extent. Liver and lymphoid systems are usually extensively involved, and the lung regularly has varying degrees of interstitial pneumonitis, diffuse alveolar damage and hemorrhage. The inflammatory response is usually minimal. Argentine hemorrhagic fever during pregnancy is rare; however, congenital malformations, fetal death and death of neonates have been reported [5]. Children tend to have a milder clinical course but severe, and even fatal, disease has been seen.

CLINICAL FEATURES

PATIENT EVALUATION, DIAGNOSIS AND DIFFERENTIAL DIAGNOSIS

South American hemorrhagic fevers resemble one another but Argentine hemorrhagic fever is the best described. The onset of clinical disease is insidious, with malaise, anorexia, chills, headache, myalgias and fever (38–39 °C). A few days later, patients develop constitutional, gastrointestinal, neurologic and cardiovascular signs and symptoms. Low backache, retro-orbital pain, nausea or vomiting, epigastric pain, photophobia, dizziness, and constipation or mild diarrhea might be present in patients. Common absence of productive cough or nasal congestion is helpful in distinguishing the initial symptoms of Argentine hemorrhagic fever from those of influenza or other acute respiratory infections.

As with many other infectious diseases, the first clinical manifestations of South American hemorrhagic fevers are nonspecific and can be confused with several acute febrile conditions, therefore the history of potential exposure to infected rodents is critical in the case of South American hemorrhagic fevers. Among the infectious diseases, the differential diagnosis includes typhoid fever, hepatitis, infectious mononucleosis, leptospirosis, hantavirus pulmonary syndrome, dengue, dengue hemorrhagic fever and rickettsioses. Malaria should also be considered in endemic areas. Diseases presenting with hematologic or neurologic alterations, such as intoxications, rheumatic diseases and blood dyscrasias may also be mistaken for hemorrhagic fever. In the respective endemic areas, or in patients with a history of travel to the specific geographic regions, a febrile syndrome with proteinuria, leukopenia and thrombocytopenia is suspicious of one of the South American hemorrhagic fever [6, 7].

Laboratory diagnosis. Final diagnosis depends on demonstration of the infecting virus, or one of its products, in acute serum samples. Reverse transcription-PCR is usually the most sensitive and produces amplicons that can be sequenced for genetic analysis. In general, viremia and antigenemia are readily detected during the acute phase and disappear as the patient recovers. The presence of viral nucleic acid can be detected during the same period and, perhaps, one or two days afterwards. Seroconversion, mainly IgM antibodies, may be detectable during illness and usually appears early in convalescence. Diagnosis of initial patients in any outbreak, particularly if there are unusual features, benefits from the study of virus isolates and classic serology. Most of the hemorrhagic fever viruses are hazardous and should only be isolated or studied under biosafety level 4 (BSL4) containment. Ideally, blood samples from patients should be collected early in the course of illness, and both serum and blood clot should be frozen as soon as possible. A second sample should be obtained before discharge for comparative serology. In fatal cases, a full autopsy should be performed, if possible, with a complete set of organ biopsy material collected in formalin for diagnostic studies: spleen, liver and lymph nodes should be collected frozen for virus isolation. Classic histopathology is often useful if yellow fever, Rift Valley fever or a filovirus infection are suspected as it can distinguish between them; it is also helpful in diagnosing some of the confounding diseases. Immunohistochemistry on fixed tissues can usually make a definitive diagnosis possible.

Precautions appropriate to each virus should be taken to prevent infection while processing samples or performing a necropsy. Frozen samples should be appropriately packed and, whenever possible, shipped on dry ice, although diagnoses can sometimes be made on mishandled specimens. The receiving laboratory should be advised of the shipment, its estimated time of arrival and the waybill number to allow for tracing the materials if, as often happens, there is a delay *en route*.

TREATMENT

Argentine hemorrhagic fever has a 6–14-day prodromic phase and 8–12 days following its onset, about 20–30% of patients advance to the neurologic and hemorrhagic phase which involves symptoms such as confusion, convulsions, coma and bleeding from body orifices [6, 7]. At this point, the case fatality rate can be variable but overall it is 10–30% and survivors of this phase enter a long convalescence period of 1–3 months' duration [6, 7]. Current recommended therapy of Argentine hemorrhagic fever involves treatment with immune plasma from convalescent patients; this is very effective if started in the first week of disease.

SUPPORTIVE TREATMENT

Supportive treatment consists of adequate hydration, symptomatic measures and proper management of the neurologic alterations, blood loss, shock and additional, superimposed infections. Intramuscular and subcutaneous injections are contraindicated because of the risk of hematomas.

In the Argentine hemorrhagic fever-endemic area, several observations have been made. Pneumonia is the most common secondary bacterial infection and is often accompanied by radiographic changes and an increase in fever, but not by leukocytosis; it usually responds to antibiotics. Transfusions are occasionally required but most of the severe forms are neurologic. It is useful to sedate agitated patients with diphenhydramine or diazepam; diazepam also gives some protection against seizures. Cerebral edema may require both steroids and mannitol.

ANTIVIRAL THERAPY

Immune plasma therapy can ameliorate the immediate disease symptoms and reduce mortality if administered during the prodromic phase but in about 10% of cases it results in a late neurologic syndrome caused by unknown mechanisms [6, 7]. Further limitations to the current use of this treatment are dictated by a short supply of plasma. Both *in vitro* and *in vivo* studies have documented the prophylactic and therapeutic value of the nucleoside analogue ribavirin against several arenaviruses, including JUNV [8, 9]. Importantly, ribavirin reduced both morbidity and mortality in humans associated with JUNV infections if given early in the course of clinical disease [10]. The mechanisms by which ribavirin exerts its anti-arenaviral action remain poorly understood, but likely involve targeting different steps of the virus life cycle. Some limitations of the use of ribavirin are: (i) its often, and significant side effects, including anemia and congenital disorders; and (ii) the need for intravenous administration for optimal efficacy. Several inhibitors of inosine monophosphate dehydrogenase, the S-adenosylhomocysteine hydrolase, a variety of sulfated polysaccharides, phenotiazine compounds, brassinosteroids and myristic acid have been reported to have anti-arenaviral activity. However, these compounds display only modest and rather non-specific effects associated with significant toxicity.

PREVENTIVE MEDICINE

The observation that the prototype XJ strain of JUNV lost virulence for guinea pigs after serial passages in newborn mice led to efforts aimed at developing a live-attenuated vaccine against Argentine hemorrhagic fever. This resulted in the generation of Candid1, which was derived from the 44th mouse brain passage of the XJ strain of JUNV and found to be attenuated in guinea pigs. Preclinical studies at the United States Army Medical Research Institute for Infectious Diseases (USAMRIID) supported the safety, immunogenicity and protective efficacy of Candid1 in both guinea pigs and rhesus macaques, showing median protective doses of 34 and <16 plaque forming units (pfu) in guinea pigs and rhesus macaques, respectively. Subsequent clinical studies involving agricultural workers in the JUNV endemic area have shown Candid1 to be an effective and safe vaccine in humans [11]. In 2006, the regulatory agency of Argentina granted this Candid 1 vaccine approval for human use exclusively in Argentina.

Studies addressing long-term immunity and safety have not been conducted in the USA. Experimental data also exist that would support the cross-protection of this vaccine against Machupo virus; however, no clinical studies were performed.

REFERENCES

1. Mills,JN, Ellis BA, Childs JE, et al. Prevalence of infection with Junin virus in rodent populations in the epidemic area of Argentine hemorrhagic fever. Am J Trop Med Hyg 1994;51:554–62.
2. Johnson KM, Halstead SB, Cohen SN. Hemorrhagic fevers of Southeast Asia and South America: a comparative appraisal. Prog Med Virol 1967;9: 105–58.
3. Douglas R, Wiebenga N, Couch R. Bolivian hemorrhagic fever probably transmitted by personal contact. Am J Epidemiol 1965;82:8591.
4. Salas R, Pacheco ME, Ramos B, et al. Venezuelan haemorrhagic fever. Lancet 1991;338:1033–6.
5. Briggiler A, Levis S, Enria DA, Maiztegui JI. Argentine hemorrhagic fever in pregnant women. Medicina (Buenos Aires) 1990;50:443.

6. Enria DA, Barrera Oro, JG. Junin virus vaccines. Curr Top Microbiol Immunol 2002;263:239–61.
7. Peters CJ. Human infection with arenaviruses in the Americas. Curr Top Microbiol Immunol 2002;262: 65–74.
8. Damonte EB, Coto CE. Treatment of arenavirus infections: from basic studies to the challenge of antiviral therapy. Adv Virus Res 2002;58:125–55.
9. Andrei G, De Clercq E. Molecular approaches for the treatment of hemorrhagic fever virus infections. Antiviral Res 1993;22:45–75.
10. McKee KT, Jr, Huggins JW, Trahan CJ, Mahlandt BG. Ribavirin prophylaxis and therapy for experimental argentine hemorrhagic fever. Antimicrob Agents Chemother 1988;32:1304–9.
11. Maiztegui JI, Kelly T, McKee KT, Jr, et al. Protective efficacy of a live attenuated vaccine against Argentine hemorrhagic fever. AHF Study Group. J Infect Dis 1998;177:277–83.

33.4 Ebola and Marburg Virus Infections

Amy L Hartman

Key features

- The filoviruses Ebola and Marburg cause sporadic outbreaks of severe viral hemorrhagic fever
- Mortality among infected patients ranges from 40–90%
- Filoviruses are transmitted by contact of mucous membranes with infected bodily fluids
- Disease begins abruptly with high fever, myalgia and possible hemorrhagic symptoms, including rash and bleeding from mucosal and venipuncture sites. Late-stage symptoms include delirium, convulsions, shock and coma
- Isolation of suspected patients and barrier nursing practices should be strictly followed to prevent nosocomial transmission. Samples from suspected patients should be handled following Biosafety Level (BSL)-3 precautions. Once filovirus infection is confirmed, both patients and samples should only be handled under BSL-4 conditions
- Supportive therapy and maintenance of fluid and electrolyte balance are the only recommended treatments at this time

INTRODUCTION

Ebola and Marburg viruses are the causative agents of a severe form of viral hemorrhagic fever. Both viruses belong to the *Filoviridae* family, which contains two genera and a newly proposed 3rd genus: *Ebolavirus, Marburgvirus,* and *Cuevavirus* (tentative) [1]. The genome of all filoviruses is a linear, non-segmented, single-stranded RNA molecule that is of a negative polarity. The *Ebolavirus* genus consists of five species: *Zaire, Sudan, Reston, Tai Forest* and the newly discovered *Bundibugyo;* the *Marburgvirus* genus contains only one species, termed *Marburg marburgvirus* (MARV) [2, 3]. The proposed *Cuevavirus* genus contains one species (*Lloviu cuevaviru*).

All filoviruses are classified as Category A Select Agent pathogens in the USA owing to the fact that they are easily transmitted between humans, cause high mortality with the potential for major public health impact, can cause public panic and disruption, and require special action for public health preparedness. Filoviruses are also infectious by aerosol under experimental settings, which adds to the concern for their use as a bioterror weapon [4, 5]. Possession and use of these viruses in the research setting is tightly regulated in the USA by the Centers for Disease Control and Prevention (CDC) Select Agent Program following the guidelines of the Select Agent Regulations. As a result of these biosafety concerns, research with filoviruses is approved for use only at Biosafety Level (BSL)-4, which provides the highest level of protection for both the laboratory worker and the environment.

EPIDEMIOLOGY

Filovirus outbreaks occur sporadically in Africa and are characterized by high mortality and a high incidence of nosocomial transmission (Table 33.4-1)[2]. The first disease caused by a filovirus was Marburg hemorrhagic fever, which broke out in 1967 in Germany and Yugoslavia after laboratory workers contracted the virus from infected primates recently imported from Uganda. A total of 31 cases were identified and the mortality among these cases was 23%. Outbreaks of Marburg hemorrhagic fever have occurred sporadically since the original discovery. The largest known Marburg hemorrhagic fever outbreak occurred in northeastern Angola in the spring of 2005, with over 250 cases identified and 90% mortality.

Ebola hemorrhagic fever was first identified in two separate large outbreaks occurring simultaneously in 1976—one in the Democratic Republic of the Congo and the other in Sudan. These two initial outbreaks were later identified as being caused by two separate species of virus: *Zaire ebolavirus* (EBOV) and *Sudan ebolavirus* (SUDV). These two viruses have been responsible for the majority of Ebola outbreaks since 1976, with EBOV generally being the most deadly of all Ebola species (Table 33.4-1).

The remaining three species of Ebola virus (*Tai Forest ebolavirus* (TAFV), *Reston ebolavirus* (RESTV), and *Bundibugyo ebolavirus* (BDBV)) have occurred less frequently. TAFV has only been known to cause a single nonfatal infection acquired during the necropsy of a dead chimpanzee. The newly identified, and genetically distinct, BDBV was responsible for an outbreak in 2007–2008 in Uganda, resulting in over 100 cases with a fatality of 42% [6].

RESTV was discovered during an investigation of hemorrhagic fever deaths in primates in a quarantine facility in Reston, Virginia in 1989. Primates imported from a single export facility in the Philippines were responsible for this and several subsequent outbreaks in primate facilities in the USA and Italy. Nine workers in the affected USA and Filippino facilities were identified as having been infected with the virus, but none of the workers developed disease, suggesting that RESTV may be less virulent or non-pathogenic in humans. RESTV was also recently detected in pigs on commercial farms in the Philippines, with no known cases of disease in humans.

The natural reservoir for filoviruses has remained elusive for some time, but, historically, bats have been a suspected reservoir. A number

TABLE 33.4-1 List of Filovirus Outbreaks

Year	Location	# of Cases	Fatality (%)
Zaire ebolavirus			
1976	Democratic Republic of the Congo	318	88
1977	Democratic Republic of the Congo	1	100
1994	Gabon	49	65
1995	Democratic Republic of the Congo	315	88
1996 (spring)	Gabon	37	57
1996 (autumn)	Gabon	60	75
2001–02	Gabon	123	79
2003 (spring)	Republic of Congo	143	90
2003 (autumn)	Republic of Congo	35	83
2005	Republic of Congo	12	75
2007	Democratic Republic of the Congo	264	71
2008	Democratic Republic of the Congo	32	47
Sudan ebolavirus			
1976	Sudan	284	53
1979	Sudan	34	65
2000–01	Uganda	425	53
2004	Sudan	17	42
Tai Forest ebolavirus			
1994	Cote d'Ivoire	1	0
Bundibugyo ebolavirus			
2007–08	Uganda	131	42
Reston ebolavirus			
1989–90	USA	4	0
1992	Italy	0	0
1996	USA	0	0
2008	Philippines	6	0
Marburg marburgvirus			
1967	Germany/Yugoslavia	31	23
1975	South Africa	3	33
1980	Kenya	2	50
1987	Kenya	1	100
1998–2000	Democratic Republic of the Congo	154	83
2005	Angola	252	90
2007	Uganda	4	25
2007	Uganda	1	0
2008	Uganda	1	100

of outbreaks of EBOV and MARV in humans have been associated with bat caves in both Uganda and Gabon. Recently, MARV was isolated from Egyptian fruit bats in a cave in Uganda; the circulating bat isolates were genetically similar to the virus found in humans infected in that region [7]. While EBOV has not yet been isolated from bats, Ebola genetic sequences have been detected by PCR and Ebola-specific IgG antibodies have been detected in a number of bat species [8, 9]. The mechanism by which bats shed and transmit the viruses to humans is currently under investigation.

NATURAL HISTORY, PATHOGENESIS AND PATHOLOGY

Filoviruses spread through the human population by close contact with sick patients [10]. Virus-containing bodily fluids include blood, vomitus, saliva, stool, semen, breast milk and tears. Transmission of filoviruses requires close proximity, such as handling fomites or direct contact with blood or bodily fluids leading to mucous membrane exposure. No true aerosol transmission between humans has been documented, but both viruses cause disease in primates after experimental aerosol infection [4, 5]. Virus transmission has not been documented during the asymptomatic incubation period.

In Africa, deficient barrier nursing practices, poor sanitary conditions and frequent re-use of needles has caused transmission of filoviruses to healthcare workers. Unfortunately, nosocomial transmission has contributed significantly to the spread of filovirus outbreaks [11]. In addition, traditional healers have been implicated in the spread of both Ebola and Marburg viruses through the use of unsterilized blades or needles [11, 12]. Another potential source of virus transmission during filoviral outbreaks is known to occur during traditional burial ceremonies [11, 12], as family members wash and prepare the deceased body for burial.

The severe disease caused by filoviruses can be attributed to rapid viral replication, host immune suppression induced by the virus and vascular dysfunction [13]. Macrophages and dendritic cells appear to play a key role because they support high levels of virus replication and initiate virus dissemination from the site of infection to the lymph nodes. The virus replicates rapidly in a variety of organs, including the liver and spleen, causing extensive cell death. Infected dendritic cells are dysfunctional in their ability to present viral antigens and co-stimulate T cells. Infected macrophages secrete high levels of inflammatory cytokines, resulting in immune dysregulation. Finally, macrophages over-express tissue factor which is thought to contribute to disseminated intravascular coagulation and the vascular impairment seen in filovirus-infected patients [14].

Pathologic investigations performed on patients with Ebola and Marburg infection all reveal extensive necrosis in a variety of organs, including the liver, spleen, kidney, thymus, lymph nodes and reproductive organs [15]. In the liver, hepatocellular necrosis is widespread and an exceedingly large number of virus particles are present. Inclusion bodies are often visible in intact cells.

CLINICAL FEATURES

The incubation period for filoviruses can be as short as 2 days or as long as 21 days [3]. Illness begins abruptly with nonspecific flu-like symptoms (chills, fever, myalgia, general malaise) (Fig. 33.4.1). Subsequent symptoms often include lethargy, nausea, vomiting, abdominal pain, anorexia, diarrhea, coughing, headache and hypotension. Hemorrhagic manifestations are not universal and generally develop during the time of peak illness. These include a rash, easy bruising, nosebleeds, bleeding from venipuncture sites and bleeding from mucosal sites, especially the gastrointestinal and genitourinary tracts.

Early symptoms are similar in survivors and non-survivors. Subsequently, fatal cases progress to more severe symptoms by 7–14 days after the onset of illness, while survivors begin to recover at this time. Survivors also have 100- to 1000-fold lower levels of viremia and higher levels of virus-specific antibodies compared with fatal cases. Shock and coma often precede death in fatal cases.

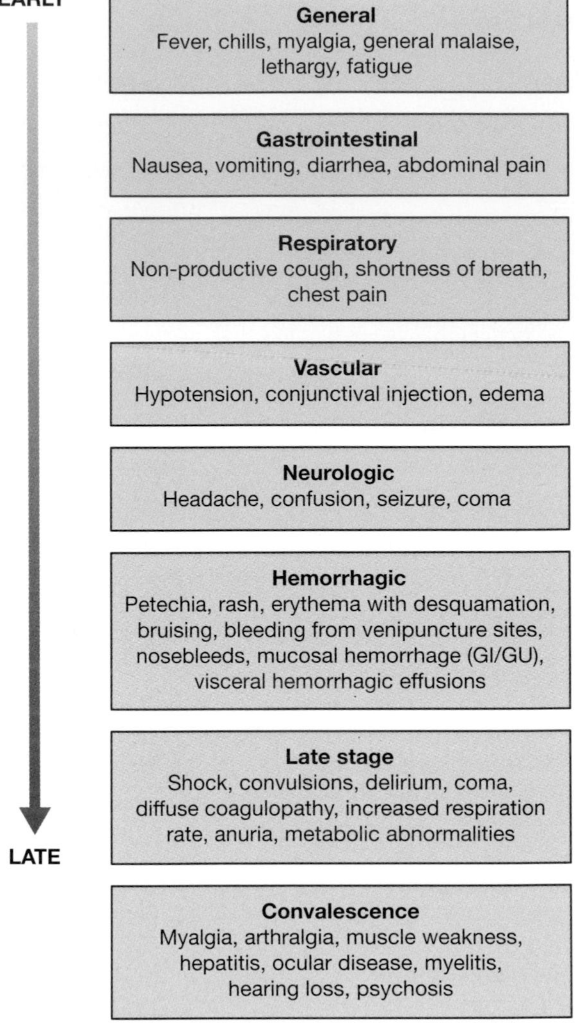

FIGURE 33.4.1 Symptoms of viral hemorrhagic fever caused by Ebola and Marburg Viruses.

Survivors of filoviral infections experience a prolonged convalescence which is characterized by myalgia, arthralgia, muscle weakness, hepatitis, ocular disease, myelitis, hearing loss and even psychosis. During early convalescence, virus can be detectable in immunologically protected sites of the body, particularly the uveal and seminal tracts. While long-term viral shedding is not thought to occur in filovirus-infected patients, infectious virus can be detected in genital secretions for up to 80 days post-onset of illness [3]. Recovering patients should be counseled to take adequate precautions to prevent sexual transmission during this time period.

PATIENT EVALUATION, DIAGNOSIS, AND DIFFERENTIAL DIAGNOSIS

In patients presenting with a history of travel to an area of Africa with an ongoing filovirus outbreak, the following clinical criteria should be considered in suspected cases: high fever (>38°C for less than 3 weeks' duration), muscle pain and at least two of the following hemorrhagic symptoms: rash, nosebleed, vomiting of blood, coughing of blood, or blood in stools [16]. Laboratory workers with a known occupational exposure (needlestick, animal bite) should be isolated until further testing can be conducted.

As nosocomial transmission of filoviruses is a primary mechanism of outbreak amplification [11], the utmost caution should be used when treating suspected cases. Clinical care of suspected filovirus patients should follow BSL-3 practices at a minimum, which requires the use of barrier gowns, two pairs of gloves, eye protection and a mask or N95 respirator. Airborne precautions and negative-pressure rooms should be used, if available. The use of double-gloves followed by hand-washing immediately after interaction with patients is critical in preventing potential exposure of mucous membranes. Impermeable liquid-barrier gowns should be worn along with leg and shoe covers. The use of face shields and/or eye goggles is highly recommended. Surgical masks and/or N95 respirators should be used, if available. Splashes of bodily fluids to the eyes or mouth have proven to be the unfortunate source of many nosocomial transmission events.

Local and state health departments should be notified of suspected cases. Diagnostic confirmation can only be obtained by sending samples to an international reference laboratory. Samples from suspected patients should be handled minimally and with the utmost caution. A class II biosafety cabinet should be used to process clinical specimens and, at a minimum, BSL-3 practices should be used. Once filovirus infection is confirmed by a reference laboratory, samples should be handled only at BSL-4.

International reference laboratories have a range of assays available for testing and identifying filovirus samples [2]. Routine laboratory tests used to diagnose suspected patients include ELISA (to detect viral antigen or the presence of IgM or IgG antibodies), virus isolation and reverse transcription (RT)-PCR. Blood and serum are the samples most preferred for diagnostic testing; however, oral and nasal swabs are sufficient [17].

DIFFERENTIAL DIAGNOSIS

The differential diagnosis for filovirus infections is extensive as a result of the generalized early symptoms. Malaria, shigellosis and typohoid fever are the most common causes of acute febrile illness in the areas of sub-Saharan Africa where filoviruses are endemic. Other diagnoses to consider include yellow fever, chickungunya fever, fulminant viral hepatitis, plague, typhus, leptospirosis and meningococcal septicemia.

TREATMENT

There are currently no licensed vaccines or therapeutic treatments available for filovirus infections. To date, strategies for treating filovirus-infected patients in an outbreak setting have proven unsuccessful [18]. Ribavirin has been shown to be an ineffective treatment. In animal models, a number of therapies have been tried, but none have been able to reverse the fatal outcome once disease has begun. Recent research studies have identified a number of promising filovirus vaccine candidates [19], although none have yet become licensed as either a preventative or post-exposure vaccine.

Until an effective vaccine or post-exposure therapy is licensed, the prognosis for patients infected with Ebola and Marburg is grim. Based on the known outbreaks, the case fatality ratios range from 42–90%, depending on the viral species and outbreak. Filovirus-infected patients should be monitored closely with supportive care, including providing supplemental oxygen and monitoring hydration, circulatory volume and blood pressure. Administration of steroids, non-steroidal anti-inflammatory drugs (NSAIDs), aspirin and anticoagulant therapies are contraindicated [16].

REFERENCES

1. Kuhn JH, Becker S, Ebihara H, et al. Proposal for a revised taxonomy of the family *Filoviridae:* classification, names of taxa and viruses, and virus abbreviations. Arch Virol 2010;155(12)2083–103.
2. Hartman AL, Towner JS, Nichol ST. Ebola and marburg hemorrhagic fever. Clin Lab Med 2010;30:161–77.
3. Sanchez A, Geisbert TW, Feldmann H. Filoviridae: Marburg and Ebola Viruses. In: Knipe BM, Howley PM, Griffen DE, et al. eds. Fields Virology, 5th edn. Philadelphia: Lippincott-Raven; 2007:1409–48.
4. Alves DA, Glynn AR, Steele KE, et al. Aerosol exposure to the angola strain of marburg virus causes lethal viral hemorrhagic fever in cynomolgus macaques. Vet Pathol 2010;47:831–51.
5. Geisbert TW, Daddario-Dicaprio KM, Geisbert JB, et al. Vesicular stomatitis virus-based vaccines protect nonhuman primates against aerosol challenge with Ebola and Marburg viruses. Vaccine 2008;26:6894–900.
6. Towner JS, Sealy TK, MKhristova ML, et al. Newly discovered ebola virus associated with hemorrhagic fever outbreak in Uganda. PLoS Pathog 2008;4: e1000212.
7. Towner JS, Amman BR, TSealy TK, et al. Isolation of genetically diverse Marburg viruses from Egyptian fruit bats. PLoS Pathog 2009;5:e1000536.
8. Pourrut X, Souris M, Towner JS, et al. Large serological survey showing cocirculation of Ebola and Marburg viruses in Gabonese bat populations, and a high seroprevalence of both viruses in *Rousettus aegyptiacus*. BMC Infect Dis 2009;9:159.
9. Towner JS, Pourrut X, Albarino CG, et al. Marburg virus infection detected in a common African bat. PLoS ONE 2007;2:e764.
10. Bausch DG, Towner JS, Dowell SF, et al. Assessment of the risk of Ebola virus transmission from bodily fluids and fomites. J Infect Dis 2007;196(suppl. 2):S142–7.
11. Georges AJ, Leroy EM, Renaut AA, et al. Ebola hemorrhagic fever outbreaks in Gabon, 1994–1997: epidemiologic and health control issues. J Infect Dis 1999;179(suppl. 1):S65–75.
12. World Health Organization. Marburg Hemmorrhagic Fever in Angola–Update 26. 2005. Available at: http://www.who.int/csr/don/2005_11_07a/en/index.html.
13. Mohamadzadeh M, Chen L, Schmaljohn AL. How Ebola and Marburg viruses battle the immune system. Nat Rev Immunol 2007;7:556–67.
14. Geisbert TW, Young HA, Jahrling PB, et al. Mechanisms underlying coagulation abnormalities in ebola hemorrhagic fever: overexpression of tissue factor in primate monocytes/macrophages is a key event. J Infect Dis 2003;188: 1618–29.
15. Zaki SR, Goldsmith CS. Pathologic features of filovirus infections in humans. Curr Top Microbiol Immunol 1999;235:97–116.
16. Borio L, Inglesby T, Peters CJ, et al. Hemorrhagic fever viruses as biological weapons: medical and public health management. JAMA 2002;287:2391–405.
17. Towner JS, Khristova ML, Sealy TK, et al. Marburgvirus genomics and association with a large hemorrhagic fever outbreak in Angola. J Virol 2006;80: 6497–516.
18. Bausch DG, Sprecher AG, Jeffs B, Boumandouki P. Treatment of Marburg and Ebola hemorrhagic fevers: a strategy for testing new drugs and vaccines under outbreak conditions. Antiviral Res 2008;78:150–61.
19. Reed DS, Mohamadzadeh M. Status and challenges of filovirus vaccines. Vaccine 2007;25:1923–34.

33.5 Crimean-Congo Hemorrhagic Fever

Christine E Mathews, Susan Fisher-Hoch

Key features

- Crimean-Congo hemorrhagic fever (CCHF) is a tick-borne, viral hemorrhagic fever found in more than 30 countries throughout Eastern Europe, Asia the Middle East and Africa
- Transmission primarily occurs through bites of infected ticks or through contamination by blood or infected material from infected ticks, animals or other humans. This disease is known for causing nosocomial outbreaks
- Incubation can last 1–6 days depending on host, viral load and route of exposure, and is followed by pre-hemorrhagic and hemorrhagic phases
- Case fatality rates usually range from 30–50%, although rates as high as 90% have been reported in outbreaks
- The use of ribavirin (oral or injectable) for treatment of CCHF is currently recommended by the World Health Organization (WHO)
- Synonyms include: *khungribta, khunymuny* or *karakhalak* in Uzbekistan, and Xinjiang fever in China

INTRODUCTION

DEFINITION AND HISTORY

Crimean-Congo hemorrhagic fever (CCHF) is a tick-borne viral disease first described in the 1940s during an outbreak among 200 Soviet military recruits in the Crimean peninsula following World War II. The earliest accounts of CCHF are believed to be traced back to a 12th century physician from what is currently known as Tajikistan. Reports of a disease that matches CCHF have been described for centuries in present Southern Uzbekistan under the names *khungribta, khunymuny* and *karakhalak*. A virus isolated in 1967 from an ill child in what is now Kisangani, Democratic Republic of Congo, was later found to be identical to a virus from the Crimea, hence the name Crimean-Congo hemorrhagic fever virus. This disease is now known to occur in 30 countries from Eastern Europe through Asia, the Middle East, the steppes and dry subtropics of middle Asia, and all of Africa. In China, the Xinjiang strain of CCHF virus causes the disease known locally as Xinjiang fever [1–4].

ETIOLOGY

CCHF virus is a member of the *Nairovirus* genus of the *Bunyaviridae*; like other nairoviruses it contains three segments of negative-sense RNA. There are 34 viral strains of nairoviruses, with the CCHF serogroup being the most important in relation to human disease. Surface glycoproteins may play a role in the pathogenicity of CCHF virus in humans, as a highly variable region of the glycoprotein precursor resembles a domain found to be associated with increased vascular permeability and hemorrhage in Ebola hemorrhagic fever [4–6].

EPIDEMIOLOGY

VECTORS AND RESERVOIRS

CCHF virus is a zoonotic agent naturally found in a cycle between ixodid ticks and vertebrates. CCHF viruses have been isolated from 31 species and subspecies of ixodid ticks, as well as one species of biting midge (*Culicoides* spp.). The best-studied tick hosts and most important vectors to humans are *Hyalomma* spp., which appear to be the most efficient transmitters of the virus. The worldwide distribution of CCHF appears to closely mirror the geographic distribution of *Hyalomma* species.

Tick bites are the source of CCHF virus for many domestic and wild animals, in all of which the infections are apparently asymptomatic. Transport of infectious ticks by birds may have contributed to the migration of CCHF virus over a wide geographic distribution [3, 4, 7, 8].

TRANSMISSION

Transmission of CCHF virus to humans occurs from bites of infected ticks or through contamination by blood or infected material from infected ticks, animals or other humans. In endemic areas, the high prevalence of anti-CCHF antibodies in domestic animals and the relatively lower prevalence in humans indicates transmission from animals to humans is infrequent. Although tick bites are frequent in those living among domestic animals in CCHF endemic areas, the relatively low frequency of primary human CCHF infection suggests that a minority of these bites result in infection [9, 10]. Avoidance of tick bites or contact with blood from infected, engorged ticks is the most effective strategy to prevent infection.

PREVALENCE OF DISEASE

Most primary CCHF infections are sporadic and can be traced to agricultural practices. Increases in prevalence of CCHF have been proposed to be caused by changes in climate and agricultural land use. Prevalence may also be influenced by the spread of immature ticks via migratory birds or movements of wild mammals [4, 11]. Seasonality of CCHF depends on climate and local tick hosts [4, 10, 12].

HUMAN DISEASE

Most primary infections are from tick bites or animal blood exposure. Case fatality rates are usually described as ranging from 30–50%, but these rates appear to vary in different locations reflecting, in part, a variable availability of medical and diagnostic services. Case fatality rates of 72.7% were documented during a 1994–1995 outbreak in the United Arab Emirates. In southern Russia, where disease surveillance is more complete, milder disease forms are often noted and case fatality rates rarely exceed 5–10%. In South Africa from 1981–1986, the case-fatality rate ranged up to 90% in some reports [2, 10, 12–14].

OCCUPATIONAL EXPOSURE

Occupational exposure is greatest for those involved in agricultural practices handling cattle or sheep, including milking, slaughtering, shearing, castrating or tail docking. Owing to the peridomestic nature of the disease, CCHF equally infects males and females and persons of all age groups in central Asia and Iraq.

Although they constitute only a minority of cases, the most noticeable infections result from nosocomial transmission. CCHF has repeatedly infected unwary surgeons, nursing staff and other medical attendants. In all reported outbreaks, direct contact with blood, needlestick or other injury, or failure to observe simple barrier techniques were recorded. Airborne spread in a hospital setting is not considered a risk [2, 3, 7, 15–17].

NATURAL HISTORY, PATHOGENESIS AND PATHOLOGY

The mechanisms of CCHF pathology have yet to be well described. Historically, outbreaks of CCHF have occurred sporadically and in areas where facilities cannot support laboratory diagnosis in required Biosafety Level 4 (BSL-4) containment facilities. As humans and suckling mice are the only known hosts to display disease pathology, research has been limited because of a lack of an appropriate animal model for disease. Thus, most information on disease pathology has been determined from observational data and data collected from CCHF patients [3].

NATURAL HISTORY

Incubation can last 1–6 days depending on the host, viral load and route of exposure. Exposure through an infected tick has the shortest incubation time (1–3 days) while incubation after exposure to human blood can last 5–6 days. Nosocomial infections generally have an incubation period of 4–9 days, but there is at least one report of as few as 48 hours elapsing between medical personnel administering mouth-to-mouth resuscitation to a bleeding patient and onset of fever. Incubation is often much shorter in fatal cases.

The pre-hemorrhagic phase lasts 3–6 days and is characterized by sudden onset of severe headache, high fever, chills, myalgia strongly localized to the lower back, joint pains and epigastric pain. Conjunctivitis and a mild flushing of the face and chest, pharyngeal hyperemia, and petechiae on the palate are frequent; bradycardia is typical.

The hemorrhagic phase is characterized by petechiae and ecchymoses, hematuria, nosebleeds and bleeding from the gut. In severe cases, hemorrhage may begin as early as 3–5 days. Bleeding may occur at any mucosal surface, as well as from venipuncture sites. Some patients develop uncontrolled bleeding and may have severe hepatic impairment. Hemorrhages are widely distributed in many organs and death may be partially attributable to blood loss. Pulmonary edema and hypovolemic shock, caused by capillary leakage and blood loss, portend a fatal outcome.

The pathology of CCHF most closely resembles that of Marburg and Ebola, both of which can be considered differential diagnoses, along with other diseases listed in Table 33.5-1. As with other viral hemorrhagic fevers, marked weight loss with generalized muscle wasting occurs over a period of just a few days. The convalescent recovery phase can be slow and prolonged, with disease sequelae affecting vision, hearing or memory. Relapse is not known to occur [4, 12, 18].

TABLE 33.5-1 Differential Diagnoses of Crimean-Congo Hemorrhagic Fever Based on Region of Patient Presentation

Geographic region of patient presentation	Differential diagnoses of consideration
Global	Q-fever
	Leptospirosis
	Brucellosis
	Viral hepatitis (HAV, HBV, HCV, HEV)
	Seoul virus—hemorrhagic fever with renal syndrome
Northern hemisphere	Tick-borne encephalitis
North America	Hantavirus pulmonary syndrome (HPS)
South America	South American hemorrhagic fevers
Eastern and Western Europe, Russia, China	Lyme disease
Scandinavia, western Europe and Russia	Puumala virus—hemorrhagic fever with renal syndrome
Balkans	Dobrava virus—hemorrhagic fever with renal syndrome
Western Siberia	Omsk hemorrhagic fever
Eastern Asia (China, Russia, Korea)	Hantavirus—hemorrhagic fever with renal syndrome
Africa	Yellow Fever
Africa (Democratic Republic of the Congo, Gabon, Sudan, the Ivory Coast (broad leaf tropical rainforest regions), Uganda, and the Congo)	Ebola
Africa (Uganda, Zimbabwe, the Democratic Republic of the Congo, Kenya and Angola (savannah regions))	Marburg
West Africa	Lassa fever
Africa, Saudi Arabia, Yemen	Rift Valley fever
Africa, Middle East, Asia	Malaria
Southern India	Kyasanur Forest disease

HAV, hepatitis A virus; HBV, hepatitis B virus; HCV, hepatitis C virus; HEV, hepatitis E virus.

PATIENT EVALUATION, DIAGNOSIS AND DIFFERENTIAL DIAGNOSIS

PATIENT EVALUATION

The white blood cell count is low ($<2000/mm^3$) early in illness with proteinuria and hematuria. Lymphopenia persists throughout the illness and a later rise in neutrophils may be observed. Severe thrombocytopenia with counts of $<20,000/mm^3$ is encountered in 60–100% of cases. Aspartate transaminase (AST) is always raised. Prothrombin times and alanine transaminase (ALT) are generally normal, underscoring that the disease process is not primarily hepatic, despite liver involvement. Factors that have been associated with fatal outcome include: a platelet count of $\leq 20 \times 10^9/L$; partial thromboplastin time of ≥60 seconds; AST of ≥200 IU/L; ALT of ≥150 IU/L; hematemesis; melena; somnolence; and a low-to-complete absence of measurable anti-CCHF virus IgM and IgG antibodies [4, 17, 18].

DIAGNOSIS

CCHF is a disease that develops rapidly following infection and patients frequently die before the development of an antibody response. Rapid diagnosis of acute disease rests on detection of the agent in blood or biopsy material. The use of reverse transcription (RT)-PCR techniques (RT-PCR) to amplify relatively well-conserved sequences in the S segment allows for rapid diagnosis with both high sensitivity and specificity, even in seronegative cases. Real-time PCR provides even more sensitive and specific results than conventional RT-PCR within an hour.

VIRUS DETECTION

Intracerebral inoculation of suckling mice is the most reliable method for primary virus isolation. In comparison, virus isolation in cell culture is faster and more easily accomplished, although generally regarded as less sensitive as it can only detect high levels of virus. Virus can be isolated from blood and organs (e.g. liver biopsy) in susceptible cell lines including Vero-E6, LLC-MK2, BHK-21 and SW-13. The virus is fairly stable but only in blood for up to 10 days at 4 °C. Transport at −70 °C or lower is important for preservation of live virus or RNA for PCR [4, 7].

ANTIBODY DETECTION

Virus-specific IgM or IgG antibodies in survivors may be present 7–10 days after infection with CCHF virus. Neutralizing antibodies appear by days 14–16 and persist for many years. Recently, a new method of detecting CCHF IgG antibodies was developed using a recombinant nucleoprotein-IFA and ELISA and may prove useful for CCHF diagnosis or epidemiologic studies [4].

TREATMENT

SPECIFIC MEASURES

Ribavirin, a drug that is effective against several RNA viruses, is active against CCHF virus *in vitro* and *in vivo* and has been used to treat acute CCHF. The use of ribavirin is currently recommended by the WHO for treatment of CCHF. Treatment regimens should deliver an initial 30 mg/kg dose followed by 15 mg/kg every 6 hours for 4 days, then 7.5 mg/kg every 8 hours for 6 days. The dose can be tolerated over a short period, given the life-threatening nature of this disease.

CCHF-specific purified immunoglobulin has been successful in a small number of patients in Bulgaria and type I interferon has shown promise in patients and animal models for other hemorrhagic fevers. Immune plasma therapy has not been found to be efficacious.

Efficacy of the antiviral depends on rapid institution of therapy. A delay in referral for antiviral treatment was found to be significantly associated with CCHF fatality rates in Turkey during 2004–2008 [19]. Care should be taken to encourage awareness of CCHF clinical signs, symptoms and treatment options for healthcare practitioners, particularly in endemic areas [14, 17, 20–21].

SUPPORTIVE

In addition to the careful management of fluid and electrolyte dynamics during the acute stages of disease, whole blood, platelets and fresh plasma may be indicated. Care must be taken to avoid over-hydrating patients because the disease may be associated with a leaky capillary syndrome [17, 20].

PATIENT ISOLATION

Together with Lassa, Marburg and Ebola viruses, CCHF is the hemorrhagic fever virus best known for nosocomial and intrafamilial secondary infections. Infectious blood and vomitus are the most likely vehicles of such transmission. Surgery and needlestick injuries must be avoided. Strict isolation, restriction and education of attendant personnel and visitors combined with observance of simple precautions are the essentials. Procedures, including mouth-to-mouth resuscitation, that have been featured in published reports of CCHF outbreaks must be avoided. In poor communities where families are culturally and out of necessity involved in direct patient care, time must be given to educating and equipping people to protect themselves [7, 15, 16].

PROPHYLAXIS

Post-exposure prophylaxis with oral ribavirin should be offered to anyone with a high-risk history of exposure to CCHF virus. High risk constitutes direct exposure to blood, either on cuts or abrasions, mucous membranes, or by needlestick or other penetrating injury [4, 7, 17].

VACCINE

A formalin-inactivated CCHF vaccine produced from brains of suckling mice has been used in Bulgaria in high-risk groups, such as farmers and border guards. The vaccine was found to produce high antibody titers; however, no efficacy trials have been performed to date [22].

REFERENCES

1. Yen YC, Kong LX, Lee L, et al. Characteristics of Crimean-Congo hemorrhagic fever virus (Xinjiang strain) in China. Am J Trop Med Hyg 1985;34:1179–82.
2. Hoogstraal H. The epidemiology of tick-borne Crimean-Congo hemorrhagic fever in Asia, Europe, and Africa. J Med Entomol 1979;15:307–417.
3. Flick R, Whitehouse CA. Crimean-Congo hemorrhagic fever virus. Curr Mol Med 2005;5:753–60.
4. Whitehouse CA. Crimean–Congo hemorrhagic fever. Antiviral Res 2004;64:145–60.
5. Haferkamp S, Fernando L, Schwarz TF, et al. Intracellular localization of Crimean-Congo Hemorrhagic Fever (CCHF) virus glycoproteins. Virol J 2005;2:42.
6. Weber F, Mirazimi A. Interferon and cytokine responses to Crimean Congo hemorrhagic fever virus; an emerging and neglected viral zonoosis. Cytokine Growth Factor Rev 2008;19:395–404.
7. Vorou R, Pierroutsakos IN, Maltezou HC. Crimean-Congo hemorrhagic fever. Curr Opin Infect Dis 2007;20:495–500.
8. Shepherd AJ, Swanepoel R, Leman PA, Shepherd SP. Field and laboratory investigation of Crimean-Congo haemorrhagic fever virus (Nairovirus, family Bunyaviridae) infection in birds. Trans R Soc Trop Med Hyg 1987;81:1004–7.
9. Mild M, Simon M, Albert J, Mirazimi A. Towards an understanding of the migration of Crimean-Congo hemorrhagic fever virus. J Gen Virol 2010;91:199–207.
10. Swanepoel R, Shepherd AJ, Leman PA, et al. Epidemiologic and clinical features of Crimean-Congo hemorrhagic fever in southern Africa. Am J Trop Med Hyg 1987;36:120–32.
11. World Health Organization. Crimean-Congo haemorrhagic fever. 2001. Available at: http://www.who.int/mediacentre/factsheets/fs208/en/, 2010.
12. Schwarz TF, Nsanze H, Ameen AM. Clinical features of Crimean-Congo haemorrhagic fever in the United Arab Emirates. Infection 1997;25:364–7.
13. Swanepoel R, Shepherd AJ, Leman PA, et al. A common-source outbreak of Crimean-Congo haemorrhagic fever on a dairy farm. S Afr Med J 1985;68:635–7.
14. Sharifi-Mood B, Metanat M, Ghorbani-Vaghei A, et al. The outcome of patients with Crimean-Congo hemorrhagic fever in Zahedan, southeast of Iran: a comparative study. Arch Iran Med 2009;12:151–3.
15. Centers for Disease Control (CDC). Management of patients with suspected viral hemorrhagic fever. MMWR Morb Mortal Wkly Rep 1988;37(suppl. 3):1–16.
16. Centers for Disease Control and Prevention (CDC). Update: management of patients with suspected viral hemorrhagic fever—United States. MMWR Morb Mortal Wkly Rep 1995;30;44:475–9.
17. Fisher-Hoch SP, Khan JA, Rehman S, et al. Crimean Congo-haemorrhagic fever treated with oral ribavirin. Lancet 1995;346:472–5.
18. Swanepoel R, Gill DE, Shepherd AJ, et al. The clinical pathology of Crimean-Congo hemorrhagic fever. Rev Infect Dis 1989;11(suppl. 4):S794–800.
19. Ergonul O, Celikbas A, Dokuzoguz B, et al. Characteristics of patients with Crimean-Congo hemorrhagic fever in a recent outbreak in Turkey and impact of oral ribavirin therapy. Clin Infect Dis 2004;39:284–7.
20. Ergonul O. Treatment of Crimean-Congo hemorrhagic fever. Antiviral Res 2008;78:125–31.
21. Tasdelen Fisgin N, Ergonul O, Doganci L, Tulek N. The role of ribavirin in the therapy of Crimean-Congo hemorrhagic fever: early use is promising. Eur J Clin Microbiol Infect Dis 2009;28:929–33.
22. Vassilenko SM, Vassilev TL, Bozadjiev LG, et al. Specific intravenous immunoglobulin for Crimean-Congo haemorrhagic fever. Lancet 1990;335:791–2.

33.6 Diseases Caused by Hantaviruses

Tony Schountz

Key features

- Hantaviruses are estimated to cause about 150,000 cases of disease each year
- Two diseases are caused by hantaviruses: hantavirus pulmonary syndrome (HPS, sometimes also known as hantavirus cardiopulmonary syndrome) and hemorrhagic fever with renal syndrome (HFRS), which, in its milder form, is known as nephropathia epidemica
- Pathogenic hantaviruses are hosted by multiple rodent reservoirs
- The most important ones are Hantaan (HTNV) virus, found across Asia and central Europe; Seoul virus (SEOV), which is found in many port cities because of its reservoir *Rattus norvegicus*; Dobrava virus (DOBV); and Puumala virus (PUUV)
- The diseases are principally immune-mediated inflammation

INTRODUCTION

During the Korean War (1950–1953) more than 3000 United Nations personnel developed Korean hemorrhagic fever, now termed hemorrhagic fever with renal syndrome (HFRS). Early efforts to identify the etiologic agent suggested a virus, which was first isolated in 1978 [1]. The virus, named Hantaan virus (HTNV) after the Hantan River valley in South Korea, defined a new genus, *Hantavirus*, in the family *Bunyaviridae*. Hantaviruses are enveloped, negative-strand RNA viruses with tripartite genomes. Historical descriptions of diseases with features similar to HFRS date back more than a millennia to ancient China; the earliest documented cases were described in 1913 in Russia [2]. Reports of other diseases associated with 20th century warfare suggest that hantaviruses caused substantial morbidity and mortality during such conflicts. It is likely that hantaviruses have caused substantial morbidity and mortality for much of human history [3].

The natural host for HTNV is the striped field mouse (*Apodemus agrarius*) that is found in Asia and through central Europe. It is thought that transmission between rodents occurs through aggressive male behaviors (e.g. biting) and aerosols during communal nesting. Seoul virus (SEOV), the agent of urban HFRS, is found in many port cities throughout the world as maritime commerce resulted in the dissemination of its reservoir—the brown or Norway rat (*Rattus norvegicus*). Two other hantaviruses are agents of HFRS: Dobrava virus and Puumala virus, which cause a typically milder form of the disease, nephropathia epidemica. It is thought that about 150,000 cases of HFRS occur globally each year, the majority of which are in East Asia [4].

In 1993, an outbreak of a highly fatal, acute respiratory distress syndrome, termed hantavirus (cardio-)pulmonary syndrome (HPS or HCPS) occurred in the Four Corners region of the USA [5, 6]. A novel hantavirus, Sin Nombre virus, was identified as the etiologic agent, with its reservoir host being the deer mouse (*Peromyscus maniculatus*). In South America, most HPS cases are caused by the related Andes virus, which is hosted by the long-tailed pygmy rice rat (*Oligoryzomys longicaudatus*). Several other New World hantaviruses have been discovered, many of which cause HPS and are hosted by rodents of the Neotominae and Sigmodontinae subfamilies (Table 33.6-1) [4].

EPIDEMIOLOGY

Most cases of hantavirus disease occur in rural settings near agricultural communities and where rodents are abundant; however, urban HFRS is associated with Seoul virus because its principal reservoir, *R. norvegicus*, was introduced to port cities by the shipping trade and has since become established in most urban areas [4]. Transmission to humans is thought to primarily occur through inhalation of dried rodent excrement—peri-domestic contact with rodents usually occurs in outbuildings and other permanent structures. A significant risk factor is the cleaning of rodent-infested buildings without proper decontamination procedures and respiratory protection. Humans are terminal hosts for hantaviruses; however, Andes virus has had demonstrated nosocomial and person-to-person transmission (and possibly sexual transmission) that caused several deaths from HPS [7].

NATURAL HISTORY, PATHOGENESIS AND PATHOLOGY

Hantaviruses have been isolated on all continents except Australia (where seropositive rodents have been identified) and Antarctica [5]. Most are not known to cause human disease. Pathogenic hantaviruses are hosted by rodent reservoirs, while hantaviruses hosted by shrews and moles, which are substantially divergent from rodents, are not known to be pathogenic to humans. Each hantavirus species is associated with a single reservoir host species, although spillover events have been documented with several hantaviruses. Infection of reservoir rodents (and presumably shrews and moles) appears to be lifelong and apathogenic, likely because of favorable regulatory immune responses that permit persistence without pathology to the host [8, 9]. As in humans, the principal target of infection in reservoirs is the capillary endothelium, without conspicuous cytopathic effects; virus can be detected in many tissues, with shedding through excrement. For the reservoir hosts and their hantaviruses, this relationship may have evolved to limit inflammatory pathology but also compromise the antiviral immune response to an innocuous infection, thus contributing to persistence and ecology of the viruses.

Human infection follows inhalation of virus. Inhalation introduces virus to the alveoli of the lungs, but how it transits to the vascular endothelium is unknown. Entry into vascular endothelial cells is thought to be via β3-integrin (CD61), a surface transmembrane protein found on several cell types, including capillary endothelial cells. Some dendritic cells are susceptible to hantavirus infection and it may be that pulmonary dendritic cells become infected and traffic to regional lymph nodes and further replication introduces virus to its principal target, capillary endothelial cells [10]. In contrast to the natural rodent hosts, pathology in humans is largely immune-mediated, with the production of pro-inflammatory cytokines that lead to vascular leakage and severe hypotension.

CLINICAL FEATURES

Infection leads to vascular leakage, edema, severe hypotension, hemoconcentration, vasodilation, thrombocytopenia, mobilization of $CD8^+$ T cells and increased leukocyte counts with increased numbers of immature leukocytes; the epithelium remains intact with no histologic evidence of viral damage to the cells [10]. It is evident that the host immune response is substantially involved in the pathogenesis of hantavirus diseases, but a principal difficulty in understanding pathogenic mechanisms is the lack of suitable animal models. While reservoir models are readily available, they do not have pathogenic

TABLE 33.6-1 Pathogenic Hantaviruses

Host subfamily	Rodent species	Virus	Abbreviation	Distribution	Disease
Murinae	*Apodemus agrarius*	Hantaan virus	HTNV	China, South Korea, Russia	HFRS
	Apodemus flavicollis	Dobrava-Belgrade virus	DOBV	Balkans	HFRS
	Rattus norvegicus	Seoul virus	SEOV	Worldwide	HFRS
	Apodemus agrarius	Saaremaa virus	SAAV	Europe	HFRS
	Apodemus peninsulae	Amur virus	AMRV	Far East Russia	HFRS
Arvicolinae	*Clethrionomys glareolus*	Puumala virus	PUUV	Europe, Asia, Americas	HFRS/NE
Neotominae	*Peromyscus maniculatus*	Sin Nombre virus	SNV	North America	HPS
	Peromyscus leucopus	Monogahela virus	MGLV	North America	HPS
	Peromyscus leucopus	New York virus	NYV	North America	HPS
Sigmodontinae	*Sigmodon hispidus*	Black Creek Canal virus	BCCV	North America	HPS
	Oryzomys palustris	Bayou virus	BAYV	North America	HPS
	Olygoryzomys fulvescens	Choclo virus	(not assigned)	Panama	HPS
	Oligoryzomys longicaudatus	Andes virus	ANDV	Argentina, Chile	HPS
	Oligoryzomys chocoenis	Bermejo virus	BMJV	Argentina	HPS
	Oligoryzomys flavescens	Lechiguanas virus	LECV	Argentina	HPS
	Bolomys obscurus	Maciel virus	MCLV	Argentina	HPS
	Oligoryzomys longicaudatus	Oran virus	ORNV	Argentina	HPS
	Calomys laucha	Laguna Negra virus	LANV	Paraguay, Bolivia, Argentina	HPS
	Bolomys lasiurus	Araraquara virus	(not assigned)	Brazil	HPS
	Oligoryzomys nigripes	Juquitiba virus	(not assigned)	Brazil	HPS

NE, neuropathica epidemica.
Adapted from Jonsson CB, Figueiredo LT, Vapalahti O. A global perspective on hantavirus ecology, epidemiology, and disease. Clin Microbiol Rev 2010;23:412–41.

outcomes. The Syrian golden hamster (*Mesocricetus auratus*) infected with Andes or Maporal viruses is a model for HPS; however, very little work has been conducted to assess the role of immuopathology because of a lack of hamster-specific reagents. In addition, both models must be conducted at Biosafety Level (BSL)-4, which limits research activity and productivity. Small animal models for HFRS are currently unavailable.

PATIENT EVALUATION, DIAGNOSIS AND DIFFERENTIAL DIAGNOSIS

HEMORRHAGIC FEVER WITH RENAL SYNDROME

The range of disease is from febrile to acute hemorrhagic shock and death. HFRS occurs in five phases: febrile (3–5 days); hypotensive (hours to two days); oliguric (days to two weeks); polyuric; and convalescent phase. Manifestations of HFRS initiate as a febrile illness and, for many patients, progresses no further. Patients with severe HFRS usually present with an erythematous flush of the face and upper torso, with blanching on pressure. The disease is preceded by a 2–3 week incubation followed by flu-like symptoms of the febrile phase, including fever, chills, dizziness, nausea, vomiting, headache and myalgia. Conjunctivitis and blurred vision are reported by some patients. Petechiae, ecchymoses, hematemesis, epitaxis, hematuria, melena and intracranial hemorrhages are common, and disseminated intravascular coagulation occurs in some patients. The vascular syndrome is followed by the hypotension and shock that can lead to death. Long-term sequelae in some surviving patients include renal dysfunction.

Laboratory findings of acute severe HFRS show development of progressive thrombocytopenia and leukocytosis during the febrile phase that continues into the hypotensive phase. Proteinuria with isosthenuria (production of urine with the specific gravity of plasma) is usually detected within the first five days of onset and hemoconcentration occurs, followed by electrolyte abnormalities and renal insufficiency during the oliguric phase.

The milder nephropathia epidemica shares many of the features of HFRS, including sudden onset of fever, chills, nausea and headache, but is rarely fatal; those that are fatal are usually associated with leukocytosis and shock [11]. Urban HFRS is also a less severe disease, with a fatality rate of about 1% [12]. However, as it is found in urban areas, it is possible that large outbreaks could occur and is thus a public health concern.

At presentation, patients typically have developed an immune response and IgM is usually detectable; neutralizing antibodies to the viral N- and C-terminal glycoproteins (G_N/G_C) are often found in convalescent sera [13]. Neutralizing antibodies to N are not found;

however, protective N-specific cytotoxic T cells have been isolated from blood. Inflammatory cytokines, including tumor necrosis factor (TNF), interleukin-6 (IL-6) and IL-10 have been detected, which are thought to contribute to vascular permeability. The presence of TNF in kidney biopsy samples has been shown to correlate with leukocyte infiltrates. Collectively, these data suggest a prominent role for the immune response in HFRS.

HANTAVIRUS PULMONARY SYNDROME (HPS)

Because of the non-descript symptoms of HPS, it is essential that clinicians consider hantavirus infection in regions where the viruses are endemic [14]. Thrombocytopenia occurs in nearly 80% of HPS patients at presentation and all patients during the course of disease. Leukocytosis with left shift and increased white blood cell counts also occur, and the circulating immunoblastoid lymphocytes include plasma cells. Hemoconcentration is thought to result from the plasma leakage. Chest radiography usually reveals interstitial edema and peribronchial cuffing; many patients develop hypoxemia. All patients develop pleural effusions as the disease progresses. Patients that develop these symptoms should be presumed to have HPS because of the rapid progression of the disease and appropriate treatment regimens employed. An IgM ELISA is used to confirm infection.

HPS typically follows a pattern of four phases: prodrome, pulmonary edema and shock, diuresis and convalescence. Clinical symptoms appear between 10 days to several weeks, with a prodromal period of 3–6 days that includes symptoms of other less severe infectious diseases, such as fever, chills, cough, tachypnea, tachycardia, nausea, headache, myalgia and gastrointestinal symptoms; dyspnea can occur and is often an indicator of imminent respiratory failure [14, 15]. While a small number of individuals recover from acute infection without cardiopulmonary disease, most patients rapidly progress from the prodrome to cardiopulmonary manifestations, with most deaths occurring within 24 hours. This phase typically lasts 3–6 days, followed by rapid progression through diuresis in 24–48 hours. During this phase, patients exhibit high urine flow rates and enter convalescence. Most patients that survive to this phase have a full recovery in a few weeks; however, some patients require up to two years for recovery.

The infected vascular endothelium presents with a capillary leak syndrome and edema. Conspicuous cytopathic effects are not usually present but most cases present with interstitial pneumonitis and mononuclear infiltrates, including immunoblasts (Fig. 33.6.1). Several pro-inflammatory cytokines, including TNF, lymphotoxin, IL-4, interferon-γ and IL-1 are detected in many of these cells at autopsy and suggest a prominent role for the immune response in the pathology of the disease [16]. Collectively, it appears that inflammatory cells recruited from the pulmonary vasculature induce immunopathology to an otherwise seemingly innocuous infection. Convalescence occurs slowly, with weakness and fatigue commonly reported. Without intervention, the mortality rate can be 70% or more, while early diagnosis and treatment results in survival of most patients.

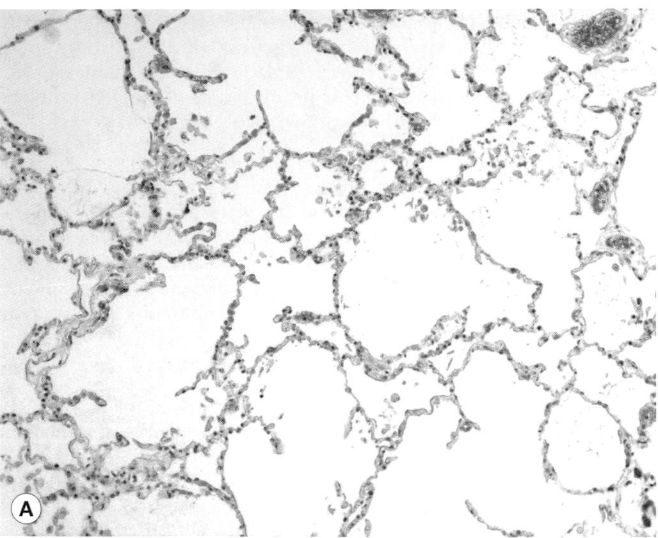

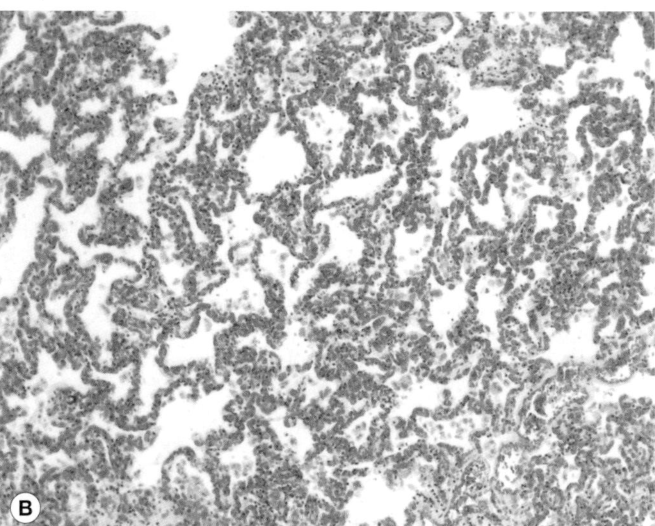

FIGURE 33.6.1 Histologic features of post-mortem lung sections. **(A)** Section from autopsy of normal lung. **(B)** Section from HPS autopsy lung.

TREATMENT

Treatment is principally supportive, with strict management of fluid balance, avoiding dangerous over-hydration in particular, and electrolytes to minimize the inflammatory process [12]. Ribavirin therapy has been shown to reduce the risk of death from HTNV-associated disease when administered early in infection. Intensive care of patients with severe HFRS has reduced fatalities and, when severe hypotension occurs, the use of vasopressor agents and colloidal solutions can maintain blood pressure. Drugs that impact renal function should be avoided and dialysis may be required.

No antiviral or immunosuppressive therapy is currently available for HPS and treatment is largely supportive [14]. The use of extracorporeal membrane oxygenation (ECMO) has dramatically improved survival rates. ECMO supports the heart and lungs and, with pharmacologic intervention, facilitates patient survival during transition to convalescence. Patients must be carefully monitored for shock and respiratory failure, for which an arterial catheter is required to monitor blood pressure. Unlike HFRS, vassopressors should be avoided for HPS because they increase cardiac afterload. Patients should be intubated if a downward trend in arterial blood gases occurs.

DISEASE CONTROL

IMMUNIZATION

Most efforts for hantavirus vaccine development have focused on HFRS because of the substantially greater impact the disease has relative to the fewer cases of HPS [17]. A HTNV formalin-inactivated suckling-mouse brain vaccine, Hantavax, has been available in Korea for more than 10 years. While the vaccine elicits antibody responses, it fails to produce neutralizing antibodies in about half of immunized individuals and its efficacy is unknown. In China, formalin-inactivated cell culture-derived vaccines for HTNV and SEOV induce neutralizing antibody responses in the great majority of recipients who received two or three doses.

Recent approaches in vaccine development have focused on genetically engineered vaccines. A recombinant vaccinia virus expressing the S and M segments of HTNV was developed, but, in trials, many vaccinia virus-immune recipients failed to produce a neutralizing antibody response to HTNV and further work with the vaccine has ceased.

Another molecular approach uses DNA vaccines delivered by gene gun. This technology is attractive because of the rapidity of vaccine development, the potential ability to mix cocktails of plasmids containing genes of various hantaviruses and the relative ease of producing large quantities of vaccine DNA. A significant limitation of this technology is its cost to implement, thus it will be necessary to devise economic strategies for its use in the developing world, where many are at risk of hantavirus diseases. A Phase 1 clinical study is currently being conducted with volunteers receiving multiple doses of DNA coated gold beads into dermal tissue.

Another study demonstrated a neutralizing antibody response in Rhesus macaques immunized with an Andes virus M segment DNA vaccine [18]. While not a pathology model, the level of antibodies produced was similar to those found in convalescent serum samples of HPS survivors. The antibodies also neutralized Sin Nombre virus and suggest the vaccine may be cross-protective. Of note, the vaccine did not protect hamsters from challenge with Andes virus; however, post-infection adoptive transfer of macaque antibodies to hamsters protected them from Andes virus-induced death, suggesting passive antibody therapy may also be useful.

Considering the immunopathologic nature of human hantavirus infections, careful assessment of candidate vaccines will be required to ensure immunization does not prime a pathogenic immune response after natural infection. There is no evidence of such responses with the current Hantavax vaccine, suggesting the risk of such adverse events may be minimal. With HCPS, a strong neutralizing antibody response is associated with favorable outcome, while low titer responses are associated with severe disease [19]. Because hantaviruses replicate slowly, the presence of neutralizing antibodies from immunization will likely confer protection without pathogenic inflammatory responses.

REFERENCES

1. Lee HW, Lee PW, Johnson KM. Isolation of the etiologic agent of Korean Hemorrhagic fever. J Infect Dis 1978;137:298–308.
2. Lee HW. Korean hemorrhagic fever. Prog Med Virol 1982;28:96–113.
3. Johnson KM. Hantaviruses: history and overview. Curr Top Microbiol Immunol 2001;256:1–14.
4. Jonsson CB, Figueiredo LT, Vapalahti O. A global perspective on hantavirus ecology, epidemiology, and disease. Clin Microbiol Rev 2010;23:412–41.
5. Duchin JS, Koster FT, Peters CJ, et al. Hantavirus pulmonary syndrome: a clinical description of 17 patients with a newly recognized disease. The Hantavirus Study Group. N Engl J Med 1994;330:949–55.
6. Nichol ST, Spiropoulou CF, Morzunov S, et al. Genetic identification of a hantavirus associated with an outbreak of acute respiratory illness. Science 1993;262:914–17.
7. Ferres M, Vial P, Marco C, et al. Prospective evaluation of household contacts of persons with hantavirus cardiopulmonary syndrome in chile. J Infect Dis 2007;195:1563–71.
8. Easterbrook JD, Zink MC, Klein SL. Regulatory T cells enhance persistence of the zoonotic pathogen Seoul virus in its reservoir host. Proc Natl Acad Sci USA 2007;104:15502–7.
9. Schountz T, Prescott J, Cogswell AC, et al. Regulatory T cell-like responses in deer mice persistently infected with Sin Nombre virus. Proc Natl Acad Sci USA 2007;104:15496–501.
10. Schonrich G, Rang A, Lutteke N, et al. Hantavirus-induced immunity in rodent reservoirs and humans. Immunol Rev 2008;225:163–89.
11. Valtonen M, Kauppila M, Kotilainen P, et al. Four fatal cases of nephropathia epidemica. Scand J Infect Dis 1995;27:515–17.
12. Linderholm M, Elgh F. Clinical characteristics of hantavirus infections on the Eurasian continent. Curr Top Microbiol Immunol 2001;256:135–51.
13. Vapalahti O, Lundkvist A, Vaheri A. Human immune response, host genetics, and severity of disease. Curr Top Microbiol Immunol 2001;256:153–69.
14. Simpson SQ, Spikes L, Patel S, Faruqi I. Hantavirus pulmonary syndrome. Infect Dis Clin North Am 2010;24:159–73.
15. Zaki SR, Greer PW, Coffield LM, et al. Hantavirus pulmonary syndrome. Pathogenesis of an emerging infectious disease. Am J Pathol 1995; 146:552–79.
16. Mori M, Rothman AL, Kurane I, et al. High levels of cytokine-producing cells in the lung tissues of patients with fatal hantavirus pulmonary syndrome. J Infect Dis 1999;179:295–302.
17. Schmaljohn C. Vaccines for hantaviruses. Vaccine 2009;27(suppl. 4):D61–4.
18. Custer DM, Thompson E, Schmaljohn CS, et al. Active and passive vaccination against hantavirus pulmonary syndrome with Andes virus M genome segment-based DNA vaccine. J Virol 2003;77:9894–905.
19. Bharadwaj M, Nofchissey R, Goade D, et al. Humoral immune responses in the hantavirus cardiopulmonary syndrome. J Infect Dis 2000;182:43–8.

33.7 Rift Valley Fever

Brian H Bird, Jean-Marc Reynes, Stuart T Nichol

The opinions expressed herein are those of the authors alone and not necessarily those of the Centers for Disease Control and Prevention.

Key features

- Mosquito-borne viral zoonosis found in Africa and the western Arabian Peninsula
- A high-consequence disease of livestock (sheep and cattle); wild ruminants are also affected, but to a lesser extent
- Contact with sick animals and animal tissues (especially aborted fetuses and fluids) are major risk factors for human infection
- Human infections are generally self-limiting, but can progress to hepatitis, retinitis or a hemorrhagic syndrome
- Hospitalized case fatality can be 10–30%; high virus loads are predictive of fatal outcomes
- Delayed-onset neurologic signs (confusion, ataxia, seizures, coma) can present 7–28 days after resolution of acute illness

INTRODUCTION

Rift Valley fever virus (RVFV) is a mosquito-borne pathogen of livestock and humans that has historically been responsible for widespread outbreaks of severe livestock and human disease throughout Africa and the western Arabian Peninsula [1]. Rift Valley fever outbreaks often occur in arid or semi-arid regions following unusually heavy rainfall and flooding, allowing the abundant emergence of mosquito vectors. Hallmarks of Rift Valley fever epizootics/epidemics include extensive losses of livestock due to abortion "storms" and neonatal mortality approaching 100% in sheep and cattle that often go unreported and precede large numbers of human cases.

EPIDEMIOLOGY

RVFV is a notorious cause of illness among herdsmen, veterinarians and others with direct contact with infected animals, especially during routine slaughtering, veterinary post-mortem and obstetric procedures. Men and working-aged persons are at greater risk of infection because of higher occupational exposure to livestock and mosquitoes. Wildlife could be affected by the virus, especially wild ruminants, even during interepizootic periods [2, 3]. Although abortion "storms" are a hallmark of livestock infections, there have been no reported cases of human abortion caused by RVFV infection. However, vertical transmission of virus to two newborn infants has been recently reported [4, 5]. Nosocomial transmission has not been documented, but patients often have high viremias, suggesting that standard barrier nursing techniques and universal blood precautions be followed, especially during invasive procedures or while attending births from infected mothers.

NATURAL HISTORY, PATHOGENESIS AND PATHOLOGY

The RVFV (family *Bunyaviridae;* genus *Phlebovirus*) is an enveloped virus with a segmented RNA genome. RVFV was first isolated in the 1930s following a large outbreak among sheep in the Rift Valley of Kenya. Today, it is found in over 30 countries where significant outbreaks occur periodically (Fig. 33.7.1) Human infections can result in isolated individual cases or extensive epidemics with infections numbering tens of thousands. Mosquitoes are the primary vector, although experimental infection of sandflies and ticks has been documented. Humans can be directly infected by mosquito bite or via contact with infected animals (especially livestock) and animal fluids and tissues, including: aborted fetuses, amniotic fluids, uncooked meat and possibly unpasteurized milk [6].

The primary target tissue for the virus is the liver. In fatal cases, extensive hepatocellular necrosis is evident with or without focal inflammatory cell infiltrates [7]. Generally, positive immunostaining for virus antigen can be found in hepatocytes and Kupffer cells and renal tubular epithelial cells. However, RVFV is promiscuous and can infect a wide variety of cell types and tissues. There are no detailed pathologic descriptions of human Rift Valley fever neurologic disease. Experimental animal studies suggest that direct neuron infection and cellular infiltrates contribute to the disease process. In hemorrhagic cases, the exact molecular mechanisms causing alterations in vascular permeability are unknown but are likely mediated by secondary cytokine/chemokine perturbations of endothelial cell barrier functions rather than direct virus infection and the cytopathic effect of endothelial cells. Among fatal RVFV human cases, RVFV does not appear to widely infect endothelial cells, even in the later stages of the disease, unlike some other hemorrhagic fever viruses (e.g. Ebola, Marburg, Crimean-Congo hemorrhagic fever, and the arenavirus hemorrhagic fevers) [3].

CLINICAL FEATURES

Following an incubation period of 2–6 days, most cases present with abrupt onset of fever, malaise, myalgia and arthralgia. A high proportion of patients report nausea, vomiting, abdominal pain and diarrhea; symptoms can clinically resemble other acute viral infections, thus complicating early differential diagnosis [8]. (Fig. 33.7.2, Table 33.7-1). Upper respiratory signs are notably absent in Rift Valley fever cases. A small percentage of infected individuals (1–2%), may develop jaundice, hepatitis, and/or a hemorrhagic syndrome. Case fatalities among hospitalized patients with coagulopathy range from 10–30%. In some patients, retinitis may develop with potential long-term sequelae including scotomas, other vision abnormalities or total blindness [9]. In the largest reported study of laboratory-confirmed hospitalized patients (n = 683, Saudi Arabia 2000–2001) hemorrhagic complications included: thrombocytopenia (38.4%); hematemesis (3.6%); petechiae (2.8%); melena (1.8%); epistaxis (1.2%); excessive bleeding from puncture sites (2.4%); and disseminated intravascular coagulation with multiple organ dysfunction, including renal failure (7.5%) [10]. Laboratory abnormalities included marked elevations of serum transaminases [aspartate transaminase (AST), alanine transaminase (ALT), gamma-glutamyl transferase (GGT)], lactate dehydrogenase (LDH), creatinine phosphokinase (CPK) and creatinine with moderate-to-severe anemia and marked thrombocytopenia. High virus loads (mean titer, $>1.0 \times 10^6$ plaque-forming units/mL of blood) are significantly linked to fatal outcomes [11]. Resolution of the acute phase can be followed 7–28 days later by delayed-onset encephalitis.

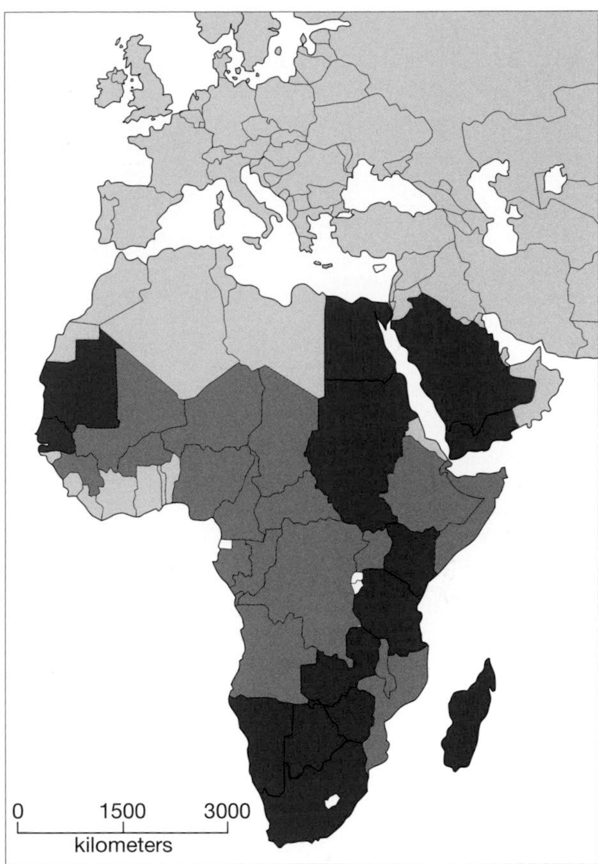

FIGURE 33.7.1 Rift Valley fever geographic distribution. Countries highlighted in dark blue have periodic widespread epidemics of human and/or livestock disease. Countries highlighted in mid-blue have occasional reports of Rift Valley fever virus infection.

PATIENT EVALUATION, DIAGNOSIS AND DIFFERENTIAL DIAGNOSES

Frequent mosquito exposure and/or contact with sick livestock in sub-Saharan Africa or the western Arabian Peninsula should raise a

TABLE 33.7-1 Clinical Signs among Hospitalized Rift Valley Fever Cases (Percent Affected)

	Sudan 2006–07*	Saudi Arabia 2000–01†
General signs		
Fever	90	93
Nausea	n.r	60
Vomiting	0	53
Abdominal pain	2	38
Diarrhea	3	22
Jaundice	35	18
Central nervous system abnormalities	11	17
Confusion	5	8
Vertigo	n.r.	3
Ataxia	n.r.	0.6
Convulsions	1	0.6
Coma	11	3
Hemorrhagic manifestations	36	7
Hematemesis	36	4
Petechiae	2	3
Gingival bleeding	21	1.4
Epistaxis	36	1.2
Conjunctival hemorrhage	10	1.2
Hematuria	16	n.r.

*N=194 patients [14].

†N varies between 475 to 532 patients depending on clinical sign [10].

n.r., not reported.

high index of suspicion for Rift Valley fever [12]. Initial Rift Valley fever presentation is often nonspecific and similar to severe malaria, leptospirosis or other viral hemorrhagic fevers, including Ebola, Marburg, Crimean-Congo hemorrhagic fever, Lassa fever, Yellow fever or Dengue fever. Patient contact with ticks, rodents, bats and nonhuman primates are not thought to be significant risk factors for Rift Valley fever and may be more indicative of Crimean-Congo hemorrhagic fever (ticks) or leptospirosis and Lassa (rodents), Ebola and Marburg (bats and nonhuman primates).

Diagnosis can be accomplished by serology and nucleic acid amplification testing [reverse transcription (RT)-PCR] or virus isolation from whole blood or serum. Post-mortem tissues can be submitted for immunohistochemical staining. Owing to safety concerns, post-mortem examinations should be performed only after consultation with national diagnostic reference centers. Handling of laboratory specimens and virus culture should only be performed in Biosafety Level (BSL)-3+- or BSL-4-capable laboratories by trained personnel. RVFV is labile and decontamination can be accomplished by use of strong detergents or 10% solutions of sodium hypochlorite (bleach).

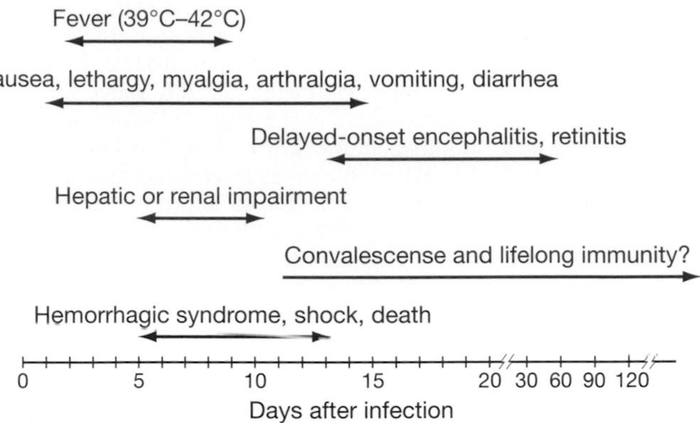

FIGURE 33.7.2 A timeline indicating the onset and duration of the major expected clinical signs of Rift Valley fever.

TREATMENT AND PREVENTION

Treatment of Rift Valley fever patients is primarily symptomatic. For the majority of patients, the disease is self-limiting. Drugs that may have potential hepatotoxic, nephrotoxic or negative effects on coagulation factors and platelet function should be avoided. Ribavirin, a guanosine analogue, is a potent antiviral drug and may be of benefit among severely affected Rift Valley fever patients [13]. However, an efficacy trial undertaken during the Rift Valley fever outbreak in Saudi Arabia in 2000 was terminated because of adverse events. The data were suggestive that ribavirin may potentiate the neurologic form of Rift Valley fever. Pharmacokinetic studies have shown that the drug has poor central nervous system penetration and Rift Valley fever animal models also suggest that treatment increases the risk of delayed-onset neurologic complications. A safe and effective formalin-inactivated vaccine was developed for human use in the 1970s, but is no longer available. There are no currently licensed veterinary vaccines for use in North America or the European Union. Live-attenuated vaccines are available for use in endemic areas, but are contraindicated in young or pregnant animals as a result of teratogenic and abortifacient properties. Several novel human and veterinary vaccine candidates (recombinant live-attenuated, virus-like particle, DNA-based and subunit approaches) are under development, but none are commercially available at this time.

REFERENCES

1. Bird BH, Ksiazek TG, Nichol ST, Maclachlan NJ. Rift Valley fever virus. J Am Vet Med Assoc 2009;234:883–93.
2. Evans A, Gakuya F, Paweska JT, et al. Prevalence of antibodies against Rift Valley fever virus in Kenyan wildlife. Epidemiol Infect 2008;136:1261–9.
3. Swanepoel R, Coetzer JAW. Rift Valley fever. In: Infectious diseases of livestock. Oxford: Oxford University Press; 2004:1037–70.
4. Adam I, Karsany MS. Case report: Rift Valley Fever with vertical transmission in a pregnant Sudanese woman. J Med Virol 2008;80:929.
5. Arishi HM, Aqeel AY, Al Hazmi MM. Vertical transmission of fatal Rift Valley fever in a newborn. Ann Trop Paediatr 2006;26:251–3.
6. Pepin M, Bouloy M, Bird BH, et al. Rift Valley fever virus (Bunyaviridae: Phlebovirus): an update on pathogenesis, molecular epidemiology, vectors, diagnostics and prevention. Vet Res. 2010;41:61.
7. Shieh WJ, Paddock CD, Lederman E, et al. Pathologic studies on suspect animal and human cases of Rift Valley fever from an outbreak in Eastern Africa, 2006–2007. Am J Trop Med Hyg 2010;83(suppl. 2):38–42.
8. Kahlon SS, Peters CJ, Leduc J, et al. Severe Rift Valley fever may present with a characteristic clinical syndrome. Am J Trop Med Hyg 2010;82:371–5.
9. Al-Hazmi A, Al-Rajhi AA, Abboud EB, et al. Ocular complications of Rift Valley fever outbreak in Saudi Arabia. Ophthalmology 2005;112: 313–18.

10. Madani TA, Al-Mazrou YY, Al-Jeffri MH, et al. Rift Valley fever epidemic in Saudi Arabia: Epidemiological, clinical, and laboratory characteristics. Clin Infect Dis 2003;37:1084–92.
11. Bird BH, Bawiec DA, Ksiazek TG et al. Highly sensitive and broadly reactive quantitative reverse transcription-PCR assay for high-throughput detection of Rift Valley fever virus. J Clin Microbiol 2007;45:3506–13.
12. Anyangu AS, Gould LH, Sharif SK, et al. Risk factors for severe Rift Valley fever infection in Kenya, 2007. Am J Trop Med Hyg 2010;83(suppl. 2):14–21.
13. Peters CJ, Reynolds JA, Slone TW. Prophylaxis of Rift Valley fever with antiviral drugs, immune serum, an interferon inducer, and a macrophage activator, Antiviral Res 1986;6:285–97.
14. El Imam MM, El Sabiq M, Omran A, et al. Acute renal failure associated with the Rift Valley fever: a single center study. Saudi J Kidney Dis Transpl 2009;20: 1047–52.

34 Viral CNS Infections

34.1 Rabies and Related Viruses

Mary J Warrell, David A Warrell

Key features

- The genus *Lyssavirus* of the *Rhabdoviridae* includes rabies and rabies-related viruses, causing at least 55,000 human deaths annually, mainly in Asia and Africa
- The greatest threat of rabies to man is the persistent cycle of infection in stray dogs, but several other terrestrial mammal species are reservoirs and there is evidence of widespread infection in bats. In the Americas, bat viruses are classic genotype 1 rabies. Elsewhere, all bat lyssaviruses are other genotypes (rabies-related viruses)
- Rabies virus can penetrate broken skin and intact mucosae. Humans are usually infected when virus-laden saliva is inoculated through the skin by the bite of a rabid animal
- After a variable, often prolonged, incubation period, signs of furious or paralytic rabies portend a rapidly fatal course. The mechanism of neuronal dysfunction is unknown
- In developing countries, diagnosis relies on recognition of hydrophobic spasms or other clinical features. Paralytic disease is less easily identified and is misdiagnosed globally. The diagnosis can be made during life, but lack of facilities often hampers confirmation of disease
- An unvaccinated patient bitten by a bat in North America has recovered from rabies encephalitis following intensive care. Clinically and experimentally the American bat strains of rabies genotype 1 viruses are less pathogenic; dog rabies virus infection remains universally fatal in humans. No treatment has proved effective experimentally and intensive care therapy is rarely indicated
- Ninety-nine percent of human deaths could be prevented by controlling the transmission of dog rabies, but education and resources are lacking. Combined pre- and post-exposure prophylaxis has proved 100% effective in humans. Pre-exposure immunization should be encouraged, but the cost may be prohibitive. Intradermal post-exposure vaccine regimens could increase the affordability of treatment

INTRODUCTION

Rabies is a zoonosis of wild and domestic mammals that may be transmitted to humans, usually by the bite of a rabid dog. Rabies viruses are bullet-shaped, single-stranded, negative-sense RNA viruses.

Encephalitis caused by dog rabies virus is invariably fatal in humans. The disease is enzootic in certain carnivore and bat species throughout most parts of the world. The highest human rabies mortality is in developing countries where rabies is uncontrolled in domestic dogs. Rabies and six genotypes of rabies-related viruses comprise the genus *Lyssavirus* of the Rhabdoviridae.

EPIDEMIOLOGY

Rabies is enzootic worldwide [1] with the exception of Antarctica and a number of islands, including Iceland, Ireland, New Guinea, New Zealand, Japan, Taiwan, Singapore and some Mediterranean and Caribbean islands. Western Europe and Australia are free of rabies in terrestrial mammals but bats may harbor rabies-related lyssaviruses. Human rabies is generally under-reported. A conservative estimate of annual mortality in Asia and Africa is 55,000. Countries with a high incidence of human rabies include India, Pakistan and Bangladesh. In the USA, 42 cases were recognized in the last 15 years; 21% were infected abroad. Ninety-seven percent of indigenous infections were due to bat rabies viruses.

The major reservoir and vector of rabies is the domestic dog, causing >99% of human infections. Sylvatic rabies occurs predominantly in skunks, raccoons, foxes and insectivorous bats in North America; foxes in the Arctic; mongooses in some Caribbean islands; vampire bats in Latin America and Trinidad; jackals, wolves and small carnivores in Africa and Asia; and foxes, wolves and raccoon dogs in Europe. Transmission occurs to vectors, for example cats which may infect humans, but there is no cycle of infection within vector species. Vampire bats (*Desmodontinae*) are confined to southern Texas, Mexico, Central and South America, and some Caribbean islands. They feed on, and infect cattle, resulting in the loss of 100,000 cattle per year. Recent outbreaks of vampire bat rabies in humans occurred in Peruvian jungle areas, possibly as a result of disturbances of bat ecology. The reservoirs and distribution of rabies-related viruses [1] are listed in Table 34.1-1.

In dogs, the incubation period is usually between 2 weeks and 4 months. The symptoms include a change in behavior, fever and intense irritation at the site of the bite. Dogs can become aggressive or, more often, have paralytic or "dumb" rabies with dysphagia and drooling of saliva. Virus may be excreted in the saliva for 2 or 3 days before there are signs of rabies and the animal usually dies within the next 7 days. Hydrophobia is not seen in animals but the inability to drink is a common symptom of rabies.

Human rabies usually results from inoculation of virus-bearing saliva through the skin by the bite of a rabid dog. Scratches, abrasions and

TABLE 34.1-1 Lyssaviruses Causing Human Disease

Lyssavirus genotype	Virus	Where virus found	Geographic range	Human disease (number of reported cases)
1	Rabies	Terrestrial mammals and bats in Americas	Widespread	Furious or paralytic
3	Mokola*	Shrew, mouse, cat, dog	Nigeria, Cameroon, Central African Republic, Ethiopia, Zimbabwe, Southern Africa	
		Human	Nigeria	Febrile convulsion, pharangitis† Fatal paralytic encephalitis† (1, 2)
4	Duvenhage	Insectivorous bat, fruit bat	South Africa, Zimbabwe	
		Human	South Africa, Kenya	Furious rabies (1, 2, 6)
5	European bat lyssavirus 1	Insectivorous bat	Across Continental Europe into Russia	
		Human	Russia	Furious/paralytic rabies (2)
6	European bat lyssavirus 2	Insectivorous bat	Netherlands, Ukraine, Germany, UK, Switzerland, Finland	
		Human	Finland, UK	Furious/paralytic rabies (2)
7	Australian bat lyssavirus	Fruit bats, insectivorous bat	Australia	
		Human	Australia	Furious/paralytic rabies (2)

*Mokola virus is in a separate phylogroup, less pathogenic than other genotypes and does not cross-neutralize with rabies, or rabies vaccines.
†Questionable diagnosis.

other wounds (also intact mucosal membranes) can be contaminated with infected saliva. Rare modes of infection are: transplantation of infected organ grafts from donors who had died of unsuspected rabies [2]; inapparent contact with bats in caves; and inhalation of virus aerosols as a result of laboratory accidents. Despite a single report of congenital or neonatal infection, many infants of infected mothers have remained healthy. No transmission of infection to hospital staff or other carers has been recorded [3].

NATURAL HISTORY, PATHOGENESIS AND PATHOLOGY

Following inoculation, rabies virus may replicate locally in myocytes before entering peripheral motor neurons by endocytosis. It is conveyed by the retrograde axonal transport mechanism towards the central nervous system (CNS) via transsynaptic spread. The virus remains intraneuronal, with massive replication in the brain [4]. Centrifugal spread of virus from the CNS along nerves infects the salivary glands (where it is shed and, in infected animals, spread by the bite), lacrimal glands, skin, respiratory tract, myocardium and many other tissues. In animals, virus is detectable in the skin before the development of symptoms.

Histopathologic changes may be surprisingly mild in victims. In furious rabies, the midbrain and medulla are mainly involved, and, in paralytic rabies, the spinal cord. Changes include ganglion cell degeneration, perineural and perivascular mononuclear cell infiltration, neuronophagia and the formation of glial nodules. Negri bodies, the characteristic intracytoplasmic inclusion bodies, are viral factories containing RNA and accumulated viral proteins.

In unvaccinated patients with rabies encephalomyelitis, no antibody response is detectable in serum or cerebrospinal fluid (CSF) until the second week of illness and may not appear before death. Experimentally, neutralizing antibody in the brain is associated with survival. Following vaccination, viral glycoprotein induces neutralizing antibody, which is protective against disease.

CLINICAL FEATURES

CLINICAL MANIFESTATIONS

The incubation period is usually between 20 and 90 days (extreme range, 4 days to >19 years). Relatively short incubation periods are observed after facial and severe multiple bites. The prodromal symptom most suggestive of rabies encephalitis is paresthesia, especially itching, at the site of the healed bite wound. Other early symptoms include fever, mood changes and nonspecific upper respiratory tract or gastrointestinal symptoms. The determinants of the clinical forms of rabies, furious (agitated) and paralytic (dumb) are unknown, but both viral and host factors, and possibly the route of infection, are suspected.

Furious Rabies [5]

This is the more commonly recognized presentation. After a few days of prodromal symptoms, the pathognomonic symptom and sign of hydrophobia or aerophobia develops (Fig. 34.1.1). A series of forceful, jerky, inspiratory spasms is provoked either by attempts to drink water or by a draft of air on the face. Both reflexes are associated with a compelling, but inexplicable terror. Splashing water on the skin, irritation of the respiratory tract, or, by conditioning, the sight, sound, or even the mention of water may provoke a hydrophobic spasm. Patients also experience episodic generalized arousal during which they become wild, hallucinated and sometimes aggressive. During lucid intervals, they cerebrate normally and are aware of their terrible predicament. Neurologic abnormalities include meningism, cranial nerve lesions, upper motor neuron lesions, fasciculation and involuntary movements. Generalized hyperesthesia or hyperacusis is described. Hypersalivation, lacrimation (Fig. 34.1.2), sweating, fluctuating blood pressure and body temperature, and diabetes insipidus, or rarely, inappropriate secretion of antidiuretic hormone, suggest disturbances of the hypothalamus. Lesions of the amygdaloid nuclei probably account for increased libido, priapism and spontaneous orgasms. Without intensive care, most patients die within a few days

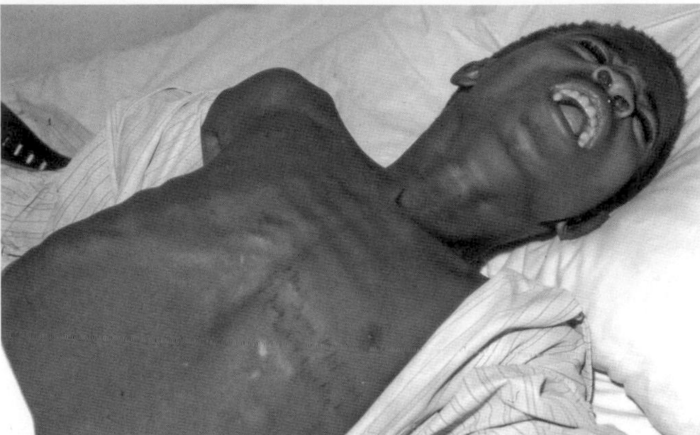

FIGURE 34.1.1 Hydrophobic spasm ending in opisthotonos in an African boy with furious rabies. *(Courtesy of David A Warrell)*

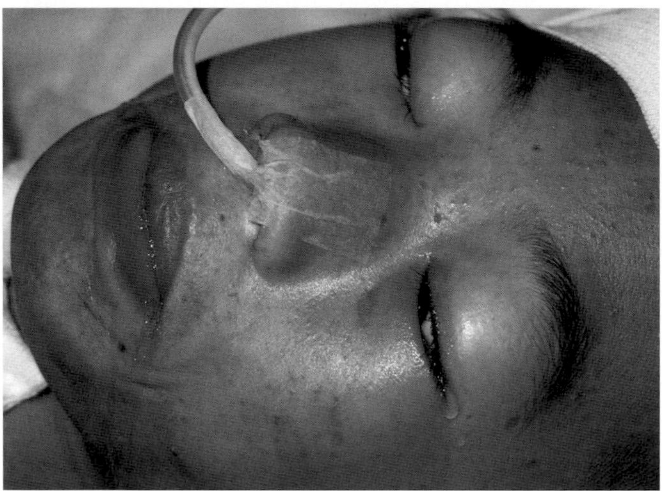

FIGURE 34.1.2 Hypersalivation, lacrimation and sweating in a Thai man with furious rabies. *(Courtesy of David A Warrell)*

of developing hydrophobia. About a third of patients die during a hydrophobic spasm, whereas the others lapse into coma with various abnormalities of respiratory rhythm.

Paralytic Rabies [5]

This is less distinctive and is undoubtedly under-diagnosed. Almost all the cases of rabies transmitted by vampire and other bats in the Americas were of this type. After the usual prodromal symptoms, especially fever, headache and local paresthesia, flaccid paralysis develops (usually in the bitten limb) and ascends symmetrically or asymmetrically with pain and fasciculation in the affected muscles and mild sensory disturbance. Paraplegia and sphincter involvement then develop and finally fatal paralysis of deglutitive and respiratory muscles. Hydrophobia is rare. Patients may survive for a month, even without intensive care.

Complications of Prolonged Survival [5]

Patients with rabies whose lives are prolonged by intensive care may develop a wide range of complications, including: aspiration pneumonia; pneumothorax; respiratory failure; cardiac arrhythmias; hypotension; pulmonary edema; myocarditis with congestive cardiac failure; generalized convulsions; cerebral edema; polyneuropathy; and hematemesis associated with ulceration or tears in the mucosa of the upper gastrointestinal tract.

Infections by Rabies-Related Viruses

(Table 34.1-1) [1, 2, 6]

These are clinically indistinguishable from rabies genotype 1 encephalitis, but they are unlikely to be recognized, as rabies is almost always diagnosed clinically in Asia and Africa. The diagnostic rabies immunofluorescent antigen test (IFAT) may be weakly positive or negative. Few laboratories are equipped to identify other genotypes.

PATIENT EVALUATION, DIAGNOSIS AND DIFFERENTIAL DIAGNOSIS [4]

Rabies should be suspected in any patient who develops neurologic symptoms more than a week after being bitten by a mammal, but there may be no history of exposure, especially after bat contact. Rabies is often misdiagnosed. In patients with furious rabies, the alteration in mood, hallucinations and bizarre behavior may raise suspicions of psychiatric disease, hysteria, malingering or rabies phobia. Other patients are referred to otolaryngologists. The spasms of tetanus may resemble hydrophobia, especially if they involve the pharyngeal muscles (cephalic tetanus). The combination of severe brain stem encephalitis with full consciousness in rabies is rare in other encephalitides, but has been described in serum sickness. Various poisons, drugs and plant toxins, including strychnine, phenothiazines, atropine-like compounds, cannabis and ethanol, can produce syndromes of muscle spasm, agitation, hallucinations, psychiatric disturbances, signs of autonomic nervous system stimulation and convulsions. Paralytic rabies should be considered in patients with rapidly ascending (Landry type) flaccid paralysis, suspected Guillain-Barré syndrome and transverse myelitis. Poliomyelitis is distinguished by the lack of sensory abnormalities. *Cercopithecine herpesvirus* encephalomyelitis, very rarely transmitted by monkey bites, has an incubation period of only a few days.

DIAGNOSIS

In humans, rabies encephalitis can be best confirmed rapidly during life by tests on skin biopsy or saliva samples (Table 34.1-2) [2, 3]. Rabies virus may be isolated early in the illness, before antibody appears. Pleocytosis may be absent initially. Brain imaging gives variable results.

PROGNOSIS

In unvaccinated people infection with canine rabies virus remains universally fatal. However, prolonged survival or recovery from rabies [2] has been reported in eight patients. All were diagnosed serologically and no virus or antigen was identified. Five had been given pre- or post-exposure vaccine and survived months or years with profound neurologic impairment.

A boy bitten by a bat in Ohio in 1970, was vaccinated late, treated with intensive care and made a complete recovery. The first unvaccinated patient to survive rabies was bitten by a bat in Milwaukee, Wisconsin in 2004 [7]. She developed typical encephalitis, without hydrophobia. Rabies antibody was already detectable on the sixth day of illness. Following intensive care treatment (ICT), including coma induction and nonspecific antiviral therapy, she recovered with only minimal neurologic deficits. Both these patients are likely to have had antibody at an early stage of the disease, and treatment probably maintained vital functions until the immune response, including neutralizing antibody, eliminated the virus, with some loss of infected neurons. Experimental evidence suggests that American bat rabies viruses are less pathogenic than canine and other terrestrial mammal strains—although they are all Genotype 1 viruses, they form a genetically distinct group.

In a remarkable report, a teenager in Texas in 2009 mentioned bats hitting her in a cave. Two months later, headaches, photophobia, vomiting and parasthesiae of face and forearms developed, with right-sided weakness. She had lymphocytic pleocytosis and a trace of rabies antibody was detected in serum and CSF but no antigen or virus was

TABLE 34.1-2 Laboratory Diagnostic Methods

Sample		Method
Full thickness skin* punch biopsy	Antigen detection	IFA test on frozen section[†] RT-PCR
Saliva or throat swab* Tears CSF	Virus isolation and antigen detection	Tissue culture Mouse inoculation test RT-PCR
Serum	Antibody test [‡]	Presence of antibody is diagnostic in unvaccinated patients If previously vaccinated, save sample for comparison later
CSF	Antibody test [‡]	Test in parallel with serum
Brain post-mortem: needle necropsy[§] or autopsy sample brain stem and cerebellum	Virus isolation and antigen detection	Tissue culture mouse inoculation test IFA test on impression smear RT-PCR

*Most useful samples for antigen detection, repeat daily until a diagnosis is confirmed.
[†]Rabies antigen seen in nerve twiglets around the base of hair follicles by immunofluorescence (IFA) test.
[‡]Immunofluorescent antibody test is rapid and sensitive. Neutralizing antibody test takes ≥2 days.
[§]Necropsies are taken with a long biopsy needle via the medial canthus of the eye; through the superior orbital fissure; via the nose through the ethmoid bone; or through the foramen magnum or open fontanelles in children.

found. She recovered from presumed mild American bat rabies virus encephalitis, but has been lost to follow-up.

TREATMENT AND PREVENTION

Experimentally, no treatment has proved effective and several other patients, bitten by bats or dogs, were treated with the Milwaukee ICT regimen without recovery. Hence, unvaccinated patients infected by dog rabies should be given palliation with heavy sedation and analgesia to relieve the agonizing symptoms and post-exposure prophylaxis offered to contacts [2]. Previously vaccinated patients given ICT have a remote chance of survival with severe neurologic sequelae. ICT should, however, be considered for American bat infections at an early stage of disease, especially if rabies antibody is present. Otherwise, it is advisable to palliate until new antiviral methods prove effective in animals.

PRE-EXPOSURE PROPHYLAXIS [8]

Immunization is recommended for anyone at risk of exposure to infection, for example veterinarians, laboratory workers, dog catchers, zoologists, other field workers, cave explorers and people visiting or resident in dog rabies-enzootic countries. An intramuscular (IM) dose of tissue culture vaccine (Table 34.1-3) is given on days 0, 7 and 28 [9]. The final dose can be advanced towards day 21 if necessary, but the antibody level may wane more rapidly. Booster doses are given according to the level of risk, from every 6 months in some laboratory workers, to 5 years if lower risk, for example animal handlers. If neutralizing antibody is detectable, boosting is unnecessary. In the USA, no boosters are recommended for travelers [10]. Further vaccine is needed urgently following possible exposure (see below). If vaccine is scarce or unaffordable, an alternative intradermal (ID) dose of 0.1 ml over the deltoid is immunogenic and also economical if more than one person can be immunized on the same day. This has been previously used in the USA and pharmaceutical regulations might permit its re-introduction. ID pre-exposure immunization should not be used for immunosuppressed people or those taking chloroquine medication.

POST-EXPOSURE PROPHYLAXIS (Table 34.1-3)

To evaluate the risk of exposure, ask about the local epidemiology; the appearance, behavior, fate and vaccination status of the animal involved and also the precise nature and severity of the wounds. Unusual contact with a bat anywhere should be considered as a possible exposure. If treatment is indicated, start immediately, even if the incident was many months ago.

TABLE 34.1-3 Post-Exposure Prophylaxis for Use in a Rabies-Enzootic Area*

Exposure	Treatment
Minor Exposure Minor scratches or abrasions without bleeding	*Start vaccine*[†]: stop treatment if animal remains healthy for 10 days or if laboratory test on animal's brain proves negative
Major Exposure Licks of mucosa or broken skin Transdermal bites or scratches Contact with suspect bat	*Rabies immunoglobulin*[‡] *and vaccine*: stop if domestic cat or dog remains healthy for 10 days or if laboratory test on animal's brain proves negative

*Following an unprovoked attack by cat or dog or an attack by wild animal. Adapted from World Health Organization: Expert Consultation on Rabies. First Report. Technical Report Series 931. Geneva, WHO 2005.
[†]Human diploid cell vaccine (Sanofi Pasteur, Lyon, France) and purified chick embryo cell vaccine (Rabavert™/Rabipur™; Novartis) are used in the USA. Purified Vero cell vaccine (Verorab™; Sanofi Pasteur) may be also available elsewhere, but a single dose vial contains 0.5 ml, whereas the other two are in 1 ml vials. See text for vaccine regimens.
[‡]Rabies immunoglobulin (RIG) is most important for severe rabies exposure (bites on the head, neck or hands, or multiple bites). Injection into and around the wound should neutralize the virus, providing some protection during the first week until the vaccine induces immunity. If local infiltration is anatomically impossible, give the rest intramuscularly at a site remote from the vaccine, but not into gluteal adipose tissue. The dose of 20 units/kg body weight of human RIG (or 40 units/kg equine RIG in some countries) must not be exceeded.

Local Measures

Bite wounds, scratches, or abrasions that may have been contaminated by infected saliva should be scrubbed with soap or detergent and rinsed energetically, using analgesia if necessary. Wounds should be irrigated with povidone-iodine or 40–70% alcohol. Suturing should be avoided, or delayed, wherever possible. The risk of other pathogens associated with mammal bites, especially tetanus, should be considered. Intact skin is a barrier to infection, but lesions from bats may be undetectable.

Specific prophylaxis aims to deliver rabies neutralizing antibody rapidly at the wound site. Passive immunization with rabies immunoglobulin (RIG) provides immediate temporary therapy until the immune response to primary vaccination appears. Cell culture vaccines (Table 34.1-3) are recommended, but the obsolete Semple and suckling mouse brain vaccines are still used.

Post-exposure Vaccine [8]

The five-dose IM post-exposure vaccine regimen comprises: one dose, injected into the deltoid or anterolateral thigh area (not the gluteal region), on days 0, 3, 7, 14 and 28 [9, 10]. In the USA, if there is a vaccine shortage, the final dose can be omitted, providing that RIG was given and the patient is otherwise healthy. An alternative four-dose IM regimen is: two doses on day 0, and one dose on days 7 and 21 [9].

A new, economical post-exposure four-site ID regimen [8] is as immunogenic as the five-dose IM regimen. It uses a whole ampoule of vaccine, divided between four ID injections over the deltoid and either the thigh or suprascapular areas on day 0. The volume per site is about 0.1 ml for vaccines containing 0.5 ml/ampoule and the equivalent dose for vaccines of 1 ml/ ampoule is 0.2 ml. On day 7, two ID injections (0.1/ 0.2 ml as above) are followed by a single ID dose on day 28. If a 1 ml/ampoule vaccine is used when resources are limited and more than one patient is treated on the same day, an alternative half ID dose of 0.1 ml/ ID site can be given on each occasion (days 0, 7 and 28). Ampoules of vaccine are shared, but remaining vaccine must be kept in the fridge and discarded at the end of the day. A two-site ID regimen is ID doses at two sites on days 0, 3, 7 and 28 [9].

Those who have received pre- or post-exposure vaccination do not require passive immunization. If they are then exposed to rabies, IM cell culture vaccine is given on days 0 and 3. An alternative, single-day regimen requires only one ampoule of vaccine divided between four ID injections over the deltoid and the thigh or suprascapular areas (the same as the initial dose of the four-site ID regimen). If a 1 ml/ ampoule vaccine is used, sharing between two is still immunogenic as above [8].

Passive immunization is recommended with primary post-exposure treatments (see Table 34.1-3).

Efficacy of Post-exposure Prophylaxis

Combined active and passive immunization given on the day of the bite, with optimum wound care, can reduce the risk of rabies from between 15 to 60% in untreated cases to practically zero with tissue culture vaccines. The risk varies with the biting species, the site and severity of the bites. Prophylaxis may fail if treatment is delayed, inadequate or if the vaccinee is immunosuppressed. Rabies vaccines may be less effective against the rabies-related viruses and ineffective against Mokola virus. Pre-exposure immunization has proved universally effective if followed by a booster vaccination after exposure.

Complications of Rabies Vaccines

Tissue culture vaccines cause mild local reactions or transient, influenza-like symptoms in a small minority of vaccinees. Intradermal injections may cause transient irritation. Pre-exposure booster injections have caused a mild allergic urticarial rash, angioedema and arthralgia within 2 weeks, which responds to symptomatic treatment.

CONTROL OF ANIMAL RABIES

Rabies can be controlled effectively in stray dogs by campaigns of vaccination, contraception and reducing available food and shelter. Control of wildlife rabies has been achieved by oral, live-attenuated or vaccinia recombinant rabies vaccines in baits. Fox rabies has been eliminated from Western Europe and recombinant vaccines have produced promising results in foxes, raccoons and coyotes in the USA. Oral vaccines for a variety of other species in America (e.g. skunks) and Africa (e.g. black-backed jackals) are being developed. Oral vaccines for stray dogs have not been practicable to date.

REFERENCES

1. Nel LH, Markotter W. Lyssaviruses. Crit Rev Microbiol 2007;33:301–24.
2. Jackson AC. Human disease. In: Jackson AC, Wunner AH, eds. Rabies, 2nd edn. London: Elsevier, Academic Press; 2007:309–40.
3. Helmick CG, Tauxe RV, Vernon AA. Is there a risk to contacts of patients with rabies? Rev Infect Dis 1987;9:511–18.
4. Schnell MJ, McGettigan JP, Wirblich C, Papaneri A. The cell biology of rabies virus: using stealth to reach the brain. Nat Rev Microbiol 2010;8:51–61.
5. Warrell DA. The clinical picture of rabies in man. Trans R Soc Trop Med Hyg 1976;70:188.
6. van Thiel PP, de Bie RM, Eftimov F, et al. Fatal Human Rabies due to Duvenhage Virus from a Bat in Kenya: Failure of Treatment with Coma-Induction, Ketamine, and Antiviral Drugs. PLoS Negl Trop Dis 2009;3(7):e428.
7. Willoughby RE Jr, Tieves KS, Hoffman GM, et al. Survival after treatment of rabies with induction of coma. N Engl J Med 2005;352:2508–14.
8. Warrell MJ. Current rabies vaccines and prophylaxis schedules: preventing rabies before and after exposure. Travel Med Inf Dis 2012 (in press) doi:10.1016/j.tmaid.2011.12.005.
9. World Health Organization. Expert Consultation on Rabies. First Report. Technical Report Series 931. Geneva: World Health Organization; 2005.
10. Human rabies prevention—United States, 2008: recommendations of the Advisory Committee on Immunization Practices. MMWR Recomm Rep 2008;57(RR-3):1–28.

34.2 Enterovirus Infections That Cause Central Nervous System Disease (including Poliomyelitis)

Peter C McMinn, Phan Van Tu

Key features

- Enteroviruses are among the most common human pathogens and cause a wide array of clinical syndromes, ranging from the trivial to severe and life-threatening
- The virtual eradication of epidemic poliomyelitis by an international vaccination campaign coordinated by the World Health Organization is a major achievement in public health
- Enterovirus 71, which causes hand-foot-and-mouth diseases and epidemic encephalomyelitis, has recently emerged as a new public health threat in the Asia-Pacific region
- Currently, there are no licensed antiviral agents available to treat severe enterovirus infections and no vaccines are available to prevent non-polio enterovirus infections.

INTRODUCTION

Enteroviruses are among the most common of human infections and are estimated to infect 50 million people annually in the USA and one billion annually worldwide. Although the majority (~90%) of infections are asymptomatic, enteroviruses are associated with a wide spectrum of disease manifestations, including: fever and rash; acute hemorrhagic conjunctivitis; upper respiratory tract infection; myocarditis and pericarditis; pleurodynia; aseptic meningitis, encephalitis; poliomyelitis; severe neonatal infection; and chronic infection in immunocompromised patients. The majority of acute enterovirus infections (>80%) occur in children below 15 years of age, owing, in part, to a lack of immunologic experience and cross-protective immunity to enterovirus infection, and to childhood behaviors that promote fecal–oral and person-to-person transmission of infection.

Human enteroviruses are small, positive-sense RNA viruses that belong to the family *Picornaviridae* and have traditionally been grouped into the echoviruses, coxsackie A and B viruses, and polioviruses based on their growth properties in cell culture and in infant mice. As this system of classification is somewhat arbitrary, since the mid-1960s newly identified enteroviruses have simply been assigned a numerical designation, the first example being "enterovirus 68." The number of individual enterovirus strains now recognized is greater than 100 [1]. Recent molecular analysis of the enterovirus genome has led to the adoption of a new taxonomy in which enteroviruses are divided into four species: human enterovirus A, B, C and D.

In this chapter, the epidemiology, pathophysiology, clinical presentation, differential diagnosis and management of enterovirus infections that cause neurologic diseases, in particular polioviruses and enterovirus 71, are presented. Enteroviruses that predominantly cause mucocutaneous disease only are discussed in Chapter 28.3.

EPIDEMIOLOGY

Enterovirus infections occur in all human populations. Enterovirus infections occur throughout the year but are more highly prevalent in summer and autumn in temperate regions. More than 80% of enterovirus infections occur in children younger than 15 years of age and attack rates are highest in infants under the age of 1 year old. The prevalence of enterovirus infections is greater in situations of poverty, overcrowding and poor personal hygiene.

The frequency with which individual enterovirus serotypes cause infection varies markedly. Some enterovirus serotypes are continuously isolated from year-to-year, whilst others may temporarily emerge after years of relative inactivity. Individual enterovirus serotypes tend to circulate for a variable period of time before they are replaced by new serotypes. Typically, 5–10 serotypes are responsible for >85% of enterovirus infection at any one time, with considerable differences in serotype distribution between geographic locations. Occasionally, global epidemics may occur, such as hemorrhagic conjunctivitis pandemics caused by enterovirus 70 or coxsackievirus A24.

Virtually all enterovirus serotypes have been associated with aseptic meningitis. In the pre-polio vaccine era, polioviruses were the most common cause of aseptic meningitis. In the post-polio vaccine era, non-polio enteroviruses, in particular, echovirus types 4, 6, 9, 11, 13, 16 and 30, coxsackievirus B2-5, coxsackievirus A9 and enterovirus 71 have been the most frequently identified pathogens.

Poliomyelitis is thought to have been associated with humanity since antiquity (Fig. 34.2.1). The first clinical descriptions of poliomyelitis date from the early 19th century and its transmissibility was established in the late 19th century. In the pre-industrial era, poliovirus infection occurred most commonly in infants and young children in situations of poverty and overcrowding and was associated with endemic circulation and a low prevalence of paralytic poliomyelitis. Improvements in hygiene and standards of living in North America and Western Europe in the late 19th century resulted in exposure to poliovirus later in life, which was associated with an increased incidence of paralytic poliomyelitis and with the onset of the large urban poliomyelitis epidemics that occurred in industrialized countries in the first half of the 20th century.

Enterovirus 71 was first isolated from a child with encephalitis in California in 1970. From 1970 until 1997, enterovirus 71 was found to be the cause of occasional outbreaks of the childhood vesicular exanthem, hand-foot-and-mouth disease and/or the enanthem herpangina associated with acute neurologic disease, including aseptic meningitis, poliomyelitis-like paralysis and brainstem encephalitis. Since 1997, large outbreaks of enterovirus 71 infection have occurred in the Asia-Pacific region in association with the generation of new, and genetically distinct, virus genotypes [2, 3].

NATURAL HISTORY, PATHOGENESIS AND PATHOLOGY

Transmission of enterovirus infection is by the fecal–oral route as a result of person-to-person contact or indirectly via fomites. The incubation period for most enterovirus infections has not been accurately determined. In the case of poliovirus, the incubation period is typically 3–5 days but may occasionally extend up to 2 weeks. Virus is shed in the respiratory secretions for 1 week and in the feces for 2–4 weeks or longer. People are most infectious during the incubation period and for the first 2–3 days after the onset of symptoms. It is considered that 80–95% of enterovirus infections are completely asymptomatic and that people who develop asymptomatic infection

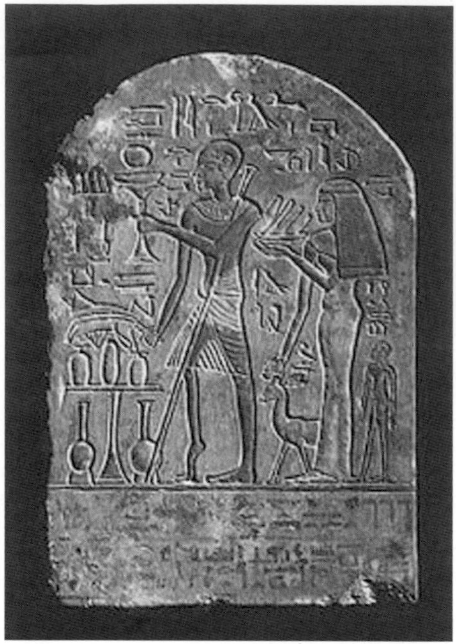

FIGURE 34.2.1 The earliest evidence of human poliomyelitis-like disease can be found in an Egyptian stele dating from 1350 BC, which depicts a young man with typical asymmetric flaccid paralysis and atrophy of the lower limb. Poliomyelitis is characterized by fever, malaise, headache, nausea, vomiting, muscle pain, stiffness of the neck and back followed by flaccid paralysis 1–3 days later.

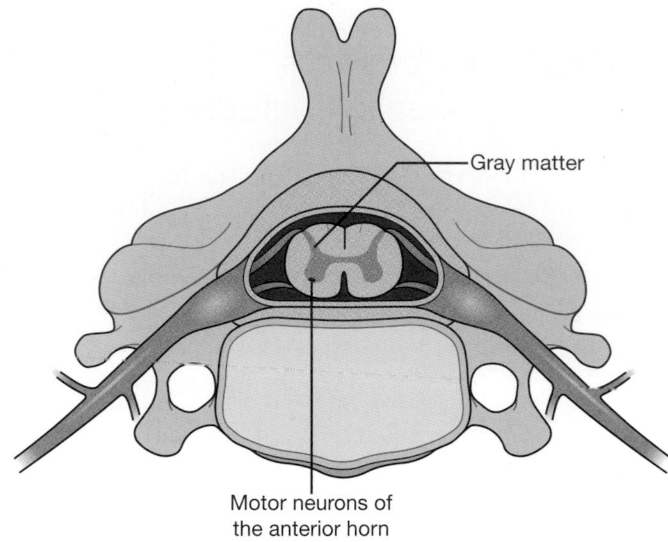

FIGURE 34.2.2 Location of motor neurons in the anterior horns of the spinal cord. After gaining entry into the CNS, poliovirus causes lytic infection of anterior horn motor neurons of the spinal cord, resulting in flaccid paralysis. Within the brain, the reticular formation, vestibular nuclei, cerebellar vermis and deep cerebellar nuclei are most often infected by poliovirus (bulbar poliomyelitis).

are the primary reservoir of enterovirus infection within the community.

Enteroviruses are the responsible pathogen in more than 90% of cases of aseptic meningitis.

Poliovirus types 1, 2 and 3 are the causative agents of acute poliomyelitis; poliovirus type 1 is most frequently associated with poliomyelitis, followed by type 3 and type 2. Enteroviruses 70, 71 and several coxsackievirus A strains are also associated with acute flaccid paralysis mimicking poliomyelitis and numerous case reports have linked other enteroviruses with this syndrome.

Most of what is understood about the pathogenesis of enterovirus infection has resulted from research on poliovirus and it is widely accepted that the early pathophysiologic events in non-polio enterovirus infections are similar. After ingestion, poliovirus first multiplies in the tonsils and Peyer's patches of the small intestine before spreading to regional lymph nodes and thence to the bloodstream as a "minor" viremia, which is transient and usually undetectable. During this phase, virus spreads to cells of the reticulo-endothelial system. In asymptomatic infection, viral replication is terminated by host defense mechanisms at this point in the infection cycle. In a small proportion of cases, infection develops within the reticulo-endothelial system leading to a sustained ("major") viremia, which coincides with the onset of symptoms. The major viremia results in the dissemination of virus to target organs, such as the central nervous system (CNS) or the skin. Infection at these sites induces host inflammatory responses and tissue necrosis; the severity of inflammation and necrosis generally corresponds to the titer of infectious virus present in the affected tissue.

The mechanism of enterovirus invasion from the bloodstream into the CNS is unknown but may either involve virus traversing the blood–brain barrier during the major viremia (the most likely mechanism in the pathogenesis of aseptic meningitis) or by retrograde axonal transport (which has recently been suggested for enterovirus 71 [4]). The primary targets of poliovirus infection in the CNS are anterior horn motor neurons of the spinal cord (Fig. 34.2.2). Enterovirus 71 infects the CNS more widely than poliovirus, including the hypothalamus, brainstem and cerebellar dentate nucleus in addition to spinal cord anterior horn motor neurons.

CLINICAL FEATURES

ASEPTIC MENINGITIS

Aseptic meningitis is a syndrome characterized by clinical signs and symptoms of meningitis with negative bacterial cultures obtained from cerebrospinal fluid (CSF) specimens. Aseptic meningitis occurs most commonly in children but is also frequently reported in adults. The illness commences with fever and headache followed by signs of meningismus (neck stiffness, positive Kernig's sign), which may range from mild to severe. The illness is occasionally biphasic, with a brief prodromal febrile illness and recovery followed by a recurrence of fever accompanied by meningismus.

POLIOMYELITIS

Infection with poliovirus may have one of several outcomes: (i) inapparent infection, which accounts for 90–94% of all infections; (ii) abortive or minor illness, which occurs in 4–8% of cases and is associated with symptoms of upper respiratory tract infection, gastrointestinal upset or influenza-like illness; (iii) non-paralytic poliomyelitis (1–2%), with clinical features similar to aseptic meningitis (see above) and from which patients usually recover fully within a few days; and (iv) paralytic poliomyelitis (0.1–2%), characterized by flaccid paralysis, which is usually asymmetric and with the lower limbs more frequently involved than the upper limbs (Fig. 34.2.3A). Cases of paralytic poliomyelitis may recover completely or be left with permanent paralysis and muscular atrophy. It may be fatal, especially when the brainstem is involved (bulbar poliomyelitis) (Fig. 34.2.3B).

ENTEROVIRUS 71 INFECTION OF THE CENTRAL NERVOUS SYSTEM (CNS)

Enterovirus 71 and coxsackievirus A16 are the commonest causes of hand-foot-and-mouth disease and herpangina. In contrast to

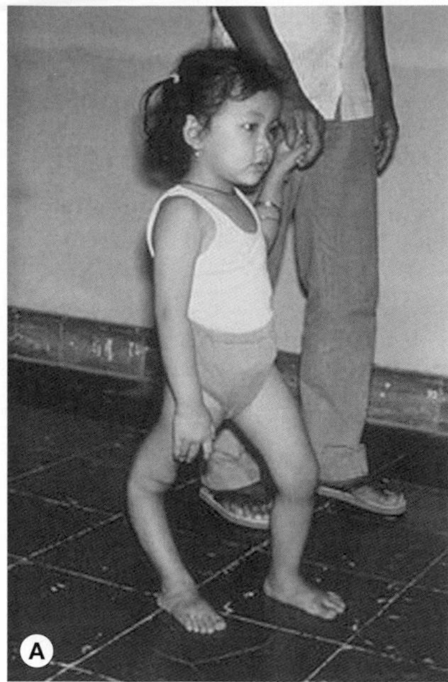

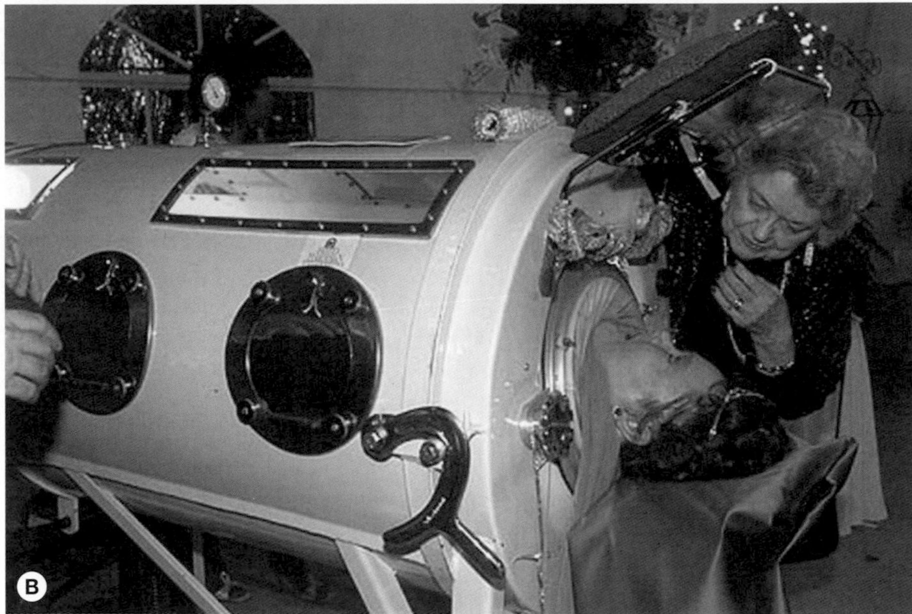

FIGURE 34.2.3 Clinical features of poliomyelitis. **(A)** A child with a deformity of her right leg caused by poliomyelitis. **(B)** A patient being treated in a negative pressure ventilator ("iron lung") because of bulbar poliomyelitis.

coxsackievirus A16, enterovirus 71 infection can be complicated by acute neurologic disease, including aseptic meningitis, poliomyelitis-like paralysis and brainstem encephalitis. Brainstem encephalitis caused by enterovirus 71 infection occurs mostly in children under 4 years of age and is associated with a high mortality as a result of a rapid onset neurogenic pulmonary edema and cardiovascular collapse.

HAND-FOOT-AND-MOUTH DISEASE

Hand-foot-and-mouth disease occurs most often in children under 10 years of age. The illness commences with fever (>38.5 °C) and sore throat. The fever lasts 1–2 days during which time vesicles appear on the anterior buccal and gingival mucous membranes and tongue. Cutaneous vesicles occur most frequently on palms of the hands and soles of the feet, but may also occur on the buttocks and extensor surfaces of the elbows and knees. The skin lesions of hand-foot-and-mouth disease are typically tender vesicles with a surrounding zone of erythema (Fig. 34.2.4).

HERPANGINA

Herpangina often occurs in outbreaks involving young children. Herpangina is a vesicular enanthem of the soft palate and fauces accompanied by fever, sore throat and painful swallowing. The illness often commences abruptly, with fever and myalgia preceding the enanthem by 24 hours. The lesions develop into 2–4 mm papules that vesiculate and ulcerate. The fever subsides in 2–4 days and the ulcers heal over 6–7 days. Herpangina is generally a mild illness and requires only symptomatic treatment.

PATIENT EVALUATION, DIAGNOSIS AND DIFFERENTIAL DIAGNOSIS

The vesicles of hand-foot-and-mouth disease can be distinguished from herpetic vesicular rashes (caused by herpes viruses) by the highly characteristic distribution of the vesicles and because the number of lesions is generally fewer than that seen in varicella (which typically spares the palms and soles). Primary herpetic gingivostomatitis is characterized by the presence of vesicular lesions within the anterior oral cavity in patients who are generally more unwell and have higher fever and regional lymphadenopathy than children with hand-foot-and-mouth disease.

It is important to distinguish herpangina from bacterial tonsillitis and other viral causes of pharyngitis. The vesicles associated with herpangina are generally located in the posterior pharynx, in contrast to other vesicular enanthems, such as herpes simplex gingivostomatitis and hand-foot-and-mouth disease, which typically occur in the anterior oral cavity, and to aphthous ulceration, which appears as large ulcers on the lips, tongue and buccal mucosa. Herpangina can generally be diagnosed confidently on clinical criteria alone.

It is of critical importance to distinguish bacterial meningitis from aseptic meningitis, which can be achieved by lumbar puncture and CSF microscopic examination and culture. However, it should be noted that partially treated bacterial meningitis may mimic aseptic meningitis in terms of the CSF profile. Aseptic meningitis caused by enteroviruses also requires differentiation from other infectious and non-infectious causes of this syndrome [5].

CSF examination is critically important in the diagnosis of meningitis. In aseptic meningitis, the CSF usually appears clear and has a low-to-moderate leukocyte count (10–500/mL) that only occasionally exceeds 1000/mL; the cell count is typically pleomorphic with a predominance of lymphocytes. However, CSF examination within the first 24 hours of illness may demonstrate a predominance of neutrophils. In general, the CSF glucose is within normal range and the CSF protein may be normal or slightly elevated. Although enteroviruses can be isolated in the CSF by cell culture, this method is slow, expensive and has a low (35%) sensitivity compared with newer molecular diagnostic methodologies (see below), which have largely replaced cell culture in the diagnosis of aseptic meningitis. Most patients with aseptic meningitis are sufficiently unwell to require hospital admission.

Poliomyelitis caused by poliovirus infection needs to be distinguished from paralysis caused by other enteroviruses, such as echovirus 6, 9, coxsackievirus A7, A9, B2-5, enterovirus 70 and enterovirus 71, Guillain-Barré syndrome, transverse myelitis, disorders of fluid and electrolyte balance, vitamin B1 deficiency, and other causes, such as the neurologic complications of diphtheria and botulism.

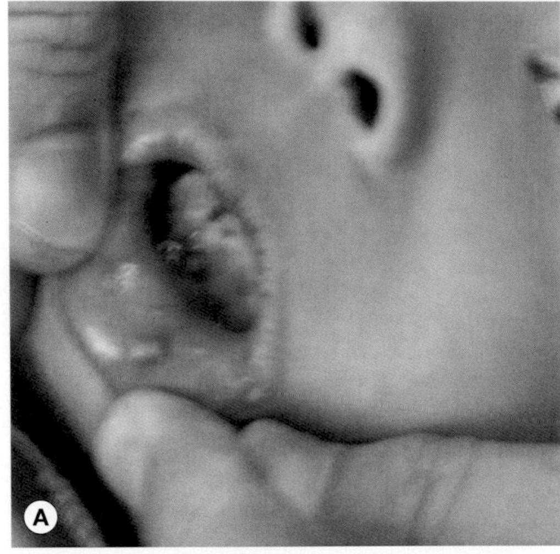

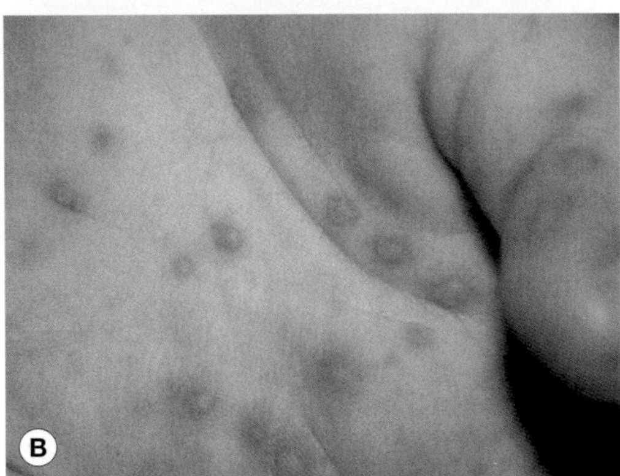

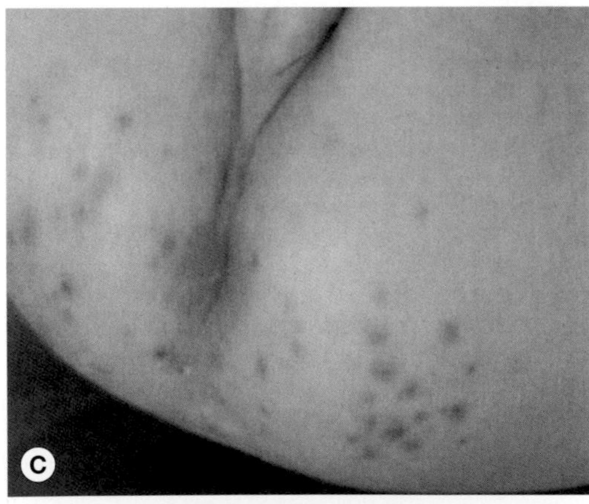

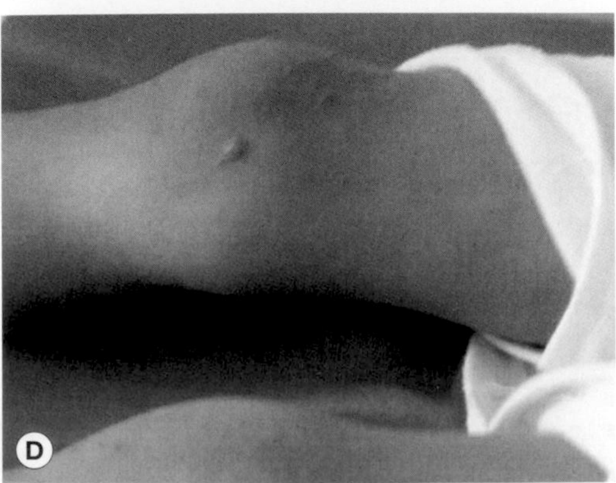

FIGURE 34.2.4 Hand-foot-and-mouth disease. **(A)** Mouth. **(B)** Palms of the hands. **(C)** Buttocks. **(D)** Extensor surface of the knee.

LABORATORY DIAGNOSIS OF ENTEROVIRUS INFECTIONS

The most readily obtainable specimens for the identification of enteroviruses include feces, and rectal and throat swabs. Although these specimens generally provide a high yield in the presence of enterovirus infection, they are usually remote from the site of disease and thus only provide indirect evidence of the causative organism. Vesicle fluid may be collected from patients presenting with hand-foot-and-mouth disease and is useful in providing a more specific diagnosis.

Although the identification of enteroviruses in CSF provides a specific diagnosis in aseptic meningitis, the sensitivity of detection is much lower than for other specimens (throat swab, feces). Paired acute and convalescent sera (at least 7 days apart) may be collected to test for the presence of enterovirus-specific antibodies.

The most widely available laboratory techniques for the identification of enterovirus infections include virus isolation in cell culture and identification of specific enterovirus serotypes using immunologic techniques (neutralization with serotype-specific antisera, immunofluorescence with serotype-specific monoclonal antibodies) or molecular techniques, in particular, the reverse-transcription (RT)-PCR assay, which have largely replaced cell culture as the primary means of enterovirus identification [6]. An excellent overview of the diagnostic modalities used in the diagnosis of poliovirus infection is provided in the World Health Organization (WHO) Polio Laboratory Manual [7].

RT-PCR assays capable of amplifying genomic material from all known enteroviruses have been developed to screen for the presence of enteroviruses in cell culture supernatants or directly from patient specimens. As these assays generally target the conserved 5′ untranslated region of the viral genome, they are not capable of distinguishing individual enterovirus strains. More recently, RT-PCR assays that target variable regions of the genome, principally the VP1 structural protein gene, have been used to identify enterovirus genomic RNA in cell culture supernatants or directly from patient specimens. Furthermore, nucleotide sequencing of the amplified RT-PCR product and searching of genetic databases, such as GenBank, allows the identification of individual infecting enterovirus strains. A number of enterovirus type-specific RT-PCR assays, such as enterovirus 71- and coxsackievirus A16-specific assays, have been developed for use in regions of the world where these viruses cause a high level of endemic infection. The main reason to seek a laboratory diagnosis in cases of herpangina or hand-foot-and-mouth disease is to distinguish enterovirus 71 from the other coxsackie A viruses, as the former is more frequently associated with acute neurologic sequelae (see above).

Although several assays for the serologic diagnosis of enterovirus infections are available, they are generally considered impractical because of the large number of virus strains and the extensive serologic cross-reactivity between them, but also because serologic diagnosis is generally retrospective and thus not useful in patient management. However, serologic assays are frequently used for seroepidemiologic investigations.

TREATMENT AND PREVENTION

No specific treatment is available for hand-foot-and-mouth disease and herpangina, which are generally mild and self-limited infections and require only symptomatic treatment. As with all other enteroviruses, infection can be prevented by hand-washing after contact with infected patients and by social distancing measures, such as closing nursery schools.

Empirical antibiotic therapy is often commenced early in aseptic meningitis and until bacterial meningitis has been positively excluded. The advent of rapid diagnostic assays for enteroviruses has proven beneficial in limiting the duration of empirical antibiotic therapy and hospital admission in many cases of aseptic meningitis. Full recovery generally occurs rapidly in young children although older children and adults may experience a longer convalescence in which subtle disturbances in motor function, coordination, learning and concentration may persist for weeks to months.

No specific antiviral treatment for poliovirus infection is available. Intensive care support is often needed for patients with bulbar poliomyelitis and/or respiratory failure. Physical therapy is used to assist with the regaining of limb function and to minimize deformities caused by contractures. Similarly, treatment for enterovirus 71 brainstem encephalitis is symptomatic and supportive, as specific antiviral therapy is not available.

The molecular characterization of enteroviruses has led to the development of novel compounds that inhibit viral replication [8]. However, very few have been found to be sufficiently selective to be useful as drug candidates. Several "WIN" compounds, which specifically bind to the enterovirus capsid and inhibit viral uncoating, have been investigated [9]. One compound, pleconaril [10], has been found to inhibit more than 90% of circulating enteroviruses, to be nontoxic in humans, and to provide significant therapeutic benefit in aseptic meningitis [5] and chronic meningoencephalitis [11]. Compassionate use of pleconaril in cases of severe neonatal enterovirus infection has also demonstrated the promise of significant therapeutic benefit [11]. Unfortunately, pleconaril has been found to have limited activity against enterovirus 71. A summary of the clinical trials undertaken to investigate pleconaril is provided in [12]. An excellent review of many experimental antiviral agents relevant to enterovirus infection is provided in [8].

Poliovirus vaccines against all three serotypes are available as either a formalin-inactivated poliovirus vaccine (IPV) or as a live-attenuated, oral poliovirus vaccine (OPV). IPV is injected intramuscularly and provides individual protection by inducing circulating antibody that blocks the spread of virus to the CNS. OPV was first licensed in 1962. The advantages of OPV are that it induces both humoral (IgM, IgG) and mucosal (IgA) immunity and is able to interrupt wild poliovirus circulation. OPV is also less costly than IPV and does not require injection by trained vaccinators. Consequently, OPV is more suitable for mass immunization campaigns. However, OPV has several disadvantages: (i) the vaccine requires the maintenance of a cold chain; (ii) interference between OPV and other enteric viruses can lead to vaccine failure; (iii) OPV is contraindicated in persons with congenital or acquired immunodeficiency; and (iv) OPV may revert to virulence and cause paralytic poliomyelitis in vaccine recipients or their contacts (vaccine-associated poliomyelitis) at a rate of approximately 1 case in every 2.5 million doses administered. Despite these disadvantages, mass immunization with OPV has formed the basis of the WHO coordinated Global Poliomyelitis Eradication Program, which had resulted in the near eradication of poliomyelitis by early 2012 and is regarded as a major achievement in global public health.

With the notable exception of poliovirus, vaccines are not yet available to prevent the most severe forms of non-poliovirus enterovirus infection. However, given the success of polio vaccination, it is reasonable to assume that the development of vaccines against non-polio enteroviruses that cause epidemics of severe neurologic disease, such as enterovirus 71, will also be successful in preventing infection. Indeed, a large effort is currently being made to develop vaccines to prevent enterovirus 71 infection (reviewed in [13]).

Currently, the only means of preventing non-polio enterovirus infections is through avoidance of contact between infected and susceptible individuals (reviewed in [3]). Realistically, this can only be achieved through infection control actions of limited efficacy, such as hand-washing and reducing contact between infected and susceptible people during epidemics. Indeed, if these actions are to have any effect, it is imperative that adequate surveillance of enterovirus activity be maintained in the community to provide early warning of impending epidemics, which is not the case in many countries.

REFERENCES

1. Oberste MS, Maher K, Nix WW, et al. Molecular identification of 13 new enterovirus types, EV79-88 and EV100-101, members of the species Human Enterovirus B. Virus Res 2007;128:34–42.
2. McMinn PC. An overview of the evolution of enterovirus 71 and its clinical and public health significance. FEMS Microbiol Rev 2002;26:91–107.
3. Solomon T, Lewthwaite P, Perera D, et al. Virology, epidemiology, pathogenesis, and control of enterovirus 71. Lancet Infect Dis 2010;10:778–90.
4. Wong KT, Munisamy B, Ong KC, et al. The distribution of inflammation and virus in human enterovirus 71 encephalomyelitis suggests possible viral spread by neural pathways. J Neuropathol Exp Neurol 2008;67:162–9.
5. Lee BE, Davies HD. Aseptic meningitis. Curr Opin Infect Dis 2007;20:272–7.
6. Oberste MS, Maher K, Kilpatrick DR, Pallansch MA. Molecular evolution of the human enteroviruses: correlation of serotype with VP1 sequence and application to picornavirus classification. J Virol 1999;73:1941–8.
7. World Health Organization. Polio Laboratory Manual, 4th edn. Geneva: Switzerland; 2004. Available at: (www.who.int/vaccines/en/poliolab/webhelp/whnjs.htm).
8. De Palma AM, Vliegen I, De Clercq E, Neyts J. Selective inhibitors of Picornavirus replication. Med Res Rev 2008;6:823–84.
9. Pevear DC, Tull TM, Seipel ME, Groarke JM. Activity of Pleconaril against enteroviruses. Antimicrob Agents Chemotherapy 1999;43:2109–15.
10. Rotbart HA, Webster AD. Treatment of potentially life-threatening enterovirus infections with Pleconaril. Clin Infect Dis 2001;32:228–35.
11. Webster ADB. Pleconaril—an advance in the treatment of enteroviral infection in immuno-compromised patients. J Clin Virol 2005;32:1–6.
12. Abzug MJ. Presentation, diagnosis and management of enterovirus infections in neonates. Pediatr Drugs 2004;6:1–10.
13. Bek EJ, McMinn PC. Recent advances in research on human enterovirus 71. Future Virol 2010;5:453–68.

34.3 Venezuelan, Eastern and Western Equine Encephalitis

Scott C Weaver, Angelle D LaBeaud

Key features

Venezuelan equine encephalitis

- Acute "flu-like" febrile illness is usually self-limited
- Mosquito-borne transmission to humans during epidemics typically follows encephalitis in equids, which are efficient amplification hosts
- Lymphotropic replication leads to immune suppression and secondary infections
- Can progress to neurologic disease, especially in children (5–15% of cases)

Key features—cont'd

- Neurologic disease typically begins with convulsions and can progress to fatal coma, or survivors can suffer permanent neurologic sequelae
- During epidemics, attack rates are typically 30–50% and overall case fatality rate is approximately 0.5%
- Synonyms: sleeping sickness, "peste loca" (Spanish)

Eastern equine encephalitis

- Prodromal, acute "flu-like" febrile illness is often undiagnosed
- Mosquito-borne transmission to humans during epidemics typically follows encephalitis cases in equids
- Symptomatic infections often progress to neurologic disease, with overall case-fatality rates of approximately 33%
- Young children and the elderly are most likely to develop severe disease, and many survivors have permanent neurologic sequelae
- Epidemiologic studies suggest that the vast majority of human infections are inapparent; an average of about five human cases is diagnosed annually
- Virus strains that circulate in the tropics are probably relatively avirulent for humans
- Synonyms: sleeping sickness

Western equine encephalitis

- Prodromal, acute "flu-like" febrile illness is often undiagnosed
- Mosquito-borne transmission to humans during epidemics typically follows encephalitis cases in equids
- Most western equine encephalitis virus infections are inapparent or present as a mild, nonspecific illness
- Symptomatic infections often progress to neurologic disease, with overall case-fatality rates of 40–80%
- High inapparent : apparent infection ratio, no human cases diagnosed since 1986
- Case fatality rate is approximately 4% and is highest in persons >75 years of age
- Synonyms: sleeping sickness

INTRODUCTION

These three closely related alphaviruses (genus *Alphavirus*, family *Togaviridae*) cause encephalitis in humans and horses, and are known as New World alphaviruses because they occur only in the Americas (Fig. 34.3.1). In contrast, the Old World alphaviruses include chikungunya, which is found in Africa, Asia and southern Europe, and causes large outbreaks of fever, arthralgia and rash (see Chapter 32.2). Venezuelan equine encephalitis virus (VEEV) is the most common arboviral cause of encephalitis in Latin America along with eastern (EEEV) and western (WEEV) equine encephalitis viruses that cause human disease mainly in temperate regions of the Americas [1]. VEEV is particularly devastating because of its ability to generate equine-amplified, mosquito-borne epidemics of mostly febrile illness that involve up to hundreds-of-thousands of people and spread over large geographic distances (Fig. 34.3.2) [2]. Endemic Venezuelan equine encephalitis has a significant human health impact, but is often unrecognized because the signs and symptoms are often indistinguishable from those of dengue and other tropical infectious diseases. Human cases of eastern and western equine encephalitis are rare in the tropics—most cases occur in North America; eastern equine encephalitis is notable for causing sporadic cases of an especially severe encephalitis, whilst WEE is notable for the fact that it has not been seen for many years.

EPIDEMIOLOGY

VEEV and closely related alphaviruses, such as Everglades and Mucambo, occur from the southern USA to northern Argentina in humid tropical forest and swamp foci [2]. Spillover infections of humans occur regularly and can be fatal. Major Venezuelan equine encephalitis epidemics occur periodically, usually every 10–20 years, after equine herd immunity declines and enzootic strains in subtype ID that normally replicate poorly in equids mutate to gain equine amplification potential. Exposure and immunity generated during previous epidemics create age-related susceptibility and infants may be protected by maternal antibodies. There is no difference in incidence between the sexes or among races, although Native American populations in Colombia and Venezuela tend to be at higher risk of infection because they live in association with domesticated and feral burros that serve as amplification hosts (Fig. 34.3.2).

EEEV infections are rarely diagnosed in the tropics and mostly occur near the Atlantic and Gulf coasts of the USA near enzootic swamp habitats (Fig. 34.3.2) with an average of six human cases diagnosed annually [1, 2]. Most cases occur in late summer or early autumn in temperate areas, but can occur throughout the year in subtropical areas of the southeast. Human infections occur in all age groups, but clinical attack rates tend to be higher in children younger than 4 years old and adults older than 55 years old.

WEEV circulates from southern Canada to Argentina. Large equine epizootics have occurred in temperate regions of Argentina and North America, but infections of both humans and equids have declined dramatically since the 1980s for unknown reasons. Like eastern equine encephalitis, the risk of western equine encephalitis is highest in the very young and very old, and most infections are inapparent [1, 2].

NATURAL HISTORY, PATHOGENESIS AND PATHOLOGY

VEEV transmission normally occurs in tropical forest or swamp foci and involves rodent reservoir hosts and mosquitoes in the subgenus *Culex* (*Melanoconion*) (Fig. 34.3.2). Major epidemics principally occur in agricultural areas where equids are abundant [2]. EEEV occupies humid tropical forest and swamp habitats in the tropics but in North America it circulates among birds in hardwood swamps inhabited by the ornithophilic (bird-biting) mosquito vector, *Culiseta melanura*. However, most transmission to mammals, including humans, probably involves other mosquitoes that feed on birds and humans and serve as bridge vectors (Fig. 34.3.3). WEEV uses birds as its reservoir hosts throughout its geographic range; in North America, epidemic transmission usually occurs in agricultural habitats where the mosquito vector *Culex tarsalis* exploits irrigated farmland for its larval habitat (Fig. 34.3.4). VEEV and WEEV can also be transmitted transplacentally and cause premature abortions, stillborn births and teratogenic effects. Unlike WEEV and EEEV, VEEV reaches sufficiently high

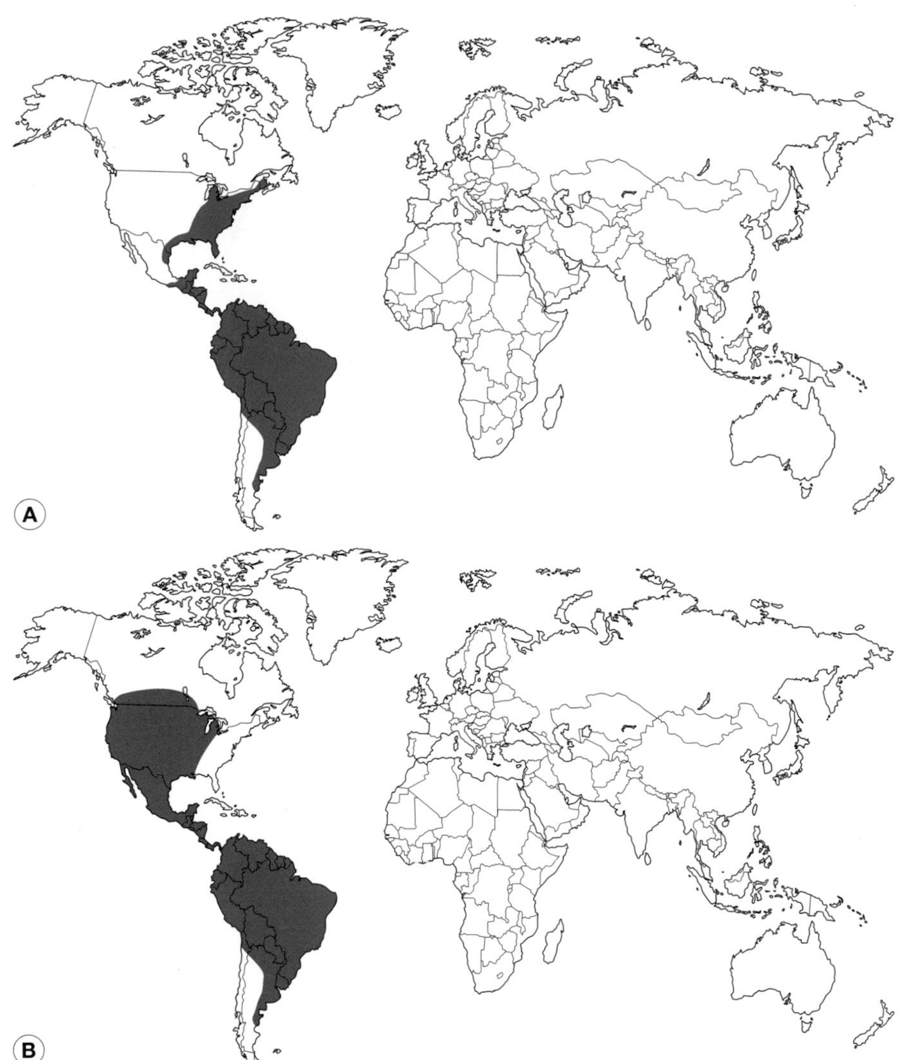

FIGURE 34.3.1 Known distribution of eastern **(A)** and western **(B)** equine encephalitis viruses.

viremia in humans to infect biting mosquitoes, suggesting that humans may not always be dead-end hosts.

CLINICAL FEATURES

Most patients with VEE have a history of exposure to mosquitoes in regions of humid tropical forests or have been present during an equine epizootic [2]. Following an incubation period of 1–5 days, chills, headache, fever, body aches and prostration begin abruptly [3]. Asthenia, dizziness and acute discomfort are incapacitating. Lumbosacral pain is common, along with nausea, vomiting, diarrhea and a sore throat. After defervescence, a dull headache and weakness may persist for several days; fever and symptoms occasionally recrudesce. Although signs of mild neurologic involvement are common, only about 4% of infected children progress to frank neurologic disease; adults rarely do. Signs include nuchal rigidity, stupor, coma, delirium, seizures, cranial nerve palsies, motor weakness, paralysis, nystagmus, pathologic reflexes and spastic paralysis. Elevated intracranial pressure and meningismus occur in most childhood cases. Approximately 0.5% of all symptomatic cases are fatal, nearly all in children. However, many survivors of neurologic disease experience sequelae, including memory problems, nervousness, asthenia, recurrent seizures, motor impairment, psychomotor retardation and behavioral disorders.

Eastern equine encephalitis typically begins after 3–10 days of incubation with the sudden onset of headache, fever, chills, photophobia, dysethesias, myalgia, malaise and vomiting [1, 2, 4]. In infants, encephalitis caused by eastern equine encephalitis virus is characterized by abrupt onset, but in older children and adults is manifested after a few days of systemic illness. Patients may recover or can progress to more severe neurologic illness beginning with a worsening headache, dizziness, vomiting, lethargy and progressing to neck stiffness, confusion and convulsions. Severe cases requiring hospitalization may involve seizures, disorientation and coma. The course of illness may be rapid in infants; infants are most likely to suffer neurologic sequelae, such as motor weakness, paralysis, aphasia, mental retardation and seizures. Many patients with permanent sequelae die a few years later.

Western equine encephalitis begins after an incubation period of 2–10 days with the sudden onset of severe headache, often followed by drowsiness, dizziness, chills, fever, myalgias, malaise, tremor, irritability, photophobia and neck stiffness [1, 2]. Neurologic signs are usually limited to generalized weakness and tremulousness, especially of the hands, tongue and lips. A minority of patients develop cranial nerve palsy, motor weakness, spasticity, convulsions and seizures. Clinical progression in infants is more rapid. Overall, stupor or coma develop in <10% of cases, sometimes accompanied by respiratory failure. The overall case fatality rate is around 4% and is highest in persons older than 75 years of age. Five to thirty percent of recovered children are left with permanent sequelae. Infants younger than 1 year old are at particularly high risk for morbidity.

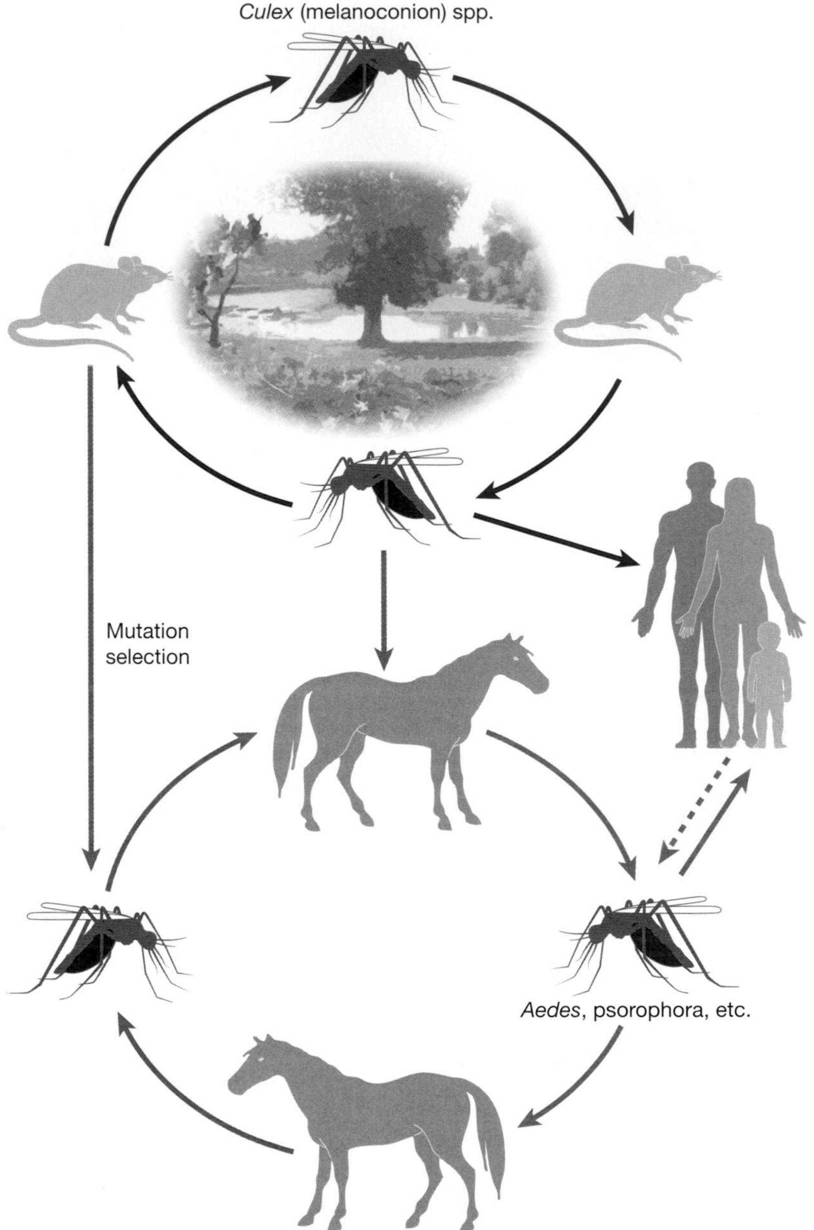

FIGURE 34.3.2 Enzootic (upper) and epizootic/epidemic (lower) transmission cycles of Venezuelan equine encephalitis viruses.

PATIENT EVALUATION, DIAGNOSIS AND DIFFERENTIAL DIAGNOSIS

The differential diagnosis of acute encephalitis is broad and includes non-infectious and infectious etiologies (Table 34.3.1) [1, 2]. Patients with non-infectious causes of altered mental status are usually afebrile. Because the infectious etiologies of encephalitis lead to nonspecific signs and symptoms, a thorough diagnostic approach is needed. Even then, only about 50% of infection-related encephalitis cases have a specific etiology determined. Initially, treatable causes, such as herpes simplex viruses (HSV), bacterial meningitis and brain abscess, should be excluded. All patients who present with signs and symptoms of encephalitis, including fever, headache, irritability, restlessness, drowsiness, anorexia, vomiting, seizures, and coma, warrant complete blood cell counts, electrolyte testing and thorough cerebrospinal fluid (CSF) evaluation, including culture and molecular diagnostic testing for common viral causes (HSV and enterovirus PCR).

Viral encephalitides often manifest as mildly elevated protein levels and mild pleocytosis which is usually lymphocyte predominant for WEEV and VEEV infection, but can be neutrophil-predominant in eastern equine encephalitis. CSF glucose levels are usually normal. Peripheral leukocytosis and hyponatremia as a result of the syndrome of inappropriate antidiuretic hormone may occur, but are nonspecific. Neuroimaging may reveal vasculitis and destruction of neurons with resultant edema [4]. Magnetic resonance imaging (MRI) with gadolinium may show enhancement of the basal ganglia and thalami, which may suggest an arboviral cause; electroencephalography (EEG) may be abnormal with diffuse slowing.

Eastern, western and Venezuelan equine viruses should be suspected in patients who have febrile illness with central nervous system (CNS)

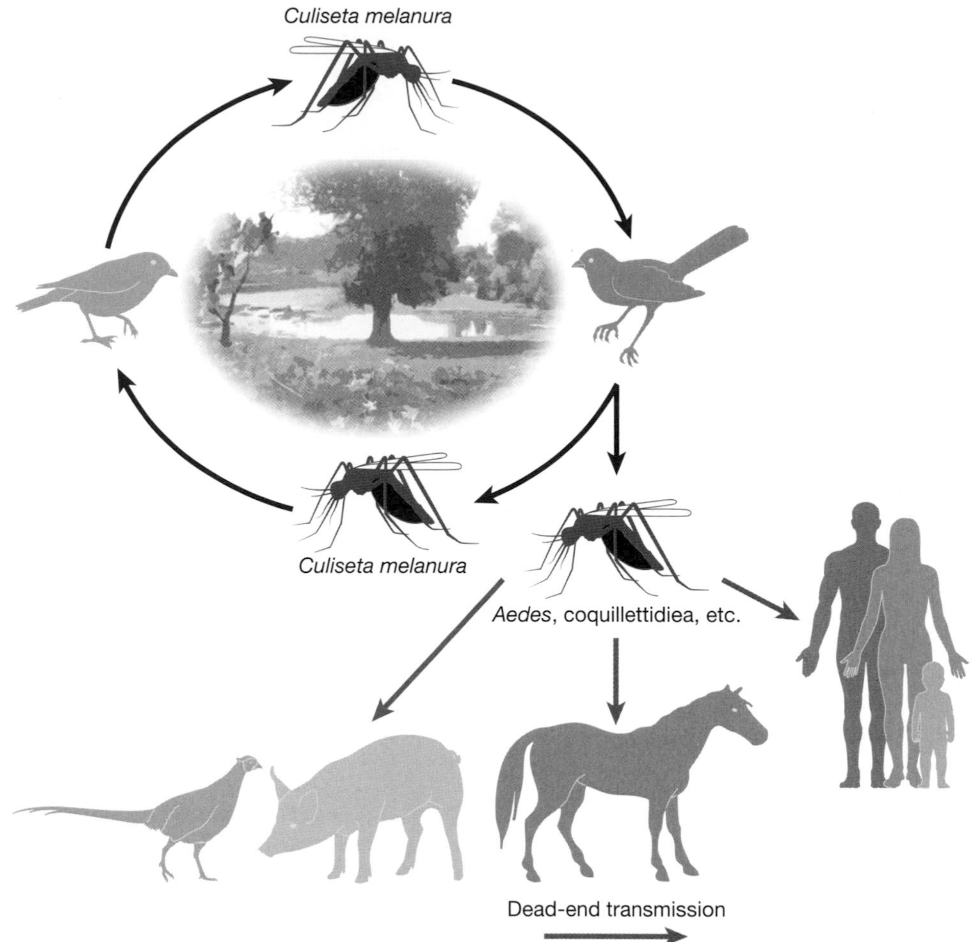

FIGURE 34.3.3 Enzootic transmission cycles of eastern equine encephalitis virus and spillover transmission to humans and domestic animals.

TABLE 34.3.1 Differential Diagnosis of Acute Encephalitis

Noninfectious causes	Infectious causes
Stroke	Herpes simplex viruses (HSV)
Tumor	Bacterial meningitis
Non-infectious CNS disorders	Brain abscess
Creutzfeldt-Jakob disease	Enteroviruses
Alzheimer's disease	Influenza
Long-term alcohol abuse	Adenovirus
Other dementias	Epstein Barr virus
	Mycoplasma
	Arboviruses
	Respiratory syncytial virus
	Rabies
	Bartonella henselae
	Lymphocytic choriomeningitis virus
	Rocky Mountain spotted fever
	Leptospirosis
	Lyme disease
	HIV
	Syphilis
	Tuberculosis
	Other mycobacterial diseases
	Fungal diseases

involvement and a history of travel to, or residence in, endemic areas [2]. Patients with Venezuelan equine encephalitis may manifest with flu-like illness without CNS involvement. VEEV produces viremia and is found in throat washings during the acute phase, whereas EEEV and WEEV are difficult to isolate from clinical samples. Therefore, serologic testing is a primary detection method, and IgG and IgM levels should be tested in both CSF and serum. In a patient with a consistent clinical picture, serum or CSF IgM positivity provides a specific diagnosis; a fourfold rise between acute and convalescent IgG titers, which can persist for life, can confirm the diagnosis. IgG ELISA should be confirmed with plaque reduction neutralization testing, which is more specific. PCR-based testing on CSF or brain tissue may also confirm the diagnosis, and may be helpful in immmunocompromised individuals who cannot manifest an appropriate antibody response, or in those who have succumbed to infection.

TREATMENT

No licensed vaccines or antiviral treatments are currently available for EEEV, WEEV or VEEV in the USA [1, 2]. Patient management focuses on supportive care and treatment of acute complications, such as seizures and increased intracranial pressure, and long-term sequelae.

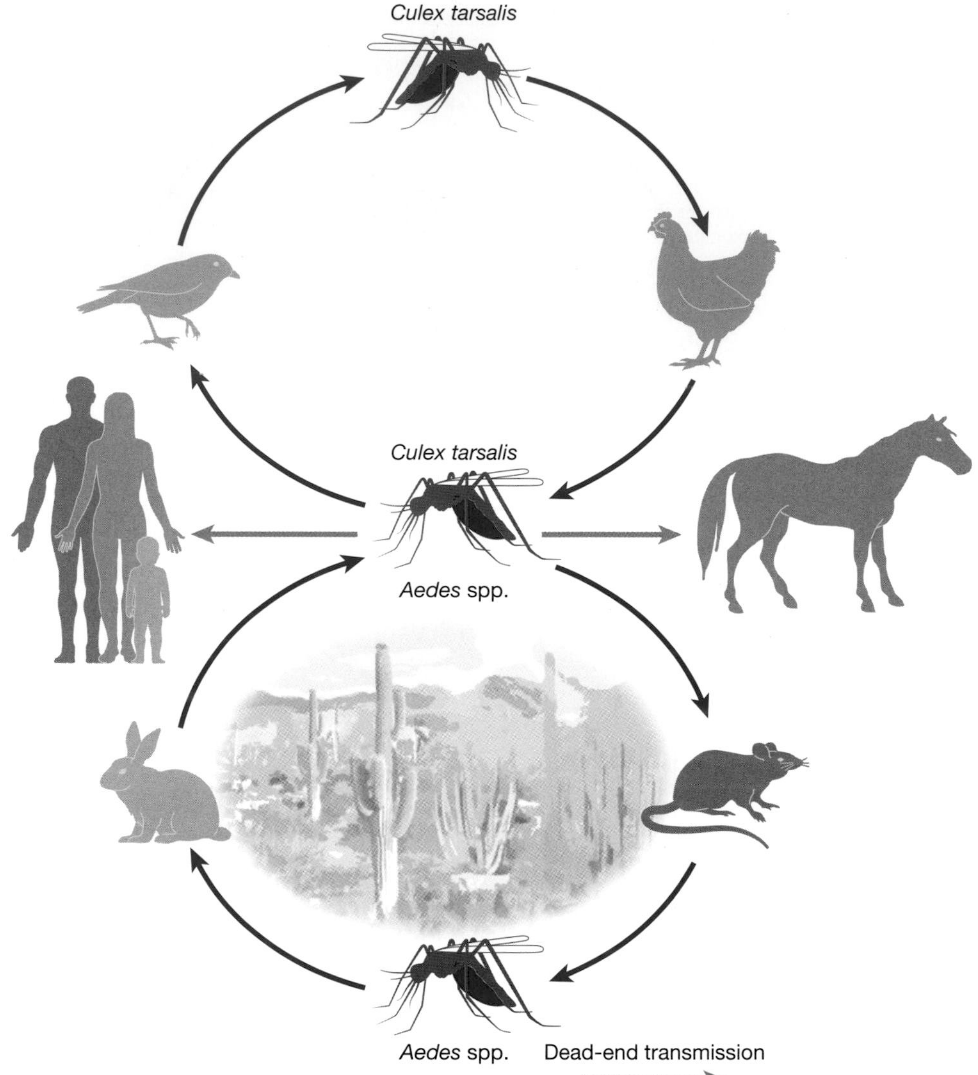

FIGURE 34.3.4 Enzootic transmission cycles of western equine encephalitis virus and spillover transmission to humans and domestic animals.

REFERENCES

1. Davis LE, Beckham JD, Tyler KL. North American encephalitic arboviruses. Neurol Clin 2008;26:727–57, ix.
2. Smith DW, Mackenzie JS, Weaver SC. Alphaviruses. In: Richman DD, Whitley RJ, Hayden FG, eds. Clinical Virology. Washington: ASM Press; 2009:1241–74.
3. Rivas F, Diaz LA, Cardenas VM, et al. Epidemic Venezuelan equine encephalitis in La Guajira, Colombia, 1995. J Infect Dis 1997;175:828–32.
4. Deresiewicz RL, Thaler SJ, Hsu L, Zamani AA. Clinical and neuroradiographic manifestations of eastern equine encephalitis. N Engl J Med 1997;336:1867–74.

34.4 Japanese Encephalitis

Tom Solomon

Key features

- This mosquito-borne flavivirus is endemic across the Asia-Pacific region and is spreading
- The disease primarily affects children, with 30,000–50,000 cases annually, 10,000–15,000 deaths and sequelae common among survivors
- Clinical features range from a nonspecific febrile illness to aseptic meningitis and severe encephalitis
- There is no specific antiviral treatment, but attention should be paid to the complications of infection, such as seizures and raised intracranial pressure
- Available vaccines include killed, live-attenuated and live-chimeric vaccines

INTRODUCTION

Outbreaks of encephalitis were first described in Japan in the 1870s and the disease now occurs across most of the Asia-Pacific region (Fig. 34.4.1). It is numerically one of the most important causes of encephalitis globally. Japanese encephalitis virus (JEV) is a member of the genus *Flavivirus*, family *Flaviviridae*, and is related to West Nile virus, tick-borne encephalitis virus, and dengue. The virus is zoonotic, being transmitted between wading birds and pigs, and by rice paddy-breeding *Culex* mosquitoes which feed in the evenings and at night (Fig. 34.4.2). There have been recent large Japanese encephalitis outbreaks in India and neighboring countries, but disease control efforts by governments, supported by the World Health Organization (WHO), the Bill and Melinda Gates Foundation, and other partners, are having some impact [1].

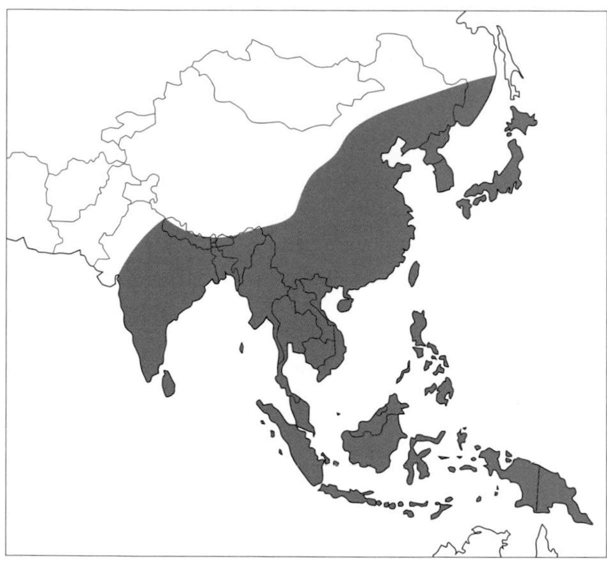

FIGURE 34.4.1 Current distribution of Japanese encephalitis.

EPIDEMIOLOGY

The geographical area affected by JEV includes most countries of the Asia-Pacific region, from Pakistan in the west and China in the north, to Australia in the southeast (Fig. 34.4.1). In northern, temperate regions, the virus causes large outbreaks in the summer months, after the start of the rainy season. In equatorial, tropical regions the virus causes sporadic, year-round disease, typically with a peak in the summer months [2].

Because the enzootic cycle is almost impossible to avoid in rural parts of Asia, almost everyone is infected during childhood, but only a small proportion develops disease—estimated to range from about 1 in 300 to 1 in 1000 [3]. An annual incidence of 30–50,000 cases of Japanese encephalitis is often quoted, but the figure may be as high as 175,000 [4]. Previously, there have been very large outbreaks in China, but these have been reduced following more widespread use of vaccines (see below). In recent years, there have been large outbreaks in northern India and Nepal.

The incidence of Japanese encephalitis varies across Asia from approximately 7 per 100,000 children in southern equatorial regions (e.g. Malaysia), to as high as 50 per 100,000 in northern regions (e.g. northern Thailand) [5–7]. Although mostly a disease of children, when the virus arrives in new regions adults are also affected because they are immunologically naïve; similarly, adult travelers visiting Japanese encephalitis endemic areas are at risk. Some of the most important research on Japanese encephalitis occurred during American military activity in Asia through various conflicts. With more widespread use of vaccines, the epidemiology is changing.

NATURAL HISTORY, PATHOGENESIS, AND PATHOLOGY

Following the bite of an infected mosquito there is viremia followed by spread into the central nervous system (CNS). Viral replication in

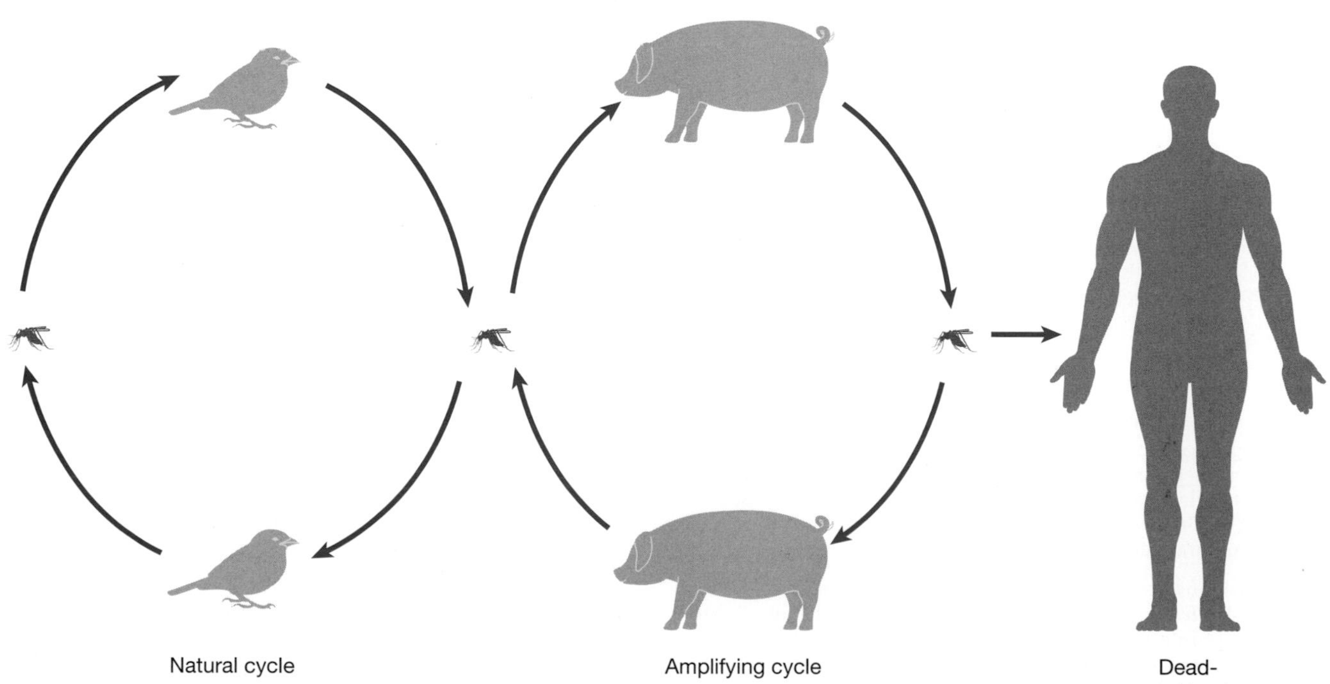

FIGURE 34.4.2 The transmission cycle of Japanese encephalitis virus.

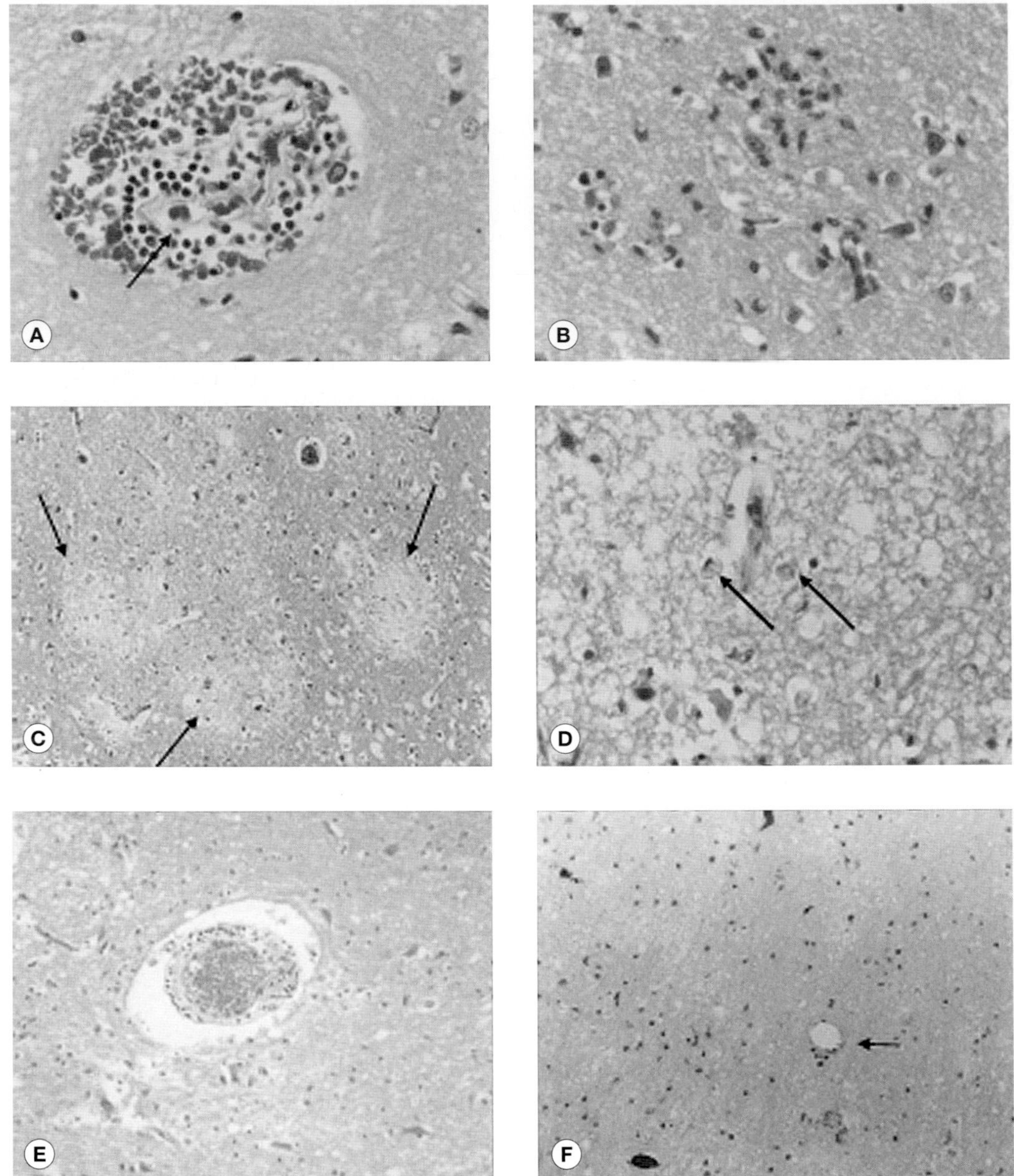

FIGURE 34.4.3 Pathological images *(From German AC, Myint KS, Mai NT, et al. A preliminary neuropathological study of Japanese encephalitis in humans and a mouse model. Transactions of the Royal Society of Tropical Medicine and Hygiene. 2006;100:1135–45).* Histopathologic alterations in patients with Japanese encephalitis (hematoxylin and eosin). **(A, B)** PIF 44, cortical tissue; **(C, D)** CNS 307 frontal cortex; **(E, F)** CNS 307, pons. **(A)** Moderate perivascular mononuclear cuffing and hemorrhage (arrow; OM ×400). **(B)** Small glial nodule (OM ×400). **(C)** Necrotic foci within the white matter (arrows; OM ×200). **(D)** Necrotic focus with gitter cells (arrows; OM ×400). **(E)** Perivascular lymphocytic infiltrate around a vein containing a fibrin plug (OM ×100). **(F)** Immunohistochemical stain for JEV antigen. Note the presence of viral antigen in the vascular endothelium (arrow; OM ×100).

neurons is accompanied by an inflammatory perivascular infiltrate with microglial cell activation, formation of glial nodules and necrotic "Swiss cheese" lesions (Fig. 34.4.3). Pathologic changes are especially marked in the deep gray matter of the basal ganglia and the anterior horn cells of the spinal cord, thus giving correlates for the Parkinsonism and flaccid paralysis often seen clinically.

The host response is thought to include an innate response, which may control infection even before viremia occurs, and thus lead to asymptomatic infection followed by antibody- and cell-mediated immunity. By the time most patients arrive at hospital, the virus cannot be detected in the blood or cerebrospinal fluid (CSF), but neutralizing antibody is detectable at admission or soon after. There is a strong pro-inflammatory cytokine and chemokine response, both in the peripheral and central nervous systems. Twenty to thirty percent of children with Japanese encephalitis die, depending on the clinical setting. Approximately 50% of survivors have obvious neurologic and/or psychiatric sequelae; many others have subtle difficulties, including personality and behavioral changes and poor school performance [6].

CLINICAL FEATURES

In taking the history, establish whether a patience comes from a rural area where Japanese encephalitis occurs and also whether there is an

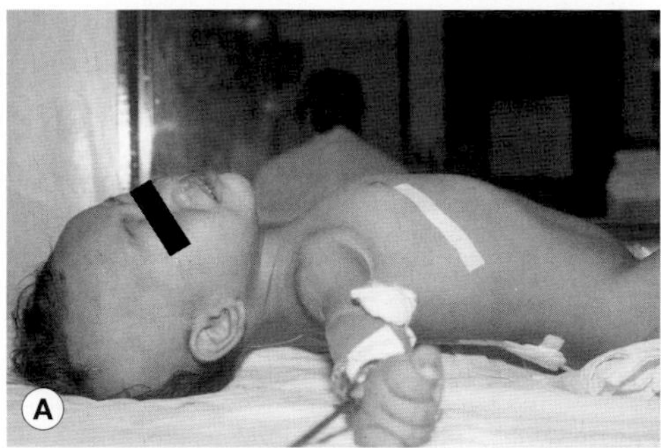

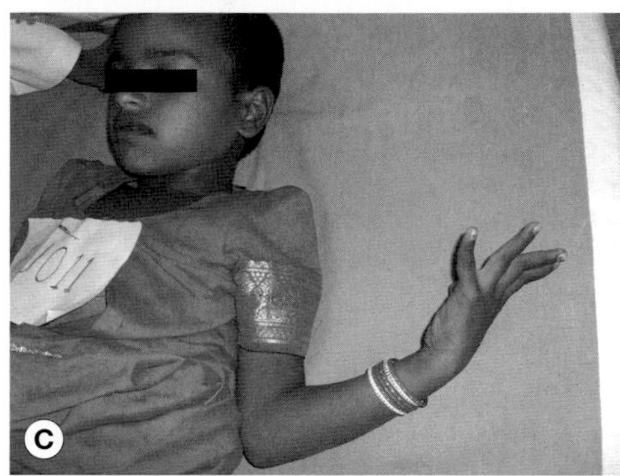

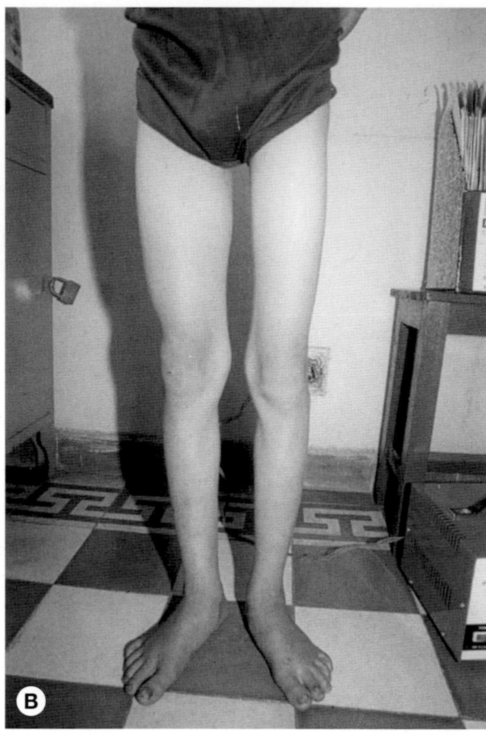

FIGURE 34.4.4 (A) Opisthotonus and other movement disorders are common in Japanese encephalitis *(photo courtesy of T. Solomon, reproduced from Solomon T. Japanese encephalitis. In: Gilman S, Goldstein GW, Waxman SG, eds. Neurobase. San Diego: Medlink Publishing; 2000.* **(B)** Poliomyelitis-like acute flaccid paralysis. This child has marked weakness and wasting one year after the initial presentation *(photo courtesy of T. Solomon, reproduced from Solomon T, Kneen R, Dung NM, et al. Poliomyelitis-like illness due to Japanese encephalitis virus. Lancet 1998;351:1094–7.)* **(C)** Sequelae of Japanese encephalitis—flexion deformities are apparent in this child 2 months after the initial illness *(photo courtesy of T. Solomon, reproduced from Solomon T. Japanese encephalitis. In: Gilman S, Goldstein GW, Waxman SG, eds. Neurobase. San Diego: Medlink Publishing; 2000..*

ongoing outbreak of encephalitic illness or other disease, such as hand, foot and mouth disease caused by enterovirus 71. Ask if the child has been vaccinated against Japanese encephalitis and whether this was recent (as it could complicate the interpretation of serological tests—see below).

Clinical presentations may range from a nonspecific febrile illness to aseptic meningitis, febrile seizures, febrile encephalopathy (with no inflammatory cells in the CSF) or a severe encephalitis (with a CSF pleocytosis or inflammation on imaging); this latter is the most common presentation [6]. Typically, children with encephalitis present with a few days history of flu-like illness, usually involving a severe headache, and may include coryza, diarrhea, and vomiting. This is followed by a reduction in the level of consciousness, often heralded by a seizure.

Seizures are more common in children with Japanese encephalitis than in adults, occurring in up to 80% of cases, and are occasionally the first symptom [3]. They may be multiple, or prolonged and status epilepticus is common. In addition to convulsive status epilepticus, some patients have subtle motor status epilepticus in which the only clinical manifestation of seizure activity may be twitching of a digit or eyebrow, ocular bobbing, or eye deviation [8]. Other patients, especially adults, may have subtle abnormalities of behavior that may be mistaken for psychiatric illness.

Neurologic signs may include pyramidal, extra-pyramidal, cranial nerve and lower motor neuron signs (Fig. 34.4.4). They may evolve rapidly over hours or even minutes, resulting in bizarre fluctuations. Pyramidal (long tract) signs are common, causing a hemiparesis. Extrapyramidal features include a Parkinsonian movement disorder with tremors, cog-wheel rigidity, and mask-like facies with a wide palpebral angle and infrequent blinking. In addition, there may be orofacial dyskinesias, dystonic posturing, spasms, opisthotonus, cerebellar signs, choreoathetosis and, occasionally, hemibalismus. Cranial nerves commonly affected in Japanese encephalitis include the third, the seventh and the bulbar nerves thus leading to an impaired, or absent, gag reflex. Lower motor neuron involvement following JEV infection may result in a poliomyelitis-like, acute flaccid paralysis. Lower motor neuron damage can also affect the bladder to cause retention and the respiratory muscles to cause ventilator dependence.

In severe disease, there are clinical signs of brainstem damage, including abnormalities in the papillary and oculovestibular reflexes, the respiratory pattern and abnormal flexor or extensor responses to pain. These may be directly caused by viral invasion and inflammation in the brainstem, or indirectly by swelling and shift of brain compartments leading to transtentorial herniation (see Fig. 10.1, Chapter 10).

PATIENT EVALUATION, DIAGNOSIS, AND DIFFERENTIAL DIAGNOSIS

The differential of Japanese encephalitis is broad and includes a range of other infectious and non-infectious causes (Table 34.4-1 and Table 10-1 in Chapter 10).

INVESTIGATIONS

A full blood count often shows a neutrophil leukocytosis and most patients have hyponatremia. A lumbar puncture usually shows a mild pleocytosis of a few hundred cells, which is predominantly lymphocytic. However, if it is performed in the first couple of days of illness, there may be a predominance of neutrophils, or even no

TABLE 34.4-1 Differential Diagnosis of Japanese Encephalitis

Viral	Comments
Arboviruses	
West Nile virus	Some overlap in geographical area, especially India
Dengue	Causes fever, arthralgia, rash and hemorrhagic disease, occasional CNS disease
Chikungunya	Causes fever, arthralgia, rash, occasional CNS disease
Chandipura virus	A vesiculovirus that has caused outbreaks in India
Other zoonotic viruses (not arthropod-borne)	
Rabies, other lyssaviruses	From rabid dogs, cats and bats
Enteroviruses	
Enterovirus 71	Epidemic hand, foot and mouth disease with aseptic meningitis, brainstem encephalitis, myelitis
Poliovirus	Principally causes myelitis, still circulating in parts of Asia
Coxsackieviruses, echoviruses, parechovirus	Mostly cause aseptic meningitis
Herpes viruses	
Herpes simplex virus type 1	Most commonly diagnosed sporadic encephalitis
Herpes simplex virus type 2	Causes meningitis (especially recurrent); meningoencephalitis occurs in the immunocompromised or in neonates
Paramyxoviruses (family Paramyxoviridae)	
Nipah virus	A zoonotic paramyxovirus, transmitted in feces of fruit bats in Malaysia and Bangladesh
Measles virus	Causes acute post-infectious encephalitis, subacute encephalitis and subacute sclerosing panencephalitis
Mumps virus	Parotitis, orchitis, pancreatitis
Bacterial	
Partially treated bacterial meningitis	
Tuberculous meningitis	
Typhoid	
Leptospirosis	
Abscess	
Para-/post-infectious	
Viral illnesses with febrile convulsions	
Acute disseminated encephalomyelitis	
Metabolic	
Reye's syndrome	
Hypoglycaemia	
Toxic encephalopathy (alcohol, drugs)	
Other	
Epilepsy	
Hysteria	

Only the most common, or important, differential is included here. For a full differential see Chapter 10. CNS, central nervous system.

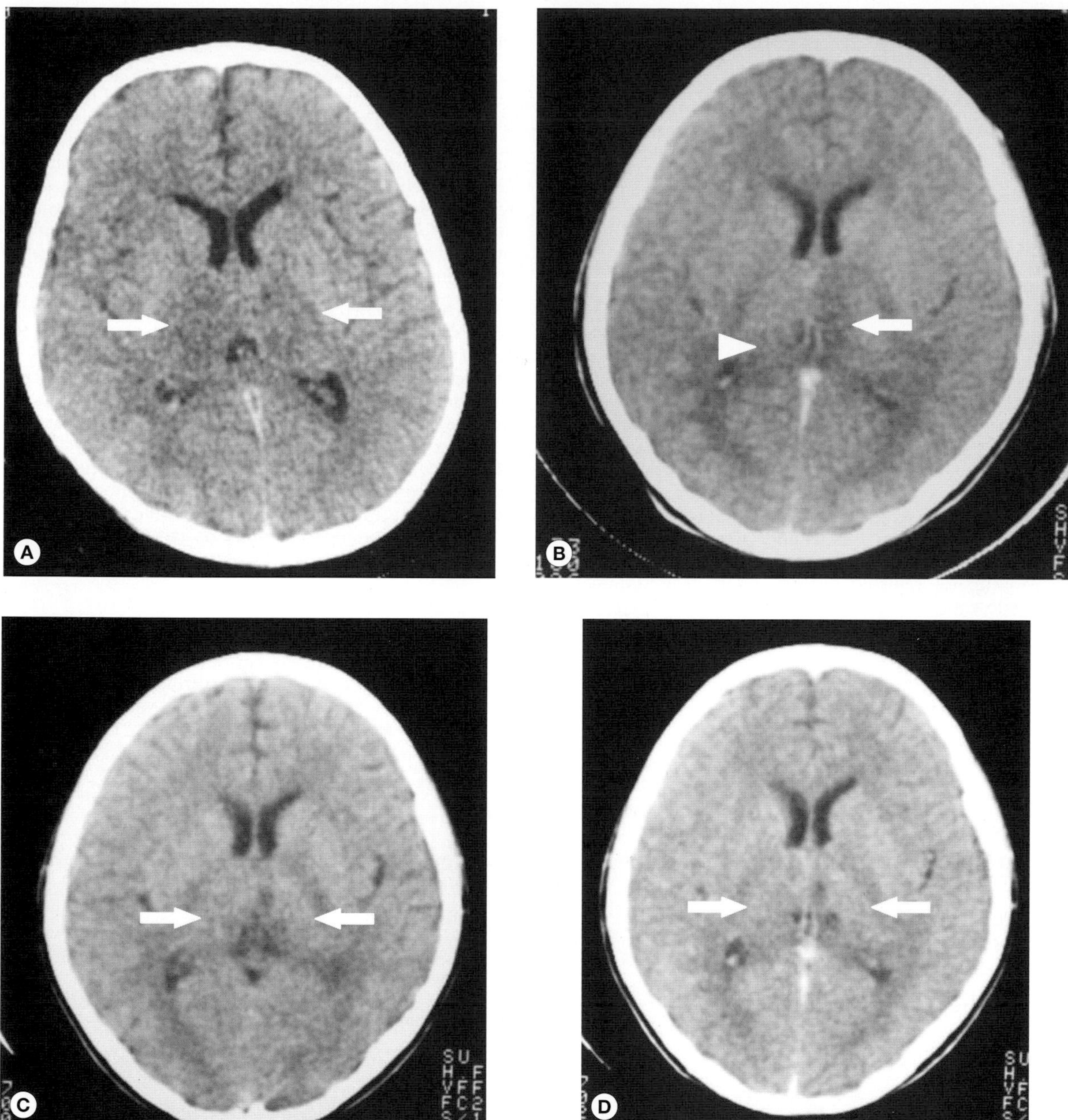

FIGURE 34.4.5 CT scans of patients with Japanese encephalitis. **(A)** Unenhanced CT of case PIF4 on day 9 of illness showing bilateral hypodense lesions in the thalamus (arrows). **(B)** Unenhanced CT of case PIF18 on day 13 showing hypodense lesions in the left medial thalamus (arrow) and the right posterior thalamus (arrowhead). **(C, D)** Pre- and post-contrast images of the same patient (case PIF18) on day 32 of illness. The hypodense thalamic lesions, although less clear, are still visible and do not enhance with contrast. *(From Dung NM, Turtle L, Chong WK, et al. An evaluation of the usefulness of neuroimaging for the diagnosis of Japanese encephalitis. Journal of neurology. 2009 Dec;256(12):2052–60.)*

pleocytosis. The glucose ratio is usually normal and the CSF protein moderately elevated. Although there is overlap between these findings and those of partially treated meningitis or tuberculous meningitis, the epidemiologic context, length of history, whether any antibiotics have been given and careful attention to the glucose ratio allow the distinction to be made in most patients. However, appropriate antibiotics must be given if there is any doubt.

Computer tomography (CT) scans of the brain may show low-density lesions caused by inflammation in the thalamus and other basal ganglia (Fig. 34.4.5). These are also seen on magnetic resonance images (MRI) as high signal intensities on T-2 weighted images; this, more sensitive, investigation may also show inflammation in the pons and medulla, as well as the anterior horns of the spinal cord [9].

DIAGNOSIS OF JAPANESE ENCEPHALITIS

The virus is hard to detect in peripheral blood or CSF by virus isolation or PCR because it has usually cleared by the time patients present to hospital. The virus is occasionally isolated in patients who have failed to make antibody—a poor prognostic sign. Newer, real-time PCR methods are proving more sensitive at detecting virus and ELISAs that capture the viral non-structural (NS)-1 protein are also in development; however, in most settings, IgM antibody detection in the CSF or serum using an ELISA is the most appropriate test because of its high sensitivity, specificity and reliability [10]. A range of diagnostic kits for Japanese encephalitis are commercially available and a laboratory network has been established across Asia to standardize testing. Detection of IgM in the CSF is preferable to serum as it confirms CNS infection. Detection of antibody in the serum may only reflect recent, coincidental, asymptomatic infection or, possibly, recent vaccination. Because in many parts of Asia JEV co-circulates with other flaviviruses, such as dengue, with which there is cross-reactivity, ELISAs for JEV and dengue are often performed in parallel and the ratio is used to help determine which was the infecting virus. Where there is uncertainty, the plaque reduction neutralization assay is the definitive specific antibody test for distinguishing flaviviruses but it is only performed in specialized laboratories. If this is a patient's first flavivirus infection, the rapid rise in serum IgM is followed by a slower rise in IgG. In contrast, if they have been previously infected with a different flavivirus, IgG rises first. Thus, the ratio of IgM to IgG can be used to distinguish primary from secondary flavivirus infection.

TREATMENT

The initial evaluation includes assessment of the airways, breathing and circulation, and examination for seizures, including subtle motor status epilepticus, as described above. Patients failing to maintain their airway and oxygenation may need immediate intubation and ventilation in an intensive care unit, although the facilities for this are often limited in areas where Japanese encephalitis occurs. Ideally, seizures should be treated with a benzodiazepine, such as diazepam or lorazepam, followed by intravenous phenytoin and then ventilation if needed (see Box 10.9 in Chapter 10). In some parts of Asia where phenytoin is not available, phenobarbitone is used, initially with a loading dose.

Fluid management is also an issue in many patients with encephalitis and is discussed in Chapter 10. Corticosteroids are also often given in Japanese encephalitis, although one small, randomized, placebo-controlled trial failed to show any benefit [11]. The antiviral drugs interferon alpha and ribavirin have also both been evaluated in clinical trials, but did not improve outcome [12, 13].

Many patients with Japanese encephalitis are tachypnoeic; this may be caused by poor respiratory effort as a result of flaccid paralysis of the respiratory muscles, brainstem damage, pneumonia or all three of these processes. The clinical clue to paralyzed respiratory musculature is paradoxical movement of the chest wall, with all the inspiratory draw being provided by the diaphragm. If tachypnea is caused by damage in the mid-brain, pons, or medulla, this is usually accompanied by other brainstem signs, such as abnormal papillary or oculovestibular reflexes. Pneumonia is typically aspiration pneumonia, with changes in the right upper lobe.

Contractures and bed sores are common, but simple techniques may reduce the risk of these. Although specialist beds and physiotherapists are not widely available in most of the areas where Japanese encephalitis occurs, nurses and family members can be taught how to gently keep joints mobile and the importance of changing position to minimize the risk of bed sores; splints may also help prevent contractures [14]. The child who survives Japanese encephalitis is left with a whole catalog of difficulties and disabilities that would prove challenging, even in a Western, industrialized setting. In poor Asian countries, rehabilitation is even harder but some simple tools for assessing disability and overcoming some of the obstacles are becoming available [15, 16].

PREVENTION OF JAPANESE ENCEPHALITIS

Measures to reduce the risk of Japanese encephalitis include avoiding the bites of infected mosquitoes by wearing long sleeves and trousers, and applying insecticide. There are several vaccines against Japanese

TABLE 34.4-2 Summary of Vaccines Against Japanese Encephalitis*

Description	Virus strain	Common name	Manufacture/ developer	Notes
Inactivated vaccines				
Mouse brain	Nakayama	BIKEN	BIKEN, Japan	Manufactured until 2006 for international distribution, but may still be some availability
Mouse brain	Nakayama	Green Cross	Green Cross, South Korea	Some available internationally under the Green Cross partnership
Vero cell	Beijing-1	BK-VJE	Japan	In development; targeted for Japanese market
Vero cell	SA14-14-2	JE-PIV (IC51) IXIARO®	WRAIR, Intercell	Distributed by Novartis in the USA, Europe and some Asian and Latin American markets, by Biological E. Ltd (India) in India and parts of Asia, and by CSL Biotherapies (Australia) in Australia, New Zealand, Papua New Guinea and Pacific Islands. The vaccine is not currently licensed for use in children, but one pediatric study has been completed and further studies are planned
Live attenuated vaccines				
Primary hamster kidney	SA14-14-2		China	Widely used in China, also in Nepal, India, South Korea and planned for Sri Lanka
Recombinant vaccines				
17-D yellow fever vectored	SA14-14-2	Chimerivax-JE	Acambis	Marketing and distribution agreements with Sanofi Pasteur and Bharat Biotech International Ltd (Indian subcontinent)

*Only the most widely available vaccines, and those in advanced development are shown. Additional, inactivated vaccines include a mouse-brain-derived vaccine manufactured in Japan and vero cell and primary hamster kidney-derived vaccines produced in China.

Modified from Beasley DW, Lewthwaite P, Solomon T. Current use and development of vaccines for Japanese encephalitis. Expert Opin Biol Ther 2008;8:95–106; Solomon T. Vaccines against Japanese encephalitis.In: Jong EC, Zuckerman JN eds. Travelers' Vaccines. Hamilton: BC Decker; 2004: 219–56.

BOX 34.4.1 Emergency Evaluation and Treatment of a Patient with Japanese Encephalitis

Assess airways, breathing and circulation

Look for abnormal movements:
- seizures, including subtle motor seizures
- tremors of dyskinesias

Treat seizures/status epilepticus with (flow chart as per Japanese encephalitis World Health Organization clinical care guidelines):
- diazepam
- phenytoin
- paraldehyde
- phenobarbitone (loading dose of 20 mg/kg, followed by 10 mg/kg)
- intubation and ventilation

Assess hydration:
- rehydrate gently if needed

Tachypnea. Look for:
- pneumonia
- respiratory muscle paresis
- brainstem signs

BOX 34.4.2 Adult Considerations in Japanese Encephatlitis

In endemic areas, adults are at low risk of Japanese encephalitis as they have already been exposed to the virus as children and have developed natural immunity. However, adults are at risk in three circumstances:

- when Japanese encephalitis virus (JEV) spreads to new areas for the first time, adults are at risk because they are immunologically naïve;
- adult travelers to Japanese encephalitis endemic areas are also at risk as they do not have prior immunity;
- there is a small increase in incidence in the elderly, which may reflect waning immunity or other risk factors, such as cerebrovascular disease or hypertention.

Compared to children, adults with Japanese encephalitis are:

- less likely to present with seizures;
- more likely to present with abnormal behavior and are thought to have psychiatric illness.

encephalitis [2] (Table 34.4-2). Formalin-inactivated, mouse-brain-derived vaccines were used routinely in wealthier Asian countries and for travelers. Production of the most widely available one (Biken) has ceased. In some Asian countries it is being replaced by a tissue culture-derived, inactivated vaccine.

A live attenuated vaccine (SA-14-14-2) developed in China has been used since the late 1980s. Its use beyond China had been limited by issues over the novel cell line used (primary hamster kidney) but, in recent years, these issues have been resolved and the vaccine has now been licensed across Asia [17]. An inactivated vaccine (Ixiaro), based on 14-14-2, developed by the Walter Reed Army Institute and then Intercell in Austria, is also becoming more widely available for travelers [18]. A chimeric vaccine, in which the structural genes of JEV strain 14-14-2 are inserted into the backbone of the live attenuated yellow fever vaccine strain 17D, is close to approval for marketing (Boxes 34.4.1 and 34.4.2).

REFERENCES

1. Solomon T. Control of Japanese encephalitis—within our grasp? N Engl J Med 2006;355:869–71.
2. Beasley DW, Lewthwaite P, Solomon T. Current use and development of vaccines for Japanese encephalitis. Expert Opin Biol Ther 2008;8:95–106.
3. Solomon T, Dung NM, Kneen R, et al. Japanese encephalitis. J Neurol Neurosurg Psychiatry 2000;68:405–15.
4. Tsai TF. New initiatives for the control of Japanese encephalitis by vaccination: minutes of a WHO/CVI meeting, Bangkok, Thailand, 13–15 October 1998. Vaccine 2000;18(suppl. 2):1–25.
5. Jmor F, Emsley HCA, Fischer M, et al. The incidence of acute encephalitis syndrome in Western Industrialised and Tropical Countries. Virol J 2008; 5:134.
6. Ooi MH, Lewthwaite P, Lai BF, et al. The epidemiology, clinical features, and long-term prognosis of Japanese encephalitis in central Sarawak, Malaysia, 1997–2005. Clin Infect Dis 2008;47:458–68.
7. Hoke CH, Nisalak A, Sangawhipa N, et al. Protection against Japanese encephalitis by inactivated vaccines. N Engl J Med 1988;319:608–14.
8. Solomon T, Dung NM, Kneen R, et al. Seizures and raised intracranial pressure in Vietnamese patients with Japanese encephalitis. Brain 2002;125: 1084–93.
9. Dung N M, Turtle L, Chong WK, et al. An evaluation of the usefulness of neuroimaging for the diagnosis of Japanese encephalitis. J Neurol 2009;256: 2052–60.
10. Solomon T, Thao TT, Lewthwaite P, et al. A cohort study to assess the new WHO Japanese encephalitis surveillance standards. Bull World Health Organ 2008;86:178–86.
11. Hoke CH, Vaughn DW, Nisalak A, et al. Effect of high dose dexamethasone on the outcome of acute encephalitis due to Japanese encephalitis virus. J Infect Dis 1992;165:631–7.
12. Solomon T, Dung NM, Wills B, et al. Interferon alfa-2a in Japanese encephalitis: a randomised double-blind placebo-controlled trial. Lancet 2003;361: 821–6.
13. Kumar R, Tripathi P, Baranwal M, et al. Randomized, controlled trial of oral ribavirin for Japanese encephalitis in children in Uttar Pradesh, India. Clin Infect Dis 2009;48: 400–6.
14. http://www.liv.ac.uk/media/livacuk/infectionandglobalhealth/docs/long-term-care.pdf
15. Lewthwaite P, Ravikumar R, et al. A simple tool for assessing disability in Japanese encephalitis. American Society of Tropical Medicine and Hygiene 54th Annual Meeting, Washington; 2005.
16. http://www.liv.ac.uk/neuroscience/brain_infections_group/education_presentations.htm
17. Hennessy S, Strom BL, Bilker WB, et al. Effectiveness of live-attenuated Japanese encephalitis vaccine (SA14-14-2): a case-control study. Lancet 1996;347: 1583–6.
18. Tauber E, Kollaritsch H, Korinek M, et al. Safety and immunogenicity of a Vero-cell-derived, inactivated Japanese encephalitis vaccine: a non-inferiority, phase III, randomised controlled trial. Lancet 2007;370:1847–53.
19. German AC, Myint KS, Mai NT, et al. A preliminary neuropathological study of Japanese encephalitis in humans and a mouse model. Transactions of the Royal Society of Tropical Medicine and Hygiene 2006;100:1135–45.
20. Solomon T. Japanese encephalitis. In: Gilman S, Goldstein GW, Waxman SG, eds. Neurobase. San Diego: Medlink Publishing; 2000.
21. Solomon T, Kneen R, Dung NM, et al. Poliomyelitis-like illness due to Japanese encephalitis virus. Lancet 1998;351:1094–7.
22. Dung NM, Turtle L, Chong WK, et al. An evaluation of the usefulness of neuroimaging for the diagnosis of Japanese encephalitis. Journal of neurology 2009 Dec;256(12):2052–60.
23. Solomon T. Vaccines against Japanese encephalitis. In: Jong EC, Zuckerman JN, eds. Travelers' Vaccines. Hamilton: BC Decker; 2004: 219–56.

34.5 West Nile Virus

Marc Fischer, J Erin Staples, Grant L Campbell

Key features

- West Nile virus (WNV) is transmitted to humans primarily through bites of infected mosquitoes
- WNV has been documented on all continents except Antarctica, but has most recently caused large seasonal outbreaks in the Middle East, Europe, and North America
- Most human WNV infections are asymptomatic (~80%) but clinical illness ranges from a systemic febrile illness (~20%) to severe neurologic disease (<1%)
- The incidence of WNV encephalitis and death increase with age
- As there is no treatment or vaccine for WNV disease, prevention depends on community-level mosquito control programs, avoiding exposure to infected mosquitoes and screening blood and organ donors

INTRODUCTION

West Nile virus (WNV) is a mosquito-borne, single-stranded, positive-sense RNA flavivirus (family *Flaviviridae*, genus *Flavivirus*), that was first isolated in Uganda in 1937 [1–4]. For the next 50 years, WNV received little attention as a cause of epidemics of febrile illness and sporadic encephalitis in parts of Africa, Asia and Europe. Beginning in the 1990s, WNV outbreaks with a higher incidence of neurologic disease were identified in the Mediterranean Basin and Eastern Europe [1]. WNV was first detected in the western hemisphere in New York City in 1999 where it subsequently spread across the continental USA and Canada, resulting in large seasonal outbreaks of both systemic febrile illness and neuroinvasive disease [5]. More recently, WNV disease has re-emerged in eastern and southern Europe [6].

EPIDEMIOLOGY

WNV is the most widely distributed arthropod-borne virus (arbovirus) in the world, with transmission documented on every continent except Antarctica [1, 2]. Since the 1990s, the largest outbreaks of WNV neuroinvasive disease have occurred in the Middle East, Europe, and North America [6]. In temperate and subtropical regions, most human WNV infections occur in summer or early autumn. In the tropics, the incidence is likely greatest during the rainy season, but data are scarce. Although all age groups and both sexes are equally susceptible to WNV infection, the incidence of encephalitis and death increase with age.

NATURAL HISTORY, PATHOGENESIS, AND PATHOLOGY

WNV is primarily transmitted to humans through bites of infected *Culex* mosquitoes. Birds are the primary amplifying hosts. Mosquitoes acquire WNV by feeding on infected birds and transmit the virus to humans and other vertebrates during subsequent feeding. Infected humans usually have <7 days of low-level viremia that is insufficient to transmit WNV to feeding mosquitoes. Nevertheless, human-to-human WNV transmission can occur through blood transfusion and organ transplantation [4, 5]. Intrauterine and probable breastfeeding transmission have also been rarely described. Percutaneous and aerosol transmission have occurred in laboratory workers—an outbreak among turkey handlers suggested WNV transmission via aerosol.

CLINICAL FEATURES

Approximately 80% of human WNV infections are asymptomatic [7]. In clinical infections, the incubation period usually is 2–6 days, but can be up to 21 days in immunocompromised people. Most symptomatic persons experience an acute systemic febrile illness that often includes headache, myalgia or arthralgia; gastrointestinal symptoms and a transient maculopapular rash also are commonly reported. Less than 1% of infected people develop neuroinvasive disease, which typically manifests as meningitis, encephalitis, or acute flaccid paralysis. Patients with encephalitis may present with seizures, mental status changes, focal neurologic deficits or movement disorders. WNV acute flaccid paralysis is often clinically and pathologically identical to poliomyelitis caused by polioviruses, with damage of anterior horn cells in the spinal cord (anterior myelitis); it may progress to respiratory paralysis requiring mechanical ventilation. WNV-associated Guillain-Barré syndrome has also been reported and can be distinguished from WNV myelitis by clinical manifestations and electrophysiologic testing. Cardiac dysrhythmias, myocarditis, rhabdomyolysis, optic neuritis, uveitis, chorioretinitis, orchitis, pancreatitis and hepatitis have been rarely described after WNV infection.

Most patients with WNV non-neuroinvasive disease or meningitis recover completely, but fatigue, malaise and weakness can linger for weeks or months [7, 8]. Patients who recover from WNV encephalitis or myelitis often have residual neurologic deficits. Among patients with neuroinvasive disease, the overall case-fatality rate is approximately 10%, but it is significantly higher in WNV encephalitis and myelitis than in WNV meningitis. Risk factors for developing neuroinvasive disease include older age and history of solid organ transplantation; other immunocompromising conditions, diabetes, and hypertension are suspected risk factors.

PATIENT EVALUATION, DIAGNOSIS, AND DIFFERENTIAL DIAGNOSIS

Routine clinical laboratory results are generally nonspecific in WNV infections. In patients with central nervous system disease, cerebrospinal fluid (CSF) examination generally shows lymphocytic pleocytosis, but neutrophils may predominate early in the illness [7]. Brain magnetic resonance imaging (MRI) is frequently normal, but signal abnormalities may be seen in the basal ganglia, thalamus and brainstem with WNV encephalitis, and in the spinal cord with WNV myelitis.

WNV infections are most frequently confirmed by detection of anti-WNV IgM antibodies in serum or CSF [1, 7]. The presence of anti-WNV IgM is usually good evidence of recent WNV infection, but may indicate infection with another closely related flavivirus. As anti-WNV IgM can persist in some patients for >1 year, a positive test result occasionally may reflect past, rather than recent, WNV infection. Serum collected within 10 days of illness onset may lack detectable IgM; the test should be repeated on a convalescent-phase sample. Plaque-reduction neutralization tests can be performed to confirm recent infection by demonstrating a ≥fourfold change in WNV-specific neutralizing antibody titers between acute- and convalescent-phase serum samples and to rule-out primary infection with a closely related flavivirus. In patients who have been previously infected by another flavivirus or vaccinated with a flavivirus vaccine (e.g. Japanese encephalitis), broadly cross-reactive antibodies may make it difficult to incriminate a specific flavivirus.

Viral culture and nucleic acid amplification tests for WNV RNA can be performed on acute-phase serum, CSF, or tissue specimens; immunohistochemical staining can detect WNV antigens in fixed tissue, but the sensitivity of these tests is low and negative results are not definitive.

WNV disease should be considered in the differential diagnosis of febrile or acute neurologic illnesses associated with recent exposure to mosquitoes, blood transfusion, or organ transplantation, and of illnesses in neonates whose mothers were infected with WNV during pregnancy or while breastfeeding. In addition to other more common causes of encephalitis and aseptic meningitis (e.g. herpes simplex virus and enteroviruses), other arboviruses should also be considered in the differential etiology of suspected WNV illness.

TREATMENT

No specific antiviral treatment for WNV disease exists [3]. Therapy consists of supportive care and management of complications. Several vaccines against WNV are licensed for use in horses; candidate human WNV vaccines are being evaluated. Information regarding the latest WNV treatment and vaccine trials can be found at: http://clinicaltrials.gov/ct2/home.

In the absence of a human vaccine, prevention of WNV disease depends on screening blood and organ donors, community-level mosquito control programs and avoiding exposure to infected mosquitoes [2]. Personal protective measures include the use of mosquito repellents, wearing long-sleeved shirts and long pants, and limiting outdoor exposure from dusk to dawn. Using air conditioning, installing window and door screens, and reducing peri-domestic mosquito breeding sites, can further decrease the risk for WNV exposure. Additional information on prevention of WNV infection is available at: http://www.cdc.gov/ncidod/dvbid/westnile/index.htm.

REFERENCES

1. Campbell GL, Marfin AA, Lanciotti RS, Gubler DL. West Nile virus. Lancet Infect Dis 2002;2:519–29.
2. Kramer LD, Styer LM, Ebel GD. A global perspective on the epidemiology of West Nile virus. Annu Rev Entomol 2008;53:61–81.
3. Diamond MS. Progress on the development of therapeutics against West Nile virus. Antiviral Res 2009;83:214–27.
4. Hayes EB, Komar N, Nasci RS, et al. Epidemiology and transmission dynamics of West Nile virus disease. Emerg Infect Dis 2005;11:1167–73.
5. Lindsey NP, Staples JE, Lehman JA, Fischer M. Surveillance for West Nile Virus Disease – United States, 1999–2008. Surv Summ, April 2, 2010. MMWR 2010; 59(SS-2).
6. Reiter P. West Nile virus in Europe: understanding the present to gauge the future. Euro Surveill 2010;15:19508. Available at: http://www.eurosurveillance.org/ViewArticle.aspx?ArticleId=19508.
7. Davis LE, DeBiasi R, Goade DE, et al. West Nile virus neuroinvasive disease. Ann Neurology 2006;60:286–300.
8. Sejvar J. The long-term outcomes of human West Nile virus infection. Clin Infect Dis 2007;44:1617–24.

34.6 Saint Louis Encephalitis and Rocio Encephalitis

James J Sejvar

Key features

- Saint Louis encephalitis virus and Rocio virus are transmitted to humans by infected *Culex* mosquitoes
- Both Saint Louis encephalitis virus and Rocio virus cause central nervous system disease, including meningitis and encephalitis
- Saint Louis encephalitis virus causes illness primarily in periodic large urban outbreaks throughout the USA
- Rocio virus resulted in a large outbreak of encephalitis in coastal Brazil from 1975–1977; it has rarely been identified since then
- There is no specific treatment for Saint Louis encephalitis virus or Rocio virus infections; management is symptomatic

INTRODUCTION

Saint Louis encephalitis virus and Rocio virus are arthropod-borne viruses (arboviruses) of the *Flavivirus* genus (family *Flaviviridae*) which can produce acute febrile illness and central nervous system (CNS) disease. Saint Louis encephalitis virus was named following the first recognized outbreak in St Louis, Missouri, USA. Rocio virus was first isolated from a fatal case of encephalitis in the Rocio district, São Paulo, Brazil. The two viruses, which are closely related, are maintained in enzootic cycles between birds and mosquitoes and transmitted to humans by infected mosquitoes. *Culex* mosquitoes, which breed in dirty water, are the most important vectors. Since it was first identified in the 1930s, Saint Louis encephalitis virus has caused periodic large outbreaks throughout the USA. In contrast, Rocio virus was first identified as the cause of an outbreak of encephalitis in Brazil in the 1970s and has rarely been detected since.

EPIDEMIOLOGY

Transmission of Saint Louis encephalitis virus and Rocio virus involves mosquito vectors and avian hosts. The geographic range of Saint Louis encephalitis virus extends from southern Canada to Argentina, but human cases have been identified primarily in the USA. Saint Louis encephalitis typically occurs in periodic large outbreaks during the late summer and early autumn. From 1960–1990, these outbreaks primarily occurred in urban areas in the southeastern and central USA, with a more sporadic disease pattern in the southwest (Fig. 34.6.1) [1, 2]. A large outbreak of Saint Louis encephalitis in the central USA in 1975 resulted in more than 2000 neuroinvasive cases and approximately 185 deaths; subsequent focal outbreaks of Saint Louis encephalitis have occurred in Florida in 1990, Louisiana in 2001 and Argentina in 2005. The factors controlling these large period outbreaks are poorly understood.

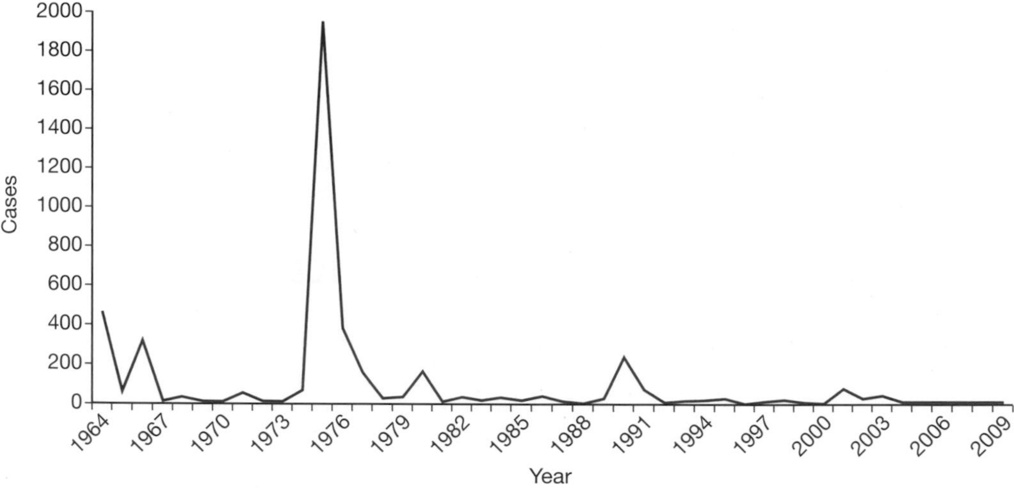

FIGURE 34.6.1 Saint Louis encephalitis virus neuroinvasive disease cases reported by state, United States, 1964–2009.

NATURAL HISTORY, PATHOGENESIS AND PATHOLOGY

Most infections with Saint Louis encephalitis virus are asymptomatic [1]. While serologic surveys suggest that all age groups are at roughly equal risk of infection, clinical illness is more frequent and more severe in older age groups.

Between 1975 and 1977, over 1000 cases of Rocio virus disease were reported in São Paulo state, Brazil [3]. Subsequently, only sporadic cases have been reported, although asymptomatic infections have been identified during serosurveys. To date, Rocio virus has not been detected outside of Brazil.

CLINICAL FEATURES

The incubation period for Saint Louis encephalitis virus is estimated to be 4–14 days. Aseptic meningitis and encephalitis are the most commonly described clinical syndromes following infection; nonspecific febrile illness likely also occurs. Saint Louis encephalitis virus meningitis is clinically similar to other viral meningitides, with clinical features including fever, headache, neck stiffness and other meningeal signs. Cerebrospinal fluid (CSF) shows a moderately elevated white cell count and protein. Outcome is generally favorable. Encephalitis caused by Saint Louis encephalitis virus infection may result in altered mental status, ataxia, tremors, seizures or other neurologic signs. The syndrome of inappropriate secretion of antidiuretic hormone (SIADH) causing hyponatremia has been described. Mortality following Saint Louis encephalitis virus encephalitis ranges from 5–20%; the case-fatality is higher in older age groups.

Clinical illness from Rocio virus is essentially the same as that described for Saint Louis encephalitis virus. The Rocio virus outbreak in 1975–1977 was associated with severe illness observed both in younger children and in older individuals.

PATIENT EVALUATION, DIAGNOSIS, AND DIFFERENTIAL DIAGNOSIS

The diagnosis of Saint Louis encephalitis should be considered in patients with fever, aseptic meningitis or encephalitis in the setting of known Saint Louis encephalitis virus transmission, or during the appropriate season in endemic areas. In patients presenting with signs of meningitis or encephalitis, CSF examination should be performed to exclude bacterial meningitis and assess for CNS inflammation. Patients should also be evaluated for possible metabolic causes of acute encephalopathy and other common viral etiologies of acute encephalitis, such as herpes simplex virus. As Saint Louis encephalitis virus and West Nile virus co-circulate in largely the same areas and are clinically nearly identical, both viruses should be considered in tandem.

Laboratory confirmation of Saint Louis encephalitis virus infection is most commonly made by detection of virus-specific IgM antibodies by enzyme immunoassay (EIA) in acute serum or CSF, or demonstration of at least a fourfold rise in Saint Louis encephalitis virus-specific antibodies between acute- and convalescent-phase serum specimens collected 2–3 weeks apart. Antibodies to Saint Louis encephalitis virus and Rocio virus may be cross-reactive with those against closely related flaviviruses (e.g. West Nile and dengue viruses) or flavivirus vaccines (e.g. yellow fever and Japanese encephalitis vaccines). In these situations, plaque-reduction neutralization testing (PRNT) may discriminate between cross-reacting antibodies. Viral culture or Saint Louis encephalitis virus-specific PCR testing may be performed on acute-phase serum, CSF, or tissue, but the sensitivity is low.

TREATMENT AND PREVENTION

There is no specific treatment for Saint Louis encephalitis virus or Rocio virus infection; management of clinical illness is supportive. Interferon- α2b has been reported to reduce the severity and duration of complications from Saint Louis encephalitis in some patients, but randomized controlled trials have not been conducted (Category 4 evidence). Corticosteroids and intravenous immune globulin have been used on an anecdotal basis to treat Saint Louis encephalitis with no clear benefit (Category 5 evidence). Preventing infection through protection from mosquito bites is of primary importance.

REFERENCES

1. Reisen WK. Epidemiology of St. Louis encephalitis virus. Adv Virus Res 2003;61:139–83.
2. Reimann CA, Hayes EB, DiGuiseppi C, et al. Epidemiology of neuroinvasive arboviral disease in the United States, 1999–2007. Am J Trop Med Hyg 2008;79:974–9.
3. de Souza Lopes O, Coimbra TL, de Abreu Sacchetta L, et al. Emergence of a new arbovirus disease in Brazil. I. Isolation and characterization of the etiologic agent, Rocio virus. Am J Epidemiol 1978;107:444–9.

34.7 Other Arboviral Encephalitides

James J Sejvar, Grant L Campbell

Key features

- Arboviruses (arthropod-borne viruses) that cause encephalitis are seasonally transmitted by insect or tick vectors, and are found worldwide
- Many arboviruses are only associated with sporadic cases of human illness
- The arboviral encephalitides are clinically indistinguishable from the other viral encephalitides
- There is no specific treatment for any arboviral disease, and management is supportive
- Recognition of the presence of these arboviruses, and avoidance of exposure to insect or tick vectors, is key to prevention of disease

TABLE 34.7-1 Selected characteristics of other arboviruses known to cause neuroinvasive illness in humans*

Family/Virus	Primary vector(s)	Vertebrate amplifying host(s)	Known geographic range
Bunyaviridae			
Cache Valley	Mosquitoes	Large mammals (?)	North America
California serogroup†	Mosquitoes	Mammals	Europe, North America
Toscana	Sandflies	Unknown	Southern Europe
Flaviviridae			
Kunjin	Mosquitoes	Birds	Australia, Southeast Asia
Kyasanur Forest disease	Ticks	Mammals (?)	India, China (?), Saudi Arabia (?)
Louping ill	Ticks	Large mammals	UK
Murray Valley encephalitis	Mosquitoes	Birds	Australia, New Guinea
Powassan	Ticks	Small mammals	North America, Russia
Tick-borne encephalitis	Ticks	Small mammals	Europe, Asia
Reoviridae			
Banna	Mosquitoes (?)	Unknown	Asia
Colorado tick fever	Ticks	Small mammals	North America
Kemerovo serogroup§	Ticks	Unknown	Europe, Middle East
Rhabdoviridae			
Chandipura	Sandflies (?)	Unknown	South Asia, West Africa

*Excluding viruses covered in other chapters.
†Includes California encephalitis, Jamestown Canyon, La Crosse, Snowshoe hare and Tahyna viruses.
§Includes Kemerovo, Lipovnik and Tribec viroses.

INTRODUCTION

Arboviruses (arthropod-borne viruses) are seasonally vectored by insects or ticks. Medically important arboviruses are found in at least five viral families (*Bunyaviridae, Flaviviridae, Reoviridae, Rhabdoviridae,* and *Togaviridae*) and are distributed worldwide. Several arboviruses associated with large numbers of cases of human neurologic disease (e.g. Japanese encephalitis, West Nile, St Louis encephalitis and the equine encephalitis viruses) are covered in earlier chapters. Many others, however, have been recognized as causing only sporadic human disease or small and infrequent outbreaks, or have been associated only with laboratory-acquired infection [1, 2]. Table 34.7-1 lists some of these viruses known to cause encephalitis and not covered in earlier chapters. Additional information on selected viruses listed in Table 34.7-1 is included below. In addition to viruses listed in Table 34.7-1, several known, or suspected, arboviruses in the families *Bunyviridae* (Bhanja, Bwamba, Erve, Oropouche and Wanowrie viruses), *Flaviviridae* (Langat and Omsk hemorrhagic fever viruses), *Orthomyxoviridae* (Thogoto virus), *Reoviridae* (Eyach virus) and Togaviridae (Semliki Forest virus) have been associated with rare, unproven, or laboratory-associated cases of neuroinvasive disease in humans.

FAMILY BUNYAVIRIDAE

La Crosse virus in the California serogroup is endemic to the deciduous forests of rural and suburban eastern North America, where its primary vector is *Ochlerotatus triseriatus* (the eastern treehole mosquito), its main amplifying hosts are small mammals (e.g. squirrels and chipmunks) and it overwinters in mosquito eggs (transovarial transmission) deposited in treeholes and artificial containers (e.g. discarded tires). In the USA, an average of 80 cases of La Crosse encephalitis are reported annually, with a case-fatality of 1–3%. Risk factors include young age (median, 8 years), male sex (60%) and living in high-incidence areas (e.g. some counties in West Virginia, North Carolina, Ohio, Tennessee, and Wisconsin). Other, less-studied, North American bunyaviruses known to cause sporadic cases of encephalitis include Jamestown Canyon, Snowshoe hare, and California encephalitis viruses in the California serogroup and Cache Valley virus in the Bunyamwera serogroup. In Europe and Asia, Tahyna virus, and possibly Inkoo virus in the Calfornia serogoup, also cause sporadic encephalitis cases. In the Phlebotomus fever serogroup, Toscana virus has recently been recognized as an important cause of summertime meningitis and, to a lesser extent, encephalitis in southern Europe from Spain to Turkey; Italy has had several outbreaks in recent years. Young adults are predominately affected; fatalities are rare. Toscana virus is vectored by sandflies, probably including *Phlebotomus perniciosus* and *Phlebotomus perfiliewi*. The role of vertebrates in the amplification or maintenance of Toscana virus is unknown; the vectors themselves may serve as the reservoir via transovarial transmission.

FAMILY FLAVIVIRIDAE

Encephalitogenic tick-borne flaviviruses include the following closely related members of the genus *Flavivirus*: tick-borne encephalitis; Kyasanur Forest disease; Louping ill; and Powassan viruses. Of these, tick-borne encephalitis virus (TBEV) is of greatest public health importance, with an average of approximately 9000 cases reported in Europe per year. TBEV includes the European, Siberian and Far Eastern subtypes. All are amplified in rodents and other small mammals and primarily vectored by *Ixodes* species: *Ixodes ricinus* for the European subtype and *Ixodes persulcatus* for the other two subtypes. Disease caused by all three TBEV subtypes is most common in people aged 15–40 years. The Far Eastern subtype is generally associated with more severe human disease, a case-fatality rate of approximately 20% and a frequency of permanent sequelae in survivors of up to 80%. In addition to encephalitis, acute flaccid paralysis caused by lower motor neuron involvement has been described. The European and Siberian subtypes are generally associated with milder disease and lower case-fatality (1–3%). The European subtype is associated with biphasic illness in approximately one-third of encephalitis cases and, uncommonly, infection may be acquired through consumption of unpasteurized cow, sheep, or goat milk. Kyasanur Forest disease virus occurs in India and the Middle East, but associated human disease has only been recognized in India. *Haemaphysalis spinigera* is considered the primary vector and rodents the principal amplifying hosts. The predominant clinical syndrome associated with Kyasanur Forest disease virus is hemorrhagic fever, but a few such cases are complicated by encephalitis. Louping ill virus is endemic to the British Isles, where it is primarily vectored by *Ix. ricinus* and amplified in sheep. Louping ill disease mainly affects sheep, but rare, sporadic cases of human encephalitis have been described, including several in laboratory workers. Powassan virus has been associated with approximately 40 sporadic cases of human encephalitis, often severe, most in North America and a few in Russia. In North America, it is primarily vectored by *Ixodes cookei* and amplified in medium-sized mammals such as woodchucks.

Murray Valley encephalitis and Kunjin viruses are mosquito-borne members of the Japanese encephalitis serologic complex of the genus *Flavivirus*. While both are endemic to Australia, Murray Valley encephalitis virus has also been identified in New Guinea and Kunjin virus in Southeast Asia. Their primary vector is *Culex annulirostris* and they are mainly amplified in birds. Although Murray Valley encephalitis virus has caused significant epidemics of encephalitis in Australia in the past, since 1974 only sporadic cases have been reported annually. A total of 5–10 sporadic cases of Kunjin encephalitis have been reported in Australia, including at least one laboratory-associated case; virologically it is closely related to West Nile virus.

FAMILY REOVIRIDAE

Colorado tick fever virus (genus *Coltivirus*) is transmitted to humans by *Dermacentor andersonii* (the Rocky Mountain wood tick) in the western USA. Its main amplifying hosts are small mammals such as squirrels and chipmunks. Although Colorado tick fever is usually a mild, generalized illness without apparent neuroinvasion, meningitis is not uncommon and encephalitis has been documented in a few cases. Banna virus is an emerging mosquito-borne reovirus in the genus *Seadornavirus*. It is endemic to China and Southeast Asia, and has been implicated as the cause of sporadic human encephalitis cases in China. Kemerovo virus in Asia and Tribec and Lipovnik viruses in Europe are tickborne members of the genus *Orbivirus* that have also been implicated in the etiology of sporadic cases of human encephalitis.

FAMILY RHABDOVIRIDAE

Chandipura virus is a sandfly-transmitted member of the genus *Vesiculovirus*. It was first isolated from a febrile adult in India in 1965. Since then, few human Chandipura virus infections have been documented. Although the recognized geographic range of Chandipura virus includes the Indian subcontinent, Africa, and Sri Lanka, associated human illness has only been described in India. Beginning in 2003, large outbreaks of "epidemic brain attack" were reported in several northern Indian states, especially Andhra Pradesh and Uttar Pradesh, where large seasonal outbreaks have continued to occur. Isolation of Chandipura virus from several of these case-patients with apparent encephalitis led to two competing hypotheses, i.e. that Chandipura virus infection was either etiologic or an incidental finding in these cases. Further research is needed.

CLINICAL FEATURES, DIAGNOSIS, TREATMENT AND PREVENTION

The encephalitic arboviruses have variable incubation periods typically ranging from 3–14 days. Most infections are silent or cause mild, self-limited febrile illness, while a minority cause neuroinvasive disease, including meningitis, encephalitis, or myelitis [3]. The arboviral encephalitides are generally not distinguishable from the other viral encephalitides, either clinically or on the basis of routine laboratory test results. Parenchymal central nervous system lesions may be seen on computed tomography or magnetic resonance imaging; there are no pathognomonic features, though involvement of the deep gray matter may be a clue to an arboviral etiology. Definitive diagnosis is substantiated by identification of live virus, viral antigens, viral nucleic acids in tissue specimens or bodily fluids or identification of virus-specific antibodies in sera or cerebrospinal fluid (CSF). Diagnostic techniques include viral culture; antigen-detection assays; PCR assays conducted on acute-phase serum, CSF, or tissue specimens; and enzyme immunoassays or neutralization tests of acute- and convalescent-phase serum or CSF. Laboratory testing for many uncommon arboviruses is available only at select reference laboratories. No proven, specific treatment is available for any arboviral infection. Clinical management is supportive only. Neurologic complications such as seizures and cerebral edema should be managed accordingly. With the exception of TBEV vaccines, vaccines to prevent infection with any of the viruses covered in this chapter are unavailable. Therefore, the cornerstones of prevention of these infections are vector avoidance, vector barriers (e.g. clothing, mosquito screens, and mosquito nets) and the use of repellents. Inactivated TBEV vaccines are available in Europe, Russia, and Canada (for travelers). Vaccination is recommended for residents in high-incidence areas and for travelers to endemic areas who plan to participate in activities with a high risk of tick exposure.

REFERENCES

1. Monath TP, ed. The Arboviruses: Epidemiology and Ecology, Vol. I-V. Boca Raton: CRC Press, Inc.; 1988–1989.
2. Gubler DJ. The global emergence/resurgence of arboviral diseases as public health problems. Arch Med Res 2002;33:330–42.
3. Rennels MB. Arthropod-borne virus infections of the central nervous system. Neurol Clin 1984;2:241–54.

34.8 Prion Disease

Richard Knight, Victor Javier Sanchez Gonzalez

Key features

- Prion diseases are also known as transmissible spongiform encephalopathies (TSEs)
- They are rare, progressive, fatal, and untreatable encephalopathies of animals and man
- Creutzfeldt-Jakob disease (CJD) is the commonest human disease
- Human prion diseases exist in idiopathic, genetic, and acquired forms
- Kuru, confined to Papua New Guinea, largely of historical interest, was transmitted by cannibalism
- The acquired forms have significant public health implications
- One disease, variant CJD, originated as a zoonotic infection via dietary contamination
- Variant CJD poses further risks via secondary transmission, particularly via blood and blood products

INTRODUCTION

Transmissible spongiform encephalopathies (TSEs), or prion diseases, are a group of rare neurodegenerative encephalopathies affecting animals and humans (Table 34.8-1). There is a common molecular pathology (involving a post-translational conformational change in the prion protein) and a potential transmissibility [1,2]. Some human prion diseases are acquired (as zoonotic or iatrogenic infections); others are genetic or idiopathic. They form part of the differential diagnosis of subacute brain disease and rapidly progressive dementia. The relevant agent (termed the prion) is incompletely characterized but is thought to represent a new class of infective agent, consisting mostly, or entirely, of protein, without constituent DNA or RNA [1,2].

EPIDEMIOLOGY

The overall annual mortality rate for human prion diseases is around 1–2/million in countries where it has been studied [3].

Sporadic Creutzfeldt-Jakob disease (sCJD) is the most common prion disease, accounting for 80–85% of cases with a worldwide distribution. It is predominantly a disease of mid- and late-life (Fig. 34.8.1).

TABLE 34.8-1 Prion Diseases of Animals and Man

Disease	Affected species	Comments
Scrapie	Sheep and goats	Naturally occurring disease, recognized since 17th century. Another form recently identified termed 'Atypical Scrapie'
Bovine spongiform encephalopathy (BSE)	Cattle	Transmitted to felines, certain exotic ungulates and humans. Originated in UK in the 1980s. Effective control measures in various countries, especially in the European Union. Two new forms recently identified, of uncertain significance, termed "H-BSE" and "L-BSE"
Feline spongiform encephalopathy (FSE)	Domestic and large cats	BSE infection via diet
Transmissible mink encephalopathy (TME)	Mink	Seen in farmed mink, of uncertain cause
Chronic wasting disease (CWD)	Cervid species	Naturally occurring disease
Kuru	Man	Confined to Papua New Guinea. Transmitted via cannabilistic mourning rituals
Sporadic CJD	Man	Worldwide with annual mortality rate of ~1–2 per million. Unknown cause. Although ~80% of cases have a relatively uniform clinical picture, there is significant clinicopathologic heterogeneity and atypical cases occur
Iatrogenic CJD	Man	Accidental human-to-human transmission of other forms of CJD via medical or surgical practice
Variant CJD	Man	Primarily a zoonotic disease caused by BSE contamination of human diet, found mostly in UK and France. Risk categorization of countries see www.oie.int/. Secondary transmission via blood transfusion
Genetic CJD	Man	CJD phenotypic illness caused by pathogenic mutations of *PRNP*
Gerstmann Sträussler Scheinker syndrome (GSS)	Man	A *PRNP* mutation disease with relatively distinct clinicopathologic phenotype
Fatal familial insomnia (FFI)	Man	A distinctive clinical phenotype related to D178N *PRNP* mutation

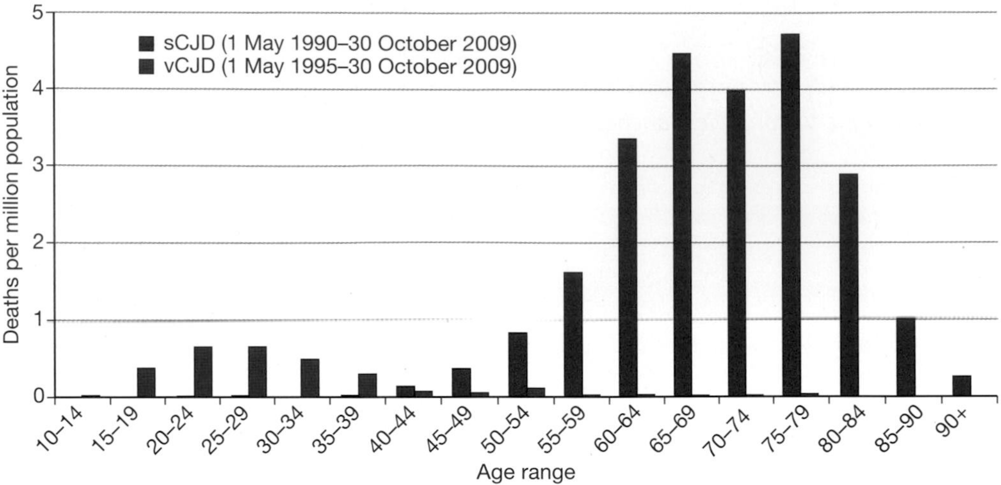

FIGURE 34.8.1 Age-specific mortality rates for sporadic and vCJD (UK).

TABLE 34.8-2 Acquired Forms of Human Prion Disease

Disease	Countries which have reported cases (numbers for those reporting five or more)	Risk period (where known–may be approximate)	Total numbers and notes
Dura mater cases	Argentina, Australia (5), Austria, Canada, Croatia, France (13), Germany (8), the Netherlands, Republic of Ireland, Italy, Japan (123), New Zealand, South Africa, Spain (10), Switzerland, Thailand, UK (7), USA	<1987	Total: 196 Nearly all cases linked to Lyodura brand of dura mater
Cadaveric-derived human growth hormone cases	Australia, Brazil, France (107), Netherlands, New Zealand (6), Qatar, UK (51), USA (26)	<1985	Total: 194
Cadaveric-derived gonadotrophin hormone cases	Australia		Total: 4
Depth EEG electrodes	Switzerland		Total: 2
Neurosurgical instruments	France, UK		Total: 4
Corneal transplants	Germany, USA		Total: 2
Kuru	Papua New Guinea		
Variant CJD	UK, France	1980–1996 (for primary cases)	

Genetic cases (gPD) comprise three clinicopathologic phenotypes (discussed below), all resulting from pathogenic mutations of *PRNP*. They account for 10–15% of prion disease cases and are found in many countries [4].

Acquired prion disease (iatrogenic and variant CJD; iCJD, vCJD) accounts for only a few percent of cases; their details are summarized in Table 34.8-2. vCJD arose from bovine spongiform encephalopathy (BSE) contamination of human food (with an estimated dietary exposure risk period of 1980–1996 in the UK) but secondary, human-to-human, transmission has been reported via blood and blood products [5]. It has a relatively young age of illness onset (Fig. 34.8.1). Most iatrogenic CJD has arisen from cadaveric-derived human growth hormone and dura mater grafts [6].

Kuru, geographically confined to certain areas of Papua New Guinea, is of largely historical importance, being transmitted from human-to-human via exposure during ritual mourning cannibalistic feasts (now discontinued).

NATURAL HISTORY, PATHOGENESIS, AND PATHOLOGY

Prion diseases are named after the prion protein which plays a pivotal pathologic role. The precise role of normal prion protein (designated PrP^C) is uncertain; it is a transmembrane glycoprotein encoded by *PRNP* (on chromosome 20) in humans. Prion diseases are characterized by a post-translational misfolding of PrP^C; the disease-related conformation (designated PrP^{Sc}) aggregates and accumulates in tissue [1, 2]. The disease process is confined to the nervous system—a progressive neurodegenerative change involves neuronal loss, spongiform change and gliosis. The precise relationship between the abnormal PrP accumulation and neuronal dysfunction is uncertain. In sporadic and genetic forms, the disease process is apparently spontaneous. The inheritance of gPD is autosomal dominant with variable (generally high) penetrance. However, a family history is absent in around 40% of cases [4]. The cause of sporadic CJD remains unknown, with the possibility that it is a heterogenous entity and with some cases even being covertly acquired. Acquired prion disease requires an infective agent and this has been termed the 'prion'. In acquired disease, the incubation period is potentially long, typically measured in years, but this varies with cause with means of 11–15 years. The figure for dietary-acquired vCJD is unknown, but the minimum is thought to be 5 years; reported incubation periods in secondary transmission via blood transfusion are around 7–8 years.

Non-pathogenic *PRNP* polymorphisms are potentially important, particularly the *PRNP* codon 129 methionine/valine (M/V) polymorphism. In acquired forms, this may affect susceptibility or incubation period and may affect the clinicopathologic expression of all forms of prion disease. All tested cases of vCJD classified as definite or probable on the WHO-adapted diagnostic criteria have been codon 129 MM, but one likely case has been reported as MV [7].

Prion diseases are universally progressive (often rapidly so), fatal and currently untreatable illnesses.

CLINICAL FEATURES

The clinical features vary somewhat between the different diseases, but encephalopathic illness with dementia, cerebellar ataxia, and myoclonus is typical.

Sporadic CJD, sCJD, the commonest form, affects the middle-aged and elderly (median age at death is around 65 years) (Fig. 34.8.1). Cases below the age of 40 years are exceptionally rare. It typically presents as a rapidly progressive dementia with cerebellar ataxia, visual disturbances, and myoclonus terminating in an akinetic mute state. The median survival is only around 4 months. Two well-described variations are presentation with a pure cerebellar syndrome and pure visual impairment leading to cortical blindness, although they progress to a similar preterminal state as in typical sCJD. These clinicopathologic variations correlate to some degree with *PRNP* codon 129 polymorphism and the prion protein type.

Genetic prion disease (gPD) has a very varied clinicopathologic phenotype, partly dependent on the underlying *PRNP* mutation. The division of gPD into gCJD, Gerstmann Sträussler Scheinker syndrome (GSS) and fatal familial insomnia (FFI) is arguably now historical, predating mutation characterization, but classical GSS presents as a progressive cerebellar ataxia with relatively late cognitive features and FFI begins with prominent sleep and autonomic disturbances. In gCJD, the mean age at onset is slightly younger and illness duration is longer than in sCJD. The commonest mutation disease is E200K-CJD which typically clinically resembles sCJD, although a polyneuropathy may be present [4].

In general, iCJD resembles sCJD with age at onset reflecting the age of exposure and the incubation period. Human growth hormone-related CJD tends to have a relatively young age at onset, reflecting the age at which hormone treatment is given, and presents differently as a progressive cerebellar syndrome with relatively minor and late cognitive features [6].

vCJD has affected a significantly younger age group and progresses more slowly (in the UK: mean age at onset, 28 years; mean duration of illness, 14 months) (Fig. 34.8.1). The initial symptoms are prominently psychiatric and behavioral, sometimes with painful sensory symptoms. As the illness progresses, cerebellar ataxia becomes prominent with cognitive impairment and involuntary movements, including myoclonus [5].

PATIENT EVALUATION, DIAGNOSIS, AND DIFFERENTIAL DIAGNOSIS

With no simple, absolute clinical diagnostic test for prion disease, definitive diagnosis requires neuropathology, i.e. autopsy or brain biopsy (the main justification for which being its necessity to diagnose an alternative, treatable, condition). However, relatively highly reliable diagnosis can be made based on the clinical features. The potentially wide differential diagnosis of prion disease varies with the clinical presentation, the age of the affected individual and the local context, for example the differential diagnosis of subacute dementia in Western industrialized nations and the tropics is different. There are no systemic abnormalities caused by prion disease: no pyrexia or other index of infection and routine hematology, biochemistry and immunologic tests are normal. Prion disease may be excluded relatively early in the diagnostic process if there are such features or the cerebrospinal fluid (CSF) contains excess white cells or cerebral imaging shows white matter abnormalities or mass lesions. The overall diagnostic process is essentially the suspicion of prion disease based on clinical pattern, the exclusion of other diagnoses and supportive investigation findings. The role of the supportive diagnostic tests in prion disease is summarized below and in Table 34.8-3. The electroencephalography (EEG), CSF, and magnetic resonance imaging (MRI) findings are not prion-disease-specific; it is important to appreciate that, while the sensitivity of such tests depends on the nature of prion disease, their specificity also depends on the testing context. They are, therefore, essentially supportive tests when prion disease is already reasonably suspected; positive results must be viewed in the light of the overall clinical situation.

SPORADIC CJD

In around two-thirds of cases, the EEG shows characteristic periodic bi- or triphasic complexes at some stage of the illness (Fig. 34.8.2). The CSF 14-3-3 protein test is positive in the majority of cases [8]. The cerebral frequently shows basal ganglia (putamen and caudate)

TABLE 34.8-3 Diagnosis of Prion Disease

Investigation	sCJD	vCJD	gPD	iCJD
EEG	Periodic discharges in many cases	Periodic discharges not typical (may occur preterminally)	Periodic discharges in some cases	Periodic discharges in some cases
CSF 14-3-3	Positive in most cases	Positive in under half of cases	Variable results	Variable results
Cerebral MRI	Hyperintensity in putamen, caudate, and some cortical areas	Hyperintensity in posterior thalamus	Variable findings, may be similar to sCJD	Variable findings, may be similar to sCJD
Tonsil biopsy	No abnormal PrP	Disease-related, abnormal PrP may be found	No abnormal PrP	No abnormal PrP
PRNP sequencing	No pathogenic mutations, but codon 129 genotype may help diagnosis	No pathogenic mutations, but codon 129 genotype may help diagnosis	Pathogenic *PRNP* mutations are detected from blood samples	No pathogenic mutations, but codon 129 genotype may help diagnosis

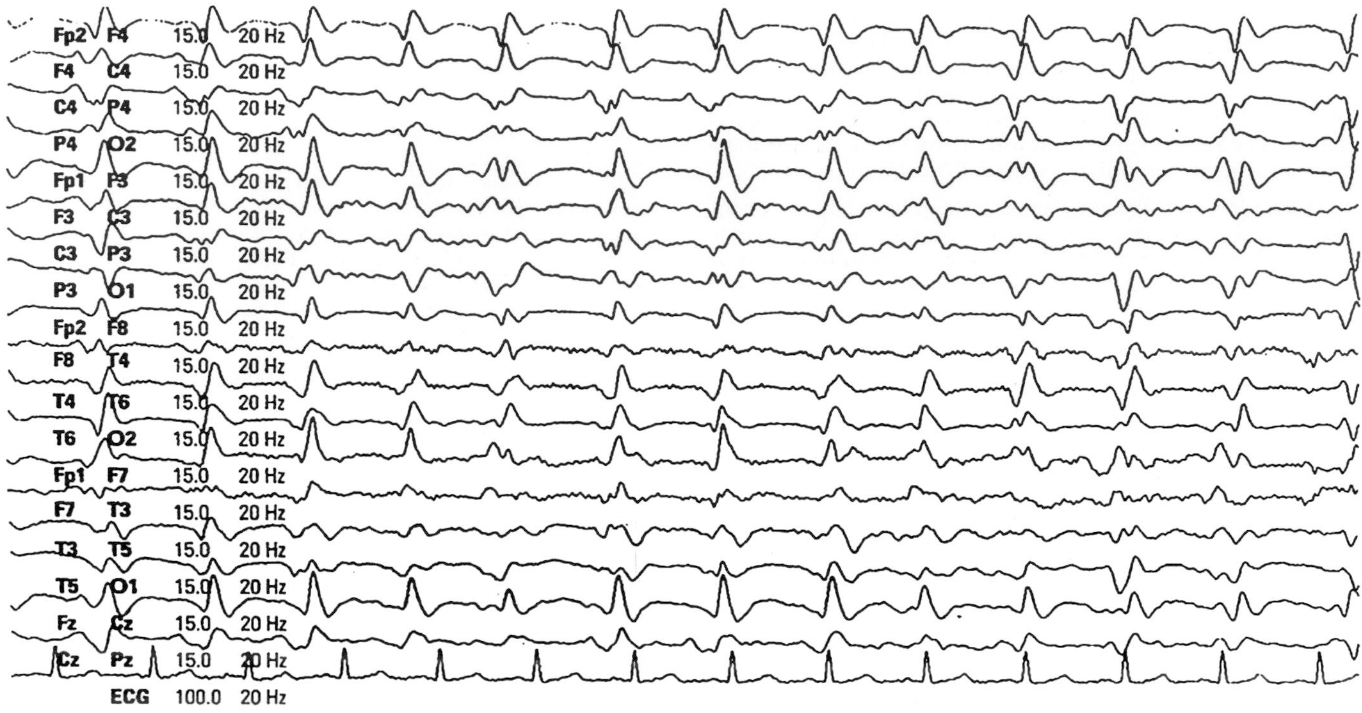

FIGURE 34.8.2 Periodic discharges in the EEG in sporadic CJD.

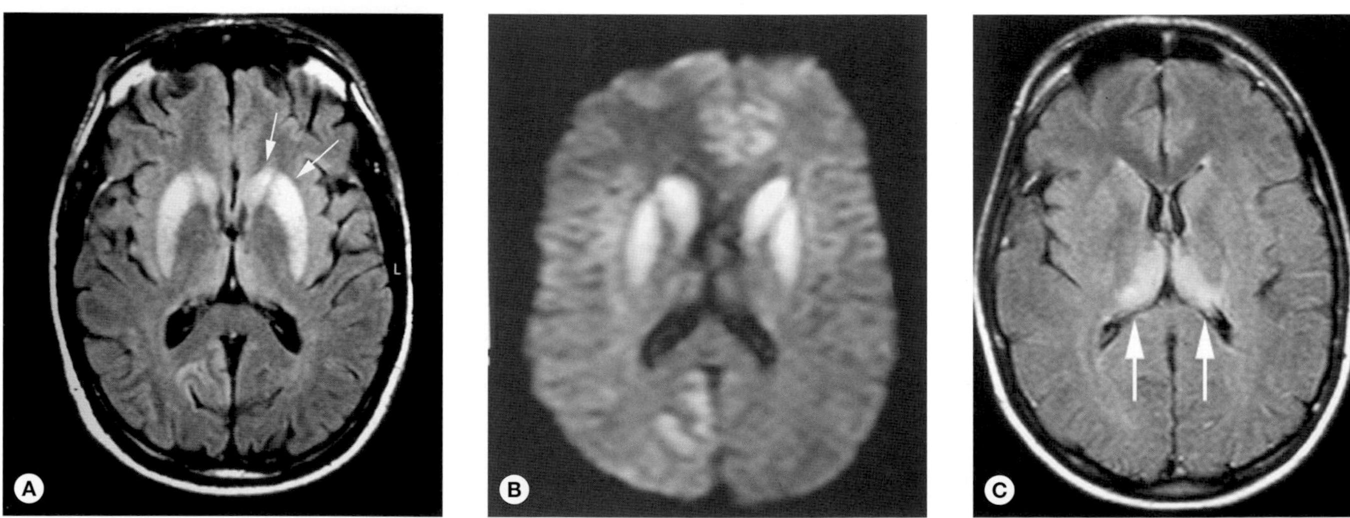

FIGURE 34.8.3 (A) Brain MRI (FLAIR) in sporadic CJD showing hyperintensity of the caudate and putamen (arrowed). **(B)** Brain MRI (DWI) in sporadic CJD showing hyperintensity of the caudate and putamen with hyperintensity in some cortical areas. **(C)** Brasin MRI in variant CJD showing the pulvinar sign (arrowed).

and cortical hyerperintensity, especially on fluid-attenuated inversion recovery (FLAIR) and diffusion weighted imaging (DWI) sequences (Figure 34.8.3) [9].

VARIANT CJD

The EEG does not usually show the periodic activity seen in sCJD. The CSF 14-3-3 is positive in less than half the cases. Cerebral MRI shows hyperintensity in the posterior thalamus (the "Pulvinar Sign") in over 90% of cases, especially on FLAIR and DWI sequences (Fig. 34.8.3) [10]. In vCJD, in contradistinction to other prion diseases, a tonsil biopsy may show the disease-specific abnormality of PrP^{Sc}.

OTHER FORMS OF PRION DISEASE

There are no abnormalities specific to other prion diseases except for genetic forms, where *PRNP* mutation testing can be undertaken on a blood sample. Given the variable clinical phenotypes of gPD, the potential similarity to sCJD and the frequently absent family history, *PRNP* mutation testing is necessary to definitively distinguish gPD and sCJD. Such testing should be considered in a wide variety of neuropsychiatric illnesses where no other diagnosis is made. Given the variability of sCJD and gCJD and the polymorphism background of vCJD (as discussed above), determining the *PRNP* 129 polymorphism may help in the diagnosis of a suspect prion disease.

TREATMENT

There is no proven disease-modifying treatment for prion disease.

In many prion diseases, particularly sCJD, the rapid progression and the lack of any simple absolute diagnostic test means that most individuals are severely neurologically impaired at the time of diagnosis and, therefore, arguably beyond the point of useful therapy. There are potential treatment approaches but, given the incomplete understanding of pathogenesis in prion diseases, it is difficult to know if these will lead to actual therapies [11]. A range of treatments have been tried including quinacrine, pentosan polysulphate, flupirtine, but none has so far proved to be unequivocally of benefit [12].

Symptomatic treatment should focus on pain relief, distress, behavioral difficulties, and involuntary movements. As disability and dependency increase, measures such as urinary catheterization and nasogastric tube/gastrostomy feeding may be appropriate. All management decisions need to be undertaken in the light of the inevitable, and ultimately fatal, progressive nature of the illness and tailored to the individual circumstances.

REFERENCES

1. Prusiner SB. An Introduction to Prion Biology and Diseases. In: Prusiner SB, ed. Prion Biology and Diseases. New York: Cold Spring Harbour Laboratory Press; 2004:1–87.
2. Brown P. Transmissible spongiform encephalopathy in the 21st century: Neuroscience for the clinical neurologist. Neurology 2008;26;70:713–22.
3. Ladogana A, Puopolo M, Croes EA, et al. Mortality from Creutzfeldt-Jakob disease and related disorders in Europe, Australia and Canada. Neurology 2005;64:1586–91.
4. Kovacs GG, Puopolo M, Ladogana A, et al. Genetic prion disease: the EUROCJD experience. Hum Genet 2005;118:166–74
5. Hewitt PE, Llewelyn CA, Mackenzie J, Will RG. Creutzfeldt–Jakob disease and blood transfusion: results of the UK Transfusion Medicine Epidemiological Review study. Vox Sang 2006;91:221–30.
6. Brown P, Brandel J-P, Preese M, Sato T. Iatrogenic Creutzfeldt–Jakob disease. The waning of an era. Neurology 2006;67:389–93.
7. Parchi P, Giese A, Capellari S, et al. Classification of sporadic Creutzfeldt-Jakob disease based on molecular and phenotypic analysis of 300 subjects. Ann Neurol 1999;46:224–33.
8. Zerr I, Pocchiari M, Collins S, et al. Analysis of EEG and CSF 14-3-3 proteins as aids to the diagnosis of Creutzfeldt-Jakob disease. Neurology 2000;55: 811–15.
9. Collie DA, Sellar RJ, Zeidler M, et al. MRI of Creutzfeldt-Jakob disease: imaging features and recommended MRI protocol. Clinical Radiology 2001;56:726–39.
10. Collie DA, Summers DM, Sellar RJ, et al. Diagnosing variant Creutzfeldt-Jakob disease with the pulvinar sign: MR imaging findings in 86 neuropathologically confirmed cases. Am J Neuroradiol 2003;24:1560–9.
11. Weissmann C., Aguzzi A. Approches to therapy of prion diseases. Annu Rev Med 2005;56:321–44.
12. Stewart L, Rydzewska L, Keogh G, Knight R. A systematic review of clinical studies of therapeutic interventions for human prion disease. Neurology 2008;70:1272–81.

34.9 Human T-Lymphotropic Virus Type I and II Infection

Nicholas J van Sickels, Susan LF McLellan

Key features

- Human T-lymphotropic viruses (HTLV I and HTLV II) are seen worldwide, with an estimated 10–20 million individuals infected
- Most persons infected will remain asymptomatic
- The majority of disease burden is from HTLV I, which is known for its association with adult T-cell leukemia/lymphoma (ATLL) and HTLV-associated myelopathy, also known as tropical spastic paraparesis (HAM/TSP)
- Other infectious diseases, such as strongyloidiasis, tuberculosis, and infective dermatitis are seen in association with HTLV-1 infection
- Both HTLV-1 and HTLV-2 are associated with an increased incidence of neurologic and autoimmune syndromes, as well as routine infections (urinary and respiratory infections)
- Treatment options for the virus itself are lacking, though options for management for ATLL and HAM/TSP are evolving

INTRODUCTION

Human T-cell lymphotrophic viruses were first described in 1979 and are best known for their propensity to cause cancer and lead to devastating neurologic disease. Human T-cell lymphotrophic virus type-I (HTLV-I), the first recognized human retrovirus, infects and stimulates proliferation of CD4 T-lymphocytes. The most severe sequelae of infection are adult T-cell leukemia/lymphoma (ATLL) and HTLV-associated myelopathy, also known as tropical spastic paraparesis (HAM/TSP). ATLL was first described in Japan and the link with HTLV-I was recognized in 1982. HAM/TSP, which is more frequently seen in the tropics, was recognized as a clinical entity some 30 years before the link with HTLV-1 was established in 1985. Infection with HTLV-I is also associated with a more aggressive course of certain other infectious pathogens, including strongyloidiasis, scabies, leprosy, and tuberculosis.

The closely related human T-lymphotrophic virus type II (HTLV-II) was discovered in 1981 and infects CD4 and CD8 T-cells, as well as monocytes. While HTLV-II infection is not associated with ATLL, cases of HAM/TSP, other neurologic manifestations (without overt myelopathy), and increased overall rates of infections have been reported [1–3].

EPIDEMIOLOGY

An estimated 10–20 million people worldwide are infected with HTLV-I . It is highly endemic in Japan and the Caribbean, with pockets of infection in Central and South America. Infection is associated with female sex and increasing age—a pattern seen in all populations affected. The virus is transmitted via the passage of infected lymphocytes, which can occur from mother to child, during sexual intercourse and with the exchange of blood products via transfusion or the sharing of infected needles.

HTLV-I is divided into six subtypes labeled A–F based on differences in proviral DNA and in long terminal repeat sequences; there is no association with specific clinical manifestations [4].

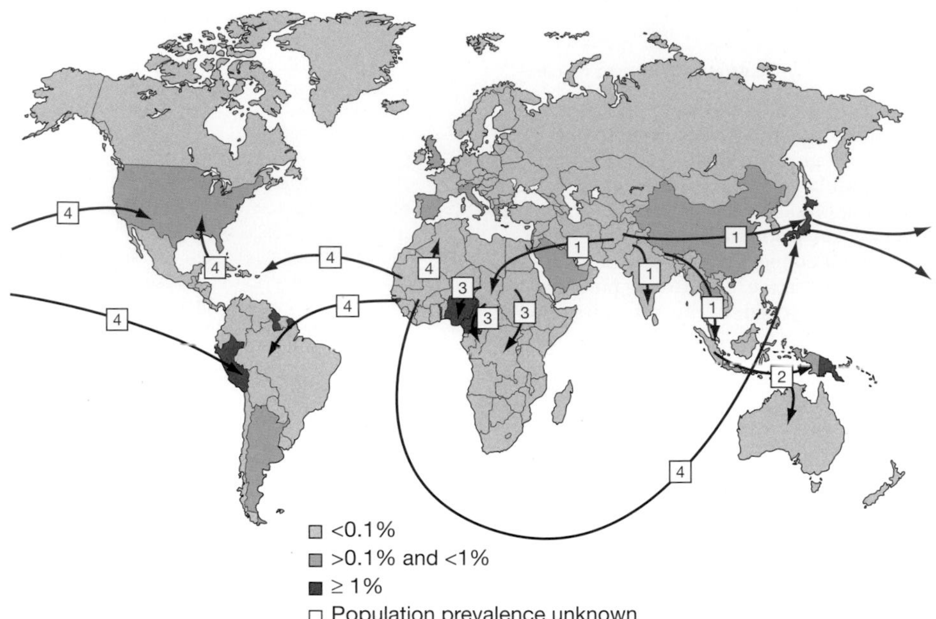

FIGURE 34.9.1 Origin and spread hypothesis based on phylogenetic and anthropological data. Primate T lymphotropic virus (PTLV) originated in African primates and migrated to Asia where it evolved into Simian T-cell leukemia virus (STLV)-1. This early STLV-1 lineage spread to India, Japan, Indonesia, and back to Africa (arrows 1). It crossed the simian–human barrier in Indonesian human beings who migrated to Melanesia, resulting in the HTLV-1c subtype (arrows 2). In Africa, STLV-1 evolved through several interspecies transmissions into HTLV-1a, HTLV-1b, and HTLV-1d, HTLV-1e, and HTLV-1f (arrows 3). As a result of the slave trade and increased mobility, HTLV-1a was introduced in the New World, Japan, the Middle East, and north Africa (arrows 4). Colors indicate current prevalence estimates based on population surveys and on studies in pregnant women and blood donors. In some countries, HTLV-1 infection is limited to certain population groups or areas. *Reprinted from Verdonck K, Gonzalez E, Van Dooren S, et al. Human T-lymphotropic virus 1: recent knowledge about an ancient infection. Lancet Infect Dis 2007;7:266–81, with permission from Elsevier and Lancet.*

Infected mothers will transmit the virus to their children 20% of the time, with most of that transmission from breastfeeding. In areas of the world where formula feeding is feasible, refraining from breastfeeding leads to a significant reduction in HTLV-I transmission.

Like HTLV-I, HTLV-II is divided into subtypes; unlike HTLV-I these subtypes are fairly closely linked to specific geographic populations or risk behaviors (Fig. 34.9.1). Worldwide prevalence estimations of HTLV-II infection are in the millions, with an estimated 200,000 infected in the USA [5].

Since the late 1980s, the US Food and Drug Administration (FDA) has recommended screening of whole blood for HTLV I/II antibodies.

NATURAL HISTORY, PATHOGENESIS, PATHOLOGY

Initial infections with HTLV-I/II are asymptomatic. Antibodies develop within 1–2 months after exposure to the virus and the latency period between seroconversion to development of disease varies from years to decades. Most patients with HTLV will remain asymptomatic throughout their lives; however, individuals with higher HTLV antibody levels and proviral load have an increased incidence of overt disease manifestations.

HTLV-I and II primarily infect CD4 and CD8 cells respectively. Cell-to-cell transmission of HTLV occurs via a viral synapse, avoiding production of extracellular virions. Once local infection takes place, viral propagation occurs at regional lymphatics and disseminates to skin, spleen, liver, and lymph nodes. Because of this, plasma viral load is undetectable and lifelong infection occurs.

ADULT T-CELL LEUKEMIA PATHOGENESIS

The most severe illnesses associated with HTLV-1 are ATLL and HAM/TSP. Lymphoproliferation is key in the pathogenesis of ATLL, and is mediated by the highly conserved tax gene and its protein, which is thought to enhance viral transcription, repression of genes responsible for apoptosis and DNA repair, and binding to tumor suppressor proteins [6].

HAM/TSP PATHOGENESIS

HAM/TSP likely occurs as a result of both immunologic and genetic factors. HTLV-1-specific cytotoxic T-cells control infection by destroying infected CD4 cells. These cells are unable to eradicate the infection and a steady state of immune activation is established. Patients with HAM/TSP have increased pro-inflammatory cytokines, high levels of HTLV-1-specific CD8+ T-cells and higher proviral loads. In Japanese populations, genomic alterations involving cytokines have also been shown to be associated with an increased incidence of HAM/TSP [6, 7].

CLINICAL FEATURES

While most patients with HTLV infection will remain asymptomatic, certain individuals are at higher risk for infectious, neurologic, dermatologic, rheumatologic, autoimmune, and malignant diseases.

ATLL

HTLV-1-associated adult T-cell leukemia/lymphoma (ATLL) tends to occur mainly in adults, usually 20–30 years after HTLV-1 infection. The yearly incidence of disease in Japan is estimated at about 0.6/1000. ATLL is divided into four categories: acute, chronic, smoldering, and lymphoma-type. Recently a fifth type, primary cutaneous tumoral ATLL, has been proposed. The acute type is the most common, followed by lymphomatous, chronic, and then smoldering. ATLL is most commonly seen in southwestern Japan, with vertical transmission and breastfeeding posing the highest risk for disease development [6].

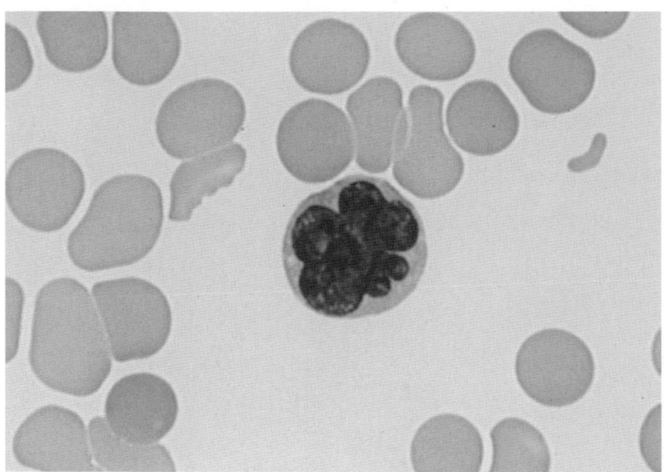

FIGURE 34.9.2 White blood cell with hyperlobulated nucleus "flower cell" *(photo courtesy of John Krause MD, Tulane University Department of Pathology).*

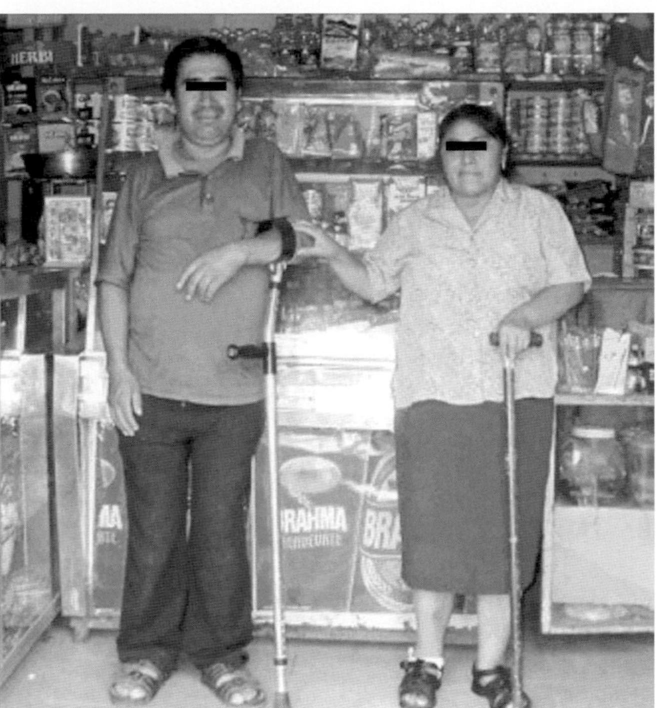

FIGURE 34.9.3 Husband and wife with HAM/TSP in Peru *(photo reprinted from Verdonck K, Gonzalez E, Van Dooren S, et al. Human T-lymphotropic virus1: recent knowledge about an ancient infection. Lancet Infect Dis 2007;7:266–81, with permission from Elsevier and the Lancet).*

Symptoms

Most patients will present with lymphadenopathy and half have hepatosplenomegaly. Skin involvement, in the form of a nodular, indurated rash, is seen in up to a third of cases. With metastasis, ATLL can affect the lungs, gastrointestinal tract, central nervous system, and musculoskeletal system. Median survival times for the acute, lymphoma-type, and chronic forms are 6, 10, and 24 months respectively. Smoldering disease has a 66% 4-year survival rate. Despite more favorable prognoses, chronic and smoldering forms retain the ability to transform into acute ATLL [6, 7].

Diagnosis

Diagnosis is suspected with clinical findings of lymphadenopathy, rash, and hepatosplenomegaly. Early in the disease, complete blood counts reveal leukocytosis without anemia or thrombocytopenia, owing to a lack of bone marrow involvement in ATLL. Acute and lymphomatous ATLL are strongly suspected when characteristic flower cells are seen on blood smear (Fig. 34.9.2)—these are atypical multilobulated, pleomorphic lymphoid cells with abnormal-appearing nuclei. HTLV-1 provirus can be detected in these abnormal nuclei. Metabolically, hypercalcemia is common (30–60%) and is caused by both parathyroid hormone-related peptide overproduction by Tax protein and liberation of calcium from lytic bony lesions [7].

Treatment

Treatments for ATLL include conventional and intensive chemotherapeutic regimens, allogenic hematopoietic stem cell transplantation, antivirals, and anti-retrovirals. Novel therapies currently under investigation include combination zidovudine and interferon-α, arsenic trioxide, monoclonal antibodies, and retinoid derivatives. As a result of immunosuppression, patients often succumb to opportunistic illness such as *Pneumocystis jirovecii* pneumonia, cryptococcal meningitis, and disseminated herpes zoster. These illnesses, as well as pulmonary and liver dysfunction, uncontrolled hypercalcemia, and sepsis, are the main causes of mortality [7, 8].

HAM/TSP

General

HAM/TSP develops in 1–4% of individuals infected with HTLV-1 over their lifetime and is the most common neurologic manifestation of HTLV-1 infection. Although most cases are caused by HTLV-I, a small number of patients infected with HTLV-II have also developed HAM/TSP. HAM/TSP presents as an indolent and progressive spastic paraparesis with bladder disturbances and sensory signs. For unknown reasons, women progress faster than men, especially those who develop disease prior to menopause. Other risk factors for more rapid progression include older age at disease onset and increased HTLV-1 proviral loads [6, 9, 10]. HTLV-II-associated disease appears to be milder and have a more slowly progressive course.

The association of HTLV-1 and HAM/TSP was first noted in tropical regions of the Caribbean and South America (hence the original name: tropical spastic paraparesis). While HAM/TSP is most commonly seen in the Caribbean, South America, and southern Japan, the relative risk of developing HAM/TSP seems to be higher in Latin America than in Japan [3, 11].

Symptoms

HAM/TSP is a chronic, subacute, and progressive disease. Neurologic findings are often the first manifestations of the disease or appear within the first year. In 60% of patients, weakness in the lower limbs is the first symptom (Fig. 34.9.3), followed by spasticity with hyperreflexia and extensor plantar responses. Urologic symptoms are common and vary from urgency and frequency to incontinence and retention. Other symptoms include back pain, constipation, and paresthesias in the lower limbs [1, 12]. Of note, significant pain is frequently described, adding to the disability of this disease.

Diagnosis

Symptoms of HAM/TSP can mimic other diseases and pursuance of this diagnosis requires their exclusion. The differential includes spinal cord tumors or compressive lesions, multiple sclerosis, toxic neuropathies (for example, B12 and folate deficiencies), and amyotrophic lateral sclerosis. In resource-poor or environmentally distraught areas of the world, dependence on the potentially toxic food substances grass pea and cassava root can lead to the neurodegenerative syndromes Lathyrism and Konzo, respectively.

Monitoring and Treatment

Patients with HAM/TSP should be monitored on a regular basis for any change in symptoms and function. Laboratory markers available for disease monitoring are the HTLV-I proviral load and HTLV-1 *tax* mRNA by PCR.

Many treatments have been attempted, but none has proven to decrease long-term disability. However, therapy with interferon-α has led to both clinical and virologic improvements; this drug is considered standard of care for HAM/TSP patients in Japan. The use of corticosteroids, plasmapheresis, and intravenous immune globulin have all been associated with transient improvements. Anti-retrovirals, disappointingly, have not shown any benefit. Current and emerging therapies are focused on modifying immune responses to infection and increasing host ability to target infected cells. Examples include humanized anti-Tac (anti-CD25 monoclonal antibody), which has been shown to reduce disability and decrease proviral load in one small trial, and a monoclonal antibody targeting interleukin-15 in phase I/II of clinical studies. Finally, the use of valproic acid may induce viral expression of HTLV from quiescent cells, making them vulnerable to destruction by the immune system [13].

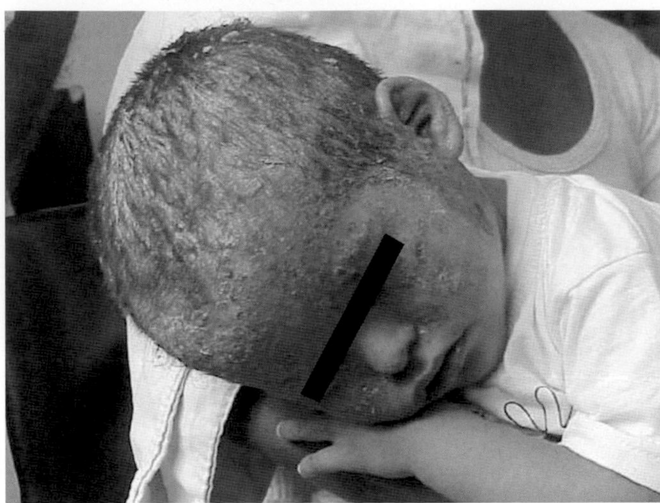

FIGURE 34.9.4 Child with infective dermatitis. Symptoms include eczema about the scalp, ears, and face, with nasal crusting and a fine papular rash. Children typically have chronic watery discharge and their anterior nares are frequently colonized with *Staphylococcus aureus* or β-hemolytic streptococci. Infective dermatitis responds rapidly to antibiotics and topical steroids only to relapse chronically once these treatments are withdrawn [14]. The presence of infective dermatitis in children has been implicated as a marker of risk for development of HAM/TSP [15] *(photo courtesy of David Barnes MD).*

OTHER CONDITIONS RELATED TO HTLV INFECTION

A myriad of infectious diseases including Norwegian scabies, molluscum contagiosum, extrapulmonary histoplasmosis, tuberculosis, leprosy, and strongyloidiasis are described in case reports and series of HTLV-1-infected persons. A review of over 1200 blood donors in the USA revealed a significantly higher incidence of kidney and bladder infections with HTLV-I infection. HTLV-II-infection was associated with higher incidence of bronchitis, bladder or kidney infections, and oral herpes. There was also a trend toward higher incidence of pneumonia in HTLV-II patients [2].

Dermatologic alterations are commonly seen in the setting of HTLV infection and include dermatophyte infections, seborrheic dermatitis, acquired ichthyosis, infective dermatitis (Fig. 34.9.4), scabies, and others.

Patients with HTLV-1 also have an increased incidence of pulmonary tuberculosis and *Mycobacterium avium* infections, as well as decreased skin response rates to purified protein derivative. Increased rates of HTLV-1 infections are also seen among residents of Hansen's disease sanatoriums in Africa [16].

Other neurologic syndromes, which do not meet the case definition of HAM/TSP, include leg weakness, impaired gait, hyper-reflexia, impaired vibratory sense, and urinary tract abnormalities [1].

A myriad of rheumatologic conditions are described with HTLV-1 detected in target tissues. These conditions include polymyositis, bronchioalveolar pneumonitis, Sjögren's syndrome autoimmune thyroiditis, uveitis, and arthropathy [6, 7].

PATIENT EVALUATION, DIAGNOSIS AND DIFFERENTIAL DIAGNOSIS

HTLV infection should be in the differential diagnosis when patients from endemic areas present with ATLL, HAM/TSP, neurologic syndromes, or any of the infectious syndromes outlined above. Recommendations for counseling of patients presenting with positive HTLV-I/II serology have been previously published [17]. Healthcare workers should inform patients that HTLV is not the virus that causes AIDS, as this is a source of common confusion and anxiety for patients. Secondarily, patients should be screened for risk factors for HTLV-infection, including: living in an endemic area, sexual partners from an endemic area (e.g. Japan or Jamaica), blood transfusions, history of injection drug use, sexual partners with histories of injection drug use, or having sex with multiple partners without condom use. Patients with a history of drug use or unprotected sex should also undergo HIV testing.

Confirmed cases of HTLV infection should be referred to a physician with experience in the field. A complete physical examination, with special attention to the lymphatics, skin, liver, spleen, and neurologic system, should be completed. Baseline laboratory evaluation includes a complete blood count with differential, serum chemistries, investigation for sexually transmitted infection (syphilis, gonorrhea, chlamydia and HIV), hepatitis serologies, purified protein derivative testing, and chest radiography.

HTLV-I-infected individuals should be informed of their increased risk for autoimmune disease, HAM/TSP and malignancy. These patients should be followed regularly, with prompt referrals to specialists if neurologic, skin, or hematologic findings appear.

HTLV-II-infected patients can be reassured that their risk of major illness is low, but they should understand the increased risk of urinary, kidney, and upper and lower respiratory tract infections. Clinicians should counsel patients about smoking cessation to reduce the risk of the latter. If abnormal findings develop, referral to a neurologist is appropriate [7].

TREATMENT

Therapies for the more severe manifestations of HTLV-I/II infection are discussed above. No definitive treatment for primary HTLV infection is available or currently recommended. The nucleoside analogues zidovudine and lamivudine have both been shown to decrease proviral loads in small *in vitro* and *in vivo* trials; however, no change in clinical outcome has been demonstrated from small studies [18, 19]. Prevention measures (refraining from breastfeeding and blood donation, condom use) are recommended to avoid transmission of the virus to others.

REFERENCES

1. Biswas HH, Engstrom JW, Kaidarova Z, et al. Neurologic abnormalities in HTLV-I- and HTLV-II-infected individuals without overt myelopathy. Neurology 2009;73:781–9.
2. Murphy EL, Glynn SA, Fridey J, et al. Increased incidence of infectious diseases during prospective follow-up of human T-lymphotropic virus type II- and

I-infected blood donors. Retrovirus Epidemiology Donor Study. Arch Intern Med 1999;159:1485–91.

3. Gotuzzo E, Cabrera J, Deza L, et al. Clinical characteristics of patients in Peru with human T cell lymphotropic virus type 1-associated tropical spastic paraparesis. Clin Infect Dis 2004;39:939–44.
4. Proietti FA, Carneiro-Proietti AB, Catalan-Soares BC, Murphy EL. Global epidemiology of HTLV-I infection and associated diseases. Oncogene 2005;24:6058–68.
5. Roucoux DF, Murphy EL. The epidemiology and disease outcomes of human T-lymphotropic virus type II. AIDS Rev 2004;6:144–54.
6. Verdonck K, Gonzalez E, Van Dooren S, et al. Human T-lymphotropic virus 1: recent knowledge about an ancient infection. Lancet Infect Dis 2007;7:266–81.
7. Shuh M, Beilke M. The human T-cell leukemia virus type 1 (HTLV-1): new insights into the clinical aspects and molecular pathogenesis of adult T-cell leukemia/lymphoma (ATLL) and tropical spastic paraparesis/HTLV-associated myelopathy (TSP/HAM). Microsc Res Tech 2005;68:176–96.
8. Tobinai K. Current management of adult T-cell leukemia/lymphoma. Oncology 2009;23:1250–6.
9. Nakagawa M, Izumo S, Ijichi S, et al. HTLV-I-associated myelopathy: analysis of 213 patients based on clinical features and laboratory findings. J Neurovirol 1995;1:50–61.
10. Takenouchi N, Yamano Y, Usuku K, et al. Usefulness of proviral load measurement for monitoring of disease activity in individual patients with human T-lymphotropic virus type I-associated myelopathy/tropical spastic paraparesis. J Neurovirol 2003;9:29–35.
11. Gotuzzo E, Arango C, de Queiroz-Campos A, Isturiz RE. Human T-cell lymphotropic virus-I in Latin America. Infect Dis Clin North Am 2000;14:211–39, x–xi.
12. Araujo AQ, Silva MT. The HTLV-1 neurological complex. Lancet Neurol 2006;5:1068–76.
13. Oh U, Jacobson S. Treatment of HTLV-I-associated myelopathy/tropical spastic paraparesis: toward rational targeted therapy. Neurol Clin 2008;26:781–97, ix–x.
14. La Grenade L, Manns A, Fletcher V, et al. Clinical, pathologic, and immunologic features of human T-lymphotrophic virus type I-associated infective dermatitis in children. Arch Dermatol 1998;134:439–44.
15. Kendall EA, Gonzalez E, Espinoza I, et al. Early neurologic abnormalities associated with human T-cell lymphotropic virus type 1 infection in a cohort of Peruvian children. J Pediatr 2009;155:700–6.
16. Marinho J, Galvao-Castro B, Rodrigues LC, Barreto ML. Increased risk of tuberculosis with human T-lymphotropic virus-1 infection: a case-control study. J Acquir Immune Defic Syndr 2005;40:625–8.
17. Recommendations for counseling persons infected with human T-lymphotrophic virus, types I and II. Centers for Disease Control and Prevention and U.S. Public Health Service Working Group. MMWR Recomm Rep 1993;42:1–13.
18. Macchi B, Faraoni I, Zhang J, et al. AZT inhibits the transmission of human T cell leukaemia/lymphoma virus type I to adult peripheral blood mononuclear cells in vitro. J Gen Virol 1997;78:1007–16.
19. Machuca A, Rodes B, Soriano V. The effect of antiretroviral therapy on HTLV infection. Virus Res 2001;78:93–100.

PART

3

BACTERIAL INFECTIONS

SECTION

A

INFECTIONS OF THE EYE & THROAT

35 Trachoma and Inclusion Conjunctivitis

Hugh R Taylor, Anu Mathew

35.1 Trachoma

Key features

- Trachoma is the leading infectious cause of blindness
- Caused by *Chlamydia trachomatis* serotypes A–C, a Gram-negative, intracellular bacterium
- Repeated episodes of infection result in scarring of the tarsal conjunctiva which leads to in-turning of the eyelashes that rub against the surface of the globe. The constant abrasion subsequently leads to corneal scarring and blindness
- Diagnosis requires a 2.5 × magnifying glass and a flashlight for illumination. The surface of the globe should be examined, followed by eversion of the upper eyelid
- The major risk factor is poor facial hygiene. Other factors associated with poor hygiene and trachoma include overcrowding, inadequate water supply, lack of latrines and flies
- Trachoma is clustered among the most impoverished communities of the world and in those with the most disadvantaged families
- The trachoma control strategy recommended by the World Health Organization is the SAFE strategy: **S**urgery, **A**ntibiotics, **F**acial cleanliness and **E**nvironmental improvement. Without a coordinated public health approach incorporating all these components, the treatment of individuals with trachoma is futile

INTRODUCTION

Trachoma is the leading cause of infectious blindness in the world. It is caused by *Chlamydia trachomatis*, an obligate, intracellular bacterium that has existed since the Jurassic period [1]. Trachoma began to manifest when humans congregated into the first settlements, spreading rapidly until populations in North America and Europe were widely affected. Trachoma slowly disappeared from the developed world and is even continuing to disappear from the developing world with socioeconomic development and improvements in sanitation and hygiene. Though the estimated proportion of blindness worldwide owing to trachoma has decreased from 15.5% in 1996 to 4% in 2004, trachoma still causes significant economic losses in affected countries.

EPIDEMIOLOGY

Trachoma is endemic in 57 countries, with an estimated 40.6 million people suffering from active disease and 8.2 million people afflicted with trachomatous trichiasis (in-turning of eyelashes that abrade the surface of the globe) [2]. Africa bears the highest load of active trachoma, but countries in the Middle East, Asia, Latin America and the Western Pacific also have areas of endemic trachoma (Fig. 35.1) [3,4]. However, half the global burden of trichiasis is concentrated in China, Ethiopia and Sudan (Fig. 35.2) [4].

Trachoma perpetuates the cycle of poverty and blindness. Trachomatous blindness and low vision not only lead to poverty from loss of productivity (US$3.5 billion annually—year of costing: 2003) [5], but impoverished communities are where risk factors for trachoma, such as overcrowding and poor sanitation facilities, exist.

Poor access to, or inappropriate use of, water for hygiene purposes leads to dirty faces with bacteria-loaded secretions. Infected facial secretions are spread through close contact secondary to overcrowding or by flies that thrive on poor sanitation conditions. The relative importance of different risk factors may vary from one community to another, although the lack of clean faces in children appears to be the final, common pathway.

Young children, especially preschool children, are the reservoir for *C. trachomatis* which causes episodes of chronic conjunctivitis. With increasing age, children appear to be re-infected less often, leading to a reduction in both the duration and cumulative incidence of active disease. Repeated episodes of infection eventually cause blinding sequelae in older age groups (Fig. 35.3) [6]. Females are usually at higher risk of blinding trachoma as a result of their roles as child caregivers that increases their exposure to active infection. It is estimated that the global disability adjusted life years (DALYs) lost by females are at least 25% more than those lost by males. This gender bias is not universal and is less pronounced or nonexistent in some populations where the division of labor is not as distinct, such as in Australian Aboriginal populations.

NATURAL HISTORY, PATHOGENESIS AND PATHOLOGY

Trachoma is caused by infection with *C. trachomatis*, almost exclusively with serotypes A, B, Ba and C. A single episode of infection results in a self-limiting episode of chlamydial conjunctivitis (inclusion conjunctivitis). Infection with *C. trachomatis* occurs in the conjunctival epithelium and active inflammation involves all layers of the conjunctiva. It has been recognized that chlamydia itself is not intrinsically toxic, but trachoma is a result of the immune response to chlamydial antigens [7]. This immune response is characterized by a

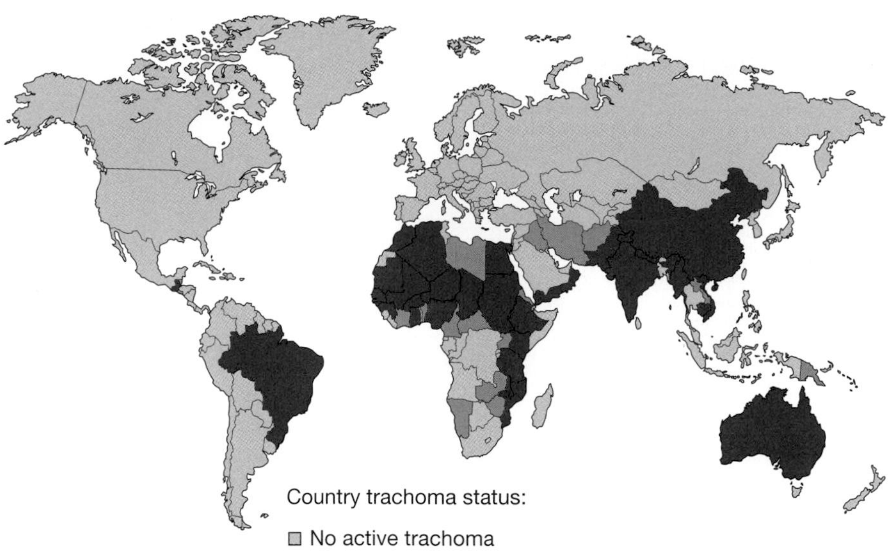

FIGURE 35.1 Map of available active trachoma data in children. *Redrawn with permission from Polack S. Maps of the Global Distribution of Trachoma: International Centre for Eye Health © 2005, International Centre for Eye Health. All right reserved.*

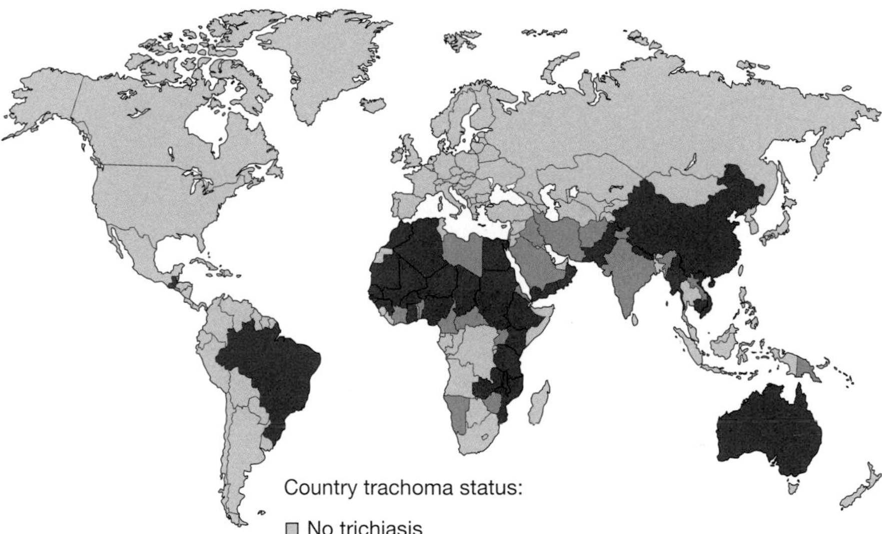

FIGURE 35.2 Map of available trichiasis data in adults >15 years. *Redrawn with permission from Polack S. Maps of the Global Distribution of Trachoma: International Centre for Eye Health © 2005, International Centre for Eye Health. All right reserved.*

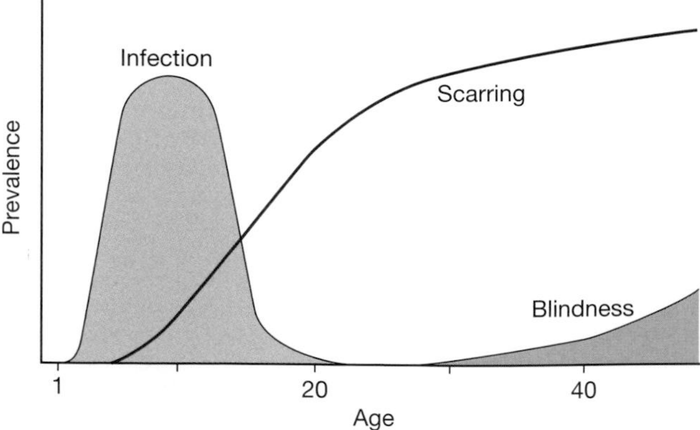

FIGURE 35.3 Relationship of trachoma and age. *Redrawn with permission from Wright HR, Keeffe JE, Taylor HR. Trachoma and the need for a coordinated community-wide response: a case-based study. PLoS Med 2006;3:186–90 (reproduced under the Creative Commons Attribution License).*

delayed-type hypersensitivity reaction. The typical clinical feature of the disease is the lymphoid follicle in the stroma surrounded by an infiltrate consisting of T cells, B cells, plasma cells, dendritic cells, macrophages and leukocytes [8]. During the initial stages of each episode of infection, laboratory tests are more likely to be positive because of the presence of the organism. However, the destructive immune response can continue for months after the infection has cleared and is observed clinically as active trachoma. Repeated episodes of infection lead to long-term, sustained inflammation. This intense inflammation leads to the formation of fibrous tissue and scarring in the subepithelium of the tarsal conjunctiva [9]. This scarring distorts the upper eyelid and insidiously progresses to the in-turning of eyelashes: trichiasis. The scar tissue can also result in loss of mucus-secreting glands, causing a dry eye and/or blockage of the nasolacrimal duct resulting in a watery eye and bacterial conjunctivitis [10]. If untreated, trichiasis leads to irreversible opacity of the cornea and blindness [11].

TRACHOMA GRADING CARD

- Each eye must be examined and assessed separately.
- Use binocular loupes (x 2.5) and adequate lighting (either daylight or a torch).
- Signs must be clearly seen in order to be considered present.

The eyelids and cornea are observed first for inturned eyelashes and any corneal opacity. The upper eyelid is then turned over (everted) to examine the conjunctiva over the stiffer part of the upper lid (tarsal conjunctiva).

The normal conjunctiva is pink, smooth, thin and transparent. Over the whole area of the tarsal conjunctiva there are normally large deep-lying blood vessels that run vertically.

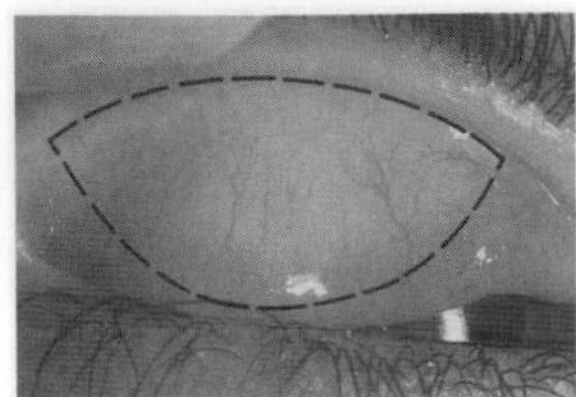

Normal tarsal conjunctiva (x 2 magnification). The dotted line shows the area to be examined.

TRACHOMATOUS INFLAMMATION – FOLLICULAR (TF): *the presence of five or more follicles in the upper tarsal conjunctiva.*

Follicles are round swellings that are paler than the surrounding conjunctiva, appearing white, grey or yellow. Follicles must be at least 0.5mm in diameter, i.e., at least as large as the dots shown below, to be considered.

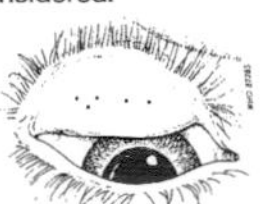

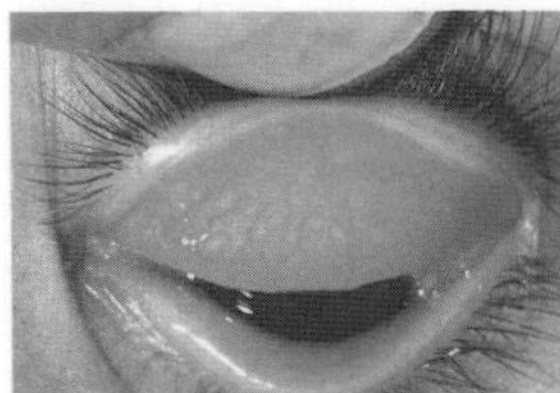

Trachomatous inflammation – follicular (TF).

TRACHOMATOUS INFLAMMATION – INTENSE (TI): *pronounced inflammatory thickening of the tarsal conjunctiva that obscures more than half of the normal deep tarsal vessels.*

The tarsal conjunctiva appears red, rough and thickened. There are usually numerous follicles, which may be partially or totally covered by the thickened conjunctiva.

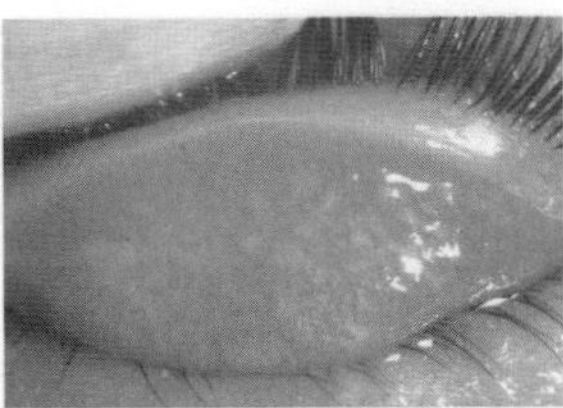

Trachomatous inflammation – follicular and intense (TF + TI).

TRACHOMATOUS SCARRING (TS): *the presence of scarring in the tarsal conjunctiva.*

Scars are easily visible as white lines, bands, or sheets in the tarsal conjunctiva. They are glistening and fibrous in appearance. Scarring, especially diffuse fibrosis, may obscure the tarsal blood vessels.

Trachomatous scarring (TS)

TRACHOMATOUS TRICHIASIS (TT): *at least one eyelash rubs on the eyeball.*

Evidence of recent removal of inturned eyelashes should also be graded as trichiasis.

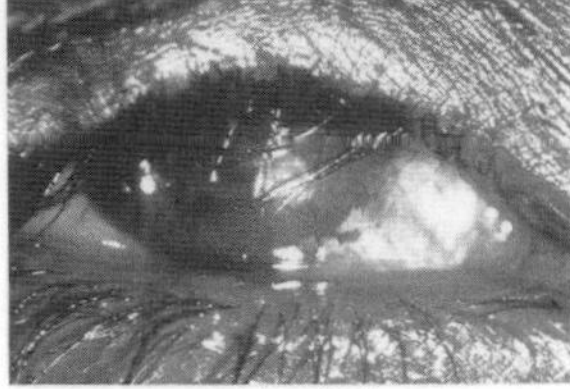

Trachomatous trichiasis (TT)

CORNEAL OPACITY (CO): *easily visible corneal opacity over the pupil.*

The pupil margin is blurred viewed through the opacity. Such corneal opacities cause significant visual impairment (less than 6/18 or 0.3 vision), and therefore visual acuity should be measured if possible.

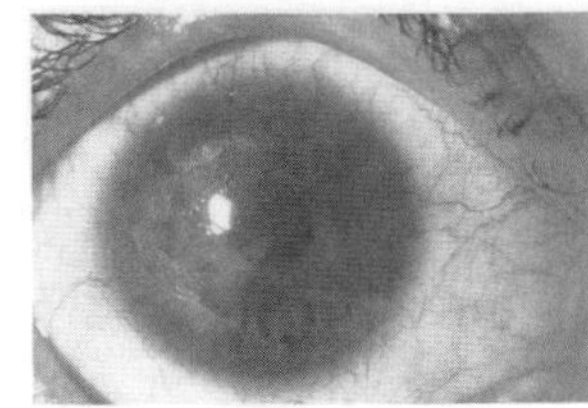

Corneal opacity (CO)

TF:– give topical treatment (e.g. tetracycline 1%).
TI:– give topical and consider systemic treatment.
TT:– refer for eyelid surgery.

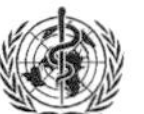

WORLD HEALTH ORGANIZATION
PREVENTION OF BLINDNESS AND DEAFNESS

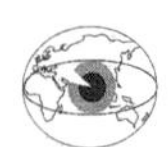

Support from the partners of the WHO Alliance for the Global Elimination of Trachoma is acknowledged.

FIGURE 35.4 Trachoma grading card. *Reproduced with permission from Negrel AD, Taylor HR, West S. Guidelines for Rapid Assessment for Blinding Trachoma. Report No.: WHO/PBD/GET/00.8. Geneva: World Health Organization; 2001.*

CLINICAL FEATURES

Most cases of active disease are asymptomatic and only a minority present with mucopurulent discharge. Therefore, trachoma is often only diagnosed on routine screening. The clinical signs of the disease are illustrated by the World Health Organization's (WHO) simplified trachoma grading classification system (Fig. 35.4) [12,13]. The five signs of the disease are independently assessed, but are not mutually exclusive, and two or more features can coexist in the same eye.

Active inflammation is characterized by follicles on the upper tarsal conjunctiva (trachomatous inflammation follicular). If the inflammation is severe, the conjunctiva becomes thickened and intensely red, obscuring the underlying vessels (trachoma inflammation intense). Scarring appears as fine, white fibrous bands across the upper tarsal conjunctiva (trachomatous conjunctival scarring). The late stages of the disease appears as in-turning of the eyelashes with at least one eyelash rubbing against the surface of the eyeball (trachomatous trichiasis) and an eventual white corneal opacity obscuring view of the pupil margin (corneal opacity).

Examination for trachoma should be performed with a 2.5 × loupe (magnifying lens) for magnification and a pocket flashlight/pentorch for illumination. In children, the upper eyelid needs to be gently everted to expose the upper tarsal conjunctiva using your thumb or another small object, such as a cotton bud. The tarsal surface should then be examined for signs of active inflammation and scarring. In adults, the lid margin of the upper lid should be gently lifted from the eye to identify any corneal opacity prior to eversion of the upper lid. Visual acuity should be measured to document the effects of trichiasis and corneal opacity. A grading of corneal opacity is usually associated with vision of less than 6/12 or 20/40.

PATIENT EVALUATION, DIAGNOSIS AND DIFFERENTIAL DIAGNOSIS

Trachoma is usually diagnosed using clinical grading based on the WHO's simplified grading classification system. Clinical diagnosis is easily learnt by health workers and has been shown to be highly reproducible [12]. There are a number of laboratory tests that have been used to detect *C. trachomatis* (Table 35-1) [14] and the tests of highest sensitivity and specificity for the detection of trachoma at present are nucleic acid amplification tests, such as PCR. However, the correlation between clinical and laboratory methods is quite variable, ranging from 10–70%. Clinically active trachoma has been shown to resolve more slowly than laboratory evidence of infection with follicles persisting for 3–6 months after the infection has resolved. Also, more severe inflammation is associated with a high rate of detectable infection as a result of higher levels of organism being shed. The use of laboratory methods is often limited by high cost and accessibility issues in trachoma-endemic areas. Until an inexpensive, reliable, rapid, field-based assay is developed, clinical grading appears to be the best method of trachoma diagnosis in operational conditions.

There are differential diagnoses to consider in the diagnosis of both active trachoma and trachomatous scarring (Table 35-2). However, in the absence of laboratory tests, cases of follicular conjunctivitis and/or conjunctival scarring in an area of known trachoma

TABLE 35-1 Methods Used for Laboratory Diagnosis of Trachoma

Method	Description	Comments
Microscopy	Identifies typical intracytoplasmic inclusions using Giemsa staining	Requires conjunctival scrapings that can be traumatic May be the least sensitive test Inexpensive
Direct fluorescent antibody (DFA)	Detects cellular proteins using fluorescent-labeled antibodies	Requires conjunctival scrapings Specificity dependent on user expertise
Culture	Uses egg yolk or other suitable cell-culture systems to grow the bacteria	Requires conjunctival scrapings High specificity and moderate sensitivity Time-consuming and expensive Dependent on user expertise
Enzyme immunoassay (EIA)	Involves binding antichlamydial antibodies to specific chlamydial antigens that produce an enzyme-triggered color change	Requires conjunctival scrapings Moderate to high specificity Sensitivity limited by type of kits used
Nucleic acid amplication techniques (NAAT)	Identifies unique chlamydial DNA or RNA via probing or amplification techniques	Requires conjunctival scrapings High sensitivity and specificity Expensive
Serology	Measure antichlamydial antibodies in host serum or secretions	Poor reproducibility Limited diagnostic value

Reproduced from Wright HR, Taylor HR. Clinical examination and laboratory tests for estimation of trachoma prevalence in a remote setting: what are they really telling us? Lancet Infect Dis 2005;5:313–20.

TABLE 35-2 Differential Diagnosis and Distinguishing Features of Follicular Conjunctivitis and Conjunctival Scarring

Follicular conjunctivitis*	
Trachoma	Likely diagnosis in an area of known endemicity or high-risk factors. Can be confirmed by laboratory evidence of *C. trachomatis*
Viral conjunctivitis	Self-limiting resolving in approximately two weeks. Often associated with mucopurulent discharge
Hypersensitive conjunctivitis	History will often reveal chronic exposure to ocular drugs or cosmetics
Vernal conjunctivitis	Usually associated with history of atopy and seasonal recurrences
Toxic conjunctivitis secondary to molluscum contagiosum	Associated with multiple nodules on eyelid or eyelid margin
Perinaud's oculoglandular syndrome	Rare condition resulting in granulomatous nodules on the palpebral conjunctiva, pre-auricular and submandibular lymphadenopathy, fever, malaise and a rash. Associated with a number of infections including bartonella, tularemia, tuberculosis, glandular fever or syphilis
Inclusion conjunctivitis	Sexually transmitted and may be associated with a history of vaginits, cervicitis or urethritis. Can be confirmed by laboratory evidence of *C. trachomatis*
Conjunctival scarring	
Repeated episodes of trachomatous inflammation	Likely diagnosis in an area of known endemicity or high-risk factors
Previous severe bacterial conjunctivitis	Associated with history of conjunctivitis with purulent discharge
Previous chalazion	Associated with history of lump on lid
Trauma	Associated with history of trauma

*Follicles found in the fornices without associated inflammation and not involving the superior tarsus, especially in young children, may occur independently of any other pathology—a condition known as folliculosis.

endemicity or that has risk factors for trachoma should be regarded as trachoma.

TREATMENT

ACTIVE TRACHOMA (TRACHOMATOUS INFLAMMATION FOLLICULAR AND/OR TRACHOMA INFLAMMATION INTENSE)

The isolated antibiotic treatment of individuals with trachoma is inappropriate and antibiotic treatment should be incorporated into a broader intervention strategy, as outlined below.

Owing to its high tissue selectivity, long half-life and effectiveness against *Chlamydia*, azithromycin is the most appropriate antibiotic for the treatment of individuals with active trachoma (Table 35-3) [15–26]. Azithromycin also has relatively little interaction with other medications and is well tolerated by the elderly, those with mild-to-moderate renal or hepatic impairment, young children and pregnant women. A single oral dose of 20 mg/kg (maximum 1 g) should be used and repeated every 6–12 months, as required.

An alternative recommended by the WHO is topical tetracycline ointment applied to both eyes 2–4 times a day for 6 weeks. Although tetracycline has been shown to be as effective as azithromycin in treating active trachoma [27], the effectiveness of tetracycline is reduced, in operational conditions, by issues with compliance as a result of its long dosing regimen and possible discomfort and blurring of vision [28].

TABLE 35-3 The Evidence-Based Role of Azithromycin in the Eradication of Blinding Trachoma

Treatment considerations	Evidence recommendations	Clinical caveat	Highest evidence category*	References
Dosing requirements	1 oral dose of 20 mg/kg (up to a maximum of 1 g)	Short course of topical drops may be as effective	1	[15]
How to treat?	Mass, community-based treatment is as effective as targeted household treatment	Cost-benefit depends upon baseline community prevalence	2	[16–19]
Who to treat?	Children (<10 years old) and people with intense inflammatory trachoma	These people represent the major source of *C. trachomatis* infection	4	[20–22]
How often to treat?	Annual treatment in endemic and biannual treatment in hyperendemic areas	Single mass-treatment will not eliminate trachoma	2	[23–25]
When to stop treatment?	When the prevalence is reduced to 5%	Complete community-wide elimination is achievable	2	[23,26]

*Category 1, double masked study; 2, clinical trial >20 subjects; 3, clinical trial <20 subjects; 4, case series; 5, anecdotal case reports.

The WHO guidelines suggest tetracycline ointment be used in children <6 months of age and in pregnant women [29]. However, azithromycin is the treatment of choice for pertussis prophylaxis in children <1 month of age and it is also the first line of treatment for genital chlamydial infection during pregnancy recommended by the Centers for Disease Control and Prevention (CDC) [30]. Many trachoma control programs use azithromycin to treat individuals of all ages.

Treating only a single case of infection is usually futile, as re-infection is almost inevitable from other infected children in the household. Treatment should be given to all members of a household where a child with active trachoma resides. For logistical reasons, the WHO recommends community-wide treatment when more than 10% of children in the community aged 1–9 years have active trachoma. Trachoma is not likely to have been eliminated in less than three years and, so, annual mass treatment should be continued for at least that time and until the prevalence of trachoma on re-assessment is less than 5%. However, as mentioned, successful trachoma control requires that antibiotic treatment be implemented as part of a public health initiative that addresses the environmental and hygiene risk factors for trachoma.

COMPLICATIONS FROM CHRONIC DISEASE

Trichiasis, whether in the early or late stages, should be treated not only to reduce the blinding complications of the disease and sometimes to improve visual acuity, but also to improve quality of life through relief of symptoms, including photophobia and eye pain [31].

The surgical technique recommended for correction of trichiasis by the WHO is the bilamellar tarsal rotation procedure [32]. Trichiasis is the end-stage of the disease and, despite corrective surgery, recurrent trichiasis is a problem. The lowest reported rates of recurrence at one year are in the order of 5% but, with less meticulous surgery, may be over 40%. Recurrence rates have reduced by adhering to high surgical standards, operating during the early stages of trichiasis and reducing risk of secondary infection with the use of antibiotics at the time of surgery. Azithromycin has been shown to be equal to, if not more effective than, tetracycline in reducing the risk of recurrence in randomized, controlled trials [33,34].

Epilation maybe used in the short-term, while awaiting surgery or to remove recurrent lashes post-surgery. However, care should be taken not to break the lashes which can cause more damage from abrasion with the stiff, remaining part of the lash.

PREVENTION AND CONTROL

The integrated trachoma control strategy recommended by the WHO is the SAFE strategy [29]: Surgery, Antibiotics and Facial cleanliness and Environmental improvement. The SAFE strategy is being implemented globally to eliminate trachoma as a cause of blindness by the year 2020, and has already proven to be effective in countries such as the Islamic Republic of Iran, Morocco, Oman and Ghana.

Surgery using the bilamellar tarsal rotation procedure is recommended to decrease the risk of blindness [32]. The finding of active trachoma in children should prompt the search for trichiasis in adults, especially in women and those over the age of 40.

Antibiotics are required to decrease the load of infection in the community. Previously, the use of azithromycin in mass community treatment strategies was limited by cost. However, large-scale donation programs by the manufacturer of azithromycin (Pfizer Inc.) [35] and more affordable, generic production of azithromycin since patent-expiry (US$0.50/single dose course in India; year of costing: 2005) have enabled the antibiotic component to be more cost-effective.

The promotion of facial cleanliness may be the most important component of the SAFE strategy, as poor facial hygiene appears to be the final common pathway of a number of environmental risk factors, such as crowding, poor water accessibility and presence of flies. Together, facial hygiene promotion and environmental improvement decrease the risk of disease transmission and are thus important for sustainable trachoma control. Behavioral changes may be difficult to achieve, but studies where facial hygiene promotion has been implemented have shown additional reductions in rates of active trachoma over antibiotics alone [36]. For sustainable change to hygiene behaviors, community-specific attitudes to hygiene need to be addressed.

Environmental improvements should address the situation-specific risk factors for trachoma, such as water accessibility, the availability of latrines, refuse disposal and animal pens. Attention should focus on specific conditions that prevent every child from having a clean face. These undertakings are usually expensive, but the effects of addressing these risk factors are often far-reaching, as a number of health issues share these risk factors.

Although it may be impossible to eradicate *Chlamydia*, correct implementation of the evidence-based, integrated SAFE strategy that addresses the behavioral, medical and surgical aspects of trachoma could well mean that eliminating this blinding disease is achievable.

35.2 Inclusion Conjunctivitis

Key features

- Caused by *Chlamydia trachomatis*, serotypes D–K, a Gram-negative, intracellular bacterium
- Infection is by inoculation of infected genital secretion into the eye: in adults, this occurs during sexual contact; in neonates, this occurs during vaginal delivery
- If untreated, serious complications of conjunctivitis are uncommon; however, systemic considerations require oral treatment: in adults to minimize the risk of infertility from concomitant genital chlamydial infection and in neonates to treat possible chlamydial pneumonia
- Treatment of adult inclusion conjunctivitis is with a single dose of oral azithromycin. Examination and treatment of sexual contacts is important. Treatment of neonatal chlamydial conjunctivitis is with a 14-day course of oral erythromycin, although one study has shown oral azithromycin to be safe and effective

INTRODUCTION

Inclusion conjunctivitis is an acute conjunctivitis usually caused by "genital" serotypes of *Chlamydia trachomatis*. It is typically found in young adults and is usually associated with urogenital infection. Neonates may be exposed to the infection during the birth process and subsequently develop a severe, purulent conjunctivitis, pneumonia, or both.

EPIDEMIOLOGY

Similar to the distribution of genital chlamydial infection, inclusion conjunctivitis is prevalent worldwide [37]. Adolescents or young adults are at highest risk of chlamydial inclusion conjunctivitis. Infection usually results from inoculation of infected genital secretions into the eye; the incubation period is 7–14 days. *Chlamydia trachomatis* is the most common sexually transmitted bacterium. Symptoms of urogenital infection are often absent or minimal; thus, a large reservoir of the pathogen goes undetected in the community. Chronic, silent urogenital infection is a leading cause of infertility.

The risk of transmission of *C. trachomatis* to an infant born through an infected birth canal is reported to be as high as 70%, with the risk of chlamydial conjunctivitis being 20–50% [38,39]. However, the prevalence of neonatal chlamydial conjunctivits is lower in areas where routine screening and treatment of chlamydial infection in pregnant women occurs. Neonatal chlamydial conjunctivitis usually develops 5–21 days after birth. Pneumonia may develop later, between 4 and 12 weeks after birth.

NATURAL HISTORY, PATHOGENESIS AND PATHOLOGY

The "genital" serotypes of *C. trachomatis* causing inclusion conjunctivitis are serotypes D–K. However, there may be some overlap between "genital" and "ocular" serotypes. The pathogenesis of the conjunctivitis is similar for both "genital" and "ocular" serotypes. If untreated, cases of both neonatal and adult inclusion conjunctivitis usually resolve spontaneously with few complications. However, scarring, similar to that seen in trachoma, has been noted, but the clinical changes tend to be more marked in the lower eyelid.

CLINICAL FEATURES

In adults, inclusion conjunctivitis usually presents as acute follicular conjunctivitis with mucopurulent discharge. The infection is often initially unilateral and frequently associated with pre-auricular lymphadenopathy. Superficial punctuate keratitis or peripheral subepithelial infiltrates may occur.

Signs of neonatal chlamydial conjunctivitis include a mucopurulent disharge, conjunctival injection, diffuse papillary reaction of the tarsal conjunctiva and lid swelling. If severe, pseudomembranes may develop and, rarely, untreated cases may develop conjunctival scarring and corneal pannus.

PATIENT EVALUATION, DIAGNOSIS AND DIFFERENTIAL DIAGNOSIS

Inclusion conjunctivitis is usually diagnosed clinically and confirmed by laboratory testing (Table 35-1). Culture from a swab containing conjunctival epithelial cells was the "gold standard" for diagnosis, with high specificity and moderate sensitivity, dependent on user expertise. Enzyme immunoassay (EIA) and direct fluorescent antibody assays (DFA) have high specificity, but sensitivity may be limited by the type of kit used. Nucleic acid amplification techniques (e.g. PCR) have higher sensitivity than culture methods while retaining high specificity and thus have replaced the other techniques [40]. If resources are limited, Giemsa-stained conjunctival scrapings can be examined for the presence of blue-stained intracytoplasmic inclusions within epithelial cells.

The differential diagnosis of adult inclusion conjunctivitis is similar to the differential of active trachoma (Table 35-2). The most important differential diagnosis in neonates is conjunctivitis caused by *Neisseria gonorrhoea*. However, gonococcal ophthalmia usually occurs earlier (2–5 days after birth) and is more rapidly progressive. Gonococcal ophthalmia and other pyogenic conjunctivitis, such as staphylococcal conjunctivitis, can be differentiated on Gram stain and subsequent culture.

TREATMENT

In adults with inclusion conjunctivitis, 1g of oral azithromycin as a single dose is now standard treatment [41]. Alternatives include doxycycline 100 mg twice daily for seven days, or erythromycin 500 mg four times a day for seven days. Topical erythromycin, tetracycline or sulfacetamide ointment can be given as an adjunct if there is marked ocular discharge. Most importantly, sexual partners need to be examined and treated because of the risk of silent infection and subsequent infertility.

Chlamydial infection in neonates is potentially serious and should be treated with a systemic antibiotic. Oral erythromycin base or ethysuccinate, 50 mg/kg/d in four divided doses for 14 days is standard therapy; however, there are compliance and tolerance issues with this regimen [41]. Oral azithromycin, 50 mg/kg/d as one daily dose for three days has been shown to be safe and effective in the treatment of neonatal chlamydial conjunctivitis in one small study [42].

PREVENTION AND CONTROL

Screening and treatment for *C. trachomatis* is recommended for all pregnant women as early as possible before delivery [43]. Erythromycin (500 mg four times a day for seven days) or amoxicillin (500 mg three times a day for seven days) is the WHO recommended first-line antimicrobial for the treatment of genital *Chlamydia* infection in pregnancy [41,44]. However, azithromycin (1 g as a single dose) has been shown to be safe and effective in a small number of studies, and is recommended as first-line treatment by the CDC [30]. Silver nitrate drops given topically to prevent gonococcal ophthalmia at birth do not prevent *Chlamydia*. Betadine eye drops (2.5%) have been shown to be cheaper and more effective than silver nitrate in preventing both chlamydial and gonococcal ophthalmia, and is associated with appreciably less chemical conjunctivitis [45]. There is no evidence that prophylactic treatment should be given to infants born to mothers with untreated chlamydial infection and there is also no evidence that infants with chlamydial infections should be isolated (standard hygiene precautions are recommended).

REFERENCES

1. Taylor HR. Trachoma: A Blinding Scourge from the Bronze Age to the Twenty-First Century. Melbourne: Centre for Eye Research Australia; 2008.
2. Mariotti SP, Pascolini D, Rose-Nussbaumer J. Trachoma: global magnitude of a preventable cause of blindness. Br J Ophthalmol 2009;93:563–8.
3. Polack S, Brooker S, Kuper H, et al. Mapping the global distribution of trachoma. Bull World Health Organ 2005;83:913–19.
4. Polack S. Maps of the Global Distribution of Trachoma: International Centre for Eye Health; 2005.
5. Frick KD, Hanson CL, Jacobson GA. Global burden of trachoma and economics of the disease. Am J Trop Med Hyg 2003;69(suppl. 5):1–10.
6. Wright HR, Keeffe JE, Taylor HR. Trachoma and the need for a coordinated community-wide response: a case-based study. PLoS Med 2006;3:186–90.
7. Brunham RC, Peeling RW. *Chlamydia trachomatis* antigens: role in immunity and pathogenesis. Infect Agents Dis 1994;3:218–33.
8. El-Asrar AMA, Van Den Oord JJ, Geboes K, et al. Immunopathology of trachomatous conjunctivitis. Br J Ophthalmol 1989;73:276–82.
9. West SK, Munoz B, Mkocha H, et al. Progression of active trachoma to scarring in a cohort of Tanzanian children. Ophthalmic Epidemiol 2001;8:137–44.
10. Guzey M, Ozardali I, Basar E, et al. A survey of trachoma: The histopathology and the mechanism of progressive cicatrization of eyelid tissues. Ophthalmologica 2000;214:277–84.
11. Bowman RJ, Jatta B, Cham B, et al. Natural history of trachomatous scarring in the Gambia: Results of a 12-year longitudinal follow-up. Ophthalmology 2001;108:2219–24.
12. Thylefors B, Dawson C, Jones B, et al. A simplified system for the assessment of trachoma and its complications. Bull World Health Organ 1987;65: 477–83.
13. Negrel AD, Taylor HR, West S. Guidelines for Rapid Assessment for Blinding Trachoma.Report No.: WHO/PBD/GET/00.8. Geneva: World Health Organization; 2001.
14. Wright HR, Taylor HR. Clinical examination and laboratory tests for estimation of trachoma prevalence in a remote setting: what are they really telling us? Lancet Infect Dis 2005;5:313–20.
15. Cochereau I, Goldschmidt P, Goepogui A, et al. Efficacy and safety of short duration azithromycin eye drops versus azithromycin single oral dose for the treatment of trachoma in children: a randomised, controlled, double-masked clinical trial. Br J Ophthalmol 2007;91:667–72.
16. Hoechsmann A, Metcalfe N, Kanjaloti S, et al. Reduction of trachoma in the absence of antibiotic treatment: Evidence from a population-based survey in Malawi. Ophthalmic Epidemiol 2001;8:145-53.
17. Frick KD, Lietman TM, Holm SO, et al. Cost-effectiveness of trachoma control measures: comparing targeted household treatment and mass treatment of children. Bull World Health Organ 2001;79:201–7.
18. Holm SO, Jha HC, Bhatta RC, et al. Comparison of two azithromycin distribution strategies for controlling trachoma in Nepal. Bull World Health Organ 2001;79:194-200.
19. Schemann JF, Guinot C, Traore L, et al. Longitudinal evaluation of three azithromycin distribution strategies for treatment of trachoma in a sub-Saharan African country, Mali. Acta Trop 2007;101:40–53.
20. Solomon AW, Holland MJ, Burton MJ, et al. Strategies for control of trachoma: observational study with quantitative PCR. Lancet 2003;362:198–204.
21. West ES, Munoz B, Mkocha H, et al. Mass treatment and the effect on the load of *Chlamydia trachomatis* infection in a trachoma-hyperendemic community. Invest Ophthalmol Vis Sci 2005;46:83–7.
22. Burton M, Holland MJ, Faal N, et al. Which members of a community need antibiotics to control trachoma? Conjunctival *Chlamydia trachomatis* infection load in Gambian villages. Invest Ophthalmol Vis Sci 2003;44:4215.
23. Melese M, Alemayehu W, Lakew T, et al. Comparison of annual and biannual mass antibiotic administration for elimination of infectious trachoma. JAMA 2008;299:778–84.
24. Lietman T, Porco T, Dawson C, Blower S. Global elimination of trachoma: how frequently should we administer mass chemotherapy? Nat Med 1999;5: 572–6.
25. Biebesheimer JB, House J, Hong KC, et al. Complete local elimination of infectious trachoma from severely affected communities after six biannual mass azithromycin distributions. Ophthalmology 2009;116:2047–50.
26. Ray KJ, Lietman TM, Porco TC, et al. When can antibiotic treatments for trachoma be discontinued? Graduating communities in three African countries. PLoS Negl Trop Dis 2009;3:e458.
27. Mabey D, Fraser-Hurt N. Antibiotics for trachoma. Cochrane Database of Syst Rev 2005:CD001860.
28. Bowman RJ, Sillah A, Van Dehn C, et al. Operational comparison of single-dose azithromycin and topical tetracycline for trachoma. Invest Ophthalmol Vis Sci 2000;41:4074–9.
29. World Health Organization, London School of Hygiene & Tropical Medicine, International Trachoma Initiative. Trachoma control—A guide for programme managers. Geneva: World Health Organization, London School of Hygiene & Tropical Medicine, International Trachoma Initiative; 2006.
30. Centers for Disease Control and Prevention. Sexually Transmitted Diseases Treatment Guidelines. MMWR Recomm Rep 2006:55.
31. Dhaliwal U, Bhatia M. Health-related quality of life in patients with trachomatous trichiasis or entropion. Ophthalmic Epidemiol 2006;13: 59–66.
32. Reacher M, Foster A, Huber J. Trichiasis Surgery for Trachoma: The Bilamellar Tarsal Rotation Procedure. Report No.: WHO/PBL/93.29. Geneva: World Health Organization; 1993.
33. Burton MJ, Kinteh F, Jallow O, et al. A randomised controlled trial of azithromycin following surgery for trachomatous trichiasis in the Gambia. Br J Ophthalmol 2005;89:1282–8.
34. West SK, West ES, Alemayehu W, et al. Single-dose azithromycin prevents trichiasis recurrence following surgery: randomized trial in Ethiopia. Arch Ophthalmol 2006;124:309–14.
35. Pfizer Inc. Partnership to End Blinding Trachoma through the International Trachoma Initiative. Available at: http://www.pfizer.com/responsibility/global_health/international_trachoma_initiative.jsp.
36. West S, Munoz B, Lynch M, et al. Impact of face washing on trachoma in Kongwa, Tanzania. Lancet 1995;345:155–8.
37. World Health Organization, Department of HIV/AIDS. Global prevalence and incidence of selected curable sexually transmitted infections: overview and estimates. Report No.: WHO/CDS/CSR/EDC/2001.10. Geneva: World Health Organization; 2001.
38. Darville T. *Chlamydia trachomatis* infections in neonates and young children. Semin Pediatr Infect Dis 2005;16:235–44.
39. Schachter J, Grossman M, Sweet RL, et al. Prospective study of perinatal transmission of *Chlamydia trachomatis*. JAMA 1986;255:3374–7.
40. Skidmore S, Horner P, Mallinson H. Testing specimens for *Chlamydia trachomatis*. Sex Transm Infect 2006;82:272–5.
41. World Health Organization, Department of Reproductive Health and Research. Guidelines for the management of sexually transmitted infections 2003. Report No.: WHO/RHR/01.10. Geneva: World Health Organization; 2003.
42. Hammerschlag MR, Gelling M, Roblin PM, et al. Treatment of neonatal, Chlamydial conjunctivitis with azithromycin. Pediatr Infect Dis J 1998;17: 1049–50.
43. World Health Organization, Department of Reproductive Health and Research. Global strategy for the prevention and control of sexually transmitted infections: 2006–2015. Breaking the chain of transmission. Geneva: World Health Organization; 2007.
44. Brocklehurst P, Rooney G. Interventions for treating genital *Chlamydia trachomatis* infection in pregnancy. Cochrane Database Syst Rev 1998:CD000054.
45. Schaller UC, Klauss V. Is Crede's prophylaxis for ophthalmia neonatorum still valid? Bull World Health Organ 2001;79:262–3.

Group A *Streptococcus* 36

Thomas L Snelling, Jonathan R Carapetis

Key features

- Group A *Streptococcus* or *Streptococcus pyogenes* is the predominant global cause of bacterial pharyngitis and skin infection
- Group A *Streptococcus* is also a cause of severe invasive, necrotizing and toxin-mediated syndromes and debilitating non-suppurative sequelae, including rheumatic fever and acute post-streptococcal glomerulonephritis
- Group A *Streptococcus* is estimated to result in over 500,000 deaths annually, mostly in developing countries and mostly because of invasive infection or from rheumatic heart disease and its complications
- Group A *Streptococcus* remains universally sensitive to penicillin which remains the mainstay of treatment of Group A Streptococcus infections and the prevention of rheumatic heart disease

INTRODUCTION

Group A *Streptococcus* causes a diverse spectrum of disease, ranging from benign and self-limited infection of the throat or skin, to lethal soft tissue infections accompanied by multi-organ failure. Until the advent of the antibiotic era, Group A *Streptococcus* was a major cause of death in industrialized countries as a result of sepsis, rheumatic heart disease and fatal epidemics of scarlet fever [1, 2]. The 1980s saw an increase in rheumatic fever cases in the Rocky Mountain states of the USA, along with an apparent resurgence in severe Group A *Streptococcus* disease in industrialized countries. The resultant increased attention paid to Group A *Streptococcus* disease in recent years has also brought to focus the continuing high burden of Group A *Streptococcus* disease in developing countries, particularly those in tropical regions [3].

EPIDEMIOLOGY

The burden of all Group A *Streptococcus* infections is highest in resource-limited settings, most of which are in tropical regions. It is assumed that the major reasons for this relate to poverty, overcrowded living conditions and limited access to medical care, although geography and climate may also play a role. The estimated number of cases and deaths of Group A *Streptococcus* diseases is shown in Table 36-1. Of the more severe diseases, 79% of rheumatic heart disease cases, 95% of acute rheumatic fever cases, 97% of acute post-streptococcal glomerulonephritis cases and 97% of invasive Group A *Streptococcus* cases come from less developed countries [3].

Pharyngitis is the most common manifestation of Group A *Streptococcus* disease—its incidence is highest in school-aged children. One episode occurs every 1–2 child years in some resource-limited settings, while only 1 episode every 7–8 child years has been observed in developed urban settings. Limited data on the incidence of Group A *Streptococcus* pharyngitis in tropical areas suggest significant variability, with rates comparable to temperate climates in some settings but, in others, the documented rate is considerably lower. Transmission is higher in winter months. Impetigo is common in childhood; transmission occurs readily in school and preschool care settings, especially in the summer months. In tropical settings where the burden is particularly high, the majority of children in some communities have impetigo at any one time.

Cellulitis and erysipelas are the most frequent manifestations of invasive Group A *Streptococcus* infection and, in contrast to pharyngitis and impetigo, incidence increases with age. In the mid-1980s, reports emerged from industrialized countries of both increasing numbers of severe necrotizing Group A *Streptococcus* infections and of streptococcal toxic shock syndrome [4]. Group A *Streptococcus* strains belonging to *emm* types 1 and 3, in particular, have been implicated in this rise. Most cases of severe invasive Group A *Streptococcus* disease are sporadic, but secondary cases and case clusters have been reported. Limited data suggest that both the incidence and case-fatality of invasive Group A *Streptococcus* disease in resource-limited countries is several-fold higher than in industrialized countries.

Acute rheumatic fever and rheumatic heart disease continue to result in a substantial component of Group A *Streptococcus*-related morbidity and mortality in resource-limited settings. Of the 517,000 Group A *Streptococcus*-related deaths each year, it is estimated that two thirds are caused by rheumatic heart disease or its complications [3]. The true prevalence of rheumatic heart disease remains uncertain, with estimates of at least 1.3 per 1000 school-aged children in developing countries based on auscultatory screening, while estimates based on echocardiography suggest the true prevalence may be more than 10 times higher [5]. Acute rheumatic fever has become uncommon in industrialized settings, although the incidence remains high among indigenous populations in Australia and New Zealand.

The incidence of acute post-streptococcal glomerulonephritis appears to be declining in industrialized settings, but sporadic cases still occur. Acute post-streptococcal glomerulonephritis continues to occur both sporadically and in epidemics in tropical climates (where Group A *Streptococcus* pyoderma is also common); limited data suggest that acute mortality and chronic morbidity from acute post-streptococcal glomerulonephritis may be higher in developing settings.

NATURAL HISTORY, PATHOGENESIS AND PATHOLOGY

The oropharynx and the skin of humans are the only recognized ecologic niches for Group A *Streptococcus* and they represent the major entry sites for both local and invasive infection [6] (see Fig. 36.1). Up to 20% of school-aged children may be colonized in the oropharynx in temperate and some tropical regions, although in many tropical settings, less than 5% of children carry Group A *Streptococcus* (with groups C and G streptococci being more common). Surface proteins facilitate specific adhesion of Group A *Streptococcus* to either the mucosal epithelium of the throat or to the skin (or both).

TABLE 36-1 Summary of Estimated Global Burden of Group A Streptococcal Diseases

Disease	Number of existing cases	Number of new cases each year	Number of deaths each year
Rheumatic heart disease (RHD)	15.6 million	282,000*	233,000†
History of acute rheumatic fever without carditis, requiring secondary prophylaxis	1.88 million	188,000*	
RHD-related infective endocarditis		34,000	8,000
RHD-related stroke	640,000	144,000	108,000
Acute post-streptococcal glomerulonephritis	§	472,000	5,000
Invasive group A streptococcal diseases		663,000	163,000
Total severe cases	**18.1 million**	**1.78 million**	**517,000**
Pyoderma	111 million		
Pharyngitis		616 million	

All estimates rounded-off. Note that these estimates assume constancy of incidence and prevalence over time.
*New RHD cases were calculated based on the proportion of incident acute rheumatic fever cases expected to develop RHD. The remainder of incident acute rheumatic fever cases are included in the "History of acute rheumatic fever without carditis" row. Therefore, the total number of new acute rheumatic fever cases each year is 282,000 + 188,000 = 470,000.
†Includes acute rheumatic fever deaths. RHD deaths are based on proportion of existing RHD cases expected to die each year.
§No attempt has been made to quantify the prevalence of acute post-streptococcal glomerulonephritis-induced chronic renal impairment or end-stage renal failure.
Reproduced with permission from Carapetis JR, Steer AC, Mulholland EK, Weber M. The global burden of group A streptococcal diseases. Lancet Infect Dis 2005;5:685–94.

Asymptomatic colonization of the oropharynx may persist at low levels for weeks without eliciting a host immune response. Colonization of the skin is more transient, becoming established only days before inoculation (e.g. by insect bite) and subsequent pyoderma.

Local infection of the oropharynx (pharyngitis) or skin (pyoderma) is mostly benign with spontaneous resolution usually within days. Invasion of Group A *Streptococcus* into normally sterile sites occurs less commonly, but is often severe with clinical manifestations arising from complex host–pathogen interactions. Preceding viral infection, in particular with varicella or influenza A, has been implicated as a frequent antecedent to invasive infection. The skin and throat are the major portals for entry, after which Group A *Streptococcus* evades host defenses by elaborating a number of virulence factors, chief of which is M protein that extends as hair-like filaments from the cell surface. M protein (together with the hyaluronic acid capsule and other surface proteins) enables Group A *Streptococcus* to evade phagocytosis by multiple mechanisms, including preventing opsonization by blocking complement fixation to the bacterial cell wall.

A number of additional cellular products appear to facilitate direct spread of the invading organism through tissue planes and bacteremia can result in hematogenous dissemination. Some strains have the capacity to elaborate pyrogenic exotoxins that may act as "superantigens", leading to polyclonal proliferation of subsets of T lymphocytes, massive cytokine production and shock [7].

Antibodies against Group A *Streptococcus* proteins (in particular antibodies against serotype-specific epitopes on the M protein) are important in providing protection against subsequent infection. However, aberrant immune responses to otherwise benign Group A *Streptococcus* pharyngitis or impetigo can result in the immune-mediated manifestations, acute rheumatic fever and acute post-streptococcal glomerulonephritis. In acute rheumatic fever, cross-reactive antibodies are thought to arise in genetically predisposed individuals infected with rheumatogenic Group A *Streptococcus* strains. These strains elicit immune responses to antigens with a similarity between epitopes on the M protein and certain host proteins contained within endocardial, synovium and neural tissues.

CLINICAL FEATURES

Group A *Streptococcus* pharyngitis may be mild or associated with high fever, tender anterior cervical lymphadenopathy, tonsillar exudates and raised peripheral white cell count. Symptoms usually resolve after 3–5 days, although suppurative complications (which are now uncommon in industrialized settings) include peritonsillar and retropharyngeal abscess, suppurative lymphadenitis, otitis media, mastoiditis and meningitis. Non-suppurative complications include scarlet fever, acute rheumatic fever or acute post-streptococcal glomerulonephritis. Scarlet fever is characterized by a diffuse blanching rash that spreads from the chest to the abdomen and extremities leaving a sandpaper-like texture to the skin. Desquamation of the fingers, toes, groin and axilla occurs one or more weeks later. The tongue is frequently coated in a white film (white strawberry tongue) that eventually gives way to a beefy red appearance (red strawberry tongue). While most cases are benign, scarlet fever was often lethal in the pre-antibiotic era. Many cases likely represented what would be regarded today as streptococcal toxic shock syndrome (STSS).

In simple impetigo, infection is confined to the epidermis with the formation of superficial crusted lesions on the face or other exposed body parts. In tropical and impoverished settings "pyodermatous" lesions may be pustular and ulcerative. Children are usually afebrile and otherwise well, although resolution of pyoderma may take many days and result in scarring. Erysipelas, which typically affects the face or an extremity, is a painful infection of the dermis resulting in a clearly demarcated red and raised area of inflammation and often formation of superficial bullae. Cellulitis involves the deeper subcutaneous tissues causing a more diffuse and less clearly demarcated area of inflammation. Infection of the draining lymphatic tracts (lymphangitis) results in tender linear streaks extending from the site of infection. Unlike impetigo, cellulitis and erysipelas are usually associated with fever and systemic toxicity.

Necrotizing fasciitis is a rapidly progressing infection of the subcutaneous fat, the superficial fascia and deeper structures, including muscle. Shock, multi-organ failure and death may ensue within hours

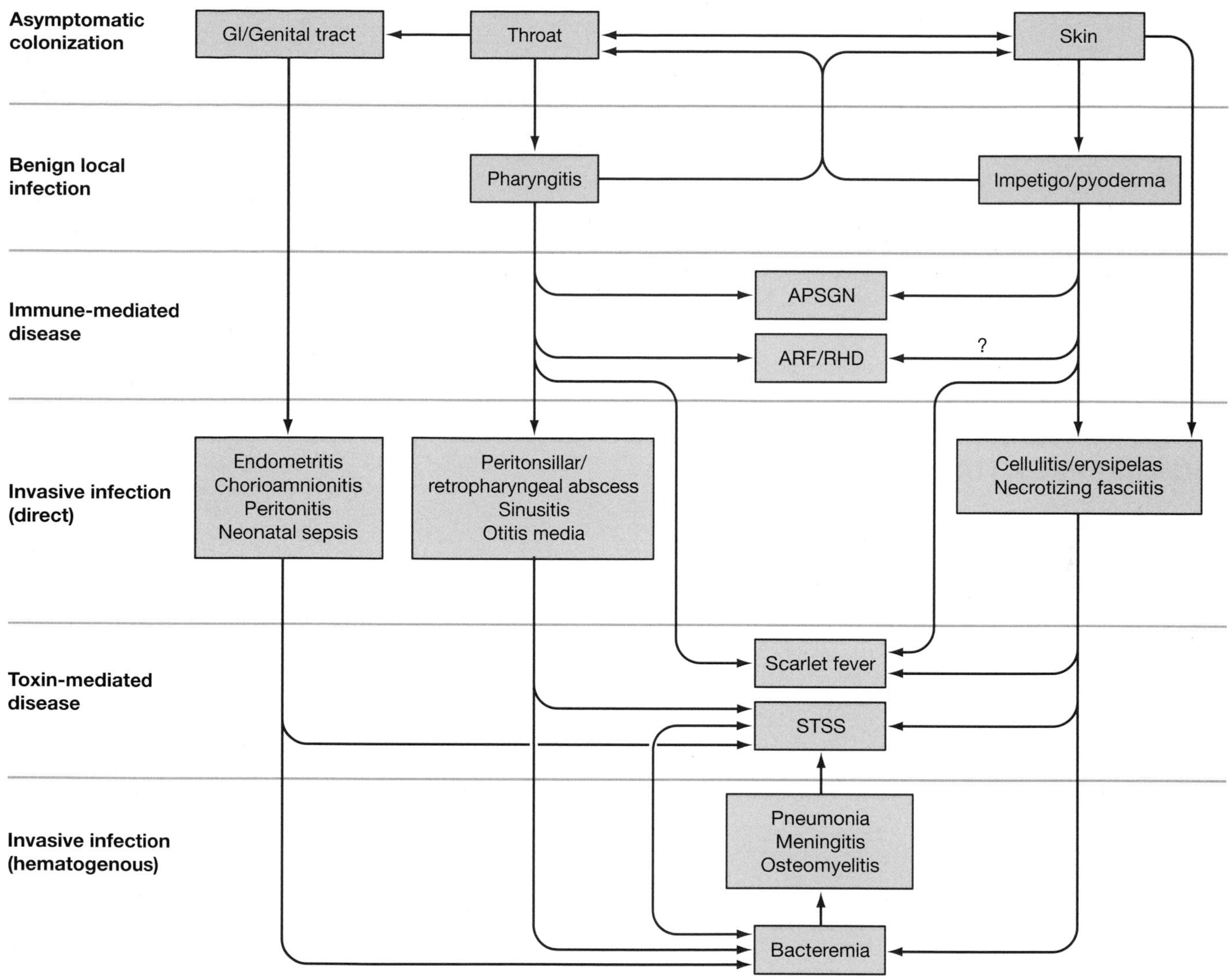

FIGURE 36.1 The inter-related manifestations of Group A *Streptococcus* colonization and local and invasive infection, including immune-mediated and toxin-mediated syndromes. ARF, acute rheumatic fever; RHD, rheumatic heart disease.

or days of onset. Initially, the overlying skin is relatively spared and severe escalating pain may be disproportionate to clinical findings. The skin subsequently becomes violaceous and bullae may form and then slough. STSS is characteristically associated with Group A *Streptococcus* necrotizing fasciitis, although it may arise in the setting of other invasive Group A *Streptococcus* infections. The case definition of STSS requires the confirmation of Group A *Streptococcus* infection, along with hypotension and two or more features of multi-organ involvement: rash, coagulopathy, respiratory distress syndrome, renal failure or hepatic impairment [8].

Otitis media, retropharyngeal and peritonsillar abscess, sinusitis, meningitis, pneumonia, bacteremia and endocarditis may arise either as a complication of tonsillopharyngitis, following surgery or trauma (including burns), following varicella infection, or without apparent antecedent. Historically, outbreaks of Group A *Streptococcus* pneumonia were reported among previously healthy adults, although more recent reports have described the highest risk amongst the elderly and those with underlying medical conditions; infection in these individuals is often associated with high case fatality [9]. A viral prodrome is often reported, although the onset of fever, chest pain and dyspnea is characteristically rapid. Group A *Streptococcus* pneumonia may be necrotizing with pleural effusions frequently present early and early complications include lung abscess formation, mediastinitis and pericarditis. Group A *Streptococcus* is an uncommon cause of meningitis in children and adults, with most reports arising in individuals with a pre-existing focus of Group A *Streptococcus* infection (e.g. pharyngitis, otitis media) or with other risk factors (e.g. skull defect or post-cranial surgery) [10]. Puerperal sepsis caused by Group A *Streptococcus* was a frequent cause of death in the pre-antibiotic era with outbreaks resulting from nosocomial transmission. A study in four tropical developing countries (Papua New Guinea, Ethiopia, The Gambia and The Philippines) during the 1990s found that Group A *Streptococcus* was one of the three leading causes of bacteremia in children aged <90 days, suggesting that Group A *Streptococcus* puerperal sepsis and septic abortion remain common in less developed, tropical countries [11]. Unlike Group B *Streptococcus*, Group A *Streptococcus* more commonly affects the mother than the infant, manifesting as post-partum endometritis, peritonitis, septic thrombophlebitis or bacteremia without focus [12]. However, chorioamnionitis and neonatal sepsis are also reported.

Acute rheumatic fever is characterized by various combinations of fever, polyarthritis or arthralgias, carditis, characteristic rash (erythema marginatum), chorea and subcutaneous nodules [13] (Table 36-3). Chorea and insidious carditis can occur as a manifestation of acute rheumatic fever in the absence of other features. Severe or recurrent episodes of acute rheumatic fever may result in progressive damage to the mitral valve (and sometimes the aortic valve) resulting in incompetence and progressive heart failure (rheumatic heart disease). Over several years, the valve may eventually become stenotic. Acute post-streptococcal glomerulonephritis can occur 1–2 weeks after throat infection or a few weeks after Group A *Streptococcus* skin infection. The features are hematuria (microscopic or gross), edema (which may be most evident peri-orbitally) and hypertension. Severe cases can also be complicated by encephalopathy. The illness is generally benign in childhood, but there may be an appreciable mortality among adults as a result of renal and congestive cardiac failure. Pediatric autoimmune neuropsychiatric disorders associated with streptococcal infections (PANDAS) is a term used to describe some children with tic or obsessive compulsive disorders in whom symptoms appear to develop or worsen following Group A *Streptococcus* infection. The existence of PANDAS is controversial [14]. Post-streptococcal reactive arthritis describes a syndrome of polyarthritis that differs from acute rheumatic fever by affecting a range of smaller joints, being relatively resistant to anti-inflammatory treatment and not being associated with carditis, although cases of acute rheumatic fever have been misdiagnosed as post-streptococcal reactive arthritis [15, 16].

PATIENT EVALUATION, DIAGNOSIS AND DIFFERENTIAL DIAGNOSIS

Viruses account for most episodes of acute pharyngitis in all age groups. Group A *Streptococcus* is isolated in only 20–40% of cases of exudative pharyngitis in school-aged children and an even lower proportion of cases in younger children and adults. Recovery of the organism may not represent infection, but colonization. The distinguishing features of Group A *Streptococcus* pharyngitis and scarlet fever, and differential diagnoses, are detailed in Table 36-2.

Staphylococcus aureus is a major cause of community-acquired pyogenic infection and an important differential diagnosis for invasive Group A *Streptococcus* infection, especially for skin and osteoarticular infections and necrotizing pneumonia. The features which may help to distinguish Group A *Streptococcus* from *S. aureus* and other skin infections are listed in Table 36-2. In addition, a form of toxic shock syndrome (TSS) may complicate *S. aureus* infection, and shares many features with STSS with the exception that it is more frequently associated with colonization rather than bacteremia or severe underlying infection.

Invasive infections resulting from trauma or bites, exposure to water or soil, or involving immunocompromised hosts (including diabetic foot infections) may be caused by a more expanded array of pathogens and therefore require broader empirical therapy and heightened efforts to obtain a microbiologic diagnosis [17].

The arthritis of acute rheumatic fever may be mistaken for septic arthritis (e.g. the polyarthritis of disseminated gonococcosis or multifocal *S. aureus* infection), rheumatologic causes of polyarthritis, including juvenile rheumatoid arthritis, and post-streptococcal reactive arthritis (see Table 36-2). Acute rheumatic fever is the most common cause of chorea in most populations with a high incidence of acute rheumatic fever—particularly those in tropical, less-developed countries—and can occur in the absence of other features of acute rheumatic fever or serologic evidence of Group A *Streptococcus* infection. However, chorea may also be a manifestation of systemic lupus erythematosus, neurovascular disease, drugs, thyrotoxicosis, Wilson's disease and a number of genetic neurodegenerative diseases that must be considered, especially where acute rheumatic fever is uncommon.

Group A *Streptococcus* pharyngitis may be diagnosed presumptively by culturing colonies of Gram-positive cocci displaying surrounding

TABLE 36-2 Differential Diagnosis for Selected Group A *Streptococcus* Infections and Group A *Streptococcus*-Related Syndromes

Group A *Streptococcus* pharyngitis		
Primary	Rhinoviruses Coronaviruses Adenoviruses Epstein-Barr virus (EBV) Enteroviruses	• Coryza, rhinorrhea and hoarseness are prominent features of rhinovirus and coronavirus-associated pharyngitis, which is usually non-exudative • Adenovirus may be exudative and associated with conjunctivitis, i.e. "pharyngoconjunctival fever" • EBV-associated pharyngitis is often part of "infectious mononucleosis" and is associated with prominent lymphadenopathy and systemic features, e.g. myalgias and atypical lymphocytosis +/– elevated transaminases • CMV and HIV may both cause a "mononucleosis-like" illness • HIV seroconversion illness may occur in the window period before ELISA tests become positive • Enterovirus "herpangina" is associated with discrete ulcerative lesions of the posterior pharynx • Group C and G streptococci are not thought to cause acute rheumatic fever or acute post-streptococcal glomerulonephritis • *Arcanobacterium haemolyticus* is more common in adolescence and associated with a pleomorphic rash affecting the extensor surfaces and spreading to the neck and trunk • *Neisseria gonorrhoeae* throat infection is more frequently asymptomatic, but should be considered in sexually active individuals • *Mycoplasma pneumoniae* and *C. pneumoniae* produce pharyngitis accompanied by lower respiratory symptoms • Diphtheria is marked by extreme toxicity and the development of a thick pharyngeal exudate. Death is commonly caused by toxin-mediated cardiac suppression or direct invasion of local structures and asphyxiation. Remains a risk in settings where vaccination programmes are poorly established or have been interrupted • Primary HSV gingivostomatitis results in ulcerative lesions of the lips, tongue and buccal mucosa associated with fever, pain and drooling • Acute necrotizing ulcerative gingivitis is caused by infection with mixed anaerobes and oral spirochetes results in painful inflammation and sloughing of the gums. Associated with limited nutrition and dental hygiene
Secondary	Group C and G streptococci Cytomegalovirus (CMV) Human immunodeficiency virus (HIV)	
Other	*Arcanobacterium haemolyticus* *Neisseria gonnorhoeae* *Mycoplasma pneumoniae* *Chlamydophila pneumoniae* *Corynebacterium diphtheriae* Herpes Simplex Virus (HSV) *Yersinia enterocolitica* *Francisella tularensis* Mixed anaerobes and spirochetes	

TABLE 36-2 Differential Diagnosis for Selected Group A *Streptococcus* Infections and Group A *Streptococcus*-Related Syndromes—cont'd

Scarlet fever		
Primary	Measles Rubella Roseola EBV Parvovirus B19	• Measles and rubella should be considered, especially if unvaccinated or history of recent contact • Measles is associated with prodromal conjunctivitis and coryzal symptoms and Koplik spots. Rubella is associated with post-auricular lymphadenopathy • Parvovirus "fifth disease or erythema infectiosum" associated with distinctive "slapped cheek" rash of face and reticular rash of limbs appearing after fever resolution • Roseola rash associated with defervescence and affects younger children (infants) more than scarlet fever • Kawasaki disease (KD) and Still's disease (SD; systemic-onset juvenile rheumatoid arthritis) associated with multiple symptoms and prolonged fever (>5 days). KD is also associated with conjunctivitis, edema of the hands and feet, and stomatitis. SD is associated with transient or "evanescent" rash, lymphadenopathy, hepatosplenomegaly, uveitis, +/– arthritis
Secondary	Kawasaki disease Still's disease Enteroviruses Drug eruption Anticonvulsant hypersensitivity syndrome	
Impetigo		
Primary	*Staphylococcus aureus* Group C and G beta-hemolytic streptococci Scabies Tinea	• *Staphylococcus aureus* impetigo is more commonly (but not always) bullous and may co-infect with Group A *Streptococcus* in pyodermatous impetigo • Non-group A beta-hemolytic streptococci may cause clinically indistinguishable lesions to Group A Streptococci, but are not associated with acute rheumatic fever or acute post-streptococcal glomerulonephritis • Scabies may result in crusted lesions and burrows that are itchy and involve the interdigital spaces or diffusely involving the trunk. Infestation may predispose to pyoderma • Tinea causes superficial scaly non-exudative lesions frequently with central sparing
Cellulitis and erysipelas		
Primary	*S. aureus* Group B, C and G *Streptococcus*	• *Staphylococcus aureus* usually associated with clear portal of entry, e.g. wound • Enterobacteriacae, pseudomonas and anaerobes more common in immunocompromised hosts, e.g. diabetic foot infections, neutropenic hosts • HSV associated with vesicular lesions • *Pasteurella multocida*, *E. corredens* and anaerobes following human or animal bites • *Aeromonas* species may be rapidly progressive and associated with water exposure • *Erysipelothrix rhusiopathiae* and contact dermatitis are not associated with toxicity and may be suspected because of distribution (e.g. on hands) and exposure history (e.g. meat-worker)
Secondary	Enterobacteriacae *Pseudomonas aeruginosa* HSV Anaerobes	
Other	*Aeromonas* species *Pasteurella multocida* *Eikenella corredens* *Erysipelothrix rhusiopathiae* Contact dematitis	
Necrotizing fasciitis		
Primary	Polymicrobial *Clostridium perfringens*	• Unlike other forms of necrotizing fasciitis, Group A *Streptococcus* necrotizing fasciitis is rarely associated with gas formation • Polymicrobial infection may be associated with abdominal surgery or an occult colonic source, typically involving the perineum and abdominal wall (Fournier's gangrene) and in patients with diabetes or peripheral vascular disease • Clostridial "gas gangrene": usually secondary to traumatic interruption of vascular supply to affected limb or a colonic pathology in case of *C. septicum* • *Vibrio vulnificus* associated with underlying illnesses and water exposure
Secondary	*Vibrio vulnificus*	
Other	*Clostridium septicum*	

Continued

TABLE 36-2 Differential Diagnosis for Selected Group A *Streptococcus* Infections and Group A *Streptococcus*-Related Syndromes—cont'd

Acute rheumatic fever		
Primary	*S. aureus* Post-streptococcal reactive arthritis (PSRA)	• *Staphylococcus aureus* is usually monoarticular. Associated with sepsis and moderate-to-severe toxicity if multifocal. Effusions are purulent and usually (but not always) culture-positive • PSRA associated with small joints and absence of other clinical features of acute rheumatic fever or a propensity to rheumatic heart disease. A diagnosis of PSRA should rarely be made in populations with a high incidence of acute rheumatic fever, and all cases should be given at least 12 months of penicillin prophylaxis before re-evaluation • *Neisseria gonorrhoeae* may be multifocal and migratory, and must be considered if sexually active. Also associated with cutaneous lesions in disseminated disease. Culture of joint fluid is frequently negative • Juvenile rheumatoid arthritis (JRA) arthritis is usually symmetrical, non-migratory and has a more gradual onset. Other features, e.g. iritis and serositis, may be present • Transient synovitis more frequent occurs in younger children, affects the hips, is self- resolving and less associated with raised inflammatory markers and fever • SLE associated with raised antinuclear antibodies and dsDNA • Reactive arthritis is associated with rash of palms and soles, conjunctivitis and urethritis
Secondary	*N. gonorrhoeae* Rheumatoid arthritis Transient synovitis	
Other	Systemic lupus erythematosus (SLE) Reactive arthritis	
Acute post-streptococcal glomerulonephritis		
Primary	SLE IgA nephropathy Mesangiocapillary glomerulonephritis (MCGN) Rapidly progressive glomerulonephritis	• Post-streptococcal glomerulonephritis distinguished by complement profile (low C3, normal C4) and raised streptococcal serology titers, although these may be coincidentally raised in non-post-streptococcal glomerulonephritis. Also anti-streptolysin O titer (ANA) may be normal if post-streptococcal glomerulonephritis secondary to impetigo • SLE, MCGN and glomerulonephritis of chronic disease are also associated with low C3 which resolves only slowly if untreated (8 weeks or more) • SLE is associated with depressed C4 and other manifestations, e.g. arthritis and/or iritis, positive antinuclear antibodies (ANA) and double-stranded DNA (dsDNA) autoantibodies • MCGN more frequently associated with heavy proteinuria and nephrotic syndrome • Glomerulonephritis of chronic disease is associated with endocarditis, chronic hepatitis B or C, syphilis and malaria. Distinguished from post-streptococcal glomerulonephritis by other features, e.g. fever, positive blood cultures, hepatitis, etc. • Rapidly progressive glomerulonephritis is associated with progression to end-stage renal failure. Occasionally secondary to post-streptococcal glomerulonephritis but may be secondary to SLE (ANA positive) or Wegeners granulomatosis (antineutrophil cytoplasmic antibody (ANCA) positive)
Secondary	Benign familial hematuria Henoch-Schonlein purpura Sickle cell nephropathy Subacute endocarditis	
Other	Hemolytic-uremic syndrome Trauma Congenital anomalies Tumor	

zones of beta-hemolysis on blood agar. Other beta-hemolytic streptococci may colonize the oropharynx (e.g. Group C and G streptococci), and differentiation requires the demonstration of growth inhibition by bacitracin or the use of commercially available, group-specific antigen detection kits. Rapid diagnostic tests have been developed to allow clinicians to reliably distinguish Group A *Streptococcus* from viral pharyngitis at the point of care. Evaluations of these tests suggested variable sensitivity of earlier generation kits (~85%), but improved sensitivity of later-generation optical immunoassay-based kits and good specificity.

Group A *Streptococcus* cellulitis and erysipelas are clinical diagnoses that are only occasionally confirmed by positive blood cultures. Culture of percutaneous aspirates is helpful if positive, but is usually negative. The clinical suspicion of necrotizing fasciitis or myonecrosis must be confirmed promptly by the demonstration of nonviable tissue at surgery. Imaging results are frequently nondefinitive and may inadvertently delay the diagnosis and institution of appropriate treatment. Group A *Streptococcus* can usually be cultured from operative specimens, if not from blood in patients with necrotizing fasciitis.

The diagnosis of a primary episode of acute rheumatic fever is based on the most recent version of the Jones' criteria—currently the 1992 version (Table 36-3). These clinical and investigational criteria have been repeatedly revised since the original 1944 version to maintain their positive predictive value in settings where incidence is decreasing. As a result, some high-burden settings have chosen to modify the revised criteria to retain their sensitivity and negative predictive value [18].

In acute post-streptococcal glomerulonephritis, activation of the alternative complement pathway results in a depressed C3 level (usually with a normal C4) that resolves after several weeks. Diagnosis generally rests on the presence of signs and symptoms, together with serologic evidence of recent Group A *Streptococcus* infection and a compatible complement profile. Biopsy is reserved for atypical features, such as anuria or failure of renal function, hypertension or depressed complement that does not improve after several weeks.

TABLE 36-3 World Health Organization 2002–2003 Criteria for the Diagnosis of Rheumatic Fever and Rheumatic Heart Disease

The Jones Criteria (1992 update):		
Major manifestations	Carditis Polyarthritis Chorea Erythema marginatum Subcutaneous nodules	
Minor manifestations	Clinical:	Arthralgia Fever
	Laboratory:	Elevated acute phase reactants (ESR, leukocyte count)
	ECG:	Prolonged PR interval
Evidence of antecedent Group A *Streptococcus* infection	Elevated or rising streptococcal antibody titers (anti-streptrolysin O or anti-DNase B titer) Positive throat culture or rapid streptococcal antigen test Recent scarlet fever	
Diagnostic categories:		
Primary episode of acute rheumatic fever	Two major manifestations, or one major and two minor manifestations plus evidence of antecedent Group A *Streptococcus* infection	
Recurrent attack of acute rheumatic fever in a patient with established rheumatic heart disease	Two minor manifestations plus evidence of antecedent Group A *Streptococcus* infection	
Recurrent attack of acute rheumatic fever in a patient with established rheumatic heart disease	Two major manifestations, or one major and two minor manifestations plus evidence of antecedent Group A *Streptococcus* infection	
Rheumatic chorea Insidious onset rheumatic carditis	Other major manifestations or evidence of Group A streptococcal infection not required	
Chronic valve lesions of rheumatic heart disease (patients presenting for the first time with pure mitral stenosis or mixed mitral valve disease and/or aortic valve disease)	Do not require any other criteria to be presenting for the first time with pure diagnosed as having rheumatic heart disease	

Reproduced with permission from World Health Organization. Rheumatic Fever and Rheumatic Heart Disease: Report of a WHO Expert Consultation. Report No. 923. Geneva: World Health Organization; 2004.

TREATMENT

Penicillin remains the antibiotic of choice for most Group A *Streptococcus* infections. Group A *Streptococcus* remains universally sensitive to penicillin and, while treatment failures occur, they invariably relate to lack of *in vivo* efficacy rather than *in vitro* non-susceptibility. As penicillins target cell wall synthesis, they may be less effective in the stationary phase of bacterial growth as they may occur in severe infections complicated by large bacterial loads [19]. However, even in instances where alternative antibiotics may be preferred because of differing mechanisms of action, they are generally used as an adjunct to—rather than in replacement of—penicillin therapy. Erythromycin and the newer macrolides have been used for Group A *Streptococcus* disease where individuals have immediate hypersensitivity to penicillin. Macrolide resistance is common in some settings and can arise abruptly, apparently related to the population level of macrolide consumption. Some mutations confer resistance to both macrolides and clindamycin, but these remain uncommon.

The use of antibiotics for the routine treatment of Group A *Streptococcus* pharyngitis is contentious because of the usually self-limiting nature of the illness. Studies suggest that treatment reduces the average duration of sore throat by 16 hours and decreases the risk of rheumatic fever and otitis media by around 70%, and the risk of peritonsillar abscess by around 85% [20]. In low-incidence settings, the numbers needed to treat to prevent complications is likely to be very large, so the main aim of antibiotic treatment, if chosen to be used, is alleviation of symptoms and shortening of the duration of illness. However, antibiotic treatment of Group A *Streptococcus* pharyngitis is essential in populations with a high incidence of acute rheumatic fever and, if diagnostic facilities are limited, empirical treatment of all sore throat cases may be justified. There is little evidence that antibiotics reduce the risk of subsequent acute post-streptococcal glomerulonephritis.

Treatment recommendations are detailed in Table 36-4. Ten days of twice-daily oral penicillin V or a single dose of intramuscular benzathine pencillin G are the preferred treatment for Group A *Streptococcus* pharyngitis, although once-daily oral amoxicillin appears to be effective for symptom resolution and Group A *Streptococcus* eradication [21]. Short courses (up to 5 days) of macrolides and some cephalosporins have been shown to have equivalent clinical and short-term microbiologic cure rates, but the risk of late microbiologic failure may be higher. There are insufficient data regarding the efficacy of short-course or non-penicillin regimens in preventing acute rheumatic fever. Treatment of impetigo may be with oral or topical antibiotics—options are given in Table 36-4.

Penicillin is the treatment of choice for invasive infection where Group A *Streptococcus* is confirmed or highly likely (e.g. erysipelas or perianal cellulitis). Because of the narrow spectrum of penicillin, empirical treatment prior to microbiologic confirmation is generally with one or more alternative antimicrobials. For example, an anti-staphylococcal penicillin or a first-generation cephalosporin is required to cover both Group A *Streptococcus* and *S. aureus* in cellulitis (see Table 36-4). Where methicillin-resistant *S. aureus* (MRSA) is prevalent, clindamycin may be an acceptable alternative if prevailing MRSA strains are susceptible. Suppurative diseases frequently seen as complications of Group A *Streptococcus* infection (e.g. peritonsillar abscess) may also be caused by organisms other than Group A *Streptococcus*.

As necrotizing soft tissue infections may be polymicrobial, broad-spectrum cover (e.g. with a carbapenem) is recommended until the microbiologic cause is confirmed.

Urgent and aggressive debridement of nonviable tissues has been the cornerstone of management of Group A *Streptococcus* necrotizing fasciitis, along with intensive supportive care and antibiotics. However, some authorities have suggested that a less aggressive approach may be acceptable if antibiotics and adjunctive therapy with intravenous immunoglobulin (IVIG) are instituted early [22]. Clindamycin is recommended as an adjunct to penicillin for the treatment of severe invasive Group A *Streptococcus* disease, including necrotizing infections, during the first few days of treatment—this is supported by the superior activity of clindamycin over penicillin in animal models [19]. However, penicillin should always be given unless there is a history of hypersensitivity. Although supportive data are limited, administration of 1 or 2 doses of IVIG early in the course of STSS is widely recommended. A multicenter, randomized, controlled trial revealed a trend toward a reduction in mortality among recipients, but the study was terminated early because of slow recruitment [23]. IVIG is also recommended by some as adjunctive treatment in severe invasive Group A *Streptococcus* infections, even in the absence of toxic shock.

TABLE 36-4 Antibiotic Treatment Guidelines for Selected Group A *Streptococcus* Infections

Rationale	Medication	Evidence*	Dose	Comments
Group A Streptococcus pharyngitis				
• Prevention of acute rheumatic fever in moderate-to-high endemic settings • Prevention of suppurative complications • Alleviation of symptoms • Prevent secondary cases	Oral phenoxymethylpenicillin (penicillin V)	1	10 mg/kg up to 500 mg BD for 10 days	Treatment may be primarily for symptom alleviation unless the risk of sequelae is high
	Oral amoxicillin	1	≤30 kg: 750 mg daily for 10 days >30 kg: 1500 mg daily for 10 days	Not proven to prevent acute rheumatic fever
	IM benzathine penicillin G	1	3–6kg: 225 mg 6–10kg: 337.5 mg 10–15kg: 450 mg 15–20kg: 675 mg 20+ kg: 900 mg as a single dose	Preferred where risk of rheumatic fever is high and adherence to oral therapy not assured
	Oral roxithromycin[†]	1	20 mg/kg up to 500 mg daily for 3 days	If hypersensitive to penicillin
Impetigo				
• Alleviate symptoms • Prevent secondary cases • Possibly prevent invasive complications	Topical mupirocin 2% ointment	1	8-hourly for 7 days	Preferred for mild disease, but not proven in high-endemic settings. Use saline, soap water or 0.1% potassium permanganate to remove crusts prior to applying. Strains of *Staphylococcus aureus* may be resistant or may acquire resistance to topical antibiotics
	Oral di/flucloxacillin	1	12.5 mg/kg up to 500 mg q 6-hourly for 10 days	First-line treatment if multiple lesions and *S. aureus* is likely
	IM benzathine penicillin G	1	3–6kg: 225 mg 6–10kg: 337.5 mg 10–15kg: 450 mg 15–20kg: 675 mg 20+ kg: 900 mg as a single dose	Preferred in endemic settings where risk of acute post-streptococcal glomerulonephritis is high and/or adherence to oral therapy not assured. Exclude *S. aureus* infection if refractory to treatment
	Oral erythromycin	1	12.5 mg/kg up to 500 mg TDS for 10 days	If hypersensitive to penicillin
Erysipelas and cellulitis mild/early				
• Alleviate symptoms • Prevent progression • Prevent complications	Oral di/flucloxacillin	1	12.5 mg/kg up to 500 mg q 6-hourly for 7–10 days	Switch to IV therapy if failure to respond and consider resistant pathogens, e.g. methicillin-resistant *Staphylococcus aureus* (MRSA)
	Oral phenoxymethylpenicillin (penicillin V)	2	10 mg/kg up to 500 mg BD for 10 days	If *S. aureus* is unlikely (e.g. early erysipelas or perianal cellulitis) or if Group A *Streptococcus* confirmed on culture. Exclude *S. aureus* infection if refractory to treatment
	Oral cephalexin	1	12.5 mg/kg up to 500 mg q 8hourly for 7–10 days	If non-immediate type hypersensitivity to penicillins
	Oral clindamycin	1	10 mg/kg up to 450 mg q 8-hourly for 7–10days	If immediate type hypersensitivity to penicillin or infection with clindamycin-sensitive MRSA likely

TABLE 36-4 Antibiotic Treatment Guidelines for Selected Group A *Streptococcus* Infections—cont'd

Rationale	Medication	Evidence*	Dose	Comments
Erysipelas and cellulitis moderate-to-severe				
• Alleviate symptoms • Prevent complications	IV di/flucloxacillin	1	50 mg/kg up to 2 g q 6-hourly	Preferred treatment unless MRSA is likely
	IV cephalothin	2	50 mg/kg up to 2 g q 6-hourly	If non-immediate type hypersensitivity to penicillin
	IV/Oral clindamycin	1	10 mg/kg up to 450 mg q 8-hourly for 7–10 days	If immediate type hypersensitivity to penicillin or infection with clindamycin sensitive MRSA likely. Bioavailability of clindamycin is high so oral clindamycin can be considered except in infants
	IV vancomycin	1	25 mg/kg (<12 yr use 30 mg/kg) up to 1g BD	If infection with clindamycin-resistant MRSA likely. Adjust dose on basis of trough blood levels
Necrotizing fasciitis§				
Prevent death Prevent complications Alleviate symptoms Minimize disfigurement	IV meropenem	5	25 mg/kg up to 1 g q 8-hourly	Broad-spectrum cover is recommended in addition to surgical debridement until Group A *Streptococcus* infection is confirmed, thereafter penicillin + clindamycin is recommended
	IV benzylpenicillin	2	45 mg/kg up to 1.8 g q 4-hourly	If Group A *Streptococcus* infection is confirmed. Use in addition to surgical debridement
	IV cephalothin	5	50 mg/kg up to 2 g q 6-hourly	If GAS confirmed and non-immediate type hypersensitivity to penicillin. If there is a history of immediate-type hypersensitivity to ß-lactams, seek expert advice
	+ IV clindamycin	2	15 mg/kg up to 600 mg q 8-hourly	Use as an adjunct to meropenem or penicillin if Group A *Streptococcus* infection is suspected or confirmed
Streptococcal toxic shock syndrome (STSS)§				
• Prevent death • Minimize complications	Intravenous immunoglobulin (IVIG)	4	2 g/kg as an immediate infusion, repeated once in 48–72 h if necessary	Use as an adjunct to penicillin and clindamycin therapy +/– debridement as recommended above for necrotizing fasciitis

Continued

TABLE 36-4 Antibiotic Treatment Guidelines for Selected Group A *Streptococcus* Infections—cont'd

Rationale	Medication	Evidence*	Dose	Comments
Acute rheumatic fever treatment				
• Alleviate symptoms • Prevent death from acute cardiac failure	Aspirin	1	80–100mg/kg/day (up to 4–8 g/day) in 4–5 divided doses	For the control of pain of acute rheumatic fever arthritis. Duration dependent on clinical response
	IM benzathine penicillin G	5	≤20 kg: 450 mg as a single dose >20 kg: 900 mg as a single dose	Preferred where adherence to oral therapy not assured. Treatment should focus on pain relief with salicylates and management of cardiac failure
	Oral phenoxymethylpenicillin (penicillin V)	5	250 mg BD for 10 days	An acceptable alternative to benzathine penicillin if adherence can be assured, e.g. in hospital
	Oral prednisolone	5	1–2 mg/kg/day (up to 80 mg/day)	Not routinely recommended for carditis, but may be considered for severe carditis if surgery is not an option
	Carbamazepine	3	7–10 mg/kg/day in 3 divided doses	Not routinely recommended for management of chorea, but may be considered in severe cases
Acute rheumatic fever prophylaxis				
• Prevent further episodes of acute rheumatid fever • Prevent progressive carditis	IM benzathine penicillin G	1	<20 kg: 450 mg >20 kg: 900 mg every 3–4 weeks	Preferred regimen. Should be continued for at least 10 years and at least until patient is 21 years old. Patients with established valve disease may require longer duration. Four-weekly injections satisfactory if a good control programme is in place
	Oral phenoxymethylpenicillin (penicillin V)	1	250 mg BD	Associated with inferior adherence. Only where IM injections are refused or risk of progressive carditis very low
	Oral erythromycin	5	250 mg BD	If hypersensitive to penicillin. Dose for erythromycin ethyl succinate is 400 mg BD

*Level of evidence: 1=randomized controlled trial, 2=comparative clinical study > 20 patients, 3=comparative clinical study < 20 patients, 4=case series, 5=expert opinion on basis of *in vitro* data or animal studies.

†Roxithromycin, semi-synthetic macrolide not commercially available in the USA.

§Intravenous immune globulin (IVIG) 2 g/kg as a single infusion, repeated if necessary 24–48 hours later is also recommended for necrotizing fasciitis or other severe invasive Group A *Streptococcus* infections (e.g. impending STSS). If indicated, IVIG should be administered as early as possible.

Management of acute rheumatic fever is primarily symptomatic. Penicillin is generally given to eradicate colonization, although acute infection has usually passed by the time symptoms of acute rheumatic fever develop. Salicylates are used to relieve fever and the pain from arthritis that is often severe. Where necessary, cardiac failure is managed with diuretics and angiotensin-converting enzyme (ACE) inhibitors. Steroids are sometimes used in cases of severe carditis, although there is no evidence that they improve the long-term outcome in RHD. Mitral valve repair, balloon valvuloplasty, or valve replacement may be required to manage patients with severe valve disease in rheumatic heart disease.

Management of acute post-streptococcal glomerulonephritis is based on control of hypertension with fluid restriction and use of a loop diuretic such as furosemide. ACE inhibitors may also be needed as an adjunct. Dialysis is occasionally required to manage severe hyperkalemia or symptomatic uremia.

Contacts of patients with Group A *Streptococcus* infection may be colonized with the same Group A *Streptococcus* strain, but primary prophylaxis of contacts is rarely indicated for simple Group A *Streptococcus* pharyngitis. Even for contacts of severe invasive infections, it is estimated that around 2000 contacts would need to receive prophylaxis in order to avoid a single, severe infection—opinion on the value of treating contacts is divided [24]. If prophylactic treatment of contacts is attempted, regimens combining rifampin with penicillin, or using alternative antibiotics such as cephalosporins or azithromycin, are usually recommended as a result of the increasing failures of penicillin alone in eradicating carriage.

However, regular secondary prophylaxis *is* recommended for all children and adults with previous acute rheumatic fever or established rheumatic heart disease. Monthly intramuscular benzathine penicillin G is central to the management of children and adults with acute rheumatic fever and rheumatic heart disease (see Table 36-4).

During outbreaks of acute post-streptococcal glomerulonephritis secondary to Group A *Streptococcus* pyoderma, community-based treatment of infected individuals and their contacts with benzathine penicillin G appears to decrease the transmission of acute post-streptococcal glomerulonephritis-producing Group A *Streptococcus* strains. In addition to treating infected individuals, reducing the transmission of Group A *Streptococcus* pyoderma in resource-limited settings is likely to require skin hygiene measures, including the control of scabies.

After a century of research, the development of a vaccine against Group A *Streptococcus* disease is at last showing promise. The most advanced of the current candidates is a multivalent vaccine including 26 of the most common Group A *Streptococcus emm* types encountered in North America and Europe. Unfortunately, there is a limited match of these strains with prevalent *emm* types in Africa and the Pacific, where *emm* types are more variable [25]. Other candidate vaccines, containing antigens conserved among most, or all, Group A *Streptococcus* strains, are approaching clinical trials.

REFERENCES

1. Katz AR, Morens DM. Severe streptococcal infections in historical perspective. Clin Infect Dis 1992;14:298–307.
2. Ellis H. The last year before the dawn of antibiotics. Br J Hosp Med (Lond) 2009;70:475.
3. Carapetis JR, Steer AC, Mulholland EK, Weber M. The global burden of group A streptococcal diseases. Lancet Infect Dis 2005;5:685–94.
4. Stevens DL, Tanner MH, Winship J, et al. Severe group A streptococcal infections associated with a toxic shock-like syndrome and scarlet fever toxin A. New Engl J Med 1989;321:1–7.
5. Steer AC, Carapetis JR. Prevention and treatment of rheumatic heart disease in the developing world. Nat Rev Cardiol 2009;6:689–98.
6. Bessen DE. Population biology of the human restricted pathogen, *Streptococcus pyogenes*. Infect Genet Evol 2009;9:581–93.
7. Fraser JD, Proft T. The bacterial superantigen and superantigen-like proteins. Immunological Rev 2008;225:226–43.
8. WGoSS I. Defining the group A streptococcal toxic shock syndrome. Rationale and consensus definition. The Working Group on Severe Streptococcal Infections. JAMA 1993;269:390–1.
9. Barnham M, Weightman N, Anderson A, et al. Review of 17 cases of pneumonia caused by *Streptococcus pyogenes*. Eur J Clin Microbiol Infect Dis 1999;18:506–9.
10. Mathur P, Arora NK, Kapil A, Das BK. *Streptococcus pyogenes* meningitis. Ind J Pediatr 2004;71:423–6.
11. Bacterial etiology of serious infections in young infants in developing countries: results of a multicenter study. The WHO Young Infants Study Group. Pediatr Infect Dis J 1999;18(suppl. 10):S17–S22.
12. Chuang I, Van Beneden C, Beall B, Schuchat A. Population-based surveillance for postpartum invasive group a streptococcus infections, 1995–2000. Clin Infect Dis 2002;35:665–70.
13. Special Writing Group of the Committee on Rheumatic Fever E, and Kawasaki Disease of the Council on Cardiovascular Disease in the Young of the American Heart Association. Guidelines for the diagnosis of rheumatic fever. Jones Criteria, 1992 update. JAMA 1992;268:2069–73.
14. Kurlan R, Johnson D, Kaplan EL. Streptococcal infection and exacerbations of childhood tics and obsessive-compulsive symptoms: a prospective blinded cohort study. Pediatrics 2008;121:1188–97.
15. De Cunto CL, Giannini EH, Fink CW, et al. Prognosis of children with post-streptococcal reactive arthritis. Pediatr Infect Dis J 1988;7:683–6.
16. Shulman ST, Ayoub EM. Poststreptococcal reactive arthritis. Curr Opin Rheumatol 2002;14:562–5.
17. Stevens DL, Bisno AL, Chambers HF, et al. Practice guidelines for the diagnosis and management of skin and soft-tissue infections. Clin Infect Dis 2005; 41:1373–406.
18. National Heart Foundation of Australia (RF/RHD guideline development working group) and the Cardiac Society of Australia and New Zealand. Diagnosis and management of acute rheumatic fever and rheumatic heart disease in Australia—an evidence-based review; 2006.
19. Stevens DL, Gibbons AE, Bergstrom R, Winn V. The Eagle effect revisited: efficacy of clindamycin, erythromycin, and penicillin in the treatment of streptococcal myositis. J Infect Dis 1988;158:23–8.
20. Del Mar CB, Glasziou PP, Spinks AB. Antibiotics for sore throat. Cochrane Database Syst Rev; 2006:CD000023.
21. Lennon DR, Farrell E, Martin DR, Stewart JM. Once-daily amoxicillin versus twice-daily penicillin V in group A beta-haemolytic streptococcal pharyngitis. Archives of disease in childhood. 2008;93:474–8.
22. Norrby-Teglund A, Muller MP, McGeer A, et al. Successful management of severe group A streptococcal soft tissue infections using an aggressive medical regimen including intravenous polyspecific immunoglobulin together with a conservative surgical approach. Scand J Infect Dis 2005;37:166–72.
23. Darenberg J, Ihendyane N, Sjolin J, et al. Intravenous immunoglobulin G therapy in streptococcal toxic shock syndrome: a European randomized, double-blind, placebo-controlled trial. Clin Infect Dis 2003;37:333–40.
24. Smith A, Lamagni TL, Oliver I, et al. Invasive group A streptococcal disease: should close contacts routinely receive antibiotic prophylaxis? Lancet Infect Dis 2005;5:494–500.
25. Steer AC, Law I, Matatolu L, et al. Global emm type distribution of group A streptococci: systematic review and implications for vaccine development. Lancet Infect Dis 2009;9:611–16.
26. World Health Organization. Rheumatic Fever and Rheumatic Heart Disease: Report of a WHO Expert Consultation. Report No. 923. Geneva: World Health Organization; 2004.

37 Diphtheria

Tejpratap SP Tiwari

Key features

- Diphtheria is a vaccine-preventable bacterial communicable disease caused by toxin-producing strains of *Corynebacterium diphtheriae*
- Transmission is person-to-person via respiratory droplets from the throat through coughing or sneezing, or by close contact with a skin lesion
- The incubation period is usually 1–5 days
- The disease is characterized by the presence of a tough pseudomembrane over the mucous membrane of the upper respiratory tract (nose, uvula, tonsils, pharynx, and larynx) or in skin ulcers in cutaneous diphtheria
- Symptoms and manifestations range from a moderately sore throat, to difficulty in swallowing and mild fever, to life-threatening airway obstruction, to toxin-related systemic complications, for example myocarditis and polyneuropathy (cranial and peripheral nerves)
- Early diagnosis and treatment with diphtheria antitoxin and antibiotics (penicillin, erythromycin) prevent complications and death
- Fatality rate ranges between 5 and 10 percent, even if properly treated, and can exceed 50% among untreated patients
- Diphtheria is preventable by vaccination and diphtheria-pertussis-tetanus (DPT) vaccines are recommended for all children, with booster vaccinations being administered to older children and adults

INTRODUCTION

Diphtheria is an acute infectious disease that is caused by toxin-producing strains of *Corynebacterium diphtheriae,* a Gram-positve rod [1]. Two other zoonotic corynebacterial species, *Corynebacterium ulcerans* and *Corynebacterium pseudotuberculosis,* can also produce diphtheria toxin. Human infections by toxigenic *C. ulcerans* can lead to clinical disease indistinguishable from that caused by *C. diphtheriae.* Infections with *C. pseudotuberculosis* can cause caseous lymphadenitis in humans. Although diphtheria is an ancient communicable disease, its etiology was not discovered until the late 19th century (Box 37.1). Throughout history, and well into the first half of the 20th century, diphtheria was a fearful scourge and a major cause of death in children. From the late 1940s, widespread and routine use of diphtheria toxoid vaccine as a preventive tool led to a dramatic decline in reported diphtheria worldwide (Fig. 37.1). Diphtheria is now virtually eliminated from industrialized countries as a result of sustained, high childhood vaccination coverage rates. However, the disease remains endemic in countries with sub-optimal childhood vaccination coverage rates and poses a threat for importation into countries with good childhood programs but low booster immunization rates, or with significant clusters of susceptible populations [2].

EPIDEMIOLOGY

Humans are the only known natural reservoir of *C. diphtheriae,* although the organism has been isolated from animals, including horses. The organisms may survive for weeks on environmental surfaces, dust and fomites. In countries with a temperate climate, respiratory disease predominates, with a peak incidence during the autumn/winter season. Transmission of *C. diphtheriae* occurs among close and susceptible contacts, and generally occurs through inhalation of respiratory droplets or through direct contact with respiratory secretions, infected skin lesions or fomites. While the majority of nasopharyngeal infections do not result in disease, transient carriage may occur and persist for several weeks, particularly in immunized persons. Asymptomatic carriers play an important role in maintaining transmission in the population. Patients with untreated clinical respiratory disease usually remain infectious for two weeks or less, but chronic carriage may occasionally occur after recovery. Individuals with symptomatic illness become non-infectious approximately two days after initiating effective antibiotic treatment; persistent carriage rarely occurs following completion of appropriate antibiotic therapy. In tropical countries, cutaneous disease is more common and serves as an important reservoir for maintaining transmission. However, in industrialized countries, including the USA, small clusters of cutaneous disease have occurred among homeless individuals and alcoholic adults.

In the pre-vaccine era, diphtheria was a major cause of childhood morbidity and mortality. Following widespread improvements in vaccine coverage in most industrialized countries, disease caused by toxigenic *C. diphtheriae* has been virtually eliminated. In the USA, reported cases declined dramatically from 147,991 in 1920, to 18,675 in 1945. Following the introduction of universal vaccination recommendations in the mid-1940s and improving vaccine coverage, reported cases (irrespective of infection site) dropped precipitously to 59 in 1979. From 1980–2003, 55 cases of respiratory diphtheria were reported and, since 2003, no indigenous case has been reported in the USA. Although diphtheria has become rare in the USA and other developed countries, a large epidemic of diphtheria occurred in the newly independent states of the former Union of Soviet Socialist Republics (USSR) with more than 157,000 cases and 5000 deaths reported between 1989 and 1998. The major factors that contributed to the propagation of the outbreak included a decline in vaccination coverage among children, a mobile population, delayed recognition and response, and poor health infrastructure. The outbreak was controlled by campaigns of mass immunization with diphtheria toxoid to the entire population. Similarly, in developing countries, reported cases have dramatically declined since 1980 following the implementation of the World Health Organization (WHO) Expanded Program for Immunization. However, significant disparities exist among countries, with some countries achieving control of diphtheria similar to industrialized countries and others having endemic disease and periodic outbreaks. Vaccine-induced immunity to diphtheria wanes over time and, in the absence of booster immunizations, the number of susceptible persons in the population increases. Serologic surveys among adults in industrialized countries indicate that 20–60% have diphtheria antibody levels below minimal protective levels. A level of 0.01 IU/mL from an *in vitro* neutralization assay is considered the lower limit of protection. When a critical proportion of the population becomes susceptible, there exists the danger of re-introduction or re-emergence of diphtheria and outbreaks [3].

BOX 37.1 Historical timeline

- Hippocrates provided the earliest historical description in the 5th century BC but *Corynebacterium* species were recovered from a mummified Egyptian woman buried about 3500 years ago.
- Pierre Bretonneau provided the first clear description of the disease in 1826, pioneered tracheostomy as treatment and gave the disease its name.
- *Corynebacterium diphtheria*, the etiologic agent, was identified in 1883 by Edwin Klebs in smears from diphtheritic membranes, and isolated from culture by Frederick Loeffler in 1884.
- In 1888, Roux and Yersin demonstrated that the sterile filtrate from cultured bacteria contained a heat-labile toxin and that diphtheria toxin that was capable of producing identical diphtheria lesions.
- On Christmas Eve of 1891, Emil Adolf Behring demonstrated the protective value of diphtheria antitoxin in a severely ill boy with diphtheria.
- In 1901, Behring received the Nobel Prize for work on the use of diphtheria immune serum (diphtheria antitoxin). Over 100 years later, equine diphtheria antitoxin continues to be the hallmark of treatment for this once dreaded disease.
- In 1923, Ramon demonstrated the immunizing property of diphtheria toxin inactivated by heat and formalin to protect against disease and paved the way for the use of diphtheria toxoid (formalin-inactivated diphtheria toxin) as a vaccine.

NATURAL HISTORY, PATHOGENESIS AND PATHOLOGY

Corynebacterium diphtheriae is a Gram-positive, slender, nonmotile, nonsporulating rod. Based on colony morphology and biochemical characteristics, four biotypes of *C. diphtheriae* (gravis, mitis, intermedius and belfanti) are recognized. Some strains produce a powerful diphtheria exotoxin. Before *C. diphtheriae* becomes toxigenic, it must be lysogenized by a specific bacteriophage. The corynebacteriophage carries the structural gene for the toxin (*tox*). Toxin-producing strains of all biotypes produce an identical diphtheria exotoxin [1]. No consistent difference in pathogenicity or severity of disease has been demonstrated among the biotypes. Toxigenic strains of *C. diphtheriae* are not invasive but cause localized toxin-mediated disease in susceptible persons by colonizing the mucosa of the upper respiratory tract, or skin wounds and ulcers. Rarely, other mucosal sites, for example conjunctiva, ear and vagina may be infected. After inhalation, the organisms proliferate at the colonized site and induce an inflammatory reaction in the mucosa of the nasopharynx, oropharynx, larynx or trachea. Inflammation is characterized by marked neutrophilic infiltration, vascular congestion, and interstitial edema. Lysogenized organisms produce diphtheria toxin that inhibits intracellular protein synthesis and causes local epithelial necrosis with thick fibrinosuppurative exudation. Necrotic debris, exudate, white and red blood cells, fibrin and bacteria coagulate to form a dirty gray and adherent pseudomembrane over the mucosa. Expansion of the pseudomembrane may lead to life-threatening respiratory tract obstruction. Attempts to remove the pseudomembrane usually result in bleeding at the site. With treatment or control of infection, the membrane may slough off from its vascular mucosal bed and result in bleeding and asphyxiation, or it may be coughed up. Diphtheria toxin may be absorbed from the site of infection into the bloodstream and transported to distant sites. Systemic absorption increases with expansion of the local inflammatory site and enlargement of pseudomembrane. In the absence of circulating neutralizing antibodies to diphtheria toxin, extensive toxin-mediated end-organ damage may occur, particularly in the heart and peripheral neural tissue. Myocardial damage manifests as myocarditis that is characterized by edema, mononuclear cell infiltration and fatty changes, and focal necrosis in the myocardium and its conducting system. Polyneuropathy results from degeneration of the myelin sheath and axis cylinder of the cranial or peripheral nerves. Occasionally, in the kidneys, acute tubular necrosis may lead to renal failure [4, 5].

Infection by nontoxigenic *C. diphtheriae* may be associated with sore throat without pseudomembrane formation, but with invasive disease. Bacteremia, endocarditis, aneurysms, osteomyelitis and septic arthritis have been reported among clusters of drug addicts, alcoholics, homeless individuals and Australian aboriginals.

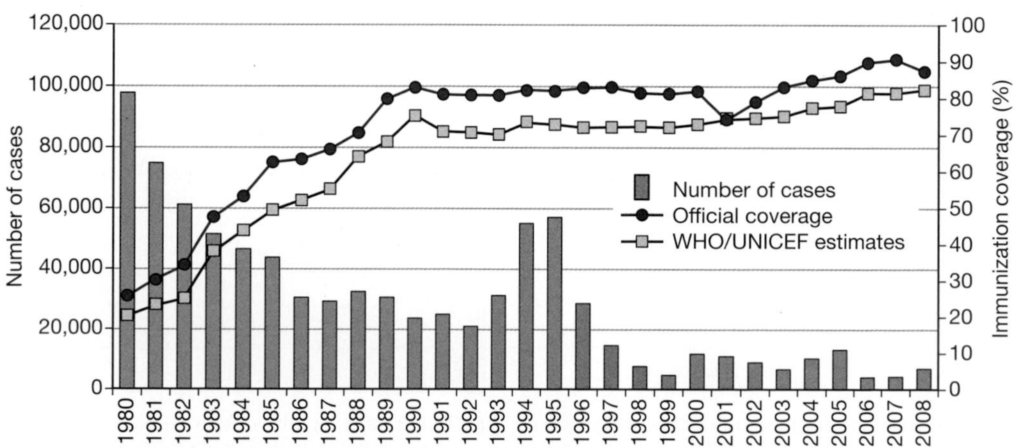

FIGURE 37.1 Diphtheria global reported incidence and DTP3 coverage, 1980–2008.

CLINICAL FEATURES

Infection usually results from exposure to respiratory secretions from cases or carriers, or exudates from cutaneous lesions. The incubation period is usually from 1–5 days, but occasionally can be longer. The frequency and severity of clinical symptoms and signs depend on the site of infection, size of the pseudomembrane and the patient's immunization history. However, regardless of the site of infection, systemic manifestations are similar and consequent to absorption of diphtheria toxin from these sites. The disease is usually localized to mucous membrane in the upper respiratory tract, the skin, or both. Symptoms and signs can develop at multiple sites in the upper respiratory tract, including the nose, pharynx, tonsils and larynx [5]. The characteristic feature of diphtheria is the formation of a tough, dirty-gray, leather-like pseudomembrane at the site of infection.

The most common site for respiratory diphtheria is the faucial area including the posterior pharynx, soft palate, periglottal area, uvula and tonsillar mucosa (Fig. 37.2). The onset is usually insidious and patients usually present with a low-grade fever (<103 °F), sore throat, pain on swallowing, hoarseness of voice, pharyngeal injection, nasal discharge, cough, malaise and prostration [5, 6]. The pulse is usually more rapid than the fever would justify. On initial examination, the pharynx is injected, but patches of exudates may appear a day after illness onset. These patches may expand and coalesce to form a white-to-dirty-gray, tenacious membrane over one or both tonsils, the nasopharynx, uvula and soft palate, and can extend downward into the larynx and trachea. The edge of the membrane is surrounded by a narrow zone of erythema and a broader zone of mucosal edema. Cervical lymph nodes are usually tender and enlarged and, along with cervical soft tissue edema, gives rise to the so-called bull-neck appearance and may cause respiratory stridor. Extension of the pseudomembrane from the pharynx to the larynx can result in life-threatening airway obstruction.

The laryngeal or tracheobronchial mucosa may be the primary site of infection in 5% of patients. However, tonsillopharyngeal membrane may extend downward into the larynx in about 10% of patients. Laryngeal diphtheria typically presents with hoarseness and stridor, dyspnea and a brassy cough. Edema and membrane formation involving the larynx, or trachea and bronchi may narrow the lumen of the airways, particularly in infants and young children, and progress to dyspnea, exhaustion and death.

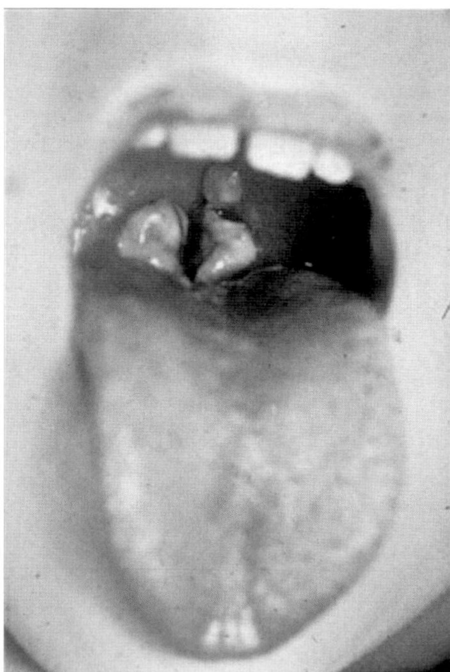

FIGURE 37.2 Faucial diphtheria showing gray pseudomembrane over tonsils and pharynx *(photo courtesy of the Public Health Image Library, Centers for Disease Control and Prevention, Atlanta, GA, USA).*

Nasal diphtheria is more frequent among infants and young children who usually present with a profuse mucoid, serosanguineous, or mucopurulent nasal discharge that can cause an erosive reaction on the external nares and upper lip. A dirty-white membrane is usually present on the nasal septum. The symptoms are generally mild and manifestations of systemic toxicity are rare.

Cutaneous diphtheria is usually more common in warm, tropical climates and is normally associated with colonization of pre-existing skin lesions, such as surgical wounds, pyoderma, eczema, burns, impetigo, psoriasis and insect bites. Co-infection with *Staphylococcus aureus* and group A *Streptococcus pyogenes* is typical. Outbreaks of cutaneous diphtheria have occurred among impoverished or indigent populations, homeless individuals and alcoholics, and in environments with overcrowding and unhygienic living arrangements. The disease classically presents as single or multiple punched-out ulcers with rolled-out margins and a dirty gray or black adherent pseudomembrane over the base. Common sites for cutaneous lesions include the lower legs (Fig. 37.3), feet and hands. Lesions from which *C. diphtheriae* are isolated are indolent, nonprogressive, superficial and indistinguishable from those caused by other bacteria. Although systemic complications rarely occur from local absorption of toxin in cutaneous diphtheria, sufficient toxin may be absorbed to act as a natural immunizing event to induce production of high antitoxin levels and protective immunity. If untreated, cutaneous diphtheria may persist for months. Shedding of *C. diphtheria* from skin lesions occurs over a longer time period than from respiratory tract colonization, and exudates from cutaneous diphtheria can contaminate the environment and may be an important and efficient means of person-to-person spread in tropical countries [7].

Rarely, the primary site of infection may be the mucous membranes at other localized sites, such as the conjunctiva, external auditory canal and vulva [5]. A local ulcer with exudate or pseudomembrane may be present and, in the ear, diphtheria may manifest as a chronic purulent discharge. However, lesions are self-limiting and rarely associated with systemic toxicity.

Complications frequently result from systemic absorption of diphtheria toxin, particularly in the heart, nerves and kidneys. Cardiac manifestations generally occur during the second week, but may occasionally be present from the first week or manifest as late as the sixth week of illness. The risk of myocarditis directly correlates with the duration, extent and severity of disease, and delay in initiating treatment with diphtheria antitoxin [5]. Diphtheritic myocarditis can

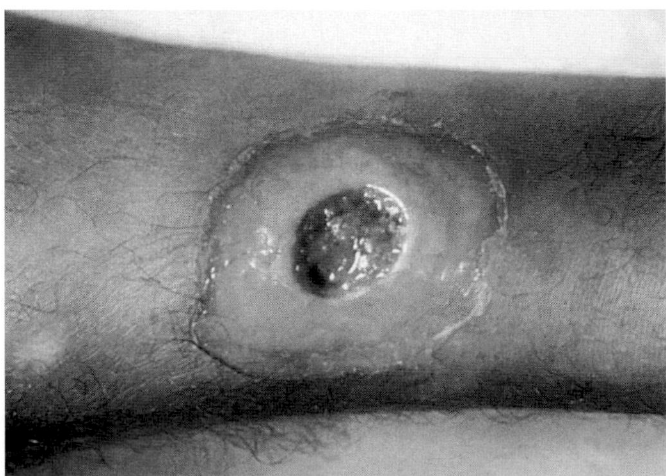

FIGURE 37.3 A diphtheria skin lesion on the leg *(photo courtesy of the Public Health Image Library, Centers for Disease Control and Prevention, Atlanta, GA, USA).*

present as a wide variety of abnormalities that includes dyspnea, angina, syncope, diminished heart sounds, new or altered murmurs, conductive disturbance arrhythmias, ectopic beats, a gallop rhythm, cardiac enlargement, low cardiac output or hypotension. Although up to 65% of patients have electrocardiographic (ECG) evidence of myocarditis after 1–2 weeks from onset, most are asymptomatic. Clinically significant myocarditis develops in 7–20% of patients with respiratory diphtheria compared with 0–5% with cutaneous diphtheria. Abnormalities in ECG pattern, particularly ST-T wave changes and first-degree heart block, can progress to more severe forms of block, atrioventricular dissociation and other arrhythmias that carry a poor prognosis. Patients with ECG findings that do not exceed ectopic supraventricular beat, sinus bradycardia, prolonged P-R interval and minor T-wave changes generally do well and are associated with little, if any, increased risk of death. Patients with single bundle branch blocks, QRS widening, ST-T segment shifts, T wave inversions, prolonged QT wave intervals or supraventricular tachycardias are associated with a 10–50% mortality. The fatality rate exceeds 90% in patients with third-degree block, more than two ventricular premature contractions, ventricular tachycardia and congestive cardiac failure. Cardiac pacing appears to be of little value in patients with third-degree block. These patients have severe cardiac injury and die from congestive cardiac failure or ventricular tachycardia. Death from myocarditis occurs within two weeks of illness onset. Abatement of ECG abnormalities reflects improving cardiac function and favors survival. Elevations of serum creatine kinase and serum aspartate aminotransaminase/serum glutamic oxaloacetic transaminase (AST/SGOT) concentration closely parallel the intensity of myocarditis and so may be used to monitor its course. Detectable cardiac injury may completely resolve over months, or even years, but some survivors are left with persistent conduction defects requiring long-term follow-up [8].

Approximately two-thirds of individuals with severe diphtheria develop neuropathy. Affected patients develop palatine and posterior pharyngeal wall paralysis and cranial neuropathies involving muscles of the eye, face, pharynx and larynx, causing dysphagia and predisposing these patients to nasal regurgitation and aspiration. The ocular manifestations of diphtheria include blurred vision and failure of accommodation. Later, several weeks after the sore throat, a peripheral motor demyelinating neuritis can occur, beginning in the proximal muscle groups in the extremities and progressing distally. In the lower extremity, the dorsiflexors of the feet may be particularly affected. Occasionally, motor nerves of the trunk, neck and upper extremity are involved (as are sensory nerves) resulting in a glove-and-stocking neuropathy. Generally, there is slow but total resolution of the limb weakness [9, 10].

Less commonly, renal failure and pneumonia may occur in severe cases. Rare instances of encephalitis and cerebral infarction have been documented. Case fatality rates have remained stable at ~10% in developed countries over the past five decades and are highest in the very young and very old; fatal outcomes are rare in fully vaccinated persons [11].

PATIENT EVALUATION, DIAGNOSIS AND DIFFERENTIAL DIAGNOSIS

Respiratory diphtheria should be suspected in the presence of a gray pseudomembrane in a patient with sore throat, mild fever, cervical lymphadenopathy, neck swelling, hoarseness of voice and signs of systemic toxicity. The diagnosis is confirmed by culturing toxigenic *C. diphtheriae* from swabs taken from the throat, respiratory tract or membrane [12, 13]. Throat swab specimens should be taken before administration of antibiotics to increase the chance of a positive culture and immediately transported to the laboratory. If clinical specimens cannot be immediately transported, they should be sent in a transport medium or, if a long delay is anticipated, in silica gel. Specimen culture optimally requires the use of a tellurite-containing medium. Identification of *C. diphtheriae* and its biotypes is made from colony morphology (black colonies with a surrounding halo) and from biochemical tests. Toxigenicity of *C. diphtheriae* can be determined by *in vivo* (guinea pig) or *in vitro* (Elek) testing. PCR tests for gene coding for the A and B fragments of the exotoxin can confirm the presence of toxigenic organisms, but not toxin. PCR testing is sensitive and rapid and is most useful in specimens taken from patients who received antibiotics. However, it is currently only available at some reference laboratories. Molecular subtyping of *C. diphtheriae* strains shows considerable promise in aiding epidemiologic investigations and is available at some reference laboratories [13].

The differential diagnosis includes streptococcal or viral tonsillopharyngitis, infectious mononucleosis, Vincent's angina, herpetic tonsillitis, thrush and acute epiglottitis.

TREATMENT

The hallmark of treatment of respiratory diphtheria is prompt administration of diphtheria antitoxin to neutralize free circulating diphtheria toxin; diphtheria antitoxin cannot neutralize cell-bound toxin. The antitoxin, an equine antiserum, is critical in the management of respiratory diphtheria and is effective in reducing the extent and severity of local disease, as well as the risk of systemic complications, such as myocarditis and polyneuropathy. As the patient's condition may deteriorate rapidly, a single dose of diphtheria antitoxin should be promptly administered if diphtheria is strongly suspected, without awaiting laboratory confirmation of the clinical diagnosis [12]. Early institution of antitoxin therapy is associated with a significant reduction in mortality risk. As diphtheria antitoxin is an equine product, skin testing should be performed prior to administration to rule out immediate-type hypersensitivity. Patients who exhibit hypersensitivity require desensitization before a full therapeutic dose of antitoxin is administered. Irrespective of the patient's age, the Centers for Disease Control and Prevention (CDC) recommend intravenous administration of 20,000–40,000 units of diphtheria antitoxin for pharyngeal or laryngeal disease of less than 2 days' duration, 40,000–60,000 units for cases with nasopharyngeal pseudomembrane formation, and 80,000–100,000 units for disease with duration of 3 days or more or extensive disease with neck swelling. A repeat dose is of no benefit and may increase the risk of anaphylaxis to horse serum protein. In the USA, diphtheria antitoxin is no longer manufactured or licensed for use. However, it is available from CDC under a Food and Drug Administration (FDA)-approved investigational new drug protocol. Physicians in the USA may obtain diphtheria antitoxin by calling the Emergency Operations Center of the Centers for Disease Control and Prevention at 770-488-7100; additional information may be obtained from the CDC website http://www.cdc.gov/vaccines/vpd-vac/diphtheria/dat/dat-main.htm. Diphtheria antitoxin may be produced and available locally outside the USA.

The administration of recommended antibiotic therapy serves to eliminate the organism, thereby stopping toxin production, improving local symptoms and signs of infection, and preventing spread of the organisms to susceptible contacts. Patients should be maintained in strict droplet isolation throughout therapy. Respiratory diphtheria should be treated with penicillin or erythromycin – the antibiotics of choice [12, 14, 15]. Both drugs are equally effective in resolving local symptoms and disappearance of the pseudomembrane. Procaine penicillin G is given at a dosage of 600,000 units (for children, 12,500–25,000 IU/kg) intramuscularly (IM) every 12 h until the patient can swallow comfortably, after which oral penicillin V is given at 125–250 mg four times daily to complete a 14-day course. Alternatively, erythromycin is given at a dosage of 500 mg IV every 6 h (for children, 40–50 mg/kg per day IV in two or four divided doses) until the patient can swallow comfortably, after which 500 mg is given PO four times daily to complete a 14-day course. A single, IM dose of benzathine penicillin G (600,000–1,200,000 units) may be considered when compliance with oral therapy is uncertain. Erythromycin is marginally superior to penicillin in eradicating the carrier state and may be preferred for initial treatment; however, there is increased risk of gastrointestinal irritation and intolerance when given orally and thrombophlebitis when administered intravenously. Alternative agents for patients who are allergic to penicillin or cannot take erythromycin include rifampin and clindamycin. Cutaneous diphtheria should be treated with antibiotics as described for respiratory disease, but patients seldom require antitoxin. It is important to treat the underlying cause of the dermatoses in addition to the co-infection with *C. diphtheriae*.

Following therapy, eradication of *C. diphtheriae* should be documented by two consecutive negative cultures at 24-hour intervals and taken at least 1 day after antimicrobial therapy is complete. A repeat throat culture two weeks later is recommended. For patients in whom the organism is not eradicated after a 14-day course of erythromycin or penicillin, an additional 10-day course followed by repeat culture is recommended. Treatment of acute diphtheria with prednisone is of limited, or no, value and does not reduce the incidence of myocarditis or polyneuropathy [12].

Supportive care is very important. Patients in whom diphtheria is confirmed should be hospitalized in respiratory-droplet isolation rooms. Bed rest is recommended during the acute phase of illness (the first 2–3 weeks from onset of illness), but proof of its benefit once the patient feels able to ambulate is lacking. Early in the disease, cardiac and respiratory complications can occur. ECG abnormalities secondary to myocarditis can occur within three days from onset of disease and progress to cardiogenic shock within a week. As significant ECG abnormalities may develop in patients without clinical evidence of myocarditis, it is important to routinely monitor their cardiograms. Cardiac complications can be detected and minimized by close ECG monitoring and initiation of indicated supportive care, including inotropy, after-load reduction and pacing. From a prognostic standpoint, patients with ECG changes of myocarditis have a mortality rate 3–4 times higher than those with normal tracings. Airway obstruction can result from aspiration of dislodged pharyngeal membrane, its direct extension into the larynx or from external compression by enlarged nodes and edema. Consultation with an anesthesiologist or an ear, nose and throat specialist is recommended because of the possibility that tracheostomy or intubation will be required to access and remove tracheobronchial membranes and to eliminate the risk of sudden asphyxia. Patients should also be monitored for development of primary or secondary pneumonia. While awaiting return of neurologic function in patients with neuropathies, physical therapy is indicated to maintain range of motion in paretic extremities. In addition, nasogastric tube-feeding may be required in patients who have palatine or pharyngeal paralysis to prevent aspiration. Protective or long-term immunity may not occur in cases of diphtheria – diphtheria toxoid is administered during the convalescent phase to boost immunity and prevent recurrence [11, 12, 14, 15].

PREVENTION

Immunization with diphtheria toxoid is the most effective means of primary prevention. Diphtheria toxoid is available in combination with tetanus toxoid (DT) and whole-cell pertussis (DTwP) or acellular pertussis antigens (DTaP) for use in children <7 years of age; the antigenic content of diphtheria toxoid in these preparations ranges from 6.7–15 limit of flocculation (Lf) units. Because the frequency and severity of local reactions from diphtheria toxoid increases with age, a combination vaccine (Td or Tdap) with lower antigenic content (≤2 Lf units) is used in children ≥7 years or older and adults. In the USA, the Advisory Committee on Immunization Practices recommends that three doses of diphtheria toxoid-containing vaccine (DTaP, DTwP or DT) be given to children at 4- to 8-week intervals beginning at 2 months of age, a fourth dose at 15–18 months, and a preschool booster dose at 4–6 years of age. An adolescent booster with tetanus toxoid and a reduced diphtheria toxoid and acellular pertussis antigens (Tdap) is recommended at 11–12 years of age, followed thereafter by a decennial Td booster dose. For added protection against pertussis in adults, a Td booster dose may be substituted with Tdap if they have not previously received a Tdap dose. For persons in whom pertussis vaccine is contraindicated, DT and Td should be used instead of DTaP/DTwP and Tdap respectively. Unvaccinated individuals who are ≥7 years of age should receive a three-dose primary series with Td with the first two doses given at 4–8-week intervals and the third dose 6–12 months later. Booster doses are recommended at 10-year intervals [15, 16].

The childhood vaccination schedule varies in developing countries. The WHO's Expanded Program on Immunization recommends a three-dose primary immunization series with combined diphtheria and tetanus toxoids and pertussis vaccines (DTwP) starting at six weeks of age and administered at least four weeks apart. Some countries recommend one or two additional booster doses to be given at 12 months of age and at school entry. The vaccination strategy for decennial booster doses varies by country and depends on vaccine resources, the capacity of immunization services and the epidemiologic pattern of diphtheria. While some developed countries routinely offer an adolescent dose, most countries do not recommend an adult booster dose [17].

REFERENCES

1. Funke F, von Graevenitz A, Clarridge JE, Bernard KA. Clinical microbiology of coryneform bacteria. Clin Microbiol Rev 1997;10:125–59.
2. World Health Organization. WHO vaccine preventable diseases monitoring system: 2009 global summary. Geneva: World Health Organization; 2009. Available at: http://www.who.int/immunization/documents/WHO_IVB_2009/en/index.html.
3. Galazka AM. The changing epidemiology of diphtheria in the vaccine era. J Infect Dis 2000;181(suppl. 1):S2–9.
4. Hadfield TL, McEvoy P, Polotsky Y, et al. The pathology of diphtheria. J Infect Dis 2000;181(suppl. 1):S116–20.
5. Naiditch MJ, Bower AG. Diphtheria: a study of 1,433 cases observed during a ten-year period at the Los Angeles County Hospital. Am J Med 1954;17: 229–45.
6. Dobie RA, Tobey DN. Clinical features of diphtheria in the respiratory tract. JAMA 1979;242:2197–201.
7. Belsey MA, Sinclair M, Roder MR, LeBlanc DR. *Corynebacterium diphtheriae* skin infections in Alabama and Louisiana. A factor in the epidemiology of diphtheria. N Engl J Med 1969;280:135–41.
8. Celik T, Selimov N, Vekilova A, et al. Prognostic significance of electrocardiographic abnormalities in diphtheritic myocarditis after hospital discharge: A long-term follow-up study. Ann Noninvasive Electrocardiol 2006;11:28–33.
9. Logina I, Donaghy M. Diphtheritic polyneuropathy: a clinical study and comparison with Guillain-Barre syndrome. J Neurol Neurosurg Psychiatry 1999;67:433–8.
10. Piradov MA, Pirogov VN, et al. Diphtheritic polyneuropathy – Clinical analysis of severe forms. Arch Neurol 2001;58:1438–42.
11. Wharton M, Vitek CR. Diphtheria Toxoid. In: Plotkin SA, Orenstein WA, eds. Vaccines, 4th edn. Philadelphia: W.B. Saunders; 2004:211–28.
12. Farizo KM, Strebel PM, Chen RT, et al. Fatal respiratory disease due to *Corynebacterium diphtheriae*: case report and review of guidelines for management, investigation, and control. Clin Infect Dis 1993;16:59–68.
13. Efstratiou A, Engler KH, Mazurova IK, et al. Current approaches to the laboratory diagnosis of diphtheria. J Infect Dis 2000;181(suppl. 1):S138–45.
14. Begg N. Diphtheria: manual for the management and control of diphtheria in the European Region. Copenhagen: World Health Organization; 1994: WHO ICP/EPI 038 (B).
15. American Academy of Pediatrics. Diphtheria. In: Pickering LK, Baker CJ, Long SS, McMillan JA, eds. Red Book: 2009 Report of the Committee on Infectious Diseases, 28th edn. Elk Grove Village: American Academy of Pediatrics; 2009: 280–3.
16. Centers for Disease Control. Preventing tetanus, diphtheria, and pertussis among adolescents: use of tetanus toxoid, reduced diphtheria toxoid and acellular pertussis vaccines: recommendations of the Advisory Committee on Immunization Practices (ACIP). MMWR 2006;55(RR-3):1–50.
17. World Health Organization. Diphtheria vaccine: WHO position paper. Wkly Epidemiol Rec 2006;81:24–32.

SECTION

B

RESPIRATORY TRACT INFECTIONS

38 Bacterial Pneumonia

W Abdullah Brooks

Key features

- Pneumonia is the leading global cause of death among children younger than 5 years of age
- Bacterial causes of pneumonia include *Streptococcus pneumoniae*, *Haemophilus influenzae*, *Staphylococcus aureus*, mycoplasma, chlamydia and *Mycobacterium tuberculosis*, among others
- Pneumonia should be suspected in patients with tachypnea and cough
- Signs of severe pneumonia include grunting, lower chest wall in-drawing, central cyanosis, inability to drink or feed (or vomiting anything ingested), lethargy, obtundation and convulsions
- Children with pneumonia should be categorized as not severe, severe and very severe based on established criteria, and treatment targeted appropriately
- It is estimated that appropriate administration of currently available vaccines would decrease global mortality from pneumonia by 50%

INTRODUCTION

Pneumonia is a syndrome of inflammation, congestion and compromise of gas exchange in the lungs that disproportionately affects children, but affects all ages, and can lead to severe illness, hospitalization and death [1]. It is usually caused by infection, although it may be caused by non-infectious exposures and aspiration. Bacteria are among the leading infectious causes of pneumonia, with many being vaccine-preventable. Pneumonia is currently the leading cause of child death worldwide [2], excluding neonatal deaths, with most deaths occurring in low- and middle-income countries (see Fig. 38.1). Although pneumonia was once the leading cause of child death in children in high income countries [1], the introduction of vaccines and improvements in overall living standards have substantially reduced infection and mortality rates. Similar reductions are possible in the developing world, although important knowledge gaps remain for optimal disease control.

EPIDEMIOLOGY

A review of 28 longitudinal, community-based studies conducted between 1969 and 1999 estimated the median incidence of clinical pneumonia in the developing world to be 0.28 episodes per child-year (interquartile range of 0.21–0.71 episodes/child-year) [3]. This translates into 151.8 million cases of pneumonia per year from developing countries alone, of which, 13.1 million (8.7%) are of hospitalizable severity. An additional 4 million cases are estimated to arise in wealthier countries, for a total global burden of 156 million pneumonia cases per year. Over 97% of incident pneumonia cases among children occur among tropical and subtropical developing countries, and over 50% occur in India, China, Pakistan, Bangladesh, Indonesia and Nigeria. Across the six World Health Organization (WHO) regions (see Fig. 38.2), the average pneumonia incidence rates (in episodes/child-year) are: Southeast Asia (0.36), Africa (0.33), Eastern Mediterranean (0.28), Western Pacific (0.22), the Americas (0.10) and the European Regions (0.06). In terms of pneumonia mortality, over 70% of deaths from clinical pneumonia occur in developing countries, primarily in the tropical/subtropical belt [3], with two-thirds of pneumonia deaths occurring in 10 countries. Pneumonia mortality has been associated with a number of risk factors, but the strongest include malnutrition, low birth weight, absence of breastfeeding, lack of measles vaccination, indoor air pollution and over-crowding [1, 3].

THE BACTERIAL ETIOLOGY OF PNEUMONIA

There are several bacterial agents associated with pneumonia. The evidence for these has been reported by two classes of studies, each with important limitations. One type of study is the prospective observational study (in some cases, simply surveillance). These have been primarily hospital-based and have primarily relied on blood cultures for etiologic detection. One limitation is that blood culture is insensitive. Typically, microbiologic analysis of blood is less than 15% sensitive for establishing a causative agent during pneumonia [1]; this sensitivity falls further by pre-culture antibiotic exposure. Moreover, some pathogens are fastidious and do not grow well in standard media. Lung aspirates, though somewhat more sensitive, are considered too invasive for most investigations. Sputum is difficult to obtain from young children and its interpretation is controversial, while nasopharyngeal swabs and aspirates may demonstrate carriage, which is common in young children in developing countries, but does not necessarily confirm invasive disease. Thus, nearly all bacterial pneumonia pathogens are substantially under-estimated. Another limitation is that, as most of these studies were of hospitalized children, they were at the more severe spectrum of illness and may not be representative of most incident pneumonia cases. The second type of study is vaccine trials – often referred to as probe studies – where the attributable burden from a particular pathogen is estimated from the proportion of pneumonia prevented by a vaccine specific for that organism. An important caveat is that bacterial and viral pathogens have both been shown to interact [4], and pneumococcal vaccine, in particular, has been shown to reduce influenza-positive pneumonia [5], thus, not all pneumonia prevented by a vaccine may be caused by the specific pathogen targeted by the vaccine.

Nonetheless, both types of studies appear to support *Streptococcus pneumoniae* (pneumococcus) as being the main bacterial cause of childhood pneumonia (30–50%), with *Haemophilus influenzae* being the second most common (10–30%) [3]. These two agents account for approximately 50% of cases of children hospitalized with pneumonia in developing countries [1]. Other bacteria that have been reported in young children include *Staphylococcus aureus*, *Klebsiella pneumoniae* and non-typable *H. influenzae* (Papua New Guinea and The Gambia). Of note, although non-typhoidal *Salmonella* spp.

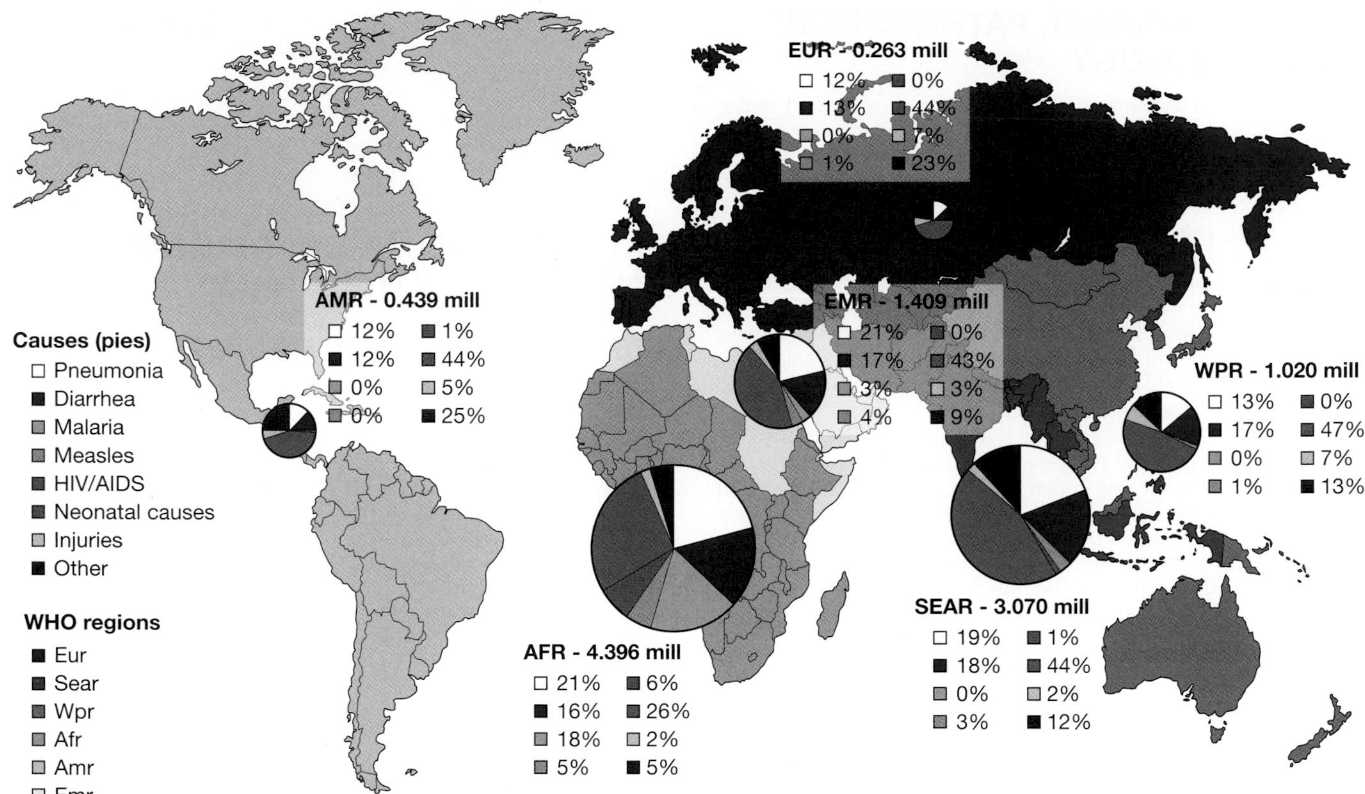

FIGURE 38.1 Global distribution of deaths from pneumonia and other causes among children <5 years old *(courtesy of Igor Rudan; redrawn with permission from Rudan I, Boschi-Pinto C, Biloglav Z, et al. Epidemiology and etiology of childhood pneumonia. Bull World Health Organ 2008;86:408–16.)*

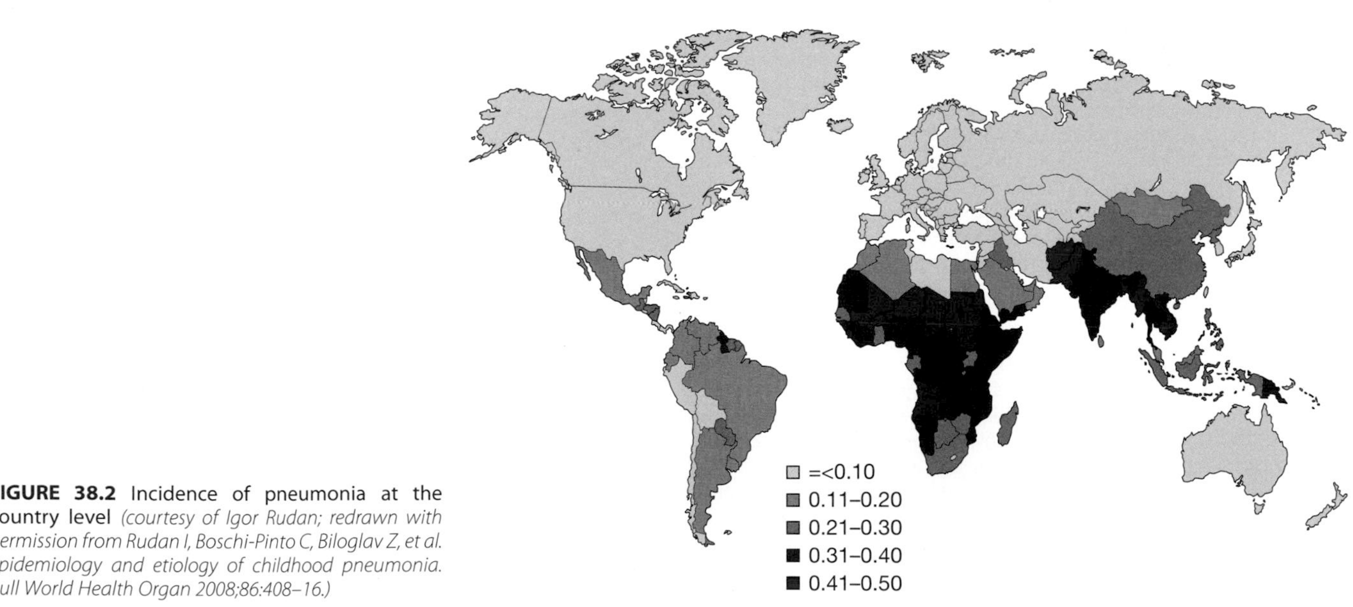

FIGURE 38.2 Incidence of pneumonia at the country level *(courtesy of Igor Rudan; redrawn with permission from Rudan I, Boschi-Pinto C, Biloglav Z, et al. Epidemiology and etiology of childhood pneumonia. Bull World Health Organ 2008;86:408–16.)*

(sub-Saharan Africa), and *Salmonella* Typhi (South Asia) have been isolated from the blood of children with pneumonia in Africa and Asia, this may represent co-infection, rather than imply causation. *Mycobacterium tuberculosis, Mycoplasma pneumoniae* and *Chlamydia* spp. have also been reported as causes of acute childhood pneumonia; however, there is little consensus regarding their relative importance to acute childhood pneumonia [3]. Viral etiologies are also common causes of acute childhood pneumonia and include influenza virus, respiratory syncytial virus, parainfluenza virus, metapneumonia virus, adenoviruses and others (discussed elsewhere), and bacterial supra-infection of lung tissue following viral infection is common, with *S. pneumoniae, S. aureus, Streptococcus* spp., and *H. influenzae* being the most commonly associated supra-infecting agents. The causes of acute bacterial pneumonia in children infected with HIV mirror those seen in HIV non-infected children, with *S. pneumoniae* and *H. influenzae* being the most commonly reported. Children co-infected with HIV are more likely to develop acute bacterial pneumonia than HIV non-infected children.

NATURAL HISTORY, PATHOGENESIS AND PATHOLOGY

Pathogen invasion and entry into the respiratory tract is poorly understood, although animal studies suggest that, at least in the case of pneumococcus, it is receptor mediated [6]. The syndrome of pneumonia, however, is one in which the alveoli and interstitium become inflamed, and fluid and cells fill the alveolar air sacs. Because liquids have surface tension, the fluid in the alveolar sacs draws the walls of the alveoli together, collapsing the alveoli. During inspiration, these alveolar air sacs are forcibly re-opened against this surface tension, giving rise to the crackling sound heard during inspiration by auscultation with a stethoscope. In turn, this surface tension creates lower airway obstruction. Normally, the alveolar air sac is only one cell layer thick, allowing for easy gas exchange. Transudate fluid and debris in the alveolar air sac compromises oxygenation (air entry into the lung) and respiration (gas exchange or the transfer of CO_2 in exchange for oxygen). The body's initial compensatory reaction is increased respiratory rate (tachypnea). This is, perhaps, the most sensitive indicator of lower airway obstruction [7]. As more alveoli become fluid filled, lower air obstruction becomes more severe and effort shifts to keeping the alveoli open. This is appreciated clinically by the use of accessory muscles – initially the intercostal muscles (intercostal retractions) – and, as obstruction progresses, the diaphragm contracts with greater force to overcome inertia, producing lower chest wall in-drawing (primarily noted in children less than three years old whose chest walls are relatively soft because of a greater cartilage/bone ratio). Other compensatory mechanisms at this stage include grunting, which is a sound produced by exhaling against a partially closed glottis or "laryngeal braking" [8]. This maintains positive pressure in the airway by retaining inspired air in the alveolar sac longer in order to prevent alveolar collapse [9]. This increases lung volume and functional residual capacity, the effect of which is to increase alveolar ventilation (the amount of air that reaches the alveoli such that oxygen can be exchanged for CO_2 per unit time), which results in a measurable increase in arterial oxygen tension (PaO_2) and a decrease in arterial carbon dioxide ($PaCO_2$). The respiratory muscles in a young child, particularly the diaphragm, have little reserve and are prone to fatigue and respiratory failure. Laryngeal braking (grunting) decreases diaphragmatic work by keeping more alveoli open at the end of expiration and improving gas exchange. Additional accessory muscles of the upper and lower thorax may be recruited in more advanced stages of lower airway obstruction, resulting in the clinical signs of "head-bobbing" and chest–abdomen "see-sawing". Clinically, these changes are seen as "respiratory distress". Maladaptive compensatory responses to obstruction include cessation of feeding, resulting in the WHO danger sign of "inability to feed or drink" [10]. As the child is fighting to prevent alveolar collapse and maintain positive pressure at the end of the respiratory cycle, as well as maximize alveolar ventilation, it opts against breath holding, which is necessary for swallowing during feeding. The effect is to deprive the child's respiratory muscles of needed fuel, which will hasten respiratory fatigue and failure, and is thus a danger sign. As lower airway obstruction continues without intervention, diaphragmatic and accessory muscle fatigue set in and respiratory rate and effort fall. This can be misinterpreted as evidence that lower airway obstruction is not severe, rather than as decompensation and impending respiratory failure. As $PaCO_2$ rises, the child may become initially agitated; as it rises further, the child may convulse. As PaO_2 falls and the child's brain is progressively deprived of oxygen, the child may, at first, become less active, then lethargic or obtunded. These are terminal phases before complete respiratory failure and death.

CLINICAL FEATURES

The clinical features of pneumonia follow from the underlying pathophysiology of infection followed by inflammation and congestion in the lower airway. There is a range of symptoms that may vary somewhat with age [7]. The most consistent feature is tachypnea, or rapid breathing, the underlying pathophysiology of which is described above. This is age-dependent and the WHO have established age-specific cut-offs as follows (breaths/minute): age <2 months ≥60/minute; age 2–11 months ≥50/min; children 12–59 months ≥40/min [10]. In addition to tachypnea, a history and presentation of cough is nearly universal. These two signs, fast breathing and cough should place pneumonia at the top of a differential diagnosis until proven otherwise by systematic exclusion. Other clinical features are discussed below in patient evaluation.

PATIENT EVALUATION, DIAGNOSIS AND DIFFERENTIAL DIAGNOSIS

CLINICAL EXAMINATION FINDINGS

A thorough history should precede the examination, with emphasis on the initial symptom onset, progression of other symptoms and their duration prior to seeking medical care. During the history, the clinician should observe the patient, specifically looking for rate and effort of breathing, cyanosis, level of alertness and responsiveness to the caretaker. These should be evaluated in the context of the patient's age (the younger the patient is, the more vulnerable they are to respiratory failure) and nutritional status (if severe malnutrition is present, hospitalize – even if pneumonia signs are not severe). The interview should solicit any history of convulsions, feeding behavior, and responsiveness to the caregiver.

A systematic clinical examination is necessary, with emphasis on key organ systems that may be compromised by the underlying pathophysiology. These include: (i) the respiratory tract, with emphasis on the effort of breathing, the quality of breath sounds and investigation for hypoxia; (ii) neurologic status, with emphasis on level of alertness and responsiveness to external stimuli; and (iii) supportive findings suggestive of severe bacterial infection, including temperature, perfusion, the presence of skin lesions and an ability to drink or feed.

Pneumonia is graded according to three levels of severity: non-severe, severe and very severe (Table 38-1). It is important to note that even non-severe pneumonia is a severe illness, as anything that compromises breathing in a small child is potentially life-threatening and should prompt intervention. *Non-severe pneumonia* is characterized by age-specific tachypnea and history of cough. The child may be irritable or less active than normal, but should otherwise be alert and responsive. On auscultation, crepitations (short, fine crackles on inspiration) or reduced breath sounds should be appreciated. This requires that the health provider time the breath sound with the breathing cycle in order to minimize confusion with other adventitious breath sounds, such as wheezing (long, high-pitched whistling sounds primarily on expiration that originate in the bronchioles). Chest-wall percussion is less diagnostic in young children than in adults. *Severe pneumonia* is characterized by tachypnea, with cough and at least one of the following signs: lower chest wall in-drawing (not to be confused with intercostal retractions), nasal flaring or grunting (primarily in young infants <24 months old). Of these, lower chest wall in-drawing is the most obvious. This is the collapse of the lower chest wall during inspiration and is caused by a sharp decrease in intrathoracic pressure as the child forcibly contracts the diaphragm to overcome lower airway obstruction. The external atmospheric pressure subsequently collapses the chest wall, much like the effect on a paper straw when one forcibly sucks against resistance. The chest wall of a young child, particularly less than three years old, is composed of more cartilage than that of an older child and is thus softer and more collapsible. Chest wall in-drawing may not be consistently appreciated in children older than three years of age [11]. *Very severe pneumonia* is characterized by tachypnea and cough plus at least one of the classic WHO danger signs: central cyanosis; inability to drink or feed (or vomiting anything ingested); lethargy or obtundation; convulsions; and other signs of severe respiratory distress such as head nodding and chest–abdominal see-sawing. As noted above, tachypnea may not be present in the later stages of very severe pneumonia as the patient begins to decompensate; however, the other danger signs will be present, particularly a decline in mental status (lethargy,

TABLE 38-1 Evidence for Case-Management Ordered by Strength of Study Design

Study type	Objective	Size	Outcome	Significance	Interpretation
Category 1: double-blind studies					
Multicenter double-blind efficacy [29]	3 vs 5 days amoxicillin for non-severe pneumonia	2000	Treatment failure: 21% 3-day vs 20% 5-day	Difference 0.7% (95% CI: 1.8, 3.2)	3-days equally effective as 5-days*
Double-blind randomized multi-site controlled trial [16]	To compare a 3-day course of standard dose (45 mg/kg/day) or double-dose (90 mg/kg/day) amoxicillin in the management of non-severe pneumonia	876 children aged 2–59 months	Treatment failure by day 5 and at 14 day follow-up	4.5% in standard vs 5.7% in double-dose regimen failed treatment by day 5; and 5.9% vs 7.9%, respectively by day 14 p = 0.55 p = 0.29	Non-severe pneumonia can be treated effectively with a standard dose 3-day course of amoxicillin
Category 2: partially blinded and non-blinded multicenter studies					
Multi-center open-label randomized efficacy [30]	Chloramphenicol vs ampicillin and gentamicin x 5 days	956	Treatment failure at 5 days: 16% failed chloramphenicol vs 11% ampicillin/gentamicin[†]	RR 1.43 (95% CI 1.03, 1.97)[§]	Ampicillin plus gentamicin is superior to chloramphenicol for very severe pneumonia
Open-label randomized efficacy [31]	Penicillin/gentamicin vs parenteral amoxicillin/clavulanic acid	72	Respiratory rate, oxygen saturation, chest wall in-drawing	76 h (±25) vs 75 h (±24) p > 0.100	Parenteral amoxicillin clavunate followed by oral amoxicillin/clavulanic is as effective as penicillin/gentamicin followed by oral amoxicillin for severe pneumonia
Randomized multicenter open-label study [32]	To determine the efficacy of parenteral-oral antimicrobial switch in treating severe (hospitalized) lobar or segmental pneumonia	177	Treatment failure	100% of patients on 2 days parenteral ceftriaxone vs 96% on 1 day ceftriaxone were cured (failure 0% vs 4%)	Parenteral oral switching is feasible for serious pediatric community-acquired pneumonia
Randomized multisite open-label trial [20]	To determine whether chloramphenicol vs combination benzyl penicillin plus gentamicin is better as first-line parenteral therapy for severe pneumonia in children	1116 (1 month–5 years)	Adverse outcome (treatment failure or relapse)	All adverse outcomes chloramphenicol vs penicillin/gentamicin: RO 1.25; 95% CI 0.95, 1.67; p = 0.11 Death: 1.25; 95% CI 0.74, 2.15; p = 0.44	Outcomes for severe pneumonia treated by either chloramphenicol or combination benzyl penicillin/gentamicin are similar
Randomized multisite open label trial [19]	To determine whether home-management with high-dose oral amoxicillin (80–90 mg/kg/day ÷ BID) and inpatient parenteral ampicillin were equivalent in the management of severe pneumonia	2037 children aged 3–59 months	Treatment failure by day 6	Risk difference 1.1%, 95% CI 1.3–3.5	Home treatment with high-dose oral amoxicillin is equivalent to hospital management with parenteral ampicillin. WHO recommendations for severe pneumonia should be revised
Category 3: non-randomized observational studies					
Multicenter prospective observational study [22]	To determine whether *in vitro* penicillin-resistant *Streptococcus pneumoniae* increases the risk of clinical failure in children hospitalized with severe pneumonia	240 children aged 3–59 months	Treatment failure	(adjusted) RR 1.03; 95% CI 0.49–1.90	No association between treatment failure and *in vitro* resistance. Penicillin remains drug of choice for treating penicillin-resistant pneumococcal pneumonia where MIC ≤2μg/ml

Continued

TABLE 38-1 Evidence for Case-Management Ordered by Strength of Study Design—cont'd

Study type	Objective	Size	Outcome	Significance	Interpretation
Category 4: pooled analyses					
Pooled analysis of prospective double-blind randomized and non-comparative studies [21]	To determine the efficacy of enhanced amoxicillin/ clavulanate to treat penicillin-resistant *S. pneumoniae*	5531	Treatment failure	Success rate pooled comparator arm: 86.5% Penicillin-resistant *S. pneumoniae* arm: 98.2%	Enhanced amoxicillin/ clavulanate twice daily is effective as empirical treatment of respiratory infections in children at risk for resistant *S. pneumoniae*
Category 5: reviews					
Review [17]	To review recommendations for first-line treatment of non-severe pneumonia, targeting *S. pneumoniae* and *Haemophilus influenzae* type b				Best first-line agent for non-severe childhood pneumonia is amoxicillin twice daily for 3–5 days with antibiotic change (e.g. high-dose amoxicillin/clavulanate or macrolide) for failure to improve after 48–72 hours
Review [33]	Determine the efficacy of ß-lactams for CAP				ß-lactams good for sensitive and intermediate resistant pneumococci. For hospitalized patients with CAP, recommend combination therapy (ß-lactam plus macrolide)
Review [34]	Evaluate amoxicillin/ clavulanate extended release against ß-lactamase-producing pathogens (*H. influenzae, Moraxella catarrhalis, Haemophilus parainfluenzae, Staphylococcus aureus*) and *S. pneumoniae* with reduced susceptibility (MIC 2.0 µg/ml)				Amoxicillin/clavulanate ER effective in outpatient CAP against these pathogens
Review [35]	To evaluate the efficacy of new respiratory fluoroquinolones against resistant organisms				Gemifloxacin given twice daily for 5–7 days is non-inferior and even superior to other standard agents
Category 6: animal studies					
In vivo and *in vitro* multiarm study	Evaluate synergy between amoxicillin and gentamicin vs amoxicillin against highly resistant vs susceptible *S. pneumoniae* serotype 19	Amoxicillin/ gentamicin more effective than amoxicillin alone after single injection and on repeated doses. Cumulative survival rate superior with amoxicillin/ gentamicin than amoxicillin alone	Single dose: ($p < 0.001$) Repeated doses: ($p < 0.05$)	Combination therapy with amoxicillin/ gentamicin may be a viable alternative for highly penicillin-resistant pneumococcal pneumonia	*In vivo* and *in vitro* multi-arm study

*Treatment failure more likely in noncompliant children and those aged <12 months ($p < 0.001$), and those with illness ≥3 days ($p = 0.004$).

†Of 112 bacterial isolates from blood and lung aspirates in 110 children (11.5% of total) 47 were *S. aureus* and 22 were *S. pneumonia.*

§Bacteremia with any organism increased treatment failure in the chloramphenicol group (2.09, 1.41–3.10), but not in the ampicillin/gentamicin group (1.12, 0.59–2.13).

CAP, community-acquired pneumonia; CI, confidence interval; ER, extended release; MIC, minimum inhibitory concentration; RR, relative risk; WHO, World Health Organization.

obtundation). This combination should prompt immediate intervention (Table 38-1).

SUPPORTIVE CLINICAL FINDINGS

Hypoxia is an under-appreciated feature of pneumonia with prognostic significance. Up to 59% of children admitted to hospital with pneumonia have oxygen saturation <90% (moderate hypoxia) or even less (severe hypoxia; SPO_2 at elevation can be lower than 50%) [1]. The risk of mortality is substantially increased (by up to four times in certain settings) among hypoxic children. Clinical signs for identifying hypoxia have proven less reliable than pulse oxymetry. The use of pulse oxymetry has been shown to reduce mortality by up to 35% compared with clinical criteria [1]. Continuous oxygen therapy by nasal prongs or nasal cannula is recommended for all children with moderate or greater hypoxia, as well as those with cyanosis, inability to drink or feed, or a respiratory rate >60/minute.

LABORATORY INVESTIGATIONS

Blood cultures are insensitive at establishing an etiologic agent [1]. Nasopharyngeal swabs are indicative of carriage, but do not establish invasiveness. A number of rapid antigen assays to detect respiratory viruses in nasopharyngeal washes or swabs are available in industrialized countries, but these are not readily available in resource-limited settings. Outside of intensive care settings, lung aspirates are considered too invasive as a general diagnostic approach. As such, there is currently no gold standard for etiologic diagnosis of acute pneumonia, although a positive blood culture with a potentially causative agent is, in most cases, considered conclusive of invasive disease. Newer technologies to identify invasive pathogens include assays resting on antigen detection and/or amplification, but none of these have, as yet, become a standard.

CHEST ROENTGENOGRAMS (CHEST X-RAYS)

Abnormal chest roentgenograms (CXRs) show reasonable sensitivity but poor specificity for bacterial pneumonia [12]; however, many children with pneumonia initially have normal chest radiographs. One reason is that CXR findings can lag behind clinical presentation [13], and CXRs are often not repeated. Current emphasis is on empirical therapy, rather than radiographic diagnosis [7].

MISCELLANEOUS CLINICAL FINDINGS

Staphylococcal pneumonia may be associated with rapid illness progression in the presence of treatment, and can result in lung cavitation, pneumatocele, pneumothorax, pleural effusions and empyema.

Tuberculosis is often a diagnosis of exclusion in the absence of available laboratory support. If children have fever for >14 days and clinical pneumonia, health providers should consider tuberculosis. If other causes of fever cannot be identified, then anti-tuberculosis therapy should also be considered based on national epidemiology and guidelines.

Pneumocystis (carinii) jiroveci infection should be considered in HIV-infected children, especially in the setting of hypoxia, respiratory distress and interstitial infiltrates on CXR. Therapy should be tailored accordingly.

DIFFERENTIAL DIAGNOSIS

The signs and symptoms of clinical pneumonia are designed to be maximally sensitive (include the largest possible fraction of true pneumonia-positive cases), while sacrificing specificity (inclusion of false-positives – children without pneumonia) in order to ensure that the largest possible fraction of true pneumonia patients receive antimicrobial treatment. Although there are regional differences in the prevalence of other diagnoses and comorbidities, some of the more important syndromes to consider include the following, listed below.

Reactive Airways Disease (RAD or Asthma)

This is reversible lower airway obstruction, associated with history of cough (particularly at night), with or without wheezing on auscultation (long, musical, high-pitched whistling sound on expiration originating in the bronchioles) and can be differentiated from crepitations (short crackling sounds on inspiration associated with pneumonia) in the alveoli by both the quality of the sound and particularly by the timing in the respiratory cycle. RAD may follow, or accompany, a viral infection, but often persists after the viral infection has resolved, and may be triggered by other causes (e.g. indoor air pollution). Fever is often not present. Cough, particularly night-time coughing may be the primary sign. This may be diagnosed by a beta-agonist challenge, such as with an albuterol nebulizer and is appreciated by a decrease in respiratory rate (by ≥5 breaths/minute) and effort, and improved oxygen saturation.

Bronchiolitis

This is usually, but not always, viral in origin and is commonly caused by respiratory syncytial virus (RSV), but is associated with many respiratory viruses. It is characterized by cough and wheezing on expiration, along with signs of viral infection – notably fever and often rhinorrhea. Children tend to be <2 years of age and may present with wheezing for the first time. Children may or may not respond to beta-agonist challenge, but young age and febrile wheezing are strongly suggestive.

Tuberculosis

Tuberculosis has been discussed above, but should also be considered in children who have been successfully treated for pneumonia who then return with subsequent pneumonia re-diagnoses. These may occur within days or weeks of prior successful treatment. Tuberculosis should also be considered in children who do not respond completely to conventional antibiotic therapy and/or have weight loss or failure-to-thrive (failure to appropriately gain weight), and/or have a known exposure or other suggestive history. Sputum for acid fast bacilli (AFB) is difficult to obtain in children, but gastric lavage, tuberculous skin testing (e.g. Mantoux) and CXR may all be considered.

Malaria

Malaria has been shown to present with many of the same signs and symptoms as severe pneumonia in high malaria endemic areas. Pallor (signs of anemia) and hemorrhagic skin lesions favor malaria [10]. Blood smears will identify malaria parasites, but may not always be diagnostic. Intervention in these cases should follow local or national guidelines.

Foreign Body Aspiration

This can mimic infectious pneumonia and can be identified by patient history if ingestion was observed or suspected by a missing object. Auscultation findings can include either crepitations and/or wheezing depending on the location of the foreign body. A CXR can be diagnostic and treatment often requires bronchoscopy, where available.

Pertussis

Pertussis is a vaccine-preventable infection that may present with a paroxysmal cough followed by a "whoop" on inhalation. The infection is primarily in the bronchi. Fever may or may not be present. Other indicators suggestive of pertussis include: subconjunctival hemorrhages (from extreme Valsalva-straining during paroxysms); apnea following cough; and an absence of diphtheria-pertussis-tetanus immunization.

Diphtheria

Diphtheria is a vaccine-preventable infection that is characterized by fever, a gray membrane in the posterior pharynx and enlarged cervical lymph nodes often resulting in a "bull neck".

TREATMENT

Early intervention with appropriate antibiotics is associated with a 36% reduction in pneumonia mortality [14]. Although there are general guidelines for treatment [7, 10], these should be tailored to local data on antimicrobial resistance. Table 38-1 includes recent supportive evidence, ranked by strength of study design, for current standard guidelines. The treatment regimens follow general principles of oral therapy for non-severe and even severe pneumonia in some cases, and parenteral antimicrobials for severe and very severe pneumonia, with two important caveats. Children with non-severe pneumonia who are less than 2 months old [7] and those who are severely malnourished [10] should be referred to hospital because of their high risk of progressing to severe illness. Coverage for pneumonia should at least target *S. pneumoniae* and *H. influenzae*. The current guidance for first-line therapy for outpatient, non-severe, childhood pneumonia is to use standard dose amoxicillin (45 mg/kg divided into two daily doses) for 3–5 days. Evidence suggests that high-dose oral amoxicillin should be effective against pneumococci with a minimum inhibitory concentration (MIC) of ≤4 μg/ml [15]. Current evidence also suggests that a three-day regimen of double-dose amoxicillin may be as effective as a five-day regimen of standard dose amoxicillin for pediatric community-acquired pneumonia [16]. Cotrimoxazole (20 mg/kg sulfamethoxazole divided into two daily doses for five days) may be used as an alternative agent. If a child fails to improve by 48–72 hours, then change to high-dose amoxicillin/clavulanate (90 mg/kg ÷ BID) for up to seven days or a macrolide such as azithromycin [17]. Additionally, the cause for treatment failure should be systematically determined.

The current practice for *very severe pneumonia* remains hospital treatment with either ampicillin with or without gentamicin or a third-generation cephalosporin (e.g. ceftriaxone IV at 50 mg/kg/day). Chloramphenicol resistance remains high and its clinical performance in multicenter evaluation has been inferior [18]. The optimal treatment of children with *severe pneumonia* is less established. Historically, international guidance was that children <5 years old with severe pneumonia should be hospitalized for parenteral therapy [10]; however, recent evidence suggests that children treated for severe pneumonia on an outpatient basis with double-dose amoxicillin for five days recovered as well as hospitalized children treated for two days with ampicillin followed by three days with high-dose amoxicillin [19]. Combination benzyl penicillin and gentamicin and chloramphenicol have shown equivalent efficacy in the treatment of severe pneumonia [20].

For outpatient *non-severe pneumonia*, enhanced amoxicillin/clavulanate twice daily is effective in treating penicillin-resistant *S. pneumoniae* [21] and parenteral benzyl penicillin remains the drug of choice for treatment of *S. pneumoniae* where the penicillin MIC is ≤2μg/ml [22]. Limited data indicate that both *severe* and *very severe pneumonia* can be managed on an outpatient basis in a daycare clinical facility [23]; however, further studies on the management of severe pneumonia are needed to determine optimal treatment guidelines.

If staphylococcal pneumonia is suspected, which is suggested by rapid clinical deterioration in the presence of standard antimicrobial therapy, by CXR findings of a pneumatocele or pneumothorax with pleural effusion, by skin pustules, soft tissue infection, or heavy growth of *S. aureus* in sputum, blood or empyema cultures, a regimen of cloxacillin (50 mg/kg IM or IV every six hours) and gentamicin (7.5 mg/kg IM or IV once daily) is recommended [10].

In addition to antimicrobial coverage, patients with moderate or severe hypoxia (≤90% SPO_2 on room air) should be provided continuous supplemental oxygen [24]. Flow rates are limited to ≤2 L/min by nasal prongs. If greater oxygenation is required, continuous positive air pressure (CPAP) or intubation in very severe cases should be considered, if feasible.

Another important support for improving pneumonia case management is breastfeeding, which has been shown to have a strong effect on both pneumonia prevention and case-management, and should be encouraged as part of all management regimens for children up to 12 months of age [10].

Other supplemental support includes beta-agonist inhaler use for children who are wheezing and antipyretics for fever. Adequate hydration support is also important, as both tachypnea and fever increase insensible water loss [10]. This raises the possibility of using oral rehydration solution as a hydration choice both because many children with pneumonia have diarrhea and also because of its ease of absorption; however, there is currently no evidence that oral rehydration solution versus other liquids is superior in treating children with pneumonia.

GOOD CLINICAL PRACTICE

Once the patient has begun treatment and is stabilized, it is good clinical practice to review with the parent the signs and symptoms of pneumonia and the indications for future clinical referral by illustrating these in the child. Many parents in high pneumonia endemic areas are poor at recognizing these signs, despite the high incidence of pneumonia [7] – presentation to a clinic may provide a "teachable moment". All patients managed on an outpatient basis should be advised to return to the clinic if they fail to improve by 72 hours, or worsen at any time. The physician should follow-up all outpatients at least once to assess their status [25].

PREVENTION AND CONTROL

Immunization with *H. influenzae* B (Hib) and protein-conjugate pneumococcal vaccines may be able to prevent up to 50% of all pneumonia-related child mortality [26]. Currently, the Hib vaccine is used in over 100 countries and 61 out of 72 (85%) countries eligible for Global Alliance for Vaccines and Immunizations (GAVI) funding have agreed to introduce the Hib vaccine [27]. As of January 2009, 42 GAVI-eligible countries (58%) expressed interest in introducing pneumococcal vaccine [28]. Current recommendations include Hib, pneumococcal protein-conjugates, measles, and pertussis vaccines to decrease the global burden of pneumonia [7]. In addition to these vaccines, other interventions for which there is strong preventive evidence include zinc and hand-washing [1, 7]. Exclusive breastfeeding for the first six months of life reduces pneumonia mortality fivefold, while continuation of breastfeeding for infants aged 6–11 months further reduces pneumonia mortality and should be encouraged [7]. Finally, as malnutrition is estimated to contribute an additional 1 million child deaths per year and complicates over 50% of all less-than-five-year-old mortality [2], long-term solutions and programs to reduce pneumonia mortality should include ensuring adequate nutrition.

REFERENCES

1. Scott JA, Brooks WA, Peiris JS, et al. Pneumonia research to reduce childhood mortality in the developing world. J Clin Invest 2008;118: 1291–300.
2. Bryce J, Boschi-Pinto C, Shibuya K, et al. WHO estimates of the causes of death in children. Lancet 2005;365:1147–52.
3. Rudan I, Boschi-Pinto C, Biloglav Z, et al. Epidemiology and etiology of childhood pneumonia. Bull World Health Organ 2008;86:408–16.
4. McCullers JA. Insights into the interaction between influenza virus and pneumococcus. Clin Microbiol Rev 2006;19:571–82.
5. Madhi SA, Klugman KP. A role for *Streptococcus pneumoniae* in virus-associated pneumonia. Nat Med 2004;10:811–13.
6. McCullers JA, Bartmess KC. Role of neuraminidase in lethal synergism between influenza virus and *Streptococcus pneumoniae*. J Infect Dis 2003;187: 1000–9.
7. Wardlaw T, Johansson EW, Hodge M. Pneumonia: The Forgotten Killer of Children. New York, Geneva: The United Nations Children's Fund (UNICEF)/ World Health Organization (WHO); 2004:1–44.
8. Davis GM, Bureau MA. Pulmonary and chest wall mechanics in the control of respiration in the newborn. Clin Perinatol 1987;14:551–79.
9. Knelson JH, Howatt WF, DeMuth GR. The physiologic significance of grunting respiration. Pediatrics 1969;44:393–400.

10. World Health Organization. Management of the child with a serious infection or severe malnutrition: guidelines for care at the first-referral level in developing countries. Geneva: World Health Organization and UNICEF; 2000:162.
11. Harari M, Shann F, Spooner V, et al. Clinical signs of pneumonia in children. Lancet 1991;338:928–30.
12. Ferrero F, Torres F, Noguerol E, et al. Evaluation of two standardized methods for chest radiographs interpretation in children with pneumonia. Arch Argent Pediatr 2008;106:510–14.
13. Redd SC, Patrick E, Vreuls R, et al. Comparison of the clinical and radiographic diagnosis of paediatric pneumonia. Trans R Soc Trop Med Hyg 1994;88:307–10.
14. Sazawal S, Black RE. Effect of pneumonia case management on mortality in neonates, infants, and preschool children: a meta-analysis of community-based trials. Lancet Infect Dis 2003;3:547–56.
15. Klugman KP. Bacteriological evidence of antibiotic failure in pneumococcal lower respiratory tract infections. Eur Respir J 2002;36(Suppl.):3s–8s.
16. Hazir T, Qazi SA, Bin Nisar Y, et al. Comparison of standard versus double dose of amoxicillin in the treatment of non-severe pneumonia in children aged 2–59 months: a multi-centre, double blind, randomised controlled trial in Pakistan. Arch Dis Child 2007;92:291–7.
17. Grant GB, Campbell H, Dowell SF, et al. Recommendations for treatment of childhood non-severe pneumonia. Lancet Infect Dis 2009;9:185–96.
18. Asghar R, Banajeh S, Egas J, et al. Chloramphenicol versus ampicillin plus gentamicin for community acquired very severe pneumonia among children aged 2–59 months in low resource settings: multicentre randomised controlled trial (SPEAR study). BMJ 2008;336:80–4.
19. Hazir T, Fox LM, Nisar YB, et al. Ambulatory short-course high-dose oral amoxicillin for treatment of severe pneumonia in children: a randomised equivalency trial. Lancet 2008;371:49–56.
20. Duke T, Poka H, Dale F, et al. Chloramphenicol versus benzylpenicillin and gentamicin for the treatment of severe pneumonia in children in Papua New Guinea: a randomised trial. Lancet 2002;359:474–80.
21. File TM Jr, Jacobs MR, Poole MD, et al. Outcome of treatment of respiratory tract infections due to *Streptococcus pneumoniae,* including drug-resistant strains, with pharmacokinetically enhanced amoxycillin/clavulanate. Int J Antimicrob Agents 2002;20:235–47.
22. Cardoso MR, Nascimento-Carvalho CM, Ferrero F, et al. Penicillin-resistant pneumococcus and risk of treatment failure in pneumonia. Arch Dis Child 2008;93:221–5.
23. Ashraf H, Jahan SA, Alam NH, et al. Day-care management of severe and very severe pneumonia, without associated co-morbidities such as severe malnutrition, in an urban health clinic in Dhaka, Bangladesh. Arch Dis Child 2008; 93:490–4.
24. Subhi R, Adamson M, Campbell H, et al. The prevalence of hypoxaemia among ill children in developing countries: a systematic review. Lancet Infect Dis 2009;9:219–27.
25. Lanata CF, Rudan I, Boschi-Pinto C, et al. Methodological and quality issues in epidemiological studies of acute lower respiratory infections in children in developing countries. Int J Epidemiol 2004;33:1362–72.
26. Madhi SA, Levine OS, Hajjeh R, et al. Vaccines to prevent pneumonia and improve child survival. Bull World Health Organ 2008;86:365–72.
27. PneumoADIP. Hib Vaccines. 2009 Available at: http://www.preventpneumo.org/vaccine_status/hib_vaccines/index.cfm.
28. PneumoADIP. Pneumococcal Vaccines. 2009. Available at: http://www.preventpneumo.org/vaccine_status/pneumococcal_vaccines/index.cfm.
29. Pakistan Multicentre Amoxycillin Short Course Therapy (MASCOT) pneumonia study group. Clinical efficacy of 3 days versus 5 days of oral amoxicillin for treatment of childhood pneumonia: a multicentre double-blind trial. Lancet 2002;360:835–41.
30. Asghar R, Banajeh S, Egas J, et al. Chloramphenicol versus ampicillin plus gentamicin for community acquired very severe pneumonia among children aged 2–59 months in low resource settings: multicentre randomised controlled trial (SPEAR study). BMJ 2008;336:80–4.
31. Bansal A, Singhi SC, Jayashree M. Penicillin and gentamicin therapy vs amoxicillin/clavulanate in severe hypoxemic pneumonia. Indian J Pediatr 2006;73:305–9.
32. Dagan R, Syrogiannopoulos G, Ashkenazi S, et al. Parenteral–oral switch in the management of paediatric pneumonia. Drugs 1994;47(Suppl. 3):43–51.
33. Aspa J, Rajas O, de Castro FR. Pneumococcal antimicrobial resistance: therapeutic strategy and management in community-acquired pneumonia. Expert Opin Pharmacother 2008;9:229–41.
34. Benninger MS. Amoxicillin/clavulanate potassium extended release tablets: a new antimicrobial for the treatment of acute bacterial sinusitis and community-acquired pneumonia. Expert Opin Pharmacother 2003;4: 1839–46.
35. Blondeau JM, Tillotson G. Role of gemifloxacin in the management of community-acquired lower respiratory tract infections. Int J Antimicrob Agents 2008;31:299–306.

39 Tuberculosis

Sonya S Shin, Kwonjune J Seung

Key features

- Tuberculosis (TB) is the second leading infectious cause of death and the leading killer of people with HIV
- TB is a disease of poverty, with the vast majority of cases occurring in low- or lower middle- income countries
- HIV infection greatly increases the risk of developing active TB for people infected with latent TB
- Multidrug-resistant TB (MDR-TB) is on the rise and is associated with lower cure rates compared with susceptible TB
- Most TB involves the lung, but extra-pulmonary involvement is more common among immunocompromised individuals and children
- Pulmonary TB radiographic findings can be subtle, mimic community-acquired pneumonia or show severe disseminated or cavitary disease
- Extra-pulmonary TB commonly involves the lymph nodes, pleural space, central nervous system (CNS), bones or gastrointestinal tract
- TB diagnosis is particularly difficult in immunocompromised individuals or children, and a clinical diagnosis of active TB and MDR-TB with empiric treatment is often necessary
- Combination therapy is necessary to avoid selection of drug-resistant pathogens

INTRODUCTION

Tuberculosis (TB) is an ancient infection of humanity. DNA-confirmed cases date to 9000 years ago and suspected TB lesions have been described in *Homo erectus* bones from 500,000 years ago. Ironically, TB remains a global public health threat as the second leading single pathogen infectious cause of death after HIV. Since the advent of effective anti-tuberculosis agents in the 1950s, TB has come to epitomize diseases of poverty: a curable disease that continues to kill 2 million people per year. As TB predominantly affects working-age populations, the macro-economic impact of TB in developing countries is also immense, with a 0.2–0.4% decrease in annual economic growth for every 10% increase in TB incidence [1]. Despite global efforts to eliminate TB, prevalence continues to rise and, in Eastern Europe and Africa, incidence is also on the rise. This reversal of trends is due, in large part, to "deadly synergies" with other chronic diseases, the emergence of strains resistant to anti-TB agents and deepening social inequality in both developed and developing countries.

EPIDEMIOLOGY

About two billion people – one-third of the world's population – have *Mycobacterium tuberculosis* infection. Among the 22 countries identified by the World Health Organization (WHO) as high TB burden countries, 19 are low- or lower middle-income countries defined by the World Bank. Of the 9.27 million new TB cases reported in 2007, 2.98 million (32%) occurred in sub-Saharan Africa and 13 of the 15 countries with the highest TB incidence are in Africa (Table 39-1, Fig. 39.1) [2].

High rates of TB incidence in African countries are attributed to the heavy burden of TB/HIV co-infection. Approximately 80% of HIV co-infected TB patients live in sub-Saharan Africa. In 2007, an estimated 14.8% of incident TB cases were HIV-positive. TB is the leading cause of death among HIV-positive people – 23% of all TB deaths occurred in HIV-positive people. Although TB typically affects men more than women over the age of 14, in countries with an HIV prevalence of greater than 1%, this ratio is reversed as a result of biologic and social factors that contribute to increased vulnerability to HIV infection and more rapid disease progression among women [2].

Another concerning trend is the increase in multidrug-resistant TB (MDR-TB, resistant to at least isoniazid and rifampin), which is associated with lower cure rates than cases of pan-susceptible TB. In 2007, MDR-TB incidence was estimated at 500,000 cases, comprising approximately 3% of new TB cases and 19% of previously-treated TB cases (Table 39-1) [3]. China and India account for about half of new MDR-TB cases. The Russian Federation and countries of the former Soviet Union have the highest proportion of MDR-TB among TB cases, estimated at 18–22.2% [4]. Recently, the term "extensively drug-resistant TB" (XDR-TB) was established to refer to MDR-TB strains that are also resistant to fluoroquinolones and at least one second-line injectable agent. Outbreaks of XDR-TB have been associated with lethal clinical outcomes, particularly among HIV co-infected cases. To date, 55 countries have reported XDR-TB cases, with the highest reported rates of XDR-TB – 13.6% of all MDR-TB cases – in the region of Eastern Europe and Russia. However, the epidemiology of XDR-TB is greatly underestimated because drug susceptibility testing (DST) is not available in many countries [5].

NATURAL HISTORY, PATHOGENESIS, AND PATHOLOGY

TB is an airborne pathogen. A cough or sneeze from an infectious host emits thousands of aerosolized droplet nuclei that are much smaller than respiratory droplets (approximately 1–5 μm). Bacilli-containing droplets remain airborne for hours to days and are small enough to be inhaled into the terminal alveoli.

Following inhalation, bacilli may extend via lung lymphatics to other areas of the lungs and to other organs throughout the body. Cellular immunity develops after approximately 6–12 weeks, resulting in either eradication of bacilli or the formation of granulomas around the sites of infection. This cellular immunity is the basis for the tuberculin skin test (TST; described below). Cell-mediated immunity

TABLE 39-1 Estimated Burden of Tuberculosis (TB) in 2008

	Incidence, 2008					**Prevalence, 2008**		**TB mortality, 2008***		**MDR-TB**	
	All forms †		***All forms HIV+***			***All forms*** †		***All forms*** †		***All cases***	
	Number	*Rate*	*% Among incident TB cases*	*Number*	*Rate*	*Number*	*Rate*	*Number*	*Rate*	*Number*	*%*
African Region (AFR)	2,828,485	351	38	1,074,824	134	3,809,650	473	385,055	48	69,000	2
American Region (AMR)	281,682	31	13	36,619	4	221,354	24	29,135	3	8,200	3
Eastern Mediterranean Region (EMR)	674,585	115	2.2	14,841	3	929,166	159	115,137	20	24,000	4
European Region (EUR)	425,038	48	5.6	23,802	3	322,310	36	55,688	6	81,000	17
South East Asian Region (SEAR)	3,213,236	183	5.7	183,154	10	3,805,588	216	477,701	27	130,000	5
Western Pacific Region (WPR)	1,946,012	109	2.3	44,758	3	2,007,681	112	261,770	15	120,000	6
Global	**9,369,038**	**139**	**15**	**1,374,048**	**21**	**11,095,750**	**164**	**1,324,487**	**20**	**440,000**	**5**

*Mortality excluding HIV, according to International Classification of Diseases (ICD)-10.
†Incidence, prevalence and mortality estimates include patients with HIV. Estimates labeled "HIV+" are estimates of HIV+ TB cases in all people. Estimates for all years are re-calculated as new information becomes available and techniques are refined.
http://www.who.int/tb/publications/global_report/2009/xls/annex3_regional_summary.xls
http://www.who.int/tb/publications/global_report/2009/update/en/index.html
http://whqlibdoc.who.int/publications/2010/9789241599191_eng.pdf
http://www.who.int/whosis/whostat/EN_WHS09_Table2.pdf
MDR-TB, multi-drug resistant-tuberculosis.
Data from World Health Organization. WHO Report 2009: Global Tuberculosis Control. Geneva: World Health Organization; 2009.

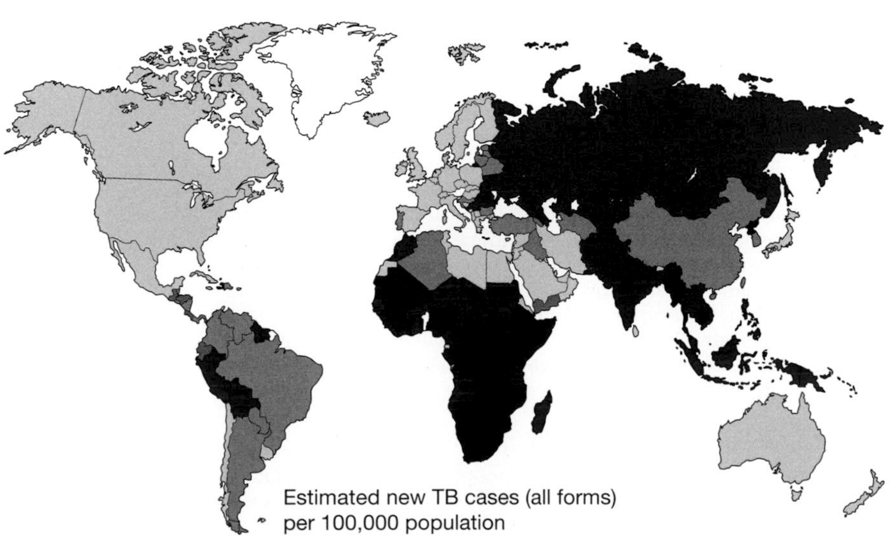

FIGURE 39.1 Estimated TB incidence rates by country, 2008 *(from World Health Organization. WHO Report 2009: Global Tuberculosis Control. Geneva: World Health Organization; 2009.)*

prevents progression to symptomatic disease in the majority of infected individuals who are considered to have latent infection. However, approximately 10% of infected individuals will develop active disease in the acute setting; in such cases, the bacilli proliferate within macrophages, provoking local inflammation and progression of lesions which can become necrotic and, ultimately, cavitary. Individuals who develop active disease within 1–2 years of infection are considered to have primary TB. Re-activation TB, or the development of active disease more than two years after infection, occurs in approximately 5–10% of infected individuals over their lifetime. HIV infection increases this risk to approximately 5–10% per year. Without anti-tuberculous chemotherapy, approximately 50% of patients with active disease die within 5 years, 30% recover spontaneously and 20% remain infectious [6].

CLINICAL FEATURES

The diverse breadth of clinical presentations is a result of the bacilli's ability to infect virtually every organ. Approximately 70–90% of active cases involve the lung, while the remaining 10–30% of cases are extrapulmonary (Fig. 39.2) [7]. Up to 15% of cases have both pulmonary and extrapulmonary involvement, although this may be an underestimate because of subclinical extra-pulmonary infection. Extrapulmonary involvement is more frequent among immunocompromised individuals and children. Among patients with AIDS, up to 70% have extrapulmonary involvement. The diagnosis of extrapulmonary TB requires a high index of suspicion. The paucity of sensitive diagnostic methods for TB and limited capacity to sample suspected sites of involvement, in particular in resource-poor settings, means that many diagnoses are based solely on clinical features. It is important to conduct a detailed survey for "subclinical" or subtle findings suggestive of additional organ involvement among individuals presenting with a predominant site of involvement, such as pulmonary TB.

Manifestations of active TB are often subacute or chronic, typically developing over weeks to months. Constitutional symptoms include fever, night sweats, anorexia and weight loss. With increasing chronicity, the classic finding of "consumption", or generalized wasting, may be observed, regardless of organ involvement. However, the blunted inflammatory response of immunosuppressed individuals can result in attenuated or absent signs and symptoms – in particular those associated with local pathology.

PULMONARY TUBERCULOSIS

Primary pulmonary TB is often characterized by lower lobe infiltrates (Fig. 39.3) and/or hilar adenopathy, reflecting the site of inoculation and early spread via lymphatics. Symptoms and radiographic findings can be subtle or mimic community-acquired pneumonia. Inquiry into recent TB contacts is important to increase the index of suspicion. Immunosuppressed individuals, such as infants and HIV-positive individuals are less able to contain the infection and therefore more likely to present with primary TB. Cavitary lesions are frequently associated with hemoptysis. Physical findings may include the use of accessory muscles, tachycardia with a widely split S2, as well as clubbing, pale conjunctiva and slow capillary refill. Lung auscultation can vary widely, ranging from a normal exam to focal râles, generalized wheezing or focally absent breath sounds. A cavitary lesion may emit a hollow, tubular low-pitched sound, sometimes producing a "waterfall" sound if fluid is present in the cavity.

TUBERCULOUS ADENITIS

Lymphadenitis is the most common extra-pulmonary manifestation of TB. As with all forms of extra-pulmonary TB, adenitis has classically been a pediatric presentation, but is increasingly observed in adults co-infected with HIV. Cervical lymphadenopathy (scrofula) is the most common (Fig. 39.4), while generalized lymphadenopathy may reflect disseminated infection. When computerized tomography (CT) or magnetic resonance imaging (MRI) is available, other sites of involvement, such as intra-abdominal and retroperitoneal lymph nodes may be identified. Single or multiple lymph nodes may be enlarged; the lympadenopathy is usually painless, unless super-infection occurs.

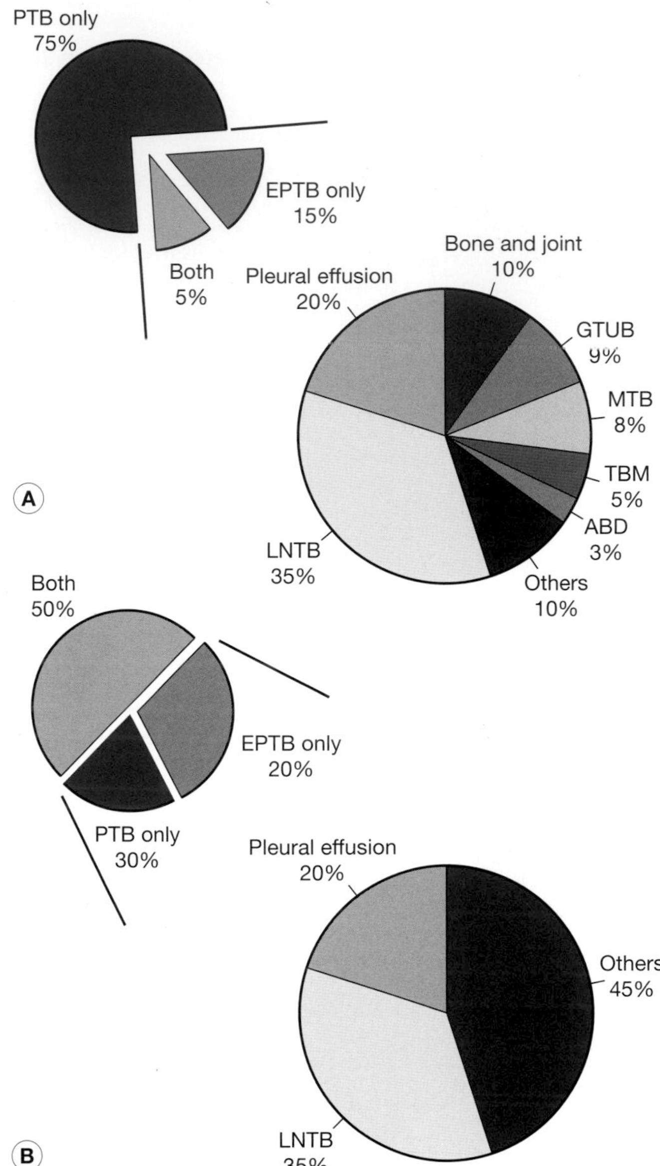

FIGURE 39.2 Distribution of TB presentation, by HIV status. (A) Distribution of TB cases by anatomical site in HIV-negative patients. (B) Distribution of TB cases by anatomical site in HIV-positive patients PTB pulmonary TB; EPTB extrapulmonary TB; GUTB genitourinary TB, MTB miliary TB; TBM tuberculosis meningitis; ABD abdominal TB; LNTB lymph node tuberculosis *(redrawn from Sharma SK, Mohan A. Extrapulmonary tuberculosis. Indian J Med Res 2004; 120:316–53.)*

Bilateral involvement is not uncommon. Chronic progression can lead to suppuration and formation of sinus tracts. Up to half of TB adenitis cases may present without systemic symptoms.

PLEURAL TUBERCULOSIS

TB pleurisy is commonly a manifestation of primary disease, although it can also be seen in the context of re-activation. In many developing countries, TB is the most common cause of pleural effusions. Symptoms may be acute or subacute, and include pleuritic chest pain, nonproductive cough and progressive dyspnea. Effusions are exudative and more than 90% are unilateral. Approximately 20–40% of cases are associated with ipsilateral parenchymal involvement. Effusions are usually small-to-moderate in size – up to 30% may be loculated. Less commonly, active infection within the pleural space results in TB empyema, which can be associated with a bronchopleural fistula or empyema necessitatis, extending into the extra-pleural space.

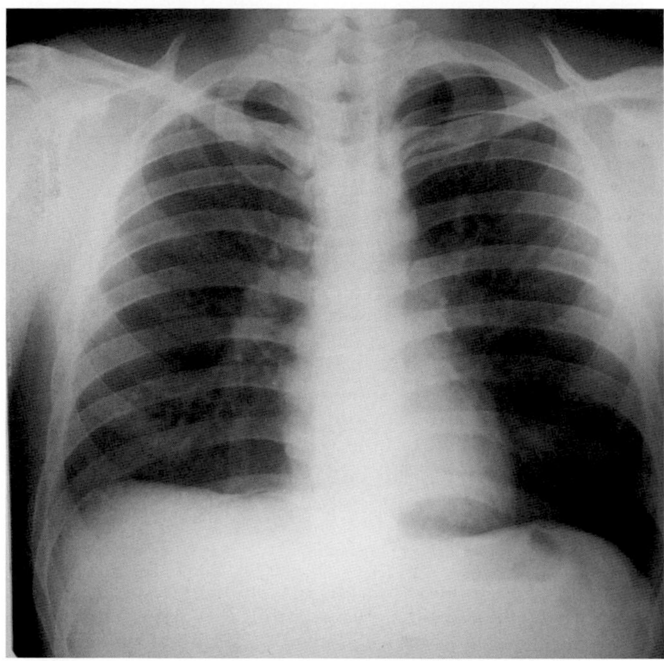

FIGURE 39.3 Chest radiograph of primary TB. Primary TB with right lower lobe infiltrate and right hilar adenopathy in a HIV-positive patient.

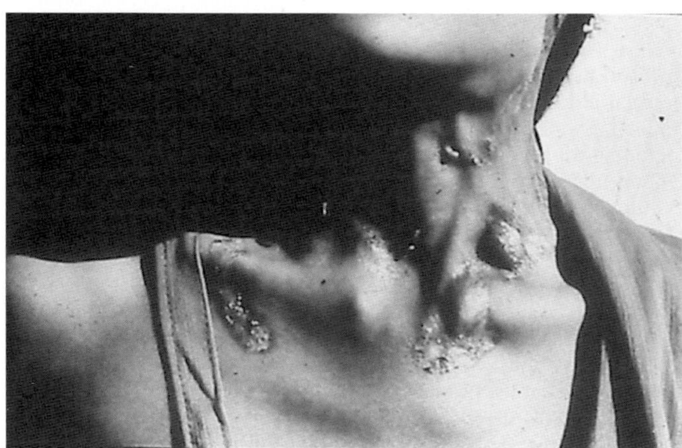

FIGURE 39.4 TB adenitis. Suppurative cervical lymphadenopathy (scrofula).

TUBERCULOSIS OF THE CENTRAL NERVOUS SYSTEM

CNS TB may present as a mass lesion (tuberculoma or abscess) or meningoencephalitis. Some estimate that up to 10% of all TB cases have CNS involvement, although many such cases may go undiagnosed or be diagnosed post-mortem. Focal lesions are often subacute and present with focal neurologic defects, seizures or symptoms caused by increased intracranial pressure as a result of mass effect. Subacute-to-chronic in tempo (usually lasting more than five days), meningoencephalitis presents with fever, headache and nuchal rigidity. Altered sensorium and cranial nerve involvement are not uncommon. Choroid tubercules may be visualized on fundoscopic exam.

OSTEOARTICULAR TUBERCULOSIS

Approximately 50% of osteoarticular TB involves the spine, although virtually any bone or joint can be involved. TB of the spine (Pott's disease) typically involves the thoracic spine and can present with chronic back pain, neurologic defects and tender spinal deformities (gibbus). Neurologic compromise and kyphotic deformities can develop if untreated. Chronic arthritis typically presents with pain and

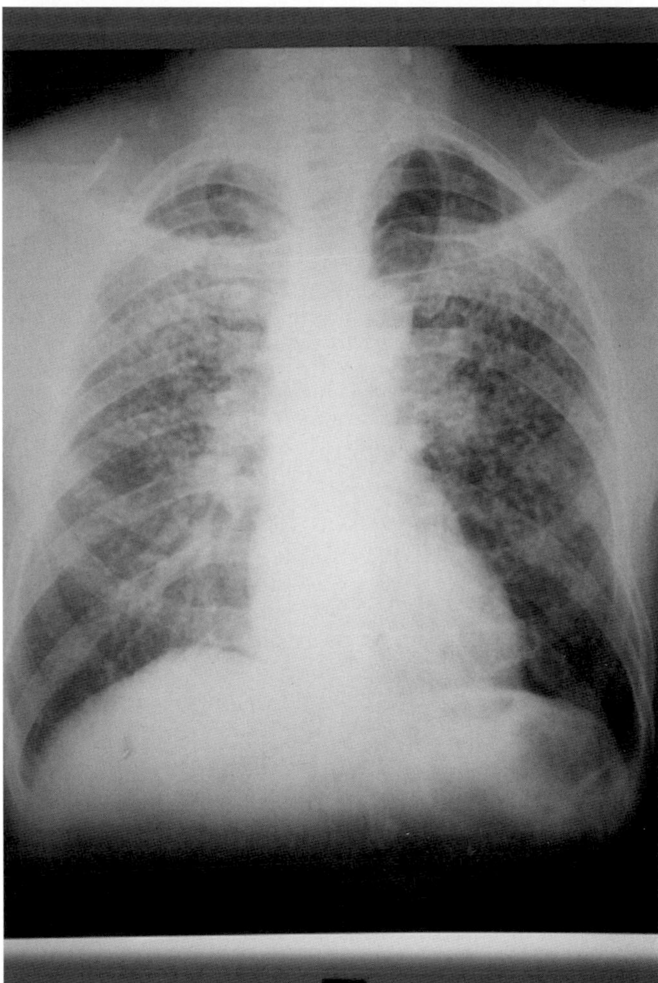

FIGURE 39.5 Miliary TB. Micronodular infiltrates resembling millet seeds represent miliary tuberculosis.

swelling of the involved joint. Bone involvement may be associated with an overlying skin lesion. Such cases are often treated with broad-spectrum antibiotics, to which the lesion may partially respond. Progression of osteoarticular TB can lead to bone and joint destruction.

OTHER MANIFESTATIONS

Gastrointestinal TB commonly presents with diffuse ascites or abdominal pain and palpable mass caused by intestinal involvement, in particular the jejunoileum and ileocecum. Individuals with TB-associated granulomatous hepatitis may present with jaundice and disproportionately elevated alkaline phosphatase values. The presence of hepatosplenomegaly should raise the suspicion of disseminated TB. Genitourinary TB includes renal involvement, orchiitis, endometritis and tubo-ovarian masses. Symptoms of pelvic inflammatory disease that are refractory or partially responsive to treatment should raise suspicion for TB in endemic areas. Renal TB may present with flank pain, dysuria, hematuria and pyuria. Imaging can reveal hydronephrosis, fibrosis and scarring, enlarged ureters and pelvic masses. Cutaneous TB may be ulcerative or nodular; lupus vulgaris, more common in women, refers to painful nodular lesions, often on the face. Other sites of involvement include the pericardium, larynx, adrenal glands and eye (including endophthalmitis, uveitis, iritis, episcleritis and choroidal tubercles). In many developing countries, ascites, pericardial effusions and sterile pyuria are considered TB until proven otherwise. Multi-organ or disseminated TB may be associated with bacteremia and the presence of a miliary pattern on chest radiograph, consisting of homogeneously-distributed micronodular infiltrates (Fig. 39.5). Lack of focal symptoms associated with disseminated

TB may result in delayed diagnosis. Advanced disseminated disease may be associated with polyserositis or acute respiratory distress syndrome. TB is also associated with rheumatologic manifestations, such as erythema nodosum and aseptic reactive polyarthritis (known as Poncet's disease).

PATIENT EVALUATION, DIAGNOSIS AND DIFFERENTIAL DIAGNOSIS

That the mainstay of TB diagnosis is an insensitive assay developed more than a century ago is testament to the urgent need for accurate diagnostics. In particular, smear-negative pulmonary TB and extrapulmonary TB remain predominantly clinical diagnoses. Among immunosuppressed individuals who present with attenuated manifestations of disease, under-diagnosis is still the norm, as evidenced by undiagnosed TB identified post-mortem in 14–54% of HIV-positive individuals and in 20% of children (Box 39.1). Diagnostic delays or failure to obtain diagnostic confirmation should not preclude initiation of appropriate therapy.

BOX 39.1 Diagnosis of Pediatric Tuberculosis

- History: cough, fever, night sweats, failure to thrive, weight loss, age (TB presentation is similar to adults among children over 4 years old).
- Physical examination: weight for age, mid-upper arm circumference, lymphadenopathy.
- Diagnostics:
  - evidence of TB infection [tuberculin skin test (TST) or interferon-gamma release assays (IGRA)] helpful;
  - radiology: atypical presentations (i.e. lymphadenopathy, miliary) more common;
  - sputum smear microscopy and culture: often negative because of difficulty producing sample and low bacillary load – gastric lavage or bronchoscopy can improve yield;
  - extra-pulmonary sites: aggressive efforts to aspirate or biopsy suspected sites helpful.
- Response to empiric therapy may provide diagnostic confirmation.

SPUTUM SMEAR MICROSCOPY

Sputum smear microscopy is often the only diagnostic test available in resource-limited settings. Smear microscopy should be performed for all suspected cases of TB, including individuals with cough lasting more than two weeks and cases of suspected extrapulmonary TB. Ideally, two or three sputum samples should be collected on consecutive mornings. The sensitivity of a single smear microscopy is 22–43%, with a mean incremental yield in sensitivity of 9% with a second sample and 4% with a third sample. Unfortunately, 20–60% of HIV-negative patients with pulmonary TB are sputum smear-negative. HIV-positive patients and children are more likely to have clinically significant disease at early stages, when the bacillary burden is still low, and therefore present with smear-negative or paucibacillary microscopy [8]. For individuals with minimal pulmonary involvement and/or scant sputum production, induced sputum, gastric lavage or broncoscopy can increase test sensitivity. Sputum processing, such as liquefaction or concentration by centrifugation, and the use of fluorescence microscopy can also increase the sensitivity of smear microscopy.

RADIOGRAPHY

Chest radiograph and fluorography are commonly used to diagnose pulmonary TB. Because there are numerous other pulmonary diseases that look similar to active TB (Table 39-2), clinical findings must complement radiographic findings to make the clinical diagnosis of TB. Re-activation TB – more frequently observed among HIV-negative cases – classically presents with apical involvement because of the high oxygen tension in the upper lung zones. Chronic findings include cavities, fibrosis, collapse of upper lobes and retraction of the mediastinal structures (Fig. 39.6). Atypical presentations, such as miliary features, intrathoracic adenopathy, pleural effusions and lower lobe infiltrates are common in HIV-positive patients. Chest radiographs are particularly useful for "ruling out" pulmonary TB before starting treatment for latent TB infection. However, chest radiographs may be normal in up to 14% of HIV-positive individuals with culture-confirmed pulmonary TB. CT and ultrasound are useful for evaluating patients with suspected extrapulmonary TB, although findings are often nonspecific and can include organomegaly, lymphadenopathy, ascites and abscesses. Plain radiographs may reveal bony destruction or compression fractures at sites of bony involvement. CT or MRI in suspected cases of CNS TB may reveal basilar meningeal enhancement and hydrocephalus, and can be helpful in ruling out alternative diagnoses in HIV-positive individuals, such as lymphoma and toxoplasmosis. In Pott's disease, compression fractures, disciitis and adjacent soft tissue involvement with cold abscesses may be revealed on imaging.

TABLE 39-2 Differential Diagnosis for Chest Radiograph Features

Presentation	Alternative diagnoses	Notes
Cavities	Fungal infections (e.g. aspergilloma), old TB, acute bacterial infection	Active TB cavities typically presents in upper lobes with adjacent infiltrates
Infiltrate	Bacterial pneumonia, aspiration (can present in upper lobes)	Alternative diagnoses more acute in presentation
Fibrosis	Silicosis and other occupational exposures, idiopathic pulmonary fibrosis, old TB	Consider exposure history and location of lesions (TB presents as apical fibrosis or fibrothorax)
Pleural effusion	Parapneumonic effusion, neoplastic, congestive heart failure	Consider comorbid conditions, constitutional symptoms; sampling of pleural fluid often informative
Lymphadenopathy	Neoplastic, other mycobacterial infections	Consider comorbid conditions, regional epidemiology of other mycobacterial infections. Tissue sampling often informative.
Miliary/disseminated	Pneumocystis jovecii, lymphocytic interstitial pneumonitis, endemic fungi (e.g. histoplasmosis)	Consider exposure history and regional epidemiology. Bronchoalveolar lavage often informative.

Data from World Health Organization. WHO Report 2009: Global Tuberculosis Control. Geneva: World Health Organization, 2009 and World Health Organization. Multidrug and extensively drug-resistant TB (M/ XDR-TB): 2010 Global Report on Surveillance and Response. Geneva: World Health Organization, 2010.

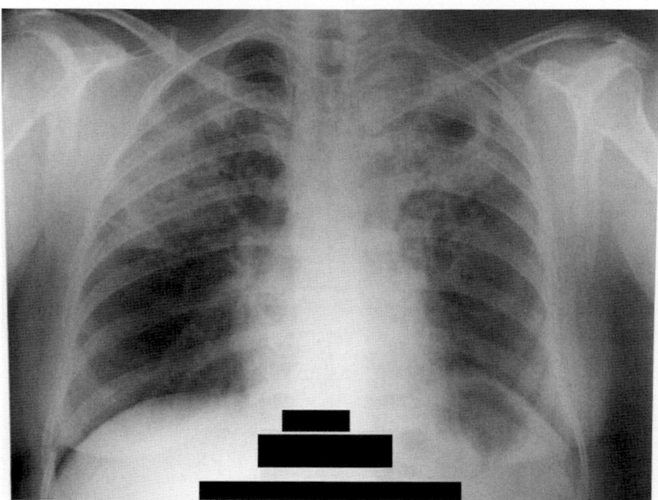

FIGURE 39.6 Re-activation TB. Extensive bilateral apical lesions include air bronchograms in the right upper lobe and a cavitary lesion in the left upper lobe.

TUBERCULOSIS CULTURE

Although considered the "gold standard" for TB diagnosis, mycobacterial culture still misses up to 20% of pulmonary cases that are confirmed based on clinical findings and response to TB therapy. Sputum culture is technically difficult and is not widely available in resource-limited settings. *Mycobacterium tuberculosis* is also slow-growing with solid culture results in 6–8 weeks. Liquid media assays (e.g. mycobacteria growth incubator) have greater sensitivity than culture on solid media and reduce the time to detection (8–16 days). However, contamination rates may be higher and commercial assays using liquid media are much more costly. One important advantage of mycobacterial culture is that additional testing, in particular drug susceptibility testing, can be performed on positive isolates.

ANALYSIS OF OTHER BODILY FLUIDS AND TISSUE SAMPLES

If extrapulmonary TB is suspected, every effort should be made to obtain a relevant sample (Table 39-3). Smear microscopy and TB culture are performed when available, but are often insensitive because of low bacillary load. The primary utility in sampling extrapulmonary sites is to quickly differentiate between non-infectious and infectious etiologies, while differentiating among infectious etiologies is more difficult. A variety of commercial nucleic acid amplification tests (e.g. PCR) have a potential role in the diagnosis of extrapulmonary TB. Although highly specific, the sensitivity of these assays is not adequate for reliably diagnosing TB in extrapulmonary samples. When available, they should be used along with clinical findings and conventional tests and are best used to confirm, rather than "rule out", the diagnosis of extrapulmonary TB. Elevated levels of adenosine deaminase (ADA) in pleural fluid is reasonably specific and sensitive for TB, but other types of effusions with a lymphocytic predominance, such as lymphoma or rheumatologic disorders can also have an elevated ADA and should be considered [9].

OTHER DIAGNOSTIC TESTS

In areas with significant rates of MDR-TB, regional or individual resistance data are crucial for designing regimens for treatment failure cases. Drug susceptibility testing (DST) methods include both phenotypic and genotypic methods (Table 39-4) [10–12]. DST may be performed directly on clinical samples or indirectly on cultured isolates. In resource-poor settings, indirect conventional DST on solid culture media is most common. Genotypic DST methods are increasingly popular, even in resource-limited settings, because they have excellent sensitivity and specificity for isoniazid and rifampin, and rapid processing times. Although the yield of direct DST on smear-positive samples is excellent, to date there are no molecular DST methods that perform well on smear-negative samples.

TABLE 39-3 Diagnostic Features of Extrapulmonary Samples

Bodily fluid or tissue sample	Findings associated with tuberculosis (TB) infection
Pleural fluid	Exudative effusion, elevated adenosine deaminase (ADA), lymphocytic predominance, pH 7.3–7.4. ADA sensitivity and specificity in pleural fluid of 58–92% and 60–90% respectively. Combined analysis of pleural fluid and pleural biopsy may increase diagnostic yield to 95%, compared with 25–75% for fluid alone
Cerebrospinal fluid (CSF)	Low glucose, high protein, usually $\leq$1000 cells/mm^3 with $\geq$50% lymphocytes. Positive acid-fast bacilli in 10–40%. TB PCR on CSF has a sensitivity of 73–100%. Neutrophilic predominance may be seen in up to one third of cases, particularly in early stages of infection. Centrifuged samples, large volume (i.e. 10 ml), and serial exams may increase diagnostic confirmation
Ascitic fluid	Lymphocytic predominance; a third may have positive smear or culture. CA-125 may be elevated in TB patients
Lymph node aspirate or biopsy	Granulomas in biopsy; AFB and/or culture often confirmatory. TB PCR may be positive in up to one third of samples
Pleural, periteoneal or pericardial biopsy	Granulomas; presence of AFB is rare; culture confirmation may be obtained in up to 66%
Blood culture	Greater yield with disseminated disease; positive in 19–96% of HIV-positive individuals
Urine	Large volume (at least 80 ml) of first morning void optimizes yield. Urine PCR has good sensitivity and specificity

TESTS FOR TUBERCULOSIS INFECTION

There are two classes of tests to diagnose TB infection: tuberculin skin test (TST) and interferon-gamma release assays (IGRA). Both tests are unable to distinguish between latent and active infection. The TST (also called the Mantoux test) involves the intradermal injection of TB antigens (i.e. purified protein derivatives, PPD) and evaluation after 48–72 hours for the presence of a local inflammatory response. The transverse diameter of the induration (not erythema) is measured and interpreted based on pretest probabilities (Box 39.2) [13]. IGRAs are *in vitro* blood tests that measure the T-lymphocyte response to *M. tuberculosis*-specific antigens [14]. Because these tests are relatively new, data on risk-stratified cut-offs and performance in high-risk populations are lacking. Although more costly than TST, IGRAs have greater specificity.

EMPIRIC TREATMENT OF TUBERCULOSIS

Given the challenges in diagnosing smear-negative TB, it is sometimes necessary to initiate empiric TB treatment. In such cases, TB treatment should be started if the patient reports a subacute history of constitutional symptoms and radiographic and diagnostic tests are consistent

TABLE 39-4 Characteristics of Novel Methods to Diagnose Tuberculosis (TB) and Drug-resistant TB

Method	Characteristics
Nitrate reductase method	Low-cost, simple assay in which *Mycobacterium tuberculosis* reduces nitrate to nitrate, resulting in color change when detection reagent added to tube. Pooled sensitivity/specificity for direct drug susceptibility testing (DST) 99%/100% for Rifampin (R) and 94%/100% for Isoniazid (H). Pooled sensitivity/specificity for indirect DST 97%/100% for R and 96%/99% for H. Turn-around time 14–21 days.
Microscopic observation drug susceptibility assay (MODS)	Low-cost, simple assay in which liquid culture allows early visualization of cord-like structures using inverted microscope. Performs well on smear-negative samples. Pooled sensitivity/specificity for direct DST for detecting resistance to R and H: 96%/96% and 92%/96% respectively. Turn-around time approximately 21 days.
Genotype MTBDRplus (Hain Life Sciences, Nehren, Germany)	Molecular test similar to Genotype MTBDR, but detects a wider array of *rpoB* and *katG/inhA* mutations associated with resistance to R and H. Specialized equipment required. Risk of DNA contamination in laboratory. Pooled sensitivity/specificity for direct DST for detecting resistance to R and H: 99%/99% and 96%/100% respectively; turnaround time 1–2 days.
INNO-LiPA Rif TB assay (Immunogenetics, Ghent, Belgium)	Line probe assay to detect most common *rpoB* mutations associated with R resistance. Specialized equipment required. Risk of DNA contamination in laboratory. Pooled sensitivity/specificity of both direct and indirect assays were 97%/99% for detecting R resistance. Turnaround time 1–2 days.

BOX 39.2 Criteria for Positive Tuberculin Skin Test (TST) by Risk Group

Response with ≥5 mm induration

HIV positive persons

Recent contacts of TB case patients

Fibrotic changes on chest X-ray consistent with TB

Patients with organ transplants and other immunosuppressed patients receiving the equivalent of 15 mg/dl of prednisone for 1 month or more*

Response with ≥10 mm induration

Recent immigrants (i.e., within the last 5 years) from high prevalence countries

Injection drug users

Residents or employees† of the following high-risk congregate settings: prisons and jails, nursing homes and other long-term facilities for the elderly, hospital and other health care facilities, residential facilities for patients with AIDS, and homeless shelters

Mycobacteriology laboratory personnel

Persons with the following clinical conditions that place them at high risk: silicosis, diabetes mellitus, chronic renal failure, some hematologic disorders (e.g., leukemias and lymphomas), other specific malignancies (e.g., carcinoma of the head, neck and lung), weight loss ≥ 10% of ideal body weight, gastrectomy, and jejunoileal bypass

Child younger than 4-years of age or infants, children, and adolescents exposed to adults at high risk

Response with ≥15 mm induration

Persons with no risk factors for TB

Source: American Thoracic Society. Targeted tuberculin testing and treatment of latent tuberculosis infection. American Thoracic Society. MMWR Recomm Rep. 2000 Jun 9;49(RR-6):1–51.

*Risk of TB in patients treated with corticosteroids increases with a higher dose and longer duration.

†For persons who are otherwise at low risk and are tested at the start of employment, a 15 mm induration response or higher is considered positive.

with TB, and alternative diagnoses are not obvious. For individuals with chronic cough, a trial of antibiotic therapy may be attempted prior to empiric TB treatment. In such cases, agents with anti-mycobacterial activity, such as fluoroquinolones, should be avoided. In high-burden TB settings, there should be a low threshold for empiric TB treatment, especially if the patient is ill or HIV-positive.

MONITORING TREATMENT RESPONSE

With effective treatment, patients experience rapid improvement in constitutional symptoms followed by a gradual decrease in cough and sputum production. Smear microscopy is a simple way to monitor treatment for cases with initially smear-positive disease. Sputum is generally smear-negative by the end of the first month of treatment; over 90% will be smear-negative after two months of regular treatment.

Any suggestion that the patient is not responding to treatment by the second month of treatment should trigger immediate re-evaluation (Table 39-5). Adherence to treatment can be assessed by careful, non-judgemental inquiry of the patient, family and providers. Drug-resistant TB should be considered, especially in settings with significant rates of primary TB and/or individuals with suboptimal treatment adherence. Patients with drug-resistant TB, even MDR-TB, may initially respond favorably to first-line TB drugs. Paradoxical worsening soon after the start of therapy may be observed. This is more common among HIV-positive individuals, in particular shortly after initiation of anti-retroviral therapy (i.e. immune reconstitution syndrome [15, 16]). However, paradoxical responses can be observed in immunocompetent individuals, including up to 10% of individuals with CNS TB. HIV-positive patients may also have other AIDS-related complications that confuse the clinical picture. More than one issue can contribute to failure to clinically respond to TB treatment in a single patient. Furthermore, in smear-negative disease, confirming a definitive diagnosis can be challenging. It is often necessary to provide empiric treatment for several likely diagnoses. In patients who are clinically unstable, hospitalization may be necessary to assess the patient carefully and quickly.

TREATMENT

TB treatment has been extensively studied in controlled clinical trials, which support the use of multidrug regimens along with measures to ensure optimal treatment adherence [17–19]. Therapy generally consists of an "intensive phase" with daily administration of at least four anti-tuberculous drugs, followed by "continuation phase" involving daily or intermittent therapy with a reduced number of drugs. A summary of anti-tuberculosis drugs and drug interactions is provided in Tables 39-6–39-12, which appear online [20, 21].

TABLE 39-5 Common Causes of Failure to Respond to Tuberculosis (TB) Treatment

Causes	Evaluations	Action
Poor adherence	Interview patient, family, health workers; count pills; verify signs and symptoms associated with drug ingestion (e.g. dark urine – rifampin)	Reinforce education, directly observed treatment (DOT)
Drug-resistant TB	Repeat culture and drug susceptibility testing (DST); close clinical monitoring	Empiric second-line TB treatment if patient is clinically unstable or once drug-resistance confirmed
HIV-related opportunistic infections	HIV testing; CD4; viral load; symptom-directed diagnosis of opportunistic infections	Early initiation of HAART; treatment of opportunistic infections
Malnutrition	Close monitoring of weight (and height in children); serum albumin	Nutritional supplementation
Paradoxical response	Rule out other causes of deterioration	Continue with treatment; for HIV-positive individuals consider use of corticosteroids

HAART, highly active anti-retroviral therapy.

TABLE 39-6 Anti-tuberculous Medications and their Side Effects

Drug name (abbreviation)	Description and adult dose	Side effects	Monitoring requirements and comments
Isoniazid (H)	Description: bactericidal; inhibits mycolic acid synthesis most effectively in dividing cells; hepatically metabolized Dose: 300 mg/day or 900 mg/day twice or thrice weekly	Common: hepatitis (10–20% have elevated of transaminases), peripheral neuropathy (dose-related; increased risk with malnutrition, alcoholism, diabetes, concurrent use of aminoglycoside (AG) or ethionamide (ETO) Less common: gynecomastia, rash, psychosis, seizure	Monitoring: consider baseline and monthly aspartate aminotransferase (SGOT), especially if age greater than 50 years Comments: give with pyridoxine 50 mg/day if using large dose or if patient is at risk for peripheral neuropathy (diabetes, alcoholism, HIV, etc.)
Rifamycins Rifampicin (R) (Rifampin) Rifabutin (Rfb)	Description: bactericidal; inhibits protein synthesis by blocking mRNA transcription and synthesis; hepatically metabolized Dose: R: 600 mg/ day; Rfb 300 mg/day	Common: orange-colored bodily secretions, transient transaminitis, hepatitis, gastrointestinal (GIT) distress Less common: cholestatic jaundice	Monitoring: baseline SGOT and bilirubin, repeat if symptoms (jaundice, fatigue, anorexia, weakness, or nausea and vomiting for more than three days)
Pyrazinamide (Z)	Description: bactericidal; mechanism unclear; effective in acidic milieu (e.g. cavitary disease, intracellular organisms); hepatically metabolized, renally excreted Dose: 15–30 mg/kg/day	Common: arthritis/arthralgias, hepatotoxicity, hyperuricemia, adominal distress Less common: impaired diabetic control, rash	Monitoring: Baseline and monthly SGOT; uric acid can be measured if arthalgias, arthritis, or symptoms of gout are present Comments: usually given once daily, but can split dose initially to improve tolerance
Ethambutol (E)	Description: bacteriostatic at conventional dosing (15 mg/kg); inhibits lipid and cell wall metabolism; renally excreted Dose: 15–25 mg/kg, consider decreasing to 15 mg/kg once patient is culture-negative	Common: generally well-tolerated Less common: optic neuritis, GI distress, arthritis/arthralgia	Monitoring: baseline and monthly visual acuity and red/green color vision test when dosed at greater than 15 mg/kg/day (more than 10% loss is considered significant); regularly question patient about visual symptoms

TABLE 39-6 Anti-tuberculous Medications and their Side Effects—cont'd

Drug name (abbreviation)	Description and adult dose	Side effects	Monitoring requirements and comments
Aminoglycosides (AG) Amikacin (AMK) Kanamycin (K) Streptomycin (S) Polypeptides: Capreomycin (CM) Viomycin (VM)	Description: bactericidal; aminogycosides inhibit protein synthesis through disruption of ribosomal function; less effective in acidic, intracellular environments; polypeptides appear to inhibit translocation of the peptidyl-tRNA and the initiation of protein synthesis; renally excreted Dose: 15–20 mg/kg/day	Common: pain at injection site, proteinuria, serum electrolyte disturbances Less common: cochlear otoxocity (hearing loss, dose-related to cumulative and peak concentrations, increased risk with renal insufficiency, may be irreversible), nephrotoxicity (dose-related to cumulative and peak concentrations, increased risk with renal insufficiency, often irreversible), peripheral neuropathy, rash, vestibular toxicity (nausea, vomiting, vertigo, ataxia, nystagmus), eosinophilia Otoxocity potentiated by certain diuretics, especially loop diuretics	Monitoring: baseline and then bi-weekly creatinine, urea, and serum potassium; more frequently in high risk patients. If potassium is low, check magnesium and calcium. Baseline audiometry and monthly monitoring in high risk patients (high risk patients – elderly, diabetic or HIV-positive patients, or patients with renal insufficiency) Comments: observe for problems with balance; increase dosing interval or reduce dose and monitor serum drug concentrations as needed to control side effects Electrolyte disturbances are more common in patients receiving CM
Fluoroquinolones Ciprofloxacin (CPX) Ofloxacin (OFX) Levofloxacin (LFX) Moxifloxacin (MFX)	Description: bactericidal; DNA-gyrase inhibitor; renally excreted Dose: Ciprofloxacin 1500 mg/day Ofloxacin 800 mg/day Levofloxacin 750 mg/day Moxifloxacin 400 mg/day	Common: generally well-tolerated, well-absorbed Less common: diarrhea, dizziness, GI distress, headache, insomnia, photosensitivity, rash, vaginitis, psychosis, seizure [central nervous system (CNS) effects seen almost exclusively in elderly]; synotenovitis	Monitoring: no laboratory monitoring requirements Comments: do not administer with antacids, sucralfate, iron, zinc, calcium, or oral potassium and magnesium replacements; LFX, MFX have the most activity against *Mycobacterium tuberculosis*
Cycloserine (CS)	Description: bacteriostatic; alanine analogue; interferes with cell-wall proteoglycan synthesis; renally excreted Dose: 500–1000 mg/day (initiate at 500 mg/day for 2–3 days then gradually increase to full dose)	Common: neurologic and psychiatric disturbances, including headaches, irritability, sleep disturbances, aggression, and tremors Less common: psychosis, peripheral neuropathy, seizures (increased risk of CNS effects with concurrent use of ethanol, H, ETO, or other centrally-acting medications), hypersensitivity	Monitoring: consider serum drug monitoring to establish optimal dosing Comments: give 50 mg for every 250 mg of CS (to lessen neurologic adverse effects)
Thiamides Ethionamide (ETO) Prothionamide (PTO)	Description: may be bactericidal or bacteriostatic depending on susceptibility and concentrations attained at the infection site; the carbotionamide group, also found on thiacetazone, and the pyridine ring, also found on H, appear essential for activity; hepatically metabolized, renally excreted Dose: 500–1000 mg/day (initiate at 500 mg/day for 2–3 days then gradually increase to full dose)	Common: GI distress (nausea, vomiting, diarrhea, abdominal pain, loss of appetite), dysgeusia (metallic taste), hypothyroidism (especially when taken with PAS) Less common: arthralgias, dermatitis, gynecomastia, hepatitis, impotence, peripheral neuropathy, photosensitivity	Monitoring: consider baseline and monthly SGOT Comments: may split dose or give at bedtime to improve tolerability; ETO and PTO efficacies are considered similar; PTO may cause fewer GI side effects
Para-aminosalicylic acid (PAS)	Description: bacteriostatic; disrupts folic acid metabolism (thought to inhibit the biosynthesis of co-enzyme F in the folic acid pathway); hepatic acetylation, renally excreted. Dose: 150 mg/day divided into 3 doses	Common: GI distress (nausea, vomiting, diarrhea), hypersensitivity, hypothyroidism (especially when taken with ETO) Less common: hepatitis, electrolyte abnormalities Drug interactions: decreased H acetylation, decreased R absorption in non-granular preparation, decreased B12 uptake	Monitoring: no laboratory monitoring requirements Comments: some formulas of enteric coated granules need to be administered with an acidic food or beverage (i.e. yogurt or acidic juice)

Adapted from PIH Guide to the Medical Management of Multidrug-Resistant Tuberculosis. Boston: Partners In Health; 2004. Available at: http://ftp.pih.org/inforesources/pihguide-mdrtb.html

TABLE 39-7 Pediatric Dosing of Tuberculosis Drugs

Medication (abbreviation)	Dose	Maximum daily dose
Isoniazid (H)	4–6 mg/kg daily or 8–12 mg 3 × wk	300 mg
Rifampin (R)	10–20 mg/kg daily	600 mg
Ethambutol (E)	25 mg/kg daily	1200 mg
Pyrazinamide (Z)	30–40 mg/kg daily	1500 mg
Streptomycin (S)	20–40 mg/kg daily	1000 mg
Kanamycin (Km)	15–30 mg/kg daily	1000 mg
Capreomycin (Cm)	15–30 mg/kg daily	1000 mg
Ofloxacin (Ofx)	15–20 mg/kg daily	800 mg
Levofloxacin (Lfx)	15–25 mg/kg daily	1000 mg
Moxifloxacin (Mfx)	7.5–10 mg/kg daily	400 mg
Ethionamide (Eto)	15–20 mg/kg daily	1000 mg
Cycloserine (Cs)	10–20 mg/kg daily	1000 mg
Para-aminosalicylic acid (PAS)	150 mg/kg daily	8 g (PASER™)

PASER, C.
From the World Health Organization's Guidelines for the Programmatic Management of Drug-resistant Tuberculosis, , Emergency Update 2008.

TABLE 39-8 World Health Organization(WHO) Recommended Use of Fixed-dose Combinations for First-line Treatment for Adults

Weight	Initial phase (two months)	Continuation phase (four months)
	2 (HRZE)	4 (HR)
	Daily 56 total doses	Daily 112 total doses
	(Isoniazid 75 mg + rifampin 150 mg + pyrazinamide 400 mg + ethambutol 275 mg)	(Isoniazid 75 mg + rifampin 150 mg)
30–39 kg	2	2
40–54 kg	3	3
55–70 kg	4	4
Over 70 kg	5	5

HR, Isoniazid & Rifampin; HRZE, Isoniazid, Rifampin, Pyrazinamide, Ethambutol.
From WHO Tuberculosis Care with TB-HIV Co-management, 2007.

TABLE 39-9 Recommendations for Concomitant Treatment of Tuberculosis (TB) and HIV Infection

Combined regimen for treatment of HIV and tuberculosis	PK effect of the rifamycin	Tolerability/ toxicity	Antiviral activity when used with rifampin	Recommendation (comments)
Efavirenz-based ART* with rifampin-based TB treatment	Well-characterized, modest effect	Low rates of discontinuation	Excellent	Preferred (efavirenz should not be used during the first trimester of pregnancy)
PI-based ART* with rifabutin-based TB treatment	Little effect of rifabutin on PI concentrations, but marked increases in rifabutin concentrations	Low rates of discontinuation (if rifabutin is appropriately dose-reduced)	Favorable, though published clinical experience is not extensive	Preferred for patients unable to take efavirenz†
Nevirapine-based ART with rifampin-based TB treatment	Moderate effect	Concern about hepatotoxicity when used with isoniazid, rifampin and pyrazinamide	Favorable	Alternative for patients who cannot take efavirenz and if rifabutin not available
Zidovudine/ lamivudine/ abacavir/ tenofovir with rifampin-based TB treatment	50% decrease in zidovudine, possible effect on abacavir not evaluated	Anemia	No published clinical experience	Alternative for patients who cannot take efavirenz and if rifabutin not available
Zidovudine/ lamivudine / tenofovir with rifampin-based TB treatment	50% decrease in zidovudine, no other effects predicted	Anemia	Favorable, but not evaluated in a randomized trial	Alternative for patients who cannot take efavirenz and if rifabutin not available
Zidovudine/ lamivudine/ abacavir with rifampin-based TB treatment	50% decrease in zidovudine, possible effect on abacavir not evaluated	Anemia	Early favorable experience, but this combination is less effective that efavirenz-based regimens in persons not taking rifampin	Alternative for patients who cannot take efavirenz and if rifabutin not available
Super-boosted lopinavir-based ART with rifampin-based TB treatment	Little effect	Hepatitis among healthy adults, but favorable experience among young children (<3 years)	Good among young children (<3 years)	Alternative if rifabutin not available; preferred for young children when rifabutin not available

*with two nucleoside analogues.
†includes patients with non-nucleoside reverse transcriptase inhibitor (NNRTI)-resistant HIV, those unable to tolerate efavirenz, women during the first 1–2 trimesters of pregnancy.
ART, antiretroviral therapy.
Managing Drug Interactions in the Treatment of HIV-related Tuberculosis. Centers for Disease Control and Prevention; 2007. Available at: www.cdc.gov/tb/publications/guidelines/TB_HIV_Drugs/default.htm

TABLE 39-10 Recommendations for Co-administration of Antiretroviral Drugs with Rifampin

Non-nucleoside reverse transcriptase inhibitors			
	Recommended change in dose of antiretroviral drug	***Recommended change in dose of rifampin***	***Comments***
Efavirenz	None (some experts recommend 800 mg for patients >60 kg)	No change (600 mg/day)	Efavirenz AUC ↓ by 22%; no change in rifampin concentration. Efavirenz should not be used during the first trimester of pregnancy
Nevirapine	No change	No change (600 mg/day)	Nevirapine AUC ↓ 37–58% and Cmin ↓ 68% with 200 mg 2x/day dose
Delavirdine	Rifampin and Delavirdine should not be used together		Delavirdine AUC ↓ by 95%
Etravirine	Rifampin and x should not be used together		Marked decrease in etravirine predicted, based on data on the interaction with rifabutin
Single protease inhibitors			
	Recommended change in dose of antiretroviral drug	***Recommended change in dose of rifampin***	***Comments***
Ritonavir	No change	No change (600 mg/day)	↓ by 35%; no change in rifampin concentration. Monitor for antiretroviral activity of ritonavir.
fos-Amprenavir	Rifampin and fos-Amprenavir should not be used together		
Atazanavir	Rifampin and Atazanavir should not be used together		Atazanavir AUC ↓ by >95%
Indinavir	Rifampin and Indinavir should not be used together		Indinavir AUC ↓ by 89%
Nelfinavir	Rifampin and Nelfinavir should not be used together		Nelfinavir AUC ↓ by 82%
Saquinavir	Rifampin and Saquinavir should not be used together		Saquinavir AUC ↓ by 84%
Dual protease-inhibitor combinations			
	Recommended change in dose of antiretroviral drug	***Recommended change in dose of rifampin***	***Comments***
Saquinavir/ ritonavir	Saquinavir 400 mg plus ritonavir 400 mg twice daily	No change (600 mg/day)	Use with caution; the combination of saquinavir (1000 mg twice daily), ritonavir (100 mg twice daily), and rifampin caused unacceptable rates of hepatitis among healthy volunteers.
Lopinavir/ ritonavir (Kaletra™)	Increase the dose of lopinavir/ ritonavir (Kaletra™) – 4 tablets (200 mg of lopinavir with 50 mg of ritonavir) twice daily	No change (600 mg/day)	Use with caution; this combination resulted in hepatitis in all adult healthy volunteers in an initial study
"Super-boosted" lopinavir/ ritonavir (Kaletra™)	Lopinavir/ ritonavir (Kaletra™) – 2 tablets (200 mg of lopinavir with 50 mg of ritonavir) + 300 mg of ritonavir twice daily	No change (600 mg/day)	Use with caution; this combination resulted in hepatitis among adult healthy volunteers. However, there are favorable pharmacokinetic and clinical data among young children
CCR-5 receptor agonists			
	Recommended change in dose of antiretroviral drug	***Recommended change in dose of rifampin***	***Comments***
Maraviroc	Increase maraviroc to 600 mg twice-daily	No change (600 mg/day)	Maraviroc Cmin ↓ by 78%. No reported clinical experience with increased dose of maraviroc with rifampin
Integrase inhibitors			
	Recommended change in dose of antiretroviral drug	***Recommended change in dose of rifampin***	***Comments***
Raltegravir	No change	No change (600 mg/day)	No clinical experience; raltegravir concentrations ↓ by 40–61%

Managing Drug Interactions in the Treatment of HIV-related Tuberculosis. Centers for Disease Control and Prevention; 2007. Available at: www.cdc.gov/tb/publications/guidelines/TB_HIV_Drugs/default.htm

TABLE 39-11 Recommendations for Co-administration of Anti-retroviral Drugs with Rifabutin

Non-nucleoside reverse-transcriptase inhibitors			
	Antiretroviral dose change	*Rifabutin dose change*	*Comments*
Efavirenz	No change	↑ to 450–600 mg (daily or intermittent)	Rifabutin AUC ↓ by 38%. Effect of efavirenz + protease inhibitor(s) on rifabutin concentration has not been studied. Efavirenz should not be used during the 1st trimester of pregnancy.
Nevirapine	No change	No change (300 mg daily or thrice weekly)	Rifabutin and nevirapine AUC not significantly changed.
Delavirdine	Rifabutin and delavirdine should not be used together		Delavirdine AUC ↓ by 70%; rifabutin AUC ↑ by 100%.
Etravirine	No change	No change (300 mg daily or thrice weekly)	No clinical experience; etravirine Cmin ↓ by 45%, but this was not thought to warrant a change in dose
Single protease inhibitors			
	Antiretroviral dose change	*Rifabutin dose change*	*Comments*
fos-Amprenavir	No change	↓ to 150 mg/day or 300 mg 3x/week	No published clinical experience
Atazanavir	No change	↓ to 150 mg every other day or 3x/week	No published clinical experience. Rifabutin AUC ↑ by 250%
Indinavir	1000 mg every 8 hours	↓ to 150 mg/day or 300 mg 3x/week	Rifabutin AUC ↑ by 170%; indinavir concentrations ↓ by 34%
Nalfinavir	No change	↓ to 150 mg/day or 300 mg 3x/week	Rifabutin AUC ↑ by 207%; insignificant change in nelfinavir concentration
Dual protease-inhibitor combinations			
	Recommended change in dose of antiretroviral drug	*Recommended change in dose of rifampin*	*Comments*
Lopinavir/ ritonavir (Kaletra™)	No change	↓ to 150 mg every other day or 3x/week	Rifabutin AUC ↑ by 303%; 25-O-des-acetyl rifabutin AUC ↑ by 47.5 fold.
Ritonavir (any dose), with saquinavir, indinavir, amprenavir, fos-amprenavir, atazanavir, tipranavir or darunavir	No change	↓ to 150 mg every other day or 3x/week	Rifabutin AUC ↑ and 25-O-des-acetyl rifabutin AUC ↑, by varying degrees
CCR-5 receptor agonists			
	Recommended change in dose of antiretroviral drug	*Recommended change in dose of rifampin*	*Comments*
Maraviroc	No change	No change	No clinical experience; a significant interaction is unlikely, but this has not yet been studied
Integrase inhibitors			
Raltegravir	No change	No change	No clinical experience; a significant interaction is unlikely, but this has not yet been studied

Managing Drug Interactions in the Treatment of HIV-related Tuberculosis. Centers for Disease Control and Prevention; 2007. Available at: www.cdc.gov/tb/publications/guidelines/TB_HIV_Drugs/default.htm

TABLE 39-12 Overlapping Toxicities of Anti-retroviral and Tuberculosis (TB) Drugs

Toxicity	Anti-retroviral agent (ARV)	Anti-tuberculosis agent	Comments
Peripheral neuropathy	**Stavudine (D4T), didanosine (ddI), zalcitabine (ddC)**	**Linezolid (Lzd), Cs, H,** Aminoglycosides, Eto/Pto, E	Avoid use of D4T, ddI and ddC in combination with Cs or Lzd because of theoretically increased peripheral neuropathy. If these agents must be used and peripheral neuropathy develops, replace the antiretroviral agent with a less neurotoxic agent.
Central nervous system (CNS) toxicity	**Efavirenz (EFV)**	**Cs**, H, Eto/Pto, Fluoroquinolones	Efavirenz has a high rate of CNS side-effects (confusion, impaired concentration, depersonalization, abnormal dreams, insomnia, and dizziness) in the first 2–3 weeks, which typically resolve on their own. If the CNS side-effects do not resolve on their own consider substitution of the agent. At present, there are limited data on the use of EFV with Cs; concurrent use is accepted practice with frequent monitoring for CNS toxicity. Frank psychosis is rare with EFV alone.
Depression	**EFV**	**Cs**, Fluoroquinolones, H, Eto/Pto	Severe depression can be seen in 2.4% of patients receiving EFV*; Consider substituting EFV if severe depression develops. The severe socioeconomic circumstances of many patients with chronic disease can also contribute to depression.
Headache	**Zidovudine (AZT), EFV**	**Cs**	Rule out more serious causes of headache such as bacterial meningitis, cryptococcal meningitis, CNS toxoplasmosis, etc. Use of analgesics (ibuprofen, paracetamol) and hydration may help. Headache secondary to AZT, EFV and Cs is usually self-limited.
Nausea and vomiting	**Ritonavir (RTV), D4T**, nevirapine (NVP), and most others	**Eto/Pto, PAS, H, E, Z** and others	Nausea and vomiting are common adverse effects and can be managed. Persistent vomiting and abdominal pain may be a result of developing lactic acidosis and/or hepatitis secondary to medications.
Abdominal pain	**All HAART has been associated with abdominal pain**	**Eto/Pto, PAS**	Abdominal pain is a common adverse effect and often benign; however, abdominal pain may be an early symptom of severe adverse effects such as pancreatitis, hepatitis or lactic acidosis.
Pancreatitis	**D4T, ddI, ddC**	**Lzd**	Avoid use of these agents together. If an agent causes pancreatitis suspend it permanently and do not use any of the pancreatitis-producing anti-HIV medications (D4T, ddI, or ddC) in the future. Also consider gallstones or alcohol as a potential cause of pancreatitis.
Diarrhea	**All protease inhibitors, ddI (buffered formula)**	**Eto/Pto, PAS**, Fluoroquinolones	Diarrhea is a common adverse effect. Also consider opportunistic infections as a cause of diarrhea or *Clostridium difficile* (a cause of pseudomembranous colitis).
Hepatotoxicity	**NVP, EFV, all protease inhibitors (RTV > other protease inhibitors), all nucleoside reverse transcriptase inhibitors (NRTIs)**	**H, R, E, Z,** PAS, Eto/Pto, Fluoroquinolones	Also consider TMP/SMX as a cause of hepatotoxicity if the patient is receiving this medication. Also rule out viral etiologies as cause of hepatitis (Hepatitis A, B, C, and cytomegalovirus).
Skin rash	**Abacavir (ABC), NVP, EFV, D4T** and others	**H,R, Z, PAS,** Fluoroquinolones, and others	Do not re-challenge with ABC (can result in life threatening anaphylaxis). Do not re-challenge with an agent that caused Steven-Johnson syndrome. Also consider TMP/SMX as a cause of skin rash if the patient is receiving this medication. Thioacetazone is contraindicated in HIV because of life-threatening rash.
Lactic acidosis	**D4T, ddI, AZT, lamuvidine (3TC)**	**Lzd**	If an agent causes lactic acidosis replace it with an agent less likely to cause lactic acidosis.
Renal toxicity	Tenofovir (TDF) (rare)	**Aminoglycosides, Cm**	TDF may cause renal injury with the characteristic features of Fanconi syndrome, hypophosphatemia, hypouricemia, proteinuria, normoglycemic glycosuria and in some cases acute renal failure. There are no data on the concurrent use of TDF with aminoglycosides or Cm. Use TDF with caution in patients receiving aminoglycosides or Cm. Even without the concurrent use of TDF, HIV-infected patients have an increased risk of renal toxicity secondary to aminoglycosides and Cm. Frequent creatinine and electrolyte monitoring every 1–3 weeks is recommended. Many antivirals and anti-tuberculosis medications need to be dose adjusted for renal insufficiency.

Continued

TABLE 39-12 Overlapping Toxicities of Anti-retroviral and Tuberculosis (TB) Drugs—cont'd

Toxicity	Anti-retroviral agent (ARV)	Anti-tuberculosis agent	Comments
Nephrolithiasis	**Indinavir (IDV)**	None	No overlapping toxicities regarding nephrolithiasis have been documented between anti-retroviral therapy (ART) and anti-tuberculosis medications. Adequate hydration prevents nephrolithiasis in patients taking IDV. If nephrolithiasis develops while on IDV, substitute with another protease inhibitor if possible.
Electrolyte disturbances	TDF (rare)	**Cm, Aminoglycosides**	Diarrhea and/or vomiting can contribute to electrolyte disturbances. Even without the concurrent use of TDF, HIV-infected patients have an increased risk of both renal toxicity and electrolyte disturbances secondary to aminoglycosides and Cm.
Bone marrow suppression	AZT	**Lzd**, R, Rfb, H	Monitor blood counts regularly. Replace AZT if bone marrow suppression develops. Consider suspension of Lzd. Also consider TMP/SMX as a cause if the patient is receiving this medication. Consider adding folinic acid supplements, especially if receiving TMP/SMX.
Optic neuritis	ddl	**E**, Eto/Pto (rare)	Suspend agent responsible for optic neuritis permanently and replace with an agent that does not cause optic neuritis.
Hyperlipidemia	**Protease inhibitors, EFV**	None	No overlapping toxicities regarding hyperlipidemia have been documented between ART and anti-tuberculosis medications. Follow World Health Organization (WHO) ART guidelines for management of hyperlipidemia.
Lipodystrophy	**NRTIs (especially D4T and ddl**	None	No overlapping toxicities regarding lipodystrophy have been documented between ART and anti-tuberculosis medications. Follow WHO ART guidelines for management of lipdystrophy.
Dysglycemia (disturbed blood sugar regulation)	**Protease inhibitors**	**Gatifloxacin (Gfx)**, Eto/Pto	Protease inhibitors tend to cause insulin resistance and hyperglycemia. Eto/Pto tend to make insulin control in diabetics more difficult, and can result in hypoglycemia and poor glucose regulation. Gatifloxacin is no longer recommended for use in treatment of TB because of this side-effect.
Hypothyroidism	D4T	**Eto/Pto, PAS**	There is potential for overlying toxicity; however, evidence is mixed. Several studies show subclinical hypothyroidism associated with HAART, particularly stavudine. PAS and Eto/Pto, especially in combination, can commonly cause hypothyroidism.

*Bristol-Myers Squibb, letter to providers, March 2005.
HAART, highly active anti-retroviral therapy; TMP/SMX, trimethoprim-sulfamethoxazole; Lzd, linezolid, sometimes used to treat drug-resistant TB given in vitro activity against *Mycobacterium* tuberculosis.
Adapted from PIH Guide to the Medical Management of Multidrug-Resistant Tuberculosis. Boston: Partners In Health; 2004. Available at: http://ftp.pih.org/inforesources/pihguide-mdrtb.html.

TREATMENT OF PATIENTS WITH DRUG-SUSCEPTIBLE TUBERCULOSIS

Patients without a history of prior TB treatment and no risk factors for drug-resistant TB should be started on standard first-line treatment, i.e. "Category I" treatment (Table 39-13). Category I treatment is effective for almost all types of patients, including pregnant women, children, HIV-positive patients and patients with extrapulmonary TB. Use of isoniazid and ethambutol in the continuation phase is less effective than isoniazid/rifampin and should not be used. Fixed-dose combination tablets can simplify dosing and reduce the risk of partial nonadherence. In some cases, therapy should be prolonged. For individuals with baseline cavitary disease and positive culture at two months, the continuation phase should be extended by three additional months. Individuals with disseminated TB and/or involvement of bone or the CNS should receive a total of 9–12 months of therapy. Principles of TB treatment in HIV-positive individuals [22], children [23, 24] and pregnant women are outlined in Boxes 39.3, 39.4 and 39.5, respectively [25]. Most resource-poor settings use WHO criteria in determining treatment outcomes [18].

RETREATMENT REGIMENS AND THE TREATMENT OF INDIVIDUALS WITH DRUG-RESISTANT TUBERCULOSIS

Ideally, all individuals with TB and a history of prior TB treatment should be tested for drug resistance. If drug susceptibility testing (DST) is not available, prior treatment history and regional resistance data should inform the choice of empiric retreatment regimens. Individuals who were fully adherent to prior treatment and those who relapsed more than a year after treatment completion may still have drug-susceptible disease. For such individuals, Category I or Category II treatment, with aggressive measures to optimize adherence, may be appropriate.

For individuals with prior self-administration or nonadherence to TB treatment, acquired drug-resistance is a concern. Those who failed to respond to prior therapy (i.e. treatment failure, relapse within a year of treatment completion) are also likely to have drug resistance. In addition, treatment-naïve patients with strong epidemiologic risk factors for MDR-TB – such as close contact with a confirmed, or

TABLE 39-13 Common First-line Tuberculosis (TB) Treatment Regimens

World Health Organization diagnostic category	Types of TB patients in which it is commonly used	Initial phase	Continuation phase	Notes
Category I	New pulmonary and extrapulmonary TB, with or without HIV infection	2HRZE	4HR or $4(HR)_3$	
		$2(HRZE)_3$	$4(HR)_3$	Thrice-weekly administration in the intensive phase may be associated with increased risk of acquired drug resistance
		2HRZE	6HE	Associated with increased risk of death and treatment failure in clinical trials compared to rifampin used throughout the continuation phase
Category II	Previously treated sputum smear-positive pulmonary TB: relapse or treatment after default	2HRZES/1HRZE	5HRE	
		$2(HRZES)_3$/ $1(HRZE)_3$	$5(HRE)_3$	Thrice-weekly administration in the intensive phase has been associated with increased risk of acquired drug resistance in clinical trials.

Adapted from World Health Organization. Treatment of Tuberculosis: guidelines for national programmes. Geneva: World Health Organization; 2003.

BOX 39.3 Tuberculosis Treatment in HIV-Positive Individuals

- All individuals starting TB therapy should be tested for HIV.
- For cases with smear-negative disease, treatment should be initiated as soon as TB is suspected, even if bacteriologic confirmation is not possible.
- Drug interactions and overlapping toxicities among anti-retroviral and anti-tuberculosis drugs must be considered (see Tables 39-9 through 39-12). Efavirenz-containing anti-retroviral therapy (ART) with standard Category I treatment with rifampin is most commonly used.
- The following regimens for the continuation phase of Category I treatment should be avoided because of an increased risk of rifamycin resistance and treatment failure and/or relapse:
  - once-weekly isoniazid and rifapentine;
  - twice-weekly isoniazid and rifampin or twice-weekly isoniazid and rifabutin (strongest data for adverse outcomes if CD4 cell count <100 cells/μl).
- Duration of therapy is generally same as that for HIV-negative individuals; however, if slow clinical response, prolongation of continuation phase to seven months suggested.
- ART reduces mortality in TB patients. Regarding timing of ART initiation, studies support the initiation of ART as soon as possible after start of TB treatment to minimize morbidity and mortality regardless of CD4 cell count.
- Immune reconstitution syndrome – paradoxical exacerbation of TB symptoms, including unmasking of clinical symptoms associated with previously asymptomatic extrapulmonary sites. Although data from controlled trials are lacking, prednisone (e.g. 1–2 mg/kg per day for 1–2 weeks then tapered) for immune reconstitution syndrome may decrease morbidity, once alternative causes (e.g. other AIDS-related complications, drug-resistant TB, etc.) are ruled out.
- Thiazetazone should be avoided because of an increased risk of Stevens Johnson syndrome.

BOX 39.4 Tuberculosis Treatment in Children

- In children under four years of age, treatment should be initiated as soon as TB is suspected, even if bacteriologic confirmation is not possible.
- Ethambutol at 15–20 mg/kg per day can be used safely, even in young children. Four-drug regimens, rather than Isoniazid, Rifampin, and Pyrazinamide, should be used in circumstances where drug-resistance is a concern.
- For children with household contacts who: (i) have confirmed multidrug-resistant TB (MDR-TB); (ii) failed, or are failing, TB therapy; or (iii) died while receiving TB therapy, suspicion of primary drug-resistance should be high. In such cases, children should receive empiric MDR-TB therapy based on resistance and treatment data of the contact.

suspected, MDR-TB patient – should be considered for empiric MDR-TB therapy. For such cases, Category II treatment is unlikely to be effective and may even amplify resistance to first-line drugs by adding a "single drug to a failing regimen." Instead, such patients should receive empirical MDR-TB treatment (Box 39.6).

ADJUNCTIVE TREATMENTS

Systematic reviews of controlled trials demonstrate that steroids reduce mortality and long-term neurologic disability caused by meningeal TB [26]. Steroids for pleural TB bring about more rapid improvement, but do not have an impact on mortality or long-term outcomes [27]. Sufficient data to confirm the efficacy of steroids in other extra-pulmonary manifestations are lacking, but steroids are often used for cases of pericardial TB and non-meningeal manifestations of CNS TB. Based on anecdotal experience, steroids, in cases of laryngeal and ocular TB, are also selectively used. Steroids may also be used when paradoxical worsening is suspected to be caused by an inflammatory response. In these cases, every effort must be made to first rule-out drug-resistant TB, which can have an identical clinical presentation.

Surgery is another important adjunct to chemotherapy in the management of patients with TB, where resources are available. Debridement should be considered in cases of osteoarticular TB and extensive

BOX 39.5 Tuberculosis Treatment During Pregnancy and Breastfeeding

- Isoniazid, rifampin and ethambutol are considered safe during pregnancy and breastfeeding. Although detailed data for PZA are lacking, most consensus guidelines recommend its use during pregnancy and breastfeeding.
- Aminoglycosides (streptomycin, kanamycin and amikacin) and capreomycin can cause ototoxicity in the fetus and are not recommended during the first 20 weeks of pregnancy. These medications have minimal gastrointestinal absorption and are therefore considered safe during breastfeeding.
- Limited data are available on second-line anti-tuberculosis drugs. The fluoroquinolones, cycloserine and para-aminosalicylic acid have not been associated with teratogenic defects in human or animal studies at therapeutic doses. Teratogenic defects, including central nervous system defects, from thiamides have been observed in animal studies.
- Pyridoxine (25 mg/day) should be co-administered.
- Breastfeeding should not be discouraged in women who are smear-negative.

soft-tissue involvement (e.g. paraspinal cold abscess, TB of the breast). Finally, for individuals with a poor prognosis with chemotherapy alone (e.g. MDR-TB and XDR-TB), resection of localized lung lesions is recommended.

ADHERENCE

Patient adherence is the most important factor associated with success of TB treatment. Adherence is difficult because of the heavy pill burden and prolonged treatment. Patients should be educated before starting treatment about the importance of adherence and the danger of treatment failure and drug resistance. International consensus endorses the use of directly observed treatment (DOT), although efficacy data from controlled trials are equivocal [28]. DOT varies widely by program [29]. Patients may travel to a health facility for DOT; community health workers or outreach teams may visit patients to observe treatment; or community volunteers or family members may be trained to observe and record doses. Enhanced-DOT includes additional adherence strategies and has been shown to be more effective than DOT alone or self-administration [30]. Incentives and enablers include transportation reimbursement, cash transfers, case-management and outreach support. Nutritional supplementation can also increase adherence and may have an independent effect on treatment success, particularly in resource-limited settings where chronic malnutrition is rampant.

TREATMENT OF LATENT TUBERCULOSIS INFECTION

A number of regimens for treatment of patients with latent TB infection (LTBI) help prevent the development of active TB disease [31, 32]. The standard of care for treatment of latent TB infection – isoniazid 300 mg daily for 6–9 months – has been shown to be effective in preventing progression to active TB and has not been associated with the development of isoniazid resistance. Latent TB infection treatment policies vary widely. In settings with low TB prevalence, latent TB infection treatment is often recommended for all individuals with a positive tuberculin skin test (TST). In most high TB-prevalence settings, latent TB infection treatment is often limited to HIV-positive patients and pediatric household contacts of active TB cases. For

BOX 39.6 Principles of Treatment of Drug-Resistant Disease

- Individuals with drug resistance, excluding resistance to rifampin, can usually be treated with rifampin-containing multidrug regimens lasting nine months.
- For individuals with rifampin-resistance and/or multidrug-resistant TB (MDR-TB) [including extensively drug-resistant TB (XDR-TB)]:
  - consider individual or regional resistance patterns and prior treatment history when designing a regimen;
  - design a treatment regimen that includes at least four drugs that are likely to be effective, according to drug susceptibility testing (DST) and by treatment history. If the patient has advanced disease (e.g. extensive parenchymal destruction), consider use of 5–7 drugs;
  - use any oral first-line drugs to which the strain is susceptible and have not been used extensively in an previous regimen;
  - include an injectable drug to which the strain is susceptible. If resistant to all injectable drugs, use one the patient has never used before (expert opinion);
  - include a higher generation fluoroquinolone. If there is fluoroquinolone resistance, use a late-generation agent, such as moxifloxacin (expert opinion);
  - use any bacteriostatic, second-line drug (thiamides, cycloserine, or para-aminosalicylic acid) that are likely to be effective;
  - If four effective drugs are not available, consider other drugs with limited evidence of anti-TB activity (amoxicillin-clavulanic acid, linezolid, clarithromycin, etc.);
  - intensive phase (with daily injectable) should last ≥6 months from time of culture-conversion but can be prolonged if the patient has a highly resistant strain or slow clinical response. The continuation phase should last ≥12 months from time of culture-conversion;
  - pyridoxine should be co-administered.
- Consider adjunctive surgery if there is localized disease.
- Provide comprehensive monitoring and adherence support.

HIV-positive individuals, repeated or prolonged LTBI treatment may be useful in preventing re-infection. Furthermore, consensus on treatment of individuals at risk of latent MDR-TB infection is lacking. Some experts recommend the use of at least two drugs to which the infecting isolate is likely to be susceptible (based on contact or regional resistance data).

REFERENCES

1. Skolnik R. Essentials of Global Health. Sudbury: Jones & Bartlett Publishers; 2008.
2. World Health Organization. WHO Report 2009: Global Tuberculosis Control. Geneva: World Health Organization; 2009.
3. World Health Organization. Anti-Tuberculosis Drug Resistance in the World. Geneva: The WHO/IUATLD Global Project on Anti-Tuberculosis Drug Resistance Surveillance; 2008.
4. World Health Organization. Anti-tuberculosis Drug Resistance in the World: Report No. 4. Geneva: World Health Organization; 2008.
5. Senior K. Relentless spread of extensively drug-resistant tuberculosis. Lancet Infect Dis 2009;9:403.

6. Grzybowski S. Natural history of tuberculosis. Epidemiology. Bull Int Union Tuberc Lung Dis 1991;66:193–4.
7. Sharma SK, Mohan A. Extrapulmonary tuberculosis. Indian J Med Res 2004; 120:316–53.
8. Colebunders R, Bastian I. A review of the diagnosis and treatment of smear-negative pulmonary tuberculosis. Int J Tuberc Lung Dis 2000;4:97–107.
9. Goto M, Noguchi Y, Koyama H, et al. Diagnostic value of adenosine deaminase in tuberculous pleural effusion: a meta-analysis. Ann Clin Biochem 2003;40:374–81.
10. Bwanga F, Hoffner S, Haile M, Joloba ML. Direct susceptibility testing for multi drug resistant tuberculosis: a meta-analysis. BMC Infect Dis 2009;9:67.
11. Nyendak MR, Lewinsohn DA, Lewinsohn DM. New diagnostic methods for tuberculosis. Curr Opin Infect Dis 2009;22:174–82.
12. Ling DI, Zwerling AA, Pai M. GenoType MTBDR assays for the diagnosis of multidrug-resistant tuberculosis: a meta-analysis. Eur Respir J 2008;32: 1165–74.
13. Targeted tuberculin testing and treatment of latent tuberculosis infection. American Thoracic Society. MMWR Recomm Rep 2000;49:1–51.
14. Mazurek GH, Jereb J, Lobue P, et al. Guidelines for using the QuantiFERON-TB Gold test for detecting *Mycobacterium tuberculosis* infection, United States. MMWR Recomm Rep 2005;54:49–55.
15. Meintjes G, Rabie H, Wilkinson RJ, Cotton MF. Tuberculosis-associated immune reconstitution inflammatory syndrome and unmasking of tuberculosis by antiretroviral therapy. Clin Chest Med 2009;30:797–810.
16. Leone S, Nicastri E, Giglio S, et al. Immune reconstitution inflammatory syndrome associated with Mycobacterium tuberculosis infection: a systematic review. Int J Infect Dis 2010;14:e283–91.
17. Blumberg HM, Leonard Jr MK, Jasmer RM. Update on the treatment of tuberculosis and latent tuberculosis infection. JAMA 2005;293:2776–84.
18. World Health Organization. Treatment of Tuberculosis: guidelines for national programmes. Geneva: World Health Organization; 2003.
19. American Thoracic Society, Center for Disease Control and Prevention, Infectious Diseases Society of America. Treatment of Tuberculosis. MMWR Recomm Rep 2003;20;52:1–77.
20. Managing Drug Interactions in the Treatment of HIV-related Tuberculosis. Centers for Disease Control and Prevention; 2007. Available at: www.cdc.gov/tb/publications/guidelines/TB_HIV_Drugs/default.htm
21. PIH Guide to the Medical Management of Multidrug-Resistant Tuberculosis. Boston: Partners In Health; 2004. Available at: http://ftp.pih.org/inforesources/pihguide-mdrtb.html
22. El-Sadr WM, Tsiouris SJ. HIV-associated tuberculosis: diagnostic and treatment challenges. Semin Respir Crit Care Med 2008;29:525–31.
23. Marais BJ. Tuberculosis in children. Pediatr Pulmonol 2008;43:322–9.
24. Marais BJ, Gie RP, Schaaf HS, et al. Childhood pulmonary tuberculosis: old wisdom and new challenges. Am J Respir Crit Care Med 2006;173:1078–90.
25. Centers for Disease Control and Prevention. Prevention and treatment of tuberculosis among patients infected with human immunodeficiency virus: principles of therapy and revised recommendations. MMWR Recomm Rep 1998;47:1–58.
26. Prasad K, Singh MB. Corticosteroids for managing tuberculous meningitis. Cochrane Database Syst Rev 2008:CD002244.
27. Engel MF, Matchaba PT, Volmink J. Corticosteroids for tuberculous pleurisy. Cochrane Database Syst Rev 2007:CD001876.
28. Volmink J, Garner P. Directly observed therapy for treating tuberculosis. Cochrane Database Syst Rev 2007:CD003343.
29. Kangovi S, Mukherjee J, Bohmer R, Fitzmaurice G. A classification and meta-analysis of community-based Directly observed therapy programs for tuberculosis treatment in developing countries. J Community Health 2009;34: 506–13.
30. Chaulk CP, Kazandjian VA. Directly observed therapy for treatment completion of pulmonary tuberculosis: Consensus Statement of the Public Health Tuberculosis Guidelines Panel. JAMA 1998;279:943–8.
31. Prevention, C.f.D.C.a. Latent TB Infection (LTBI) Guideline Updates. 2009. Available at: http://www.cdc.gov/tb/publications/reportsarticles/mmwr/mmwr_updates.htm.
32. Marais BJ, Ayles H, Graham SM, Godfrey-Faussett P. Screening and preventive therapy for tuberculosis. Clin Chest Med 2009;30:827–46.
33. World Health Organization. Multidrug and extensively drug-resistant TB (M/XDR-TB): 2010 Global Report on Surveillance and Response. Geneva: World Health Organization; 2010.

Pertussis 40

Kevin Forsyth

Key features

- Pertussis (also called "whooping cough") is a highly contagious respiratory infection caused by *Bordetella pertussis* or *parapertussis*
- These organisms produce a potent toxin that causes disease
- Classically, pertussis manifests as a respiratory infection with a chronic cough that comes in paroxsyms, followed by post-tussive vomiting or an inspiratory "whoop"
- Young children can develop pneumonia, apnea and encephalopathy
- Pertussis affects 30–50 million humans each year, killing at least 200,000—mostly young children
- Diagnosis is usually based on a combination of clinical recognition, serology, PCR and culture
- Treatment does not usually affect the clinical course of pertussis, but treatment can interrupt transmission. Treatment usually involves macrolide antimicrobial such as erythromycin or a derivative
- A highly effective vaccine exists for all age groups and immunization is the primary mechanism of controlling pertussis
- Unfortunately, the World Health Organization (WHO) estimates that only 80% of children receive three doses of anti-pertussis vaccines, and very few adults in resource-limited settings receive anti-pertussis vaccines

INTRODUCTION

Pertussis is a debilitating respiratory disease that can affect humans throughout life, but pertussis has a particularly high mortality in infants less than 6 months of age. The mainstay of public health management is for widespread immunization approaches. This not only reduces individual cases of disease, but avoids epidemic disease.

Pertussis, commonly referred to as "whooping cough", is a highly contagious respiratory infection. It is caused by *Bordetella pertussis* or *Bordetella parapertussis* and is transmitted by respiratory droplets. It most commonly presents as a respiratory illness with rhinorrhea and fever, and can lead to pneumonia. A paroxysmal cough is common, often associated with an inspiratory "whoop". In young children, the clinical picture can be complicated by apnea, seizures and encephalopathy. The cough can become chronic, especially in older children and adults.

Control of pertussis rests largely upon immunization programs. Whole cell (wP) and acellular (aP)-based anti-pertussis vaccines exist in the form of combination anti-diphtheria and anti-tetanus vaccines (DTwP, DTaP). All infants should receive three doses of such vaccines in infancy, a booster at around 18 months and a further booster at pre-school age. Older children and adults should receive regular 10 year boosters with Tdap (the size of the letters corresponds with the amount of antigen contained in the vaccine). The WHO estimates that global vaccine coverage of young children with DTP-3 (completion of three doses) approximates 80%, and global coverage of older children and adults with Tdap is significantly lower [1] (Fig. 40.1).

EPIDEMIOLOGY

Pertussis is an important cause of vaccine-preventable deaths with approximately 200,000 deaths in children worldwide in 2008 [1]. Despite the fact that fewer than 150,000 cases are officially reported to the WHO each year, it is thought that globally, 30–50 million cases occur annually, 90% of which are in developing countries; many of the deaths occur during infancy. The very young, particularly those less than 6 months of age, are at particular risk from pertussis.

Global reported pertussis disease incident rates (some based on clinical confirmation only in those countries with limited access to laboratory services) are provided from WHO data in Table 40-1. These data will significantly under-represent actual cases.

In the USA, approximately 30,000 cases of pertussis are reported each year. Over the last 30 years, there has been an increase in reported cases of pertussis in the USA, especially among older children, teenagers and young adults, and also among children younger than 6 months of age [2].

Within Australia, a developed country of 20 million people with high vaccination rates, there is a national notifiable disease surveillance system that provides active surveillance data. During the period 1991–1996 there were 19,815 notifications of pertussis, which yielded a pertussis rate of 22–57.6 notifiable cases per 100,000 Australian populations [3]. Given that this estimate is for notifiable cases only, the real figure could be considerably higher (it is thought that true versus notified cases is in the order of up to 300-fold higher).

At a global level, there are, for example, a considerable number of cases identified in Afghanistan [4]. Pertussis is endemic in school age children in the UK where, in a prospective analysis of 172 children aged 5–16 years who presented at a general practitioner with a cough lasting 14 days or more, 37% had serologic evidence of a recent pertussis infection; of these, 86% had been fully immunized [5]. There are only occasional confirmed cases from China, although the true burden is not known [6].

In an analysis of immunization rates in the African region of the Expanded Immunization programme, DPT-3 coverage increased by 15% from 54% in 2000 to 69% in 2004, resulting in a decline in non-immunized children from 1.4 million in 2002 to 900,000 in 2004 [7] (Fig. 40.2).

There is increasing evidence that pertussis remains an active problem in communities whose young children are well immunized with DTP-3. In 2004, the Centers of Disease Control and Prevention

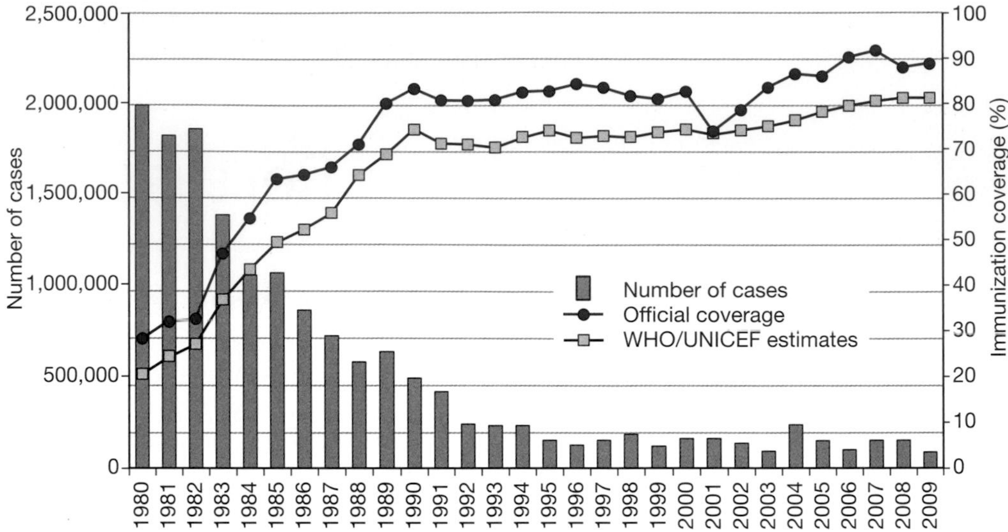

FIGURE 40.1 Pertussis global annual reported cases and DTP3 coverage (1980–2009).

TABLE 40-1 World Health Organization Regional and Global Summaries of Pertussis Incidence, 1980, 1990 and 1996–2005

	Year											
Location	1980	1990	1996	1997	1998	1999	2000	2001	2002	2003	2004	2005
Africa	367,961	89,515	35,682	12,101	38,961	11,066	52,008	50,386	19,452	16,418	26,335	22,139
Americas	123,763	38,009	17,901	16,496	28,375	22,089	18,144	12,811	15,162	12,756	26,194	8747
Eastern Mediterranean	171,631	27,437	2823	3210	4367	2840	2112	4257	2650	1161	81,987	5164
Europe	90,546	129,735	54,745	67,307	56,317	48,897	53,675	31,084	25,176	25,530	42,220	26,425
Southeast Asia	399,310	156,028	22,479	41,940	46,666	127,76	34,930	37,813	43,250	39,371	39,002	37,764
Western Pacific	829,173	35,653	8009	25,953	15,875	17947	25,282	32,182	30,682	11,348	21,106	21,560
Global	1,982,384	476,377	141,339	167,007	185,561	115,615	186,151	168,533	13,6372	106,584	236,844	121,799
Noumber of countries	151	164	155	163	151	156	159	162	162	150	165	156

(CDC) noted a 19-fold increase in the number of cases reported in individuals aged 10–19 years and a 16-fold increase in persons over 20 years of age. Data such as these are what has prompted the recommendation that anti-pertussis immunization not stop in young childhood (which was the previous recommendation).

NATURAL HISTORY, PATHOGENESIS AND PATHOLOGY

Following a usual incubation period of 5–10 days, individuals with clinical pertussis may manifest with a prodromal period lasting a few days to one week with upper respiratory symptoms (rhinorrhea, fever), followed by a hacking, paroxysmal cough. The second phase—the characteristic phase of pertussis with its coughing paroxysms—lasts 2–6 weeks, while the third phase—convalescence —may last up to 4 months: this phase is characterized by gradual reduction in coughing. The organisms of pertussis, *B. pertussis* and *B. parapertussis* (and, less commonly, *Bordetella bronchiseptica*) infect respiratory mucosa, leading to mucus hypersecretion and cilial paresis. The organisms release a number of toxins, the most important of which is the pertussis toxin. It is possible that the pertussis toxin acts within the central nervous system to exacerbate coughing fits. Hence, there are both central and local factors inducing cough.

CLINICAL MANIFESTATIONS

Pertussis is essentially a disease of the respiratory system. Initial symptoms consist of a runny nose and perhaps mild fever, but are quite nonspecific. This is considered the early phase of the disease, generally up to one week, followed by persistent coughing, which is the key feature of pertussis. The cough has a characteristic repetitive nature to it, with bursts of coughing triggered by a number of external factors, including cold air, exercise and inhaled irritants, or it can just occur spontaneously. One of the traps for the unwary clinician is that a parent can give a history typical of pertussis, describing particularly in a young infant a terrible repetitive cough. When examined by the doctor the child may appear to have no respiratory signs whatsoever and can be dismissed from the doctor's room only to have a spasm of coughing on going outside after receiving a blast of cold air as an irritant. Hence, history is critical in this condition—a history characterized by repetitive spasmodic coughing.

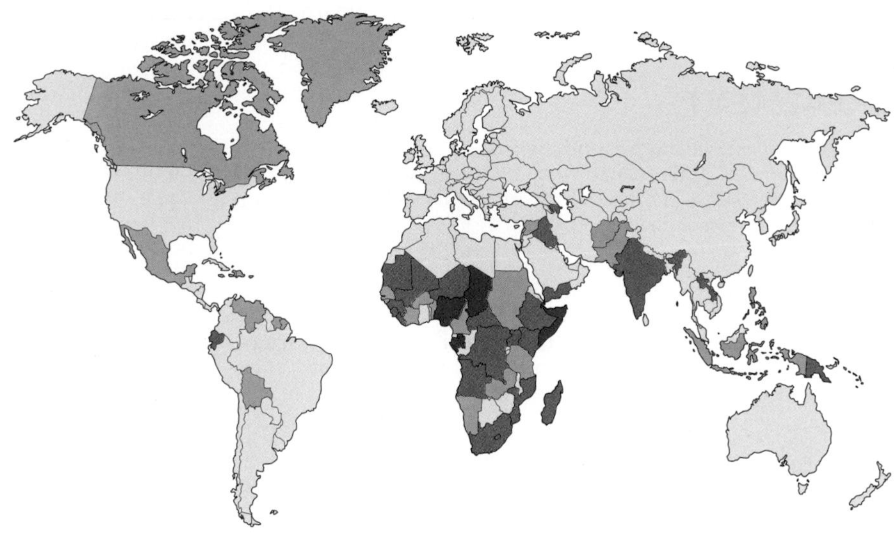

FIGURE 40.2 Immunization coverage with DTP3 vaccines in infants (2009).

The cough will, at times, lead to vomiting in a younger child, typically at the end of a period of coughing. At the end of a coughing bout there may be a sharp inspiration of air with the characteristic "whoop" sound. Any history of prolonged paroxysmal coughing followed by vomiting or whooping is highly characteristic of pertussis disease. The pertussis cough is sometimes colloquially termed "the 100 day cough". Interestingly, this cough may appear to disappear and then reoccur within six months or so of the primary infection when the patient is exposed to certain irritants or another unrelated respiratory infection.

It is important to emphasize that pertussis disease is particularly problematic in infants. Mortality rates for infants are high; they can present with atypical forms of the disease, such as apnea, encephalopathy or even multisystem organ failure unrelated to respiratory disease. Hence, early immunization of infants is critical. It is considered that three doses of vaccine are required to provide significant immunity to younger children. Three doses are not normally achieved until 5 or 6 months of age. Hence, infants in their first six months of life have little protection. In addition, they have small airways and appear highly vulnerable to the effects of pertussis toxin.

In addition to the clear respiratory manifestations of pertussis disease, there are also multiple side effects from this disease, for example subconjunctival hemorrhages caused by the force of the coughing, is characteristic of pertussis. There can also be pneumonia, encephalopathy and seizures.

PATIENT EVALUATION

CLINICAL DIAGNOSIS

There have been a number of different criteria used for the clinical definition of pertussis. The WHO definition of pertussis illness requires a paroxysmal cough lasting for at least 21 days and laboratory confirmation or contact with a culture-positive case. Unfortunately, this rather strict definition requires a fairly severe form of illness given the 21-day cough requirement and availability of laboratory diagnostics. Another definition that is in common use is of 14 days of cough, which can have a sensitivity of 84–92% and a specificity of 63–90% [8].

There may need to be different clinical criteria used for episodic cases in contrast to epidemic cases.

Given the elasticity in clinical case definition, where there are available laboratory diagnostics, a more substantive approach to diagnosis can be made through appropriate use of laboratory investigations.

LABORATORY DIAGNOSIS

The classical way to provide laboratory confirmation of *B. pertussis* is through the collection of a nasopharyngeal swab plated onto appropriate media. Although this approach gives high specificity, it has low sensitivity and is not practical for rapid diagnoses.

SEROLOGY

Serological diagnosis of pertussis by ELISA (using specific *B. pertussis* proteins as antigens) using paired sera with demonstration of a rise in antibodies of fourfold from the first sample to the second sample is the classical way to confirm infection by serology. However, this requires two blood tests and a delay in time which is not helpful for the acute diagnosis of pertussis. Hence, there have recently been moves to look at single serology estimates for the diagnosis of pertussis. Although different laboratories achieve different results, in general a single measurement of IgG ≥27 IU/ml can be considered appropriate for laboratory confirmation of clinical pertussis in adults in the first three weeks of an outbreak [9].

A more recent study [10] comparing high-sensitivity real time PCR assays and single serum pertussis serology showed that single serology was the most efficient diagnostic test with relatively high sensitivity (greater than 64%) and high specificity (greater than 90%). Using PCR, it was found that this was the second most efficient tool. An advantage of PCR is utilizing nasopharyngeal aspirates compared with blood.

The precision (sensitivity and specificity) in the diagnosis of pertussis is, however, laboratory dependent. It is recommended that practitioners become familiar with the laboratory diagnostic test offered by their local laboratory service. All of these tests are ancillary and helpful in the diagnosis but need to be interpreted with some degree of caution. Clinicians need to be respectful of the overall clinical and laboratory setting in which the patient presents and the stability of the source material as it is transferred to the laboratory.

TREATMENT

Bordetella pertussis and *B. parapertussis* are susceptible to a range of antibiotics *in vitro*. Antibiotics to which these organisms are sensitive include the penicillins, the macrolides, tetracyclines, chloramphenicol and trimethoprim-sulfamethoxazole.

Unfortunately, the antibiotics make no difference to the course or outcomes of pertussis disease. What they are effective at is eliminating the organism from the nasopharynx. This is an important consideration. Efforts to reduce transmission to other people, particularly infants, require prioritization. Hence, if a case is confirmed, it is advised that elimination of the organism may reduce spread of this disease.

The most commonly recommended antimicrobial to use is erythromycin estolate because of its higher levels of active antibiotic in the secretions of the respiratory tract. However, other forms of erythromycin are also considered to be acceptable.

Short-term antibiotics (azithromycin for 3 to 5e days, or clarithromycin or erythromycin for 7 days) are as effective as long-term (erythromycin for 10 to 14 days) in eradicating *B. pertussis* from the nasopharynx but has fewer side effects. Trimethoprim/sulfamethoxazole for seven days is also effective. Contact prophylaxis of contacts older than 6 months of age with antibiotics does not significantly improve clinical symptoms or the number of cases developing culture-positive B. pertussis [11].

If there is an outbreak of pertussis, then immunization is the first step in management. Close contacts of an infected case can be treated with erythromycin or azithromycin, as recommended. However, most countries only recommend the use of antimicrobial prophylaxis for those at greatest risk from pertussis disease, i.e. young infants. Erythromycin treatment is not recommended for infants younger than 2 weeks of age.

IMMUNIZATION STRATEGIES

Given that antimicrobial treatment can eliminate the organism and, hence, transmission to others, but has no impact on the course of disease in an individual patient, primary prevention through the use of immunization becomes paramount. The mainstay of immunization for pertussis over the years has been the whole cell pertussis vaccine. Three immunizations with the vaccine afford approximately 90% protective efficacy that lasts throughout infancy, but whole cell vaccines are associated with common moderate and severe local reactions and fever.

"Acellular" vaccines contain subsets of immunogenic antigens from *Bordetella* and are much better tolerated, although they are more expensive. In resource-limited settings, childen often receive DTwP. In resource-rich settings, children usually receive DTaP. For children, as part of the Expanded Program in Immunization, most countries use a 2, 3, 4-, or 2, 4, 6-month immunization regimen of DTwP or DTaP.

Historically, adults and older children did not receive booster immunizations. This was owing, in part, to the assumption that adults were unlikely to get pertussis and the high adverse event profile of the whole-cell pertussis-based vaccines in older children and adults. As mentioned above, however, cases of pertussis among older children and adults has been increasing. This fact, and the development of safe, effective and well-tolerated acellular pertussis vaccine products has subsequently led to the endorsement of broader pertussis immunization programs for older children and adults with Tdap. Unfortunately, most older children and adults in resource-limited settings do not have access to, or the ability to receive, such vaccines. As a starting point, the Global Pertussis Initiative has recommended that a number of strategies that may be adopted at a country level in resource-limited settings to supplement the Expanded Program in Immunization program. In addition to adherence to standard immunization schedules, the Global Pertussis Initiative recommends that there be universal adolescent immunization of an anti-pertussis vaccine, that there be selective immunization of new mothers, family and close contacts of newborns (the cocoon strategy), that a preschool booster at 4 years of age be administered, that there be selective immunization of healthcare workers and childcare workers, and, possibly, a move towards a universal adult immunization strategy [12].

For public health benefits against pertussis to be realized, there needs to be a clear public health strategy at a country level. Such a public health strategy should include an effective vaccine delivery mechanism. This may be through regional child health clinics, family medicine clinics and local hospitals. Utility can only be measured through adequate surveillance processes.

REFERENCES

1. World Health Organisation. World Health Report 2011. Available at: http://www.who.int/immunization_monitoring/diseases/pertussis/en/index.html (accessed March 3, 2012).
2. Centres for Disease Control and Prevention. Pertussis—United States. 2011. Available at: http://www.cdc.gov/pertussis/about/index.html (accessed March 3, 2012).
3. NNDSS Reports. Annual Reports. CDI 1999;23:11.
4. Kakar RM, Mojadidi MK, Mofleh J. Pertussis in Afghanistan 2007–2008. Emerg Infect Dis 2009;15:501.
5. Harnden A, Grant C, Harrison T, et al. Whooping cough in school age children with persistent cough: prospective cohort study in primary care. BMJ 2006; 333:174–7.
6. Wang J, Yang Y, Li J, et al. Infantile pertussis re-discovered in China. Emerg Infect Dis 2002;8:859–61.
7. Arevshatian L, Clements CJ, Lwanga SK, et al. An evaluation of infant immunization in Africa: is a transformation in progress? Bull WHO 2007;85: 449–57.
8. Patriarca P, Biellik R, Sanden G, et al. Sensitivity and specificity of clinical case definitions of pertussis. Am J Public Health 1998;78:833–6.
9. Mertens P, Stals F, Steyerbeg E, Richardus J. Sensitivity and specificity of single IGA and IGG antibody concentrations for early diagnosis of pertussis in adults: an evaluation for outbreak management in public health practice. DMC Infect Dis 2007;7:53.
10. Andre P, Caro V, Njamkepo E, et al. Comparison of serological and real-time PCR assays to diagnose *Bordetella pertussis* infection in 2007. J Clin Micro 2008;45:1672–7.
11. Altunaiji S, Kukuruzovic R, Curtis N, Massie J. Antibiotics for whooping cough (pertussis). Cochrane Database Syst Rev. 2007 Jul 18;(3):CD004404.
12. Forsyth K, Tan T, Wirsing Von Konig C-H, et al. Potential strategies to reduce the burden of pertussis paediatric. Infect Dis J 2005;24:S69–S74.

SECTION

C

GASTROINTESTINAL TRACT INFECTIONS

41 *Helicobacter pylori* Infection

Caroline M den Hoed, Ernst J Kuipers

Key features

- Occurs worldwide
- Prevalence in developing countries >80%
- Mainly acquired in childhood, persisting for life
- Associated with chronic gastritis, peptic ulcer disease, gastric cancer and gastric mucosa-associated lymphoid tissue (MALT) lymphoma
- Defined by the World Health Organization (WHO) as class I carcinogen
- Diagnosed by variety of invasive and noninvasive methods
- Consensus guidelines exist regarding indications for treatment and treatment regimens
- Treatment requires multiday combination antibiotic therapy
- No vaccine is currently available

INTRODUCTION

The presence of spiral, Gram-negative bacteria on the human gastric mucosa was recognized in the late 19th century and related to peptic ulcer disease and gastric cancer. In 1983, Warren and Marshall were the first to successfully culture *Helicobacter pylori* from gastric biopsy samples. Through self-ingestion, they confirmed that this bacterium caused gastro-duodenal disorders [1]. Today, *H. pylori* is known to be the main cause of chronic gastritis, peptic ulcer disease, gastric carcinoma and gastric mucosa-associated lymphoid tissue (MALT) lymphoma and has been declared by the WHO, for these reasons, as a class I carcinogen. It is estimated that more than half of the world's population is colonized with *H. pylori*, with the vast majority becoming infected in childhood.

EPIDEMIOLOGY

H. pylori is allegedly one of the world's most common infections, if not the most common (see Fig. 41.1). The bacterium is present in human populations throughout the world, and phylogeographic studies indicate that humans have been colonized by *H. pylori* since their ancestral migration from east Africa more than 50,000 years ago. There are substantial differences in its prevalence, both within, and between, countries. In industrialized countries, the overall prevalence of *H. pylori* generally varies between 30 and 40 percent and increases with age. This is related to an age-cohort effect with decreasing infection rates in subsequent generations because of improved hygiene and housing conditions. In developing countries, however, *H. pylori* prevalence rises rapidly during the first 5 years of life often to 80% or more, and then remains constant thereafter. This indicates that *H. pylori* is mostly acquired early in childhood [2]. Once acquired, colonization persists throughout life in the absence of antibiotic therapy. The infection rate is thus inversely related with socioeconomic development and is a direct reflection of living conditions during childhood. In Western countries, prevalence remains considerably higher among first- and second-generation immigrants [3].

H. pylori has a narrow host range and is almost exclusively found in humans. The exact mechanisms whereby *H. pylori* is acquired are largely unknown. New infections are thought to occur as a consequence of direct human-to-human transmission, either via the oral–oral or fecal–oral route, or both [1].

NATURAL HISTORY, PATHOGENESIS AND PATHOLOGY

H. pylori is a spiral, Gram-negative bacterium with flagella. It is microaerophilic, requiring low levels of oxygen. Although its natural habitat is the acidic gastric lumen and it can resist brief exposure to pH levels below 4, growth only occurs at a pH between 5.5 and 8.0. Intragastric survival occurs within the protective mucus layer, with local acid-buffering by the high bacterial urease activity. The associated gastritis also impairs acid production and thus enhances bacterial survival [1].

PATHOGENESIS

H. pylori colonization induces chronic active gastritis in virtually all infected subjects. Colonization is accompanied by a persistent immune response, but this is ineffective in clearing the bacterium. Only a minority of colonized subjects develop overt disease, in particular, peptic ulcer disease and gastric cancer. The risk of disease development in the presence of *H. pylori* is related to a combination of factors, including bacterial strain differences, host susceptibility and environmental factors. *H. pylori* exhibits a high level of genetic diversity which translates into major differences in virulence. Two main virulence factors are the *cagA* and *vacA* genes. The *cagA* pathogenicity island is present in some 40–60% of strains, and is strongly associated with the development of peptic ulcers, as well as gastric cancer. The *vacA* gene is present in all strains, but has polymorphisms which translate into differences of expression. Host susceptibility is influenced by genetic polymorphisms in various cytokine genes that affect the level and profile of the inflammatory response to colonization with *H. pylori*. Furthermore, environmental factors play a role in *H. pylori*-related pathogenesis. Smoking increases the risk of ulcers, while diets high in salt and low in antioxidants and vitamin C increase cancer risk.

Finally, the pattern of *H. pylori* colonization also determines disease risk. Subjects with normal-to-high acid output have an antral-predominant gastritis and are most at risk for duodenal ulceration. Subjects with low acid output demonstrate pan-gastritis and are most at risk for gastric ulceration and cancer [1, 4].

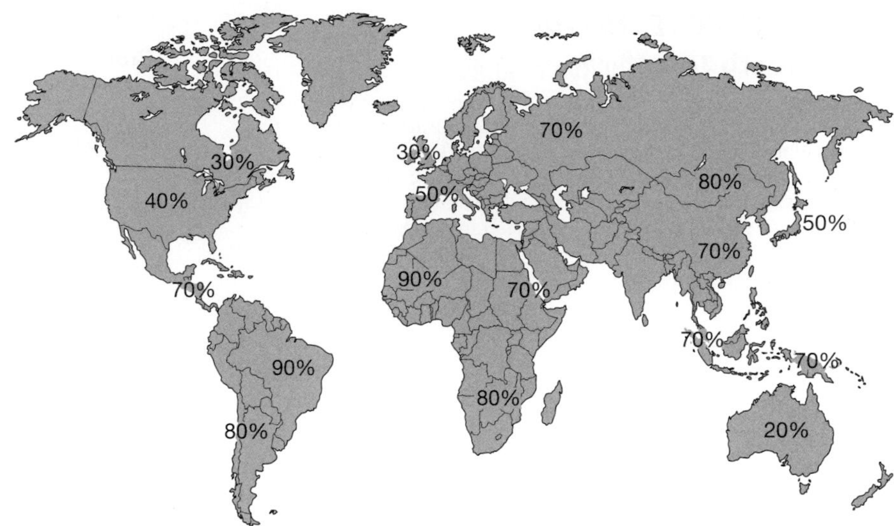

FIGURE 41.1 World map with *Helicobacter pylori* infection prevalence [2, 3, 8]. Percentages on the map are the *H. pylori* infection rates in the specific regions.

CLINICAL FEATURES

H. pylori infection is associated with chronic gastritis, peptic ulcer disease, distal gastric adenocarcinoma, gastric MALT lymphoma and Ménétrier's disease.

GASTRITIS

Colonization with *H. pylori* is in the first weeks can be associated with acute gastritis, which can be accompanied by transient, nonspecific dyspepsia symptoms, such as fullness, nausea and vomiting. The majority of subjects do not clear the infection, despite the humoral and cellular response, and continue to develop chronic colonization with chronic active gastritis [1].

PEPTIC ULCER DISEASE

It is estimated that approximately 20% of *H. pylori*-positive subjects develop peptic ulcer disease during their lifetime, and those with an ulcer have a more than 50% risk for recurrent ulcer disease in the years thereafter. Ulcers may be associated with intestinal bleeding and perforation and, in some cases, stricture formation. Eradication of *H. pylori* prevents recurrence of ulcers and their complications in most patients, unless they have a second risk factor for ulceration, in particular use of nonsteroidal anti-inflammatory drugs (NSAIDs) or aspirin. This strong association exists for both duodenal ulcers and gastric ulcers [1, 5].

GASTRIC CANCER

H. pylori infection is the starting point in a cancer-associated cascade that passes through the stages of chronic gastritis, atrophic gastritis, intestinal metaplasia and dysplasia, and cancer. *H. pylori* may initiate this process by causing chronic cellular proliferation, increasing the likelihood of mutagenic processes in the presence of carcinogenic substances. Although development of the initial stages of this progressive cascade (in particular atrophic gastritis and intestinal metaplasia) are common in *H. pylori*-positive individuals, only 1–2% of *H. pylori*-infected patients eventually develop gastric carcinoma as a result of lifelong infection [4–8].

MUCOSA-ASSOCIATED LYMPHOID TISSUE (MALT) LYMPHOMA

Healthy gastric mucosa normally does not contain lymphoid follicles, but lymphocytes are inevitably present in the gastric mucosa in all *H. pylori*-positive individuals. In rare cases, this eventually leads to the development of MALT B-cell lymphomas (usually low-grade). Close to 100% of patients with low-grade gastric MALT lymphoma have evidence of *H. pylori* infection. *H. pylori* eradication is the primary treatment for these patients, as it leads to partial, or complete, regression in more than 70% of patients [5, 8].

MÉNÉTRIER'S DISEASE

Ménétrier's disease, also called hypertrophic gastropathy, is a rare condition of unknown etiology. However, a majority has evidence of *H. pylori* infection; successful eradication can lead to major improvement of symptoms and should therefore always be considered [5, 8].

GASTROESOPHAGEAL REFLUX DISEASE (GERD)

Although *H. pylori* has been clearly demonstrated as a cause of the above-mentioned diseases, discussion remains as to whether it also carries potential beneficial effects. This discussion, in particular, focuses on the negative association between *H. pylori* colonization and the development of gastroesophageal reflux disease (GERD) and its sequelae, including esophageal cancer [5, 8].

H. PYLORI *INFECTION IN CHILDREN*

H. pylori infection in children may be associated with recurrent abdominal pain, iron deficiency and, during conditions of nutritional limitation, with growth retardation; however, the incidence of peptic ulcer disease is lower than in adults. In contrast, there are reports which suggest that *H. pylori* protects children from developing asthma and atopy [2, 5, 8].

PATIENT EVALUATION, DIAGNOSIS AND DIFFERENTIAL DIAGNOSIS

H. pylori can be diagnosed by various methods, each with advantages and disadvantages. Noninvasive testing is recommended for primary screening of young individuals and children who present with upper abdominal complaints. These tests are based on the detection of *H. pylori* enzyme activity, antigen or antibodies. Invasive testing is usually reserved for patients undergoing diagnostic or therapeutic upper intestinal endoscopy as part of a broader evaluation, and involves sampling of mucosal tissue for evaluation of presence of *H. pylori* through direct detection of measuring enzyme activity. As *H. pylori* may not be evenly spread throughout the stomach in infected individuals, multiple biopsy samples from various locations are required for optimal sensitivity [8, 9].

NONINVASIVE TESTS [10]

Urea Breath Tests

Urea breath tests (UBT) are based on the large urease production by all *H. pylori* strains. UBTs are very reliable, low-burden tests that have been validated both in adults and children. Fasting patients consume a small amount of either ^{14}C or ^{13}C-labeled urea. Urease degrades urea, releasing labeled carbon dioxide which enters the blood stream via the gastric mucosa and can be detected in a breath sample.

Serology

Serum antibodies (especially IgG) against *H. pylori* can easily be detected. The main disadvantage of serology is that antibodies can still be detected for a considerable period after eradication of *H. pylori*. Furthermore, as the antigenic properties of *H. pylori* strains vary between countries, the tests should be locally standardized.

Fecal Antigen Testing

H. pylori specific antigens (*Hp*SA) can be detected in diluted stool samples. This is an attractive test for use in small children, as obtaining breath samples can be difficult and serum sampling can be burdensome.

INVASIVE TESTS [10]

Culture

In reference microbiologic laboratories, culturing for 3–7 days at 37°C under microaerophilic conditions can be performed, enabling detection of *H. pylori* and determination of antimicrobial resistance.

Histology

H. pylori can be identified by hematoxylin-eosin staining and histopathologic examination. When performed by an experienced pathologist, it is highly reliable and often considered the gold standard for diagnosing *H. pylori*. Special stains enhance detection, but are not necessary.

TABLE 41-1 International Recommendations for *Helicobacter pylori* Eradication in Infected Patients

Recommendations	Grade of recommendation
Non-ulcer dyspepsia (test and treat)	Strongly recommended
Un-investigated dyspepsia for populations with a prevalence of *H. pylori* >20%	Strongly recommended
Duodenal and gastric ulcer	Strongly recommended
Atrophic gastritis	Advisable
Gastric MALT lymphoma	Strongly recommended
After gastric cancer resection	Advisable
First-degree relatives of patients with gastric cancer	Advisable
In patients on long-term NSAIDs treatment and who have peptic ulcer and/or ulcer bleeding, *PPI maintenance treatment is better than* H. pylori *eradication in preventing ulcer recurrence and/or bleeding*	Strongly recommended
Patient requests (after explanation of risks and benefits)	Strongly recommended

Reprinted with permission from Malfertheiner P, Megraud F, O'Morain C, et al. Current concepts in the management of Helicobacter pylori infection: the Maastricht III Consensus Report. Gut 2007;56:772–81.

TABLE 41-2 Overview of Antibiotics Used for *Helicobacter pylori* Eradication (Adapted from [8] and [11])

Drug class	Drug	Triple therapy* Dose	Quadruple therapy† Dose	Sequential therapy§ Dose
Acid suppression	Proton pump inhibitor	20–40 mg bid¶	20–40 mg bid¶	20-40 mg bid¶
Standard antimicrobials	Bismuth compound**	2 tablets bid	2 tablets bid	
	Amoxicillin	1 g bid		1 g bid
	Metronidazole††	500 mg bid	500 mg tid	500 mg bid
	Clarithromycin	500 mg bid		500 mg bid
	Tetracycline		500 mg qid	
Salvage antimicrobials	Levofloxacin	300 mg bid		
	Rifabutin	150 mg bid		
	Furazolidone	100 mg bid		

*Triple therapy consists of a protein pump inhibitor (PPI) or bismuth compound, together with two of the listed antibiotics, usually given for 7–14 days.
†Quadruple therapy consists of a PPI plus bismuth compound with two antibiotics, as listed, given for 4–10 days.
§Sequential therapy consists of 10 days of treatment with a PPI plus amoxicillin for the first 5 days, and a combination of clarithromycin and metronidazole for the second 5 days [9].
¶PPI dose equivalent to omeprazole 20 mg bid.
**Bismuth subsalicylate or subcitrate.
††Alternative = tinidazole 500 mg bid.
Adapted from Malfertheiner P, Megraud F, O'Morain C, et al. Current concepts in the management of Helicobacter pylori infection: the Maastricht III Consensus Report. Gut 2007;56:772–81 and Vakil N, Vaira D. Sequential therapy for Helicobacter pylori: time to consider making the switch? JAMA 2008;300:1346–7.

Rapid Urease Test

Probably the most widely used invasive test is the rapid urease test, which is based on bacterial urease. Urea degradation is accompanied by a pH increase that is detected by a color change of an indicator. It is an easy and low-cost test, but also has the lowest sensitivity and specificity of the invasive assays.

TREATMENT

INDICATIONS

Indications for treatment are still evolving (Table 41-1). Consensus exists for the treatment of individuals with *H. pylori*-associated peptic ulcer disease and gastric MALT lymphoma. Treatment of individuals with non-ulcer dyspepsia is more controversial. Most authorities would treat *H. pylori*-infected individuals thought to be at increased risk of gastric carcinoma, including those with a family history of gastric cancer and those with gastric dysplasia. Individuals with Ménétrier's disease and *H. pylori* should be treated [8].

ANTIMICROBIALS

In vitro, H. pylori is susceptible to most antimicrobials, but *in vivo* only a few antimicrobials can be used to cure infected patients. This is related to limited drug levels within the gastric mucus layer. Metronidazole, clarithromycin, amoxicillin and tetracycline are the most widely used antimicrobial drugs used to treat individuals with *H. pylori* infection. None of the above-mentioned antibiotics is effective enough to eliminate *H. pylori* when given as monotherapy. Successful eradication of *H. pylori* requires a combination of drugs, consisting of two antibiotics in combination with an acid-suppressive drug. Current guidelines for the treatment of *H. pylori* are given in Table 41-2.

In general practice, 20–30% of the treatment regimens fail, usually because of insufficient patient compliance or the presence of antibiotic resistance. Patients who fail treatment are usually retreated with another antimicrobial combination (Table 42-2) [8, 9].

ALTERNATIVES

Increasing antibiotic resistance among *H. pylori* is occurring worldwide. Research efforts are focusing on the development of an effective vaccine, with the hope that prophylactic, as well as therapeutic, vaccination could potentially save millions of lives and reduce the costs related to the treatment of *H. pylori*-associated diseases [1, 9].

REFERENCES

1. Kusters JG, van Vliet AH, Kuipers EJ. Pathogenesis of *H. pylori* infection. Clin microbiol Rev 2006;19:449–90.
2. Cover TL, Blaser MJ. *H. pylori* in health and disease. Gastroenterology 2009;136:1863–73.
3. The EUROGAST Study Group. Epidemiology of, and risk factors for *H. pylori* infection among 3194 asymptomatic subjects in 17 populations. Gut 1993;34:1672–6.
4. Peek RM Jr, Crabtree JE. Helicobacter infection and gastric neoplasia. J Pathol 2006;208:233–48.
5. Kuipers EJ, Blaser MJ. *H. pylori* and gastroduodenal disorders. In: Scheld WM, Armstrong D, Hughes JM, eds. Emerging Infections. ASM Press, Washington; 1998:191–205.
6. de Vries AC, van Grieken NC, Looman CW, et al. Gastric cancer risk in patients with premalignant gastric lesions: a nationwide cohort study in the Netherlands. Gastroenterology 2008;134:945–52.
7. Correa P, Haenszel W, Cuello C, et al. A model for gastric cancer epidemiology. Lancet 1975;2:58–60.
8. Malfertheiner P, Megraud F, O'Morain C, et al. Current concepts in the management of H. pylori infection: the Maastricht III Consensus Report. Gut 2007;56:772–81.
9. Gerrits MM, van Vliet AH, Kuipers EJ, et al. *H. pylori* and antimicrobial resistance: molecular mechanisms and clinical implications. Lancet Infect Dis 2006;6:699–709.
10. Kuipers EJ, Kusters JG, Blaser MJ. Clinical approach to the *H. pylori* positive patient. In: Blaser MJ, ed. Infections of the Gastroinestinal Tract. Lippincott Williams & Wilkins, Philadelphia, PA; 2002:495–529.
11. Vakil N, Vaira D. Sequential therapy for *H. pylori*: time to consider making the switch? JAMA 2008;300:1346–7.

42 *Escherichia coli* Diarrhea

Jorge J Velarde, Myron M Levine, James P Nataro

Key features

- *Escherichia coli*, typically part of the normal intestinal flora, can cause distinct diarrheal syndromes when they harbor specific virulence factors
- The unique pathogenic mechanisms of each pathotype of diarrheagenic *E. coli* give rise to the specific clinical syndromes they cause
- Clinical syndromes caused by diarrheagenic *E. coli* include watery, short-lived diarrhea (ETEC, EPEC, EAEC, DAEC), persistent infant diarrhea (EPEC and EAEC), invasive inflammatory diarrhea (EIEC, EHEC) and hemorrhagic colitis and the hemolytic uremic syndrome (EHEC)
- Definitive microbiologic diagnosis of diarrheagenic *E. coli*, other than Shiga toxin-producing *E. coli*, is not usually possible using routine laboratory methods and requires specific assays to identify pathogenic mechanisms performed in a reference or research laboratory
- Despite limitations of diagnostic testing, most cases of illness caused by diarrheagenic *Escherichia coli* are self-limited, requiring only supportive care with appropriate hydration and can be managed empirically based on clinical presentation
- Individuals with enterohemorrhagic *E. coli* (EHEC) should not be treated with antimicrobial agents, as such use markedly increases the risk for hemolytic uremic syndrome (HUS) and renal failure. Individuals with EHEC usually present with bloody diarrhea and low or absent fever

INTRODUCTION

The bacterial species *E. coli* plays an important role in maintaining normal gut physiology in humans. Nevertheless, there exist within this species primary pathogens that cause various syndromes of diarrheal disease, including watery diarrhea, dysentery and hemorrhagic colitis in different age groups under distinct epidemiologic settings.

EPIDEMIOLOGY

ETIOLOGIC AGENTS

Escherichia coli are motile, Gram-negative, rod-shaped bacteria within the family Enterobacteriaceae. Strains of *E. coli* that cause diarrhea are of six major categories: enterohemorrhagic (EHEC), enterotoxigenic (ETEC), enteroinvasive (EIEC), enteropathogenic (EPEC), enteroaggregative (EAEC) and diffuse-adherent (DAEC). More than 170 O serogroups and more than 60 H types (based on the scheme proposed by Kauffman in the 1940s) are currently recognized. Each category of diarrheagenic *E. coli* comprises a separate set of O:H serotypes, and has distinct virulence attributes resulting in distinctive clinical syndromes and characteristic epidemiologic patterns [1, 2].

First described in the 1940s and 1950s was EPEC, associated with sporadic cases of infant summer diarrhea and epidemic gastroenteritis in hospital nurseries. ETEC was first described in the 1950s in cases of severe, cholera-like, watery diarrhea on the Indian subcontinent. In the early 1970s, *E. coli* strains were isolated from patients with clinical dysentery; such strains were designated EIEC and these are now known to behave like *Shigella*, particularly in their ability to invade epithelial cells and induce inflammation. A multistate outbreak of hemorrhagic colitis in the USA in the early 1980s caused by organisms of serotype O157:H7 led to the discovery of enterohemorrhagic *E. coli* (EHEC). *Escherichia coli* strains that exhibit a unique pattern of adherence to HEp-2 cells, so-called aggregative adherence, and associated with diarrheal disease in infants in developing countries were coined enteroaggregative *E. coli* (EAggEC or EAEC) in the 1980s. In some epidemiologic studies, *E. coli* strains that manifest a diffuse pattern of adherence to HEp-2 cells, diffuse-adherent *E. coli* (DAEC), have also been associated with non-bloody diarrheal illness in young children in developing countries [1–5].

DISTRIBUTION AND INCIDENCE

ETEC, EPEC, EIEC and EAEC are commonly isolated as agents of diarrheal disease among infants and young children in less developed countries. In many developing countries, ETEC is the second most common cause (after rotavirus) of significant diarrheal dehydration in infants. ETEC is also the most common cause of traveler's diarrhea in adults [1, 2, 5, 6]. As a contrast in epidemiologic pattern, EHEC is an emerging cause of diarrheal illness, hemorrhagic colitis and hemolytic-uremic syndrome (HUS) in industrialized countries (North America, Europe, Japan, Australia). EHEC disease is considered rare in developing countries, although outbreaks of EHEC in Africa suggest that the relevance of this pathogen in the developing world may be underestimated [1, 2, 7, 8].

EPEC is no longer a major cause of diarrheal disease in industrialized countries, but remains an important cause of diarrhea in infants in many developing and newly industrializing countries [1, 2]. EAEC has been identified as an important cause of persistent diarrhea among infants in Asia and South America. More recent data suggest that EAEC may also be common in some industrialized countries [9]. The geographic distribution of DAEC diarrhea is the least well mapped, with the most incriminating studies coming from Latin America. In some epidemiologic studies in developing countries, DAEC was more common in children >1 year of age [2, 10], in contrast with EPEC, ETEC and EAEC which manifest the highest incidence in the first year of life.

TRANSMISSION

ETEC is transmitted by contaminated food and water vehicles; relatively large inocula (circa 10^8 organisms) are required to cause illness [2, 5]. Classic EPEC is mostly associated with bottle-feeding infants

TABLE 42-1 Pathogenetic mechanisms of diarrheagenic *E. coli*

Category	Typical size of virulence plasmid	Proteins promoting interaction with mucosa	Characteristic pattern of attachment to HEp-2 cells	Toxins
ETEC	60 MDa	CFA fimbriae	None	LT, ST
EPEC	60 MDa	BFP; intimin	Localized adherence	None, T3SS effectors
EIEC	140 MDa	IPAs	Invasion	ShET-2, T3SS effectors
EHEC	60 MDa	Novel fimbriae; intimin	None	Shiga toxin 1 & 2, T3SS effectors
EAggEC	65 MDa	AAF fimbriae	Aggregative adherence	EAST1, 108 kda toxin
DAEC	60 MDa	F1845 fimbriae; AIDA-I outer membrane protein	Diffuse adherence	Sat

AAF, aggregative adherence fimbriae; BFP, bundle forming pili; CFA, colonization factor antigen; DAEC, diffusely adherent *E. coli*; EAggEC, enteroaggregative *E. coli*; EAST1, enteroaggregative heat-stable enterotoxin 1; EHEC, enterohemorrhagic *E. coli*; EIEC, enteroinvasive *E. coli*; EPEC, enteropathogenic *E. coli*; ETEC, enterotoxigenic *E. coli*; IPAs, invasion plasmid antigens; LT, heat-labile enterotoxin; ShET2, *Shigella* enterotoxin 2; ST, heat-stable enterotoxin.

in developing countries [2, 8, 11]. EHEC can be transmitted by low inocula (10^1-10^2 organisms) and is primarily transmitted by ingestion of contaminated food vehicles, although it can also be transmitted directly by contact spread [2, 12, 13]. The modes of transmission of EAEC and DAEC are not yet clearly defined.

NATURAL HISTORY, PATHOGENESIS AND PATHOLOGY

Different categories of diarrheagenic *E. coli* have certain pathogenesis motifs in common. A brief summary of these properties for each category of diarrheagenic *E. coli* is shown in Table 42-1.

ENTEROTOXIGENIC ESCHERICHIA COLI *(ETEC)*

ETEC carry one or two plasmids circa 60 MDa in size that encode heat-labile (LT) or heat-stable (ST) enterotoxins (or both). These also encode one or more fimbrial colonization factor antigens (CFAs) and genes encoding the regulatory protein necessary for the high-level expression of CFAs. LT closely resembles cholera enterotoxin and has a similar mode of activity (ADP ribosylation of Gs protein). ST, which consists of peptides of 18 or 19 amino acids in length, activates guanylate cyclase, which results in an intracellular accumulation of cyclic GMP that leads to secretion [1, 5]. Genomic studies suggest that ETEC strains share a very small number of genes in addition to these primary virulence factors [14].

ENTEROPATHOGENIC ESCHERICHIA COLI *(EPEC)*

In contrast to ETEC, EPEC strains harbor a large array of virulence-associated genes, which execute a complex and finely orchestrated pathogenetic strategy (reviewed in [15]). All classic EPEC strains carry a circa 60 MDa plasmid which encodes the bundle-forming pilus (BFP); BFP mediates initial attachment and microcolony formation on the small intestinal mucosa. The plasmid also encodes PerC, a transcriptional activator for the BFP and for a large number of chromosomal genes. One such gene encodes intimin, a 94 kd protein that mediates intimate attachment to enterocytes. The receptor for intimin is the translocated intimin receptor (Tir), which is injected directly into the target cell cytoplasm via an extraordinarily complex organelle called a type III secretion system (T3SS). In addition to Tir, the EPEC T3SS additionally injects more than 20 additional protein toxins into the enterocyte. In aggregate, this panoply of toxins leads to cytoskeletal changes in the target enterocyte, the consequence of which is a pathognomonic "attaching and effacing" intestinal lesion observed by electron microscopy Other phenotypes induced by the T3SS include loss of tight junction integrity, release of pro-inflammatory cytokines and conversion of the cell from a net absorptive state to a net secretory state [1, 2, 16].

ENTEROINVASIVE ESCHERICHIA COLI *(EIEC)*

EIEC closely resembles *Shigella* in its pathogenesis, involving an early step of enterotoxin production leading to intestinal secretion and invasion of intestinal epithelium. EIEC possesses virtually the identical 140 MDa virulence plasmid as *Shigella flexneri*. Many of the pathogenic effects of EIEC are mediated through a T3SS which injects a distinct set of toxins that mediate invasion. The bacteria disseminate in the epithelial layer, are taken up into enterocytes, spread intracellularly and intercellularly, and cause death of the enterocytes. EIEC infection is characterized by an influx of polymorphonuclear leukocytes into the lamina propria of affected intestinal mucosa [1, 2, 17].

ENTEROHEMORRHAGIC ESCHERICHIA COLI *(EHEC)*

EHEC carries an ~60 MDa plasmid that appears to be involved in the expression of adherence fimbriae. Phages carried by EHEC encode the powerful cytotoxins, Shiga toxin 1 or 2. EHEC express the 94-kd intimin protein and harbor a T3SS homologous to that expressed by EPEC. EHEC expressing these proteins can cause attaching and effacing lesions of the colon, whereas EPEC induces these lesions in the small intestine [1, 2].

ENTEROAGGREGATIVE ESCHERICHIA COLI *(EAEC)*

EAEC harbors a plasmid of ~60 MDa in size that encodes fimbrial colonization factors that mediate the pathognomonic aggregative adherence to HEp-2 cells. EAEC expresses at least two enterotoxins that may contribute to pathogenesis, including the Pet cytotoxin and the plasmid-encoded EAEC heat-stable enterotoxin (EAST) [1, 9].

DIFFUSE-ADHERENT ESCHERICHIA COLI *(DAEC)*

The characteristic diffuse adherence to epithelial cells is mediated by fimbriae. Some DAEC strains produce a protease called Sat which may disrupt tight junctions and induce cytoskeletal alterations [1, 18, 19].

CLINICAL FEATURES

The different categories of diarrheagenic *E. coli* cause distinct clinical syndromes, closely related to their virulence mechanisms, which are summarized in Table 42-2.

TABLE 42-2 Clinical and epidemiologic characteristics of diarrheagenic *E. coli*

Category	Characteristic clinical syndrome*	Predominant geographic distribution	Peak age incidence of disease	Molecular diagnostic targets
ETEC	Watery diarrhea	Developing world	Infants, adult travelers	ST, LT genes
EPEC	Watery diarrhea	Developing world	Very young infants	EAF plasmid, BFP and intimin genes
EIEC	Dysentery[†]	Worldwide	Toddlers, preschool children	Inv plasmid
EHEC	Hemorrhagic colitis, HUS	Developed world, Latin America	Children 2–7 years of age	EHEC plasmid; intimin and Shiga toxin genes
EAggEC	Persistent diarrhea	Worldwide	Mainly infants	AA plasmid
DAEC	Watery diarrhea	Unknown	Preschool children	F1845 fimbrial genes

*In mild cases, the clinical illness caused by any of the categories of diarrheagenic *E. coli* consists of watery diarrhea, low-grade fever, nausea and mild abdominal cramps and is indistinguishable.
[†]Dysentery occurs in only 10% of patients; the other 90% exhibit watery diarrhea without blood.
AA, aggregative adherence; BFP, bundle forming pili; DAEC, diffusely adherent *E. coli*; EAF, EPEC adherence factor; EAggEC, enteroaggregative *E. coli*; EHEC, enterohemorrhagic *E. coli*; EIEC, enteroinvasive *E. coli*; EPEC, enteropathogenic *E. coli*; ETEC, enterotoxigenic *E. coli*; LT, heat-labile enterotoxin; ST, heat-stable enterotoxin.

ENTEROTOXIGENIC ESCHERICHIA COLI *(ETEC)*

Clinical ETEC infection exhibits a wide range of severity in infants in developing countries and in adult travelers. Mild illness presents as diarrhea, sometimes with low-grade fever, nausea and mild abdominal cramps, and gurgling. Severe ETEC diarrhea closely resembles cholera, although more curtailed, with voluminous rice-water stools rich in electrolytes; like cholera, severe ETEC diarrhea can rapidly lead to dehydration [2, 5, 20].

ENTEROPATHOGENIC ESCHERICHIA COLI *(EPEC)*

Fulminant EPEC disease, typically occurring in the first 12 months of life, is characterized by watery diarrhea with prominent mucus, toxemia, fever and rapid onset of dehydration [2, 20].

ENTEROINVASIVE ESCHERICHIA COLI *(EIEC)*

EIEC has a predilection for colonic mucosa as the favored site of host–pathogen interaction. The illness is marked by fever, abdominal cramps, malaise, toxemia and watery diarrhea. In under 10% of individuals, overt dysentery occurs, manifested by scanty stools with blood and mucus [1, 2, 20].

ENTEROHEMORRHAGIC ESCHERICHIA COLI *(EHEC)*

EHEC exhibits a wide spectrum of clinical illness. Mild cases manifest as diarrhea indistinguishable from that caused by many other agents. A high percentage of infections progress to hemorrhagic colitis, characterized by severe abdominal cramps and copious bloody diarrhea, with most patients not exhibiting fever (Table 42-2). The absence of fever and fecal leukocytes help to differentiate EHEC from dysentery caused by EIEC and *Shigella* [2, 20]. Between 3 and 20 percent of EHEC infections may result in hemolytic-uremic syndrome (HUS). In HUS, a disseminated intravascular coagulopathy occurs with massive hemolytic anemia, the presence of fragmented erythrocytes (schistocytes) in the peripheral blood smear, severe thrombocytopenia and acute renal failure. This is an emerging health problem in industrialized and rapidly industrializing countries, but not in developing countries, where HUS is more often seen second to *Shigella*-associated dysentery, although the contribution from EHEC may be underestimated in the developing world [8, 21].

ENTEROAGGREGATIVE ESCHERICHIA COLI *(EAEC)*

EAEC strains induce watery diarrhea among patients of all ages without frank evidence of inflammation (i.e. fever, fecal leukocytes). However, subtle signs of inflammation may be seen, including the presence of mucus in stools and fecal lactoferrin. Though most are brief (1–3 days) and self-limiting, infection may persist for >14 days and can be a cause of persistent diarrhea among infants and children which then predisposes them to malnutrition and immune compromise [2, 9, 22, 23].

DIFFUSE-ADHERENT ESCHERICHIA COLI *(DAEC)*

DAEC infection is associated with a fairly nonspecific clinical picture of watery diarrhea and low-grade fever occurring in developing countries and more commonly involves preschool children rather than infants [1, 24].

PATIENT EVALUATION, DIAGNOSIS AND DIFFERENTIAL DIAGNOSIS

In most clinical scenarios the management of diarrheal illness is empiric and the identification of a specific underlying etiologic agent is unnecessary. Because diarrheagenic *E. coli* are not usually distinguishable from non-pathogenic *E. coli* using routine microbiology tests, the definitive identification of diarrheagenic *E. coli* requires assays that identify specific virulence properties of *E. coli* isolated from the stool, normally performed in a research or reference laboratory. Multiplexed molecular diagnostic techniques are under development to greatly facilitate the detection of diarrheagenic *E. coli* infections in situations where this is important to case management or epidemiology.

INDICATIVE CLINICAL FEATURES

ETEC

Copious purging of rice-water stools should lead to a suspicion of severe ETEC infection, as well as cholera [5, 25].

EPEC

The presence of prominent mucus in the diarrheal discharges of a young, bottle-fed infant less than 6 months of age with toxemia should raise suspicion of EPEC (rotavirus would be the other main suspect) [2, 20].

EIEC

With the absence of overt dysentery, clinical EIEC infection exhibits no characteristic clues. On the other hand, among patients with overt dysentery, EIEC must be one of the agents considered in the differential diagnosis [1, 20]. If mucus from a diarrheal stool with or without gross blood is stained and microscopic examination reveals large numbers of fecal leukocytes, EIEC should be considered in the differential diagnosis along with *Shigella*, *Salmonella* and *Campylobacter jejuni*; *Yersinia enterocolitica*, which also results in many fecal leukocytes, is rarely diagnosed in the tropics.

EHEC

The occurrence of hemorrhagic colitis is indicative of EHEC infection. In the tropics, HUS is more likely to be caused by *Shigella dysenteriae* serotype 1; nevertheless, EHEC must be considered in the differential diagnosis [20].

EAEC

Persistent diarrhea in young infants without other defined etiology should lead the clinician to consider EAEC [23, 26].

DAEC

There are no characteristic clinical features of DAEC-associated diarrhea.

LABORATORY TESTS

Stool Culture

Some EIEC are late lactose fermenters (or even fail to ferment lactose) [27], and some EHEC, particularly of serotype O157:H7, do not ferment sorbitol [28]. All other diarrheagenic *E. coli* are visually indistinguishable on the usual enteric media from normal flora strains of *E. coli*.

Immunoassays

ELISAs have been described to identify ETEC, EPEC, EIEC and EHEC using colony blots or culture supernatants [2, 5, 28]. ELISAs that can be used directly on stool extracts are available to identify heat-labile (LT), heat-stable (ST) and Shiga toxins [5, 28].

DNA Probes and PCR

Molecular diagnostic methods are widely used in the detection of diarrheagenic *E. coli.* Polynucleotide and oligonucleotide assays are typically employed in epidemiologic studies. Using this method, large numbers of *E. coli* can be tested at one time for several different gene targets. PCR for detection of pathogen-specific genes may be more difficult to perform in the setting of a very large epidemiologic study. In contrast, for the processing of a single clinical stool specimen, it is typically more efficient to run a panel of PCR reactions using primers against diarrheagenic *E. coli* target genes. PCR assays have been described using primers specific for ETEC, EIEC, EHEC, EPEC and EAggEC [2, 5, 26, 28].

Adherence to HEp-2 cells

The HEp-2 assay is one of the most useful phenotypic assays used in the detection of diarrheagenic *E. coli* (Figs 42.1, 42.2 and 42.3). The presence of the distinctive adherence pattern visualized by light microscopy after 3-hour co-incubation of bacteria with HEp-2 cells correlates well with the EPEC (localized), EAggEC (aggregative) and DAEC (diffuse) categories [2].

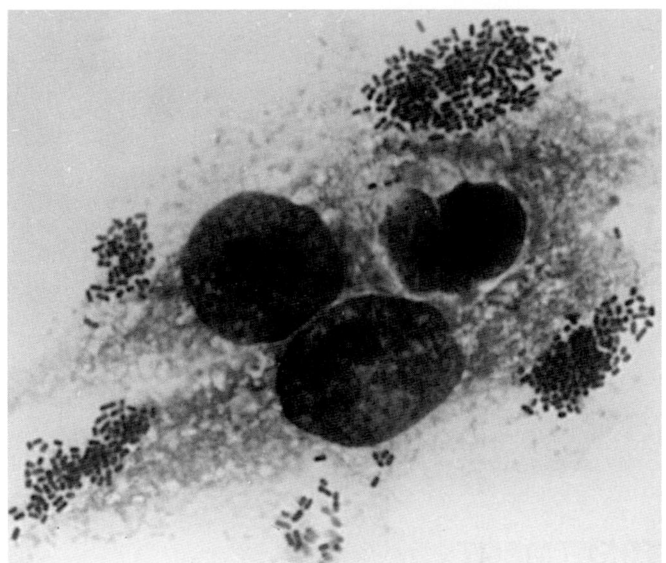

FIGURE 42.1 The localized adherence pattern of enteropathogenic *E. coli* (EPEC) to HEp-2 cells in tissue culture. Focal clusters of bacteria are seen attached to one portion of the HEp-2 cells.

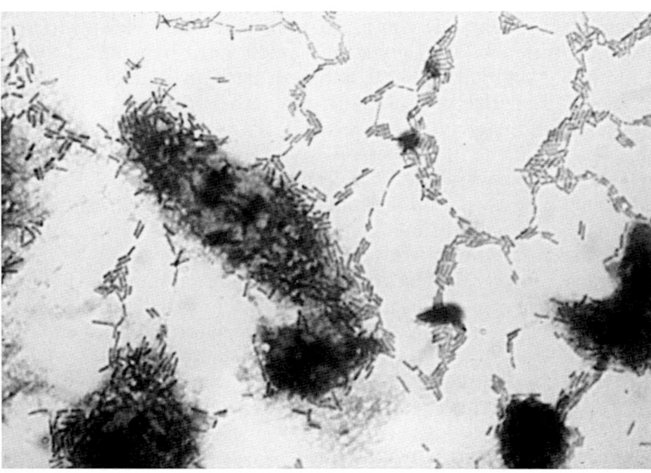

FIGURE 42.2 The aggregative pattern of adherence to HEp-2 cells diagnostic of enteroaggregative *E. coli* (EAggEC). Note the stacked brick appearance of bacteria attaching both to the tissue culture cells and to the glass slide in between the cells.

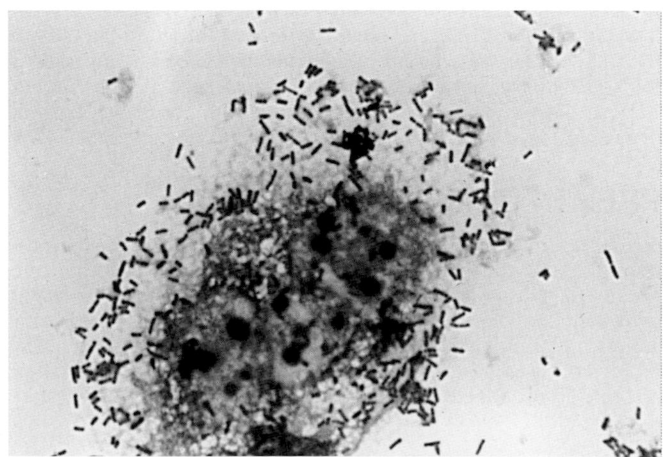

FIGURE 42.3 The diffuse pattern of adherence to HEp-2 cells that identifies diffuse adherence *E. coli* (DAEC). The bacteria are attached individually, interspersed over the surface of the entire HEp-2 cell.

Serology

Following diarrheal infection with *E. coli*, rises in serum antibody against the O antigen of the infecting strain can be demonstrated. Many of the virulence attributes of the different categories are also immunogenic, although in almost all instances these remain research tools available only in reference laboratories.

Stool microscopy

Patients with dysentery or suspected EIEC infection should have a drop of stool mucus fixed, stained and examined by light microscopy for the presence of fecal leukocytes. Many patients with EIEC will have numerous polymorphonuclear leukocytes [27]. Although nonspecific, this test provides evidence that a bacterial pathogen has invaded the intestinal mucosa. Other bacterial enteropathogens that cause a dysenteric syndrome and are associated with abundant fecal leukocytes are *Shigella* spp., *Campylobacter jejuni* and *Salmonella* causing nontyphoidal infections. *Yersinia enterocolitica*, which also results in many fecal leukocytes, is rarely diagnosed in the tropics.

TREATMENT

Assessment of hydration status and appropriate rehydration should be the critical first step in management of diarrheagenic *E. coli*. In patients with mild and moderate dehydration, oral rehydration usually suffices; intravenous rehydration may be necessary in more severe cases. In the few controlled trials reported, EPEC-associated diarrhea in infants was significantly ameliorated by treatment with appropriate antibiotics [2, 29], although rigorous comparative effectiveness clinical trials of antibiotic regimens have not been performed. Importantly, EPEC is not associated with adult diarrhea. ETEC diarrhea in infants in developing countries responds adequately to rehydration therapy alone. Traveler's diarrhea caused by EAEC and ETEC can be treated with antibiotics (fluoroquinolones, azithromycin, rifaximin) early in the course of clinical illness, which significantly diminishes the severity and duration of illness [5, 30]. Without treatment, however, traveler's diarrhea is usually self-limited. Antibiotics are indicated in the treatment of persistent diarrhea in children caused by EAEC, although the optimal regimen is not known and can be appropriately guided by results of susceptibility testing. It is likely that the same antibiotics effective for ETEC will also be effective for EAEC infections. Although there are no controlled trials of EIEC antibiotic management, because of its close resemblance clinically to shigellosis it is usually treated with the same antibiotics as used for *Shigella* infections, including oral azithromycin, or cefixime, or parenteral ceftriaxone in young children, and oral fluoroquinolones, such as ciprofloxacin, in adults [17]. Of note, resistance to these antibiotics has been documented and it is crucial to understand local resistance patterns. Current data would strongly support that administration of most antibiotics to individuals with EHEC can markedly increase the risk of HUS and renal failure, and antibiotics should not routinely be administered to individuals with bloody diarrhea and low or absent fever who may have EHEC-associated diarrhea [21, 31, 32]. It is not known if antibiotics affect the course of DAEC diarrheal disease.

PREVENTION AND CONTROL

Adequate sanitation and proper personal and food hygiene practices minimize the chance of acquiring *E. coli* diarrheal infection. To prevent ETEC-associated diarrhea, travelers must be assiduous about what they eat and drink. There is limited evidence for non-absorbable antimicrobial prophylaxis (rifaximin) for adults in situations where prophylaxis is required to prevent ETEC-associated traveler's diarrhea, but this agent is ineffective against many other causes of traveler's diarrhea [30].

Considerable progress has been made to develop vaccines to prevent ETEC diarrhea. These vaccines aim at stimulating protective immune responses of both an antitoxin and an anticolonizing nature. The most advanced candidate vaccines under development include: (i) inactivated ETEC-expressing colonization factor antigens (CFAs) combined with B subunit of cholera toxin or heat-labile (LT) toxin; (ii) attenuated *Shigella* or *Salmonella typhi* live vectors expressing CFAs and LT B subunit or a mutant LT; and, (iii) transcutaneous patch delivery LT, mutant LT, and/or fimbrial antigens [5, 33].

EHEC-associated diarrhea is most commonly reported from industrialized countries, largely because of food production and distribution systems. Cattle can act as a reservoir source; prevention of EHEC infection of humans usually involves proper food processing, preparation and food surveillance.

REFERENCES

1. Kaper JB, Nataro JP, Mobley HL. Pathogenic *Escherichia coli*. Nat Rev Microbiol 2004;2:123–40.
2. Nataro JP, Kaper JB. Diarrheagenic *Escherichia coli*. Clin Microbiol Rev 1998;11142–201.
3. Marier R, Wells J, Swanson RC, et al. An outbreak of enteropathogenic *Escherichia coli* foodborne disease traced to imported French cheese. Lancet 1973;302:1376–8.
4. Neter E, Korns RF, Trussel RE. Association of *Escherichia coli* serogroup 0111 with two hospital outbreaks of epidemic diarrhea of the newborn infant in New York State during 1947. Pediatrics 1953;12:377–83.
5. Qadri F, Svennerholm AM, Faruque AS, Sack RB. Enterotoxigenic *Escherichia coli* in developing countries: epidemiology, microbiology, clinical features, treatment, and prevention. Clin Microbiol Rev 2005;18: 465–83.
6. Shah N, DuPont HL, Ramsey DJ. Global etiology of travelers' diarrhea: systematic review from 1973 to the present. Am J Trop Med Hyg 2009; 80:609–14.
7. Mark Taylor C. Enterohaemorrhagic *Escherichia coli* and *Shigella dysenteriae* type 1-induced haemolytic uraemic syndrome. Pediatr Nephrol 2008;23: 1425–31.
8. Okeke IN. Diarrheagenic *Escherichia coli* in sub-Saharan Africa: status, uncertainties and necessities. J Infect Dev Ctries 2009;3:817–42.
9. Flores J, Okhuysen PC. Enteroaggregative *Escherichia coli* infection. Curr Opin Gastroenterol 2009;25:8–11.
10. Spano LC, Sadovsky AD, Segui PN, et al. Age-specific prevalence of diffusely adherent *Escherichia coli* in Brazilian children with acute diarrhoea. J Med Microbiol 2008;57:359–63.
11. Ochoa TJ, Barletta F, Contreras C, Mercado E. New insights into the epidemiology of enteropathogenic *Escherichia coli* infection. Trans R Soc Trop Med Hyg 2008;102:852–6.
12. Grif K, Orth D, Lederer I, et al. Importance of environmental transmission in cases of EHEC O157 causing hemolytic uremic syndrome. Eur J Clin Microbiol Infect Dis 2005;24:268–71.
13. Orth D, Grif K, Zimmerhackl LB, Wurzner R. Prevention and treatment of enterohemorrhagic *Escherichia coli* infections in humans. Expert Rev Anti Infect Ther 2008;6:101–8.
14. Sahl JW, Steinsland H, Redman JC, et al. A comparative genomic analysis of diverse clonal types of enterotoxigenic *Escherichia coli* reveals pathovar-specific conservation. Infect Immun 2011;79:950–60.
15. Dean P, Kenny B. The effector repertoire of enteropathogenic *E. coli*: ganging up on the host cell. Curr Opin Microbiol 2009;12:101–9.
16. Lapointe TK, O'Connor PM, Buret AG. The role of epithelial malfunction in the pathogenesis of enteropathogenic *E. coli*-induced diarrhea. Lab Invest 2009;89:964–70.
17. Kosek M, Yori PP, Olortegui MP. Shigellosis update: advancing antibiotic resistance, investment empowered vaccine development, and green bananas. Curr Opin Infect Dis 2010;23:475–80.
18. Guignot J, Chaplais C, Coconnier-Polter MH, Servin AL. The secreted autotransporter toxin, Sat, functions as a virulence factor in Afa/Dr diffusely adhering *Escherichia coli* by promoting lesions in tight junction of polarized epithelial cells. Cell Microbiol 2007;9:204–21.
19. Servin AL. Pathogenesis of Afa/Dr diffusely adhering *Escherichia coli*. Clin Microbiol Rev 2005;18:264–92.
20. Chao HC, Chen CC, Chen SY, Chiu CH. Bacterial enteric infections in children: etiology, clinical manifestations and antimicrobial therapy. Expert Rev Anti Infect Ther 2006;4:629–38.
21. Scheiring J, Andreoli SP, Zimmerhackl LB. Treatment and outcome of Shiga-toxin-associated hemolytic uremic syndrome (HUS). Pediatr Nephrol 2008; 23:1749–60.
22. Harrington SM, Dudley EG, Nataro JP. Pathogenesis of enteroaggregative *Escherichia coli* infection. FEMS Microbiol Lett 2006;254:12–18.

23. Okhuysen PC, Dupont HL. Enteroaggregative *Escherichia coli* (EAEC): a cause of acute and persistent diarrhea of worldwide importance. J Infect Dis 2010;202:503–5.
24. Scaletsky IC, Fabbricotti SH, Carvalho RL, et al. Diffusely adherent *Escherichia coli* as a cause of acute diarrhea in young children in Northeast Brazil: a case-control study. J Clin Microbiol 2002;40:645–8.
25. Sanchez J, Holmgren J. Virulence factors, pathogenesis and vaccine protection in cholera and ETEC diarrhea. Curr Opin Immunol 2005;17:388–98.
26. Weintraub A. Enteroaggregative *Escherichia coli*: epidemiology, virulence and detection. J Med Microbiol 2007;56:4–8.
27. Echeverria P, Sethabutr O, Pitarangsi C. Microbiology and diagnosis of infections with *Shigella* and enteroinvasive *Escherichia coli*. Rev Infect Dis 1991; 13(suppl. 4):S220–5.
28. Kehl SC. Role of the laboratory in the diagnosis of enterohemorrhagic *Escherichia coli* infections. J Clin Microbiol 2002;40:2711–15.
29. Thoren A, Wolde-Mariam T, Stintzing G, et al. Antibiotics in the treatment of gastroenteritis caused by enteropathogenic *Escherichia coli*. J Infect Dis 1980;141:27–31.
30. DuPont HL. Therapy for and prevention of traveler's diarrhea. Clin Infect Dis 2007;45 (suppl. 1):S78–84.
31. Bitzan M. Treatment options for HUS secondary to *Escherichia coli* O157:H7. Kidney Int 2009;Feb(suppl.):S62–6.
32. Wong CS, Jelacic S, Habeeb RL, et al. The risk of the hemolytic-uremic syndrome after antibiotic treatment of *Escherichia coli* O157:H7 infections. N Engl J Med 2000;342:1930–6.
33. Hill DR, Beeching NJ. Travelers' diarrhea. Curr Opin Infect Dis 2010; 23:481–7.

43 Cholera and Other Vibrios

Debasish Saha, Regina C LaRocque

Key features

- *Vibrio* species are environmental organisms that are found in fresh- and marine-water habitats around the world
- Cholera is caused by *Vibrio cholerae* O1 and O139 strains that carry the genes encoding cholera toxin
- Cholera is spread by contaminated water and food
- Cholera can spread rapidly in areas with unsafe water and food, and can lead to epidemics
- Cholera is endemic in over 50 countries and regularly causes outbreaks and epidemics in these settings
- Treatment of cholera is inexpensive, simple and life-saving
- Other Vibrio species ("non-cholera" Vibrios) are less common pathogens and may cause septicemia, soft tissue infection and gastrointestinal illness

VIBRIO CHOLERAE

INTRODUCTION

Cholera has been one of the great scourges of mankind. Seven global pandemics have occurred since the early 19th century and each has been associated with a tremendous human death toll [1]. The current seventh global pandemic of cholera, caused by *Vibrio cholerae* O1 biotype El Tor, began in Sulawesi, Indonesia in 1961.

The history of cholera is closely tied to the history of medicine. In 1854, John Snow made the seminal observation that sewage-contaminated municipal water was the source of cholera in a London community—a key contribution to the germ theory of disease. Robert Koch isolated the causative bacterium during the fifth pandemic in 1883. Oral rehydration solution (ORS), originally developed for the treatment of cholera, has saved millions of lives and is one of the landmark medical achievements of the 20th century.

EPIDEMIOLOGY

Cholera is a substantial health burden in the developing world. The disease is endemic in Africa, Asia and Central and South America. In particular, the Ganges River Delta is the ancestral epicenter of cholera ("Asiatic cholera"), and predictable seasonal outbreaks occur in this region. Explosive epidemics can occur in under-developed areas with inadequate sanitation, poor hygiene and limited access to clean drinking water. The most recent example of this is the outbreak of cholera that began in Haiti in October 2010.

Precise estimates of global cholera incidence are lacking; the World Health Organization (WHO) estimates that less than 10% of cholera cases are reported, despite the fact that it is a notifiable disease [2]. Limitations in local surveillance and reporting systems and economic disincentives contribute to the global underreporting of cholera. Figure 43.1 shows the global distribution of cholera based on cases reported to the WHO in 2008.

In endemic areas, cholera exhibits a seasonal pattern with periods of high and low incidence. The highest incidence of cholera in endemic regions is among children aged 1–9 years old. In both endemic and epidemic settings, individuals of blood group O with cholera are at much higher risk of developing severe disease (cholera gravis) than persons of other blood groups [3].

NATURAL HISTORY, PATHOGENESIS AND PATHOLOGY

Vibrios are curved, rod-shaped, Gram-negative bacteria that are highly motile owing to the presence of a single polar flagellum. They are found in brackish water environments around the world, often closely associated with zooplankton and other fauna with chitinous exoskeletons [4]. Humans become infected after drinking contaminated water (Fig 43.2). An extremely high concentration of organisms (up to 100 million bacteria per milliliter) is found in cholera stool. Stool-shed organisms are transiently hyperinfectious for the next host—this may contribute to the explosive nature of cholera epidemics [5].

Strains of *V. cholerae* are differentiated serologically on the basis of the lipopolysaccharide O antigen. To date, more than 200 serogroups have been identified. Historically, the O1 serogroup has caused the vast majority of disease. The O1 serogroup is subdivided into two phenotypically distinct biotypes: El Tor and classical. Both biotypes can be further subdivided into two serotypes: Inaba and Ogawa. In the past 20 years, the El Tor biotype has largely replaced the classical biotype and is the cause of the current seventh global pandemic. The O139 serogroup emerged as a cause of disease in 1992, but has remained limited to areas of Asia.

Pathogenic strains of *V. cholerae* O1 and O139 possess two key virulence factors—cholera toxin and the toxin co-regulated pilus (TCP) [7]. TCP is a surface pilus that aggregates organisms together on the surface of the small intestine. Cholera toxin is a prototypical AB subunit toxin. The B subunit binds the toxin to the surface of epithelial cells, while the enzymatically active A subunit is translocated into the cell. The A subunit increases cyclic AMP activity, leading to the massive fluid and electrolyte efflux that is the hallmark of the disease.

CLINICAL FEATURES

The clinical features of cholera caused by *V. cholerae* O1 and O139 are similar. The incubation period varies with host susceptibility and inoculum size; it can range from several hours to as long as 3–5 days. Most cases are mild or asymptomatic, especially in endemic settings.

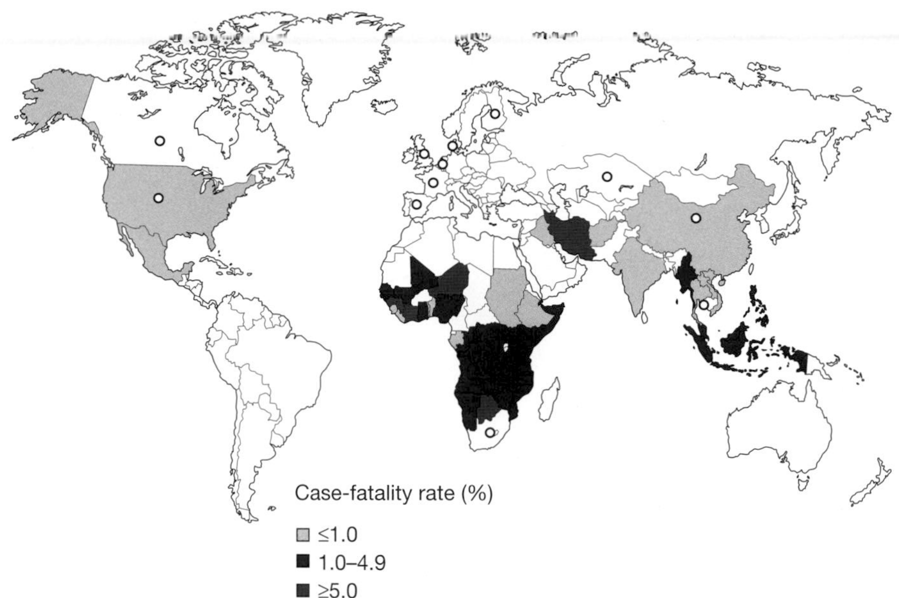

FIGURE 43.1 Global distribution of cholera based on cases reported to the WHO in 2008 (http://gamapserver.who.int/gho/interactive_charts/atlas.html).

In severe cholera (cholera gravis), the characteristic symptom is the frequent passage of profuse "rice-water" stool (Fig. 43.3)—a watery stool with flecks of mucus and a typical fishy odor. Stool output can reach as high as 1 liter per hour in the most severe cases. Abdominal discomfort, borborygmi and vomiting are other common symptoms, particularly in the early phases of disease. Fever is rare.

Dehydration and electrolyte abnormalities are the most important complications of cholera. Examination may reveal sunken eyes (Fig. 43.4), dry mouth, cold clammy skin, decreased skin turgor, or wrinkled hands and feet ("washer woman's hands"). Patients are frequently apathetic and lethargic. Kussmaul breathing may occur as a result of acidosis. The peripheral pulse is rapid and initially thready; it may become difficult to palpate as blood pressure drops. Urine output decreases with time and renal failure with acute tubular necrosis may occur. Muscle cramping and weakness caused by the loss of potassium and calcium are common. In children, depletion of glycogen stores and inadequate gluconeogenesis can lead to severe hypoglycemia or even coma. Aspiration pneumonia is a common comorbidity in children. There are no long-term complications of cholera when it is appropriately treated. Blood stream invasion by the organism is rare. Laboratory testing of cholera patients, when performed, may reveal hypokalemia, hyponatremia, hypocalcemia and acidosis.

"Cholera sicca" is an unusual form of the disease whereby fluid accumulates in the intestinal lumen. Circulatory collapse and even death can occur in the absence of diarrhea.

PATIENT EVALUATION, DIAGNOSIS AND DIFFERENTIAL DIAGNOSIS

Cholera often occurs in outbreaks and hence the diagnosis should be quickly suspected in the appropriate epidemiologic setting. Mild-to-moderate cases of *V. cholerae* may be indistinguishable from infection with other pathogens, such as enterotoxigenic *Escherichia coli*, *Campylobacter* spp. or *Salmonella* spp.

Vibrio cholerae O1 or O139 infection is confirmed by the isolation of the organism in stool culture, followed by biochemical tests and serogrouping with specific antisera. Thiosulfate citrate bile salts sucrose (TCBS) agar or tellurite taurocholate gelatin agar (TTGA) are used for the selective isolation of *V. cholerae*. Cholera can be more rapidly diagnosed using direct dark field microscopy of stool where motile *Vibrio* organisms appear like "shooting stars". An immunochromatographic dipstick test specific for *V. cholerae* has also been developed for rapid testing in field settings without access to laboratory facilities.

TREATMENT

Treatment of cholera is simple and inexpensive. Most importantly, the fluid deficit and ongoing fluid loss must be corrected. Antibiotics, although not necessary, can be administered to stop multiplication of the organism and to decrease the duration of illness. Complications need to be recognized and addressed in a timely manner.

CORRECTION OF FLUID LOSS

Correction of dehydration through fluid replacement and maintenance remains the cornerstone of cholera treatment. A cholera patient can lose between 5 and 10 percent of their body weight in fluid during the course of the illness. Fluid therapy rests upon assessing the level of dehydration (Fig. 43.5). Fluid replacement occurs in two phases. In the **rescue phase**, aggressive fluid replacement, usually administered intravenously, is given in a short period of time to replace the fluid deficit. In the **maintenance phase**, intravenous fluid or ORS is given to replenish ongoing fluid losses. Frequent assessment of ongoing fluid loss is necessary. Stool output should be measured every 4–6 hours during the maintenance phase. Such measurement can be facilitated by the use of a cholera cot: a simple plastic cot with a central hole to facilitate collection of stool in a bucket. Intravenous and oral rehydration fluids are designed to correct the water and electrolyte loss in cholera stool (Table 43-1). The most commonly used intravenous solution is commercially available Ringer's lactate. Locally prepared "Dhaka fluid", which contains more potassium than Ringer's lactate, is used in endemic countries like Bangladesh.

The use of ORS, a readily prepared sugar and salt solution, has revolutionized the treatment of cholera, as well as dehydration caused by other organisms [7]. ORS takes advantage of the fact that glucose-mediated cotransport of sodium and water across the mucosal surface of the small intestine remains intact during cholera. Rice-based ORS involves the use of rice powder instead of glucose and has been shown to be equally effective as standard ORS in adults. Recently, a reduced osmolar ORS that is better tolerated has been developed and is associated with lower rates of associated hypernatremia. Hypo-osmolar ORS (Box 43.1) is currently recommended by the WHO.

Packets for the easy preparation of ORS are widely available in developing countries. If ORS packets are not available, dehydration can

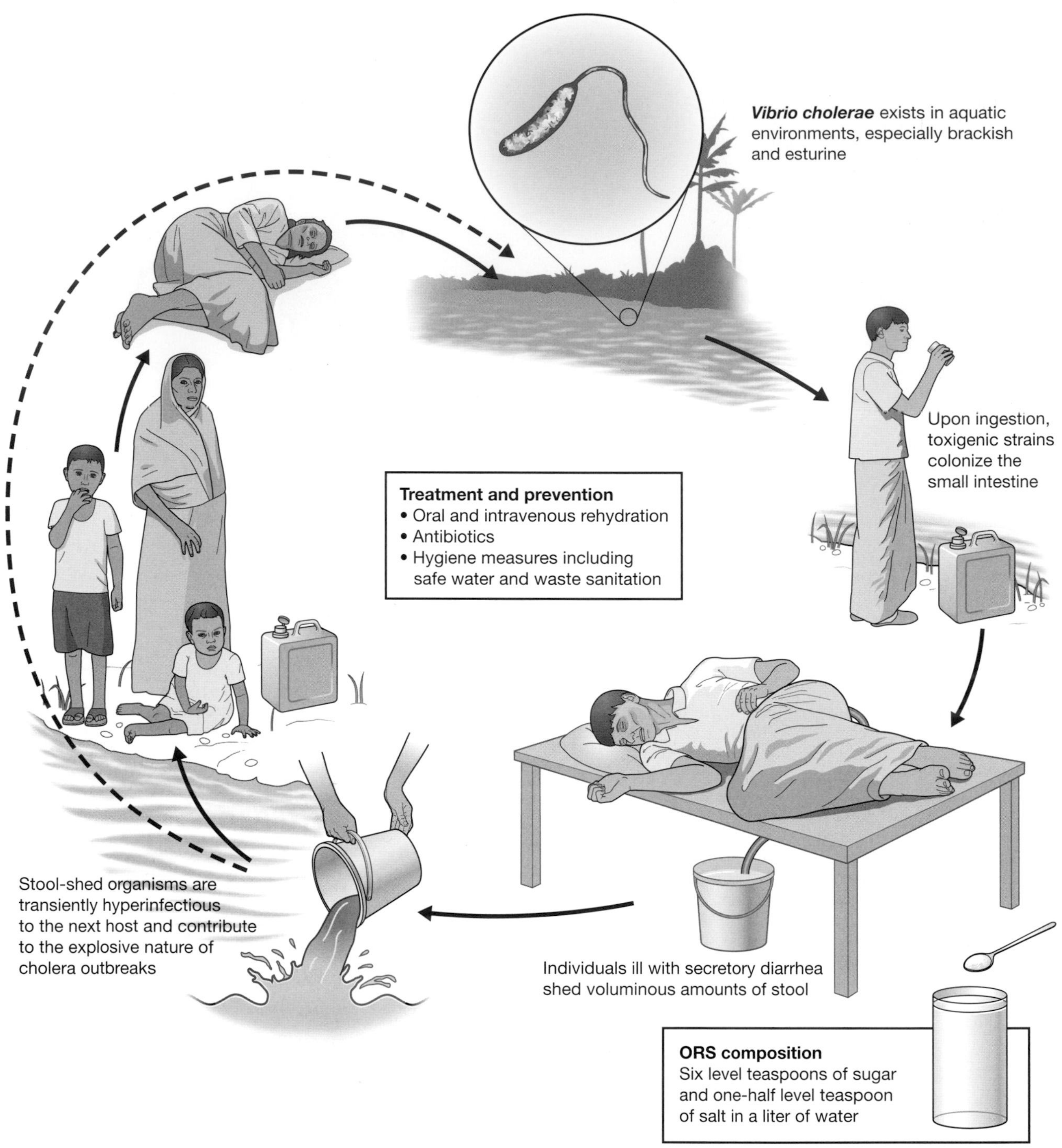

FIGURE 43.2 Cholera lifecycle.

be treated with a solution made with six level teaspoons of sugar and one-half level teaspoon of salt dissolved in one liter of clean water.

Multiple intravenous lines may be required to infuse an adequate amount of fluid to a cholera patient during the rescue phase of rehydration. If an intravenous line cannot be established, fluid should be introduced through a nasogastric tube. In children, an interosseous line in the medial aspect of the tibia can be considered.

Apart from fluid replacement, the intake of freshly prepared food is encouraged when tolerated and breastfeeding should be continued where appropriate. For children up to 5 years of age, supplementary administration of zinc (10 mg/day x 2 weeks in children < 6 months; 20 mg/day x 2 weeks in children 6 months–5 years) has proven effective in reducing the duration of diarrhea, as well as reducing successive diarrhea episodes [8].

ANTIBIOTICS

Antimicrobial therapy is an adjunct to fluid therapy in cholera and has been shown to reduce the duration and volume of diarrheal stool by half. The WHO advocates the use of antibiotics for individuals with severe dehydration, basing choice on local availability and susceptibility pattern [2]. A wide range of antibiotics, both in single- and

TABLE 43-1 Electrolyte content of cholera stool and fluids used in the treatment of cholera

Stool or solution	Electrolyte concentration (mmol/L)				
	Sodium	*Potassium*	*Chloride*	*Acetate/lactate*	*Other*
Cholera stool (adult)	135	15	100	40	–
Cholera stool (child)	100	30	90	30	–
Ringer's lactate	130	4	111	29	3 (calcium)
Dhaka solution	133	13	98	48	–
Standard ORS	90	20	80	10	111 (glucose)
Rice-based ORS	90	20	80	10	88 (rice powder)
Hypo-osmolar ORS	75	20	65	10	75 (glucose)

ORS, oral rehydration solution.

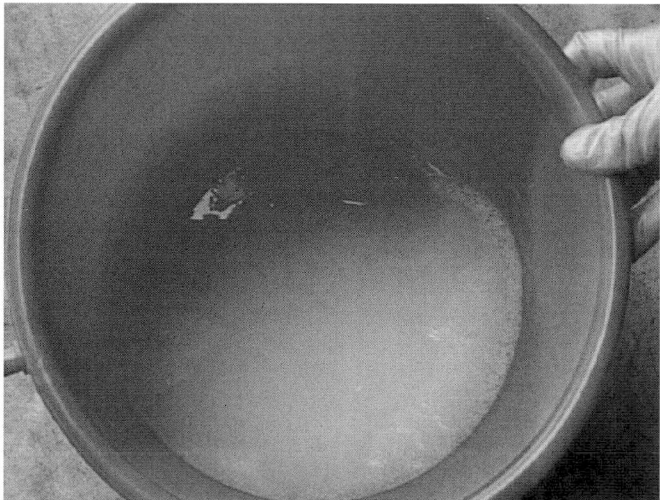

FIGURE 43.3 Rice-water stool.

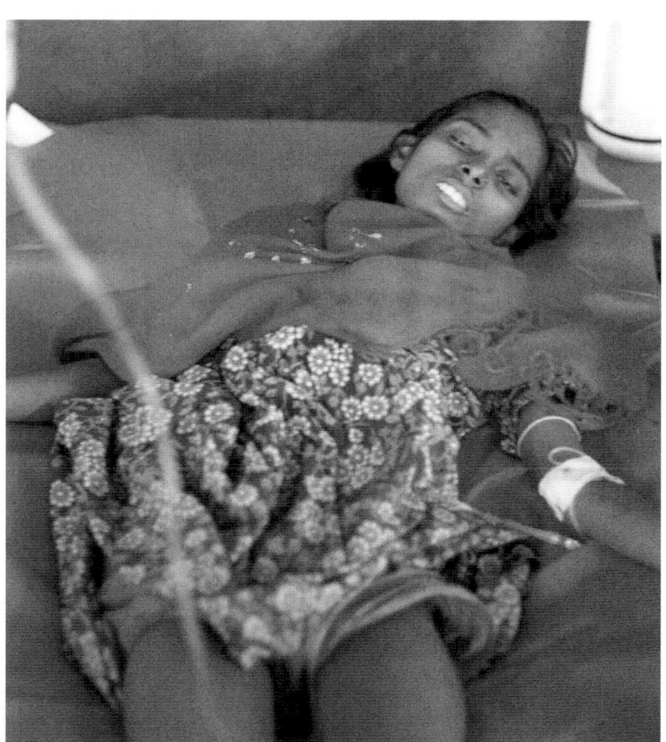

FIGURE 43.4 A cholera patient with sunken eyes.

multiple-dose regimens, are used for the treatment of cholera, as shown in Table 43-2. Resistance of *V. cholerae* O1 and O139 to many commonly used antibiotics is an emerging problem and, thus, knowledge of the local resistance pattern is mandatory. Single-dose regimens are particularly preferred in outbreak settings where healthcare personnel are scarce.

PREVENTION

A clean water supply and appropriate sanitation are essential to the prevention of cholera. Breastfeeding is protective for young infants in endemic settings. Filtering water through a sari cloth before drinking has been demonstrated to be effective in lessening the likelihood of *V. cholerae* infection acquired from surface water sources, probably through removal of *V. cholerae* adherent to particulates. Two oral, killed cholera vaccines are currently available in various countries. These vaccines are usually administered in 1–3 doses 10–15 days apart and are given in 150 milliliters of safe water. The WHO recommends use of cholera vaccines in select situations in conjunction with improved water supplies, adequate sanitation and health education [9].

BOX 43.1 Recipe for Making one Liter of Hypo-osmolar ORS [10]

Sodium chloride (NaCl)	2.6 g
Sodium citrate	2.9 g
Potassium chloride (KCl)	1.5 g
Glucose	13.5 g

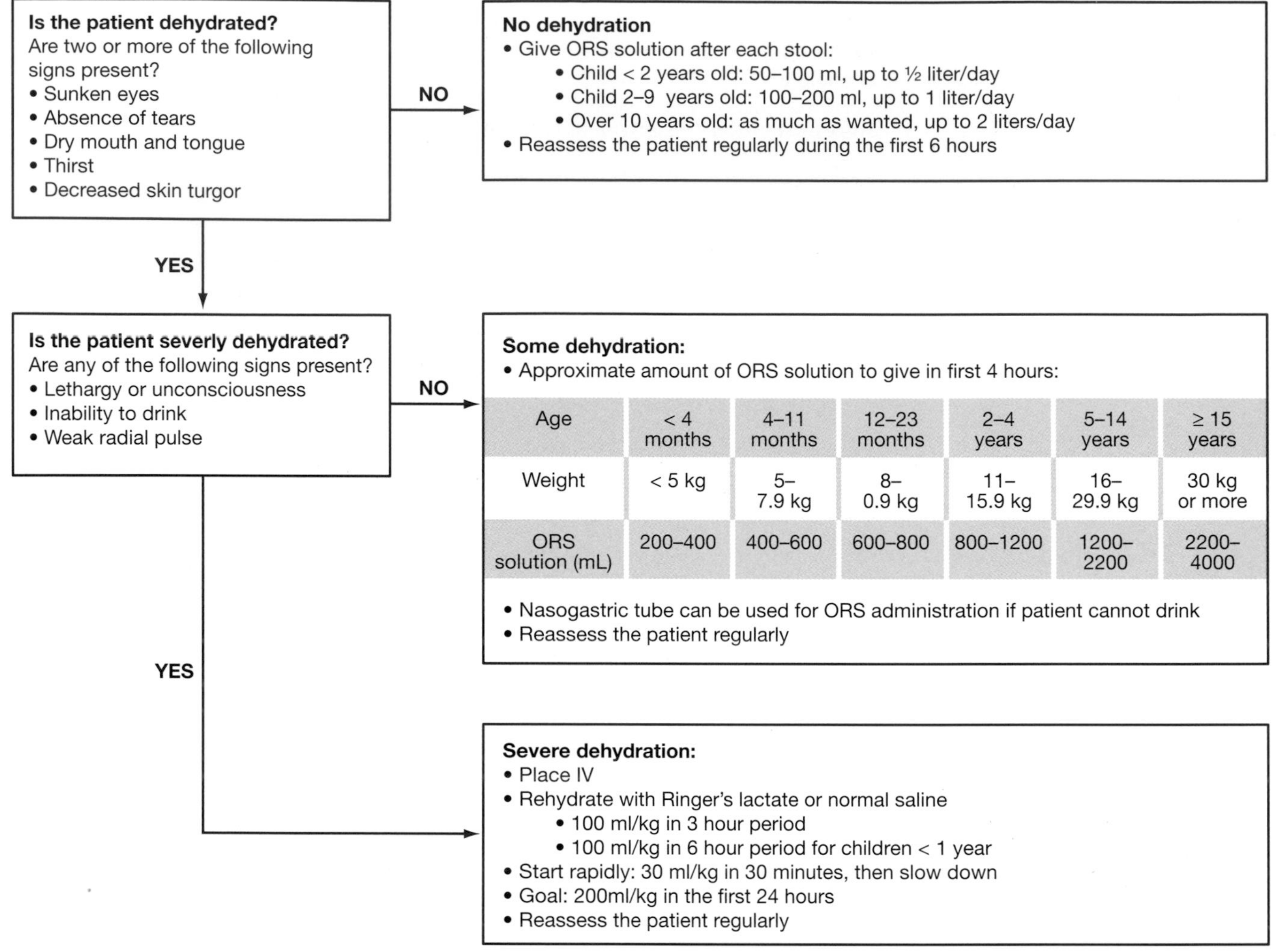

FIGURE 43.5 Approach to fluid management in patients with dehydration.

TABLE 43-2 Antibiotics for the management of cholera

Antibiotic	Older children and adults	Child*	Comments
Tetracycline	500 mg every 6 hours for 3 days	50 mg/kg/day divided every 6 hours for 3 days	Reports of resistance. Contraindicated in pregnant women. Short course precludes teeth staining in children.
Doxycycline	300 mg single dose	4–6 mg/kg single dose	Same as above
Erythromycin	500 mg every 6 hours for 3 days	50 mg/kg/day divided every 6 hours for 3 days	Widely used in pediatric population
Azithromycin	1 g single dose	20 mg/kg single dose	
Ciprofloxacin	500 mg once daily for 3 days OR 1 g single dose	20 mg/kg body weight single dose	

Trimethoprim/sulfamethoxazole, ampicillin, chloramphenicol and furazolidone have previously been used for the treatment of cholera, but are no longer preferred because of resistance patterns and side effect profiles.
*Not to exceed adult dose.

OTHER VIBRIOS

VIBRIO PARAHAEMOLYTICUS

Vibrio parahaemolyticus is the most commonly isolated noncholera vibrio. Like *V. cholerae*, it is found in marine environments. *Vibrio parahaemolyticus* causes gastroenteritis as a result of consumption of raw or partially cooked food, particularly seafood. *V. parahaemolyticus* accounts for a large proportion of food-borne illness in Japan, where consumption of seafood is common. The incubation period for *V. parahaemolyticus* ranges from 4 to 48 hours. Clinical illness tends to be mild, with gastroenteritis symptoms including nausea, vomiting, abdominal pain and diarrhea. The disease is usually self-limiting. Oral rehydration is typically adequate and tetracycline or ciprofloxacin can be administered in severe cases.

VIBRIO VULNIFICUS

Vibrio species have been isolated from wounds exposed to seawater. *Vibrio vulnificus* is a particularly important pathogen in *Vibrio*-associated soft tissue infections and sepsis. Immunocompromised individuals and those with underlying liver disease are especially prone to septicemia with *V. vulnificus*. Thrombocytopenia and disseminated intravascular coagulation are common, along with characteristic bullous skin lesions. The mortality rate is greater than 50%. Tetracycline appears to be effective in conjunction with other supportive treatments. In severe infection, tissue debridement and amputation of the affected limb may be required.

REFERENCES

1. Sack DA, Sack RB, Nair GB, Siddique AK. Cholera. Lancet 2004;363:223–33.
2. The Global Task Force on Cholera Control. Available at: http://www.who.int/cholera/en/.
3. Harris JB, Khan AI, Larocque RC, et al. Blood group, Immunity, and risk of infection with *Vibrio cholerae* in an area of endemicity. Infect Immun 2005;73:7422–7.
4. Colwell RR. Infectious disease and environment: cholera as a paradigm for waterborne disease. Int Microbiol 2004;7:285–9.
5. Nelson EJ, Harris JB, Morris JG Jr, et al. Cholera transmission: the host, pathogen and bacteriophage dynamic. Nat Rev Microbiol 2009;7:693–702.
6. Matson JS, Withey JH, DiRita VJ. Regulatory networks controlling *Vibrio cholerae* virulence gene expression. Infect Immun 2007;75:5542–9.
7. Guerrant RL, Carneiro-Filho BA, Dillingham RA. Cholera, diarrhea, and oral rehydration therapy: triumph and indictment. Clin Infect Dis 2003;37:398–405.
8. Roy SK, Hossain MJ, Khatun W, et al. Zinc supplementation in children with cholera in Bangladesh: randomised controlled trial. BMJ 2008;336:266–8.
9. Cholera Vaccines: WHO Position Paper. Wkly Epidemiol Rec 2010;85:117–28.
10. World Health Organization. The International Pharmacopoeia, 4th edn. Geneva: World Health Organization; 2008.

44 Shigellosis

Michael L Bennish, Wasif Ali Khan

Key features

- Shigellosis is caused by an invasive Gram-negative bacteria, *Shigella*, which destroys ilieal and colonic epithelium and elicits a local and systemic inflammatory response
- Four distinct *Shigella* species cause infection, with clinical presentations varying by species and serotype. Of these, *Shigella dysenteriae* type 1 is associated with epidemic disease and the highest risk of mortality
- Humans are the only reservoir for *Shigella* and infection occurs by fecal–oral or human-to-human transmission where hygiene and sanitation are problematic, such as in developing countries or in daycare centers
- Patients with severe shigellosis have tenesmus, cramps, passage of bloody-mucoid stools, and high fever
- Patients with dysentery or systemic symptoms require antimicrobial therapy, while those with less severe symptoms may be managed symptomatically
- Because of lack of microbiology facilities in most developing country settings, the decision to initiate treatment with an antimicrobial agent should be empiric, based upon a presumptive clinical diagnosis
- A number of complications may occur in patients with shigellosis, including hemolytic uremic syndrome (with *S. dysenteriae* type 1), reactive arthritis and seizures
- Synonyms: bacillary dysentery

INTRODUCTION

Epidemic dysentery has been known since antiquity. The causative organism, *Shigella dysenteriae* type 1, a Gram-negative bacillus, was identified by the pioneering Japanese microbiologist Kiyoshi Shiga in 1897 [1]. Subsequently, other species of *Shigella* causing endemic dysentery or diarrhea were identified and received eponymous species names (*Shigella flexneri, Shigella boydii* and *Shigella sonnei*). These species vary in their virulence, with *S. dysenteriae* type 1, the only species that produces Shiga toxin, being the most virulent, and *S. sonnei* generally the least virulent.

Shigellosis is associated with poor hygiene and under-development, and continues to be an important health problem in developing countries. Although efforts to develop an effective vaccine are ongoing, none have yet been marketed. Thus, control of shigellosis continues to require improvement in hygienic conditions and appropriate identification and treatment of those who are infected.

EPIDEMIOLOGY

Shigellosis remains an important cause of morbidity and mortality worldwide. Although estimates of disease burden are hampered by limited surveillance and reporting [2], it is estimated that more than 150 million clinical infections with *Shigella*, and more than 200,000 deaths, occur annually. Approximately two-thirds of these infections and deaths occur in children less than 5 years of age [3]. However, mortality, if not incidence, may currently be less given a recent decline in the number of *S. dysenteriae* type 1 epidemics.

Although shigellosis can occur in all ages, infection predominantly occurs in young children. This may be a result of both the less fastidious hygiene habits of the young and the lack of protective immunity in infants and young children, which may result from previous exposure. Although many areas with high rates of endemic shigellosis also have a high prevalence of HIV, there is little evidence that those with HIV are disproportionally at risk of *Shigella* infection in developing countries [4].

The geographic distribution of *Shigella* infections varies by species (Fig. 44.1). In wealthy, industrialized countries *S. sonnei* is the predominant cause of infection; the more virulent *S. flexneri* is less common. The reverse is true in relatively poor countries in the tropics, where *S. flexneri* predominates (Fig. 44.1) [2, 5]. Indeed, the switch from a preponderance of *S. flexneri* infections to *S. sonnei* infections (as has recently occurred in Thailand) [5] may be a marker of a country's social and economic development.

Epidemics of dysentery, especially those with high mortality rates, are usually the result of *S. dysenteriae* type 1 infections. In recent decades, endemic and epidemic *S. dysenteriae* type 1 infections have most commonly occurred in South Asia and central and east Africa. Since 2000, *S. dysenteriae* type 1 infections have become uncommon in these regions. Infections with *S. boydii* have, historically, been most common in South Asia and have also been reported from Africa, but never account for a majority of infections [2]. Infections with *S. dysenteriae* other than type 1 are even less common.

Humans are the only natural reservoir of *Shigella* and infections usually result from either fecal–oral or direct person-to-person transmission. Transmission by water or by commercial food products is less common but does occur. Transmission of *Shigella* can occur with a low inoculum—less than 10 organisms have been shown to be able to transmit infection.

NATURAL HISTORY, PATHOGENESIS AND PATHOLOGY

Shigellosis is an infection of the distal ileum and colon. Shigellae are enteroinvasive, i.e. they invade, multiply within and destroy colonic epithelial cells resulting in tissue destruction, mucosal ulceration, disruption of small vessels and hemorrhage, and microabscesses in the colon (Fig. 44.2). Infection and inflammation is most severe in the rectosigmoid and less severe proximally [6]. There may also be involvement of the distal ileum.

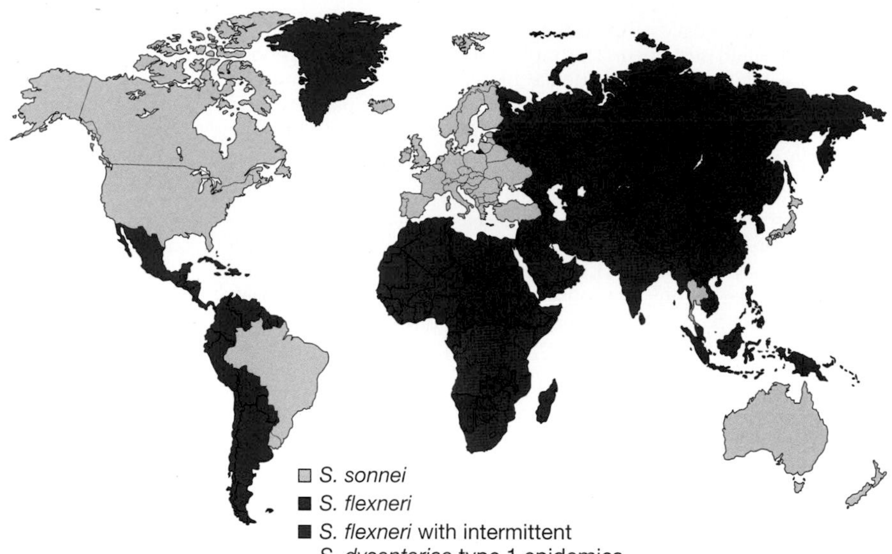

FIGURE 44.1 Geographic distribution of Shigella by species and serotype.

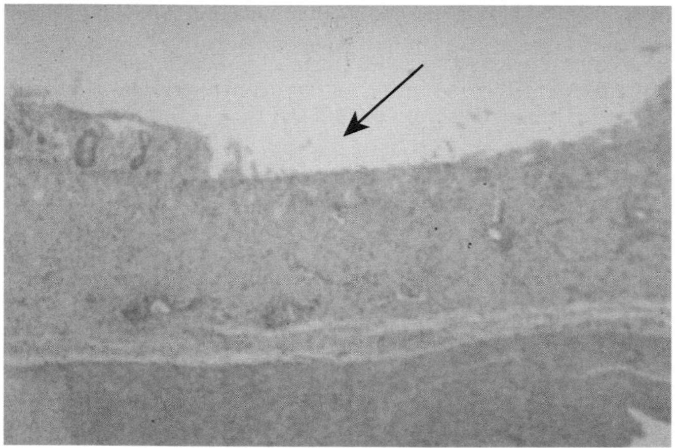

FIGURE 44.2 Microscopic view of colonic epithelium obtained from descending colon of patient with shigellosis showing extensive ulceration to the level of the lamina propria (arrow).

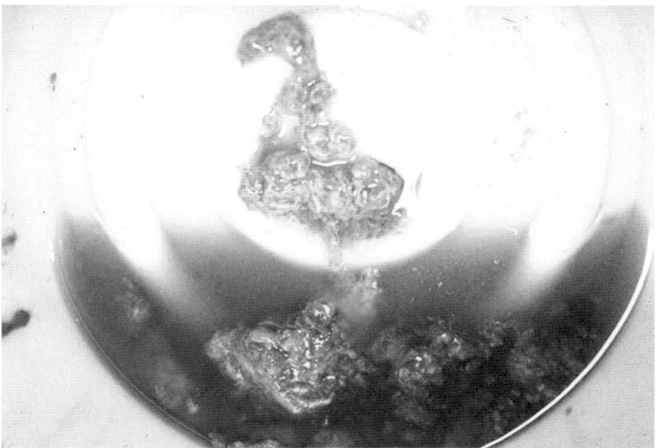

FIGURE 44.3 Characteristic dysenteric stool of a patient with shigellosis containing blood, mucus, and small amounts of fecal matter.

Infection elicits—both locally and systemically—a profound inflammatory response with an outpouring of polymorphonuclear cells and mucus. This, along with the blood from the ulceration and destruction of small vessels in the colonic epithelium, results in the characteristic dysenteric stool (Fig. 44.3). The systemic inflammatory response is reflected in the chills, fever, and malaise that often precede the dysentery.

Virulence in *Shigella* is primarily controlled by a 220-kb virulence plasmid that has genes encoding adherence and invasion of colonic epithelial cells, and spread within and between cells [7]. It is this plasmid that makes *Shigella* distinct from *Escherichia coli*, which it otherwise closely resembles genetically.

Shigella dysenteriae type 1 produces an exotoxin, Shiga toxin, which inhibits protein synthesis. It role in the pathogenesis of infection remains unclear, but *S. dysenteriae* infections are associated with a more severe colitis than seen in other infections, and systemic complications, including hemolytic-uremic syndrome (HUS) and leukemoid reaction, that almost never occur with other species or serotypes of *Shigella*. Additional enterotoxins—*Shigella* enterotoxins (ShET) 1 and 2—have been identified more recently and are implicated in the watery diarrhea that is often the presenting feature of shigellosis.

CLINICAL FEATURES

The hallmark of *Shigella* infections is dysentery, which consists of the frequent, painful passage of small volume stools that consist of mucus, blood, inflammatory cells, and fecal matter (Fig. 44.3). The passage of stools is accompanied by tenesmus and cramping. All of these features are a result of the inflammatory and ulcerative changes in the colon. In children with severe colitis, the repeated straining that is associated with the tenesmus can result in rectal prolapse (Fig. 44.4).

Watery diarrhea, rather than dysentery, can often be the presenting intestinal symptom. In some patients, especially those with *S. sonnei* infection, the diarrhea remains watery and dysentery never occurs.

Intestinal complications (Table 44-1) include toxic colitis [8], which causes obstruction and systemic toxicity, and mimics the toxic colitis seen with ulcerative colitis (Fig. 5A, B), a disease with a similar pathology, if different etiology, from shigellosis. Other intestinal complications include perforation and a protein-losing enteropathy.

A host of systemic, nonintestinal complications can occur with shigellosis, most of which appear to be more common and more severe among malnourished children in developing countries (Table 44-1).

Fever is a characteristic of most *Shigella* infections and can often be high (40°C) and sustained. The rapid rise of fever with shigellosis leads to a relatively high incidence of seizures in young children who are infected (≈ 5% in one study of hospitalized patients) and can occur with infection of any of the species of *Shigella* [9]. The metabolic complications described below can also produce seizures (Fig. 44.6).

Patients, especially children, may also develop encephalopathy. Lethargy and confusion are common in severe shigellosis; obtundation and coma may also occur. These mental status changes may result from the metabolic complications described below or because shigellosis, especially *S. dysenteriae* type I, induces more generalized, but poorly understood, neurologic complications.

Metabolic complications (Table 44-1) include hypoglycemia from inadequate gluconeogenesis [10] and hyponatremia, presumably from inappropriate antidiuretic hormone (ADH) secretion. Though the blood loss from the intestinal microhemorrhages is usually not severe enough to cause anemia, it may exacerbate pre-existing anemia, or cause anemia in those with underlying hepatic or clotting abnormalities. Hypoproteinemia can occur, presumably resulting from a combination of protein loss in the gut, diminished nutrition during illness and systemic inflammation causing diminished protein synthesis [11].

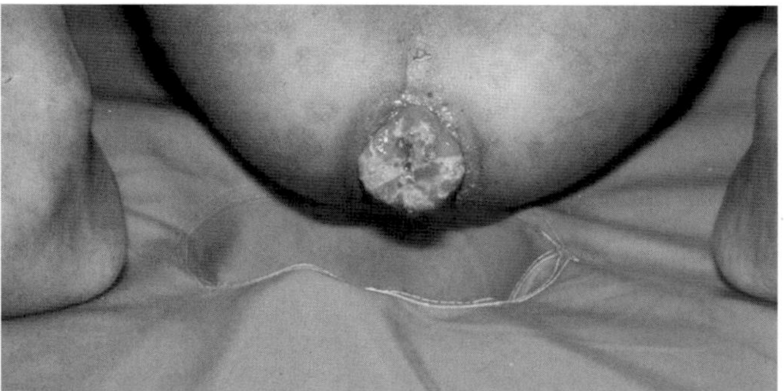

FIGURE 44.4 Child with complete rectal prolapse.

Shigella may also cause infection of epithelial surfaces outside the gut, including the cornea and the vagina [12, 13], and may also be systemically invasive, causing bacteremia and sepsis [14]. Bacteremia with other bacterial pathogens may also occur during *Shigella* infection, presumably from the translocation of gut bacteria across a damaged epithelium or from iatrogenic causes, including contaminated intravenous fluids and catheter-related infections [15].

Perhaps the most serious complication of *Shigella* infection is the development of HUS [16]. This complication occurs with *S. dysenteriae* type 1 infection, which, like enterohemorrhagic *E. coli* (EHEC), produces an exotoxin—Shiga toxin (Shiga-like toxin in EHEC)—that is thought to be related to the development of HUS. In addition to the microangiopathic anemia and renal failure, leukemoid reaction (peripheral blood polymorphonuclear cell count > 50,000 mm^3) and thrombocytopenia may occur in association with HUS, or separately as a "forme fruste" of HUS.

PATIENT EVALUATION, DIAGNOSIS, AND DIFFERENTIAL DIAGNOSIS

The diagnosis of shigellosis is important because, unlike watery diarrhea caused by noninvasive enteric pathogens (rotavirus, other enteric diarrheogenic viruses, enterotoxigenic *E. coli*), patients with dysentery caused by *Shigella* require antimicrobial therapy, rather than simply fluid therapy to prevent, or treat, dehydration. Antimicrobial therapy is important both to relieve the suffering that occurs from the primary disease—tenesmus is an agonizing condition —and to prevent complications from occurring [17].

Although isolation of *Shigella* from stool is required for the definitive diagnosis of shigellosis, the time required for isolation—48 hours—the lack of diagnostic microbiologic facilities at most health facilities in developing countries and the insensitivity of current culture methods [6], make such an approach not particularly useful in the management of individual patients. The initiation of treatment must be empiric, based upon a presumptive clinical diagnosis.

The distinguishing feature of shigellosis is dysentery. In developing countries where shigellosis is endemic, children with dysentery (bloody-mucoid stools and tenesmus) have a high probability of

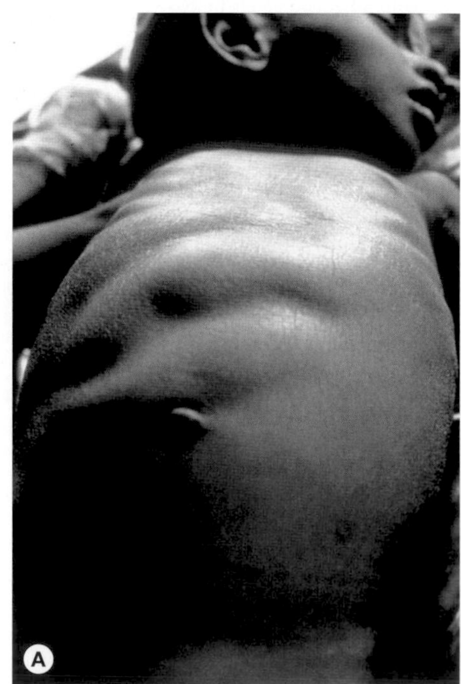

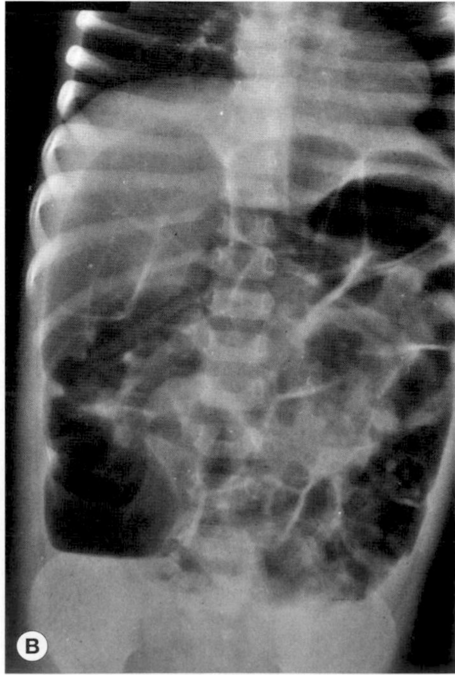

FIGURE 44.5 (A, B) Child with toxic megacolon showing dilated loops of bowel; obstruction and air fluid levels on abdominal radiograph.

TABLE 44-1 Complications associated with shigellosis

Complication	Species most common with	Etiology and pathogenesis	Management	Outcome
Intestinal complications				
Rectal prolapse	*Shigella dysenteriae* type 1, *Shigella flexneri*	Increased intra-abdominal pressure associated with repeated tenesmus and straining, Most common in infants and children because of lack of development of musculature	Magnesium sulfate compresses to reduce edema; gentle re-insertion for grade 1–2 prolapse	Usually recovers completely, but often recurs if diarrhea recurs
Toxic megacolon	*S. dysenteriae* type 1	Transmural inflammation of colon, possibly increase in nitric oxide production in colonic musculature inhibiting motility	Supportive. Intravenous fluids, no oral intake, antibiotics for sepsis and for treatment of primary infection. In poor countries where complications are most common, colectomy often not available and long-term care after colectomy is problematic	Ominous complication often associated with leukemoid reaction or HUS. Mortality rate >33%
Intestinal perforation	*S. dysenteriae* type1	Transmural ulcer from severe colonic inflammation	Surgical repair if possible; broad-spectrum antimicrobial therapy for sepsis. Medical management if surgery not possible	Less ominous outcome than toxic megacolon
Extraintestinal complications				
Metabolic complications				
Dehydration	*Shigella sonnei*, other species	Watery diarrhea, with or without dysentery, can be a feature of all *Shigella* infections. Watery diarrhea maybe caused by *Shigella* enterotoxins 1 and 2. Also increased fluid loss because of fever. Decreased fluid intake because of anorexia	Severe dehydration uncommon. Oral or intravenous fluid as appropriate	Rarely lethal alone, no long-term sequelae if managed appropriately
Hyponatremia	*S. dysenteriae* type 1, less commonly *S. flexneri*	Probable inappropriate secretion of antidiuretic hormone	If severe (Na <120 mmol/L) with altered consciousness infusion of 3% NaCl (12 ml/kg over a 4-hour period); less severe episode (Na; 120–130 mmol/L), infusion of 0.9% NaCl; restriction of water intake	If treated, no long-term complications. If not recognized, can cause seizures, unconsciousness
Hypoglycemia	*S. dysenteriae* type 1	Depleted glycogen stores; impaired gluconeogenesis	Intravenous infusion of dextrose (2.0 ml/kg of 25% glucose)	No long-lasting complications if recognized early
Hypoproteinemia	*S. dysenteriae* type 1, *S. flexneri*	Protein loss in stool; decreased protein synthesis because of inflammation	High-protein diet; management of edema	Pulmonary edema, ascites. Complications will resolve if hypoproteinemia is corrected
Other systemic complications				
Seizures and encephalopathy	*S. sonnei*, other *Shigella* species	Seizures may be febrile in origin in young children; encephalopathy may be caused by metabolic aberrations or sepsis. Shiga toxin produced by *S. dysenteriae* type 1 known to be neurotoxic in animals—no evidence it causes neurotoxicity in humans	Correction of metabolic disorder if present; reduction of fever; anticonvulsant treatment, if required	Mortality usually not directly related to altered consciousness; rarely long-term sequelae if recognized and treated
Septicemiae	*S. dysenteriae* type 1, other *Shigella* species less commonly	Colonic perforation or leakage because of transmural inflammation; iatrogenic from contamination of intravenous solutions or needle	Broad-spectrum antibiotic; infusion of intravenous fluid to combat shock	High mortality if not recognized; no long-term sequelae if treated appropriately

TABLE 44-1 Complications associated with shigellosis—cont'd

Complication	Species most common with	Etiology and pathogenesis	Management	Outcome
Hemolytic uremic syndrome (HUS)	*S. dysenteriae* type 1	Related to Shiga toxin production	Fluid restriction; peritoneal or hemodialysis if required and facilities available; blood transfusion for anemia	In developing country settings associated with high risk of mortality because of lack of appropriate treatment. Usually no long-term severe renal impairment if patient recovers from acute phase
Leukemoid reaction	*S. dysenteriae* type 1	Feature of HUS, but may occur alone—also presumably related to Shiga toxin	Treat primary infection	No long-term sequelae
Reactive arthritis	*S. flexneri, S. sonnei*	Autoimmune reaction with genetic susceptibility (persons with HLA-B27)	Anti-inflammatory treatment, symptomatic relief of pain, rest	Usually occurs during second or third week of illness. Usually monoarticular or migrating arthritis affecting large joints without redness or rise of temperature at the site; may be associated with conjunctivitis and urethritis. Little long-term follow-up reported, but can persist or recur
Infection at other epithelial sites (conjunctiva, vagina)	All species	*Shigella* occasionally infect other epithelial sites	Systemic antimicrobial therapy	Resolves with appropriate therapy
Malnutrition	*S. dysenteriae* type 1, *S. flexneri*	Decreased food intake because of anorexia; increased protein loss in gut; increased metabolism from fever, inflammation; decreased protein synthesis because of inflammation	Ensure adequate feeding. Use nasogastric tube if required. High-protein diet	Post-infectious malnutrition puts children at risk of other infections. Associated with high mortality if not corrected

HLA, human leukocyte antigen.

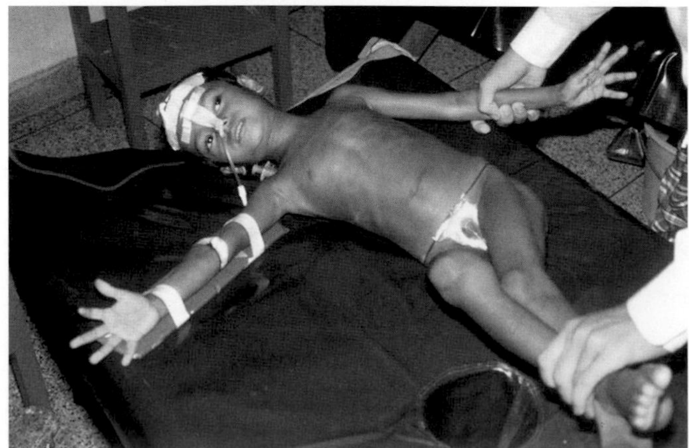

FIGURE 44.6 Child with seizures occurring in conjunction with hyponatremia.

being infected with *Shigella*. In adults, other causes of dysentery are more common than in children, but all patients with severe dysentery in the tropics still have a high probability of having shigellosis.

In addition to the dysenteric stool, other features supportive of the diagnosis of shigellosis include abdominal tenderness, fever (though less common in malnourished children), and rectal prolapse. During a *S. dysenteriae* type 1 epidemic, the probability that dysentery is a result of *Shigella* infection is even greater.

The laboratory test that is likely to be most immediately available in developing countries is microscopic examination of the stool using either a wet mount or Gram-stain. Either will show large numbers of polymorphonuclear cells and erythrocytes. Other supportive laboratory tests include a peripheral blood leukocyte count with leukocytosis. Though rapid bedside tests for identification of *Shigella* infection have been developed [18], none are commercially available. Rapid tests for the identification of Shiga toxin exist, and could, presumably, be of help in the diagnosis of *S. dysenteriae* type 1 infections. However, the diagnosis of shigellosis primarily remains a clinical one based on the patient having the classic signs of dysentery.

If microbiologic laboratory facilities are available, definitive diagnosis is done by isolation of *Shigella* from the stool. Shigellae are not hardy, thus cultures are best done by plating a stool sample at the bedside or immediately transporting a sample to the laboratory. If stools samples cannot be immediately processed, they should be transported in a buffered-glycerol saline media, which has a higher yield than the more commonly available Cary-Blair transport media. Stool samples are plated upon media selective for Gram-negative organisms. *Shigella* does not ferment lactose and thus appear white or colorless on selective media containing acid-sensitive indicator dyes. Non-lactose-fermenting colonies are then further analyzed using biochemical tests for definitive confirmation that they are *Shigella*.

Another important cause of dysentery in developing countries—intestinal amebiasis caused by *Entamoeba histolytica* infection—is a much less frequent cause of the dysentery syndrome, especially in children. When compared with patients with shigellosis, patients with amebiasis are less likely to have fever, have fewer white cells in their stool and are generally less toxic [19]. If direct microscopy is available, the finding of enterophagocytic trophozoites of *E. histolytica* on examination of stool is characteristic of amebiasis—the presence of *E. histolytica* cysts is not. *Campylobacter jejuni* infections, though common in children, are less often symptomatic; cramping is more common than tenesmus and stools are less bloody than in shigellosis. Ulcerative colitis is exceedingly rare in comparison with shigellosis. The chronicity of ulcerative colitis will, in time, distinguish it from shigellosis.

Patients suspected of having shigellosis should be evaluated for complications of the disease (Table 44-1). Rectal prolapse (Fig. 44.4) will be self-evident on cursory examination, but may be only intermittently present. Patients with suspected hypoglycemia—either because of alteration in consciousness or preceding severe anorexia—should be monitored using simple finger-prick blood glucose monitoring. Other metabolic abnormalities, including hyponatremia, should also be suspected in patients with altered consciousness and require laboratory monitoring. The development of toxic-megacolon is best identified by physical examination showing signs of obstruction: distended abdomen (Fig. 44.5A) accompanied by vomiting and often hyperactive bowel sounds. Abdominal radiographs will show ileus and findings of obstruction (Fig. 44.5B).

If *S. dysenteriae* type 1 infection is suspected, there should be monitoring of hematocrit or hemoglobin, and renal function. If severe anemia or diminished renal function (measured either by an increase in blood creatinine or urea nitrogen and diminished urine output) occurs, such patients should be transferred to a facility (if available) capable of conducting renal dialysis.

TREATMENT

ANTIMICROBIAL THERAPY

Antimicrobial drugs are the definitive treatment for shigellosis and all patients with dysentery symptoms should receive antimicrobial therapy. Controlled studies from the 1950s onward established the value of antimicrobial therapy in children and adults with shigellosis. In those early studies, a number of children receiving placebo died [20] and, since that time, appropriately few placebo controlled trials have been conducted in shigellosis. Virtually all the randomized controlled trials have compared two or more agents that were thought to be effective.

Drugs that are effective, and useful, in the treatment of shigellosis have the following characteristics [21]:

- are effective *in vitro* against *Shigella*;
- achieve concentrations in the blood stream in excess of the minimum inhibitory concentration (MIC) of the infecting strain of *Shigella*;
- are effective when given orally because of the difficulties of providing parenteral therapy where the majority of *Shigella* infections occur;
- are preferably available in a liquid formulation suitable for use in children;
- are inexpensive.

A wide variety of drugs have proven effective in the treatment of shigellosis. Previous mainstays of therapy included ampicillin, trimethoprim-sulfamethoxazole, and nalidixic acid. However, widespread resistance to all three drugs limits their current usefulness for treating shigellosis. Despite good serum concentrations and *in vitro* activity, amoxicillin [22] and oral cephalosporins have not been effective in the treatment of shigellosis [23, 24].

Optimally, the choice of antibiotic is based upon knowledge of local resistance patterns—information that is all too often lacking. Because of current widespread resistance to the previous mainstays of therapy, fluoroquinolones and azithromycin are the current drugs of choice for treating shigellosis. Both fluoroquinolones and azithromycin have been demonstrated to be effective in well-conducted, randomized, controlled trials. However, resistance to these newer agents is now starting to appear—particularly with *S. dysenteriae* type 1, but also with other *Shigella* species. Treatment doses and recommendations are shown in Table 44-2.

Patients with *Shigella* infection but without dysentery or systemic signs of illness do not require antimicrobial therapy. However, such mild cases of *Shigella* infection are unlikely to be identified as stool cultures are not usually obtained from such patients [25].

SUPPORTIVE THERAPY AND TREATMENT OF COMPLICATIONS

Severe dehydration is not a common feature of shigellosis and, thus, intravenous therapy is rarely required in conscious patients [26]. Patients should receive oral rehydration therapy to replace those fluids that are lost.

Equally important is early feeding [27]. Because of the anorexia, protein loss in the gut and increased metabolism, the development of malnutrition (or exacerbation of pre-existing malnutrition) can be an important complication of shigellosis. Aggressive feeding with a high-protein diet if possible, can ameliorate the nutritional deterioration that follows dysentery with *Shigella* and also help prevent hypoglycemia. In infants, frequent breastfeeding (or formula-feeding) should be encouraged throughout the course of the illness while, in older children, additional, high-protein meals can be initiated while the patient remains symptomatic. Nasogastric feeding and intravenous dextrose can be used for those who are severely anorexic.

Supplemental zinc reduces the severity and duration of the acute infection and also reduces the incidence and severity of diarrhea in the 3 months after infection. Thus, 20 mg of elemental zinc once daily for 10–14 days for children 7–59 months old and 10 mg per day for infants aged 6 months or less is recommended for children with shigellosis in developing countries. Vitamin A supplementation during the acute illness does not reduce the severity or duration of the acute infection, nor has it been proved to reduce the incidence of new infections. It may be useful in malnourished children, however, and the practice at some centers of excellence is to give a single dose of vitamin A to severely malnourished children who have not received vitamin A in the last 6 months (50,000 units for those below 6 months of age; 100,000 units for infants aged 6–12 months; 200,000 units for children aged 1–5 years).

Rectal prolapse is best treated with warm magnesium sulfate compresses to reduce edema and definitive treatment of the infection to lessen the tenesmus that causes the prolapse. Convulsions that occur in the absence of any metabolic derangements, such as hypernatremia or hypoglycemia are usually not complex or sustained and are best managed using local protocols for the management of febrile convulsions in children, including the provision of antipyretics.

TABLE 44-2 Current options for antimicrobial therapy of shigellosis

Antimicrobial agent		Pediatric			Adult			Comment
		Dose/route of administration	*Frequency*	*Duration*	*Dose/route of administration*	*Frequency*	*Duration*	
Drugs of choice								
Ciprofloxacin	Multiple dose	15 mg/kg orally to maximum adult dose	Every 12 h	3 days	500 mg	Every 12 h	3 days	Single-dose therapy is not effective in treatment of *Shigella dysenteriae* type 1 infections and may not be effective in the treatment of infections caused by other *Shigella* species that are not highly susceptible to ciprofloxacin (MIC <0.004 μg/ml)
	Single dose	Not evaluated			1 g	Upon diagnosis	Single dose	
Azithromycin		15 mg/kg orally to maximum adult dose as initial dose, followed by 10 mg/kg day to maximum adult dose on subsequent days	Every 24 h	5 days	500 mg day 1 followed by 250 mg on subsequent days	Every 24 h	5 days	
Alternative drug therapies								
Pivmecillinam (registered as amdinocillin pivoxcil in the USA, where it currently is not available)		20 mg/kg orally to maximum adult dose	Every 6 h	5 days	400 mg	Every 6 h	5 days	In contrast to ampicillin, pivmecillinam selectively binds to penicillin-binding protein 2 and is relatively resistant to many common β-lactamases, thus may be effective in treatment of strains resistant to ampicillin
Ceftriaxone		50 mg/kg intravenously or intramuscularly to maximum individual dose of 1.5 g	Every 24 h	2–5 days	Not evaluated			Because this agent must be administered parenterally, it is reserved for use in patients who are infected with strains of *Shigella resistant to* first-line oral drugs or are severely ill and need parenteral drugs in hospital. It has not been evaluated in controlled studies for treatment of *S. dysenteriae* type 1. For infection with other species of *Shigella*, both two-dose 2-day and five-dose 5-day courses of therapy have proven successful. Although not evaluated in adults, there is no reason to believe it would not be effective. In controlled trials, oral cephalosporins have been ineffective in the treatment of shigellosis and should not be used

MIC, minimum inhibitory concentration.

REFERENCES

1. Trofa AF, Ueno-Olsen H, Oiwa R, Yoshikawa M. Dr. Kiyoshi Shiga: discoverer of the dysentery bacillus. Clin Infect Dis 1999;29:1303–6.
2. Ram PK, Crump JA, Gupta SK, et al. Part II. Analysis of data gaps pertaining to Shigella infections in low and medium human development index countries, 1984–2005. Epidemiol Infect 2008;136:577–603.
3. Kotloff KL, Winickoff JP, Ivanoff B, et al. Global burden of Shigella infections: implications for vaccine development and implementation of control strategies. Bull World Health Organ 1999;77:651–66.
4. van Eijk AM, Brooks JT, Adcock PM, et al. Diarrhea in children less than two years of age with known HIV status in Kisumu, Kenya. Int J Infect Dis 2010;14:e220–5.
5. von Seidlein L, Kim DR, Ali M, et al. A multicentre study of Shigella diarrhoea in six Asian countries: disease burden, clinical manifestations, and microbiology. PLoS Med 2006;3:e353.
6. Speelman P, Kabir I, Islam M. Distribution and spread of colonic lesions in shigellosis: a colonoscopic study. J Infect Dis 1984;150:899–903.
7. Parsot C. Shigella spp. and enteroinvasive *Escherichia coli* pathogenicity factors. FEMS Microbiol Lett 2005;252:11–8.
8. Bennish ML, Azad AK, Yousefzadeh D. Intestinal obstruction during shigellosis: incidence, clinical features, risk factors, and outcome. Gastroenterology 1991;101:626–34.
9. Khan WA, Dhar U, Salam MA, et al. Central nervous system manifestations of childhood shigellosis: prevalence, risk factors, and outcome. Pediatrics 1999;103:E18.
10. Bennish ML, Azad AK, Rahman O, Phillips RE. Hypoglycemia during diarrhea in childhood. Prevalence, pathophysiology, and outcome. N Engl J Med 1990;322:1357–63.
11. Bennish ML, Salam MA, Wahed MA. Enteric protein loss during shigellosis. Am J Gastroenterol 1993;88:53–7.
12. Murphy TV, Nelson JD. Shigella vaginitis: report of 38 patients and review of the literature. Pediatrics 1979;63:511–6.
13. Macdonald R Jr, Edwards WC. Shigella corneal ulcer. Am J Ophthalmol 1965;60:136–9.
14. Duncan B, Fulginiti VA, Sieber OF Jr, Ryan KJ. Shigella sepsis. Am J Dis Child 1981;135:151–4.
15. Struelens MJ, Patte D, Kabir I, et al. Shigella septicemia: prevalence, presentation, risk factors, and outcome. J Infect Dis 1985;152:784–90.
16. Rahaman MM, Jamiul Alam AK, Islam MR, Greenough WB III. Shiga bacillus dysentery associated with marked leukocytosis and erythrocyte fragmentation. Johns Hopkins Med J 1975;136:65–70.
17. Bennish ML, Khan WA, Begum M, et al. Low risk of hemolytic uremic syndrome after early effective antimicrobial therapy for *Shigella dysenteriae* type 1 infection in Bangladesh. Clin Infect Dis 2006;42:356–62.
18. Nato F, Phalipon A, Nguyen TL, et al. Dipstick for rapid diagnosis of *Shigella flexneri* 2a in stool. PLoS One 2007;2:e361.
19. Speelman P, McGlaughlin R, Kabir I, Butler T. Differential clinical features and stool findings in shigellosis and amoebic dysentery. Trans R Soc Trop Med Hyg 1987;81:549–51.
20. Haltalin KC, Nelson JD, Ring R III, et al. Double-blind treatment study of shigellosis comparing ampicillin, sulfadiazine, and placebo. J Pediatr 1967;70:970–81.
21. Salam MA, Bennish ML. Antimicrobial therapy for shigellosis. Rev Infect Dis 1991;13:S332–S341.
22. Nelson JA, Haltalin KC. Amoxicillin less effective than ampicillin against Shigella in vitro and in vivo: relationship of efficacy to activity in serum. J Infect Dis 1974;129(suppl.):S222–7.
23. Salam MA, Seas C, Khan WA, Bennish ML. Treatment of shigellosis: IV. Cefixime is ineffective in shigellosis in adults. Ann Intern Med 1995;123:505–8.
24. Nelson JD, Haltalin KC. Comparative efficacy of cephalexin and ampicillin for shigellosis and other types of acute diarrhea in infants and children. Antimicrob Agents Chemother 1975;7:415–20.
25. World Health Organization. Guidelines for the control of shigellosis, incuding epidemics due to *Shigella dysenteriae* 1. Geneva: World Health Organization; 2005. Available at: *http://whqlibdoc.who.int/publications/2005/9241592330.pdf*.
26. Bennish ML, Harris JR, Wojtyniak BJ, Struelens M. Death in shigellosis: incidence and risk factors in hospitalized patients. J Infect Dis 1990;161:500–6.
27. Kabir I, Malek MA, Mazumder RN, et al. Rapid catch-up growth of children fed a high-protein diet during convalescence from shigellosis. Am J Clin Nutr 1993;57:441–5.

45 Nontyphoid *Salmonella* Disease

Melita A Gordon, Nicholas A Feasey, Stephen M Graham

Key features

- The importance of nontyphoid Salmonellae (NTS) as a cause of invasive disease in Africa has overtaken their importance as a cause of diarrheal illness and enterocolitis
- Invasive NTS disease disproportionately affects very young children and HIV-infected adults with CD4 <200 cells/μl, in whom it is considered an AIDS-defining illness
- The decision to initiate antibiotic therapy for invasive NTS disease is usually based on clinical suspicion alone
- The nonspecific clinical presentation of invasive NTS disease and frequent occurrence of co-infections such as pneumonia, malaria, and tuberculosis (TB) presents diagnostic challenges and complicates treatment decisions
- The widespread emergence of multidrug-resistant NTS presents additional management challenges and further emphasizes the need for evidence to guide optimal choice and duration of antibiotic treatment
- High mortality rates and frequent recurrence after discontinuation of therapy underscore the importance of invasive NTS infection

INTRODUCTION

The importance of nontyphoid Salmonellae (NTS) as a cause of invasive disease in Africa has overtaken their importance as a cause of diarrheal illness and enterocolitis. NTS have been a significant cause of invasive bacterial disease among children in the tropics, particularly in sub-Saharan Africa, for many decades, pre-dating the HIV epidemic. In 1983, the first six cases of AIDS presenting among African adults were described, three of whom had *Salmonella* Typhimurium bacteremia [1, 2]. Invasive NTS (iNTS), associated with AIDS in Africa, was first described as being predominantly caused by *S.* typhimurium, with an absence of diarrhea and a high recurrence rate [3] now all well-recognized features of this illness. Recurrent NTS bacteremia was added to the CDC case definition of AIDS in 1987. As the HIV epidemic has evolved, iNTS disease has become one of the commonest causes of febrile adult admission in sub-Saharan Africa. iNTS in children and HIV-infected adults carries a high mortality and, even with appropriate antibiotic treatment, there is a 30–50% rate of recurrence. Empiric diagnosis and management remain challenging, and multidrug antimicrobial resistance is a rapidly developing problem.

EPIDEMIOLOGY

Blood culture series of febrile adults and children in HIV-endemic Africa have consistently shown that NTS are one of the commonest causes of invasive bacterial infection together with *Streptococcus pneumoniae* and *Mycobacterium tuberculosis* (see Fig. 45.1) [4]. In sub-Saharan Africa, the incidence of iNTS far exceeds that of invasive disease caused by *Salmonella* Typhi [5]. *Salmonella* Typhimurium and *Salmonella* Enteritidis are the most commonly isolated serovars. In contrast, in North Africa, where HIV prevalence is lower and malaria is not endemic, *Salmonella* Typhi is often the commonest blood isolate [6]. An increase in iNTS disease coincided with an increase in HIV prevalence in Thailand, but iNTS remains much less common in Asia than *S.* Typhi and *S.* Paratyphi in all ages.

There are very few estimates of the burden of NTS diarrheal disease in Africa [7]. Most healthy African children appear to have been exposed to *Salmonella*, presumably during early intestinal infection, and acquired killing antibodies by the age of 16 months [8]. Among African children, the rate of asymptomatic carriage in the stool may be nearly as high as the rate of detection during diarrheal disease [9], but this is not a universal finding.

iNTS occurs in a bimodal age distribution in Africa, peaking among young children, aged 6–24 months and among adults aged 20–45 years (see Fig. 45.2) [5]. Conservative estimates of the incidence of pediatric iNTS in sub-Saharan Africa range from 170–388 per 100,000 person years in children under the age of 3 years; this drops to

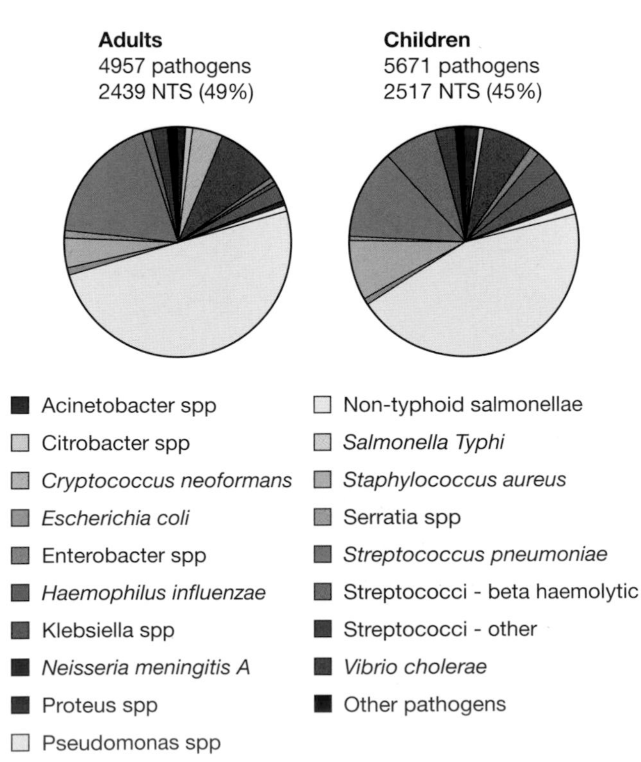

FIGURE 45.1 Pathogens isolated from blood cultures among febrile adults and paediatric admissions in Blantyre, Malawi, 1998–2004 (listed from the 12 o'clock position on the pie-chart).

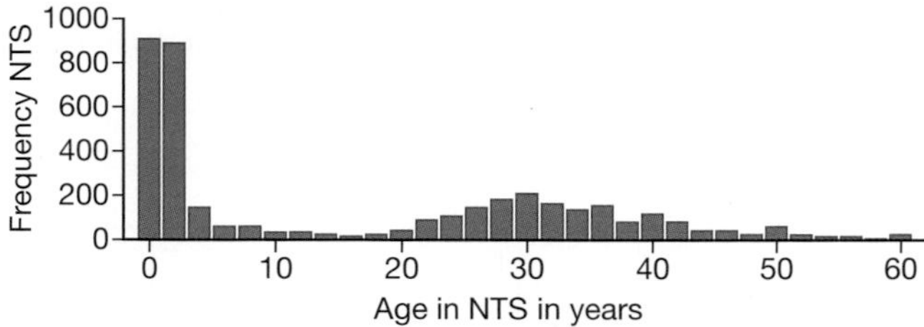

FIGURE 45.2 The distribution of cases of invasive NTS disease by age in Blantyre, Malawi.

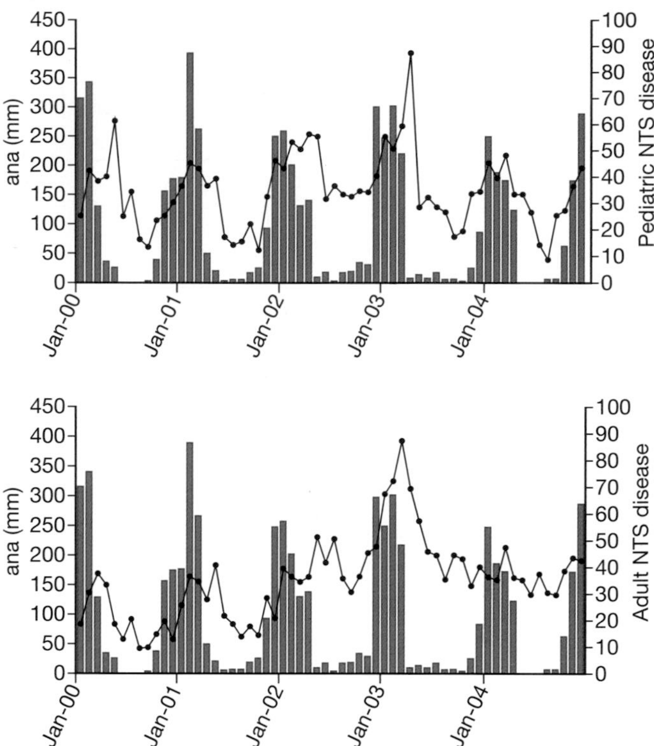

FIGURE 45.3 The relationship between rainy season and incidence of invasive NTS in adults and children, by month, in Malawi, 2000–2004.

6/100,000 over the age of 5 years [10–12]. There is a lower incidence among infants in the first 4 months of life, consistent with protection from maternal IgG or from secretory IgA in breastmilk [8], but NTS may, nonetheless, be a significant cause of neonatal sepsis and meningitis [13].

In children, severe malaria and malnutrition are associated with an increased risk of invasive bacterial disease, including iNTS. Compared with other bacterial pathogens in children, iNTS is associated with severe anemia, often in the context of malaria [14–18]. Sickle cell anemia is strongly associated with iNTS in African children, but this is not a common risk factor. HIV infection also confers an increased risk of iNTS in African children but, in contrast to adults, most cases of iNTS in African children are not HIV-related.

In adults, there is a close association between iNTS and advanced HIV disease in sub-Saharan Africa, with over 95% of cases occurring in HIV-infected individuals [6, 19]. The incidence of iNTS in HIV-infected adults ranges from 2000–8500/100,000 person years of observation. Events are rare at high CD4 counts, but rise up to 9000/100,000 when CD4 <200 cells/µl [20]. The impact of widely available anti-retroviral treatment (ART) in Africa is not yet clear.

Other conditions predisposing adults to invasive NTS disease include diabetes, long-term steroid use, hematologic or solid cancers, autoimmune disease, advanced liver disease (particularly alcoholic liver disease), renal or other transplantation, and the use of other immunosuppressive drugs, including anti-tumor necrosis factor (TNF) antibody treatment. Invasive NTS disease is also seen in children with specific primary immunodeficiencies, including chronic granulomatous disease and rare genetic deficiencies of cytokine subunits or receptors in the interleukin (IL)12/IL23 pathway [20].

iNTS incidence in both adults and children is associated with seasonal rainfall (see Fig. 45.3), although it is uncertain whether this results from increased waterborne transmission, or whether it is because it coincides with the peak period for malaria and malnutrition, which are also risk factors. The relationship between invasive disease, diarrheal disease, and stool carriage of NTS is poorly understood and transmission routes are not well-defined. In contrast to the well-known role of infected food-animals or contaminated food items in diarrheal *Salmonella* disease in industrialized countries, studies have failed to identify a major animal, food, or environmental reservoir of iNTS in Africa, and person-to-person spread may play a relatively greater role in transmission [21]. The conditions in many hospitals in tropical Africa may also support nosocomial transmission, especially in the emergence of drug-resistant NTS.

NATURAL HISTORY, PATHOGENESIS, AND PATHOLOGY

DIARRHEAL DISEASE

Diarrheal disease caused by NTS in immunocompetent individuals is characterized by inflammatory mucosal disease, with inflammatory infiltrates in the lamina propria of the ileum and colon, and crypt abscess formation (enterocolitis). A lack of colonic crypt architectural disturbance may be helpful in distinguishing infective colitis from idiopathic inflammatory bowel disease on biopsy. Asymptomatic carriage in the stool may continue for several months. Antibiotic treatment is known to increase the rate and duration of carriage in the stool after an episode of *Salmonella* diarrhea.

INVASIVE DISEASE

NTS causing invasive disease likely invade through the small bowel mucosa causing a primary bacteremia. As many patients do not report gastrointestinal symptoms, such as pain or diarrhea, this may occur without overt inflammation. The lack of inflammation and diarrhea in HIV-infected patients may be because of a loss of mucosal Th17 T cells, leading to a lack of recruitment of neutrophils [22]. By the time patients present with fever, they usually already have an established disseminated intracellular infection with replication in the bone marrow and reticuloendothelial system, as well as bacteremia (see Fig. 45.4) [23, 24]. This may be the explanation for the high rate of recrudescence, even after antibiotic treatment. Although the pathogenesis of iNTS is reminiscent of that of enteric fever, classic complications of enteric fever such as small bowel perforation and hemorrhage are not usually seen in iNTS disease.

MICROBIOLOGY

Salmonella is a genus of motile, facultative anerobic Gram-negative bacilli closely related to *Escherichia coli*. Definitive diagnosis of iNTS disease is by aerobic blood culture, and of diarrheal NTS disease by stool culture in appropriate selective broth and plates. There are two species, *S. enterica* and *S. bongori;* all Salmonellae causing human disease fall within the species *S. enterica*, which has six subspecies. Human isolates usually fall within the subspecies *enterica*. A serologic method of typing devised by Kaufman and White, based on lipopolysaccharide (LPS) somatic cell wall O antigens, envelope antigens (eg Vi antigen) and phase 1 and phase 2 flagellar H antigens enables differentiation of *Salmonella* into serovars, designated with names describing clinical syndromes (e.g. Choleraesuis, Typhimurium, Enteritidis), or the place where the organism was described (e.g.

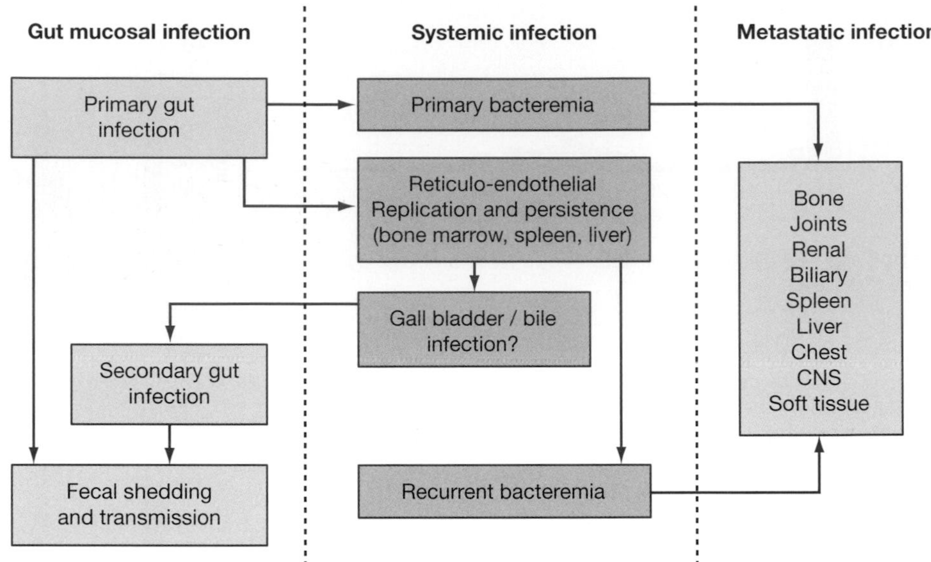

FIGURE 45.4 A scheme to illustrate the pathogenesis of invasive NTS disease in HIV.

Dublin, Newport). To distinguish serovars from species and subspecies, they are notated in non-italicized text with a capital letter (e.g. *Salmonella enterica* subsp. *enterica* serovar Typhimurium, usually shortened to *S.* Typhimurium).

Among human isolates, *Salmonella* Typhi and Paratyphi are considered "typhoidal" and cause a human-restricted illness called enteric fever. All other serovars, which have a wider vertebrate host range, are considered "non-typhoid Salmonellae", or NTS.

The vast majority of diarrheal illness is caused by only a few serovars, with *S.* Enteritidis, *S.* Typhimurium, *S.* Virchow, *S.* Newport, *S.* Hadar, *S.* Heidelberg, *S.* Agona, and *S.* Indiana being the most common globally, although data from the tropics are scanty.

Invasive *Salmonella* disease in the industrialized world is typically, but not exclusively, associated with serotypes *S.* Cholerasuis, *S.* Virchow, and *S.* Dublin. Invasive disease in tropical settings is most commonly caused by *S.* Typhimurium and *S.* Enteritidis. A novel sub-Saharan African variant of *S.* Typhimurium, designated ST313 has emerged, which has loss of genes required for an enteric lifestyle, similar to that seen in *S.* Typhi, suggesting recent evolution of *S.* Typhimurium towards a more human-adapted invasive lifestyle [24].

Antibiotic resistance is an emerging problem among Salmonellae worldwide including among iNTS. Plasmid-borne multidrug resistance to chloramphenicol, cotrimoxazole and ampicillin is now documented from many sites in Africa. Resistance to fluoroquinolones or cephalosporins is not yet widespread in Africa, but is emerging and likely to continue and spread, given the increasing empiric use of these agents for bacterial infections during HIV infection [25].

CLINICAL FEATURES

DIARRHEAL NTS DISEASE

NTS enterocolitis presents with abdominal cramps, nausea and vomiting, and watery diarrhea, which may also be bloody in severe cases. Patients may be febrile, and 1–4% of adults have a transient bacteremia, which may lead to focal or metastatic infection, particularly in elderly patients. In severe cases, enterocolitis may be accompanied by shock related to dehydration or to associated sepsis. Diarrheal illness usually lasts 2–5 days, resolving spontaneously. Complications including toxic colonic dilatation and perforation may be heralded by a prolonged disease course, severe pain, abdominal tenderness, signs of peritonitis or shock. Diarrheal disease may be followed by seronegative reactive arthritis or Reiter's syndrome.

INVASIVE DISEASE (iNTS)

The usual presentation of iNTS is a nonspecific febrile illness and the frequency of common presenting clinical features is shown in Table 45-1. As these data show, the clinical picture is heterogeneous and there may be no obvious clinical focus. Diarrhea is often absent. The clinical picture may be complicated by co-infections—especially in HIV-infected patients—including respiratory, such as tuberculosis (TB), *S. pneumoniae* or *Klebsiella* spp. A concurrent respiratory infection may cause a simultaneous intravascular Gram-negative sepsis to be overlooked [19]. In young children especially, there is clinical overlap with the presentation of pneumonia, severe malaria, and anemia [26]. This means that clinical diagnosis is especially difficult in the resource-limited setting and that empiric antibiotic treatment must have broad coverage (see below). Mortality associated with an index event of iNTS is very high (25–50%), even in microbiologically confirmed cases with appropriate antibiotic treatment [19, 25, 27].

In adults, iNTS generally presents during stage 4 HIV disease and 80% of patients at index presentation have a CD4 count of below 200 cells/μl. Features of advanced HIV disease may be present. Other causes of immunosuppression should be sought in the absence of HIV in adults.

RECURRENT iNTS DISEASE

Recurrence of NTS bacteremia occurs in 30–40% of survivors, even after 2 weeks of antibiotic treatment. Relapse is typically seen after 2–6 weeks and represents a recrudescence with the same index isolate. The number of viable bacteria is higher in bone marrow at relapse compared with the first presentation, suggesting an established intracellular niche. Re-treatment with antibiotics is not always successful, and 25% of patients with one recurrence go on to have multiple recurrences [19]. If ART is available, successful immune reconstitution appears to greatly reduce the risk of iNTS recurrence.

FOCAL AND SUPPURATIVE NTS DISEASE

Salmonellae have a capacity to cause focal suppurative disease [28]. This is a problem in the elderly, in young children with diarrheal disease and transient bacteremia, in immunosuppressed patients, and in children with invasive NTS infection. There is a particular predilection to cause osteomyelitis and pyogenic arthritis, particularly in sickle cell disease [29]. Intravascular infections at structurally damaged sites, such as atheroma, aneurysms, or damaged heart valves cause persistent bacteremia, usually require combined surgical and medical therapy, and have a poor outcome. Focal infections during HIV are

TABLE 45-1 Clinical features of invasive nontyphoid *Salmonella* (NTS) disease among adults and children in sub-Saharan Africa

Clinical feature	Children	Adults	Comment
Age of peak incidence	6–36 months	20–45 years	
Fever	97%	95%	May be absent in malnourished children
Diarrheal illness	30–50%	20–40%	Often absent, or not a prominent feature
Respiratory illness	50–60%	30%	With abnormalities on physical examination or chest radiogram, often attributable to a second pathogen
No obvious focus	25–40%	20–30%	
Splenomegaly	45%	30–40%	An independent predictor of iNTS in febrile adults
Hepatomegaly	35%	15%	
Severe anemia	25–35%	50%	A predictor of poor outcome
Malaria slide positive	25–40%	15%	Acute high parasitemia, and recent malaria episodes are risk factors for iNTS among children
HIV co-infection	20–25%	95%	
Case definition of AIDS	–	50–80%	iNTS is an event defining stage 4 HIV disease
Relapse rate	–	30–43%	Relapse is usually from an intracellular sanctuary site, and difficult to treat, but may be prevented by prompt effective anti-retroviral treatment
Mortality	22–25%	25–50%	

also described in the chest (empyema and, rarely, primary pneumonia), renal tract, genital tract, and hepatobiliary tract [20].

NTS meningitis in adults and children in Africa has a very poor outcome (60% mortality among children, 80% mortality among adults) [13, 30], and subdural or epidural empyema are also described. Of particular note in the tropics is a phenomenon where active schistosomiasis is associated with persistent or recurrent NTS bacteremia among children, despite antibiotic treatment. This occurs because the bacterium is able to adhere to the adult helminth's tegument using a bacterial pilus, providing it with a sanctuary where it can evade antimicrobial treatment. Treatment with praziquantel kills the adult helminth, and allows effective antibiotic eradication of the *Salmonella* with prompt resolution of fever [31].

PATIENT EVALUATION, DIAGNOSIS, AND DIFFERENTIAL DIAGNOSIS

The two most common clinical syndromes arising from NTS are enterocolitis with diarrheal disease or invasive disease with sepsis. In resource-limited settings it is usually necessary to take a syndromic approach to evaluating these two modes of presentation.

DIARRHEAL DISEASE

Acute febrile diarrheal disease is usually presumed to be infective unless specific features suggest other diagnoses or complications. Evaluation should include assessment of history, duration, fever, pain, shock, dehydration, urine output, and careful examination of the abdomen. The abdominal pain may be severe and the clinical picture may resemble one of appendicitis. Simple stool microscopy may show polymorphic inflammatory cells. Stool may be positive for occult or occasionally frank blood, but this is not diagnostically helpful. Plain abdominal film or sigmoidoscopy are necessary only if toxic dilatation, other complications, or alternative diagnoses are suspected.

INVASIVE DISEASE

The nonspecific clinical features seen in iNTS (Table 45-1), limited access to laboratory and microbiology facilities, and the emergence of multi-drug resistance make iNTS a challenging illness to diagnose and manage in resource-limited settings. Although definitive diagnosis of iNTS is by blood culture, these facilities are not widely available in sub-Saharan Africa. Therefore, an empiric approach to diagnosis and management is often necessary.

An approach often used among children is to "rule out" malaria through blood film or malaria antigen card test. However, because of the association of pediatric malaria with iNTS, malaria parasitemia does not rule out iNTS or other co-infections. Differential diagnosis of patients presenting in the tropics with fever as their primary complaint must include malaria, TB, and pneumococcal sepsis in addition to iNTS. Among adults, HIV testing and staging is essential, and presentation with iNTS defines stage 4 HIV disease. Given the strong association of iNTS with advanced HIV disease, co-infection with any, and all, of these pathogens must also be considered. Presentation with NTS bacteremia and concomitant pneumonia caused by a second pathogen is particularly diagnostically challenging among both adults and children. Many children with iNTS also meet the World Health Organization (WHO) case definition for acute lower respiratory tract infection (LRTI), and empiric treatment for pneumonia may not cover NTS disease [26].

In a study of clinical predictors of blood stream pathogens among febrile admissions in Africa, splenomegaly with high fever (>39 °C) conferred a high independent odds ratio (4.9) for NTS bacteremia. Surprisingly, splenomegaly did not predict malaria or TB. Splenomegaly may, therefore, be a useful clinical marker of iNTS disease in adults in an HIV-prevalent setting [32], but it is only found in 30–40% of cases.

TREATMENT

DIARRHEAL DISEASE

Management of enterocolitis caused by NTS should be supportive; antibiotic treatment is not indicated except in severe, or complicated, cases. In cases of dysentery (grossly bloody diarrhea), where an etiologic agent is not sought or identified, empiric antibiotic therapy should be directed against *Shigella* species, which are more common causes of dysentery and also derive a clear benefit from treatment. In contrast, antibiotics do not reduce the duration of diarrheal illness caused by NTS, and they prolong stool shedding and increase the risk of side effects from treatment itself (evidence grade 1).

INVASIVE DISEASE

The choice of empiric therapy for febrile patients requiring hospital admission in an HIV-endemic area is difficult. Reliance on narrow-spectrum penicillin, even if respiratory features are prominent, may miss cases of iNTS. There is also widespread resistance of iNTS to chloramphenicol, ampicillin and co-trimoxazole. Broader-spectrum cover (see below) may be considered necessary and judged according to known local antimicrobial resistance patterns and local availability of antimicrobials. If an antibiotic or combination of antibiotics inactive against iNTS fails to cause defervescence and clinical improvement in febrile patients after 48 hours, consideration should be given to changing to a regimen with activity against NTS.

Antibiotics which may be available and effective against NTS include third-generation cephalosporins (such as ceftriaxone), fluoroquinolones (such as ciprofloxacin), and the macrolide azithromycin. However, there have been no clinical trials for iNTS disease to provide guidance. Fluoroquinolones probably offer superior intracellular penetration and reduce the risk of recurrence (evidence grade 4), but the risks of using fluoroquinolones include partial treatment of disseminated TB which may obscure the diagnosis and generate drug resistance. Short courses of fluoroquinolones, as are used in typhoid fever, should be avoided in iNTS because of the high rate of recurrence seen in this disease. If a microbiologic diagnosis of iNTS is confirmed, then a course of 14 days of an effective antimicrobial should be used.

Failure to improve on an effective agent should lead the clinician to consider TB as an alternative or additional diagnosis. However, in some cases of iNTS, even in the setting of appropriate therapy, resolution of fever may take several days. A clinical search should also be made for focal suppurative complications. Prolonged antibiotic treatment, for at least 6–8 weeks, is required for focal sepsis, along with drainage of any pus collection. Needle aspiration of infected large joints is an acceptable first step, but formal surgical drainage may be necessary if there is a poor response (evidence grade 2). Joints should not be immobilized during treatment, but movement allowed as pain permits. Outcomes for septic arthritis can be excellent if well-managed. Our experience of NTS empyema is that prolonged chest drainage is required, with antibiotic treatment, but results were disappointing. Treatment of infected heart valves and vascular structures frequently requires a combination of surgical and prolonged antibiotic treatment, and outcomes following mycotic aneurysm infection are especially poor. Treatment with praziquantel to eradicate possible live schistosomal helminths in endemic areas is safe and may be helpful (evidence grade 4).

PREVENTION OF RECURRENCE

iNTS frequently recrudesces from an intracellular site of persistence in HIV-positive adults [19, 23]. Although prolonged courses of fluoroquinolones (i.e. 4–6 weeks of ciprofloxacin) have been suggested for treatment and secondary prevention in guidelines from industrialized countries (evidence grade 5), this is based on expert opinion in settings with low prevalence of TB and in the pre-ART era. Prolonged therapy has not been subject to clinical trials or cost–benefit analysis, and its impact on broader antimicrobial resistance has not yet been assessed. This is particularly important as fluoroquinolones are a mainstay of treatment for multidrug-resistant TB.

The impact of ART and cotrimoxazole preventive therapy on preventing recurrence in HIV-infected adults and children remains unknown. However, as recrudescence is often early, resistance to cotrimoxazole and logistical difficulties in early initiation of ARVs may reduce the impact of these interventions. Clinical trials of strategies to prevent recurrence without compromising antimicrobial efficacy are urgently needed. As there are no satisfactory evidence-based options for prevention, expectant management with retreatment of iNTS with an effective agent as it recurs remains the best option (evidence grade 5).

VACCINATION

There is currently no vaccine for NTS. Antibody is likely to be protective, and a deficiency of antibody against NTS has been shown in susceptible African children [8]. Among some HIV-infected adults, however, the observation has been made that there is an excess of inhibitory anti-*Salmonella* antibodies directed again LPS, that compete with killing antibodies. This raises the possibility that a vaccine directed against LPS might do harm, so a vaccine directed against *Salmonella* membrane proteins or other targets would be more appropriate [33].

REFERENCES

1. Clumeck N, Mascart-Lemone F, de Maubeuge J, et al. Acquired immune deficiency syndrome in Black Africans. Lancet 1983;1:642.
2. Offenstadt G, Pinta P, Hericord P, et al. Multiple opportunistic infection due to AIDS in a previously healthy black woman from Zaire. N Engl J Med 1983;308:775.
3. Sperber SJ, Schleupner CJ. Salmonellosis during infection with human immunodeficiency virus. Rev Infect Dis 1987;9:925–34.
4. Reddy EA, Shaw AV, Crump JA. Community-acquired bloodstream infections in Africa: a systematic review and meta-analysis. Lancet Infect Dis 2010;10: 417–32.
5. Feasey NA, Archer BN, Heyderman RS, et al. Typhoid fever and invasive nontyphoid salmonellosis, Malawi and South Africa. Emerg Infect Dis 2010; 16:1448–51.
6. Morpeth SC, Ramadhani HO, Crump JA. Invasive non-Typhi Salmonella disease in Africa. Clin Infect Dis 2009;49:606–11.
7. Majowicz SE, Musto J, Scallan E, et al. International Collaboration on Enteric Disease 'Burden of Illness' Studies. Clin Infect Dis 2010;50:882–9.
8. MacLennan CA, Gondwe EN, Msefula CL, et al. The neglected role of antibody in protection against bacteremia caused by nontyphoidal strains of Salmonella in African children. J Clin Invest 2008;118:1553–62.
9. Valentiner-Branth P, Steinsland H, Fischer TK, et al. The global burden of nontyphoidal Salmonella gastroenteritis. J Clin Microbiol 2003;41:4238–45.
10. Berkley JA, Lowe BS, Mwangi I, et al. Bacteremia among children admitted to a rural hospital in Kenya. N Engl J Med 2005;352:39–47.
11. Sigauque B, Roca A, Mandomando I, et al. Community-acquired bacteremia among children admitted to a rural hospital in Mozambique. Pediatr Infect Dis J 2009;28:108–13.
12. Enwere G, Biney E, Cheung YB, et al. Epidemiologic and clinical characteristics of community-acquired invasive bacterial infections in children aged 2-29 months in The Gambia. Pediatr Infect Dis J 2006;25:700–5.
13. Raffatellu M, Santos RL, Verhoeven DE, et al. Simian immunodeficiency virus-induced mucosal interleukin-17 deficiency promotes Salmonella dissemination from the gut. Nat Med 2008;14:421–8.
14. Mabey DC, Brown A, Greenwood BM. *Plasmodium falciparum* malaria and Salmonella infections in Gambian children. J Infect Dis 1987;155:1319–21.
15. Brent AJ, Oundo JO, Mwangi I, et al. Salmonella bacteremia in Kenyan children. Pediatr Infect Dis J 2006;25:230–6.
16. Graham SM, Molyneux EM, Walsh AL, et al. Nontyphoidal Salmonella infections of children in tropical Africa. Pediatr Infect Dis J 2000;19:1189–96.
17. Graham SM, Walsh AL, Molyneux EM, et al. Clinical presentation of non-typhoidal Salmonella bacteraemia in Malawian children. Trans R Soc Trop Med Hyg 2000;94:310–4.
18. Bronzan RN, Taylor TE, Mwenechanya J, et al. Bacteremia in Malawian children with severe malaria: prevalence, etiology, HIV co-infection and outcome. J Infect Dis 2007;195:895–904.
19. Gordon MA, Banda HT, Gondwe M, et al. Non-typhoidal salmonella bacteraemia among HIV-infected Malawian adults: high mortality and frequent recrudescence. AIDS 2002;16:1641.
20. Gordon MA. Salmonella infections in immunocompromised adults. J Infect 2008;56:413–22.
21. Kariuki S, Revathi G, Kariuki N, et al. Invasive multidrug-resistant non-typhoidal Salmonella infections in Africa: zoonotic or anthroponotic transmission? J Med Microbiol 2006;55:585–91.
22. Milledge J, Calis JC, Graham SM, et al. Aetiology of neonatal sepsis in Blantyre, Malawi: 1996-2001. Ann Trop Paediatr 2005;25:101–10.
23. Gordon MA, Kankwatira AM, Mwafulirwa G, et al. Invasive non-typhoid salmonellae establish systemic intracellular infection in HIV-infected adults: an emerging disease pathogenesis. Clin Infect Dis 2010;50:953–62.
24. Kingsley RA, Msefula CL, Thomson NR, et al. Epidemic multiple drug resistant Salmonella Typhimurium causing invasive disease in sub-Saharan Africa have a distinct genotype. Genome Res 2009;19:2279–87.
25. Gordon MA, Graham SM, Walsh AL, et al. Epidemics of invasive *Salmonella enterica* serovar Enteritidis and *Salmonella enterica* serovar Typhimurium infection associated with multidrug resistance among adults and children in Malawi. Clin Infect Dis 2008;46:963–9.

26. Graham SM, English M. Nontyphoidal salmonellae: a management challenge for children with community acquired invasive disease in tropical African countries. Lancet 2009;372:267–9.
27. Gordon MA, Walsh AL, Chaponda M, Soko D, Mbvwinji M, Molyneux ME, et al. Bacteraemia and mortality among adult medical admissions in Malawi—predominance of non-typhi salmonellae and *Streptococcus pneumoniae*. J Infect 2001;42:44–9.
28. Cohen JI, Bartlett JA, Corey GR. Extra-intestinal manifestations of Salmonella infections. Medicine 1987;66:349–88.
29. Lavy CM. Septic arthritis in Western and sub-Saharan African children—a review. Int Orthop 2007;31:137–44.
30. Molyneux EM, Walsh AL, Malenga G, et al. Salmonella meningitis in children in Blantyre, Malawi, 1996–1999. Ann Trop Paediatr 2000;20:41–4.
31. Gendrel D, Kombila M, Beaudoin-Leblevec G, Richard-Lenoble D. Nontyphoidal salmonellal septicemia in Gabonese children infected with Schistosoma intercalatum. Clin Infect Dis 1994;18:103–5.
32. Peters RPH, Zijlstra EE, Schijffelen MJ, et al. A prospective study of bloodstream infections as a cause of fever in Malawi - clinical predictors and implications for management. Trop Med Int Health 2004;9:928–34.
33. MacLennan CA, Gilchrist JJ, Gordon MA, et al. Dysregulated humoral immunity to nontyphoidal Salmonella in HIV-infected African adults. Science 2010;328:508–12.

46 *Campylobacter* Infections

Paola J Maurtua-Neumann, Richard A Oberhelman

Key features

- *Campylobacter* species are microaerophilic, small, curved Gram-negative rods associated with diarrhea in both developed and developing countries
- Commonly colonizes gastrointestinal tract of chickens and other animals, which serve as reservoirs
- Major cause of pediatric diarrhea and traveler's diarrhea in resource-poor countries, presenting as dysentery or as watery diarrhea
- Usually presents as bloody diarrhea and dysentery in higher-income country populations
- Associated with post-infectious inflammatory conditions, including post-infectious arthropathy, Reiter's sundrome and Guillain-Barré syndrome (GBS)
- Diagnosed by stool culture, using special techniques developed specifically for this organism
- Macrolide antibiotics or fluoroquinolones are usually used for cases requiring antibiotic therapy

INTRODUCTION

Campylobacter jejuni is currently the leading identified cause of bacterial gastroenteritis in the developed world and of significant prevalence in developing countries. Young children are the most susceptible group, in both the developing and the developed world [1]. Most *Campylobacter* infections are caused by *C. jejuni* or *Campylobacter coli*. These organisms are motile, comma-shaped, microaerophilic, Gram-negative rods with a corkscrew-like motion produced by a polar, unsheathed flagellum. They commonly occur as commensals in warm-blooded animals, especially poultry [2]. *Campylobacter jejuni* strains can be differentiated by using two different serotyping schemes, one based on heat-labile flagellar protein, referred to as Lior serotypes (there are over 100 Lior serotypes), the other based on heat-stable flagellar proteins referred to as Penner serotypes (there are over 60 Penner serotypes).

Campylobacter was first identified in 1916 when two British veterinary surgeons reported a peculiar organism in the uterine mucus of pregnant sheep. In 1947, Vincent et al. isolated the organism from the blood of three pregnant women with sepsis and spontaneous abortion. The organism was most probably *Campylobacter fetus*, a common cause of veterinary disease but uncommon in humans. Later, *Campylobacter*-like organisms were associated with other infections, including endocarditis, meningitis and gastroenteritis. The association between *Campylobacter* and diarrhea was not made until the 1970s; this link was challenging to prove because of the fastidious nature of the organism and because of the stringent culture conditions required to isolate the organism from stool [3].

EPIDEMIOLOGY

Campylobacter infection is a zoonotic disease, observed in most parts of the world. Animals (fowl, swine, cattle, sheep, dogs, cats and rodents) are the major reservoir for the bacteria and are usually asymptomatic. *Campylobacter* enteritis has no seasonal preference in developing countries in contrast with developed countries, where epidemics occur in summer and early autumn.

In higher-income countries, acquisition of organisms results from the handling or consumption of poultry in about 50% of cases. Other causes include the consumption of beef, pork, raw milk and contaminated water, and contact with pets and farm animals. In the USA, surveillance studies showed a 30% decrease in incidence of culture-confirmed *Campylobacter* infections from 1996 to 2006, with an average of 13.9 cases per 100,000 in 2006. In New Zealand, incidence has been increasing since the 1980s, with almost 400 cases per 100,000 persons in 2003. Europe reported 45 per 100,000 persons in 2005 and in Canada the rate in 2004 was 30 cases per 100,000. The variations in incidence between countries may be caused, in part, by differences in surveillance systems [1, 4].

In studies from resource-poor countries in Latin America and Africa, *Campylobacter* is the most commonly isolated bacterial pathogen among children with diarrhea. The incidence of *Campylobacter* enteritis among children younger than 5 years old in these areas is as high as 40,000/100,000. Although these rates seem extraordinarily high, they are substantiated by *Campylobacter* diarrhea rates in travelers to these countries of 27,000–38,000/100,000 per year. In developing parts of Asia, Africa and Latin America, *Campylobacter* isolation rates have ranged from 5–20% in surveys performed in children with diarrhea. Older children and adults are infected less frequently because acquired immunity increases with age. Healthy children living in tropical countries frequently have asymptomatic infection. Infections caused by *C. coli* are more likely to be asymptomatic than ones caused by *C. jejuni* [1, 4].

Well-documented risk factors for *Campylobacter* infections include drinking well-water, visiting or living on a farm, and having exposure to pets with diarrhea and exposure to chickens living in the household. Studies of fecal output of household chickens of peri-urban shantytowns in Lima, Peru, demonstrated that up to 61% of chickens were colonized with *Campylobacter*. Viable bacteria can survive in chicken droppings for about 4 days. Contact with cats and dogs is also significant. Secondary spread of infection from person to person has not been documented, although household contacts have higher rates of infection than persons living in houses without cases of infection. This increased rate of infection is attributable to common sources of exposure [1, 5, 6].

TRAVELER'S DIARRHEA

Campylobacter species are important causes of diarrhea in travelers to the developing world. Isolation rates vary by geographic location but tend to be highest in travelers returning from South America, North and East Africa, the Middle East, and South and Southeast Asia. In a study in Sweden, researchers found that the highest risk was seen in

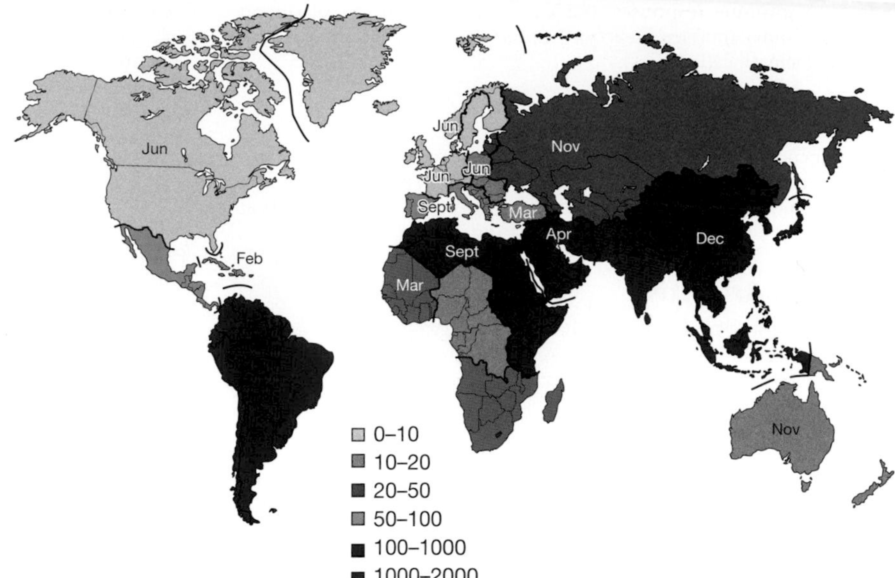

FIGURE 46.1 Map showing *Campylobacter* risk per 100,000 returning travellers to Sweden from different regions of the world. In regions with a distinct seasonality, the month with the highest risk (OR) is given. *Reproduced with permission from Ekdahl K, Andersson Y. Regional risks and seasonality in travel-associated campylobacteriosis. BMC Infect Dis 2004;4:54.*

returning travelers from the Indian subcontinent (1253 cases/100,000 travelers) and the lowest in travelers from the other Nordic countries (3/100,000 travelers). In Africa, there are large differences in risk between regions (502/100,000 in travelers from East Africa compared with 76/100,000 from West Africa and 50/100,000 from Central Africa) (Fig. 46.1) [6, 7].

NATURAL HISTORY, PATHOGENESIS AND PATHOLOGY

Campylobacter infection causes local acute inflammatory changes in both the small and large bowel. The organism is able to invade and replicate in gut epithelia, causing interleukin-8 (IL 8) production, activation of the innate immune system via Toll-like receptors (TLR)-2 and TLR-4, and disruption of the integrity of the epithelial barrier. The induction of IL-8 causes the recruitment of dendritic cells, macrophages and neutrophils that interact with *C. jejuni*. These interactions result in a massive pro-inflammatory response and increases in corresponding cytokines [8].

After 6 months of age, baseline levels of serum antibody increase. Higher antibody responses in older children correlate with excretion of few organisms and with the presence of milder, non-bloody diarrhea—findings consistent with the development of immunity [9].

BREASTFEEDING AND INFECTION

The protection in breast-fed infants against *Campylobacter* appears to occur through acquired and innate defense factors found in human milk, including antibodies, oligosaccharides and their glycolconjugates. Milk glycans prevent *Campylobacter* infections and decrease its disease severity [10].

CLINICAL FEATURES

In humans, the infective dose for *Campylobacter jejuni* is between 500 and 10,000 organisms. Symptoms occur 1–7 days following ingestion. Disease usually manifests as self-limited gastroenteritis lasting up to 7 days. Excretion of *Campylobacter* organisms typically lasts 2–3 weeks without treatment [2].

The clinical spectrum ranges from watery diarrhea to dysentery and may include mesenteric adenitis—giving a clinical picture that mimics appendicitis. Post-infectious complications include irritable bowel syndrome, post-infectious arthropathy, Reiter's syndrome and Guillain-Barré syndrome (GBS). Post-infectious inflammatory complications usually present within 1–6 weeks after ingestion [3].

In the developed world, *Campylobacter jejuni* enteritis can be quite severe in children and adults. The most prominent features among patients who seek medical attention are bloody diarrhea, abdominal pain and fever. Abdominal pain is the most characteristic manifestation of illness. In hospital surveys, bloody diarrhea occurs in about half of the patients [3, 6].

In developing countries, *Campylobacter jejuni* enteritis is milder than in patients in developed countries. In Thailand, about one-third of symptomatic infections are bloody, one-third are watery and one-third are mucoid. In the developing world, bloody diarrhea is most often seen with *Shigella* infections. In one study in Thailand, *Shigella* organisms were associated with grossly bloody diarrhea in 37% of cases, whereas *Campylobacter* and *Salmonella* organisms were associated with bloody stools in 14% and 26%, respectively. More than 10 fecal leukocytes per high-power microscopic field (an indicator of invasive diarrheal disease) were present in 24–36% of patients infected with *Campylobacter* species. The incidence of bloody diarrhea and the duration of illness decrease with age among children from most developing countries [6].

TRAVELER'S DIARRHEA

Campylobacter species is an important cause of traveler's diarrhea. Most *Campylobacter* infections in travelers cause symptoms, although frank dysentery is rare. In a study of Spanish travelers with *Campylobacter* enteritis acquired in developing countries, only 4% had dysentery. Abdominal cramps were present in 83% of cases, fever in 46%, nausea and vomiting in 42%, and grossly bloody diarrhea in only 3% of cases [6, 7].

POST-INFECTIOUS INFLAMMATORY COMPLICATIONS

Guillain-Barré Syndrome

GBS is an acute, immune-mediated flaccid paralysis frequently associated with *Campylobacter* infection. GBS is the most serious complication of *Campylobacter* infection and *C. jejuni* is the most frequently observed antecedent infection in cases of GBS. Its incidence is about 1/1000 infections, and 1 in 3 GBS cases is associated with a preceding *C. jejuni* infection. Symptoms of GBS usually occur 1–3 weeks after the onset of *Campylobacter* enteritis. GBS cases associated with *Campylobacter* infection are usually more severe than non-*Campylobacter*-associated cases. The association of GBS and *Campylobacter* infection relates to immune responses that target surface antigens of certain *C. jejuni* strains and cross-reactive human antigens on the surface of neuronal sheath cells [3, 11].

Irritable Bowel Syndrome

Post-infectious irritable bowel syndrome can occur following *Campylobacter* enteritis and usually manifests as persistent abdominal discomfort, bloating and diarrhea, alternating with constipation, that continue even with clearance of the inciting pathogen [12].

Reactive Arthritis

Reactive arthritis is a spondyloarthropathy—a group of diseases with a strong association with HLA-B27, absence of rheumatoid factor, family aggregation and frequent extra-articular symptoms. Acute reactive arthritis is characterized by sterile joint inflammation. It typically develops within 4 weeks following an intestinal or urogenital infection with obligate or facultative intracellular bacteria, such as *Salmonella, Shigella, Yersinia* and *Campylobacter*. The joint symptoms vary from mild mono- or oligo-arthralgia, to severely disabling polyarthritis. The arthritis has a predilection for joints of the lower extremity, particularly knees and ankles [13].

Campylobacter infection can lead to reactive arthritis with conjunctivitis and urethritis (Reiter's syndrome).

DIAGNOSIS

Transport of stool samples from patients with diarrhea looking for *Campylobacter* can be done in conventional containers but if delay is anticipated, samples should be placed in transport medium, such as Cary-Blair medium and kept cool. Transport medium should also be used to transport rectal swabs. Some studies suggest that *Campylobacter* enteritis can be diagnosed by direct microscopic examination of fresh liquid feces, either with Gram stain or a phase-contrast optical system by observing typical curved small bacilli in the stool [3]. However, if available, confirmation by stool culture is advisable.

Stool culture is the primary method for diagnosis of *Campylobacter*-related diarrhea. Isolation of *C. jejuni* and *C. coli* requires specialized, enriched, selective media incubated at 42°C under microaerophilic conditions [3]. Selective media for *Campylobacter* can be divided into two main groups: blood-containing media (e.g. Preston agar, Skirrow agar, Butzler agar, Campy-cefex) and charcoal-containing media (e.g. modified charcoal cefoperazone deoxycholate agar, Karmali agar or charcoal-selective medium). Most selective media also include antibiotic mixtures to suppress the growth of other contaminating flora [14].

Passive filtration is another isolation method—it takes advantage of *Campylobacter*'s high motility, obviates the need for selective media and can be used in resource-limited settings. Use of both selective media and a filter method is associated with maximal sensitivity [15].

Campylobacter species can also be detected directly in stool specimens by commercially available enzyme immunoassay or in research laboratories by PCR. Serology may be used to assess previous exposure in individuals with reactive arthritis, or Guillain Barré syndrome (GBS) [15].

TREATMENT

The most important treatment for a patient with diarrhea is rehydration therapy, which can usually be accomplished by the oral route. *Campylobacter* enteritis is often a self-limited infection not requiring antimicrobials, although antibiotic therapy is indicated for pregnant women and for patients with *Campylobacter* infection who are acutely ill, have persistent fever, bloody diarrhea or are immune-compromised individuals, including those with HIV infection [3].

For confirmed *C. jejuni* infection, macrolide antibiotics such as erythromycin, azithromycin or clarithromycin are the antibiotics of choice. Treatment courses are usually for 3–7 days [16, 17]. Unfortunately, resistance of *C. jejuni* to fluoroquinolones is now common, especially in Southeast Asia, markedly limiting the utility of these agents in treating individuals with campylobacteriosis. Owing to widespread resistance, tetracyclines should also not be used.

In patients with bacteremia, treatment should be based on the identity of the infecting species and susceptibilities when available. *Campylobacter fetus* is the most common species associated with bacteremia and it is generally susceptible to aminoglycosides, extended-spectrum cephalosporins, meropenem and imipenem [16, 17].

PREVENTION AND CONTROL

Appropriate precautions in the handling and preparation of foods of animal origin reduce cross-contamination. Raw meat and poultry should be cooked adequately. Hands should be washed thoroughly with soap after handling raw foods of animal origin and before touching anything else. Chopping boards used for raw meats should not be used for preparing other foods and should be cleaned well with soap and hot water. No vaccine is commercially available to prevent disease in humans.

REFERENCES

1. Allos BM. *Campylobacter jejuni* infections: update in emerging issues and trends. Clin Infect Dis 2001;32:1201–6.
2. Snelling WJ, Matsuda M, Moore JE, Dooley JS. Campylobacter jejuni. Lett Appl Microbiol 2005;41:297–302.
3. Butzler JP. *Campylobacter*, from obscurity to celebrity. Clin Microbiol Infect 2004;10:868–76.
4. Ailes E, Demma L, Hurd S, et al. Continued decline in the incidence of *Campylobacter* infections, FoodNet 1996–2006. Foodborne Pathogen Dis 2008;5:329–37.
5. Black RE, Lopez de Romana G, Brown KH, et al. Incidence and etiology of infantile diarrhea and major routes of transmission in Huascar, Peru. Am J Epidemiol 1989;129:785–99.
6. Oberhelman R, Taylor DE. *Campylobacter* infections in developing countries. In: Nachamkin I, Blaser MJ, eds. Campylobacter. Washington: ASM Press; 2000:139–53.
7. Al-Abri SS, Beeching NJ, Nye FJ. Traveller's diarrhoea. Lancet Infect Dis 2005;5:349–60.
8. Young KT, Davis LM, DiRita VJ. *Campylobacter jejuni*: molecular biology and pathogenesis. Nat Rev Microbiol 2007;5:665–79.
9. Martin PMV, Mathiot J, Ipero J, et al. Immune response to *Campylobacter jejuni* and *Campylobacter coli* in a cohort of children from birth to 2 years of age. J Clin Microbiol 1989;57:2542–6.
10. Morrow AL, Ruiz-Palacios GM, Jiang X, Newburg DS. Human-milk glycans that inhibit pathogen binding protect breast-feeding infants against infectious diarrhea. J Nutr 2005;135:1304–7.
11. Chowdhury D, Arora A. Axonal Guillain Barre syndrome: a critical review. Acta Neurol Scand 2001;103:267–77.
12. Thabane M, Kottachchi DT, Marshall JK. Systematic review and meta-analysis: The incidence and prognosis of postinfectious irritable bowel syndrome. Aliment Pharmacol Ther 2007;26:535–44.
13. Pope JE, Krizova A, Garg AX, et al. Campylobacter reactive arthritis: a systematic review. Semin Arthritis Rheum 2007;37:48–55.
14. López L, Castillo FJ, Clavel A, Rubio MC. Use of a selective medium and a membrane filter method for isolation of Campylobacter species from Spanish paediatric patients. Eur J Clin Microbiol Infect Dis 1998;17:489–92.
15. World Organisation for Animal Health. *Campylobacter jejuni* and *Campylobacter coli*. In: Wagenaar JA, Jacobs-reitson WF (eds) Manual of Diagnostic Tests and Vaccines for Terrestrial Animals. 2009. Paris: Office Internationale Des Epizooties.
16. Gibreel A, Taylor DE. Macrolide resistance in *Campylobacter jejuni* and *Campylobacter coli*. J Antimicrob Chemother 2006;58:243–55.
17. Moore JE, Barton MD, Blair IS, et al. The epidemiology of antibiotic resistance in Campylobacter. Microbe Infect 2006;8(7):1955–66.
18. Ekdahl K, Andersson Y. Regional risks and seasonality in travel-associated campylobacteriosis. BMC Infect Dis 2004;4:54.

Miscellaneous Bacterial Enteritides 47

47.1 *Yersinia enterocolitica*

Farah Naz Qamar, Anita KM Zaidi

Key features

- *Yersinia enterocolitica* is a Gram-negative rod found in dairy products, meats (e.g. pork and poultry) and vegetables
- *Yersinia enterocolitica* is primarily associated with gastrointestinal disease, but can cause extraintestinal infections in immunocompromised hosts, especially in conditions of iron overload
- Young adults may present with acute abdominal pain mimicking appendicitis (pseudo-appendicitis) and surgery may be inadvertently performed for suspected appendicitis
- Secondary immune-mediated sequelae, such as arthritis, glomerulonephritis, myocarditis, Reiter's syndrome and erythema nodosum can occur following *Y. enterocolitica* infection in individuals
- Fluoroquinolone therapy can be used to treat individuals with severe enteritis. Cefotaxime and ceftriaxone alone, or in combination with aminoglycosides, are effective in the treatment of individuals with *Y. enterocolitica* bacteremia

INTRODUCTION

Yersinia enterocolitica is a facultatively anaerobic, nonlactose-fermenting, Gram-negative rod belonging to the family *Enterobacteriaceae*. It is motile at 25°C, but non-motile at 37°C. *Yersinia enterocolitica* lacks a siderophore and growth is enhanced in the presence of a heme-rich environment with high concentrations of iron. The organism primarily causes gastrointestinal disease but can cause extraintestinal infections, particularly in immunocompromised hosts and in conditions associated with iron overload.

EPIDEMIOLOGY

The natural reservoir of *Y. enterocolitica* is the intestinal tracts of farm animals, especially pigs, cows and goats. The bacteria can also be isolated from the feces of dogs and cats. There are over 60 serogroups of *Y. enterocolitica*, but only 11 are implicated in human disease. *Yersinia enterocolitica*-associated gastroenteritis is reported worldwide, most commonly from northern European countries. Infection is uncommonly reported from tropical environments. A major source of infection in humans is ingestion of improperly cooked swine products, such as chitterlings (pig intestines). Nosocomial, as well as food-borne, outbreaks have been described [1].

NATURAL HISTORY, PATHOGENESIS AND PATHOLOGY

Infection with *Y. enterocolitica* occurs after ingestion of contaminated food or water. *Yersinia* species have a marked tropism for lymphoid tissue and bacteria migrate to the terminal ileum where they adhere to M cells in the Peyer's patches and penetrate through these cells to colonize lymphoid follicles. Continued proliferation of bacteria in the lamina propria enables the bacteria to survive and spread to other organs, such as the liver, spleen and mesenteric lymph nodes. Virulence is associated with three chromosomally encoded proteins (Invasin, Ail and YadA) that promote adherence to (YadA) and invasion (invasin) of M cells. Additionally, several plasmid-mediated outer member proteins (Yops) act synergistically to block various steps in the phagocytic pathway. Non-pathogenic strains of *Yersinia* are Yops negative and are rapidly phagocytized [2].

An association of *Y. enterolitica* sepsis in patients with hematologic dyscrasias, such as thalassemia or aplastic anemia requiring frequent transfusions and desferrioxamine as an iron-chelating agent, is well-established. This propensity is related to the ability of *Y. enterocolitica* to use ferrioxamine as a growth factor [3].

CLINICAL FEATURES

GASTROENTERITIS

Yersinia enterocolitica can cause illness ranging from acute watery diarrhea or dysentery to fatal necrotizing enterocolitis. Infection is more common in children and often associated with fever and vomiting. The illness may last for 3–28 days. Exposure to the small intestines of pigs, especially when steamed or fried for food (also known as chitterlings or chitlins), has been associated with a high risk of *Y. enterocolitica* enteritis in children. Infants younger than 3 months old are at risk of developing bacteremia and sepsis. Infections with serogroup O:8 may be severe and can cause extensive ulceration of the gastrointestinal tract and death. In young adults, *Y. enterolitica* infection can present with acute terminal ileitis and mesenteric lymphadenitis mimicking appendicitis (pseudoappendicitis). Surgery may be inadvertently performed for suspected appendicitis. Infected individuals may shed *Y. enterocolitica* in stools for weeks after resolution of symptoms. Treatment with antibiotics shortens the duration of bacterial shedding [4–6].

SEPTICEMIA

Septicemia is reported in patients with predisposing conditions, such as alcoholism, diabetes mellitus, immune deficiency and iron overload. Invasion of the bloodstream may result in abscess formation in the liver or spleen, pneumonia, septic arthritis, meningitis, panophthalmitis, osteomyelitis and endocarditis, or localize in a major blood vessel leading to a mycotic aneurysm. Occasionally, sepsis may be acquired through transfusion of contaminated blood that has been stored for long periods [7–10].

POST-INFECTIOUS SEQUELAE

Yersinia enterocolitica can cause post-infectious inflammatory conditions, such as reactive arthritis. Individuals with the HLA-B27 haplotype are particularly susceptible and can develop arthritis, Reiter's syndrome, glomerulonephritis, myocarditis and erythema nodosum following *Y. enterocolitica* infection. Joint symptoms occur in up to 2% of patients, usually 1–2 weeks after gastrointestinal illness. The large joints of the lower extremities are most commonly involved and symptoms usually persist for 1–4 months, although prolonged syndromes can occur. Erythema nodosum manifests as painful raised red or purple lesions on the lower extremities within three weeks of infection and usually resolves spontaneously [9, 11].

MISCELLANEOUS INFECTIONS

Yersinia enterocolitica has rarely been reported to cause urinary tract infections, conjunctivitis, localized skin abscess, intussusception and appendicitis. Pharyngitis after oral ingestion of the organism has also been reported.

DIAGNOSIS

Definitive diagnosis usually rests on isolating the organism from stool, blood or other specimens. *Yersinia enterocolitica* grow as small, nonlactose-fermenting colonies on MacConkey agar kept at 25°C for 48 hours. Growth can be enhanced by use of differential agar such as cefsulodin-irgasin novbiocin (CIN) agar, as well as cold enrichment techniques. High levels of antibodies to *Yersinia* may be helpful in the diagnosis of post-infectious complications. Ultrasound or computed tomography (CT) scanning may be useful in differentiating *Yersenia* mesenteric adenitis from acute appendicitis [5, 11].

TREATMENT

Yersinia enterocolitica are usually susceptible to cotrimoxazole, fluoroquinolone, aminoglycosides, chloroamphenicol, third-generation cephalosporins, aztreonam and imipenem. Cefotaxime and ceftriaxone are the most active third-generation cephalosporins against *Y. enterocolitica*.

Use of antibiotics in uncomplicated enteritis is controversial; hydration is the mainstay of therapy. Antibiotics are indicated in immunocompromised individuals to prevent or mitigate bacteremia and sepsis. For severe gastrointestinal infections, doxycycline and aminoglycoside (in combination), or fluoroquinolone therapy is indicated. Antimotility agents are contraindicated in the treatment of *Y. enterocolitica* enteritis. Cefotaxime and ceftriaxone, alone or in combination with aminoglycosides, are effective in the treatment of *Y. enterocolitica* bacteremia. Deferoxamine therapy should be discontinued during treatment of *Yersinia* bacteremia [12–14].

REFERENCES

1. Bottone EJ. *Yersinia enterocolitica*: overview and epidemiologic correlates. Microbes Infect 1999;1:323–33.
2. Grosdent N, Maridonneau-Parini I, Sory MP, Cornelis GR. Role of Yops and adhesins in resistance of *Yersinia enterocolitica* to phagocytosis. Infection Immunity 2002;70:4165–76.
3. Robins-Browne RM, Prpic JK. Effects of iron and desferrioxamine on infections with *Yersinia enterocolitica*. Infection Immunity 1985;47:774–9.
4. Abdel-Haq NM, Asmar BI, Abuhammour WM, Brown WJ. *Yersinia enterocolitica* infection in children. Pediatr Infect Dis J 2000;19:954–8.
5. Zartash Zafar Khan MRS, Johnston MH, Martin GJ. Yersinia Enterocolitica. 2009. Available at: http://emedicine.medscape.com/article/232343-overview.
6. Puylaert J, der Zant FMV, Mutsaers J. Infectious ileocecitis caused by *Yersinia*, *Campylobacter*, and *Salmonella*: clinical, radiological and US findings. European Radiol 1997;7:3–9.
7. Haditsch M, Binder L, Gabriel C, et al. *Yersinia enterocolitica* septicemia in autologous blood transfusion. Transfusion 1994;34:907–9.
8. Melby K, Slordahl S, Gutteberg TJ, Nordbo SA. Septicaemia due to *Yersinia enterocolitica* after oral overdoses of iron. BMJ 1982;285:467–85.
9. Smego RA, Frean J, Koornhof HJ. Yersiniosis I: microbiological and clinicoepidemiological aspects of plague and non-plague *Yersinia* infections. Eur J Clin Microbiol Infect Dis 1999;18:1–15.
10. Van Noyen R, Peeters P, Van Dessel F, Vandepitte J. Mycotic aneurysm of the aorta due to *Yersinia enterocolitica*. Contrib Microbiol Immunol 1987;9: 122–6.
11. Bottone EJ. *Yersinia enterocolitica*: The charisma continues. Clin Microbiol Rev 1997;10:257–76.
12. Thielman NM, Guerrant RL. Acute infectious diarrhea. N Engl J Med 2004;350:38–47.
13. Capilla S, Goni P, Rubio MC, et al. Epidemiological study of resistance to nalidixic acid and other antibiotics in clinical *Yersinia enterocolitica* O: 3 isolates. J Clin Microbiol 2003;41:4876–8.
14. Abdel-Haq NM, Papadopol R, Asmar BI, Brown WJ. Antibiotic susceptibilities of *Yersinia enterocolitica* recovered from children over a 12-year period. Int J Antimicrobial Agents 2006;27:449–52.

47.2 *Clostridium* Infections

S Asad Ali, Anita KM Zaidi

Key features

- *Clostridium* spp. are ubiquitous Gram-positive spore-forming bacteria that cause a wide range of diseases, including botulism, tetanus, soft tissue infections, neonatal sepsis and enteric infections
- *C. perfringens* causes gas gangrene and self-limited food poisoning syndrome associated with eating contaminated beef, poultry and precooked foods that undergo slow cooling
- *C. botulinum* causes botulism, a cause of flaccid paralysis
- *C. tentani* causes tetanus, a cause of rigid paralysis

Key features—cont'd

- *C. difficile* is a frequent cause of hospital-associated diarrhea or diarrhea that develops after receiving antibiotics [*C. difficile*-associated diarrhea (CDAD)]
- Offending antibiotics should be discontinued as soon as possible and clinically indicated if a patient develops *C. difficile*-associated illness. Patients with CDAD should be treated with oral vancomycin or oral or intravenous metronidazole; additional agents may also be effective

INTRODUCTION

Clostridium spp. are Gram-positive, anaerobic, spore-forming bacteria that are found widely in nature, especially in soil, sewage, decaying tissue and the gastrointestinal tracts of humans and other animals. Of the more than 80 species of clostridia, at least 14 are pathogenic in humans, where they cause diseases such as botulism, tetanus, soft tissue infections, neonatal sepsis and enteric infections.

EPIDEMIOLOGY

Two species of clostridia, *C. perfringens* and *C. difficile* are most commonly associated with enteric illness. Both these organism and their associated syndromes have worldwide distribution. *C. perfringens* is frequently present in contaminated raw meat and poultry. *C. difficile* is commonly present in soil and in the hospital environment. In many hospitals in industrialized countries, *C. difficile* gastroenteritis has become a major infection control challenge [1].

NATURAL HISTORY, PATHOGENESIS AND PATHOLOGY

C. perfringens-associated enteritis occurs when foods (usually beef, poultry, gravy, dried or precooked foods) heavily contaminated with *C. perfringens* type A are ingested. Spores of *C. perfringens* can survive cooking; these spores germinate and multiply during slow cooling and storage at temperatures from 20–60°C. Infection is usually acquired at banquets or institutions where food is prepared in large quantities and kept warm for prolonged periods. The organism produces an enterotoxin in the colon which causes crampy abdominal pain and diarrhea. Illness is not transmitted from person to person.

C. difficile is often present in hospitals and children's facilities, largely because of its ability to form spores that are resistant to many common disinfectants. It does not usually affect healthy individuals unless the normal intestinal flora is disrupted by the use of antibiotics. *C. difficile* produces two primary toxins—A and B—which produce enterotoxic and cytotoxic effects respectively [2].

CLINICAL FEATURES

C. perfringens-associated food poisoning usually occurs as part of an outbreak. The incubation period ranges from 6–24 hours—usually 8–12 hours. Major symptoms are crampy, mid-epigastric pain, nausea and non-bloody diarrhea. Vomiting and fever are generally absent. In rare instances, a more severe form of enteritis occurs called 'enteritis necroticans'. It is caused by *C. perfringens* type C that produces a beta toxin. Enteritis necroticans is characterized by abdominal cramps, vomiting, diarrhea (which may be bloody), shock and acute inflammation of small intestine with areas of necrosis and gangrene. This condition is seen more often after consumption of large quantities of contaminated meat by people who generally consume low-protein diets and hence produce limited amounts of digestive proteases. In New Guinea, this condition is called "pigbel" enteritis where it is associated with traditional pig feasting activities in which large quantities of pork are consumed [3].

C. difficile causes a wide variety of gastrointestinal symptoms ranging from asymptomatic colonization or mild diarrhea to pseudomembranous colitis, or even illness resembling an intra-abdominal catastrophe. Pseudomembranous colitis is characterized by profuse watery diarrhea, abdominal cramps, fever and small (2–5 mm), raised, yellowish plaques on the colonic mucosa.

PATIENT EVALUATION, DIAGNOSIS AND DIFFERENTIAL DIAGNOSIS

C. perfringens food poisoning is usually seen in the setting of an outbreak. The shorter incubation period (usually 8–12 hours) of *C. perfringens*-associated food poisoning and complete resolution of symptoms usually by 24 hours, and absence of fever in most patients differentiates this syndrome from shigellosis and salmonellosis. On the other hand, this incubation period is longer compared with some other causes of food-borne illnesses, such as heavy metal poisoning, *Staphylococcus aureus* enterotoxin-associated food poisoning, and shellfish toxins. The diarrheal illness caused by *Bacillus cereus* enterotoxin is quite similar to that caused by *C. perfringens*. As the fecal flora of healthy individuals often includes *C. perfringens*, counts of *C. perfringens* spores $>10^6$/g of feces obtained within 48 hours of illness in acutely ill patients are required to presumptively confirm the diagnosis. Enterotoxins can also be detected in the stool of affected individuals. In order to confirm *C. perfringens* as a cause of an outbreak, demonstration of large numbers of *C. perfringens* ($>10^5$/g) in the implicated food and/or demonstration of the same serotype of *C. perfringens* in the implicated food and the stools of affected individuals may be used.

C. difficile should be suspected in patients with diarrhea who have received antibiotics in the previous 2 months, or whose diarrhea starts 72 hours after hospitalization. Typically, toxin testing of a single stool specimen by enzyme immunoassay (EIA) or tissue culture assay establishes the diagnosis. However, repeat testing may be required. Although *C. difficile* can be easily isolated from the stools by the use of selective media, distinction between toxigenic and non-pathogenic strains cannot be made and *C. difficile* can be isolated in the stool of many asymptomatic individuals. Neonates, young infants and toddlers are very commonly colonized with *C. difficile*, which may or may not produce toxins; however, *C. difficile*-associated diarrhea is rarely seen in this age group.

TREATMENT

Food poisoning caused by *C. perfringens* is self-limited and does not require any specific therapy beyond oral rehydration or, in some cases, intravenous fluid and electrolyte replacement. Antimicrobial agents are not indicated. For enteritis necroticans, a specific antitoxin to the beta toxin produce by *C. perfringens* type C offers significant benefit. Treatment for *C. difficile*-associated disease requires discontinuation of the causative antibiotic regimen when feasible. Antibiotics against *C. difficile* are also indicated. Oral or intravenous metronidazole is the drug of choice for initial treatment of mild disease. Oral vancomycin has been shown to be more effective than metronidazole, but should be reserved for more severe or refractory cases as it may increase the recovery of vancomycin-resistant enterococci. Intravenous vancomycin is not effective as it does not enter the colonic lumen. Newer investigational therapies for *C. difficile*-associated disease include antimicrobials such as nitazoxanide, rifamixin and tinadozole, as well as alternative therapeutic approaches using immune globulin therapy, toxin binders and restoring intestinal tract flora.

REFERENCES

1. American Academy of Pediatrics. Clostridial Infections. In: Pickering LK, Baker CJ, Kimberlin DW, Long SS, eds. Red Book: 2009 Report of the Committee on Infectious Diseases, 28th ed. Elk Grove Village: American Academy of Pediatrics; 2009:263–6.
2. Kelly CP, LaMont JT. *Clostridium difficile*—more difficult than ever. N Engl J Med 2008;359:1932–40.
3. Murrell TG, Walker PD. The pigbel story of Papua New Guinea. Trans R Soc Trop Med Hyg 1991;85:119–22.

47.3 *Aeromonas*

Farah Naz Qamar, Anita KM Zaidi

Key features

- *Aeromonas* spp. are Gram-negative rods that can cause infections in healthy, as well as immunocompromised, hosts
- Predominantly, three serotypes (*Aeromonas hydrophila, Aeromonas caviae,* and *Aeromonas veronii*) are of clinical significance
- Gastroenteritis is the major clinical illness associated with *Aeromonas* species, although causation and estimates of disease burden are controversial
- Diarrhea associated with *Aeromonas* spp. is usually self-limited, but cases of dysentery, cholera-like illness and chronic diarrhea have also been associated
- *Aeromonas* species can cause wound and soft tissue infections and septicemia and have been associated with pneumonia and peritonitis
- *Aeromonas*-associated bacteremia and sepsis in immunocompromised patients can have a high mortality
- *Aeromonas* are resistant to ampicillin. Aminoglycosides and quinolones can be used to treat *Aeromonas* infections. Third-generation cephalosporins should be used carefully, as increasing resistance is being reported

INTRODUCTION

Aeromonas are motile, Gram-negative facultatively anaerobic rods in the family *Aeromonadaceae. Aeromonas* are commonly isolated in diarrheal specimens in tropical countries, but causation is controversial. *Aeromonas* species can cause wound infections and septicemia. *Aeromonas* spp. exist in aquatic environments and can cause disease in amphibians, reptiles and fish [1, 2].

MICROBIOLOGY

Aeromonas are flagellated, Gram-negative rods. There are currently 17 recognized species of *Aeromonas*. Only three species are of major clinical importance: *Aeromonas hydrophila, Aeromonas caviae* and *Aeromonas veronii*. The other species are predominantly found in the environment [3, 4].

EPIDEMIOLOGY

Aeromonas hydrophila has been recognized as a pathogen of amphibians, reptiles, snails, cows and humans. It has been found in soil, as well as a variety of aquatic environments, including lakes, rivers, streams, springs, rainwater, swimming pools, seawater and tap water. Relative resistance to chlorine, unlike other enteropathogens, is a potential public health hazard. *Aeromonas* have been isolated from a wide variety of foods, such as vegetables, raw milk, ice cream, meat and seafood. Despite being prevalent in the environment, reported outbreaks of gastroenteritis caused by this organism are rare.

Aeromonas are isolated with increased frequency during warmer months. Illness can occur in healthy, as well as in immunocompromised hosts, especially those with hematological malignancies and liver cirrhosis. Infections in immunocompromised individuals may be severe and associated with a high case fatality rate [2, 5].

NATURAL HISTORY, PATHOGENESIS AND PATHOLOGY

Aeromonas can form biofilms, which can assist in adherence in pipes and can help the organism survive exposure to chlorine. *Aeromonas* secrete at least two hemolysins: an alpha hemolysin causes hemorrhagic enteritis and increased secretion in the rabbit ileum and is lethal if injected intraperitoneally in experimental animals; a beta hemolysin, also known as aerolysin or cytotoxic toxin, encoded by the *Act* gene, has both hemolytic and cytotoxic activity. Both the alpha and beta hemolysins cause dermonecrosis if injected in animal skin. The enterotoxins secreted by *Aeromonas* have been broadly divided into cytotonic and cytotoxic types. Cytotonic enterotoxins are encoded by two genes *Ast* (thermo-stable) and *Alt* (thermo-labile), which are genetically different from cholera toxin, but function by increasing secretion of cAMP.

The cytotonic enterotoxin genes encoding Alt and Ast were found in 16% of isolates from diarrheal stools from Bangladeshi children, whereas the cytotoxic gene encoding Act was not identified in any of the isolates. The presence of all three genes in clinical isolates may be associated with dysentery [6–8].

CLINICAL FEATURES

Aeromonas species have been associated with a wide variety of intestinal, as well as extraintestinal, infections, although the burden of diarrheal illness that can be ascribed to *Aeromonas* spp. is controversial. Asymptomatic carriage, as well as failure to produce disease in healthy volunteers, has raised questions regarding its enteropathogenicity [9].

When *Aeromonas* spp. are detected in diarrheal stools, the diarrhea is usually acute and watery, with vomiting and abdominal pain. *Aeromonas* spp. may also be associated with dysentery, especially in children [10]. Cases with severe dehydrating cholera-like illness and rice-water stools associated with *A. veroni* biovar sobria and *A. caviae* have also been reported. These organisms have also been associated with traveler's diarrhea. In most cases, *Aeromonas*-associated diarrhea is self-limiting, but cases of chronic diarrhea have been reported [11].

Aeromonas have been implicated as causative agents in wound infections and can also cause bacteremia and sepsis. Pneumonia, meningitis, urinary tract infections, endocarditis, endophthalmitis, and bone and joint infections have also been reported. Wound infections caused by *Aeromonas* usually occur in healthy young individuals following trauma or abrasions. Infections result from exposure to contaminated water or soil. *Aeromonas* species were among the most commonly isolated organisms from tsunami victims with skin and soft tissue infections in southern Thailand in 2004. Many of these infections were polymicrobial [12]. Cases have also been reported following bites of snakes and reptiles, in burn patients, and following pelvic and abdominal surgeries. *Aeromonas veronii* biovar *sobria* is a normal component of leech flora, and wound infections in both adult and pediatric patients have been described following leech therapy. Soft tissue infections caused by *Aeromonas* may be fulminant and even lead to gas gangrene. *Aeromonas* septicemia mainly occurs in older males with underlying liver cirrhosis, malignancies, diabetes, or other underlying chronic infections. Mortality during *Aeromonas*-associated septicemia ranges from 24–68% [13–15].

PATIENT EVALUATION, DIAGNOSIS AND DIFFERENTIAL DIAGNOSIS

Diagnosis can be made by isolation of *Aeromonas* spp. from clinical specimens in culture. *Aeromonas* species grow well on blood agar, MacConkey and xylose, lysine, deoxycholate (XLD) agar. Selective media incorporating ampicillin in blood agar (ABA) can be used to aid isolation of *Aeromonas* species. Further identification can be performed using the API (analytical profile index) 20E system or more sophisticated PCR techniques [5].

Aeromonas infection should be suspected in any patient with injuries and exposure to water, as well as in immunocompromised individuals with Gram-negative shock, especially those with underlying liver disease.

TREATMENT

Aeromonas species are sensitive to tetracycline, chloramphenicol, trimethoprim-sulfamethoxazole, third-generation cephalosporins, aminoglycosides (except streptomycin) and fluoroquinolones. Most species are resistant to ampicillin, ticarcillin, amoxicillin-clavulanate and first-generation cephalosporins. Increasing antimicrobial resistance among *Aeromonas* species has been observed worldwide. The increasing resistance amongst *Aeromonas* spp. is not only caused by increased use of antibiotics in the clinical setting, but increasing use of antibiotics in animal husbandry and fish-farming also play a role. Chromosomally encoded, inducible ß-lactamase production has been observed among *Aeromonas* species [16].

Most diarrhea associated with *Aeromonas* species is self-limited and does not require antimicrobial therapy. Fluoroquinolones may be used in chronic diarrhea, dysentery or diarrhea in travelers. Immunocompromised patients with *Aeromonas* diarrhea may be at increased risk of complications and may benefit from treatment. For extraintestinal infections and septicemia, aminoglycosides or fluoroquinolones can be used for empiric therapy, and antimicrobial susceptibility can guide further treatment decisions [17, 18].

REFERENCES

1. Figueras MJ, Guarro J, Martínez-Murcia A. Clinically relevant *Aeromonas* species. Clin Infect Dis 2000;30:988–9.
2. Khalifa Sifaw Ghenghesh SFA, El-Khalek RA, Atef Al-Gendy JK. *Aeromonas*-associated infections in developing countries. J Infect Developing Countries 2008;2:81–98.
3. Garrity GM, Bell JA, Lilburn TG. Taxonomic outline of the prokaryotes. Bergey's manual of systematic bacteriology. Bergey's Manual Trust; 2004. New York: Springer.
4. Colwell RR, MacDonell MT, De LEY. Proposal to recognize the family *Aeromonadaceae* fam. nov. Int J Systematic Evolutionary Microbiology 1986; 36:473.
5. Janda JM, Abbott SL. The genus *Aeromonas*: taxonomy, pathogenicity, and infection. Clin Microbiol Rev 2010;23:35–73.
6. Khardori N, Fainstein V. *Aeromonas* and *Plesiomonas* as etiological agents. Ann Rev Microbiol 1988;42:395–419.
7. Chopra AK, Houston CW. Enterotoxins in *Aeromonas*-associated gastroenteritis. Microbes Infect 1999;1:1129–37.
8. Albert MJ, Ansaruzzaman M, Talukder KA, et al. Prevalence of enterotoxin genes in *Aeromonas* spp. isolated from children with diarrhea, healthy controls, and the environment. J Clin Microbiol 2000;38:3785.
9. Morgan DR, Johnson PC, DuPont HL, et al. Lack of correlation between known virulence properties of *Aeromonas hydrophila* and enteropathogenicity for humans. Infection Immunity 1985;50:62.
10. Mm SD, Moezardalan K. Aeromonas spp associated with childrens diarrhoea in Tehran: a case-control study. Ann Trop Paediatr Int Child Health 2004;24: 45–51.
11. Von Graevenitz A. The role of *Aeromonas* in diarrhea: a review. Infection 2007;35:59–64.
12. Hiransuthikul N, Tantisiriwat W, Lertutsahakul K, et al. Skin and soft tissue infections among tsunami survivors in southern Thailand. Clin Infect Dis 2005;41:e93–6.
13. Ouderkirk JP, Bekhor D, Turett GS, Murali R. *Aeromonas* meningitis complicating medicinal leech therapy. Clin Infect Dis 2004;38:36–7.
14. Ko WC, Chuang YC. *Aeromonas* bacteremia: review of 59 episodes. Clin Infect Dis 1995;20:1298–304.
15. Stano F, Brindicci G, Monno R, et al. *Aeromonas sobria* sepsis complicated by rhabdomyolysis in an HIV-positive patient: case report and evaluation of traits associated with bacterial virulence. Int J Infect Dis 2009;13:113–8.
16. Vivekanandhan G, Savithamani K, Hatha AAM, Lakshmanaperumalsamy P. Antibiotic resistance of *Aeromonas hydrophila* isolated from marketed fish and prawn of South India. Int J Food Microbiol 2002;76:165–8.
17. Guerrant RL, Van Gilder T, Steiner TS, et al. Practice guidelines for the management of infectious diarrhea. Clin Infect Dis 2001;32:331–51.
18. Oldfield EC, Wallace MR. The role of antibiotics in the treatment of infectious diarrhea. Gastroenterology Clinics North America 2001;30:817–35.

SECTION

D

SEXUALLY TRANSMITTED DISEASES

48 Chlamydial Infections

David Mabey, Rosanna Peeling

Key features

- The most common bacterial sexually transmitted infection
- Most prevalent in younger, sexually active age groups
- Often asymptomatic
- A cause of reproductive sequelae, such as infertility and ectopic pregnancy
- Controlled by case finding, screening and prompt treatment of patients and their sexual partners
- Usually diagnosed by sensitive nucleic acid amplification tests which can be performed on urine samples or self-administered vaginal swabs

The *Chlamydiae* are pathogenic bacteria that can only replicate inside eukaryotic host cells. Their unique developmental cycle involves alternation between a metabolically inert, infectious, spore-like elementary body that can survive in the extracellular environment, and a metabolically active, replicating reticulate body that cannot. The *Chlamydiae* have their own order (*Chlamydiales*) and family (*Chlamydiaceae*).

CLASSIFICATION

The *Chlamydiae* have been classified as four species belonging to a single genus, *Chlamydia*: *C. trachomatis,* a human pathogen causing ocular and genital infections; *C. pneumoniae* causing mainly human respiratory disease; *C. psittaci* which infects birds and other animals; and *C. pecorum*, a pathogen of cattle and sheep. The latter two occasionally affect humans. A recent taxonomic re-classification based on ribosomal DNA sequence data has not been widely adopted. *Chlamydiae* have one of the smallest bacterial genomes, containing around 1 million base pairs [1]. Virtually all strains of *C. trachomatis* also contain a 4.4 MDa plasmid of unknown function. Genomes of *C. trachomatis* serovars D, A, B and L2 have been sequenced, and show a high level of conservation of gene order and content (>99%) [2]. A high degree of genetic conservation is also seen across *Chlamydia* species.

BIOLOGY

The elementary body is approximately 300 nm in diameter, binds to the host cell and enters by "parasite-specified" endocytosis. Fusion of the chlamydia-containing endocytic vesicle with lysosomes is inhibited, and the elementary body differentiates into the larger, metabolically active reticulate body which divides by binary fission. By 20 hours post-infection, a proportion of reticulate bodies has begun to re-organize into a new generation of elementary bodies. These reach maturity up to 30 h after entry into the cell and accumulate within the endocytic vacuole, which typically contains more than 1000 organisms. These are released by lysis of the host cell 30–48 h after the start of the cycle. *Chlamydia trachomatis* contains two biovars: the more invasive lymphogranuloma venereum (LGV) biovar and the more common trachoma biovar, which is largely confined to squamo-columnar epithelial cells of the eye and genital tract. Both contain several serovars defined by the presence of serovar-specific epitopes on the major outer membrane protein (MOMP). Serovars D–K cause genital and oculo-genital infections.

PATHOGENESIS AND IMMUNITY

After an incubation period of 5–10 days, *C. trachomatis* elicits an acute inflammatory response with a purulent exudate. A period of chronic inflammation ensues, with the development of sub-epithelial follicles; this eventually leads, in some cases, to fibrosis and scarring, which is responsible for much of the morbidity associated with *C. trachomatis*. It is particularly likely to be seen after repeated infections.

Genital *C. trachomatis* infection is most prevalent in the youngest sexually active age groups, suggesting that infection elicits a degree of protective immunity—the chlamydial isolation rate for men with non-gonococcal urethritis is lower in those who have had previous episodes. In animal models and human ocular infection, cell-mediated immune responses mediated by CD4+ lymphocytes are important for the clearance of infection. Trachoma vaccine trials showed that killed, whole organism vaccines provided some degree of protection against ocular *C. trachomatis* infection in humans and non-human primates [3], but also suggested that vaccination could provoke more severe, immunopathologic disease on subsequent challenge [4]. This would be in keeping with the histopathology of *C. trachomatis* infection, in which the lymphoid follicle is the hallmark. A chlamydial heat-shock protein (hsp 60), homologous with the GroEL protein of *Escherichia coli,* elicits antibody responses that are associated with the damaging sequelae of *C. trachomatis* infections. In recent years, research has focused on the development of a subunit vaccine against *C. trachomatis*. Purified preparations of MOMP were protective in murine models, provided the native trimeric structure of the protein was maintained. In non-human primates, a similar preparation reduced peak shedding from the ocular surface, but had no effect on the duration of infection or on ocular disease [5, 6].

EPIDEMIOLOGY

Chlamydia trachomatis is the most common bacterial sexually transmitted infection (STI) [7]. It is common in all sexually active populations; prevalence is usually highest in the young. The World Health Organization estimates that 101 million new cases of genital chlamydial infection occur annually worldwide.

CLINICAL MANIFESTATIONS

The clinical manifestations of genital *C. trachomatis* infection are similar to those of gonorrhea, but are usually less severe (Table 48-1). Many chlamydial infections are asymptomatic. Long-term sequelae,

TABLE 48-1 Human Diseases Caused by *Chlamydiae*

Species	Serovars	Disease
C. trachomatis	A, B, Ba, C	Trachoma
	D-K	Urethritis, epididymitis
		Cervicitis, pelvic inflammatory disease
		Curtis-Fitz-Hugh syndrome
		Adult and neonatal conjunctivitis
		Neonatal pneumonia
		Reactive arthitis
	L_1, L_2, L_3	Lymphogranuloma venereum
		Proctocolitis
C. psittaci	Many	Pneumonia, endocarditis, abortion
C. pneumoniae	Only one	Community-acquired pneumonia
		Bronchitis

such as infertility are generally caused by fibrosis and scarring following prolonged or repeated infections and may develop even in those with few, or no, symptoms.

CLINICAL MANIFESTATIONS IN MEN

URETHRITIS

Chlamydia trachomatis is detectable in the urethra of up to 50% of men with symptomatic non-gonococcal urethritis. Patients present with a history of dysuria, usually accompanied by a mild-to-moderate mucopurulent urethral discharge. As mixed infections are common, patients with gonococcal urethritis should also be treated for chlamydial infection. Failure to do so may result in chlamydial post-gonococcal urethritis.

EPIDIDYMITIS

Chlamydia trachomatis is responsible for a high proportion of cases of acute epididymitis in young men presenting with unilateral scrotal pain, swelling and tenderness, often accompanied by fever. Most give a history of current or recent urethral discharge.

PROCTITIS

Proctitis in men who practice receptive anal intercourse may be caused by LGV or non-LGV strains of *C. trachomatis*. The non-LGV strains cause a milder disease that may be asymptomatic or give rise to rectal pain, bleeding and mucopurulent anal discharge.

CLINICAL MANIFESTATIONS IN WOMEN

CERVICITIS

Chlamydia trachomatis typically infects the columnar epithelial cells of the endocervix, but not the squamous epithelium of the vagina. *Chlamydia trachomatis* is associated with a mucopurulent discharge from the cervix, visible on speculum examination, and with hypertrophic cervical ectopy that tends to bleed on contact. The prevalence of cervical *C. trachomatis* infection is no higher among women who complain of vaginal discharge than among those who do not, suggesting that it is not a major cause of symptomatic vaginal discharge.

URETHRITIS

Chlamydia trachomatis is a cause of the urethral syndrome, characterized by dysuria, frequency and sterile pyuria. Clinical signs of urethritis, such as urethral discharge or meatal redness, are not usually found.

PELVIC INFLAMMATORY DISEASE

Chlamydia trachomatis may spread from the endocervix to the endometrium and fallopian tubes, causing pelvic inflammatory disease (PID). This is more likely to occur after trauma to the cervix as a result of, for example, termination of pregnancy, insertion of an intrauterine contraceptive device, or delivery. Classical signs of PID may be present (fever, lower abdominal pain and tenderness, and cervical motion tenderness), but chlamydial PID may be subclinical. Spread to the peritoneum may result in perihepatitis (Curtis Fitz-Hugh syndrome). Infertility may be the first indication of asymptomatic tubal disease, resulting from endometritis, blocked or damaged fallopian tubes, or abnormalities of ovum transportation. Other consequences of PID are chronic pelvic pain and ectopic pregnancy.

PREGNANCY OUTCOME

Some studies have shown *Chlamydia trachomatis* infection in pregnancy to be associated with low birth weight and preterm delivery, but others have failed to confirm this [8]. In general, *C. trachomatis* was diagnosed and treated at a later stage of gestation in those studies which found a correlation between infection and adverse birth outcome than in those that did not.

OTHER CONDITIONS OF THE FEMALE GENITAL TRACT

A significant association between cervical chlamydial infection and cervical squamous cell carcinoma has been established. It has been suggested that chlamydial infection may enhance the effect of oncogenic papillomaviruses.

CLINICAL MANIFESTATIONS OCCURRING IN BOTH SEXES

ADULT PARATRACHOMA (INCLUSION CONJUNCTIVITIS) AND OTITIS MEDIA

Adult chlamydial ophthalmia commonly results from the accidental transfer of infected genital discharge to the eye, presenting as a unilateral follicular conjunctivitis with swollen lids, mucopurulent discharge, papillary hyperplasia, follicular hypertrophy and, occasionally, punctate keratitis. About one-third of patients have otitis media.

REACTIVE ARTHRITIS

Arthritis occurring with, or soon after, non-gonococcal urethritis is termed "sexually acquired reactive arthritis". Conjunctivitis and other features characteristic of Reiter's syndrome are seen in about a third of patients. Evidence of chlamydial infection (a specific serologic response, or *C. trachomatis* DNA or antigen in the joints) is found in at least one-third of cases.

NEONATAL INFECTIONS

Conjunctivitis occurs in 20–50% of infants exposed to cervical *C. trachomatis* infection at birth. A mucopurulent discharge occurs 1–3 weeks later. About half of infants with chlamydial conjunctivitis also develop pneumonia, usually presenting between the fourth and eleventh weeks of life [9]. There is tachypnea and prominent, staccato cough, but usually no fever. Radiographs show hyperinflation of the lungs with bilateral diffuse, symmetrical, interstitial infiltration and scattered areas of atelectasis.

DIAGNOSIS

An endocervical swab is needed for the diagnosis of *C. trachomatis* infection by culture or antigen detection assay. However, the greater sensitivity of nucleic acid amplification tests (NAATs) for *C. trachomatis* means that vaginal swabs (which may be self-administered) and "first-catch" urine specimens give equivalent results to endocervical swabs when using these assays [10].

CULTURE

Cell-culture techniques are no more than 70% sensitive when compared to NAATs. They are expensive and labor-intensive. As culture is essentially 100% specific, it still has a role in medico-legal cases.

DIRECT IMMUNOFLUORESCENCE

Detection of elementary bodies using species-specific fluorescent monoclonal antibodies is rapid and highly sensitive and specific in the hands of skilled observers. However, it is subjective and not suitable for high-throughput testing.

ENZYME IMMUNOASSAYS

Enzyme immunoassays that detect chlamydial antigens, usually the group-specific lipopolysaccharide, were widely used before NAATs became available. However, the lower limit of detection is 1000 organisms or more and these tests are only about 70% sensitive compared to the now more widely used NAATs.

NUCLEIC ACID AMPLIFICATION TESTS (NAATs)

The PCR assay, the strand displacement assay (SDA) and the transcription-mediated amplification (TMA) technique are extremely sensitive, detecting 10–100 organisms. Commercial assays based on each of these three amplification methods are widely used. The first two assays amplify nucleotide sequences of the cryptic plasmid present in multiple copies in each chlamydial elementary body. A recently described Swedish variant of *C. trachomatis* harbors a deletion in the plasmid, which gives rise to false-negative results with these assays [11, 12]. The TMA reaction is directed against rRNA, which is also present in multiple copies. These assays are now the "gold standard" for the diagnosis of *C. trachomatis* infection.

POINT-OF-CARE TESTS

Several point-of-care antigen detection tests are available for the diagnosis of *C. trachomatis* infection, but they are less sensitive than NAATs and cannot be used on vaginal swabs or urine samples.

SEROLOGIC TESTS

Serologic tests may be helpful in the diagnosis of PID, LGV and in Curtis Fitz-Hugh syndrome, as antibody titers tend to be higher in these conditions than in uncomplicated cervical infections. *Chlamydia trachomatis* IgM antibody is the gold standard for the diagnosis of chlamydial pneumonia in babies.

TREATMENT OF *CHLAMYDIA TRACHOMATIS* INFECTION

Tetracyclines and macrolides are the mainstay of treatment for *C. trachomatis* infections. Treatment is often started before a microbiologic diagnosis can be established, so additional broad-spectrum antibiotics are needed to cover gonococcal and, in the case of PID, anaerobic infections. Treatment of patients' partners is essential to prevent re-infection.

Uncomplicated *C. trachomatis* infections are treated with a single dose of azithromycin 1 g or with doxycycline 100 mg twice daily for 7 days. Chlamydial PID is treated with a 14-day course of doxycycline 100 mg twice daily. Doxycycline is contraindicated in pregnancy. Azithromycin 1 g as a single dose and amoxicillin 500 mg three times daily for 7 days have both been shown to be safe and effective in pregnant women. Ophthalmia neonatorum and neonatal pneumonia caused by *C. trachomatis* should be treated with erythromycin syrup by mouth, 50 mg/kg/day divided into four doses, for 14 days [13].

REFERENCES

1. Stephens RS, Kalman S, Lammel C, et al. Genome sequence of an obligate intracellular pathogen of humans: *Chlamydia trachomatis*. Science 1998; 282:754–9.
2. Carlson JH, Porcella SF, McClarty G, Caldwell HD. Comparative genomic analysis of *Chlamydia trachomatis* oculotropic and genitotropic strains. Infection and Immunity 2005;73:6407–18.
3. Wang SP, Grayston JT, Alexander ER. Trachoma vaccine studies in monkeys. American Journal of Ophthalmology 1967;63:1615–20.
4. Brunham RC, Rey-Ladino J. Immunology of Chlamydia infection: implications for a *Chlamydia trachomatis* vaccine. Nature Reviews Immunology 2005; 5:149–61.
5. Kari L, Whitmire WM, Carlson JH, et al. Pathogenic diversity among *Chlamydia trachomatis* ocular strains in non-human primates is affected by subtle genomic variations. J Infect Dis 2008;197:449–56.
6. Kari L, Whitmire WM, Crane DD, et al. *Chlamydia trachomatis* native major outer membrane protein induces partial protection in nonhuman primates: implication for a trachoma transmission blocking vaccine. J Immunol 2009;182:8063–70.
7. www.who.int/topics/sexually_transmitted_infections/en/
8. Silveira MF, Ghanem KG, Erbelding EJ, et al. *Chlamydia trachomatis* infection during pregnancy and the risk of preterm birth: a case-control study. Int J STD AIDS 2009;20:465–9.
9. Beem MO, Saxon EM. Respiratory tract colonisation and a distinctive pneumonia syndrome in infants infected with *Chlamydia trachomatis*. N Engl J Med 1977;296:306–10.
10. Cook RL, Hutchison SL, Østergaard L, et al. Systematic review: noninvasive testing for *Chlamydia trachomatis* and *Neisseria gonorrhoeae*. Ann Intern Med 2005;142:914–25.
11. Seth-Smith HMB, Harris SR, Persson K, et al. Co-evolution of genomes and plasmids within *Chlamydia trachomatis* and the emergence in Sweden of a new variant strain. BMC genomics 2009;10:239.
12. Watson EJ, Templeton A, Russell I, et al. The accuracy and efficacy of screening tests for *Chlamydia trachomatis*: a systematic review. J. Med. Micro 2002; 51:1021–31.
13. www.cdc.gov/std/treatment/2010/default.htm

Lymphogranuloma Venereum 49

August Stich

Key features

- Lymphogranuloma venereum (LGV) is a sexually transmitted disease caused by the invasive intracellular bacteria *Chlamydia trachomatis* serotypes L1–L3
- LGV is a systemic disease with an aggressive nature and initially presents as a painless genital papule or ulcer leading to excessive regional lymphadenopathy, sometimes even resulting in lymphedema or elephantiasis
- Diagnosis is best done by PCR
- Doxycycline is the treatment of choice, and is highly effective when given early in the course of the disease

INTRODUCTION

Lymphogranuloma venereum (LGV), along with gonorrhea, syphilis, chancroid and donovanosis, is one of the five classic venereal diseases. There is considerable confusion about terminology, especially between the latter and LGV (Table 49-1).

EPIDEMIOLOGY

GEOGRAPHICAL DISTRIBUTION

LGV has a worldwide distribution but is more prevalent in tropical and subtropical areas. LGV is sporadic in North America and Europe, where recent outbreaks have been reported among men who have sex with men [1, 2]. LGV remains endemic in parts of Africa, India, Southeast Asia, the Caribbean and Brazil. Prevalence depends on the quality of diagnostic facilities and the training of health personnel.

TRANSMISSION

LGV is a sexually transmitted infection (STI). Major sources are asymptomatic carriers, especially women with LGV endocervicitis. The frequency of infection following exposure seems to be relatively low, although the actual risk of infection is unknown. Extragenital transmission, mostly in laboratory infections, occasionally occurs. Autoinfection (conjunctivitis) is possible.

LGV is six times more frequently observed in men. However, delayed complications, such as lymphedema or rectal strictures, are more commonly reported among women.

ETIOLOGY AND PATHOLOGY

A relationship between inguinal bubos and granulomas was first observed in the 18th century. The first description of LGV was by Wallace in 1833. With the introduction of the first serologic tests for venereal diseases by Wassermann in 1906, separation of syphilis from other ulcerative STIs became possible. The first full description of LGV was given in 1913 by Durand, Nicolas and Favré. The introduction of an intradermal skin test by Frei in 1925 allowed a distinct diagnosis of lesions, formerly called "climatic" or "tropical bubo" and connected the late complications of elephantiasis and rectal stricture with LGV. With the isolation and culture of chlamydiae in the 1930s and the introduction of specific serologic tests in the 1960s, the natural history of LGV could be fully described. Advances in immunology and molecular biology in the last decades of the 20th century led to a new understanding of the disease. DNA amplification tests began to replace cell culture as the gold standard of diagnosis.

Chlamydiae are highly specialized, obligate, intracellular Gram-negative bacteria, with a unique reproductive cycle (see Chapter 48, "Chlamydial infections"). Whereas the other serotypes of *C. trachomatis* all produce superficial epithelial infections of mucous membranes in the eyes, genitalia or respiratory system, serotypes L1–L3 (the "LGV strains") display a distinct invasive behavior in lymphatic tissue. They grow rapidly in cell culture, show enhanced resistance to phagocytosis and kill mice after intracerebral inoculation.

LGV is primarily a lymphatic disease. *Chlamydia* gain access to lymphatic vessels through microtrauma of the skin or mucous membranes. Being partly the result of an excessive T-cell mediated immune response, the leading pathologic feature of LGV is a progressive thrombolymphangitis. Endothelial cells along the lymphatic vessel walls proliferate, finally causing stenosis and obstruction, and the inflammatory reaction spreads to the surrounding tissue. Regional lymph nodes are invaded by neutrophils and mononuclear macrophages, leading to granuloma formation and the characteristic three- or four-cornered "stellate" microabscesses, finally resolving in progressive fibrosis and scarring. Although the immune system is capable of suppressing chlamydial replication, it usually cannot completely eradicate the organism that can persist for decades in local lesions [3].

CLINICAL FEATURES

LGV is a systemic disease with three distinct stages. The clinical features vary according to gender and sexual practices of the patient. Immunosuppression, for example underlying HIV disease, seems to result in more severe and prolonged symptoms.

PRIMARY LYMPHOGRANULOMA VENEREUM (LGV)

A small papule, erosion or ulcer develops at the site of infection (usually penis, labia, vulva or cervix) after an incubation period varying from 3 to 30 days. The initial lesion is inconspicuous and may resemble herpes simplex infection, but is usually painless. It is more often seen in men, with a ratio of four men to every woman, and heals spontaneously after a few days.

Other locations of primary LGV are the anus, rectum or urethra. Extragenital manifestations are rare—the best known being a conjunctivitis with pre-auricular lymphadenopathy and lymphedema of the eyelid ("Parinaud's oculoglandular syndrome"), usually following autoinfection.

TABLE 49-1 Terminology of Donovanosis and Lymphogranuloma venereum

Accepted terminology	Donovanosis	Lymphogranuloma venereum
Infectious agent	*Calymmatobacterium granulomatis*	*Chlamydia trachomatis* L1, L2, L3
Synonyms	Granuloma inguinale Granuloma venereum	Lymphopathia venereum Lymphogranuloma inguinale Tropical bubo, climatic bubo Durand-Nicolas-Favré disease

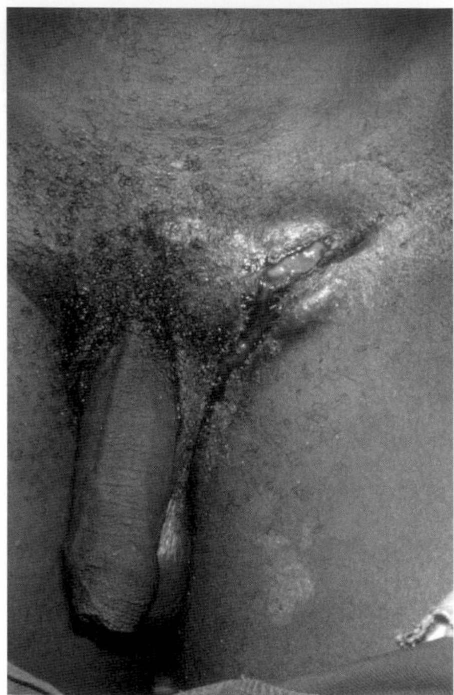

FIGURE 49.1 Lymphogranuloma venereum. Bilateral inguinal buboes with separation of the matted left inguinal and femoral lymph nodes by the inguinal ligament, creating the pathognomonic sign of the "groove".

SECONDARY LYMPHOGRANULOMA VENEREUM (LGV)

From the site of the primary lesion, the infection reaches the neighboring lymph nodes, resulting in an extensive inflammation of the regional lymphatic tissue. This feature is often the first noted presentation of the disease and seen at a time when the primary lesion has already healed.

Inguinal Syndrome

Most commonly, patients present with an "inguinal syndrome", a painful inguinal lymphadenopathy that usually develops 2–6 weeks after the initial infection. The inflammation starts unilaterally but tends to spread to the other side in about a third of cases. Progressive periadenitis involves the overlying skin. Small abscesses coalesce, forming bubos that may rupture spontaneously. Multiple fistulae and sinuses break open and discharge purulent fluid. The enlargement of lymph nodes above and below the inguinal ligament results in a characteristic "groove sign" (Fig. 49.1).

After several months, spontaneous healing occurs leaving extensive scars and masses of fibrotic granulomatous tissue. Relapse occurs in about 20% of untreated cases.

Constitutional symptoms are common during the secondary stage of LGV, indicating dissemination of the infection. Fever, malaise and myalgia are reported by most patients. Meningism, arthralgia and other extra-genital manifestations are less frequent. Severe systemic infection following hematogenous spread is usually a feature of severely immunosuppressed patients.

Anorectal Syndrome

An LGV-associated anorectal syndrome is most commonly reported in men who have anally receptive sex with men. Patients present with a hemorrhagic proctitis or proctocolitis resembling histologically chronic ulcerative bowel disease. Extensive lymphadenopathy may develop in the pelvic, obturator or iliac area, leading to complaints of lower abdominal or back pains. When left untreated, the condition may result in rectal fistulae, perirectal abscess formation, adhesion of the rectum to the pelvic wall and rectal strictures, usually with a long and tubular appearance.

TERTIARY LYMPHOGRANULOMA VENEREUM (LGV)

Late complications of untreated LGV may appear months or years after the initial infection in about 25% of inappropriately treated patients. Obstruction of lymphatic vessels results in lymphedema and elephantiasis of the external genitalia and sometimes the lower limbs. Patients with these presentations are rare except in areas with very limited health facilities.

DIAGNOSIS

MICROSCOPIC DIAGNOSIS

LGV cannot be diagnosed exclusively on clinical grounds; specialized laboratory examinations are required. Smears, scrapings, aspirated material or biopsies can be Giemsa-stained and examined for inclusion bodies in the cytoplasm of macrophages or stellate abscesses in tissue sections. Microscopic examination has a low sensitivity and specificity that can be enhanced by using fluorescein-conjugated monoclonal antibodies and immunofluorescence.

MOLECULAR DIAGNOSIS

Isolation and strain differentiation in cell culture is an expensive and technically demanding method that was formerly the gold standard for the diagnosis of LGV. This method has now been largely replaced by nucleic acid amplification techniques (NAAT) that enable direct pathogen detection in smears and affected tissues. The diagnosis of a *C. trachomatis* infection can be established by sequencing the *outer membrane protein A* (*ompA*) gene. However, NAAT have not been approved by the United States Food and Drug Administration (FDA) for the diagnosis of rectal chlamydial infection.

ANTIBODY DETECTION TESTS

Antibody detection tests are of limited value for diagnosing LGV. Normally, a fourfold or greater increase in a specific titer is considered to be diagnostic. Several test assays are available based on ELISA, complement fixation or indirect immunofluorescence techniques.

The intradermal skin test (Frei test) is historical and no longer in use.

TREATMENT

ANTIBIOTIC TREATMENT

Antibiotics can stop progressive inflammation, but cannot prevent tissue destruction and scarring. The treatment of choice for LGV is doxycycline 100 mg b.i.d. for 21 days. Alternatively, tetracycline 500 mg q.i.d. can be used. Resistance to these antibiotics is not known. Treatment failure is usually a result of misdiagnosis, poor compliance or re-infection.

Should tetracyclines be contraindicated, erythromycin (500 mg q.i.d. for 21 days), azithromycin (1 g daily for 21 days), rifampicin or chloramphenicol can be used. Comparative studies have not been done. The activity of fluoroquinolones is uncertain. Penicillins, cephalosporines and aminoglycosides are not effective [4].

SURGICAL TREATMENT

Pus from bubos should be aspirated and drained and fistulas should receive clean dressings. The severe deformities of tertiary LGV can only be treated with plastic surgery, which should only be performed after a prolonged course of antibiotics. Patients with extensive scarring should be monitored at least annually and, if necessary, suspicious lesions should be biopsied to assess for presence of malignancy.

REFERENCES

1. Kapor S. Re-emergence of lymphogranuloma venereum. JEADV 2008; 22:409–16.
2. Stary G, Stary A. Lymphogranuloma venereum outbreak in Europe. JDDG 2008;6:935–9.
3. Perine PL, Stamm WE. Lymphogranuloma venereum. In: Holmes KK, ed. Sexually Transmitted Diseases, 3rd edn. New York: McGraw-Hill; 1999: 423–32.
4. Mabey D, Peeling RW. Lymphogranuloma venereum. Sex Transm Infect 2002;78:90–2.

50 Gonorrhea

Ronald C Ballard

Key Features

- Gonorrhea is caused by *Neisseira gonorrhoeae*, a Gram-negative diplococcus that infects columnar epithelial surfaces often resulting in extensive mucopurulent discharge
- In contrast to men, many women with gonococcal infection are asymptomatic or minimally symptomatic
- Gonorrhea is usually transmitted sexually
- Gonorrhea can cause urethritis, endocervical infection, pelvic inflammatory disease, proctitis, pharyngitis, ocular infection and disseminated infection
- Neonates can become infected by passage through the birth canal, and infected neonates may present with purulent ocular discharge (ophthalmia neonatorum)
- Diagnosis of gonococcal infection is usually based on syndromic recognition, or culture or non-culture assays
- Antibiotic resistance is problematic and of growing concern
- Treatment often involves the use of single dose parenteral ceftriaxone (to target gonorrhea) together with a 7-day course of a tetracycline or a macrolide antibiotic (to empirically treat possible chlamydial co-infection)
- Metronidazole is often added to the above regimwen to treat women with pelvic inflammatory disease (PID)
- Newborns with gonoccocal ophthalmia neonatorum need systemic parenteral treatment, usually with ceftriaxone
- Prevention of gonorrhea involves adherence to safer sex practices and tracing and treating of contacts and partners
- Individuals with gonorrhea should be evaluated and treated for other sexually transmitted diseases

INTRODUCTION

Gonorrhea is caused by *Neisseria gonorrhoeae*, a Gram-negative diplococcus that can infect a variety of mucosal surfaces lined by columnar epithelial cells. It remains the second most commonly reported notifiable disease in the USA. Following a significant decline in incidence during the last three decades of the 1990s, probably as a result of successful implementation of control activities, rates have essentially stabilized over the past 10 years. Elsewhere in the industrialized world, the decline in gonorrhea has also been precipitous, with the disease nearing eradication in some Scandinavian countries. Gonorrhea remains a significant public health problem in many developing countries.

Gonorrhea is transmitted almost exclusively by sexual contact, with adults under 30 years of age who have unprotected sex with multiple sexual partners at highest risk of infection. The sites most affected are the urethra in men and the uterine cervix and urethra in women. Rectal infection is common in both women and men who have sex with men, and gonococcal pharyngitis can occur in both sexes following orogenital contact. Although gonococcal vulvovaginitis in prepubertal girls can be the result of contact with fomites, sexual transmission is the most frequent cause of infection, even in young children. Vertical transmission can result in conjunctivitis and infection of the pharynx, vagina and rectum of babies born to infected mothers.

ETIOLOGY

Neisseria gonorrhoeae is a Gram-negative diplococcus that forms small, mucoid, oxidase-positive colonies on chocolate agar. It is differentiated from other species of *Neisseria* by its ability to ferment glucose, but not lactose, sucrose or maltose. Confirmatory tests include co-agglutination with monoclonal antibodies and DNA hybridization. The ultrastructure of the gonococcal cell envelope is similar to that of other Gram-negative bacteria. Notably, the cell wall contains a number of antigenic proteins, lipopolysaccharide and pili (which are filamentous structures that aid attachment to cell surfaces and enhance resistance to phagocytosis and killing by neutrophils).

ANTIGENS AND IMMUNITY

The gonococcal pili, lipopolysaccharide and the outer membrane proteins are antigenic; IgG and IgA antibodies to homologous isolates have been detected in mucosal secretions following uncomplicated infections [1]. However, in practice, natural, uncomplicated gonococcal infections do not confer any significant immunity and re-infections are common. Patients with a congenital deficiency in one of the terminal components of complement (C7, C8, C9) may experience recurrent episodes of disseminated gonococcal infection. A variety of methods for gonococcal typing have been developed, including auxotyping (which is dependent upon determining requirements for growth), or protein I serotyping. By using both auxotyping and serovar analysis, gonococci have been divided into a large number of classes that have been widely used as a tool for the epidemiologic study of gonococcal infections. More recently, molecular methods, such as pulsed field gel electrophoresis, *opa*-typing and, particularly, *Neisseria gonorrhoeae* Multi-Antigen Sequence Typing (NG-MAST) have been used to elucidate the epidemiologic linkages of gonococcal infections in various sexual networks.

ANTIBIOTIC-RESISTANT STRAINS

Plasmids encoding for the production of ß-lactamases were first demonstrated in gonococci in 1976. These penicillinase-producing *N. gonorrhoeae* (PPNG) are now commonly encountered around the world. High-level resistance to tetracyclines associated with the acquisition of a 25.2 MDa tet-M plasmid (TRNG) was initially detected in 1985 and has subsequently spread around the world [1]. In addition, gonococci may be resistant to many antibiotics as a result of chromosomal mutations. Strains showing chromosomal resistance to penicillin/ampicillin/amoxicillin may also show decreased susceptibility to cephalosporins, tetracycline and macrolide antibiotics. Decreased susceptibility and high-level chromosomal resistance of gonococcal strains to the fluoroquinolone antibiotics emerged more recently in many countries. Such resistance is thought to be the result of the acquisition of point mutations in genes encoding gonococcal DNA gyrase (*gyr*A) and topoisomerase IV (*par*C) enzymes, and changes in bacterial cell membrane permeability. These mechanisms of resistance can occur in combination, rendering most treatment options ineffective. Where fluoroquinolone resistance is common, the only class of antibiotic that can be used with confidence is the cephalosporins. Even here, problems have emerged with oral cephalosporin treatment failures being recorded in the Far East. It is clear that, barring the development of a new class of antibiotic active against *N. gonorrhoeae,* the era of single-dose, single-agent treatment for gonorrhea may be coming to an end, and that combination therapy may become routine in the near future.

CLINICAL MANIFESTATIONS

URETHRITIS

The clinical features of gonococcal urethritis in men are a urethral discharge, which is often profuse and purulent (Fig. 50.1), dysuria and frequency of micturition [2]. The onset of symptoms is often sudden following an incubation period of 1–10 days but, in a minority of cases, the disease may be asymptomatic. In rare cases, *N. gonorrhoeae* may spread to the epididymis and testis, the prostate, or Skene's and Littré's glands.

ENDOCERVICAL INFECTION

In contrast to men, most women with gonococcal infection are asymptomatic or minimally symptomatic. Those with symptoms may complain of a vaginal discharge or dysuria, which may be associated with infection of the urethra. On speculum examination, a purulent discharge may be seen arising from the endocervical canal but, in many cases, no visible endocervical mucus can be detected on visual inspection. If left untreated, these infections may progress to salpingitis without any obvious symptoms.

GONOCOCCAL PELVIC INFLAMMATORY DISEASE

Neisseria gonorrhoeae may ascend from the endocervical canal to the endometrium, fallopian tubes and, eventually, the peritoneal cavity, causing endometritis, salpingitis and pelvic peritonitis. Symptomatic patients may report lower abdominal pain which is usually bilateral. The severity of the condition may vary from being virtually asymptomatic to life-threatening. A profuse vaginal discharge, often with an offensive odor, is commonly noted and is often associated with dysuria. Abnormal uterine bleeding occurs in 35–40% of patients, probably as a result of endometritis. Patients with gonococcal pelvic inflammatory disease (PID) may have associated chlamydial infection, while anaerobic super-infection may contribute to disease etiology, particularly in severe cases [3].

Clinical findings include pyrexia, tachycardia, lower abdominal tenderness and pelvic, or even generalized, peritonitis. Vaginal examination reveals cervical excitation tenderness and, frequently, adnexal tenderness. Adnexal masses may be formed from tubo-ovarian abscesses or from omentum and bowel adherent to the inflamed tubes and ovaries. Occasionally, a patient may present *in extremis*, with features of generalized peritonitis, septicemic shock and disseminated intravascular coagulopathy. In some severe cases, the liver capsule can become inflamed and attached to the peritoneum by fine "violin-string" adhesions. This perihepatitis is also known as Fitz-Hugh-Curtis syndrome. Resolution of tubal infections may result in formation of fine scars that are associated with increased risk of ectopic pregnancy and tubal infertility.

GONOCOCCAL PROCTITIS

Most cases of gonococcal proctitis are asymptomatic, but may be associated with an anal discharge, blood and/or mucus in stools, and pain during defecation. Gonococcal proctitis is common in men who have sex with men who practice anal-receptive intercourse; the disease is frequently associated with other sexually acquired enteric infections. Women may acquire gonococcal proctitis from heterosexual anal intercourse or as a result of spread from the adjacent vagina.

GONOCOCCAL PHARYNGITIS

Pharyngeal gonococcal infection, in common with rectal infection, tends to be asymptomatic. However, a minority of patients may complain of a sore throat and, on examination, a mucopurulent exudate may be present. Pharyngeal infections occur in those patients practicing fellatio or cunnilingus.

OCULAR INFECTIONS

Ocular infections occur in neonates born to infected mothers. It is characterized by edema of the lids and a profuse purulent discharge (Fig. 50.2). The incubation period is usually short (normally 1–4 days). Occasionally, a severe, purulent keratoconjunctivitis is seen in adults following accidental exposure of the eye to genital secretions. Both neonatal and adult eye infections require prompt diagnosis and treatment in order to prevent sight-threatening sequelae that may ensue as a result of corneal opacities, scarring, or panophthalmitis and perforation.

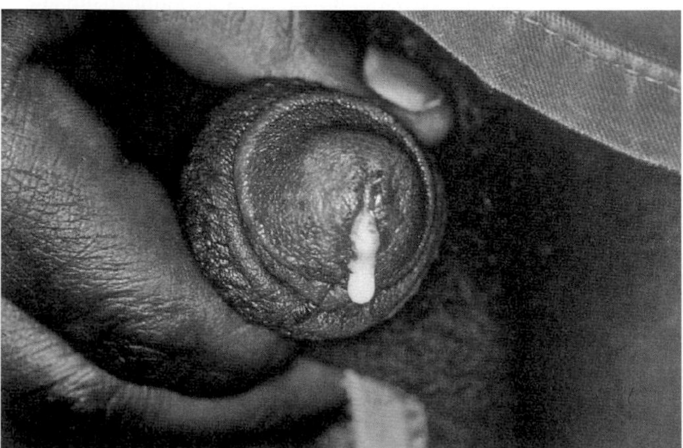

FIGURE 50.1 Purulent urethral discharge associated with gonococcal urethritis.

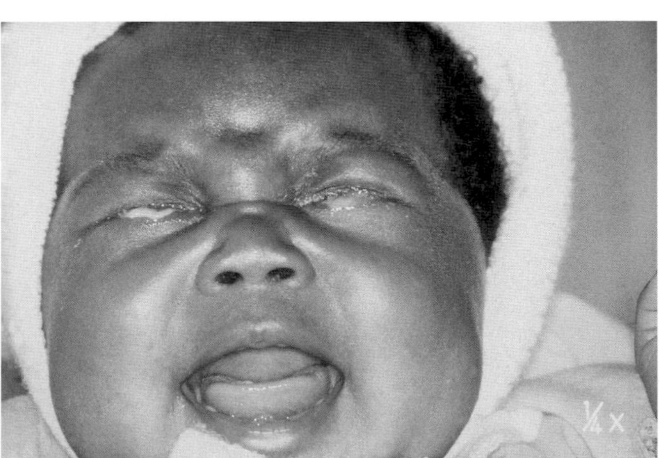

FIGURE 50.2 Gonococcal ophthalmia neonatorum.

DISSEMINATED GONOCOCCAL INFECTION

Disseminated gonococcal infection (DGI) occurs as a result of gonococcal bacteremia. The source of infection tends to be asymptomatic endocervical, pharyngeal, rectal or urethral disease. The most common form of DGI is the dermatitis-arthritis syndrome, in which patients, usually women, develop arthralgias and macular, pustular, hemorrhagic or necrotic skin lesions on the distal extremities. A minority of patients develops septic joints with a purulent effusion and associated fever. The disease normally affects isolated joints. Other manifestations of gonococcal bacteremia include endocarditis and meningitis. Fortunately, these complications are extremely rare.

LABORATORY DIAGNOSIS

THE GRAM STAIN

The finding of intracellular Gram-negative diplococci in Gram-stained smears of urethral or conjunctival material is generally regarded as sufficient evidence for a presumptive diagnosis of gonococcal infection in symptomatic men with acute urethritis and in patients with conjunctivitis (Fig. 50.3). However, whenever possible, the exudate should be cultured on a selective medium to confirm the diagnosis. Owing to the presence of large numbers of bacteria that can be mistaken for (or mask) *N. gonorrhoeae* in the female genital tract and rectum, or the presence of other *Neisseria* spp., especially in the oropharynx, Gram-stained smears of genital secretions from women and from the rectum or pharynx of patients with suspected gonococcal infection are of questionable diagnostic value.

CULTURE

Urethral swabs should be taken from men and endocervical, urethral and rectal swabs from women to optimize isolation rates. Pharyngeal swabs should be taken from patients with a history of recent orogenital contact.

Specimens for culture of *N. gonorrhoeae* should be plated directly onto a selective medium such as Thayer-Martin or New York City medium, each of which is composed of a gonococcal, or equivalent, agar base, with additional growth supplements and antibacterial and antifungal agents. If the specimen is obtained from a site that is usually sterile (e.g. blood or synovial fluid), it can be inoculated directly onto plates of nonselective chocolate agar. Inoculated plates can be stored at room temperature in a candle extinction jar for up to 6 hours without significant loss of viability. Alternatively, specimens may be sent to the laboratory in Stuart's or Amies' transport medium. After incubation for 24–48 hours at 35–36.5 °C in an atmosphere of 10% carbon monoxide, in air, isolated colonies can provisionally be identified on the basis of a Gram stain, oxidase test and sugar fermentation reactions. *Neisseria gonorrhoeae* produces oxidase and ferments glucose, but not sucrose, lactose or maltose. Alternatively, isolated organisms can be identified by using monoclonal antibodies in commercial co-agglutination tests.

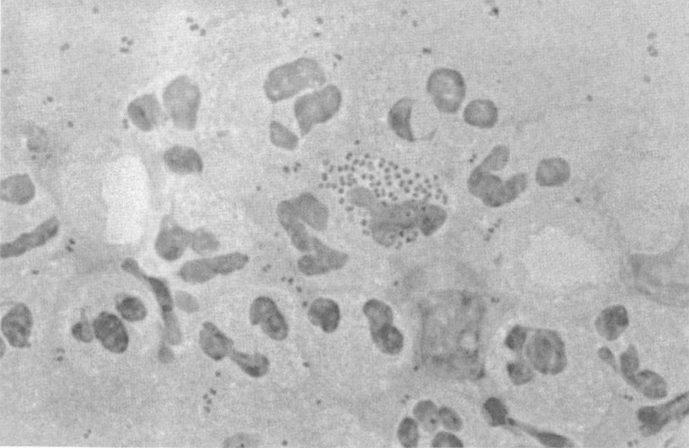

FIGURE 50.3 Gram-stained smear of urethral exudate showing Gram-negative intracellular diplococci.

While culture is largely being replaced by nonculture methods for the diagnosis of gonorrhea in many industrialized countries, it is essential to maintain culture capability for *N. gonorrhoeae* in order to perform antimicrobial susceptibility testing where necessary.

NONCULTURE TESTS

Commercially available nonculture tests for the diagnosis of gonorrhea include antigen detection tests, for example ELISA assays, non-amplified nucleic add probes and nucleic acid amplification tests (NAATs), such as PCR, strand displacement amplification (SDA), transcription-mediated amplification (TMA) and real-time PCR tests. These amplified tests, although relatively expensive, are more sensitive than culture and have the advantage that they can be applied to "noninvasive" specimens, such as self-administered vaginal swabs in women and first-catch urine in men—making them ideal for screening applications. Despite the emergence of NAATs as the diagnostic tests of choice for gonorrhea, false-positive results are known to occur, particularly when testing specimens obtained from nongenital sites. It is therefore recommended that positive gonococcal NAAT results should be confirmed with another NAAT which uses an alternative target sequence in order to reduce the possibility of false-positive results that are known to occur with related *Neisseria* spp. Unfortunately, all nonculture tests share the disadvantage that they can detect nonviable *N. gonorrhoeae*. Therefore, they cannot be recommended for evaluation of tests of cure following treatment.

TREATMENT

UNCOMPLICATED GONOCOCCAL INFECTIONS

Single-dose therapy is preferred to overcome problems associated with patient compliance. However, in many countries where gonorrhea is common, the choice of treatment is limited by financial constraints and the availability of antibiotics. The likelihood of concurrent infection justifies the use of combination therapies active against all possible causes of the presenting disease "syndrome". This "syndromic approach" to the management of sexually transmitted infections has been advocated by the World Health Organization (WHO) [4]. Since 1985, the treatment guidelines for gonorrhea published by the Centers for Disease Control (CDC) have recommended that single-dose treatments effective for eradication of *N. gonorrhoeae* be automatically followed by a 7-day course of a tetracycline or a macrolide antibiotic, which would be expected to eradicate concomitant *Chlamydia trachomatis* infection and other causes of nongonococcal urethritis. In many countries with few laboratory facilities, routine treatment of acute urethritis in men is achieved with such dual therapy, while routine therapy of sexually acquired vaginal discharge and PID is achieved by addition of multidose metronidazole to this regimen to eradicate trichomoniasis, bacterial vaginosis and anaerobes associated with pelvic infection.

In the few regions of the world where antimicrobial resistance of *N. gonorrhoeae* is not a problem, single-dose treatment with either ciprofloxacin 500 mg or ofloxacin 400 mg, by mouth, remains acceptable, followed by a 7-day course of doxycycline 100 mg twice daily or tetracycline 500 mg four times daily, both by mouth. In areas where fluoroquinolone resistance is common, cefixime 400 mg as a single oral dose or ceftriaxone 250 mg or spectinomycin 2 g as a single, intramuscular injection (IM) may precede the 7-day treatment for other infections. Less expensive, and possibly less effective, alternatives used in some developing countries include combining anti-chlamydial therapy with either kanamycin 2 g or gentamicin 240 mg as a single, intramuscular injection. Sexual partners of patients with gonorrhea should be treated simultaneously, regardless of the results of laboratory investigations.

EPIDIDYMO-ORCHITIS

As this is usually caused by *N. gonorrhoeae* or *C. trachomatis*, the treatment for this complication is identical to that of uncomplicated disease.

PELVIC INFLAMMATORY DISEASE (PID) AND OTHER GENITAL COMPLICATIONS

Empirical therapy for PID is complicated by the diversity of organisms isolated from specimens obtained from the upper genital tract. The presence of *N. gonorrhoeae* in the endocervix does not automatically indicate that it is the main etiologic agent of any associated PID. Hospital admission is warranted for a temperature >38°C, pelvic or abdominal peritonitis, or pelvic masses, or when the diagnosis is in doubt. Outpatient therapies recommended by the WHO for treatment of PID in areas where gonococcal resistance is common include: single-dose therapy normally recommended for uncomplicated gonorrhea plus doxycycline, 100 mg orally twice daily, or tetracycline, 500 mg orally four times daily for 14 days, plus metronidazole, 400–500 mg orally, twice daily for 14 days.

In cases of severe PID requiring hospitalization, the spectrum of causative organisms is even broader. To provide adequate antimicrobial cover for *N. gonorrhoeae, C. trachomatis,* anaerobic bacteria (*Bacteroides* spp. and Gram-positive cocci), facultative Gram-negative rods, and *Mycoplasma hominis,* the WHO recommends one of the following treatment regimens [4].

1. Ceftriaxone, 500 mg by IM injection, once daily, plus doxycycline, 100 mg orally or by intravenous (IV) injection, twice daily, or tetracycline, 500 mg orally four times daily, plus metronidazole, 400–500 mg orally or by IV injection, twice daily, or chloramphenicol, 500 mg orally or by IV injection, four times daily.
2. Clindamycin, 900 mg by IV injection, every 8 hours, plus gentamicin 1.5 mg/kg by IV injection every 8 hours.
3. Ciprofloxacin 500 mg orally, twice daily, or spectinomycin 1g by IM injection, four times daily, plus doxycycline, 100 mg orally or by IV injection, twice daily, or tetracycline, 500 mg orally, four times daily, plus metronidazole 400–500 mg orally or by IV injection, twice daily, or chloramphenicol, 500 mg orally or by IV injection, four times daily.

For all three regimens, therapy should be continued until at least 2 days after the patient has improved and should then be followed by either doxycycline 100 mg orally, twice daily for 14 days, or tetracycline, 500 mg orally, four times daily for 14 days.

As intrauterine devices (IUDs) are recognized as a risk factor for PID, removal of the IUD is recommended soon after initiation of antimicrobial chemotherapy. When the IUD has been removed, appropriate contraceptive counseling should be provided.

DISSEMINATED GONOCOCCAL INFECTION

Prolonged therapy with ceftriaxone or spectinomycin has been recommended by the WHO: ceftriaxone, 1g by IM or IV injection, once daily for 7 days; or spectinomycin, 2g by IM injection, twice daily for 7 days.

Repeated aspiration of fluid from any septic joint is recommended. For gonococcal meningitis and endocarditis, treatment with either of the above regimens is recommended, but the duration of therapy should be extended to 14 days in the case of meningitis and 4 weeks in the case of endocarditis.

GONOCOCCAL EYE INFECTIONS

Ocular infections in adults should be treated as for uncomplicated infections of the genital tract. In addition, the eyes should be irrigated frequently with sterile saline to prevent accumulation of purulent discharge. Topical antibiotics alone are not considered sufficient therapy. Neonates with gonococcal ophthalmia should, ideally, be hospitalized and isolated for 24 hours after initiation of therapy. Ceftriaxone 50 mg/kg (maximum 125 mg), spectinomycin 25 mg/kg (maximum 75 mg) or kanamycin 25 mg/kg (maximum 75 mg) can all be given as a single IM injection. As with adults, the eyes of babies should be irrigated with sterile saline hourly to prevent accumulation of discharge. Topical antibiotic preparations alone are not sufficient for therapy. Both parents of neonates with gonococcal ophthalmia must receive appropriate treatment.

PREVENTION AND CONTROL

Prevention strategies for gonorrhea are identical to those used for other sexually transmitted infections, namely, rapid diagnosis and provision of effective therapy together with early partner notification, condom promotion and patient education programs. In developing countries, targeted interventions, such as periodic preventive therapy and outreach aimed at high-risk populations, for example sex workers, military personnel and migrant workers, may be productive. Broad-based case-finding programs using noninvasive techniques, for example testing of self-administered vaginal swabs or first-catch urine for specific gonococcal nucleic acid sequences by PCR, SDA or TMA, may be cost-effective in more affluent settings.

Gonococcal ophthalmia neonatorum may be prevented by the instillation of 1% silver nitrate eye drops at birth (Credé prophylaxis). However, as many cases of chemically- induced conjunctivitis have been recorded following this procedure, many centers routinely use topical tetracycline, chloramphenicol or erythromycin eye ointment for ocular prophylaxis.

REFERENCES

1. Sparling PF. Biology of *Neisseria gonorrhoeae*. In: Holmes KK, Sparling PF, Stamm WE, et al, eds. Sexually Transmitted Diseases, New York: McGraw-Hill; 2008:607–26.
2. Hook EW III, Handsfield HH. Gonococcal Infections in the Adult. In: Holmes KK, Sparling PF, Stamm WE, et al, eds. Sexually Transmitted Diseases, New York: McGraw-Hill; 2008: 627–45.
3. Ison CA, Lewis DA. Gonorrhea. In: Morse SA, Ballard RC, Holmes KK, Moreland AA, eds. Atlas of Sexually Transmitted Diseases and AIDS, 4th edn. London: Mosby; 2010.
4. World Health Organization. Guidelines for the Management of Sexually Transmitted Infections. Geneva: World Health Organization; 2010.

51 Chancroid

Allan R Ronald

> **Key features**
>
> - A painful ulcerative sexually transmitted infection (STI) caused by *Haemophilus ducreyi*
> - A disease of core groups, especially sex workers and their clients
> - Diagnosed by PCR or by culture, but culture is difficult owing to the fastidious growth requirements of *H. ducreyi*
> - Was the leading cause of genital ulceration in Africa in the 1980s, but its incidence has fallen in recent years and *Herpes simplex* now causes a much greater proportion of genital ulcers

DEFINITION

In 1889, Ducrey described the etiologic agent, *Haemophilus ducreyi*, responsible for the genital ulcerating disease, chancroid. Classic chancroid is an acutely painful, irregular genital ulcer with associated inguinal lymphadenitis that may proceed to bubo formation.

ETIOLOGY

Haemophilus ducreyi is a small, Gram-negative, bipolar staining organism that often has a "school of fish" arrangement on stained microscopy. The organism requires hemin and the amino acids glutamine and cystine. Its taxonomic placement is controversial, but it is more closely related to the *Actinobacillus* than to the *Haemophilus* genus. *Haemophilus ducreyi* replaces nitrate and produces alkaline phosphatase. It possesses several characteristics that appear important for virulence including pili, a hemolysin, several toxins and a hemoglobin receptor [1].

PATHOGENESIS

As few as 30 *H. ducreyi* organisms can produce ulceration following inoculation on the forearms of healthy human volunteers [1]. Immunohistochemical analysis of the ulcerating lesions has shown that a cell-mediated Th1 response consisting predominantly of T lymphocytes and macrophages is present interstitially and perivascularly [2]. Presumably, cytotoxins and hemolysins produced by *H. ducreyi* cause tissue destruction [1]. The pathogenesis of the lymphadenitis and bubo formation is not understood.

EPIDEMIOLOGY

Chancroid was endemic in many developing countries with frequent introductions, often at seaports, in the developed world. However, since the year 2000, chancroid has largely disappeared from East Africa and many areas of Asia where it once accounted for 50% or more of genital ulcerating disease (GUD). In 2007, *H. ducreyi* still caused about 15% of GUD in Malawi, but less than 1% in South Africa and Botswana [3–6]. Studies in the 1980s demonstrated that chancroid flourishes in societies in which men are uncircumcised, where many men have sex with a few women (most of whom are commercial sex workers) and where sexually transmitted disease (STD) control programs are ineffective [7, 8]. The disappearance of chancroid has not been carefully studied, but it may be occurring because of improved STD control during the HIV era and the widespread use of quinolones for the treatment of STIs. Although accurate incidence figures are not available, in 2010 chancroid occurs in only a few countries, and even in these countries the incidence is falling [3, 4, 6].

RESERVOIR

The reservoir for *H. ducreyi* is presumed to be sexually active persons with genital ulcers [7]. The attack rate following unprotected intercourse is high, with at least 50% of men acquiring genital ulcers [7]. Secondary attack rates are also substantial, with at least half of subsequent partners infected.

INTERACTION WITH HIV

Numerous studies have demonstrated that *H. ducreyi* and HIV infection interact to increase heterosexual transmission of HIV, while concomitantly altering chancroid [9–11]. HIV sero-negative men with chancroid have a fivefold greater risk of HIV seroconversion than men with urethritis following exposure to HIV-infected women [9]. Women with genital ulcers who sell sex are at greater risk of acquiring HIV. The immune response to *H. ducreyi* recruits and activates macrophages and T-helper lymphocytes, which may predispose individuals with ulcers to susceptibility of HIV infection. Excretion of HIV in genital discharge is increased; as a result, genital ulcers become both the portal of HIV entry and exit. Patients with chancroid who are HIV-infected more commonly fail treatment or relapse. As a result of these interactions, a cycle of amplification between *H. ducreyi* and HIV occurs that markedly increases the risk of transmission of HIV [8,10].

CLINICAL FEATURES

After an incubation period of 3–7 days, a rapidly eroding genital ulcer develops. About 50% of chancroid ulcers are classic and present as irregular, non-indurated, very painful lesions of variable depth with an undermined edge and yellow-gray purulent exudative base that bleeds readily. The skin surrounding the ulcer is usually not inflamed. Other presentations include: giant ulcers formed when several smaller ones merge (Fig. 51.1); dwarf ulcers, which are tiny, shallow, round ulcers that mimic genital herpes; transient superficial ulcers that resemble lymphogranuloma venereum; single, painless ulcers that can be confused with syphilis; and beefy, raised indurated lesions that clinically appear to be granuloma inguinale. The sensitivity and specificity of the clinical diagnosis depends on the relative proportion of genital ulcers caused by *H. ducreyi* in the population [12].

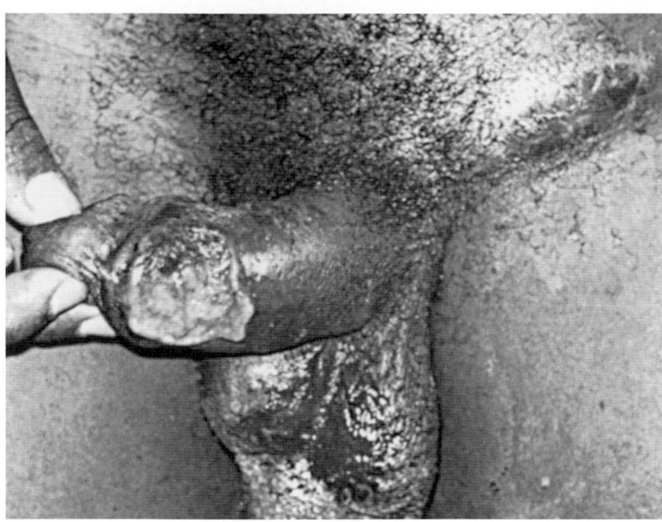

FIGURE 51.1 Chancroid. Large penile ulceration with a suppurative left inguinal bubo.

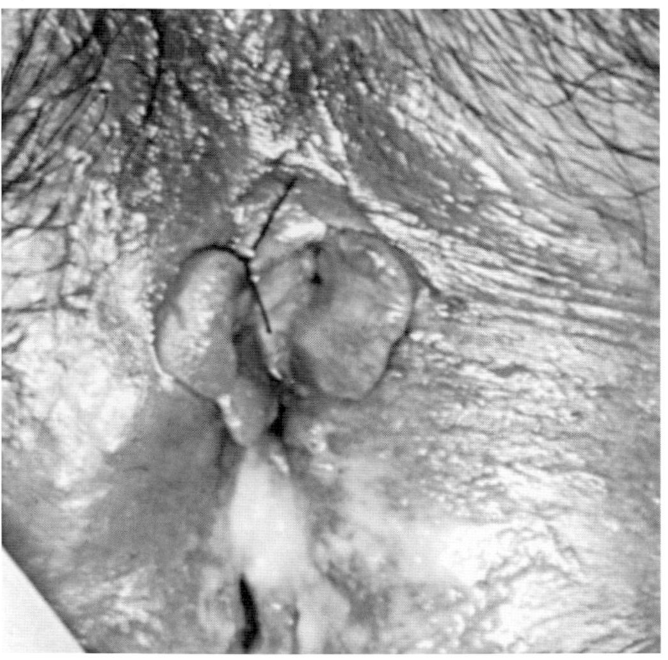

FIGURE 51.2 Chancroid. Labial lesion. *(Courtesy of the Armed Forces Institute of Pathology, Photograph Neg. No. 82-9102)*

The site of ulceration on the genitalia varies, with about half the lesions occurring on the prepuce in uncircumcised men. Kissing lesions are common on adjacent cutaneous surfaces. In women, the majority of lesions are on the fourchette, labia and perineal area (Fig. 51.2). About 40% of patients develop painful inguinal adenitis that can progress to bubo formation with overlying erythema; buboes may rupture and produce an inguinal abscess.

Careful, definitive laboratory studies suggest that about 10–15% of patients with chancroid also have a second ulcerating pathogen, usually either herpes simplex or *Treponema pallidum*.

Two recent reports, both from the South Pacific Islands, have identified *H. ducreyi* in children presenting with chronic cutaneous infections [13, 14].

LABORATORY DIAGNOSIS

Specimens should be either plated directly or swabs transported at 4° and plated within 24 hours [15]. The culture should be plated on gonococcal agar with added vancomycin (3 mg/L) to inhibit the growth of Gram-positive bacteria, 2% hemoglobin, 1% vitamin enrichment and 0.25% charcoal [15]. Incubation should be carried out at 32° in a 100% humidity, CO_2-enriched environment. A candle extinction jar with a moist paper towel is adequate. After 2–5 days, small, yellow-gray colonies of varying size appear on the culture plate. The colonies can be moved intact with a straight wire [15].

Nucleic acid technologies are sensitive and specific for the diagnosis of *H. ducreyi* infection [16]. Serologic studies have been used for the diagnosis of *H. ducreyi*, but these are insensitive and best reserved for seroimmunologic investigation of populations.

TREATMENT

Haemophilus ducreyi acquires plasmids readily and antimicrobial resistance develops and spreads quickly. In most of the world, *H. ducreyi* is resistant to tetracycline, ampicillin, sulfonamides and trimethoprim. In addition, plasmids that mediate resistance to kanamycin, streptomycin and chloramphenicol have been described.

Erythromycin 500 mg three times daily for 7 days or azithromycin as a single, 1-g dose are equally effective treatment regimens. Ceftriaxone as a single 250-mg dose administered intramuscularly is effective but treatment failures occur in patients concomitantly infected with HIV. Ciprofloxacin and other fluoroquinolones are very effective, with cure rates of 95% following a 3-day regimen.

Fluctuant buboes should be incised or aspirated.

PREVENTION

With the evidence that links chancroid to explosive heterosexual transmission of HIV, control and elimination of chancroid from populations should be a priority [17]. Enhanced STD control strategies to include effective treatment regimens based on syndromic diagnosis at the point of first contact with the health care system, the increased use of condoms (particularly by female sex workers), programs to provide care and treatment for prostitutes, and partner referral can all successfully control and regionally eliminate chancroid [17]. A rapid response to outbreaks should be included in all national STD control programs to ensure that chancroid, once eliminated from a country or region, is not re-introduced and allowed to become endemic again. Strategies for surveillance and expedited control with a goal of maintaining societies free of chancroid should be part of all national and international STD programs. Chancroid is the one STD that is susceptible to rapid control strategies with the goal of elimination. Its proven role in facilitating HIV transmission requires continued efforts to ensure its control [17].

REFERENCES

1. Janowicz DM, Ofner S, Katz BP, Spinola S. Experimental infection of human volunteers with *Haemophilus ducreyi*: Fifteen years of clinical data and experience. J Infect Dis 2009;199:1671–80.
2. King R, Gough J, Ronald A, et al. An immunohistochemical analysis of naturally ccurring chancroid. J Infect Dis 1996;174:427–30.
3. Freeman EE, Orroth KK, White RG, et al. Proportion of new HIV infections attributable to herpes simplex 2 increases over time: simulations of the changing role of sexually transmitted infections in sub-Saharan African HIV epidemics. Sex Trans Infect 2007;83(suppl.1):i17.
4. Hoffman I, Kamanga G, Mapanj E, et al. The etiology of GUD in Malawi 1992–2007. Abstract P-318. International Society for Sexually Transmitted Diseases Research, June 2009.
5. Jaiswal AK, Banerjee S, Matety AR, Grover S. Changing trends in sexually transmitted diseases in North Eastern India. Indian J Dermatol Venereol Leprol 2002;68:65–6.
6. Paz-Bailey G, Rahman M, Chen C, et al. Changes in the etiology of sexually transmitted diseases in Botswana between 1993 and 2002: implications for

the clinical management of genital ulcer disease. Clin Infect Dis 2005;41: 1304–12.

7. Plummer FA, D'Costa LJ, Nsanze H, et al. Epidemiology of chancroid and *Haemophilus ducreyi* in Nairobi. Lancet 1983;322:1293–5.
8. Weiss HA, Thomas SL, Munabi SK, Hayes RJ. Male circumcision and risk of syphilis, chancroid, and genital herpes: a systematic review and meta-analysis. Sex Transm Infect 2006;82:101–10.
9. Cameron DW, Simonsen JBN, D'Costa IJ, et al. Female to male transmission of human immunodeficiency virus type 1: risk factors for seroconversion in men. Lancet 1989; 334:403–7.
10. Jessamine P, Ronald AR. Chancroid and the role of genital ulcer disease in the spread of human retroviruses. Med Clin N Amer 1990;74:1417–32.
11. Orroth KK, White RG, Korenromp EL, et al. Empirical observations underestimate the proportion of human immunodeficiency virus infections attributable to sexually transmitted diseases in the Mwanza and Rakai sexually transmitted disease treatment trials: simulation results. Sex Transm Dis 2006;33:536–44.
12. Ndinya-Achola JO, Kihara AN, Fisher LD, et al. Presumptive specific clinical diagnosis of genital ulcer disease (GUD) in a primary health care setting in Nairobi. Int J STD AIDS 1996;7:201–5.
13. McBride WJ, Hannah RC, LeCornec GM, Bletchly C. Cutaneous chancroid in a visitor from Vanuatu. Australas J Dermatol 2008;49:98–9.
14. Ussher JE, Wilson E, Campanella S, et al. *Haemophilus ducreyi* causing chronic skin ulcerations in children visiting Samoa. Clin Infect Dis 2007;4:e85–7.
15. Alfa M. The laboratory diagnosis of *Haemophilus ducreyi*. Can J Infect Dis Med Microbiol 2005;16:31–4.
16. Orle KA, Gates CA, Martin DH, et al. Simultaneous PCR detection of *Haemophilus ducreyi, Treponema pallidum*, and herpes simplex virus types 1 and 2 from genital ulcers. J Clin Microbiol 1996;34:49–54.
17. Steen R. Eradicating chancroid. Bull World Health Organ 2001;79:818–26.

Granuloma Inguinale 52

John Richens

Key features

- A rare ulcerative sexually transmitted infection caused by intracellular *Klebsiella granulomatis*
- Encountered mainly in Papua New Guinea, India, South Africa, and South America
- Usually manifests as beefy red genital ulcers or inguinal lesions erupting through overlying skin
- Complications include lymphedema, internal spread in women and, rarely, hematogenous dissemination
- Diagnosed by clinical recognition or by detection of intracellular Donovan bodies with closed safety-pin appearance on smears of ulcer fluid on biopsy
- Treatment usually involves azithromycin; or possibly doxycycline, fluoroquinolone, or ceftriaxone

INTRODUCTION

Granuloma inguinale (donovanosis) is the sexually transmitted infection with the most clearly tropical geographical distribution. The first published case series came from British Guiana in 1876. Recognition of the hallmark diagnostic sign of intracellular inclusion (Donovan) bodies was made independently in India (Donovan), Surinam (Flu), and German New Guinea (Siebert). The causative organism was first isolated in chick yolk-sac by Anderson in 1942. Recent work has led to reclassification of the organism as *Klebsiella granulomatis* [1].

EPIDEMIOLOGY

Most recent published research on granuloma inguinale has come from India, Australia, and South Africa. In all of these countries, the disease is in decline and in Australia a successful eradication campaign has recently been concluded. The disease continues to be reported from Papua New Guinea, Brazil, and the Guianas. Large epidemics linked to ritual sexual practices are unique to Papua New Guinea, the last being reported in the 1950s. The disease is observed most commonly in young, sexually active male and female adults. Infections in Caucasians are conspicuously rare. In the countries where it is seen, the disease is strongly associated with poverty, prostitution, and marginalized communities. The predominance of genital lesions and association with other sexually transmitted infections point strongly to sex as the main mode of transmission.

NATURAL HISTORY, PATHOGENESIS AND PATHOLOGY

Lesions of granuloma inguinale are predominantly genital, but primary lesions of the anus and mouth are also seen. A small nodule develops at the point of inoculation, later breaking down to form an ulcer. Neglected ulcers tend to extend slowly along skin folds (Fig. 52.1). The infection reaches local lymph nodes via the lymphatics, leading to adenopathy, occasionally abscess formation (the "pseudobubo") and, more commonly, to the development of inguinal ulceration. In women, primary lesions of the cervix may lead to ascending infection of uterus and tubes. Tearing of cervical lesions in labor can precipitate dangerous hematogenous dissemination to liver, spleen, and bone with potentially fatal outcome. Internal lesions in males are very uncommon and involvement of the rectum is exceptional. Chronic infections may be accompanied by scarring, lymphedema, fistula formation, and genital mutilation (auto-amputation of penis). Squamous carcinoma can develop as a late complication of chronic ulceration. Congenitally infected infants show a tendency to develop granulomatous lesions involving the ears and post-auricular nodes.

CLINICAL FEATURES

The incubation period reported by Clark was between 3 and 40 days in 92% of 60 patients. The most common sites of infection are the distal penis in men (Fig. 52.1) and vulva in women (Fig. 52.2). The ulcers are rarely painful. Lesions may be solitary or multiple. A characteristic pungent odor is associated with larger ulcers. Morphologic types of lesion include: (1) a beefy red, flat ulcer with a rolled margin (Fig. 52.2); (2) pale, hypertrophic lesions where granulomatous tissue pouts from the base of the ulcer (Fig. 52.1); and (3) cicatricial lesions where extensive scar tissue formation is seen alongside areas of extending ulceration. Most patients with inguinal pathology show firm nodes or ulcerative lesions in the skin overlying the nodes. The term pseudobubo was introduced by Greenblatt to describe unruptured fluctuant inguinal lesions. These are comparatively rare. A comparable form of ulcer-adenopathy syndrome has been observed in association with primary oral lesions. In women, lesions of the cervix may masquerade as cervical carcinoma and pelvic lesions can mimic pelvic cancers, including the development of hydronephrosis. The clinical picture of congenitally transmitted donovanosis is unusual and appears to result from infectious material being squeezed into the external auditory meatus during birth. Involvement of the ears and local nodes has been reported several times and may take a number of weeks to appear.

PATIENT EVALUATION, DIAGNOSIS, AND DIFFERENTIAL DIAGNOSIS (see Table 52-1)

Donovanosis should be considered in any patient with a genital ulcer and inguinal signs who reports unprotected sexual exposure in one of the regions where the disease remains endemic, particularly if more common causes of genital ulceration have been ruled out. The disease should be considered in any patient with ulcerating adenopathy involving inguinal or cervical nodes. The differential diagnosis includes other sexually transmitted diseases that produce genital lesions, especially primary and secondary syphilis, chancroid and lymphogranuloma venereum, squamous carcinoma involving cervix,

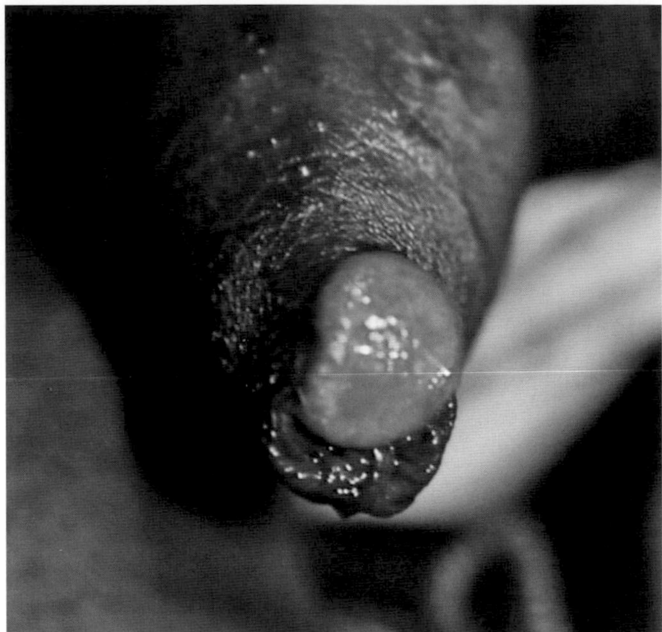

FIGURE 52.1 Typical hypertrophic lesion of donovanosis in a male.

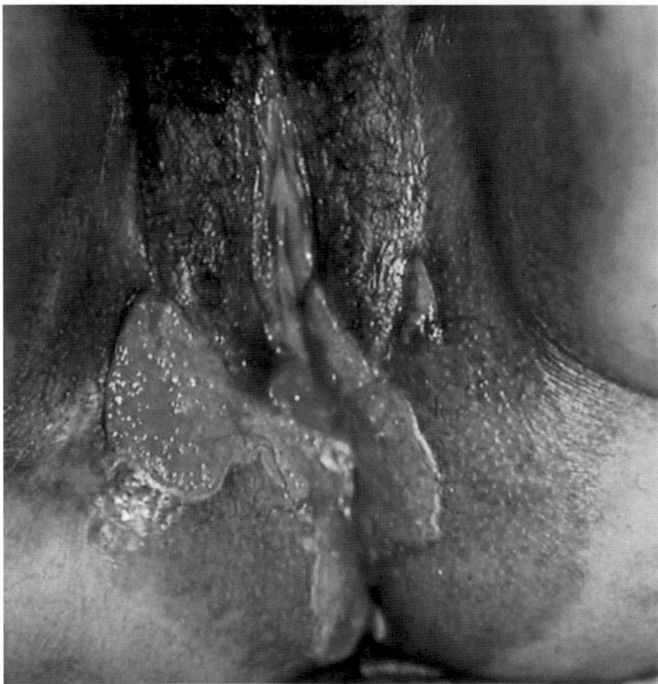

FIGURE 52.2 Extensive vulval and perineal ulceration caused by donovanosi, showing characteristic beefy red color and serpiginous outline. This patient was the sexual partner of the patient shown in Figure 52.1.

glans penis or anus, tuberculous lesions of genitalia, and ulceration caused by *Entamoeba histolytica*. Co-infection with other sexually transmitted infections, notably syphilis, is commonly reported.

The mainstay of diagnosis is the demonstration of characteristic Donovan bodies (Fig. 52.3) within histiocytes obtained by smear or biopsy of ulcers and stained with Giemsa. When organisms are plentiful, it is sufficient to roll a swab across the ulcer to obtain a smear. A better preparation can be made by nipping off a small fragment of tissue and crushing it between two glass slides. *Klebsiella granulomatis* cannot be grown on solid media. PCR methods of diagnosis have been developed, but are not commercially available [2]. Screening for other sexually transmitted infections, including HIV, is recommended for the patient and recent sexual partners [3].

Table 52-1 Differential Diagnosis of Donovanosis

Diagnosis	Distinguishing features
Common differential diagnoses	
Primary syphilis	Similar to early lesion of donovanosis. Diagnosis by demonstration of spirochetes or PCR
Secondary syphilis (condylomata lata)	Close resemblance to hypertrophic lesions of donovanosis. Mixed infections common. Diagnosis by demonstration of additional clinical features of secondary syphilis, laboratory detection of spirochetes, serology or PCR
Chancroid	Ulcers are usually more painful than donovanosis; inguinal lesions have greater tendency to abscess formation. Diagnosis by culture of *H. ducreyi* or PCR
Lymphogranuloma venereum (LGV)	Large inguinal lesions and lymphedema of genitalia similar to donovanosis. Ulcers small and transient. Systemic symptoms more prominent. Diagnosis by PCR, confirmed by type-specific PCR for LGV strains
Less common differential diagnoses	
Squamous carcinoma	Close resemblance between cervical lesions of donovanosis and carcinoma. Ureteric obstruction also possible with pelvic donovanosis. Failure to identify donovanosis has on occasion led to penile amputation for supposed squamous carcinoma
Genital tuberculosis	Tuberculous lesions of the cervix and glans closely resemble donovanosis

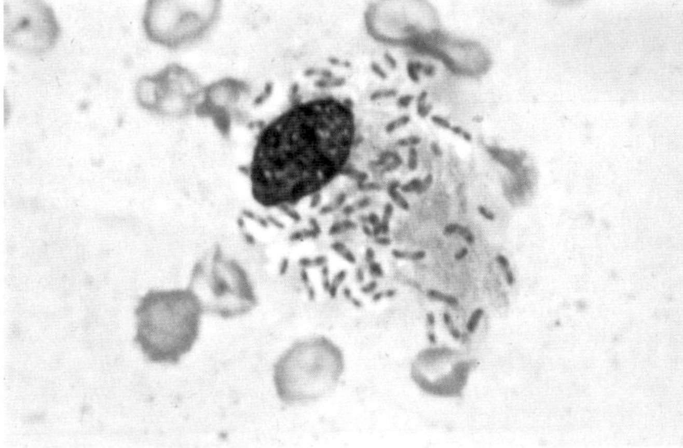

FIGURE 52.3 Intracellular Donovan bodies showing characteristic "close safey pin" appearance.

TREATMENT (see Table 52-2)

Donovanosis has been shown to respond to a wide variety of different antibiotics [4]. No recent head-to-head comparisons have been

Table 52-2 Recommendations For the Treatment of Donovanosis from International Guidelines

Drug	Dosage	Strength of evidence
Azithromycin	1 g weekly, until lesions have healed	Ib
Doxycycline	100 mg twice daily, until lesions have healed	IIb
Ceftriaxone	1 g daily intramuscular	IIb
Ciprofloxacin	750 mg twice daily, until lesions have healed	IIb
Erythromycin base	500 mg four times daily, until lesions have healed	IV

reported. As it is not practical to isolate the organism in culture, investigation of antibiotic sensitivity is not currently feasible. The most recent trials have evaluated the use of azithromycin, comparing daily and weekly regimens and showing excellent results with both [5]. One of the attractions of azithromycin is its good penetration into cells. Alternative agents include tetracyclines, fluoroquinolones, and third-generation cephalosporins.

The development of chronic genital lymphedema is not uncommon in neglected cases, especially in females. Plastic surgical operations may be of help to correct such deformities.

REFERENCES

1. Carter JS, Bowden FJ, Bastian I, et al. Phylogenetic evidence for reclassification of *Calymmatobacterium granulomatis* as *Klebsiella granulomatis* comb. nov. Int J Syst Bacteriol 1999;49:1695–1700.
2. Carter J, Kemp D. A colorimetric detection system for *Calymmatobacterium granulomatis*. Sex Transm Inf 2000;76:134–6.
3. Hoosen AA, Mphatsoe M, Kharsany AB. Granuloma inguinale in association with pregnancy and HIV infection. Int J Gynecol Obstet 1996;53:133–8.
4. Richens J. The diagnosis and treatment of donovanosis (granuloma inguinale). Genitourin Med 1991;32:441–52.
5. Bowden FJ, Mein J, Plunkett C, Bastian I. A pilot study of azithromycin in the treatment of genital donovanosis. Genitourin Med 1996;7217–19.

53 Syphilis and the Endemic Treponematoses

David Mabey, John Richens

Key features

- Syphilis is an ulcerative treponematosis transmitted through sexual contact caused by *Treponema pallidum* subsp. *pallidum*
- Characterized at microscopic level by obliterative endarteritis
- A triphasic natural history passing from primary ulcer (chancre) to a secondary stage dominated by florid skin symptoms and a tertiary stage involving the cardiovascular and nervous systems
- A major cause of abortion, stillbirth, and low birth weight in developing countries
- Diagnosis is usually based on clinical recognition and serology
- Treatment involves the use of penicillin
- There is no commercially available vaccine
- Non-venereal treponematoses respond to penicillin treatment and include yaws, pinta, and endemic syphilis

INTRODUCTION

The treponematoses form an interesting group of infections caused by a group of closely related spirochetes found in humans and primates. At present, the bacteria responsible for the treponematoses are all classified as subspecies of *Treponema pallidum*; commercially available serologic tests remain incapable of differentiating between venereal and non-venereal infections. Some authorities believe that venereal syphilis and the endemic treponematoses are essentially the same disease, with the route of transmission explaining the differences in epidemiology and clinical features. Nonetheless, the treponematoses show distinct differences in clinical features and the propensity for visceral involvement and vertical transmission. Recent research points to small, but important, genetic differences and tissue tropisms in strains associated with different clinical variants. The Columbian hypothesis posits that syphilis was a new disease introduced to Europe from North America in 1493. A recent phylogenetic study has provided support for both hypotheses by showing a close similarity between sexually transmitted strains of *T. pallidum* worldwide and two strains obtained from cases of yaws in Guyana [1]. The findings of this study suggest the Old World treponematoses represent the earliest of the treponematoses, and that venereal syphilis evolved from American strains of yaws before being exported back to Europe (Fig. 53.1). In affluent countries, syphilis is predominantly found among men who have sex with men and migrants from the tropics. In the tropics, it remains highly endemic in many countries, contributing significantly to fetal and neonatal morbidity and mortality, and challenging physicians with a notoriously diverse array of clinical presentations in adults.

EPIDEMIOLOGY

Syphilis is found throughout the world (Fig. 53.2), but prevalence studies indicate marked distinctions between high- and low-income settings. In developing countries, a prevalence of 2–5% is often reported in pregnant women (Fig. 53.3) and even higher levels are often observed among female sex workers. Prevalence peaks at the age of greatest sexual activity, i.e. young adults. In high-income countries, syphilis rates are notably higher in white Caucasian males, largely linked to homosexual behavior. Within individual countries, syphilis has shown marked fluctuations over time, with notable peaks occurring at times of war, in the period following the introduction of the oral contraceptive pill until the emergence of HIV and, most recently, following the fall in AIDS mortality that followed improvements in HIV treatment. There have been suggestions that syphilis fluctuates within populations over an 8–11-year cycle, correlating with the rises and falls of herd immunity.

Among adults, syphilis usually presents with either a primary chancre, skin lesions of secondary syphilis or as a latent infection detected serologically [2]. Presentations with neurologic or cardiovascular manifestations of tertiary syphilis (common prior to the introduction of penicillin treatment) are now rarely encountered, although an exception could be made for the early development of neurologic involvement among HIV co-infected patients.

Congenital syphilis remains a significant public health problem in settings where effective screening and treatment for syphilis in pregnancy are not implemented. This results in significant levels of fetal wastage, low birth weight, stillbirth, and congenital syphilis.

Transmission of syphilis via blood transfusion is prevented by screening donated blood and storage at low temperature.

NATURAL HISTORY, PATHOGENESIS, AND PATHOLOGY

Treponema pallidum is remarkable for its ability to survive for extended periods in humans. Recent research suggests that the evasion of an effective immune response is attributable to a well-developed mechanism for antigenic variation in the face of immunologic attack. These events are believed to underlie the emergence of secondary syphilis shortly after the clearance of bacteria from the primary lesion and similarly in the transition from secondary to late syphilis. The key pathologic feature of syphilis, observable at all stages, is an obliterative endarteritis and periarteritis. Depending on the location, the endarteritis can engender the formation of ulcers, gummata, aneurysms, and lesions of the nervous system.

Syphilis is usually initiated when a susceptible individual is exposed to the spirochetes of a sexual partner. After 9–90 days of incubation, primary lesions develop—most commonly genital—but lesions of the mouth, breast, and anus are also well known. A clean, indurated, painless ulcer (termed the primary chancre), accompanied by local adenopathy constitutes the primary stage of infection. Cerebrospinal fluid (CSF) studies at this stage show the presence of spirochetes in

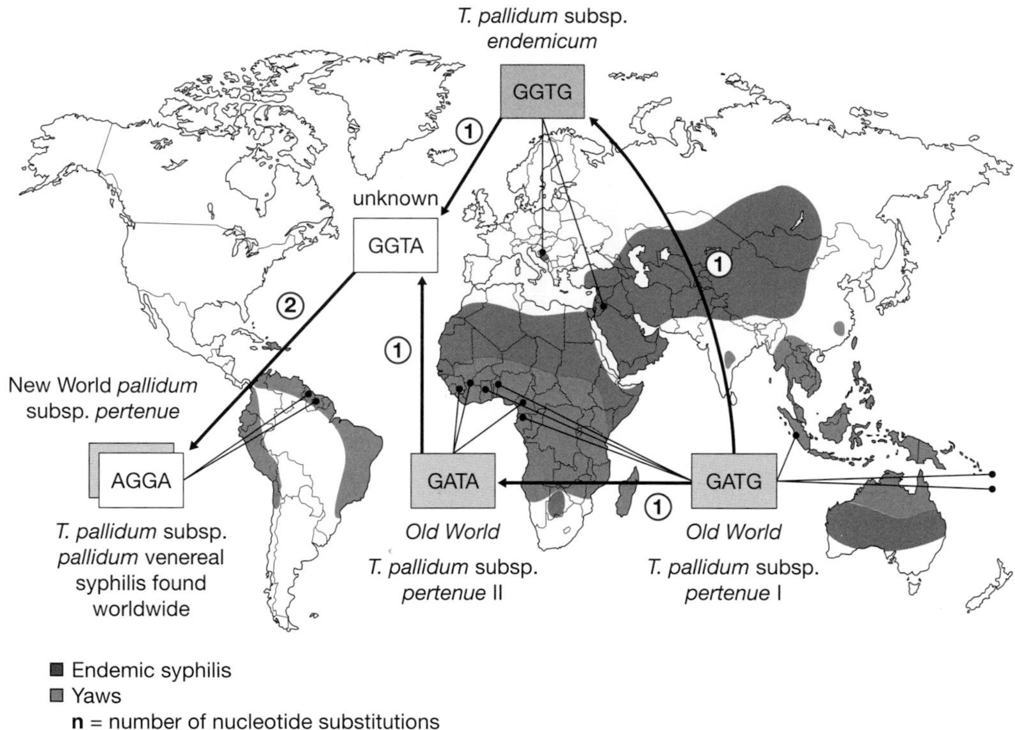

FIGURE 53.1 A network path for four informative substitutions shows that New World subsp. *pertenue*, or yaws-causing strains, are the closest relatives of modern subsp. pallidum strains. The geographical distribution of the endemic treponemal diseases c.1900 is shown based on a map created by Hackett. Each polymorphism pattern is linked to the sites where the strains that contain it were gathered. Arrows convey the directionality of change, determined from phylogenetic trees. The four substitutions were located in two genes located on separate sides of the genome, *tprl* and *gpd*. *(Reproduced with permission from Harper KN, Ocampo PS, Steiner BM, et al. On the origin of the treponematoses: a phylogenetic approach. PLoS Negl Trop Dis 2008;2:e148.)*

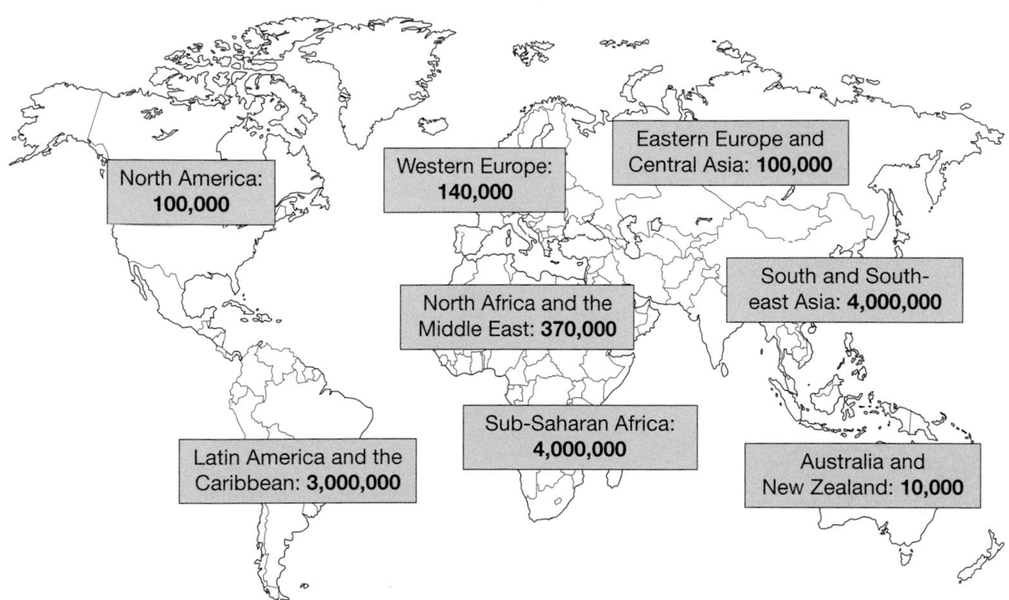

FIGURE 53.2 Estimated new cases of syphilis among adults by region for 1999. *Data from the World Health Organization.*

about 25% of patients, indicating rapid, early dissemination of infection. In the absence of treatment, the primary chancre usually heals spontaneously by 6 weeks. As a new generation of spirochetes evolves, syphilis moves into the secondary stage, during which skin manifestations predominate, including widespread rashes, mucosal lesions, and condylomata lata. Untreated, this phase can last up to 2 years, with alternating periods of activity and latency.

The final, tertiary stage of syphilis is seldom encountered nowadays. Data from the famous Oslo natural history study suggest that late-stage disease may take 10–30 years to emerge. The so-called "benign" tertiary syphilis is characterized by gumma formation affecting skin, bone, or viscera. Cardiovascular syphilis shows a predilection for the ascending aorta, resulting in aneurysm formation and aortic incompetence. The attack of syphilis on the nervous system can take many forms. The classic forms affect the spinal cord (tabes dorsalis) and brain (general paresis), with psychosis, seizures, and dementia as prominent components, and the eye (optic neuritis and Argyll-Robertson pupils).

Untreated, syphilis in pregnancy can lead to a combined fetal and perinatal mortality of around 40%. The risk of vertical transmission

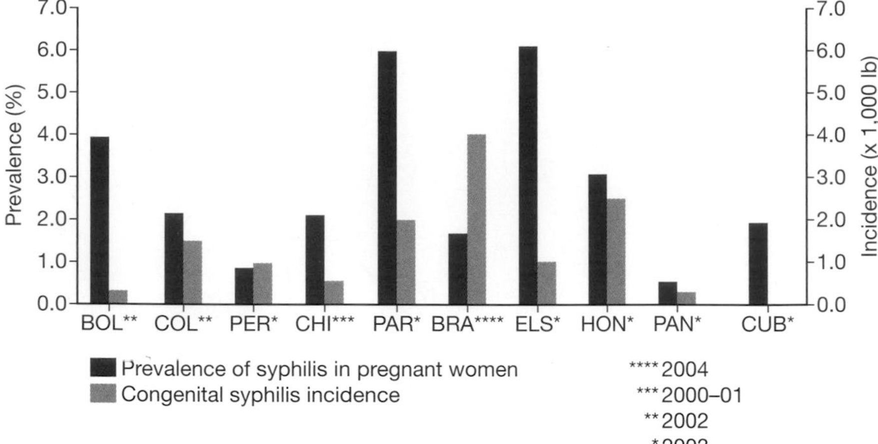

FIGURE 53.3 Prevalence of syphilis among pregnant women and incidence of congenital syphilis per 1000 live births (lb) in countries of South America. BOL, Bolivia; COL, Colombia; PER, Peru; CHI, Chile; PAR, Paraguay; BRA, Brazil; ELS, El Salvador; HON, Honduras; PAN, Panama; CUB, Cuba.

is highest during secondary syphilis, but can linger on into late syphilis. The natural history of congenital syphilis varies from a fulminating early infection leading to rapid death, to an indolent late presenting form, including keratitis, deafness, dental and nasal anomalies, and arthritis.

It is important to stress that the natural history of syphilis shows much variation from person to person. Infection may terminate at any stage, and a significant number of persons acquire latent infection without manifesting any outward signs. Onward progression, particularly to late syphilis, occurs in a minority (about 30%) of untreated persons. Since the advent of HIV, is has become apparent that immunosuppression can alter clinical presentation, for instance in delaying resolution of chancres, overlap of primary and secondary stages, and higher frequency and earlier presentation of neurosyphilis and gumma formation.

CLINICAL FEATURES (ADULTS)

Among all diseases, syphilis has a unique reputation for a diversity of clinical manifestations affecting all organ systems of the body and an extraordinary ability to mimic a wide range of other conditions.

An important distinction is made between early syphilis (primary, secondary and latent syphilis of less than 2 years' duration) and late syphilis (post-secondary or of unknown duration) because the single-dose treatments recommended for early syphilis are not considered sufficient for later-stage infection where organisms are believed to have slower division times. Neurosyphilis can present early during the secondary phase or as a component of late syphilis.

PRIMARY SYPHILIS

The most characteristic lesion (Fig. 53.4) is a painless, solitary, genital ulcer of up to 3 centimeters in diameter with an indurated base accompanied by non-tender rubbery inguinal adenopathy. The classic locations are the distal penis or vulva, but lesions of the mouth, lips, fingers, anus, and cervix also occur. Occasionally, more than one primary lesion is seen (notably in the presence of HIV) [3]. Extragenital chancres are more likely to be painful.

SECONDARY SYPHILIS

A florid, non-pruritic, maculo-papular rash involving the trunk, palms (Fig. 53.5), and soles is characteristic. The morphology of the rash is highly variable. In moist skin folds, especially in the ano-genital area, broad-based condylomata lata may develop (Fig. 53.6). Mucosal lesions may be seen on the buccal mucosa ("snail-track ulcers") and genitalia. Non-specific systemic symptoms are common; among the wide array of rarer symptoms described are: patchy alopecia, uveitis, hepatitis, nephritis, gastritis, proctitis, and meningitis.

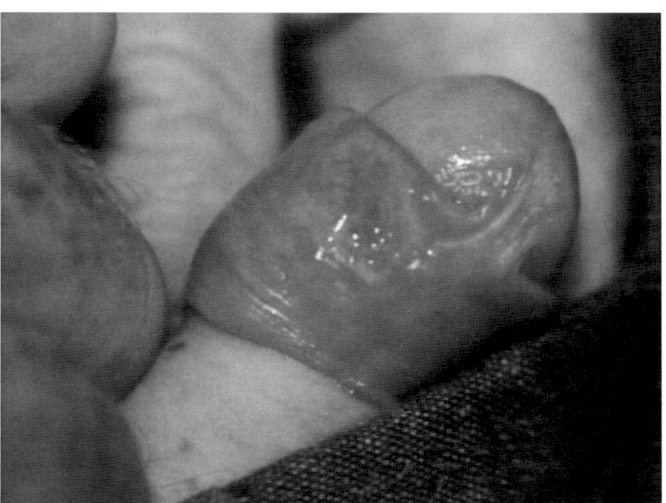

FIGURE 53.4 Primary chancre of syphilis.

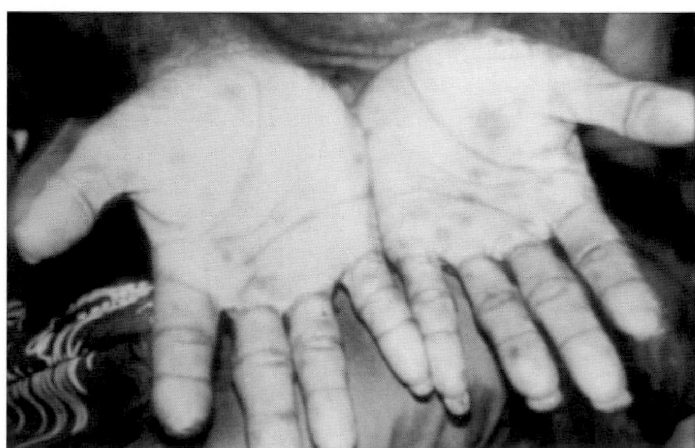

FIGURE 53.5 Classic palmar rash of secondary syphilis.

TERTIARY SYPHILIS

Gummata ("benign" tertiary syphilis)

The gumma is a necrotic mass lesion that may involve skin (causing ulceration), or bone, joints, cartilage, or viscera (mostly liver or heart) where it may mimic neoplasia.

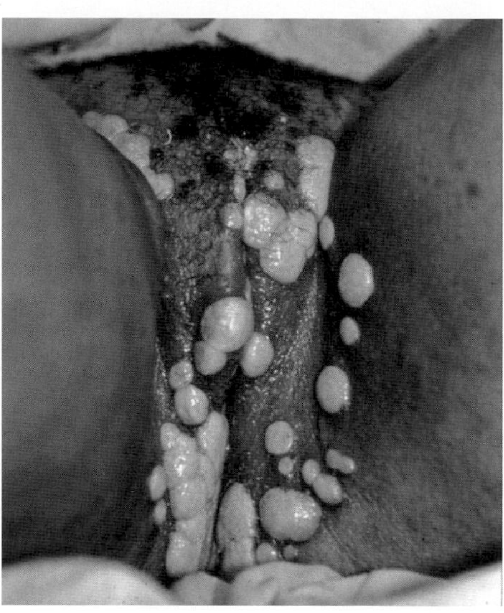

FIGURE 53.6 Condylomata lata of secondary syphilis.

BOX 53.1 Classic Features of Neurosyphilis

Meningovascular syphilis:
Headache
Meningitis
Hemiplegia
Cranial palsies (especially oculomotor, auditory)

Parenchymatous neurosyphilis and tabes dorsalis:
Dementia
Seizures
Psychosis
Argyll-Robinson pupils: irregular pupils, accommodation preserved, light reflexes lost
Optic neuritis
Paraesthesiae, lightning pains, ataxia in lower limbs
Charcot joints
Trophic ulcers of feet
Paroxysmal visceral pain (tabetic crises)

Cardiovascular syphilis

Syphilitic endarteritis involving vasa vasorum of the aorta leads to aneurysm formation in the ascending aorta, aortic incompetence and cardiac hypertrophy ("cor bovinum"). Treatment of patients with syphilitic aortitis carries a risk of reactive coronary ostial occlusion.

NEUROSYPHILIS

Features of neurosyphilis are listed in Box 53.1. Meningovascular syphilis can develop in association with secondary syphilis.

CLINICAL FEATURES (CHILDREN AND NEONATES)

The clinical spectrum encountered in congenital syphilis shows some notable departures from syphilis in adults. Many infections result in abortion, stillbirth, or hydrops fetalis. Infants born alive with severe infection show low birth weight, failure to thrive, and multi-organ involvement, including hepatosplenomegaly, rhinitis, and anemia.

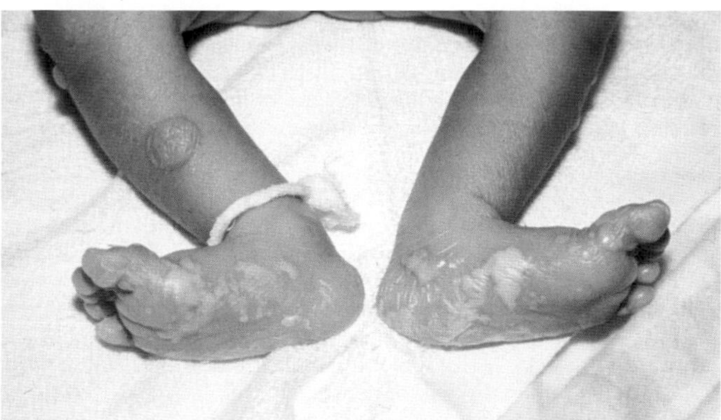

FIGURE 53.7 Severe congenital syphilis in a neonate showing bullous lesions present from birth *(photo courtesy of D. McGregor).*

Skin lesions may display an atypical bullous character (Fig. 53.7). More commonly, congenital syphilis presents some weeks after birth. Desquamating plantar and palmar lesions similar to those of adults are common. Painful periostitis presenting as "pseudoparalysis" of a limb may develop. Late congenital syphilis is rarely encountered nowadays. The classic features are band keratitis, deafness, notched incisors, "mulberry" molars, saddle-nose, and knee effusions.

HISTORY AND EXAMINATION

A careful sexual history is required when syphilis is under diagnostic consideration to determine whether unprotected sexual exposure has occurred with a person at risk of having syphilis, or in a country where syphilis is prevalent. It is important to ascertain the dates of any prior positive or negative serologic testing or treatment for syphilis. Any history of penicillin allergy should be noted. Examination should be thorough, taking in the ano-genital area with regional lymph nodes, and full examination of skin and mouth.

PATIENT EVALUATION, DIAGNOSIS, AND DIFFERENTIAL DIAGNOSIS

The first consideration in syphilis diagnosis is whether there are any infectious lesions that could be sampled for the presence of spirochetes. Such lesions might be primary chancres, condylomata lata, or enlarged lymph nodes. The best sample consists of 1–2 mL of serum expressed from the lesion with minimal blood contamination. A secure diagnosis requires a trained technician using a dark-ground microscope. A more sensitive (but more time-consuming) option is to use a syphilis PCR test on lesion material. PCR testing is more reliable for extragenital sites that can be colonized by non-treponemal spirochetes. Serologic testing for syphilis is recommended for all patients. Confirming a diagnosis of syphilis requires combining a specific treponemal antibody test (e.g. enzyme immunoassay, *T. pallidum* particle agglutination or chemiluminescent assay) with a cardiolipin (reagin) test which uses the antigen "cardiolipin", a normal constituent of mammalian cells. The treponemal test alone is insufficient to diagnose a new, active infection, as treponemal bodies are highly persistent. The reagin tests (most commonly the Venereal Disease Research Laboratory test [VDRL] or rapid plasmin reagin [RPR]) provide a useful marker of active early syphilis and are repeated following treatment to check for a decline in titer. All types of serologic tests can be negative in the earliest stages of primary infection or as a result of the prozone phenomenon, when high titer samples misleadingly test negative when not diluted. Repeat screening at 6 and 12 weeks should be considered after negative tests in patients with significant risks. For syphilis screening in pregnancy, a new generation of rapid treponemal immunoassays offers new scope for programs to control congenital syphilis in developing countries. In patients presenting with neurologic signs, brain imaging followed by evaluation of CSF cytology with serologic tests performed on CSF is recommended in order to determine whether an intensive neurosyphilis treatment regimen is indicated. Patients diagnosed as having late, latent syphilis are advised to have electrocardiography (ECG) and chest x-ray performed to exclude evidence of syphilitic aortitis, which carries potential hazards during treatment. It is recommended that all patients diagnosed with syphilis are also screened for co-infection with gonorrhea, chlamydia, and HIV.

A definitive diagnosis of congenital syphilis requires demonstration of spirochetes within lesions or a positive test for treponemal IgM antibodies. Treponemal IgG antibodies may come from the mother and can only be considered significant if the titer is four or more times higher than in the mother. Infants testing positive should undergo further assessment, including CSF studies and x-rays of the long bones. To minimize the risk of congenital syphilis, repeat testing or presumptive treatment should be considered.

DIFFERENTIAL DIAGNOSIS

Primary syphilis needs to be distinguished from the other ulcerative STIs, namely herpes, chancroid, donovanosis, and lymphogranuloma venereum. Pointers to diagnosis are summarized in Table 53-1.

Secondary syphilis on the trunk is mimicked most strongly by pityriasis rosea. The palmar and plantar lesions may resemble a pompholyx. The broad-based condylomata lata are liable to be confused with condylomata acuminata caused by human papilloma virus, particularly when these occur in the peri-anal area.

Syphilis has a certain notoriety for presenting in unusual or unexpected ways. Good examples of this are syphilis presenting as deafness, uveitis, organic psychosis, gastritis, hepatitis, proctitis, or a cerebrovascular accident in a young person.

TREATMENT

After many decades of use, penicillin remains the mainstay of syphilis treatment. Resistance to penicillin has not been demonstrated, although individual instances of treatment failure are not uncommon. There have been many debates about how to optimize penicillin treatment, particularly in patients with neurologic disease and those co-infected with HIV. Nonetheless, a single dose of benzathine penicillin is suitable for early syphilis in the vast majority of patients and prevents adverse pregnancy outcomes caused by syphilis if given before 28 weeks' gestation [4]. Specific multidose regimens of penicillin are recommended for patients with late syphilis, neurosyphilis and congenital syphilis. Whenever treatment for syphilis is administered, patients should be advised about the likelihood of the Jarisch-Herxheimer reaction which causes flu-like symptoms and can aggravate syphilis lesions for around 24 hours. Prednisolone 40–60 mg daily for 3 days starting 24 hours prior to antibiotic therapy is sometimes used to ameliorate the reaction in patients with advanced pregnancy and those with eye or aortic involvement; however, steroid use in the first trimester carries risks of teratogenicity. Benzathine penicillin is a painful injection and some clinicians co-administer the dose with 8 ml of 1% lidocaine. In patients with penicillin allergy, desensitization according to careful protocols is the preferred option in some centers. Doxycycline is the most favored alternative except for in pregnant women. Pregnant women with an allergy to penicillin can be desensitized to penicillin or receive treatment with erythromycin. There is now considerable treatment experience with erythromycin and azithromycin, but an important point mutation that causes full resistance to these drugs has recently emerged on such a significant scale that these drugs can no longer be recommended as a first-line treatment [5]. Patients with late syphilis are given more extended forms of treatment as spirochetes are believed to replicate more slowly. Some experts argue in favor of adopting a similar approach for any patients co-infected with HIV. For further details of recommended treatments see Tables 53-2 and 53-3. Post-treatment serologic follow-up should start at one month and continue until reagin titers have reverted to a negative or stable, low level. CSF examination is advised in patients failing to respond to treatment.

THE ENDEMIC TREPONEMATOSES

INTRODUCTION

The endemic treponematoses are caused by *T. pallidum* transmitted by non-sexual contact, mainly between children living in poor hygienic conditions. The epidemiology and clinical features depend on geography, with yaws being found in hot humid climates and endemic syphilis in dry climates. Pinta, a milder disease, has been described among indigenous people in the Amazon region and Central America [6]. Yaws is caused by *T. pallidum* subsp. *pertenue*, endemic syphilis is caused by *T. pallidum* subsp. *endemicum* and pinta is caused by *T. pallidum* subsp. *carateum*; however, few isolates of these have been obtained and it is not clear that they are distinct subspecies.

EPIDEMIOLOGY

Between 1952 and 1964, the treponematoses control program of the World Health Organization (WHO) treated more than 50 million people in 46 tropical countries with penicillin for endemic treponematoses, reducing the overall disease prevalence by more than 95%. Since the 1960s, when surveillance and treatment were discontinued, there has been a resurgence of yaws in a number of countries in Africa, Asia and South America [7]. The WHO estimates that there are currently 2.5 million cases of yaws and endemic syphilis, of which almost 500,000 are infectious. Most cases of yaws are in West and Central

TABLE 53-1 Differential Diagnosis of Genital Ulcer

Infection	Ulcer characteristics	Pattern of regional node involvement	Other clinical clues to diagnosis
Syphilis	Painless, usually solitary, 3 mm–3 cms, induration	Painless, firm, rubbery nodes	Features of secondary syphilis may be apparent
Chancroid	Usually painful, purulent with undermined edge, often multiple lesions	Tender nodes, inguinal abscess formation	Rare outside of areas where these infections remain endemic
Donovanosis	Hypertrophic granulomatous lesions common	Ulceration of skin overlying node is common	
Lymphogranuloma venereum	Small, transient ulcer with nonspecific appearance	Large, tender nodes, sometimes sinus formation	Systemic symptoms common
Herpes simplex virus (HSV)	Multiple small, superficial, painful, itchy ulcers	Small tender nodes	Systemic symptoms with primary episode, history of prior episodes with recurrent disease

TABLE 53-2 Antibiotics Recommended for Treatment of Syphilis in Adults

Stage/type of syphilis	Recommendation	Strength of evidence (key to grades: see Table 53-4)	Notes
Early syphilis including HIV co-infected patients, epidemiologic treatment	Benzathine penicillin 2.4 megaunits IM single dose	Ib	Co-administration with 1% lidocaine may relieve pain. Alternative regimes use amoxycillin or procaine penicillin.
	Doxycycline 100 mg twice by mouth for 14 days	III	Used when allergy to penicillin or injection not feasible
	Azithromycin 2 g single dose	Ib	Resistance identified in some regions
Late syphilis	Benzathine penicillin 2.4 megaunits IM weekly x 3	III	
	Doxycycline 100 mg twice by mouth for 28 days	IV	
Neurosyphilis	Procaine penicillin 1.8–2.4 MU IM plus probenecid 500 mg four times daily for 17 days	III	
	Doxycycline 200 mg twice by mouth for 28 days	III	
Syphilis in pregnancy	Benzathine penicillin 2.4 megaunits IM single dose	II	A second dose may be given if patient is in the third trimester. Fetal monitoring advised if treatment is given after 26 weeks gestation.
	Erythromycin 500 mg four times daily for 14 days	III	Inferior to penicillin in crossing placenta and blood brain barrier. Treatment of neonate with penicillin recommended.

Note: this is an abbreviated summary. For fuller recommendations readers should consult STI treatment guidelines, such as those published by Centers for Disease Control and Prevention or by the British Assocation for Sexual Health and HIV.

TABLE 53-3 Treatment of Congenital Syphilis and Infants Born to Mothers with Syphilis

Clinical scenario	Treatment	Strength of evidence (see Table 53-4)	Notes
Congenital syphilis	Procaine penicillin 50,000 units/kg IM for 10 days	III	These regimes are targeted against CNS involvement; less intensive treatments may suffice for mild disease
	Benzyl penicillin sodium 100,000–150,000 units/kg daily i.v. (in divided doses given as 50,000 units/kg 12-hourly in the first 7 days of life and 8-hourly thereafter) over 10 days	III	
Infants born to mother's treated for syphilis in last trimester or with non-penicillin regimens	Benzathine penicillin 50,000 units/kg IM		May be administered to any infant where congenital syphilis has not been diagnosed but where risk is considered high

Africa, Indonesia, Papua New Guinea, and Timor L'Este, with smaller foci in Central and South America.

CLINICAL FEATURES

Clinical features of endemic treponematoses can be divided into primary, secondary, and tertiary stages, as with venereal syphilis, but congenital infection rarely, if ever, occurs.

Yaws

The primary lesion starts as a papule at the site of inoculation, usually on the foot, leg, or buttocks. This enlarges to form a papilloma, which is typically painless, may ulcerate and persists for 3–6 months; there may be regional lymphadenopathy. Secondary lesions may appear before the primary lesion has resolved, or up to 2 years later. They consist of papules and papillomas that exude highly infectious serum, a variety of squamous macular lesions and hyperkeratotic lesions on the palms and soles. The clinical appearance varies by season, with lesions being less profuse during the dry season and more likely to be restricted to moist areas such as the axillae or perineum. Early bone lesions, such as painful osteo-periostitis affecting the arms, legs, or fingers may occur at this stage. Secondary lesions resolve spontaneously over a period of weeks or months, but relapses may occur.

Tertiary lesions (gummas) appear in about 10% of cases after a period of latency, involving the skin, subcutaneous tissues (e.g. palmoplantar hyperkeratosis), bones, and joints. Involvement of the facial bones may lead to swelling and destruction of the nose and palate, and chronic osteitis of the tibia may lead to characteristic curvature (sabre tibia). De-pigmentation of the skin, especially affecting the hands, is

TABLE 53-4 Key to Levels of Evidence for Treatments

Level	Type of evidence
Ia	Evidence from meta-analysis of randomized controlled trials
Ib	Evidence from at least one randomized controlled trial
IIa	Evidence from at least one controlled study without randomization
IIb	Evidence from at least one other type of quasi-experimental study
III	Evidence from non-experimental descriptive studies, such as comparative studies, correlation studies and case-control studies
IV	Evidence from expert committee reports or opinions and/or clinical experience of respected authorities

another characteristic late feature of yaws. There is some evidence that late yaws may cause aortitis and lesions of the central nervous system (CNS) [8].

Clinically milder forms of yaws (attenuated yaws) have been described in areas of reduced transmission. Secondary lesions are fewer and smaller, and resolve more rapidly. Subclinical infection is common in yaws-endemic communities.

Endemic syphilis

Primary lesions are rarely seen, but may be seen on the lips. Secondary lesions of the skin and mucous membranes resemble those seen in venereal syphilis, and bone involvement may be seen, as in yaws. Tertiary lesions are similar to those of yaws, predominantly affecting the skin and bones.

Pinta

Primary lesions are papules or squamous plaques that enlarge over a period of weeks or months and become hypopigmented at the center. There may be regional lymphadenopathy. Secondary lesions, which appear months or years later, are scaly papules that enlarge and coalesce to form psoriasiform plaques ("pintids") that may last for months or years, leaving characteristic hypopigmented scars. The late stage of pinta only involves the skin.

DIAGNOSIS

The clinical features of endemic treponematoses resemble those of venereal syphilis; the diseases can be impossible to distinguish clinically or microbiologically in endemic communities. *Treponema pallidum* can be found by dark-field microscopy in serum from primary or secondary lesions; both treponemal and non-treponemal serologic tests are positive after the early primary stage in all the treponemal diseases.

TREATMENT

Benzathine penicillin by intramuscular injection remains highly effective, as in venereal syphilis. A total of 2.4 million units are given as a single dose to adults, and 1.2 million units to children under 10 years of age. Because of the high prevalence of latent infection, mass treatment has been used to control yaws in communities where the prevalence exceeds 10% and selective mass treatment (patients and their household contacts) where the prevalence is lower. Doxycycline (as for venereal syphilis) is also effective.

REFERENCES

1. Harper KN, Ocampo PS, Steiner BM, et al. On the origin of the treponematoses: a phylogenetic approach. PLoS Negl Trop Dis 2008;2:e148.
2. Singh AE, Romanowski B. Syphilis: review with emphasis on clinical, epidemiologic and some biological features. Clin Microb Rev 1999;12:187–209.
3. Rompalo AM, Joesoef MR, O'Donnell JA, et al. Clinical manifestations of early syphilis by HIV status and gender. Sex Transm Dis 2001;28:158–65.
4. Watson-Jones D, Gumodoka B, Weiss H, et al. Syphilis in pregnancy in Tanzania. II. The effectiveness of antenatal syphilis screening and single-dose benzathine penicillin treatment for the prevention of adverse pregnancy outcomes. J Infect Dis 2002;186:948–57.
5. Lukehart SA, Codornes C, Molini BJ, et al. Macrolide resistance in *Treponema pallidum* in the United States and Ireland. New Engl J Med 2004;351:154–8.
6. Antal GM, Lukehart SA, Meheus AZ. The endemic treponematoses. Microbes Infect 2002;4:83–94.
7. Gerstl S, Kiwila G, Dhorda M, et al. Prevalence study of yaws in the Democratic Republic of Congo using the lot quality assurance sampling method. PLoS One 2009;4:e6338.
8. Roman GC, Roman LN. Occurrence of congenital, cardiovascular, visceral, neurologic and neuro-ophthalmologic complications in late yaws: a theme for future research. Rev Infect Dis 1986;8:760–70.

SECTION

E

INFECTIONS CAUSING NEUROLOGIC MANISFESTATIONS

54 Acute Bacterial Meningitis

Rathi Guhadasan, Enitan D Carrol

Key features

- Bacterial meningitis is a medical emergency. Prompt administration of parenteral antibiotics saves lives
- Symptoms of bacterial meningitis may be nonspecific, especially in infants and young children
- Bacterial meningitis may be caused by hematogenous seeding or spread from contiguous sites (otitis, sinusitis)
- The gold standard for the diagnosis of bacterial meningitis is lumbar puncture with Gram stain and culture
- Common causative agents include *Streptococcus pneumoniae, Haemophilus influenzae* and *Neisseria meningitidis.* Causative agents in neonates includes Group B streptococci and Gram-negative organisms. *Listeria monocytogenes* can cause meningoencephalitis, usually in immunocompromised, elderly and pregnant individuals
- In patients with HIV infection, acute bacterial meningitis may present with similar clinical features to that of cryptococcal meningitis and tuberculous meningitis, i.e. a more indolent presentation
- Adjunctive dexamethasone appears to be of no benefit in low-income countries
- Treatment of bacterial meningitis should target the (likely) causative agent(s), but in resource-limited settings usually involves the use of a third-generation cephalosporin such as ceftriaxone or the use of oral chloramphenicol. In non-resource-limited settings, ampicillin should also be administered to individuals at risk of listeriosis, and vancomycin should be added in areas with ceftriaxone-resistant pneumococci. Neonates in non-resource-limited settings are usually treated with ampicillin and gentamycin, ceftriaxone or cefotaxime
- Many of the causative agents of bacterial meningitis are preventable by currently available vaccines but use of these vaccines is not universal in resource-limited settings

INTRODUCTION

Acute bacterial meningitis is defined as inflammation of the meninges secondary to bacterial infection. Infection of the meninges arises secondary to colonization of the nasopharynx followed by mucosal invasion, bacteremic spread and finally crossing the blood-brain barrier into the subarachnoid space. The highest burden of disease from bacterial meningitis exists in tropical and resource-limited areas, where the infrequent use of vaccines targeting the common causative agents of acute bacterial meningitis, coupled with the HIV/AIDS pandemic, has amplified the problem. Bacterial meningitis is usually fatal without treatment. Therefore, prompt and accurate diagnosis, coupled with the timely administration of parenteral antibiotics, is necessary in order to save lives [1]. The presenting clinical features of bacterial meningitis may be similar to those of other central nervous system (CNS) infections, such as tuberculous meningitis, cryptococcal meningitis and viral meningitis. Historically, most reports of bacterial meningitis in sub-Saharan Africa describe epidemics of meningococcal meningitis caused by serogroup A, occurring approximately every decade. More recently, other serogroups, such as W-135, have been reported in Africa, although serogroup A continues to predominate [2].

EPIDEMIOLOGY

The annual incidence of acute bacterial meningitis is 4–6 per 100,000 in high-income countries and 10-fold higher in developing countries. There is a high case fatality rate in developing countries (10–50%) that is augmented by pre-existing comorbidities (e.g. malnutrition, HIV infection and sickle cell disease), late presentation to health services, emerging antibiotic resistance and lack of appropriate antibiotics, medical expertise and the use of conjugate vaccines against the main three pathogens: *Streptococcus pneumoniae, Haemophilus influenzae,* and *Neisseria meningitidis.*

Neisseria meningitidis-associated meningitis occurs across the globe, but *N. meningitidis* can also cause large outbreaks, especially in crowded conditions, and in the "meningitis belt" of Africa (Fig. 54.1), where epidemics occur every 5–15 years in the Harmattan season (dry and dusty with a strong wind between November and March) and are associated with up to 10% mortality [3].

The peak incidence for *S. pneumoniae* and *H. influenzae* (Hib) meningitis occurs in children. Hib meningitis is rare over the age of five years, but pneumococcal and meningococcal meningitis can occur in all age groups [3]. The predominant organism causing bacterial meningitis in children in the tropics is *S. pneumoniae* (Fig. 54.2A). The organisms that cause acute bacterial meningitis in adults in Africa are shown in Figure 54.2 (B). In Southeast Asia, *Streptococcus suis* is a cause of acute bacterial meningitis in adults.

NATURAL HISTORY, PATHOGENESIS, AND PATHOLOGY

The most common bacteria causing acute bacterial meningitis (*S. pneumoniae, N. meningitidis,* and *H. influenzae*) have neurotropic potential, which allows them to invade the host mucosal epithelium, multiply in the bloodstream and cross the blood brain barrier into the cerebrospinal fluid (CSF). The bacteria colonize the nasopharyngeal epithelium by adhering to the epithelial lining of the respiratory tract—the mechanisms of which vary depending on the organism. *Neisseria meningitidis* and other Gram-negative bacteria adhere via pili; *S. pneumoniae* binds by pneumococcal surface-associated proteins, such as pneumococcal surface adhesion A (PsaA) or choline-binding

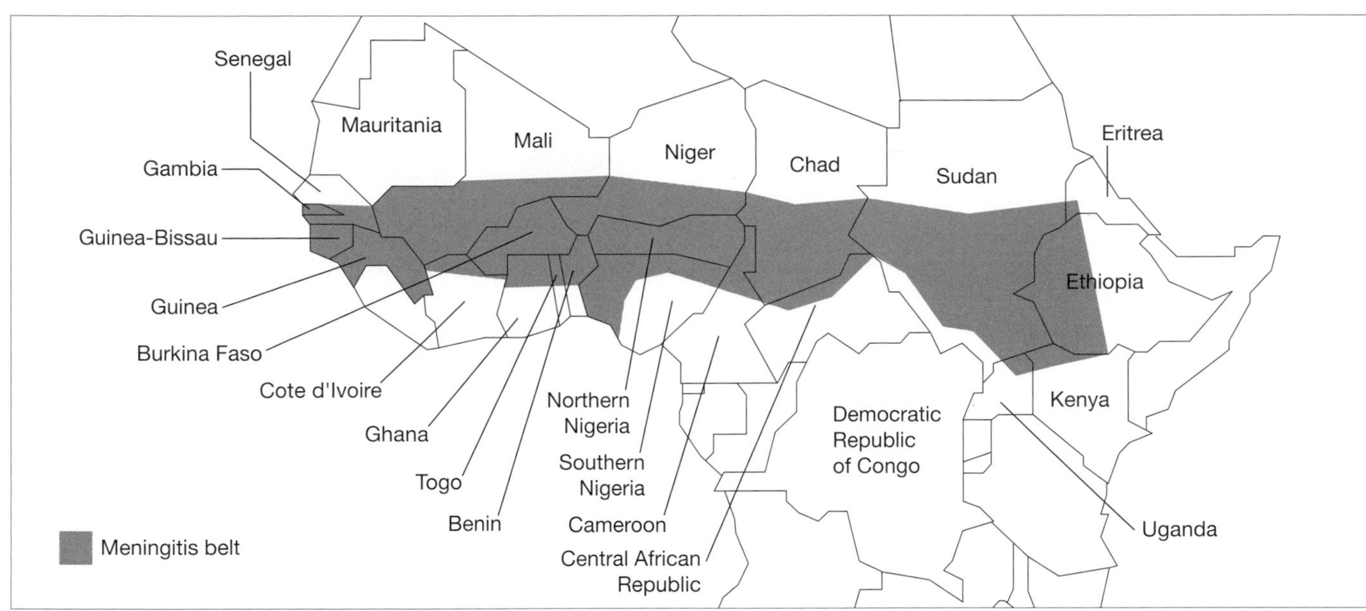

FIGURE 54.1 Map of African meningitis belt.

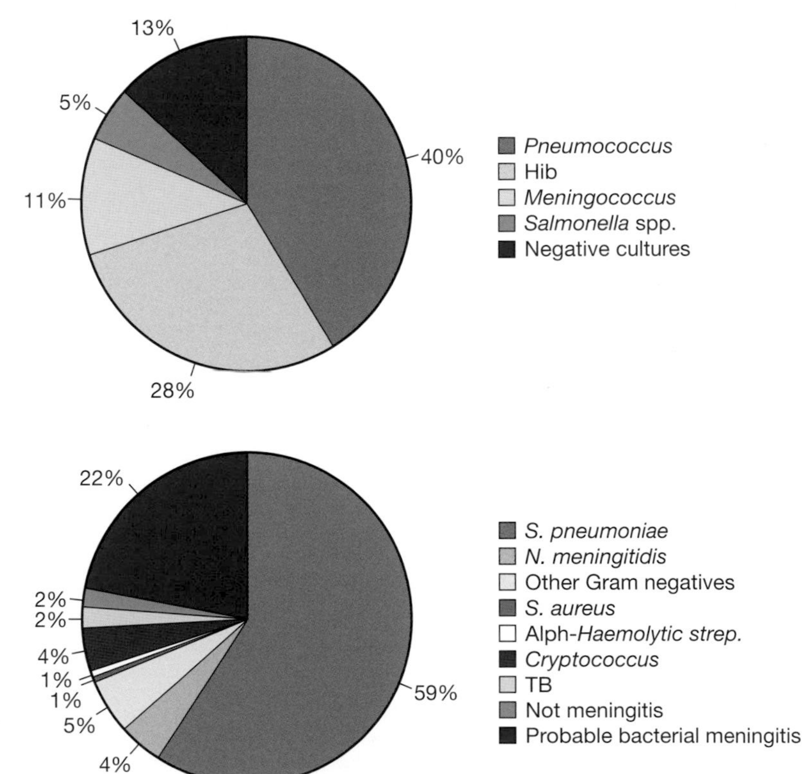

FIGURE 54.2 The proportion of acute bacterial meningitis attributed to each pathogen in children and adults in Malawi *Reproduced with permission from Lin AL, Safdieh JE. The evaluation and management of bacterial meningitis: Current practice and emerging developments. Neurologist 2010;16:143–51.* **(A)** Cause of childhood bacterial meningitis 2002. **(B)** Causes of meningitis in adults in Malawi, 2007.

protein A (CbpA) [4]. Young children mount inadequate immune responses to bacterial capsular polysaccharides, rendering them particularly vulnerable to these infections [5]. Bacteria invade the mucosal epithelium via a number of processes that include transcytosis, through phagocytes in a "Trojan horse" manner, or directly following damage to the integrity of the mucosa, such as occurs with a viral infection. Survival within the bloodstream depends on the bacteria avoiding host defence mechanisms, particularly complement-dependent killing. *Neisseria meningitidis* and *S. pneumoniae* both recruit complement factor H, the main regulator of the alternative complement pathway that controls early activation of the complement cascade. *Neisseria meningitidis* produces Factor H binding protein and the *S. pneumoniae* proteins CbpA and pneumococcal surface protein C (PspC) bind complement factor H.

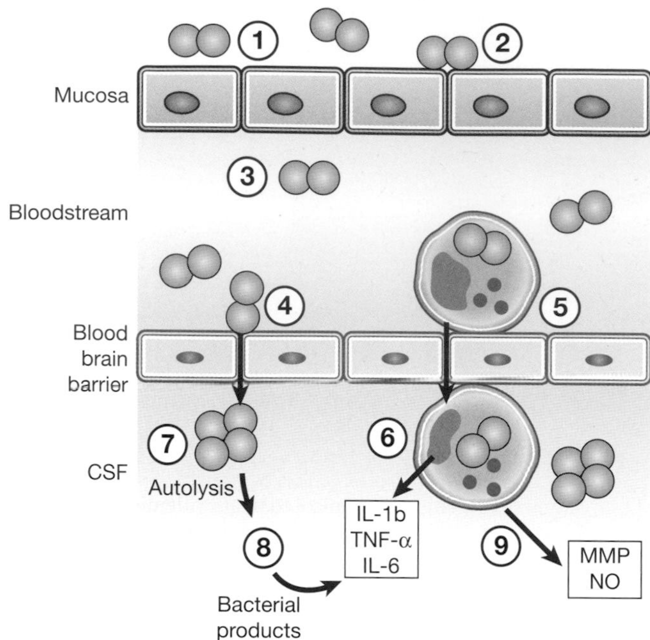

FIGURE 54.3 Pathogenesis of bacterial meningitis. **1.** Adherence and colonization of mucosa; **2.** Invasion of blood stream; **3.** Multiplication in bloodstream; **4.** Increased permeability of blood brain barrier and bacteria cross blood-brain barrier; **5.** Infiltration of CSF by white cells; **6.** Release of pro- inflammatory cytokines; **7.** Uncontrolled replication of bacteria in sanctuary site, CSF; **8.** Bacterial products stimulate inflammatory cascade; **9.** Activated leukocytes lead to production of matrix metalloproteinase (MMP) and oxidants.

Bacterial translocation of the blood brain barrier is a result of specific bacteria-host interactions involving cell signal transduction pathways with effects on actin cytoskeleton rearrangements [6]. Bacteria cross the blood brain barrier by a number of processes that include: (i) disruption of the tight junctions; (ii) transcellular migration by transcytosis; and, (iii) surviving within phagocytes using a "Trojan horse" mechanism.

Once within the CSF, bacteria enter a sanctuary site with relatively low concentrations of complement and antibody. Bacteria and bacterial products (resulting from autolysis) stimulate an inflammatory response of pro-and anti-inflammatory cytokines. In turn, the pro-inflammatory cells stimulate the release of chemokines. Neuronal cell death occurs mainly in the hippocampus, through apoptosis, and in the cortex, through necrosis. White matter injury also occurs, secondary to small-vessel vasculitis, focal ischemia or venous thrombosis. The process is summarized in Figure 54.3.

CLINICAL FEATURES

In infants and young children, clinical features are very non-specific and include fever, lethargy, irritability, poor feeding, seizures, respiratory distress, vomiting and diarrhea, and a bulging fontanelle [7, 8], while older children and adults have headache (80–95%), photophobia (30–50%), neck stiffness (50–90%), lethargy, confusion, and positive Kernig's sign (resistance to knee extension upon passive hip flexion; 5%) and Brudzinski's sign (hip flexion upon passive neck flexion; 5%) [1, 8]. Adults with acute bacterial meningitis usually present with features of fever, neck stiffness and altered mental status. However, it has recently been proposed that this triad should now become a quartet to include fever, neck stiffness, headache and altered mental status, which are present in 95% of adults with acute bacterial meningitis [9]. More advanced disease may include opisthotonus, focal neurologic deficit (20–30%), seizures (15–30%) and a reduced level of consciousness (Fig. 54.4).

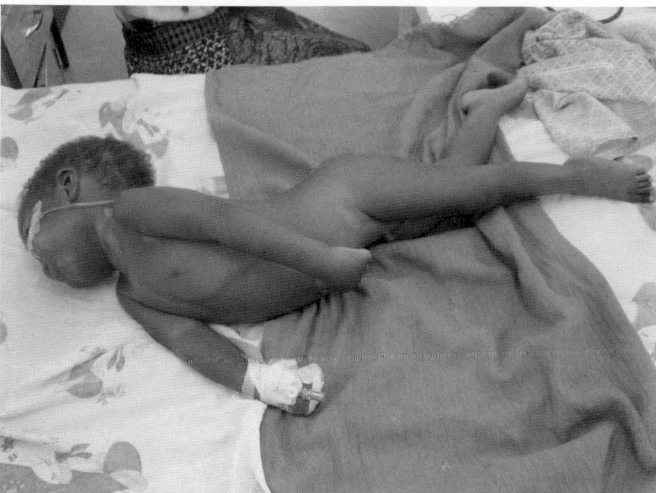

FIGURE 54.4 Opisthotonus in a Malawian child with bacterial meningitis.

A rash may be present in 10–15% of cases of acute bacterial meningitis—most commonly this is the purpuric rash of meningococcal meningitis with septicemia, but a purpuric rash may also be caused by other pathogens. Shock and disseminated intravascular coagulation occur in meningococcemia. Cushing's triad of systemic hypertension, bradycardia and respiratory depression occurs late and indicates raised intracranial pressure and shift of brain compartments [8]. HIV-positive children with acute bacterial meningitis are more likely to present in extremis and have pneumococcal meningitis, seizures or a focus of infection, such as otitis media. They take longer to defervesce and are more likely to die or experience recurrence.

Patients should be monitored closely for dehydration, shock, seizures, altered conscious level or rising intracranial pressure. Cerebrovascular events, such as infarction and/or edema, obstructive or communicating hydrocephalus, epidural abscess and subdural empyema are uncommon complications. Immune complex-mediated arthritis occurs late in Hib or meningococcal illness. Neurologic sequelae, such as deafness, cognitive impairment and developmental delay, occur in 5–40% of survivors [8].

PATIENT EVALUATION, DIAGNOSIS, AND DIFFERENTIAL DIAGNOSIS

PATIENT EVALUATION

Initial evaluation should include a thorough history to elicit information on duration of illness, history of seizures, anti-retroviral or anti-tuberculous treatment, HIV status and previous antibiotics or anti-malarials. Examination should include assessment of nutritional status, presence of a rash, examination of the fontanelle and eliciting neck stiffness. In the tropics, features of acute bacterial meningitis often overlap with those of severe malaria or cerebral malaria, leading to difficulties in the early recognition of acute bacterial meningitis in children. Several predictor algorithms to assist in establishing the diagnosis of acute bacterial meningitis have been derived, most of which include laboratory data. Only two of these have been evaluated in resource-poor settings. In children, Berkley et al. reported that the presence of one or more of the following is an indication for lumbar puncture [10]: bulging fontanelle, neck stiffness, cyanosis, impaired consciousness, partial seizures and seizures outside the febrile convulsions age range. Thwaites et al. described a weighted diagnostic score to distinguish acute bacterial meningitis from tuberculous meningitis in adults, which included age, white blood cell count, duration of history of illness, CSF white cell count and CSF percentage neutrophils [11]. In areas with a high incidence of HIV infection, *S. pneumoniae* is the commonest cause of acute bacterial meningitis; however, tuberculous meningitis and cryptococcal meningitis are also commonly associated with HIV-infection—the presenting clinical features of all three diseases are very similar [1]. A clinical algorithm for the management of CNS infections in adults has been described for use in resource-poor settings with a high prevalence of HIV; it demonstrated reduced time to diagnosis and treatment of cryptococcal meningitis.

DIAGNOSIS

The gold standard for the diagnosis of acute bacterial meningitis involves a lumbar puncture with Gram staining and culturing of CSF. Characteristic laboratory findings suggestive of acute bacterial meningitis include a CSF white cell count of >1000 cells/mm^3 with a neutrophil predominance, an elevated protein of >50 mg/dl and a CSF to blood glucose ratio of <0.6. Lower CSF cell counts are seen in children and immunocompromised patients [1]. If there has been partial pretreatment with antibiotics, there may be lymphocyte predominance in the CSF. A large study of predominantly HIV-infected adults with acute bacterial meningitis found that CSF analysis was normal in 4% of cases. CSF Gram staining is inexpensive but requires experienced staff to accurately interpret findings. The sensitivity of Gram staining is reported to be between 50–90% with a high specificity [1]. In the absence of prior antibiotic treatment, culturing of CSF is 80–85% sensitive in adults and children.

Latex agglutination tests are simple and rapid to perform, but their cost is still prohibitive for resource-limited settings and refrigeration is required for the kits. Studies have shown that they do not add much to the microbiologic diagnosis of acute bacterial meningitis in areas with microbiologic capability. In contrast, the sensitivity and specificity of cryptococcal latex agglutination tests are high and this may help to rapidly differentiate between bacterial and cryptococcal etiology in areas of high HIV incidence. A recently developed duplex rapid diagnostic test for *N. meningitidis* has been evaluated on CSF samples from Niger and reported very good sensitivities and specificities for serogroup A and serogroup W135 [12].

Nucleic acid amplification using PCR targeting bacterial DNA is sensitive but the major drawback in the tropics include the cost and requirement for specialized equipment and technical expertise.

TREATMENT

ANTIBIOTICS

In addition to airway and hemodynamic stabilization and supportive management, antibiotics are the cornerstone of acute bacterial meningitis treatment. Untreated, acute bacterial meningitis is almost always fatal; early treatment improves clinical outcome [8]. When acute bacterial meningitis is suspected, high-dose empirical intravenous antibiotic treatment based on the likely organisms for the patient's age and susceptibility patterns of that region should be commenced without delay (Table 54-1) [1, 8].

Ceftriaxone is recommended by the World Health Organization (WHO) as first-line therapy [1]. Intravenous and intramuscular administration routes are equally effective, as is once-daily dosing [1]. However, chloramphenicol (in oily suspension) remains the first choice for treatment in many low-income settings as it is cheap and readily available. It is contraindicated in infants aged below two months [8]. The WHO recommends a single intramuscular injection of ceftriaxone or oily chloramphenicol to treat epidemic meningococcal meningitis [3, 13], although longer courses are advised if the child has fever, seizures or coma after the first 24 hours of treatment [1, 3, 13]. Single dosing is reasonably safe during epidemics as 95% of cases are expected to be caused by meningococcus, which responds well to this treatment; however, single dose is absolutely contraindicated in non-epidemic situations or for babies under 2 months of age, where the risk of partial treatment of pneumococcal, Hib or Group B streptococcal meningitis is high [3]. In all categories, the WHO recommends regular clinical reassessment and referral if there is no improvement after 48 hours, or coma or repeated seizures [3]. A randomized, controlled trial compared 4- and 7-day ceftriaxone treatment courses in Chilean children and showed rapid initial recovery in both groups (the most common pathogens in this study were Hib and meningococcus) [14]. A large multicountry, double-blind, placebo-controlled, randomized equivalence study of 5 versus 10 days of treatment with ceftriaxone in 1004 children, concluded that in children beyond the neonatal age-group with purulent meningitis caused by *S. pneumoniae*, *H. influenzae* type b, or *N. meningitidis* who are stable by day 5 of ceftriaxone treatment, there was no difference in relapse or bacteriological failure rates between the two groups [15].

TABLE 54-1 WHO Recommended Empirical Antibiotic Treatment in Non-epidemic Situations in Resource-poor Settings without Laboratory Support

Age group	Likely pathogens	Treatment	Duration of treatment
0–2 months	*Streptococcus agalactiae* *Streptococcus pyogenes* Enterobacteria	Ceftriaxone 100 mg/kg/day o.d	7 days 21 days for Gram-negative bacilli (*Escherichia coli*, non-typhoidal *Salmonella*)
2–23 months	*Streptococcus pneumoniae* *Haemophilus influenzae b* *Neisseria meningitidis* Enterobacteria	Ceftriaxone 100mg/kg/day o.d	5 days 21 days
2–5 years	*S. pneumoniae* *H. influenzae b* *N. meningitidis*	Ceftriaxone 100mg/kg/day o.d	5 days
5–14 years	*S. pneumoniae* *N. meningitidis*	Ceftriaxone 100mg/kg/day o.d (max. 2 g)	5 days
>14 years	*S. pneumoniae* *N. meningitidis*	Ceftriaxone 2 g/day o.d	5 days
Elderly	*S. pneumoniae* *N. meningitidis*	Ceftriaxone 2 g/day	5 days

o.d., once daily.

Source from World Health Organization. Standardised treatment of bacterial meningitis in Africa in epidemic and non-epidemic situations; 2007. Available at: http://www.who.int/csr/resources/publications/meningitis/WHO_CDS_EPR_2007_3/en/index.html.

High rates of Hib and pneumococcal chloramphenicol resistance occur in Africa (10–13%) and Southeast Asia [3, 16]. Pneumococcal resistance to cephalosporins is a growing global concern; as many as 41% of isolates worldwide (5% in Africa) demonstrate cephalosporin and penicillin resistance [1, 3, 17], necessitating the addition of vancomycin or rifampin [16].

In non-resource-limited settings, ampicillin should also be administered to individuals at risk of listeriosis; neonates in non-resource-limited settings are usually treated with ampicillin and gentamycin, cetriaxone or cefotaxime.

Epidemics are usually caused by meningococci; empiric treatment usually involves ceftriaxone in any age group and irrelevant of pregancy status, or oily chloramphenical in children over 2 years of age and non-pregnant adults [3].

ADJUVANT THERAPIES

If administered prior to the initiation of antibiotics, studies in resource-rich developed countries suggest that dexamethasone can decrease long term sequelae and mortality from Hib and pneumococcal meningitis [3, 7, 18, 19]. However, there are major differences between the cohorts of patients evaluated in these studies and patients in resource-limited settings, including late presentation for clinical care, pre-hospital antibiotic use, high HIV rates and malnutrition [7, 19].

A Vietnamese study of adults and adolescents found that dexamethasone only improved outcome (reduced death or disability) for those with microbiologically-proven disease, which, of course, is not known at the point of treatment [20, 21]. Dexamethasone was associated with increased one-month mortality in those with probable meningitis (possibly owing to tuberculous meningitis cases in that group). The most commonly isolated pathogen was *S. suis* [1, 20]. A study of Malawian adults showed no improved outcome with adjuvant dexamethasone [7]. HIV prevalence was 90%, compared with 1% in the Vietnamese study [7]. Thus, a recent review of acute bacterial meningitis in resource-poor settings was only able to recommend steroid use for HIV-negative adults with microbiologically-proven disease (presumably a positive Gram stain on initial lumbar puncture) [1]. A recent meta-analysis of individual patient data from one European and four developing country trials appears to support this [22], while a recent Cochrane review demonstrated no beneficial effect of dexamethasone in low-income countries [19].

Glycerol (1,2,3-propanetriol) is a naturally occurring osmotic agent [23] that reduces cerebral edema and improves brain perfusion. Glycerol may also reduce brain inflammation by scavenging oxygen free radicals. It is attractive to the low-income setting as it is cheap, easily available and administered orally [8, 23]. Although one study suggested that oral glycerol therapy prevented severe neurologic sequelae in childhood bacterial meningitis [23], other studies showed no benefit [24, 25].

FLUID MANAGEMENT

Routine fluid restriction is not recommended and may be detrimental [15]. A Cochrane review of three trials comparing unrestricted and restricted fluid regimens recommended maintenance of intravenous fluids in settings where children present late and where acute bacterial meningitis mortality is high [26]. A third of children with acute bacterial meningitis are hyponatremic; therefore, resuscitation with isotonic fluids is advocated where appropriate. Intravenous fluids are preferable to the nasogastric route but may be expensive and the expertise required to deliver them may be lacking in some settings. A trial in Papua New Guinea showed no significant difference in mortality whether children with acute bacterial meningitis were resuscitated with intravenous or nasogastric fluids, although other complications were higher in the nasogastric fluids group [1].

VACCINATION

Conjugate vaccines have substantially reduced the incidence of Hib, pneumococcus and Group C meningococcus meningitis in high-income countries, and of Hib and pneumococcal meningitis in the African countries where these have been introduced [1]. Conjugate vaccines are the most effective form of immunization for those under two years of age who are particularly vulnerable to bacterial meningitis. High-income countries have reported an increase in invasive pneumococcal disease from non-vaccine serotypes with the introduction of conjugate vaccines. Therefore, enhanced surveillance will be necessary for resource-poor countries when pneumococcal conjugate vaccines are introduced. Single (Group A) and quadrivalent capsular polysaccharide meningococcal vaccines have been used in the African meningitis belt; a conjugate meningococcus group A vaccine (MenAfriVac™) has been rolled out in several African countries in the meningitis belt (www.meningvax.org) [1, 7].

REFERENCES

1. Scarborough M, Thwaites GE. The diagnosis and management of acute bacterial meningitis in resource-poor settings. Lancet Neurol 2008;7:637–48.
2. Harrison LH, Trotter CL, Ramsay ME. Global epidemiology of meningococcal disease. Vaccine 2009;27(suppl. 2):B51–63.
3. World Health Organization. Standardised treatment of bacterial meningitis in Africa in epidemic and non-epidemic situations; 2007. Available at: http://www.who.int/csr/resources/publications/meningitis/WHO_CDS_EPR_2007_3/en/index.html.
4. Koedel U, Scheld WM, Pfister HW. Pathogenesis and pathophysiology of pneumococcal meningitis. Lancet Infect Dis 2002;2:721–36.
5. Riordan A. The implications of vaccines for prevention of bacterial meningitis. Curr Opin Neurol 2010;23:319–24.
6. Kim KS. Pathogenesis of bacterial meningitis: from bacteraemia to neuronal injury. Nat Rev Neurosci 2003;4(5):376–85.
7. Lin AL, Safdieh JE. The evaluation and management of bacterial meningitis: current practice and emerging developments. Neurologist 2010;16:143–51.
8. Kim KS. Acute bacterial meningitis in infants and children. Lancet Infect Dis 2010;10:32–42.
9. van de Beek D, de Gans J, Spanjaard L, et al. Clinical features and prognostic factors in adults with bacterial meningitis. N Engl J Med 2004;351:1849–59.
10. Berkley JA, Versteeg AC, Mwangi I, et al. Indicators of acute bacterial meningitis in children at a rural Kenyan district hospital. Pediatrics 2004;114:e713–9.
11. Thwaites GE, Chau TT, Stepniewska K, et al. Diagnosis of adult tuberculous meningitis by use of clinical and laboratory features. Lancet 2002;360:1287–92.
12. Chanteau S, Dartevelle S, Mahamane AE, et al. New rapid diagnostic tests for *Neisseria meningitidis* serogroups A, W135, C, and Y. PLoS Med 2006;3:e337.
13. Molyneux EM, Tembo M, Kayira K, et al. The effect of HIV infection on paediatric bacterial meningitis in Blantyre, Malawi. Arch Dis Child 2003;88:1112–8.
14. Roine I, Ledermann W, Foncea LM, et al. Randomized trial of four vs. seven days of ceftriaxone treatment for bacterial meningitis in children with rapid initial recovery. Pediatr Infect Dis J 2000;19:219–22.
15. Molyneux E, Nizami SQ, Saha S, et al. CSF 5 Study Group. 5 versus 10 days of treatment with ceftriaxone for bacterial meningitis in children: a double-blind randomised equivalence study. Lancet 2011;377(9780):1837–45.
16. Yogev R, Guzman-Cottrill J. Bacterial meningitis in children: critical review of current concepts. Drugs 2005;65:1097–112.
17. Deghmane AE, Alonso JM, Taha MK. Emerging drugs for acute bacterial meningitis. Expert Opin Emerg Drugs 2009;14:381–93.
18. van de Beek D, Farrar JJ, de Gans J, et al. Adjunctive dexamethasone in bacterial meningitis: a meta-analysis of individual patient data. Lancet Neurol 2010;9:254–63.
19. Brouwer MC, McIntyre P, de Gans J, et al. Corticosteroids for acute bacterial meningitis. Cochrane Database Syst Rev 2010:CD004405.
20. Nguyen TH, Tran TH, Thwaites G, et al. Dexamethasone in Vietnamese adolescents and adults with bacterial meningitis. N Engl J Med 2007;357:2431–40.
21. Scarborough M, Gordon SB, Whitty CJ, et al. Corticosteroids for bacterial meningitis in adults in sub-Saharan Africa. N Engl J Med 2007;357(24):2441–50.
22. van de Beek D, Farrar JJ, de Gans J, et al. Adjunctive dexamethasone in bacterial meningitis: a meta-analysis of individual patient data. Lancet Neurol 2010;9:254–63.
23. Peltola H, Roine I, Fernandez J, et al. Adjuvant glycerol and/or dexamethasone to improve the outcomes of childhood bacterial meningitis: a prospective,

randomized, double-blind, placebo-controlled trial. Clin Infect Dis 2007;45: 1277–86.

24. Peltola H, Roine I, Fernandez J, et al. Hearing impairment in childhood bacterial meningitis is little relieved by dexamethasone or glycerol. Pediatrics 2010;125:e1–8.
25. Ajdukiewicz KM, Cartwright KE, Scarborough M, et al. Glycerol adjuvant therapy in adults with bacterial meningitis in a high HIV seroprevalence setting in Malawi: a double-blind, randomised controlled trial. Lancet Infect Dis 2011;11(4):293–300.
26. Maconochie I, Baumer H, Stewart ME. Fluid therapy for acute bacterial meningitis. Cochrane Database Syst Rev 2008:CD004786.

55 Tetanus

Guy E Thwaites, C Louise Thwaites

Key features

- Tetanus is a neurologic syndrome characterized by acute skeletal muscle spasm and autonomic nervous system disturbance, caused by a neurotoxin released from *Clostridium tetani*, a ubiquitous environmental bacterium that can contaminate wounds
- Tetanus can be completely prevented by vaccination, yet more than 100,000 people develop tetanus each year, primarily in regions with inadequate vaccination programs
- Tetanus is a clinical diagnosis. The cardinal clinical features are muscle spasms, airway obstruction, and (in severe cases) autonomic dysfunction
- At diagnosis, the management priorities are to secure the airway, administer antitoxin immune globulins and debride potentially infected wounds
- Spasms can be controlled with high-dose benzodiazepines; magnesium sulfate infusions may help control spasms and autonomic dysfunction
- Disease does not confer immunity: vaccinate all survivors

INTRODUCTION

Tetanus is a vaccine-preventable disease caused by *Clostridium tetani*, a spore-forming and neurotoxin-producing bacterium. The spores of *C. tetani* are ubiquitous and can be found in soil, dust, and animal and human feces throughout the world. Therefore, tetanus can occur in any unvaccinated individual, regardless of where they live. The disease is characterized by acute skeletal muscle spasm and autonomic nervous system disturbance and, once established, is associated with a high mortality.

EPIDEMIOLOGY

It is estimated that over 100,000 individuals die of tetanus each year, with many (61,000) of these deaths being in neonates and children less than 5 years of age. Most cases of tetanus are never reported. As worldwide vaccination coverage has improved, the number of cases of tetanus has fallen, particularly in children and neonates who have been targeted by recent vaccination programs. Indeed, the elimination of maternal and neonatal tetanus by vaccination during pregnancy is one of the targets of the World Health Organization (WHO) and its partners' Expanded Program on Immunization (EPI).

Comprehensive vaccination programs in the developed world have meant tetanus is a rare disease in these settings and mostly occurs in incompletely vaccinated or unvaccinated individuals. High-risk groups include injection drug users and those aged over 60 years of age with decreased antibody concentrations [1].

Vaccination against tetanus is highly effective. The vaccine consists of an inactivated tetanus toxin, or toxoid, which induces antibody-mediated protective immunity against the toxin. The WHO guidelines for tetanus vaccination recommend a primary course of three vaccinations in infancy, then boosters at 4–7 and 12–15 years, and one in adult life. Centers for Disease Control and Prevention (CDC) recommendations in the USA suggest an additional dose at 14–16 months and boosters every 10 years. 'Catch-up' schedules recommend a three-dose primary course for non-immunized adolescents followed by two further doses. For those with a complete childhood primary course but no further boosters, two doses at least 4 weeks apart are recommended.

Standard WHO recommendations for the prevention of maternal and neonatal tetanus are of two doses of tetanus toxoid at least 4 weeks apart. However, in high-risk areas success has been achieved with a more intensive approach aiming to provide all women of childbearing age with a primary course of vaccination plus additional education on safe delivery and postnatal practices [2].

Individuals sustaining tetanus-prone wounds should also be immunized if they have incomplete or unknown vaccination status, or if a booster was given >10 years previously. In the USA, the CDC also recommends that unvaccinated individuals sustaining high risk, dirty wounds should also receive passive immunization with tetanus immune globulin (human; TIG).

NATURAL HISTORY, PATHOGENESIS, AND PATHOLOGY

Clostridium tetani is an anaerobic, Gram-positive, spore-forming rod. The spores are highly resilient, which explains their ubiquity, and can easily contaminate wounds, especially those associated with soil contamination. Once inoculated into a suitable anaerobic environment, the spores germinate to produce vegetative bacteria which release the neurotoxin. The toxin is extremely potent – only very small concentrations are required to produce disease. No entry wound or focus of infection is found in approximately 20% of cases of tetanus [3]. Superficial abrasions to the limbs are the commonest infection sites in adults. Deeper infections, for example through open fractures or drug injections, are associated with more severe disease and worse outcomes. In neonates, the umbilical stump is the usual source of infection, and contamination can result from poor umbilical cord care, cutting the cord with grass or applying animal dung to the stump. Circumcision or ear-piercing of the newborn can also result in neonatal tetanus.

Tetanus toxin (or tetanospasmin) is a 150-kDa protein closely related to botulinum toxin (the cause of botulism), the latter produced by *Clostridium botulinum*. Unlike botulinum toxin, which remains at the neuromuscular junction to cause a flaccid paralysis, tetanus toxin is transported within the motor nerves to the central nervous system (CNS). Once there, the toxin preferentially targets inhibitory gamma aminobutyric acid (GABA)-ergic interneurons and inhibits the binding and release of presynaptic vesicles containing the neurotransmitter [4].

Thus, tetanus toxin effectively blocks inhibitory interneuron discharge, which results in unregulated activity of the motor and autonomic nervous system. Hence, the characteristic clinical features seen in tetanus are skeletal muscle spasm and autonomic system disturbance.

CLINICAL FEATURES

Tetanus can produce a spectrum of clinical features depending on the site of infection and the amount of toxin produced. In its mildest form, isolated areas of the body are affected and only local muscle spasm may be apparent. In such cases, outcome is usually good, with the important exception of cephalic tetanus. In this condition, the cranial nerves are involved and phargyngeal or laryngeal muscles may spasm, leading to sudden aspiration or airway obstruction. These patients require careful observation.

Generalized muscle spasm is the most typical feature of tetanus. The muscles of the face and jaw are often affected first, producing the characteristic "risus sardonicus" and trismus (lockjaw) [3]. Many patients also experience difficulty swallowing, back pain, and generalized muscle pain and stiffness. Neonates typically present with difficulty in feeding. As the disease progresses, generalized muscle spasms develop, which can be very painful. Commonly, the laryngeal muscles are involved early, which can be life-threatening as it may lead to sudden and complete airway obstruction. Spasm of the respiratory muscles results in respiratory failure and, without mechanical ventilation, is the commonest cause of death. Spasms strong enough to produce tendon avulsions and crush fractures have been reported, but are rare.

Autonomic disturbance is maximal during the second week of the illness and can be fatal. Blood pressure, heart rate and temperature can fluctuate wildly, and can be associated with gastrointestinal stasis, sweating and increased secretions.

Rapid development of tetanus is associated with more severe disease and poor outcome. The incubation period (time from wound to first symptom) and period of onset (time from first symptom to the first generalized spasm) are of particular significance, with shorter times associated with worse outcome. Likewise, in neonatal tetanus, the younger the infant when symptoms occur, the worse the prognosis (Fig. 55.1).

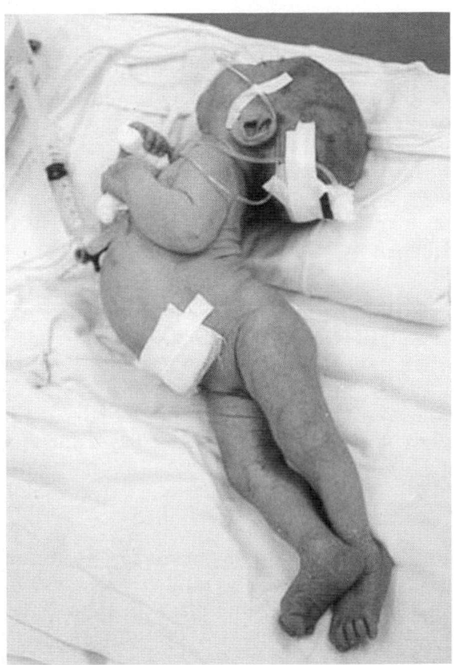

FIGURE 55.1 Opisthotonus in neonatal tetanus.

PATIENT EVALUATION, DIAGNOSIS AND DIFFERENTIAL DIAGNOSIS

The diagnosis of tetanus depends upon typical clinical features rather than the results of laboratory tests. Therefore, disease definitions exist to assist diagnosis and to enable comparative clinical and epidemiologic surveys. Tetanus is defined by "the acute onset of hypertonia, or by painful muscular contractions (usually of the muscles of the jaw and neck) and generalized muscle spasms without other apparent medical cause" [5]. Neonatal tetanus is defined by the WHO as "an illness occurring in a child who has the normal ability to suck and cry in the first 2 days of life but who loses this ability between days 3 and 28 days of life and becomes rigid and has spasms" [2]. Maternal tetanus is defined as occurring during pregnancy or within 6 weeks of the end of pregnancy (whether pregnancy ended with birth, miscarriage, or abortion) [2].

Few conditions mimic generalized tetanus, but strychnine poisoning and dystonic reactions to antidopaminergic drugs (e.g. metaclopramide) can produce similar clinical features. Continuous abdominal muscle rigidity is characteristic of tetanus, whereas it is episodic in the other two conditions. Cephalic tetanus can be confused with other causes of trismus, such as oropharyngeal infection. Hypocalcemia or meningoencephalitis can be confused with tetanus in neonates.

TREATMENT

Once the tetanus toxin has reached the inhibitory interneurons in the CNS and symptoms have begun, there is limited opportunity to affect disease progression. Wound debridement may stop the production of further toxin and neutralizing immunoglobulins (antitoxin) may limit disease severity but, in general, management strategies aim to support vital functions until the effects of the toxin have worn off.

It is important to establish a secure airway early in severe tetanus; hyperactivity and spasm of laryngeal muscles can make endotracheal intubation difficult once the disease has progressed and many advocate early tracheostomy. In addition, patients should be cared for in a quiet environment, as light and noise can trigger spasms.

If possible, the entry wound should be identified, cleaned and debrided of any necrotic material in order to remove any anaerobic focus of infection and prevent further tetanus toxin production. Failure to identify or remove the focus can be associated with prolonged or recurrent tetanus. Antibiotics may be helpful; metronidazole (400 mg rectally, or 500 mg intravenously every 6 hours for 7 days) is preferred, despite a lack of comparative studies with other antibiotics [6]. Benzylpenicillin is an alternative, although there are theoretical concerns that penicillins may exacerbate spasms.

Antitoxin should be given early in an attempt to neutralize any circulating tetanus toxin and prevent its uptake into the nervous system. Antitoxin can be given by intramuscular or intrathecal injection. A recent meta-analysis of controlled trials suggested a single 50–1500 IU intrathecal dose of human antitoxin was associated with reduced disease progression and improved outcomes in neonates and adults compared with the intramuscular route [7]. There are two antitoxin preparations available – human tetanus immune globulin and equine antitoxin. Human tetanus immune globulin is preferred because it is less likely to be associated with anaphylactic reactions. Standard intramuscular therapy is 3000–6000 IU as a single dose (or 10,000–20,000 U/kg equine preparation).

The best way to control the severe muscle spasms of tetanus has not been defined by controlled trials. Most authorities, however, use high-dose benzodiazepines (up to 100 mg/hour diazepam has been reported) in combination with other drugs, such as chlorpromazine or phenobarbitone [8]. More recently, intravenous magnesium sulfate has been used as a muscle relaxant [9].

The problem with all these treatments is that the doses necessary to control spasms also cause respiratory depression, thus controlling spasms, while maintaining adequate ventilation is a particular issue in settings without facilities for mechanical ventilation. Respiratory failure is a common cause of death in these circumstances. If mechanical ventilation is available, severe spasms are best dealt with using a combination of benzodiazepines, magnesium, and relatively short-acting, cardiovascularly inert, nondepolarizing neuromuscular blocking agents, as they allow titration against spasm intensity. Infusions of propofol have also been used successfully to control spasms and provide sedation.

The autonomic disturbance of severe tetanus is notoriously difficult to treat. A recent, double-blind, placebo-controlled trial of intravenous magnesium sulfate (plasma concentrations 2–4 mmol/l) for severe tetanus found treatment with magnesium was associated with reduced requirements for benzodiazepines, nondepolarizing muscle relaxants (pipecuronium), and verapamil (used for the control of tachycardia) [10]. In addition to magnesium, morphine and drugs acting specifically on the cardiovascular system (e.g. esmolol, calcium antagonists, and inotropes) may be required.

Complications arising from the treatment of tetanus are common. Ventilator-associated pneumonia, central venous catheter infections, and septicemia are particularly important. In some centers, prophylaxis against deep vein thrombosis and thromboembolism is routine.

Recovery from tetanus may take 4–6 weeks with prolonged immobility secondary to muscle stiffness. In addition, patients must be given a full primary course of immunization, as tetanus toxin is poorly immunogenic and does not provoke a protective immune response.

REFERENCES

1. McQuillan GM, Kruszon-Moran D, Deforest A, et al. Serologic immunity to diphtheria and tetanus in the United States. Ann Intern Med 2002;136: 660–6.
2. Roper MH, Vandelaer JH, Gasse FL. Maternal and neonatal tetanus. Lancet 2007;370:1947–59.
3. Thwaites CL, Yen LM, Nga NTN, et al. Impact of improved vaccination programme and intensive care facilities on incidence and outcome of tetanus in southern Vietnam, 1993–2002. Trans R Soc Trop Med Hyg 2004;98: 671–7.
4. Caleo M, Schiavo G. Central effects of tetanus and botulinum neurotoxins. Toxicon 2009;54:593–9.
5. Bardenheier B, Prevots DR, Khetsuriani N, Wharton M. Tetanus surveillance – United States, 1995–1997. Mor Mortal Wkly Rep CDC Surveill Summ 1998;47:1–13.
6. Farrar JJ, Yen LM, Cook TF, et al. Tetanus. J Neurol Neurosurg Psychiatry 2000;69:292–301.
7. Kabura L, Ilibagiz D, Menten J, Van den Ende J. Intrathecal vs. intramuscular administration of human antitetanus immunoglobulin or equine tetanus antitoxin in the treatment of tetanus: a meta-analysis. Trop Med Int Health 2006;11:1075–81.
8. Okoromah CNLF. Diazepam for treating tetanus (Cochrane Review). The Cochrane Library. Chichester: John Wiley & Sons; 2004.
9. Attygalle D, Rodrigo N. Magnesium as first line therapy in the management of tetanus: a prospective study of 40 patients. Anaesthesia 2002;57: 811–17.
10. Thwaites CL, Yen LM, Loan HT, et al. Magnesium sulphate for treatment of severe tetanus: a randomised controlled trial. Lancet 2006;368:1436–43.

Botulism 56

Stephen J Aston, Nicholas J Beeching

Key features

- Botulism is a rare paralytic illness caused by potent neurotoxins produced by *Clostridium botulinum*
- Botulism typically presents with bilateral cranial nerve palsies followed by symmetrical descending flaccid paralysis and occasional progression to respiratory muscle weakness. The four "Ds" are the key clues—dysphonia, dysphagia, dysarthria and descending paralysis
- Clostridial spores are ubiquitous in the environment and botulism is presumed to occur worldwide, but under-reporting is significant
- Several naturally occurring forms are recognized: food-borne botulism, wound botulism, infant botulism and adult intestinal toxemia botulism
- Food-borne disease remains a significant problem in countries where home-preservation of food is popular
- Wound botulism has increased in recent years as a result of an epidemic among injecting drug users

INTRODUCTION

Botulism is a rare, naturally-occurring paralytic illness caused by potent neurotoxins produced by *Clostridium botulinum* and, rarely, other *Clostridium* species. It manifests as a characteristic syndrome of symmetrical cranial nerve palsies followed, to a varying extent, by symmetrical descending paralysis of voluntary muscle that can progress to respiratory compromise and death. Botulinum spores are ubiquitous in the natural environment and cases occur worldwide, although they are probably greatly under-reported.

The first complete clinical description of botulism was published by Kerner in 1822 who termed the disease "sausage poisoning", having observed outbreaks associated with the consumption of spoiled meat. The early 20th century saw a massive rise in cases of botulism owing to the increasing popularity of food canning. Following the elucidation of its mechanism of action in the mid-20th century, the potential therapeutic use of botulinum toxin has been exploited [1–3].

EPIDEMIOLOGY

Attempts to describe the global epidemiology of botulism are hampered by the lack of detailed incidence data [4]. In particular, there is a complete absence of data from Africa. As *C. botulinum* spores are ubiquitous in the environment, it is presumed that cases occur globally, although rates may vary with dietary customs and food handling practices.

Food-borne Botulism

Food-borne botulism is caused by consumption of food contaminated with preformed botulinum toxin. It is usually associated with uncooked food products as heating food to >85 °C for more than five minutes inactivates toxin. Although botulinum spores may potentially contaminate many foodstuffs, germination and toxin production only occur when spores are incubated in an anaerobic, low-salt milieu at greater than 4 °C. The processes of canning and fermentation of foods are particularly conducive to producing such conditions. Effective methods of inactivating spores introduced in the early 20th century mean that outbreaks of food-borne botulism attributable to commercially canned foods are now rare. However, home-canned foods continue to be a major source of intoxication, especially in Eastern Europe and the southern USA [5]. There is an exceptionally high incidence of food-borne botulism in Alaska attributable to the widespread consumption of fermented aquatic mammal meat [6].

Wound Botulism

Wound botulism follows the absorption of toxin produced by organisms contaminating a wound site, so clinical incubation periods are longer than for botulism caused by food which contains preformed toxin. Cases have increased in developed countries in recent years, driven by an epidemic among injecting drug-users and strongly associated with the practice of injecting into the subcutaneous tissues or muscle, known as "skin-" or "muscle-popping". The majority of cases occur in the USA [7]. Sporadic cases of botulism associated with contaminated compound fractures are occasionally reported.

Infant Botulism

Infant botulism is caused by the endogenous production of toxin by *C. botulinum* that has colonized the infant gastrointestinal tract following the germination of ingested spores [8]. In 2008, 83 cases, representing 70% of total botulism cases, were reported in the USA. Ingestion of honey, which is often contaminated by *C. botulinum* spores, was implicated in the majority of early cases. More recently, concerns have been raised over the potential for contamination of commercial powdered infant formula and corn-syrup. A few cases of a similar syndrome have been described in adults and has been termed *"adult intestinal toxemia botulism"*, and is associated with gastrointestinal surgery, inflammatory bowel disease and/or antimicrobial use.

Iatrogenic botulism following the direct inoculation of concentrated botulinum toxin preparations for cosmetic purposes has been reported. Intoxication following absorption of toxin across the respiratory mucosa, termed inhalational botulism, has also been rarely reported.

NATURAL HISTORY, PATHOGENESIS AND PATHOLOGY

Clostridium botulinum are anaerobic, Gram-positive, spore-forming bacilli that are found in soils and aquatic sediments. Strains of *C. botulinum* are classified into seven types, designated A to G, according to the antigenic properties of the botulinum toxin they produce. Human botulism is caused by types A, B, E and, rarely, type F. Some strains of *Clostridium baratii* and *Clostridium butyricum* can also produce botulinum neurotoxin and have been implicated in human disease. The spores of *C. botulinum* are highly resistant. Under appropriate conditions, they germinate to release vegetative organisms that produce neurotoxin. Following absorption and hematogenous dissemination, botulinum toxin exerts its effects at the presynaptic terminals of cholinergic nerve junctions by blocking neurotransmitter release.

CLINICAL FEATURES

The clinical presentation of all forms of botulism is dominated by neurologic features resulting from the toxin-induced blockade of voluntary motor and autonomic cholinergic junctions.

In adults, cranial nerve palsies are almost always the initial presenting symptoms. Extraocular muscle paresis results in blurred, or double, vision. Marked ptosis is usually evident and pupillary responses may also be depressed. The face may appear expressionless as a consequence of bilateral facial nerve dysfunction. Involvement of lower cranial nerves causes dysphonia, dyarthria and dysphagia. Early autonomic involvement causes anhydrosis leading affected individuals to complain of extremely dry, and often painful, mouth, tongue and throat.

Disease progression manifests as a symmetrical, flaccid, descending paralysis of voluntary muscles associated with loss of deep tendon reflexes. Involvement of the diaphragm and accessory thoracic muscles may result in respiratory compromise and death unless supportive care is provided. Because of the generalized lack of motor function, respiratory failure often occurs without apparent features of respiratory distress and may be overlooked until very advanced. Significant pharyngeal muscle weakness causing airway compromise may necessitate intubation and ventilation, even in the absence of respiratory muscle weakness. Progressive autonomic involvement leads to constipation, urinary retention and hemodynamic dysregulation.

Fever is usually absent, except in some cases of wound botulism when it probably indicates concurrent wound infection with other bacteria. Sensory nerves are unaffected by botulinum toxin. Similarly, there is no effect on level of consciousness or cognitive function, although the features of expressionless facies and dysarthria are often mistaken for alcohol or drug intoxication.

The extent, severity and rate of progression of clinical features vary, and not all untreated cases progress to respiratory muscle paralysis. Some affected individuals only develop cranial nerve palsies that gradually resolve without any other features of botulism becoming evident. Botulinum toxin binding is irreversible, and recovery of function depends on nerve terminal regeneration. Individuals with respiratory compromise typically require ventilatory support for 2–8 weeks, although, occasionally, recovery is much more protracted.

In food-borne disease, the neurologic features of botulism may be preceded by abdominal pain, nausea, vomiting and diarrhea, although at the time of neurologic manifestation, constipation is common. Such gastrointestinal disturbance has not been reported in wound botulism and probably represents the effect of other bacteria and their toxins co-contaminating the causative improperly preserved food. Clinical effects of botulinum toxin usually become evident 18–36 hours after consumption of the implicated foodstuff.

PATIENT EVALUATION, DIAGNOSIS AND DIFFERENTIAL DIAGNOSIS

In the context of a large outbreak in which multiple patients present with combinations of cranial nerve palsies and subsequent development of descending flaccid paralysis, botulism is easily recognizable. However, it is a rare condition, and the majority of cases occur singularly, meaning that the diagnosis is often delayed or missed altogether.

Botulism should be suspected in any adult with acute-onset gastrointestinal, autonomic and cranial nerve dysfunction. The four "Ds" are the key clues: dysphonia, dysphagia, dysarthria and descending paralysis. Demonstration of bilateral cranial nerve findings and evidence of neurologic progression increase the level of suspicion. Reported recent consumption of home-canned foods or similar illness in family members or close contacts provides further supporting evidence for the diagnosis. Alternatively, features of injecting drug use are highly suggestive.

Important differential diagnoses to consider when botulism is suspected include alcohol or drug misuse, Guillain-Barré syndrome

TABLE 56-1 Differential diagnoses (in alphabetical order)

Differential diagnosis	Distinguishing features
CNS infections	Altered mental status; abnormal CSF; EEG changes
CNS space-occupying lesion	Asymmetrical weakness and upper motor neurone signs; abnormal brain imaging
Diabetic neuropathy	Sensory features; limited cranial nerve involvement
Diphtheria	Antecedent pharyngitis; sensory features; associated cardiac complications
Eaton-Lambert syndrome	Similar EMG findings; often evidence of underlying lung cancer
Electrolyte disturbances (e.g. hypermagnesemia)	Abnormal serum electrolytes
Guillain-Barré syndrome	Ascending paralysis with early areflexia; history of antecedent infection; raised CSF protein; abnormal nerve conduction studies
Hyperthyroidism	Thyrotoxic features; abnormal thyroid function tests
Inflammatory myopathy	Elevated creatine kinase; EMG findings
Intoxication (e.g. alcohol, drugs, carbon monoxide)	History of exposure; CNS features; elevated serum drug levels
Myasthenia gravis	Fatiguable muscle weakness with positive response to edrophonium; acetylcholine receptor antibodies; decrease in muscle action potentials with repetitive stimulation
Organophosphate poisoning	History of exposure; prominent cholinergic features (e.g. rhinorrhea, excess salivation, bronchospasm) before onset of paralysis
Paralytic shellfish poisoning	History of shellfish ingestion; rapid disease onset; sensory findings
Poliomyelitis	Travel to endemic region; antecedent febrile illness; asymmetrical weakness; CSF pleocytosis and elevated protein
Psychiatric conversion disorder	Normal EMG; atypical or inconsistent neurologic signs
Stroke	Asymmetrical weakness and upper motor neurone signs; abnormal brain imaging
Tick paralysis	Resident or traveler to endemic areas; ascending paralysis often with paresthesiae; tick attached to skin; abnormal nerve conduction

CNS, central nervous system; CSF, cerebrospinal fluid; EEG, electroencephalography; EMG, electromyography.

(GBS), myasthenia gravis, stroke syndromes, Eaton-Lambert syndrome and tick paralysis. Table 56-1 includes other differential diagnoses with important distinguishing features.

GBS typically presents as an ascending paralysis and there is often a history of antecedent infection. Distinguishing botulism from the triad of ophthalmoplegia, ataxia and areflexia that characterize the Miller Fisher variant, is often more difficult. However, in contrast to botulism, areflexia typically precedes the onset of significant muscle weakness in GBS. Fatiguable muscle weakness is the hallmark of myasthenia gravis. A marked improvement with administration of edrophonium is highly suggestive of myasthenia gravis, although about 25% of patients with botulism show some response. Patients with Eaton-Lambert syndrome usually have clinically apparent lung cancer, although electromyographic findings are indistinguishable from botulism. The asymmetrical weakness and upper motor neurone signs caused by most stroke syndromes should be readily distinguishable from botulism on clinical examination. Tick paralysis causes paresthesiae and ascending paralysis; the diagnosis is particularly apparent if the tick is still attached.

Cerebrospinal fluid analysis may be useful; protein levels are normal in botulism compared with GBS, where they are typically raised, although this may not be apparent until several days after symptom onset. Electromyography (EMG) may also be helpful. In particular, repetitive stimulation at high frequencies shows facilitation of muscle action potentials in botulism that is not evident in either GBS or myasthenia gravis. EMG is best performed and interpreted by an experienced operator, as results may vary between muscle groups. To avoid false-negative results, it is essential that clinically affected muscle groups are tested. Brain imaging by computed tomography (CT) or magnetic resonance imaging (MRI) should be used to uncover the rare brain stem stroke syndromes that produce symmetrical bulbar palsies.

Definitive laboratory confirmation of botulism requires the demonstration of toxin in specimens of patient serum, gastric secretions or stool or, in the case of food-borne botulism, a food sample. The standard method for the demonstration of botulinum toxin is the mouse lethality bioassay in which mice are observed for the presence of botulism-specific symptoms following intraperitoneal injection of extracts of clinical specimens. It is performed in only a limited number of laboratories and there is a significant false-positivity rate. Moreover, it cannot be used as a basis for clinical management decisions as results may not be available for up to four days. Several rapid *in vitro* assays are currently in development, but none are yet widely standardized as adequate replacements for mouse bioassays to confirm botulism diagnosis.

TREATMENT

The core principles of botulism management are the early administration of antitoxin and the prompt recognition of respiratory compromisation, allowing the timely implementation of ventilatory support. Having been as high as 70%, the current mortality rate from botulism is less than 5% where adequate intensive care is available.

Most antitoxin preparations contain combinations of equine-derived antibodies directed against specific botulinum toxin serotypes [9]. The only preparation for which there is prospective comparative trial-based evidence of effectiveness is the use of human-derived botulinum immune globulin for the treatment of infant botulism [3]. Systemic administration of antitoxin neutralizes botulinum toxin that is not yet bound to nerve terminals and thus arrests further disease progression. In retrospective series of food-borne botulism, its early use is associated with a reduction in mortality and shortening of the duration of respiratory failure requiring ventilatory support. Hypersensitivity reactions, including anaphylaxis, have previously been a significant concern, although using currently recommended dosing schedules serious reactions are seen in <1% patients.

The use of antitoxin is indicated on the basis of clinical suspicion of botulism and treatment should not be delayed while waiting for the results of laboratory investigations. Botulinum antitoxins are generally given by slow intravenous infusion. Vital signs should be monitored carefully during administration and medication for the management of acute allergic reactions should be readily available. Some national guidelines recommend repeat treatment within 24 hours if the patient continues to deteriorate.

All patients with botulism should be managed in a high-dependency setting to facilitate close monitoring. Ventilatory support should be promptly instituted upon development of respiratory compromisation, indicated by diminishing vital capacity; up to 50% of patients with food-borne botulism require ventilatory support. Meticulous attention should be paid to the prevention and early treatment of nosocomial infection and to the maintenance of adequate nutritional status. Attendants should remember that, unlike many patients on ventilatory support, patients with botulism are fully awake and have no sensory deficits, unless they have specifically received sedation.

In wound botulism, appropriate management of the wound is also essential in order to prevent relapse caused by ongoing toxin production by persisting vegetative organisms after antitoxin has been cleared from the body. All wounds should be surgically debrided and treated with antibiotics until completely healed. Relevant wounds may appear trivial or innocuous, and the presence of deep-seated abscesses should be always considered.

Upon suspicion of a diagnosis of botulism, the local public health authorities should be contacted immediately. Investigations should be undertaken to rapidly identify other possible cases and suspected food exposures, as rapid control measures such as impounding home-canned foods or emergency products recalls may need to be instigated.

PEDIATRIC CONSIDERATIONS

CLINICAL FEATURES

Constipation is usually the first manifestation of infant botulism. Over 1–2 weeks, neurologic features develop leading to presentations with a weakened cry, diminished feeding and an increasingly "floppy" infant as descending paresis occurs. Examination reveals hypotonia, loss of facial expression, extraocular muscle weakness and dilated pupils. The extent and severity of clinical features is highly variable, ranging from mild hypotonia to severe flaccid paralysis. Up to 70% of patients require intubation and ventilation, although mortality rates are <1%.

TREATMENT

Historically, equine-derived antitoxin has not been used to treat infant botulism because of concerns regarding serious hypersensitivity reactions and an inadequate duration of therapeutic effect. A human-derived antitoxin product, known as BabyBIG, has been recently developed. A randomized, controlled trial demonstrated that when administered early in the disease course it significantly reduces the duration of mechanical ventilation and length of hospital stay [3].

REFERENCES

1. Sobel J. Botulism. Clin Infect Dis 2005;41:1167–73.
2. Centers for Disease Control and Prevention: Botulism in the United States, 1899–1996. Handbook for Epidemiologists, Clinicians, and Laboratory Workers. Atlanta: Centers for Disease Control and Prevention; 1998.
3. Chalk C, Benstead TJ, Keezer M. Medical treatment for botulism. Cochrane Database Syst Rev 2011;3:CD008123.
4. Reller ME, Douce RW, Maslanka SE, et al. Wound botulism acquired in the Amazonian rain forest of Ecuador. Am J Trop Med Hyg 2006;74:628–31.
5. Sobel J, Tucker N, Sulka A, et al. Food-borne botulism in the United States, 1990–2000. Emerg Infect Dis 2004;10:1606–11.
6. Fagan RP, McLaughlin JB, Castrodale LJ, et al. Endemic foodborne botulism among Alaska Native persons—Alaska, 1947–2007. Clin Infect Dis 2011; 52:585–92.
7. Werner SB, Passaro D, McGee J, et al. Wound botulism in California, 1951–1998: Recent epidemic in heroin injectors. Clin Infect Dis 2000;31:1018.
8. Brook I. Infant botulism. J Perinatol 2007;27:175–80.
9. Tacket CO, Shandera WX, Mann JM, et al. Equine antitoxin use and other factors that predict outcome in type A food-borne botulism. Am J Med 1984;76:794–8.

SECTION

F

INFECTIONS OF SKIN AND SOFT TISSUES

Bacterial Skin and Soft Tissue Infections in the Tropics

Aisha Sethi

Key features

- Pyodermas or bacterial skin infections are a major cause of morbidity throughout the tropical world and in resource-limited countries
- Heat, humidity, poor host nutrition, and hygiene are contributing factors for increased bacterial skin and soft tissue infections in the tropics
- Staphylococcal infections of the skin and soft tissues include: impetigo (bullous and non-bullous), folliculitis, furuncles, carbuncles, and cellulitis
- Streptococcal infections include: ecthyma infectiosum, gas gangrene and necrotizing fasciitis
- Tropical ulcer and tropical pyomyositis are also important bacterial skin infections seen in the tropics
- Antibiotic resistance, inadequate therapy and high cost of new antibiotics hinder therapy of cutaneous skin infections in the tropics

IMPETIGO

Impetigo is a very common and contagious bacterial skin infection that characteristically involves the face, and classically manifests as honey-colored crusted erosions and scabs. There are two forms, bullous and non-bullous, with the non-bullous form being more common in children. Impetigo is especially common in hot, humid, tropical climates and the peak number of cases are seen in the summer and rainy season. Nasal, axillary, pharyngeal and/or perineal *Staphylococcus aureus* colonization imparts an increased risk for developing impetigo [1].

Worldwide, non-bullous impetigo is most commonly caused by *S. aureus*, while a minority of cases are caused by *Streptococcus pyogenes* (group A beta-hemolytic Streptococci) or a mixed infection. In 5% of cases, non-bullous impetigo is caused by *S. pyogenes* (serotypes 1, 4, 12, 25 and 49) and can result in acute post-streptococcal glomerulonephritis (APSG) (http://www.expertconsultbook.com/expertconsult/b/linkTo?type=bookPage&isbn=978-1-4160-2999-1&eid=4-u1.0-B978-1-4160-2999-1..50078-3--cetablefn3&appID=NGE), [2].

Bullous impetigo is exclusively caused by the exfoliatin toxin-secreting strain of *S. aureus* and is most commonly seen in children under the age of 2 years. Bullous impetigo is considered a localized form of staphylococcal scalded skin syndrome (SSSS).

Clinically, impetigo classically manifests as grouped fragile vesicles that proceed to become cloudy pustules that easily rupture (Fig. 1). After rupture, the lesions become crusted, honey-colored erosions. The most common areas of involvement are the face and neck, and sometimes the extremities. In contrast to non-bullous impetigo, bullous impetigo can occur on intact skin. Initially, small vesicles and pus-filled bullae are seen. The lesions enlarge and become flaccid, transparent bullae measuring up to 3–5 cm in diameter with a collarette of scale. Exfoliative toxin may disseminate and cause SSSS [3].

Treatment involves local hygiene with soap and water, followed by application of an antibacterial agent. In resource-limited settings, topical 0.5% Gentian Violet (GV) paint is commonly available as a cheap and effective anti-bacterial agent. For extensive disease, oral antibiotics, such as cloxacillin, erythromycin or trimethoprim-sulfamethoxazole may be used. To reduce the risk of relapse, it is important to note that impetigo may be a secondary complication of other underlying dermatoses, such as scabies, insect bites, atopic dermatitis and dermatophytosis.

ECTHYMA

Ecthyma is considered to be the ulcerated form of bullous impetigo and is usually caused by *S. pyogenes* [4]. It initially presents as a vesicle that develops into a shallow "punched out" ulcer with a necrotic base, usually on the lower extremities (Fig. 2). The ulcers are usually multiple and smaller in size than tropical ulcer. The most common locations are the backs of legs, thighs and buttocks, and, occasionally, on the trunk and arms. In the tropics, ecthyma usually occurs in those working in damp, swampy and humid environments, for example rice paddy workers. Treatment includes systemic antibiotics in conjunction with topical antibiotics, such as fusidic acid or topical 0.5% GV paint application daily, along with leg elevation.

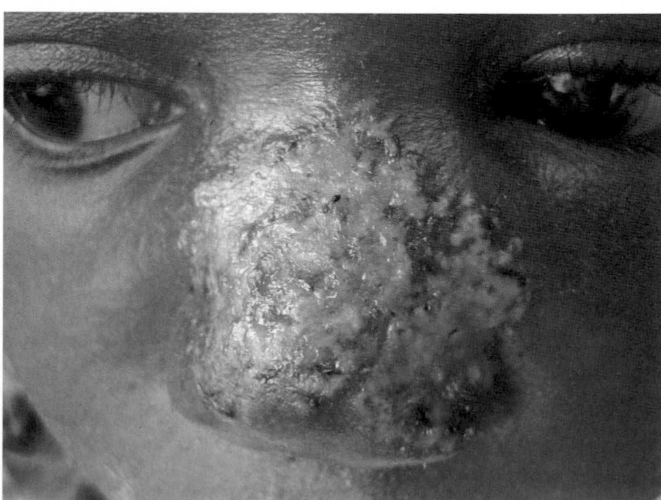

FIGURE 1 Impetigo with cloudy pustules and erosions clustered on the nose.

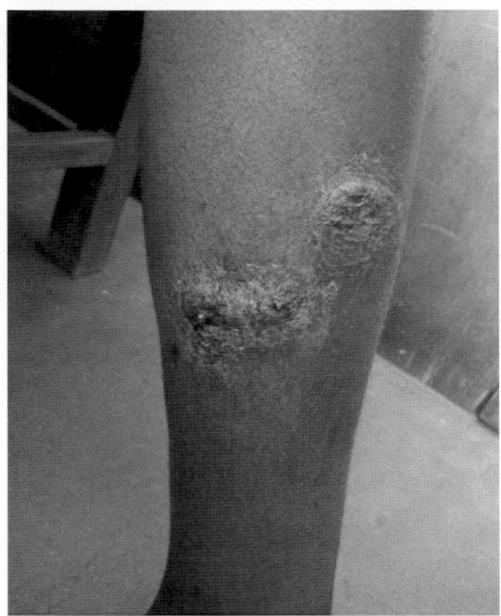

FIGURE 2 Ecthyma lesions on the lower leg.

FOLLICULITIS, FURUNCLES AND CARBUNCLES

Folliculitis usually presents as papules and pustules centered around a hair follicle. Furuncles are acute, inflammatory, deep abscesses of the hair follicles and begin as a hard, tender, red nodule that becomes painful and fluctuant. *Staphylococcus aureus* is the most common causative organism, although anaerobes are implicated in recurrent furuncles in the anogenital region. It is also important to note that furuncular myiasis should be considered in the differential diagnosis in some tropical areas.

Carbuncles are collections of furuncles that extend deep into the subcutaneous tissue with overlying sinus tracts. Systemic symptoms are usually present and carbuncles usually heal with residual scarring.

For simple furuncles, warm compresses may promote resolution, while fluctuant lesions require incision and drainage. Systemic antibiotics should be used for large and recurrent lesions.

CELLULITIS

Cellulitis is a bacterial infection of the deep dermis and subcutaneous tissue. It is most commonly caused by *S. pyogenes* and *S. aureus* [5]. Bacteria may gain access to the dermis via a break in the skin barrier in healthy adults, while the hematogenous route is more common in immunocompromised patients.

The affected skin is usually erythematous, swollen, painful and warm to the touch. Severe cellulitis can be complicated by bullae, pustules or necrotic tissue. Damage to lymphatic vessels can lead to recurrent episodes of cellulitis [6]. In areas of the world endemic for lymphatic filariasis, it is important to rule out filariasis in cases of recurrent bouts of lower extremity cellulitis and lymphangitis.

The differential diagnosis of lower extremity cellulitis includes deep vein thrombosis, superficial thrombophlebitis and lipodermatosclerosis. It is also important to rule out necrotizing fasciitis, especially when the cellulitis is associated with the presence of anesthesia and bullae.

Patients with a mild case of cellulitis can usually be treated with an oral antibiotic targeting Gram-positive organisms. Intravenous therapy and hospitalization should be considered for patients who have facial cellulitis, underlying diabetes, or cellulitis surrounding decubitus ulcers, and those with progressive systemic symptoms. Specific types of cellulitis (e.g. those caused by *Erysipelothrix rhusiopathiae* and *Vibrio vulnificus*) may present with overlying hemorrhagic bullae [7].

GAS GANGRENE

This is a rare infection of the skin produced by exotoxin-producing *Clostridial* species. The most common type is traumatic gas gangrene, which occurs via direct inoculation of a contaminated ischemic wound with soil or fecal matter, or sometimes following an abdominal surgical procedure. The causative organism is *Clostidium perfringens* in about 80–95% of cases. The infection is rapidly progressive with symptoms of sepsis, myonecrosis and gas production; this condition counts as an infectious disease emergency.

The key feature is pain out of proportion to the physical cutaneous findings. Light-to-dark brown discoloration of the skin with associated crepitus and bullae may be accompanied by a foul-smelling serosanguinous drainage. The patient may exhibit other signs of toxemia. The crepitus is an important clinical clue and, if available, plane radiograph may reveal the presence of gas in the soft tissue.

The mainstay of treatment is wide surgical excision and debridement in conjunction with systemic antibiotic therapy (high dose penicillin often with an agent that inhibits bacterial protein synthesis such as clindamycin may be used). In severe cases, amputation may be necessary.

NECROTIZING FASCIITIS

Necrotizing fasciitis is a rapidly progressive inflammatory infection of the deep fascia associated with a high morbidity and mortality. The infection may follow trauma or occur around foreign bodies in surgical wounds. The initiating bacteria are usually group A hemolytic streptococci and *S. aureus*. Resolving varicella is a risk factor for bacterial superinfection. Necrotizing fasciitis caused by mixed aerobic and anaerobic infection is associated with involvement of the pelvic and abdominal areas [8].

The presence of anesthesia suggests deeper extension of a soft tissue infection. Clinical clues that suggest necrotizing fasciitis include severe pain, rapidly spreading tense edema, hemorrhagic bullae formation, crepitance, gray-blue discoloration, "dish-water" discharge and elevated creatine phosphokinase level.

Successful management demands early diagnosis, rapid resuscitation and aggressive surgical excision and debridement coupled with high doses of broad-spectrum antibiotics targeting the causative agents [9]. Penicillin G is the drug of choice for streptococcal causes, often given in conjunction with clindamycin to inhibit bacterial protein synthesis. If a causative agent is not know, broad spectrum antibiotics that target methicillin-resistant *S. aureus* (MRSA), Gram-negative organisms and anaerobes should be administered. High dose intravenous immunoglobulin may be some benefit to patients with streptococcal-associated necrotizing fasciitis. Hyperbaric oxygen therapy, when available, has also been utilized in combination with aggressive surgical debridement and antibiotics.

TROPICAL (PHAGADENIC) ULCER

The term "tropical ulcer" is used to denote ulcers of the lower legs which occur in people in the tropics, especially during the rainy season. Young children are affected more frequently and the ulcers are usually a polymicrobial infection.

Clinically, the ulcer starts off as a fairly well-demarcated painful round ulcer with surrounding erythema on the lower legs. Exposure of the injured skin to mud and slow-moving fresh water has also been implicated [10]. Over the course of a few weeks, the ulcer becomes less painful and may heal with residual scarring.

If the ulcer has purulent discharge, then treatment should include systemic antibiotics. The ulcer base should be cleaned and leg elevation advised. Topical treatments include daily cleaning of the ulcer with 1–6% hydrogen peroxide solution or GV paint and covering the ulcer with moist gauze.

TROPICAL PYOMYOSITIS

Pyomyositis is a primary bacterial infection of the skeletal muscles most commonly caused by *S. aureus* and, less commonly, *S. pyogenes*. Early diagnosis is vital as untreated disease can progress to septicemia and septic shock. Once referred to as "tropical myositis", it is becoming more prevalent in temperate climates. Patients may give a history of trauma or recent travel to a tropical area, but pyomyositis in temperate climates is also associated with HIV infection, intravenous drug abuse, immunosuppression and diabetes mellitus. Pyomyositis may complicate influenza.

Diagnosis is often difficult, as patients frequently present with nonspecific signs and symptoms, including myalgias and low-grade fever. Progressive induration, pain and enlargement of a soft tissue mass over 10–14 days is characteristic. A "woody" induration is observed on palpation of involved soft tissues. Muscle abscess formation occurs during the second stage of disease and septic shock may follow.

Magnetic resonance imaging (MRI), although recommended, is not readily available in many locations. In some cases, pyomyositis can be confirmed by ultrasound-guided aspiration. Treatment includes surgical incision and drainage, and appropriate intravenous antibiotics until clinical improvement is noted, followed by oral antibiotics for a total of 1–3 weeks.

Large muscles of the trunk and proximal compartments of the limbs are usual sites of involvement.

REFERENCES

1. Noble W. Skin bacteriology and the role of *Staphylococcus aureus* in infection. J Dermatol 1998;139:9–12.
2. Darmstadt G, Lane A. Impetigo: an overview. Pediatr Dermatol 1994;11: 293–303.
3. Shriner D, Schwartz R, Janniger C. Impetigo. Cutis 1994;45:30–2.
4. Carroll J. Common bacterial pyodermas. Postgrad Med 1996;100:311–22.
5. Koning S, Verhagen AP, van Suijlekom-Smit LW, et al. Interventions for impetigo. Cochrane Database Syst Rev 2004;CD003261.
6. Lewis R. Soft tissue infections. World J Surg 1998;22:146–151.
7. Sachs M. Cutaneous cellulitis. Arch Dermatol 1991;124:493–500.
8. Davidson A, Rotstein O. The diagnosis and management of common soft-tissue infections. Can J Surg 1988;31:333–6.
9. McGeehan DF. Necrotising fasciitis: a biological disaster. Today's Emergency 1999;5:27–8.
10. Robinson DC, Adriaans B, Hay RJ, Yesudian P. The clinical and epidemiologic features of tropical ulcer (tropical phagedenic ulcer). Int J Dermatol 1988; 27:49–53.

Leprosy 57

Diana NJ Lockwood, Saba Lambert

Key features

- Leprosy, also known as Hansen's disease, is a chronic granulomatous bacterial infection principally affecting skin and peripheral nerves. It is caused by *Mycobacterium leprae*
- Following contact with an infective dose of *M. leprae*, most people will develop adequate protective immunity. Only a small percentage of individuals will develop clinical disease. Patients can present with manifestations that represent a spectrum of disease and host-pathogen interactions, ranging from heavy and diffuse organism loads and minimal host reactions, to pauci-bacillary disease and prominent host immune responses
- A patient with Hansen's may present with a macular hypo-pigmented skin lesion, weakness or pain in the hand because of nerve involvement, facial palsy, acute foot drop, or a painless burn or ulcer in an anesthetic hand or foot. Patients may also present with painful eyes as a first indication of lepromatous leprosy. The diagnosis of leprosy should be considered in anyone from an endemic area who presents with typical skin lesions, neuropathic ulcers, or a peripheral neuropathy (sensory loss and/or weakness)
- Diagnosis is usually based on clinical recognition and/or detection of acid-fast bacilli (AFB) in skin smears/biopsies
- Treatment is based on the World Health Organization (WHO) multidrug therapy regimens (MDT) and involves months of treatment
- Leprosy may be complicated by immunologic phenomena called "reactions". These sudden episodes of acute inflammation are a medical emergency and occur in approximately 30% of leprosy patients. The inflammation is a result of immune reactions against *M. leprae* antigens. These immunologic reactions cause neurologic damage that leads to subsequent tissue damage and eventual deformity. Treatment often involves steroids
- Physiotherpay, education, early wound care, and behavioral modifications to minimize risk of trauma are important components of the long-term care of individuals with complications of leprosy

Leprosy, also known as Hansen's disease, is a chronic granulomatous bacterial infection principally affecting skin and peripheral nerves [1].

In 2010, 228,474 new cases were registered worldwide and reported to the WHO. The top six endemic countries are: India, Brazil, Indonesia, Democratic Republic of Congo, Nigeria, and Bangladesh [2]. Most cases occur in resource-poor countries and leprosy continues to be a significant public health problem and a stigmatizing disease (Fig. 57.1).

THE CAUSATIVE ORGANISM AND HOST RESPONSE

Mycobacterium leprae is an acid-fast, rod-shaped, Gram-positive organism. It is an obligate intracellular pathogen and it has not been grown in axenic medium since being identified as the causative organism of leprosy by Armauer Hansen in 1874. It can be harvested after prolonged incubation in the mouse footpad and occurs by natural infection in the nine-banded armadillo, which is a reservoir for the organism in the states of Texas and Louisiana in the USA.

In 2001, the genome of *M. leprae* was sequenced. The organism appears to have undergone extensive reductive evolution with considerable downsizing of its genome compared with *Mycobacterium tuberculosis*. Almost half of the genome is occupied by pseudogenes [3].

Transmission is thought to occur mainly through aerosolized nasal droplets, spread when coughing or sneezing takes place. Forty-eight percent of lepromatous patients compared with 3% of borderline patients have nasal discharge containing *M. leprae*. The number of acid-fast bacilli in a single nasal blow averaged 1.1×10^8 in a study of 17 patients [4]. Contacts of leprosy patients are at higher risk of developing the disease than the general population. There are case reports of leprosy occurring following presumed inoculation through the skin during surgical procedures, tattooing, or accidental trauma [5]. The organism can persist outside the body under various environmental conditions for up to 5 months [6].

Following contact with an infective dose of *M. leprae*, most people will develop adequate protective immunity (Fig. 57.2). Only a small percentage of individuals will develop clinical disease. Infecting organisms are taken up by histiocytes in the skin and by Schwann cells in the peripheral nerves. This usually elicits an inflammatory response of histiocytes and lymphocytes. The earliest clinical sign is a vague, small hypo-pigmented macule, described as indeterminate leprosy; over 70% of these heal spontaneously. If bacillary growth outstrips the defense mechanism, then the condition progresses to one of the patterns that make up the spectrum of disease in leprosy. The incubation period can range between 2 and 12 years. Inflammation plays an important role in the neurologic damage that leads to subsequent tissue damage and eventual deformity.

DIAGNOSIS OF LEPROSY

The basis of clinical diagnosis of leprosy is the presence of one of the three cardinal signs:

- hypo-pigmented/reddish skin lesions with possible sensory loss;
- thickened peripheral nerves;
- acid-fast bacilli (AFB) seen in skin smears/biopsies.

A patient may present with a macular hypo-pigmented skin lesion (Fig. 57.3), weakness or pain in the hand owing to nerve involvement,

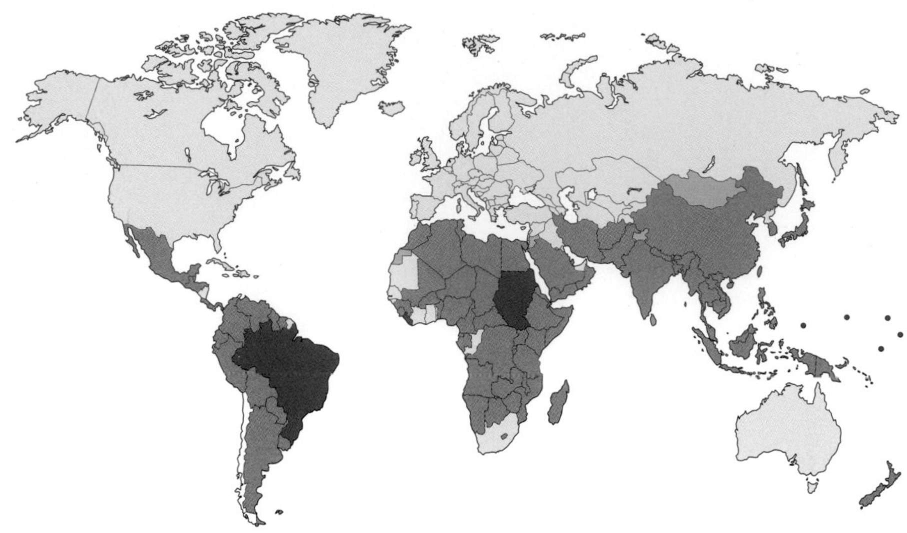

FIGURE 57.1 Leprosy global prevalence map (2011).

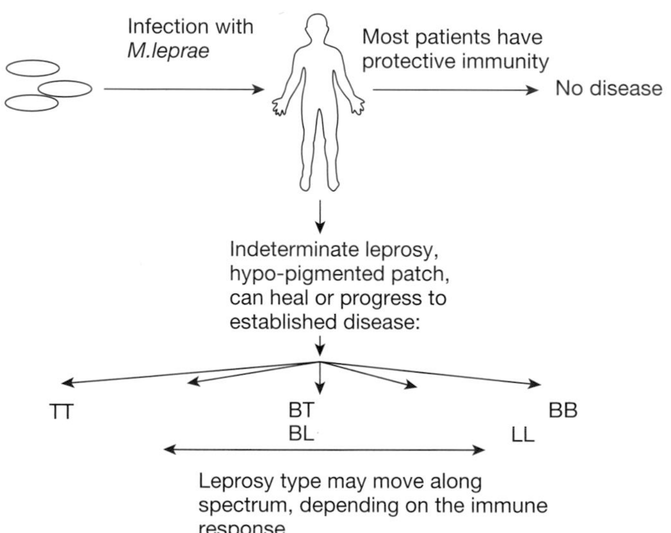

FIGURE 57.2 Relationshionship between *M. leprae* Infection and clinical leprosy.

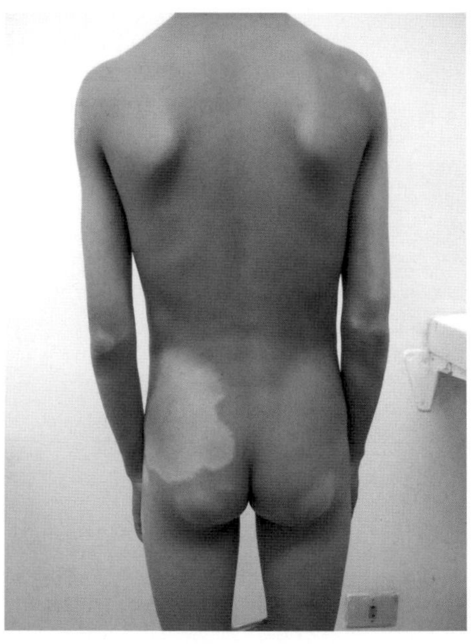

FIGURE 57.3 Young patient with extensive leprosy patches (BT) that are hypo-pigmented, dry, hairless and anesthetic. There are several lesions with a well-defined, but irregular, edge; a few satellite lesions are visible.

facial palsy, acute foot drop, or a painless burn or ulcer in an anesthetic hand or foot. Patients may also present with painful eyes as a first indication of lepromatous leprosy. The diagnosis of leprosy should be considered in anyone from an endemic area who presents with typical skin lesions, neuropathic ulcers, or a peripheral neuropathy (sensory loss and/or weakness).

LABORATORY TESTS

The presence of AFB in skin smear examination or biopsy material examination can provide supporting evidence for the diagnosis. The Bacterial Index gives a measure of bacterial density in the skin sample under examination on a logarithmic scale ranging from 0 to 6. Histopathologic evaluation is essential for accurate classification of leprosy lesions and is the best diagnostic test in a well-resourced setting, both for confirming and excluding the diagnosis of leprosy.

Recent advances have been made in serologic diagnostic test. Antibodies to the *M. leprae*-specific antiphenolic glycolipid (PGL-1) are present in 90% of patients with untreated lepromatous disease, but only 40–50% of patients with paucibacillary disease and 1–5 % of healthy controls [7]. An easy to use immunohistochromatographic assay, the ML flow test, based on PGL-1 detection, is being assessed by a Brazilian team [8]. PCR for detection of *M. leprae*-encoding specific genes or repeat sequences is potentially highly sensitive and specific, as it detects *M. leprae* DNA in 95% of multibacillary and 55% of paucibacillary patients. PCR is currently not used in clinical practice [7].

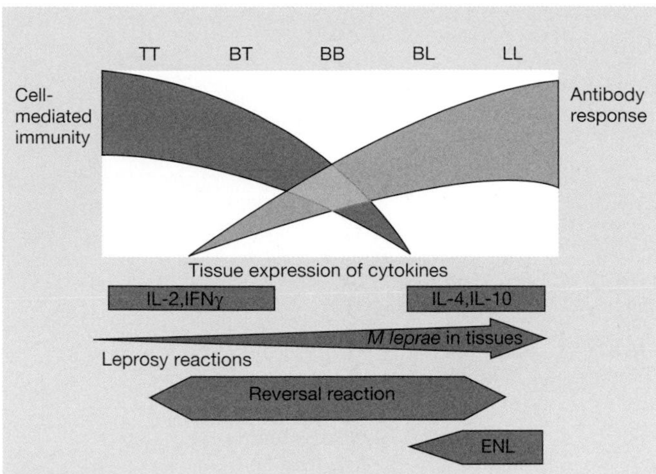

FIGURE 57.4 The Ridley-Jopling Classification and the relationship with host immunity.

CLASSIFICATION OF LEPROSY

Leprosy may be considered an immunologic disease. Immunity defines susceptibility to leprosy, type of clinical leprosy, pathology and major clinical complications of leprosy. Classification of the disease is important to determine prognosis, patients at higher risk of reactions and nerve damage, as well as select appropriate treatment. Leprosy patients can be classified using two systems: the Ridley-Jopling system and the WHO system.

The Ridley-Jopling system [9] (Fig. 57.4) uses clinical and histopathologic features and the Bacterial Index. Leprosy manifests in a spectrum of disease forms, ranging from the tuberculoid to the lepromatous. The clinical manifestations of leprosy are determined by the host's response to the leprosy bacillus: tuberculoid (TT) patients have a strong cell-mediated immune response manifesting as limited clinical disease, granuloma formation and no detectable mycobacteria; lepromatous (LL) patients have no cell-mediated immunity to *M. leprae* and have widespread disease and a high bacterial load. Between these two extremes there is a range of variations in host response; these comprise borderline cases (BT, borderline tuberculoid; BB, borderline borderline; BL, borderline lepromatous). Immunologically, borderline cases are unstable and polar tuberculoid and lepromatous cases are stable. Patients can move along the spectrum in the absence or presence of treatment.

The WHO classification is a simplified version that can be used in the field when slit skin smears are not available. Patients with fewer than six lesions are classified as paucibacillary and those with six or more lesions (Fig. 57.5) are classified as multi-bacillary. This is a quick and useful tool that can be employed by a wide variety of healthcare workers as it provides a low-cost strategy for leprosy diagnosis, without the need for skilled neurologic assessment and slit skin smear examination.

CLINICAL FEATURES

The cardinal signs of leprosy are anesthetic skin lesions, numbness or weakness as a result of damage to sensory and motor nerves and ulcers or burns in an anesthetic hand or foot. However, the clinical presentation ultimately depends on the host's immunity to *M. leprae* and clinical features can be divided into the disease spectrum classified according to Ridley-Jopling (Table 57-1).

TREATMENT

The management of leprosy consists of treating the *M. leprae* infection with antibiotic chemotherapy, managing the immune-mediated reactions (discussed separately), preventing nerve damage and educating the patient.

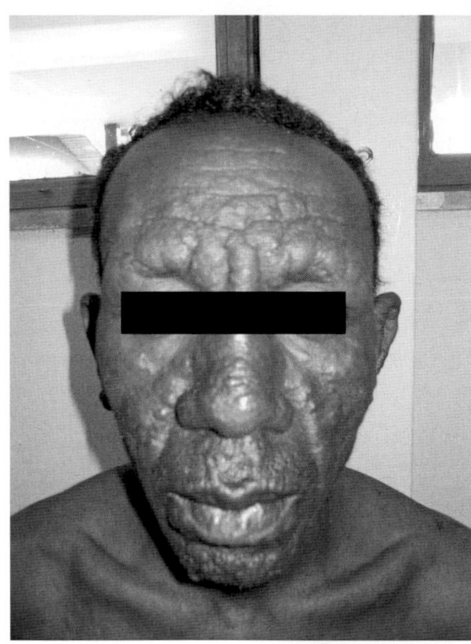

FIGURE 57.5 A 25-year-old man with lepromatous leprosy. The skin is heavily infiltrated and multiple nodules are present, giving a leonine appearance. Partial madurosis and nodules on the ears are present.

Antibiotic chemotherapy is based on the WHO multidrug therapy regimens (MDT) (Table 57-2).

Over the past 20 years, more than 14 million people have received MDT and have been cured of *M. leprae* infection. Relapse rates following treatment with MDT vary from 0–2.5% in paucibacillary disease. In multi-bacillary disease, the published rates of relapse are between 0 and 7.7% (www.clinical evidence.com). The study with the highest relapse rate in multi-bacillary patients demonstrated that 90% of relapses occurred in patients who had an initial Bacterial Index of >4 [10]. Leprosy can occur in children and the doses of medication will be lower. Consultation with a specialist is recommended.

In the USA, treatment regimens vary from the WHO-MDT (Table 57-3). The more common side effects of the WHO MDT drugs are summarized in Table 57.4.

ALTERNATIVE ANTI-MICROBIAL AGENTS

Minocycline 100 mg daily can be used as a substitute for Dapsone in individuals who do not tolerate this drug. It can also be used instead of clofazimine, although currently there is no evidence that minocycline protects patients against developing erythema nodosum leprosum (ENL).

Clarithromycin 500 mg daily is also effective against *M. leprae*, and can be used as a substitute for any of the other drugs in a multi-drug regimen.

Ofloxacin 400 mg daily may also be used in place of clofazimine for adults.

REACTIONS

Leprosy is complicated by immunologic phenomena called "reactions". These sudden episodes of acute inflammation are a medical emergency and occur in approximately 30% of leprosy patients. The inflammation is caused by immune reactions against *M. leprae* antigens. Patients can present in reaction before MDT treatment, and a significant proportion of patients develop reactions within the first six months of treatment. There is also an increase in the incidence of reactions in post-partum patients. However, reactions can also occur after successful MDT treatment and are probably caused by the persistence of *M. leprae* antigens. Patients may experience repeated

TABLE 57-1 Major Clinical Features of the Disease Spectrum in Leprosy

Classification		Bacterial Index	Skin lesions	Nerve involvement	Systemic features
Ridley- Jopling	*WHO*				
Indeterminate	PB	0	Solitary hypo-pigmented 2–5cm lesion. May become TT-like	None clinically detectable	Nil
Tuberculoid (TT)	PB/MB	0–1	Few, often one macule or plaque with well-defined border and sensory loss. The patch is dry (loss of sweating) and hairless	May have one peripheral nerve enlarged. Occasionally presents as a mono-neuropathy	Nil
Borderline tuberculoid (BT)	MB	0–2	Several larger irregular plaques with partially raised edges. Satellite lesions at the edges	Asymmetrical multiple nerve involvement	Nil
Borderline (BB)	MB	2–3	Many macular lesions and infiltrated lesions with punched out centers	Asymmetrical multiple nerve involvement	
Borderline lepromatous (BL)	MB	1–4	Many small macular lesions and multiple nodules and papules	Widespread nerve thickening. Sensory and motor loss	
Lepromatous (LL)	MB	4–6	Numerous nodular skin lesions in a symmetrical distribution, not dry or anesthetic. May present as many confluent macular lesions. There are often thickened shiny earlobes, loss of eyebrows and diffuse skin thickening	Widespread nerve enlargement. Glove and stocking anesthesia occurs late in disease	Nasal stuffiness, epistaxis. Testicular atrophy. Ocular involvement. Bones and internal organs can be affected

MB, multi-bacillary; PB, paucobacillary; TT, tuberculoid.

Table 57-2 World Health Organization (WHO)-Recommended Multidrug Therapy (MDT) Regimes for Adults

Type of leprosy	Drug treatment		Duration of treatment
	Monthly supervised	*Daily, self-administered*	
Paucibacillary (TT and BT)	Rifampin 600 mg	Dapsone 100 mg	6 months
Multibacillary (BB,BL and LL)	Rifampin 600 mg, clofazimine 300 mg	Clofazimine 50 mg Dapsone 100 mg	12 months

BT, borderline tuberculoid; BB, borderline borderline; BL, borderline lepromatous; LL, lepromatous; TT, tuberculoid.

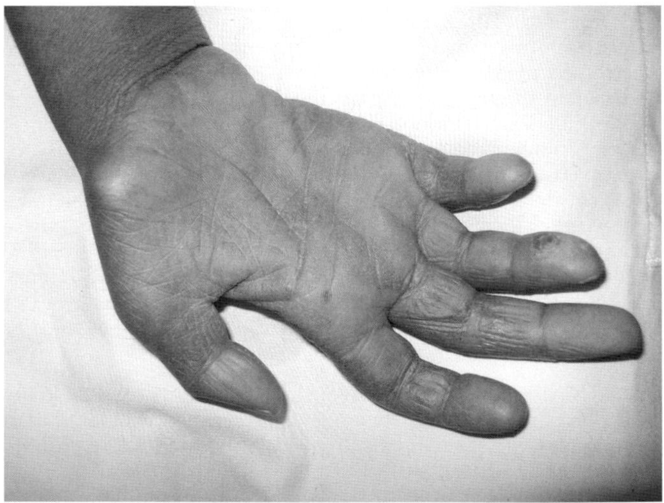

FIGURE 57.6 Median and ulnar nerve damage in leprosy: dry skin, muscle wasting, mobile clawing of fourth and fifth finger, desensitization and painless burn on the fourth finger.

reactions after treatment, resulting in increased suffering and disability. These immunologic reactions and the influx of inflammatory cells cause nerve damage through demyelination. It is this neurologic damage that leads to subsequent tissue damage and eventual deformity (Fig. 57.6).

Nerve function impairment (NFI) is defined as clinically-detectable impairment of motor, sensory or autonomic nerve function [11]. NFI may occur in the absence of symptoms and may go unnoticed by the patient, i.e. "silent neuropathy". NFI is detected clinically by testing the sensation in the patient's hands and feet with graded monofilaments and testing the small muscles' power.

Patients seen with NFI of recent onset (less than 6 months) should be given a course of prednisolone therapy and physiotherapy. Some of these patients will recover function of the affected part.

MANAGEMENT OF TYPE 1 REACTIONS

The clinical manifestations of these reactions are edema and erythema of skin lesions, and neuritis. Acute neuritis (defined as spontaneous nerve pain, paraesthesia or tenderness with new sensory or motor impairment of recent onset) may also occur without evidence of skin inflammation (Fig. 57.7).

Corticosteroids are used to treat moderate and severe reactions, where pain is severe and NFI is present. Prednisolone 40–60mg daily should be started and tapered down after clinical improvement to the minimal effective dose until the reaction subsides. There is no clear consensus on the optimum dose of corticosteroids or the length of

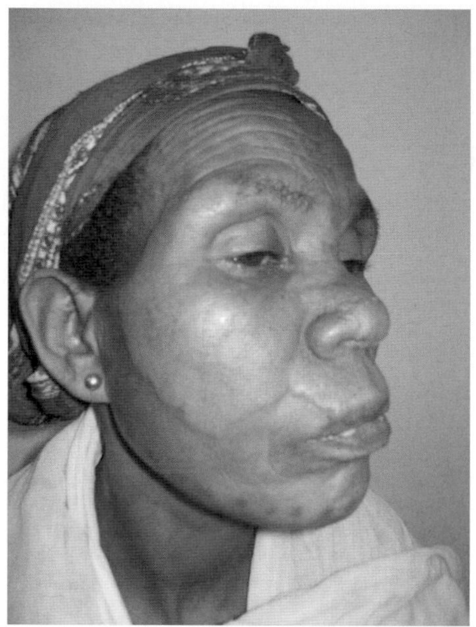

FIGURE 57.7 Female patient diagnosed with paucibacillary leprosy with single facial lesion showing Type 1 reaction. The lesion has become acutely inflamed, swollen and tender.

TABLE 57-3 Centers for Disease Control and Prevention (CDC) Recommended Multidrug Therapy (MDT) Regimens for Adults in the USA

Type of leprosy	Drug treatment *Daily, self-administered*	Duration of treatment
Paucibacillary (TT and BT)	Rifampin 600 mg and dapsone 100 mg	12 months
Multibacillary (BB,BL and LL)	Rifampin 600 mg, dapsone 100 mg and clofazimine 50 mg	24 months

BT, borderline tuberculoid; BB, borderline borderline; BL, borderline lepromatous; LL; lepromatous; TT, tuberculoid.

TABLE 57-4 Side Effects of Multidrug Therapy (MDT) Drugs

Drug	Side effect
Dapsone	Hemolytic anemia Exfoliative dermatitis Fixed drug eruption Psychosis
Clofazimine	Severe dryness of skin Brownish or reddish discoloration of skin and patch Abdominal pain—sign of acute abdomen Pigmentation of conjunctiva
Rifampin	Flu-like syndromes (dose-dependent hypersensitivity reaction) Liver dysfunction Abdominal pain Loss of appetite Red urine, stool, saliva

TABLE 57-5 Comparison of Clinical Features of Type 1 and Type 2 Leprosy Reactions

Parameter	Type 1	Type 2 (ENL)
Patients at risk	BL, BB, BT	LL, BL
Onset of reaction	Gradual, over a few weeks	Sudden, "overnight"
Cutaneous lesions	Increased erythema and induration of previously existing or new lesions	Numerous erythematous, tender nodules on face, extremities, or trunk, without relationship to prior lesions
Neuritis	Frequent, often severe	Frequent, often severe
Systemic symptoms	Afebrile, mild malaise	Fever, malaise, lymph node enlargement, arthritis, iritis, orchitis
Histopathologic features	CD4 cell↑, granuloma edema, ↑ giant cell size and numbers, dermal oedema and HLA-DR expression	Polymorphonuclear cell infiltrates in lesions 24 h old,
Treatment	Corticosteroids	Corticosteroids, thalidomide
Recurrence	Approx. 30%	Approx. 65 %

BT, borderline tuberculoid; BB, borderline borderline; BL, borderline lepromatous; ENL, erythema nodosum leprosum; HLA-DR, human leukocyte antigen-DR; LL; lepromatous; TT, tuberculoid.

treatment although a recent study has shown that a longer period of treatment (5 months) was more beneficial that the 3 months often used [12] (Table 57-5).

MANAGEMENT OF ERYTHEMA NODOSUM LEPROSUM (ENL) REACTIONS

Type 2 leprosy reactions (i.e. ENL) present as a systemic illness: a patient with ENL may be very sick, with high temperatures, painful subcutaneous nodules, peripheral edema, and inflammation of the nerves, eyes, joints, muscles, bones, and testes. The onset of ENL is acute, but it may pass into a chronic phase and is often recurrent (Table 57-5).

For mild ENL, aspirin may be used. Patients with severe ENL require hospitalization and treatment with high-dose prednisolone (starting at 60 mg). The efficacy is variable and some patients with chronic, or recurrent, ENL may need to take prednisolone for several years [13]. These long, high doses of steroids are associated with steroid side effects, such as hypertension, diabetes, cataracts, and acne [14]. Thalidomide, starting at a dose of 100–400 mg daily and tapering down, is the treatment of choice for severe ENL. It controls ENL symptoms rapidly and prevents recurrences but its availability and teratogenicity limits its use. Clofazimine (up to 300 mg) is effective against ENL, although it takes 4–6 weeks of continuous use for the anti-inflammatory effect to manifest.

Other alternatives to prednisolone, such as azathioprine and cyclosporine, are being studied.

ONGOING MANAGEMENT AND PREVENTION OF COMPLICATIONS

Education concerning factual information, such as mode of transmission, infectivity, treatment, and complications, is essential for all patients and health providers. Patients should be taught self-examination of the hands and feet with early medical review if signs of inflammation or trauma occur. Adequate footwear or other protective devices should be made available to those with insensitive or deformed feet. Ulcers in anesthetic feet are the most common cause of hospitalization. Ulcers are treated by rest and cleaning, although any signs of osteomyelitis need to be referred for surgical debridement. Appropriate early physiotherapy must be instituted and patients must be referred to the appropriate specialist for evaluation and correction of deformity. Leprosy still elicits stigma in many communities and the patient will benefit from social and psychological support.

Chemoprophylaxis and Immunotherapy

To date, no specific vaccine has been developed to prevent infection by *M. leprae*, although there is good evidence that Bacillus Calmette-Guérin (BCG) has protective efficacy. A meta-analysis of 26 studies demonstrated an overall protective effect between 26% and 61%. The age at vaccination did not predict the protective effect of BCG [15].

A Bangladeshi study showed that the overall reduction in incidence of leprosy using a single dose of rifampin in the first 2 years was 57% [16]. However, the difference was no longer significant in the third and fourth years.

Leprosy and HIV

There were concerns that an interaction between HIV and *M. leprae* infection would result in an increased incidence of leprosy cases. However, studies in Uganda, Mali, Ethiopia, and South India have not shown an increased prevalence of leprosy cases associated with HIV infection [17–19].

An association has been found between HIV infection and complications of leprosy. In a case-controlled study in Uganda, HIV seropositivity was found to be a significant risk factor for developing reactions and neuritis; an unusual finding because reversal reactions are associated with an increase in CD4 cells. Similarly, Sampaio et al. found that HIV-infected patients with low CD4 counts had normal granuloma formation with numerous CD4 cells [20].

Treatment of a leprosy patient with concurrent HIV infection does not differ from that of a seronegative leprosy patient and reactions should be managed with corticosteroids or thalidomide as appropriate.
Since the introduction of highly active anti-retroviral therapy (HAART) in the management of HIV, leprosy is being increasingly reported as part of the immune reconstitution inflammatory syndrome (IRIS) [21]. It is possible that the immune response to *M. leprae* in an HIV-infected person is suppressed before starting HAART and that leprosy manifests as IRIS with the sudden reversal of this suppression and the rise of CD4 [22]. Further studies are needed to understand the clinical and pathologic features in HIV and leprosy co-infection.

CONCLUSION

Since the implementation of MDT in 1982 in endemic areas, more than 90% of registered cases have received treatment, 14 million patients have been cured and global prevalence has declined. The continuation of surveillance and leprosy control programs are essential.

The current treatment for leprosy reactions is still not optimal, with a significant number of patients not responding to prednisolone and some ENL patients requiring chronic thalidomide therapy. Researchers are still looking for different immunosuppressant drugs with efficacy in the treatment of reactions (e.g. azathioprine [23] and cyclosporine [24]).

The stigma associated with the diagnosis of leprosy is still a very real problem and the management of someone with the disease should include discussion of their psychosocial status and education for the patient and their family.

REFERENCES

1. Walker SL, Lockwood DN. Leprosy. Clin Dermatol 2007;25:165–72.
2. World Health Organization. Leprosy Update 2011. Weekly Epidemiological Record No. 36 2011;86:389–400.
3. Cole ST, Eiglmeier K, Parkhill J, et al. Massive gene decay in the leprosy bacillus. Nature 2001; 409:1007–11.
4. Davey TF, Rees RJW. The nasal discharge in leprosy: clinical and bacteriological aspects. Lepr Rev 1974;45:135–44.
5. Brandsma JW, Yoder Land Macdonald M. Leprosy acquired by inoculation from a knee injury. Lepr Rev 2005;76:175–9.
6. Desikan KV, Sreevatsa. Extended studies on the viability of *M. leprae* outside the human body. Lepr Rev 1995;66:287–95.
7. Britton WJ, Lockwood DNJ. Leprosy. Lancet 2004;363:1209–19.
8. Lyon S, Lyon AC, Castorina Da Silva R, et al. A comparison of ML Flow serology and slit skin test smears to assess the bacterial load in newly diagnosed leprosy patients in Brazil. Leprosy Review 2008;79:162–70.
9. Ridley DS, Jopling WH. Classification of leprosy according to immunity. A five-group system. Int J Lepr Other Mycobact Dis 1966;34:255–73.
10. Deshpande J, Chougule SG, Thakar UH, Revankar CR. Rate of relapse and reactions in MB leprosy patients after 24 and 12 months of MDT in Maharashtra. Indian J Lepr 2004;76:229–30.
11. Van Brakel WH, Khawas IB. Nerve damage in leprosy: an epidemiological and clinical study of 396 patients in west Nepal—Part 1. Definitions, methods and frequencies. Lepr Rev 1994;65:204–21.
12. Sandor Rao PSS, Sugamaran DST, Richard J, Smith WCS. Multi-centre, double blind, randomized trial of three steroid regimens in the treatment of type-1 reactions in leprosy. Lepr Rev 2006;77:25–33.
13. Pocaterra L, Jain S, Reddy R, et al. Clinical course of erythema nodosum leprosum: an 11-year cohort study in Hyderabad, India. Am J Trop Med Hyg 2006;74:868–79.
14. Richardus JH, Withington SG, Anderson AM, et al. Adverse events of standardized regimens of corticosteroids for prophylaxis and treatment of nerve function impairment in leprosy: results from the 'TRIPOD' trials. Lepr Rev 2003; 74:319–27.
15. Setia MS, Steinmaus C, Ho CS, et al. The role of BCG in prevention of leprosy: a meta-analysis. Lancet Infect Dis 2006;6:162–70.
16. Moet FJ, Pahan D, Oskam L, Richardus JH. Effectiveness of single dose rifampicin in preventing leprosy in close contacts of patients with newly diagnosed leprosy: cluster randomised controlled trial. BMJ 2008;336: 761–4.
17. Kawuma HJS, Bwire R, Adatu-Engwau F. Leprosy and infection with the human immunodeficency virus in Uganda.; a case-control study. Int J Lepr 1994;62:521–6.
18. Lienhardt C, Kamate B, Jamet P et al. Effect of HIV infection on leprosy: a three year survey in Bamako, Mali. Int J Lepr Other Mycobact Dis 1996; 64:383–91.
19. Sekar B, Jayasheela M, Chattopadhya D, et al. Prevalence of HIV Infection and high-risk characteristics among leprosy patients of South India; a case-control study. Int J Lepr 1994;62:527–31.
20. Sampaio EP, Caneshi JRT, Nery JAC, et al. Cellular immune response to *Mycobacterium leprae* infection in human immunodeficiency virus infected individuals. Infect Immun 1995;63:18848–54.
21. Deps PD, Lockwood DNJ. Leprosy occurring as immune reconstitution syndrome. Trans R Soc Trop Med Hyg 2008;102:966–8.
22. Ustianowski AP, Lawn SD, Lockwood DNJ. Interactions between HIV infection and leprosy: a paradox. Lancet Infect Dis 2006;6:350–60.
23. Marlowe SN, Hawksworth RA, Butlin CR, et al. Clinical outcomes in a randomized controlled study comparing azathioprine and prednisolone versus prednisolone alone in the treatment of severe leprosy type 1 reactions in Nepal. Trans R Soc Trop Med Hyg 2004;98:602–9.
24. Marlowe SN, Leekassa R, Bizuneh E, et al. Response to ciclosporin treatment in Ethiopian and Nepali patients with severe leprosy Type 1 reactions. Trans R Soc Trop Med Hyg 2007;101:1004–12.

Buruli Ulcer 58

Mark H Wansbrough-Jones, Richard O Phillips

Key features

- *Mycobacterium ulcerans* causes chronic skin ulcers, referred to as Buruli ulcers
- Common in parts of rural West Africa, but the mode of transmission is unknown
- Subcutaneous necrosis is caused by secretion of mycolactone toxin, a plasmid-encoded polyketide molecule
- Treatment includes 8 weeks of rifampin and streptomycin
- Early recognition and treatment including physiotherapy can prevent disabilities

INTRODUCTION

Buruli ulcer is the accepted name for a disease caused by skin infection with *Mycobacterium ulcerans*, an unusual mycobacterium that secretes a toxin that causes disease. Infections can be successfully treated with rifampin and streptomycin. Current challenges include educating individuals in endemic zones to recognize infection early and delivering treatment to affected individuals in rural tropical areas.

EPIDEMIOLOGY AND TRANSMISSION

Buruli ulcer is a disease of high focal prevalence mainly within countries in West Africa (Fig. 58.1), but sporadic cases have been reported in many countries with high humidity in tropical wetlands. Buruli ulcer has been seen among people living in more than 30 countries around the world (Fig. 58.2), including French Guiana, Peru, Mexico, Papua New Guinea, Japan, and Southern China. Outbreaks are also observed in temperate South Eastern Australia, where the association of *M. ulcerans* with Buruli (Bairnsdale) ulcer was first recognized in 1948. Disturbance of water systems by mining, deforestation or flooding has been associated with increased incidence of disease. Newly arrived migrants in endemic zones are susceptible to infection, as demonstrated by the occurrence of Buruli ulcer among displaced Rwandans in the Kinyara refugee camps in Uganda in the 1960s. These refugees were displaced from a non-endemic zone and developed ulcers within 4–10 weeks of arrival, suggesting the disease's incubation period.

Mycobacterium ulcerans has been identified in wild koalas and ringtail possums. It is difficult to culture, although it has been isolated from fresh water bugs in endemic zones following serial passage in mice [1]. *Mycobacterium ulcerans* probably exists in an ecologic niche related to slow-flowing or stagnant water in West Africa, but how it is transmitted to humans remains unknown. Experimental evidence shows that it can be transmitted from infected water bugs to mice by biting [2]. In Australia, DNA from *M. ulcerans* was detected in mosquitoes from an affected area, but not in mosquitoes from a non-infected area, as well as in possum feces; however, the significance of these observations is unclear. To date, *M. ulcerans* has not been detected in African mammals.

Buruli ulcer can affect people of all ages but, in West Africa, it predominantly affects children aged 5 to 15 years, and in Southeast Australia, it affects elderly residents in retirement towns.

CLINICAL PRESENTATION

Most patients with Buruli ulcer present with a chronic ulcer, often of a few months' duration. Patients fail to present early because the lesions are painless and affected individuals often live in remote rural areas lacking easy access to affordable health care [3]. The disease manifests as a 1–5 cm painless subcutaneous nodule attached to the overlying skin (Fig. 58.3A). In Australia, early lesions are often papular. More extensive indurated plaques may also occur, the margins of which are difficult to define. Nodules, plaques, and ulcers may be associated with edema in surrounding tissue (10–15% in Ghana) which spreads outwards (Fig. 58.3B). Ulceration spreads from the initial lesion into edematous areas. The patient remains well and there is no fever or pain unless secondary bacterial infection occurs. Occasionally, osteomyelitis occurs in bone adjacent to a skin lesion, but involvement of other organs is rare.

The distinguishing features of Buruli ulcers are that they are painless and that the edges are undermined so that a swab can be pushed a few millimeters (or sometimes centimeters) under the surrounding skin (Fig. 58.3C). The ulcer border is not raised. Tissue destruction is caused by cytotoxic mycolactone toxin that also prevents the development of an inflammatory response [4]. The process is chronic and histologic examination of affected tissue often shows a mixture of scar formation, featureless necrosis around clumps of proliferating acid-fast mycobacteria, and acute, chronic and granulomatous inflammation. Organisms are rarely seen within macrophages in untreated lesions but careful immunohistologic studies have demonstrated that intracellular organisms can be observed during antibiotic treatment when the effect of mycolactone is lost [5].

In 90% of cases, ulcers involve the limbs but they can also involve the head, neck, or trunk. When scarring occurs close to a joint, there is often limitation of joint movement; large lesions on the trunk may inhibit spinal movement. Buruli ulcers recognize no anatomic boundaries and may involve critical sites, such as the face, breast, and genital area.

DIAGNOSIS

Diagnosis is usually based on clinical recognition. Buruli ulcers on the lower extremities may be difficult to distinguish from diabetic or venous stasis ulcers. Acid-fast bacilli can be detected in about 40% of ulcers when a swab is taken from the base, close to undermined areas. Cultures (on Löwenstein Jensen medium at 32°C) are more sensitive (up to 60% positive), yielding mycobacterial growth when performed in a laboratory near the endemic area, but it can take 6 weeks or more for mycobacterial growth to be detectable. Histologic examination

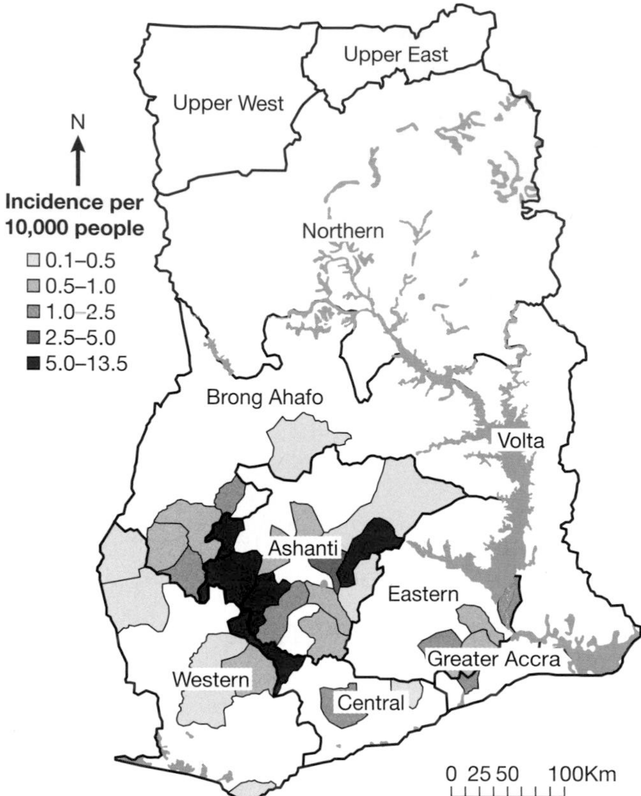

FIGURE 58.1 Buruli ulcer incidence in Ghana during 2008 (map created by Julie Clennon, Rollins School of Public Health from data provided by Edwin Ampadu and William Opare, Ghana National BU Control Programme. Funded by: National Institute of Environmental Health Sciences grants #R01ES015525 and #T32ES012160).

can be 85% sensitive but is not available in many endemic areas. The most sensitive diagnostic test (98%) is PCR for the IS2404 repeat sequence of *M. ulcerans*. PCR can be applied to swabs, punch biopsies (3–4mm diameter) and fine needle aspirates. The latter approaches may be helpful in diagnosing individual nodules, plaques, and edematous lesions that have not yet ulcerated [6].

MANAGEMENT

Commonly used treatments for Buruli ulcer are unknown compounds in traditional topical applications, many of which may be harmful, and none of which have been shown to be beneficial. Their use delays diagnosis and effective treatment. Daily treatment under observation with rifampin 10 mg/kg orally and streptomycin 15 mg/kg intramuscularly for 8 weeks results in healing of all forms of *M. ulcerans* disease with few exceptions [7]. Recurrence after antibiotic treatment is rare (0–2.5%).

Further studies of antibiotic therapy are in progress. A small study has shown that intramuscular injections of streptomycin can be given 5 days per week instead of 7 without apparent loss of efficacy. The 8-week duration of treatment was recommended by the World Health Organization (WHO) expert advisors after a study showed that *M. ulcerans* organisms were still viable in early lesions excised after 2 weeks of treatment, whereas cultures were sterile when treatment was extended to 4, 8, or 12 weeks [8]. Thus, treatment for 8 weeks allows a wide safety margin; it may be possible to treat some lesions for a shorter period. Recently, a large, controlled trial has shown that clarithromycin can be substituted for streptomycin in the second 4 weeks of treatment without loss of efficacy [9].

COMPLICATIONS

Chronic ulceration leads to disfiguring scars and significant loss of tissue. Extensive ulcers on the limbs sometimes require amputation, particularly when there is concurrent osteomyelitis. Secondary bacterial infection of a Buruli ulcer may cause life-threatening septicemia.

Paradoxical reactions, characterized by increased inflammation and lesion size or the appearance of new lesions, occur in up to 10% of patients. A fluctuant mass may appear close to the initial lesion during antibiotic treatment and purulent discharge that is usually sterile can be aspirated. These lesions resolve without additional antibiotic treatment.

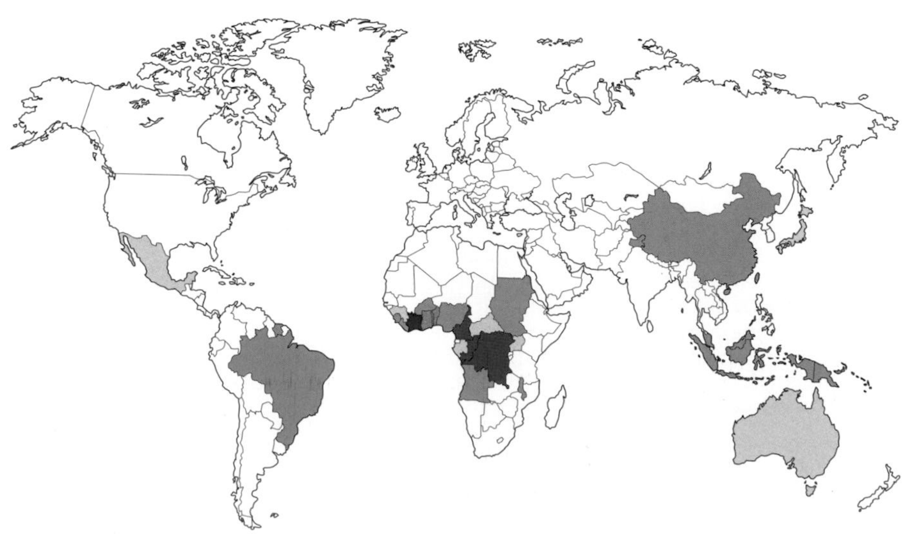

FIGURE 58.2 New cases of Buruli ulcer reported to the WHO in 2008. Provided by Dr Kingsley Asiedu, WHO.

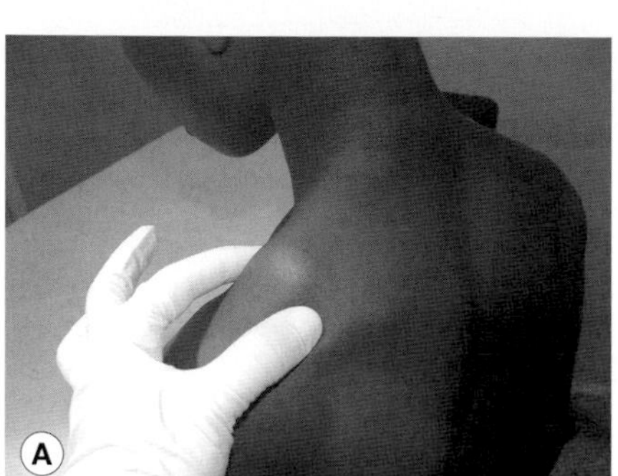

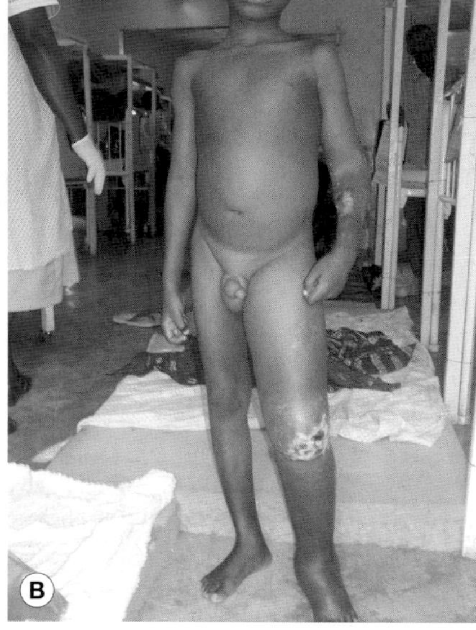

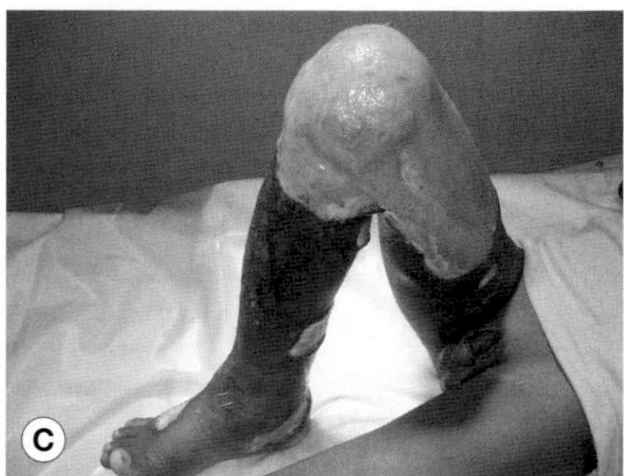

FIGURE 58.3 Clinical forms of Buruli ulcer disease. **(A)** Subcutaneous firm, painless nodule attached to the skin. **(B)** Extensive edema of the left arm and leg and genitalia with ulceration on the left arm and knee. **(C)** Partially debrided ulcer on the right knee with further ulceration on the leg and foot. All the ulcers were probably connected subcutaneously.

When a Buruli ulcer is close to a joint there may be limitation of joint movement, and an increased risk of scarring. Functional limitation can be prevented by simple physiotherapy that can be taught to the patient and family when treatment is started.

PREVENTION

Understanding how *M. ulcerans* infection is transmitted to humans is a priority as this information could lead to preventative strategies. Epidemiologic studies have shown that exposure to water sources near endemic villages is a risk factor for developing Buruli ulcer but reducing exposure, particularly of children, to such sources is impractical in rural West Africa.

No effective vaccine is currently available, although Bacillus Calmette-Guérin (BCG) vaccine has been associated with short-lived protection in small trials.

REFERENCES

1. Portaels F, Meyers WM, Ablordey A, et al. First Cultivation and Characterization of Mycobacterium ulcerans from the Environment. PLoS Negl Trop Dis 2008;2:e178.
2. Marsollier L, Robert R, Aubry J, et al. Aquatic insects as a vector for *Mycobacterium ulcerans*. Appl Environ Microbiol 2002;68:4623–8.
3. Asiedu K, Etuaful S. Socioeconomic implications of Buruli ulcer in Ghana: a three-year review. Am J Trop Med Hyg 1998;59:1015–22.
4. Demangel C, Stinear TP, Cole ST. Buruli ulcer: reductive evolution enhances pathogenicity of *Mycobacterium ulcerans*. Nat Rev Microbiol 2009;7: 50–60.
5. Schutte D, Um-Boock A, Mensah-Quainoo E, et al. Development of highly organized lymphoid structures in buruli ulcer lesions after treatment with rifampicin and streptomycin. PLoS Negl Trop Dis 2007;1:e2.
6. Phillips R. O, Sarfo FS, Osei-Sarpong F, et al. Sensitivity of PCR targeting *Mycobacterium ulcerans* by use of fine needle aspirates for diagnosis of Buruli ulcer. 2009. J Clin Microbiol 2009;47:924–26.
7. Chauty A, Ardant MF, Adeye A, et al. Promising clinical efficacy of streptomycin-rifampin combination for treatment of buruli ulcer (*Mycobacterium ulcerans* disease). Antimicrob Agents Chemother 2007;51:4029–35.
8. Etuaful S, Carbonnelle B, Grosset J, et al. Efficacy of the combination rifampin-streptomycin in preventing growth of *Mycobacterium ulcerans* in early lesions of Buruli ulcer in humans. Antimicrob Agents Chemother 2005;49:3182–6.
9. Nienhuis WA, Stienstra Y, Thompson WA, et al. Antimicrobial treatment for early, limited Mycobacterium ulcerans infection: a randomised controlled trial. Lancet 2010;375:664–72.

59 *Mycobacterium marinum* Infection

Francisco Vega-López

Key features

- This condition is suspected following a history of exposure to water in a fish tank, swimming pool, aquarium or seawater with infected fish and/or amphibians
- Clinical signs manifest 2–8 weeks after exposure to infected fish or water. The "sporotrichoid" distribution of non-healing nodules frequently involves fingers, hands and upper limbs unilaterally and with proximal dissemination
- Severe and chronic nodular lesions unresponsive to treatment occur in the immunocompromised host
- Investigate and exclude sporotrichosis, cutaneous leishmaniasis, nocardiosis, sarcoidosis and cutaneous tuberculosis. Diagnosis rests on a history of exposure, typical skin lesions and granulomatous inflammation on histology. Laboratory isolation of *Mycobacterium marinum* from a clinical specimen confirms the diagnosis
- *Mycobacterium marinum* is a multi-drug-resistant organism; however, cure can be achieved in ~85% of cases with combinations of clarithromycin, rifampin, ethambutol, tetracyclines and/or trimethoprim-sulfamethoxazole. Relapse can occur

INTRODUCTION

Mycobacterium marinum is an environmental mycobacterium ubiquitous in fresh, brackish and sea water. It infects more than 150 species of fish and also causes clinical illness in frogs, eels, oysters, toads and snakes. It is responsible for human granulomatous cutaneous infection through direct inoculation into the skin. Currently, it is an uncommon human disease and most patients respond to treatment with combinations of anti-mycobacterial drugs.

EPIDEMIOLOGY

The disease is uncommon and usually presents as sporadic individual cases, although outbreaks have been reported. The disease is associated with exposure to fresh- or seawater; *M. marinum* can infect fish and amphibians.

NATURAL HISTORY, PATHOGENESIS AND PATHOLOGY

Inoculation of *M. marinum* takes place through skin abrasion or injury while handling infected fish or water. Skin lesions appear on the inoculation site 2–8 weeks later and spread proximally on the affected limb to dermal and lymphatic tissue. Infection is often chronic, lasting months. Lymphangitic (sporotrichoid) spread can occur. Spontaneous resolution has been observed and relapse is not uncommon after weeks or months of apparently successful treatment. The clinical features can last for many years if left untreated.

Histologic examination of a lesion biopsy reveals either chronic, non-specific inflammation or a mixed inflammatory response with granuloma formation. In advanced cases, well-formed epithelioid tuberculoid granuloma and intracellular acid-fast bacilli can be observed.

CLINICAL FEATURES

A single, erythematous, papule or small nodule with a smooth or warty surface appears at the inoculation site – commonly the dorsal aspect of a finger. Proximal spread then slowly progresses over the next few weeks and nodular lesions can involve the lymphatic track (Fig. 59.1). The lesions are commonly asymptomatic but may become tender or with pyogenic features from secondary bacterial infection (Fig. 59.2). Cutaneous lesions can affect the whole limb. Deep extension can lead to involvement of bone or tendons in more than 2% of cases. Disease severity is increased in immunocompromised individuals.

PATIENT EVALUATION, DIAGNOSIS AND DIFFERENTIAL DIAGNOSIS

A history of exposure to infected water, fish or amphibians, together with a typical clinical picture allow for high diagnostic suspicion. This, together with a compatible histologic picture, can be used to recommend a therapeutic course. Definitive diagnosis rests on identifying the organism, but microbiologic culturing is insensitive (approximately 50%). In the laboratory, *M. marinum* is an intermediate grower and develops best at lower temperatures of between 30° and 33°C.

Differential diagnosis includes sporothrichosis, nocardiosis, cutaneous leishmaniasis, cutaneous tuberculosis and cutaneous sarcoidosis.

TREATMENT

Mycobacterium marinum is a multi-drug-resistant organism and is often best treated with combinations of two or three anti-mycobacterial drugs. *Mycobacterium marinum* is susceptible to anti-mycobacterial drugs, including clarithromycin, rifampin, ethambutol, minocycline and trimethoprim-salfamethoxazole. Susceptibility to fluoroquinolones is variable. Most current treatment regimens include clarithromycin, often with rifampin and ethambutol. Treatment is usually for months. The length of optimal treatment is uncertain; many authorities treat for a minimum of 4 weeks after clinical resolution (Fig. 59.3). Paradoxical worsening after initiation of therapy has been noted in some patients. Surgical debridement is required if there is involvement of tendon or bone. Therapeutic failure has to be considered after 4–6 weeks of treatment without improvement; a different drug combination should be tried at this stage.

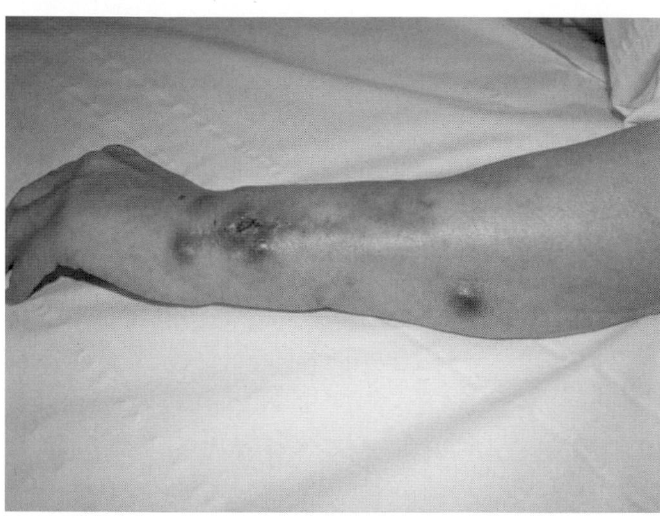

FIGURE 59.1 Sporotrichoid dissemination in fish tank granuloma following dog bite.

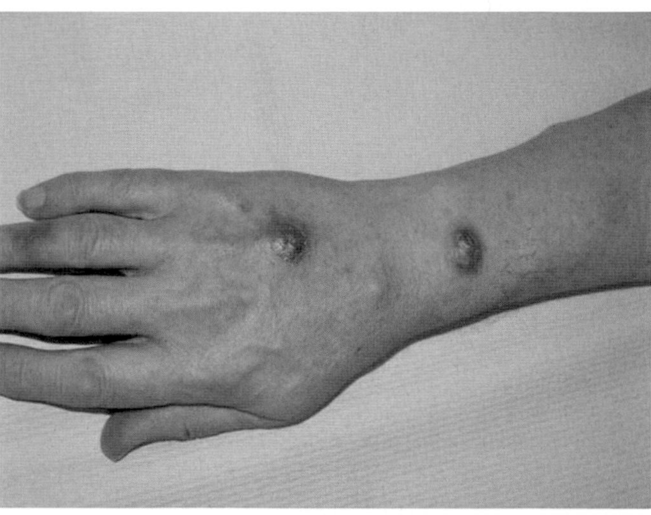

FIGURE 59.2 Erythematous and flesh-colored nodules on the right upper limb in a fish tank owner.

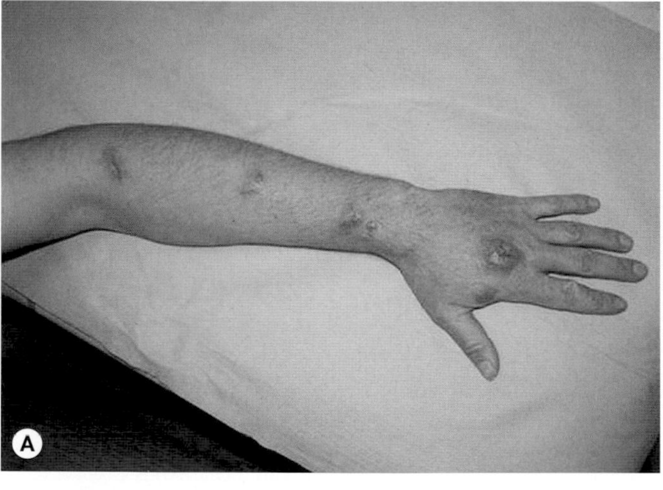

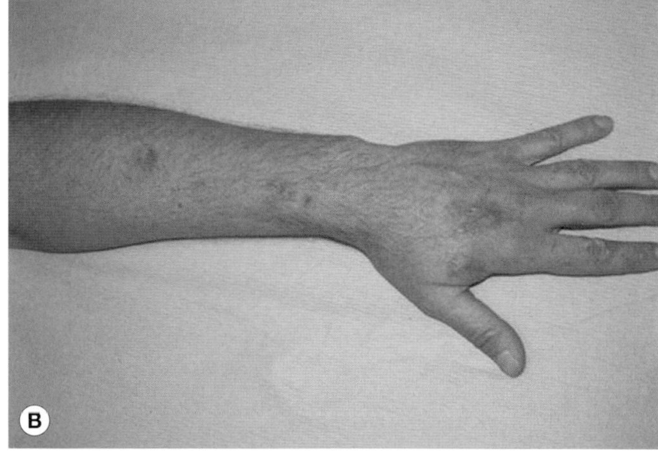

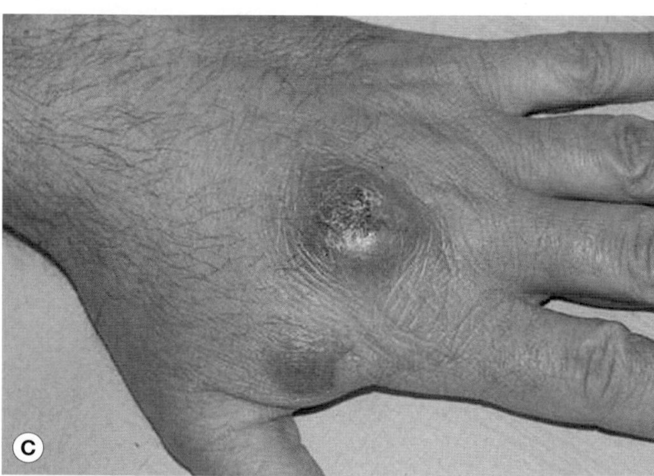

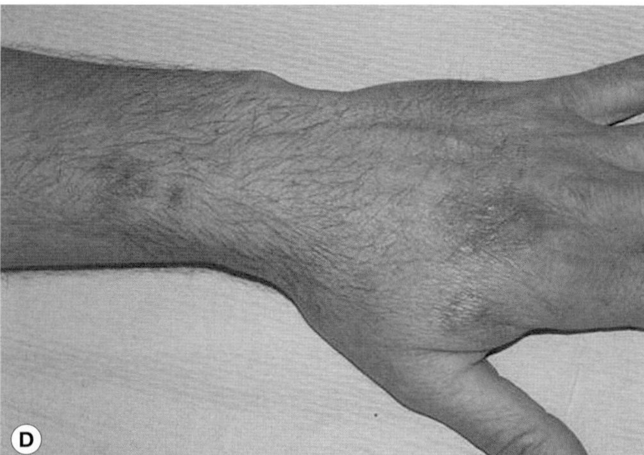

FIGURE 59.3 Fish tank granuloma erythemato-violaceous nodules before and after treatment.

60 Anthrax

Arthur M Friedlander, Nicholas J Vietri

Key features

- Anthrax is an acute bacterial zoonosis predominantly of herbivorous animals
- It is caused by *Bacillus anthracis* that persists in the environment as dormant spores and may be transmitted to humans by inoculation, inhalation, or ingestion
- The majority of naturally occurring human cases involve the skin; only very rarely are the respiratory and gastrointestinal tracts affected
- Cutaneous anthrax is characterized by the development of a papule followed by a black eschar, often surrounded by significant edema. It may be complicated by septicemia and death in 5–20% of untreated cases
- Inhalational anthrax and gastrointestinal anthrax, both characterized by regional lymphadenitis and septicemia, have a mortality rate approaching 100% if untreated and ~50% even with antimicrobial therapy and supportive care
- Vaccines are available

INTRODUCTION

Anthrax is an acute bacterial zoonosis, predominantly of herbivores, caused by *Bacillus anthracis*. Animal anthrax is rare in developed nations as a result of intensive surveillance and control. However, the disease remains endemic in animals and not uncommon in humans in many developing countries. Humans become infected after contact with infected animals or contaminated animal products by inoculation, ingestion, or inhalation. A major concern is the use of anthrax to intentionally cause disease, as occurred in 2001 with the mailing of letters containing anthrax spores.

EPIDEMIOLOGY

INCIDENCE OF HUMAN ANTHRAX

Human infection with *B. anthracis* is infrequent in developed countries. Approximately 20,000–100,000 cases of human anthrax are estimated to occur annually worldwide, although accurate figures are impossible to obtain. However, anthrax is ubiquitous in agricultural nations dependent on animal husbandry. Epidemics of human anthrax are rare. Large outbreaks of cutaneous anthrax occurred during wars in Zimbabwe in 1978–1980 and in Chad in 1988. The largest epidemic of inhalational anthrax occurred in 1979 in Sverdlovsk (Ekaterinburg), Russia resulting from the accidental release of spores from a military facility. In 2001, 22 cases of bioterrorism-related anthrax (11 inhalational) occurred after envelopes containing spores were mailed through the United States Postal Service.

ZOONOTIC ANTHRAX

Anthrax is chiefly a disease of herbivores. Animals are infected via the gastrointestinal tract by grazing on contaminated pasture and rarely by contact with other infected animals. Before death, animals often contaminate the soil with infected saliva, blood, urine, or feces. Soil, forage and, to a lesser extent, groundwater are major reservoirs of anthrax.

GEOGRAPHIC OCCURRENCE

Outbreaks are sporadic in developed nations, while disease remains endemic in parts of Africa, India, Southeast Asia, the Middle East, Greece, Albania, southern Italy, Romania, the former Soviet Union, and Central and South America (Fig. 60.1). *Bacillus anthracis* spores germinate in soil at 20–44 °C in areas with >85% humidity. Germinated bacilli are destroyed by other soil microbes. Therefore, in many tropical regions, animal anthrax occurs predominantly in the dry season, with some persistence into the wet season. It is likely that persistence in soil results from amplification caused by growth in infected animals and sporulation in animal carcasses with subsequent contamination of the soil. Vultures and non-biting flies may be responsible for dissemination of anthrax.

HUMAN ANTHRAX

Human anthrax is traced to agricultural, industrial or, rarely, laboratory acquisition. Only two cases of human-to-human transmission have been reported involving contact with a cutaneous case.

INDUSTRIALLY ACQUIRED ANTHRAX

In economically developed countries, industrial acquisition accounts for ~80% of cutaneous anthrax and almost all inhalational anthrax, and occurs predominantly among tanners or leather, hair, wool, or bone-meal fertilizer workers. Subclinical infection and seroconversion among workers in these industries may be more common than overt illness. Infections in developed countries are acquired from contaminated animal hides, hair, or bones imported from developing countries with zoonotic anthrax. Leather goods and drums from Haiti and West Africa have been vehicles of anthrax transmission. Recently, cutaneous cases have been seen in heroin addicts in the UK and Germany.

AGRICULTURAL ANTHRAX

In developed countries, contact with infected animals by farmers, butchers, and veterinarians is implicated in ~20% of cutaneous cases. Transmission by biting insects has been suspected and bone-meal fertilizer implicated in sporadic cases of inhalational anthrax among gardeners.

NATURAL HISTORY, PATHOGENESIS, AND PATHOLOGY

Anthrax bacilli are large (1.0–1.5 μm by 3–8 μm), non-motile, Gram-positive rods. Abundant in smears of blood and tissues, bacilli occur

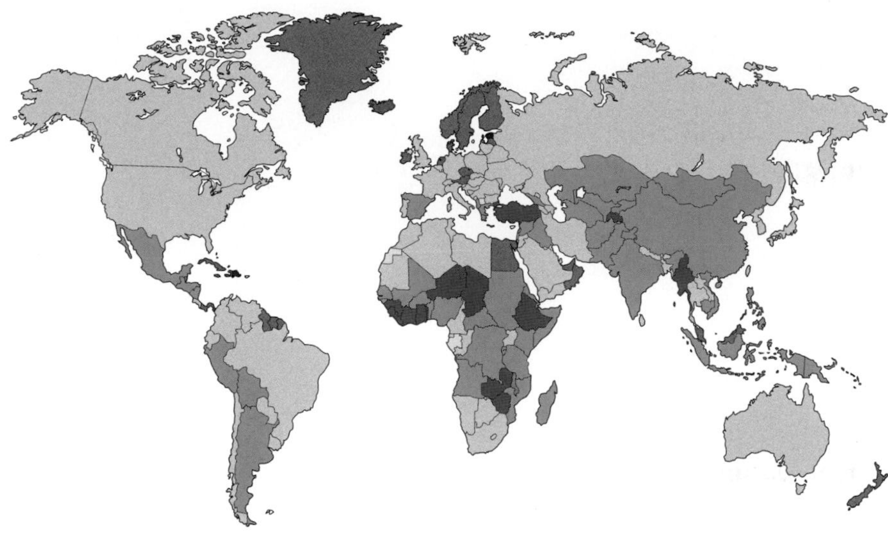

FIGURE 60.1 Geographic distribution of anthrax *(reproduced with permission from World Health Organization,* http://www.vetmed.lsu.edu/whocc/mp_world.htm*).*

singly or in short chains. *Bacillus anthracis* also develops spores in culture or soil, but not *in vivo* unless exposed to ambient air. Spores are resistant to heat and many disinfectants. They are destroyed by boiling for 10 min, dry heat (140 °C) for 3 h or autoclaving (121 °C) for 15 min, but remain viable for years in dry soil. Cattle have become infected by grazing in fields where animals died of anthrax decades before [1].

BACILLUS ANTHRACIS *VIRULENCE FACTORS*

Bacillus anthracis possesses three major virulence factors: a poly-γ-D-glutamic acid capsule and two protein exotoxins. The capsule is antiphagocytic, enabling the bacillus to resist killing by leukocytes. The anthrax toxins are composed of a eukaryotic cell receptor-binding protein and a second protein possessing cytotoxic activity. The cell receptor-binding protein protective antigen combines with edema factor, a calmodulin-dependent adenylate cyclase, to produce edema toxin or with lethal factor, a zinc metalloprotease, to produce a lethal toxin. Protective antigen is necessary for binding and translocation of the cytotoxic proteins. Edema toxin raises intracelluar levels of cyclic adenosine monophosphate (cAMP), interfering with cell function, while lethal factor inactivates mitogen-activated protein (MAP) kinases, interfering with signal transduction [2]. The toxins interfere with innate immunity, having been shown *in vitro* to impair the function of neutrophils, macrophages, lymphocytes, and dendritic cells. Additional effects of the toxins occur *in vivo* because of the fact that the toxin receptors are expressed on a wide variety of cells.

CUTANEOUS ANTHRAX

Cutaneous anthrax follows inoculation of spores into skin. Spores then germinate and the bacilli multiply and elaborate their virulence factors. Hematogenous dissemination follows in 5–20% of untreated cases. Cutaneous lesions may demonstrate satellite bullous lesions in which Gram-positive bacilli can be observed; pus is not present.

INHALATIONAL ANTHRAX

Inhalational anthrax follows the inhalation of spores of 1–5 μm in diameter. Larger particles are cleared by the mucociliary mechanism of the lungs. Spore aerosols may be encountered by workers handling contaminated batches of hair, wool, or bone-meal fertilizer. The aerosol infective dose for human infection is high – in wool mills, non-immune workers inhaled as many as 510 spores of 5 μm or less in diameter per 8-hour shift without becoming ill. Animal studies indicate that inhaled spores are ingested by alveolar phagocytes and carried to tracheobronchial and mediastinal lymph nodes. There, the spores germinate into bacilli with the production of capsule and toxins. Hemorrhagic edema and necrosis of mediastinal lymph nodes ensue. Alveoli show a hemorrhagic exudate and only rarely bacilli; neutrophils are usually absent. Alveolar capillaries contain fibrin thrombi and bacilli [3]. Hemorrhagic pleural effusions commonly occur. Hematogenous dissemination to the meninges, spleen, and intestine can occur.

GASTROINTESTINAL ANTHRAX

Oropharyngeal and intestinal anthrax follow ingestion of poorly cooked, contaminated meat [4]. An ulcer in the stomach, terminal ileum, or cecum may be present, and hemorrhage and edema of regional lymphatics occurs.

SEPTICEMIC ANTHRAX

Generalized sepsis may follow cutaneous anthrax and, almost invariably, accompanies inhalational and gastrointestinal anthrax. Vascular injury may result from the proliferation of bacteria in the blood and effects of the exotoxins acting directly on the endothelium or indirectly through other mediators. Widespread capillary thrombosis, circulatory failure, and shock occur prior to death. Adrenocortical hemorrhage can occur. In addition, anthrax bacteremia may lead to hemorrhagic meningitis. The leptomeninges reveal scant inflammation but widespread hemorrhages. The brain has hemorrhages and generalized cerebral edema. Subarachnoid hemorrhage may also occur.

CLINICAL FEATURES

CUTANEOUS ANTHRAX

Cutaneous anthrax accounts for >95% of human infections and commonly involves areas of the face, neck, hands, and arms [5]. The incubation period is 12 hours to 7 (mean 3) days. The initial lesion is a small, erythematous macule or papule. It turns brown and develops a ring of erythema and a vesicle. Vesicular satellite lesions may appear (Fig. 60.2) and, after a few days, the clear, vesicular fluid becomes blue-black from hemorrhage. The papule ulcerates, developing a black eschar by the fifth to seventh day. Non-pitting, gelatinous edema may be prominent, occasionally extending to the iliac crest from lesions of the head and neck. This so-called "malignant edema", together with a black eschar, is pathognomonic for anthrax. Patients

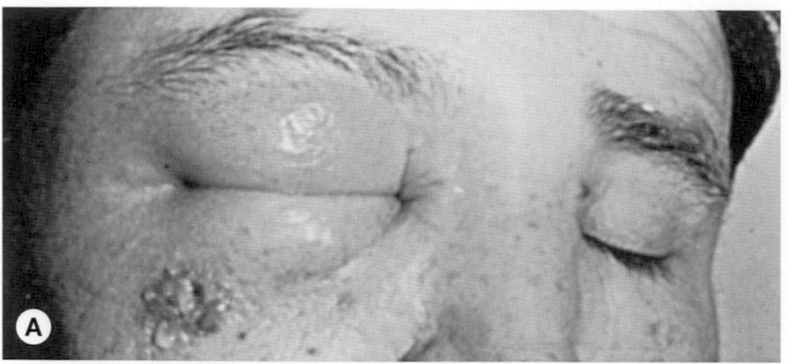

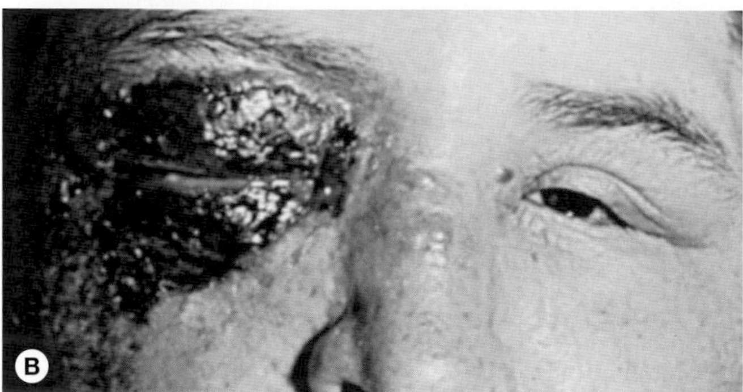

FIGURE 60.2 Cutaneous anthrax in a 45-year-old cattleman. **(A)** Early facial lesion with prominent edema and vesicular satellite lesions that revealed abundant anthrax bacilli on Gram-stain and culture. **(B)** Evolution of the cutaneous eschar despite antimicrobial therapy *(courtesy of Dr Alejandro Morales).*

have few symptoms, for example malaise, headache, and low-grade fever.

INHALATIONAL ANTHRAX

Inhalational anthrax accounts for <5% of reported cases. Nonspecific symptoms of mild fever, malaise, fatigue, and myalgia develop 1–5 days after exposure; nonproductive cough is often reported. In cases occurring in the 2001 epidemic, nausea or vomiting was common [6] and some had extreme fatigue and severe headache. Patients may have transient improvement after several days or may directly develop severe respiratory distress with cyanosis, diaphoresis, increased fever, and tachycardia. Stridor, diffuse rales, and basilar dullness may be heard. Chest radiographs reveal symmetric, characteristic mediastinal widening, pleural effusions and, in some cases, patchy infiltrates (Fig. 60.3). Massive, superficial edema of the head and neck may occur. Meningitis, often hemorrhagic, occurs in ~50% of cases. Pleural effusions may also be hemorrhagic. *Bacillus anthracis* is usually isolated in cultures of blood, pleural fluid, and cerebrospinal fluid.

GASTROINTESTINAL ANTHRAX

Oropharyngeal and gastrointestinal anthrax account for <5% of cases. Oropharyngeal anthrax presents with sore throat, an ulcer in the oral cavity, dysphagia, cervical and submandibular lymphadenopathy, and often dramatic neck edema. Gastrointestinal anthrax develops after an incubation period of 2–5 days. Patients have generalized abdominal pain, anorexia, nausea, vomiting and, in some cases, hematemesis. Severe prostration accompanies the development of ascites, bloody diarrhea, toxemia, and shock. Subcutaneous edema may extensively involve the lower trunk.

CENTRAL NERVOUS SYSTEM (CNS) ANTHRAX

Anthrax meningitis follows bacteremia from a cutaneous, pulmonary or intestinal source. Patients usually present with fever, meningismus, and rapidly deteriorating mental status. Lumbar puncture reveals spinal fluid containing Gram-positive rods and is often hemorrhagic. Bacteremia occurs in 70% of patients; the usual survival is 2–4 days.

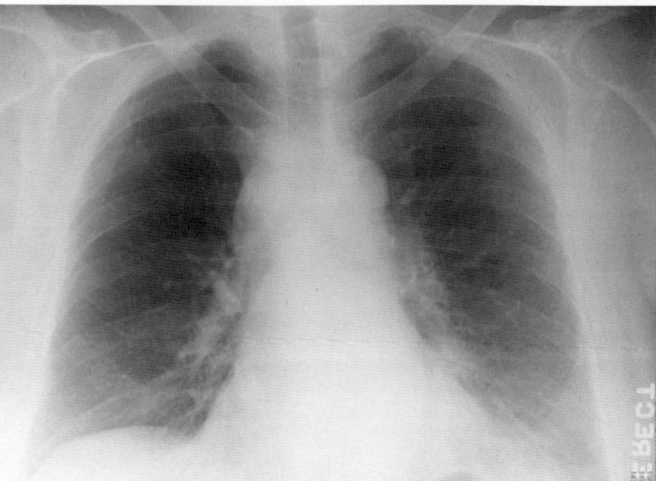

FIGURE 60.3 Chest x-ray of a case of inhalational anthrax showing mediastinal widening and a small left pleural effusion *(reproduced with permission from Jernigan JA, Stephens DS, Ashford DA, et al. Bioterrorism-related inhalational anthrax: the first 10 cases reported in the United States. Emerg Infect Dis 2001;7:933–44.)*

In very rare cases, patients present with isolated meningitis without other evidence of disease.

PATIENT EVALUATION, DIAGNOSIS, AND DIFFERENTIAL DIAGNOSIS

DIFFERENTIAL DIAGNOSIS

The epidemiologic background of an industrial or agricultural exposure, the evolution of a pruritic then painless lesion without cellulitis or lymphangitis, and the dramatic appearance of the black eschar and extensive non-pitting edema help to distinguish anthrax from other skin infections. The initial, nonspecific symptoms of inhalational anthrax may resemble influenza, bronchitis, or the common cold; however, there are no upper respiratory symptoms in inhalational anthrax [7]. The later stage may mimic congestive cardiac failure but should be suggested by mediastinal widening on chest radiographs in the setting of occupational exposure. Anthrax meningitis may be confused with other forms of bacterial meningitis or subarachnoid hemorrhage. Intestinal anthrax with fever and severe abdominal pain will only be recognized pre-surgery or premortem if the appropriate epidemiologic history is obtained.

DIRECT SMEAR AND CULTURE DIAGNOSIS

In cutaneous anthrax, encapsulated bacilli can be identified on Gram- or Giemsa-stained smears and readily cultured. Bacilli may also be abundant in cerebrospinal or pleural fluid in cases of inhalational anthrax. Direct fluorescent antibody stains for cell wall and capsule are available for definitive, early identification of *B. anthracis* from vesicular fluid, tissue or culture. On sheep blood agar, 3- to 5-mm, gray-white, opaque, rough, non-hemolytic colonies become evident within 24 h. In the presence of carbon dioxide, the organism produces a capsule and the colony is round and mucoid. Identification is confirmed immunologically by the presence of the capsule, susceptibility to specific bacteriophage and testing by PCR for toxin and capsule genes.

SEROLOGIC DIAGNOSIS

Antibody to protective antigen or capsule, measured by ELISA, develops in 67–94% of cases of cutaneous or oropharyngeal anthrax and in 100% of inhalational anthrax cases, but is only useful retrospectively. Rapid diagnostic tests for the detection of protective antigen, lethal factor, and capsule in body fluids have been developed and shown to be of value in nonhuman primate models and one human case.

TABLE 60-1 Treatment of Anthrax in Adults and Children

Cutaneous anthrax in adults*	**Inhalational, gastrointestinal or severe cutaneous anthrax in adults***
Ciprofloxacin, 500 mg PO twice daily **or** Doxycycline, 100 mg PO twice daily **or** Levofloxacin, 500 mg PO once daily	Ciprofloxacin, 400 mg IV every 12 h **or** Levofloxacin, 500 mg IV every 24 h
	plus
	one or two additional antibiotics with good CNS penetration and in vitro activity against *B. anthracis* such as rifampin, 300 mg IV every 12 h; meropenem, 2 g IV every 8 hours; ampicillin, 2 g IV every 6 h; penicillin G, 4 million units IV every 4 h; vancomycin, 15–20 mg/kg IV every 8 to 12 h **plus** clindamycin, 900 mg IV every 8 h
Cutaneous anthrax in children*	**Inhalational, gastrointestinal or severe cutaneous anthrax in children***
Ciprofloxacin, 15 mg/kg PO twice daily (max. 1 g/day) **or** Doxycycline, >8 yrs and >45 kg: 100 mg PO twice daily; >8 yrs and ≤45 kg: 2.2 mg/kg PO twice daily; ≤8 yrs: 2.2 mg/kg PO twice daily (max. 200 mg/day) **or** Levofloxacin, ≥6 months and <50 kg: 8 mg/kg PO twice daily (max. 500 mg/day); >50 kg: 500 mg PO once daily	Ciprofloxacin, 15 mg/kg IV every 12 h (max. 1 g/day) **or** Levofloxacin, ≥6 months and <50 kg: 8 mg/kg IV every 12 h (max. 500 mg/day); >50 kg: 500 mg IV every 24 h
	plus
	one or two additional antibiotics with good CNS penetration and in vitro activity against *B. anthracis* such as rifampin, 20 mg/kg IV every 24 h (max 600 mg/day); meropenem, 40 mg/kg IV every 8 h (max. 6 g/day); ampicillin, 50–100 mg/kg IV every 6 h (max. 12 g/day); penicillin G, 250,000–400,000 units/kg/day IV in divided doses every 4–6 h (max. dose 24 million units/day); vancomycin, 15 mg/kg IV every 6 h **plus** clindamycin, 25–40 mg/kg/day IV divided doses every 6–8 h

*For disease associated with a bioterrorism event, total duration of oral and IV treatment combined should be 60 days and levofloxacin should be considered a second-line antibiotic because of limited long-term safety data.

TREATMENT

Consensus treatment recommendations are available (Table 60-1) [8].

CUTANEOUS ANTHRAX

Untreated cutaneous anthrax can progress to septicemia, shock, renal failure and, in 5–20% of cases, death. Almost all cutaneous cases are cured with effective antimicrobial therapy. Treatment with oral ciprofloxacin, doxycycline, or levofloxacin for 7–10 days is recommended by the United States Centers for Disease Control and Prevention (CDC) for uncomplicated cases of naturally acquired cutaneous anthrax [8], although a recent study conducted in Turkey suggests that antibiotic treatment for 3–5 days is as effective as 7–10 days. Oral therapy with penicillin can be used for penicillin-sensitive isolates. If severe systemic symptoms, extensive edema, or lesions on the head or neck are present, intravenous therapy with ciprofloxacin for 7–10 days is preferred. For cutaneous anthrax associated with a bioterrorism attack, but without systemic symptoms, lesions on the head or neck, or extensive edema, the guidelines recommend oral ciprofloxacin or doxycycline for 60 days because of the potential exposure to airborne spores. Levofloxacin is recommended as a second-line antibiotic as a result of limited long-term safety data. Amoxicillin can be used to complete the 60-day course for penicillin-sensitive isolates. Treatment for severe cutaneous anthrax with bacteremia is the same as for inhalational and gastrointestinal anthrax, which require intravenous antibiotics as described below.

OTHER ANTHRAX SYNDROMES

Historically, the treatment for inhalational or gastrointestinal anthrax was high-dose intravenous penicillin. However, current CDC treatment guidelines for inhalational or gastrointestinal anthrax, based on experience derived from the 2001 cases, recommend a multidrug regimen of either intravenous ciprofloxacin or levofloxacin, combined with one or two additional intravenous antibiotics with penetration into the CNS and *in vitro* activity against *B. anthracis*, such as rifampin, vancomycin, meropenem, penicillin G, or ampicillin. Clindamycin is also recommended as an additional antibiotic because of its ability to rapidly inhibit protein and, presumably, toxin synthesis. A recent CDC update gives preference to ciprofloxacin or other fluoroquinolones with similar activity over doxycycline as the primary antimicrobial agent, because of the high likelihood of clinical or subclinical meningitis in patients with inhalational anthrax [8]. To complete a 60-day course of therapy, treatment can be switched to oral medicines when the patient is stable. There are no controlled-treatment studies for inhalational anthrax – the suggested 60-day course of antibiotics is based on the possible germination of retained dormant spores late after infection. While the prolonged course of antibiotics is necessary for post-exposure prophylaxis (PEP) as described below, recent studies in nonhuman primates demonstrated that a 10-day course of antibiotics is sufficient to treat established inhalational anthrax. Although historically viewed as invariably fatal, data from the 2001 inhalational anthrax cases showed that a multidrug antibiotic regimen combined with supportive therapy reduced mortality to 45% [9].

SUPPORTIVE THERAPY

The evolution of the anthrax skin lesion is not modified by antimicrobial treatment. Pleural fluid drainage was likely associated with decreased mortality in the 2001 anthrax cases.

ISOLATION OF PATIENTS

Human-to-human transmission has not been observed in inhalational or gastrointestinal anthrax. Therefore, standard infection control precautions should suffice. However, if bloody sputum is present, respiratory isolation should be instituted. Because of the potential infectious nature of an untreated cutaneous anthrax lesion or gastrointestinal anthrax, contact and secretion precautions should be used.

POST-EXPOSURE PROPHYLAXIS (PEP)

PEP requires a different therapeutic approach compared with treatment of established disease (Table 60-2). Most spores deposited into the alveolar spaces germinate within a few days. However, germination is not synchronous. Studies have demonstrated viable spores in the lungs of rhesus macaques 100 days after exposure and anthrax has occurred several months after exposure in animals given antibiotics for short periods. As spores can remain dormant for long periods and antibiotics act only after spores have germinated, PEP to prevent disease from dormant spores that may subsequently germinate requires either a prolonged course of antibiotics or antibiotics plus vaccination. The current CDC recommendation for PEP for exposure to aerosolized *B. anthracis* spores is 60 days of oral antibiotics combined with anthrax vaccine (BioThrax) 0.5 ml given subcutaneously at 0, 2 and 4 weeks [10]. Antibiotics recommended for PEP include ciprofloxacin or doxycycline. Levofloxacin is recommended as a second-line antibiotic owing to limited long-term safety data. Penicillin should not be used presumptively for PEP of anthrax. Although not US Food and Drug Administration (FDA)-approved, amoxicillin can be used to complete the 60-day course of therapy once the strain is proven to be penicillin-susceptible. Other antibiotics to be considered for off-label use in patients unable to tolerate first-line antibiotics include other fluoroquinolones, clindamycin, rifampin, and chloramphenicol [8].

TABLE 60-2 Post-exposure Prophylaxis after *Bacillus anthracis* Exposure in Adults and Children*

Adults
Ciprofloxacin, 500 mg PO twice daily **or** Doxycycline, 100 mg PO twice daily **or** If intolerant to ciprofloxacin or doxycycline, use levofloxacin, 500 mg PO once daily
Children
Ciprofloxacin: 15 mg/kg PO twice daily (max. 1 g/day) **or** Doxycycline, >8 yrs and >45 kg: 100 mg PO twice daily; >8 yrs and ≤45 kg: 2.2 mg/kg PO twice daily; ≤8 yrs: 2.2 mg/kg PO twice daily (max. 200 mg/day) **or** If intolerant to ciprofloxacin or doxycycline, use levofloxacin, ≥6 months and <50 kg: 8 mg/kg PO twice daily (max. 500 mg/day); >50 kg: 500 mg PO once daily
Once the organism is shown to be susceptible to penicillin, amoxicillin 15 mg/kg PO three times daily (max. 1500 mg/day) can be used

*The PEP antimicrobial regimen should continue for 60 days, combined with three doses of anthrax vaccine (BioThrax).

REFERENCES

1. Turnbull PCB. Anthrax in Humans and Animals, 4th edn. Geneva: World Health Organization; 2008.
2. Montecucco C, Mock M. Anthrax. Mol Aspects Med 2009;30:345–6.
3. Grinberg LM, Abramova FA, Yampolskaya OV, et al. Quantitative pathology of inhalational anthrax I: quantitative microscopic findings. Mod Pathol 2001;14:482–95.
4. Kunanusont C, Limpakarnjanarat K, Foy HM. Outbreak of anthrax in Thailand. Ann Trop Med Parasitol 1990;84:507–12.
5. Friedlander AM. Anthrax – Clinical features, pathogenesis, and potential biological warfare threat. In: Remington JS, Swartz MN, eds. Current Clinical Topics in Infectious Diseases. Malden: Blackwell Science; 2000:335.
6. Jernigan JA, Stephens DS, Ashford DA, et al. Bioterrorism-related inhalational anthrax: the first 10 cases reported in the United States. Emerg Infect Dis 2001;7:933–44.
7. Kuehnert MJ, Dolye TJ, Hill HA. Clinical features that discriminate inhalational anthrax from other acute respiratory illnesses. Clin Infect Dis 2003;36:328–36.
8. Stern EJ, Uhde KB, Shadomy SV, et al. Conference report on public health and clinical guidelines for anthrax. Emerg Infect Dis 2008;14:e1.
9. Holty JE, Bravata DM, Lui H, et al. Systematic review: a century of inhalational anthrax cases from 1900 to 2005. Ann Intern Med 2006;144:270–80.
10. Centers for Disease Control and Prevention. Use of anthrax vaccine in the United States. Recommendations on the Advisory Committee on Immunization Practices (ACIP), 2009. MMWR 2010;59(No. RR-6):1–29.

SECTION

G

FEBRILE SYSTEMIC SYNDROMES WITH OR WITHOUT LYMPHADENOPATHY

61 Epidemic Louse-borne Typhus

Aurélié Renvoise, Didier Raoult

Key features

- The etiological agent of epidemic louse-borne typhus is *Rickettsia prowazekii*
- Epidemic typhus is transmitted by body lice and largely affects impoverished or displaced people
- Epidemic typhus manifests as an acute febrile illness with headache and myalgia. Neurologic manifestations, rash, vasculitis, and gangrene of extremities can occur. In untreated cases, mortality is high
- Diagnosis is usually based on clinical suspicion, especially in the right epidemiologic situation. Serology is available
- Treatment is simple, safe and inexpensive, and usually involves a single 200-mg dose or short course of doxycycline
- Relapses years after initial infection are termed Brill-Zinsser disease
- Synonyms: epidemic typhus, louse-borne typhus, exanthematic typhus, jail fever
- Control efforts should focus on de-lousing both individuals and populations and providing hygienic conditions

INTRODUCTION

Epidemic typhus is transmitted by human body lice from infected patients (during acute infection or relapse) to naïve people. It is one of the major threats to public health during civil unrest, displacement, and war. Typhus has probably caused more deaths than wars in the history of humanity; it remains a permanent public health problem, as poor sanitary conditions can lead to epidemic outbreaks, such as in Burundi in 1997 [1].

Epidemic typhus may have been the cause of the Athens plague described by Thucydides, but it may also have been typhoid fever. The first account of typhus may have been recorded during the civil wars of Grenada 1489–90. In 1739, Huxham made the first distinction between typhus and typhoid; in 1760 Boissier de Sauvage quoted the name "typhus", which is Greek for "smokey/cloudy", and refers to the mental status changes associated with typhus. "Typhoid" was an illness that had many features of typhus, but was distinct. In 1909, Charles Nicolle showed the role of body lice in the transmission of epidemic typhus; in 1910, Brill described the recrudescent form; finally, in 1916, Rocha Lima described the bacterium and named it *Rickettsia prowazekii* in honor of previous researchers who both died of typhus [2].

EPIDEMIOLOGY

Epidemic typhus has been traditionally associated with wars and other catastrophic conditions that lead to poor sanitary conditions with lice infestation. It has been described as a disease of the highlands, cold areas, poverty, imprisonment and civil unrest, when people are forced to repetitively wear the same clothing, often in crowded and unhygienic conditions; however, epidemic typhus has a potentially worldwide repartition. Incidence of epidemic typhus is highest in colder months (it mainly occurs during the winter and spring). Men and women are equally affected [3]. Brill-Zinsser disease (the relapsing form of the disease) can occur up to 40 years after primary infection under stress conditions or in immunocompromised hosts. Sylvatic forms associated with flying squirrels and the presence of *R. prowazekii* in ticks suggest that reservoirs and transmission dynamics of *R. prowazekii* are more complex than previously described [4].

In 1997, a large outbreak of typhus was reported in Burundi during the civil war; 100,000 people were estimated to be infected and the case fatality rate was 15% [1]. Small outbreaks and sporadic cases have also been reported in different regions of the world since 1997, including Russia, Peru, Northern Africa, the USA, and France (Fig. 61.1). This highlights the persistent threat of epidemic typhus. Eradication of epidemic typhus appears to be difficult because of possible recrudescence of *R. prowazekii* in infested people which is associated with Brill-Zinsser disease, and the unknown contribution of nonhuman reservoirs.

NATURAL HISTORY, PATHOGENESIS, AND PATHOLOGY

In1909, Charles Nicolle observed the role of the body louse *Pediculus humanus* subsp. *corporis* (or *P. humanus* subsp. *humanus*) in the transmission of epidemic typhus. Lice become infected when feeding on the blood of a bacteremic patient. Transmission between human hosts is associated with close human contacts; primary infection occurs when *R. prowazekii* is transmitted from the vector to the host, not by louse bites, but by contamination of bite sites, conjunctivae and mucous membranes (including the respiratory tract) with the infectious feces or crushed bodies of infected lice. These infested aerosols constitute a source of infection of typhus for clinicians in contact with lice-infested patients. In the case of Brill-Zinsser disease, recrudescent infection of the human host is associated with bacteremia; if louse infestation of the patient occurs at the same time, lice become infected through host feeding and, if appropriate conditions exist, an outbreak can occur [3].

It was previously thought that humans were the only reservoir of *R. prowazekii* and human body lice the only vectors. But since the 1950s, specific antibodies have been detected in, and the bacterium isolated from, several domestic and wild animals. Ticks might be a reservoir for *R. prowazekii*, as *Amblyomma* spp. and *Hyalomma* spp. were found to be infected in Mexico and Ethiopia, respectively [3]. Of particular

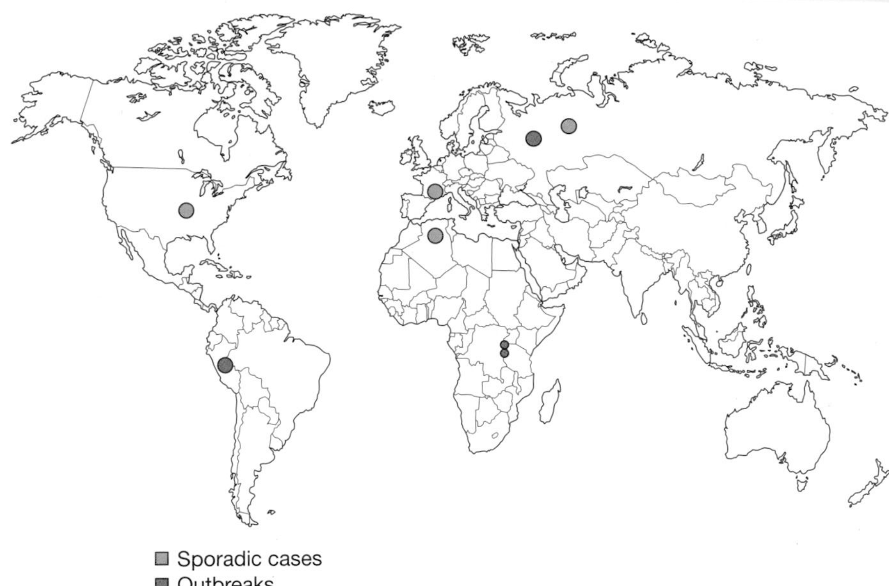

FIGURE 61.1 Cases of epidemic typhus reported in the world since 1997.

interest is the reservoir formed by flying squirrels (*Glaucomys volans*). Reported cases of epidemic typhus in the USA have been associated with contact with flying squirrels [4]. The role of animal reservoirs in the global burden of typhus is currently not well-defined. After entering the body of an infected human, the bacteria spread through blood and lymph, then they infect endothelial cells of the small capillaries. Rickettsial infection leads to endothelial damage, which is associated with widespread vasculitis; the clinical signs and symptoms relate to the affected organs. Endothelial injury can also lead to micro- and macroscopic foci of hemorrhages. Vasculitis can also be associated with thrombi in small vessels and surrounding inflammatory infiltrates. These correspond to typhus nodules and may occur focally throughout the central nervous system (CNS); these lesions explain the neurologic features commonly associated with epidemic typhus [3]. The vasculitis of *R. prowazekii* infection is generalized and, thus, any organ may be involved.

CLINICAL FEATURES

Clinical features of epidemic typhus are nonspecific and consequently not easy to differentiate from other infectious processes. The incubation period is usually 10–14 days, but may be as short as 6 days. A prodromal malaise may pre-date the onset of fever by 1–3 days. Onset of typhus is usually abrupt and manifested by fever (which continues until death or recovery), severe headaches, severe myalgias, abdominal pain, arthralgias, malaise, anorexia, chills, photophobia, and nonproductive cough. Facial flushing and conjunctival suffusion can occur, as can nausea, vomiting, diarrhea, or constipation. During a 1997 outbreak in Burundi [1], a crouching attitude named "sutama" was reported, caused by myalgia and severe fatigue.

In untreated cases, as the illness progresses, neurologic manifestations become more common. In up to 80% of untreated cases, CNS manifestations, such as delirium that interrupts stupor, coma, seizures, and hearing loss, can occur. Rash is often present, although difficult to discern in individuals with dark skin. The rash is initially nonconfluent, with erythematous and blanching areas; macules, petechiae, and purpura can occur. It begins on the trunk and the axilla and may spread centrifugally. It is not found on the face, palms, or soles, except in severely ill patients. In mild cases, it may fade in 1 or 2 days. Cough is reported in 38–70% of patients. Primary pulmonary involvement, as well as secondary bacterial pneumonia, can occur during epidemic typhus. In severe cases, symptoms secondary to vasculitis can provoke cerebral thrombosis, gangrene (that can require amputation), and multiple organ dysfunction, shock, and death [3].

Prior to the development of antimicrobial treatment, mortality could reach 60%. With appropriate antibiotics, mortality of approximately 4% is now common. Severity is associated with malnutrition and advanced age.

Brill-Zinsser disease usually occurs with advancing age and waning immunity. Cases are sporadic and unrelated to recent louse infestation. Compared with acute infection, Brill-Zinsser disease is shorter and its clinical features are usually mild, although fatal cases can occur. Rashes are reported to be less frequent.

Cases of typhus related to flying squirrels are sporadic. These cases may clinically present as meningitis. This form of typhus is poorly understood.

PATIENT EVALUATION, DIAGNOSIS, AND DIFFERENTIAL DIAGNOSIS

Clinical diagnosis of sporadic cases is difficult, although clinically diagnosing a compatible case during a known epidemic is less uncertain. Taken in isolation, differentiating the clinical signs of typhus from those of other infections is not easy. This underscores the importance of obtaining a thorough history of animal and lice or arthropod contact in patients with acute febrile illness. However, a cluster of sudden onset of severe pyrexia among louse-infested people living in cold, crowded and unhygienic conditions should immediately alert the clinician to possible typhus. Any severe outbreak of unexplained fever in unhygienic environments should also evoke consideration of epidemic typhus.

The main differential diagnoses that should be considered when considering louse-borne typhus are typhoid (these diagnoses have been clinically confused for centuries), murine typhus, other riskettsioses, malaria, and hemorrhagic fevers. Finally, lice transmit three diseases which must be suspected in case of fever in louse-infested patients as they can occur simultaneously [1]: relapsing fever, trench fever, and epidemic typhus. The fever pattern in epidemic typhus is daily or continuous, while in the other two entities it is often more cyclical.

Laboratory findings during epidemic typhus include thrombocytopenia (40% of cases), increased hepatic transaminase activity (up to 60%; although jaundice is rare), hyperbilirubinemia (20%) and increased blood urea nitrogen concentrations (31%). Oliguria and proteinuria are common. In the early phase, leukopenia can be observed.

The reference method for diagnosis is serologic testing using an indirect immunofluorescence assay. Fresh blood, as well as blood dried on blotting paper, can be used. Both acute- and convalescent-phase serum should be assayed. However, there is cross-reactivity mainly with *R. typhi*. Western blotting with cross-adsorption is required to differentiate between these typhus group *Rickettsia* and to diagnose epidemic typhus rather than endemic typhus. It is also difficult to differentiate between primary infection and Brill-Zinsser disease solely based on serologic results. Usually in Brill-Zinsser disease, no specific IgM are recovered, but the diagnosis cannot solely be based on this feature [3].

Cell culture can be used to isolate *R. prowazekii* from samples, but this approach is not clinically practical and requires Biosafety Level-3 laboratories with an experienced staff. Molecular detection of *R. prowazekii* has been developed and is becoming increasingly clinically useful. Real-time PCR assays are especially useful, because they are rapid, sensitive and specific [5]. Molecular detection can be performed on several types of human samples (blood, skin biopsy, etc.) and also on lice (that can be sent dry or in alcohol). The latter approach can be particularly helpful in cases of possible typhus outbreaks because detection of rickettsial DNA in lice can indicate extant human typhus (*R. prowazekii* is pathogenic for lice and provokes rapid death of lice, therefore if rickettsial DNA is detected in lice, it corresponds to an active and extensive outbreak).

TREATMENT

The treatment of typhus is safe, easy and inexpensive. A single dose of 200 mg of orally administered doxycycline will usually cure patients [6]. Early administration must be prescribed in any suspected case without waiting for laboratory confirmation. The absence of clinical response within 2–3 days of treatment strongly argues against louse-borne typhus. A 5-day therapy or a therapy lasting for 2–4 days after defervescence is often administered to preclude relapses. For Brill-Zinsser disease, doxycycline is also the recommended treatment. A single dose or short course of doxycycline in young children poses only a small risk of teeth staining, but that risk needs to be weighed against high mortality associated with advanced disease (Box 61.1). If an alternative is required, chloramphenicol is usually the recommended treatment. Doxycycline can be used intravenously or intramuscularly in case of clinical severity or if oral course is impossible. Ciprofloxacine must be avoided; indeed a patient misdiagnosed as having typhoid, died from typhus after this treatment, in spite of its *in vitro* efficiency.

In association with antibiotic treatment, de-lousing is a critical control measure, but quarantine is not necessary. Eradication of lice can be performed with an insecticide (by washing clothing and bedding with soap containing 7% dichlorodiphenyltrichloroethane [DDT]); clothing can also be washed in water hotter than 60°C and then ironed; if the previous measures are not possible, clothes must be removed and left unworn for a week, as lice die 5 days after being deprived of blood. Effective prevention also requires the application of basic hygiene and sanitary conditions. Nevertheless, it must be highlighted that de-lousing is not sufficient for eradication of epidemic typhus, because infected individuals retain *R. prowazekii* for the rest of their lives and can therefore initiate new outbreaks if a bacteremia concomitant to lice infestation occurs.

BOX 61.1 Pediatric Box

The standard regimen treatment for children is a single 100-mg doxycycline dose. Any suspected case should be treated immediately. A single dose or short course of doxycycline in young children poses only a small risk of teeth staining, and that risk needs to be weighed against the high mortality associated with advanced disease. No particular clinical or epidemiologic feature distinguishes epidemic typhus in children from that in adults.

When dealing with control at a population level, a preferred method is the blowing of insecticidal powder between humans and their underclothes, following World Health Organization (WHO) recommendations. For example, talcum powder can be used with permethrin (0.5%), DDT (10%), or lindane (1%). Application can be performed with any kind of dusting apparatus or by hand; 30–50 g of dust per person is usually needed and is blown through neck openings, up the sleeves, from all sides of the loosened waist and also into socks, headwear, and bedding. Usually one treatment is sufficient, but re-treatment may be required if infestation persists [7]. Doxycycline must be prescribed in any suspected case.

Vaccines against epidemic typhus have existed since 1920. The attenuated strain *R. prowazekii* Madrid E has been used as a vaccine; however, the limited market for vaccine and the efficacy of antibiotic treatment and other control strategies have limited vaccine development and usage. There is currently no commercially available vaccine for epidemic typhus.

REFERENCES

1. Raoult D, Ndihokubwayo JB, Tissot-Dupont H, et al. Outbreak of epidemic typhus associated with trench fever in Burundi. Lancet 1998;352:353–8.
2. Socolovschi C, Raoult D. Typhus fevers and other rickettsial diseases, Historical. In: Encyclopedia of Microbiology. Elsevier; 2009:100–20.
3. Bechah Y, Capo C, Mege JL, Raoult D. Epidemic typhus. Lancet Infect Dis 2008;8:417–26.
4. Reynolds MG, Krebs JS, Comer JA, et al. Flying squirrel-associated typhus, United States. Emerg Infect Dis 2003;9:1341–3.
5. Svraka S, Rolain JM, Bechah Y, et al. Rickettsia prowazekii and real-time polymerase chain reaction. Emerg Infect Dis 2006;12:428–32.
6. Krause DW, Perine PL, McDade JE, Awoke S. Treatment of louse-borne typhus fever with chloramphenicol, tetracycline or doxycycline. East Afr Med J 1975; 52:421–7.
7. WHO control measures: www.who.int/entity/water_sanitation_health/resources/vector262to287.pdf/.

Murine Typhus 62

Achilleas Gikas

Key features

- Synonyms: flea-borne typhus, endemic typhus
- Epidemiology: worldwide distribution, incidence affected by rat and flea population and climate
- Main pathogenic mechanism: systemic inflammatory vasculitis
- Common clinical characteristics: fever, headache, and rash
- Common laboratory abnormalities: liver enzymes elevation, hypoalbuminemia
- Disease outcome: usually favorable – low rate of complications and mortality
- Treatment: doxycycline, chloramphenicol
- Prevention: rodent-control programs

INTRODUCTION

Murine typhus is caused by an obligate intracellular Gram-negative organism, *Rickettsia typhi*, which is transmitted to humans from rodents through fleas, mainly the rat flea *Xenopsylla cheopis*. The isolation of *R. typhi* and the recognition of its lifecycle were not made until the first decades of the 20th century. Subsequent studies confirmed the worldwide presence of murine typhus. The disease is common in temperate and subtropical coastal regions during warm periods of the year, primarily in areas with low sanitation and where there is close proximity between rats and man. Although considered endemic in several countries, the nonspecific clinical features make it difficult to estimate the true incidence of the disease. The disease usually has a mild course with a low mortality rate.

EPIDEMIOLOGY

The principal vector of *R. typhi* is the rat flea *X. cheopis* [1], but the cat flea *Ctenocephalides felis*, the mouse flea *Leptopsyllia segnis*, and lice, mites, and ticks have also been implicated [1, 2]. The infection of the flea is lifelong [1–3]. The primary reservoirs are the urban rats *Rattus norvegicus* and *Rattus rattus* [1], but occasional hosts include house mice, cats, opossums, shrews, and skunks [1]. Humans are considered as accidental hosts of *R. typhi*.

The flea becomes infected after ingesting blood from an infected vertebrate host. Rickettsiae multiply in the epithelial cells of the midgut and are excreted with the feces [1, 2]. Human contamination happens when the flea is feeding on a human host. The irritation of the flea bite causes the host to scratch. In this way, rickettsia from the feces of the flea are inoculated through the skin. Other routes of infection are through the conjunctiva and via inhalation [1, 2].

On a global scale, a higher prevalence of murine typhus is recorded in warmer regions [2]. The disease is considered endemic in Mediterranean countries, in several African countries, and in Southeast Asia, mostly in areas with large rat populations [1, 3, 4]. Most cases occur late in summer or in early autumn owing to the abundance of the vector fleas [1, 5]. Rat and flea populations are directly associated with the incidence of murine typhus [1, 6]. The true incidence of the disease is probably underestimated because of its benign and nonspecific clinical presentation [2].

NATURAL HISTORY, PATHOGENESIS, AND PATHOLOGY

A number of rickettsial genes are involved in the pathogenesis of murine typhus, including hemolysins and genes involved in intracellular survival [7].

In the initial stages of infection, the rickettsiae adhere to a protein-dependent receptor on the host-cell membrane and enter the cell through induced phagocytosis [8]. The bacterium then escapes phagolysosomal fusion and acquires the essential nutrients for its multiplication in the cytosol, avoiding intracellular host-defensive mechanisms [8]. Cell membrane lysis releases the rickettsiae into the bloodstream, leading to the infection of vascular endothelial cells. Disseminated vasculitis of almost every organ can result. Pathologic examination reveals vascular injury, lymphohistiocytic inflammatory vasculitis, and increased vascular permeability with hemorrhages and petechiae affecting almost every organ, leading to interstitial pneumonitis, interstitial myocarditis, interstitial nephritis, portal triaditis, gastrointestinal tract vasculitis, and meningitis [3, 4, 9, 10].

CLINICAL FEATURES

After an incubation period of 6–14 days, the disease has an abrupt presentation [11]. Although the classic triad of fever, headache, and rash may raise suspicion, the nonspecificity of symptoms and variability in clinical manifestations often hamper early diagnosis. In general, the most common clinical features of murine typhus are fever, headache, chills, rash, malaise, anorexia, and myalgias. Other, less common features include nonproductive cough, conjuctivitis, hepatomegaly and/or splenomegaly, mild gastrointestinal disorders, and central nervous system (CNS) abnormalities [5, 6, 11, 12]. Appearance of rash varies throughout the clinical course after fever onset. The rash is mostly macular or maculopapular, papular, and rarely petechial or morbilliform, and is mainly encountered on the trunk. Presence on the palms, soles, or face is rare [5, 11].

The clinical course of murine typhus is usually mild [5]. However, in severe cases, any organ may be affected. The most frequent complication is renal insufficiency, which can be life-threatening in patients with G6PD insufficiency [13]. Other complications include CNS disorders (mental confusion, seizures, stupor, prostration, and lethargy), liver dysfunction (jaundice), pulmonary complications (pleural effusion, respiratory failure), cardiac dysfunction (benign electrocardiographic abnormalities), disseminated intravascular coagulation, and shock.

Mortality without treatment is very low (<5%); recovery usually occurs within 2–3 weeks, particularly in uncomplicated cases [5, 6, 14].

PATIENT EVALUATION, DIAGNOSIS, AND DIFFERENTIAL DIAGNOSIS

As the clinical features of the disease are nonspecific, murine typhus should be considered in a febrile patient with headache, a macular or maculopapular rash on the trunk, malaise, myalgias and related epidemiologic information, such as recent contact with animals – either directly with wild animals (mainly rats) or with pets that have been exposed to wild animals – exposure to fleas and/or residence in an area with a high prevalence of endemic typhus [2, 4, 6].

The primary laboratory findings are mildly elevated liver enzymes, elevated lactate dehydrogenase levels, and hypoalbuminemia [5, 6]. Other biochemical abnormalities include increased creatinine phosphokinase and alkaline phosphatase levels, and mild hyponatremia. Hematologic abnormalities mainly consist of thrombocytopenia, mild anemia, and leukopenia in the early stages of the disease [5, 6]. Hematuria may be present.

Diagnosis of *R. typhi* infection is confirmed through specific serologic and/or molecular methods. The indirect immunofluorescence assay (IFA) is currently the reference serologic test in most laboratories [15, 16]. With a high sensitivity and specificity, IgG and IgM antibodies can be detected 7–15 days after disease onset [15]. According to the Unité des Rickettsies (Marseille, France), diagnosis requires an IFA titer equal to or greater than >1:64 for IgG and/or >1:32 for IgM, or a fourfold rise in antibody titer to *R. typhi* antigen in acute- and convalescent-phase specimens, ideally taken 2 and 4 weeks after disease onset, respectively [15, 16]. Molecular methods are based on DNA amplification of various rickettsial genes and require an adequately equipped laboratory. PCR can give a positive result before seroconversion, and is considered the technique of choice for diagnosing early disease [15, 16].

Murine typhus should be differentiated from epidemic typhus (*R. prowazekii* infection), Rocky Mountain spotted fever, ehrlichiosis and anaplasmosis, meningococcemia, malaria, Kawasaki disease, measles, typhoid fever, viral hemorrhagic fever, secondary syphilis, leptospirosis, and toxic shock syndrome.

PEDIATRIC CONSIDERATIONS

The classic triad of symptoms, observed in adults, is not as common in children [17, 18]. The main characteristics of the disease in children include fever, rash, anorexia, and hepatosplenomegaly, accompanied by increased liver enzymes, pulmonary infiltrates on radiography, thrombocytopenia, and leukopenia. Complications are rare and, although duration is longer than in adults, disease outcome is still favorable [17, 18].

TREATMENT

The principal treatment regimens for murine typhus in adults are illustrated in Table 62-1. Antibiotics that are considered effective to treat patients with endemic typhus are doxycycline and chloramphenicol. Ciprofloxacin has been administered to a small number of patients with controversial results [19–22].

TREATMENT CONSIDERATIONS IN CHILDREN

Doxycycline is the drug of choice for children, as the risk of teeth discoloration in children younger than 8 years old is minimal when treatment duration is 7–10 days [20]. Dosage is 5 mg/kg/day in 2 doses up to a maximum 100 mg per dose [23].

Chloramphenicol could be a potential alternative in severe cases, taking into account the risk of aplastic anemia. Dosage is 150/mg/kg/day [23].

TABLE 62-1 Principal Treatment Regimens for Murine Typhus in Adults

Antibiotic	Dosage and duration	Comments
Doxycycline	Adults: 100 mg orally every 12 hours Duration of 7–15 days, or at least 48 hours after defervescence [23]	The most efficient antibiotic against *R. typhi in vitro* [24] Defervescence within mean 2.9 days [19] Drug of choice for nonpregnant adults
Chloramphenicol	50 mg/kg/day orally or intravenously in 4 doses, up to 2 g /day. Duration until 4–5 days after defervescence .	Alternative when doxycycline is contraindicated [19] Drug of choice for pregnant, but not for parturient (risk of gray baby syndrome) Defervescence within mean of 4 days [19] Risk of fatal aplastic anemia [23]
Ciprofloxacin	500 mg orally or intravenously every 12 hours	Effective *in vitro* Used on a small number of patients, with controversial results [7,20–22] Defervescence within mean 4.2 days [19]

PREVENTION

Murine typhus is best prevented through rodent and flea control measures. These measures include eliminating rodents from food depots, granaries, and residences with rodenticides, rat trapping, and dusting harborages with carbaryl or permethrin for flea control [3].

A useful way to ensure early diagnosis of murine typhus is to increase medical awareness in areas known to be endemic. Suspected cases should be reported to local health authorities because of the risk of epidemic spread.

A vaccine is not available for murine typhus.

REFERENCES

1. Azad AF. Epidemiology of murine typhus. Annu Rev Entomol 1990;35:553–69.
2. Raoult D, Roux V. Rickettsioses as paradigms of new or emerging infectious diseases. Clin Microbiol Rev 1997;10:694–719.
3. Dumler JS, Walker DH. *Rickettsia typhi* (murine typhus). In: Mandell GL, Bennett JE, Dolin R, eds. Principle and Practice of Infectious Diseases, 5th edn. Philadelphia: Churchill-Livingstone; 2000:2053–5.
4. Baxter J. The typhus group. Clin Dermatol 1996;14:271–5.
5. Dumler JS, Taylor JP, Walker DH. Clinical and laboratory features of murine typhus in Texas, 1980 through 1987. J Am Med Assoc 1991;266:1365–70.
6. Gikas A, Doukakis S, Pediaditis IJ, et al. Murine typhus in Greece: epidemiological, clinical, and therapeutic data from 83 cases. Trans R Soc Trop Med Hyg 2002;96:250–3.
7. McLeod MP, Qin X, Karpathy SE, et al. Complete genome sequence of *Rickettsia typhi* and comparison with sequences of other rickettsiae. J Bacteriol 2004;186:5842–55.
8. Walker DH, Valbuena GA, Olano JP. Pathogenic mechanisms of diseases caused by Rickettsia. Ann NY Acad Sci 2003;990:1–11.

9. Walker DH, Parks FM, Betz TG, et al. Histopathology and immunohistologic demonstration of the distribution of Rickettsia typhi in fatal murine typhus. Am J Clin Pathol 1989;91:720.
10. Binford CH, Ecker HD. Endemic (murine) typhus: report of autopsy findings in three cases. Am J Clin Pathol 1947;17:797–806.
11. Betz TG, Rawlings JA, Taylor JP, Davis BL. Endemic typhus in Texas. Tex Med 1983;79:48–53.
12. Tselentis Y, Babalis U, Chrysanthis D, et al. Clinicoepidemiological study of murine typhus on the Greek island of Evia. Eur J Epidemiol 1992;8:268–72.
13. Whelton A, Donadio JV Jr, Elisberg BL. Acute renal failure complicating rickettsial infections in glucose-6-phosphate dehydrogenase-deficient individuals. Ann Intern Med 1968;69:323.
14. Stuart BM, Pullen RL. Endemic (murine) typhus fever: clinical observations of 180 cases. Ann Intern Med 1945;23: 520–36.
15. La Scola B, Raoult D. Laboratory diagnosis of rickettsiosis: current approaches to diagnosis of old and new rickettsial diseases. J Clin Microbiol 1997;35: 2715–27.
16. Brouqui P, Bacellar F, Baranton G, et al. ESCMID Study Group on Coxiella, Anaplasma, Rickettsia and Bartonella; European Network for Surveillance of Tick-Borne Diseases. Guidelines for the diagnosis of tick-borne bacterial diseases in Europe. Clin Microbiol Infect 2004;12:1108–32.
17. Whiteford SF, Taylor JP, Dumler JS. Clinical, laboratory, and epidemiologic features of murine typhus in 97 Texas children. Arch Pediatr Adolesc Med 2001;155:396.
18. Gikas A, Kokkini S, Tsioutis C, et al. Murine typhus in children: Clinical and laboratory features from 41 cases in Crete, Greece. Clin Microbiol Infect 2009;15(suppl. 2):211–12.
19. Gikas A, Doukakis S, Pediaditis J, et al. Comparison of the effectiveness of five different antibiotic regimens on infection with *Rickettsia typhi*: therapeutic data from 87 cases. Am J Trop Med Hyg 2004;70:576–9.
20. Laferl H, Fournier PE, Seiberl G, et al. Murine typhus poorly responsive to ciprofloxacin: a case report. J Travel Med 2002;9:103–4.
21. Strand O, Stromberg A. Ciprofloxacin treatment of murine typhus. Scand J Infect Dis 1990;22:503–4.
22. Committee on Infectious Diseases of the American Academy of Pediatrics. Report of the Committee on Infectious Diseases. American Academy of Pediatrics, 22nd edn. Elk Grove Village; 1991:407.
23. Raoult D, Drancourt M. Antimicrobial therapy of rickettsial diseases. Antimicrob Agents Chemother 1991;35:2457–62.
24. Rolain JM, Stuhl L, Maurin M, Raoult D. Evaluation of antibiotic susceptibilities of three rickettsial species including Rickettsia felis by a quantitative PCR DNA assay. Antimicrob Agents Chemother 2002;46(9):2747–2751.

63 Scrub Typhus

Paul N Newton, Nicholas PJ Day

Key features

- Common, but under-recognized, cause of undifferentiated fever in Asia and Australia caused by *Orientia tsutsugamushi*, with some one billion people at risk
- May also cause severe disease, such as meningoencephalitis, pneumonitis, jaundice, hypotensive shock, and death
- Transmitted by the bite of larval trombiculid mites (chiggers) in a wider diversity of habitats than "scrub" suggests
- Can be difficult to diagnose clinically; laboratory tests are inadequate
- There is evidence for tetracycline- and chloramphenicol-resistant *O. tsutsugamushi* in northern Thailand. Elsewhere, tetracyclines, chloramphenicol, and rifampicin appear efficacious
- Synonyms: tsutsugamushi disease, chigger-borne rickettsiosis

INTRODUCTION

Scrub typhus was described in Japan in the 1800s and then in Malaysia in the 1920s, where it was distinguished from murine typhus. It was a major clinical problem in many Asian theaters of the Second World War and the Indochina Wars [1]. Management was transformed by chloramphenicol and tetracyclines. It remains a major, under-appreciated cause of undifferentiated fever in Asia. Diagnosis is greatly hampered by the lack of accurate and accessible laboratory diagnosis. Given the large populations of India and China, the numbers potentially exposed are enormous. With the growth of eco-tourism in Asia, more travelers are returning to non-endemic areas with this disease.

EPIDEMIOLOGY

Scrub typhus occurs in the most populous rural areas of the world – across 13,000,000 km^2 from the Pacific rim, Southeast Asia, northern Australia and Northeast Asia across South and Central Asia as far west as Uzbekistan and including the Maldives (Fig. 63.1) [1]. This has been conventionally called the "scrub typhus triangle", but it is more of a rhomboid than a triangle. There are no reliable estimates of community incidence and most are hospital-derived, such as recent data that 3% of patients in Nepal and 15% of patients in Laos admitted with undifferentiated fever had scrub typhus [2, 3]. It predominantly afflicts farmers, including their children, but may also affect urban populations through exposure in gardens or visits to the countryside. There are no known genetic predispositions. The name scrub typhus is misleading, as the disease can be contracted in many other habitats, including primary forest, beaches, gardens, and plantations. Indian patients with scrub typhus are more likely to have lived close to bushes and wood piles, to have worked on farms, to have seen rodents and to have reared domestic animals, but are less likely to wash or change clothes after work. For Koreans, wearing a long-sleeved shirt while working, keeping work clothes off the grass and always using a mat to rest on outdoors were protective [4].

The most commonly reported serotypes are Karp, Kato, Gilliam, and Boryong, but the wide phenotypic and genotypic diversity of *Orientia tsutsugamushi* has major implications for the design of diagnostic tests and vaccines [1].

NATURAL HISTORY, PATHOGENESIS, AND PATHOLOGY

Scrub typhus is transmitted by chiggers – the third-stage larvae of *Leptotombidium* mites (Fig. 63.2), which feed on the extracellular fluid of vertebrates such as rodents and humans. Mites are the main reservoir of *O. tsutsugamushi*, with the organisms maintained in the population by transovarial transmission. Blood transfusion and needlestick injury have been recorded as transmitting scrub typhus.

The genome of *O. tsutsugamushi* (~2 million bp) is much larger than that of other members of Rickettsiaceae and is the most highly repeated bacterial genome sequenced [1]. The median *O. tsutsugamushi* DNA load in blood is low (~13 [0–310,253] copies/ml); approximately half of patients have bacterial loads undetectable by current techniques [5]. Post-mortem examination has demonstrated *O. tsutsugamushi* in endothelial cells of major organs. Significantly higher concentrations of gamma interferon and interleukin-10 occur during the acute than the convalescent phase. Comparison of patterns of endothelial and leukocyte activation in a range of "typhus-like" illnesses suggest mononuclear cell activation in scrub typhus. Evidence is accumulating that *O. tsutsugamushi* exhibits tropism for mononuclear cells rather than endothelial cells, at least in early infection [6]. Intriguingly, evidence from Thailand suggests that HIV-1-suppressive factors are produced during some scrub typhus infections.

CLINICAL FEATURES

The incubation period is approximately 6–14 days. Ten to fifty percent of patients may have an eschar – this variability probably reflects, at least in part, the extent to which patients are examined. Eschars, which are usually single and in secluded areas such as the axilla and groin, are painless, erythematous papules that develop a central black scab, resembling a cigarette burn (Fig. 63.3). They are not pathognomonic for scrub typhus, as similar lesions may be produced by spotted fever group rickettsioses. Chiggers are minute and, unlike ticks, are not normally noticed. Patients may scratch off the characteristic black scab. Lymphadenopathy is more frequent than in sympatric murine typhus [2]. Headache, myalgia, and dry cough frequently occur; a maculopapular erythematous rash occurs in a minority of patients [1,2]. Deafness, tinnitus, and conjunctival suffusion occur. Severe

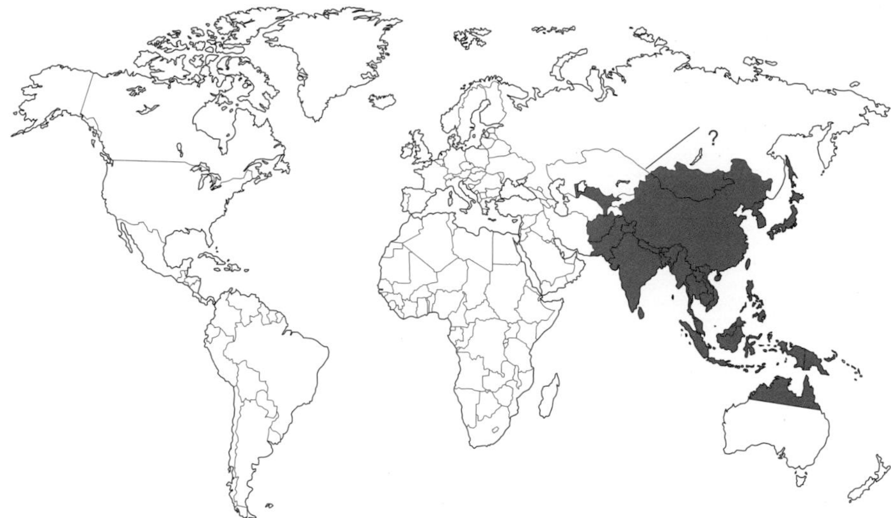

FIGURE 63.1 Map of the distribution of scrub typhus. Please note that this map disguises considerable heterogeneity between and within countries. ?, areas where the extent of scrub typhus is uncertain.

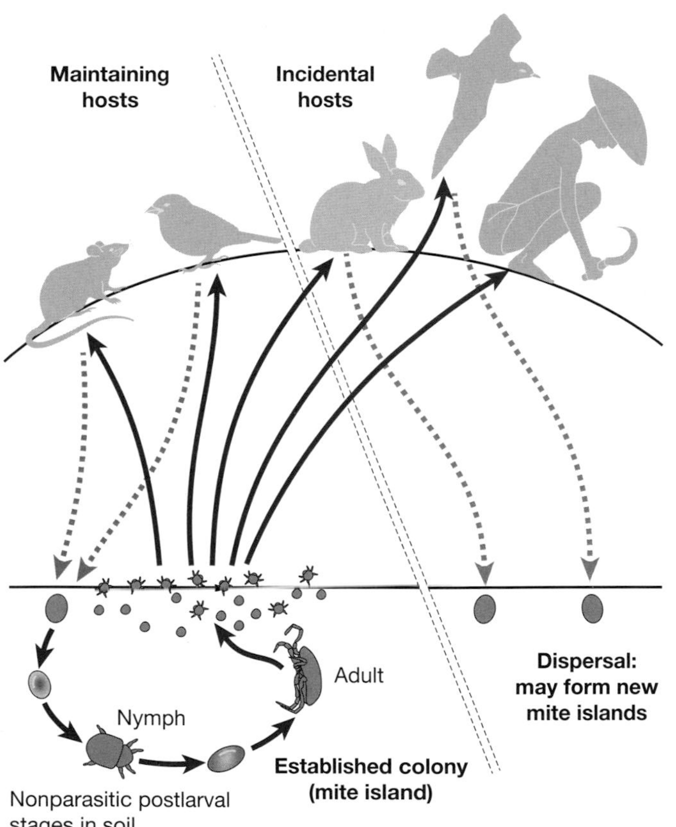

FIGURE 63.2 The life cycle of *O. tsutsugamushi*. *Reproduced with permission from Audy JR, Red Mites and Typhus. Published by The Athlone Press, University of London, 1968.*

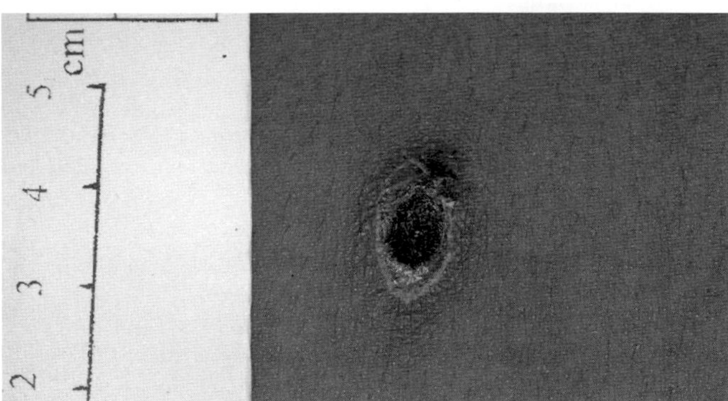

FIGURE 63.3 An eschar on a Lao patient with scrub typhus. *Taken by Dr Rattanaphone Phetsouvanh.*

disease can manifest as pneumonitis, acute respiratory distress syndrome, jaundice with mildly raised transaminases, meningoencephalitis, coagulopathy, multi-organ failure, acute renal failure, acute transverse myelitis, myocarditis, and Guillain-Barré syndrome. Why some, and not others, develop severe disease is not understood. Mortality is positively correlated with blood bacterial load [5]. *Orientia tsutsugamushi* DNA has been demonstrated in cerebrospinal fluid (CSF), with normal glucose, a mild increase in white cell density (ranging from 11–88% lymphocytes) and raised protein [7]. Scrub typhus appears to be less severe in children, but there have been no prospective comparisons between children and adults from the same population. Scrub typhus can cause serious adverse effects for mother and baby in pregnancy [8]. Although homologous strain immunity persists for at least 1–3 years, immunity to heterologous *Orientia* strains is as short as 1 month. There are few data on the dynamics of IgM/IgG responses – the annual reversion of scrub typhus patients sera back to a titer of <1:50 was 61% [9].

PATIENT EVALUATION, DIAGNOSIS, AND DIFFERENTIAL DIAGNOSIS

The majority of scrub typhus patients are not diagnosed or treated. A patient with fever, headache, and myalgia with an eschar in an endemic area is likely to have scrub typhus. The differential diagnosis would include spotted fever group rickettsiosis, which would also be expected to respond to tetracyclines. Scrub typhus eschars could be confused with the lesions of anthrax, tularemia, chancroid, lymphogranuloma venereum, and injury. In the absence of an eschar, few clinical features are helpful. Murine typhus, leptospirosis, Q fever, dengue, hemorrhagic fever with renal syndrome (HFRS), infectious mononucleosis, HIV seroconversion, septicemia (especially typhoid), and malaria are important differential diagnoses. In comparison with those with Q fever, Taiwanese patients with scrub typhus had a higher frequency of residence or travel in a mountainous region or offshore island, and skin rash. In comparison to HFRS in China, eschar, regional lymphadenopathy and maculopapular rash were more

TABLE 63-1 Clinical Trial and Clinical Case Series Evidence for Antibiotic Therapy for Scrub Typhus

Therapies	Location and sample size	Outcome	Category	Ref.
Chloramphenicol 3 g every 24 h for 3 days vs tetracycline 2 g every 24 h for 3 days	Vietnam (60)	Similar fever clearance times	3	[18]
Doxycycline 200 mg stat vs tetracycline 500 mg every 6 h for 7 days	Malaysia (55)	Similar fever clearance times	3	[14]
Doxycycline 100 mg every 12 h for 3 days vs tetracycline 500 mg every 6 h for 7 days	South Korea (116)	Similar fever clearance times	3	[19]
Doxycycline 200 mg followed by 100 mg every 12 h for 7 days vs rifampicin 300 mg every 12 h for 7 days vs rifampicin and doxycycline combined in doses as above	Northern Thailand (126)	Rifampicin and doxycycline combined inferior to the other two single-agent groups. Fewer patients febrile at 48 h in the rifampicin group compared with the doxycycline group (RR 0.41, 95% CI 0.22–0.77)	3	[20]
Doxycycline 2.5 mg/kg every 12h, chloramphenicol 50 mg/kg/d in 3–4 doses or roxithromycin 5 mg/kg every 12h	South Korea (39 children)	Fever clearance times not significantly different	4	[21]
Azithromycin single 500 mg dose vs 200 mg doxycycline every 24 h for 7 days	South Korea (93)	Fever clearance and cure rates not significantly different	3	[15]
Telithromycin 800 mg every 24 h for 5 days vs doxycycline 100 mg every 12 h for 5 days	South Korea (92)	Fever clearance and cure rates not significantly different	3	[16]
Azithromycin single 1000 mg dose followed by 500 mg every 24 h for 2 days vs 200 mg doxycycline followed by 100 mg every 12 h for 7 days	Thailand (57)	At 48 h after initiation of treatment, a significantly higher proportion of the doxycycline-treated group were afebrile than with azithromycin-treated group ($p = 0.03$)	3	[3]

Category 1, double blind study; 2, clinical trial < 20 subjects; 3, clinical trial > 20 subjects; 4, series; 5, anecdotal case reports. CI, confidence interval; RR, relative risk. All clinical trials involved random allocation of treatment.

commonly found in patients with scrub typhus. In Laos, the presence of peripheral lymphadenopathy, chest signs and eschars are clinically useful signs that suggest scrub, rather than murine, typhus [2].

Laboratory diagnosis of scrub typhus is difficult. Culture (requiring BSL3 facilities) is 100% specific, but has low sensitivity. Immunofluorescence (IFA) and immunoperoxidase IgM and IgG antibody tests have been commonly used, but these are expensive, rarely accessible and are bedevilled by subjectivity of interpretation and uncertainty as to the most appropriate cut-off titers in different communities [10]. Ideally, they should be interpreted by comparing titers between paired acute and convalescent samples. Karp, Gilliam, and Kato prototypic antigens are usually used in IFAs and therefore may not detect antibodies to other strains. The Weil-Felix OXK test is still commonly used in Asia, but has low sensitivity. Conventional and quantitative real-time PCR assays for the detection of *O. tsutsugamushi* in blood, eschar tissue, and CSF have been developed [11, 12]. However, there remain great difficulties in the accessibility of the diagnosis of scrub typhus in rural endemic areas. Mixed infections may occur with, for example, leptospirosis but, given the persistence of antibodies, distinguishing these from serial infections without culture or PCR techniques is difficult.

TREATMENT

Given the difficulties of making a timely laboratory diagnosis and the significant minority who develop severe disease, empirical treatment should be considered for all cases with scrub typhus in the differential diagnosis. The diversity of *O. tsutsugamushi* suggests it is unlikely that one treatment regimen will be appropriate across the wide distribution of this organism. Chloramphenicol- and doxycycline-resistant scrub typhus have been described in northern Thailand [13], but there are no subsequent published data on this clinical problem.

Interpretation of data informing treatment decisions is difficult, as studies are few, often of small sample size and "relapses" were usually not proven to be relapses of scrub typhus, rather than another cause of fever (Table 63-1). Current data suggest that fluoroquinolones are inferior to doxycycline as therapy for scrub typhus. For uncomplicated disease, the data available do not allow generalizable conclusions of the duration of doxycycline therapy or whether a loading dose is required. In Laos and Thailand, a 7-day treatment course of 2 mg/kg twice daily after a loading dose of 4 mg/kg is administered. There is evidence from Malaysia that shorter courses may be efficacious [14]. Upper gastrointestinal side effects are common; patients should be counseled to take doxycycline with plenty of fluid, during meals, and while sitting or standing. Chloramphenicol, telithromycin, rifampicin, and azithromycin are potential alternatives [15–20].

There are few data to guide the antibiotic treatment of severe disease – parenteral or nasogastric doxycycline or chloramphenicol are potential options. Appropriate supportive care is essential. The treatment of scrub typhus in pregnancy is problematic – chloramphenicol (although contraindicated in the last trimester), azithromycin, and rifampicin have been used. In children, the risks of short-course doxycycline are almost certainly exceeded by the benefit of effective cure. In a retrospective analysis of children with scrub typhus, no significant differences in fever clearance times were found between doxycycline, chloramphenicol, or roxithromycin therapy [21].

Mortality is very variable, ranging from 0–60% in untreated patients, for reasons that are unclear. Delayed administration of doxycycline has been associated with major organ dysfunction and prolonged hospitalization, emphasizing the importance of early empirical doxycycline therapy. Relapse was described during volunteer experiments in Malaysia, but whether this is an important phenomenon in clinical practice is uncertain. Insecticides have been used to control chiggers, both in high-risk habitats and on blankets and clothes, but neither are currently practical in rural Asia for farmers (who are at most risk of scrub typhus). For short-term adult visitors, weekly 200 mg doxycycline reduces the risk of contracting scrub typhus. There is currently no safe and effective vaccine available.

REFERENCES

1. Kelly DJ, Fuerst PA, Ching WM, Richards AL. Scrub typhus: the geographic distribution of phenotypic and genotypic variants of *Orientia tsutsugamushi*. Clin Infect Dis 2009;48(suppl. 3):S203–30.
2. Phongmany S, Rolain JM, Phetsouvanh R, et al. Rickettsial infections and fever, Vientiane, Laos. Emerg Infect Dis 2006;12:256–62.
3. Phimda K, Hoontrakul S, Suttinont C, et al. Doxycycline versus azithromycin for treatment of leptospirosis and scrub typhus. Antimicrob Agents Chemother 2007;51:3259–63.
4. Kweon SS, Choi JS, Lim HS, et al. A community-based case-control study of behavioral factors associated with scrub typhus during the autumn epidemic season in South Korea. Am J Trop Med Hyg 2009;80:442–6.
5. Sonthayanon P, Chierakul W, Wuthiekanun V, et al. Association of high *Orientia tsutsugamushi* DNA loads with disease of greater severity in adults with scrub typhus. J Clin Microbiol 2009;47:430–4.
6. Paris DH, Jenjaroen K, Blacksell SD, et al. Differential patterns of endothelial and leucocyte activation in 'typhus-like' illnesses in Laos and Thailand. Clin Exp Immunol 2008;153:63–7.
7. Pai H, Sohn S, Seong Y, et al. Central nervous system involvement in patients with scrub typhus. Clin Infect Dis 1997;24:436–40.
8. Mathai E, Rolain JM, Verghese L, et al. Case reports: scrub typhus during pregnancy in India. Trans R Soc Trop Med Hyg 2003;97:570–2.
9. Saunders JP, Brown GW, Shirai A, Huxsoll DL. The longevity of antibody to *Rickettsia tsutsugamushi* in patients with confirmed scrub typhus. Trans R Soc Trop Med Hyg 1980;74:253–7.
10. Blacksell SD, Bryant NJ, Paris DH, et al. Scrub typhus serologic testing with the indirect immunofluorescence method as a diagnostic gold standard: a lack of consensus leads to a lot of confusion. Clin Infect Dis 2007;44:391–401.
11. Paris DH, Aukkanit N, Jenjaroen K, et al. A highly sensitive quantitative real-time PCR assay based on the groEL gene of contemporary Thai strains of *Orientia tsutsugamushi*. Clin Microbiol Infect 2009;15:488–95.
12. Paris DH, Blacksell SD, Newton PN, Day NP. Simple, rapid and sensitive detection of *Orientia tsutsugamushi* by loop-isothermal DNA amplification. Trans R Soc Trop Med Hyg 2008;102:1239–46.
13. Watt G, Chouriyagune C, Ruangweerayud R, et al. Scrub typhus infections poorly responsive to antibiotics in northern Thailand. Lancet 1996;348: 86–9.
14. Brown GW, Saunders JP, Singh SL, et al Single dose doxycycline therapy for scrub typhus. Trans R Soc Trop Med Hyg 1978;72:413–6.
15. Kim YS, Yun HJ, Shim SK, et al. A comparative trial of a single dose of azithromycin versus doxycycline for the treatment of mild scrub typhus. Clin Infect Dis 2004;39:1329–35.
16. Kim DM, Yu KD, Lee JH, et al. Controlled trial of a 5-day course of telithromycin versus doxycycline for treatment of mild to moderate scrub typhus. Antimicrob Agents Chemother 2007;51:2011–5.
17. Panpanich R, Garner P. Antibiotics for treating scrub typhus. Cochrane Database Syst Rev 2002;CD002150.
18. Sheehy TW, Hazlett AD, Turk RE. Scrub typhus: A comparison of chloramphenical and tetracycline in its treatment. Arch Int Med 1973;132:77–80.
19. Song JH, Lee C, Chang LW, et al. Short course doxycycline treatment versus conventional tetracycline therapy for scrub typhus: A multiple randomized trial. Clin Infect Dis 1995;21:506–10.
20. Watt G, Kantipong P, Jongsakul K, et al. Doxycycline and rifampicin for mild scrub-typhus infections in northern Thailand: a randomised trial. Lancet 2000;356:1057–61.
21. Lee KY, Lee HS, Hong JH, et al. Roxithromycin treatment of scrub typhus (tsutsugamushi disease) in children. Pediatr Infect Dis J 2003;22:130–3.

64 Tick-borne Spotted Fever Rickettsioses

Cristina Socolovschi, Philippe Parola, Didier Raoult

Key features

- Tick-borne rickettsioses are caused by obligate intracellular bacteria belonging to the spotted fever group of the genus *Rickettsia* within the family *Rickettsiaceae* in the order *Rickettsiales*
- Ecologic characteristics of the tick vectors influence the epidemiology and clinical aspects of tick-borne diseases
- The clinical presentation of tick-borne rickettsiosis can vary from mild to very severe, with the frequency of fatality from highly virulent rickettsiae ranging from 2–6%. The main clinical signs include: fever; headache; rash that is maculopapular or sometimes vesicular; inoculation eschars at the site of the tick bite; and localized lymphadenopathy
- Early empirical treatment should be started in any suspected rickettsioses before laboratory confirmation of the diagnosis. Based on *in vitro* susceptibility and *in vivo* experience, doxycycline is the currently recommended drug for treating spotted fever group rickettsioses
- There are no vaccines commercially available to prevent tick-borne rickettsioses in humans—prevention involves minimizing exposure to ticks
- The emergence and re-emergence of these illnesses are attributed to changes in the environment and human behavior

INTRODUCTION

Tick-borne rickettsioses are caused by Gram-negative obligate intracellular bacteria belonging to the spotted fever group of the genus *Rickettsia,* in the family *Rickettsiaceae,* in the order *Rickettsiales* [1]. These zoonoses are among the oldest known vector-borne diseases. In 1899, Edward E. Maxey reported the first clinical description of Rocky Mountain spotted fever in the Snake River Valley of Idaho, USA and, in 1910, Conor and Brush described the first case of Mediterranean spotted fever in Tunis. In 1905, McCalla, an Idaho physician, demonstrated the role of the wood tick in the transmission of *Rickettsia rickettsii,* the causative agent of Rocky Mountain spotted fever. With the full consent of the participants, he attached a tick obtained from the chest of a man who was very ill with spotted fever to the arm of another patient. The tick remained on the second patient for 48 hours and was then applied to the leg of a woman, where it remained for at least 10 hours. The incubation periods were 9 and 3 days, respectively. Around 1930 the role of the brown dog tick, *Rhipicephalus sanguineus,* in the transmission of *Rickettsia. conorii,* the causative agent of Mediterranean spotted fever, was demonstrated using human models [2]. The history of tick-borne illnesses is one of constant renewal, with discoveries of new pathogens associated with descriptions of novel diseases concurrent with advances in molecular and cell-culture techniques [3].

ETIOLOGY

Rickettsiae are strictly intracellular bacteria whose sizes range from 0.3–2.0 μm. These bacteria multiply by binary fission in the cytoplasm of eukaryotic host cells. As a consequence, *Rickettsiae* must be cultivated in tissue culture, guinea pigs, or embryonated chicken eggs. *Rickettsiae* are difficult to stain with ordinary bacterial stains but, conveniently, are stained by the Gimenez method. At this time, there are 25 formally recognized species in the genus *Rickettsia,* which can be classified into four groups: the typhus group (*Rickettsia typhi* and *Rickettsia prowazekii*); the spotted fever group (21 *Rickettsiae*) (Table 64-1); *Rickettsia bellii*; and the *Rickettsia canadensis* group. Many other isolates exist, but they are not characterized. Recently, guidelines for the identification and description of new rickettsial isolates have been proposed using sequences of the 16S rRNA (rrs) gene and four protein-coding genes: *gltA, ompA, ompB,* and gene D [4]. Official criteria have been proposed for the creation of subspecies within *R. conorii* and *Rickettsia sibirica* based on epidemiologic, clinical, serotypic, and genotypic differences.

EPIDEMIOLOGY

Tick-borne rickettsioses have a global distribution. Ticks are hematophagous arthropods that parasitize every class of vertebrates in almost every region of world and occasionally bite humans. Each species has a particular set of optimal environmental conditions and biotopes that determine the geographical distribution of the ticks and, therefore, of the individual tick-borne rickettsioses (Fig. 64.1). The prevalence of *Rickettsiae* in different populations of ticks is variable—it ranges from usually less than 1% for *R. conorii* and *R. rickettsii* to 100% for *Rickettsia africae*. The tick vectors usually involved in transmission of tropical rickettsioses belong to the genera *Rhipicephalus, Ixodes, Amblyomma, Hyalomma, Haemaphysalis,* and *Dermacentor* (Table 64-1). Tick-borne rickettsioses may be transmitted among ticks transstadially (stage-to-stage) and transovarially (transfer of bacteria from adult females to the subsequent generation of ticks via the eggs). As a consequence, ticks may act as reservoirs for these bacteria, such as *Amblyomma* spp. for *R. africae,* and play a role in maintaining the agent in nature. Tick-borne diseases are emerging zoonoses with a re-emergence of "old" diseases. Increasing international travel and the possibility of the ticks being carried by hosts such as birds have resulted in a number of imported cases of tick-borne rickettsioses. An analysis of the GeoSentinel database (a worldwide communications and data collection network of travel/tropical-medicine clinics) showed that 3.1% of febrile travelers have rickettsiosis. It has also been suggested that global warming has led to a northward expansion of several tick species and to an increase in the aggressiveness of the brown dog tick, and that these have increased the incidence of *Rh. sanguineus*-transmitted pathogens, such as *R. conorii, R. rickettsii, Rickettsia massiliae,* other non-pathogenic rickettsial agents like *Rickettsia rhipicephali,* or as-yet undescribed microorganisms [2, 5].

TABLE 64-1 Tick-borne Rickettsioses throughout the World

	Disease	*Rickettsia*	Tick vector	Selected epidemiologic and clinical characteristics
Spotted fever group with inoculation eschar	Mediterranean spotted fever	*R. conorii conorii*	*Rhipicephalus sanguineus*	Disease occurs in urban (66%) and rural (33%) settings during summer months; cases generally sporadic. Classic single eschar and maculopapular, generalized rash (97%). Mortality: 2.5%
	Astrakhan fever	*R. conorii caspia*	*Rh. sanguineus*, *Rhipicephalus pumilio*	Disease occurs mostly in rural settings. Symptoms include eschar (23%), maculopapular rash (94%) and conjunctivitis (34%). No fatal cases reported
	Indian tick typhus	*R. conorii indica*	*Rh. sanguineus*	Rash frequently purpuric, eschar rarely found, no fatal forms
	Israeli spotted fever	*R. conorii israelensis*	*Rh. sanguineus*	Compared to Mediterranean spotted fever, eschars are less frequent. Mild-to-severe illness
	Siberian tick typhus	*R. sibirica sibirica*	*Dermacentor nuttalli*, *Dermacentor marginatus*, *Dermacentor silvarum*, *Haemaphysalis concinna*	Disease occurs in predominantly rural settings. Cases occur during spring and summer. Increasing reports of cases. Cases generally associated with rash (100%), eschar (77%) and lymphadenopathy
	Far-Eastern tick-borne rickettsiosis	*R. heilongjiangensis*	*D. silvarum*	Rash, eschar, and lymphadenopathy. No fatal cases reported
	Japanese or Oriental spotted fever	*R. japonica*	*Haemaphysalis flava*, *Haemaphysalis longicornis*, *Dermacentor taiwanensis*, *Ixodes ovatus*	Disease occurs mainly from April to October in predominantly rural settings. Associated with agricultural activities, bamboo cutting. Fever, macular rash (100%) and eschar (91%)
	Queensland tick typhus	*R. australis*	*Ixodes holocyclus*, *Ixodes tasmani*	Disease occurs in rural and urban areas; cases occur from June to November. Vesicular eruption (100%), eschar (65%), lymphadenopathy (71%). Few fatal cases described
	Flinders Island spotted fever	*R. honei*	*Aponomma hydrasauri*, *Aponomma cajennense*, *Aponomma granulatus*	Disease occurs mainly in rural areas and peaks between December and January. Symptoms include eruption (85%), eschar (25%) and lymphadenopathy (55%)
		R. honei marmionii	*Haemaphysalis novaeguineae*, *I. holocyclus*	Fever, headache (83%), arthralgia (50%), cough (50%), maculopapular rash (33%) and pharyngitis (33%)
	Spotted fever	*R. parkeri*	*Aponomma maculatum*, *Aponomma triste*	Fever, myalgia, malaise, headache and a maculopapular eruption. Sometimes vesicular or pustular rash
Scalp eschar and neck lymphadenopathy (SENLAT)	Spotted fever	*R. slovaca*	*D. marginatus*, *Dermacentor reticulatus*	Fever and rash rare. Typical scalp eschar with cervical lymphadenopathy. Alopecia and chronic fatigue. Illness mild
	Spotted fever	*R. raoultii*	*D. marginatus*, *D. reticulatus*	Fever, painful eschar and adenopathies, headache, asthenia. No alopecia was noted, but 50% of patients had prolonged asthenia (1–6 months) and 25% had chronic asthenia
Lymphangitis-associated rickettsioses (LAR)	Lymphangitis-associated rickettsiosis	*R. sibirica mongolitimonae*	*Haemaphysalis asiaticum*, *Haemaphysalis truncatum*, *Haemaphysalis anatolicum excavatum* *Rh. pusillus*	Sixteen confirmed cases: fever (100%), headache (50%), rash (83%), eschar (92%), multiple eschars (17%), adenopathy (58%) and lymphangitis (42%)

TABLE 64-1 Tick-borne Rickettsioses throughout the World—cont'd

	Disease	*Rickettsia*	Tick vector	Selected epidemiologic and clinical characteristics
RMSF	Rocky Mountain spotted fever	*R. rickettsii*	*Dermacentor andersoni, Dermacentor variabilis, Rh. sanguineus, Amblyomma cajennense, Aponomma aureolatum*	Peak occurrence during spring and summer. Petechial rash including palms (60%) and soles (80%). No eschar. Fatal cases 2–6%
African tick-bite fever (ATBF)	African tick-bite fever	*R. africae*	*Aponomma variegatum, Aponomma hebraeum*	Disease occurs in predominantly in rural settings. Symptoms include fever (88%), eschar (95%), multiple eschar (54%), maculopapular (49%) or cesicular (50%) eruption and lymphadenopathy (43%). No fatal cases reported
Infrequently reported tick-borne rickettsial diseases	Spotted fever	*R. aeschlimannii*	*Hyalomma marginatum marginatum, Hy. marginatum rufipes, Rhipicephalus sanguineus appendiculatus*	High fever, eschar and maculopapular generalized rash
	Spotted fever	*R. massilae*	*Rh. sanguineus, Rhipicephalus turanicus, Rhipicephalus muhsamae, Rhipicephalus lunulatus, Rhipicephalus sulcatus*	Two confirmed cases: eschar and maculopapular generalized rash; one case of chorioretinis
	Spotted fever	*R. helvetica*	*Ixodes ricinus, Ixodes ovatus, Ixodes persulcatus, Ixodes monospinus*	Although implicated in perimyocarditis and sarcoidosis, the validity of these associations has been debated or not accepted by rickettsiologists. Few cases documented by serology and PCR. Rash and eschar seldom occur
	Spotted fever	*R. monacencis*	*I. ricinus*	Two confirmed cases: fever, headache and an erythematous rash with no inoculation eschar.

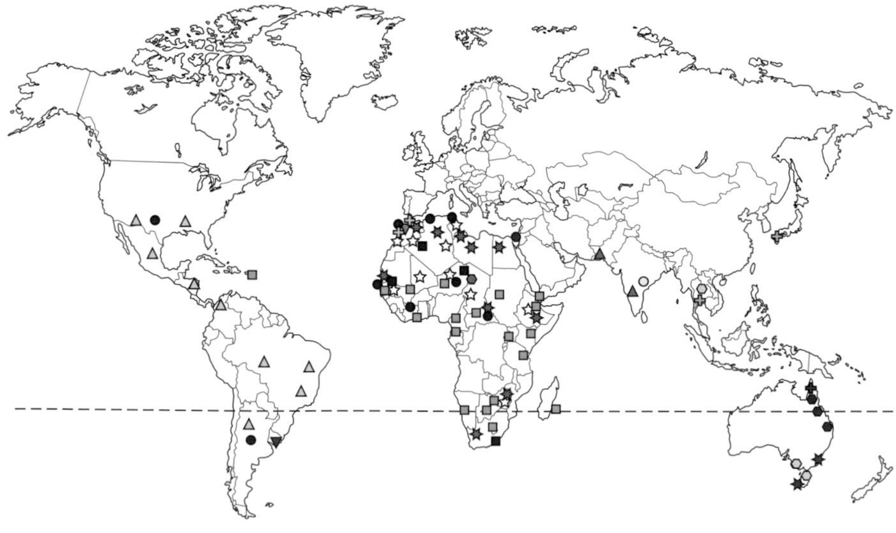

FIGURE 64.1 Tick-borne rickettsiae in tropical regions.

SPOTTED FEVER GROUP WITH INOCULATION ESCHAR

MEDITERRANEAN SPOTTED FEVER

Rickettsia conorii, the causative agent of Mediterranean spotted fever, is endemic in the Mediterranean area, including northern Africa and southern Europe; cases have also been reported sporadically in central Europe and central and southern Africa. In Italy, in 2002, the national incidence rate was 1.6 cases per 100,000 persons (although in Sicily it was 10 cases per 100,000 persons); in Portugal between 1989 and 2003, the annual incidence was 8.9 cases per 100,000 inhabitants; in Spain between 1983 an 1985, the estimated incidence was 23–45 cases per 100,000 persons—the same rate was also observed in Marseille during that time. This disease affects all age groups and occurs mainly in summer. Recently, an increased incidence of MSF was associated with warmer weather, which increases the aggressiveness and northward expansion of *Rh. sanguineus*.

The incubation period from the time of infection to onset is 6 days. Often, the patient presents with abrupt fever (100%), flu-like symptoms (headache, chills, arthromyalgias), and a *"tache noire"* at the tick-bite site. The *"tache noire"*, the hallmark of disease, is an inflamed red papule, the center of which becomes necrotic, black and indolent, usually located on the trunk, legs, or arms (in infants it is often on the scalp, in the retroauricular area). Occasionally, the eschar is not found and it is seen rarely in multiples. Unilateral or bilateral conjunctivitis may represent the eye-inoculation site of the rickettsia. A generalized maculopapular rash (97% of cases) on the extremities and then on the trunk often involves the palms, soles and, to a lesser extent, the face (Fig. 64.2). Other common clinical manifestations are myalgia (73%), headache (69%), conjunctivitis (32%), hepatomegaly (44%), and splenomegaly (19%). Gastrointestinal symptoms may be present in about 30% of patients and are more likely to be present in children [6]. Severe disease occurs in 5–6% of cases and is associated with disseminated vasculitis, with renal, neurologic and cardiovascular complications, as well as phlebitis. Recently, in a prospective study conducted in Algeria, 49% of the patients were hospitalized with a severe form. The global death rate was 3.6% but it was 54.5% in patients hospitalized with major neurologic manifestations and multi-organ involvement.

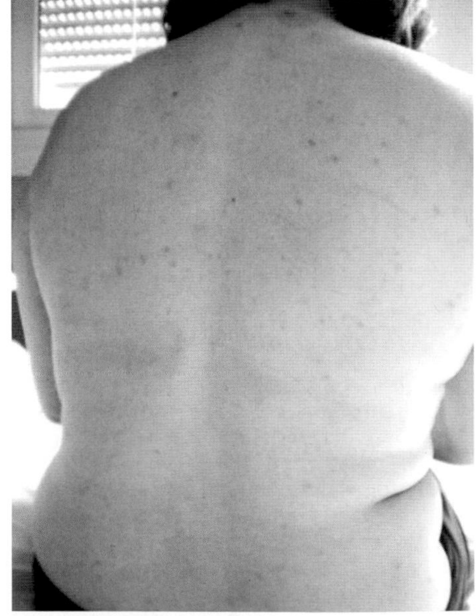

FIGURE 64.2 Rash in a patient with Mediterranean spotted fever.

ASTRAKHAN FEVER

Rickettsia conorii caspia, the infectious agent of Astrakhan fever, was described primarily in patients living in rural areas in Astrakhan, a region of Russia. *Rhipicephalus sanguineus* and *Rhipicephalus pumilio* were shown to harbor this rickettsia. Clinically, the disease is similar to Mediterranean spotted fever except for the absence of a fatal form and a lower incidence of inoculation eschar. Recently, a rickettsial isolate was obtained from a patient in Chad, Africa. The patient presented with fever, dyspnea, a maculopapular rash, an inoculation eschar on the leg, and conjunctivitis of the right eye.

INDIAN TICK-BITE TYPHUS

The etiological agent of Indian tick-bite typhus is *R. conorii indica*, prevalent in India, which has never been isolated in human samples. Indian tick-bite typhus differs from Mediterranean spotted fever by the presence of purpuric rash and, infrequently, an inoculation eschar at the bite site.

ISRAELI SPOTTED FEVER

Rickettsia conorii israelensis is the causative agent of Israeli spotted fever. The first case was described in Israel; however, this bacteria was recently isolated from human samples and ticks in Italy and Portugal. The clinical manifestations of ISF are similar to those of other spotted fever group infections, but the eschar at the inoculation site is absent in more than 90% of cases and resembles a small, pinkish papule when visible. Several fatal cases and severe forms of ISF have been described, especially in children, as well as in travelers and those with glucose-6-phosphate dehydrogenase deficiency.

SIBERIAN TICK TYPHUS

Rickettsia sibirica is the causative agent of Siberian tick typhus. It was described in southern and eastern Siberia, northern China, Mongolia, and Kazakhstan. The annual morbidity rates in the years 1995–2004 varied from 1.5 to 2.4 per 100,000 in Russia, but in the area where this disease is endemic, morbidity may reach 40–120 per 10,000. The peak of disease is noted in May and the clinical course is benign. Onset is typically abrupt, with high fever, headache, myalgia, arthralgia, digestive symptoms, an inoculation eschar (62–77%), regional adenopathy, and a cutaneous rash that appears 2 to 4 days after onset [1, 3, 7].

FAR-EASTERN TICK-BORNE RICKETTSIOSIS

The etiological agent of this disease, also named "neglected rickettsioses" is *Rickettsia heilongjiangensis*. Reported cases have occurred in far-eastern territories of Russia and in northern China. Its seasonal peak runs from the end of June through July and it mostly affects older populations; no fatal case has been reported. The clinical picture is similar to other spotted fever group rickettsioses. All reported cases had a history of tick bite, tick exposure or having visited the endemic area. Symptoms include fever, maculopapular rash, inoculation eschar, regional lymphadenopathy, and conjunctivitis [3].

JAPANESE OR ORIENTAL SPOTTED FEVER

Rickettsia japonica, the causative agent of Japanese spotted fever, is located along the coast of southwestern and central Japan and in northeastern Thailand. The onset of the disease is 2–10 days after work in the fields and is abrupt, with common symptoms of headache (81%), high fever (100%), shaking chills (87%), and tick-bite eschar (94%). A macular rash (100%) appears after 2 or 3 days, all over the body, including the palms and soles. It becomes petechial after 3 or 4 days and disappears in 2 weeks. In a series of 28 Japanese patients hospitalized from 1993 to 2002, 21% of Japanese spotted fever cases were classified as severe and included one fatality [1].

QUEENSLAND TICK TYPHUS

Rickettsia australis, the causative agent of Queensland tick typhus, occurs only down the east coast of Australia, from the tip of the continent and Torres Strait Island to the southeastern corner (Wilson's promontory in Victoria) [8]. Most cases (78%) occur between June and November. The disease is characterized by sudden onset of fever, headache and myalgia. Within 10 days, a maculopapular or vesicular rash appears. An inoculation eschar is identified in 65% of cases and lymphadenopathy in 71% of cases.

FLINDERS ISLANDS SPOTTED FEVER

Flinders Islands spotted fever, caused by *Rickettsia honei*, occurs primarily in Australia (Tasmania, South Australia, Queensland, Torres Strait Islands) and may be worldwide (Thailand, Sri Lanka, Italy) [1, 8]. *Aponomma hydrosauri*, the reptile tick, is suspected to be a vector of this disease. It is a relatively mild disease—no deaths have yet been recorded. The incidence of Flinders Islands spotted fever was estimated at 150 per 100,000 persons. It causes a summer febrile illness associated with a rash, being erythematous in the majority of cases, while it was purpuric in two severe cases associated with thrombocytopenia. An eschar typical for spotted fever group rickettsiosis (25%) and enlarged local nodes (55%) was observed. Recently, a genetic variant of *R. honei*, the "marmionii" strain transmitted by *Haemaphysalis novaeguineae* and *Ixodes holocyclus*, was reported to cause acute disease in several patients in eastern Australia.

Spotted fever related to *Rickettsia parkeri* has been described in the USA and South America. The first recognized case of infection in a human was reported in 2004, 65 years after the initial isolation of this rickettsia from ticks. This disease was previously confused with Rocky Mountain spotted fever or with Rickettsialpox. Recently, six new confirmed cases were reported. This disease is characterized by: fever; myalgia; malaise; headache; maculopapular, vesicular or pustular eruption; and inoculation eschar (sometimes multiple eschars). No deaths were reported [9].

ROCKY MOUNTAIN SPOTTED FEVER

The severity of symptoms of Rocky Mountain spotted fever caused by *R. rickettsii* separates this disease from other tick-borne rickettsioses. Rocky Mountain spotted fever is endemic to regions of North, Central and South America, in both rural and urban zones. The peak of disease occurs during the months of April to September. Since its initial description in the late 19th century, Rocky Mountain spotted fever has been considered a lethal infection. For example, from 1904 to 1913 in Montana, 96 (63%) of 153 patients diagnosed with Rocky Mountain spotted fever died from this disease. The fatality rate of Rocky Mountain spotted fever was reduced to approximately 23% by advances in supportive care and the discovery of antimicrobial therapy. In the recently published *"Summary of Notifiable Diseases—United States, 2006"*, a total of 3908 cases of Rocky Mountain spotted fever were reported in 2002–2004, including 22 deaths, making the case-fatality rate 0.7%. There are a few reasons to believe that the fatal cases are more often unreported than benign cases: (i) some cases are confounded with spotted fever caused by *R. parkeri*, *R. massiliae*, *Rickettsia amblyommi*, *Rickettsia akari*, and *Rickettsia felis*; (ii) some imported cases of rickettsioses, for example African tick-bite fever in travelers are incorrectly reported as Rocky Mountain spotted fever; and (iii) in some *R. rickettsii* strains, there are variations in virulence (for example, in an early description of Rocky Mountain spotted fever in the Idaho region, a 5% case-fatality rate was reported compared with 70–80% in Montana) [10]. In Brazil, where Rocky Mountain spotted fever is endemic to at least five states, mortality was 40% in Minas Gerais State between 1981 and 1989. The risk factors for severity are: old age; a delay between disease onset and diagnosis; wrong antibiotic choice; and no known documentation of tick bite.

Around one week after being bitten by an infected tick, the disease begins with fever, chills, myalgia and headache. During the next few days, these symptoms continue and may be accompanied by anorexia, nausea, vomiting, abdominal pain, diarrhea, photophobia and cough. The fever is typically high (39–41 °C) and associated with a severe frontal headache. Rash, considered the hallmark feature of Rocky Mountain spotted fever, appears on day three of fever as small, pink, blanching macules (typically on the wrists, ankles and forearms) that evolve maculopapules. Within 24 hours, it spreads centrally to involve the legs, buttocks, arms, axillae, trunk, neck and face. The entire body may be involved, including the mucous membranes of the palate and pharynx [11]. Characteristic of the rash are petechial lesions, in a distribution that includes the palms and soles, which occur in 36% to 82% of patients. In some severe cases, petechiae may coalesce to form large ecchymoses. No eschar at the inoculation site is visible. Severe manifestations may include pulmonary edema and hemorrhage, cerebral edema, myocarditis, renal failure, disseminated intravascular coagulopathy and gangrene. Three factors are independent predictors of failure by the physician to initiate therapy the first time a patient is seen: absence of a rash, presentation between August 1 and April 30, and presentation within the first three days of illness. In untreated patients who survive their illness, the natural course of fever terminates after two to three weeks.

SCALP ESCHAR AND NECK LYMPHADENOPATHY (SENLAT)

The tick-borne rickettsial etiological agents of scalp eschar and neck lymphadenopathy (SENLAT) are *Rickettsia slovaca* and *Rickettsia raoultii*, which are transmitted by the ticks *Dermacentor marginatus* and *Dermacentor reticulatus*. The old name of this disease is tick-borne lymphadenitis (TIBOLA) or *Dermacentor*-borne necrosis erythema lymphadenopathy (DEBONEL). Recently, the spectrum of the causative agents of SENLAT was extended, and several reports demonstrated that this syndrome can be caused by *Borrelia burgdorferi*, *Bartonella henselae*, *Coxiella burnetii*, *R. rioja*, and *Francisella tularensis*, all transmitted by the above ticks. SENLAT occurs in Europe, more frequently in women and children during the colder months. The clinical description is similar for *R. slovaca* and *R. raoultii* infection, including fever, headache, asthenia, rash, painful eschar, painful adenopathies and face edema. The difference between these two infections is that alopecia lasting for several months has been recorded in 59% or more of the cases with *R. slovaca*, but not with *R. roultii* [12, 13].

LYMPHANGITIS-ASSOCIATED RICKETTSIOSIS

Rickettsia sibirica mongolitimonae causes lymphangitis-associated rickettsiosis. It appears that the distribution of this disease corresponds to the distribution of *Hyalomma* spp. ticks. Recently, *R. sibirica mongolitimonae* was detected in *Rh. pusillus* ticks in Portugal and in France. Sixteen cases were confirmed in the literature: 13 from Europe (France, Portugal, Greece and Spain) and 3 from Africa (Algeria, South Africa and Egypt). The available clinical features for the 16 reported cases (ten men and six women) include fever in all patients (range 38–39.5 °C), chills (three patients), headache (13 patients), myalgia (13 patients), arthralgia (three patients), cutaneous rash (11 patients), enlarged lymph nodes (ten patients), lymphangitis expanding from an inoculation eschar to the draining node (six patients) and retinal vasculitis in a pregnant woman [3, 14]. Lymphangitis-associated rickettsiosis occurred primarily between March and September; a single case was reported in December in Greece.

AFRICAN TICK-BITE FEVER

African tick-bite fever is caused by *R. africae* and transmitted by *Amblyomma* ticks in rural sub-Saharan Africa and the West Indies (Fig. 64.3) [1, 15]. Some reports indicate that African tick-bite fever poses a significant problem to local populations. In Zimbabwe, the annual incidence rate of African tick-bite fever is 60–80 cases per 100,000 in areas where *Amblyomma* is endemic. Whereas reports on African tick-bite fever in indigenous populations are scarce, the number of reported cases has recently increased in travelers from Europe and elsewhere. Usually, grouped cases of African tick-bite fever are described, for example several cases in the same family or in the same travel group.

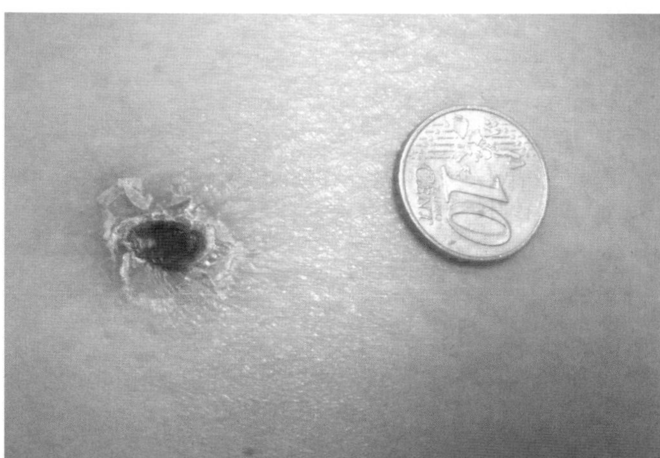

FIGURE 64.3 Eschar of African tick-bite fever

The clinical course typically comprises an abrupt onset of fever (59–10%), nausea, headache (62–83%), and neck myalgia (81%) beginning 5–10 days after a tick bite. Most patients develop an inoculation eschar (53–100%) at the site of the tick bite and up to 54% of patients have multiple eschars—a rather specific clinical sign. A painful regional lymphangitis (43–100%) is common and may be seen in the absence of an inoculation eschar. A generalized cutaneous rash, sometimes vesicular and usually most visible close to the eschar, is present in 15–46% of patients (Fig. 64.4). Less frequent clinical signs of African tick-bite fever include aphtous stomatitis (11%) and arthralgia. Complications are rarely seen, but long-lasting fever, reactive arthritis, subacute cranial or peripheral neuropathy, chronic fatigue, neuropsychiatric symptoms and myocarditis have been reported. There are no known fatal cases [15]. African tick-bite fever should be considered along with malaria and other tropical fevers in the differential diagnosis of all febrile patients returning from the tropics.

INFREQUENTLY REPORTED TICK-BORNE RICKETTSIAL DISEASES

Rickettsia aeschlimannii was detected in *Hyalomma* ticks from several African countries, southern Europe and Kazakhstan (Table 64-1) [7]. Four clinical cases were described in the literature: one patient returning from Morocco to France, one patient returning from a hunting and fishing trip in South Africa, and two cases in Algeria. All of these patients presented with typical signs of spotted fever: an inoculation eschar (in one case two inoculation eschars), fever, headache and a generalized maculopapular rash [1].

Rickettsia massiliae has been detected in several species of *Rhipicephalus* ticks in tropical African countries—the Central African Republic, Senegal, Ivory Coast and Mali—and also in southern Europe and the USA [1]. It is an emergent pathogen with only three cases of human infection described in Italy, in France, and in Argentina. These three patients presented the same clinical signs as Mediterranean spotted fever. The French patient presented acute visual loss and bilateral chorioretinitis [5].

Rickettsia helvetica has been detected in *Ixodes ricinus* in many European countries, northern Africa and Asia. Among 4604 clinical rickettsial cases reported in Italy from 1998 to 2002, three cases of a mild form of rickettsiosis were serologically attributed to *R. helvetica*. The *R. helvetica* infection presented as a mild disease in the warm season and was associated with fever, headache and myalgia, and sometimes with a cutaneous rash. Additional evaluation and isolation of the bacterium from clinical samples are needed to confirm the pathogenicity of this bacterium.

Rickettsia monacensis has been detected in Europe, northern Africa and the USA [7]. Recently, two cases were described in Spain. The clinical picture is the same as with Mediterranean spotted fever, without inoculation eschars. The strain of *R. monacensis* isolated from human samples was not analyzed by another laboratory; its epidemiology remains unknown.

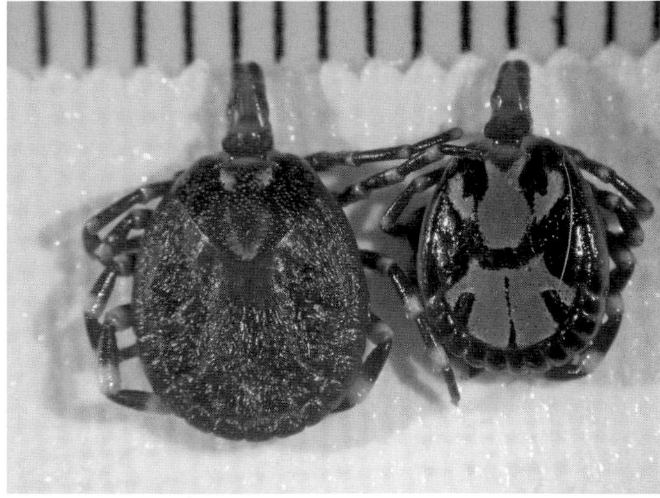

FIGURE 64.4 *Amblyomma variegatum* adult ticks (male right, female left), a vector of African tick-bite fever, the etiological agent of *Rickettsia africae*.

Candidatus Rickettsia kellyi was detected in human samples from a one-year-old boy from India. He presented with fever and maculopapular rash. To date, the rickettsial strain has not been isolated from human samples or arthropod vector. Further investigations are required for characterization of its role in human pathology [7].

DIAGNOSIS

STANDARD LABORATORY FEATURES

Hematological anomalies include anemia with thrombocytopenia, with neutropenia in the acute phase of disease and leukocytosis in the later stages. Non-specific biochemical changes include decreased levels of protein (particularly albumin), sodium, potassium and chloride, and elevated hepatic enzyme levels during the first 10 days of disease. Creatinine phosphokinase and lactic dehydrogenase are also often raised.

DIAGNOSTIC TOOLS

The diagnosis of tick-borne rickettsioses is based on clinical and epidemiologic findings. The diagnosis should be suspected in a febrile patient with a history of tick bite, headache, a rash and/or a skin lesion consisting of a black necrotic area surrounded by erythema or a pseudofurunculus or crust. The classic features of tick-borne rickettsioses may only occur in 50–75% of patients. Confirmation of the diagnosis may be assessed by specific serology or by isolation or molecular identification of the causative organism. For serologic diagnosis, one serum sample should be collected early in the course of the disease; a second sample should be obtained two to three weeks later. If antibody titers remain negative in these two samples, a later sample must be tested (4 to 6 weeks). Usually, antibodies are absent in the early phase of the disease. The presence of specific IgM antibodies or a fourfold increase in titer of IgG antibodies from acute-phase illness to the convalescent phase is considered diagnostic. The interpretation of serologic data can be confounded by the cross-reactivity that occurs among spotted fever group rickettsiae. Western blot analysis will yield false-positive results because of cross-reacting antibodies that are directed mainly against lipopolysaccharides. Western blots, particularly in conjunction with sera that have been cross-adsorbed, can also be used to identify the infecting rickettsial species, but the technique is only appropriate for reference laboratories (Fig. 64.5).

To isolate rickettsiae organisms from skin biopsy and heparin, blood specimens collected before antimicrobial therapy (preferably from

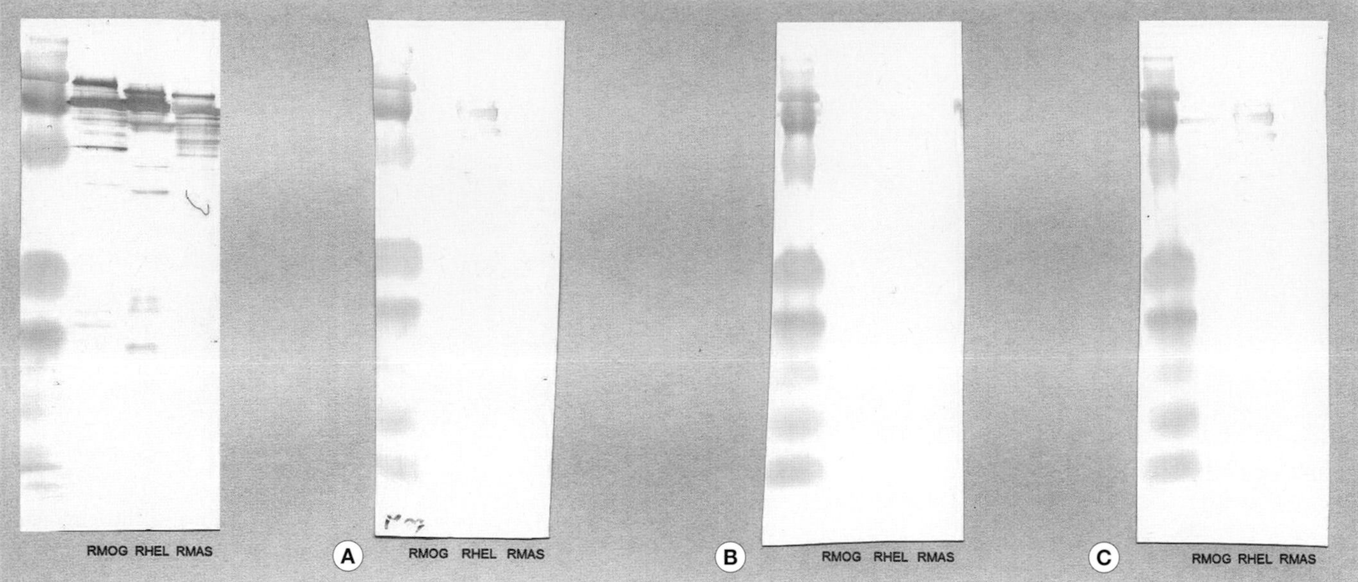

FIGURE 64.5 Western blot before and after cross-adsorption with *Rickettsia sibirica mongolitimonae* **(A)**, *R. helvetica* **(B)**, or *R. massiliae* **(C)**. When cross-adsorption is performed with *R. helvetica*, the specific antigen-corresponding line disappears—this implicates *R. helvetica* as the causative microorganism.

the site of tick attachment) must be processed in cell culture using the shell vial technique (only in Biosafety Level [BSL] 3-specialized laboratories). Shell vial culture remains the best tool for the isolation of intracellular bacteria. Several samples can be used for the diagnosis of rickettsiosis by molecular tools, such as EDTA blood sample, biopsy specimens of the eschar, swab of skin lesions, paraffin-embedded tissues and arthropods. This specimen collection should be carried out as early as possible in the course of the illness [16, 17]. Biopsy material kept in formalin can be used for immunohistochemistry.

TREATMENT

Early empirical treatment should be started in any suspected rickettsioses before laboratory confirmation of the diagnosis. Based on *in vitro* susceptibility and *in vivo* experience, doxycycline is currently the recommended drug for treating spotted fever group rickettsioses. In adults, 200 mg of doxycycline daily for 2–5 days or until 24 h after apyrexia is most commonly used, but a single 200 mg dose of doxycycline has been shown to be effective for certain spotted fever group rickettsioses [1]. In severe forms of the disease, 200 mg intravenous doxycycline per day followed by 200 mg doxycycline orally per day should be prescribed until complete recovery (10 days). In children and pregnant women, treatment with the macrolide josamycine for 5–7 days has been recommended, but a single dose of doxycycline at 5 mg/kg/d is efficient and has no side-effect of tooth coloration. In those allergic to tetracyclines, ciprofloxacin (1.5 g/day orally for 5 days) or chloramphenicol (2 g day for 7–10 days) is effective against spotted fever group rickettsiae. Treatment failure was reported for chloramphenicol and rifampin. The use of corticosteroids in severe forms is controversial. Ineffective antibiotics include β-lactams, aminoglycosides, and cotrimoxazole.

PREVENTION AND CONTROL

Prophylaxis is based on the prevention of tick bite. Early detection (within 20 h) and appropriate detachment of ticks is essential to avoid the transmission of tick-borne rickettsioses diseases. The classic method of removal is to grasp the tick mouthparts as close to the skin as possible with fine forceps or tweezers and gently lever the arthropod off. To prevent further inoculation, the body should not be squeezed. Any retained fragments should not be dug out, but the site cleaned and antiseptic applied. Antibiotic prophylaxis after tick bites is not justified, even in endemic areas.

REFERENCES

1. Parola P, Paddock CD, Raoult D. Tick borne rickettsioses around the world:emerging diseases challenging old concepts. Clin Microbiol Rev 2005;18:719–56.
2. Parola P, Socolovschi C, Raoult D. Deciphering the relationships between *Rickettsia conorii conorii* and *Rhipicephalus sanguineus* in the ecology and epidemiology of Mediterranean spotted fever. Ann N Y Acad Sci 2009;1166:49–54.
3. Renvoise A, Mediannikov O, Raoult D. Old and new tick-borne rickettsioses. International Health 2009;1:17–25.
4. Fournier PE, Dumler JS, Greub G, et al. Gene sequence-based criteria for identification of new rickettsia isolates and description of *Rickettsia heilongjiangensis* sp. nov. J Clin Microbiol 2003;41:5456–65.
5. Parola P, Socolovschi C, Jeanjean L, et al. Warmer weather linked to tick attack and emergence of severe rickettsioses. PLoS Negl Trop Dis 2008;2:e338.
6. Rovery C, Raoult D. Mediterranean spotted fever. Infect Dis Clin North Am 2008; 22:515–30.
7. Mediannikov OY, Parola P, Raoult D. Other tick-borne rickettsioses. In: Parola P, Raoult D, eds. Rickettsial diseases. New York: Informa Healthcare; 2007: 139–62.
8. Graves S, Stenos J. Rickettsioses in Australia. Ann N Y Acad Sci 2009;1166:151–5.
9. Paddock CD, Finley RW, Wright CS, et al. *Rickettsia parkeri rickettsiosis* and its clinical distinction from Rocky Mountain spotted fever. Clin infect dis 2008;47:1188–96.
10. Raoult D, Parola P. Rocky Mountain spotted fever in the USA: a benign disease or a common diagnostic error? Lancet Infect Dis 2008; 8:587–9.
11. Childs J, Paddock C. Rocky Mountain Spotted Fever. In: Raoult D, Parola P, eds. Rickettsial Diseases. New York: Informa; 2007:97–116.
12. Parola P, Rovery C, Rolain JM, et al. *Rickettsia slovaca* and *R. raoultii* in Tick-borne Rickettioses. Emerg Infect Dis 2009;15:1105–8.
13. Angelakis E, Pulcini C, Watson J, et al. Scalp eschar and neck lymphadenopathy caused by *Bartonella henselae* after tick bite. Clin Infect Dis 2010; 50:549–51.
14. Fournier PE, Gouriet F, Brouqui P, et al. Lymphangitis-associated rickettsiosis, a new rickettsiosis caused by *Rickettsia sibirica mongolotimonae*: Seven new cases and review of the literature. Clin Infect Dis 2005;40:1435–44.
15. Jensenius M, Fournier PE, Kelly P, et al. Afican tick bite fever. Lancet Infect Dis 2003;3:557–64.
16. Brouqui P, Bacellar F, Baranton G, et al. Guidelines for the diagnosis of tick-borne bacterial diseases in Europe. Clin Microbiol Infect 2004;10: 1108–32.
17. Fenollar F, Raoult D. Molecular genetic methods for the diagnosis of fastidious microorganisms. APMIS 2004;112(11-12):785–807.

Rickettsialpox 65

Christopher D Paddock

Key features

- A mite-borne zoonosis caused by *Rickettsia akari* and transmitted to humans by the house mouse mite (*Liponyssoides sanguineus*)
- Most cases originate in urban settings and are associated with house mouse infestations
- A relatively mild spotted fever rickettsiosis with a cosmopolitan distribution
- Clinical disease characterized by fever, an inoculation eschar, and a vesiculopustular rash
- Severe disease is unusual and there have been no known deaths
- Doxycycline is the therapy of choice
- Prevention usually involves anti-rodent measures

INTRODUCTION

Rickettsialpox, a mite-borne zoonosis that cycles among house mice (*Mus musculus*) and house mouse mites (*Liponyssoides sanguineus*), was discovered by physicians in 1946 in the borough of Queens, New York City, USA, during an epidemic of this disease that involved more than 120 people. Within just a few months, epidemiologists, entomologists, and microbiologists successfully identified the cause of the outbreak and isolated and described the causative agent – *Rickettsia akari* (from the Greek word for *mite*). In 1949, Soviet investigators in the Ukraine identified a large outbreak of a disease they described as "vesicular rickettsiosis", subsequently recognized as rickettsialpox. Confirmed, or probable cases, of rickettsialpox are now recognized from at least 13 countries around the world (Fig. 65.1), making this disease one of the few spotted fever rickettsioses with a cosmopolitan distribution [1–3].

EPIDEMIOLOGY

Despite its global distribution, every case series of rickettsialpox published during the last 50 years describes a patient cohort that resided within the geographical boundaries of New York City [4–8]. This observation suggests that most clinicians beyond the borders of New York City are relatively unfamiliar with rickettsialpox, despite documented occurrences of the pathogen in several other regions of the USA and in many other countries, including Ukraine, Croatia, South Korea, and Mexico [3, 9–11]. Suspect cases of rickettsialpox, identified by serologic assays, have been reported from Albania, Bosnia-Herzegovina, Costa Rica, Central African Republic, France, Germany, South Africa, and Turkey [3, 12, 13]; however, many clinically similar, eschar-associated spotted fever group rickettsioses caused by other species of spotted fever group rickettsiae occur in countries around the world; antibodies generated to any of these other agents may cross-react with antigens of *R. akari*. Rickettsialpox has been described in patients of all ages, from infants as young as 6 months, to adults as old as 92 years. In most patient series, the disease occurs equally among males and females and cases are documented from all months of the year. Cases of rickettsialpox often cluster in time and space, and simultaneous or consecutive illnesses have been identified among family members or other residents from a single common location. In contrast with many other rickettsioses, most cases of rickettsialpox are described from large metropolitan areas and urban centers, consistent with the important role of peri-domestic rodents in the distribution and occurrence of *R. akari* [1, 3–7].

NATURAL HISTORY, PATHOGENESIS, AND PATHOLOGY

Rickettsia akari is transmitted among several species of rodents by *Liponyssoides sanguineus* (Fig. 65.2A). Humans are not a regular component in the natural circulation of *R. akari* – zoonotic transmission of this pathogen occurs only when a mite infected with rickettsiae is unable to locate its natural host and is forced to obtain a blood meal from a human host. In that context, ecologic factors that govern populations of rodent reservoirs or their ectoparasites undoubtedly influence the emergence of this disease in human populations. *Rickettsia akari* has been cultured from commensal and wild rodent species, particularly the house mouse (Fig. 65.2B); however, trans-ovarial and trans-stadial transmission of rickettsiae occurs in *L. sanguineus*, implicating the mite as an important reservoir host of *R. akari*. *Liponyssoides sanguineus* is a small (approximately 400–700 μm) ectoparasite, most often found in proximity to rodent haborages that include nests and burrows, and in cracks and crevices close to nesting sites. Nymphal stages and adult mites ingest blood and can transmit *R. akari* to a susceptible host. Because of its minute size, this mite is almost never seen by patients.

Liponyssoides sanguineus has been collected from house mice and various rodent species in the USA, Eurasia, and Africa. Despite broad geographic distributions of the vector mite and the house mouse, confirmed reports of rickettsialpox are relatively sparse and sporadic, suggesting that conditions that favor the parasitism of humans by *L. sanguineus* may have the greatest impact on the epidemiologic activity of rickettsialpox. The tropical rat mite (*Liponyssus bacoti*) can also serve as an efficient vector of *R. akari* under experimental conditions and *R. akari* has been detected in trombiculid mites in South Korea, suggesting that other species of hematophagous mites are involved in the natural history of this pathogen [3, 14–19].

Rickettsia akari does not stain well with conventional Gram- or eosin-azure-based methods, but does stain with Giménez, Macchiavello's and other related techniques that use carbol basic fuchsin (Fig. 65.2C). *Rickettsia akari* is best identified in host tissues by using immunohistochemical or fluorescein stains. Using these techniques, the bacteria appear as small (approximately 0.3 μm × 1. 0 μm) rods or coccobacilli situated in the cytoplasm of the host cell. *Rickettsia akari* is predominantly found in macrophages in the perivascular and

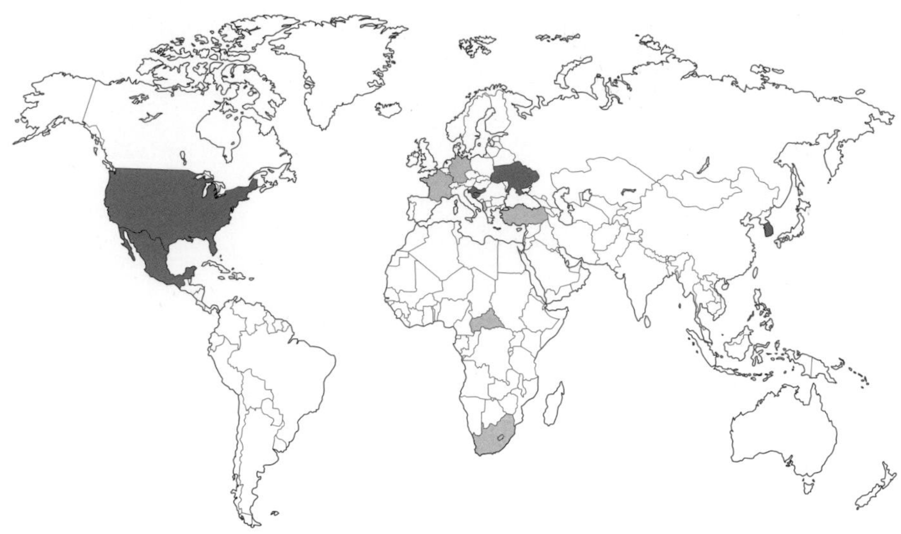

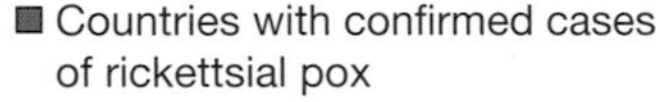

FIGURE 65.1 Global distribution of confirmed (dark green) and probable (light green) cases of rickettsialpox throughout 2009.

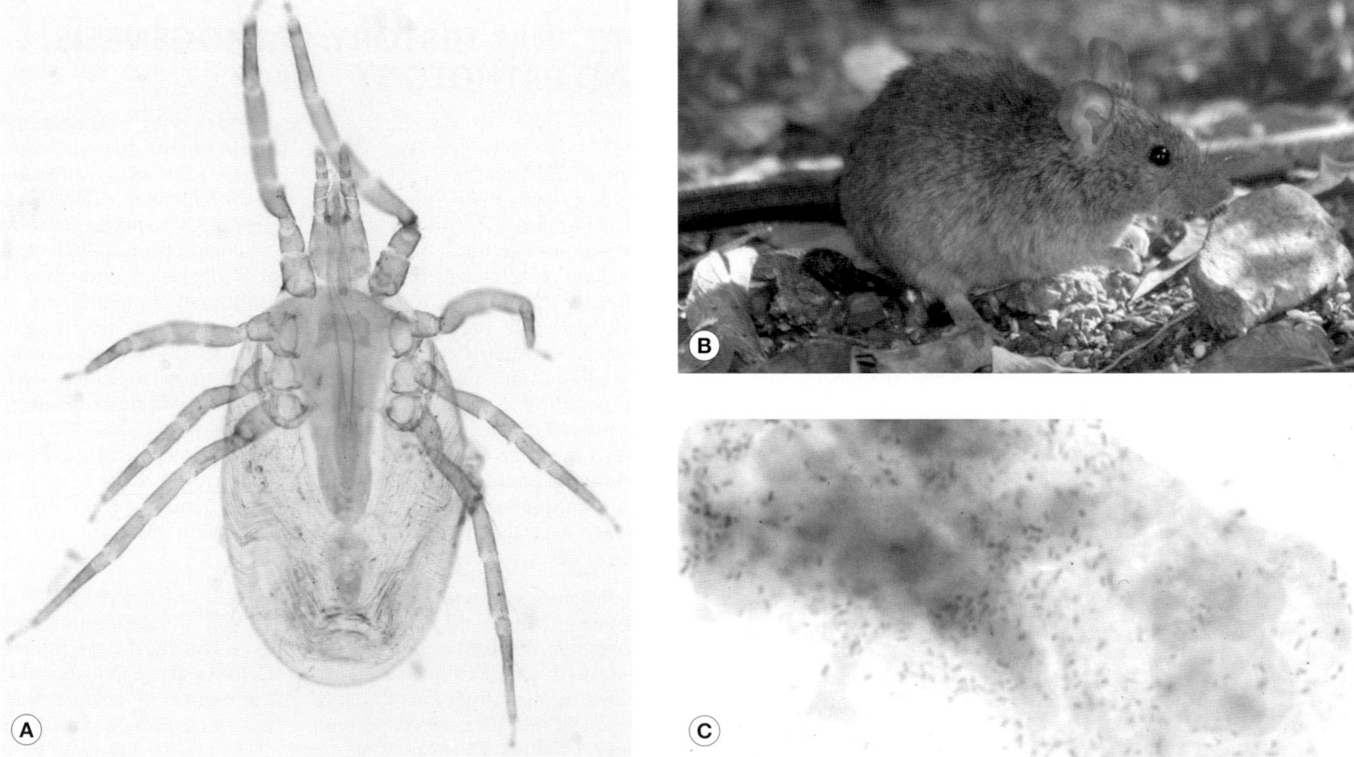

FIGURE 65.2 (A) Ventral aspect of an adult female *L. sanguineus* (Acari: Dermanyssidae), the mite vector of rickettsialpox. Cleared specimen stained with acid fuchsin. **(B)** The house mouse (*M. musculus*), an important vertebrate host involved in the epidemiology of rickettsialpox. **(C)** Giménez-stained *R. akari* bacteria in mouse peritoneal macrophages. *We gratefully acknowledge Larry Masters for image B.*

periadnexal inflammatory cell infiltrates of the cutaneous lesions and only rarely in vascular endothelial cells. The histopathology of the inoculation eschar demonstrates extensive necrosis of the epidermis and dermis, with subjacent perivascular and periadnexal inflammatory cell infiltrates and occasional panniculitis. The histopathology of the rash is typically more variable and age-dependent; however, fully developed papulovesicles show subepidermal vesicle formation that is a characteristic histopathologic feature of rickettsialpox. Inflamed blood vessels demonstrate varying degrees of endothelial swelling, blurring or obliteration of the vessel wall by inflammatory cell infiltrates, mural necrosis, extravasation of red cells, or fibrin thrombi. Lymphocytes and macrophages comprise the predominant inflammatory cell types, although neutrophils are occasionally present in, and around, necrotic foci [3, 20, 21].

CLINICAL FEATURES

Estimated limits of the incubation period range from 6 to 15 days following the bite of an infected mite. The primary lesion, or inoculation eschar, is described for 83–100% of patients in several large series (Table 65-1). In its early stages, it is a painless, non-pruritic, erythematous papule that soon enlarges and develops a central vesicle containing clear, or opaque, fluid (Fig. 65.3A). Eventually, the vesicle ruptures and a dark brown or black crust develops over the lesion, forming the characteristic eschar (Figs 65.3B, C). The eschar is often surrounded by a larger zone of erythema. Primary lesions range in size from 0.5 to 2.5 cm and are most frequently observed on the extremities, but may be found anywhere on the body. Two eschars are occasionally identified on separate anatomic sites. The eschar generally persists for 3–4 weeks and may heal to form a small, depressed scar. A cutaneous eruption develops in most patients 1–4 days following the onset of fever. This eruption is characterized by small (2–10 mm), discrete, erythematous maculopapules distributed on the extremities, abdomen, back, chest, and face, and only rarely on the palms and soles. After 2–3 days, some lesions become indurated and develop a small vesicle containing cloudy fluid at the apex. The number of papules varies from 5 to more than 100, although most patients develop approximately 20–30 of these lesions. The rash is neither painful nor pruritic and generally resolves within 7 days to leave small, hyperpigmented spots. An enanthem occurs in approximately 20–25% of patients and is characterized by small (2–4 mm) vesicles, maculopapules or erosions on the oral mucosae [2, 4–8, 22].

Patients with rickettsialpox typically develop fever, diaphoresis, lassitude, myalgias, and headache within 2–7 days after the appearance of the inoculation eschar. In patients who do not receive specific antibiotic therapy, these symptoms persist for approximately 7–10 days. The peak temperature is 38–40 °C, although it may rise to 41 °C. A headache, usually frontal and occasionally severe, is described in approximately 90–100% of patients. Myalgias are frequently reported and are most commonly described as backache. Less frequently described findings include conjunctivitis, splenomegaly, pharyngitis, nausea and vomiting. Rickettsialpox is recognized as a relatively benign, self-limited illness and, in most case series, patients are hospitalized infrequently. Moderate-to-severe manifestations are reported rarely and include hepatitis, disseminated intravascular coagulopathy with hemorrhagic diatheses, photophobia and nuchal rigidity. No deaths have been attributed to infection with *R. akari* [2, 11, 23].

PATIENT EVALUATION, DIAGNOSIS, AND DIFFERENTIAL DIAGNOSIS

The differential diagnosis of a patient with an eschar and fever includes ecthyma gangrenosum, herpetic dermatitis, aspergillosis, cutaneous leishmaniasis, tularemia, melioidiosis and cutaneous anthrax; however, several other rickettsial diseases, including African tick-bite fever, *Rickettsia parkeri* rickettsiosis, boutonneuse fever, Queensland tick typhus, scrub typhus, (Table 65-1) are, perhaps, the most likely to clinically resemble rickettsialpox [24–27]. Among these diseases, rickettsialpox is notable for the frequent occurrence of a vesicular rash and the relative infrequency of regional adenopathy. A carefully collected patient history that includes questions about area of residence, recent travel and potential exposures to rodents (particularly house mice) can provide additional diagnostic clues [3, 6, 7, 21].

Laboratory diagnosis of rickettsialpox is ascertained most often by serologic methods. Most patients with rickettsialpox, in contrast with

TABLE 65-1 Clinical and Epidemiologic Characteristics of Rickettsialpox and Other Selected Eschar-Associated Rickettsioses

Characteristic or clinical feature	Rickettsialpox (n = 197)	African tick-bite fever (n = 191)	*Rickettsia parkeri* rickettsiosis (n = 12)	Queensland tick typhus (n = 80)	Scrub typhus (n = 87)
Causative agent	*Rickettsia akari*	*Rickettsia africae*	*Rickettsia parkeri*	*Rickettsia australis*	*Orientia tsutsugamushi*
Arthropod vector	Mite	Tick	Tick	Tick	Mite
Geographic distribution	Worldwide	Sub-Saharan Africa, West Indies	Southern USA, South America	Australia	Australia, Afghanistan India, Japan, Taiwan China, Southeast Asia
Inoculation eschar(s)					
Any	92%	95%	92%	74%	46%
Multiple	14%	54%	17%	2%	NR
Rash					
Any type	100%	46%	83%	84%	34%
Maculopapules	100%	24%	83%	79%	34%
Vesiculopustules	100%	21%	42%	62%	0
Lymphadenopathy	17%	43%	25%	73%	85%
Hospitalization	18%	NR	33%	12%	100%[1]
Case-fatality ratio	0	0	0	0[2]	0[3]
Reference(s)	2, 6, 22	24	25	26	27

NR, not reported or data not available.
[1]Series selected among febrile hospitalized patients; rates of hospitalization typically lower in other studies.
[2]No deaths in this series; however, fatal disease has been described rarely.
[3]No deaths in this series; however, case-fatality ratio of untreated patients from other studies are 0.5–10%.

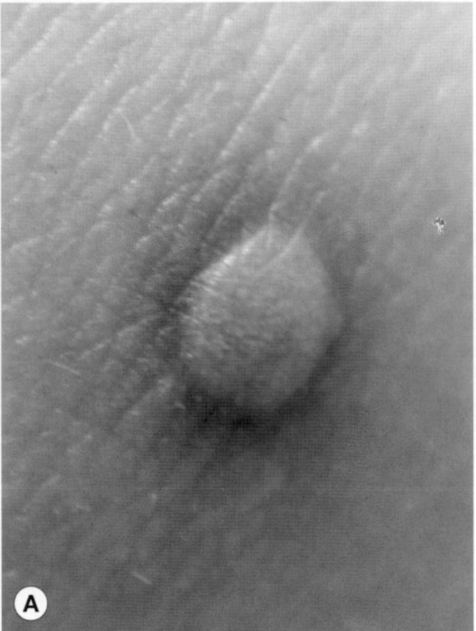
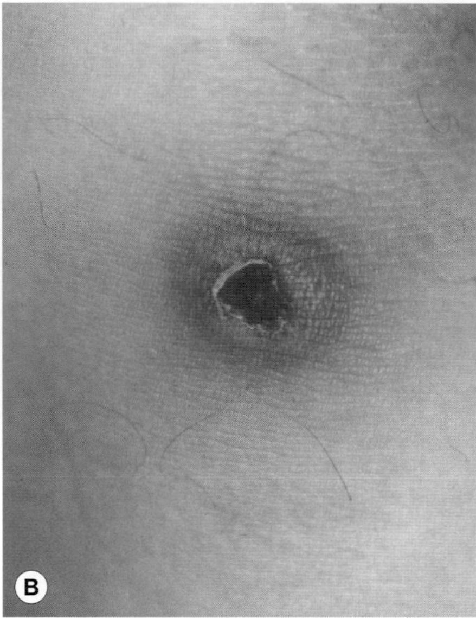
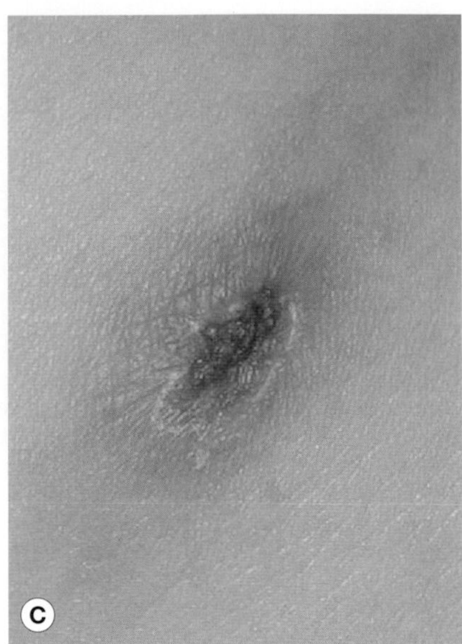

FIGURE 65.3 (A) Vesicular lesion on the ankle of a patient with rickettsialpox. **(B)** Inoculation eschar on the arm of a patient with rickettsialpox. *Rickettsia akari* was subsequently isolated in cell culture from this lesion. **(C)** Inoculation eschar on the chest of a patient approximately 2 days prior to onset of fever and headache and 6 days prior to the onset of a papulovesicular rash. We gratefully acknowledge the following individuals for their assistance: David E. Geist, M.D (University of Massachusetts Medical School) for image A, Tamara Koss, M.D. (Columbia University College of Physicians and Surgeons) for image B and Benjamin Gewurz, M.D. (Brigham and Women's Hospital) for image C.

other spotted fever rickettsioses, do not develop agglutinating antibodies against the OX-19, OX-2, and OX-K antigens of *Proteus vulgaris* (i.e. negative Weil-Felix reactions). A negative Weil-Felix test is considered a relatively consistent serologic feature of rickettsialpox, but provides only presumptive evidence. The microimmunofluorescence or indirect immunofluorescence (IFA) assay is currently the most widely available and frequently used assay to detect antibodies reactive with spotted fever group *Rickettsia* species. Major caveats in the interpretation of all commonly used and commercially-available serologic techniques include the frequent absence of diagnostic antibody titers (i.e. ≥64) during the first week of the illness and the high cross-reactivity among antigens of rickettsiae in the spotted fever group. The evaluation of serologic results should be always considered in the context of the epidemiologic situation. When possible, more specific techniques, such as cross-adsorption or Western blotting should used to corroborate the diagnosis; however, these assays are generally restricted to specialized research laboratories and reference centers [3, 7, 17].

Because rickettsiae and rickettsial antigens are distributed in great abundance in the inoculation eschar, a skin biopsy specimen of this lesion generally represents the best diagnostic sample for the confirmation of rickettsialpox. Portions from one 4-mm punch biopsy obtained from the central aspect of the lesion can be evaluated by routine histopathologic methods, stained by immunohistochemical stains for spotted fever group *Rickettsia* species, tested by PCR or used to inoculate cell cultures for attempted isolation of *R. akari*. PCR testing of swabs obtained from unroofed eschar lesions has proven to be an effective method for diagnosing other eschar-associated rickettsioses, including those caused by *Rickettsia australis*, *Rickettsia africae*, and *R. parkeri*, and may also provide a useful diagnositic adjunct for rickettsialpox if a skin biopsy is not achievable [28]. Molecular and immunohistochemical staining techniques are sensitive methods of diagnosis during the acute phase of the disease; however, the availability of these assays is generally limited to national reference centers or specialized research laboratories [3, 7, 20, 21]. The reference standard for laboratory confirmation of rickettsialpox is cultivation of *R. akari* in cell culture; *R. akari* will grow in several standard cell lines, including Vero E6 and L929 cells. In this context, Biosafety Level (BSL) 2 laboratories that routinely perform viral cultures should be able to isolate *R. akari* from clinical specimens in cell culture; however, BSL 3 practices would be required for subsequent propogation of any established isolate [9, 21].

TREATMENT

Tetracyclines, particularly doxycycline, remain the drugs of choice for the treatment of rickettsialpox. In two contemporary case series documenting antibiotic responses in 28 patients who received tetracycline or doxycycline treatment for rickettsialpox, fever and other systemic symptoms resolved in most patients within 24 hours and all patients became asymptomatic within 48 hours [5, 6]. The standard oral dose of doxycycline is 100 mg every 12 hours for 5–10 days. Despite concerns regarding dental staining after use of tetracyclines in pregnant women or in children younger than 8 years of age, a short (e.g. 5 days) course of therapy is not considered to cause dental staining. Chloramphenicol, given at a dosage of 12.5 mg/kg every 6 hours for 5–10 days can be used as alternate therapy in those patients for whom there is an absolute contraindication for receiving doxycycline.

Rickettsia akari is susceptible *in vitro* to various fluoroquinolones, including ciprofloxacin, oflaxacin and pefloxacin, and several macrolide antibiotics, including josamycin, pristinamycin, and clarithromycin and azithromycin; however, there are no clinical data to evaluate the efficacy of these drugs for the treatment of rickettsialpox [29, 30].

PREVENTION

There is no commercialy available vaccine for use in humans. Prevention usualy involves minimizing human contact with rodents and their dwellings.

REFERENCES

1. Greenberg M, Pellitteri OJ, Jellison WL. Rickettsialpox—a newly discovered rickettsial disease. III. Epidemiology. Am J Pub Health 1947;37:860–8.
2. Greenberg M, Pellitteri O, Klein IF, Huebner RJ. Rickettsialpox—a newly recognized rickettsial disease. II. Clinical observations. J Am Med Assoc 1947;133:901–6.
3. Paddock CD, Eremeeva ME. Rickettsialpox. In: Raoult D, Parola P, eds. Rickettsial Diseases. New York: Informa Healthcare; 2007:63–86.
4. Brettman LR, Lewin S, Holzman RS, et al. Rickettsialpox: report of an outbreak and a contemporary review. Medicine (Baltimore) 1981;60:363–72.
5. Kass EM, Szaniawski WK, Levy H, et al. Rickettsialpox in a New York City hospital, 1980 to 1989. N Engl J Med 1994;331:1612–17.

6. Koss T, Carter EL, Grossman ME, et al. Increased detection of rickettsialpox in a New York City hospital following the anthrax outbreak of 2001: use of immunohistochemistry for the rapid confirmation of cases in an era of bioterrorism. Arch Dermatol 2003;139:1545–52.
7. Paddock CD, Zaki SR, Koss T, et al. Rickettsialpox in New York City: a persistent urban zoonosis. Ann N Y Acad Sci 2003;990:36–44.
8. Saini R, Pui JC, Burgin, S. Rickettsialpox: report of three cases and a review. J Am Acad Dermatol 2004;51:S65–70.
9. Radulovic S, Feng HM, Morovic M, et al. Isolation of *Rickettsia akari* from a patient in a region where Mediterranean spotted fever is endemic. Clin Infect Dis 1996;22:216–20.
10. Choi YJ, Jang WJ, Ryu JS, et al. Spotted fever group and typhus group rickettsioses in humans, South Korea. Emerg Infect Dis 2005;11:237–44.
11. Zavala-Castro JE, Zavala-Velázquez JE, Peniche-Lara GF, Sulú Uicab JE. Human rickettsialpox, southeastern Mexico. Emerg Infect Dis 2009;15: 1665–7.
12. Ozturk MK, Gunes T, Coker C, Radulovic S. Rickettsialpox in Turkey. Emerg Infect Dis 2003;9:1498–9.
13. Le Gac P, Giroud P. Rickettsiose vésiculeuse en Oubangui-Chari (A.E.F.). Bull Soc Pathol Exot 1951;44:413–15.
14. Eustis EB, Fuller HS. Rickettsialpox. II. Recovery of *Rickettsia akari* from mites, *Allodermanyssus sanguineus*, from West Hartford, Conn. Proc Soc Exp Biol Med 1952;80:546–9.
15. Fuller HS, Murray ES, Ayres JC, et al. Studies of rickettsialpox. II. Recovery of the causative agent from house mice in Boston, Massachusetts. Am J Hyg 1951;54:82–100.
16. Jackson EB, Danauskas JX, Coale MC, Smadel JE. Recovery of *Rickettsia akari* from the Korean reed vole *Microtus fortis pelliceus*. Am J Hyg 1957;66: 301–8.
17. Bennett SG, Comer JA, Smith H, Webb JP. Serologic evidence of *Rickettsia akari*-like infection among wild-caught rodents in Orange County and in humans in Los Angeles County, California. J Vector Ecol 2007;32:198–201.
18. Philip CB, Hughes LE. The tropical rat mite, *Liponyssus bacoti*, as an experimental vector of rickettsialpox. Am J Trop Med 1948;28:697–705.
19. Choi YJ, Lee EM, Park JM, et al. Molecular detection of various rickettsiae in mites (Acari: Trombiculidae) in southern Jeolla province, Korea. Microbiol Immunol 2007;51:307–12.
20. Walker DH, Hudnall SD, Szaniawski WK, Feng HM. Monoclonal antibody-based immunohistochemical diagnosis of rickettsialpox: the macrophage is the principal target. Mod Pathol 1999;12:529–33.
21. Paddock CD, Koss T, Eremeeva ME, et al. Isolation of *Rickettsia akari* from eschars of patients with rickettsialpox. Am J Trop Med Hyg 2006;75:732–8.
22. Rose HM. The clinical manifestations and laboratory diagnosis of rickettsialpox. Ann Intern Med 1949:31:871–83.
23. Madison G, Kim-Schulger L, Braverman S, et al. Hepatitis in association with rickettsialpox. Vector-Borne Zoonotic Dis 2008;8:1–5.
24. Raoult D, Fournier PE, Fenollar F, et al. *Rickettsia africae*, a tick-borne pathogen in travelers to sub-Saharan Africa. N Engl J Med 2001;344:1504–10.
25. Paddock CD, Finley RW, Wright CS, et al. *Rickettsia parkeri* rickettsiosis and its clinical distinction from Rocky Mountain spotted fever. Clin Infect Dis 2008;47:1188–96.
26. Hudson BJ, Hofmeyr A, Williams E, et al. Prospective study of Australian spotted fever—clinical and epidemiological features. In: Abstracts of the 4th International Conference on Rickettsiae and Rickettsial Diseases, Logrono, La Rioja, Spain 2005 June 18–21. Abstract P-201.
27. Berman SJ, Kundin WD. Scrub typhus in South Vietnam, a study of 87 cases. Ann Intern Med 1973;79:26–30.
28. Wang JM, Hudson BJ, Watts MR, et al. Diagnosis of Queensland tick typhus and African tick bite fever by PCR of lesion swabs. Emerg Infect Dis 2009;15:963–5.
29. Rolain JM, Maurin M, Vestris G, Raoult D. In vitro susceptibilities of 27 rickettsiae to 13 antimicrobials. Antimicrob Agents Chemother 1998; 42;1537–41.
30. Ives TJ, Manzewitsch P, Regnery RL, et al. In vitro susceptibilities of *Bartonella henselae, B. quintana, B. elizabethae, Rickettsia rickettsii, R. conorii, R. akari*, and *R. prowazekii* to macrolide antibiotics as determined by immunofluorescent antibody analysis of infected Vero cell monolayers. Antimicrob Agents Chemother 1997;41:578–82.

66 Q Fever

Matthieu Million, Didier Raoult

Key features

- Q fever is a zoonosis with cattle and sheep being important reservoirs
- The causative agent is *Coxiella burnetii*, an intracellular bacterium
- Humans become infected after environmental exposure to aerosolized pseudospores
- Clinical manifestations are myriad and include pneumonia, hepatitis, prolonged fever, and endocarditis
- Diagnosis is usually one of clinical recognition and serologic analysis
- Treatment usually involves doxycycline, with or without hydroxycholoroquine, and may need to be prolonged
- Human vaccine is commercially available only in Australia
- Prevention usually involves limiting exposure to infected animals and their products, especially placental materials

INTRODUCTION

Q fever is a widespread zoonotic infection caused by the pathogen *Coxiella burnetii* that has both acute and potentially lethal chronic manifestations [1]. The designation Q fever (from Query) was made in 1935 following an outbreak of febrile illness in an abattoir in Queensland, Australia. Its agent, *C. burnetii*, a potential agent of bioterrorism (classified as Class B by the USA Centers for Disease Control and Prevention [CDC]) [2], has a worldwide distribution, including tropical areas.

EPIDEMIOLOGY

RESERVOIR

Q fever is a worldwide zoonosis and humans are incidental hosts. The reservoir includes mammals, birds, and arthropods (mainly ticks) [1]. The most commonly identified sources of human infection are farm animals, such as cattle, goats, and sheep. Infected mammals shed *C. burnetii* in urine, feces, milk, and birth products, in particular.

TRANSMISSION TO HUMANS

Human exposure results from inhalation of contaminated aerosols from parturient fluids of infected livestock [1]. Occupational exposure is a common form of acquisition [3, 4]. Transmission can also occur by the consumption of raw milk, transplacentally, via exposure to blood or through sexual intercourse [5, 6]. Exposure to soil and standing water has also been postulated as a possible source of infection in tropical areas [7].

TEMPORAL AND GEOGRAPHIC DISTRIBUTION

The geographic distribution of Q fever is worldwide. As the clinical presentation is nonspecific, the identification of cases depends upon clinical recognition and the availability of a reference laboratory. Thus, incidence figures for the disease vary widely. In southern France, the incidence of acute Q fever is approximately 50 cases per 100,000 people per year; approximately 1 case per 1,000,000 people per year are diagnosed with Q fever endocarditis. Cases of acute Q fever in Europe occur more frequently in spring and early summer [8]. Large outbreaks of Q fever have been reported in several countries in Europe and North America; cases and outbreaks are probably underestimated in resource-limited countries.

NATURAL HISTORY, PATHOGENESIS, AND PATHOLOGY

Coxiella burnetii is a short (0.3–1.0 μm), pleomorphic rod, possessing a membrane similar to a Gram-negative bacterium stained by the Gimenez method. While previously classified as a Rickettsia, *C. burnetii* has been placed into the gamma subdivision of the Proteobacteria, characterizing it closer to Legionella and Francisella than to Rickettsia [9]. *Coxiella burnetii* has a number of distinctive characteristics, including a sporulation-like process that protects the organism against the external environment, where it can survive for long periods [10]. In mammals, the usual host cell of *C. burnetii* is the macrophage, which is unable to kill the bacterium. Another important characteristic of *C. burnetii* is its antigenic variation, called phase variation. This antigenic shift can be measured and is valuable for differentiating acute from chronic Q fever [1].

CLINICAL FEATURES

Approximately half of individuals infected with *C. burnetii* will be asymptomatic and only 2% will be hospitalized [11, 12]. Symptomatic infection is more likely in adults compared with children, and in men compared with women [12]. Chronic Q fever is defined as infection lasting for more than 6 months and occurs in 5% of patients after acute Q fever [1].

ACUTE INFECTION

The incubation period is approximately 20 days [11]. Three clinical presentations are typically encountered [1]: i) the most common is a self-limited, flu-like syndrome. The onset is typically abrupt with high-grade fever (104°F/40°C), fatigue, headache, and myalgias; ii) pneumonia is very common and patients usually present with a nonproductive cough, fever, and minimal auscultatory abnormalities. Acute respiratory distress has been reported and pleural effusions may be present. Radiographic findings are non-specific and may resemble those seen with a viral or atypical pneumonia, such as that caused by *Mycoplasma pneumonia*; iii) hepatitis is also a common manifestation and may be mild, moderate or severe. Jaundice is rarely present. Chronic involvement can manifest as a granulomatous hepatitis (Fig. 66.1). Other manifestations of acute Q fever include maculopapular or purpuric rash, pericarditis, myocarditis, aseptic meningitis, and/or encephalitis and gastroenteritis. Acute acalculous cholecystitis has been reported [13], as has uveitis [14] and other rare, organ-specific immunologic manifestations [15].

CHRONIC INFECTION

Chronic Q fever may develop insidiously months or years after acute disease, especially in immunocompromised patients and in those with significant comorbidities. Chronic Q fever may include endocarditis, vascular mycotic aneurysm or infection of prosthetic devices, all with an accompanying poor prognosis [16, 17]. Other manifestations of chronic Q fever include osteoarthritis, osteomyelitis, and isolated hepatitis, possibly complicated by hepatic fibrosis and cirrhosis.

ENDOCARDITIS

Acute Q fever in patients with valvular disease, particularly a bicuspid aortic valve or a prosthetic valve, results in endocarditis in approximately 40% of patients unless proper treatment is instituted [18]. Some patients who develop Q fever endocarditis have clinically silent and previously undiagnosed valve disease. As a result, a screening echocardiography may be warranted in patients with Q fever [18]. Q fever endocarditis is often the predominant manifestation of chronic infection and can lead to heart failure or arterial embolism [19].

Q FEVER IN PREGNANCY

During pregnancy, Q fever is most often asymptomatic, but may result in obstetrical complications, such as spontaneous abortion, intrauterine growth retardation, intrauterine fetal death, oligoamnios, and premature delivery [12, 20–22]. Although intrauterine transmission of *C. burnetii* has been documented, the consequences of congenital Q fever are uncertain.

CHILDREN

In children, acute Q fever is mostly asymptomatic. Endocarditis may occur in children with congenital heart disease or in those with a history or rheumatic fever.

PATIENT EVALUATION, DIAGNOSIS, AND DIFFERENTIAL DIAGNOSIS

LABORATORY FINDINGS

The laboratory findings during acute Q fever are nonspecific and may include an elevated leukocyte count (25%), thrombocytopenia (25%), and elevated liver enzyme (85%). Autoantibodies are frequently found in Q fever, although their significance is still unknown [19].

PCR

PCR has been successfully employed to detect DNA in both cell cultures and clinical samples [19]. In addition, PCR testing is helpful in confirming the serologic diagnosis of chronic infection in patients who have persistent elevations of IgG anti-phase I titers (see below).

CULTURE

If microbiologic culturing for *C. burnetii* is to be performed, isolation must be undertaken using Biosafety Level (BSL) 3 containment because of the risk of laboratory-associated infection [19]. Shell vial culture is the best, and simplest, technique, allowing isolation of *C. burnetii* from blood or tissues, including cardiac valves.

SEROLOGY

An immunofluorescence assay (IFA) assessing IgG, IgM, and IgA levels against *C. burnetii* phase I versus phase II antigens is currently the reference method used to serodiagnose patients with Q fever. Anti-phase II IgG titers ≥200 and IgM ≥50 are indicative of recent Q fever infection, while an anti-phase I IgG titer >800 suggests chronic infection [19]. As the persistence of high levels of anti-phase I antibodies 6 months after completion of treatment, and the reappearance of previously decreasing antibody titers may signal the development of chronic infection, serologic monitoring should be performed for at least 6 months after acute Q fever, especially for immunocompromised or pregnant patients, and those with valvular or vascular abnormalities.

IMMUNOHISTOCHEMISTRY

Coxiella burnetii can be identified by immunohistochemical analysis of resected valve or liver biopsy specimens using a monoclonal antibody and hematoxylin counter-stain (Figs 66.1 and 66.2).

DIFFERENTIAL DIAGNOSIS

Many infections can manifest in ways similar to Q fever, including *Legionella* spp., *Mycoplasma* spp., and *Leptospira* spp., or viral infections such as those caused by Epstein-Barr virus, cytomegalovirus, hepatitis viruses, and HIV. In addition to *C. burnetii*, the currently recognized agents of "culture-negative" endocarditis include *Bartonella* spp.,

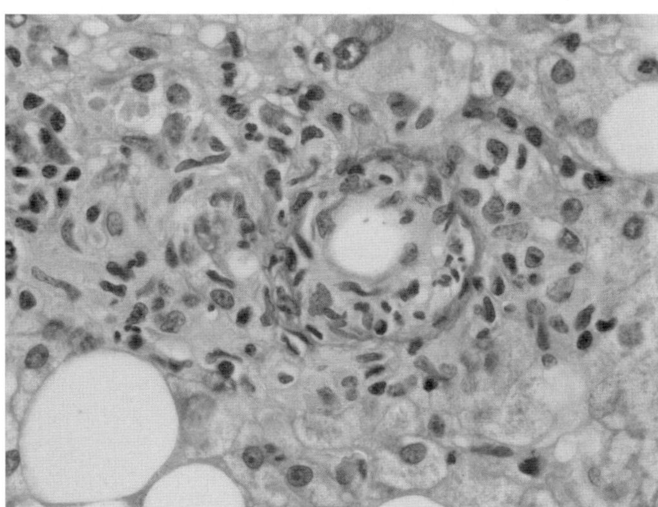

FIGURE 66.1 Histology of the liver in a patient with acute Q fever. Hepatic ring granuloma of Q fever with peripheral epithelioid macrophages and lymphocytes admixed with neutrophils, characteristic central "doughnut" hole, and ring of fibrin. Note the "fatty liver" parenchyma (hematoxylin and eosin, original magnification ×400).

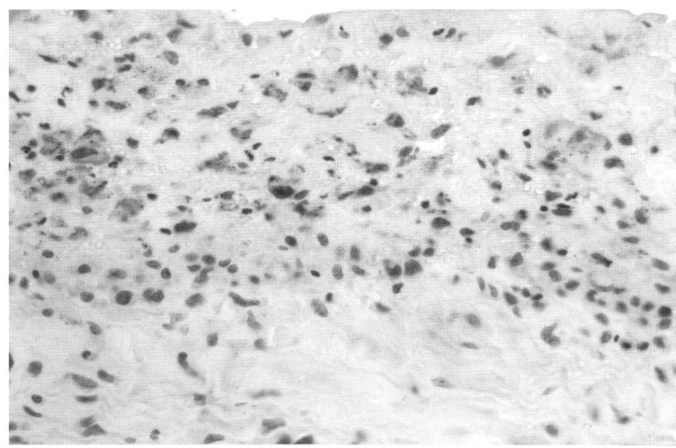

FIGURE 66.2 Immunohistochemical detection of *Coxiella burnetii* in a resected valve from a patient with Q fever endocarditis using a monoclonal antibody and hematoxylin counterstain. Note the intracellular location of the bacteria in the macrophage cytoplasm (original magnification ×400).

Tropheryma whipplei, *Abiotrophia elegans*, *Mycoplasma hominis*, and *Legionella pneumophila* [23].

TREATMENT

MEDICAL THERAPY

In acute disease, treatment of patients infected with *C. burnetii* should target only those who are symptomatic. Doxycycline therapy (100 mg PO twice daily for 14 days) is the recommended regimen for symptomatic acute Q fever [24]. Fluoroquinolones and newer macrolides may be of clinical use and can be considered as second-line agents [25].

ACUTE Q FEVER IN PATIENTS WITH UNDERLYING VALVULAR DISEASE

In patients with underlying valvular disease and acute Q fever, experts suggest that hydroxycholoroquine should be used in combination with doxycycline for 12 months [18]. This regimen may prevent endocarditis.

PREGNANCY

Treatment of pregnant women with Q fever infection is difficult. Many of the drugs used to treat Q fever are contraindicated during pregnancy (e.g. doxycycline, fluoroquinolones). The use of long-term cotrimoxazole therapy has been shown to decrease the risk of placentitis, obstetrical complications, and maternal chronic Q fever infection [26]. Newer macrolides may also be of clinical use.

Q FEVER ENDOCARDITIS

Patients with Q fever endocarditis should be treated with a prolonged course of combination therapy of hydroxychloroquine and doxycycline [27]. The optimum duration of treatment is 18 months for native valves and 24 months for prosthetic valves [28]. This duration should be extended only in the absence of favorable serological outcomes. Patients should be serologically monitored for at least 5 years because of the risk of relapse.

CHILDREN

No reliable antibiotic regimen can be recommended for children. Doxycycline should be prescribed when the disease is life-threatening.

PREVENTION

A human vaccine is commercially available in Australia (Q-VAX). Prevention usually involves limiting exposure to infected animals and their products, especially placental materials.

REFERENCES

1. Raoult D, Marrie T. Q fever. Clin Infect Dis 1995;20:489–95.
2. Raoult D, Marrie T, Mege J. Natural history and pathophysiology of Q fever. Lancet Infect Dis 2005;5:219–26.
3. Wade AJ, Cheng AC, Athan E, et al. Q fever outbreak at a cosmetics supply factory. Clin Infect Dis 2006;42:e50–2.
4. Pantanowitz L, Telford SR, Cannon ME. Tick-borne diseases in transfusion medicine. Transfus Med 2002;12:85–106.
5. Raoult D, Levy PY, Dupont HT, et al. Q fever and HIV infection. AIDS 1993;7:81–6.
6. Milazzo A, Hall R, Storm PA, et al. Sexually transmitted Q fever. Clin Infect Dis 2001;33:399–402.
7. Gardon J, Heraud JM, Laventure S, et al. Suburban transmission of Q fever in French Guiana: evidence of a wild reservoir. J Infect Dis 2001;184:278–84.
8. Tissot DH, Raoult D, Brouqui P, et al. Epidemiologic features and clinical presentation of acute Q fever in hospitalized patients: 323 French cases. Am J Med 1992;93:427–34.
9. Stein A, Saunders NA, Taylor AG, Raoult D. Phylogenic homogeneity of *Coxiella burnetii* strains as determinated by 16S ribosomal RNA sequencing. FEMS Microbiol Lett 1993;113:339–44.
10. Hackstadt T, Williams JC. Biochemical stratagem for obligate parasitism of eukaryotic cells by *Coxiella burnetii*. Proc Natl Acad Sci USA 1981;78:3240–4.
11. Dupuis G, Petite J, Peter O, Vouilloz M. An important outbreak of human Q fever in a Swiss Alpine valley. Int J Epidemiol 1987;16:282–7.
12. Tissot-Dupont H, Vaillant V, Rey S, Raoult D. Role of sex, age, previous valve lesion, and pregnancy in the clinical expression and outcome of Q fever after a large outbreak. Clin Infect Dis 2007;44:232–7.
13. Rolain JM, Lepidi H, Harle JR, et al. Acute acalculous cholecystitis associated with Q fever: report of seven cases and review of the literature. Eur J Clin Microbiol Infect Dis 2003;22:222–7.
14. Matonti F, Conrath J, Bodaghi B, et al. Uveitis in the course of Q-fever. Clin Microbiol Infect 2009;15:176–7.
15. Million M, Lepidi H, Raoult D. Q fever: current diagnosis and treatment options. Med Mal Infect 2009;39:82–94.
16. Brouqui P, Dupont HT, Drancourt M, et al. Chronic Q fever. Ninety-two cases from France, including 27 cases without endocarditis. Arch Intern Med 1993;153:642–8.
17. Botelho-Nevers E, Fournier PE, Richet H, et al. *Coxiella burnetii* infection of aortic aneurysms or vascular grafts: report of 30 new cases and evaluation of outcome. Eur J Clin Microbiol Infect Dis 2007;26:635–40.
18. Fenollar F, Thuny F, Xeridat B, et al. Endocarditis after acute Q fever in patients with previously undiagnosed valvulopathies. Clin Infect Dis 2006;42:818–21.
19. Fournier PE, Marrie TJ, Raoult D. Diagnosis of Q fever. J Clin Microbiol 1998;36:1823–34.
20. Carcopino X, Raoult D, Bretelle F, et al. Q Fever during pregnancy: a cause of poor fetal and maternal outcome. Ann NY Acad Sci 2009;1166:79–89.
21. Raoult D, Fenollar F, Stein A. Q fever during pregnancy: diagnosis, treatment, and follow-up. Arch Intern Med 2002;162:701–4.
22. Stein A, Raoult D. Q fever during pregnancy: a public health problem in southern France. Clin Infect Dis 1998;27:592–6.
23. Houpikian P, Raoult D. Blood culture-negative endocarditis in a reference center: etiologic diagnosis of 348 cases. Medicine (Baltimore) 2005;84:162–73.
24. Raoult D. Treatment of Q fever. Antimicrob Agents Chemother 1993;37:1733–6.
25. Gikas A, Kofteridis DP, Manios A, et al. Newer macrolides as empiric treatment for acute Q fever infection. Antimicrob Agents Chemother 2001;45:3644–6.
26. Carcopino X, Raoult D, Bretelle F, et al. Managing Q fever during pregnancy: the benefits of long-term cotrimoxazole therapy. Clin Infect Dis 2007;45:548–55.
27. Raoult D, Houpikian P, Tissot DH, et al. Treatment of Q fever endocarditis: comparison of 2 regimens containing doxycycline and ofloxacin or hydroxychloroquine. Arch Intern Med 1999;159:167–73.
28. Million M, Thuny F, Richet H, Raoult D. Long-term outcome of Q fever endocarditis: a 26-year personal survey. Lancet Infect Dis 2010;10:527–35.

Trench Fever 67

Barbara Doudier, Philippe Brouqui

Key features

- Trench fever is a relapsing acute febrile disease caused by *Bartonella quintana*
- Trench fever is transmitted by body lice
- Risk factors are war, famine, displacement, poverty, and crowding in resource-limited settings, and deprived social conditions and homelessness in developed countries; these conditions lead to body lice infestation
- Trench fever usually manifests as a sudden febrile illness with headache and post-orbital pain , dizziness, and bone pain, especially of the shins, and may include malaise, chills, anorexia, profuse sweating, conjunctival infection, and myalgia
- Chronic bacteremia following clinical resolution can occur
- Diagnosis is usually based on clinical recognition, serologic tests, or microbiologic culture.
- Individuals with trench fever should be treated with doxycycline and gentamycin; erythromycin may be an alternative
- There is no vaccine available. Prevention usually involves de-lousing, hygiene, and changing clothes

INTRODUCTION

Trench fever is caused by *Bartonella quintana*, a facultative intracellular bacterium transmitted by the human body louse. An estimated 1 million people were affected by trench fever during World War I [1]. It is characterized by attacks of fever that last 2–4 days and is associated with headache, pain in the shin and dizziness, which recur every 4–6 days, although each succeeding attack is usually less severe. Trench fever is now most commonly associated with conditions that predispose to louse infestation, including civil conflict, poverty, overcrowding, and displacement [2], as well as homelessness in industrialized areas, including Europe and the USA [3].

EPIDEMIOLOGY

Bartonella quintana is a cosmopolitan bacterium transmitted by the human body louse, *Pediculus humanus corporis*, which lives in clothes and is associated with poverty, lack of hygiene, and cold weather (Fig. 67.1). Pediculosis (lice infestation) is transmitted by contact with clothes or bedding and is prevalent in impoverished, as well as homeless, populations (Fig. 67.2). In San Francisco, 33.3% of body lice-infested persons and 25% of head lice-infested persons had lice pools infected with *B. Quintana* [4]. In a French cohort of 930 homeless persons, lice infestation was present in 22% of people and 25% had a recent or ongoing bacteremia with *B. quintana* [5]. In Peru, volunteers from four different villages were included in a serologic study: 20% had antibodies against *Rickettsia prowazekii* and 12% had antibodies against *B. quintana* [6].

Bacterial multiplication in body lice starts 4 days after ingestion; *B quintana* is excreted in louse feces for at least 3 weeks [7]. The number of bacteria in feces reaches 10^7 per louse by day 15. The doubling time of *B. quintana* is estimated to be approximately 20 hours. These attributes contribute to the ability of *B. quintana* to cause epidemic disease.

NATURAL HISTORY, PATHOGENESIS, AND PATHOLOGY

Bartonella quintana DNA was detected in the dental pulp of 4000-year-old human remains [8] and it was also detected in lice found in a mass grave containing remains of soldiers serving in Napoleon's army in Lithuania [9].

However, trench fever was first described as a distinct clinical entity during World War I. At this time, the causative bacteria and effective treatment were unknown, but the association with trenches, unsanitary conditions, and louse infestation led to the institution of preventive measures, including bathing and de-lousing.

Bartonella quintana multiplies in the louse's intestine and the bacterium is transmitted by contact with infected louse feces through skin breaks, not through a bite of a louse. Persistent bacteremia in human facilitates its spread back to lice. The bites of body lice can lead to pruritus and scratching, which lead to microabrasions and facilitate transmission of the bacteria. Some humans become chronically bacteremic following resolution of acute illness [10].

Bartonella quintana is also a cause of bacillary angiomatosis and peliosis hepatis. These are disorders of vascular hyperproliferation linked with endothelial cell proliferation and pseudo-tumor formation in immunocompromised persons, especially those with advanced HIV infection [11]. Variable outer membrane proteins ("VOMPS") of *B. quintana* are involved in vascular endothelial growth factor (VEGF) secretion and inducing vascular proliferation.

CLINICAL FEATURES

TRENCH FEVER

Trench fever is an acute disease characterized by sudden onset of high-grade fever, headaches, dizziness, and a characteristic pain in the shins. Dizziness and headaches are sometime so sudden that soldiers have been known to fall over in the trenches. Other symptoms include post-orbital pain (typically exacerbated by movement), pain in the lower limbs and back, constipation, a rash on the face, and a loss of appetite [12]. The first episode of fever may last 2–4 days and may be followed by relapses every 4–6 days, giving rise to trench fever's

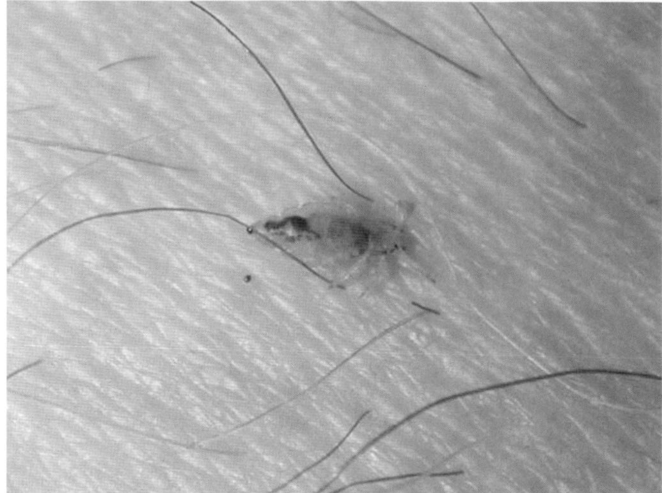

FIGURE 67.1 Body louse, a vector for *B. quintana*, sucking blood on a homeless patient.

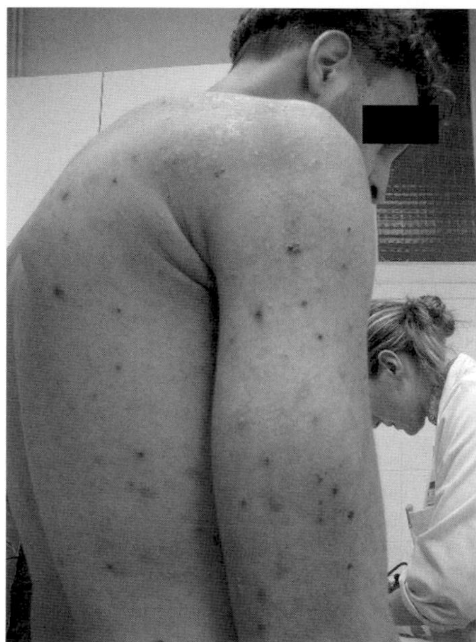

FIGURE 67.2 Pediculosis and super infection in a homeless man seeking care during a snapshot intervention in shelters. *(Reproduced with permission from Brouqui P, Stein A, Dupont HT, et al. Ectoparasitism and vector-borne diseases in 930 homeless people from Marseilles. Medicine (Baltimore) 2005;84:61–8.)*

appellation of "quintane" fever (reflected in its scientific name, *B. quintana*).

The incubation period is typically 15–25 days but may be reduced to 6 days in experimental infections. Although trench fever often results in prolonged disability, it is rarely fatal.

CHRONIC INFECTION AND COMPLICATIONS CAUSED BY B. QUINTANA

Persistent bacteremia has long been associated with *B. quintana* infection. Asymptomatic and prolonged bacteremia can be detected in 20–30% of patients; *B. quintana* has been detected in the blood of trench fever patients up to 8 years after initial infection.

Bartonella species are associated with culture-negative endocarditis. Clinical features include fever. *Bartonella* endocarditis is typically diagnosed in individuals without previous valvular abnormalities, although risk factors include homelessness, alcoholism, and body louse infestation [10].

Bacillary angiomatosis is a proliferative vascular disease of immunodeficient patients (usually individuals with advanced HIV infection), although rare cases in immunocompetent individuals have been reported. Bacillary angiomatosis can be caused by *B. quintana* and *Bartonella henselae*, the cause of cat scratch disease. Various organs may be affected, including the liver, spleen, bone marrow, and lymph nodes, but the skin is most often involved. Cutaneous lesions may be solitary or multiple and may bleed profusely when punctured.

PATIENT EVALUATION, DIAGNOSIS, AND DIFFERENTIAL DIAGNOSIS

DIAGNOSIS

Diagnosis of trench fever is usually based on clinical recognition in the setting of epidemiologic risk factors and supported by serologic analysis or, less commonly, microbiologic culture of blood. Indirect immunofluorescence (IFA) is considered the standard serologic assay. Nucleic acid amplification tests may also be used.

IMMUNOHISTOCHEMISTRY

Immunohistochemistry may also be used to detect *B. quintana* in tissue samples, such as resected cardiac valvular tissue or bacillary angiomatosis tissue.

TROPICAL AREAS

The burden of *B. quintana* infection and trench fever in resource-limited settings is uncertain. *Bartonella quintana* has a worldwide distribution: trench fever has occurred among refugees in Burundi [2]; *B. quintana*-associated endocarditis has been reported in Ethiopia, Algeria, Tunisia [13], and Senegal; and bacillary angiomatosis has been reported in HIV patients in South Africa.

PREVENTION AND TREATMENT

No vaccine to prevent *B. quintana* infection is available. Prevention usually involves de-lousing, changing clothes and blankets, bathing, and treating louse-bite associated pruritus [14].

TREATMENT

Adults with trench fever or *B. quintana* chronic bacteremia should be treated with doxycycline 200 mg orally daily for 4 weeks and gentamycin 3 mg/kg IV once a day for 2 weeks [15]. Optimal treatment for children younger than 8 years of age is unknown, but erythromycin may be an alternative. Individuals with bacillary angiomatosis or hepatic peliosis should be treated with erythromycin 500 mg orally 4 times a day for 3 and 4 months, respectively [15]. Children can be similarly treated with oral erythromycin ethylsuccinate 40 mg/kg total/day in four divided doses (maximum total daily dose, 2 g/day) for 3–4 months, respectively [15].

REFERENCES

1. Raoult D, Roux V. The body louse as a vector of reemerging human diseases. Clin Infect Dis 1999;29:888–911.
2. Raoult D, Ndihokubwayo JB, Tissot-Dupont H, et al. Outbreak of epidemic typhus associated with trench fever in Burundi. Lancet 1998;352:353–8.
3. Badiaga S, Raoult D, Brouqui P. Preventing and controlling emerging and reemerging transmissible diseases in the homeless. Emerg Infect Dis 2008; 14:1353–9.
4. Bonilla DL, Kabeya H, Henn J, et al. *Bartonella quintana* in body lice and head lice from homeless persons, San Francisco, California, USA. Emerg Infect Dis 2009;15:912–15.
5. Brouqui P, Stein A, Dupont HT, et al. Ectoparasitism and vector-borne diseases in 930 homeless people from Marseilles. Medicine (Baltimore) 2005;84: 61–8.

6. Raoult D, Birtles RJ, Montoya M, et al. Survey of three bacterial louse-associated diseases among rural Andean communities in Peru: prevalence of epidemic typhus, trench fever, and relapsing fever. Clin Infect Dis 1999;29:434–6.
7. Seki N, Kasai S, Saito N, et al. Quantitative analysis of proliferation and excretion of *Bartonella quintana* in body lice, *Pediculus humanus* L. Am J Trop Med Hyg 2007;77:562–6.
8. Drancourt M, Tran-Hung L, Courtin J, et al. *Bartonella quintana* in a 4000-year-old human tooth. J Infect Dis 2005;191:607–11.
9. Raoult D, Dutour O, Houhamdi L, et al. Evidence for louse-transmitted diseases in soldiers of Napoleon's Grand Army in Vilnius. J Infect Dis 2006;193:112–20.
10. Foucault C, Brouqui, P, Raoult D. *Bartonella quintana* characteristics and clinical management. Emerg Infect Dis 2006;12:217–23.
11. Schulte B, Linke D, Klumpp, S, et al. *Bartonella quintana* variably expressed outer membrane proteins mediate vascular endothelial growth factor secretion but not host cell adherence. Infect Immun 2006;74:5003–13.
12. Kostrzewski J. Epidemiology of trench fever. Med Dosw Mikrobiol 1950;2:19–51 [in Polish].
13. Znazen A, Rolain JM, Hammami N, et al. High prevalence of *Bartonella quintana* endocarditis in Sfax, Tunisia. Am J Trop Med Hyg 2005;72:503–7.
14. Badiaga S, Foucault C, Rogier C, et al. The effect of a single dose of oral ivermectin on pruritus in the homeless. J Antimicrob Chemother 2008;62:404–9.
15. Rolain JM, Brouqui P, Koehler JE, et al. Recommendations for treatment of human infections caused by Bartonella species. Antimicrob Agents Chemother 2004;48:1921–33.

68 Bartonellosis: Carrion's Disease and other *Bartonella* Infections

Ciro Maguiña, Eloy E Ordaya

Key features

- South American bartonellosis (Carrion's disease) is a bacterial infection caused by *Bartonella baciliformis*
- Distribution is isolated to regional highland areas in Peru, Ecuador, and Colombia
- It is transmitted by a sandfly, and includes two clinical stages: an acute hemolytic phase (Oroya fever) and a chronic verrucous form (verruga peruana)
- The acute phase is characterized by fever, pallor, and hemolytic anemia, and can be fatal
- The verrucous form has a prolonged, but more benign course, and is distinguished by erythematous skin lesions
- A number of other *Bartonella* spp. are significant causes of human disease, including *Bartonella henselae*, which causes cat scratch disease, and *Bartonella quintana*, the agent of trench fever. These *Bartonella* spp. can also cause bacillary angiomatosis, a vascular hyperproliferation disorder, particularly in patients with advanced immunosuppression, including AIDS patients

INTRODUCTION

South American bartonellosis or Carrion's disease is a biphasic bacterial infection caused by *Bartonella bacilliformis*. It is transmitted by a sandfly, *Lutzomya* spp.

It is named after the Peruvian medical student Daniel Alcides Carrión, who self-inoculated the discharge from a patient with a chronic verruga peruana skin lesion and developed the acute hemolytic phase of illness and died. This act demonstrated that both diseases had a common source [1].

EPIDEMIOLOGY

Carrion's disease had been exclusively reported in inter-Andean valleys in Peru, Ecuador, and Colombia; however, the disease has been emerging in new areas in Ecuador and in high forest areas of Peru between the jungle margin and altiplano. The changing distribution may relate, in part, to changing climate (Fig. 68.1). The majority of cases occur in Peru—Carrion's disease had an incidence in Peru in 2004 of 57 cases per 100,000.

Serologic studies suggest that more than 60% of the population in endemic areas has been infected and 0.5% of asymptomatic residents in endemic zones may be bacteremic. Bartonellosis affects males and females equally and is more common in children [2].

NATURAL HISTORY, PATHOGENESIS, AND PATHOLOGY

Humans act as a reservoir host. Whether additional reservoirs of significance exist is uncertain. *Bartonella bacilliformis* is transmitted by the bite of female New World sandflies, *Lutzomya* spp. The most effective vector in Peru is the sandfly, *Lutzomya verrucarum*, that lives in narrow river valleys between 500 and 3200 meters above sea level. In Colombia, the most significant vector is *Lutzomya columbiana*. After the inoculation of *B. bacilliformis* by the vector, the bacilli infect the endothelium of capillary vessels. They are then released to the blood and first adhere to, and then invade, erythrocytes. This process activates reticular-endothelial cells that cause systemic symptoms and destruction of infected erythrocytes; a hemolytic anemia occurs. If the patient survives, approximately 5% develop the chronic phase of illness. In this stage, the bacterium invades the endothelial cells, forms Rocha-Lima inclusion bodies and stimulates endothelial proliferation and angiogenesis. The proliferative responses leads to formation of hypervascular nodules, similar to hemangiomas, called "Peruvian warts" [3].

CLINICAL FEATURES

Classically, Carrion's disease is characterized by two sequential clinical stages: an initial hemolytic phase (Oroya fever), followed by a verrucous phase (Peruvian wart). However, individuals infected with *B. bacilliformis* may manifest only one or other of these two phases, or may have additional involvement ranging from asymptomatic bacteremia to recurrent verrucous presentations.

The incubation period for Oroya fever is usually about 3 weeks, but may range from 10 days to months. Individuals with Oroya fever usually present with a febrile illness characterized by headaches and myalgias. The hemolytic phase can be associated with severe pallor, jaundice, or hepatomegaly. Myocarditis, pericarditis, encephalopathy, seizures, retinal hemorrhages, papilledema, and multi-organ failure and death can occur. Concomitant infectious complications are common, and include *Salmonella* bacteremia, reactivation of toxoplasmosis, disseminated histoplasmosis, reactivation of pulmonary tuberculosis, leptospirosis, or pneumocystosis. Oroya fever can last for 2 to 4 weeks and, in untreated cases, is associated with up to 90% mortality, and up to 10% mortality in treated patients.

The chronic verruga peruana phase occurs several weeks or months later in a subset of patients, and is manifested by arthralgias, fever, and painless eruptive lesions that are commonly located on the face and upper and lower limbs. There are three types of lesions: miliary (multiple small, reddish papules of 3 mm or less; Fig. 68.2); mular (ulcerative or non-ulcerative angioma-like tumors of more than 5 mm; Fig. 68.3); and a nodular or sub-dermic form (Fig. 68.4). In rare cases, verruga can involve the oral, conjunctival or nasal mucosa. The lesions usually last from 3 to 6 months and can heal without therapy [4–6].

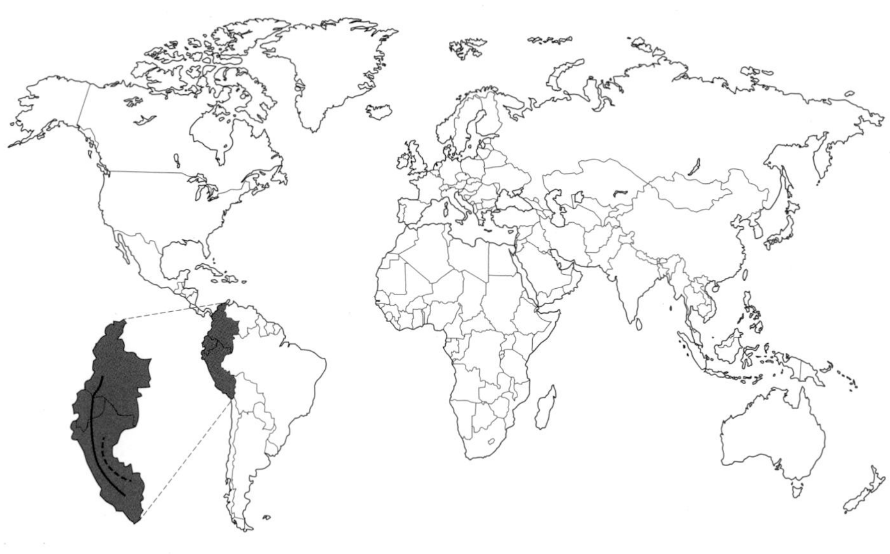

FIGURE 68.1 Global distribution of Bartonellosis or Carrion's disease.

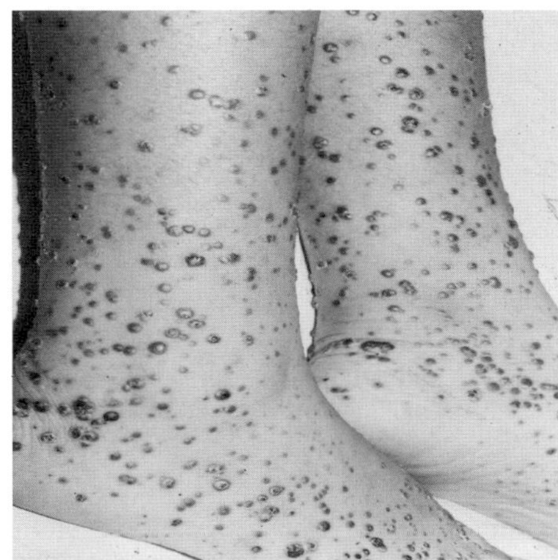

FIGURE 68.2 Peruvian wart, miliary form (small) final.

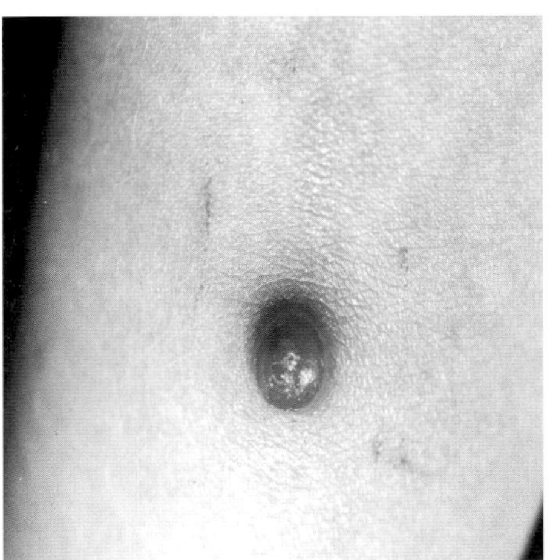

FIGURE 68.3 Peruvian wart, mular form.

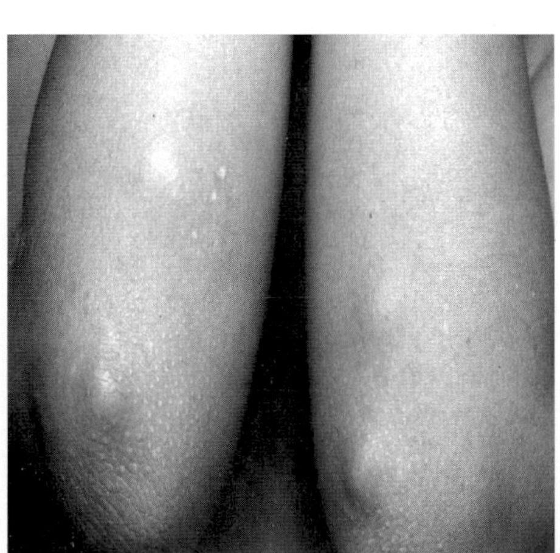

FIGURE 68.4 Peruvian wart, nodular or subdermic form final.

PATIENT EVALUATION, DIAGNOSIS, AND DIFFERENTIAL DIAGNOSIS

The differential diagnosis of Oroya fever is broad as individuals usually present with a nonspecific febrile illness (Table 68-1). Epidemiologic history and analysis of a potential incubation period are critical as South American Bartonellosis is a geographically restricted infection. The presence of hemolytic anemia assists in considering the diagnosis, as well as malaria. The diagnosis is confirmed by isolating the organism from blood, or by analysis of a peripheral blood Giemsa-Wright smear to detect erythrocyte-associated bacteria that may appear bacillary or coccoid. Analysis of a peripheral smear is, unfortunately, insensitive (approximately 30–40%), and requires an experienced microscopist able to distinguish bacteria from artifacts, basophilic stippling, and Howell-Jolly bodies. Blood cultures should be held for up to 6 weeks; recovery is highest using Columbia Agar supplemented with 5% defibrinated human blood incubated at 28°C. The differential diagnosis of verruga peruana usually involves consideration of other nodular skin lesion, although the hypervascular nature of verruga peruana assists in establishing the diagnosis. Evaluation of blood smear in this stage is very insensitive (10%); microbiologic evaluation of blood is 50% sensitive. The diagnosis of veruga peruana is usually made by histopathologic analysis of tissue, demonstrating proliferation of endothelial cells, monocytes, and macrophages, and neovascularization. Mitoses may be evident. Analysis of tissue using the Warthin-Starry stain can reveal bacteria dispersed in the tissue. Immunohistochemistry may also be used to indentify *B.* bacilliformis [7, 8].

Serologic methods like western blot or PCR are also available to diagnose individuals with Carrion's disease, but are not used widely because of their high cost and lack of standardization.

TREATMENT

In vitro, *B. bacilliformis* is susceptible to ß-lactams, tetracyclines, fluoroquinolones, macrolides, rifampin, and chloramphenicol. They are resistant to vancomycin, aminoglycosides, clindamycin, and carbapenems.

TABLE 68-1 Differential Diagnosis of Bartonellosis or Carrion's Disease

Oroya fever
Typhoid fever
Malaria
Brucellosis
Viral hepatitis
Leptospirosis
Sepsis
Systemic tuberculosis
Hematological malignancies
Parvovirus B19 infection
Hemolytic anemias
Aplastic anemia
Peruvian wart
Angioma
Bacillary angiomatosis
Granuloma Pyogenicum
Kaposi's sarcoma
Leprosy
Lymphomatoid papillomatosis
Fibrosarcoma
Cutaneous lymphoma
Reticuloendotheliosis
Molluscum contagiosum
Chickenpox
Yaws
Spitz nevus

Because of the high rate of co-infection with *Salmonella* during the acute Oroya fever phase, many experts use a fluoroquinolone, such as ciprofloxacin, or chloramphenicol as front-line therapy (Table 68-2). Amoxicillin plus clavulanic acid may be used in pregnant women; there are also anecdotal reports of clinical effectiveness with amoxicillin alone.

Dexamethasone is sometimes administered for 3–4 days in patients with severe neurologic complications in an attempt to reduce cerebral edema, but this approach has not been well studied. Blood transfusions are indicated for patients with severe anemia; pericardial effusions may require drainage.

During the chronic verruga peruana phase, chloramphenicol and ß-lactam penicillins are ineffective. Azithromycin is now the drug of choice, although ciprofloxacin or rifampin are alternatives [9, 10].

OTHER BARTONELLA *INFECTIONS*

Over a dozen *Bartonella* spp. have been identified to cause disease in humans. Beyond *B. bacilliformis*, perhaps the other two *Bartonella* of most clinical significance are *Bartonella quintana*, the agent of trench fever, and *Bartonella henselae*, a cause of cat scratch disease.

Trench fever was described in soldiers during World War I who developed a relapsing febrile illness associated with 5 days of fever. It is caused by *B. quintana* and the vector is the human body louse, *Pediculus humanus humanus*. Homelessness, poor sanitation, and lack of personal hygiene are factors associated with this condition. The clinical course varies from a mild, afebrile state, to a relapsing fever with rash, bone pain, myalgias, headaches, and marked conjunctival injection. The organism can be cultured using special media, but most cases are diagnosed on clinical grounds or serology tests including ELISA or immunofluorescent antibody (IFA) assay. Trench fever is a self-limiting disease, but chloramphenicol or tetracycline show rapid disappearance of symptoms [1, 10].

Cat scratch disease is cosmopolitan in distribution and is more common in children than adults. It is considered to be the most common *Bartonella* infection worldwide. *Bartonella henselae* is now regarded as the main etiologic agent of cat scratch disease. It is transmitted to cats through fleas. Human infection occurs after scratches, bites, or licks from infected cats or from the bite of an arthropod vector. Cat scratch disease classically presents as a chronic papular, pustular or ulcerative skin lesion and regional lymphadenopathy after a cat scratch, but, not infrequently, *B. henselae* can cause systemic manifestations including encephalitis, retinitis, non-specific fever, and Parinaud's oculoglandular syndrome. Diagnosis is usually based on

TABLE 68-2 Treatment Protocols for Bartonellosis or Carrion's Disease

Stage	Drug	Doses	Notes	Level of evidence
Oroya Fever	Ciprofloxacin	500 mg twice daily for 14 days	Drug of choice; its use has shown less complications and reduced mortality	1
	Chloramphenicol	50–75 mg per kilo (up to 3 gr/d), divided into four doses for 10–14 days	Recurrence has been described in patients who received this therapy	1
	Amoxicillin plus clavulanic Acid	1 gr (based on amoxicillin) twice daily for 14 days	Drug of choice in pregnancy	2
Peruvian wart	Azithromycin	500 mg once daily for 7 days	Drug of choice in all ages and pregnant patients	1
	Rifampin	600 mg once daily for 14–21 days	Treatment failures have been reported	1
	Ciprofloxacin	500 mg twice daily for 14 days	Added in the last Bartonellosis National Guide	2

1, Evidence from multiple time series; 2, evidence based on clinical experience or expert opinions.

clinical presentation, serology, or histopathology. Cat scratch disease is often self-limited, but patients are often treated with azithromycin or doxycycline [1, 11].

Bartonella henselae and *B. quintana* can also cause bacillary angiomatosis, a disorder of vascular hyperproliferation. The typical lesion is a reddish-purple papule, but may be a hyperkeratotic plaque, or an infiltrative or hypervascular nodule. Bacillary angiomatosis is most commonly seen in severe immunocompromised patients, especially those with advanced HIV infection. Involvement can be confined to the skin, or can involve deep organs and structures. Involvement of the liver is referred to as peliosis hepatis. Diagnosis is confirmed by histopathology using Warthin-Starry or Giemsa stain. Treatment usually involves prolonged use of erythromycin alone or combined with doxycycline in AIDS patients [1, 10, 12].

A number of *Bartonella* species can also cause "culture-negative" chronic endocarditis, which is most frequently caused by *B. quintana* or *B. henselae*, or both.

REFERENCES

1. Maguiña C, Guerra H, Ventosilla P. Bartonellosis. Clin Dermatol 2009;27:271–80.
2. Maguiña Vargas C, Ugarte-Gil C, Breña Chavez P, et al. Update of Carrion's disease. Rev Med Hered 2008;19:36–41.
3. Walker D, Maguiña C, Minnick M. Bartonelloses. In: Guerrant R, Walker D, Weller P, eds. Tropical infectious diseases: principles, pathogens, & practice, 2nd edn. Philadelphia: Elsevier Churchill Livingstone; 2006: 454–62.
4. Maguiña C, Garcia PJ, Gotuzzo E, et al. Bartonellosis (Carrion's Disease) in the modern era. Clin Inf Dis 2001;33:772–9.
5. Kosek M, Lavarello R, Gilman RH, et al. Natural history of infection with *Bartonella bacilliformis* in a nonendemic population. J Infect Dis 2000;182:865–72.
6. Maguiña Vargas C, Ordaya Espinoza E, Ugarte-Gil C, et al. Cardiovascular involvement during the acute phase of Carrion's disease or human Bartonellosis: A 20-year experience in Cayetano Heredia National Hospital. Acta Med Peruana 2008;25:30–8.
7. Birtles RJ, Fry NK, Ventosilla P, et al. Identification of *Bartonella bacilliformis* genotypes and their relevance to epidemiological investigations of human bartonellosis. J Clin Microbiol 2002;40:3606–12.
8. Henriquez C, Infante B, Merello J, et al. Identificación de *Bartonella bacilliformis* por métodos moleculares. Rev Med Hered 2002;13:58–63 [in Portuguese].
9. Tarazona A, Maguiña C, Lopez de Guimaraes D, et al. Terapia antibiótica para el manejo de la bartonelosis o enfermedad de Carrión en el Perú. Rev Perú Med Exp Salud Publica 2006;23:188–200. [in Portuguese].
10. Rolain JM, Brouqui P, Koehler JE, et al. Recommendations for treatment of human infections caused by *Bartonella* species. Antimicrob Agents Chemother 2004;48:1921–33.
11. Piérard-Franchimont C, Quatresooz P, Piérard GE. Skin diseases associated with Bartonella infection: Facts and controversies. Clin Dermatol 2010;28:483–8.
12. Maguiña C, Gotuzzo E. Bartonelose. In: Focaccia R, ed. Tratado de Infectologia, 3rd edn. Sao Paulo: Atheneu; 2006: 759–62 [in Portuguese].

69 Typhoid and Paratyphoid (Enteric) Fever

Jason B Harris, W Abdullah Brooks

Key features

- *Salmonella enterica* serotypes Typhi and Paratyphi A, B, and C are the causative agents of typhoid and paratyphoid fever, respectively. Enteric fever refers to either typhoid or paratyphoid fever
- Enteric fever is a nonspecific illness characterized by prolonged fevers and persistent bacteremia
- Life-threatening complications of enteric fever include intestinal hemorrhage, perforation, and encephalopathy
- The diagnosis of enteric fever should be considered in any patient with prolonged fever and exposure in an endemic area
- Because of the limitations of diagnostic tests, the initiation of antibiotic treatment for enteric fever is often based on a presumptive diagnosis
- The choice of empiric antibiotic therapy depends on local patterns of antibiotic resistance
- Vaccines to prevent typhoid are available

INTRODUCTION

Typhoid and paratyphoid fever are systemic febrile illnesses caused by *Salmonella enterica* serotype Typhi and serotypes Paratyphi A, B, or C, respectively. Enteric fever refers to either typhoid or paratyphoid fever. Collectively, *S.* Typhi and *S.* Paratyphi A cause approximately 27 million cases of enteric fever and over 200,000 deaths annually (Box 69.1).

Both typhoid and paratyphoid fever are characterized by prolonged fever and sustained bacteremia. The name typhoid, meaning "typhus-like", was coined in 1829 by A. Louis and reflects the difficulty physicians had in differentiating the illness from epidemic typhus. Among 19th-century American physicians, "typho-malaria" was a common diagnosis, indicative of the difficulty differentiating typhoid from other causes of persistent fever. This proved fortuitous in 1948, when two patients were referred for a study of the efficacy of chloramphenicol in scrub typhus, but were subsequently found to have *S.* Typhi bacteremia. Both patients improved rapidly after antibiotic therapy – a finding that ushered in the post-antibiotic era in typhoid fever [1].

EPIDEMIOLOGY

INCIDENCE AND DISTRIBUTION OF ENTERIC FEVER (Fig. 69.1)

Typhoid fever. *Salmonella* Typhi causes approximately 22 million cases of typhoid fever annually with an estimated mortality of 1% [2]. The regions with the highest incidence are South central Asia (~1000 cases/100,000 person-years) and Southeast Asia (~100 cases/100,000 person-years). Sub-Saharan Africa reports more non-typhoidal Salmonella bacteremia than *S.* Typhi, yet major epidemics of typhoid fever occur.

Paratyphoid fever. *Salmonella* Paratyphi A causes approximately 5 million cases of enteric fever annually [2]. The proportion of cases of enteric fever caused by *S.* Paratyphi A has increased over the past two decades, and now exceeds 50% in parts of southern Asia [3]. This is significant as current typhoid fever vaccines do not protect against *S.* Paratyphi A. Serotypes Paratyphi B and C are rare causes of enteric fever.

TRANSMISSION AND PATTERNS OF INFECTION

Source of Infection

Salmonella Typhi and *S.* Paratyphi A, B, and C are human-restricted pathogens; no known animal reservoirs exist. Enteric fever patients shed organisms in the stool during acute illness and often for months after convalescence. In the pre-antibiotic era, up to 3% of typhoid fever survivors developed chronic asymptomatic bacterial shedding in the stool. Chronic carriage can persist for life; gallbladder disease is a major risk factor for carriage. A recent study in Nepal found that 5% of individuals undergoing elective cholecystectomy for gallstones grew *S.* Typhi of *S.* Paratyphi A from biliary cultures [4]. While chronic carriers are a source of transmission where disease is sporadic, it is unclear whether carriers are an important reservoir in endemic areas.

Mode of Transmission

In endemic areas, most infections are acquired via contaminated food or water – with water playing the greater role in endemic urban settings. The inoculum required to produce disease in 50% of adult volunteers (ID_{50}) is 10^7 organisms, although as few as 10^3 organisms may produce disease. Risk factors include drinking non-boiled water and eating food prepared outside the home. While direct contact with a typhoid fever patient is an infection risk factor, more than 80% of cases occur in individuals with no known contact [5]. In South central Asia and Southeast Asia, peak transmission occurs during the monsoon season, although disease is present year-round. Large waterborne epidemics may be superimposed on endemic seasonality.

Antimicrobial Resistance

Chloramphenicol-resistant *S.* Typhi was described in 1950 – 2 years after the antibiotic was first used to treat patients with typhoid fever. Multidrug-resistant *S.* Typhi, carrying plasmid-mediated resistance to chloramphenicol, ampicillin, trimethoprim, and sulfonamides, became common in the 1980s, and nalidixic-acid-resistant *S.* Typhi and *S.* Paratyphi A in the 1990s. Nalidixic-acid-resistant strains are associated with decreased susceptibility to fluoroquinolones (an increased risk of treatment failure) and increased mortality [6]. In Asia, most *S.* Typhi and Paratyphi A strains are now nalidixic-acid-resistant. In the past decade, complete resistance to ciprofloxacin and extended spectrum cephalosporins has emerged [7]. While resistance to these newer agents is increasing, susceptibility to original first-line agents may be re-emerging, at least in some locations. Thus, antimicrobial resistance in S. Typhi and Paratyphi A varies significantly by region and patterns of antibiotic use.

Severity

The majority of cases are not severe enough to require hospitalization. Case fatality prevalence for typhoid fever patients in the pre-antibiotic era was approximately 15%. Current hospital-based mortality rates range by location (0–15%), with a median mortality rate of 2% [8]. In the USA, where disease is sporadic, the fatality rate of reported cases is 0.2% [9].

BOX 69.1 Nomenclature of *Salmonella* Infections

The multiple microbiologic, serologic and clinical designations applied to *Salmonella* infections are confusing [36]. Most pathogenic *Salmonella* belong to a single subspecies designated *Salmonella enterica* subspecies enterica. In addition to this species designation, *Salmonella* are classified serologically. The serogroup is assigned based on the O antigen alone, while the serotype designation, from which the name is derived, is based on both the O and H antigens.

Salmonella enterica subsp. enterica includes over 1400 serotypes. Although the full name of the cause of typhoid fever is ***Salmonella enterica* subsp. enterica serotype Typhi**, it is normally just shortened to: ***S.* Typhi**. While serogroup designation is performed routinely in many laboratories, the test lacks clinical utility. Complete serotype identification is often performed in a reference laboratory; however, *S.* Typhi and Paratyphi A can also be identified by biochemical tests in a routine microbiology laboratory. Identification of *S.* Typhi and Paratyphi A are reviewed in detail in the World Health Organization's "The diagnosis, treatment and prevention of typhoid fever" [22].

Clinically, *Salmonella* are classified as typhoidal or non-typhoidal. The typhoidal serotypes are *S.* Typhi and Paratyphi A, B and C. All others are classified as non-typhoidal. However, this is also misleading as many non-typhoidal strains also cause invasive infection that may mimic typhoid fever.

Age and Immunity

In the most highly endemic communities, the incidence of enteric fever is highest in children between the age 1 and 5 years old. In such areas, S. Typhi is the leading cause of bacteremia in children and may be responsible for over 75% of cases of occult bacteremia [10]. In less endemic areas, the median age of patients with typhoid fever increases. Relapse and recurrent infections among patients who have recovered from typhoid fever demonstrate that immunity is neither lifelong nor universally acquired after a single illness.

Sporadic Disease and Travelers

In countries where typhoid fever is sporadic (<1/100,000 person-years), most cases are imported through travel. In the USA, over 75% of cases are travel-related. The typhoid fever incidence is estimated at 10 per 1 million travelers arriving from Asia, but increases to 89 per 1 million travelers arriving from India. Many remaining cases can be traced to small, foodborne outbreaks and/or a chronic carrier [9]. The risk of travel-related enteric fever is higher among travelers visiting friends and relatives [11].

NATURAL HISTORY, PATHOGENESIS AND PATHOLOGY

INVASION AND LATENCY

Salmonella Typhi and S. Paratyphi A, B, and C are rod-shaped, Gram-negative bacteria that have adapted to survive and replicate in human macrophages. *Salmonella* Typhi and Paratyphi breach the intestinal barrier though specialized microfold cells (M cells) that transport the bacteria across the basolateral membrane where they are phagocytosed by macrophages in the intestinal lymphoid tissue. This invasion phase of infection is usually asymptomatic, but may be accompanied by transient diarrhea in 10–20% of patients. Latent infection typically lasts one to two weeks (range 3–60 days), depending on the number of organisms ingested.

DISSEMINATED INFECTION

Typhoidal *Salmonella* deploy an array of virulence factors that enable them to persist and replicate in an intracellular compartment [12]. Intracellular organisms disseminate throughout the reticuloendothelial tissues via the blood and lymphatic system. Infection is

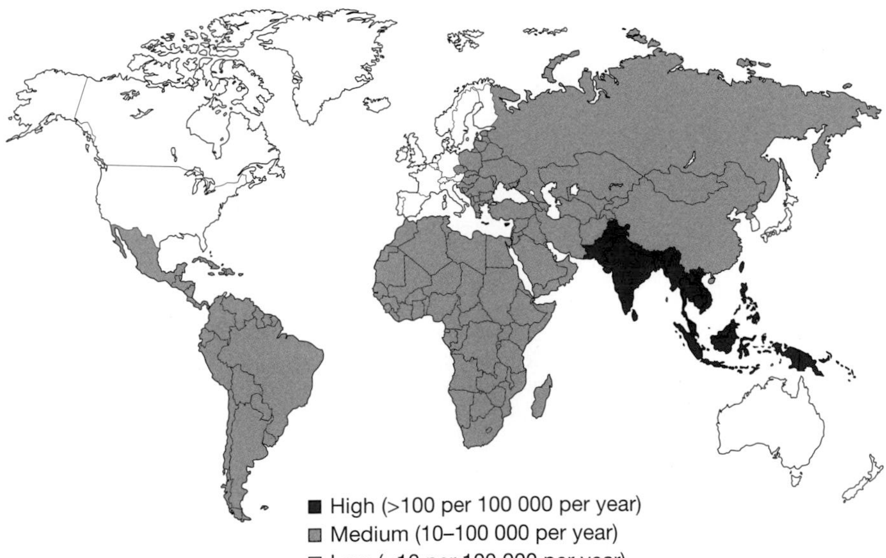

FIGURE 69.1 Global distribution of typhoid fever.

established in the intestinal lymphoid tissue, liver, spleen, gallbladder, and bone marrow.

Patients with typhoid fever generally have low-grade bacteremia. The median number of culturable bacteria is less than 1 per mL of whole blood and 10 per mL of bone marrow in patients with typhoid fever. The proportion of bacteria in the bone marrow increases over the course of the illness [13]. Infection results in the secretion of inflammatory cytokines which cause prolonged fever. However, unlike prototypical Gram-negative bacteremia, overt sepsis with hypotension and neutrophilia are rare.

PATHOLOGIC FINDINGS

Intestinal lymphoid tissue is the major site of localized inflammation in enteric fever. Peyer's patches in the terminal ileum and draining mesenteric nodes become enlarged and contain infiltrates predominantly consisting of macrophages and lymphocytes. As the disease progresses, necrosis of the intestinal lymphoid tissue may occur with ulceration of the overlying intestinal mucosa. This can lead to hemorrhage or intestinal perforation – life-threatening complications of enteric fever. Other affected organs include the spleen, with nodular monocytic infiltrates in the red pulp, and liver, with small monocytic infiltrates and foci of parenchymal necrosis ("typhoid nodules"). Monocytic infiltrates also occur in the bone marrow and gallbladder.

RELAPSE AND CHRONIC CARRIAGE

Untreated, typhoid fever may persist for three to four weeks. Relapse occurs in 5–10% of untreated cases, usually within 2 weeks of resolution of the fever. The gallbladder is the primary site of chronic carriage. The observation that *S. enterica* forms biofilms on cholesterol gallstones may explain the association between gallstones and carriage [14].

CLINICAL FEATURES

The clinical features of enteric fever are nonspecific. The major clinical findings in enteric fever are listed in Table 69-1. Fever, without localizing signs or symptoms, may be the sole manifestation of enteric fever.

TABLE 69-1 Clinical Features of Typhoid and Paratyphoid Fever

	Clinical feature	Approx. frequency (%)*
	Fever	>95
Flu-like symptoms	Headache	80
	Chills	40
	Cough	30
	Myalgia	20
	Arthralgia	<5
Abdominal symptoms	Anorexia	50
	Abdominal pain	30
	Diarrhea	20
	Constipation	20
Physical findings	Coated tongue	50
	Hepatomegaly	10
	Splenomegaly	10
	Abdominal tenderness	5
	Rash	<5
	Generalized adenopathy	<5

*The proportion of patients demonstrating these clinical features of enteric fever varies depending on the time, region and the type of clinical population (hospitalized or ambulatory) assessed. Estimates are drawn from recent case series in an endemic area presenting for ambulatory or inpatient care [16, 37].

Most enteric fever cases are diagnosed in the ambulatory setting, are mild and up to 90% are treated as outpatients [15]. In contrast, classic descriptions of typhoid fever are based on hospitalized patients with more severe disease. Although life-threatening complications of enteric fever usually occur more than a week after fever onset, both intestinal perforation and encephalopathy may occur within days of initial fever.

Historically, paratyphoid fever was considered less severe than typhoid fever. Current evidence suggests that infections caused by S. Typhi and S. Paratyphi A are clinically indistinguishable and equally severe [16].

MILD ILLNESS

Enteric fever is usually insidious. Fever may gradually increase over the first week of illness. Headache, anorexia, malaise, and other nonspecific, flu-like symptoms are common and may precede fever. Abdominal complaints including diarrhea, constipation, and nonlocalizing abdominal pain each occur in less than a third of cases, but may raise clinical suspicion [16].

Physical findings are also nonspecific. Relative bradycardia, or pulse-temperature dissociation, is considered a classic sign of enteric fever, but there is no widely accepted definition of relative bradycardia and little evidence that it is a useful predictor [17]. Rose spots are small, blanching pink macular lesions, typically 2–4 mm, that usually occur on the chest, abdomen and/or back during the second week of illness, but are infrequently observed. A white, yellow or brown coating of the tongue that spares the tongue's edges is common. Mild abdominal tenderness may be present. Hepatomegaly and splenomegaly, if present, are usually modest.

In contrast to other causes of bacteremia, patients with enteric fever rarely demonstrate leukocytosis, neutrophilia, or increased immature neutrophils. A typical leukocyte count is $5–8 \times 10^6$ cells per mL, with 60–75% neutrophils [16]. However, neither leukocytosis nor leukopenia excludes enteric fever. Hematocrit and platelet counts are usually normal or slightly low. Modest elevations, typically double the upper end of the normal range, in aspartate transaminase and alanine transaminase are common. Excessive levels of blood transaminases should prompt concern for other etiologies, including viral hepatitis.

SEVERE ILLNESS AND COMPLICATIONS

Patients with severe enteric fever are ill or toxic appearing and have generally been febrile for more than a week. They are likely to have moderate abdominal pain or tenderness, and either constipation or diarrhea. Moderate hepatomegaly and splenomegaly are also common.

The major complications of typhoid fever are listed in Table 69-2. Complications associated with increased mortality include intestinal hemorrhage and perforation, severe encephalopathy, seizures and pneumonia [18], although pneumonia has also been noted frequently in children without other complications [10].

GASTROINTESTINAL COMPLICATIONS

Some degree of intestinal hemorrhage occurs in up to 10% of hospitalized patients; this is usually self-limited. Intestinal perforation (Fig. 69.2) occurs in up to 3% of hospitalized patients and is associated

TABLE 69-2 Complications of Typhoid and Paratyphoid Fever

System	Complication	Notes
Gastrointestinal	Hemorrhage	10–15% hospitalized patients.
	Perforation	3% hospitalized patients.
Hepatobiliary	Jaundice	1–3% hospitalized patients.
	Hepatitis	Usually subclinical (↑ ALT/AST)
	Acute cholecystitis	Rare, gallbladder may perforate.
Neurologic	Mild encephalopathy	Confusion or apathy common.
	Severe encephalopathy	Delerium, stupor or coma.
	Seizures	Common in children ≤5 years old
	Meningitis	Rare, primarily infants
	Guillain-Barré syndrome	Reported
Respiratory	Bronchitis	Cough is common
	Pneumonia	May be other concomitant bacterial infection (e.g. *S. pneumoniae*)
Cardiovascular	Myocarditis	Usually subclinical (ECG changes)
	Shock	Uncommon
Hematologic	Anemia	Usually subclinical
	Disseminated intravascular coagulation (DIC)	Usually subclinical (↑ PT/PTT)
Other	Pyogenic infections	Uncommon
	Hemolytic uremic syndrome	Reported, uncertain relationship
	Miscarriage	Reported

ALT, alanine amino transferase; AST, aspartate aminotransferase; ECG, electrocardiography; PT, prothrombin time; PTT, partial thromboplastin time.

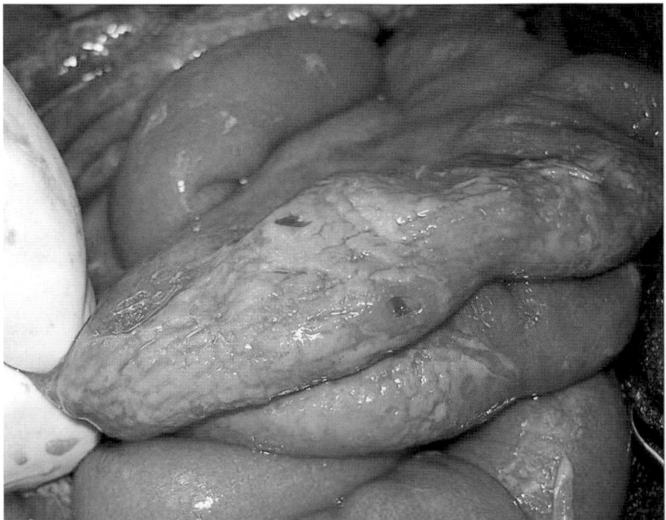

FIGURE 69.2 Intraoperative photograph of intestinal perforation caused by *S.* Typhi. A single perforation is seen on the anti-mesenteric border of the inflamed small bowel along with patchy exudates on the serosal surface *(photo courtesy of Dr Pukar Maskey, Patan Hospital, Katmandu, Nepal).*

with substantial mortality. A recent series of 27 cases of intestinal perforation demonstrated that the median length of illness preceding perforation was 9 days (range 1–22 days) from the onset of fever [19]. Perforation is suggested by clinical signs of sepsis and peritonitis, including tachycardia, leukocytosis with predominant neutrophilia, and abdominal pain with guarding and rebound tenderness. Radiographic evidence of pneumoperitoneum may be present in only 50% of cases. Perforation may be difficult to recognize, as patients may be toxic appearing with accompanying abdominal tenderness, even before perforation.

NEUROLOGIC COMPLICATIONS

Severe enteric fever may present with encephalopathy. A history of confusion is common and patients often demonstrate an apathetic affect. Severe encephalopathy manifested by delirium and stupor; coma occurs in a smaller number of hospitalized patients and is associated with a high risk of mortality [18, 20, 21]. Seizures are most common in young children and are associated with increased mortality risk [18]. Even in severe encephalopathy or seizure cases, cerebrospinal fluid (CSF) cultures are usually negative and pleocytosis, if present, reveals fewer than 35 cells per uL [20, 21]. Meningitis is uncommon and is primarily seen in infants. Focal neurologic findings have been reported but should prompt consideration of an alternative diagnosis.

OTHER COMPLICATIONS

Pneumonia is a serious comorbidity associated with severe enteric fever [18]. Although enteric fever is a disseminated bacterial infection, distal pyogenic complications are not common. This contrasts with invasive non-typhoidal *Salmonella* in which osteomyelitis and endovascular infection occur more frequently. Numerous other enteric fever complications have been reported, affecting all major organ systems [15].

PATIENT EVALUATION, DIAGNOSIS AND DIFFERENTIAL DIAGNOSIS

Enteric fever can be a life-threatening infection if not treated with appropriate antimicrobial therapy and should be suspected in any patient with prolonged fever and exposure to an endemic area. There are no reliable clinical criteria to establish the diagnosis of enteric fever, and no sensitive or specific diagnostic laboratory tests. Therefore, the diagnosis of enteric fever is usually presumptive.

CLINICAL EVALUATION

The first requirement for diagnosis is clinical suspicion. In a highly endemic area, three or more days of nonfocal fever should prompt consideration of enteric fever. Patients should undergo a routine clinical history and physical examination. Although most of the findings associated with enteric fever are nonspecific, many other causes of febrile illness will become apparent after a careful history and examination. Routine laboratory studies are also of limited value in establishing a diagnosis of enteric fever, but may be more useful in eliminating other potential causes of nonfocal fever.

In a highly endemic area, factors that should increase the clinical suspicion for enteric fever early in the course of the illness include: young age; a temperature above 39 °C; ill appearance; and any abdominal complaints, including diarrhea, constipation or abdominal pain [10]. In the most highly endemic settings, three of more days of fever without localizing signs and a combination of any of these features, in the absence of another obvious cause, may be sufficient to prompt a diagnostic evaluation for enteric fever along with the initiation of empiric therapy.

As fever duration increases, the likelihood of enteric fever increases. Any patient with seven or more days of unexplained fever from an area where enteric fever is endemic should undergo a diagnostic evaluation and empiric treatment should be considered, given the potential complications of untreated enteric fever [15].

DIFFERENTIAL DIAGNOSIS

The differential diagnosis should reflect local febrile disease prevalence. Malaria, dengue fever, influenza, leptospirosis, rickettsial infections, urinary tract infection, and other causes of childhood occult bacteremia (e.g. *Streptococcus pneumoniae*, *Haemophilus influenzae*, and *Neisseria meningitiditis*) should all be considered in the differential diagnosis of fever without localizing signs. In patients with prolonged fever (>7 days) with or without localizing signs, the infectious differential diagnosis includes malaria, Epstein–Barr virus infection, tuberculosis, brucellosis, tularemia, plague, occult abscesses (including amebic liver abscess), and typhus.

MICROBIOLOGIC DIAGNOSIS

Although presumptive diagnosis of enteric fever is sufficient justification to initiate treatment in an ill-appearing patient, a definitive diagnosis of enteric fever can only be made by detection or isolation of S. Typhi or S. Paratyphi A, B, or C from blood, bone marrow, or other normally sterile clinical specimen. The isolation of a causative organism also provides the opportunity to optimize antimicrobial therapy.

Isolation of S. Typhi or Paratyphi A is most commonly achieved by blood culture. Factors that affect the sensitivity of blood isolation include the culture medium, prior antibiotic exposure, blood volume and the duration of illness prior to sample collection. The overall sensitivity of blood culture ranges from 40–80%, reflecting the low number of organisms present in the blood and prior antibiotic use. High blood volumes optimize the yield of blood culture; the World Health Organization (WHO) recommends that 10–15 ml of blood be obtained from school-aged children and 2–4 ml of blood be used for culture in toddlers and pre-school-aged children [22]. Although alternatives to standard blood culture (e.g. direct plating of the buffy coats or the use of selective ox bile media) have been recommended, the use of routine blood cultures with standard broth media is preferable because such methods may detect other potential bacterial pathogens as well.

Bone marrow cultures have an 80–95% sensitivity for isolating S. Typhi. Bone marrow cultures may remain positive for several days after initiating antibiotics. However, the invasiveness of bone marrow culture limits its practical utility in uncomplicated cases. Under optimal conditions, a single high volume (>15 ml) blood culture in an adult has a sensitivity nearly equivalent to a 1 ml bone marrow culture [13, 23].

Stool cultures are positive in over 50% and 30% of infected children and adults, respectively. Rectal swabs are not recommended, and the yield of stool cultures is optimized by the use of >1 g of stool and a selective enrichment broth [22]. Cultures obtained from intestinal biopsies of patients with perforation are rarely positive [19].

SEROLOGIC AND MOLECULAR DIAGNOSIS

The most commonly utilized diagnostic test for enteric fever is Widal's test, which was developed in 1896 and detects agglutinating antibodies against the O and H antigens of S. Typhi. Widal's test is not sufficiently sensitive, specific or reliable enough to be an optimal diagnostic assay for typhoid fever and it does not aid in the diagnosis of paratyphoid fever, as these antibodies are not cross-reactive against S. Paratyphi A, B and C antigens. A false-negative Widal's test may result from the assay being performed early in the course of illness and a false-positive Widal's test is more likely in an area of high endemnicity where antibodies may represent past infection.

Rapid serologic tests, including the IDL Tubex® and Typhidot® assays are available. In principle, tests such as Tubex, which detects IgM antibodies to the O9 antigen – a T-cell independent response to *Salmonella* infection which is, therefore, rapid – and Typhidot, which detects both IgM and IgG to the 50kD antigen of S. Typhi, should be useful in identifying early acute infection [22]. However, in practice, these tests have met with mixed success in high endemic settings because they have not consistently demonstrated an ability to distinguish between current and past infection and, in some cases, have not consistently been as sensitive as the Widal test [24, 25]. While diagnostic approaches based on nucleic acid detection appear promising, these tests are not widely available.

TREATMENT AND PREVENTION OF ENTERIC FEVER

Appropriate antibiotics and supportive care reduce the mortality of enteric fever from 10–15% to less than 1%. Fevers resolve after an average of 3–5 days of appropriate antibiotics, compared with 3–4 weeks in untreated infections. The widespread emergence of antibiotic resistant S. Typhi and Paratyphi A complicates the choice of antibiotics. Most patients can be managed in an ambulatory setting.

ANTIBIOTICS FOR ENTERIC FEVER

Uncomplicated enteric fever is usually treated with a single antibacterial drug. Antimicrobial choice depends on patient age, their ability to take oral medications, and drug availability and cost. Knowledge of antibiotic resistance patterns is essential because, in most cases, empiric antibiotics are initiated before an isolate is obtained. Table 69-3 summarizes antibiotic therapy for enteric fever.

TABLE 69-3 Antibiotics Commonly Used to Treat Individuals with Enteric Fever

	Antibiotic	Route	Typical pediatric dosage*	Adult dosage	Typical duration	Comments
Original first-line agents	Chloramphenicol	PO/IV	12.5–25 mg/kg QID	2–3 g/day (divided QID)	14–21 days	These agents are effective for susceptible strains; however, multidrug resistance to all of these agents is common in many areas
	Amoxicillin	PO	25–45 mg/kg/day (divided q12h)	1 g TID	14 days	
	Ampicillin	IV	25–50 mg/kg q6h	2 g q6h	14 days	
	TMP/STX	PO/IV	8-–12 mg/kg/day (TMP) 40–60 mg/kg/day (STX) (divided QID)	160 mg/800 mg QID	14 days	
Fluoroquinolones [27]	Ofloxacin	PO/IV	15 mg/kg BID	400 mg PO BID	5–14 days	Ofloxacin, levofloxacin, and ciprofloxacin effective for nalidixic-acid-susceptible strains. Short courses of 5–7 days are acceptable in uncomplicated cases. Ten- to 14-day courses are recommended in patients requiring hospitalization or parenteral therapy Gatifloxacin appears effective for uncomplicated cases caused by NaR strains but was removed from the US commercial market because of the adverse event profile [28]
	Levofloxacin	PO/IV	10–15 mg/kg qD	500 mg PO QD	5–14 days	
	Ciprofloxacin	PO/IV	15 mg/kg BID	500 mg PO BID	5–14 days	
	Gatifloxacin	PO	10 mg/kg qD	10 mg/kg/day qD	7 days	
Third-generation cephalosporins	Ceftriaxone	IV	50–100 mg/kg q24h	1–2 g IV q24h	10–14 days**	These are an alternative to fluoroquinolones for NaR strains and for empiric therapy in areas where NaR is common
	Cefixime	PO	10 mg/kg BID	200 mg PO BID	7–14 days	
Macrolides [31]	Azithromycin	PO	10–20 mg/kg qD	500mg–1 g PO qD	7 days	An alternative for uncomplicated infections caused by NaR strains and for empiric therapy where multidrug resistance and NaR are common
Eradication of carriage	Ciprofloxacin	PO	–	500–750 mg BID	28 days	If eradication is indicated for public health reasons, a trial of medical therapy is justified, even in patients with evidence of cholelithiasis [34]

*Weight-based pediatric dosage should not exceed adult maximum. **Recommended that treatment continue for at least 7 days post-defervescence to minimize relapse. NaR, Nalidixic-acid resistance; STX sulfamethoxazole; TMP, trimethoprim.

CHLORAMPHENICOL, AMPICILLIN, AND TRIMETHOPRIM-SULFAMETHOXAZOLE

The original "first-line" therapies for enteric fever include chloramphenicol, ampicillin, and trimethoprim-sulfamethoxazole [26]. After decades of increasing resistance among *S.* Typhi and Paratyphi A to these antibiotics, the trend may be reversing. Chloramphenicol results in a marked decrease in mortality and clearance of fevers in 3–5 days. It is inexpensive, has excellent oral bioavailability, is available even in the poorest parts of the world and has broad-spectrum activity against other occult childhood bacterial infections (including bacteremia and meningitis caused by *H. influenzae, S. pneumoniae,* and *N. meningitides*). However, up to 1:20,000 patients develop fatal irreversible aplastic anemia. Also, chloramphenicol does not substantially reduce the risk of relapse and chronic carriage. Ampicillin, and its oral formulation amoxicillin, and trimethoprim-sulfamethoxazole are also inexpensive, broad-spectrum antibiotics that are effective against susceptible strains of *S.* Typhi and Paratyphi A.

FLUOROQUINOLONES AND NALIDIXIC-ACID-RESISTANT S. TYPHI AND S. PARATYPHI A

Widespread acquisition of resistance to chloramphenicol, ampicillin, and trimethoprim-sulfamethoxazole led to the use of fluoroquinolones as the first-line therapy. However, this approach is changing because of the emergence of strains with reduced susceptibility to fluoroquinolones. Nalidixic-acid resistance (NaR) is a marker of decreased fluoroquinolone susceptibility. Although nalidixic acid is a first-generation quinolone that is not widely used to treat enteric fever, NaR predicts an increased resistance to fluoroquinolones and the possibility of a poor clinical response to ciprofloxacin, even if the NaR strain meets the Clinical Laboratory and Standards Institute's cut-off for susceptibility to ciprofloxacin [6].

In the absence of NaR, ciprofloxacin, levofloxacin and ofloxacin are highly efficacious in the treatment of enteric fever. These agents have excellent oral bioavailability, result in rapid defervescence (an average of ~3–4 days) and decreased rates of relapse and carriage compared with chloramphenicol and ß-lactam antibiotics. Concern about fluoroquinolone-induced cartilage toxicity in children is based on animal models; however, several studies support their safety in children [27].

Gatifloxacin is a newer generation fluoroquinolone available in many countries where enteric fever is endemic, has good *in vitro* activity against NaR S. Typhi, and has demonstrated efficacy in the treatment of uncomplicated enteric fever caused by NaR Salmonella [28]. Unfortunately, gatifloxacin was associated with increased frequency of hypoglycemia and hyperglycemia compared to other fluoroquinolones and, for this reason, was withdrawn from the US market and should be used, if ever, with caution. Alternative fluoroquinolones with improved safety profiles are available.

THIRD-GENERATION CEPHALOSPORINS

The emergence of NaR stains with decreased fluoroquinolone susceptibility (and associated treatment failures) have caused a shift toward the use of third generation cephalosporins as first-line therapy in more severe cases, although this approach may result in a longer period until defervescence and has a higher relapse rate compared with the use of effective fluoroquinolones [27]. Ceftriaxone is an effective antibiotic for treating enteric fever, including cases caused by NaR isolates. However, ceftriaxone must be given parenterally and short courses (≤7 days) are associated with high rates of relapse [29]. Furthermore, clinical defervescence may be delayed and longer courses of ceftriaxone may be required, depending on the clinical response [30]. Cefixime is an oral, third-generation cephalosporin that may be used to treat enteric fever, although short courses of cefixime also result in high rates of relapse. Resistance to ceftriaxone and other extended spectrum ß-lactam antibiotics is rare, but increasing [7].

AZITHROMYCIN

Azithromycin is an effective oral treatment for uncomplicated enteric fever, including enteric fever caused by NaR and multidrug-resistant isolates [31]. A 7-day course of azithromycin appears to be as effective as gatifloxacin in the treatment of enteric fever caused by NaR isolates and results in lower rates of clinical failure and relapse compared with cefixime or ceftriaxone. Azithromycin is safe in children, has excellent bioavailability and pharmacokinetics with once-daily dosing and reaches high intracellular concentrations that may contribute to the high rates of cure seen after seven days of therapy.

SUPPORTIVE AND ADJUNCTIVE THERAPY

Adjunctive therapy is aimed at managing the inflammatory complications of infection. In a double-blind trial in Indonesia in the 1980s, a short course of high-dose intravenous dexamethasone initiated concurrently with the first dose of antibiotics significantly reduced mortality in critically ill patients with typhoid fever with shock and/or profound encephalopathy manifested as delirium or obtundation [32]. In suspected cases of severe typhoid fever with shock or encephalopathy in adults and children, dexamethasone should be administered along with intravenous antibiotics as soon as possible, usually before the results of blood cultures are obtained, and may be administered at an initial dose of 3 mg/kg IV, followed by 1 mg/kg IV every 6 hours for eight additional doses.

Supportive care, including rehydration and nutritional management, are important in patients with enteric fever. Rehydration and nutritional supplementation can be managed according to WHO standards. Despite historical concerns regarding their use, debilitating fevers and malaise can be managed safely with antipyretics [33].

MANAGEMENT OF INTESTINAL COMPLICATIONS

Prompt surgical intervention in suspected cases of perforation is the mainstay of therapy. The majority of cases involve single perforation along the anti-mesenteric border of the terminal ileum. However, careful inspection of the bowel is required, as multiple perforations are present in approximately 25% of patients and perforation can occur along the proximal or distal bowel. Surrounding tissues are usually inflamed and friable. While simple closure may be performed in some cases, wedge excision with debridement of the necrotic bowel or segmental resection is more often necessary. In cases of multiple perforations, more extensive resections and temporary ileostomy may be required. Drainage of fluid collections and peritoneal lavage should be performed prior to wound closure. Antibiotic coverage should be broadened to include other intestinal flora, including anaerobes. Perforation-associated mortality rates are variable; early recognition, surgical intervention and supportive care enhance survival [19].

Intestinal hemorrhage can usually be managed through supportive care. Blood products, including packed red cells and plasma may be needed to correct resulting anemia and optimize coagulation parameters in severe cases. Refractory bleeding and severe bleeding leading to shock suggest the need for surgical resection of the involved bowel.

TREATMENT OF RELAPSE

Relapse usually occurs within two weeks of the discontinuation of antibiotics. Isolates obtained following a relapsed infection typically have the same antibiotic susceptibility as the isolate from the primary episode. Relapsed illness is usually milder compared with the primary episode. The approach to treating a relapsed infection is the same as treating a primary episode.

TREATMENT OF CHRONIC CARRIERS

Chronic carriage is asymptomatic and not associated with recurrence of illness. Although chronic carriage is associated with an increased risk of gallbladder carcinoma, no clear, causal relationship is established and it is unknown whether the eradication of carriage reduces this risk of carcinoma. The decision to attempt to eradicate carriage is based on public health considerations and it is more difficult to eliminate carriage in patients with cholelithiasis. However, in some case-series, ciprofloxacin has demonstrated over 90% efficacy in the eradication of carriage [34]. Cholecystectomy may be necessary to eradicate carriage in persons with cholelithiasis that fail medical therapy but for whom eradication is essential for public health reasons (e.g. food-handlers).

PREVENTION

There are two licensed commercially-available vaccines for typhoid fever: the Vi (capsular) polysaccharide parenteral vaccine and a live attenuated Ty21a oral vaccine (Table 69-4). Both vaccines are primarily used by travelers; neither vaccine protects against paratyphoid fever A. Although the WHO's Strategic Advisory Group of Experts (SAGE) has recommended that typhoid vaccination programs be considered in highly endemic settings [35], these vaccines are not yet widely utilized in most endemic regions. A Vi-conjugate vaccine has also been shown to be both safe and immunogenic, including in young children in areas of the world endemic for typhoid. A previous whole-cell, killed parenteral vaccine required multiple injections, was associated with a high adverse event profile and should not be used.

Other strategies to prevent S. Typhi and Paratyphi A include interventions to reduce exposure to food- and waterborne bacteria. At a household level, strategies include boiling and storing water in narrow-mouthed, covered containers. Food safety involves handwashing with soap before preparing or consuming foods, and the avoidance of certain food types in endemic areas, such as raw foods

TABLE 69-4 Commercially Available Vaccines for Typhoid Fever [11, 22]

Vaccine	Type	Route	Dose and interval	Minimum age	Protection against S. Typhi	Boosting interval in travelers	Licensed in # countries
Ty21a	Live-attenuated	Oral	Four doses Administer one dose every other day until complete	5*	50–80%	Every five years	56**
Vi capsule antigen	Polysaccharide	Intramuscular	1	2	50–80%	Every two years	>90**

*Five years and older per WHO [22], 6 years and older per Advisory Committee on Immunization Practices [11]. **As of March 2010.

and shellfish, and consuming only foods that are thoroughly cooked and hot at the time of consumption [22]. At a community level, prevention entails ensuring reliable access to safe water and improved sanitation.

EXAMPLES OF CLINICAL AND SEROLOGIC CLASSIFICATION OF PATHOGENIC *SALMONELLA*

Clinical classification	Serotype	Formal designation	Serogroup
Typhoidal	Typhi	*S. enterica* subsp. enterica ser. Typhi	D
	Paratyphi A	*S. enterica* subsp. enterica ser. Paratyphi A	A
	Paratyphi B (schottmuelleri)	*S. enterica* subsp. enterica ser. Paratyphi B	B
	Paratyphi C (hirschfeldii)	S. enterica subsp. enterica ser. Paratyphi C	C
Non-typhoidal	Typhimurium	*S. enterica* subsp. enterica ser. Typhimurium	B
	Enteriditis	*S. enterica* subsp. enterica ser. Enteriditis	D
	Newport	*S. enterica* subsp. enterica ser. Newport	C

REFERENCES

1. Hornick RB, Woodward WE, Greisman SE. Doctor T. E. Woodward's legacy: from typhus to typhoid fever. Clin Infect Dis 2007;45(suppl. 1):S6–8.
2. Crump JA, Luby SP, Mintz ED. The global burden of typhoid fever. Bull World Health Organ 2004;82:346–53.
3. Ochiai RL, Wang X, von Seidlein L, et al. *Salmonella paratyphi* A rates, Asia. Emerg Infect Dis 2005;11:1764–6.
4. Khatri NS, Maskey P, Poudel S, et al. Gallbladder carriage of *Salmonella paratyphi* A may be an important factor in the increasing incidence of this infection in South Asia. Ann Intern Med 2009;150:567–8.
5. Vollaard AM, Ali S, van Asten HA, et al. Risk factors for typhoid and paratyphoid fever in Jakarta, Indonesia. JAMA 2004;291:2607–15.
6. Chau TT, Campbell JI, Galindo CM, et al. Antimicrobial drug resistance of *Salmonella enterica* serovar typhi in Asia and molecular mechanism of reduced susceptibility to the fluoroquinolones. Antimicrob Agents Chemother 2007;51:4315–23.
7. Kumar S, Rizvi M, Berry N. Rising prevalence of enteric fever due to multidrug-resistant Salmonella: an epidemiological study. J Med Microbiol 2008;57: 1247–50.
8. Crump JA, Ram PK, Gupta SK, et al. Part I. Analysis of data gaps pertaining to *Salmonella enterica* serotype Typhi infections in low and medium human development index countries, 1984–2005. Epidemiol Infect 2008;136:436–48.
9. Lynch MF, Blanton EM, Bulens S, et al. Typhoid fever in the United States, 1999–2006. JAMA 2009;302:859–65.
10. Brooks WA, Hossain A, Goswami D, et al. Bacteremic typhoid fever in children in an urban slum, Bangladesh. Emerg Infect Dis 2005;11:326–9.
11. Bhattarai A, Mintz E. Typhoid and Paratyphoid Fever. In: CDC Health Information for International Travel, 2010th edn. Mosby; 2010:44. Available at: http://wwwnc.cdc.gov/travel/yellowbook/2012/chapter-3-infectious-diseases-related-to-travel/typhoid-and-paratyphoid-fever.htm. Centers for Disease Control and Prevention, Atlanta, GA 30333, USA.
12. Monack DM, Mueller A, Falkow S. Persistent bacterial infections: the interface of the pathogen and the host immune system. Nat Rev Microbiol 2004;2: 747–65.
13. Wain J, Pham VB, Ha V, et al. Quantitation of bacteria in bone marrow from patients with typhoid fever: relationship between counts and clinical features. J Clin Microbiol 2001;39:1571–6.
14. Crawford RW, Rosales-Reyes R, Ramirez-Aguilar Mde L, et al. Gallstones play a significant role in Salmonella spp. gallbladder colonization and carriage. Proc Natl Acad Sci USA 2010;107:4353–8.
15. Parry CM, Hien TT, Dougan G, et al. Typhoid fever. N Engl J Med 2002;347:1770–82.
16. Maskey AP, Day JN, Phung QT, et al. *Salmonella enterica* serovar Paratyphi A and *S. enterica* serovar Typhi cause indistinguishable clinical syndromes in Kathmandu, Nepal. Clin Infect Dis 2006;42:1247–53.
17. Davis TM, Makepeace AE, Dallimore EA, Choo KE. Relative bradycardia is not a feature of enteric fever in children. Clin Infect Dis 1999;28:582–6.
18. Butler T, Islam A, Kabir I, Jones PK. Patterns of morbidity and mortality in typhoid fever dependent on age and gender: review of 552 hospitalized patients with diarrhea. Rev Infect Dis 1991;13:85–90.
19. Nguyen QC, Everest P, Tran TK, et al. A clinical, microbiological, and pathological study of intestinal perforation associated with typhoid fever. Clin Infect Dis 2004;39:61–7.

20. Punjabi NH, Hoffman SL, Edman DC, et al. Treatment of severe typhoid fever in children with high dose dexamethasone. Pediatr Infect Dis J 1988; 7:598–600.
21. Hoffman SL, Punjabi NH, Kumala S, et al. Reduction of mortality in chloramphenicol-treated severe typhoid fever by high-dose dexamethasone. N Engl J Med 1984;310:82–8.
22. World Health Organization. Background document: The diagnosis, treatment and prevention of typhoid fever. Geneva: World Health Organization; 2003.
23. Wain J, Diep TS, Bay PV, et al. Specimens and culture media for the laboratory diagnosis of typhoid fever. J Infect Dev Ctries 2008;2:469–74.
24. Naheed A, Ram PK, Brooks WA, et al. Clinical value of Tubex and Typhidot rapid diagnostic tests for typhoid fever in an urban community clinic in Bangladesh. Diagn Microbiol Infect Dis 2008;61:381–6.
25. Olsen SJ, Pruckler J, Bibb W, et al. Evaluation of rapid diagnostic tests for typhoid fever. J Clin Microbiol 2004;42:1885–9.
26. Snyder MJ, Gonzalez O, Palomino C, et al. Comparative efficacy of chloramphenicol, ampicillin, and co-trimoxazole in the treatment of typhoid fever. Lancet 1976;2:1155–7.
27. Thaver D, Zaidi AK, Critchley JA, et al. Fluoroquinolones for treating typhoid and paratyphoid fever (enteric fever). Cochrane Database Syst Rev 2008: CD004530.
28. Dolecek C, Tran TP, Nguyen NR, et al. A multi-center randomised controlled trial of gatifloxacin versus azithromycin for the treatment of uncomplicated typhoid fever in children and adults in Vietnam. PLoS One 2008;3:e2188.
29. Frenck RW, Jr, Nakhla I, Sultan Y, et al. Azithromycin versus ceftriaxone for the treatment of uncomplicated typhoid fever in children. Clin Infect Dis 2000;31:1134–8.
30. Tatli MM, Aktas G, Kosecik M, Yilmaz A. Treatment of typhoid fever in children with a flexible-duration of ceftriaxone, compared with 14-day treatment with chloramphenicol. Int J Antimicrob Agents 2003;21:350–3.
31. Effa EE, Bukirwa H. Azithromycin for treating uncomplicated typhoid and paratyphoid fever (enteric fever). Cochrane Database Syst Rev 2008:CD006083.
32. Hoffman SL, Punjabi NH, Kumala S, et al. Reduction of mortality in chloramphenicol-treated patients with severe typhoid fever by high dose dexamethasone. Trans Assoc Am Physicians 1983;96:188–96.
33. Vinh H, Parry CM, Hanh VT, et al. Double blind comparison of ibuprofen and paracetamol for adjunctive treatment of uncomplicated typhoid fever. Pediatr Infect Dis J 2004;23:226–30.
34. Zavala Trujillo I, Quiroz C, Gutierrez MA, et al. Fluoroquinolones in the treatment of typhoid fever and the carrier state. Eur J Clin Microbiol Infect Dis 1991;10:334–41.
35. Meeting of the Immunization Strategic Advisory Group of Experts, November 2007 – conclusions and recommendations. Wkly Epidemiol Rec 2008; 83:1–15.
36. Brenner FW, Villar RG, Angulo FJ, et al. Salmonella nomenclature. J Clin Microbiol 2000;38:2465–7.
37. Zimmerman MD, Murdoch DR, Rozmajzl PJ, et al. Murine typhus and febrile illness, Nepal. Emerg Infect Dis 2008;14:1656–9.

Brucellosis 70

Georgios Pappas

Key features

- Brucellosis is a common zoonotic infection worldwide with significant medical, veterinary, and economic consequences
- The disease is transmitted by direct contact with, or consumption of, products of a variety of domestic and wild animals
- Human disease can manifest in myriad ways, including prolonged fever, granulomatous hepatitis, uveitis, endocarditis, and osteoarticular or genitourinary involvement
- Infection is often characterized by its chronicity
- Treatment involves combination antimicrobial therapy and should be administered for a minimum of 6 weeks
- There is no vaccine commercially available for use in humans. Prevention is usually targeted to risk factor reduction and behavioral modifications, for example avoidance of consumption of unpasteurized dairy products
- Synonyms: Malta fever, Undulant fever, Bang's disease

INTRODUCTION

Brucellosis is a zoonotic infection with worldwide distribution that is caused by species of the genus Brucella including *Brucella melitensis, Brucella abortus, Brucella suis*, and *Brucella canis*. Brucellosis is an ancient disease with lesions attributed to possible brucellosis recently recognized in a 2.4–2.8-million-year-old hominid [1]. In the late 19th century, the pathogen was implicated in human disease and isolated from goat milk by Sir David Bruce (hence the name Brucella) and his colleagues in Malta.

EPIDEMIOLOGY

An estimated half a million new cases of brucellosis occur each year worldwide, with four major high-risk zones delineated by recent epidemiologic data [2]: the Middle East, Central Asia, parts of Latin America, and the Mediterranean, with particularly increasing trends observed in the Balkan Peninsula (Fig. 70.1). There is limited information about the extent of disease prevalence in sub-Saharan Africa because of limited veterinary surveillance and diagnostic facilities for the detection of human disease. In India, the disease remains endemic; in Southeast Asia known burden is unknown, with confirmed cases being limited to case reports. Disease distribution strongly correlates with general socioeconomic status and exposure to animals and animal products [2].

NATURAL HISTORY, PATHOGENESIS, AND PATHOLOGY

Brucella species are, in general, host-specific. The vast majority of human disease is attributed to *B. melitensis*, the natural reservoirs of which are sheep and goats. *Brucella abortus* (bovine brucellosis) causes a significant percentage of cases, particularly in countries with a tradition in cow-raising. Both these species can also reside in camels. *Brucella suis* (swine brucellosis) and *B. canis* (canine brucellosis) are rare causes of human disease, although there is concern about the former's presence in wild boars and the subsequent risk for hunters [3]. *Brucella ovis* (also found in sheep) and *Brucella neotomae* (found in rodents) are not human pathogens. Additional species have also been recently identified, including *Brucella ceti* and *Brucella pinnipedialis* (causing brucellosis in marine mammals) [4], *Brucella microti* (found in wild foxes of Central Europe) and *Brucella inopinata*, a novel species recently isolated from a human case [5].

Humans are infected through direct contact with infected animals or animal products. Shepherds and abattoir workers are at occupational risk of infection. Humans also become infected through the ingestion of contaminated animal products, such as unpasteurized dairy products, or through the inhalation of aerosolized particles [6]. The latter mode of transmission, often overlooked, lies behind the potential use of *Brucella* spp. in biological warfare (although its significance in such settings is largely historical) [7], but also explains why brucellosis remains a common laboratory-acquired infection in microbiologists and laboratory technicians [8].

Brucella reside within infected macrophages and, potentially, other phagocytes and establish latent and chronic infection [9]. The components of protective immunity are poorly understood [10].

CLINICAL FEATURES AND DIAGNOSIS

Clinical brucellosis can present in myriad ways. The commonest presentation is nonspecific, with fever and malaise. Typically, symptoms are mild and are often reported from patients for weeks prior to diagnosis. Physical examination can reveal lymphadenopathy and hepatosplenomegaly in a minority of patients. Focal disease involving osteoarticular structures is common, including peripheral arthritis or sacroiliitis (the latter predominantly in younger patients), or spondylitis. Epididymo-orchitis is common in male patients. Table 70-1 lists other clinical characteristics of uncomplicated, or focal, brucellosis.

Involvement of the bone marrow can lead to mild pancytopenia; relative lymphocytosis is common. Liver function tests are often moderately abnormal. Lactic acid levels may be increased in joint fluid of affected joints [11] and radiographic evidence of spondylitis is highly suggestive of brucellosis [12].

Definitive diagnosis rests on isolation of the pathogen, but diagnosis usually rests on serologic analysis. Blood cultures should be incubated for up to 4 weeks. Serologic analysis usually involves the use of serum agglutination tests (SAT), with a titer equal to or above 1:320

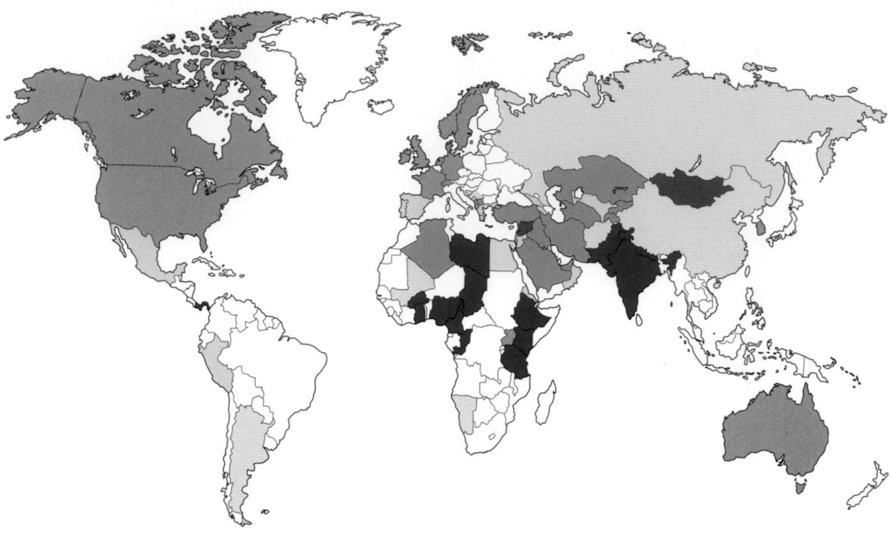

Annual incidence of brucellosis per 1,000,000 population

- >500
- 50–500 cases
- 10–50
- 2–10
- <2
- Possibly endemic, no data
- Non-endemic/no data

FIGURE 70.1 Global endemicity of brucellosis. *Reproduced from: Gutierrez Ruiz C, Miranda JJ, Pappas G (2006) A 26-year-old man with sternoclavicular arthritis. PLoS Med 3(8): e293 and derived from Ariza J, Bosilkovski M, Cascio A, et al. Perspectives for the treatment of brucellosis in the 21st century: the Ioannina recommendations. PLoS Med. 2007 Dec;4(12):e317 and Pappas G, Papadimitriou P, Akritidis N, Christou L, Tsianos EV (2006) The new global map of human brucellosis. Lancet Infect Dis 6:91-99.*

TABLE 70-1 Clinical Manifestations of Brucellosis (Focal Complications in Descending Order of Frequency)

System involved	Manifestations
General	Fever, malaise, anorexia
Reticuloendothelial system	Lymphadenopathy, hepatosplenomegaly
Osteoarticular	Spondylitis
	Peripheral arthritis
	Sacroiliitis
Genitourinary	Epididymo-orchitis in males
	Possible increased risk of abortion in pregnant females
Liver	Moderate and rarely severe hepatitis, granuloma formation, chronic suppurative disease, decompensation of pre-existing liver pathology
Hematologic	Lymphocytosis, pancytopenia, rarely hemophagocytosis
Skin	Various rashes, vasculitis
Respiratory	Pneumonia/bronchitis
Gastrointestinal	Vomiting and diarrhea, rarely peritonitis, cholecystitis, colitis
Central nervous system	Meningitis/meningoencephalitis, myelitis, radiculopathy, rarely peripheral neuropathy
Cardiovascular	Endocarditis, mycotic aneurysms
Ocular	Uveitis

TABLE 70-2 Differential Diagnosis of Brucellosis

Clinical syndrome	Differential diagnosis (in descending order of frequency)
Fever with nonspecific constitutional symptoms	Lymphoma; malaria in endemic areas; Q fever; typhoid fever; tularemia; rheumatic/autoimmune syndromes; viral infections including mononucleosis
Osteoarticular disease	Septic arthritis/spondylitis; tuberculous spondylitis; rheumatic/autoimmune syndromes
Chronic complaints with nonspecific findings	Psychiatric disorders; chronic fatigue syndrome; hypothyroidism

considered positive, even in endemic areas. ELISAs are available, but analysis has not been standardized. PCR assays for brucellosis are also available and real-time PCR, in particular, has been shown to be extremely sensitive and specific in numerous settings [8, 13, 14].

Table 70-2 summarizes important differential diagnostic considerations for the commonest clinical patterns of human brucellosis.

TREATMENT

Antibiotic regimens to treat individuals with brucellosis usually contain at least two agents and treatment should be continued for weeks. Consensus recommendations for uncomplicated disease are summarized in Table 70-3 [15]. Doxycycline and streptomycin may be microbiologically optimal but, because of convenience, doxycycline and rifampin are usually the drugs of choice for treating individuals with non-spondylitic brucellosis. Doxycycline and gentamycin are also being used.

There is evidence to suggest that doxycycline-streptomycin is the combination of choice for patients with brucellosis complicated by

TABLE 70-3 Consensus "Ioannina Recommendations" for the Treatment of Human Brucellosis

Treatment regimen	Dose	Notes
Doxycycline and streptomycin (DOX + STR)	DOX: 100 mg twice daily for 6 weeks STR: 15 mg/kg daily intramuscularly for 2–3 weeks	
Doxycycline and rifampin (DOX + RIF)	DOX: 100 mg twice daily for 6 weeks RIF: 600–1200 mg daily for 6 weeks, one morning dose	
Doxycycline and gentamycin (DOX + GENT)	DOX: 100 mg twice daily for 6 weeks GENT: 5 mg/kg daily parenterally in a single dose for 7 days	
Trimethoprim-sulfamethoxazole (TMP - SMX)-containing regimens	TMP-SMX: 800 + 160 mg twice daily for 6 weeks	Can be used in children less than 8 years old, including with aminoglycoside
Quinolone-containing combination regimens	Ofloxacin: 400 mg twice daily/ Ciprofloxacin: 500 mg twice daily, both for 6 weeks	Can be used as second agent in patients intolerant of aminoglycosides, tetracyclines or rifampin.

From Ariza J, Bosilkovski M, Cascio A, et al. Perspectives for the treatment of brucellosis in the 21st century: the Ioannina recommendations. PLoS Med 2007;4:e317.

spondylitis (but not other osteoarticular complications) and that treatment in such patients should be extended possibly to 12 weeks [16]. Many clinicians use at least three drugs to treat individuals with brucellosis involving the central nervous system and individuals with brucella-associated endocarditis usually require surgical intervention. Young children with brucellosis are usually treated with rifampin and trimethoprim-sulfamethoxazole.

Even with effective drug treatment, relapses occur in 5–10% of patients, usually in the early post-treatment period. Relapses tend to be mild and can be re-treated with the same, or another, first-line regimen.

A minority of patients complain of malaise and nonspecific depressive symptoms following completion of effective drug regimens. Brucella have occasionally been isolated from such patients years after treatment, underscoring the potential chronicity of brucellosis [9, 17]. Currently, there is no vaccine commercially available for use in humans. Prevention is usually targeted to risk factor reduction and behavioral modifications, for example avoidance of the consumption of unpasteurized dairy products.

REFERENCES

1. D'Anastasio R, Zipfel B, Moggi-Cecchi J, et al. Possible brucellosis in an early hominin skeleton from Sterkfontein, South Africa. PLoS One 2009;4:e6439.
2. Pappas G, Papadimitriou P, Akritidis N, et al. The new global map of human brucellosis. Lancet Infect Dis 2006;6:91–9.
3. Centers for Disease Control and Prevention (CDC). *Brucella suis* infection associated with feral swine hunting–three states, 2007–2008. MMWR Morb Mortal Wkly Rep 2009;58:618–21
4. Foster G, Osterman BS, Godfroid J, et al. *Brucella ceti* sp. nov. and *Brucella pinnipedialis* sp. nov. for Brucella strains with cetaceans and seals as their preferred hosts. Int J Syst Evol Microbiol 2007;57:2688–93.
5. De BK, Stauffer L, Koylass MS, et al. Novel Brucella strain (BO1) associated with a prosthetic breast implant infection. J Clin Microbiol 2008;46:43–9.
6. Almuneef MA, Memish ZA, Balkhy HH, et al. Importance of screening household members of acute brucellosis cases in endemic areas. Epidemiol Infect 2004;132:533–40.
7. Pappas G, Panagopoulou P, Christou L, Akritidis N. Brucella as a biological weapon. Cell Mol Life Sci 2006;63:2229–36.
8. Bouza E, Sánchez-Carrillo C, Hernangómez S, et al. Laboratory-acquired brucellosis: a Spanish national survey. J Hosp Infect 2005;61:80–3.
9. Vrioni G, Pappas G, Priavali E, et al. An eternal microbe: Brucella DNA load persists for years after clinical cure. Clin Infect Dis 2008;46:e131–6.
10. Pappas G, Akritidis N, Bosilkovski M, Tsianos E. Brucellosis. N Engl J Med 2005;352:2325–36.
11. Mavridis AK, Drosos AA, Tsolas O, Moutsopoulos HM. Lactate levels in Brucella arthritis. Rheumatol Int 1984;4:169–71.
12. Colmenero JD, Jiménez-Mejías ME, Sánchez-Lora FJ, et al. Pyogenic, tuberculous, and brucellar vertebral osteomyelitis: a descriptive and comparative study of 219 cases. Ann Rheum Dis 1997;56:709–15.
13. Navarro E, Segura JC, Castaño MJ, Solera J. Use of real-time quantitative polymerase chain reaction to monitor the evolution of *Brucella melitensis* DNA load during therapy and post-therapy follow-up in patients with brucellosis. Clin Infect Dis 2006;42:1266–73.
14. Queipo-Ortuño MI, Colmenero JD, Reguera JM, et al. Rapid diagnosis of human brucellosis by SYBR Green I-based real-time PCR assay and melting curve analysis in serum samples. Clin Microbiol Infect 2005;11:713–8.
15. Ariza J, Bosilkovski M, Cascio A, et al. Perspectives for the treatment of brucellosis in the 21st century: the Ioannina recommendations. PLoS Med 2007;4:e317.
16. Pappas G, Seitaridis S, Akritidis N, Tsianos E. Treatment of brucella spondylitis: lessons from an impossible meta-analysis and initial report of efficacy of a fluoroquinolone-containing regimen. Int J Antimicrob Agents 2004; 24:502–7.
17. Castaño MJ, Solera J. Chronic brucellosis and persistence of *Brucella melitensis* DNA. J Clin Microbiol 2009;47:2084–9.
18. Gutierrez Ruiz C, Miranda JJ, Pappas G. A 26-year-old man with sternoclavicular arthritis. PLoS Med 2006;3:e293.

71 Melioidosis and Glanders

Nicholas J White

Key features

- Melioidosis is an infection by *Burkholderia pseudomallei*, an environmental, saprophytic, Gram-negative bacterium found in water and soil in South and East Asia and Northern Australia. In endemic areas, it accounts for up to 20% of community-acquired septicemias
- Glanders is an infection with *Burkholderia mallei*, a pathogen of horses and other equines; it is now very rare
- Melioidosis predominantly affects adults with underlying diabetes, chronic renal disease, alcoholism, cirrhosis, or immunosuppression
- Pneumonia, septicemia, and metastatic abscess formation (often in liver, spleen, lungs, and muscle) are common; mortality approaches 50%
- In children, *B. pseudomallei* causes a unique syndrome of acute suppurative parotitis
- Treatment is with high doses of parenteral ceftazidime or a carbapenem, followed by oral doxycycline and trimethoprim-sulfamethoxazole to complete 20 weeks of antibiotic treatment

INTRODUCTION

The first description of glanders, a disease primarily of horses caused by *Burkholderia mallei*, is usually attributed to Aristotle who wrote "The ass suffers chiefly from one particular disease which they call "melis". It arrives first in the head, and a clammy humour runs down the nostrils, thick and red; if it stays in the head the animal may recover, but if it descends into the lungs the animal will die." Thereafter, the nasal and pulmonary infection (glanders) and subcutaneous abscesses (farcy) of horses, mules, and donkeys were well known as a potential threat to humans. In Rangoon in 1911, Whitmore and Krishnaswami documented a "hitherto undescribed glanders-like illness" among the ill and neglected inhabitants of the town" [1]. The disease, killing emaciated morphine addicts who languished on the streets of Rangoon, was caused by a bacterium "sufficiently peculiar to distinguish it from all pathogenic bacteria previously known to us". Whitmore demonstrated that Koch's postulates could be fulfilled and he proposed the name *Bacillus pseudomallei* for the newly discovered bacterium. By 1917, Krishnaswami had reported over 100 cases from Rangoon (5% of all post-mortem examinations). Sporadic cases were reported during, and following, the Second World War and many more cases were reported in soldiers fighting in Vietnam during the war of independence with France and the later conflict involving the USA. The Vietnam War experience skewed clinical descriptions towards more chronic forms of the infection and reactivations long after exposure. Very few cases were reported in indigenous people in South and East Asia, but with improvements in hospital microbiology facilities in some countries over the past two decades, melioidosis has been increasingly recognized throughout this populous region [2, 3]. The clinical and pathologic picture seen today is much as Whitmore originally described it. Meanwhile, glanders in equines has become a rarity and human cases are extremely unusual.

EPIDEMIOLOGY

Areas of the world endemic for melioidosis are generally within the latitudes 20°S and 20°N [2]. In recent years, there have been increasing numbers of case reports of human melioidosis from Southern China, Taiwan, many areas of Southeast Asia, and the south of India. These are areas inhabited by a significant proportion of the world's population. Cases have also been described in Brazil and Africa (Fig. 71.1). Thus, as with many tropical bacterial diseases, our current understanding of epidemiology reflects the distribution of microbiology laboratories capable of making the diagnosis. In the case of melioidosis, current estimates of the global burden are likely to be a considerable underestimate. *Burkholderia pseudomallei* is also a major veterinary pathogen in Australia and a major problem for zoos. It causes lethal infections in many species, but large primates (notably highland gorillas), certain bird species, and sea mammals are particularly vulnerable.

In endemic areas, melioidosis is a rainy season disease. It predominantly affects people who have direct contact with wet soils and who have an underlying predisposition to infection. These are patients with diabetes mellitus, renal disease (calculi, renal failure), and cirrhosis, or patients who are immunosuppressed, either as the result of disease or drug treatment [3] but, interestingly, it is not specifically associated with HIV infection. Diabetes is the most important predisposing condition, accounting for about half of cases. The infection may present at any age, with the peak incidence in the fourth and fifth decades of life, which reflects the appearance of the underlying predisposing illnesses. In northeast Thailand, where *B. pseudomallei* accounts for 20% of community-acquired septicemias, the average annual incidence (1987–1991) was estimated to be 4.4 per 100,000, but this is increasing steadily as the local population is living longer with improved health services and economic conditions. In Singapore (1991–1994), where melioidosis accounts for 7% of community-acquired pneumonias, incidence was estimated at 1.6 per 100,000 per year. In the Top End of the Northern Territory, Australia, where melioidosis is the commonest cause of fatal septicemic pneumonia, annual incidence between 1989 and 1999 was 16.5 per 100,000 [4].

Serologic studies in Thailand indicate that exposure occurs as soon as the infant makes contact with soil and water, with seroconversion of approximately 25% per year for the first 4 years of life. Exposure occurs very frequently during rice farming (a major occupation in the region). Thus, the majority of the population in endemic areas have serologic evidence of exposure, but there is no evidence that this antibody is protective. Disease either results from a failure of host defense, resulting from disease or drugs or, less commonly, a particularly large inoculum (major trauma, near drowning).

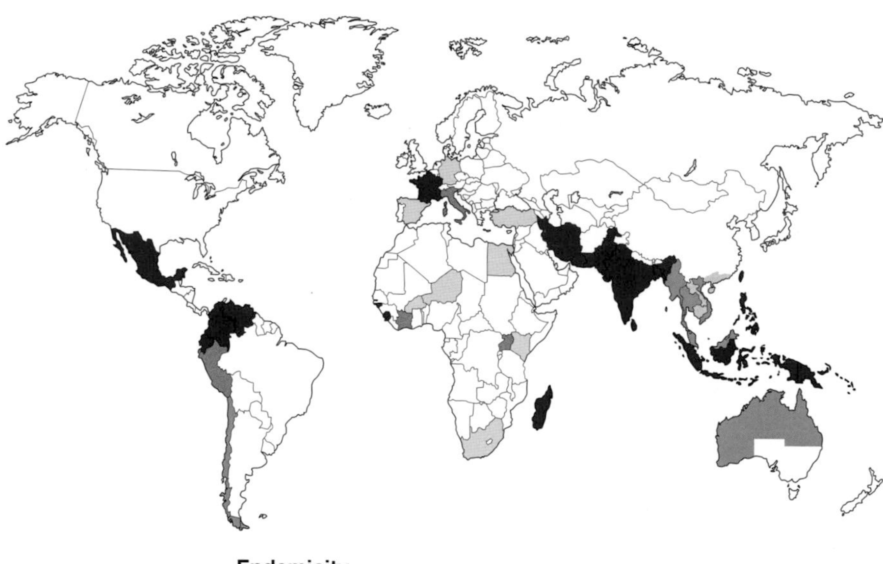

FIGURE 71.1 Global distribution of *B. pseudomallei*. *Reproduced with permission from Cheng AC, Currie BJ. Melioidosis: epidemiology, pathophysiology, and management. Clin Microbiol Rev 2005;18:383–416.*

NATURAL HISTORY, PATHOGENESIS, AND PATHOLOGY

Burkholderia pseudomallei is a soil saprophyte and can be readily recovered from water and wet soil (often rice paddy fields) in endemic areas [5]. The bacterium is a motile, aerobic, non-spore-forming, Gram-negative bacillus. In contrast, *B. mallei* is an obligate pathogen. The genome of *B. pseudomallei* is one of the largest and most complex bacterial genomes yet sequenced. It comprises 7.24 Mb, divided unequally between two circular chromosomes (4.07 Mb and 3.17 Mb) encoding ~5800 genes with an overall G + C content of 68%. The molecular and epidemiologic evidence suggests that mammalian pathogenicity is unimportant in *B. pseudomallei* ecology, whereas *B. mallei* appears to have undergone reductive evolution from a *B. pseudomallei* ancestor (they have 99% homology in conserved genes) and in adapting to its equine host has shed approximately 1.41 Mb of DNA containing the genes necessary for soil survival. *Burkholderia pseudomallei,* like many soil bacteria, is a difficult organism to kill: it can survive in triple-distilled water for years; it is resistant to complement and lysosomal defensins and cationic peptides; it survives inside several cell lines; and it produces proteases, lipase, lecithinase, catalase, peroxidase, superoxide dismutase, hemolysins, and siderophores. The genome encodes many classical virulence genes, such as adhesins, fimbriae, exopolysaccharides, and Type III secretion systems [6]. The cell wall lipopolysaccharide, which is the immunodominant antigen, is highly conserved and contains two distinct O-polysaccharides. *Burkholderia pseudomallei* produces a highly hydrated glycocalyx "capsule" – an important virulence determinant – that forms a slime. This facilitates the formation of microcolonies in which the organism is both protected from antibiotic penetration and phenotypically altered. Organisms that cause invasive disease are indistinguishable from those found in the environment.

Melioidosis in humans is usually acquired by inoculation or inhalation. There is no evidence it can be acquired by ingestion. Occasional nosocomial infections have occurred and sexual transmission has been reported twice. Rice farmers suffer repeated minor cuts and abrasions whilst immersed for much of the day in water containing *B. pseudomallei,* but they do not develop active infection unless an underlying predisposing condition develops. The risk of disease is proportional to the concentration of organisms in the soil. Neutrophils play a central role in innate host defense, which is initiated by Toll-like receptors (TLRs; principally TLR-2) [6]. In animal models, interferon-gamma is essential for host defense, but other components are also important.

Human infection with *B. mallei* has occurred rarely among laboratory workers and those in direct contact with infected animals. Person-to-person spread of *B. mallei* is extremely rare. The bacteria usually enter the body through the eyes, nose, mouth, cracked skin, or cuts. Direct contact with the skin can lead to a localized cutaneous infection. Inhalation leads to pneumonia, septicemia, or disseminated abscesses in muscle, liver, and spleen – a pattern similar to that of melioidosis. *Burkholderia mallei* is a dangerous organism in the laboratory and should be investigated only in Biosafety Level (BSL) 3 facilities. It is highly infectious as an aerosol and, as infection requires only a few organisms, it has been used as a biological warfare agent. Use during the American Civil War, World Wars I and II, and the Russian invasion of Afghanistan has all been reported.

CLINICAL FEATURES

Melioidosis presents as a febrile illness, ranging from a chronic, debilitating, localized infection to an acute, fulminant septicemia characterized by local or metastatic abscess formation [5]. Usually, there is no obvious infected wound or trauma. The majority of cases are septicemic. Nearly all clinical studies have come from Thailand, Malaysia, Singapore, and Northern Australia. The overall mortality in adults in Thailand is approximately 50%, with many deaths occurring rapidly before microbiologic confirmation. In Northern Australia, the mortality of severe melioidosis has been falling in recent years with earlier recognition and intensive care treatment [4]. The lung is the most commonly affected organ, presenting either with a lung abscess or pneumonia, or secondary multifocal "blood-borne pneumonia". Large or peripherally sited lung abscesses commonly rupture into the pleural space to cause empyema. Seeding and abscess formation may occur in any organ, although the liver, spleen, skeletal muscle, and prostate are relatively common sites. Renal abscesses are often associated with calculi and urinary infection. In nearly 3000 patients prospectively studied in Thailand, a wide variety of clinical presentations have been seen, but primary meningitis or endocarditis have not (although secondary meningitis from cerebral abscesses and mycotic aneurysms does occur). Melioidosis may present as an uncomplicated, localized infection of the skin, subcutaneous tissues, or eye. Corneal ulcers secondary to trauma and then exposure to contaminated water are rapidly destructive. Metastatic pyomyositis is relatively common. Melioidosis causes acute suppurative parotitis. This unique syndrome occurs mainly in children (29% of pediatric cases, 1% of adult cases,) with no other evidence of an underlying predisposing condition. In approximately 10% of cases, the parotitis is bilateral. The patient presents with fever, pain, and swelling over the parotid gland. In advanced cases, there may be rupture either to the skin or through to the external ear. Incision and drainage are often required; great care must be taken to avoid damaging the facial nerve. Delay in drainage may also result in a permanent Bell's palsy.

In approximately 4% of cases from Australia and, less commonly, elsewhere (<0.2% of cases in Thailand), melioidosis presents as a brainstem encephalitis with peripheral motor weakness or flaccid paraparesis. Prominent features of the brain stem syndrome on presentation are unilateral limb weakness, cerebellar signs, and cranial nerve palsies. Focal, multiple, small microabscesses in the brainstem and spinal cord are thought to be the cause. The clinical experience from Northern Australia is generally similar to that in Southeast Asia, but with two other notable differences; parotid abscess is uncommon (although children comprise only 4% of cases compared with 15% in Thailand) and genitourinary infections (commonly prostatic abscess) comprise 15% of cases compared with <2% elsewhere.

Glanders is characterized by initial onset of fever, rigors, and malaise culminating in a rapid onset of pneumonia, bacteremia, skin pustules, and disseminated abscesses. Death occurs in 7–10 days without antibiotic treatment. Even with antibiotic treatment, septicemic glanders has a mortality of 50%. The course of infection depends on the route of acquisition.

PATIENT EVALUATION, DIAGNOSIS, AND DIFFERENTIAL DIAGNOSIS

Melioidosis should be suspected in any severely ill febrile patient with an underlying predisposing condition who lives in, or has traveled from, an endemic area. The differential diagnosis includes any other bacterial cause of septicemia, cavitating pneumonia, or abscess formation. In northeast Thailand, *B. pseudomallei* is the most common cause of septicemic illness during the rainy season in adult diabetics. There is often abscess formation, either in the lungs (seen on the chest radiograph) or in the liver and spleen (seen on ultrasound examination). Splenic abscess is a pointer to melioidosis in endemic areas (in northeast Thailand, 95% of splenic abscesses are caused by *B. pseudomallei*). In up to 13% of cases with septicemia, subcutaneous abscesses are present in which Gram-negative rods can be demonstrated. *Burkholderia pseudomallei* is readily cultured from infected sites or the blood. Throat swab culture is 90% sensitive compared with sputum culture and is more easily obtained in children or debilitated patients.

In the laboratory, *B. pseudomallei* grows aerobically on most agar media producing clearly visible colonies within 48 hours at 37°C. Ashdown's selective medium (a simple agar containing crystal violet, glycerol, and gentamicin) is commonly used to culture the organism. The colonies develop a characteristic appearance (becoming rugose, or cornflower head-like, with a silvery sheen) and they take up the crystal violet dye [7]. Gram-stain reveals Gram-negative rods that are often described as bipolar staining or like safety pins – although in clinical specimens morphology and staining is extremely variable. The organism is oxidase-positive, utilizes glucose by an oxidative pathway and can be reliably identified from its biochemical profile using kit-based systems. *Burkholderia pseudomallei* is intrinsically resistant to many antibiotics. In general, it is susceptible to chloramphenicol, the tetracyclines, trimethoprim-sulfamethoxazole, ureidopenicillins, third-generation cephalosporins, carbapenems and, unusually for a "pseudomonad", amoxicillin-clavulanate. *Burkholderia pseudomallei* is intrinsically resistant to other penicillins, first- and second-generation cephalosporins, macrolides, rifamycins, colistin, and the aminoglycosides. Rare, naturally occurring mutants have been reported that lack the efflux pump and are susceptible to both macrolides and aminoglycosides. The fluoroquinolones have weak activity and have proved very disappointing in clinical trials. This unusual antibiotic, susceptibility profile (i.e. gentamicin and colistin resistance but co-amoxiclav susceptibility) in an oxidase-positive, Gram-negative rod is also useful for rapid identification. *Burkholderia mallei* generally shows a similar pattern of antimicrobial susceptibility, except that it is gentamicin-sensitive.

Cultures should be plated on routine blood agar and Ashdown's selective medium. Swabs from open, contaminated sites should also be placed in a selective pre-incubation broth. Small colonies are often evident on agar plates in 24 hours. The median time to blood culture positivity is 48 hours but is shorter with automated systems. Direct immunofluorescence on sputum, urine, or pus is 98% specific and approximately 70% sensitive compared with culture but allows a diagnosis to be made in less than 30 minutes. *Burkholderia pseudomallei* has a characteristic biochemical profile and can be rapidly identified by specific latex agglutination tests. The definitive diagnosis of melioidosis is made by isolation of *B. pseudomallei* from any site; the organism is not carried asymptomatically. In the past, serologic tests, such as the indirect hemagglutination (IHA) assay were used widely. The IHA predominantly detects antibodies directed against the remarkably conserved lipopolysaccharide – the immunodominant antigen. Serologic tests may be of value in excluding melioidosis or supporting the diagnosis in areas where prevalence is low; however, they are of less value in endemic areas where a significant proportion of the population is seropositive.

TREATMENT

Initial intensive care management of severe melioidosis is similar to that of any severe Gram-negative septicemia. Patients should be resuscitated with adequate intravenous fluids as hypovolemia is common in the acute phase. There have been eight randomized trials of parenteral antibiotic treatment and four of oral eradication therapy, all conducted in northeast Thailand. Carbapenems kill *B. pseudomallei* more rapidly than cephalosporins. Imipenem proved equivalent to ceftazidime in a large, randomized trial. Meropenem is currently being evaluated, but the most evaluated drug has been ceftazidime. Thus, the antibiotics of choice are ceftazidime or a carbapenem (meropenem or imipenem; see Table 71-1). Other third-generation cephalosporins are less effective. Parenteral co-amoxiclav was associated with a similar mortality to ceftazidime, but had a higher rate of treatment failure. Cefoperazone-sulbactam has also proved effective. Thus, co-amoxiclav is an appropriate empirical treatment for septicemia in areas where melioidosis is endemic, but treatment should be changed to ceftazidime or a carbapenem once the diagnosis of melioidosis has been confirmed. Large and accessible abscesses should be drained. Melioidosis is difficult to treat. Systemic infections respond very slowly to specific treatment. The median time to fever

TABLE 71-1 Parenteral Treatment of Melioidosis

Parenteral drug	Dose
Ceftazidime	40 mg/kg: 8-hourly*
Imipenem	20 mg/kg: 8-hourly
Meropenem	20 mg/kg: 8-hourly
Amoxicillin-clavulanate	20 mg/5mg/kg: 4-hourly

*or 19 mg/kg IV stat followed by a continuous infusion of 3.5 mg/kg/h. Parenteral treatment should continue until there is clear improvement and the patient can take oral medications. Parenteral treatment should be given for at least 10 days. The therapeutic response is very slow (median fever clearance: 9 days). Physicians often switch antibiotics prematurely, fearing the emergence of resistance (which occurs in <3% of patients). Dosages often require adjustment for renal failure. Other third-generation cephalosporins (e.g. cefotaxime, ceftriaxone) should not be used, as these have been associated with an increased mortality despite apparent *in vitro* susceptibility.

TABLE 71-2 Oral Treatment of Melioidosis

Oral drug	Dose
Doxycycline +	2 mg/kg/day 12-hourly
Trimethoprim-sulfamethoxazole	<40 kg: 5/25 mg/kg 12-hourly 40–60 kg: 240/1200 mg 12-hourly >60 kg: 320/1600 mg 12-hourly
Amoxicillin-clavulanate*	20 mg/5mg/kg: 8-hourly

The treatment of choice in adults is doxycycline plus trimethoprim-sulphamethoxazole.
*Children younger than 8 years old and pregnant women should be given amoxicillin-clavulanate. The usual total duration of treatment is 20 weeks.

resolution is 9 days. Patients with large abscesses or empyema may have high swinging fevers for more than 1 month. Inexperienced physicians commonly switch antibiotic treatment prematurely, fearing that the persistent fever reflects the emergence of drug resistance. This is rare; resistance develops to the ß-lactam antibiotic in less than 1% of treated cases. High-dose parenteral treatment should be given for a minimum of 10 days in systemic infections and the switch to oral treatment only made when there is clear evidence of clinical improvement. Enlargement of an abscess or appearance of new abscesses, particularly in skeletal muscle, or seeding to a joint, is not uncommon in the first week of treatment and it is not necessarily a sign of treatment failure. Blood cultures are usually negative by the end of the first week, whereas infected sputum or draining abscesses can remain culture-positive for 1 month in infections that are responding to treatment.

Oral treatment is with a three-drug combination of doxycycline, trimethoprim, and sulfamethoxazole continued for a full 20 weeks of treatment (see Table 71-2). Whether this regimen can be simplified to trimethoprim-sulfamethoxazole alone is currently being studied. In pregnant women or children, high-dose amoxicillin-clavulanate acid may be given as an alternative. Despite this protracted course, the recurrence rate is approximately 10%, which rises to nearly 30% if 8 weeks of antibiotic treatment or less is given. In Thailand, the median time to recurrence is 21 weeks. Two-thirds of recurrences are relapses and a third are re-infections. The prognosis of melioidosis is better in children and relapse is rare. Adult patients require life-long follow-up. The optimum duration of maintenance treatment for suppurative parotitis has not been determined but, in general, 8 weeks of treatment are sufficient. These patients do not relapse and the overall prognosis is good.

REFERENCES

1. Whitmore A, Krishnaswami CS. An account of the discovery of a hitherto undescribed infective disease occurring among the population of Rangoon. Ind Med Gaz 1912;47:262–7.
2. Dance DAB. Melioidosis: the tip of the iceberg? Clin Micro Rev 1991;4:52–60.
3. Chaowagul W, White NJ, Dance DA, et al. Melioidosis: a major cause of community-acquired septicemia in northeastern Thailand. J Infect Dis 1989;159:890–9.
4. Cheng AC, Currie BJ. Melioidosis: epidemiology, pathophysiology, and management. Clin Microbiol Rev 2005;18:383–416.
5. White NJ. Melioidosis. Lancet 2003;361:1715–22.
6. Wiersinga WJ, van der Poll T, White NJ, et al. Melioidosis: insights into the pathogenicity of *Burkholderia pseudomallei*. Nat Rev Microbiol 2006;4: 272–82.
7. Walsh AL, Wuthiekanun V. The laboratory diagnosis of melioidosis. Br J Biomed Sci 1996;53:249–53.

72 Plague

Michel Drancourt

Key features

- Plague is a deadly zoonosis caused by the bacterium *Yersinia pestis*
- Historically, the rat flea has been a prime vector for causing human plague
- Human plague most commonly manifests as febrile lymphadenitis (bubonic plague). Primary pneumonic, septicemic and ingestional plague also occur
- Untreated bubonic plague evolves toward septicemic plague and pneumonic plague with death occurring in less than seven days
- Plague has had a huge impact on humanity and resulted in the death of one third of the population of Western Europe in the Middle Ages
- The current global plague pandemic is now over a century old, and involves cases in Asia, Africa and America
- Diagnosis usually rests on clinical suspicion, antigen dipsticks and culture
- Treatment involves gentamicin, streptomicin, and/or doxycycline
- Prevention usually involves limiting human-rodent-zoonotic-ectoparasitic interactions

INTRODUCTION

Plague is a deadly zoonosis caused by *Yersinia pestis* [1], a bacterium first isolated in 1894 by Alexandre Yersin in Hong Kong at the outset of the most recent pandemic which is still ongoing [2]. Plague is a reportable and quarantinable disease covered by national and international health regulations. Plague has had a huge impact on humanity. It was probably the cause of the Justinian plague of the 6th century and was the cause of the Black Death plague in Europe in the Middle Ages that claimed one third of the population [3]. The current pandemic began in Asia in the end of the 19th century and now involves the Old and New World. *Yersinia pestis* genotyping indicates that ancient *Y. pestis* organisms belonged to the Orientalis biotype, suggesting that this biotype was responsible for all three historical pandemics and that it may have the unique capability to rapidly spread in human populations over large geographic areas [3].

EPIDEMIOLOGY

PLAGUE CYCLES

Yersinia pestis exists in a number of transmission cycles. Any of the five recognized biotypes can circulate in rodents, causing epozootics of limited geographic extension. Such epizooties can lead to sporadic human cases involving any of the five biotypes. Focal and limited human outbreaks can also occur with any of the five biotypes as a result of the exposure of humans in a limited period of time to infected animals, or because of limited direct or vector-borne inter-human transmission. In comparison, extensive and ongoing human outbreaks have been associated with the Orientalis biotype, including the current worldwide pandemic.

ANIMAL INFECTION

Yersinia pestis can persist in soil for several months; this attribute may contribute to the long-term persistence of plague foci and may be a primary source of infection for burrowing rodents [4]. More than 200 species of rodents can be infected by *Y. pestis*, with plague-resistant species being regarded as reservoirs for *Y. pestis* [1, 5]. Several ectoparasites, including ticks, have been found to be naturally infected with *Y. pestis*, but fleas are thought to be the vector of primary importance. One hundred and thirty-one species of fleas are the most common vectors of *Y. pestis* among rodents [1, 5]. Fleas are particularly effective at transmitting *Y. pestis*, as ingested *Y. pestis* bacteria express plasminogen activator Pla that leads to blockage of the flea proventriculus, facilitating both increased hunger and therefore attempted feeding of the flea, and contamination of regurgitated blood back into the bite site [1]. *Yersinia pestis* has evolved numerous mechanisms to suppress inflammatory responses in plague-resistant hosts, promoting high blood concentrations (up to 10^8 organisms/ml) and facilitating successful transmission via the small amount of blood ingested by a flea (10^{-4} ml).

Carnivores can be infected after ingestion of contaminated rodents, but dogs and canids are resistant to plague [6] (Fig. 72.1). The complex life cycle of *Y. pestis* involving soil, ectoparasites and mammals results in a variable prevalence of animal plague (enzoonosis) with sudden outbreaks of dying-off in plague-susceptible animals (epizoonoses).

HUMAN PLAGUE (FIG. 72.2)

Inoculation by an infectious flea bite can result in bubonic plague. Infectious fleas often leave dead rodents and will drink human blood if rodents are not available. Fleas must have a daily blood meal in order to survive—the risk of being bitten by infected fleas is especially high after large numbers of plague-infected rats have died [1].

Inoculation through skin lacerations may result in bubonic or septicemic plague after handling (typically skinning) of dead animals [6].

Inhalation of *Y. pestis* leads to primary pneumonic plague, and involves inhalation of large droplets after close contact (<1.5 meters) with infected cats or a patient coughing copious amounts of bloody sputum. The average number of secondary cases per primary inhalational case is 1.3 [7, 8].

Ingestion of *Y. pestis* has been observed after consumption of raw or poorly cooked contaminated food, with contaminated camel meat and liver being the most frequently reported source of food-borne transmission [6].

Human ectoparasitic transmission may be an under-appreciated route of human-to-human transmission that may have played a key

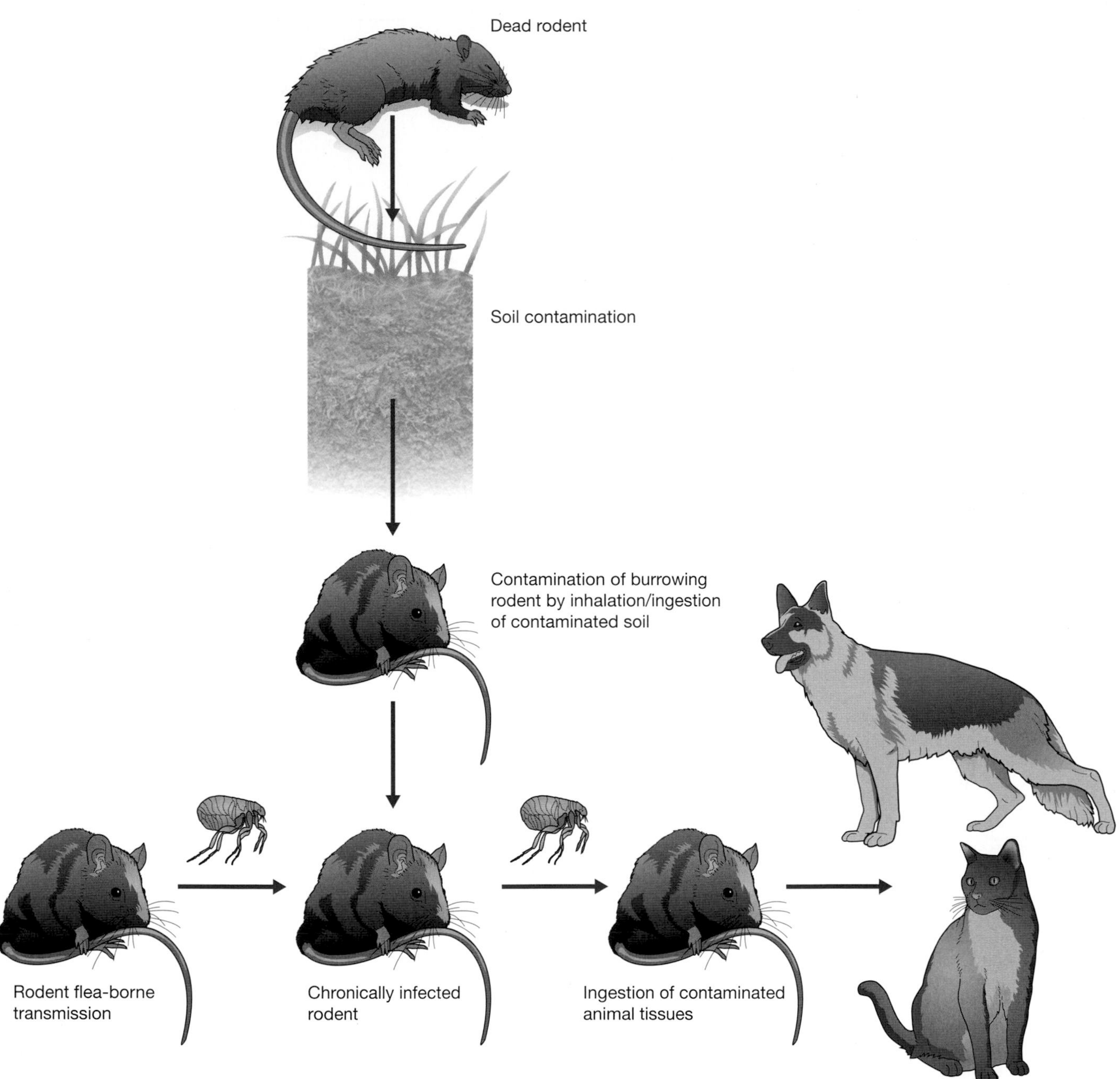

FIGURE 72.1 Reservoirs and transmission of animal plague.

role during historical epidemics [9]. Transmission by the anthropophilic flea *Pulex irritans* and by the human body-louse *Pediculus humanus* has been suggested during familial cases of plague [10], the latter being supported by experimental evidence [11].

GEOGRAPHIC DISTRIBUTION OF HUMAN PLAGUE

A soil reservoir and the relative resistance of various rodent species may explain why plague regularly re-emerges in long-lasting plague foci in all continents except Antartica and Oceania (Fig. 72.3). During the last 15 years, at least 8 geographic areas have experienced outbreaks of human plague after silent periods of 30–50 years: India in 1994, Zambia in 1996, Indonesia in 1997, Algeria in 2003 and 2009, Congo in 2005, Uganda in 2006, and Lybia and China in 2009. The World Health Organization (WHO) 2009 update indicated that, in 2007, 966 cases were reported in the Congo, 700 in Zambia, 591 in Madagascar, 257 in Uganda, 59 in Tanzania, 7 in the USA, and one in Mongolia [12] (Fig. 72.3). Plague can therefore be considered a re-emerging disease, mainly contracted during outdoor professional and recreational activities, contrary to what had been observed during the large historic urban outbreaks of the preceding centuries. In the USA, it has been shown that activities with close extended contacts with pet dogs (such as sleeping in the same bed as a pet dog) were significantly associated with plague [13]. In Europe, no human cases have been recently reported, but animal plague is still present along the western banks of the Caspian Sea. In all geographic areas, a seasonal pattern of human plague is observed, although the seasonal pattern is different from one geographic area to another, even within the same country [6].

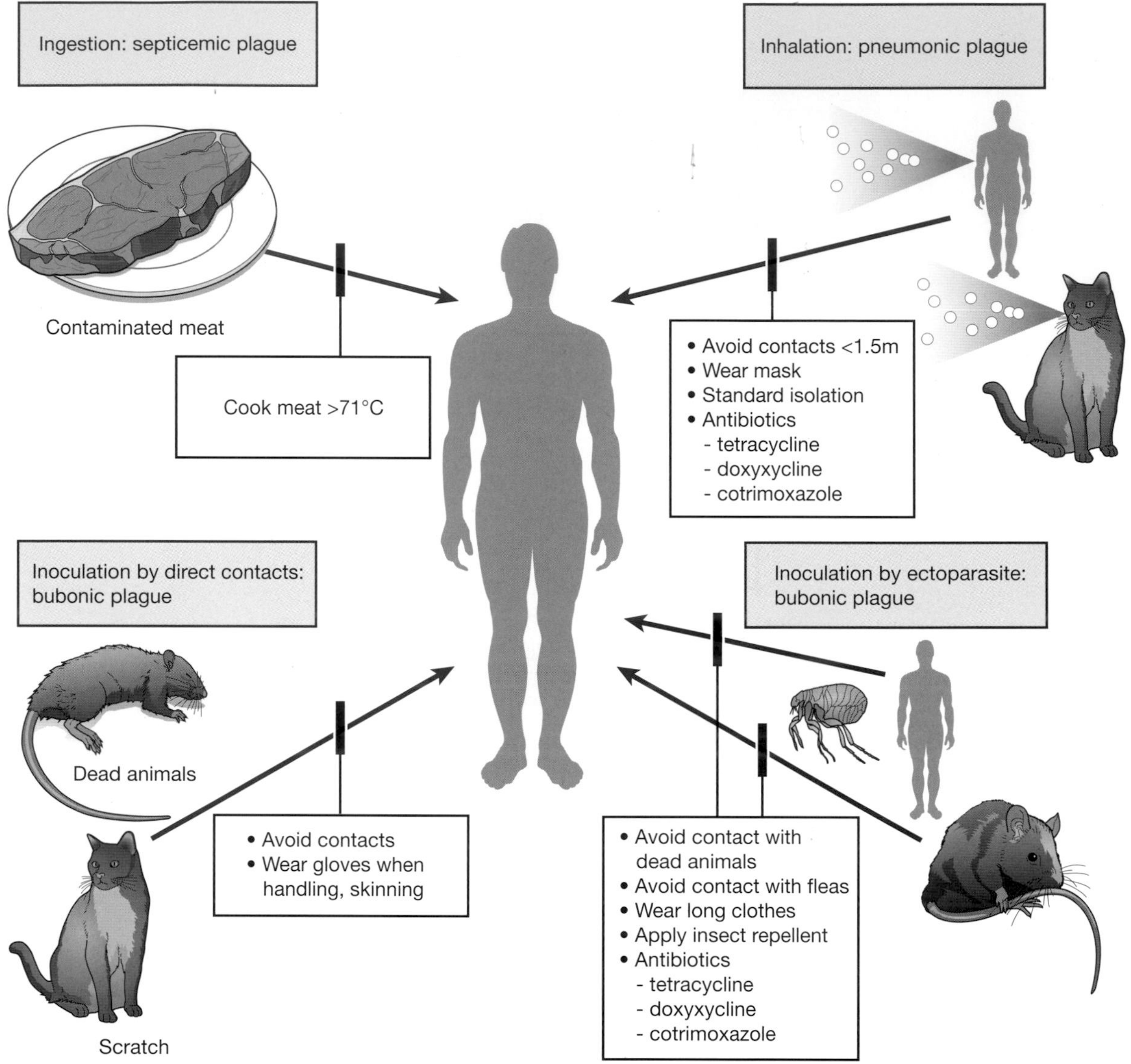

FIGURE 72.2 The sources and prevention of human plague.

NATURAL HISTORY, PATHOGENESIS AND PATHOLOGY

YERSINIA PESTIS

The gamma-proteobacteria *Y. pestis* (genome size, 4.60–4.65 Mb) may have emerged 20,000 years ago by reductive evolution from *Yersinia pseudotuberculosis* (genome size, 4.72 Mb) [14]. Genome sequencing has identified numerous insertion sequences, evidence of intragenomic recombination and lateral gene transfer, and remnants suggestive of a previous enteric lifecycle. A 70–75-kb plasmid common to all pathogenic *Yersinia* species (termed pCD1, pCad, pVW, pYV or pLcr plasmid) encodes a type III secretion system (Yops for "*Yersinia* Outer Proteins") and V antigen. A 100–110-kb plasmid (termed pFra/Tox, pFra, pTox, pMT1 or pYT plasmid) encodes the capsular F1 glycoprotein antigen and the *Yersinia* murine toxin Ymt. A 9.5-kb plasmid (termed pPst, pPla, pPCP1 or pYP plasmid) encodes the plasminogen activator Pla (which is thought to promote the systemic spread of *Y. pestis* from peripheral sites) and pesticin, a bacteriocine involved in iron capture in mammalian hosts [1]. Not all field isolates harbor the three plasmids, which are unstable during laboratory culture; new plasmids have been characterized, unsurprisingly illustrating the plasticity and ongoing evolution of *Y. pestis* [5]. Other virulence factors encoded on the chromosome are associated with the lipopolysaccharide endotoxin and with iron uptake—giving the pigmentation of colonies grown on Congo red medium. *Yersinia pestis* is a non-sporulated, aerobic, Gram-negative, oxidase-negative, urease-negative, catalase-positive bacillus growing slowly at 28°C, pH 7.4. Biochemical profiling distinguishes nine biovars which have been proposed as subspecies, including *Y. pestis* subsp. *pestis* and additional subspecies *angola, altaica, caucasica, hissarica, quinghaiensis, talassica, ulegeica* and *xilingolensis*, organisms of unknown pathogenicity isolated from various rodent species in Angola (subspecies *angola*) and Central Asia [5]. *Yersinia pestis* subsp. *pestis* organisms biotype Antiqua are glycerol and nitrate reduction-positive, Medievalis are glycerol-positive and nitrate reduction-negative, and Orientalis are glycerol-negative and nitrate reduction-positive. Microtus biotype organisms have been proposed to include rhamnose-positive rodent strains, while rhamnose-positive, Antiqua-like isolates occasionally isolated from patients in China could form a fifth biotype: Intermedium [15]. *Yersinia pestis* subsp. *pestis* Orientalis isolates are unique in their capacity to stabilize a bacteriophage contributing to the pathogenicity in their chromosome [16].

PATHOGENESIS

In humans, the ectoparasite's bite results in discrete local inflammation and spreading by the lymphatic route towards the regional

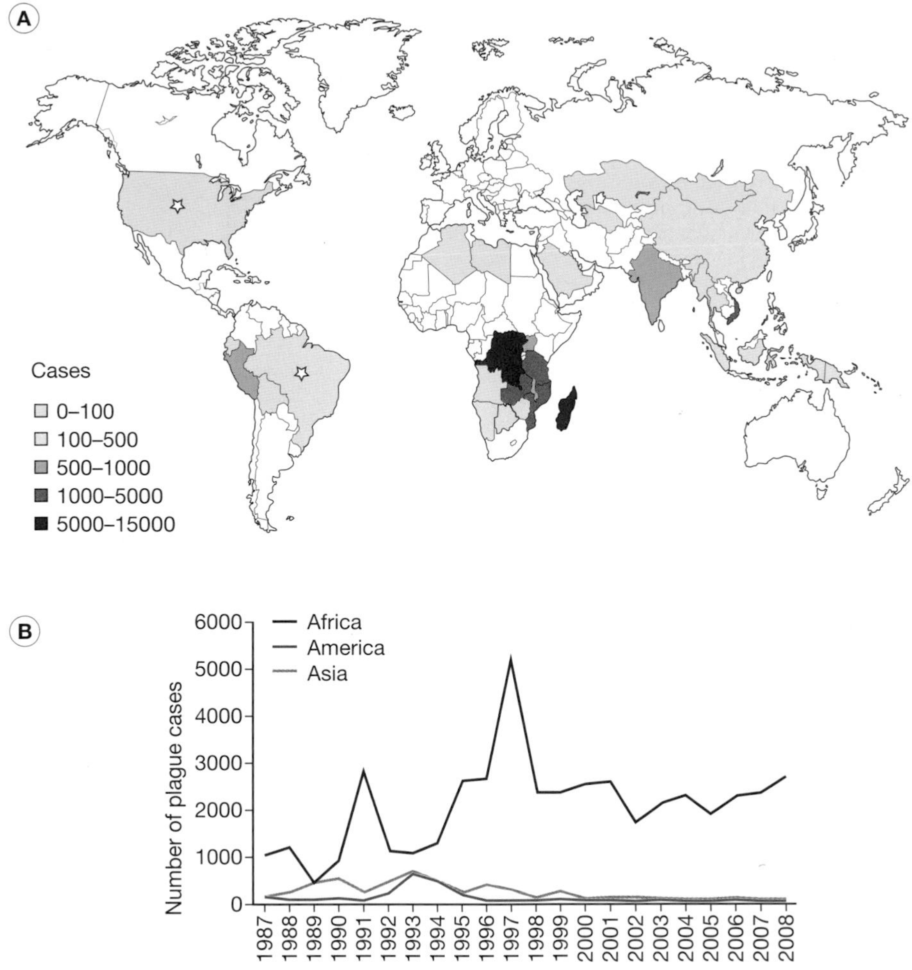

FIGURE 72.3 (A) The global distribution of plague 1994–2009, featuring the countries with known presence of plague in animal reservoirs and the countries where human plague has been either published or declared to the WHO (*, sporadic cases). Countries with human plague cases prior to 1994 are not listed. Compiled from the WHO and MedLine databases. **(B)** Annual regional incidence of human plague 1987–2008.

lymph node. Overwhelming bacterial growth in the node results in the so-called "bubo" and *Y. pestis* further disseminates via the lymphatic and blood vessels to the spleen and liver and can cause a rapidly fatal septicemia, with dissemination in the lung resulting in secondary pneumonic plague, and in the meninges and cerebrospinal fluid (CSF), causing meningitis. Hematogenous dissemination of the bacteria to other organs and tissues may cause intravascular coagulation and endotoxic shock. During this process, *Y. pestis* rapidly multiplies in human tissues because it protects itself from the human immune system by serum resistance and evasion from innate immune functions. *Yersinia pestis* is a facultative intracellular bacterium that multiples within macrophages [15].

CLINICAL FEATURES OF PLAGUE

People of all ages and both genders are susceptible to plague, although recently, most cases have been reported in children with a small predominance for males over the last decade [6]. It remains controversial whether the CCR5Delta32 mutation, the one which confers resistance to HIV infection, also confers resistance to plague [17].

Bubonic plague is the most frequent clinical form of plague, developing 2–10 days after inoculation of *Y. pestis* [6]. It features chills, fever, myalgias, arthralgias, weakness and a painful, tender, swollen, enlarged lymph node referred to as a "bubo" draining the site of inoculation (Fig. 72.4). The femoral and inguinal nodes are most

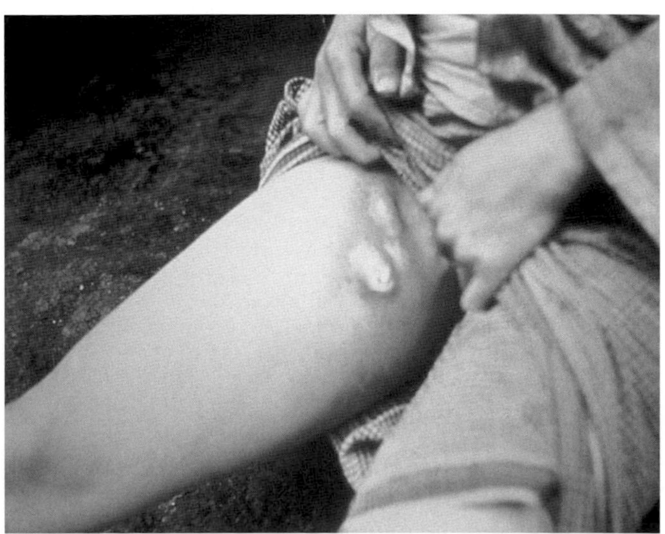

FIGURE 72.4 Patient with right inguinal and femoral buboes.

frequently involved (bubo is Greek for "groin"), followed in frequency by axillary and cervical nodes. Careful examination may reveal local skin inflammation at the site of the ectoparasite's bite with a papule, pustule, scab or ulcer. The bubo of plague is clinically distinguishable from enlarged lymph nodes owing to other causes by its association with systemic signs of toxemia and its rapid onset. Moreover, plague is the only cause of clustered cases of febrile, enlarged lymph nodes, leading to its unambiguous diagnosis in this situation. Bubonic plague usually rapidly responds to appropriate antibiotic therapy with the lymph node remaining enlarged and tender for one week. If untreated with an effective antibiotic, the patient will become increasingly toxic and will develop a septicemic form of plague, with a mortality risk of 50–90%.

Septicemic plague is usually secondary to the bubonic form and features a rapidly progressive, overwhelming toxemia. The patient may present with gastrointestinal symptoms including nausea, vomiting, diarrhea and abdominal pain which may confuse the diagnosis. In the absence of rapid supportive therapy combined with effective antibiotic treatment, septicemic plague is fulminate and fatal.

Pneumonic plague is the most rapidly fatal form; the incubation period for primary pneumonic plague is 1–3 days after contact with a coughing patient. Onset is sudden, with chills, fever, chest pain, cough, dyspnea and hemoptysis. Case fatality rates exceed 40% within three days despite treatment. Pneumonic plague has been responsible for limited outbreaks lasting a few weeks.

Other clinical forms include meningeal plague, an unusual form following insufficiently treated bubonic plague. Pharyngitis is a rare form diagnosed in patients who consumed raw or poorly cooked contaminated meat, such as camel meat, and features anterior cervical lymphadenitis. Pleuritis, endophthalmitis and myocarditis are exceptional forms of plague.

PATIENT EVALUATION, DIAGNOSIS AND DIFFERENTIAL DIAGNOSIS

Plague should be considered in any patient returning from, or living in, a country with active plague epizoonoses who presents with febrile adenitis. In this circumstance, it is useful to rapidly collect whole blood in three successive blood culture bottles, as well as sputum, urine and lymph node fluid. Lymph node fluid can be sterilely obtained using saline for aspiration [6]. More rarely, CSF could be collected if clinically indicated. Additional environmental specimens may include any ectoparasite found on the patient's body and clothes, as well as specimens from any animal suspected to be a potential source of infection. Clinical and environmental specimens should be handled in a Biosafety Level (BSL)-2 laboratory, but handling and culture of *Y. pestis* requires a BSL3 laboratory. Plague is usually a reportable and quarantinable disease covered by national and international health regulations.

Point-of-care diagnosis usually involves using a commercially-available dipstick immunochromatographic assay detecting the F1 capsular antigen [18]. This dipstick assay has been applied to urine, whole blood, bubo pus and sputum. It takes a few minutes and exhibits a 98.4% specificity and 90.1% sensitivity for serum, and 100% for bubo fluid. Direct microscopic examination of clinical specimens after Gram staining is another technique for the rapid diagnosis of plague, and involves detection of Gram-negative bacilli exhibiting a characteristic bipolar staining with a "hairpin appearance" (Fig. 72.5). PCR-based assays are also available [19].

Isolation and culture of *Y. pestis* is performed by incubating cultures at 32°C under a 5% CO_2 atmosphere for 1–4 days. Because slow growth is observed on MacConkey agar, other selective media, including the cefsulodin-Irgasan-novobiocin (CIN) and beef heart-Irgasan-novobiocin (BIN) agar have been developed [20]. The identification of *Y. pestis* can be achieved rapidly using immunochromatographic detection of the F1 antigen on colonies [21]. Rapid identification using peptidic profiling by mass spectrometry

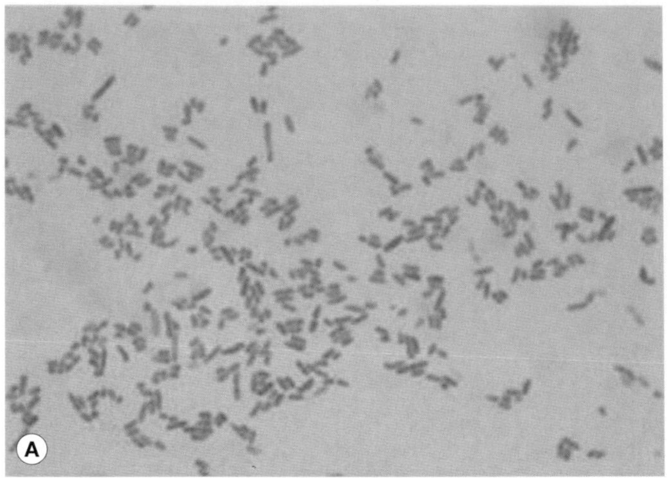

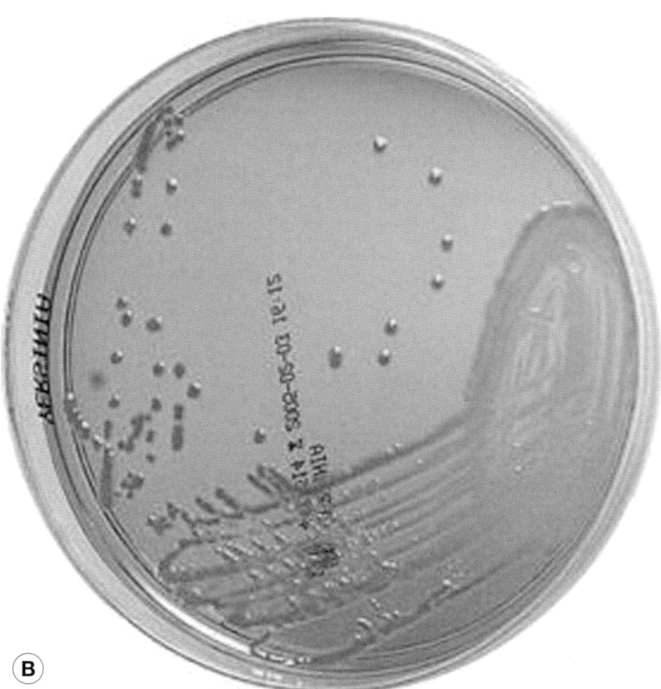

FIGURE 72.5 *Yersinia pestis*: Gram-staining appearance **(A)** and colonies grown on blood-agar **(B)**.

is also effective (M. Drancourt and D. Raoult, personal communication).

Antibiotic susceptibility testing should be performed as a few antibiotic-resistant strains have emerged in Madagascar [22]. One strain was resistant to eight antimicrobial agents, including those recommended for therapy (streptomycin, chloramphenicol and tetracycline) and prophylaxis (sulfonamide and tetracycline), as well as ampicillin, kanamycin and spectinomycin. A second strain was only resistant to streptomycin. In these strains, all of the resistance genes were carried by conjugative plasmids of approximately 150 kb and 40 kb respectively [22]. Horizontal gene transfer in the flea may be the source of antibiotic-resistant *Y. pestis* strains isolated from plague patients in Madagascar [22]. Ampicillin and tetracycline-resistant isolates have been identified in fleas and rats in Madagascar [22], whereas the 150-kd plasmid backbone was shown to be broadly disseminated among multidrug-resistant zoonotic pathogens associated with agriculture [23]. Experimental data indicate that *Y. pestis* strains resistant to fluoroquinolones could be easily selected in the laboratory, but such strains have not been found in the clinical setting.

TABLE 72-1 Antibiotic Treatment of Plague (Evidence Category: 1 = double blind study; 2 = clinical trial >20 subjects; 3 = clinical trial <20 subjects; 4 = series; 5 = anecdotal case reports)

Drug	Regimen: adults	Regimen: children	Duration (days)	Evidence
Doxycyline	100 mg orally twice a day	100 mg per os twice a day	7	2
Gentamicin	2.5 mg/kg IM twice a day	2.2 mg/kg per os twice a day	7	2
Tetracycline	1 g orally, 4 times daily	–	10	4
Streptomycin	15 mg/kg IM twice a day	as adult regimen	10	4
Trimethoprim-sulfamethoxazole	160/800 mg twice a day	as adult regimen	7–10	3, 4
Chloramphenicol	25 mg/kg IV loading dose; 15 mg/kg 4 times daily	as adult regimen	7–10	5
Ciprofloxacin	15 mg/kg 4 times daily	–	7–10	5

IM, intramuscularly; IV, intravenously.

Typing of *Y. pestis* is done by testing nitrate reduction, glycerol assimilation and rhamnose assimilation to determine biotype [15]; molecular typing can be done by single nucleotide polymorphism analysis, regions of deletion analysis, clustered regularly interspaced short palindromic repeats analysis, multiple loci variable number of tandem repeats (VNTR) analysis [15], multilocus sequence typing, restriction fragment length polymorphism (RFLP) analysis and multispacer sequence typing analysis [3]. VNTR analysis has proved useful in identifying sources of human exposure [24].

Serology using modern techniques is useful to measure seroprevalence in sentinel animals and could be used for the rapid diagnosis of patients for whom serum is the only available specimen, during outbreaks [25].

TREATMENT

Rapid administration of an effective antibiotic to patients with suspected plague is mandatory. Streptomycin, the historical reference antibiotic still used in Madagascar, is no longer available in most countries. Gentamicin alone, or in combination with a tetracycline, is an acceptable substitute [26] (Table 72.1). Gentamicin and doxycycline were shown to be equivalent in curing patients, except in terminal stage disease [27]. Fluoroquinolones, as well as cephalosporins, are effective in animal models, yet they are not recommended as, with the exception of a single reported case of plague successfully treated with ciprofloxacin [6], there are no clinical data addressing their efficacy. Antibiotic treatment should be continued for 10 days. Improvement is clinically evident 2–3 days after initiation of antibiotics, although fever may persist for a few more days.

Supportive therapy should be undertaken in case of septic shock and septicemic plague.

PREVENTION AND CONTROL

Before exposure to *Y. pestis*, primary prevention relies on: avoiding areas with known epizootic plague; avoiding apparently sick and dead animals; reporting such animals to the health department and avoiding exposure to rats and fleas from diseased rats or other rodents, including use of protective clothes and repellents to avoid exposure to ectoparasites when outdoors; applying insect repellent containing N,N-Diethyl-meta-toluamide (DEET) to legs and ankles; applying repellents and insecticides to clothes and outer bedding; using gloves for the manipulation of dead animals and carcasses, and cooking meat on an open-flame grill or on a clam-shell type electric grill [28].

Vaccines (live attenuated *Y. pestis* EV76 strain; formalin-inactivated, whole-cell plague; heat-killed whole-cell plague; F1 fraction) can be administrated by aerosol (EV76), subcutaneously (EV76; heat-killed CSL vaccine; CSL Ltd, Victoria, Australia) or intramuscularly (formalin-inactivated Greer vaccine; Greer Laboratories Inc., NC, USA) [29]. The F1 fraction vaccine appears to have low efficacy (<60%) and side effects in 35% of vaccines. There is not enough evidence to evaluate the effectiveness of any plague vaccine or the relative effectiveness between vaccines and their tolerability. Circumstantial data from observational studies suggest that killed vaccines may be more effective against bubonic plague and have fewer adverse effects than attenuated vaccines. No evidence is available regarding the long-term effects of any plague vaccine and their role in controlling plague outbreaks [29].

In the case of potential exposure to *Y. pestis*, secondary prevention relies on the administration of tetracycline or trimethoprim-sulfamethoxazole to people who are bitten by fleas during a local outbreak or who are exposed to tissues or fluids from a plague-infected animal, people living in a household with a bubonic plague patient (as they may also be exposed to infected fleas), and people in close contact with a person or pet with suspected pneumonic plague [26]. Recent evaluation indicates that doxycycline should be considered as a first-line antibiotic in the management of bioterrorism agents, including *Y. pestis* [30]. For a mass casualty situation, oral therapy with doxycycline, tetracycline or ciprofloxacin has been recommended [2], the latter option being supported by animal models. Prevention of human-to-human transmission from patients with pneumonic plague can be achieved by implementing standard isolation procedures until at least four days after the initiation of antibiotic treatment.

Control of plague is based on active surveillance of sentinel animals. In areas with epizootic outbreaks, it is mandatory to eliminate food and shelter for rodents around homes, work places, and certain recreational areas, such as picnic sites or campgrounds where people congregate. Remove brush, rock piles, junk and food sources, including pet food. Treat pets (cats and dogs) for flea control regularly. Likewise, the control of a human plague outbreak mainly relies on the rapid confirmation of the diagnosis and treatment of confirmed and suspected cases. Killing any human ectoparasite is mandatory during plague outbreak, as well as killing animal fleas using appropriate and licensed insecticides.

REFERENCES

1. Perry RD, Fetherston JD. *Yersinia pestis*—etiologic agent of plague. Clin Microbiol Rev 1997;10:35–66.
2. Inglesby TV, Dennis DT, Henderson DA, et al. Plague as a biological weapon: medical and public health management. Working Group on Civilian Biodefense. JAMA 2000;283:2281–90.
3. Drancourt M, Roux V, Dang LV, et al. Genotyping, Orientalis-like *Yersinia pestis*, and plague pandemics. Emerg Infect Dis 2004;10:1585–92.
4. Mollaret HH, Karimi Y, Eftekhari M, Baltazard M. Burrowing plague. Bull Soc Pathol Exot Filiales 1963;56:1186–93.
5. Anisimov AP, Lindler LE, Pier GB. Intraspecific diversity of *Yersinia pestis*. Clin Microbiol Rev 2004;17:434–64.
6. Butler T. Plague into the 21st century. Clin Infect Dis 2009;49:736–42.
7. Kool JL. Risk of person-to-person transmission of pneumonic plague. Clin Infect Dis 2005;40:1166–72.
8. Gani R, Leach S. Epidemiologic determinants for modeling pneumonic plague outbreaks. Emerg Infect Dis 2004;10:608–14.
9. Drancourt M, Houhamdi L, Raoult D. *Yersinia pestis* as a telluric, human ectoparasite-borne organism. Lancet Infect Dis 2006;6:234–41.
10. Blanc G, Baltazard M. Rôle des ectoparasites humains dans la transmission de la peste. Bull Acad Med 1942;125:446–8 [in French].
11. Ayyadurai S, Sebbane F, Raoult D, Drancourt M. Body lice, *Yersinia pestis* orientalis, and black death. Emerg Infect Dis 2010;16(5):892–3.
12. World Health Organization. World Health Statistics 2009. Geneva: World Health Organization; 2009:61–9.
13. Gould LH, Pape J, Ettestad P, et al. Dog-associated risk factors for human plague. Zoonoses Public Health 2008;55:448–54.
14. Achtman M, Zurth K, Morelli G, et al. *Yersinia pestis*, the cause of plague, is a recently emerged clone of *Yersinia* pseudotuberculosis. Proc Natl Acad Sci USA 1999;96:14043–8.
15. Li Y, Cui Y, Hauck Y, et al. Genotyping and phylogenetic analysis of *Yersinia pestis* by MLVA: insights into the worldwide expansion of Central Asia plague foci. PLoS One 2009;4:e6000.
16. Derbise A, Chenal-Francisque V, Pouillot F, et al. A horizontally acquired filamentous phage contributes to the pathogenicity of the plague bacillus. Mol Microbiol 2007;63:1145–57.
17. Sabeti PC, Walsh E, Schaffer SF, et al. The case for selection at CCR5-Delta 32. PLoS Biol 2005;3:e378.
18. Chanteau S, Rahalison L, Ralafiarisoa L, et al. Development and testing of a rapid diagnostic test for bubonic and pneumonic plague. Lancet 2003;361: 211–16.
19. Stewart A, Satterfield B, Cohen M, et al. A quadruplex real-time PCR assay for the detection of *Yersinia pestis* and its plasmids. J Med Microbiol 2008;57: 324–31.
20. Ber R, Mamroud E, Aftalion M, et al. Development of an improved selective agar medium for isolation of *Yersinia pestis*. Appl Environ Microbiol 2003;69:5787–92.
21. Tomaso H, Thullier P, Seibold E, et al. Comparison of hand-held test kits, immunofluorescence microscopy, enzyme-linked immunosorbent assay, and flow cytometric analysis for rapid presumptive identification of *Yersinia pestis*. J Clin Microbiol 2007;45:3404–7.
22. Galimand M, Carniel E, Courvalin P. Resistance of *Yersinia pestis* to antimicrobial agents. Antimicrob Agents Chemother 2006;50:3233–6.
23. Welch TJ, Fricke WF, McDermott PF, et al. Multiple antimicrobial resistance in plague: an emerging public health risk. PLoS One 2007;2:e309.
24. Lowell JL, Wagner DM, Atshabar B, et al. Identifying sources of human exposure to plague. J Clin Microbiol 2005;43:650–6.
25. Rajerison M, Dartevelle S, Ralafiarisoa LA, et al. Development and evaluation of two simple, rapid immunochromatographic tests for the detection of *Yersinia pestis* antibodies in humans and reservoirs. PLoS Negl Trop Dis 2009;3:e421.
26. Boulanger LL, Ettestad P, Fogarty JD, et al. Gentamicin and tetracyclines for the treatment of human plague: review of 75 cases in New Mexico, 1985–1999. Clin Infect Dis 2004;38:663–9.
27. Mwengee W, Butler T, Mgema S, et al. Treatment of plague with gentamicin or doxycycline in a randomized clinical trial in Tanzania. Clin Infect Dis 2006;42:614–21.
28. Porto-Fett AC, Juneja VK, Tamplin ML, Luchansky JB. Validation of cooking times and temperatures for thermal inactivation of *Yersinia pestis* strains KIM5 and CDC-A1122 in irradiated ground beef. J Food Prot 2009;72: 564–71.
29. Jefferson T, Demicheli V, Pratt M. Vaccines for preventing plague. Cochrane Database System Rev 1998; CD000976.
30. Brouillard JE, Terriff CM, Tofan A, Garrison MW. Antibiotic selection and resistance issues with fluoroquinolones and doxycycline against bioterrorism agents. Pharmacotherapy 2006;26:3–14.

Tularemia 73

Max Maurin

Key features

- Tularemia is a rare zoonosis caused by the Gram-negative bacterium *Francisella tularensis*, including subspecies *tularensis* (type A) and subsp. *holarctica* (type B)
- The disease is restricted to the northern hemisphere and the more virulent type A strains are mainly found in North America
- A wide spectrum of animal species are susceptible to *F. tularensis* infection, but lagomorphs and small rodents are responsible for most human infections. Humans become infected through direct contact with infected animals, through the bite of an arthropod, or after exposure to an infected environment
- Tularemia is often a systemic disease with potential spread of bacteria to the whole reticuloendothelial system as a result of the intracellular lifestyle of *F. tularensis*, which can multiply within phagocytic cells, such as macrophages
- Six main syndromes are recognized based on the bacteria's portal of entry: the ulceroglandular and glandular forms (skin); the oculoglandular form (conjunctival mucosa); the oropharyngeal and digestive form (digestive mucosa) the pneumonic form (respiratory mucosa); and the typhoidal form (severe systemic disease usually with undetermined portal of entry)
- Although usually benign, tularemia may evolve to be a chronic, disabling, and even fatal, disease. The high mortality rate of the pneumonic form of tularemia explains the potential use of *F. tularensis* for biological warfare and bioterrorism
- Patients with tularemia should be treated with fluoroquinolone or doxycycline, or gentamicin in severely diseased patients
- There is no commercially available vaccine available in the USA to prevent tularemia

INTRODUCTION

Francisella tularensis (initially named as *Bacterium tularense*), a fastidious, Gram-negative, facultative intracellular *Coccobacillus* was first isolated by McCoy and Chapin from ground squirrels in 1911 in Tulare County (California, USA) and then from a human case of tularemia in 1914 by Wherry and Lamb (Ohio, USA) [1]. The name of the bacterium emphasizes the contribution made by Edward Francis in the early 20th century to improving the knowledge of the medical, epidemiologic and diagnostic aspects of tularemia. Today's renewed medical interest in tularemia stems from the potential use of *F. tularensis* as a bioterrorism agent (Centers for Disease Control and Prevention [CDC] class A) [2]. Tularemia is currently a notifiable disease in many developed countries.

Tularemia is not normally found in the tropics or the southern hemisphere [3]. Two *F. tularensis* subspecies are responsible for human infections: subsp. *tularensis* (type A) mainly in North America, and subsp. *holarctica* (type B) throughout the northern hemisphere. Contact with infected animals, tick bites and exposure to contaminated environments are the usual mode of infection in humans. In endemic areas, farmers, hunters, trappers, veterinarians, forest workers, and recreational users of the forest are particularly at risk of acquiring tularemia. The disease is usually of mild severity, but it may be chronic, debilitating and occasionally fatal, especially when type A strains are involved. The spread of *F. tularensis*, whether intentional (bioterrorism) or not (e.g. importation of animals for hunting), in endemic or non-endemic areas is an ongoing public health threat.

EPIDEMIOLOGY

Tularemia is restricted to the northern hemisphere and predominates in North America, Russia, Scandinavia, and Japan (Fig. 73.1) [3]. However, the incidence and geographic distribution of human infections have recently increased, and unusual tularemia outbreaks have occurred in Bulgaria, Kosovo, and Turkey, but also Spain and probably northern Portugal [4, 5] – two previously non-endemic countries.

Both type A and, to a lesser extent, type B strains of *F. tularensis* cause human tularemia in North America. In the USA, most reported cases occur in mid-western states (Arkansas, Missouri, South Dakota, and Oklahoma) and in Massachusetts (particularly on Martha's Vineyard Island); cases have never been reported in Hawaii. Among type A strains, the genotype AI (or A-east) has been found in the mid-west, California, Maryland, and Massachusetts, whereas genotype AII (or A-west) has been reported in California, Nevada, Utah, and Wyoming [6]. Further genotypes have been recently described (A1a, A1b, A2a, and A2b) [7].

Only type B strains are responsible for human tularemia cases in Eurasia. In Europe, tularemia is now endemic in all countries except Iceland and the UK [8]. Classically, type B strains belong to biovar I (erythromycin-susceptible) in Western Europe and North America and to biovar II (erythromycin-resistant) in Eastern Europe and Asia. Type B strains found in Japan are genetically different and may be a new subspecies. *Francisella tularensis* subsp. *mediasiatica* has only been isolated in animals in central Asia. Recently, type A1 strains close to the American laboratory Schu4 strain have been isolated in arthropods and rodents in Slovakia and Austria.

Francisella tularensis can infect mammals, birds, amphibians, fishes, and invertebrate animals [9]. Lagomorphs (rabbits, hares) and small rodents (e.g. voles, mice, squirrels, muskrats, prairie dogs, and beavers) are considered major enzootic reservoirs of *F. tularensis*; domestic animals and pets (cats, hamsters) are occasionally infected. Many arthropods may serve as vectors for transmission of *F. tularensis* to

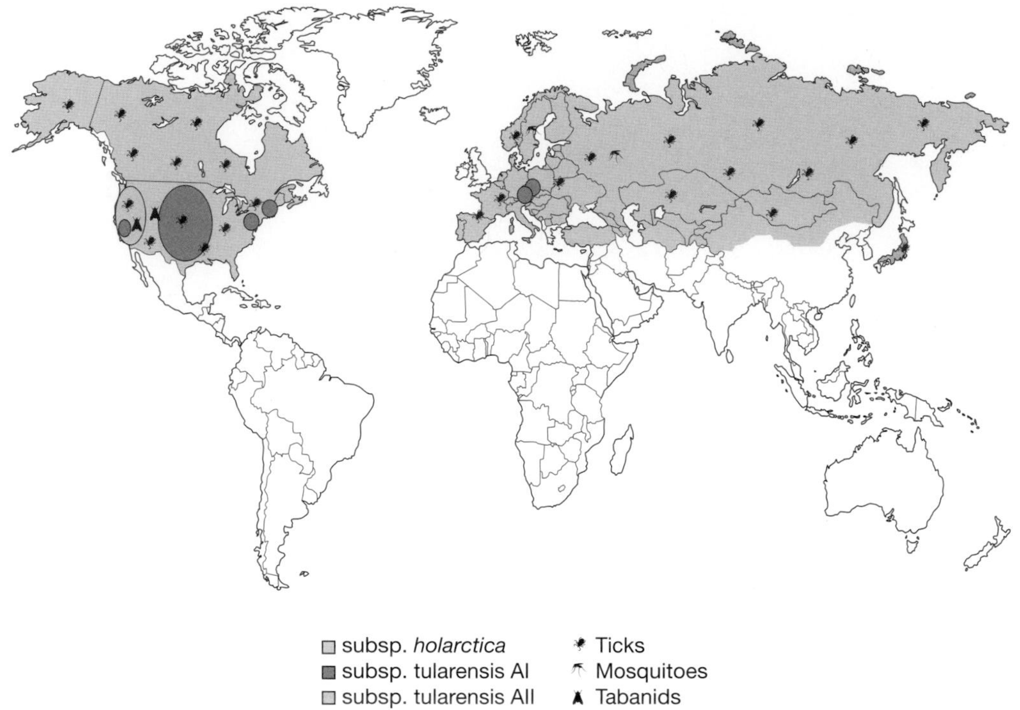

FIGURE 73.1 Geographic distribution of the *Francisella tularensis* subspecies and the main arthropod vectors.

TABLE 73-1 Epidemiologic and Clinical Aspects of Tularemia

Reservoir	Geographic distribution	Professionally or occupationally exposed persons	Modes of transmission	Most common tularemia forms
Lagomorphs, rodents, other wild and domestic animals	Entire northern hemisphere	Hunters and their households, farmers, trappers, veterinarians	Direct contact with live or dead animals, animal bites	Ulceroglandular, glandular, oculoglandular, oropharyngeal
			Ingestion	Oropharyngeal and digestive, typhoidal
			Inhalation of infected fomites	Pneumonic
Ticks*	Entire northern hemisphere	Persons walking in tick-infested areas	Tick bites, tick-crushing	Ulceroglandular, glandular, oculoglandular, typhoidal
Mosquitoes	Scandinavia	Persons walking near lakes and streams	Mosquito bites	Ulceroglandular, glandular
Tabanids	Western USA	Outdoor activities in rural areas	Tabanid bites	Ulceroglandular, glandular
Contaminated environment (water, mud, dust, grass)	Entire northern hemisphere	Water sports, landscapers	Swimming, bathing, canyoning, etc. in infected spring water	Ulceroglandular, glandular, oculoglandular, oropharyngeal
			Ingestion of contaminated water	Oropharyngeal and digestive, typhoidal
			Inhalation of infected dust, lawn mowing, brush cutting	Pneumonic

*Including *Ixodes ricinus, Ixodes persulcatus, Dermacentor reticulatus, Dermacentor marginatus, Rhipicephalus rossicus*, and *Haemaphisalis concinna* in Eurasia; *Amblyomma americanum* (Lone Star tick) in southeastern USA; *Dermacentor variabilis* (American dog tick) in eastern USA, California, and central and eastern Canada; *Dermacentor andersoni* (Rocky Mountain wood tick) in the western USA; *Haemaphisalis flava* and *Ixodes ovatus* in Japan.

animals and humans (Table 73-1). Ixodidae ticks are the primary vectors and a major reservoir of *F. tularensis* worldwide. Other potential vectors include mosquitoes (mainly in Scandinavia [10]) and tabanids (deer flies, i.e. *Chrysops* sp.) in the USA (particularly in Wyoming, Utah, Nevada, and California) [11]. *Francisella tularensis* can survive for months in humid and cold environments (e.g. water, mud), possibly in association with amebae.

Human contamination may occur directly after contact with an infected animal or animal carcass, by ingestion of contaminated water or food, by arthropod inoculation, or after contact with a contaminated environment (Table 73-1) [3]. Human-to-human transmission is considered unlikely. Farmers, hunters, trappers, meat handlers, veterinarians, animal care professionals, pet owners, and persons walking in tick-infested lands (prairies, forest, etc.) in endemic areas are considered most at risk of contracting tularemia. Arthropod-borne tularemia cases usually occur in spring, summer and early autumn during the main activity of these vectors and when persons are most exposed to their bites by wearing short clothes. In contrast, tularemia caused by direct contact with game animals usually occurs during the winter hunting season. Laboratory workers handling *F. tularensis* cultures are also at high risk of developing tularemia; laboratory staff should be notified when handling samples potentially containing *F. tularensis*. Such samples and subcultures should be handled in biosafety cabinets-hoods to minimize aerosol-based exposure.

NATURAL HISTORY, PATHOGENESIS, AND PATHOLOGY

Human inoculation with *F. tularensis* can occur through the skin, the conjunctiva, and the digestive or respiratory mucosa [12]. Local infection may lead to a cutaneous ulcer, conjunctivitis, pharyngitis, enteritis, or pneumonia. Bacteria rapidly invade the regional lymph nodes, draining the territory of the skin or mucosa lesions. Enlarged lymph nodes may develop at various sites: epitrochlear, subclavicular, axillary, cervical, pretragal, mesenteric, inguinal, mediastinal, etc. A transient bacteremia often allows *F. tularensis* to spread throughout the body, infecting reticuloendothelial cells. In most patients, the immune response will control the disease. In about 20–30% of cases, the lymphadenopathy will evolve to chronic suppuration and necrosis. Less frequently, secondary localizations may supervene (e.g. meningitis, encephalitis, pneumonia, endocarditis, osteomyelitis), possibly leading to death. Whatever the portal of entry, a fulminant course of tularemia with persistent *F. tularensis* bacteremia, delirium and septic shock is referred to as the typhoidal form of tularemia.

Francisella tularensis virulence factors have been partially characterized, but the higher virulence of type A compared with type B strains remains unexplained [13]. *Francisella tularensis* is an intracellular pathogen that predominantly grows in macrophages, but probably also in neutrophils, dendritic cells, and non-professional phagocytic cells, such as alveolar epithelial cells, endothelial cells and hepatocytes. This bacterium harbors a pathogenicity island (FPI) that includes genes necessary for intramacrophage growth and virulence, such as the intracellular growth locus operon *iglABCD* and *pdp* genes (especially *pdpA*). Bacteria phagocytized by macrophages escape the phagocytic vacuole to the cell cytosol where they multiply. *Francisella tularensis* does not trigger a high pro-inflammatory host response because of a relatively inert lipopolysaccharide (LPS) and a probable direct inhibition of pro-inflammatory cytokine signaling pathways. Type IV pili appear essential for tissue adhesion and invasion, and a surface exopolysaccharide capsule protects bacteria from the killing action of serum complement during bacteremia.

A humoral response develops within 2 weeks following infection with *F. tularensis*, with antibodies primarily directed against the bacterial LPS, but also against outer membrane proteins (OmpA, FopA) and intracellular proteins (GroEL, KatG) [14]. These antibodies probably control *F. tularensis* bacteremia and extracellular multiplication. Mucosal antibody response (mainly of IgA type) may also partially protect vaccinated or previously infected persons from re-infection. Cell-mediated immunity (i.e. $CD4^+$ and $CD8^+$ T cells) is assumed to play a major role in controlling intracellular multiplication of *F. tularensis*.

Pathologic aspects of tularemia are not specific [15]. In chronically enlarged lymph nodes, histologic lesions may range from well-defined zones of acute inflammation and necrosis located within the outer cortex of lymph nodes, to generalized necrosis that can obliterate the node. Granulomatous inflammation may also be present. Caseous necrosis is usually absent. Post-mortem examination of tissues from patients dying of tularemia may reveal lesions resembling those of tuberculosis, particularly the presence of well-developed granulomas in lungs, liver, spleen, and lymph nodes. Necrotizing pneumonia with abundant fibrin, cellular debris, edema, and neutrophils within alveolar walls and alveolar spaces may also be observed. The use of specific monoclonal or polyclonal antibodies allows visualization of *F. tularensis* within infected tissues.

CLINICAL FEATURES

The incubation period of tularemia is typically 3–5 days, but may vary from a few hours to up to 2 weeks [1, 10]. Many patients have few symptoms and remain undiagnosed. More symptomatic patients usually seek medical attention several days or weeks after symptom onset. A minority of patients experience acute, severe, and even fulminant, disease (e.g. pneumonic or typhoidal form). Infected patients usually experience a sudden onset of flu-like symptoms including fever, chills, headaches, myalgias, and arthralgias. Coughing is frequent, and mild diarrhea is found in about 10% of patients. Relative bradycardia is a classically described but uncommon finding. About 20–40% of patients develop a generalized papular or maculopapular rash that may become vesicular or pustular. Erythema nodosum has also been reported, especially in women.

The spectrum of the clinical manifestations of tularemia is wide, but six clinical syndromes are classically recognized and may occasionally be combined [1, 10]: the ulceroglandular form; the glandular form; the oculoglandular form; the oropharyngeal and digestive form; the pneumonic form; and the typhoidal form. Another classification only differentiates ulceroglandular tularemia (the three former syndromes) from typhoidal tularemia (patients without skin or lymph-node involvement and with systemic symptoms) [16].

Approximately 75–90% of patients present with an ulceroglandular form, which combines a cutaneous lesion at the site of *F. tularensis* skin inoculation and a regional lymphadenopathy (Figs 73.2 and 73.3). The skin lesion first corresponds to a small papule that develops within a few days into a pustule and then a cutaneous eschar that is typically erythematous, indurated and nonhealing. In the much rarer glandular form (about 2% of cases), a cutaneous lesion has not developed or it has healed at the time of the first medical visit. In both forms, the patient usually consults when the lymph nodes become severely enlarged and tender. The lymphadenopathy may be epitrochlear, subclavicular, axillary, cervical or inguinal, and typically lasts for several weeks, and even months. It evolves to suppuration in about 20–30% of cases, sometimes with skin fistulization, especially when adapted antibiotic therapy has been delayed for more than 2 weeks. The progression of the lymphadenopathy is poorly influenced by antibiotic therapy and surgical treatment is often needed for cure after several weeks or months of progression. However, lymph node incision should not be performed in the early stage of the disease because of the frequent spread of infection to surrounding tissues. Although rarely fatal, the glandular and ulceroglandular forms may evolve to disseminated disease and secondary localizations (e.g. spleen, liver, lung or brain).

The oropharyngeal and digestive form of tularemia (the second most frequent form) usually occurs a few days after ingestion of

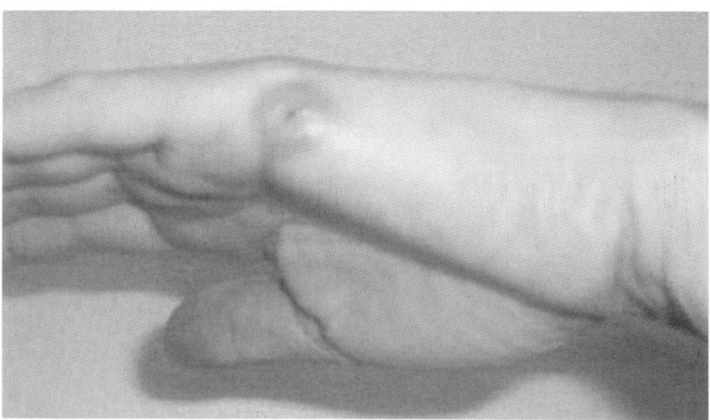

FIGURE 73.2 A tularemia skin eschar of the left hand after manipulation of a hare *(courtesy of Dr B. Castan).*

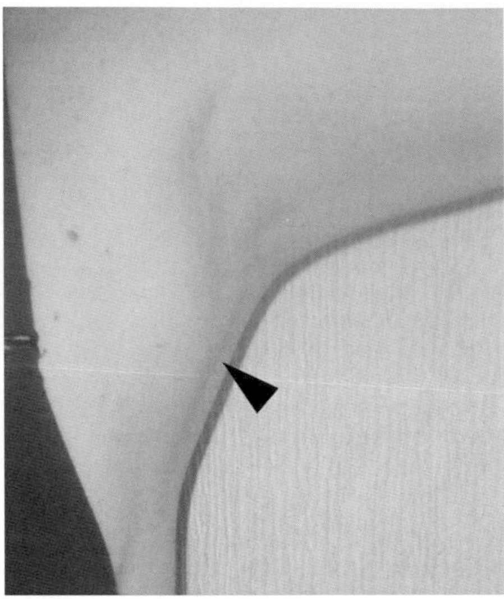

FIGURE 73.3 A left axillary lymphadenopathy in a woman with tularemia after skinning a hare *(courtesy of Dr B. Castan).*

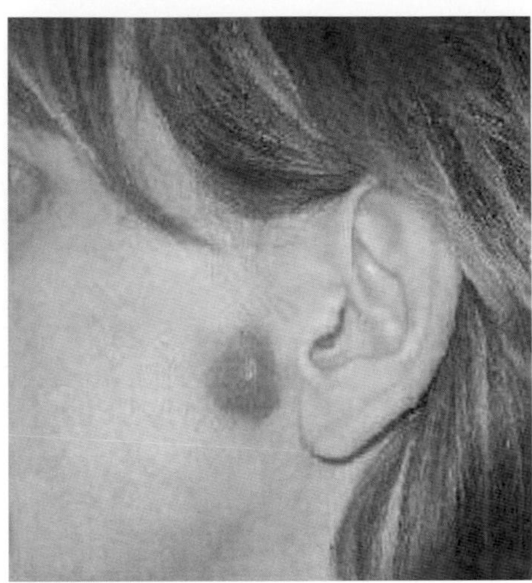

FIGURE 73.4 A pretragal inflammatory lymphadenopathy in a woman with oculoglandular tularemia *(courtesy of Dr N. Roch).*

undercooked food or water contaminated with *F. tularensis*. The disease often manifests as clustered cases, either in a family (food-borne infections) or in a localized population (water-borne infections). Large outbreaks have recently been reported in Turkey, Kosovo, and Bulgaria, with most patients presenting with oropharyngeal tularemia [17–19]. Patients with oropharyngeal involvement present with fever and acute exudative or membranous pharyngitis and rapid development of swollen cervical lymph nodes. Enlarged tonsils with yellow-white pseudomembranes may suggest diphtheria. Pharyngitis is usually severe, of prolonged duration (several weeks to months) and resists ß-lactam therapy. Complications may include cervical lymph node suppuration with skin fistulization and tonsillar phlegmon. Gastrointestinal tularemia probably develops in patients after ingestion of a high dose of bacteria and may manifest by mild diarrhea, abdominal pain, nausea, vomiting and gastrointestinal bleeding. Enlarged mesenteric lymph nodes may be found. Extensive ulceration of the bowel may lead to severe symptoms and even death.

The oculoglandular form (2–3% of cases) usually corresponds to conjunctival inoculation of *F. tularensis* by touch with a contaminated finger, for example following manipulation of an infected animal or after crushing a tick. Symptoms usually manifest early and correspond to Parinaud's oculoglandular syndrome, combining a granulomatous unilateral conjunctivitis with homolateral regional lymphadenopathy (Fig. 73.4). The inflamed conjunctiva is painful, with numerous yellowish nodules and pinpoint ulcers. Enlarged lymph nodes may be found in the pretragal, retroauricular or cervical regions. ß-lactams are not effective and the conjunctivitis may last for several weeks or months without appropriate antibiotic treatment. The most frequent complications include keratitis, sometimes with corneal perforation, lymph node suppuration and cellulitis in nearby skin tissue.

The pneumonic form may develop after inhalation of an infectious aerosol, for example during lawn mowing or brush cutting [20], following aerosolized laboratory exposure, or, alternatively, as a secondary localization of *F. tularensis* bacteremia. Symptoms are those of atypical pneumonia, including fever, a nonproductive cough, dyspnea, and pleuritic chest pain. Bilateral patchy infiltrates are found on chest radiography. Pleural effusions and empyema may develop. Mediastinal lymph nodes may develop and persist for several months after resolution of pneumonia. Pneumonia is often fulminant with lung tissue necrosis when caused by a type A strain.

The typhoidal form corresponds to a rapid systemic progression of tularemia with fever, a typhoid state and shock in the absence of apparent portal of entry (e.g. skin lesion) or lymphadenopathy. This form is often fatal.

Other rare clinical manifestations of tularemia may include meningitis, encephalitis, pericarditis, endocarditis, peritonitis, hepatitis, splenitis, osteoarticular infections, septic shock with rhabdomyolysis, and acute renal failure.

PATIENT EVALUATION, DIAGNOSIS, AND DIFFERENTIAL DIAGNOSIS

Mild-to-moderate tularemia cases are usually managed on an outpatient basis. Patients with severe clinical manifestations (pneumonia, typhoidal tularemia, severe digestive involvement, brain or cardiac involvement) should be hospitalized and possibly admitted to an intensive care unit, especially if septic shock is present.

Nonspecific biologic abnormalities may include moderate leukocytosis with granulocytosis, a relative increase in mononuclear cells, an inflammatory syndrome with mild elevation of C-reactive protein and, rarely, a mild elevation of liver enzymes.

Tularemia diagnosis is usually confirmed by serologic methods, especially the microagglutination test and, less frequently, the indirect immunofluorescence and ELISA techniques [21, 22]. These tests are both sensitive and specific, although serology may be negative in the early course of the disease. Antibody titers are usually only detected at significant levels 2–3 weeks following symptom onset, peak after 6–8 weeks progression of the disease and then decline slowly over months or years. Serologic titers of 1:160 or more are usually considered significant for the microagglutination test, but cut-off titters may vary between laboratories using different techniques and antigens. A seroconversion or a fourfold rise in antibody titers between acute-phase and convalescent-phase sera is considered diagnostic. Cross-reacting antibodies have been reported between *Francisella* sp., *Brucella* sp., *Proteus* OX19, *Yersinia enterocolitica* O:3 and *Yersinia pestis* antigens, but titers are usually low and not confounding. The Western blot technique may be used. Importantly, serologic tests cannot determine the *Francisella* subspecies and clade involved.

Francisella tularensis culture remains tedious and hazardous for laboratory personnel [21, 22]. Type A strains are class 3 pathogens, and should be grown in a Biosafety Level (BSL) 3 laboratory. Ideally, clinical samples should be transported frozen at −80 °C or directly inoculated to antibiotic-containing medium to prevent overgrowth by commensal species. Isolation of *F. tularensis* requires enriched medium containing cysteine (e.g. Thayer-Martin medium, chocolate agar supplemented with Polyvitex™ or Isovitalex™) and incubation at 37 °C for a minimum of 3–5 days. Automated blood culture systems are useful in the rare patients with bacteremia. *Francisella tularensis* may be grown from blood, skin eschar discharges, lymph node samples, conjunctival or throat swabs, cerebrospinal fluid (CSF), sputum, and other suppurations or organ biopsies. Culture sensitivity is considered low (about 25% for cutaneous and lymph node samples) and decreases significantly after administration of effective antibiotics. Suspected colonies may be rapidly identified as *F. tularensis* by using a specific antiserum or by PCR amplification of specific genes (e.g. *fopA* or *tul4*).

PCR-based techniques now provide a rapid, sensitive and specific diagnosis of tularemia and carry a much lower infection risk for laboratory personnel than culture [21, 22]. Sensitivities of 73–78% have been reported for skin samples from patients with ulceroglandular tularemia. PCR may remain positive despite previous administration of antibiotics or when testing formalin-fixed tissue specimens. PCR targets include the insertion sequence *ISFtu2*, the 16SrRNA-encoding gene, the succinate dehydrogenase gene *SdhA* and genes encoding outer membrane-associated proteins (Tul4, a 17-kDa lipoprotein encoded by the *tul4* gene; OmpA, a 43-kDa protein encoded by the *fopA* gene; and an unnamed 23-kDa protein). *Francisella tularensis* DNA has been amplified from blood, lymph nodes, skin ulcer discharge and skin biopsies, conjunctival discharge, pharynx and CSF. These PCRs are genus- or species-specific. The *F. tularensis* subspecies and clade involved may be identified by several molecular methods, including analysis of whole-genome restriction digests by pulse-field gel electrophoresis (PFGE), amplified fragment length polymorphism (AFLP), regional difference analysis (RD1 or *pdpD* locus) and multiple-locus variable number tandem repeat analysis (MLVA).

Tularemia should be systematically evoked in patients living in (or visiting) an endemic area, with compatible clinical manifestations and a potential exposure. When suggestive epidemiologic conditions are lacking, however, the differential diagnosis of tularemia may be wide because symptoms are poorly specific [21]. Ulceroglandular tularemia is the most easily diagnosed form, but atypical skin lesions associated with enlarged lymph nodes may suggest infections caused by *Staphylococcus aureus*, *Streptococcus pyogenes* or *Mycobacterium marinum*, as well as cat-scratch disease, pasteurellosis, syphilis, anthrax, rat-bite fever, rickettsiosis and sporotrichosis. The chronically-evolving lymphadenopathy of the glandular form is more challenging and may suggest other infectious diseases [tuberculosis, non-tuberculous mycobacterial diseases, cat-scratch disease, plague, lymphogranuloma venereum, Ebstein Barr virus (EBV), cytomegalovirus (CMV) or HIV infections, toxoplasmosis or histoplasmosis] and non-infectious diseases (immunologic diseases, malignant diseases including lymphoma, etc.). Oropharyngeal tularemia may suggest *S. pyogenes* (group A) infection or diphtheria in the case of pseudomembranous pharyngitis. Failure of ß-lactam therapy may prompt the clinician to make further investigations, but diagnosis is often delayed. Parinaud's oculoglandular syndrome is not specific and *Mycobacterium tuberculosis*, *Bartonella henselae* and herpes virus are more frequent etiologies of this syndrome, among others. *Francisella tularensis* pneumonia should be considered, together with other causes of atypical pneumonia, including plague and anthrax in the context of bioterrorism. Typhoidal tularemia may be observed in many other severe infectious diseases, including typhoid fever.

TREATMENT

Human tularemia cases are usually more severe in North America than in Eurasia. Respective global mortality rates for type A and type B infections changed from 5–10% and 0.5–1% before the antibiotic era, to 2–3% and close to 0% when appropriate antibiotic therapy became available [21]. Higher mortality rates have been reported in patients with the pneumonic or typhoidal forms (30–60%) and in immunocompromised patients. Recently, mortality rates of 4%, 24%, 0% and 7% have been associated in the USA with the A1a, A1b, A2 and B genotypes, respectively [7].

In vitro, most strains of *F. tularensis* are resistant to penicillin G and aminopenicillins because of the action of a ß-lactamase [21]. Susceptibility to third-generation cephalosporins (e.g. cefotaxime, ceftriaxone) varies according to the strains studied, but these antibiotics are not effective against intracellular *F. tularensis* and they are clinically unreliable [23].

Chloramphenicol, cotrimoxazole, and macrolides are poorly effective. The aminoglycosides, the fluoroquinolones, the tetracyclines, rifampin and the ketolide telithromycin display a bactericidal activity against *F. tularensis*, both in axenic medium and in cell systems.

The optimum treatment of tularemia cannot be based on randomized, controlled clinical trials because the disease is so rare. According to clinical experience, the aminoglycosides are considered the most effective antibiotics (Table 73-2) [21, 24]. Streptomycin has been used for decades with success rates of over 97%. This antibiotic is now difficult to obtain in many countries. Gentamicin is currently used as an alternative, whereas other aminoglycosides are less effective. Administration of an aminoglycoside is still recommended in severe tularemia cases, with the monitoring of antibiotic serum levels. However, aminoglycosides have many side effects (including ototoxicity and nephrotoxicity) and are only administrable parenterally.

The fluoroquinolones are now proposed as first-line drugs in the vast majority of patients with mild-to-moderate clinical manifestations, including in children, as the risk of skeletal toxicity appears low. Their clinical efficacy is better documented in type B than in type A tularemia. These antibiotics are less toxic than aminoglycosides and administrable orally. Ciprofloxacin has been used in most cases reported in the literature with success rates over 95%. Ofloxacin (200 mg twice daily) or levofloxacin (500 mg once daily) may also be effective, but clinical data are scarce.

Tetracyclines, especially doxycycline, represent a possible alternative, although more frequent relapses are observed upon antibiotic withdrawal. Gastrointestinal side effects are frequent, but may be reduced by taking the drug with food. Tetracyclines are classically contraindicated in children less than eight years old because of the

TABLE 73-2 Main Current Therapeutic Options for Tularemia

Antibiotic	Dosage and duration	References	Category*	Comments
Ciprofloxacin	750 mg per os twice a day for 10–14 days	[4, 10, 24, 27]	4	First line in adults and children, especially if type B disease
Doxycycline	100 mg per os twice a day for 10–14 days	[4, 10]	4	Adults and children > 8 years, higher relapse rate
Gentamicin	5 mg/kg IV or IM in one or two divided doses for 14 days	[1, 24, 28]	4	Adults, children and pregnant women with severe disease. Streptomycin or gentamycin are usually considered front-line effective therapy for type A disease

*Category 1, double-blind study; 2, clinical trial <20 subjects; 3, clinical trial >20 subjects; 4, series; 5, anecdotal case reports.

risk of tooth discoloration, and in pregnant women because of fetal bone toxicity.

Whatever the drug administered, 10–14 days treatment duration should be considered a minimum. Failures and relapses may still be observed in patients with severe disease and/or with delayed onset of appropriate antibiotic therapy. Suppurated lymph nodes may need to be surgically removed to obtain clinical cure. Combined therapy (e.g. an aminoglycoside with a tetracycline or a fluoroquinolone) has been occasionally used in patients with severe disease. There is no indication that it may be superior to monotherapy.

Antibiotic treatment of tularemia in pregnant women remains an unsolved problem. ß-lactams and the macrolides are considered unreliable. Rifampin is not used as monotherapy because of possible selection for resistance. Gentamicin may be used is severe cases, but exposes the mother and fetus to ototoxicity and nephrotoxicity. Telithromycin may be an interesting alternative, but clinical data are lacking and its administration in pregnant women is currently not recommended.

Prevention of tularemia in the most at-risk persons includes: (i) avoiding exposure to sick animals and wearing protective gloves when handling animal carcasses; (ii) wearing long clothing and using insect repellents when walking in endemic areas to prevent arthropod bites, as well as careful skin inspection and prompt removal of ticks; and (iii) performing *F. tularensis* cultures in a BSL 3 laboratory to prevent laboratory contamination. Post-exposure prophylaxis of tularemia may be considered in the context of bioterrorism, during food- or water-borne tularemia outbreaks, or in laboratory workers after contamination with *F. tularensis* cultures. Ciprofloxacin or doxycycline administered for 10–14 days at a full dosage is currently recommended, but clinical data supporting these recommendations are scarce.

Inactivated vaccines and purified immunogenic polysaccharide- or protein-based vaccines have not proved to be effective in preventing tularemia [25, 26]. Live attenuated vaccines were first developed in the former Soviet Union where millions of people were vaccinated with the attenuated strains 15 and 155 until 1960. The live vaccine strain developed in the USA was derived from these Russian strains. The live vaccine strain mainly protects from the occurrence of severe tularemia disease (e.g. the pneumonic and typhoidal forms), but it is less effective in preventing ulceroglandular tularemia. It has not been licensed by the Food and Drug Administration (FDA) in the USA, nor in any other country because of significant side effects and because the basis of attenuation of this strain has not been fully characterized. Construction of defined attenuated strains of *F. tularensis* is under way.

REFERENCES

1. Evans ME, Gregory DW, Schaffner W, McGee ZA. Tularemia: a 30-year experience with 88 cases. Medicine 1985;64:251–69.
2. Dennis DT, Inglesby TV, Henderson DA, et al; Working Group on Civilian Biodefense. Tularemia as a biological weapon: medical and public health management. JAMA 2001;285:2763–73.
3. Sjöstedt A. Tularemia: history, epidemiology, pathogen physiology and clinical manifestations. Ann N Y Acad Sci 2007;1105:1–29.
4. Pérez-Castrillón JL, Bachiller-Luque P, Martín-Luquero M, et al. Tularemia epidemic in northwestern Spain: clinical description and therapeutic response. Clin Infect Dis 2001;33:573–6.
5. de Carvalho IL, Escudero R, Garcia-Amil C, et al. *Francisella tularensis*, Portugal. Emerg Infect Dis 2007;13:666–7.
6. Staples JE, Kubota KA, Chalcraft LG, et al. Epidemiologic and molecular analysis of human tularemia, United States, 1964–2004. Emerg Infect Dis 2006;12:1113–18.
7. Kugeler KJ, Mead PS, Janusz AM, et al. Molecular epidemiology of *Francisella tularensis* in the United States. Clin Infect Dis 2009;48:863–70.
8. Eliasson H, Broman T, Forsman M, Bäck E. Tularemia: current epidemiology and disease management. Infect Dis Clin North Amer 2006; 20:289–311.
9. Keim P, Johansson A, Wagner DM. Molecular epidemiology, evolution, and ecology of *Francisella*. Ann NY Acad Sci 2007;1105:30–66.
10. Eliasson H, Bäck E. Tularaemia in an emergent area in Sweden: an analysis of 234 cases in five years. Scand J Infect Dis 2007;39:880–9.
11. Petersen JM, Carlson JK, Dietrich G, et al. Multiple *Francisella tularensis* subspecies and clades, tularemia outbreak, Utah. Emerg Infect Dis 2008;14:1928–30.
12. Ellis J, Oyston PC, Green M, Titball RW. Tularemia. Clin Microbiol Rev 2002; 15:631–46.
13. McLendon MK, Apicella MA, Allen LA. *Francisella tularensis*: taxonomy, genetics, and immunopathogenesis of a potential agent of biowarfare. Annu Rev Microbiol 2006;60:167–85.
14. Kirimanjeswara GS, Olmos S, Bakshi CS, Metzger DW. Humoral and cell-mediated immunity to the intracellular pathogen *Francisella tularensis*. Immunol Rev 2008;225:244–55.
15. Lamps LW, Havens JM, Sjostedt A, et al. Histologic and molecular diagnosis of tularemia: a potential bioterrorism agent endemic to North America. Mod Pathol 2004;17:489–95.
16. Nigrovic LE, Wingerter SL. Tularemia. Infect Dis Clin North Am 2008;22:489–504.
17. Helvaci S, Gediko lu S, Akalin H, Oral HB. Tularemia in Bursa, Turkey: 205 cases in ten years. Eur J Epidemiol 2000;16:271–6.
18. Reintjes R, Dedushaj I, Gjini A, et al. Tularemia outbreak investigation in Kosovo: case control and environmental studies. Emerg Infect Dis 2002;8:69–73.
19. Kantardjiev T, Ivanov I, Velinov T, et al. Tularemia outbreak, Bulgaria, 1997–2005. Emerg Infect Dis 2006;12:678–80.
20. Feldman KA, Enscore RE, Lathrop SL, et al. An outbreak of primary pneumonic tularemia on Martha's Vineyard. N Engl J Med 2001;345: 1601–6.
21. Tärnvik A, Chu MC. New approaches to diagnosis and therapy of tularemia. Ann NY Acad Sci 2007;1105:378–404.
22. Hepburn MJ, Simpson AJ. Tularemia: current diagnosis and treatment options. Expert Rev Anti Infect Ther 2008;6:231–40.
23. Cross JT, Jacobs RF. Tularemia: treatment failures with outpatient use of ceftriaxone. Clin Infect Dis 1993;17:976–80.
24. Enderlin G, Morales L, Jacobs RF, Cross JT. Streptomycin and alternative agents for the treatment of tularemia: review of the literature. Clin Infect Dis 1994;19:42–7.
25. Wayne Conlan J, Oyston PC. Vaccines against *Francisella tularensis*. Ann NY Acad Sci 2007;1105:325–50.
26. Isherwood KE, Titball RW, Davies DH, et al. Vaccination strategies for *Francisella tularensis*. Adv Drug Deliv Rev 2005;57:1403–14.
27. Johansson A, Berglund L, Gothefors L, et al. Ciprofloxacin for treatment of tularemia in children. Pediatr Infect Dis J 2000;19:449–53.
28. Cross JT Jr, Schutze GE, Jacobs RF. Treatment of tularemia with gentamicin in pediatric patients. Pediatr Infect Dis J 1995;14:151–2.

Leptospirosis 74

George Watt

Key features

- Leptospirosis is a neglected, emerging zoonosis that causes substantial morbidity and mortality in impoverished regions of the tropics
- Weil's disease is the name given to classic severe leptospirosis and is characterized by jaundice, renal failure and a high mortality rate
- Leptospirosis-associated pulmonary hemorrhage syndrome (LPHS) is a more recently recognized severe disease manifestation causing massive bleeding into the lungs and a poor clinical outcome
- The pathogenesis of leptospirosis remains largely unexplained and the key pathologic feature is a paucity of histopathologic changes in organs with marked functional impairment
- Diagnostic confirmation is rarely available in areas where most disease transmission occurs
- Individuals with leptospirosis should receive antimicrobial therapy, often oral doxycycline or intravenous penicillin, although other agents may also be effective
- There is no commercially available vaccine for use in humans to prevent leptospirosis, although prophylactic weekly doxycycline can be used to prevent disease among select at-risk populations and during outbreaks

INTRODUCTION

Leptospirosis is a worldwide zoonosis transmitted by pathogenic spirochetes of the genus *Leptospira*. The pathogenesis remains largely unexplained even though Weil published a clinical description of leptospirosis in 1886. In 1916, Inada isolated leptospires, identified them as the etiologic agent and linked rats to disease transmission [1]. The disease is of greatest public health importance in the tropics, where it is an endemic disease of rice farmers and residents of urban slums [2]. Substantial recent outbreaks superimposed on endemic disease activity were linked to the introduction of a new clone of *Leptospira* in Thailand [3] and followed severe flooding caused by two typhoons in the Philippines [4].

EPIDEMIOLOGY

Leptospirosis is caused by spirochetes of the genus *Leptospira*. This genus contains at least 18 species classified on the basis of DNA relatedness and more than 300 serovars (serovarieties) based on agglutinating antigens. Leptospires nest in the renal tubules of mammalian hosts and are shed in the urine. They can survive for several months in the environment under moist conditions, particularly in the presence of warmth (above 22 °C) and a neutral pH (pH 6.2–8.0). These conditions occur all year round in the tropics, but only during the summer and autumn months in temperate climates. Roughly 160 animal species harbor organisms, but rodents are the most important reservoir. Carrier rates of over 50% have been measured in Norway rats, which shed massive numbers of organisms for life, without showing clinical illness. Some serovars appear to be preferentially adapted to select mammalian hosts. For example, the serovar icterohaemorrhagiae is primarily associated with the Norway rat, canicola with dogs and pomona with swine and cattle. However, a particular host species may serve as a reservoir for one or more serovars and a particular serovar may be hosted by many different animal species.

The transmission of infection from animal to human usually occurs through contact with contaminated water or moist soil. Organisms enter humans through abrasions of the skin or through the mucosal surface of the eye, mouth, nasopharynx, or esophagus. Crowded cities that are flood-prone and have large rat populations provide ideal conditions for disease transmission. Escalating migration of the rural poor to urban slums is likely to further exacerbate the risks of leptospirosis transmission [2, 5]. An outbreak in Nicaragua in 1995 and an urban epidemic in Salvador, Brazil in 1999 were associated with particularly heavy rains and flooding. In 2009, two typhoons struck the Philippines and caused massive flooding. Leptospirosis was recognized as the most urgent threat to health in the aftermath of the typhoons [4]. Special clinics to treat the disease were set up in evacuation centers and an estimated 1.3 million flood survivors were given chemoprophylaxis.

Intense exposure to leptospires has been documented in rice, sugar cane, and rubber plantation workers. Less frequently, leptospirosis is acquired by direct contact with the blood, urine, or tissues of infected animals. Epidemiologic patterns in the USA and UK have changed. Recreational exposure to freshwater (e.g. canoeing, sailing, water skiing) and animal contact at home have replaced occupational exposure as the chief sources of disease in industrialized areas.

Measuring incidence by active surveillance confirms that leptospirosis is a surprisingly common disease. Antibody positivity rates of 37% have been recorded in rural Belize and 23% in Vietnam. More than 2527 human cases and 13 deaths were reported for the first 9 months of 1999 by the Ministry of Public Health in Thailand. Human leptospirosis is an important disease in China, Southeast Asia, India, Africa, and South and Central America. It is also of significance in eastern and southern Europe, Australia, and New Zealand. In the USA, the disease is primarily of veterinary importance, with only 50–150 human cases reported annually.

NATURAL HISTORY, PATHOGENESIS, AND PATHOLOGY

Infection may be asymptomatic, but 5–15% of cases are severe or fatal. Pathogenesis, particularly that of severe disease, remains poorly understood. Overall, renal failure is the most common cause of death in leptospirosis. Leptospires are frequently found in human renal tissue, but their role in mediating kidney damage is unknown. Interstitial nephritis is primarily found in individuals who have survived until inflammation has had an opportunity to develop, but is frequently absent in patients with fulminant disease. Impaired renal perfusion constitutes the fundamental nephropathic change. In some geographic areas, pulmonary hemorrhage is the principal cause of death and is associated with the linear deposition of immunoglobulins and complement on the alveolar surface [6]. It is unclear why renal failure predominates as the principal cause of death in some places, while pulmonary hemorrhage is the major cause in others, even where the most common infecting serovars are the same. There are only minor histopathologic changes in the kidneys and livers of patients with marked functional impairment of these organs. Patients who survive severe leptospirosis have complete recovery of hepatic and renal function – consistent with the lack of structural damage to these organs.

CLINICAL FEATURES

The most common clinical features of leptospirosis are summarized in Table 74-1.

Subclinical infection is common and less than 10% of symptomatic infections result in severe, icteric illness. Even relatively virulent serovars, such as icterohaemorrhagiae lead more often to anicteric than to icteric disease. Old terms such as peapicker's disease, swineherd's disease and canicola fever, which linked specific serotypes with distinct disease manifestations, are misleading and should be abandoned. The median incubation period is 10 days, with a range of 2–26 days. The duration of the incubation period has no prognostic significance. Once symptoms develop, they may follow a biphasic course: after an initial febrile illness there is defervescence of fever and symptomatic improvement followed by a second period of disease. However, a clear demarcation between the first and second stages is atypical of icteric leptospirosis and, in mild cases, the distinction can be unclear or the second stage may never occur. The diagnostic usefulness of a history of a biphasic illness has been overemphasized. HIV co-infection does not seem to affect the clinical presentation of leptospirosis in the few co-infected patients described thus far.

TABLE 74-1 The Most Common Clinical Manifestations of 208 Leptospirosis Patients in Puerto Rico

Symptoms (% of cases)	Anicteric (106 cases)	Icteric (102 cases)
Fever	100	99
Myalgia	97	97
Headache	82	95
Chills	84	90
Sore throat	72	87
Nausea	71	81
Vomiting	65	75
Eye pain	54	38
Diarrhea	23	30
Oliguria	20	30
Cough	15	32
Hemoptysis	5	14
Signs (% of cases)		
Conjunctival infection	100	98
Muscle tenderness	70	79
Hepatomegaly	60	60
Pulmonary findings	11	36
Lymphadenopathy	35	12
Petechiae, ecchymoses	4	29

Adapted from Alexander AD, Benenson AS, Byrne RJ, et al. Leptospirosis in Puerto Rico. Zoonoses Res. 1963;2:152–227.

ANICTERIC LEPTOSPIROSIS

Symptoms and Signs

Typically, the disease begins with the abrupt onset of intense headache, fever, chills, and myalgia. Fever often exceeds 40 °C (103 °F) and is preceded by rigors. Muscle pain can be excruciating and occurs most commonly in the thighs, calves, lumbosacral region, and abdomen. Abdominal wall pain accompanied by palpation tenderness can mimic an acute surgical abdomen. Nausea, vomiting, diarrhea, and sore throat are other frequent symptoms. Cough and chest pain figure prominently in reports of patients from Korea and China.

Conjunctival suffusion is a helpful diagnostic clue that usually appears two or three days after the onset of fever and involves the bulbar conjunctiva. Pus and serous secretions are absent and there is no matting of the eyelashes and eyelids. Mild suffusion can easily be overlooked. Less common and less distinctive signs include pharyngeal injection, splenomegaly, hepatomegaly, lymphadenopathy, and skin lesions. Within a week, most patients become asymptomatic. After several days of apparent recovery, the illness resumes in some individuals. Manifestations of the second stage are more variable and mild than those of the initial illness and usually last 2–4 days. Leptospires disappear from the blood, cerebrospinal fluid (CSF), and tissues, but appear in the urine. Serum antibody titers rise – hence the term "immune" phase. Meningitis is the hallmark of this stage of leptospirosis. Pleocytosis of the CSF can be demonstrated in 80–90% of all patients during the second week of illness, although only about 50% will have clinical signs and symptoms of meningitis. Meningeal signs can last several weeks, but usually resolve within a day or two. Uveitis is a late manifestation of leptospirosis, generally seen 4–8 months after the illness has begun. The anterior uveal tract is most frequently affected and pain, photophobia, and blurring of vision are the usual symptoms.

Laboratory Findings

White blood cell count varies, but neutrophilia is usually present. Urinalysis may show proteinuria, pyuria, and microscopic hematuria. Enzyme markers of skeletal muscle damage, such as creatinine kinase and aldolase are elevated in the sera of 50% of patients during the first week of illness. Chest radiographs from patients with pulmonary manifestations show a variety of abnormalities, but none is pathognomonic of leptospirosis. The most common finding is small, patchy, snowflake-like lesions in the periphery of the lung fields.

ICTERIC LEPTOSPIROSIS (WEIL'S DISEASE)

Weil's disease refers to severe, life-threatening leptospirosis and is characterized by jaundice, renal dysfunction, hemorrhagic manifestations, and a high mortality rate. Although jaundice is the hallmark of severe leptospirosis, fatalities do not occur because of liver failure. The degree of jaundice has no prognostic significance, but its presence or absence does – virtually all leptospirosis deaths occur in icteric patients. Icterus first appears between the fifth and ninth days of illness, reaches maximum intensity 4 or 5 days later and continues for an average of 1 month. Hepatomegaly is found in the majority of patients; hepatic percussion tenderness is a reliable clinical marker of continuing disease activity. There is no residual liver dysfunction in survivors of Weil's disease, consistent with the absence of structural damage seen on pathologic examination.

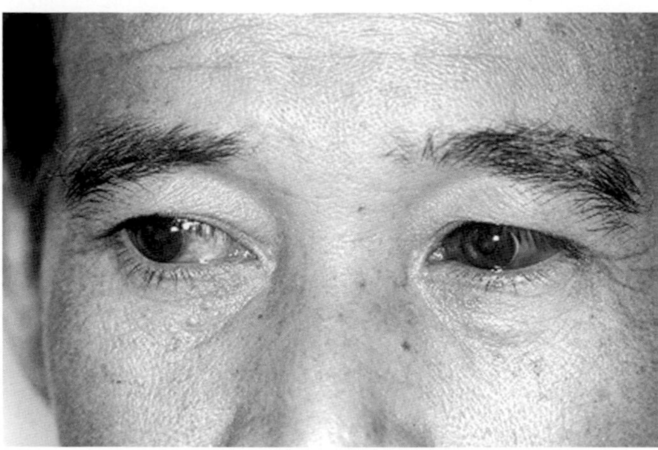

FIGURE 74.1 Jaundice, hemorrhage, and conjunctival suffusion in acute leptospirosis.

Bleeding is occasionally seen in anicteric cases but is most prevalent in severe disease. Purpura, petechiae, epistaxis, bleeding of the gums, and minor hemoptysis are the most common hemorrhagic manifestations; however, deaths occur from subarachnoid hemorrhage and exsanguination from gastrointestinal bleeding. Conjunctival hemorrhage is an extremely useful diagnostic finding and, when combined with scleral icterus and conjunctival suffusion, produces eye findings strongly suggestive of leptospirosis (see Fig. 74.1). The frequency with which severe pulmonary hemorrhage complicates leptospirosis is variable but is a cardinal feature of some outbreaks.

Life-threatening renal failure is a complication of icteric disease, although all forms of leptospirosis may be associated with mild kidney dysfunction. Oliguria or anuria usually develop during the second week of illness, but may appear earlier. Complete anuria is a grave prognostic sign often seen in patients who present late in the course of illness with frank uremia and irreversible disease. Because renal failure develops very quickly in leptospirosis, symptoms and signs of uremia are frequently encountered. Anorexia, vomiting, drowsiness, disorientation, and confusion are seen early and rapidly progress to convulsions, stupor, and coma in severe cases. Disturbances of consciousness in a patient with severe leptospirosis are usually caused by uremic encephalopathy, whereas in anicteric cases aseptic encephalitis is the usual cause. Renal function eventually returns to normal in survivors of Weil's disease, although detectable abnormalities may persist for several months.

Leptospirosis-associated severe pulmonary hemorrhage syndrome (SPHS) is now recognized as a widespread public health problem with a case fatality rate of about 50%. This lethal complication of leptospirosis can occur either with or without jaundice and renal failure. Hemoptysis is the cardinal sign but may not be apparent until patients are intubated. Real-time PCR has shown that leptospiremia is 10,000 or more bacteria per milliliter of blood in SPHS – the apparent critical threshold for severe outcomes such as SPHS and death [6].

Laboratory Features of Weil's Disease

Hyperbilirubinemia results from increases in both conjugated (direct) and unconjugated (indirect) bilirubin, but elevations of the direct fraction predominate. Prolongations of the prothrombin time commonly occur but are easily corrected by the administration of vitamin K; modest elevations of serum alkaline phosphatase are typical. There is mild hepatocellular necrosis; greater than fivefold increases of transaminase (aminotransferase) levels are exceptional. Jaundiced patients usually have leukocytosis in the range of 15,000 to 30,000 per mm^3 and neutrophilia is constant. Anemia is common and multifactorial; blood loss and renal dysfunction contribute frequently, intravascular hemolysis less often. Mild thrombocytopenia often occurs but decreases in platelet count sufficient to be associated with bleeding are exceptional. The specific gravity of the urine is high. Hypokalemia due to renal potassium wasting can occur and hypomagnesemia has been reported.

PATIENT EVALUATION, DIAGNOSIS, AND DIFFERENTIAL DIAGNOSIS

PATIENT EVALUATION

Patients who present with an undifferentiated febrile illness must be carefully evaluated for possible leptospirosis. A history of water or animal contact is particularly helpful. Key symptoms and signs are conjunctival suffusion and severe myalgia with tenderness. In the context of a known outbreak of leptospirosis, individuals must be carefully assessed for signs of severe disease. The most important signs of severity are jaundice, bleeding, pulmonary involvement, oliguria, and a raised serum creatinine level.

DIAGNOSIS

Most cases go undiagnosed because symptoms and signs are often nonspecific and serologic confirmation is rarely available where most disease transmission occurs. Failure to diagnose leptospirosis is particularly unfortunate: severely ill patients often recover completely with prompt treatment but delayed therapy is likely to result in a poor clinical outcome. Late disease can often be recognized by its typical clinical manifestations, but the presentation of early leptospirosis is usually nonspecific and is therefore difficult to identify clinically. Leptospirosis has long been acknowledged to be a frequent cause of undifferentiated febrile illness in developing countries. Co-infection with diseases such as malaria and scrub typhus has been reported and adds to the diagnostic confusion of tropical fevers.

Laboratory diagnosis of leptospirosis remains problematic. The microscopic agglutination test is considered the serodiagnostic method of choice for leptospirosis, but its complexity limits its use to reference laboratories. Dilutions of patient sera are applied to a panel of live, pathogenic leptospires. The results are viewed under dark-field microscopy and expressed as the percentage of organisms cleared from the field by agglutination. Inadequate quality controls of the live reference strain panels can lead to frequent false-negative results [7]. A new generation of commercially available, rapid serodiagnostic kits that rely on whole *Leptospira* antigen preparations have been developed. Unfortunately, these assays seem to have unacceptably low sensitivities during acute-phase illness and persistent antibody produces low specificity in regions of high endemic transmission. The need for practical, affordable diagnostic kits to be available in areas where leptospirosis is common cannot be overemphasized. PCR and urine antigen detection are research tools that would be of the greatest potential diagnostic value in patients who present early, before antibodies have reached detectable levels.

Isolation of leptospires from blood or CSF is possible during the first 10 days of clinical illness, but specialized media are necessary. Serially diluted urine provides the highest yield. Unfortunately, culture results are only known 4–6 weeks later – too late to benefit severely ill, hospitalized patients.

Several attempts have been made to formulate diagnostic algorithms by assigning points to various clinical, epidemiologic and laboratory parameters. The points are totaled and the score is then used to represent the likelihood that the patient in question has leptospirosis. An example is shown in Table 74-2. The usefulness of these scoring systems is limited by their complexity, by marked regional variability in the quality of available diagnostic tests and by regional differences in the prevalent differential diagnoses that must be considered. However, these scoring systems are useful teaching tools, and emphasize the important epidemiologic and clinical characteristics of leptospirosis.

TABLE 74-2 Modified World Health Organization (WHO) Criteria for Diagnosis of Leptospirosis

Part A Clinical signs and symptoms (score)	
• Fever >39.0°C	(2 points)
• Conjunctival suffusion	(4 points)
• Myalgias	(4 points)
• Meningeal signs	(4 points)
• Jaundice	(1 point)
• Proteinuria	(1 point)
Part B Risk factors for exposure (score)	
• Heavy rainfall	(5 points)
• Flooding	(5 points)
• Animal contact	(1 point)
Part C Laboratory test results (score)	
• Positive IgM ELISA	(15 points)
• Microscopic agglutination	(15 points)
• Test (MAT) – single high titer	
• MAT fourfold rise in titer	(25 points)

Interpretation:
Presumptive leptospirosis if score >25 points;
Possible leptospirosis if score between 20–25 points.
MAT, microscopic agglutination test.

DIFFERENTIAL DIAGNOSIS

The typical leptospirosis patient has a history of water or animal contact, conjunctival suffusion and severe myalgia. It is important to solicit these findings in both mild and severe cases of leptospirosis. Atypical or mild cases are often confused with other entities but, because of a low index of suspicion and the disease's protean manifestations, the diagnosis is often missed, even in typical cases. The most important differential diagnoses differ in mild and severe disease.

Anicteric Leptospirosis

Fever of unknown origin and aseptic meningitis are the most common clinical impressions in mild leptospirosis. Severe myalgia involving several different muscle groups – not just the abdominal wall – suggests leptospirosis rather than appendicitis. Fever and vomiting are frequently misdiagnosed as gastroenteritis.

Weil's Disease

Viral hepatitis is a common misdiagnosis in patients with Weil's disease. Leukocytosis, elevated serum bilirubin levels without marked transaminase elevations, and renal dysfunction are typical of leptospirosis, but unusual in hepatitis. Marked leukocytosis and a negative blood film argue against malaria. Jaundice, severe renal dysfunction, and leukocytosis are atypical of typhoid fever. Differentiating leptospirosis from scrub typhus and Korean hemorrhagic fever (caused by Hantaan virus) in areas where these diseases coexist is more difficult. Both are associated with animals and both can cause conjunctival suffusion. Korean hemorrhagic fever is transmitted by infected rodent urine and mixed infection with *Leptospira interrogans* and Hantaan virus has been reported. Liver disease is not usually a prominent manifestation of Korean hemorrhagic fever. Splenomegaly and generalized lymphadenopathy are characteristic of scrub typhus, but not leptospirosis. Serum creatinine levels are usually normal, even in jaundiced patients with *Orientia tsutsugamushi* infection. The myalgia of leptospirosis is usually more severe than that of scrub typhus (Box 74.1).

BOX 74.1 Clinical Pearl

Muscles of patients with leptospirosis can be exquisitely tender and painful to the touch

but.........

palpation of painful muscles in patients with scrub typhus sometimes provides pain relief.

BOX 74.2 Clinical Pearl

Kawasaki's disease (mucocutaneous lymph node syndrome) must be differentiated from leptospirosis in children <5 years old with desquamation and involvement of the gallbladder and myocardium.

Severe Pulmonary Hemorrhage Syndrome (SPHS)

Leptospirosis with prominent hemorrhagic manifestations is easily misdiagnosed as dengue virus infection. A severe outbreak of leptospirosis with SPHS in Nicaragua was initially thought to be dengue [8].

CHILDHOOD LEPTOSPIROSIS

This shares many features with adult disease; pulmonary hemorrhage occurs and severe renal dysfunction is common. Distinct clinical features include hypotension, acalculous cholecystitis, pancreatitis, and abdominal causalgia (burning pain). Skin lesions may desquamate and become gangrenous (Box 74.2).

TREATMENT

Placebo-controlled, double-blind trials have proven that doxycycline benefits patients with early, mild leptospirosis and that intravenous penicillin helps adults with severe, late disease [9]. The outcome of severe, pediatric leptospirosis is also improved by penicillin therapy. Antibiotics should therefore be given to all patients with leptospirosis, regardless of age or when in their disease course they are seen. Doxycycline is given at doses of 100 mg orally twice a day for 1 week. Patients who are vomiting or are seriously ill require parenteral therapy. Intravenous penicillin G is administered to adults as 1.5 million units every 6 h for 1 week. Recent trials from Thailand indicate that treatment with ceftriaxone, cefotaxime, and doxycycline had equivalent efficacy to penicillin in patients with mild-to-moderately severe disease. However, it is not known whether these antibiotics are as effective as high-dose penicillin for treatment of the most severely ill individuals. Doxycycline and azithromycin had comparable efficacy as presumptive treatment of mildly ill patients found later to have leptospirosis, scrub typhus, or dual infections.

There is controversy regarding the occurrence of a Jarisch–Herxheimer reaction in leptospirosis. If present, it is much less prominent in leptospirosis than in other spirochetal illnesses. The important practical consideration is that antibiotics should not be withheld because of the fear of a possible Jarisch–Herxheimer reaction.

The management of pulmonary hemorrhage often requires prompt intubation and mechanical ventilation. SPHS patients have physiologic and pathologic evidence for acute respiratory distress syndrome so ventilation using low tidal volumes and high post-expiratory end-pressures should be provided. Respiratory support to maintain adequate tissue oxygenation is essential because in nonfatal cases complete recovery of pulmonary function can be achieved. Ensuring adequate renal perfusion prevents renal failure in the vast majority of oliguric individuals. Continuous hemofiltration has been shown to be more effective than peritoneal dialysis in treating infection-associated hypercatabolic renal failure. Peritoneal dialysis, however, may be the only option in resource-limited settings. Whichever method of dialysis is chosen, it must be started promptly – delays increase mortality.

PREVENTION

Doxycycline 200 mg taken once a week prevents infection by pathogenic leptospires. Widespread use of doxycycline prophylaxis is not indicated, but it can benefit those who are at high risk for a short time, such as military personnel and certain agricultural workers. Infection by leptospires confers only serovar-specific immunity; second attacks caused by different serovars can occur. The efficacy and safety of human leptospiral vaccines have yet to be conclusively demonstrated. Prevention of leptospirosis in the tropics is particularly difficult. The large animal reservoir of infection is impossible to eliminate, the occurrence of numerous serovars limits the usefulness of serovar-specific vaccine and the wearing of protective clothing (e.g. rubber boots in rice fields) is both prohibitively expensive and impractical. Providing proper sanitation in urban slum communities would be the most effective control measure in this setting.

REFERENCES

1. Ko AI, Goarant C, Picardeau M. Leptospira: the dawn of the molecular genetics era for an emerging zoonotic pathogen. Nature 2009;7:736–47.
2. Ko AI, Galvao Reis M, Ribiero Dourado CM, et al. Urban epidemic of severe leptospirosis in Brazil. Lancet 1999; 354:820–5.
3. Thaipadungpanit J, Wuthiekanun V, Chierakul W, et al. *Leptospira interrogans* associated with an outbreak of human leptospirosis in Thailand. PLoS Negl Trop Dis 2007;1:e56.
4. McCurry J. Philippines struggles to recover from typhoons. Lancet 2009;374: 1489.
5. McBride AJ, Athanazio DA, Reis MG, et al. Leptospirosis. Curr Opin Infect Dis 2005,18:376–85.
6. Nicodemo AC, Duarte MI, Alves VA, et al. Lung lesions in human leptospirosis: microscopic, immunohistochemical, and ultrastructural features related to thrombocytopenia. Am J Trop Med Hyg 1997;56:181–7.
7. Smythe LD, Wuthiekanun V, Chierakul W, et al. The microscopic agglutination test (MAT) is an unreliable predictor of infecting *Leptospira* in Thailand. Am J Trop Med Hyg 2009;81:695–7.
8. Zaki SR, Shieh WJ, the Epidemic Working Group. Leptospirosis associated with outbreak of acute febrile illness and pulmonary haemorrhage, Nicaragua. Lancet 1996;347:535–6.
9. Watt G, Padre LP, Tuazon ML, et al. Placebo-controlled trial of intravenous penicillin for severe and late leptospirosis. Lancet 1988;1:433–5.
10. Alexander AD, Benenson AS, Byrne RJ, et al. Leptospirosis in Puerto Rico. Zoonoses Res 1963;2:152–227.

75 Relapsing Fever and Borrelioses

Michel Drancourt

Key features

- Relapsing fevers (RF) are ectoparasite-borne, tropical diseases caused by a group of related species of *Borrelia*, different from the *Borrelia* species responsible for the Lyme disease
- RF is a common and often unappreciated cause of fever in many areas of Africa and Asia
- RF can be louse-borne (LBRF) or tick-borne (TBRF)
- LBRF is a human-restricted infection caused by *Borrelia recurrentis* associated with human body lice
- TBRF is associated with a number of borreliae, including *Borrelia duttoni*, transmitted by soft ticks often associated with animal reservoirs
- RFs are characterized by recurrent/relapsing episodes of fever and spirochetemia
- RF can be severe. Mortality can exceed 30% in untreated cases of LBRF
- Rapid diagnosis usually relies on microscopic observation of borreliae on thick blood smear, but PCR-based diagnosis tests are also available
- Treatment usually involves administration of doxycycline or penicillin
- The Jarisch-Herxheimer reaction is frequent within the first 2 hours of treatment
- Prevention involves de-lousing and minimizing exposure to soft ticks; no vaccine is available

INTRODUCTION

Relapsing fevers (RF) are a group of bacterial diseases characterized by recurrent episodes of fever and spirochetemia. The true global burden of RF is uncertain, but a number of studies suggest that RF is a very common cause of fever in areas of Africa, especially among populations where louse infestation is common, or where humans are exposed to competent tick vectors. The term RF was first used to describe an illness that broke out in Edinburgh from 1843 to 1846. A causative *Borellia* agent was first observed in the blood of German patients by Otto Obermeier in the Berlin Charité Hospital in 1873 [1]. Tholozan then described RF in Eurasia in 1882 [2]. Tick transmission was demonstrated in 1905 in Western Africa by Dutton and Todd [3] after tick-borne relapsing fever (TBRF) plagued the David Livingstone expedition in Africa [4]. American cases were first documented in 1915 in Colorado [5].

RF remains a major cause of morbidity and mortality in large areas of Africa and Asia [4, 6].

EPIDEMIOLOGY

RESERVOIRS AND TRANSMISSION OF RELAPSING FEVER (RF) BORRELIAE (FIG. 75.1)

Borrelia recurrentis is unique among RF borreliae, being a human-restricted pathogen transmitted by the body louse *Pediculus humanus*; crushing the infected louse introduces *B. recurrentis* organisms into scratched skin; prolonged excretion of *B. recurrentis* in lice feces may enhance transmission [4, 7]. Other RF borreliae are responsible for TBRF transmitted from various reservoirs without any apparent adverse effects upon their vectors [4]. TBRF borreliae are transmitted by soft ticks belonging to the genus *Ornithodoros*, family Argasidae. They have nocturnal feeding habits involving painless bites. TBRF borreliae invade all tick organs, including salivary glands and excretory organs; infectious saliva and coxal fluid may contaminate the feeding site [3]. *Borrelia duttonii* was believed to predominately affect humans, but it may have other significant reservoirs, as suggested by the detection of *B. duttonii* DNA in chickens and pigs [4]. Other TBRF *Borrelia* species primarily infect rodents and insectivorous animals and are largely zoonotic [8]. Bats have been implicated as reservoirs for *Borrelia persica* in Central Asia [2], and a new, unnamed TBRF species related to *B. recurrentis* was recently identified in a bat in the UK [9]. The new TBRF, *Borrelia johnsonii*, was found in a *Carios* bat tick in the USA [10]. Competence of birds as reservoir has not been determined, but the same *Borrelia hermsii* genotype has been documented in an owl and a pine squirrel in Montana [11], and seabirds infested with *Carios* ticks in Japan were found to be infected by a new TBRF [12]. TBRF borreliae can survive in ticks for up to 7 years after feeding, and some ticks demonstrate transovarial transmission [2, 4].

GEOGRAPHIC DISTRIBUTION (FIG. 75.2)

Each RF *Borrelia* species is considered to be vector-specific [3]. In Europe, a few cases have been related to an unnamed TBRF *Borrelia* most closely related to *Borrelia hispanica* in Spain [13]. In Africa, *Ornithodoros erraticus* transmits *B. hispanica* in coastal areas of Morocco, Algeria, and Tunisia, *Ornithodoros sonrai* (formerly *Alectorobius sonrai*) transmits *Borrelia crocidurae* in West Africa and several arid areas of Northern Africa, *Ornithodoros moubata*/*Ornithodoros porcinus* transmit *B. duttonii* in Central, Eastern and Southern Africa, whereas *B. recurrentis* persists only in Ethiopia [3, 4, 14]. In Tanzania, molecular studies have identified a non-cultured *Borrelia* species most closely related to North America TBRF borreliae; its role in human infection is unknown [4]. In Central Asia, *B. persica* is transmitted by *O. tholozani* [15, 16]. In North America, *B. hermsii* is the main cause of TBRF in western areas, extending from southern British Columbia down to Los Angeles county [17]; *Borrelia turicatae* is transmitted by *O. turicatae* in Texas and *Borrelia lonestari* has been isolated only from *Amblyomma americanum* ticks in the south-eastern and south-central USA, where it is a putative agent of the "Southern tick-associated rash illness" (STARI) [18, 19]. Among TBRF borreliae of unknown pathogenicity in humans, *Borrelia anserina* is recognized as the agent of fowl spirochetosis [20] and *Borrelia coriaceae* is a putative agent of epizootic bovine abortion [21].

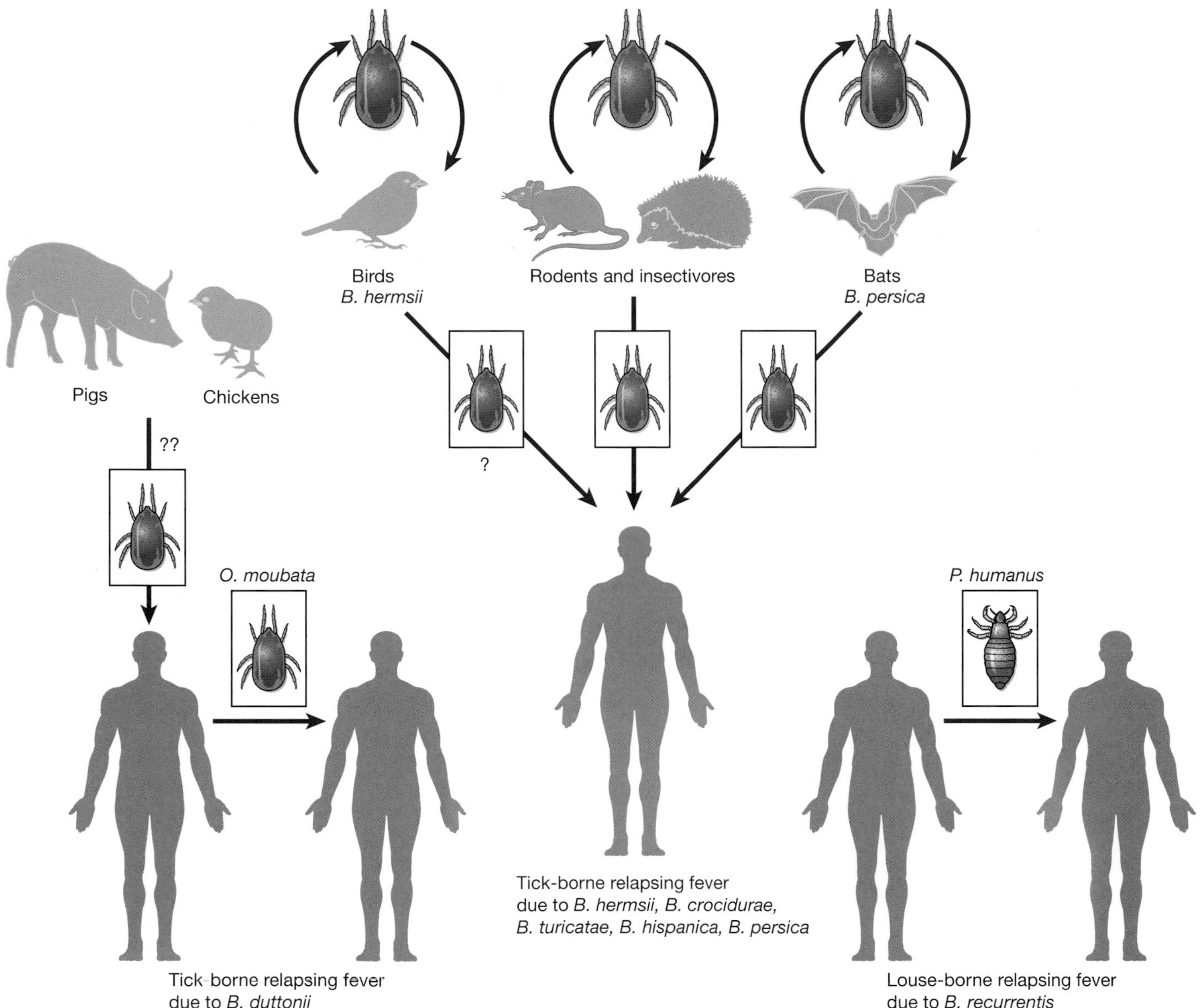

FIGURE 75.1 Reservoirs and epidemiologic cycle for RF borreliae. Question mark indicates that the reservoir/vector is putative in the absence of reproducible, firm data.

The rate of TBRF transmission following the feeding of an infectious tick has been estimated to be of 50%, with an incubation period of 2–18 days [16], but the epidemiology of RF borrelioses is poorly understood as most data are specific to louse-borne RF and TBRF estimates have been made on the basis of sporadic localized studies [4]. Moreover, routine microscopic examination of blood does not allow distinguishing between the various *Borrelia* species [4]. Interestingly, TBRF was found to be the most common bacterial infection in Senegal [22], to be responsible for 27% of hospital admission in Ethiopia [4] and was diagnosed in 21% of patients with unexplained fever in Morocco [23]. In the Democratic Republic of Congo, TBRF was found in 4.3–7.4% of outpatients [14]. In Tanzania, it is responsible for perinatal mortality with rates of 463/1000 in endemic regions [4].

Seasonality of human RF seems to be driven by human activities; in Ethiopian rural settings, a recent study indicated that louse-borne RF (LBRF) was more frequent in the dry season, possibly associated with the seasonal migration of highlanders [4]. In North America, cases are more frequent during spring and summer, in line with vacation periods, [5], and are associated with activities that expose individuals to infectious ticks, including overnight stays in mountain recreational cabins, caves, and crawl spaces under buildings [17, 24, 25].

NATURAL HISTORY, PATHOGENESIS, AND PATHOLOGY

RELAPSING FEVER (RF) BORRELIAE

The genus *Borrelia*, phylum *Spirochetae*, includes a number of borreliae, including Lyme disease borreliae, about 20 species of RF borreliae and reptile-associated borreliae without current medical interest [26] (Fig. 75.3). RF borreliae feature a spiroid morphology and contain a 1.2–1.5 Mb, linear and fragmented genome comprised of one chromosome and 7–16 plasmids [27]. Genomic analyses indicate that RF borreliae have several silent variable membrane protein gene copies kept in a plasmidic library, only one of these being expressed on the chromosome at any given time. Analyses indicate that *B. recurrentis* is a louse-borne derivative of *B. duttonii* undergoing genomic decay [27].

PATHOGENESIS

After inoculation into blood, RF organisms are cleared by an IgM-mediated, complement-independent mechanism targeting the

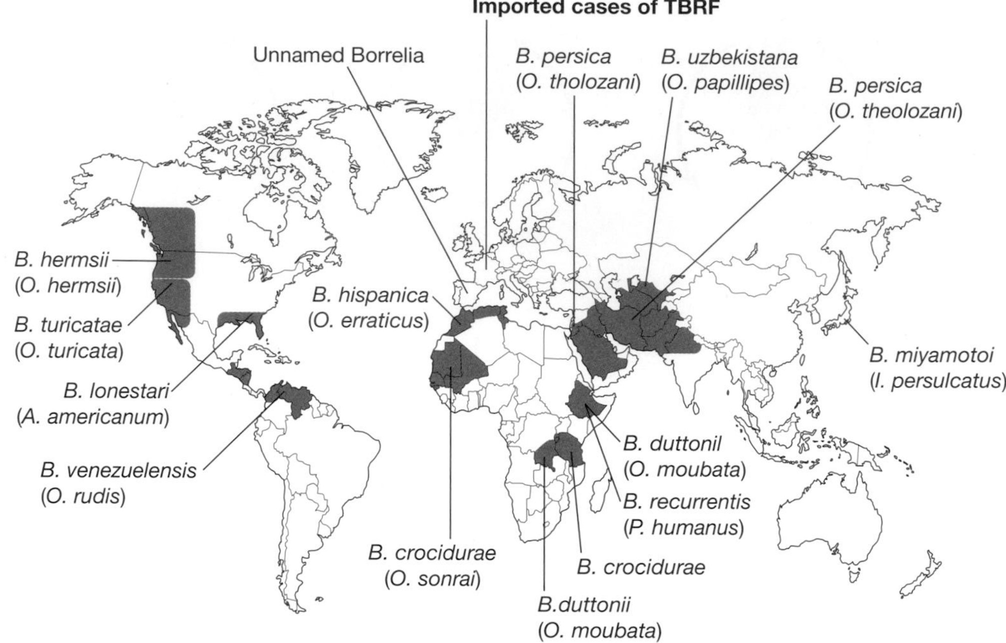

FIGURE 75.2 Geographic distribution of RF borrelioses.

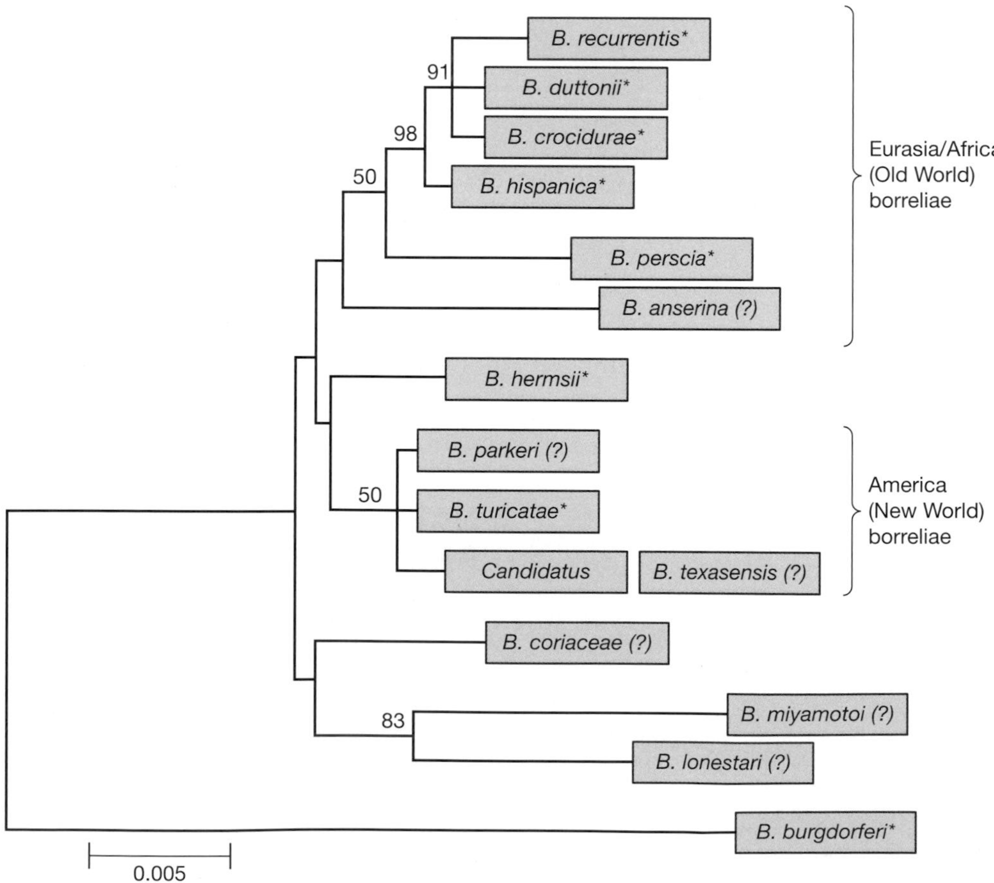

FIGURE 75.3 The various RF borreliae as depicted by analysis of the 16S rDNA gene. Number at node indicates the bootstrap value. *Borrelia burgdorferi*, the Lyme disease *Borrelia*, was put as an outgroup to root the tree. Pathogenicity for human is either certain (*) or unknown (?) when the TBRF has been characterized only in ticks.

expressed variable membrane protein, as well as antibody-independent splenic phagocytosis [28]. The organism undergoes antigen variation, with the expression of a new variable membrane protein resulting in evasion of the immune system, the expansion of a new *Borrelia* clone and an illness characterized as a RF. *Borrelia duttonii* and *B. crocidurae* (but not *B. recurrentis*) bind to erythrocyte neolactoglycans (leading to erythrocyte rosetting), providing borreliae with essential purine metabolites and contributing to immune system evasion, hemorrhages, reduced tissue blood perfusion and tissue invasiveness [4, 29]. Bacteremia results in multisystemic infection of the skin, joints, heart, and the central nervous system, but RF borreliae have never been observed intracellularly. Systemic dissemination results in complications and even death. Congenital TBRF may result from transplacental transmission or may possibly be caused by infection while traversing the birth canal [30]. The brain can remain infected weeks after blood clearance and borreliae entrapped in the brain can re-seed blood in the case of immunosuppression [31]. A Jarisch-Herxheimer reaction is often observed in patients within hours of initiation of treatment with penicillin or tetracyclines and is linked to the lysis of intravascular borreliae with subsequent activation of cytokine cascades and a transient elevation of plasma tumor necrosis factor, interleukin (IL) 6, and IL8 [32].

CLINICAL FEATURES

LBRF is characterized by high fevers that can relapse up to four times (five fever episodes in total); *Borrelia crocidurae* and *B. hispanica* infection have been associated with up to 13 recurrences of fever observed over several months [4]. Fever is accompanied by a flu-like syndrome with rigors, headache, myalgia, and arthralgias in >90% patients [4]. North American TBRF is associated with nausea and vomiting [17]. Evidence of a tick-bite can be found in only 25% of patients, although clinical examination may reveal a transient, erythematous macular lesion at the site of the tick bite [17], tachycardia occurs in >95% of patients, conjunctivitis in >90% of *B. recurrentis*-infected patients, and hepatosplenomegaly in >65% patients [4]. Although TBRF patients may have thrombocytopenia, bleeding complications have been specifically observed in almost a third of LBRF patients and may include epistaxis, purpura, hemoptysis, hematemesis, bloody diarrhea, hematuria, subarachnoidal and cerebral hemorrhages, and retinal hemorrhage [4, 5]. In North American TBRF, dysuria occurs in over 10% of patients, microhematuria in 30% and proteinuria in 46% [5].

Neurologic manifestations are observed in 10–80% patients with *B. duttonii, B. turicatae*, and *B. recurrentis* infection, and in <5% patients with *B. persica, B. hermsii, B. hispanica*, and *B. recurrentis* infection [24]. Neurologic involvement may include meningismus and normal or slightly abnormal cerebrospinal fluid (CSF) in the case of TBRF, but not in the case of LBRF [24]. TBRF borreliae have been isolated from the CSF in African patients. Cranial neuritis and febrile facial palsy have been observed during the second or subsequent relapses with *B. duttonii* and *B. turicatae*, but not in LBRF. Encephalitis may manifest as extreme somnolence, seizures, or hemiplegia for a few weeks. Less common manifestations include myelitis, radiculitis, and neuropsychiatric disturbances.

Ocular complications observed after the third relapse of *B. duttonii, B. hermsii, B. turicatae*, and *B. hispanica* infection (but not LBRF) include iritis, cyclitis, choroiditis, and optic neuritis. Ocular involvement impairs vision [24, 33]. Myocarditis and liver dysfunction are rare. Infection with *B. crocidurae* and *B. hispanica* are associated with a low mortality (<0.2%) [22], but mortality can exceed 30% during untreated LBRF *B. recurrentis* infection [4]. Even with appropriate treatment, mortality can reach 2–6% in LBRF [4].

RF during pregnancy can be severe. *Borrelia crocidurae* provoked one early delivery among 16 women in Senegal [22] and, in one study in the Democratic Republic of Congo, *B. duttonii* was diagnosed in 6.4% of hospitalized pregnant women and was associated with maternal death and spontaneous abortion [14]. In Africa, mortality of TBRF is higher among pregnant women than in the general population [34]. In North America, infection of four pregnant women by *B. hermsii* resulted in congenital TBRF in one case [5].

PATIENT EVALUATION, DIAGNOSIS, AND DIFFERENTIAL DIAGNOSIS

The diagnosis of RF should be considered in any patient presenting with a febrile flu-like syndrome returning from, or living in, a country endemic for RF. In Africa, the diagnosis must be considered in a patient presenting with "*Plasmodium*-negative malaria" or "treatment-resistant malaria" [35]; moreover, malaria co-infection has been reported [4]. A history of tick-bite and a history of RF increase the predictive value of the diagnosis, but bites of soft ticks are usually unnoticed by patients.

Diagnosis usually involves microscopic examination of a blood smear after Giemsa, Wright or Gram staining, or using dark-field microscopy. Thick blood smears should be performed (thin smears are only 20% as sensitive as thick blood smears) [22, 23]. Spirochetemia is usually <200 borreliae/μL in most of *B. crocidurae* and *B. hispanica* cases. It is ten times higher in *B. duttonii* patients and even higher in *B. recurrentis* cases [4]. Quantitative buffy coat (QBC) analysis is effective in the detection of blood *B. crociduare*, but requires a fluorescence microscope [36].

Molecular detection can be performed using whole blood using 16S rDNA-derived primers [23], the noncoding intergenic 16S-23S rDNA spacer [23] or the flagellin-encoding gene *fla* [2] which are common to Lyme disease and TBRF borreliae, whereas the *glp*Q gene is specific for TBRF borreliae [37]. Semi-nested and nested PCR both carry a high risk of contamination and should be avoided. Nested PCR-based detection must be interpreted with caution.

Isolation and culture of borreliae is very sensitive and involves inoculating decontaminated ticks or human blood or CSF into Barbour-Stonner-Kelly (BSK)-H medium [38] complemented by 12% rabbit serum, or into modified Kelly's medium [37] or tick cell line [18]. Inoculation with 200 μL patients' whole blood, the platelet-rich fraction of plasma or the buffy coat is the most sensitive method [36]. Antibiotic susceptibility testing is not a routine test. Animal models indicate that TBRF could be treated with tetracyclines, penicillin, cephalosporins, including ceftriaxone, and aminoglycosides; the latter results disagree with *in vitro* data [24]. Animal studies indicate that chloramphenicol is not effective [24].

Serologic assays are complicated by the fact that RF borreliae extensively alter their surface proteins and by the fact that >10 proteins cross-react with Lyme disease borreliae [5]. As RF borreliae are not widely available, a standardized ELISA for *Borrelia burgdorferi* could be used as a first-line serologic test with Western blot allowing discriminating between cross-reacting RF borreliae, Lyme disease borreliae, and syphilis. A GlpQ assay specific for RF borreliae has also been used [39].

TREATMENT

Rapid administration of an effective antibiotic is mandatory in suspected cases of RF. Patients are most commonly treated with doxycycline (200 mg per day; 1–2 mg/kg/day in children aged >8 years); short-course treatment could be used for LBRF, whereas a 7–21-day treatment is recommended for TBRF in order to prevent relapses [6, 23]. In children <8 years and in pregnant women, 1.5 g/day amoxicillin for 7–21 days could be used. Patients with neurologic involvement may be treated with 2 g ceftriaxone/day for 14 days. A Jarisch-Herxheimer reaction with sudden fever, rigors, and hemodynamic instability has been observed with β-lactams, tetracyclines, erythromycin, and ciprofloxacin [40]; it was reported in almost all patients with LBRF, in up to 59% in *B. duttonii* patients and in up to 54% *B. hermsii* patients, but not in *B. crocidurae* patients [5, 32]. Patients should be observed for at least 2 hours after initiation of antibiotic treatment [5].

Supportive therapy should be undertaken including for patients developing the Jarisch-Herxheimer reaction.

PREVENTION AND CONTROL

Primary prevention of TBRF relies on public education regarding the risk of minimizing rodent exposure, rodent nest manipulation and visiting caves and similar sites [25]. Advice should be given on minimizing exposed skin and pretreating bed nets and clothes with an insecticide such as permethrine or dimethyltoluamide to prevent the attachment of all stages of *Argasidae* ticks to humans [41]. Pre-exposure prophylaxis with amoxicillin has been successfully used [2].

Primary prevention of LBRF relies on cloth hygiene aimed at avoiding body louse infestation [4].

There is no vaccine against RF.

In the case of potential exposure to ticks in high-risk environments, secondary prevention by pre-emptive administration of oral doxycycline (200 mg on day 1 and then 100 mg per day for 4 days) has been demonstrated to be effective and safe [16]. Doxycycline prophylaxis has, however, been associated with photo-allergic rash, photo-onycholysis, nausea, diarrhea, and vaginal itch [41]. People should be informed of these potential side effects and advised to minimize sun exposure.

REFERENCES

1. Obermeier O. Vorkommen feinster eine eigenbewegung zeigender faden im blute von rekurrenskranken. Zentralbl Med Wiss 1873;11:145–5 [in German].
2. Assous MV, Wilamowski A. Relapsing fever borreliosis in Eurasia—forgotten, but certainly not gone! Clin Microbiol Infect 2009;15:407–14.
3. Parola P, Raoult D. Ticks and tick-borne bacterial diseases in humans: an emerging infectious threat. Clin Infect Dis 2001;32:897–e928.
4. Cutler SJ. Relapsing fever—a forgotten disease revealed. J Appl Microbiol 2010;108:115–22.
5. Dworkin MS, Anderson DE Jr, Schwan TG, et al. Tick-borne relapsing fever in the Northwestern United States and Southwestern Canada. Clin Infect Dis 1998;26:122–1.
6. Larsson C, Andersson M, Bergstrom S. Current issues in relapsing fever. Curr Opinion Infect Dis 2009;22:443–9.
7. Houhamdi L, Raoult D. Excretion of living *Borrelia recurrentis* in feces of infected human body lice. J Infect Dis 2005;191:1898–906.
8. Barbour AG. Relapsing fever. In: Goodman JL, Dennis DT, Sonenshine DE, eds. Tick-borne diseases of humans. Washington: ASM Press; 2005:268–91.
9. Evans NJ, Bown K, Timofte D, et al. Fatal borreliosis in bat caused by relapsing fever spirochete, United Kingdom. Emerg Infect Dis 2009;15:1331–33.
10. Gill JS, Ullmann AJ, Loftis AD, et al. Novel relapsing fever spirochetes in bat tick. Emerg Infect Dis 2008;14:522–3.
11. Fischer RJ, Johnson TL, Raffel SJ, Schwan TG. Identical strains of *Borrelia hermsii* in mammal and bird. Emerg Infect Dis 2009;15:2064–6.
12. Takano A, Muto M, Sakata A, et al. Relapsing fever spirochete in seabird tick, Japan. Emerg Infect Dis 2009;15:1528–30.
13. Anda P, Sanchez-Yebra W, del Mar Vitutia M, et al. A new *Borrelia* species isolated from patients with relapsing fever in Spain. Lancet 1996;348:162–5.
14. Tissot Dupont H, La Scola B, Williams R, Raoult D. A focus of tick-borne relapsing fever in Southern Zaire. Clin Infect Dis 1997;25:139–44.
15. Moemenbellah-Fard MD, Benafshi O, Rafinejad J, Ashraf H. Tick-borne relapsing fever in a new highland endemic focus of western Iran. Ann Trop Med Parasitol 2009;103:529–37.
16. Hasin T, Davidovitch N, Cohen R, et al. Postexposure treatment with doxycycline for the prevention of tick-borne relapsing fever. N Engl J Med 2006; 355:148–55.
17. Schwan TG, Raffel SJ, Schrumpf ME, et al. Tick-borne relapsing fever and *Borrelia hermsii*, Los Angeles county, California, USA. Emerg Infect Dis 2009; 15:1026–31.
18. Varela AS, Luttrell MP, Howerth EW, et al. First culture isolation of *Borrelia lonestari*, putative agent of southern tick-associated rash illness. J Clin Microbiol 2004;42:1163–9.
19. James AM, Liveris D, Wormser GP, et al. *Borrelia lonestari* infection after a bite by an *Amblyomma americanum* tick. J Infect Dis 2001;183:1810–14.
20. Lisboa RS, Teixeira RC, Rangel CP, et al. Avian spirochetosis in chickens following experimental transmission of *Borrelia anserina* by *Argas* (*Persicargas*) *miniatus*. Avian Dis 2009;53:166–8.
21. LeFebvre RB, Perng GC. Genetic and antigenic characterization of *Borrelia coriaceae*, putative agent of epizootic bovine abortion. J Clin Microbiol 1989;27:389–93.
22. Vial L, Diatta G, Tall A, et al. Incidence of tick-borne relapsing fever in West Africa: longitudinal study. Lancet 2006;368:37–43.
23. Sarih M, Garnier M, Boudebouch N, et al. Molecular detection of *Borrelia hispanica* relapsing fever in Morocco. Emerg Infect Dis 2009; 15:1626–9.
24. Cadavid D, Barbour AG. Neuroborreliosis during relapsing fever: review of the clinical manifestations, pathology, and treatment of infections in humans and experimental animals. Clin Infect Dis 1998;26:151–64.
25. Maupin WSP, Scott-Wright AO, Craven RB, Dennis DT. Outbreak of tick-borne relapsing fever at the North Rim of the Grand Canyon: evidence for effectiveness of preventive measures. Am J Trop Med Hyg 2002;66:71–5.
26. Takano A, Goka K, Une Y, et al. Isolation and characterization of a novel *Borrelia* group of tick-borne borreliae from imported reptiles and their associated ticks. Environ Microbiol 2010;12:134–46.
27. Lescot M, Audic S, Robert C, et al. The genome of *Borrelia recurrentis*, the agent of deadly louse-borne relapsing fever, is a degraded subset of tick-borne *Borrelia duttonii*. PLoS Genet 2008;4:e1000185.
28. Connolly SE, Benach JL. Cutting edge: the spirochetemia of murine relapsing fever is cleared by complement-independent bactericidal antibodies. J Immunol 2001;167:3029–32.
29. Guo BP, Teneberg S, Münch R, et al. Relapsing fever *Borrelia* binds to neolacto glycans and mediates rosetting of human erythrocytes. Proc Natl Acad Sci USA. 2009;106:19280–5.
30. Fuchs PC, Oyama AA. Neonatal relapsing fever due to transplacental transmission of *Borrelia*. JAMA 1969;208:690–2.
31. Larsson C, Andersson M, Pelkonen J, et al. Persistent brain infection and disease reactivation in relapsing fever borreliosis. Microbes Infect 2006;8: 2213–19.
32. Negussie Y, Remick DG, DeForge LE, et al. Detection of plasma tumor necrosis factor, interleukin 6, and 8 during the Jarisch-Herxheimer reaction of relapsing fever. J Exp Med 1992;175:1207–12.
33. Lim LL, Rosenbaum JT. *Borrelia hermsii* causing relapsing fever and uveitis. Am J Ophthalmol 2006;142:348–9.
34. Barclay A, Coulter J. Tick-borne relapsing fever in central Tanzania. Trans Roy Soc Trop Med Hyg 1990;84:852–6.
35. Nordstrand A, Bunikis I, Larsson C, et al. Tickborne relapsing fever diagnosis obscured by malaria, Togo. Emerg Infect Dis 2007;13:117–23.
36. van Dam AP, van Gool T, Wetsteyn JCFM, Dankert J. Tick-borne relapsing fever imported from West Africa: diagnosis by quantitative buffy coat analysis and in vitro culture of *Borrelia crocidurae*. J Clin Microbiol 1999;37: 2027–30.
37. Halperin T, Orr N, Cohen R, et al. Detection of relapsing fever in human blood samples from Israel using PCR targeting the glycerophosphodiester phosphodiesterase (GlpQ) gene. Acta Trop 2006;98:189–95.
38. Barbour AG. Isolation and cultivation of Lyme disease spirochetes. Yale J Biol Med 1984;57:521–5.
39. Schwan TG, Schrumpf ME, Hinnebusch BJ, et al. GlpQ: an antigen for serological discrimination between relapsing fever and Lyme borreliosis. J Clin Microbiol 1996;34:2483–92.
40. Webster G, Schiffman JD, Dosanjh AS, et al. Jarisch-Herxheimer reaction associated with ciprofloxacin administration for tick-borne relapsing fever. Pediatr Infect Dis J 2002;21:571–3.
41. Croft, AM, Jackson CJ, Darbyshire AH. Doxycycline for the prevention of tick-borne relapsing fever. N Engl J Med 2006;355:1614.

PART

4

THE MYCOSES

76 General Principles

Roderick J Hay

Key features

- Mycoses are diseases caused by fungi and are among the most common microorganisms. Fungi are highly successful organisms that have spread widely; they affect humans both indirectly and directly
- As agents of spoilage and destruction they cause serious losses to crops and stored foodstuffs
- Several fungi can cause disease by invasion of external or internal body surfaces. The type of infection varies from localized superficial colonization of hair shafts to invasive disease with a high mortality
- Fungi may also produce toxins that can be highly potent. Outbreaks of mycotoxicoses have been reported in the tropics where individuals or communities consume grain or other produce that has become moldy
- Fungi may produce airborne spores, sometimes in very large numbers, that can sensitize atopic subjects, causing symptoms of respiratory allergy after inhalation
- Fungal infections are diagnosed by staining and microscopic examination of scrapings, exudates or biopsies, or by culture on specialized media; serology may also be useful
- Management may be the simple application of topical therapies or requires prolonged, complex, and often toxic, systemic treatment

DISTRIBUTION AND MEDICAL IMPORTANCE

Some mycoses are restricted to certain geographic areas; others are worldwide. Their recognition may be comparatively simple but, in many instances, the full spectrum of diagnostic aids, including microscopy, culture, gene analysis and serology are necessary before an etiology can be established. Mycoses do not rank with parasites or bacteria as causes of mortality in the tropics, but they are common causes of morbidity, and individual patients can develop progressively disabling or disseminated disease. Although most fungal infections are acquired exogenously, some mycoses, for example candidosis, are initiated by fungi that are a part of the normal human microflora.

MORPHOLOGY

The basic vegetative organization of most pathogenic fungi is filamentous. In substrates supporting growth, the cells and hyphae are cylindrical or branching, usually about 3–5 μm in diameter, bound by a rigid carbohydrate cell wall. They may have septa along their length. Hyphae increase in length only at their tips. Because they regularly send out side branches, new growing tips are constantly formed and the rate of colonization of host substrate can increase rapidly.

For many fungi, growth of the vegetative phase in artificial media and in the natural environment is followed by development of a reproductive phase. Fungi produce an enormous range of spore types that are useful in distinguishing different species. Spores are also the means by which the pathogen can gain access to its host. Many spores (conidia) are dispersed in the air and infection is acquired by the respiratory route. Some fungi, for example yeasts, are unicellular and reproduce via production of daughter cells by budding.

In several of the more important pathogenic species, fungi may assume one form when growing in their natural habitat (e.g. soil, decaying vegetation) or in culture media, and a different form in parasitized tissue (dimorphism). The saprophytic and pathogenic phases in several species, for example *Histoplasma capsulatum* and *Blastomyces dermatidis*, correspond to filamentous (hyphal) and yeast-like (budding) growth respectively.

DIAGNOSIS

Isolation and identification of the causal agent are valuable laboratory procedures. Serologic tests can be helpful, although they may yield equivocal results. Direct microscopy of skin fragments or scrapings, sputum or examination of tissue sections stained with special fungal stains [e.g. methenamine silver, Grocott modification or periodic acid-Schiff (PAS)] can provide unequivocal evidence of fungal etiology and identity. A feature of most mycoses is the development of a host immune response, including the appearance of specific antibodies. Immunologic tests may therefore be of value in epidemiologic studies (using skin tests to assess previous infection) and in diagnosis (using serologic procedures to detect and quantitate specific antibodies). Increasingly, genetic methods are used in diagnosis, epidemiology and for the investigation of pathogenesis, although there are few commercial diagnostic tests.

DISEASE CLASSIFICATION

Traditionally, mycoses have been classified according to their route of infection and body site [1-4].

SUPERFICIAL MYCOSES (see Chapter 77)

These mycoses, for example pityriasis versicolor, affect only the outer layers of the epidermis. Living tissues are seldom invaded. Some of these mycoses, for example tinea, although confined to keratinized parts of the body, can elicit acute or chronic inflammatory changes in the skin. These changes can be painful, unsightly or disfiguring. Invasion of nails can result in dystrophy. Superficial mycoses can be acute or chronic, inflammatory or non-inflammatory, and – unusually among fungal infections – acquired via person-to-person transmission.

SUBCUTANEOUS MYCOSES OR MYCOSES OF IMPLANTATION (see Chapter 78)

These diseases, for example mycetoma, are introduced through the skin surface by a penetrating wound, such as a thorn prick or splinter wound. The agents are usually environmental saprophytes. Once established they provoke an intense and destructive host response. The lesions tend to be localized and progressive, usually without a tendency to heal spontaneously.

SYSTEMIC MYCOSES (see Chapters 79, 80)

Some of the respiratory mycoses, for example histoplasmosis, are acquired by inhalation of airborne spores, with the initial site of multiplication in the lung. While most infections are self-limiting, serious progressive or disseminated disease occurs in a small proportion of patients, particularly those who are immunocompromised. Opportunistic mycotic infections (see Chapter 79), for example zygomycosis, are able to infect because of the susceptibility of the host, rather than an inherent pathogenicity of the fungus. They occur in patients whose normal defenses have been compromised by AIDS, leukemia, diabetes, and malnutrition, for example, or by defects in the immune system, by cancer or transplantation chemotherapy, or by treatment with broad-spectrum antibiotics.

REFERENCES

1. Chandler F, Kaplan W, Ajello L. A Color Atlas and Textbook of the histopathology of mycotic diseases. London: Wolfe Medical Publications; 1980.
2. Merz WG, Hay RJ, eds. Medical Mycology. In: Topley and Wilson's Microbiology and Microbial Infections. London: Hodder Arnold; 2005.
3. Kibbler CC, McKenzie DWR, Odds FC. Principles and Practice of Clinical Mycology. Chichester: Wiley; 1996.
4. Dismukes WE, Pappas PG, Sobel JD. Clinical Mycology. New York: Oxford University Press; 2003.

77 Superficial Mycoses

Roderick J Hay

77.1 Dermatophyte Infection (Ringworm, Tinea)

Key features

- Filamentous fungal infections of skin, hair, and nails
- Acquired from animals, other humans, or soil
- Cause tinea or ringworm infections
- Scalp, groin, and body infections common in tropics
- Respond to topical azoles or oral antifungal drugs such as terbinafine, griseofulvin, or itraconazole

INTRODUCTION

The dermatophytes cause infections (ringworm or tinea) that are confined to the superficial stratum corneum, as well as keratinized structures, for example hair or nail arising from skin [1]. In temperate climates, tinea pedis affects the interdigital spaces on the feet and is the most common symptomatic form of ringworm in the tropics, however, groin, body, and scalp infections are more prevalent. Infections are derived from three main sources – humans (anthropophilic), animals (zoophilic), and soil (geophilic). Zoophilic infections tend to produce lesions of the scalp or body and are often highly inflammatory. The anthropophilic organisms can cause lesions in any site and, depending on the species involved, the inflammatory response is often minimal. Organisms originating from soil are uncommon. The fungi that cause dermatophyte infections in humans are confined to three genera, defined by culture or genetic characteristics: *Trichophyton*, *Microsporum*, and *Epidermophyton*.

EPIDEMIOLOGY

The most common cause of ringworm worldwide is *Trichophyton rubrum* (Table 77-1). *Trichophyton violaceum* has been isolated predominantly from patients in India and the Far and Middle East.

Distribution of agents of scalp ringworm throughout the tropical world is complex [2]. In sub-Saharan Africa, there is considerable variation in the types of scalp ringworm. Frequently, small pockets of infection with distinct organisms occur, for example *Microsporum audouinii* in West Africa and *T. violaceum* in North Africa, India, East Africa, and the Middle East. The factors underlying this pattern include the stability of the population, absence of control measures and, on occasion, spread via external agents, such as hairdressers' equipment [3].

TINEA IMBRICATA

Trichophyton concentricum is the cause of the tropical infection known as tinea imbricata or tokelau. It is characterized by the appearance of homogeneous sheets or concentric rings of scaling that may cover large areas of the body (Fig. 77.1). Tinea imbricata is best known in the Pacific Islands and Melanesia, but reports of the disease in isolated populations, often living in primitive conditions, have been reported from Malaysia, India, Brazil, and Mexico.

NATURAL HISTORY, PATHOLOGY, AND PATHOGENESIS

Infection follows transfer from an individual or animal source by contact. Host resistance to dermatophytosis depends on several innate and acquired immunologic factors. These include increased epidermal turnover, locally produced peptides and fatty acids, and transferrin. In addition, acquired immunity mediated through T lymphocyte (Th1) cytokines is critical, although its effectiveness is reduced in non-inflammatory infections, for example the soles of the feet and tinea imbricata.

CLINICAL MANIFESTATIONS

The clinical features of dermatophytosis depend on the site of infection. In temperate areas, occluded surfaces, such as the groin, toe webs, and axillae are most often infected, but in the tropics any site can be involved.

FOOT INFECTIONS

Athlete's foot or tinea pedis is a term used to describe scaling and maceration accompanied by itching between the toes, particularly the fourth interdigital space. It is a syndrome that may be caused by *Candida* species, erythrasma or Gram-negative bacteria, as well as by dermatophytes. In dermatophyte infections, the area between the toes may be wet or dry and, in some infections, particularly those caused by *Trichophyton interdigitale*, vesicular. Involvement of the dorsum of the foot or the sole may occur. The commonest cause is *T. rubrum*.

Symptoms may be minimal. It is more common in people who wear shoes and socks and is therefore associated with urban areas in the tropics.

Tinea pedis in tropical areas must be distinguished from eczema and, less commonly, plantar psoriasis [4]. The interplay between bacteria and fungi is poorly understood but, in the tropics, secondary Gram-negative bacterial infection on top of interdigital dermatophytosis can occur.

TABLE 77-1 The Most Common Dermatophyte Fungi in the Tropics

Genus	Species	Source
Trichophyton		
	T. rubrum	Humans
	T. mentagrophytes	Humans, rodents, cats, dogs
	T. tonsurans	Humans
	T. concentricum	Humans
	T. violaceum	Humans
Microsporum	*T. soudanense*	Humans
Epidermophyton	*M. audouinii*	Humans
	M. canis	Cats, dogs
	M. gypseum	Soil
	E. floccosum	Humans

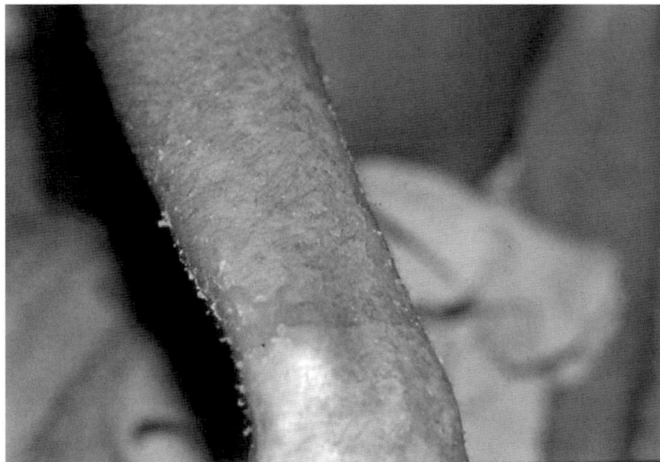

FIGURE 77.1 Tinea imbricata, caused by *T. concentricum*, is characterized by concentric rings of scales *(image courtesy of the Armed Forces Institute of Pathology, Photograph Neg. No. 39237).*

Two non-dermatophyte fungi (*Scytalidium dimidiatum* and *Scytalidium hyalinum*) cause infections that closely resemble the dry type of palmar, plantar, interdigital and nail infections caused by *T. rubrum* [5].

TINEA CRURIS (RINGWORM OF THE GROIN)

Dermatophyte infections of the groin are frequently seen in the tropics. A ring of itchy erythema with a scaling margin radiates from the groin down the inner border of the thigh (Fig. 77.2). Tinea cruris is more common in males and may extend posteriorly to include the intergluteal cleft. In women in tropical areas, an extensive form of ringworm may be found in the waist area that involves a large part of the skin surface around the hip girdle. *Candida* intertrigo may closely resemble tinea cruris.

TINEA CORPORIS (RINGWORM OF THE BODY)

The characteristic lesion of dermatophyte infection on trunk or limbs is an annular plaque with a varying degree of erythema and a prominent edge (kerion) (Fig. 77.3). Scaling is most prominent at this margin [6]; however, appearance varies with the organism and host. Particularly in the tropics, *T. rubrum* can be associated with persistent and minimally inflammatory tinea corporis. Discoid eczema, impetigo, psoriasis, and discoid lupus erythematosus can be mistaken for ringworm.

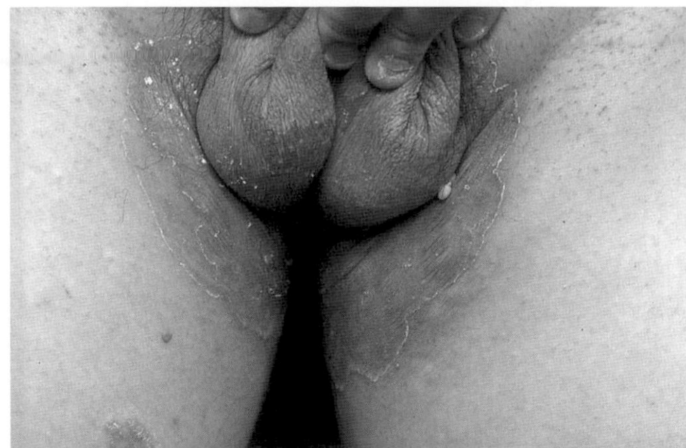

FIGURE 77.2 Tinea cruris caused by *T. rubrum* *(image courtesy of the St John's Institute of Dermatology, London).*

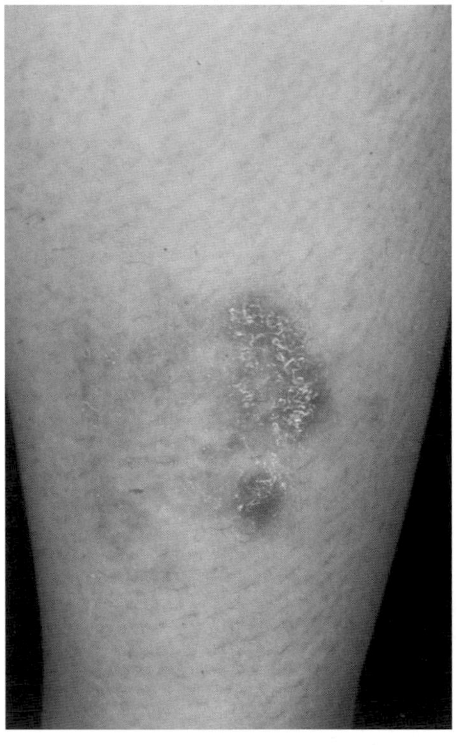

FIGURE 77.3 Tinea corporis caused by *T. rubrum* *(image courtesy of the St John's Institute of Dermatology, London).*

TINEA CAPITIS (RINGWORM OF THE SCALP)

Invasion of scalp hairs is seen with certain dermatophytes. In some, particularly those spread from animals, scalp hairs often break several millimeters above the skin surface. There can be considerable exudation and erythema. In other infections, including many of those spread from child to child, the onset is insidious. Hairs break at scalp level and inflammation can be minimal. Most cases present with hair loss, usually in patches, and a varying degree of scaling (Fig. 77.4). However, kerions (very inflammatory pustular lesions) can develop.

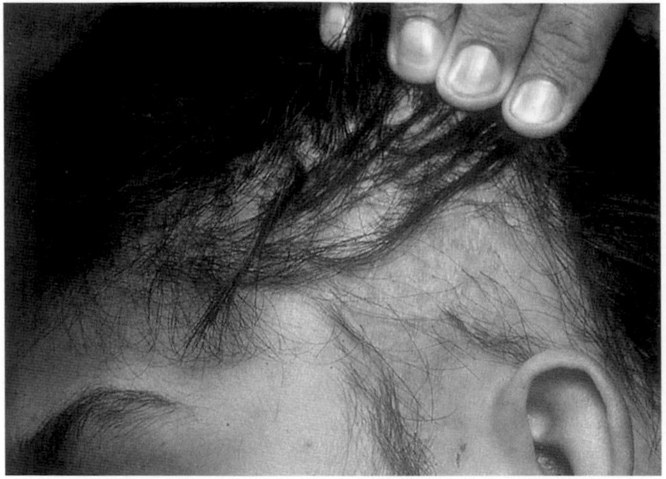

FIGURE 77.4 Tinea capitis, caused by *Microsporum audouinii*, presents with multiple patches of alopecia with scaling in this boy *(image courtesy of the Armed Forces Institute of Pathology, Photograph Neg. 7–6860).*

Favus, a scalp infection seen in some parts of Africa, for example Ethiopia, presents with hair loss accompanied by the formation of crusts or scutula. These tend to coalesce to form a dense mat in patches or large areas of the scalp. The diagnosis of tinea capitis is facilitated by filtered ultraviolet light examination (Wood's light), although only *Microsporum* species fluoresce under these conditions. Ringworm of the scalp must be distinguished from seborrheic dermatitis, psoriasis, or cicatricial alopecia. The last may be produced in end-stage favus.

ONYCHOMYCOSIS

Dermatophyte invasion of the nails is uncommon in the tropics. The nail plate is invaded from the distal border and lateral surfaces, usually from the underside. The affected nail becomes thickened and opaque with a varying degree of onycholysis. Patients often have infection of other sites, such as the soles or toe webs. In addition to psoriasis, other fungal infections, for example candida or *Scytalidium*, must be differentiated from onychomycosis caused by dermatophytes [7].

DERMATOPHYTOSIS OF OTHER SITES

Dermatophytosis of the beard area (tinea barbae) may be highly inflammatory and persistent. Involvement of the palms is most commonly with *T. rubrum*. Often, only one hand is involved and the fingernails on that side may be invaded. The palm shows mild scaling similar to the dry type of sole infection.

DIAGNOSIS

Although not essential, laboratory diagnosis is helpful as the clinical diagnosis is not always reliable – particularly in scalp ringworm. Scrapings or a hair sample can be taken from the lesion with a scalpel, mounted in 10% potassium hydroxide and examined with a microscope.

CULTURE

Scrapings or hairs can be plated onto Sabouraud's agar. Their gross and microscopic appearance, as well as nutritional requirements, are used in identification. Molecular probes can identify and type organisms.

TREATMENT

TOPICAL THERAPY

Dermatophytoses can be treated topically. Topically applied dyes are known to have weak antifungal properties and may be sufficient to treat some dermatophytes, for example tinea cruris. Gentian violet and magenta paint are examples. Whitfield's ointment (BPC), which contains 3% salicylic acid and 3% benzoic acid, is a weak antifungal agent but is inexpensive and effective in treating all dermatophyte infections apart from scalp or nail disease, or kerion.

TOPICAL ANTIFUNGALS

Antifungal compounds include imidazole creams or ointments (miconazole, clotrimazole, econazole, and bifonazole) and terbinafine [8]. All are available for topical therapy in 1–2% concentration. Many are also effective against candidiasis and pityriasis versicolor. Topical antifungals have no place in the management of tinea capitis.

SYSTEMIC THERAPY

For nail and scalp disease, or extensive or severe infections, including kerion, systemic treatment is necessary. Griseofulvin is given in a daily dose of 500–1000 mg in adults or 10 mg/kg in children. For scalp infections, 6–8 weeks of treatment are usually necessary. More rapid treatment for these indications is provided by terbinafine (250 mg daily) and itraconazole (100–400 mg daily) [9]. These agents shorten the treatment period and provide effective therapy; however, they are more expensive than griseofulvin.

77.2 Superficial Candidiasis

Key features

- Caused by yeast fungi
- Patients, apart from those with vulvo-vaginal infection, usually have a predisposing reason for candidiasis
- Oral infection can be an early sign of AIDS
- Avoid long-term treatment (more than 1 month) with fluconazole if the infection is not responding as drug resistance can develop

DEFINITION

Superficial infections caused by species of the genus *Candida*. They include thrush and vaginal candidiasis, as well as interdigital candidiasis [10].

EPIDEMIOLOGY

Candidiasis occurs throughout the world. *Candida albicans* is the organism most commonly associated with superficial candidiasis; however, other species, such as *Candida tropicalis* or *Candida guilliermondii*, can be involved. *Candida albicans* is a common saprophyte on mucosal surfaces, particularly in the mouth, gastrointestinal tract, and

TABLE 77-2 Predisposing Factors in Superficial Candidiasis

Infancy, pregnancy, old age
Occlusion of epithelial surfaces, for example by dentures, occlusive dressings
Disorders of immune function
- Primary, for example chronic granulomatous disease
- Secondary, for example HIV/AIDS, leukemia, corticosteroid therapy

Chemotherapy
- Immunosuppressive
- Antibiotic

Endocrine disease, for example diabetes mellitus
Carcinoma
Miscellaneous, for example damaged nail folds

vagina. Oral colonization may begin in infancy, although its incidence is increased by a number of factors, including hospitalization and bottle-feeding. *Candida albicans* can be isolated from the environment, often where contact with humans is frequent, such as wash basins and drinking bowls.

NATURAL HISTORY AND PATHOGENESIS

When *C. albicans* causes infection as opposed to colonization, it is usually in individuals with predisposing factors (Table 77-2). Some of these factors are systemic and others relate to local conditions on the skin or mucosa. The effect of climate on infection is unknown, although in the tropics there is a high incidence of saprophytic carriage of *Candida* species.

CLINICAL MANIFESTATIONS

ORAL CANDIDIASIS (THRUSH)

This is common, particularly in the elderly, infants, and denture wearers [11]. It can follow immunosuppression or antibiotic therapy and is an important marker of AIDS. Infection presents with solitary or confluent white plaques on the oral mucosa (pseudomembranous candidiasis). Alternatively, the mucosa may appear glazed and erythematous (erythematous candidiasis). Oral candidiasis in AIDS patients in the tropics is often accompanied by esophageal infection [12]. One of the earliest features of oral candidiasis is the appearance of cracking at the angles of the mouth, or angular cheilitis.

VAGINAL CANDIDIASIS

Vaginal infection with *Candida* is common and although it can be associated with diabetes and the third trimester of pregnancy, the majority of those affected have no obvious underlying abnormality. The symptoms of vaginal candidiasis are irritation and discomfort associated with a creamy discharge. Similar to oral infection, the vaginal mucosa can be covered with small white plaques or become red and friable. Infection must be distinguished from *Trichomonas* and gonorrhea. Candidiasis of the groin is erythematous with a prominent border. Small "satellite" pustules or crusts are often seen outside this border.

PARONYCHIA AND CANDIDA ONYCHOMYCOSIS

Infection of the nail folds by *Candida* species is a cause of paronychia. The periungual skin is raised and painful, and a prominent gap develops between the fold and the nail plate. Rarely, invasion of the nail plate with onycholysis occurs. The condition is caused by a number of factors, including bacterial infection, although women with heavy domestic responsibilities (e.g. washing, cooking) seem to be predisposed. Superficial erosion on the web space between the fingers can also be caused by *Candida* infection in the tropics.

CANDIDA INTERTRIGO

Candida intertrigo is the name given to a painful or irritative inflammatory dermatosis confined to body folds; secondary bacterial infections can contribute to the process. Infection is most common in overweight or diabetic subjects.

DIAGNOSIS

Laboratory diagnosis is made by demonstration of *Candida* in potassium hydroxide wet mounts. Yeast and hyphal forms are both seen. *Candida* can be cultured on Sabouraud's agar.

TREATMENT

Topical treatment with gentian violet is effective in some patients. However, locally applied amphotericin, nystatin, or an imidazole preparation is preferable, and powders, lotions, and/or pessaries (vaginal tablets) are available. Oral treatments for superficial candidiasis are fluconazole, itraconazole, voriconazole, posaconazole, and ketoconazole. These are best reserved for severe oral or chronic forms of candidiasis. AIDS patients with oral candidiasis should usually be treated with fluconazole, but may respond to topical therapy [13]. Resistance to fluconazole can develop if the drug is continuously employed in clinically unresponsive infection. Vaginal infections respond to intensive topical therapy given for 3–5 days using a combination of cream and pessaries; however, a single dose of fluconazole is more effective and convenient.

77.3 Pityriasis (Tinea) Versicolor

Key features

- Very common in the tropics
- Diffuse hypo- or hyper-pigmented non-itchy scales on upper trunk
- Responds to selenium sulfide or topical azole creams
- Relapse is common

INTRODUCTION

Pityriasis versicolor is caused by the lipophilic yeast, *Malassezia*, and is widespread in the tropics. *Malassezia* species are present as saprophytes on normal skin. There are at least six species commonly found. Development of pityriasis versicolor lesions is usually accompanied by the formation of short, stubby hyphae. Rarely, disease can occur in immunocompromised individuals, although seldom in HIV infection.

EPIDEMIOLOGY

Infection occurs throughout the world and is extremely common in the tropics where, in some areas, 60% of the population may be infected.

PATHOLOGY AND PATHOGENESIS

Malassezia normally inhabits the superficial layers of keratin, particularly around the orifices of hair follicles [14].

The development of hyphal forms can be observed during immunosuppressive therapy, which suggests that immune factors play a role in preventing infection. Exposure to sunlight, heat, and humidity, as well as locally applied oils, have been thought to be risk factors.

CLINICAL MANIFESTATIONS

The lesions of pityriasis versicolor are small, scaling macules that are hypopigmented or hyperpigmented (Fig. 77.5) [15]. Scaling is usually not prominent but can be elicited by scratching affected areas. This feature is helpful in distinguishing this infection from other types of macular pigmentary disorders, for example vitiligo. Under Wood's light, the patches can fluoresce pale yellow. The areas most commonly infected are the upper trunk, neck, and upper arms. In the tropics, infection can extend beyond these areas to involve the face, abdomen, lower arms, and penis. The rash is rarely symptomatic but may cause concern because of its superficial resemblance to certain types of leprosy.

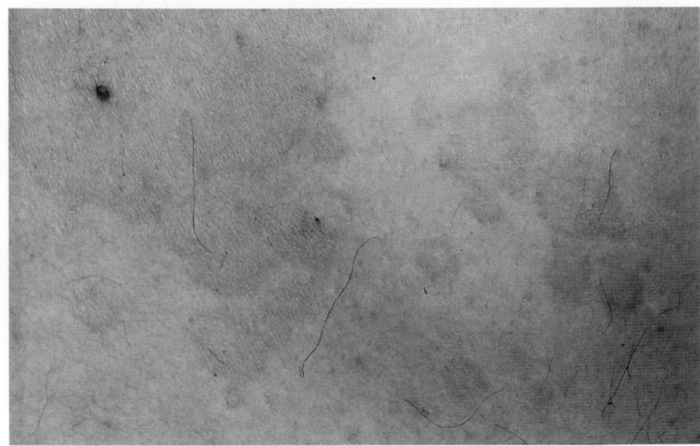

FIGURE 77.5 Pityriasis (tinea) versicolor on the chest *(image courtesy of the St John's Institute of Dermatology, London).*

DIAGNOSIS

The diagnosis can be confirmed by demonstration of clusters of yeast and pseudo-hyphae in potassium hydroxide mounts. Recognition of the fungi is facilitated by the addition of equal quantities of blue-black ink to the potassium hydroxide.

TREATMENT

Application of 2.5% selenium sulfide twice daily for 7–10 days is usually effective. The response to a topical imidazole may be more rapid, and 5 days of 200 mg itraconazole is also reported to be effective.

77.4 Other Superficial Mycoses

BLACK PIEDRA

Black piedra is an uncommon, persistent infection confined to hair shafts and is seen in small endemic areas in the tropics, for example Latin America or Central Africa. Individual or case clusters can occur. The hallmark of this condition is the presence of small, gritty nodules on hair shafts. These represent areas of hyphal invasion in which characteristic spores (ascospores) of the organism *Piedraia hortae* can be found.

WHITE PIEDRA

White piedra is caused by the yeasts *Trichosporon inkin, Trichosporon ashasii*, or *Trichosporon mucoides*. The clinical appearances are similar to those of black piedra, although the swellings are "softer" and pale [16]. The infected sites may involve hair on the scalp, groin or, rarely, the axillae. Infections are not commonly diagnosed, but have been recognized in different climates, from temperate to tropical.

TINEA NIGRA

Tinea nigra is a superficial tropical infection caused by a black yeast, *Phaeoanellomyces werneckii* and is associated with focal areas of hyperpigmentation, usually on the palms or soles [17]. Infection is primarily in Central and South America, as well as in the Far East. Characteristically, the lesion is a dark brown or black stain that appears on the palms or the soles and, on rare occasions, elsewhere. There is little scaling and multiple lesions are rare. The diagnosis can be confirmed by demonstration of characteristic darkly pigmented arthrospores in scrapings. The infection responds well to Whitfield's ointment.

REFERENCES

1. Graser Y, de Hoog GS, Summerbell RC. Dermatophytes: recognizing species of clonal fungi. Med Mycol 2006;44:199–209.
2. Elewski BE. Tinea capitis: a current perspective. J Am Acad Dermatol 2000;42:1–20.
3. Gugnani HC, Njoku-Obi ANU. Tinea capitis in school children in East Nigeria. Mykosen 1986;29:132–44.
4. Howell SA, Clayton YM, Phan QG, Noble WC. Tinea pedis: The relationship between symptoms, organisms and host characteristics. Microbiol Ecol Health Dis 1988;1:131–5.
5. Hay RJ, Moore MK. Clinical features of superficial fungal infections caused by *Hendersonula toruloidea* and *Scytalidium hyalinum*. Br J Dermatol 1984;110: 677–83.
6. Hay RJ. Fungal infections. Clin Dermatol 2006;24:201–12.
7. Roberts DT. Onychomycosis: current treatment and future challenges. Br J Dermatol 1999;141(suppl. 56):1–4.
8. Wright S, Robertson VJ. An institutional survey of tinea capitis in Harare, Zimbabwe and a trial of miconazole cream versus Whitfield's ointment in its treatment. Clin Exp Dermatol 1986;11:371–7.
9. Fuller LC, Smith CH, Cerio R, et al. A randomized comparison of 4 weeks of terbinafine vs. 8 weeks of griseofulvin for the treatment of tinea capitis. Br J Dermatol 2001;144:321–7.
10. Edwards JE. *Candida* species. In: Mandell GL, Bennett JE, Dolin R, eds. Principles and Practice of Infectious Diseases, 7th edn. Philadelphia: Churchill Livingstone; 2010:3225–40.
11. Samaranayake LP, Yaacob HB. Classification of oral candidiasis. In: Samaranayake LP, MacFarlane TW, eds. Oral Candidiasis. London: Wright; 1990.

12. Khongkunthian P, Grote M, Isaratanan W. Oral manifestations in 45 HIV-positive children from Northern Thailand. J Oral Pathol Med 2001; 30:549–52.
13. Mofenson LM, Brady MT, Danner SP, et al. Guidelines for the Prevention and Treatment of Opportunistic Infections among HIV-exposed and HIV-infected children: recommendations from CDC, the National Institutes of Health, the HIV Medicine Association of the Infectious Diseases Society of America, the Pediatric Infectious Diseases Society, and the American Academy of Pediatrics. MMWR Recomm Rep 2009;58:1–166.
14. Ashbee HR. Recent developments in the immunology and biology of *Malassezia* species. FEMS Immunol Med Microbiol 2006;47:14–23.
15. Crespo Erchiga V, Delgado Florencio V. *Malassezia* species in skin diseases. Curr Opin Infect Dis 2002;15:133–42.
16. Therizol-Ferly M, Kombila M, Gomez de Diaz M, et al. White piedra and *Trichosporon* species in equatorial Africa: 1. History and clinical aspects: an analysis of 449 superficial inguinal specimens. Mycoses 1994;37:249–53.
17. Perez C, Colella MT, Olaizola C, et al. Tinea nigra: report of twelve cases in Venezuela. Mycopathologia 2005;160:235–8.

78 Subcutaneous Mycoses: General Principles

Roderick J Hay

INTRODUCTION

Subcutaneous mycoses are chronic fungal infections resulting from the percutaneous inoculation of agents from an exogenous source. The primary site of multiplication is the dermis or subcutis and although lesions generally remain localized to the site of inoculation, there is slow and inexorable spread to surrounding tissue. Lesions usually do not undergo spontaneous remission and, if unchecked, tissue destruction can be severe. Dissemination is rare.

78.1 Mycetoma (Maduromycosis, Madura foot)

Key features

- Caused by either fungi (eumycetoma) or filamentous bacteria (actinomycetoma)
- Mainly seen in dry tropics
- Present with draining sinuses
- Discharge of one or more grains from lesions is key to the diagnosis
- Actinomycetomas usually respond to antibiotics but eumycetomas are seldom curable with antifungals alone

INTRODUCTION

Mycetoma is a chronic, localized, slowly progressive, subcutaneous infection caused by species of actinomycetes or fungi [1]. It is characterized by destructive granulomatous and suppurative responses, and by draining sinus tracts that can communicate with each other and with the skin surface. In affected tissues, filaments of the causal agents form compact grains or granules.

Mycetoma has multiple etiologies, with more than 20 species of fungi or bacteria implicated. About 60% of infections are caused by actinomycetes (actinomycetoma) and 40% by filamentous fungi (eumycetoma) (Table 78-1). It is important to know whether the cause is a fungus or bacterium in order to determine the correct therapy.

EPIDEMIOLOGY

Mycetoma is endemic in many tropical countries and is most commonly reported from Africa, Central and South America, India, and the Far East. It occurs in regions with a short rainy season of 4–6 months, daily temperature range of 30–37°C, and a humidity of 60–80%, alternating with a dry season.

Areas of endemicity are characterized by savannah or forest and the presence of thorny trees or bushes, such as Acacia scrub. Many of the agents causing mycetoma have been isolated from soil, local plants, or trees. Patients are often field laborers or herdsmen whose occupation exposes them to minor penetrating injuries.

NATURAL HISTORY, PATHOGENESIS, AND PATHOLOGY

Infection is initiated by traumatic implantation, often by the piercing of skin or mucosal surfaces with thorns or wood splinters [2]. Once introduced subcutaneously, the agent begins to grow, eliciting a suppurative inflammatory response that is predominantly neutrophilic but can be accompanied by a granulomatous reaction. The agent appears in infected tissues as compact grains or granules up to 5 milimeters in diameter whose microscopic appearance may be diagnostic of the infecting species. A key feature is the formation of sinuses and fistulae that interconnect and erupt onto the skin surface.

CLINICAL FEATURES

The initial lesion, which appears several months after the traumatic incident, is a small, firm, painless subcutaneous nodule or plaque that progressively increases in size. The evolution of eumycetoma and actinomycetoma can differ. Lesions of eumycetoma are firm, remain localized and progress slowly. Skin papules or nodules form pustular lesions discharging sanguinous or purulent exudates. As it progresses, there is deformity and the production of draining sinus tracts through which fungal grains are expelled (Fig. 78.1). In actinomycetoma, progression is often rapid. Lesions have less well-defined margins, sinus tracts are prominent and involvement of bone is earlier and more extensive than in eumycetomas.

Most mycetomas are painless, even when well established. Mycetoma can result in loss of function of an infected limb and consequent inability to work as the condition does not spontaneously remit. The foot is the most common site involved with about 70% of infections affecting the lower limbs. Other sites include the buttocks and perineum, hands, back, and scalp.

DIAGNOSIS AND DIFFERENTIAL DIAGNOSIS

IMAGING

X-ray, ultrasound, and magnetic resonance imaging (MRI) scanning are useful in delineating the extent and presence of bone invasion. Cavities, periosteal spicule, and proliferation formation are present [3].

TABLE 78-1 Macro- and Microscopic Features of Mycetoma Grains

Organism	Size (mm)	Consistency	Appearances in hematoxylin and eosin-stained sections
Eumycetoma			
1. Dark grains			
Madurella mycetomatis	0.2–5.0	Hard, brittle	Cement, compact, vesicles sometimes
Madurella grisea	0.34–5.0	Soft	Cement lacking, compact outer layer
Leptosphaeria senegalensis	0.44–6.0	Soft	Cement, dark periphery with vesicular center
Exophiala jeanselmei	0.24–3.0	Soft	Cement absent, often hollow
Pyrenochaeta romeroi	0.34–6.0	Soft	Cement lacking, compact outer layer
2. Pale grains			
Fusarium species	0.1–2.0	Soft	Compact, pigment lacking, interwoven fungal filaments
Acremonium species	0.1–2.0	Soft	Compact, pigment lacking, interwoven fungal filaments
Scedosporium apiospermum	0.1–2.0	Soft	Compact, pigment lacking, interwoven fungal filaments
Aspergillus nidulans	0.1–2.0	Soft	Compact, pigment lacking, interwoven fungal filaments
Neotestudina rosatii	0.1–2.0	Soft	Compact, pigment lacking, interwoven fungal filaments
Actinomycetoma			
1. Pale (white-to-yellow) grains			
Actinomadura madurae	0.14–5.0	Soft	Variegated
Nocardia brasiliensis	0.04–1.0	Soft	Small, pale blue, eosinophilic
2. Yellow-to-brown grains			
Streptomyces somaliensis	0.24–6.0	Soft	Grains fractured, basophilic
3. Red-to-pink grains			
Actinomadura pelletieri	0.064–2.0	Soft	Small, basophilic

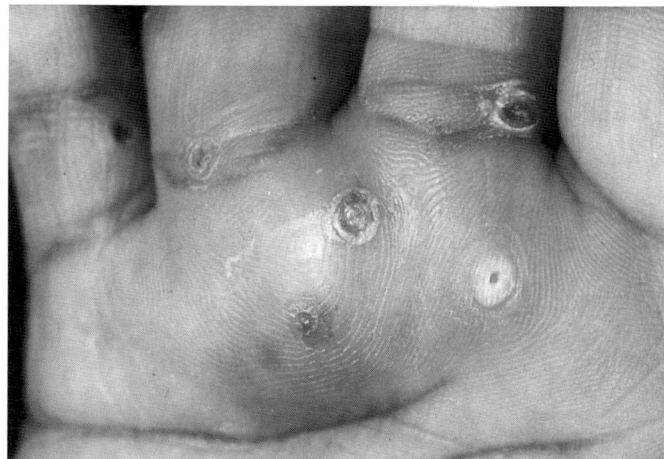

FIGURE 78.1 Mycetoma (eumycetoma) affecting the palm *(image courtesy of the St John's Institute of Dermatology, London).*

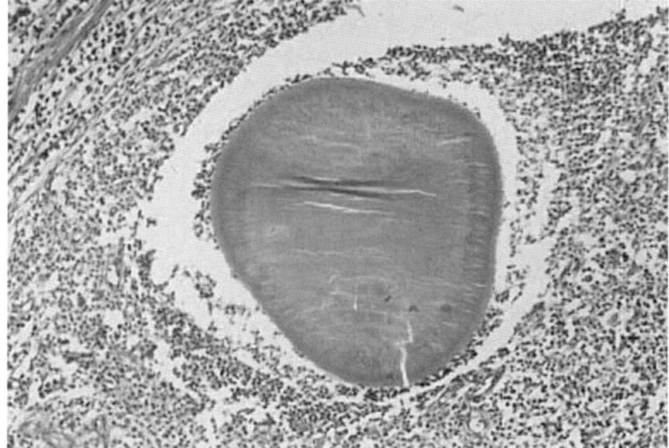

FIGURE 78.2 Grain of *Streptomyces somaliensis* surrounded by acute inflammatory cells (hematoxylin and eosin stain, magnification ×360; *image courtesy of the St John's Institute of Dermatology, London).*

DIAGNOSIS

Grains produced by different agents may be distinctive enough for the diagnosis to be made by examination of hematoxylin and eosin-stained tissue sections (Fig. 78.2). Fungal grains have a coarser texture and may be pigmented, consisting of a dense mass of interwoven filaments (hyphae) 2–5 μm in diameter. Actinomycete grains are more finely textured – the filaments are 1 μm or less in diameter – and are not individually distinguishable.

DIRECT EXAMINATION

Exudates should be examined for the presence of grains. Opening a surface pustule over a sinus tract with a sterile needle may reveal them.

Differentiation of fungal and actinomycete grains is readily achieved by crushing the grain between two glass slides and examining it microscopically with 10% potassium hydroxide.

CULTURE OR MOLECULAR DETECTION

In view of the multiple etiologies, a range of culture media and conditions of incubation should be employed. There are no commercially available molecular tests.

DIFFERENTIAL DIAGNOSIS

Chronic osteomyelitis of bacterial etiology, for example syphilitic, actinomycotic or tuberculous may resemble mycetoma, particularly in the early stages. Botryomycosis, in which persistent bacterial infection is associated with granule and sinus formation, must also be distinguished.

TREATMENT

EUMYCETOMA

Eumycetoma is poorly responsive to chemotherapy; however, a trial of chemotherapy may be justified. Some *Madurella mycetomatis* infections respond to ketoconazole or itraconazole, and voriconazole is active in some cases [4]. Radical surgical removal is an alternative. In advanced cases of eumycetoma, amputation may be the only way to achieve eradication.

ACTINOMYCETOMA

Medical treatment with trimethoprim/sulfamethoxazole (co-trimoxazole) and streptomycin or rifampin is often effective. Good results have been claimed with a combination of dapsone and streptomycin. Alternatives include amikacin and fusidic acid.

78.2 Sporotrichosis

Key features

- Tropics and subtropics
- Occasionally can appear in small epidemics
- Diagnosis can be confirmed by culture
- Common differentials – *Mycobacterium marinum* and leishmaniasis
- Responds to potassium iodide, itraconazole, and terbinafine

INTRODUCTION

Sporotrichosis is a chronic fungal infection principally affecting the skin, lymphatics, and subcutaneous tissues. Pulmonary and disseminated forms, with involvement of the lungs, osteoarticular and musculoskeletal tissues, viscera, mucous membranes, and central nervous system (CNS), are uncommon. Sporotrichosis is caused by a single species, *Sporothrix schenckii,* which is widely distributed as a soil saprophyte. It is dimorphic, existing as a mold in nature and a yeast in infected tissue.

EPIDEMIOLOGY

Sporotrichosis occurs worldwide but is most common in warm, temperate or tropical countries, and has typically been reported from Central and South America, Africa, and Australasia [5]. Most cases are sporadic, but epidemics can occur in hyperendemic areas. A large outbreak that occurred in Rio de Janeiro state, Brazil, was attributed to spread from infected cats [6]. The disease affects individuals whose occupation brings them into contact with soil, plants, or plant materials, such as straw, wood, or reeds.

NATURAL HISTORY, PATHOGENESIS AND PATHOLOGY

The agent is rarely seen in histopathologic material from primary infections. When present, it is often pleomorphic, appearing as small, round, oval or cigar-shaped budding yeast cells, 2–3 μm wide by 3–8 μm long. In some instances, a central fungal cell is surrounded by radiating eosinophilic material (asteroid body).

CLINICAL FEATURES

The route of entry is via minor traumatic subcutaneous inoculation. The incubation period varies from 1–4 weeks and, rarely, up to 6 months. About 75% of infections affect an upper extremity. There is evidence to suggest that some patients have self-limited infections [7].

CUTANEOUS SPOROTRICHOSIS

The most common form of sporotrichosis is lymphangitic, in which a small, firm, movable subcutaneous nodule develops at the site of inoculation. The nodule later becomes soft and breaks down to form a persistent friable ulcer or chancre. Subsequently, additional nodules develop along the draining lymphatics that progress to ulceration. The presence of a persistent ulcer on a finger or hand and a chain of swollen lymph nodes extending up the arm is suspicious for sporotrichosis. In about a quarter of cutaneous infections, the lesion remains "fixed", without lymphatic spread. Fixed infections are more common in children and in Latin America. Less commonly, lesions may present as chronic ulcers, mycetoma-like lesions, or well-defined granulomas. Disseminated cutaneous lesions have been reported in patients with AIDS.

PULMONARY SPOROTRICHOSIS

Primary pulmonary infection is rare. It can be asymptomatic but, in individuals with a low level of immunity, it can progress to disseminated disease.

DISSEMINATED SPOROTRICHOSIS

This is uncommon and is generally seen in persons with underlying disease or a predisposition, such as alcoholism [8]. It originates by hematogenous spread, usually from the lung. Sites affected include skin, joints, lungs, bone, mucous membranes, and the CNS.

DIAGNOSIS AND DIFFERENTIAL DIAGNOSIS

Classic cutaneous lymphatic sporotrichosis is distinct, but the variability of other forms can make diagnosis difficult. Direct examination of pus or skin is seldom helpful and *Sporothrix schenckii is* usually absent, or rare, in tissue sections. Culture is of the greatest value – *S. schenckii is* readily isolated from clinical material on a variety of culture media.

Sporotrichosis must be distinguished from other mycoses and from infective skin lesions, such as tularemia, leishmaniasis, anthrax, tuberculosis, and pyogenic infection. Lymphatic spread similar to that of sporotrichosis can occur in *Mycobacterium marinum* and some South American forms of cutaneous leishmaniasis.

TREATMENT

The usual treatment for cutaneous infection is orally administered potassium iodide (KI) in saturated solution, which usually produces a cure within 3 months. An adult can be given 1 ml of KI three times daily, with drops in incremental increases to a maximum of 4–6 ml 3 times daily after 1 month. To increase palatability, the drug may be administered with milk. Treatment should be continued for 3–4 weeks after clinical cure. Alternatives include itraconazole 100–200 mg daily or terbinafine 250 mg daily.

78.3 Chromoblastomycosis

Key features

- Seen in humid tropical regions
- Presents with verrucous (warty) or flat plaques
- Diagnosis depends on histopathology with demonstration of pigmented fungal cells
- Responds to itraconazole or terbinafine

INTRODUCTION

Chromoblastomycosis (chromomycosis) is a chronic mycosis affecting skin and subcutaneous tissues characterized by slow-growing verrucous nodules that coalesce and form hyperkeratotic plaques [9]. It is caused by several species of related fungi; the most common are: *Fonsecaea pedrosoi, Fonsecaea compactum, Phialophora verrucosa,* and *Cladophialophora carriomi.* Irrespective of the species, each has an identical appearance in infected tissues, i.e. single or clustered, rounded or angular, thick-walled and dark-brown bodies ("sclerotic or muriform cells"). Like saprophytes, the organisms are commonly found in soil and wood.

EPIDEMIOLOGY

Chromoblastomycosis is a tropical mycosis diagnosed more frequenlty in males than in females and is more prevalent in rural than urban areas. The disease has a worldwide distribution with a high prevalence in Costa Rica (1/21,000 population) and Madagascar (1/30,000 population).

NATURAL HISTORY, PATHOGENESIS, AND PATHOLOGY

The disease follows implantation from the environment and is seen in healthy individuals.

CLINICAL MANIFESTATIONS

The initial lesion is a warty papule on an exposed site, for example leg or arm, that enlarges slowly to form a verrucous plaque. In some instances, the primary lesion is a pustule, a flat plaque, or an ulcer [10]. As infection progresses, ulceration and serous exudation occur (Fig. 78.3). Non-painful, large hyperkeratotic plaques up to 3 cm thick with central scar formation occur. Super-infection may be responsible for lymphostasis and resultant elephantiasis, and secondary-infected lesions have an unpleasant smell.

DLAGNOSIS AND DIFFERENTIAL DIAGNOSIS

Clinical history and manifestations are often diagnostic. Lesions are usually hyperkeratotic and characterized by pseudoepitheliomatous hyperplasia with microabscess formation. On microscopy of scrapings, distinctive brown fungal cells can be identified in 20% potassium hydroxide (Fig. 78.4). In tissue sections, fungal cells, i.e. muriform cells or sclerotic bodies, are 5–12 µm in diameter, common in some sections and rare in others. Culture and identification of the

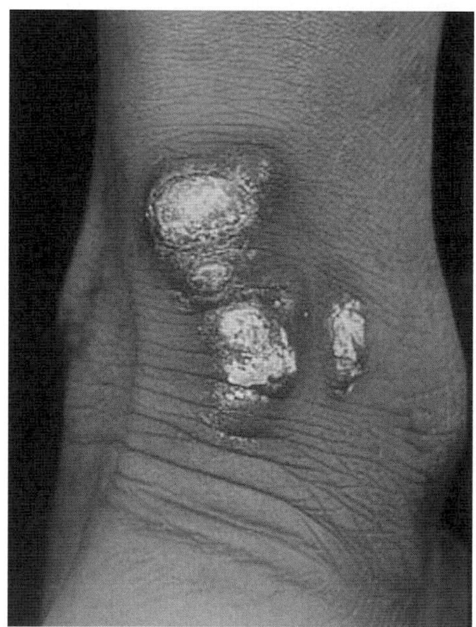

FIGURE 78.3 Chromoblastomycosis – an early lesion on the ankle *(image courtesy of the St John's Institute of Dermatology, London).*

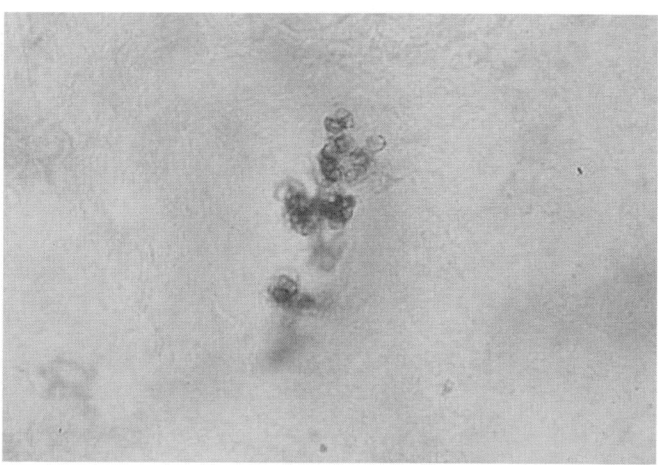

FIGURE 78.4 Scraping of chromoblastomycosis mounted in 20% potassium hydroxide. Note the thick-walled, pigmented fungal cells *(image courtesy of the St John's Institute of Dermatology, London).*

specific etiologic agent can be time-consuming and should always be done by a specialist laboratory because the polymorphic appearance of many isolates makes their positive identification difficult.

Chromoblastomycosis can resemble cutaneous tuberculosis, leishmaniasis, syphilis, and yaws.

TREATMENT

No antifungal regimen is universally satisfactory, although itraconazole (200–400 mg/d) and terbinafine (500 mg/d) have been effective. In extensive lesions, amphotericin B should be given intravenously (Chapter 84) at the outset of treatment; in some cases flucytosine is given in addition. Local application of heat may be effective.

78.4 Rhinosporidiosis

INTRODUCTION

Rhinosporidiosis is a chronic, localized granulomatous condition that presents with polyp-like lesions. The causative organism has been identified by genetic techniques as a member of the aquatic Protista [11]. There are no experimental models and the organism cannot be cultured. Disease has been reported from many tropical countries, but 90% of reported cases are from India and Sri Lanka.

Rhinosporidiosis is most commonly seen in children and young adults, and in males more than females (three to one).

The most common site of rhinosporidiosis is the nose (70% of cases), with sessile or pedunculated polyps affecting the nostrils. Lesions can affect the conjunctiva and, rarely, the larynx, genitals, and skin. Dissemination has been reported, but is exceptional.

DIAGNOSIS AND DIFFERENTIAL DIAGNOSIS

Examination of hematoxylin and eosin-stained sections reveals sporangia of varying sizes and stages of development. Culture serologic tests are not helpful. Nasal lesions must be distinguished from polyps and lesions in other sites, particularly in the perianal region, must be distinguished from warts, condylomata and hemorrhoids

TREATMENT

Chemotherapy is of little proven value. The treatment of choice is surgical excision.

78.5 Entomophthoromycosis caused by *Basidiobolus*

INTRODUCTION

Entomophthoromycosis (subcutaneous phycomycosis, subcutaneous zygomycosis) is a localized mycoses of the nasal mucosa and surrounding tissue. It causes a firm, progressive swelling of subcutaneous tissues. The causal fungus is *Basidiobolus haptosporus*, a mucormycete. Cases are usually reported from India and sub-Saharan Africa. The condition affects children and adolescents rather than adults, and boys rather than girls.

PATHOGENESIS AND PATHOLOGY

The mode of entry has not been established but most likely follows implantation from an exogenous source.

CLINICAL MANIFESTATIONS

Subcutaneous swelling is firm, movable and well-defined; satellite lesions may be palpable at the advancing margins [12].

The overlying skin is usually intact and may be tense, edematous, hyperpigmented or normal in color. Ulceration occurs but is uncommon, and pain and tenderness are usually absent. Any part of the body may be affected, but the most common sites are the limbs, buttocks, and neck. Regional lymph nodes are rarely affected.

DIAGNOSIS AND DIFFERENTIAL DIAGNOSIS

Histology shows strands of broad 5–15 μm thin-walled, branching and generally non-septate hyphae toward the edge of the lesions, each with an eosinophilic sheath several micrometers wide (Splendore-Hoepple phenomenon). It is characterized by eosinophil infiltration and granuloma formation. Cutaneous lymphoma can be similar to subcutaneous zygomycosis, but is characterized by a more rapid onset. Other differentials include scleroderma and pretibial myxedema.

TREATMENT

The most effective treatment is itraconazole in doses of 100–200 mg daily. An alternative is oral potassium iodide (KI) in saturated solution in doses up to 10 ml three times daily for 3 months. Amphotericin B has been used in patients refractory to treatment.

78.6 Entomophthoromycosis caused by *Conidiobolus*

INTRODUCTION

Infections caused by *Conidiobolus coronatus* (rhinoentomophthoromycosis) lead to a chronic, localized subcutaneous infection affecting tissues of the nose, cheek, and upper lip [13].

EPIDEMIOLOGY

Conidiobolus coronatus is a mucormycete found in tropical rain forest areas. In contrast to zygomycosis caused by *Basidiobolus*, rhinoentomophthoromycosis is a disease of young adults, rather than children.

Males are more commonly affected than females. Most infections are reported from West Africa, particularly Nigeria, but cases have been recognized in India and South America.

The mode of infection is unknown, but is probably inoculation of contaminated soil or vegetable matter through minor trauma or insect bites.

CLINICAL MANIFESTATIONS

Infection apparently originates in the nasal mucosa, leading to nasal obstruction, which may be unilateral. Tissue swelling becomes pronounced affecting the nose and nasolabial folds, cheeks, and upper lip, eventually producing gross facial distortion (Fig. 78.5). The infected areas have distinct margins but the mass is not movable over the underlying tissues. There are few symptoms.

DIAGNOSIS AND DIFFERENTIAL DIAGNOSIS

The clinical features are distinctive, i.e. localized swelling of the nose and face in tropical countries. Biopsy may be diagnostic when characteristic hyphae are present and associated with an eosinophilic sheath and eosinophilic granuloma, as with *Basidiobolus* infections. *Conidiobolus* and *Basidobolus* infections can be differentiated by the site involved.

TREATMENT

Treatment is the same as for *Basidiobolus* (Chapter 78.5).

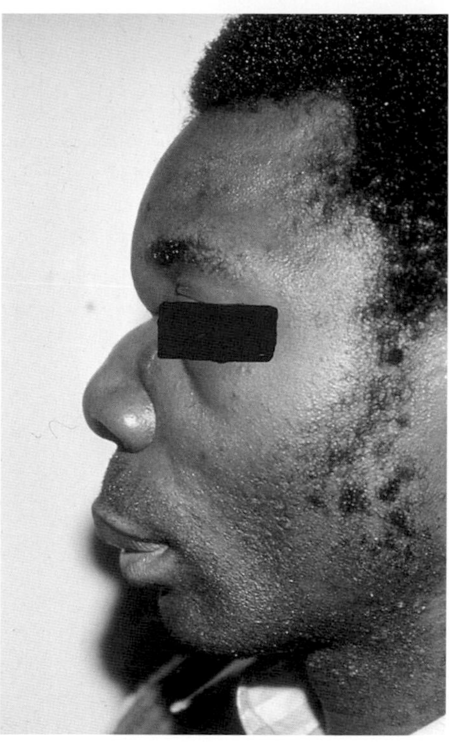

FIGURE 78.5 Nigerian patient with subcutaneous zygomycosis caused by *Conidiobolus* *(image courtesy of the Armed Forces Institute of Pathology, Photograph Neg. No. 76-6165).*

78.7 Other Subcutaneous Mycoses

PHAEOHYPHOMYCOSIS

INTRODUCTION AND EPIDEMIOLOGY

Phaeohyphomycosis describes infections with dark-pigmented fungi that are clinically and pathologically distinct from chromoblastomycosis or mycetoma and where the organisms are present as irregular hyphae in tissue. The range of causal organisms is wide, embracing some 16 genera and almost 30 species.

CLINICAL MANIFESTATIONS AND TREATMENT

Lesions are usually solitary and circumscribed, occurring on the feet, legs, hands, and other body sites [14]. Over a period of months or years, the lesions may increase in size, producing a crusted or cystic mass that remains localized. Diagnosis depends on the recognition of brown fungal elements by direct microscopy or in tissue sections, which may be filamentous, irregularly swollen or yeast-like, and by isolation and identification of the agents in a specialist laboratory. The treatment for localized forms of the disease is surgical excision.

LOBOMYCOSIS

Lobomycosis or Lobo disease is a chronic, localized mycosis of skin and subcutaneous tissues characterized by keloidal or verrucoid lesions that contain abundant or lemon-shaped cells. The disease is rare and only recorded in remote and tropical areas of South and Central America. It has also been described in freshwater dolphins. The causative organism, *Lacazia loboi*, has not been isolated and its habitat is unknown [15].

Patients present with circumscribed plaques or keloid-like lesions usually on exposed areas such as the face, ears, or trunk. These may slowly increase in size and plaques can cover wide areas of the body. They are usually asymptomatic. The diagnosis is made by biopsy and histopathology of the lesions. The organisms are present as chains of cells, each with a short, tube-like connection between individual cells.

The best treatment is excision.

REFERENCES

1. Fahal AH. Mycetoma: a thorn in the flesh. Trans Roy Soc Trop Med Hyg 2004;98:3–11.
2. Ahmed A, Adelmann D, Fahal A, et al. Environmental occurrence of *Madurella mycetomatis*, the major agent of human eumycetoma in Sudan. J Clin Microbiol 2002;40:1031–6.
3. Abd El Bagi ME. New radiographic classification of bone involvement in pedal mycetoma. Am. J Roentgenol 2003;180:665–8.
4. Lacroix C, de Kerviler E, Morel P, et al. *Madurella mycetomatis* mycetoma treated successfully with oral voriconazole. Br J Dermatol 2005;152:1067–8.
5. Bustamante B, Campos PE. Endemic sporotrichosis. Curr Opin Infect Dis 2001;14:145–9.
6. da Rosa AC, Scroferneker ML, Vettorato R, et al. Epidemiology of sporotrichosis: a study of 304 cases in Brazil. J Am Acad Dermatol 2005;52:451–9.
7. Ramos-e-Silva M, Vasconcelos C, Carneiro S, Cestari T. Sporotrichosis. Clin Dermatol 2007;25:181–7.
8. Kauffman CA. Sporotrichosis. Clin Infect Dis 1999;29:231–6.
9. López Martínez R, Méndez Tovar LJ. Chromoblastomycosis. Clin Dermatol 2007;25:188–94.

10. Minotto R, Bernardi CD, Mallmann LF, et al. Chromoblastomycosis: a review of 100 cases in the state of Rio Grande do Sul, Brazil. J Am Acad Dermatol 2001;44:585–92.
11. Arseculeratne SN. Rhinosporidiosis: what is the cause? Curr Opin Infect Dis 2005;18:113–8.
12. Gugnani HC. A review of zygomycosis due to *Basidiobolus ranarum*. Eur J Epidemiol 1999;15:923–9.
13. Prabhu RM, Patel R. Mucormycosis and entomophthoramycosis: a review of the clinical manifestations, diagnosis and treatment. Clin Microbiol Infect 2004;10(suppl. 1):31–47.
14. Rinaldi MR. Phaeohyphomycosis. Dermatol Clin 1996;14:147–53.
15. Paniz-Mondolfi AE, Reyes Jaimes O, Dávila Jones L. Lobomycosis in Venezuela. Int J Dermatol 2007;46:180–5.

Protothecosis 79

Ann M Nelson, Ronald C Neafie

Key features

- Rare disease caused by achlorophyllic algae of the genus *Prototheca*
- Infection via direct contact with organism in environment, often associated with trauma
- Three clinical pathologic syndromes:
  - localized olecranon granulomatous bursitis in immunocompetent individuals
  - eczematoid dermatitis and soft tissue infection in immunosuppressed individuals
  - life-threatening disseminated infections in severely immunosuppressed patients
- Skin scrapings, culture and biopsy used for diagnosis
- Surgical resection adequate for olecranon bursitis
- Amphotericin B and azole antifungals have some effect but the organism responds poorly to most local and systemic therapy

INTRODUCTION

Protothecosis is a rare human infection caused by achlorophyllic algae belonging to the genus *Prototheca* [1, 2]. Infections have involved skin, subcutaneous tissue, olecranon bursa and, rarely, lymph nodes or deep organs [3, 4]. Slightly more than 100 cases have been reported in the world literature from temperate and tropical areas of all continents, with no clear geographic distribution [2]. As a veterinary infection, such as bovine mastitis, becomes more frequent, prothecosis takes on greater economic and public health importance.

EPIDEMIOLOGY, NATURAL HISTORY, PATHOGENESIS, AND PATHOLOGY

The index case of protothecosis in humans (Fig. 79.1) was caused by *Prototheca zopfii* [3]. With a few exceptions, all other infections in humans where the species was determined have been caused by *Prototheca wickerhamii* [2, 4]. *Prototheca wickerhamii* and *P. zopfii* are ubiquitous achloric algae usually found in soil and contaminated water. Both are spherical unicellular organisms, 3–30 μm in diameter with hyaline sporangia and asexual reproduction by internal septation and cytoplasmic cleavage. *Prototheca* are thought to be mutant strains of chlorophyllic (green) algae. *Prototheca wickerhamii* divides to form characteristic morulas (Fig. 79.2), a form described rarely in *P. zopfii*. Infections by both organisms have been reported in a variety of animals. Animal pathogens, *Prototheca stagnora*, and *Prototheca blaschkeae*, are not known to cause disease in humans [2].

Chlorella is similar to *Prototheca* and must be differentiated in tissue sections. Both *Prototheca* and *Chlorella* are distinct from fungi and bacteria by size, morphology, and type of reproduction. In addition, *Prototheca* and *Chlorella* lack the glucosamine of the fungal cell wall and the muramic acid of bacteria [2]. Although infections by *Chlorella* have been described in several animals, there is only one published report involving a human [4].

Very little is known about the pathogenesis of protothecosis. Recent evidence suggests that neutrophil and natural killer cell dysfunction increases susceptibility.

CLINICAL FEATURES

There are two clinical syndromes associated with *Prototheca* infection: a localized infection of the olecranon bursa in patients with normal immunity and an eczematoid dermatitis/soft tissue infection in immunosuppressed individuals [4, 5]. Some infections have been associated with trauma and/or contact with contaminated water; others are iatrogenic from contaminated catheters, peritoneal dialysis or following orthopedic procedures. A third clinical syndrome, involvement of internal organs or systemic infection, has been reported in several patients with severe immune suppression (AIDS, chemotherapy, and post-transplantation) [6–8].

Protothecosis of the olecranon bursa develops several weeks after injury to the elbow. The lesions are localized to the bursa, but there may be epithelial hyperplasia and underlying sinus tracts. The bursa is thickened and histopathologic changes include areas of caseation necrosis surrounded by epithelioid cells, Langhan's giant cells, and fibrosis. *Prototheca* organisms are scattered throughout the areas of necrosis and in the wall of the granuloma.

In the cutaneous and subcutaneous forms, there are single or multiple lesions on the skin or within the subcutaneous tissue, usually over an exposed portion of the body, such as a limb or the face. The lesions are papulomacular to plaque-like and may have an overlying crust or focal ulceration; they spread slowly, often in a centrifugal pattern, and do not resolve. The inflammatory response varies from minimal to necrotizing granulomatous reaction and appears related to the depth of the invasion. The organisms may be in any or all layers of the skin and may be single or in clusters, extracellular or within giant cells. These lesions must be differentiated from other chronic granulomatous diseases of the skin and soft tissue. In the few reported cases of systemic infection, affected tissue showed fibrosis and eosinophilia.

PATIENT EVALUATION, DIAGNOSIS, AND DIFFERENTIAL DIAGNOSIS

Scrapings of the skin, biopsy specimens, and aspirates can be cultured on Sabouraud's medium and require 1–2 days for growth [2]. Typical sporulating forms are identified on stained wet-mounts. Although the

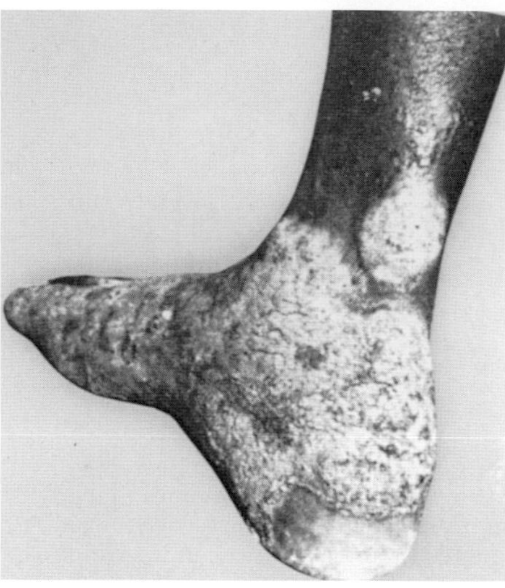

FIGURE 79.1 Protothecosis of the foot of a rice farmer from Sierra Leone. The lesion began as a papule on the instep 9 years earlier. It now encircles the foot and there is a satellite lesion *(Armed Forces Institute of Pathology, Neg. No. 75-12872-2. Photograph courtesy of Dr P.O. Wakelin).*

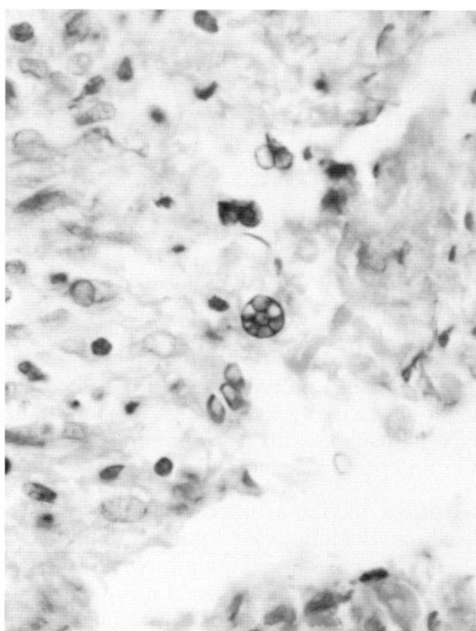

FIGURE 79.2 Characteristic morula of *P. wickerhamii* in subcutaneous tissue of the wrist *(courtesy of the Armed Forces Institute of Pathology, Photograph Neg. No. 86-7088).*

organisms are usually apparent with routine staining by hematoxylin-eosin, they are much better seen with fungal stains, such as Gomori methenamine-silver, periodic acid-Schiff, and Gridley fungus. *Prototheca species* are distinguished from *Cryptococcus, Coccidioides, Blastomyces,* and other fungi by the type of division. Sugar assimilation tests and fluorescent immunoassay aid in species determination.

TREATMENT

Simple bursectomy cures protothecosis of the olecranon bursa. The cutaneous lesions in immunosuppressed patients resist treatment and may persist for several years, eventually spreading to other sites [2]. Topical treatments, including Castellani's paint, saturated copper sulfate, potassium permanganate and amphotericin B, as well as systemic griseofulvin, penicillin, emetine hydrochloride, 5-fluorouricil, and pentamidine isothionate, have not been effective. *In vitro* studies have demonstrated sensitivity to amphotericin B, tetracycline, gentamicin, and ketoconazole [2]. Combined therapy with tetracycline and amphotericin B may be effective. Isolated cutaneous, bursal and soft tissue lesions are best treated with local excision and ketoconazole. Infections that are multifocal, visceral or occur in immunocompromised hosts require amphotericin-B or combined therapy.

REFERENCES

1. Chandler FW, Watts JC. Protothecosis and infections caused by green algae. In: Pathologic Diagnosis of Fungal Infections, 2nd edn. Chicago: American Society of Clinical Pathologists; 1987:43–53.
2. Lass-Flörl C, Mayr A. Human protothecosis. Clin Microbiol Rev 2007;20: 230–42.
3. Connor DH, Gibson DW, Zeifer AM. Diagnostic features of three unusual infections: Micronemiasis, pheomycotic cyst, and protothecosis. In: Manjo G, Cotran RS, eds. Current Topics in Inflammation and Infection. Baltimore: William and Wilkins; 1982:205–39.
4. Nelson AM, Neafie RC, Connor DH. Cutaneous protothecosis and chlorellosis, extraordinary :aquatic-borne" algal infections. In Mandojano RM, ed. Clinic in Dermatology (Aquatic Dermatology). Philadelphia: J. B. Lippincott; 1987: 76–8.
5. Kuo TT, Hsueh S, Wu JL, et al. Cutaneous protothecosis: a clinicopathologic study. Arch Pathol Lab Med 1987;111:737–40.
6. Lanotte P, Baty G, Senecal D, et al. Fatal algaemia in patient with chronic lymphocytic leukemia. Emerg Infect Dis 2009;15:1129–30.
7. Luong-Player AT, Romansky SG. Human protothecosis: Lethal, disseminated infection by *Prototheca zopfii in* a pediatric patient with leukemia. Arch Pathol Lab Med 2009;133:1709.
8. Woolrich A, Koestenblatt E, Don P, et al. Cutaneous protothecosis and AIDS. J Am Acad Dermatol 1994;31:920–4.

Histoplasmosis 80

Eileen E Navarro, Thomas J Walsh, Roderick J Hay

Key features

- Histoplasmosis is a widely distributed infection caused by *Histoplasma capsulatum*, a dimorphic fungus
- Individuals from endemic areas are often infected subclinically, whereas symptomatic disease depends upon interplay between the intensity of infection and the host's immune status
- Clinical syndromes include acute pulmonary infection following heavy exposure, chronic cavitary pulmonary infection in persons with underlying chronic obstructive pulmonary disease and disseminated infection usually in immunosuppressed individuals. In Central and West Africa, a variety of histoplasmosis due to *Histoplasma duboisii* causes skin and bone infection
- Diagnosis is through demonstration of typical budding yeast in sputum or biopsy, culture, DNA probes, or antigen detection
- Although an immunocompetent person with mild-to-moderate pulmonary infection can be managed symptomatically, those with severe pulmonary infection or disseminated disease should be treated with amphotericin flowed by itraconazole

INTRODUCTION

Histoplasmosis is a widely distributed infection caused by *Histoplasma capsulatum*, a dimorphic fungus. Darling, who first described the pathology of histoplasmosis in 1905, named the organism *Histoplasma capsulatum* because the small yeasts within the cytoplasm of macrophages resembled encapsulated parasites.

Histoplasma capsulatum var. *capsulatum* generally causes subclinical infection in persons from endemic areas [1]. However, following high exposure, symptomatic pulmonary infection can occur and debilitated or immunocompromised persons can present with disseminated disease. Infections caused by *H. capsulatum* var. *duboisii* are restricted to West and Central Africa [2]. African histoplasmosis classically presents with cutaneous and skeletal involvement.

EPIDEMIOLOGY

In the USA, the Mississippi and Ohio river valleys are endemic. Infections are associated with outdoor activities and exposure to starling roost or soil upheaval.

The tropical presence of *H. capsulatum* was established from a description of the post-mortem pathology of construction workers building the Panama canal. Skin testing [3] indicates high prevalence throughout Latin America; however, few population-based studies are available from other tropical areas. In the tropics, conditions that support the growth of *H. capsulatum* occur in bat roosting sites, including caves, where exposure in the confined space has resulted in epidemics.

With the environmental isolation of *H. capsulatum* in Southeast Asia, the Indian continent, and the Middle East, the increase in immunocompromising therapies in the developing world and the AIDS pandemic, there has been a rise in symptomatic histoplasmosis in all areas in the tropics including sub-Saharan Africa [4, 5]. Imported infections have also been acquired by travellers.

NATURAL HISTORY, PATHOGENESIS, AND PATHOLOGY

Histoplasma capsulatum grows in its mycelial form at lower temperatures (25–30 °C) [1]. This phase, characterized by hyphae with slender conidiophores and characteristic tuberculate macroconidia, is the saprobic state found in the environment. When incubated at 37 °C on an enriched medium, the conidia germinate into yeast – the phase also found in host tissue.

Histoplasmosis is acquired by the respiratory route; conidia are aerosolized from soil containing bat or bird guano and inhaled into alveoli. Alveolar macrophages, modulated by T lymphocytes, contain this initial infection, resulting in localized granulomatous inflammation. This self-limiting process is evidenced by the development of delayed-type skin reactions and the production of specific antibodies, as well as asymptomatic calcification in the lung, spleen, and mediastinal lymph nodes. A small percentage of these episodes advance to progressive pulmonary or disseminated infection, often in the immunocompromised [6].

CLINICAL FEATURES

Histoplasmosis can be classified by site (pulmonary, extrapulmonary, or disseminated), by duration (acute, subacute, and chronic) and by pattern (primary versus reactivation). Most infections in normal hosts are asymptomatic; even symptomatic primary infection can be underdiagnosed given its brief, mild nature [7].

Asymptomatic fungemia occurs with the primary infection, as evidenced by splenic and pulmonary calcifications. Unrecognized dissemination permits subsequent reactivation at pulmonary and extrapulmonary sites if the host becomes immunocompromised [8]. Acute disseminated disease is often reported in young children and infants, or in patients with cellular immune deficiency, and can be a fulminant, fatal disease.

PULMONARY HISTOPLASMOSIS

Acute primary pulmonary histoplasmosis (APPH) develops in immunocompetent hosts exposed to a heavy inoculum. A history of environmental exposure should be sought and public health authorities notified if a source is identified. Symptoms of APPH often resemble those of an influenza-like illness [7]. The sudden onset of fever, erythema nodosum or multiforme, and a brassy cough secondary to airway compression from lymphadenopathy can be accompanied, in severe cases, by pericarditis, nights sweats, cyanosis, hemoptysis, or disseminated disease. Chest x-ray demonstrates a diffuse alveolar-interstitial infiltrative or reticulonodular pattern. Radiographic changes resolve slowly or leave a miliary pattern. Features that can differentiate this from tuberculosis are the pattern of grouped calcification in paratracheal nodes and larger calcifications (>4 mm in the parenchyma and >1 cm in the mediastinum). In patients with active pulmonary histoplasmosis, yeast can be observed on direct examination of sputum, often within pulmonary alveolar macrophages.

CHRONIC CAVITARY PULMONARY HISTOPLASMOSIS (CCPH)

This is an indolent, progressive respiratory infection of patients with underlying chronic obstructive pulmonary disease that is rarely described in the tropics. These patients are usually elderly, cigarette-smoking males who suffer progressive deterioration of pulmonary function, most likely caused by a combination of chronic lung disease and histoplasmosis [7].

DISSEMINATED HISTOPLASMOSIS

Acute Disseminated Histoplasmosis

This can occur with primary infection, often in young children or infants, or in the immunosuppressed host. The disease varies in severity, clinical manifestations and course from a fulminant, fatal disease marked by shock, to a subacute disease with little systemic inflammation and focal, organ-specific signs and symptoms [1].

The most severely compromised hosts present with hectic fever, cough, dyspnea, and pulmonary infiltrates and adenopathy. Weight loss, infiltration of the reticuloendothelial system and bone marrow, diffuse cutaneous lesions and central nervous system (CNS) involvement reflect systemic spread. Rapidly fatal overwhelming infections marked by disseminated intravascular coagulation (DIC), adult respiratory distress syndrome (ARDS), bone marrow suppression and multi-organ failure occur in a minority. Children often have marked hepatosplenomegaly, gastrointestinal bleeding, and anemia. AIDS patients present with lymphadenopathy, CNS manifestations, and skin lesions that vary from erythematous macules, purpura and ulcers, to papules resembling molluscum contagiosum [6, 9].

Chronic Progressive Disseminated Histoplasmosis

Patients have wasting and fatigue with painful nodules on the tongue or gingiva and ulcers in the buccal mucosa or nasal vestibule that can be mistaken for malignancy. Biopsy reveals abundant yeast with very little granulomatous reaction. In subacute forms, constitutional symptoms are prominent, with abdominal pain and diarrhea, masses in the terminal ileum and cecum, bowel obstruction or perforation and, occasionally, massive bleeding. Chronic basilar leptomeningitis with vasculitis and small cerebral granulomas or ring-enhancing cerebral mass lesions characterize CNS involvement. Endocarditis with large vegetations of the aortic and mitral valve can occur. Histopathology of valvular lesions reveals extracellular yeast and mycelial elements. Adrenal involvement is common [8].

PATIENT EVALUATION, DIAGNOSIS, AND DIFFERENTIAL DIAGNOSIS

COLLECTION AND TRANSPORT OF SPECIMENS [1]

Most diagnostic specimens will be sputum, bronchoalveolar lavage, transtracheal aspirates, or lung biopsy. Specimens should be transported and processed promptly to avoid overgrowth by bacteria or saprophytic fungi. Mycelial conidia are highly infectious and easily transmissible by aerosolization. When cultures are handled for identification or sent to reference laboratories, they must be sealed.

DIRECT EXAMINATION

Histoplasma capsulatum should be examined with special stains. The budding yeast of *H. capsulatum* (2–4 μm) in a calcofluor white or potassium hydroxide preparation of sputum can be too small for reliable detection and can be confused with *Candida glabrata* (Fig. 80.1).

Bone marrow aspirates, buffy coat smears and peripheral blood smears are valuable in disseminated disease. Touch preparations of bone marrow biopsies, lymph nodes, and other tissues can also detect fungi. Giemsa or Wright stain reveals yeast within circulating monocytes or tissue macrophages. Staining of a paraffin-embedded clot section of bone marrow aspirate by periodic acid-Schiff (PAS), Gomori methenamine stain (GMS), Giemsa and Wright stains allows visualization in granulomas.

CULTURE [10]

Plating and study of cultures should be performed within a biosafety cabinet. Isolation media for sputum samples should contain

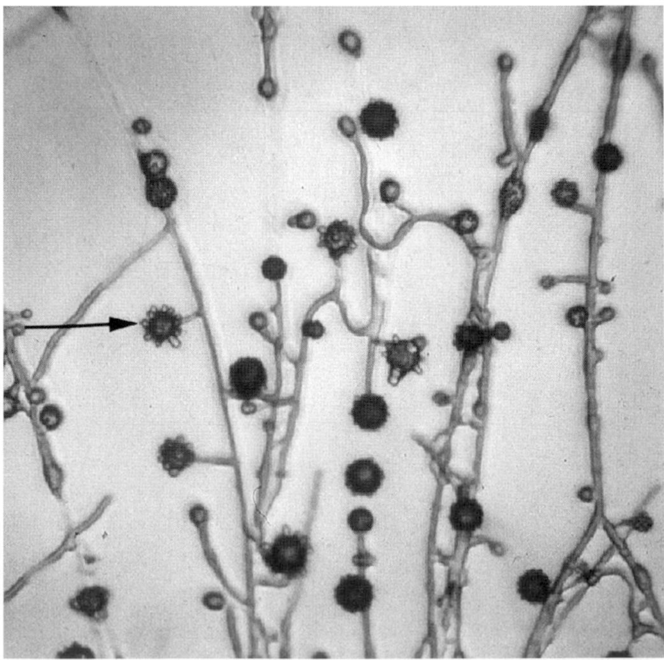

FIGURE 80.1 *Histoplasma capsulatum*. Slender conidiophore bearing characteristic tuberculate macroconidia (arrow) may be mistaken for *Sepedomium* spp. The occurrence of microconidia and the dimorphic nature of *H. capsulatum* differentiates it from *Sepedomium* (Sabouraud dextrose agar, x600).

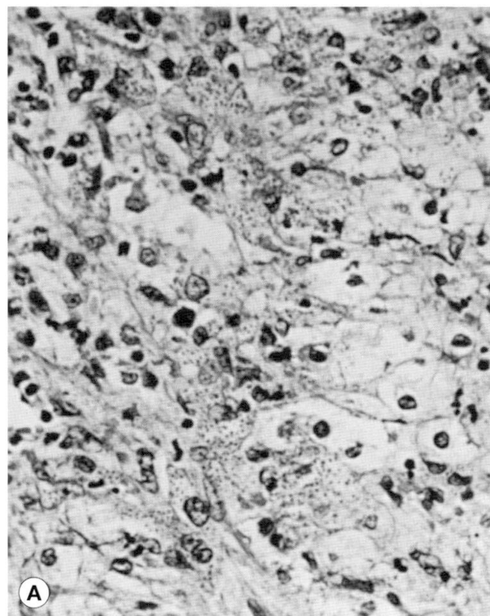

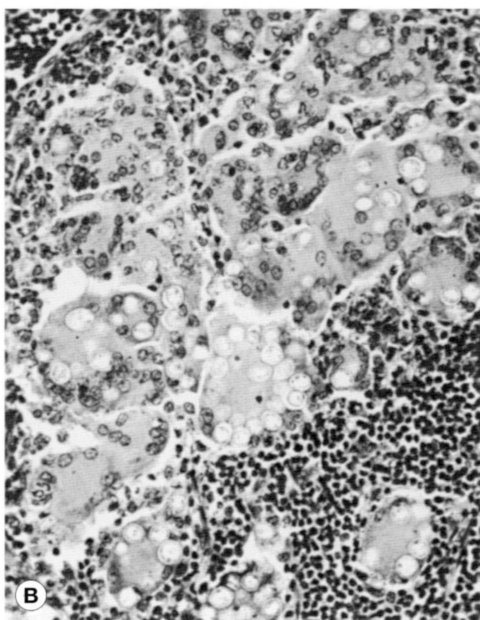

FIGURE 80.2 (A) Small, intracellular yeasts packed in tissue macrophages from a patient with classic histoplasmosis (*Histoplasma capsulatum* var. *capsulatum*; hematoxylin and eosin, X 400). **(B)** *Histoplasma capsulatum* var. *duboisii* infection revealing aggregates of giant cells with large ovoid yeast cells (hematoxylin and eosin, x310) *(images courtesy of the Armed Forces Institute of Pathology Photograph Neg. Nos. 54-17185 and 54-19426, respectively).*

antibiotics and cycloheximide to inhibit saprophytic fungi. Normally, sterile specimens can be inoculated directly onto blood agar, brain-heart infusion (BHI) agar, Sabouraud glucose agar (SGA) and enriched broth, such as BHI broth. Cultures should be incubated at 25–30°C under humidified, aerobic conditions for 4–8 weeks.

Cultures at 25–30°C reveal a slowly growing colony with aerial mycelia that vary in color from white to buff to brown. During early growth, microconidia (2–5 μm in diameter) are present and, with continued growth, the mold develops slender conidiophores and characteristic macroconidia (Fig. 80.2) measuring 8–16 μm in diameter. Conversion to the yeast occurs after incubating mycelia at 37°C on enriched medium, such as BHI agar with cysteine. Spherical-to-oval budding yeast cells (2–5 μm in diameter) develop in 7–10 days. Yeast can also be isolated on blood agar or other enriched media incubated at 37°C.

NUCLEIC ACID PROBES

A recent advance in the identification of *H. capsulatum* from cultures, are nucleic acid probes, commercially available in kit format (e.g. AccuProbe). The procedure takes approximately 1 hour and provides early testing on young cultures, rapid processing, easy interpretation of results and high accuracy.

ANTIGEN DETECTION [10]

Detection in serum and urine of a galactomannan of *H. capsulatum* can be used in the diagnosis and therapeutic monitoring of disseminated histoplasmosis, particularly in HIV-infected patients.

SEROLOGY AND SKIN TESTING

Of the serologic tests, complement fixation against the yeast phase is more sensitive and immunoprecipitating antibodies to the H antigen are more specific [1]. Antibodies become positive weeks after infection and titers generally wane several months after uncomplicated infection, correlate with severity of illness and are present in low levels in the general population in an endemic area. The utility of skin testing is limited to documentation of prior exposure to *H. capsulatum*.

DIFFERENTIAL DIAGNOSIS

Histoplasmosis can resemble tuberculosis and other granulomatous pulmonary processes, such as sarcoidosis. Cutaneous lesions have been mistaken for molluscum contagiosum or varicella, *Leishmania, Rochalimea*, herpes simplex, and systemic mycoses such as *Penicillium marneffei* and *Cryptococcus neoformans*. The reticuloendothelial proliferation and bone marrow infiltration can suggest neoplasia, visceral leishmaniasis, brucellosis, or malaria.

TREATMENT

Treatment of pulmonary histoplasmosis depends on the immune status of the host and extent of disease [1, 11].

While amphotericin B continues to be the drug of choice for severe, refractory or relapsing infections, the azoles (particularly itraconazole) have expanded the treatment alternatives for milder infections and suppressive therapy (see Chapter 87).

Immunocompetent patients with mild-to-moderate acute pulmonary histoplasmosis usually have self-limiting disease that can be managed with supportive care [12]. Patients with acute pulmonary histoplasmosis who are elderly, less than 2 years old, debilitated or immunocompromised can be treated with itraconazole (administered as a loading dose of 400 mg b.i.d. for 3 days followed by 200 mg b.i.d.).

Itraconazole (200 mg t.i.d. daily for 3 days, then 200 mg qd or b.i.d.) for 6- to 12-month courses is the preferred agent for chronic cavitary histoplasmosis.

Profoundly immunocompromised patients, those with severe pulmonary histoplasmosis or life-threatening extrapulmonary disease are treated with amphotericin B at a dose of 0.7–1.0 mg/kg/day (or a lipid formulation) for 1–2 weeks followed by itraconazole. Short-term corticosteroid therapy can be considered for patients with severe respiratory compromise.

Patients with acute disseminated histoplasmosis and AIDS should be treated with amphotericin B 1 mg/kg/day (or liposomal amphotericin B) until stable, followed by itraconazole at 200 mg twice a day for prevention of relapse. Patients with AIDS and mild-to-moderate disseminated histoplasmosis have been successfully treated with itraconazole alone; ketoconazole has been associated with failure and relapse. Therapeutic response, particularly in HIV-infected patients who have a high *H. capsulatum* antigen burden, can be monitored by serial urine and serum samples.

Histoplasma meningitis can be refractory to treatment with frequent relapses, even with intrathecal amphotericin B. Surgical resection of valves in endocarditis with systemic amphotericin B affords the best chance for cure.

PREVENTION

There is no practical environmental control, although it is useful to post warning notices in caves known to contain the organism. Spraying contaminated soil with 3% cresol or formalin may eliminate viable organisms

AFRICAN HISTOPLASMOSIS

African histoplasmosis is an uncommon illness restricted to the African continent. It is most prevalent in West Africa and has not been recognized north of the Sahara Desert or in countries south of the Zambesi River [2]. Although the portal of entry is presumed to be respiratory, cases with pulmonary involvement are rare. Histoplasmin surveys cannot estimate the risk of subclinical exposure because classic histoplasmosis can be endemic in the same areas and both organisms are antigenically related.

The most common clinical sites for African histoplasmosis are skin and bone [2, 13]. Skin lesions present as small papules that can develop an umbilicated center, nodules, abscesses, or ulcers. With larger lesions, underlying bone deposits are common. Bone deposits are well circumscribed and lytic, and typically found in the long bones and skull. Patients presenting with African histoplasmosis should be investigated radiologically for occult bone foci. Involvement of lung, lymph nodes, and gastrointestinal tract is less common. Multi-organ invasion rarely occurs and is associated with a poor prognosis.

The diagnosis is made by biopsy, smears, and cultures taken from skin or bone lesions. *Histoplasma duboisii* are larger than *H. capsulatum* measuring 8–15 μm in diameter, round or oval in shape with thick walls, and located within giant cells (Fig. 80.2B). The place of serology in African histoplasmosis is not established.

Solitary cutaneous lesions can be surgically removed and, in many cases, do not recur. Oral itraconazole (200–600 mg daily) is effective in most cases [13], either on its own or in addition to surgery. In widespread infection, amphotericin B may be necessary (Chapter 87). Reasonable responses have also been seen with ketoconazole. Relapse after therapy is common.

REFERENCES

1. Kauffman CA. Histoplasmosis: a clinical and laboratory update. Clin Microbiol Rev 2007;20:115–32.
2. Cockshott WP, Lucas AO. Histoplasma duboisii. Q J Med 1964;33:223–38.
3. Edwards PQ, Billings EL. Worldwide pattern of skin sensitivity to histoplasmosis. Am J Trop Med Hyg 1971;20:288–319.
4. Ajello L, Manson-Bahr PEC, Moore JC. Amboni caves, Tanganyika, a new epidemic area for *Histoplasma capsulatum*. Am J Trop Med Hyg 1960;9:633–8.
5. Suzuki A, Kimura M, Kimura S, et al. An outbreak of acute pulmonary histoplasmosis among travellers to a bat inhabited cave in Brazil. J Jpn Assoc Infect Dis 1995;69:444–6.
6. Wheat JD, Connolly-Springfield PA, Baker RL, et al. Disseminated histoplasmosis in the acquired immune deficiency syndrome; Clinical findings, diagnosis, and treatment, and review of the literature. Medicine 1990;69:361–74.
7. Goodwin RA, Lloyd JE, Des Prez RM. Histoplasmosis in normal hosts. Medicine 1981;60:231–66.
8. Wang TL, Cheah JS, Holmberg K. Case report and review of disseminated histoplasmosis in South East Asia: Clinical and epidemiological implications. Trop Med Internal Health 1996;1:35–42.
9. Barton EN, Roberts L, Ince WE, et al. Cutaneous histoplasmosis in the acquired immunodeficiency syndrome: a report of three cases from Trinidad. Trop Geogr Med 1988;40:153–7.
10. Wheat JD, Kohler R, Tewari L. Diagnosis of disseminated histoplasmosis detection of *Histoplasma capsulatum* antigen in serum and urine specimens. N Engl J Med 1986;314:83–8.
11. Wheat JD, Hafrier R, Korzun AH, et al. Itraconazole treatment of disseminated histoplasmosis in patients with the acquired immunodeficiency syndrome. Am J Med 1995;98:336–42.
12. Wheat LJ, Freifeld AG, Kleiman MB, et al. Clinical practice guidelines for the management of patients with histoplasmosis: 2007 update by the Infectious Diseases Society of America. Clin Infect Dis 2007;45:807–25.
13. Velho GC, Cabral JM, Massa A. African histoplasmosis: therapeutic efficacy of itraconazole. J Eur Acad Dermatol Venereol 1998;10:77–80.

Coccidioidomycosis 81

Gregory M Anstead, John R Graybill

Key features

- One of the major endemic mycoses. Occurs primarily in the Western hemisphere (south-western USA, Mexico, Argentina)
- Infection by inhalation of conidia. Vulnerable patient groups include African Americans, Filipinos, native Americans, women in the third trimester of pregnancy and the immunosuppressed, especially persons with AIDS
- Infection manifests as acute or chronic pneumonia, soft tissue verrucous lesions or abscesses, meningitis and osteomyelitis, especially of the spine
- Readily diagnosed by culture, serologic testing (antibody and antigen detection) and histopathology
- Treatment is with triazoles (fluconazole, itraconazole) or amphotericin B, depending on disease site and severity. *In vitro* susceptibility testing is not helpful
- Treatment is prolonged, with responses of 50–70%, and relapses in up to a third of patients who initially respond

INTRODUCTION

This fungal infection was first described in an Argentine soldier in 1892. Initially, the fungus in tissue was mistaken for a coccidian protozoan, hence the name *Coccidioides immitis*. Coccidioidomycosis is now recognized as an important health problem in the southwestern USA and Mexico, with 150,000 cases occurring in the USA annually [1].

EPIDEMIOLOGY

On the basis of molecular genetics, *C. immitis* has recently been divided into *C. immitis* (California isolates) and *Coccidioides posadasii* (other regions); both species are similarly pathogenic [2], and herein will be referred to as *C. immitis*. The fungus grows in mycelial form just beneath the soil surface and is made up of arthroconidia intercalated with nonviable segments.

The endemic area is the Lower Sonoran Life Zone, marked by arid or semi-arid climates, sandy soil and mild winters [2]. These conditions are found in the southwestern USA (primarily Arizona, California, New Mexico, and Texas), the Gran Chaco region of Bolivia, Paraguay, and Northern Argentina, and much of northern Mexico (Fig. 81.1). Rare cases occur in other areas of Central America (Guatemala, Honduras, Nicaragua) and South America (Venezuela, Brazil, Colombia).

Outbreaks of coccidioidomycosis often occur after spring rains or major disturbance of the soil. Between 1995 and 2005, the incidence of coccidioidomycosis gradually increased in the USA, rising from 12 to more than 58 cases/100,000 residents of Arizona/year [2]. Agricultural and rural construction workers are among those most vulnerable to infection. In California, the annual incidence of severe coccidioidomycosis (requiring hospitalization) is 3.7/100,000, with about 70 patients dying of coccidioidomycosis in the state per year [3]. This increase may reflect the rising population in endemic regions with new housing construction.

Patients of African, native American, or Filipino descent are more vulnerable to symptomatic and disseminated disease, as are those with immunosuppression, such as persons with AIDS and pregnant women [1,2]. Coccidioidomycosis also infects many other species of mammalian species, ranging from zoo primates to cattle, cats, and dogs.

NATURAL HISTORY, PATHOGENESIS, AND PATHOLOGY

When disturbed, the fragile mycelia break up into a cloud of infectious conidia which can be carried for miles by the wind; these infect the host following inhalation. Inhaled conidia are phagocytosed by alveolar macrophages and, over the course of several days, convert into the characteristic large (8–24 μm diameter) spherule. The spherules elaborate small endospores, which multiply, and after 3–4 days, hundreds of endospores burst out of the mature spherule. The endospores are ingested by neutrophils, but are not killed. These gradually enlarge into the next generation of spherules [2].

Early in the course of infection, *Coccidioides* can hematogenously disseminate to the skin, bones, and central nervous system (CNS). Clinical manifestations of these remote lesions can appear soon after the acute infection or after many months, sometimes without clinical evidence of the primary infection. Uncontrolled infection often presents as suppurating abscesses, with draining exudates containing abundant neutrophils and spherules (Fig. 81.2A), whereas chronic low-grade infection manifests as better-formed granulomas containing few organisms (Fig. 81.2B). Both B- and T-lymphocytes are essential for host defense, suggesting that a balanced Th1/Th2 response is necessary for protective immunity [4].

CLINICAL FEATURES

The course of coccidioidomycosis is asymptomatic in over half of patients, from inhalation to resolution of primary pulmonary sites of infection. Such individuals were detected in earlier years by skin testing, using either coccidioidin (derived from the mycelia phase) or spherulin (spherule phase origin). Skin test surveys defined the major endemic zones of coccidioidomycosis, but the skin-testing reagents are no longer available.

PRIMARY INFECTION

A variety of hypersensitivity reactions can occur with primary infection. These include fever, erythema nodosum, erythema multiforme, and migratory arthralgias. They are collectively known as "Valley

Fever" after the San Joaquin Valley of California, a focus of coccidioidomycosis [2]. These may be the only manifestations of primary coccidioidomycosis, or may blend into invasive forms of disease.

PULMONARY INFECTION

Most symptomatic patients have a transient pulmonary infection occurring 1–3 weeks after exposure, which manifests as fever, dry cough, and pleuritic chest pain. Although this is usually indistinguishable from community-acquired pneumonia, it is commonly accompanied by hilar or paratracheal lymphadenopathy [2]. In studies of community-acquired pneumonia in Arizona, serologic studies demonstrated that coccidioidomycosis is the etiology in 15% of patients [5].

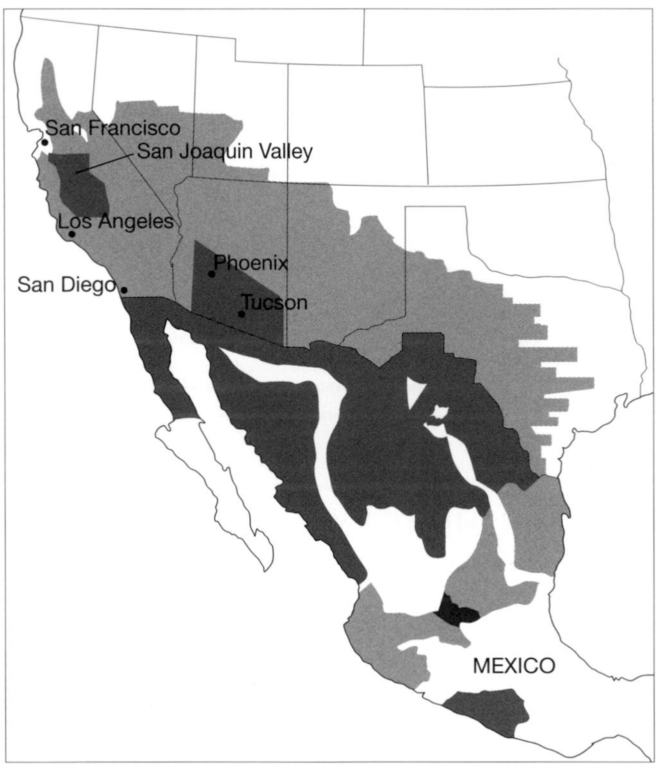

FIGURE 81.1 Endemic range of coccidioidomycosis in North America.

Typically, the symptoms of acute pulmonary coccidioidomycosis resolve spontaneously in less than a month. Alternatively, the pulmonary infiltrates may condense into nodules that may resolve or persist asymptomatically. While primary pneumonia usually resolves, in 5–19% of patients, the disease may linger for months, with chronic pulmonary infiltrates, cough and pleuritic chest pain. Pulmonary infiltrates can also undergo cavitation. Cavitary disease can be asymptomatic or cause chronic productive cough and occasional hemoptysis, or rupture into the pleura [2]. Cavities may also develop secondary bacterial or *Aspergillus* (fungus ball) infection. Small cavities (<5 cm diameter) are more likely to resolve spontaneously than large ones. Chronic pulmonary coccidioidomycosis may follow an intermittent waxing and waning course or be slowly progressive over years [6].

Uncommonly, patients have fulminating pneumonia, with diffuse reticulonodular infiltrates, fever, and hypoxia (Fig. 81.3). Aggressive pulmonary disease can occur in pregnancy, especially the last trimester, and in other immunosuppressive conditions, such as AIDS, or treatment with corticosteroids or tumor necrosis factor-alpha antagonists [6].

EXTRAPULMONARY DISEASE

Extrapulmonary coccidioidomycosis usually presents as skin lesions (papules, nodules, abscesses, verrucous plaques, ulcers), lymphadenitis, deep abscesses, osteoarticular disease (manifested by lytic bone lesions and thickened synovium), or CNS disease [2, 6]. Nearly any organ can be involved in coccidioidomycosis [6].

MENINGITIS

Coccidioidal meningitis manifests as progressive headache, cranial neuropathies, and altered mental status [2]. Granuloma formation causes a variety of focal neurologic signs. The cerebrospinal fluid (CSF) is characteristic of granulomatous meningitis, with lymphocytosis and hypoglycorrachia. CSF eosinophilia, if present, is a helpful diagnostic characteristic and the CSF is usually positive for IgG antibody. CSF cultures are positive in <50% of cases. Untreated, coccidioidal meningitis is lethal within 2 years [6].

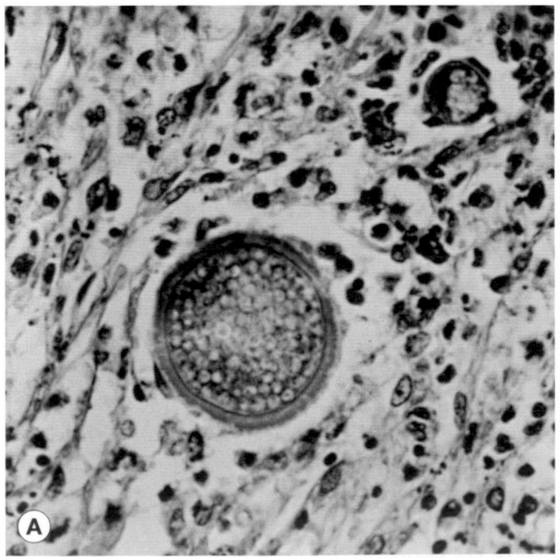

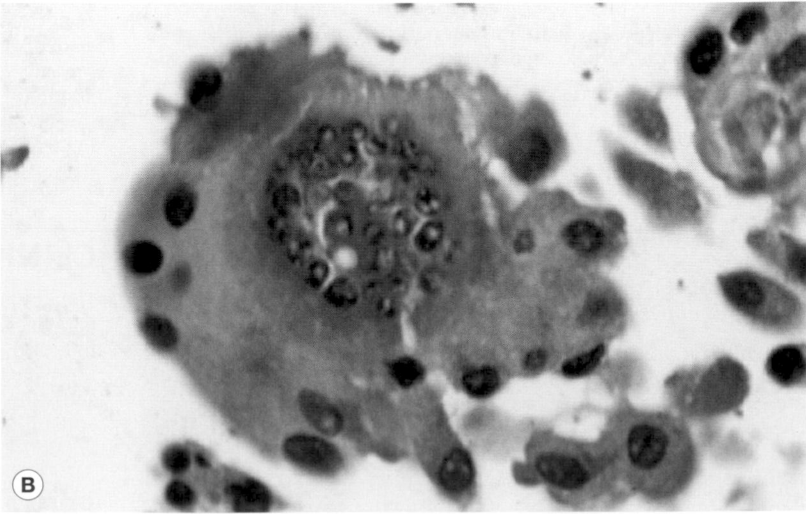

FIGURE 81.2 (A) Lesion with *Coccidioides immitis* spherule within a collection of neutrophils in an abscess (poor immune response; *Courtesy of the Armed Forces Institute of Pathology, Photograph Neg. No. 59-5706*). **(B)** Giant cell with intracellular spherule and endospores. The spherule has a poorly defined cell wall (better immune response).

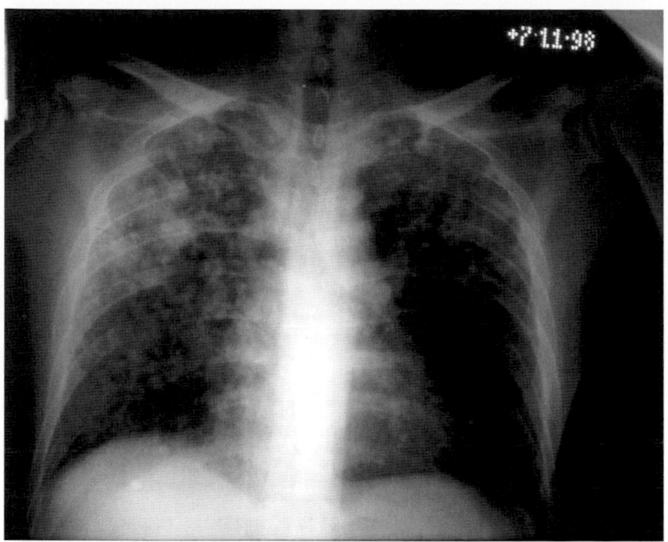

FIGURE 81.3 Chest radiograph showing diffuse reticulonodular infiltrates in an AIDS patient with coccidioidomycosis.

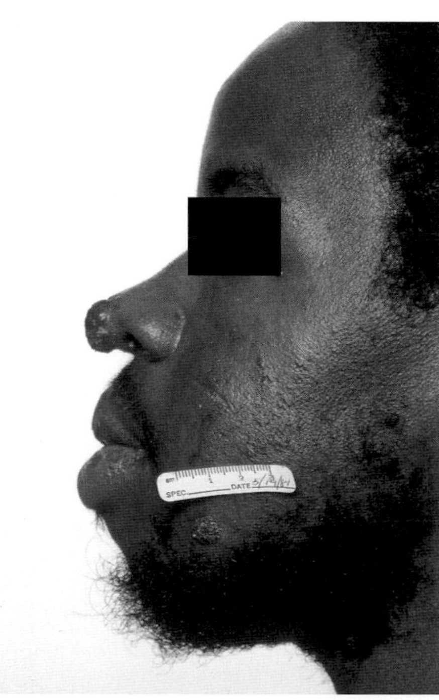

FIGURE 81.4 Verrucous skin lesions on the nose and cheek in a patient with coccidioidomycosis.

SOFT TISSUE AND OSTEOARTICULAR DISEASE

Soft tissue involvement in coccidioidomycosis ranges from scattered chronic verrucous granulomatous lesions to multiple abscesses draining pus, containing large numbers of spherules (Fig. 81.4). In general, lesions with purulent drainage are associated with a worse prognosis. Lesions may be cutaneous or internal along lymph node chains. Coccidioidal osteomyelitis often involves the vertebrae and may be associated with compression fractures (Fig. 81.5). Synovial involvement of large joints is common: *Coccidioides* can be cultured from a synovial biopsy specimen more frequently than from joint fluid. Blood cultures can also be positive in widely disseminated disease; this is an indicator of poor prognosis.

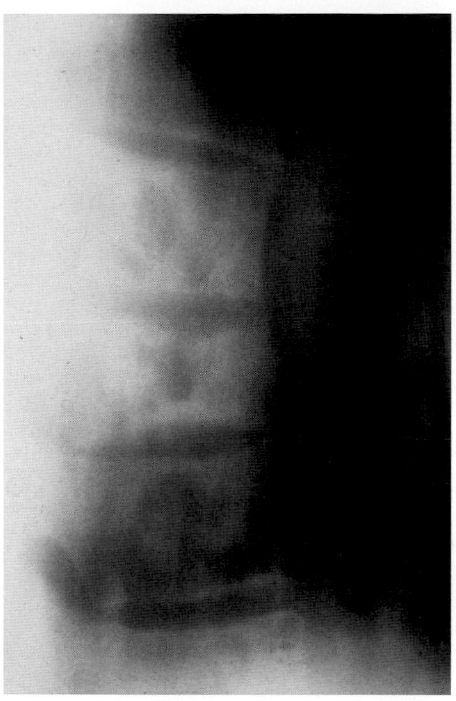

FIGURE 81.5 Radiograph showing lytic vertebral lesions of skeletal coccidioidomycosis.

PATIENT EVALUATION, DIAGNOSIS, AND DIFFERENTIAL DIAGNOSIS

The physician should think of coccidioidomycosis with a compatible illness occurring in a resident or visitor to an endemic region. Rapid diagnostic methods are direct examination of sputum or exudates from purulent lesions, or detection of spherules on histopathologic exam of cutaneous lesions, bronchoscopy specimens, or lymph nodes. The morphology of *Coccidioides* spherules is nearly pathognomonic. Although the spherule can resemble the adiaspore of adiaspiromycosis (a rare infection), the two diseases are distinguished by culture and mycologic expertise [6]. Fresh tissue samples from *Coccidioides*-infected patients are not directly hazardous, but must be disposed of or rendered nonviable quickly.

Coccidioides immitis is cultured in its mycelial form on a variety of media. The spherules found in sputum and tissue convert to mycelia, which grow in 7–10 days. There is nothing characteristic in the appearance of the mycelia to distinguish *Coccidioides* from non-pathogenic fungi, and thus plates with fungal mycelia should be sealed and opened only in biohazard facilities. Careless handling of culture plates has caused several cases of coccidioidomycosis in laboratory personnel [6]. In the USA, *C. immitis* and *C. posadasii* have been designated as potential agents of bioterrorism (a questionable designation) and so the organisms must be killed promptly after identification [6].

IgM antibodies develop within weeks after infection but are not sustained. IgG antibodies take 1–2 months to appear (in blood and CSF) and persist for many months. Titers >1 : 16 correlate with increased severity of illness and declining titers reflect clinical improvement. However, in practice, following the level of antibody titers has not been useful in assessing the course of illness because these titers respond slowly to the clinical status of the patient. Also, in severe immunodeficiency, antibody titers may be low, or even negative [2]. An assay to detect urinary antigen is available from MiraVista Laboratories (Indianapolis, IN), with 71% sensitivity for patients with moderate-to-severe disease, versus 87% for culture. There is also some cross-reactivity in this assay with *Histoplasma capsulatum* antigens [7].

TREATMENT

Treatment guidelines were published in 2005 [1]. *In vitro* susceptibility testing is not helpful; *Coccidioides* isolates are generally susceptible to amphotericin B and multiple triazoles *in vitro*, but treatment responses are highly dependent on host factors, such as immunocompetence and race/ethnicity [1, 2, 6]. Mycelia of *Coccidioides* are susceptible to echinocandins but the spherules can be less vulnerable and clinical experience is limited [6]. Treatment courses are prolonged and should continue many months after clinical improvement. Because some lesions can progress while others wane, a scoring system has been developed. This initially included scoring for symptoms and signs, cultures, radiographically apparent lesions and serologic titers, with a reduction of a cumulative score to less than 50% of baseline considered to be the criterion of response to therapy [6]. As cultures are often not repeated (especially if invasive methods are required) and serologic titers change very slowly, the burden of disease has recently been measured using clinical signs and symptoms and radiographic evaluation of lesion size. In coccidioidal meningitis, normalization of CSF findings can be used as an indicator of treatment response.

Selection of the antifungal agent depends, in part, on the involved site and the severity of disease [1]. No treatment is recommended for asymptomatic coccidiomas, which have been resected during a search for presumptive lung cancer. The nephrotoxicity of amphotericin B initially discouraged physicians from treating primary coccidioidal pneumonia, which usually resolves spontaneously in most patients. However, all patients require observation for at least 2 years to document resolution of infection and to promptly identify complications. With the efficacy of triazoles demonstrated in a variety of the manifestations of coccidioidomycosis, fluconazole has been increasingly deployed to treat primary coccididioidal pneumonia. Nevertheless, there are no clear data to indicate the efficacy of fluconazole in the treatment of primary coccidioidal pneumonia or the prevention of later dissemination [1].

For patients at risk for disseminated disease (the immunosuppressive conditions and ethnic/racial groups listed above), antifungal treatment of primary coccidioida pneumonia is appropriate. Other indications for treatment are severe disease: infiltrates involving both lungs or more than half of one lung, or significant hilar or mediastinal lymphadenopathy; IgG titers >1:16; highly symptomatic disease (weight loss >10%; night sweats >3 weeks; symptoms >2 months) [1]. Signs of chronic infection, such as weight loss, night sweats, persistent multi-lobar infiltrates and symptoms of more than 2 months duration suggest progression to the chronic pulmonary form. These patients should also be treated.

Based on excellent tolerability, linear renal clearance, limited drug interactions and good efficacy, fluconazole has become the drug of choice for less severely ill patients. In a clinical trial, the response rate in chronic pulmonary and disseminated disease was 50% for fluconazole versus 63% for itraconazole ($p = 0.08$) [8]. Fluconazole doses of 400 mg/day are used initially, but slow responses and clinical failures in meningitis have led physicians to use initial doses as high as 1000 mg per day for meningitis [1]. A course of treatment for 6 months has been suggested for primary pneumonia and treatments of greater than 12 months *after* response of chronic, or severe pulmonary or disseminated, disease [1].

Although itraconazole is slightly superior to fluconazole in some patients, the less predictable pharmacokinetics and more frequent adverse events (gastrointestinal intolerance, hepatotoxicity, heart failure, and an occasional syndrome of hypertension, edema and hypokalemia) have made itraconazole a secondary drug [6]. Itraconazole is administered either as capsules with a lipid-containing meal or orally as a solution in the fasted state, at 400–600 mg per day. The largest comparative studies have been done with the capsule form, which is better tolerated but less predictably absorbed [8]. It is conceivable that itraconazole solution might give better results as a result of its higher oral bioavailability, but intolerance has been a problem. Itraconazole inhibits and is metabolized by cytochrome 3A4, so its drug interactions are extensive and problematic [9]. Tacrolimus and cyclosporine (among other drugs) doses must be reduced and rifampin can induce metabolism to the degree that itraconazole is unmeasurable in the serum. There is much less experience with itraconazole in the treatment of coccidioidal meningitis [6].

For life-threatening coccidioidomycosis, amphotericin B desoxycholate or a lipid formulation of amphotericin B should be used [1]. The latter is generally preferred because of the need for prolonged therapy and its decreased risk of nephrotoxicity. There is no evidence that high doses of the lipid formulations (e.g. 10 mg/kg) are more effective than doses of 3–6 mg/kg. Responses to amphotericin therapy on the order of 50–70% are seen [6]. When the patient has improved or when nephrotoxicity occurs, treatment is shifted to triazoles for the remainder of the therapy.

Because the triazoles may be teratogenic, another indication for amphotericin B is coccidioidomycosis during pregnancy [1]. If a pregnant patient develops severe nephrotoxicity, one may be forced to use a triazole for at least a limited time, preferably later in pregnancy [6].

A challenge in the management of coccidioidomycosis is treatment when initial therapy fails, or when the patient relapses (which may be years later). At present, there are two options for salvage. The first is voriconazole at 400–600 mg/day, which has proven successful in six of seven patients with refractory disease [10]. However, we have seen one patient respond well to voriconazole given as a "last ditch" effort, only to have her relapse more than a year after treatment was stopped. Another salvage option is posaconazole, 200 mg four times per day with a fatty meal. More than half of patients who have failed other treatments respond to posaconazole [11, 12]. Posaconazole has also been used as primary therapy with responses in 85% of 20 patients [13]. Unfortunately, the trial was terminated at 6 months of therapy, with relapses later appearing in a third of 15 patients who initially responded.

For coccidioidal meningitis, there is the additional option of intrathecal amphotericin B. However, intrathecal amphotericin B can cause arachnoiditis and vasculitis and should be administered with corticosteroids to suppress these inflammatory adverse events; it is seldom used in the post-fluconazole era [6]. Voriconazole has also been used successfully in salvage treatment of coccidoidal meningitis [10]. Hydrocephalus may require ventriculoperitoneal shunting. Occasionally, hydrocephalus may recur with granuloma formation at the distal shunt orifice causing obstruction. Reduction of immunosuppression is an important adjunct to antifungal therapy, including the initiation of antiretroviral therapy if the patient has AIDS. It is unclear when to terminate antifungal treatment of patients with AIDS, though some have considered this when the CD4 count is above 250 cells/mm^3 [1]. It has been increasingly appreciated that patients with coccidioidal meningitis require lifelong antifungal therapy [1, 2, 6]. This may also apply to patients with relapsing non-meningeal disease.

There are other measures which have been used in the treatment of coccidioidomycosis, such as surgical debulking of large abscesses or granulomatous lesions, but these have no proven efficacy. Treatment for vertebral osteomyelitis may require surgical stabilization [2].

During recent decades, there have been multiple efforts to develop a vaccine against coccidioidomycosis. Although there are many vaccine candidates, there is no clearly efficacious vaccine.

REFERENCES

1. Galgiani JN, Ampel NM, Blair JE, et al. Coccidioidomycosis. Clin Infect Dis 2005;41:1217–23.
2. Parish JM, Blair JE. Coccidioidomycosis. Mayo Clin Proc 2008;83:343–48.
3. Flaherman VJ, Hector R, Rutherford GW. Estimating severe coccidioidomycosis in California. Emerg Infect Dis 2007;13:1087–90.
4. Hung C-Y, Xue J, Cole GT. Virulence mechanisms of *Coccidioides*. Ann NY Acad Sci 2007;1111:225–35.
5. Chang DC, Anderson S, Wannemuehler K, et al. Testing for coccidioidomycosis among patients with community-acquired pneumonia. Emerg Infect Dis 2008;14:1053–9.

6. Anstead GM, Graybill JR. Coccidioidomycosis. Infect Dis Clin N Amer 2006;20:621–43.
7. Durkin M, Connolly P, Kuberski T, et al. Diagnosis of coccidioidomycosis with use of the *Coccidioides* antigen enzyme immunoassay. Clin Infect Dis 2008;47:e69–73.
8. Galgiani JN, Catanzaro A, Cloud GA, et al. Comparison of oral fluconazole and itraconazole for progressive, nonmeningeal coccidioidomycosis – a randomized, double-blind trial. Ann Intern Med 2000;133:676–86.
9. Graybill JR, Galgiana JN, Stevens DA, et al. Itraconazole treatment of coccidiodomycosis. Am J Med 1990;89:292–300.
10. Freifeld A, Proia L, Andes D, et al. Voriconazole use for endemic fungal infections. Antimicrob Agents Chemother 2009;53:1648–51.
11. Stevens DA, Rendon A, Gaona-Flores V, et al. Posaconazole therapy for chronic refractory coccidioidomycosis. Chest 2007;132:952–8.
12. Anstead GM, Corcoran G, Lewis J, et al. Refractory coccidioidomycosis treated with posaconazole. Clin Infect Dis 2005;40:1770–6.
13. Catanzaro A, Cloud GA, Stevens DA, et al. Safety, tolerance, and efficacy of posaconazole therapy in patients with nonmeningeal disseminated or chronic pulmonary coccidioidomycosis. Clin Infect Dis 2007;45:562–8.

82 Blastomycosis

Keyur S Vyas, Robert W Bradsher Jr

Key features

- Endemic mycosis caused by the dimorphic fungus *Blastomyces dermatitidis*
- Most often reported from the Mississippi, Ohio, and St Lawrence river basin areas of North America, with occasional cases reported in Central and South America, Africa, and Europe
- Pulmonary infection is common and may be subclinical or present as an acute or chronic pneumonia, or chronic mass lesions; skin lesions are also common
- Direct visualization of the organism by microscopic examination of stained histopathology or cytology specimens and culture of secretions or tissue remains the cornerstone of diagnosis
- Itraconazole is the treatment of choice for most manifestions. Amphotericin B is reserved for initial treatment of life-threatening or central nervous system infection

INTRODUCTION

Blastomycosis is caused by the dimorphic fungus *Blastomyces dermatitidis*, one of the endemic mycoses. Historically, this disease was termed "North American blastomycosis". This terminology has been abandoned as there have been increasing reports of blastomycosis from other parts of the world and the term paracoccidioidomycosis has become accepted for the disease previously called "South American blastomycosis", which is caused by *Paracoccidioides brasiliensis* [1]. Infection typically presents as an acute or indolent pulmonary process, or as a chronic skin lesion, although infection of almost any site can occur. The disease may often be misdiagnosed as another type of infection or malignancy. Treatment with antifungal agents is usually successful.

EPIDEMIOLOGY

Most reported cases of blastomycosis have been from North America, concentrated in the Mississippi, Ohio, and St Lawrence River basins and the Great Lakes region of the USA and Canada [2]. Occasional cases have been reported from Africa, Central America, northern South America, and the Mediterranean basin. Unlike other endemic mycoses, such as histoplasmosis or coccidioidomycosis, *B. dermatitidis* has not been consistently isolated from the soil, although epidemiologically, this is the source [3]. There have been common-source outbreaks reported in the literature, and Klein and coworkers provided strong evidence of *B. dermatitidis* in the soil by culturing the organism in association with an epidemic of infection [4]. In this report, there was an association of exposure to beaver dams. However, this epidemic was more likely because of the presence of moist soil, highly enriched with organic material that provided favorable conditions for the organism to grow. In this outbreak, it was noted that many patients with infection did not have signs and symptoms characteristic of blastomycosis, supporting the existence of subclinical or self-limited infection, as occurs in histoplasmosis and coccidioidomycosis.

Although there is no particular predisposition to developing blastomycosis, many patients have a history of recreational or occupational exposure to wooded areas, and often to soil associated with animals or bodies of freshwater such as lakes and rivers [1, 3]. A review of 1114 cases from the literature revealed that 87% of patients were between 20 and 69 years of age [5]. The male to female ratio is at least 4:1, probably owing to differences in exposure risk [1]. While infection in children is rare, it is well documented [6].

Infection has occurred in dogs, cats, cows, and other mammals, but zoonotic spread to humans has not occurred, except in very rare cases of dogs with oral lesions transmitting infection via bites. Likewise, person-to-person transmission is rare, with a single case of a man with genitourinary disease transmitting pelvic blastomycosis to his wife [7], and rare cases of intrauterine transmission from mother to child [8].

Unlike other endemic mycoses, such as histoplasmosis, coccidioidomycosis or penicilliosis, blastomycosis has only occasionally been reported as a significant pathogen in patients with AIDS. When it does occur in this setting, it is typically during advanced stages of AIDS with very low CD4 lymphocyte counts. The disease tends to be rapidly progressive, widely disseminated and usually fatal [9]. If response to antifungal agents occurs, the patient should be maintained on chronic secondary prophylaxis until immune reconstitution occurs [10]. Blastomycosis has been reported in patients with other immunosuppressive conditions such as organ transplantation, hematologic malignancies, corticosteroid use and, more recently, tumor necrosis factor inhibitor use.

NATURAL HISTORY, PATHOGENESIS, AND PATHOLOGY

The portal of infection is the lung, via inhalation of infective conidia, which are taken up by bronchopulmonary phagocytes. It is here that the fungus undergoes transformation into the yeast phase. Pulmonary infection may be asymptomatic, present like an acute bacterial pneumonia, or a more indolent chronic pneumonia with pulmonary nodules or cavitation. Presenting signs and symptoms are generally nonspecific, but referable to sites of hematogenous seeding in the skin, bone, prostate, epididymis, or other organs. The inflammatory response is a mixture of granulomatous and pyogenic elements. Collections of neutrophils range in size from microscopic to large abscesses (Fig. 82.1). Pseudoepitheliomatous hyperplasia and acanthosis is found in skin and mucous membrane lesions that has prompted misdiagnosis of squamous cell carcinoma or keratoacanthoma in some patients [2].

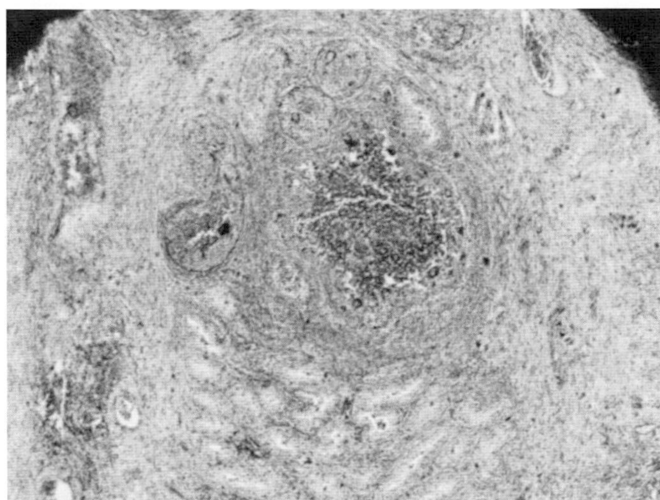

FIGURE 82.1 Testicular blastomycosis (hematoxylin and eosin stain, ×23). Note the microscopic abscess surrounded by granulomatous inflammation.

CLINICAL FEATURES

LUNG LESIONS

Acute pulmonary blastomycosis can present as an asymptomatic radiographic infiltrate or as a pneumonia that is indistinguishable from acute bacterial pneumonia with fever, chills, and productive cough with or without hemoptysis. Another presentation is several months of fever, nightsweats, productive cough, and chest pain; this is typical for patients with chronic pulmonary blastomycosis. Adult respiratory distress syndrome can manifest in patients with miliary or endobronchial spread of infection and is associated with a high mortality. Pulmonary findings are present radiologically in half of patients. The radiologic appearance can resemble bacterial pneumonia in patients who present more acutely (Fig. 82.2) or as a mass lesion in patients with a more indolent course [11]. Chronic pulmonary lesions may show fibrosis and cavitation. Calcification, pleural effusion or hilar adenopathy are rarely encountered.

SKIN LESIONS

The skin is the most common extrapulmonary site of infection, with 40–80% of patients having skin involvement [12]. Lesions are often multiple and tend to be located on the face and extremities (Fig. 82.3). They are typically erythematous, well-circumscribed, hyperkeratotic, crusted nodules or plaques that enlarge over weeks. These lesions may ulcerate to leave an undermined edge (Fig. 82.4). Some central healing can occur in chronic cases forming a hypopigmented, atrophic, fibrotic area. Lesions may also occur in the mucous membranes of the nose, lips, larynx, and vagina.

BONE LESIONS

Osteomyelitis occurs in up to 25% of patients, affecting essentially any bone [2]. Osteolytic lesions and an adjacent cold abscess are typical features. In the majority, concomitant skin or lung infection allows the diagnosis to be made. The treatment course is usually of longer duration for bone infection [10].

SYSTEMIC INFECTIONS

Almost every organ has been reported to be infected with *B. dermatitidis*. Systemic signs of fever and weight loss are mild early in the course, but become progressively more severe with disease extension. After a period of time ranging from weeks to years, chronic infection may disseminate to multiple organs and cause death if unrecognized. Spontaneous remission is rarely observed once infection has progressed beyond the lung.

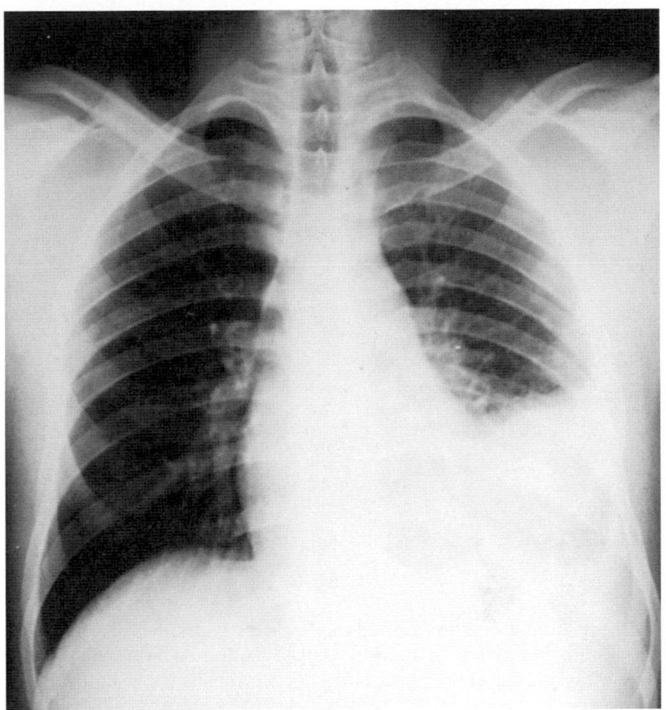

FIGURE 82.2 Blastomycosis of left lower lobe.

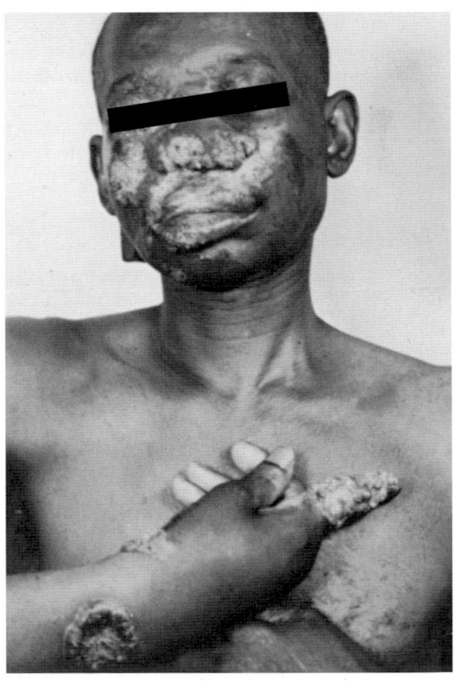

FIGURE 82.3 Cutaneous blastomycosis in a 50-year-old patient in the USPHS Hospital, New Orleans, LA, USA. No pulmonary lesions were visible radiographically *(courtesy of the Armed Forces Institute of Pathology, Photograph Neg. No. 75-9748).*

PATIENT EVALUATION, DIAGNOSIS, AND DIFFERENTIAL DIAGNOSIS

Microscopic examination of stained histopathology or cytology specimens and culture of secretions or tissues remains the cornerstone of diagnosis for blastomycosis. When clinical suspicion is high, direct microscopic examination of sputum, skin, aspirates of abscess fluid,

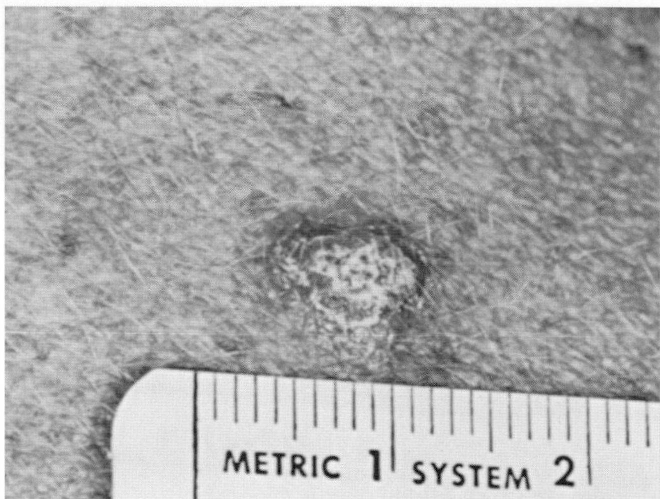

FIGURE 82.4 Small hyperkeratotic skin lesion of blastomycosis.

or body fluid following either digestion of human cells with 10% potassium hydroxide or staining with calcafluor white or Papanicolaou's stain is the most rapid and effective means for diagnosis. The organism can be visualized in tissue specimens stained with methenamine silver or periodic acid-Schiff stains [12].

Culture should be done and is positive in almost all cases. At room temperature, the organism will grow as a mold in 2–4 weeks on a wide range of culture media, including Sabouraud agar. Skin tests are not helpful and are not available. Serologic studies using a variety of antigens and methods have likewise been unreliable for diagnosis [13]. An assay to detect *B. dermatitidis* antigens in urine is available commercially and may be helpful, although significant cross-reactivity has been noted with histoplasmosis, paracoccidioidomycosis, and penicilliosis [14].

DIFFERENTIAL DIAGNOSIS

Skin lesions may be mistaken for basal or squamous cell carcinoma. Nasal lesions may resemble leishmaniasis and paracoccidioidomycosis. Laryngeal lesions mimic epidermoid carcinoma both clinically and pathologically. Pulmonary blastomycosis may resemble tuberculosis and other granulomatous infections, or bronchogenic carcinoma both symptomatically and radiographically.

TREATMENT

The vast majority of patients coming to medical attention will need antifungal chemotherapy [2]. Oral itraconazole at a dose of 200–400 mg daily is now the recommended drug for all but the most severe cases. Amphotericin B was the drug of choice for all patients in the past and continues to be initial therapy for those with life-threatening blastomycosis or central nervous system (CNS) infection [10]. The deoxycholate formulation is given intravenously at a dose of 0.7–1mg/kg daily. Alternatively, the liposomal formulation, which is preferred for CNS disease, can be given at 3–5 mg/kg daily with fewer side effects, but at greater cost. Amphotericin formulations are typically given for 1–2 weeks (4–6 weeks for CNS disease), until improvement occurs, after which therapy can be completed with oral itraconazole. Non-life-threatening infections can be treated for the entire course with itraconazole alone. Itraconazole achieves cure rates of approximately 95% in those completing therapy [15]. It also has fewer adverse effects than amphotericin B. Fluconazole has lower success rates in treatment and requires much higher doses than itraconazole. A few cases have been treated with voriconazole or posaconazole.

REFERENCES

1. Bradsher RW. Blastomycosis. Infect Dis Clin North Am 1988;2:4.
2. Bradsher RW, Chapman SW, Pappas PG. Blastomycosis. Infect Dis Clin North Am 2003;17:21–40.
3. Bradsher RW. Water and blastomycosis: Don't blame beaver. Am Rev Respir Dis 1987;136:1324–6.
4. Klein BS, Vergeront JM, Weeks RJ, et al. Isolation of B. dermatitidis in soil associated with a large outbreak of blastomycosis in Wisconsin. N Engl J Med 1986;314:529–34.
5. Furcolow ML, Chick EW, Busey JD, Menges RW. Prevalence and incidence studies of human and canine blastomycosis cases in the United States 1885-1968. Am Rev Respir Dis 1970;102:60–7.
6. Schutze GE, Hickerson SL, Fortin EM, et al. Blastomycosis in children. Clin Infect Dis 1996;22:496–502.
7. Craig MW, Davey WN, Green RA. Conjugal blastomycosis. Am Rev Respir Dis 1970;102:86–90.
8. Maxson S, Miller SF, Tryka AF, Schutze GE. Perinatal blastomycosis: a review. Pediatr Infect Dis J 1992;11:760–3.
9. Pappas PG, Pottage JC, Powderly WG, et al. Blastomycosis in patients with the acquired immunodeficiency syndrome. Ann Intern Med 1994;116: 847–53.
10. Chapman SW, Dismukes WE, Proia LA, et al. Clinical practice guidelines for the management of blastomycosis: 2008 update by the Infectious Diseases Society of America. Clin Infect Dis 2008;46:1801–12.
11. Halvorsen RA, Duncan JD, Merten DF, et al. Pulmonary blastomycosis: Radiologic manifestations. Radiology 1984;150:1–5.
12. Saccente M, Woods GL. Clinical and laboratory update on blastomycosis. Clin Micro Rev 2010;23:367–81.
13. Bradsher RW, Pappas PG. Detection of specific antibodies in human blastomycosis by enzyme immunoassay. South Med J 1995;88:1256–9.
14. Durkin M, Witt J, Lemonte A, Wheat B, Connolly P. Antigen assay with the potential to aid in diagnosis of blastomycosis. J Clin Microbiol 2004;42: 4873–5.
15. Dismukes WE, Bradsher RW, Cloud GC, et al. Itraconazole therapy of blastomycosis and histoplasmosis. Am J Med 1992;93:489–97.

Paracoccidioidomycosis 83

Ricardo Negroni

Key features

- Chronic progressive form: oropharyngeal ulcers, granulomatous laryngitis, chronic respiratory disease, skin ulcers, and adrenal insufficiency
- Acute form of juvenile type: patient of less than 30 years of age, fever, adenomegalies, hepatosplenomegaly, diarrhea, and loss of body weight
- Rural population of tropical regions in South America
- Mixed granuloma, epithelioid and suppurative, showing multibudding yeast-like cells
- Synonyms: South American blastomicosis and Lutz's mycosis

INTRODUCTION

Paracoccidioidomycosis is a systemic mycosis endemic in South and Central America caused by a dimorphic fungus, *Paracoccidioides brasiliensis.*

This mycosis was discovered by Adolfo Lutz in Brazil in 1908. Alfonso Splendore (1912) published several cases in São Paulo (Brazil) and described the etiologic agent. Floriano P. de Almeida (1930) clearly separated this mycosis from coccidioidomycosis [1–3].

EPIDEMIOLOGY

Paracoccidioidomycosis is endemic in humid tropical and subtropical areas of Latin America, from Southern Mexico to 34° South in Argentina and Uruguay (Fig. 83.1). It is frequent in Brazil, where 80% of all patients are detected, and where it is the eighth leading cause of death. This mycosis also occurs in Argentina, Colombia, Ecuador, Paraguay, and Venezuela [4].

The endemic zones have acid soils, rich in organic material, with many streams and rivers, and exuberant vegetation. The habitat of *P. brasiliensis* is not well known; it probably lives in soil near water. It has been isolated from different natural sources, but these isolations have not been replicated. Beside humans, infection has been observed in armadillos and squirrel monkeys. Animal-to-human and human-to-human transmission have not been confirmed [2–4].

Infection is most likely acquired by airborne inhalation of conidiae; primary infections of skin or mucosa are rare. Primary pulmonary infection is often asymptomatic or mild and self-limited (paracoccidioidomycosis-infection) [5].

Reactivation of latent pulmonary or extrapulmonary foci leads to progressive clinical forms that are severe (paracoccidioidomycosis disease). This presentation is frequently observed in adult males above 35 years of age, the majority of whom are rural workers; genetics, smoking and alcoholism seem to be risk factors. The juvenile type of paracoccidioidomycosis is less common (only 3–5% of clinical cases). It has an acute course and affects both sexes equally [4, 5].

The incidence and prevalence of paracoccidioidomycosis are not known because there is no compulsory reporting.

NATURAL HISTORY, PATHOGENESIS, AND PATHOLOGY

In infected tissue and culture at 37 °C, *P. brasiliensis* appears as spherical cells of 10–40 μm in diameter with a thick bi-refringent cell wall and several peripheral buds, like a pilot wheel. Mother cells with a single blastoconidium and short chains of three to four budding cells are often found (Fig. 83.2). In Sabouraud dextrose agar and in yeast extract agar at 25 °C, *P. brasiliensis* grows very slowly and yields cotton-like, whitish colonies that exhibit microscopically branched, septated and hyaline hyphae with chlamidospores and aleurioconidiae. This fungal species is genetically heterogeneous and a new species, with the same morphologic characteristics, named *Paracoccidiodes lutzi*, has been proposed [1, 3, 6]. This strain was isolated from southwest Brazil.

Infection occurs following inhalation of aleurioconidiae that turn into yeast-like elements inside alveolar macrophages. A nonspecific inflammatory reaction is initially observed. In a few days these inflammatory changes progress to epithelioid cell granuloma with giant cells, plasmacytes, and lymphocytes. Microabscesses are common and caseous necrosis is observed in lymph nodes. Tissue repair involves fibrosis. Cell-mediated immunity, with a predominant Th_1 cytokine response (INF-γ, IL_{12}, IL_2, TNF-α), is the most important defense mechanism, this type of reaction is genetically controlled. Antibodies are also produced during progressive disease but their significance in the control of the infection is not well understood [7].

Progressive paracoccidioidomycosis may be the result of reactivation of a latent focus of infection (in chronic forms) or the lack of control of the primary infection (in the acute juvenile type) [5].

CLINICAL FEATURES

NONPROGRESSIVE INFECTIONS

Primary infections are often asymptomatic or subclinical and self-limited. Symptomatic primary infections are rare, calcifications of lung or lymph node foci are infrequent and 6–50% of inhabitants of endemic regions have positive paracoccidioidin skin tests as evidence of a prior subclinical infection [5].

PROGRESSIVE FORMS

Acute form of Juvenile Type

This clinical form in children and adolescents has an acute course marked by toxemia, fever, asthenia, anorexia, weight loss, subcutaneous abscesses, diffuse lymphadenopathy, hepatosplenomegaly,

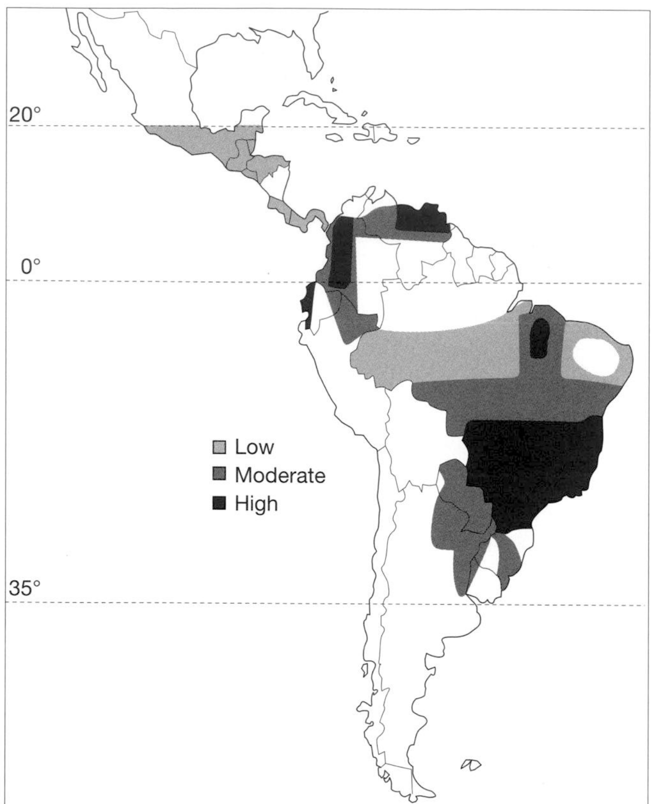

FIGURE 83.1 Geographic distribution of paracoccidiodomycosis *(courtesy of Flavio de Queiroz Telles).*

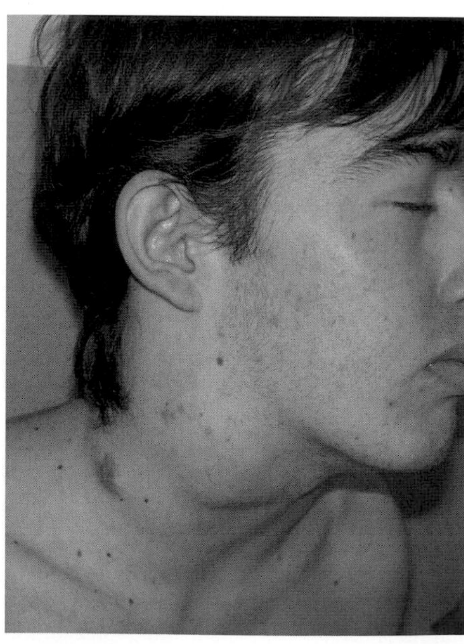

FIGURE 83.2 Acute disseminated form of juvenile type with enlarged lymph nodes in the neck.

diarrhea, jaundice, anemia, and leukocytosis with eosinophilia. Radiographic alterations of the lungs and mucous membrane lesions are rarely observed. Acneiform lesions of the skin, scrofuloderma, osteomyelitis, and gastrointestinal involvement are often present. Moderate cases with stable general condition and localized lymph node involvement occur (Fig. 83.3) [2–4].

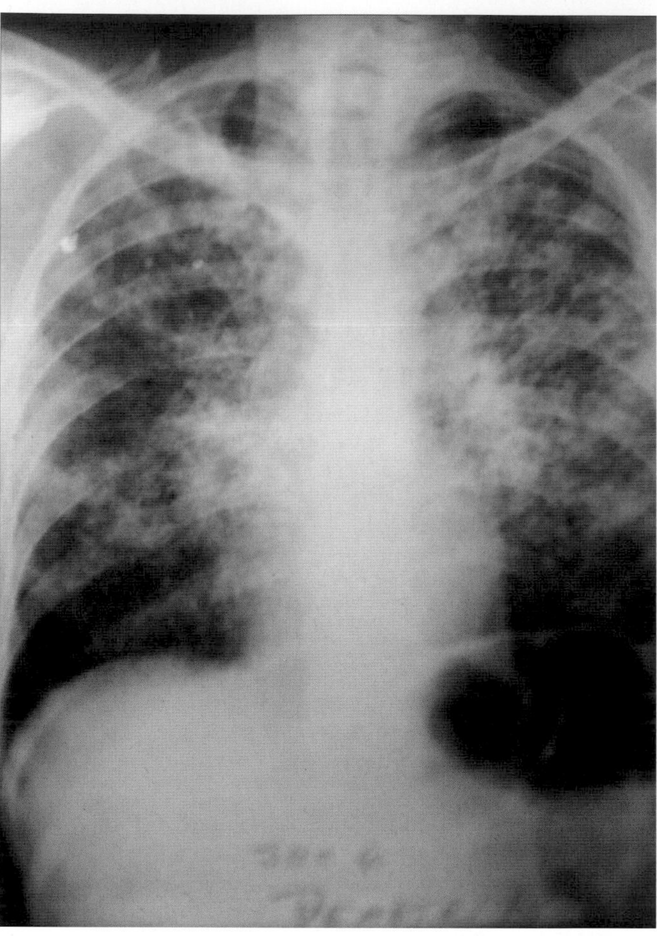

FIGURE 83.3 Chest x-ray of a patient suffering chronic adult-type paracoccidiodomycosis. Disseminated interstitial disease is observed.

Chronic form of Adult Type

This clinical form usually occurs in adult males. The onset is insidious with asthenia, loss of weight, and exertional dyspnea being the prominent features, lesions may be unifocal or multifocal [5].

In 25% of cases, only pulmonary involvement is detected, characterized by low-grade fever, cough, mucopurulent expectoration, hemoptysis, and dyspnea. Chest x-ray studies show bilateral symmetric lesions, generally perihiliar in distribution, resembling the wings of the butterfly and formed by infiltrates, micronodular and linear shadows (Fig. 83.4). Death occurs after several years, as a result of cachexia or respiratory impairments [2, 4].

Multifocal presentation is observed in more than 70% of patients; skin, mucous membranes, lungs, lymph nodes, adrenal glands, abdominal organs, and central nervous system (CNS) are often involved. Typical oropharyngeal lesions are ulcers with hemorrhagic granulomatous foci and an infiltrated hard base (mulberry-like stomatitis) (Fig. 83.5). A firm red-violet edema is frequently observed in the lips and gingival mucosa (thromboid-like lip) [2]. These lesions make eating and drinking painful. Laryngeal attacks cause dysphonia, obstructive dyspnea, and dysphagia.

Skin lesions include papules, nodules, and ulcers; they are often located at the face and neck (Fig. 83.6). Some ulcers become vegetative and papillomatous. Cervical lymph nodes are generally hypertrophic and firm, but sometimes they are suppurative or necrotic, opening to the skin and causing a scrofula-like lesion. Adrenal glands involvement occurs in more than 15% of chronic cases and when severe, causes Addisons disease. CNS compromise is observed in 10% of cases; abscessed granulomas located in the posterior fosse and

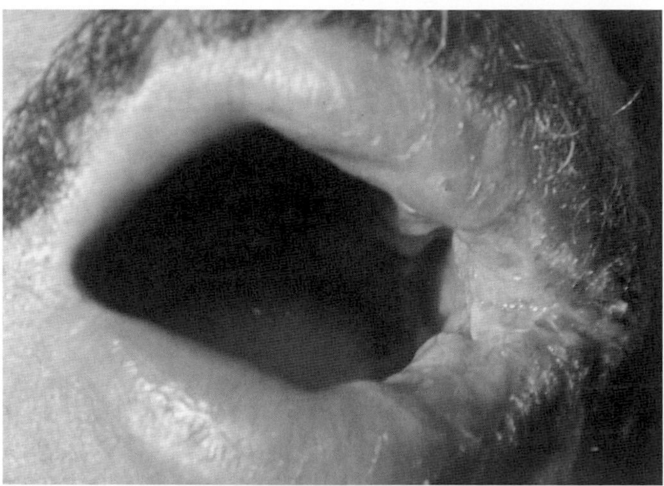

FIGURE 83.4 Granulomatous ulcerated lesion of the oral mucosa in a patient with a chronic progressive paracoccidiodomycosis.

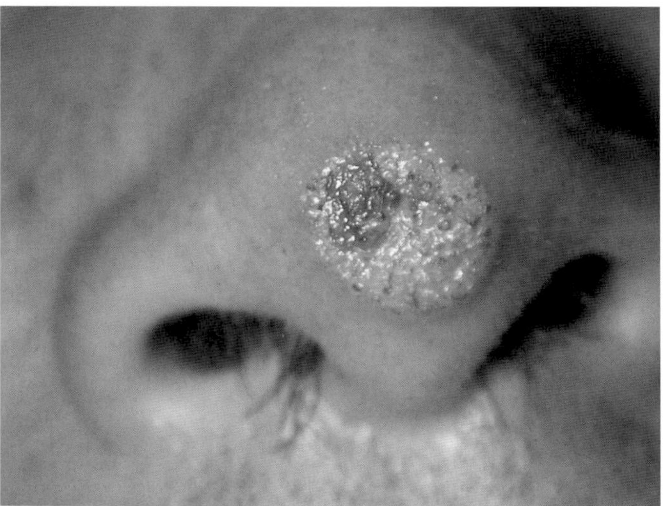

FIGURE 83.5 Ulcerated lesion of the skin, a typical granulomatous hemorrhagic lesion is observed.

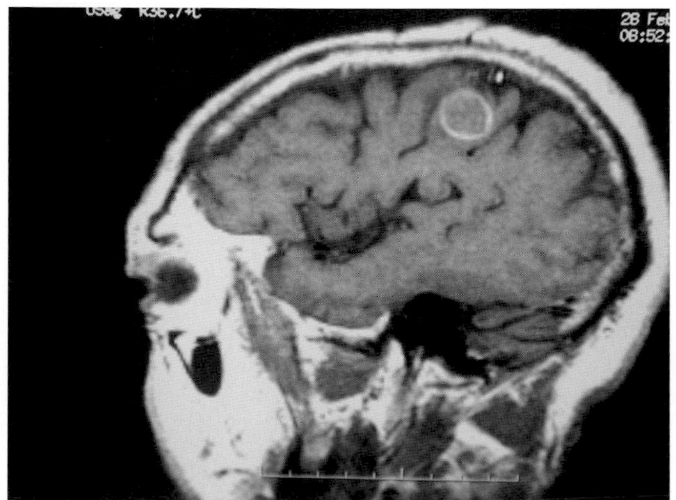

FIGURE 83.6 Computed tomography of the brain of a granulomatous lesion on the parietal lobe.

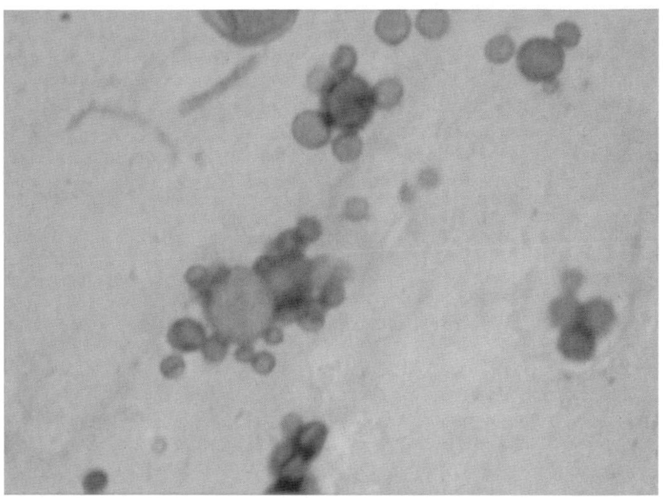

FIGURE 83.7 Bronchoalveolar lavage smear stained by Grocott methenamine silver. Typical yeast-like elements of *P. brasiliensis* are observed (400×).

subacute meningoencephalitis have been reported (Fig. 83.7). Other locations can be testicles, epidydimis, prostate, bones, liver, and spleen. Death may occur from respiratory failure, malnutrition, or intercurrent infections [2, 3, 5].

After effective treatment some lesions remain latent and relapses can occasionally occur [2].

- AIDS-related paracoccidioidomycosis. This association has been observed frequently only in Brazil. The majority of patients present with acute disseminated juvenile type; the mortality rate is approximately 30% in treated cases.
- Paracoccidioidomycosis is associated with tuberculosis in 10–12% of cases.
- The incidence of neoplasms, especially lung cancer, seems to be more common among the paracoccidioidomycosis patients [5, 8].

PATIENT EVALUATION, DIAGNOSIS, AND DIFFERENTIAL DIAGNOSIS

Diagnosis is confirmed by finding typical yeast-like elements of *P. brasiliensis* in microscopic examination of wet preparations of specimens submitted for mycologic studies (Fig. 83.2). Cultures should be done in yeast extract agar without glucose, brain-heart infusion agar and Sabouraud dextrose agar with antibiotics and incubated for 4 weeks at 25 °C and 37 °C. The fungus grows slowly and its isolation is difficult. Inoculation of clinical specimens in laboratory animals is rarely done [1, 2].

Histopathologic specimens should be stained with periodic acid Schiff or Grocott methenamine-silver [2, 5].

In the progressive forms of paracoccidioidomycosis, specific antibodies can be detected by immunodiffusion in agar gel, counterimmunoelectrophoresis, complement fixation test, and ELISA. A specific glycoprotein of 43 kDa (gp 43), as well as other antigens, have been used in these tests [9]. Titers are proportional to severity of the infection and with cure they decline or became negative. In severe cases antigen can be detected in serum and urine by ELISA using monoclonal antibodies against gp 43 [3].

Paracoccidioidin skin test has little diagnostic value for progressive paracoccidioidomycosis. It is valuable in epidemiologic studies; most infected people without active lesions have positive reactions [2].

In patients with severe disease, serology is positive with high titers, paracoccidioidin skin test is often negative, polyclonal hypergammaglobulinemia, and eosinophilia and low CD_4-positive cell counts are frequently detected. All these alterations may revert with clinical improvement [2, 3, 5, 7].

The differential diagnosis depends upon the clinical manifestation. Chronic disseminated disease can be confused with tuberculosis, histoplasmosis, leishmaniasis, carcinoma, and sarcoidosis; acute disseminated disease presents with clinical characteristics similar to tuberculosis, malaria, leukemia, and lymphomas.

TREATMENT

Sulfonamides, ketoconazole, itraconazole, and amphotericin B have been successfully used in the treatment of paracoccidioidomycosis. Accepted treatment schedules are: ketoconazole 200–400 mg/day for 12 months; itraconazole 100–200 mg/day for 6 months; and amphotericin B given intravenously at daily dose of 0.7–0.8/kg, up to a maximum total dose of 35 mg/kg. The azoles are administered by oral route after a meal. Amphotericin B is indicated in severe cases where there is malabsorption. Itraconazole is the treatment of choice and is effective in more than 95% of cases. However, its absorption requires gastric acid and its effect can be reduced by involvement of mesenteric lymph nodes, especially in acute disseminated form. It should not be used for patients with tuberculosis under treatment with rifampin.

Co-trimoxazole is still frequently used in Brazil, especially in recently diagnosed patients with no previous therapy, in chronic unifocal progressive disease, and as maintenance after a course of amphotericin B. It is given to adults every 12 hours, at a dosage of 160 mg of trimethoprim and 800 mg of sulfamethoxazole, for 2–3 years [3, 7].

Children suffering paracoccidiodomycosis are usually treated with amphotericin B intravenously at daily dose of 0.7 mg/kg of body weight or sulfadiazine 200 mg/kg/day by oral route, often because of the difficulty they have in taking oral medication and the frequent involvement of mesenteric lymph nodes [3, 7].

Other drugs that have been successfully used are voriconazole, posaconazole, and terbinafine, but clinical experience with them remains limited.

Paracoccidiodomycosis is always a severe infection that requires prolonged treatment. Relapses are common and cure often leaves incapacitating sequelae, for example laryngeal and tracheal stenosis, buccal atresia, and pulmonary fibrosis.

Although several antigens have been studied as inmunogens to prevent paracoccidiodomycosis in laboratory animals, none of them have been used in human beings and there is no measure to avoid the risk of infection [3, 7, 8].

REFERENCES

1. Brummer E, Castañeda E, Restrepo A. Paracoccidioidomycosis; an update. Clin Microbiol Rev 1993;6:89–117.
2. Negroni R. Paracoccidioidomycosis (South American blastomicosis, Lutz's Mycosis). Intern J Dermatol 1993;32:847–59.
3. Restrepo Moreno A. Paracoccidioidomycosis. In: Dismukes W, Pappas P, Sobel JD, eds. Medical Mycology. Oxford: Oxford University Press; 2003:328–45.
4. Wanke B, Londero AT. *Paracoccidioides brasiliensis*. In: Ajello L, Hay R eds. Medical Mycology. Topley and Wilson's Microbiology and Microbial Infections, 9th edn, Vol. 4. London, Sydney, Auckland: Arnold; 1998:395–407.
5. de Franco MF, Lacaz C da S, Restrepo-Moreno A, Del Negro G, eds. Paracoccidioidomycosis. Boca Raton. Ann. Arbor, London, Tokyo: C.R.C. Press; 1994.
6. Felipe MS, Teixeira MM. Is *Paracoccidioides brasiliensis* an unique species? Biomédica 2008;28:136.
7. Calich VLG, da Costa TA, Felonato M, et al. Innate immunity to *Paracoccidioides brasiliensis* infection. Mycopathologia 2008;165:223–36.
8. Negroni R. *Paracoccidioides brasiliensis*. In: Yu V, Weber R, Raoult D, eds. Antimicrobial Therapy and Vaccines, 2nd edn. New York: Apple Trees Production LLC; 2002:1097–105.
9. Camargo ZP de, Franco MF de. Current knowledge on pathogenesis and immunodiagnosis of paracoccidioidomycosis. Rev Iberoamer Micol 2000; 17:41–8.

Cryptococcosis 84

Françoise Dromer, Olivier Lortholary

Key features

- Cryptococcosis is a life-threatening infection caused by two encapsulated yeasts: mainly *Cryptococcus neoformans* but also *Cryptococcus gattii*
- *Cryptococcus neoformans* meningoencephalitis is a major opportunistic infection in anti-retroviral naïve patients with AIDS
- Severity of disease (central nervous system involvement, dissemination, high antigen titers, acute respiratory symptoms) needs to be assessed for optimization of treatment
- The most severe patients should be treated with a combination of an amphotericin B formulation and flucytosine for at least 2 weeks when possible and switched to fluconazole for a total of 10–12 weeks and then maintenance therapy with low-dose fluconazole
- Control of elevated intracranial pressure is crucial for treatment efficacy

INTRODUCTION

Cryptococcosis is a major cause of global mortality (fourth, before tuberculosis), particularly with the AIDS epidemic and the lack of availability of anti-retroviral therapy in many countries. Outbreaks caused by *Cryptococcus gattii* have recently been reported in both apparently immunocompetent and immunodeficient hosts in the Pacific Northwest of North America.

EPIDEMIOLOGY

Cryptococcus neoformans [cosmopolitan, including variety *grubii* (serotype A) and var. *neoformans* (serotype D) and *C. gattii* (serotypes B and C)] are basidiomycetous yeasts found in the environment (especially bird droppings, dust). *Cryptococcus gattii* is mostly found in tropical and subtropical areas but a highly virulent lineage has recently spread to Vancouver Island, the Canadian mainland, and Pacific Northwest.

HIV infection is a major risk factor for cryptococcosis: ~ 1 million cases/year, particularly in sub-Saharan Africa and Southeast Asia with >600,000 deaths/year [1]. The incidence rate was 95/100,000 among HIV-infected persons and 1400/100,000 among persons living with AIDS in a population-based surveillance program in South Africa [2]. The prevalence of infection was 18% among HIV-infected Cambodian patients with <200 CD4$^+$/mm^3 [3]. When available, highly active anti-retroviral therapy (HAART) decreases the incidence of cryptococcosis [4] and the associated long-term mortality and relapse rate [5]. Patients with AIDS are only rarely infected with *C. gattii*.

Risk factors for cryptococcosis in HIV-negative persons are corticosteroid therapy, chronic lymphoid malignancies, solid organ transplantation and other diseases (e.g. sarcoidosis, diabetes mellitus, liver or renal dysfunctions, idiopathic CD4 lymphopenia) [6]. About 5% of patients have no obvious risk factors.

Males are more susceptible than females, regardless of the HIV status. Cryptococcosis is rare in children, even those who are immunocompromised [7].

NATURAL HISTORY, PATHOGENESIS, AND PATHOLOGY

Infection by *C. neoformans* usually represents reactivation of a latent infection acquired early in life by inhalation [8]. However, acute pneumonia following massive inhalation of contaminated dust or primary skin infection following injury occurs. Disease with *C. gattii* is estimated to begin anywhere from 2–11 months after exposure [9].

Cryptococcus spp. are encapsulated yeasts. The capsule is composed of polysaccharides of which the main component, glucuronxylomannan, is a major virulence factor. It is secreted during growth *in vitro* and during the infection. Its detection in body fluids is used for the diagnosis of cryptococcosis with commercially available and reliable kits. Other virulence factors have been uncovered, such as the ability to grow at 37°C, melanin production and production of other enzymes [8].

Invasion of the central nervous system (CNS) following fungemia is a key feature. The term meningoencephalitis rather than meningitis is used because of frequent involvement of the brain parenchyma. The presence of polysaccharide around the pseudocysts/masses formed by dilatations of the Virchow-Robin spaces is responsible for brain edema and increased intracranial pressure (Fig. 84.1). Infection by *C. neoformans* is usually characterized by a low inflammatory response of the host, especially HIV-infected patients, in contrast to those caused by *C. gattii* where brain and lung granulomas can be observed. The immune reconstitution inflammatory syndrome (IRIS) which corresponds to a granulomatous tissue reaction induced by the restoration of a Th1 response following initiation of HAART can provoke severe symptoms requiring intensive care hospitalization [10, 11]. It has to be differentiated from cryptococcosis relapse.

CLINICAL FEATURES

CRYPTOCOCCUS NEOFORMANS *INFECTIONS*

Central Nervous System (CNS) Involvement

Meningoencephalitis is diagnosed in ≥75% of cases and more frequently in HIV-infected patients [12]. Symptoms are rarely acute. More often, patients complain of dizziness, headache, and nausea. Changes in behavior can be noted. Fever is rarely high and is usually intermittent. As infection progresses, impaired vision or hearing, coma, seizures, and other palsies can occur. Signs of meningeal irritation are often lacking. Neurologic abnormalities are present in up to

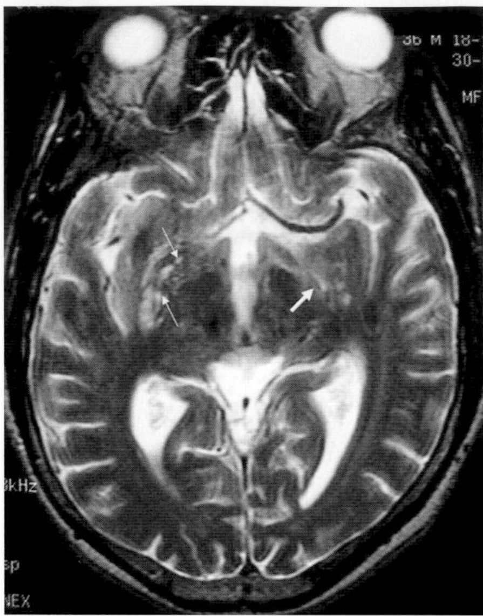

FIGURE 84.1 Magnetic resonance T2-weighted image showing dilated Virchow Robin spaces (thin arrows) and pseudocysts (thick arrow) in the basal ganglia in an HIV-infected patient with cryptococcosis.

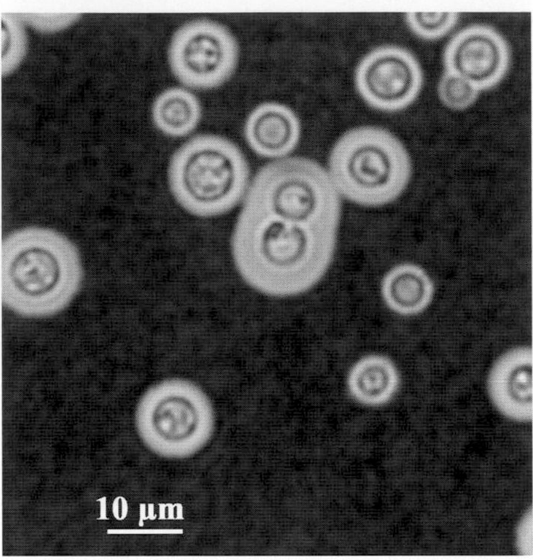

FIGURE 84.2 Visualization of the capsule surrounding *Cryptococcus neoformans* yeasts (suspension of a two-day culture in India ink, light microscopy).

50% of patients and are associated with a poor prognosis, as is a short duration (<2 weeks) between onset of symptoms and consultation. High cerebrospinal fluid (CSF) opening pressure alters the outcome and survival [13, 14].

Computed tomography (CT) and, more efficiently, magnetic resonance imaging (MRI), can detect brain edema, hydrocephalus, and mass lesions (cryptococcomas) (Fig. 84.1). Pleocytosis, elevated protein and low glucose levels associated with elevated pressure of the CSF are frequent; however, CSF findings can be normal, especially in HIV-infected individuals. A limited inflammatory reaction (<20 cells/mm^3) is associated with poor prognosis.

Lung Disease

Cryptococcal pneumonia is not distinctive clinically [15]. The presence of *Cryptococcus* spp. in a respiratory specimen should prompt investigation for dissemination and meningoencephalitis. Symptoms are low-grade fever, dull chest pain, and dry cough. Focal infiltrates are common; cavitation and pleural effusion rare. Asymptomatic pneumonia or enlarged mediastinal lymph nodes can be detected in previously healthy individuals. Diagnosis of lung colonization can only be made in immunocompetent individuals if cryptococcal disease has been ruled out (negative antigen detection and negative blood, urine and CSF cultures).

Cutaneous Infection

Skin lesions in disseminated infection exist in ~5% of patients, irrespective of their HIV status. Typical lesions are multiple and appear as ulcerated papules producing an exudate rich in cryptococci, but almost any kind of lesion can be seen. Primary cutaneous infections are rare and often associated with serotype D.

Involvement of Other Sites

Blood (up to 45%) and urine (15–30% in male patients) cultures are often positive in AIDS patients. Bones and joints can demonstrate osteolytic lesions and development of cold abscesses with *Cryptoccoccus*-rich exudates. Lymph node involvement is common. Occasional cases of keratitis (after corneal transplantation), endocarditis, peritonitis, and myositis have been reported. All localized infections should be considered as potential manifestations of disseminated disease thus requiring an extended work-up.

CRYPTOCOCCUS GATTII *INFECTIONS*

The diagnosis of *C. gattii* infection should be considered in tropical areas and the Pacific Northwest in patients (immunocompetent or not) presenting fever with cerebral and/or pulmonary masses that may suggest malignancy [16].

PATIENT EVALUATION, DIAGNOSIS, AND DIFFERENTIAL DIAGNOSIS

PATIENT EVALUATION

Investigations should include cultures of the CSF, urine, and blood, as well as sputum or bronchoalveolar lavage samples (in case of abnormal x-ray finding), together with cryptococcal antigen testing in serum and CSF [17]. The larger the volume of fluid sampled, the more likely the chance of making a diagnosis.

DIAGNOSIS

Diagnosis of cryptococcosis can be made based on the presence of encapsulated yeasts, culture of *C. neoformans* or *C. gattii* from a body site, and/or positive antigen detection in serum or CSF.

Fluids can be processed by mixing the pellet (CSF, pleural fluid, or bronchoalveolar lavage) with India ink (Fig. 84.2). Tissue sections can be stained with mucicarmine or Halcian blue to highlight the capsule.

For culture of *Cryptococcus*, which will allow speciation, specimens should be incubated on Sabouraud agar at 30–35°C (for up to 4 weeks in cases of prior antifungal treatment). Lysis centrifugation or culture of the buffy coat improves detection in blood. On agar, colonies are creamy and mucoid. The genus is identified by the presence of capsule, urease production and assimilation pattern using commercial kits. Molecular tools can be used to identify the species.

Cryptococcosis can also be diagnosed solely with detection of antigen in serum or CSF from high-risk patients. Most of the commercially available kits have an excellent performance profile. Antigen titers vary depending on the host's immune status (titers higher in AIDS), type of infection (low, and even negative, serum titers in case of localized extrameningeal infections) and the kit used. Systematic screening of serum samples from severely immunodeficient HIV-infected patients can be of value in highly endemic areas [18].

DIFFERENTIAL DIAGNOSIS

None of the clinical features is distinctive. Cryptococcal infection can appear similar to diseases ranging from lymphoma or other malignancies, to many opportunistic bacterial, fungal, viral, or parasitic infections.

TREATMENT

All patients with cryptococcal meningitis should receive antifungal therapy, as should all patients with extrameningeal cryptococcosis and an underlying risk factor. Reported case fatality rates (CFRs) despite treatment are still approximately 20%, even in patients without underlying disease. The CFRs are higher in endemic countries, possibly because of late presentation [17].

Precise guidelines for the treatment of cryptococcosis are available from the Infectious Diseases Society of America that take into consideration the immune status and the clinical presentation [19]. Treatment for severe forms of cryptococcosis (meningoencephalitis, disseminated infection, acute pneumonia) include an induction phase with amphotericin B (0.7–1.0 mg/kg/day) and flucytosine (100 mg/kg/day in four divided doses) for 2 weeks (with normal renal function) followed by fluconazole (≥400 mg/day) for an additional 8–10 weeks. When flucytosine is not available, an alternate, less validated, strategy for the induction phase may be the combination of amphotericin B and high-dose fluconazole. Lipid formulations of amphotericin B can also be used, particularly in those with renal dysfunction during treatment. Flucytosine blood levels should be monitored. Whether or not high-dose fluconazole ± flucytosine could be used as initial therapy remains to be determined.

The duration and dose of maintenance therapy depends on the immune status of the host. In milder forms of the disease, fluconazole (400 mg/d for at least 6–10 weeks) can be prescribed. In AIDS patients, long-term maintenance treatment with fluconazole (200 mg/d) should be given until immune reconstitution has occurred following institution of anti-retroviral treatment (ART) (CD4+ >100–200 cells/μL and undetectable viral load for >3 months).

Elevated intracranial pressures needs to be monitored. For patients with clinical evidence of increased intracranial pressure and a CSF pressure of ≥25 cm, daily lumbar puncture with CSF removal can be performed. CSF shunting is necessary when lumbar puncture cannot control symptoms. AIDS patients can also develop IRIS when treated concurrently with cryptococcal therapy and ART. Therapy for both infections can be continued; short-course corticosteroids may help control symptoms. Some experts recommend delaying ART until the patient has been treated for their cryptococcal disease for two or more weeks [19]. Surgical excisions for pulmonary mass lesions caused by *C. gattii* have been done.

Sterilization of all infected sites should be obtained. Encapsulated yeasts can be seen long after CSF sterilization. Serial evaluations of serum cryptococcal antigen titers may not correlate with treatment responses.

PROPHYLAXIS

Although fluconazole prophylaxis has been shown to reduce the incidence of cryptococcosis in HIV-infected patients before the HAART era in developed areas, it has not been shown to reduce the overall mortality and is thus not recommended in high-income settings [19]. In contrast, low-dosage fluconazole has been shown to be effective for the primary prophylaxis of cryptococcal meningitis in HIV-infected patients in Thailand and is recommended in the field by several public health authorities.

REFERENCES

1. Park BJ, Wannemuehler KA, Marston BJ, et al. Estimation of the current global burden of cryptococcal meningitis among persons living with HIV/AIDS. Aids 2009;23:525–30.
2. McCarthy KM, Morgan J, Wannemuehler KA, et al. Population-based surveillance for cryptococcosis in an antiretroviral-naive South African province with a high HIV seroprevalence. Aids 2006;20:2199–206.
3. Micol R, Lortholary O, Sar B, et al. Prevalence, determinants of positivity, and clinical utility of cryptococcal antigenemia in Cambodian HIV-infected patients. J Acquir Immune Defic Syndr 2007;45:555–9.
4. Mirza SA, Phelan M, Rimland D, et al. The changing epidemiology of cryptococcosis: an update from population-based active surveillance in 2 large metropolitan areas, 1992–2000. Clin Infect Dis 2003;36:789–94.
5. Lortholary O, Poizat G, Zeller V, et al. Long-term outcome of AIDS-associated cryptococcosis in the era of combination antiretroviral therapy. Aids 2006; 20:2183–91.
6. Mitchell TG, Perfect JR. Cryptococcosis in the era of AIDS – 100 years after the discovery of *Cryptococcus neoformans*. Clin Microbiol Rev 1995;8: 515–48.
7. Abadi J, Nachman S, Kressel AB, Pirofski L-A. Cryptococcosis in children with AIDS. Clin Infect Dis 1999;28:309–13.
8. Casadevall A, Perfect JR. Cryptococcus neoformans. Washington: American Society for Microbiology; 1998.
9. Lindberg J, Hagen F, Laursen A, et al. *Cryptococcus gattii* risk for tourists visiting Vancouver Island, Canada. Emerg Infect Dis 2007;13:178–9.
10. Bicanic T, Meintjes G, Rebe K, et al. Immune reconstitution inflammatory syndrome in HIV-associated cryptococcal meningitis: a prospective study. J Acquir Immune Defic Syndr 2009;51:130–4.
11. Lortholary O, Fontanet A, Memain N, et al. Incidence and risk factors of immune reconstitution inflammatory syndrome complicating HIV-associated cryptococcosis in France. Aids 2005;19:1043–9.
12. Dromer F, Mathoulin-Pelissier S, Launay O, Lortholary O. Determinants of disease presentation and outcome during cryptococcosis: the CryptoA/D study. PLoS medicine 2007;4:e21.
13. Graybill JR, Sobel J, Saag M, et al., the NIAID Mycoses Study Group and AIDS Cooperative treatment Groups. Diagnosis and management of increased intracranial pressure in patients with AIDS and cryptococcal meningitis. Clin Infect Dis 2000;30:47–54.
14. Bicanic T, Brouwer AE, Meintjes G, et al. Relationship of cerebrospinal fluid pressure, fungal burden and outcome in patients with cryptococcal meningitis undergoing serial lumbar punctures. Aids 2009;23:701–6.
15. Lortholary O, Nunez H, Brauner M, Dromer F. Pulmonary cryptococcosis. Sem Resp Crit Care Med 2004;25:145–57.
16. Chen S, Sorrell T, Nimmo G, et al. the Australasian Cryptococcal Study Group. Epidemiology and host- and variety-dependent characteristics of infection due to *Cryptococcus neoformans* in Australia and New Zealand. Clin Infect Dis 2000;31:499–508.
17. Jarvis JN, Dromer F, Harrison TS, Lortholary O. Managing cryptococcosis in the immunocompromised host. Curr Opin Infect Dis 2008;21:596–603.
18. French N, Gray K, Watera C, et al. Cryptococcal infection in a cohort of HIV-1-infected Ugandan adults. Aids 2002;16:1031–8.
19. Perfect JR, Dismukes WE, Dromer F, et al. Clinical practice guidelines for the management of cryptococcal disease: 2010 update by the Infectious Diseases Society of America. Clin Infect Dis 2010;50:291–322.

85 Penicilliosis Marneffei

Khuanchai Supparatpinyo

Key features

- Penicilliosis marneffei is a systemic fungal infection that causes morbidity and mortality in HIV-infected patients resident in or having visited Southeast Asia, northeastern India, southern China, Hong Kong, and Taiwan
- Papular skin lesions provide a clue for diagnosis. Other clinical manifestations are less specific: fever, weight loss, nonproductive cough, hepatosplenomegaly, and generalized lymphadenopathy
- Diagnosis is made by isolation of the fungus from clinical specimens or identification of organisms in tissue sections
- Mortality is high in delayed or untreated patients. Antifungal therapy with amphotericin B and itraconazole is effective in most cases
- After induction therapy, lifelong maintenance therapy is necessary; treatment can be discontinued if immune recovery occurs
- Synonyms: *Penicillium marneffei* infection, disseminated *Penicillium marneffei* infection, disseminated penicilliosis marneffei

INTRODUCTION

Penicillium are a genus of fungi that are widely distributed in the environment, but rarely cause infection in humans [1]. *P. marneffei* is the most common *Penicillium* species to cause human infection and can occur both in normal hosts but more frequently in immunocompromised hosts. At the peak of the HIV/AIDS epidemic in northern Thailand, penicilliosis marneffei was the fourth most common AIDS-related opportunistic infection, after tuberculosis, extrapulmonary cryptococcosis, and *Pneumocystis* pneumonia [2]. Cases of disseminated infection have also been reported in HIV-infected patients from other countries following visits to the endemic area [3].

P. marneffei was first isolated from the visceral organs of a bamboo rat (*Rhizomys sinensis*) in Vietnam in 1956 [4]. The first natural human infection was reported in an American missionary with Hodgkin disease who had been living in Southeast Asia for several years [5]. The first case of penicilliosis marneffei in an HIV-infected native of Southeast Asia was reported in 1989 from Bangkok, coinciding with the beginning of the AIDS epidemic in the region [6]. The number of cases has markedly increased since.

EPIDEMIOLOGY

P. marneffei is endemic in Southeast Asia and southern China [7, 8]. Although the majority of cases have been reported from northern Thailand, the prevalence of this infection has also increased in other countries in the region after the HIV/AIDS epidemic; these include Vietnam, Hong Kong, Taiwan, Malaysia, Cambodia, and the provinces of Guangxi and Guangdong in China. Recently, indigenous cases of penicilliosis marneffei have been described from Manipur State, India [9]. Figure 85.1 illustrates the current endemic areas for this fungal infection. Residents or travelers who visit these areas, in particular those with HIV infection, have a risk of acquiring this systemic fungal infection.

NATURAL HISTORY, PATHOGENESIS, AND PATHOLOGY

P. marneffei is the only species of the genus that is a dimorphic fungus. In the environment, it grows in mycelial form, and in humans or animals, it grows as a yeast-like form. Many aspects of the ecology of *P. marneffei* and the relationship to human infection remain unknown. Several studies have found that *P. marneffei* can infect four species of bamboo rats, i.e. *R. sinensis*, *R. pruinosus*, *R. sumatrensis*, and *Cannomys badius* [10]. However, attempts to link bamboo rats and human infection have been unsuccessful. The mode of transmission of *P. marneffei* is unknown; however, similar to other endemic fungal pathogens, it is likely that inhalation is the major route. A case report from France of a laboratory-acquired infection also suggests an airborne route of infection [11].

CLINICAL FEATURES

P. marneffei infection usually occurs late in the course of HIV infection. The majority of cases are observed in patients who have $CD4^+$ cell counts of <100 cells/mm^3 [12]. Clinical manifestations of penicilliosis marneffei are nonspecific, including fever, weight loss, nonproductive cough, hepatosplenomegaly, and generalized lymphadenopathy [7]. Skin lesions are seen in more than 70% of patients and, when present, are the best clues to the diagnosis. They are usually found as papules on the face, chest, and extremities. The center of the papule subsequently becomes necrotic, giving the appearance of an umbilicated papule (Fig. 85.2). Atypical presentations are osteoarthritis, lung mass or cavitary lesions, mesenteric lymphadenitis, and mucosal lesions in the oral cavity, oropharynx, hypopharynx, stomach, colon, and genitalia. Laboratory values are nonspecific and can include slight elevation of liver enzymes and bilirubin, anemia, and leukocytosis or leukopenia. Roentgenograms of the chest may show diffuse reticulonodular, localized alveolar, or diffuse alveolar infiltrates. Clinical features in children are the same as those seen in adults.

PATIENT EVALUATION, DIAGNOSIS, AND DIFFERENTIAL DIAGNOSIS

Clinical diagnosis of penicilliosis marneffei, especially in patients with advanced HIV infection, is often difficult. Differential diagnoses include disseminated fungal infection, mycobacterial infection, and other HIV-related opportunistic infections. Physician awareness and a high degree of suspicion can lead to a timely diagnosis and management. History of travel to or residence in the endemic region is

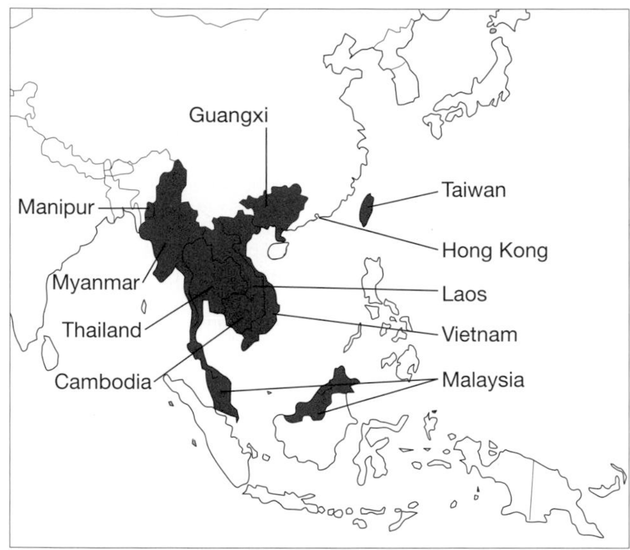

FIGURE 85.1 Endemic areas of penicilliosis marneffei.

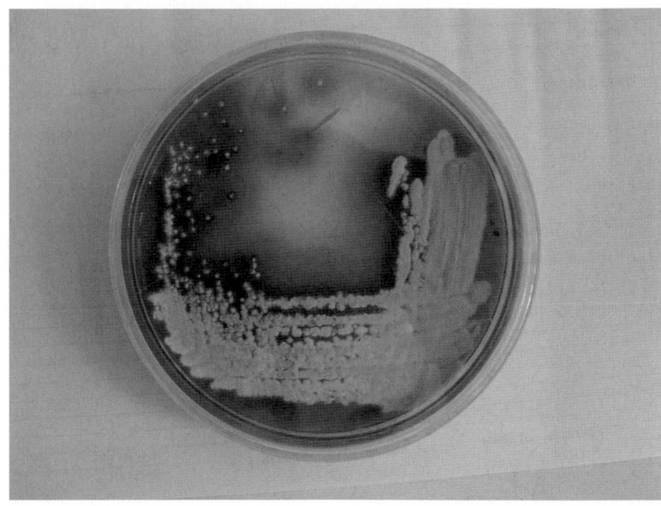

FIGURE 85.3 A blood-agar plate of a skin scraping from an HIV-infected patient with penicilliosis marneffei after incubation at 25°C for 4 days. Typical *P. marneffei* colonies have red pigment diffused into the surrounding culture media.

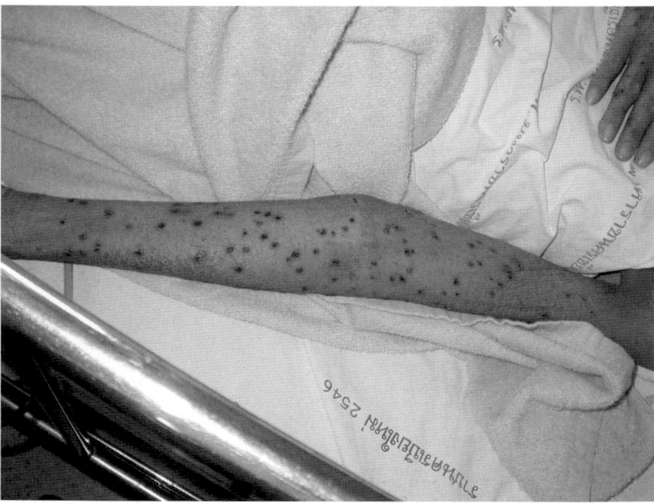

FIGURE 85.2 Typical papulonecrotic skin lesions on the arm of an HIV-infected patient with penicilliosis marneffei.

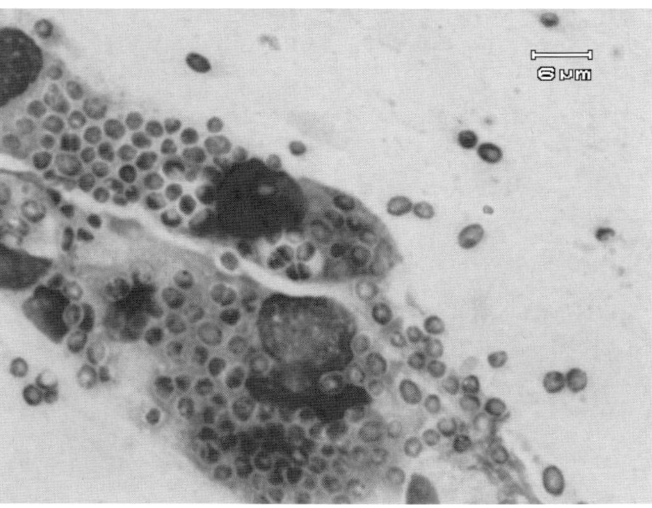

FIGURE 85.4 A photomicrograph of a Wright-stained sputum smear from an HIV-infected patient, showing numerous intracellular yeast-like organisms, some of which have the typical septate yeast forms.

essential information. The definitive diagnosis is based on isolation of organisms from culture of clinical specimens (Fig. 85.3) or by histopathologic demonstration of characteristic organisms in biopsy materials. However, these may require several days or weeks to get the results. Rapid diagnosis can be made by a bedside technique: microscopic examination of Wright-stained samples of skin scrapings, bone marrow aspirate, or lymph node biopsy touch smear. Many intracellular and extracellular basophilic, spherical, oval and elliptical yeast-like organisms are usually found. Some cells have a central septum which is a characteristic feature of *P. marneffei* (Fig. 85.4) [7]. This technique can also be used with tissue obtained by fine needle aspiration of the lymph node. It is particularly helpful in cases where there is no skin lesion or peripheral lymphadenopathy [13]. On some occasions, the fungus can be identified by microscopic examination of a Wright-stained peripheral blood smear [14]. *P. marneffei* bears a morphologic resemblance to *Histoplasma capsulatum* but tends to form more elongated yeast cells and divides by central septate fission rather than budding.

Recently, special techniques to identify organisms in tissue samples and serologic testing have been described [15, 16]. However, these tests are not widely used because commercial reagents are not available.

TREATMENT

P. marneffei is highly susceptible to itraconazole, ketoconazole, miconazole, and 5-flucytosine. Amphotericin B has intermediate antifungal activity, and fluconazole is the least active [17]. The mortality rate with delayed or no treatment is high [7,17]. In patients with severe disease, treatment with amphotericin B 0.6 mg/kg/day intravenously for 2 weeks followed by itraconazole 400 mg/day orally for 10 weeks is recommended [18]. Oral itraconazole 400 mg/day for 8 to 12 weeks can be used in patients with less severe disease [9, 19]. Voriconazole is an effective alternative; it can be given by intravenous followed by oral administration or orally from the beginning [20]. Treatment in children is similar to that in adults. Relapse of penicilliosis marneffei is common after discontinuation of antifungal therapy [19, 21]. Suppressive therapy with itraconazole 200 mg once daily after successful antifungal therapy is required lifelong or for as long as immunocompromise persists [21].

Primary prevention of *P. marneffei* with an antifungal agent in HIV-infected patients is not usually recommended. However, in areas where systemic fungal infections are common, primary prophylaxis of AIDS-associated opportunistic infections can be considered [12].

In advanced HIV disease and *P. marneffei* infection, antiretroviral therapy (ART) should be administered after 2 to 8 weeks of antifungal therapy in all patients who are clinically stable. Primary and secondary prophylaxis of penicilliosis marneffei can be discontinued in patients receiving ART and with $CD4^+$ cell counts of >100 cells/mm^3 for at least 6 months [22]. However, antifungal prophylaxis should be reintroduced if the $CD4^+$ count decreases to <100 cells/mm^3.

REFERENCES

1. Lyratzopoulos G, Ellis M, Nerringer R, Denning DW. Invasive infection due to *Penicillium* species other than *P. marneffei*. J Infect 2002;45:184–95.
2. Chariyalertsak S, Sirisanthana T, Saengwonloey O, Nelson KE. Clinical presentation and risk behaviors of patients with acquired immunodeficiency syndrome in Thailand, 1994–1998: regional variation and temporal trends. Clin Infect Dis 2001;32:955–62.
3. Walsh TJ, Groll A, Hiemenz J, et al. Infections due to emerging and uncommon medically important fungal pathogens. Clin Microbiol Infect 2004;10 (Suppl 1):48–66.
4. Capponi M, Sureau P, Segretain G. Penicillose de Rhizomys sinensis. Bull Soc Pathol Exot 1956;49:418.
5. Disalvo AF, Fickling AM, Ajello L. Infection caused by *Penicillium marneffei*: description of first natural infection in man. Am J Clin Pathol 1973;60: 259–63.
6. Sathapatayavongs B, Damrongkitchaiporn S, Saengditha P, et al. Disseminated penicilliosis associated with HIV infection. J Infect 1989;19:84–5.
7. Supparatpinyo K, Khamwan C, Baosoung V, et al. Disseminated *Penicillium marneffei* infection in southeast Asia. Lancet 1994;344:110–13.
   The first large series of HIV-infected patients with penicilliosis marneffei. Clinical manifestations and management of patients are reviewed.
8. Duong TA. Infection due to *Penicillium marneffei*, an emerging pathogen: review of 155 reported cases. Clin Infect Dis 1996;23:125–30.
   A literature review of all patients with penicilliosis marneffei, including both HIV and non-HIV cases, reported before 1996 from many countries. This emphasizes the emerging nature of this fungal pathogen.
9. Ranjana KH, Priyokumar K, Singh TJ, et al. Disseminated *Penicillium marneffei* infection among HIV-infected patients in Manipur state, India. J Infect Dis 2002;45:268–71.
10. Gugnani HC, Fisher MC, Paliwal-Johsi A, et al. Role of *Cannomys badius* as a natural animal host of *Penicillium marneffei* in India. J Clin Microbiol 2004;42:5070–5.
11. Hilmarsdottir I, Coutellier A, Elbaz J, et al. A French case of laboratory-acquired disseminated *Penicillium marneffei* infection in a patient with AIDS. Clin Infect Dis 1994;2:357–8.
12. Chariyalertsak S, Supparatpinyo K, Sirisanthana T, et al. A controlled trial of itraconazole as primary prophylaxis for systemic fungal infections in patients with advanced human immunodeficiency virus infection in Thailand. Clin Infect Dis 2002;34:277–84.
   The first double-blind, randomized, controlled trial to demonstrate the efficacy and safety of using oral itraconazole for primary prophylaxis in HIV-infected patients with $CD4^+$ cell counts of <200 cells/mm^3, in an area where Penicillium marneffei is endemic.
13. Chaiwun B, Khunamornpong S, Sirivanichai C, et al. Lymphadenopathy due to *Penicillium marneffei* infection: diagnosis by fine needle aspiration cytology. Mod Pathol 2002;15:939–42.
14. Supparatpinyo K, Sirisanthana T. Disseminated *Penicillium marneffei* infection diagnosed on examination of a peripheral blood smear of a patient with human immunodeficiency virus infection. Clin Infect Dis 1994;18:246–7.
15. Kaufman L, Standard PG, Anderson SA, et al. Development of specific fluorescent-antibody test for tissue form of *Penicillium marneffei*. J Clin Microbiol 1995;33:2136–8.
16. Sekhon AS, Li JSK, Garg AK. Penicilliosis marneffei: serological and exoantigen studies. Mycopathology 1982;77:51.
17. Supparatpinyo K, Nelson KE, Merz WG, et al. Response to antifungal therapy by human immunodeficiency virus-infected patients with disseminated *Penicillium marneffei* infections and in vitro susceptibilities of isolates from clinical specimens. Antimicrob Agents Chemother 1993;37:2407–11.
18. Sirisanthana T, Supparatpinyo K, Perriens J, et al. Amphotericin B and itraconazole for treatment of disseminated *Penicillium marneffei* infection in human immunodeficiency virus-infected patients. Clin Infect Dis 1998;26:1107–10.
   The largest therapeutic clinical trial in HIV-infected patients with penicilliosis marneffei. It demonstrates the efficacy of amphotericin B followed by oral itraconazole in the treatment of this systemic fungal infection.
19. Supparatpinyo K, Chiewchanvit S, Hirunsri P, et al. An efficacy study of itraconazole in the treatment of *Penicillium marneffei* infection. J Med Assoc Thai 1992;75:688–91.
20. Supparatpinyo K, Schlamm HT. Voriconazole as therapy for systemic *Penicillium marneffei* infections in AIDS patients. Am J Trop Med Hyg 2007; 77:350–3.
21. Supparatpinyo K, Perriens J, Nelson KE, et al. A controlled trial of itraconazole to prevent relapse of *Penicillium marneffei* infection in patients infected with the human immunodeficiency virus. N Engl J Med 1998;339:1739–43.
   The first double-blind, randomized, controlled trial to demonstrate the efficacy and safety of using oral itraconazole for the secondary prophylaxis of penicilliosis marneffei in HIV-infected patients after successful primary treatment. This resulted in the recommendation of secondary prophylaxis as a standard of care in endemic areas.
22. Chaiwarith R, Charoenyos N, Sirisanthana T, et al. Discontinuation of secondary prophylaxis against penicilliosis marneffei in AIDS patients after HAART. AIDS 2007;21:365–7.
   The first retrospective cohort study with historical control to determine the safety of discontinuation of secondary prophylaxis against penicilliosis marneffei in HIV-infected patients after having received antiretroviral therapy and with $CD4^+$ cell counts >100 cells/mm^3 for at least 6 months.

Pneumocystis Pneumonia 86

Powel Kazanjian

Key features

- *Pneumocystis jiroveci* causes an acute or subacute, potentially life-threatening pneumonia in immunocompromised individuals, typically those with AIDS
- Symptoms are dyspnea, nonproductive cough, fever, and fatigue that gradually progresses over several days to weeks
- Radiograph shows a bilateral, diffuse interstitial infiltrate in the later stage of the illness, but may be normal in early stages
- Early recognition, prompt diagnosis, and initiation of anti-pneumocystis treatment leads to the best outcome
- For patients with mild to moderate disease, oral regimens and outpatient management are often successful. For those with severe disease, intravenous regimens accompanied by adjunctive corticosteroids initiated within 24–72 hours of anti-pneumocystis therapy are indicated

INTRODUCTION

Pneumocystis pneumonia (PCP) is an acute and sometimes life-threatening pneumonia due to the fungus *Pneumocystis jiroveci* which occurs in immunocompromised people. In tropical countries, most adult patients with PCP have AIDS, whereas in developed countries it also occurs in immunocompromised patients with conditions other than AIDS, e.g. those receiving chemotherapeutic agents for hematologic malignancies, or people taking immunosuppressive drugs to prevent rejection following organ transplantation. In infants and children in developing countries, PCP may occur in those with kwashiorkor.

In children and adults with AIDS, PCP was initially thought to occur less frequently in developing regions than in industrialized countries. Autopsy reports conducted during the first decade of the pandemic showed that tuberculosis, and bacteremia with nontyphoid *Salmonella* and pneumococci occurred more often in African AIDS patients than in those living in developed countries [1]. Based on these reports, texts concluded that in the developing world, PCP was uncommon [2]. More recently, however, a higher prevalence of PCP among AIDS patients with respiratory symptoms from many regions of the developing world has been reported.

EPIDEMIOLOGY

In low-income regions of the world, there are variations in the reported prevalence of PCP in patients with AIDS. This variability may be due to differences in study design, including a lack of standardization of inclusion criteria (e.g. including patients in all stages of HIV infection vs those with AIDS), rates of PCP prophylaxis, and diagnostic tests used with differing sensitivity in detecting PCP in sputum. Furthermore, differences in ecologic factors that result in exposure to *P. jiroveci* may also influence the prevalence of PCP, even though the environmental habitat and means of transmission remain unknown. Despite these considerations, PCP now accounts for a substantial percentage of respiratory symptoms in HIV-infected patients in the developing world; in Africa, Asia, the Philippines, and Central and South America, the percentage ranges from 45% to 65% compared with earlier studies in the 1980s where the percent was 3% to 35% [3].

It is not known whether the trend towards an increase in the percentage of cases represents a true increase in prevalence or whether the early reports underestimated the actual prevalence. In contrast to the developing world, the incidence of PCP in the developed world has significantly declined due to the use of potent antiretroviral therapy (ART) and *Pneumocystis* prophylaxis. It seems likely that increased use of ART in the developing world will reduce the occurrence of PCP in tropical regions, but this remains to be demonstrated.

NATURAL HISTORY, PATHOGENESIS, AND PATHOLOGY

In asymptomatic people, a few *P. jiroveci* organisms may reside latently in the alveolar septal walls of the lung. This asymptomatic form has been recognized incidentally in specimens of lung obtained at autopsy [4]. Immunodeficiency is the common predisposing condition for developing pneumonia due to this latent infection. Although the possibility of reactivation has not been entirely discounted, more recent studies suggest that pneumonia can be due to recently acquired organisms [5].

The organism causes denudation of alveolar cells. This results in foamy, honeycombed intra-alveolar exudates consisting of masses of cysts and desquamated alveolar cells, with an interstitial infiltrate of plasma cells and lymphocytes. The number of organisms increases as pneumonia develops, accounting for the characteristic diffuse rather than localized nature of the pneumonitis [4]. Systemic dissemination of organisms is rare. It can occur in association with the use of aerosolized pentamidine, and can involve any organ, including liver, spleen, lymph node, or bone marrow. The order and level of immunodeficiency at which PCP and other opportunistic infections occur in HIV-infected people in developing regions has not been defined [6]. However, there is no evidence to support speculation that PCP occurs at an earlier stage of infection than in high-income countries. Thus, it is likely that the majority of cases in HIV-infected people worldwide occur when CD4 counts decline below 200 cells/mm^3.

CLINICAL FEATURES

PCP can have an acute onset or occur gradually. In general, in patients without HIV infection, PCP has a more fulminant course than in HIV-infected people, in whom infection is often indolent [7].

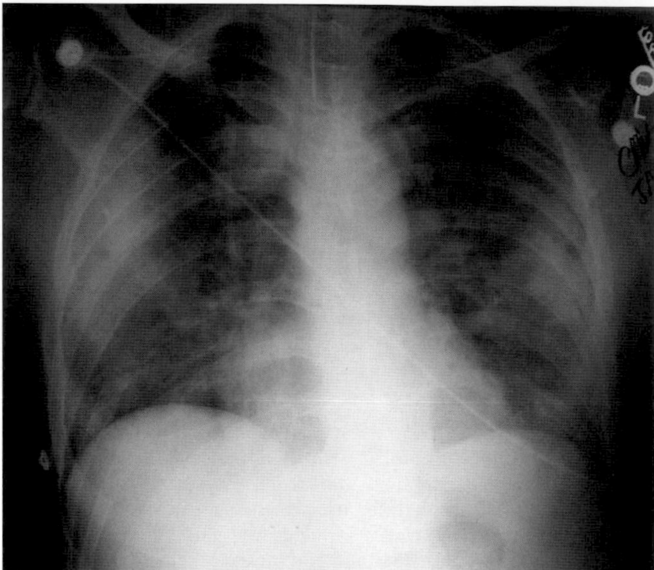

FIGURE 86.1 Chest x-ray of a patient with *Pneumocystis* pneumonia demonstrating bilateral diffuse interstitial changes occurring predominantly in the lower lung fields.

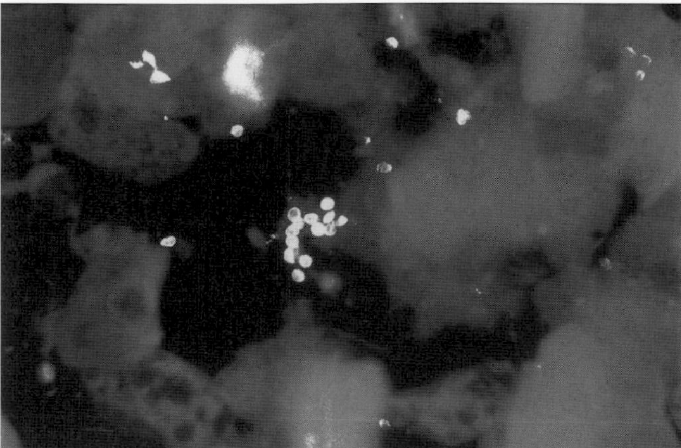

FIGURE 86.2 Immunofluorescence stain of a sputum specimen obtained by induction. The oval, cup-shaped, 4–6-µm *Pneumocystis jiroveci* organisms stain an apple green color against a red background.

Nevertheless, practicing clinicians have noted that either presentation can occur in both hosts. The usual symptoms are fever (80–100%), nonproductive or minimally productive cough (95–100%), and dyspnea (95%). Pulmonary symptoms are typically progressive over a 1- to 2-week course, and may be accompanied by systemic symptoms of fatigue, chest pain, and weight loss. On examination, the patient is usually tachypneic with either bibasilar rales or a normal lung examination. The abnormalities on examination are usually limited to the lungs, but in the unusual case of extrapulmonic pneumocystosis, there may be enlargement of lymph nodes, spleen, or liver.

Oxygen saturation, a routinely performed laboratory test available in several tropical settings, is usually low at rest and most often declines further with exertion. The arterial oxygen tension (PaO_2) is low, the carbon dioxide level normal, and the alveolar–arterial (A-a) gradient is increased. Routine chest x-rays may be normal in up to one-fourth of patients early in the course, but then evolve into a bilateral, diffuse, interstitial infiltrative pattern (Fig. 86.1) [8]. Variant x-ray findings are upper lobe involvement (especially in people receiving aerosolized pentamidine), focal consolidation, or thin-walled cavities (pneumatoceles) that can be complicated by a pneumothorax. In patients with normal x-rays, high-resolution CT scans, if available, can show patchy or nodular ground-glass attenuation, suggestive, but not diagnostic, of PCP. Lactic dehydrogenase (LDH) levels are elevated in most, but not all, patients.

These clinical features have usually been described in reports from industrialized countries, with scant literature from developing countries. Some papers from developing countries note markedly high respiratory rates, ranging from 30 to 80 per minute, and very low O_2 saturation percent (60–82%), and pO_2 (<70 mmHg) [5]. These data suggest that in some tropical regions, PCP may tend to be recognized in its more severe stage.

PATIENT EVALUATION, DIAGNOSIS, AND DIFFERENTIAL DIAGNOSIS

Although PCP can be suspected based upon typical clinical and radiologic findings, the diagnosis should be confirmed by sampling a respiratory specimen. The clinical and radiographic features of PCP overlap with viral and atypical bacterial pathogens that cause community pneumonia. Thus, if initiated empirically, a full course of anti-pneumocystis treatment should not be completed without establishing a diagnosis, given the potential toxicities from PCP regimens. Since obtaining a respiratory specimen and staining specimens are not rapid tests for *P jiroveci,* and the severity of the pneumonia can progress while awaiting specimens, it is appropriate to initiate empiric treatment pending the results of diagnostic specimens. The role of gallium-67 citrate scanning is limited by its lack of specificity. The utility of a serum assay for diagnosis, beta-D-glucan, a cell wall component of *Pneumocystis,* remains to be determined [9].

Procedures for obtaining and sampling respiratory specimens may not be available in low-income regions. Where they are available, the least invasive method of obtaining respiratory specimens for PCP analysis is sputum induced by inhaling hypertonic saline generated by a handheld nebulizer [10]. Induction is continued for 15 minutes until an adequate specimen volume (5 to 10 mL) is produced. The specimen is then stained by conventional methods: silver nitrate, toluidine blue O or Giemsa stains, indirect immunofluorescence, or PCR for *P. jirovecii* (Fig. 86.2). The sensitivity of sputum induction ranges from 55% to 92%, depending upon experience and expertise. Thus, if PCP is not identified by sputum induction, or if induced sputum is unavailable, then bronchoscopy with bronchoalveolar lavage should be performed. Lung biopsy is not required to establish the diagnosis. The utility of noninvasive tests from oropharyngeal washings (e.g. gargling) to diagnose PCP when coupled with PCR testing remains attractive in resource-limited regions [11].

TREATMENT

No prospective, controlled treatment trial to assess PCP therapy has been carried out in the developing world. Thus, it is reasonable to use the same treatment regimens that are used in industrialized countries [12]. An assessment should be made of the severity of illness to determine whether oral or intravenous regimens should be used [13]. Mild to moderate disease can be managed with one of several oral treatment regimens and without adjunctive corticosteroids. Response rates to oral drugs have been reported to be 80–95% in the developed world. Mild to moderate disease can be defined by clinical findings (absence of severe respiratory distress or pronounced tachypnea) and O_2 results (pO_2 > 70; A-a gradient <35 mmO_2). Due to its high rate of success, the regimen of choice is a 3-week course of trimethoprim–sulfamethoxazole (TMP-SMX) at a dosage of 15–20 mg (TMP)/kg/day in three divided doses (5 to 7 double-strength tablets per day) for 21 days. The major adverse reactions to TMP-SMX are rash, which may range from mild to life-threatening, cytopenias, and gastroenterologic upset. For those who develop a non-life-threatening rash to TMP-SMX, trimethoprim (300 mg three times daily) plus dapsone (100 mg/day) can be used. Seventy percent of patients who have reactions to TMP-SMX are able to tolerate TMP-dapsone, which has a similar efficacy to TMP-SMX. For those unable to tolerate TMP-dapsone, either atovaquone (750 mg twice daily, with food), or primaquine (30 mg/day) plus clindamycin (300–450 mg three times a day) can be used.

In general, intravenous regimens should be given in severe disease (pO_2 <70; A-a gradient >35 mmO_2) [14]. The agent of choice is TMP-SMX; the intravenous dose is identical to the oral regimen. For patients intolerant to or not responding to TMP-SMX after 7 days of treatment, pentamidine isethionate (3 mg/kg/day) can be used. Pentamadine is almost as effective as TMP-SMX, but it has a higher rate of serious side effects, including renal insufficiency, arrhythmias and pancreatitis. For patients with severe disease, adjunctive corticosteroids initiated within 24 to 72 hours of anti-pneumocystis therapy prevents early deterioration of oxygenation by reducing inflammation associated with lysis of *P. jiroveci* organisms. The dose is prednisone 40 mg twice daily days 1–5, 40 mg daily days 6–10, then 20 mg daily days 11–21 [15].

There are several points about treatment outcomes in developing countries. First, in adult patients, the mortality rates range from 10% to 27%, similar to those reported in the US. However, PCP mortality rates in children are higher than in industrialized countries, ranging from 10% to 80% [16]. A more rapid progression of HIV infection may be a factor contributing to mortality, since ART was not available in developing countries at the time the treatment studies were conducted. Based on the degree of oxygen exchange impairment, it is also possible that lower response rates may have been due to late initiation of anti-pneumocystis treatment. This underscores the importance of early recognition and prompt treatment for improving outcomes. Second, a full array of anti-pneumocystis regimens used in industrialized nations may not be available in developing countries. Thus, treatment options for those not responding to or intolerant to TMP-SMX may be limited.

For prophylaxis in people with AIDS and a CD4 cell count <200 cells/mm^3, TMP-SMX reduces the incidence of PCP. AIDS patients who respond to ART by increasing CD4 cell counts to >200 for more than 3 months may discontinue PCP prophylaxis.

REFERENCES

1. Lucas SB, Hounnou A, Peacock C, et al. The mortality and pathology of HIV infection in a West African City. AIDS 1993;7:1569–79.
2. Colebunders R, Quinn T. Retroviruses and HIV. In: Warren KS, Mahmoud AAF, eds. Tropical and Geographical Medicine. New York: McGraw Hill; 1990: 728–41.
3. Fisk D, Meshnick S, Kazanjian P. *Pneumocystis carinii* pneumonia in AIDS patients in the developing world. Clin Infect Dis 2003;36:70–8.
PCP is not uncommon in patients with AIDS who have respiratory symptoms in the developing world, where PCP accounted for 45% cases of respiratory symptoms in adults with AIDS.
4. Hughes WT. Pneumocystosis. In: Strickland GT, ed. Tropical Medicine and Emerging Infectious Diseases. Philadelphia: WB Saunders; 2000:701–4.
5. Beard CB, Carter JL, Keely SP, et al. Genetic variation in *Pneumocystis carinii* isolates from different geographic regions: implications for transmission. Emerg Infect Dis 2000;6:265–72.
This study examined the geographic variation of Pneumocystis genotypes from patients in differing locales, and showed that the genotypes at the time of diagnosis matched the person's place of diagnosis, not the place of birth. This supports the theory that disease results from new acquisition of Pneumocystis rather than latent reactivation.
6. Walzer P. Pneumocystosis. In: Guerrant RL, Walker DH, Weller PF, eds. Tropical Infectious Diseases: Principles, Pathogens, and Practice. Philadelphia: Churchill Livingstone; 1999:673–84.
7. Kovacs JA, Hiemenz JW, Macher AM, et al. *Pneumocystis carinii* pneumonia: a comparison between patients with the acquired immunodeficiency syndrome and patients with other immunodeficiencies. Ann Intern Med 1984; 100:663–71.
8. DeLorenzo LJ, Huang CT, Maguire GP, et al. Roentgenographic patterns of *Pneumocystis carinii pneumonia* in 104 patients with AIDS. Chest 1987; 91:323–7.
9. Marty FM, Koo S, Bryar J, et al. Beta-D-Glucan assay positivity in patients with *Pneumocystis jiroveci* pneumonia. Ann Intern Med 2007;147:70–2.
10. Metersky ML, Aslenzadeh J, Stelmach P. A comparison of induced and expectorated sputum for the diagnosis of *Pneumocystis carinii* pneumonia. Chest 1998;113:1555–9.
Sputum induction when done properly can be a simple and relatively well-tolerated procedure with a sensitivity of 55%. This method of diagnosis is important in regions in the developing world where bronchoscopic techniques are not available.
11. Wakefield AE, Miller RF, Guiver LA, et al. Oropharyngeal samples for detection of *Pneumocystis carinii* by DNA amplification. Q J Med 1993;86:401–6.
PCR technology has allowed for the use of specimens obtained from oropharyngeal gargling to diagnose PCP. This study reported a sensitivity of 84%, equivalent to that of induced sputum.
12. Kaplan JE, Benson C, Holmes KH, et al. Guidelines for prevention and treatment of opportunistic infections in HIV-infected adults and adolescents: recommendations from CDC, the National Institutes of Health, and the HIV Medicine Association of the Infectious Diseases Society of America. MMWR Recomm Rep 2009;58:1–207.
13. Safrin S, Finkelstein DM, Feinberg J, et al. Comparison of three regimens for treatment of mild to moderate *Pneumocystis carinii* pneumonia in patients with AIDS. Ann Intern Med 1996;124:792–802.
14. Sattler FR, Cowan R, Nielsen DM, et al. Trimethoprim-sulfamethoxazole or pentamidine for *Pneumocystis carinii* pneumonia in the acquired immunodeficiency syndrome. A prospective randomized trial. Ann Intern Med 1986; 105:37–44.
15. Gagnon S, Boota AM, Fischl MA, et al. Corticosteroids as adjunctive therapy for severe *Pneumocystis carinii* pneumonia in the acquired immunodeficiency syndrome. A double-blind, placebo-controlled trial. N Engl J Med 1990; 323:1444–50.
16. Zar HJ, Dechaboon A, Hanslo D, et al. *Pneumocystis carinii* pneumonia in South African children with human immunodeficiency virus. Pediatr Infect Dis J 2000;19:603–7.

87 Treatment of Systemic Mycoses

Edward C Oldfield III

Key features

- The older, inexpensive, but more toxic formulation of amphotericin B (desoxycholate) is being replaced with the more expensive, but less toxic lipid formulations
- Although well tolerated for chronic therapy, the triazoles have drug interactions due to inhibition of cytochrome P450 hepatic enzymes
- Voriconazole represents an advance in the treatment of invasive *Aspergillus* infections and has become the drug of choice
- Posaconazole is the first orally available antifungal with significant activity against the agents of mucormycosis, chromoblastomycosis, phaeohyphomycosis, mycetoma, and *Scedosporium apiospermum*
- Echinocandins are the drugs of choice for empiric treatment of *Candida* infections, pending speciation, because of their broad spectrum of activity and minimal toxicity

INTRODUCTION

Treatment of systemic mycoses is a clinical challenge. Infections are chronic, with a tendency to relapse, and the standard therapy, amphotericin B, has multiple toxicities. The introduction of azole antifungals provides relatively nontoxic long-term therapy. This chapter discusses the properties and use of the major antifungals: amphotericin B, flucytosine, triazoles, and echinocandins. Specific treatment indications, duration of therapy, and parameters indicating response are covered in the disease chapters.

AMPHOTERICIN B

Amphotericin B is a product of *Streptomyces nodosus.* Despite its toxicities, amphotericin remains the standard therapeutic agent for many of the deep mycoses.

MECHANISM OF ACTION

The polyene structure of amphotericin B is responsible for both its therapeutic and its toxic properties. Amphotericin B interacts with cell membrane sterols, leading to an alteration in the integrity of the membrane, with subsequent leakage of intracellular contents. In fungi, the interaction is with ergosterol and results in inhibition of fungal growth, whereas in human cells, the interaction is with cholesterol, resulting in toxic side effects.

SENSITIVE ORGANISMS

Most of the systemic fungi are sensitive to amphotericin B. These include *Coccidioides immitis, Cryptococcus neoformans, Histoplasma capsulatum, Blastomyces dermatitidis, Paracoccidioides brasiliensis, Candida,* and *Aspergillus* spp. There is also activity against a number of protozoan pathogens: *Entamoeba, Naegleria, Leishmania* and trypanosomes. Isolates of *Pseudallescheria boydii, Candida lusitaniae, Trichosporon beigelii,* and *Scedosporium inflatum* are commonly resistant. Because of a lack of standardization among laboratories and the variance between in vitro and clinical results, there is little value from routine in vitro susceptibility testing or measurement of serum levels of amphotericin B. Development of resistance during therapy has not been a problem.

There is synergy of amphotericin B with a number of agents. Combination therapy is most useful with flucytosine for treatment of cryptococcal meningitis.

PHARMACOLOGIC PROPERTIES

Peak serum concentrations of amphotericin B with standard therapeutic doses are 0.5 to 2.0 μg/mL. The fate of the drug is unknown, and no metabolites have been identified. There is biphasic excretion, with a rapid elimination half-life of 24 hours, followed by a prolonged terminal half-life of 15 days. Renal excretion accounts for only 3–5% of total drug elimination. For this reason, there is no accumulation of amphotericin B in serum during renal failure, and no dosage adjustment is necessary, even in the anephric patient. Amphotericin B is not removed by peritoneal dialysis or hemodialysis. Biliary excretion is 19%, but hepatic disease does not necessitate a dosage change.

Amphotericin B is available as the standard formulation with desoxycholate (AMBD, Fungizone, Squibb), which creates a colloidal dispersion of the insoluble antibiotic. The usual daily dose of 0.5–1.0 mg/kg is reconstituted with 10 mL of sterile water and then added to 5% dextrose in water. The addition of even minimal amounts of sodium or chloride will reduce bioactivity and induce turbidity in the infusion. Therefore, AMBD should not be mixed with electrolytes or acidic solutions. AMBD is light-sensitive, but during a 24-hour period there is no appreciable loss of activity; there is no need to wrap the bottle with aluminum foil. The drug is poorly absorbed from the gastrointestinal tract, and should never be used to treat systemic infections. Its only oral use is for candidal infections of the oropharynx.

Lipid formulations have been developed in an effort to reduce the nephrotoxicity of AMBD: amphotericin B lipid complex (ABLC, Abelcet, Enzon), amphotericin B cholesteryl sulfate complex (ABCS, Amphotec), and liposomal amphotericin B (AmBisome, Astellas) [1]. Each has significantly less nephrotoxicity; ABLC has similar infusion-related toxicity (see below), Amphotec may have increased, and Ambisome has less infusion-related toxicity. The lipid formulations have increased concentration in the spleen, liver, and lung. This increased uptake in the reticuloendothelial system results in decreased amphotericin in the kidneys. Because the cost is 10- to 20-fold greater than the old formulation, use of the lipid products is often reserved for patients with renal insufficiency or who are otherwise refractory to or intolerant of conventional AMBD. The recommended dose of ABLC is 5.0 mg/kg given as a single daily infusion at a rate of 2.5 mg/kg/hour. For AmBisome, the dose is 3 mg/kg/day for empiric therapy, 3–5 mg/kg/day for systemic fungal infections and 6 mg/kg/day for cryptococcal meningitis. For Amphotec, the dose is 3–4 mg/kg/day.

THERAPEUTIC USE

Amphotericin B is initiated with a 1-mg test dose in 5% dextrose in water infused over 20 minutes to evaluate the extent of the commonly encountered febrile response. Vital signs should be monitored closely. Subsequent dosage increments are determined by the severity of the toxic reactions encountered and the severity of the fungal infection. For chronic infections, the dose may be increased daily until the desired dose is reached. In severe cases, the full therapeutic dose (usually 35 to 50 mg) may be put in 500 mL of 5% dextrose. The equivalent of 1 mg is infused over 20 to 30 minutes, and if no severe reactions occur, the remainder is infused over 2 to 3 hours.

If toxic reactions are noted, hydrocortisone (25 mg) may be added to the infusion bottle to decrease the frequency, but not the severity, of fever and chills. Premedication with acetaminophen and diphenhydramine can further ameliorate toxicity. Nonsteroidal anti-inflammatory drugs should be avoided as there is a potential to enhance amphotericin nephrotoxicity. Many patients will develop tolerance to amphotericin B, and the hydrocortisone can be discontinued. During prolonged therapy, toxicity is expected and can be monitored with twice-weekly measurement of serum creatinine, blood urea nitrogen, potassium, magnesium, and hematocrit.

The total duration of therapy is variable and depends on the clinical situation. With less toxic oral triazoles, amphotericin is often used as a 14-day induction, followed by conversion to an oral triazole.

TOXICITY

With appropriate management, most patients can complete a course of therapy [2]. Infusion-related toxicities are fever, occasionally in excess of 40°C, rigors, headaches, anorexia, nausea, vomiting, dyspnea, and hypotension. Intravenous meperidine hydrochloride, in an average dose of 45 mg, can terminate rigors and chills which develop during an infusion [3]. For patients with severe rigors, the meperidine may be given prophylactically.

In some series, more than 80% of patients developed a significant alteration of renal function with AMBD, with the serum creatinine level rising to 2.0 to 3.0 mg/dL. The creatinine will often plateau at this level and therapy can be continued. Renal toxicity is enhanced by intravascular volume depletion. Infusion of 500 to 1000 mL of normal saline before each dose of amphotericin B can decrease nephrotoxicity. Lipid formulations should be considered in patients who develop progressive declines in renal function despite sodium supplementation. If a lipid product is not available, once the creatinine rises above 3.0 mg/dL, the AMBD may need to be temporarily withheld. The use of a double dose of amphotericin B on alternate days (usually not exceeding 70 mg) is as efficacious as daily therapy.

In patients who receive a total dose of less than 4 g, renal insufficiency is usually reversible; once the total dose exceeds 5 g, there will be some degree of persistent renal insufficiency.

A decrease in hematocrit of 10 units can be expected in 75% of patients; one-third will have a reduction of ≥15 units. The hematocrit decreases early in therapy and then stabilizes. Thrombocytopenia and neutropenia are rare.

Renal potassium wasting is common and oral supplementation is necessary in 25% of patients. Hypomagnesemia has also been noted.

Allergic reactions are absent with amphotericin B, and a rash that appears during therapy can usually be attributed to another cause.

Pregnancy

Amphotericin B has been used in pregnancy without evidence of teratogenesis or persistent toxicity in infants.

FLUCYTOSINE

Flucytosine (5-fluorocytosine) is a fluorinated pyrimidine, synthesized as an antitumor agent in 1957. The drug has a narrow spectrum of activity and is used because of its synergy with amphotericin B against cryptococcus.

MECHANISM OF ACTION

Flucytosine is deaminated within the fungal cell to 5-fluorouracil, which is incorporated into fungal RNA as 5-fluorouridine triphosphate. This leads to faulty protein synthesis and growth inhibition.

SENSITIVE ORGANISMS

Flucytosine is active against *Cryptococcus neoformans, Candida albicans,* other *Candida* species, and the agents of chromomycosis. When flucytosine is used alone, resistance develops during therapy in as many as two-thirds of isolates.

PHARMACOKINETICS

Oral absorption and penetration of tissue by flucytosine is excellent, resulting in tissue levels that are equal to or greater than those in serum. The concentration of flucytosine in CSF averages 75% of serum levels. Excretion is primarily renal, with minimal metabolism. The half-life of flucytosine with normal renal function is 3 to 4 hours, but even minor decreases in renal function leads to prolongation. Both peritoneal dialysis and hemodialysis remove the drug.

DOSAGE AND ADMINISTRATION

The standard daily dose of flucytosine (Ancobon, Valeant North America) is 100 mg/kg/day divided into four doses. The dose must be adjusted for renal insufficiency. In order to avoid accumulation of toxic levels in serum (>100 μg/mL), the following dosage adjustments are recommended: maintaining a normal dose of 25 mg/kg but prolonging the interval, with a 12-hour interval for creatinine clearance (CrCl) of 20 to 40 mL/min and a 24-hour interval for CrCl of 10 to 20 mL/min. For patients on hemodialysis, a dose of 25 mg/kg after each dialysis can be used. Serum levels as well as creatinine, liver function, and platelet and white blood cell counts must be monitored.

TOXICITY

In a large series, 18% of patients experienced gastrointestinal, 7% hepatic, and 18% hematologic complications. Gastrointestinal toxicity is usually not severe. However, severe colitis with multiple colonic perforations has been reported. Hepatitis can occur; abnormalities usually resolve with discontinuation of the drug.

Neutropenia is the most common hematologic adverse event; thrombocytopenia can also occur. Bone marrow toxicity usually resolves with decreased dosage or discontinuation of flucytosine; however, fatal bone marrow suppression has been reported.

Less commonly reported adverse events are maculopapular rashes and eosinophilia. Flucytosine should be used with caution in women of childbearing age because of possible teratogenicity.

THERAPEUTIC INDICATIONS

The combination of amphotericin B and flucytosine as induction therapy during the first 14 days is the treatment of choice for cryptococcal meningitis and disseminated disease. It improves cure rates and decreases relapses when compared with therapy with amphotericin B alone. The presence of amphotericin B decreases the emergence of flucytosine resistance but can lead to an increase in flucytosine toxicity.

TRIAZOLES

One of the most significant advances in the treatment of the systemic mycoses have been the azoles: the first generation (fluconazole, itraconazole, and ketoconazole) and the second generation drugs (voriconazole, and posaconazole). Albaconazole, ravuconazole, and isavuconazole are investigational.

All triazoles have a broad spectrum of activity against systemic mycoses including dimorphic fungi, yeasts, and dermatophytes. Azoles are fungistatic. Although there are few direct comparisons with amphotericin B, they are efficacious, less toxic, and more convenient, especially when chronic therapy is indicated. In-vitro sensitivity testing is available only at reference centers.

MECHANISM OF ACTION

The triazoles are potent inhibitors of ergosterol synthesis, the major membrane sterol of fungi. They block the cytochrome P450-dependent enzyme C-14 alpha-demethylase, which is needed to convert lanosterol to ergosterol. Many drug interactions and toxic effects are related to interaction with human enzymes that are dependent on cytochrome P450 [4] (Table 87-1). Itraconazole and posaconazole are more potent inhibitors of CYP3A4 than fluconazole and voriconazole. Fluconazole and voriconazole are also strong noncompetitive inhibitors of CYP2C19 and CYP2C9. Other drugs can induce production of the CYP450 enzymes, resulting in subtherapeutic azole levels and clinical failure.

The triazoles are teratogenic and embryotoxic in animals and are not recommended during pregnancy or while nursing.

The azoles are commonly used for subacute clinical presentations, chronic suppression, and meningitis (especially fluconazole), with amphotericin B often reserved for the initial management of fulminant infections.

ITRACONAZOLE

Itraconazole is the preferred agent for *Histoplasma capsulatum, Blastomyces dermatitidis, Sporothrix schenckii,* and *Paracoccidioides brasiliensis* [5]. It is supplied as 100-mg capsules, an intravenous formulation and an oral solution (Sporanox, Janssen). It is similar in many respects to ketoconazole: highly lipophilic, protein bound, achieves low CSF levels, and undergoes extensive hepatic metabolism. Gastric acidity is required for optimal absorption of the capsules, with absorption increased two- to threefold when taken with food [6]. The oral solution does not require food or acidity for absorption.

Because of the extended time to reach steady state (10 to 14 days), itraconazole therapy should be initiated with a loading dose. For serious or life-threatening infections, a loading dose of 200 mg three times a day for 3 days is given. No adjustment of dose is required with renal insufficiency; caution should be used in patients with hepatic impairment.

The most common side effects of itraconazole and ketoconazole are nausea, vomiting, and abdominal pain, that can be decreased by administration with a meal. Hepatitis has been noted with all three first-generation triazoles, and is rarely fatal. A reversible hepatitis occurs in about 1 in 800 patients on itraconazole, and asymptomatic elevation of transaminases occurs in < 3%.

Itraconazole has negative inotropic effects. Congestive heart failure and peripheral edema have been reported [7]. It should not be used in patients with ventricular dysfunction. A syndrome of severe hypokalemia, hypertension, adrenal insufficiency, and rhabdomyolysis has been reported in patients taking itraconazole at doses of 600 mg/day.

FLUCONAZOLE

Fluconazole is the preferred agent for *Coccidioides immitis, Cryptococcus neoformans,* and oropharyngeal and esophageal *Candida* [8]. The drug is available as oral and intravenous preparations. It is water-soluble, has low protein binding, achieves high levels in the urine, and has excellent CSF penetration (70–90% of peak serum concentration). These properties make fluconazole an excellent choice for treatment of urinary tract infections and meningitis. Because time to achieve a steady state is 6 to 10 days, a single loading dose of double the maintenance dose is given on the first day. Oral and intravenous doses are the same, because oral bioavailability is better than 90%. Unlike for other azoles, there is minimal hepatic metabolism, with 80% of the drug excreted unchanged in the urine. The dose of fluconazole should

TABLE 87-1 Drug Interactions With Triazoles

Fluconazole	Itraconazole	Voriconazole	Posaconazole
Avoid concomitant use unless benefits exceed risks (significant decrease in fluconazole levels): rifampin	Avoid concomitant use unless benefits exceed risks (significant decrease in itraconazole levels): isoniazid, rifampin, phenobarbital, carbamazepine, phenytoin	**Contraindicated** (significant decrease in voriconazole levels): rifampin, rifabutin, ritonavir (high dose), efavirenz, carbamazepine, phenobarbital	Avoid concomitant use unless benefits exceed risks (decreases posaconazole AUC by 39–49%): rifabutin, phenytoin, cimetidine
Contraindicated (fluconazole inhibits metabolism, risk of QT prolongation or ventricular arrhythmia): cisapride, pimozide, ergot alkaloids Generally avoid: quinidine Monitor closely: halofantrine	**Contraindicated** (itraconazole inhibits metabolism, risk of QT prolongation and ventricular arrhythmias): quinidine, cisapride, terfenadine, astemizole, pimozide, ergot alkaloids Monitor closely: halofantrine	**Contraindicated** (voriconazole inhibits metabolism, risk of QT prolongation and ventricular arrhythmias): quinidine, halofantrine, terfenadine, astemizole, cisapride, pimozide,ergot alkaloids	**Contraindicated** (posaconazole inhibits metabolism, risk of QT prolongation and ventricular arrhythmias): quinidine, halofantrine, terfenadine, astemizole, cisapride, pimozide. ergot alkaloids
Fluconazole increases drug exposure, careful monitoring/ dose adjustment may be required: warfarin, sulfonylureas (glipizide, glyburide, tolbutamide), phenytoin, cyclosporine	Itraconazole increases drug exposure, careful monitoring/dose adjustment may be required: phenytoin, digoxin, warfarin, sulfonylureas (glipizide, glyburide, tolbutamide), digoxin, cyclosporine	Voriconazole increases drug exposure, careful monitoring/dose adjustment required: warfarin, methadone, sulfonylureas (glipizide, glyburide, tolbutamide), lovastatin, simvastatin, felodipine, omeprazole, midazolam, triazolam, vinca alkaloids, cyclosporine, tacrolimus Two-way interactions: phenytoin, oral contraceptives, protease inhibitors, nevirapine	Posaconazole increases drug exposure, careful monitoring dose adjustment required: rifabutin,phenytoin, midazolam, cyclosporine, tacrolimus

be decreased by 50% and 75% when the CrCl is less than 50 and 20 mL/min, respectively. For patients on hemodialysis, a full dose is given after each dialysis.

VORICONAZOLE

Voriconazole is an advance for treatment of invasive *Aspergillus* infections and *Fusarium* and *Scedosporium apiospermum* [9]. The drug is structurally related to fluconazole and is available as an intravenous formulation, as tablets (50 and 200 mg) and an oral suspension (40 mg/mL). The oral formulations have a 96% oral bioavailability. Voriconazole is extensively metabolized by cytochrome P450 enzymes, especially CYP2C19 and to a lesser extent by CYPC2C9 and CYP3A4. Large inter-patient variability in serum levels has been reported owing to genetic polymorphisms. Low levels are associated with clinical failure, while increased levels are associated with neurologic toxicity, including encephalopathy. Monitoring of trough drug levels is recommended after 1 week of therapy, with a target of >1 to 5.5 mg/L [10].

The most frequent adverse event has been visual disturbances, occurring in 20–30% of patients. These usually start within 30 minutes of the dose, last about 30 minutes, and are described as increased brightness, blurred vision, altered color perception, and photopsia. Nausea and vomiting (6%), and diarrhea and headache can occur. Hallucinations, elevated transaminases (3%) and rare hepatic failure have been reported. Mild to moderate rashes (7%) and photosensitivity can be seen.

The intravenous dose of voriconazole is a loading dose of 6 mg/kg every 12 hours for 24 hours, followed by a maintenance dose of 4 mg/kg every 12 hours. The oral dose is 200 mg every 12 hours (1 hour before or after eating) for those weighing >40 kg and 100 mg every 12 hours for those who weigh <40 kg. For patients with a CrCl <50 mL/min, the intravenous formulation should be avoided, as the cyclodextrin used to solubilize the voriconazole will accumulate. With mild to moderate cirrhosis, patients can receive the normal loading dose, but the maintenance dose should be reduced by 50%.

POSACONAZOLE

Posaconazole is a broad-spectrum azole and the first antifungal with significant activity against the agents of mucormycosis, chromoblastomycosis, phaeohyphomycosis, mycetoma, and *Scedosporium apiospermum* [11]. The drug is available only as an oral suspension (Noxafil, Schering). It must be administered with a full meal or a liquid nutritional supplement for absorption (bioavailability increases 2.5–4.0-fold). Posaconazole is metabolized by glucuronidation, with the majority of the drug excreted unchanged in the feces. There is no dose adjustment for renal or hepatic insufficiency.

Posaconazole is well tolerated, with elevated liver function tests (3%), nausea (8%) and vomiting (6%), similar to fluconazole. The dose for invasive infections is 400 mg twice daily with a meal or nutritional supplement. If food or supplement is not tolerated, the dose should be 200 mg four times daily to optimize absorption. Proton pump inhibitors should be avoided.

ECHINOCANDINS

Echinocandins inhibit fungal cell wall glucan by inhibiting beta-1,3 glucan synthesis. The three available echinocandins, caspofungin, micafungin and anidulafungin, are therapeutically equivalent. The drugs are available only as intravenous formulations; choices between them are based upon cost or drug interactions. The major use of echinocandins is in the treatment of systemic candidal infections, especially the empiric treatment of candidemia prior to species identification. They are also used for empiric therapy in febrile neutropenia. The echinocandins are highly active against *Aspergillus* spp.

CASPOFUNGIN

Caspofungin (Cancidas, Merck) is highly protein bound and slowly cleared from plasma by distribution into tissues [12]. Metabolism is by slow peptide hydrolysis. There is no interaction with the P450 system. Tacrolimus levels are decreased by 25%. The usual loading dose is 70 mg followed by 50 mg daily. No adjustment is needed with renal insufficiency or dialysis. With moderate hepatic insufficiency, the maintenance dose is decreased to 35 mg daily. Efavirenz, nevirapine, dexamethasone, rifampin, phenytoin and carbamazepine all reduce serum levels by about 20%. When these drugs are used, a daily dose of 70 mg should be maintained. Caspofungin is well tolerated; reported adverse events include fever, headache, nausea, vomiting, phlebitis and abnormal liver function tests. Histamine-related symptoms have been noted (rash, pruritus, facial flushing).

MICAFUNGIN

Micafungin (Mycamine, Astellas) is metabolized in the liver and excreted in an inactive form in the bile and urine [13]. Drug interactions are limited as the drug is not metabolized by the P450 system. Sirolimus and nifedipine levels are increased by 20%. Micafungin is well tolerated, with a side-effect profile similar to that of caspofungin. The recommended dose is 50 mg/day for prophylaxis and 100 mg/day when used for treatment. There is no dose adjustment for renal insufficiency or mild–moderate liver disease.

ANIDULAFUNGIN

Anidulafungin (Eraxis, Pfizer) is biotransformed by biochemical degradation and excreted in the feces [14]. It is not metabolized, so there are few drug interactions, and there is no dose adjustment with renal or hepatic insufficiency. Anidulafungin is well tolerated, with only rare adverse events. The recommended dose for esophageal candidiasis is 100 mg loading dose followed by 50 mg daily. For invasive candidiasis, the loading dose is 200 mg followed by 100 mg daily.

REFERENCES

1. Wong-Beringer A, Jacobs RA, Guglielmo BJ. Lipid formulations of amphotericin B: clinical efficacy and toxicities. Clin Infect Dis 1998;27:603–18.
2. Bowler WA, Oldfield EC. New approaches to amphotericin B administration. Infections in Medicine 1992;9:17–23.
   Practical review of how to administer AMB, including management of infusion-related toxicity, premedication and nephrotoxicity.
3. Burke LC, Aisner J, Fortner CL, et al. Meperidine for the treatment of shaking chills and fever. Arch Intern Med 1980;140:483–4.
4. Lomaestro BM. Azole drug interaction update. J Invasive Fungal Infect 2007;1:122–32.
5. [Anonymous]. Itraconazole. Med Lett Drugs Ther 1993;35:7–9.
6. Chin TWF, Loeb M, Fong IW. Effects of an acidic beverage (Coca-Cola) on absorption of ketoconazole. Antimicrob Agents Chemother 39:1671–5, 1995.
7. Ahmad SR, Singer SJ, Leissa BG. Congestive heart failure associated with itraconazole. Lancet 2001;357:1766–7.
8. Kowalsky SF, Dixon DM. Fluconazole: a new antifungal agent. Clin Pharm 1991;10:179–94.
9. Johnson LB, Kauffman CA. Voriconazole: a new triazole antifungal agent. Clin Infect Dis 2003;36:630–7.
10. Pascual A, Calandra T, Bolay S, et al. Voriconazole therapeutic drug monitoring in patients with invasive mycoses improves efficacy and safety outcomes. Clin Infect Dis 2008;46:201–11.
11. Nagappan V, Deresinski S. Posaconazole: a broad spectrum triazole antifungal agent. Clin Infect Dis 2007;45:1610–17.
12. Deresinski SC, Stevens DA. Capofungin. Clin Infect Dis 2003;36:1445–57.
13. Chandrasekar PH, Sobel JD. Micafungin: a new echinocandin. Clin Infect Dis 2006;42:1171–8.
14. Vazquez JA, Sobel JD. Anidulafungin: a novel echinocandin. Clin Infect Dis 2006;43:215–22.

PART

5

PROTOZOAL INFECTIONS

88 General Principles

Alan J Magill

PARASITISM

DEFINITIONS

Parasite comes from the Greek word *parasitos* and is defined as "a plant or an animal which lives upon or within another living organism at whose expense it obtains some advantage". Parasitism is a type of *symbiosis* in which an intimate and obligatory relationship exists between two heterospecific organisms. The *parasite*, generally the smaller of the two, is usually metabolically dependent on its host. This association may be beneficial to both (*mutualism*), beneficial to one with little effect on the other (*commensalism*), or beneficial to one and detrimental to the other (*parasitism*). The term parasite is generally reserved for animal species of protozoa, helminths, and arthropods.

NATURAL HISTORY

HOST

The organism on, or within, which the parasite lives is called the *host*. The lifecycle of the parasite may take place in a single host species (e.g. *Entamoeba histolytica*—human), in two host species (e.g. *Plasmodium vivax*—human and mosquito) or in more than two host species (e.g. *Clonorchis sinensis*—human, snail, and cyprinoid fish).

A *definitive host* (e.g. humans for *Taenia saginata*) is one in which a parasite undergoes sexual reproduction. Humans may be the only definitive host for some parasites (e.g. *Trichomonas vaginalis*), whereas others may have several definitive hosts (e.g. bushbuck, other game animals, and humans for *Trypanosoma brucei rhodesiense*). Animals that harbor a parasite that is pathogenic for other animals are called *reservoir hosts* (e.g. dogs for *Leishmania infantum*). Parasites that have reservoir hosts (e.g. *Brugia malayi*) are more difficult to eradicate than those that do not (e.g. *Wuchereria bancrofti*); the reservoir host serves as an alternate in the lifecycle, thus increasing the chance of transmission and survival.

The animal in which the larval or asexual stage habitates (e.g. freshwater snail for *Schistosoma* species) is known as the *intermediate host*. A *transfer or paratenic host* (e.g. large predator fish for *Diphyllobothrium latum*) is not necessary for the completion of the lifecycle of the parasite but is utilized as a temporary refuge and vehicle for reaching the obligatory or definitive host. An *incidental host* is one that is accidentally infected and is not required for the parasite's survival or development (e.g. humans for *Toxoplasma gondii and Leshmania*).

VECTOR

A *vector* (from the Latin *vehere*, to carry), usually an arthropod, transfers an infectious agent from one host to another. The parasite may develop or multiply within the body of the vector before becoming infective, in which case the vector is called a *biologic vector*. Biologic vectors are actually hosts—definitive hosts in the case of anopheline mosquitoes for human *Plasmodium* species or intermediate hosts in the case of *Cyclops* species for *Dracunculus medinensis*. A *mechanical vector* carries a parasite from one host to another but is not essential for the parasite's life cycle (e.g. houseflies for *Entamoeba histolytica*).

PROTOZOA

DEFINITIONS

Protozoa, derived from the Greek words, *protos*, meaning first or primary, and *zoon*, meaning animal, is a phylum comprising some of the morphologically simplest organisms of the animal kingdom. Most species are unicellular, eukaryotic and microscopic in size; most are free-living and motile, but some have commensalistic, mutualistic or parasitic relationships. Approximately 10,000 of the described living species are parasitic. Protozoa infect most vertebrate and invertebrate species and have developed the capacity to adapt to living in most host organs.

The parasitic protozoa, unlike almost all helminths, can replicate (sexually, asexually or both ways) within the host's body—a phenomenon that largely explains their survival, as well as the overwhelming infections that develop from single exposures.

CLASSIFICATION

It remains convenient to divide protozoa pathogenic to man into four phyla or subphyla (or superclasses in the case of the sporozoa) according to their type of locomotion: (1) Sarcodina (amebae); (2) Mastigophora (flagellates); (3) Ciliophora (ciliates); and (4) Sporozoa.

SARCODINA

Ameboid movements produce pseudopods in the Sarcodina. Reproduction is almost exclusively asexual, usually by binary fission. Amebae that infect man include *E. histolytica* (Chapter 89). Other species of Sarcodina that can be either parasitic (e.g. *Naegleria fowleri*, normally a free-living organism), mutualistic or commensalistic (e.g., *Entamoeba hartmanni* and *Entamoeba coli*) are covered in Chapters 102 and 94. Most are parasites or commensals of the gastrointestinal tract.

MASTIGOPHORA

Flagella produce a whip-like motion. Most species, like those of the Sarcodina, have both *cysts* (transmission stage) and *trophozoites* (proliferative stage). Flagellates that infect man include *Giardia lamblia* (Chapter 90), *T. vaginalis* (Chapter 95), *Trypanosoma brucei gambiense*, *T. b. rhodesiense* and *Trypanosoma cruzi* (Chapters 97 and 98), and *Leishmania* species (Chapter 99). Species in this group are capable of infecting many different tissues and cells.

CILIOPHORA

Cilia supply the motion in this subphylum. They have two kinds of nuclei: a macronucleus and a micronucleus. Reproduction is by asexual transverse binary fission and sexual conjugation. *Balantidium coli*, the largest intestinal parasite of man, is a ciliate (Chapter 94).

SPOROZOA

Protozoa in this subphylum typically have no locomotor organs in the adult stage(s) and reproduce alternately by asexual multiplication (schizogony) and sexual multiplication (sporogony). They are exclusively parasitic. Pathogens of man in this group include *Plasmodium* species (Chapter 96), *T. gondii* (Chapter 101), *Cryptosporidium parvum* (Chapter 91), *Cyclospora* (Chapter 92), and *Isospora, Sarcospora, Microspora* and *Cystoisospora* (Chapters 93 and 104). Based upon ribosomal gene analysis, *Pneumocystis carinii* (Chapter 86) is now considered to be a fungus.

PHYSIOLOGY

With the exception of the Sarcodina trophozoites, which have an ectoplastic covering, protozoa have cell membranes.

ECTOPLASM

Across this membrane, nutrients can be actively transported, phagocytized or moved by pinocytosis. Some species have a peristome through which food passes directly into the cytosome and cytopharynx to the endoplasm.

ENDOPLASM

Protozoa are eukaryotic; some have multiple nuclei. Cytoplasmic inclusions and a variety of organelles are responsible for metabolic, reproductive and protective functions.

REPRODUCTION

Asexual or binary fission-type reproduction is characteristic of the Sarcodina, Mastigophora and Ciliophora. In some species, asexual reproduction is more complex. Sexual reproduction in the Sporozoa always takes place in the definitive host (e.g. mosquito for malarial parasites, cat for *T. gondii*); it results in the formation of a zygote. Asexual reproduction occurs in the intermediate host (e.g. humans for malarial parasites and for *T. gondii*).

TRANSMISSION

INTESTINAL PROTOZOA

These are usually transmitted from host to host by the fecal–oral route via food and water. Many species have a cystic stage that is capable of resisting adverse environmental conditions (e.g. drying, heat, and cold). *Toxoplasma gondii* is also transmitted by ingestion of undercooked meat (contaminated with cysts) or soil, food or other vehicles contaminated with cat feces (contaminated with oocysts).

BLOOD AND TISSUE PROTOZOA

Most of these have two hosts—vertebrate (man) and an invertebrate vector (arthropod). The parasite is usually transmitted by the vector's bite (e.g. in infections with *Plasmodium* species, *T. b. gambiense* and *T. b. rhodesiense, Leishmania* species, or *Babesia* species) or by exposure to contaminated vector feces (e.g. in infections with *T. cruzi*).

MAGNITUDE OF THE HEALTH PROBLEM

Protozoal infections cause man more disease and misery than any other group of infectious agents.

MALARIA

Infections with *Plasmodium* species remain one of the greatest causes of mortality and morbidity in the world today, particularly in children under 5 years of age and in pregnant women. The World Health Organization (WHO) has set a long-term goal of control of transmission with drugs, insecticide-treated bed nets and indoor residual spraying of insecticides and selected intensive efforts at local elimination. The continuing development of resistance to insecticides by the anopheline vectors has meant that new chemicals are required, and these are often too expensive to be used by those who need them most.

Multiple drug–resistant *P. falciparum* is widespread in Southeast Asia into the Indian subcontinent, the Western Pacific, in malaria-endemic areas of South America and sub-Saharan Africa. During the mid-1990s, some strains of *P. vivax* in Indonesia, New Guinea, the Solomon Islands, and northern South America developed resistance to chloroquine, complicating and increasing the cost of treatment of this species as well.

Estimates of the numbers infected and dying from malaria vary widely and are often inaccurate because of a lack of specific parasitologic conformation. Recently, the WHO has recommended that all cases of fever be confirmed as being caused by malaria prior to giving antimalarial treatments. In endemic areas, most individuals exposed to infectious bites have low levels of asexual parasites and gametocytes in the peripheral blood. The introduction of non-microscopic rapid diagnostic tests (RDTs) that can detect circulating antigens of plasmodia can provide confirmation of malaria infection where quality microscopic diagnosis is not available.

Many, frequently children, have high-level parasitemias that are often associated with illness. Severe malarial anemia kills the youngest children, whereas older children, and sometimes adults, die of cerebral malaria. Malaria also causes hypoglycemia, which is often confused with cerebral malaria and may be fatal if not specifically treated.

AFRICAN TRYPANOSOMIASIS

Infection with either *T. b. gambiense* or *T. b. rhodesiense* almost always causes severe human illness. If untreated, it is fatal; fortunately, however, relatively few people are infected. *Trypanosoma brucei brucei*, which is morphologically identical to the subspecies causing human sleeping sickness (Chapter 97), causes infection in cattle (nagana) across much of Central and East Africa. Thus, cattle-raising is limited, greatly interfering with economic development and with the nutritional status of the entire area but probably protecting the environment from overgrazing, which has occurred in much of Africa. An increase in fatal cases of African trypanosomiasis was reported in the late 1990s and early 2000s, particularly in Angola, the Democratic Republic of Congo, and southern Sudan owing to a collapse in health-care infrastructure and delivery associated with conflicts. In 2009, after intensive control efforts, the number of cases reported has dropped below 10,000 (9878) for the first time in 50 years.

AMERICAN TRYPANOSOMIASIS

Trypanosoma cruzi affects as many as 15 million people living in South and Central America. Although acute infections may be fatal, most infections are not detected (Chapter 98). Unfortunately, chronic complications years later often lead to severe disability and death from Chagas' cardiopathy and the "mega" syndromes. The poor ,who live in crudely built huts infested with the vector, "the kissing bug," contract Chagas' disease. Infection can be transmitted transplacentally from mother to fetus and by blood transfusion. Increasing immigration from Central and South America to the USA, led to concern regarding the safety of blood transfusions and Food and Drugs Administration (FDA) approval of the first blood screening tests in the USA for Chagas disease on 2006. There are still no FDA-approved efficacious and safe drugs for treating the infection, particularly the chronic form. Over 1500 confirmed positive cases of Chagas have been detected via the new blood donor screening policies as of 2011.

LEISHMANIASIS

Leishmania species infect millions worldwide and cause clinical syndromes varying from a minimal, single, self-healing chronic ulceration (urban oriental sore) to a severe, and often fatal, generalized febrile illness (kala-azar [Chapter 99]). *Leishmania* species causing these different syndromes appear morphologically identical. Polymorphisms can be detected, however, by using biochemical, immunologic and genetic techniques that correlate with epidemiologic and clinical differences. Improved diagnosis to include molecular techniques has demonstrated more cases of subclinical and mild infections than of the characteristic diseases. Patients with silent chronic infections with species causing visceral disease, i.e. *Leishmania donovani, L. infantum,* or *Leishmania chagasi,* sometimes develop visceral leishmaniasis when they become immunocompromised. Associated with the conflict in Afghanistan, tens of thousands of people have been infected with epidemic anthroponotic *Leishmania tropica* during the past 10 years.

NEW DEVELOPMENTS

There have been several developments in protozoology since the last edition of this book was published.

MALARIA

The introduction and increasing worldwide use of oral artemisinin combination treatments (ACTs) for the treatment of uncomplicated *P. falciparum* malaria has led to a decrease in the morbidity and mortality caused by malaria in many countries. In addition, two large, randomized, controlled, clinical trials—one in adults in Southeast Asia and in one children in sub-Saharan Africa—comparing intravenous artesunate with intravenous quinine for the treatment of severe and complicated malaria demonstrated the superiority of artesunate in decreasing all-cause mortality. The possible emergence of artemisinin-resistant falciparum malaria along the Thailand–Cambodian border will increase the difficulty and the cost of treating and controlling that disease. The introduction of RDTs for the diagnosis of malaria has proven to be a valuable tool for the optimal use of anti-malarial drugs. Providing useful alternative diagnostic testing for those who test negative for malaria parasites remains challenging. In general when available control interventions, such as drugs, diagnostic testing, bed nets, and vector control measures, are introduced in a malaria endemic area, especially in a coordinated and integrated manner, the reductions in disease incidence and prevalence have been striking.

AFRICAN TRYPANOSOMIASIS

The significant decline in reported cases of human African trypanosomiasis (HAT) over the last 5 years is as a result of improved case detection and management. Thanks to a partnership between Sanofi Aventis (the manufacturer of the world's supply of pentamidine, melarsoprol, and intravenous eflornithine) and the WHO, these life-saving drugs have been distributed to countries where the disease is endemic, thanks to the logistics of the association Doctors Without Borders (known as MSF—*Médecins sans Frontières*). Efforts to develop improved treatments met with some success in heroic clinical trials conducted by MSF and Drugs for Neglected Diseases Initiative (DNDi). The combination of 10 days of oral nifurtimox combined with a shorter 7-day course of intravenous eflornithine was shown to be as effective as the standard 14-day course of intravenous eflornithine. The Nifurtimox-Eflornithine Combination Therapy (NECT) significantly decreases the number of intravenous injections needed and thus is easier for field administration in endemic areas. With the inclusion in April 2009 of NECT in the WHO Essential List of Medicines, disease-endemic countries now have a new opportunity and a less complex option to treat the second stage of the Gambiense form of HAT.

AMERICAN TRYPANOSOMIASIS

There has been renewed interest in developing new efficacious and safe drugs for treating the infection, particularly the chronic form. The Benznidazole Evaluation for Interrupting Trypanosomiasis (BENEFIT) project, is a large, multicenter (most sites are in Brazil and Argentina), randomized, double-blind, placebo-controlled phase III clinical trial investigating the role of benznidazole in patients with chronic Chagas heart disease began in 2004 with initial results anticipated in 2013. This project investigates whether etiologic treatment significantly reduces parasite burden, as assessed by PCR-based techniques and also will determine the safety and tolerability profile of the trypanocidal drug in this type of chagasic population.

The non-profit drug research and development organization, DNDi, is teaming up with Eisai, a Japanese pharmaceutical company, to test the safety and effectiveness of a prodrug of the antifungal ravuconazole in patients with Chagas disease. The trial, the first in 40 years of a new drug for this disease, began in June of 2011 in South America. In addition, Schering-Plough also began a study of oral posaconazole in the treatment of asymptomatic chronic chagas disease in Argentina in July of 2011 as well.

LEISHMANIASIS

The decade between 2000 and 2010 saw a significant expansion in available drug treatments for visceral leishmaniasis, especially in the Indian subcontinent. At the beginning of the decade we faced pentavalent antimony-resistant visceral leishmaniasis in India, and had few other options. A significant expansion in the use of amphotericin B out of necessity was accompanied by a series of clinical trials demonstrating the remarkable efficacy and relative safety of liposomal amphotericin B (LAMB) when given as a single 10-mg/kg infusion. Current WHO recommendations also include intramuscular paromomycin and oral miltefosine. Optimal regimens for East Africa remain to be determined. Unfortunately there have not been significant advances for the treatment of cutaneous leishmaniasis or mucosal leishmanaisis except to show the efficacy of LAMB for both syndromes. The cost of LAMB is prohibitive in resource poor countries with endemic disease.

SECTION

A

INTESTINAL AND GENITAL INFECTIONS

89 *Entamoeba histolytica* (Amebiasis)

Eric Houpt, Chien-Ching Hung

Key features

- *Entamoeba histolytica*, the cause of amebiasis, is microscopically indistinguishable from *Entamoeba dispar* and *Entamoeba moshkovskii*, which are non-pathogenic parasites. Differentiation requires stool antigen detection or PCR
- Infections with *E. histolytica* may be asymptomatic or cause intestinal or extraintestinal amebiasis
- Clinical suspicion of amebic liver abscess can be confirmed by a positive amebic serologic test in conjunction with positive results of a sonographic or radiologic imaging procedure, followed by a response to specific therapy
- Nitroimidazoles, in particular metronidazole or tinidazole, are the mainstay of therapy for invasive amebiasis
- Nitroimidazole treatment should be followed with a luminal agent to cure intestinal infection

INTRODUCTION

Entamoeba histolytica is a protozoan parasite that accounts for an estimated 100,000 annual deaths globally [1]. Infection ranges from asymptomatic colonization of the large bowel to invasive intestinal and extra-intestinal disease, particularly liver abscess. Fedor Losch is first credited with identifying motile amebae in the stool of a patient with dysentery in 1875; however, an association between dysentery and liver disease goes back to Hippocrates. Diagnosis conventionally involves microscopic demonstration of the parasite; however, this is neither sensitive nor specific. Treatment is effective with metronidazole or tinidazole.

EPIDEMIOLOGY

Entamoeba histolytica has a worldwide distribution but is more prevalent in tropical areas. Early microscopic surveys are confounded by the re-description of *E. histolytica* into two species: *E. histolytica*, which is pathogenic, and *Entamoeba dispar*, which is not, but is ~10 times more common [1]. Further molecular studies have identified a third species, *Entamoeba moshkovskii*, which also tends to be non-pathogenic [2]. Microscopy cannot distinguish *E. histolytica* cysts or trophozoites from *E. dispar* or *E. moshkovskii*, thus previous studies on *E. histolytica* prevalence based on microscopy are likely flawed. Serologic studies are more reliable as *E. histolytica* generates a serum antibody response while *E. dispar* and *E. moshkovskii* do not. A large survey from Mexico showed that 8.4% of persons have been exposed [3]. In Dhaka, Bangladesh, an *E. histolytica*-specific fecal antigen assay revealed infection in 80% of preschool children over the course of 4 years, with an incidence of diarrhea and dysentery of 0.09 and 0.03 per child-year respectively [4]. There is little gender variation in amebiasis in children; however, in the adult population, invasive disease is more common in males than females, particularly for liver abscess, but also for colitis, with an overall male-to-female ratio between 3 and 10:1 [5]. In central Vietnam, the incidence of amebic liver abscess peaks at 125/100,000 in 40-year-old adult males [6]. Epidemiology on incidence of amebiasis in Africa is particularly limited, but appears widespread [7].

In developed countries, most cases are imported and high-risk populations include returned travelers, expatriates, and immigrants. The GeoSentinel network revealed 120/1000 (2.5% of all reported acute diarrhea) returning travelers presenting with diarrhea had amebiasis [8]. Approximately 5% of immigrants to the USA from Africa may have *E. histolytica/E. dispar/E. moshkovskii* in their stools [9]. Studies in the 1980s revealed that men who have sex with men (MSM) were at high risk of intestinal infection with *E. dispar* [10]. However, recent studies from Taiwan, Japan, Korea, and Australia have shown high rates of invasive *E. histolytica* infection in HIV-infected MSM [11]. The reasons for this are unclear, as globally and in sub-Saharan Africa it has not been appreciated that HIV-positive persons are more susceptible to amebiasis.

Although animal reservoirs of *E. histolytica* and *E. dispar* have been described, they are not thought to play a major role in transmission. Human-to-human and fecal–oral transmission are the major sources of human infections. Persons of all ages are susceptible to infection. Females are as likely to be infected as males, but invasive disease is more common in males [5].

NATURAL HISTORY, PATHOGENESIS, AND PATHOLOGY

Motile trophozoites passed with diarrheal or dysenteric stools can survive only briefly outside the body and are destroyed by gastric secretions, and therefore have no role in transmission.

Cysts are relatively hardy and can survive outside the body long enough to be ingested. They are sensitive to desiccation and to temperatures of >40°C and <5°C and are killed almost immediately by boiling. They are moderately resistant to chlorine, not being destroyed by concentrations usually used for water purification. Cysts may remain viable for 1 month at 4°C in both sewage and natural surface water. Cysts have survived for as long as 48 hours at room temperature on cheese, bread, green salads, and fruits.

After ingestion of an *E. histolytica* cyst from fecally contaminated food or water or via oral–anal sexual practices, excystment occurs in the small intestine. The resulting small metacystic trophozoites are carried into the cecum with the fecal stream where colonization and tissue invasion occur depending on the virulence of the infecting strain. Approximately 90% of individuals will remain asymptomatic and most will eventually clear. Symptoms develop after an incubation period of 2–4 weeks. Diarrhea is the most common manifestation of disease, followed by dysentery and then extra-intestinal abscess.

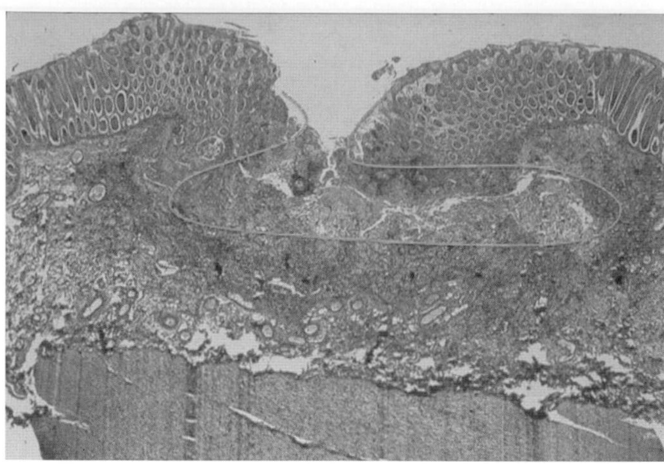

FIGURE 89.1 Flask-shape ulcer.

Prospective studies of asymptomatic carriers indicate a risk of ~9% of progressing to dysentery or liver abscess over the ensuing year [12]. This clinical variability, from asymptomatic carriage to dysentery, was captured in Walker and Sellards' human challenge studies of 1913 [13].

Pathogenesis follows an elaborate series of events beginning with parasite adherence to the colonic mucus and epithelium, host cell damage and then development of a cell-mediated immune response that can either perpetuate or clear infection [14]. After invading the epithelial layer, there is neutrophil recruitment, tissue damage and a characteristic flask-shaped ulcer may develop (Fig. 89.1).

Amebiasis is seen most frequently in the cecum and ascending colon, although the sigmoid colon, rectum, and appendix can also be involved. In a minority of infections, parasites presumably find submucosal blood vessels and embolize to produce liver abscesses. Most cases of extraintestinal abscess exist without evidence of coexisting intestinal infection, and most cases of colitis exist without extraintestinal abscess, such that stool studies are only 40% sensitive for detection of *E. histolytica* during liver abscess. Rarely, liver abscess can directly rupture into the pleura or pericardium; at other times, parasites can be carried hematogenously to distant sites such as the brain.

CLINICAL FEATURES

INTESTINAL AMEBIASIS

Intestinal amebiasis includes asymptomatic colonization or infection and symptomatic intestinal disease and its complications to include amebic colitis, fulminate colitis (toxic megacolon), intestinal perforation with or without peritonitis, intra-abdominal abscess, amebic appendicitis, hemorrhage, ameboma, amebic stricture and perianal (cutaneous) amebiasis.

Asymptomatic intestinal infection with *E. histolytica*/*E. dispar*/*E. moshkovskii* is diagnosed incidentally during stool examination for ova and parasites, for instance during post-travel screening or in immigrants. Symptomatic disease is only associated with *E. histolytica* infection.

Intestinal amebiasis presents as a spectrum of disease from acute amebic dysenteric colitis to a more chronic nondysenteric colitis that presents subacutely with a nonspecific watery diarrhea. Approximately 8% of *E. histolytica*-associated diarrhea cases will have visible blood (dysentery) [15]. Abdominal pain is seen in ~40%. Fever occurs in a minority of cases. Onset of symptoms is often gradual over several weeks and is often associated with weight loss.

Patients with extensive transmural colonic involvement may present acutely with concomitant bacterial peritonitis following intestinal perforation. These patients are toxic, febrile, hypotensive and have profuse bloody diarrhea. Fulminant colitis or toxic megacolon can occur, but is rare (<0.5% of cases), which is associated with a mortality of more than 40%; malnourished persons, pregnant women, corticosteroid users and very young children may be at increased risk. Patients typically appear very ill and have fever, profuse bloody mucoid diarrhea, diffuse abdominal pain, distended abdomen and are hypotensive with signs of peritoneal irritation. Intestinal perforation usually manifests as a slow leakage rather than an acute event. Surgical intervention is indicated for bowel perforation, although attempts to suture such necrotic bowels are usually unsuccessful.

Some report a chronic syndrome of intermittent diarrhea, abdominal pain, flatulence and weight loss for months in patients with amebas in the stool and positive anti-amebic serologic tests. Not all patients respond to anti-amebic therapy so the role of *E. histolytica* in all instances is unclear. However, a trial of therapy is reasonable, as is ruling out inflammatory bowel disease, as amebiasis may worsen if corticosteroids are started.

The formation of annular colonic granulation tissue at a single or multiple sites following the healing of amebic ulcers leads to an intestinal mass called an ameboma. It usually involves the cecum or ascending colon and may mimic carcinoma of the colon. The same fibrosis may also lead to intestinal stricture. Amebic appendicitis almost always occurs as a complication of transmural amebic colitis and should be considered in the presence of other signs of amebiasis. However, isolated amebic appendicitis has been described in a patient with a prior history of colitis [16].

Perianal amebiasis may result from extension of severe bowel disease to the skin. Lesions can be ulcerative or condylomatous, enlarge slowly over weeks to months, and result in pain and bleeding. The diagnosis of cutaneous amebiasis requires a high index of suspicion, especially primary disease not associated with intestinal symptoms. The characteristic cutaneous ulcer is well-demarcated, round or oval, with heaped-up borders and an erythematous halo. Motile trophozoites can be visualized in a fresh smear of the ulcer exudate or a scraping of the ulcer edge.

EXTRAINTESTINAL AMEBIASIS

Amebic liver abscess may occur in the presence or absence of intestinal symptoms. It often develops after a latent period following earlier diarrhea or other intestinal illness, particularly in those with a history of residence or prior travel to endemic areas. Amebic liver abscess is the most common extraintestinal manifestation of amebiasis and can present in a variety of ways (http://www.bhj.org/books/liver/). The syndrome is most often seen in adult males, aged 20–40 years old. Approximately 80% of patients in endemic areas present within 2–4 weeks [17]; however, most returning travelers present, on average, three months after leaving the endemic area. Onset can be insidious, subacute or acute. Symptoms include fever, a nonproductive cough and a constant, dull, aching pain in the right upper quadrant or epigastrium. Pleuritic pain in the right lower anterior chest or right hypochondrium is common. In a minority of patients a subacute course may present with prominent weight loss with less fever and abdominal pain. Hepatomegaly with point tenderness over the liver below the ribs or in the intercostal spaces is a typical finding. Right lobe lesions are usually single lesions and about five times more common than left lobe lesions. Right-sided pleural pain or referred shoulder pain occurs when the diaphragmatic surface of the liver is involved. Associated gastrointestinal symptoms occur in a minority of patients (10–35%) with a liver abscess. Leukocytosis in the range of 12,000–20,000/mm^3 is seen in most cases, with mild normochromic normocytic anemia in more than half. Peripheral eosinophilia is not seen in either hepatic or intestinal amebiasis. Patients with acute amebic liver abscess tend to have a normal alkaline phosphatase level and elevated transaminases [18]; the opposite is true for those with more chronic disease. Ultrasonography, abdominal computed tomography (CT) and magnetic resonance imaging (MRI) are all excellent for detecting liver abscesses.

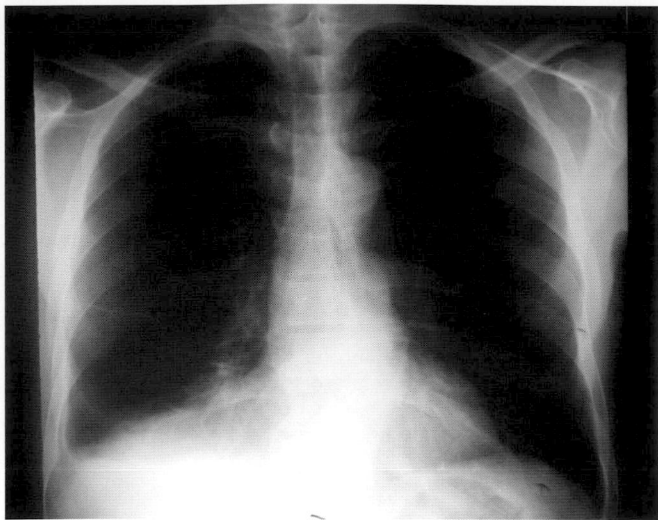

FIGURE 89.2 Amebic liver abscess. Chest x-ray shows reactive right lower lobe atelectasis and pleural effusion.

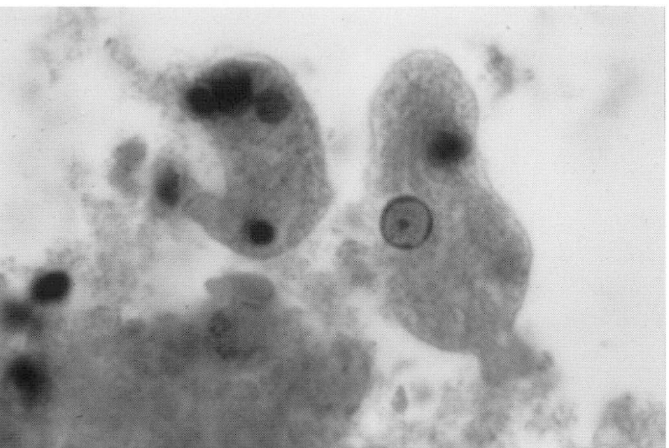

FIGURE 89.3 *Entamobea histolytica* trophozoite in stool sample showing ingested red blood cells. *Image courtesy of the Herman Zaiman collection.*

Pleuropulmonary amebiasis is the most common complication of amebic liver abscess and can take the form of pneumonitis, lung abscess or bronchohepatic fistula [19]. It generally occurs as a result of the rupture of a superior right lobe abscess with erosion through the diaphragm to involve the pleural space, lung parenchyma or bronchus. In contrast, serous pleural effusion and atelectasis are common findings and do not indicate extension of disease (Fig. 89.2). Intraperitoneal rupture occurs rarely but is associated with a high mortality. Left lobe abscesses are more likely to progress to rupture because of late clinical presentation. Pericardial amebiasis, a rare complication, usually presents with fever and abdominal pain with progression to chest pain. Signs are typical of pericarditis, including a friction rub.

Cerebral amebiasis has an abrupt onset, and progresses rapidly to death over 12–72 hours without adequate therapy [20]. Thus, when patients with known amebiasis have alteration of mental states or focal signs, amebic brain abscess or encephalitis should be considered and CT or MRI of the brain should be performed if available. Genitourinary amebiasis is rare and includes rectovaginal fistulas and vulvar lesions in women and penile amebiasis, in homosexual men in particular [21].

PATIENT EVALUATION, DIAGNOSIS, AND DIFFERENTIAL DIAGNOSIS

The differential diagnosis of nonspecific diarrhea involves a long list of bacterial, toxin, viral and parasitic causes which clinical features cannot distinguish. Consideration for amebiasis should occur when a patient has diarrhea that is not improving with conservative management. In many countries, metronidazole is used abundantly for empiric management of diarrhea, such that many cases of amebiasis are probably treated.

There are multiple ways to evaluate patients with suspected amebiasis, including microscopy, antigen detection, molecular diagnosis with PCR techniques, serology, endoscopic procedures and imaging modalities.

MICROSCOPY

Globally, the most commonly available laboratory technique is stool microscopy; typically only a saline wet mount is performed, which is only useful for visualization of motile trophozoites. Additionally, a stained slide will allow visualization of morphologic features including 10–15 μm quadrinucleate cysts and trophozoites with ingested red blood cells (Fig. 89.3), which is more compatible with *E. histolytica* than *E. dispar* or *E. moshkovskii*. Amebic cysts and trophozoites are passed intermittently in the stool and, therefore, three stools should ideally be submitted, as this has increased the sensitivity of detection by 23% [22]. In some series, 18% of stools with *E. histolytica* diarrhea will be hemoccult-positive. Fecal leukocytes are variable and Charcot-Leyden crystals have been reported. In general, microscopy is neither sensitive nor specific.

ANTIGEN DETECTION

Current antigen detection tests are a great advance over microscopy; however, they are expensive and poorly available in resource-limited settings. Presently, there are several commercially-available antigen kits for detecting *Entamoeba* (TechLab *E. histolytica* II, Blacksburg, VA, USA; Ridascreen *Entamoeba*, R-Biopharm, Darmstadt, Germany; Triage Micro Parasite Panel, Biosite Diagnostics, Inc., San Diego, CA, USA; ProSpecT *E. histolytica*, Remel Inc., Lenexa, KS; CELISA Path, Cellabs, Brookvale, Australia). Unfortunately, these tests require fresh, not fixative-preserved, stool for analysis. The TechLab and Cellabs kits report being specific for *E. histolytica* and thus offer the benefit of excluding *E. dispar* and *E. moshkovskii*.

PCR

Research laboratories can perform PCR on stool or liver abscess pus, as well as isoenzyme analysis on cultured trophozoites to confirm *E. histolytica*.

SEROLOGY

Serum antibodies should be detectable in >70% of patients with amebic colitis and >90% of patients with liver abscess and thus should be obtained on all patients when the diagnosis is being considered. Depending on the method used, the serologic response can remain positive for 5 years; thus, in an individual from an endemic area, a positive result does not ensure the diagnosis of amebiasis. However, a negative result has a strong negative predictive value. The indirect hemagglutination assay is reported to be the most sensitive; however, the ELISA is most commonly available.

ENDOSCOPIC PROCEDURES

Colonoscopy is preferred over flexible sigmoidoscopy because disease may be limited to the right side (ascending) of the colon or the cecum. Bowel cleansing with cathartics or enemas should not be done so as to optimize identification of parasites. The endoscopist should aspirate material from the ulcer base and ulcer margin. The gross appearance of the intestinal mucosa in amebic colitis is granular,

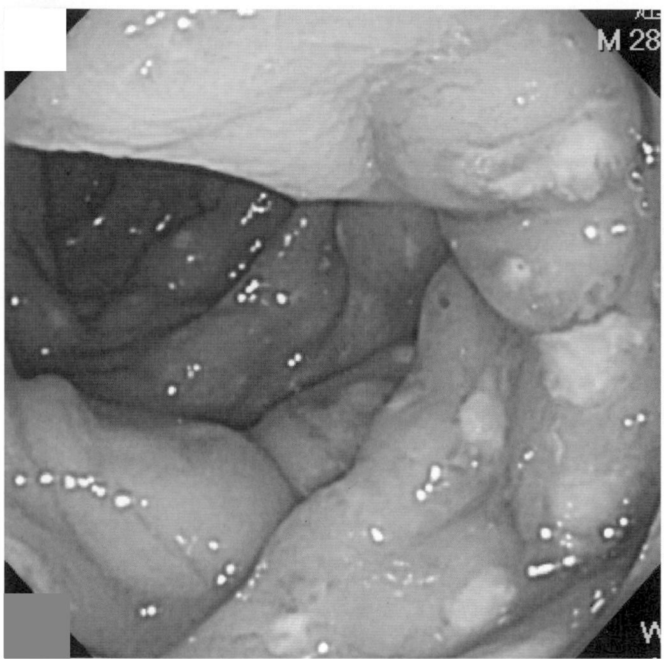

FIGURE 89.4 Colonoscopy of a 54-year-old male who presented with lower gastrointestinal bleeding caused by *E. histolytica* colitis.

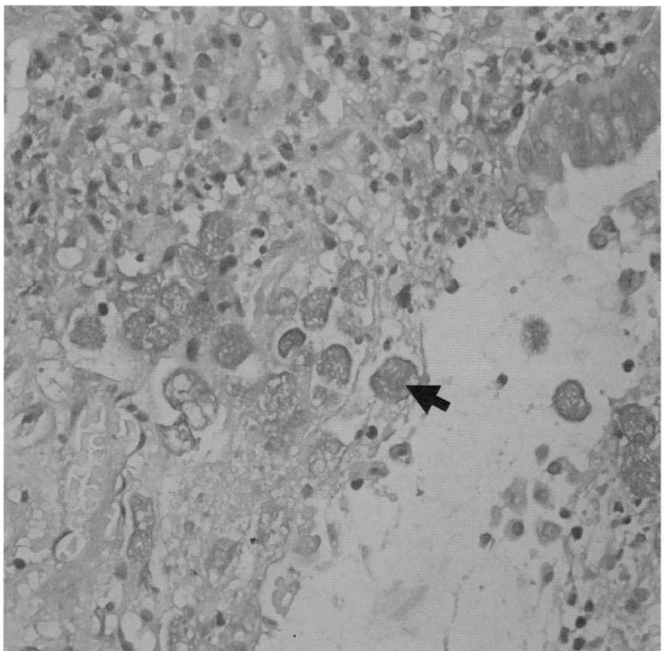

FIGURE 89.5 Numerous trophozoites shown by periodic acid-Schiff (PAS) stain of the colon biopsy (arrow).

friable and diffusely ulcerated and may be indistinguishable from that seen in IBD (Figs 89.4 and 89.5).

IMAGING PROCEDURES

Imaging of the liver can be made by ultrasonography, CT or MRI (Fig. 89.6). Ultrasonography reveals abscesses as hypoechoic lesions. CT with administration of contrast material shows the abscess center as non-enhancing, surrounded by an irregular, or rim-like, area of inflammation that shows increased enhancement (Fig. 89.7). Echinococcal cysts of the liver, which typically do not cause fever or

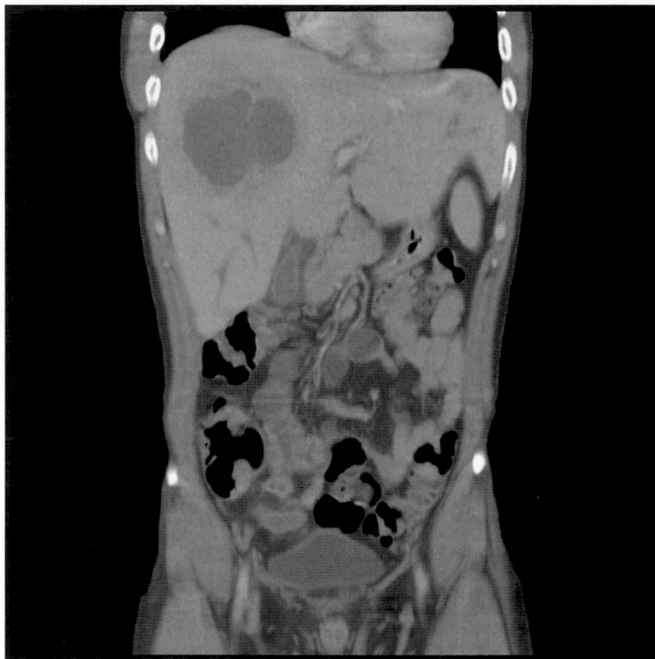

FIGURE 89.6 MRI of amebic liver abscess.

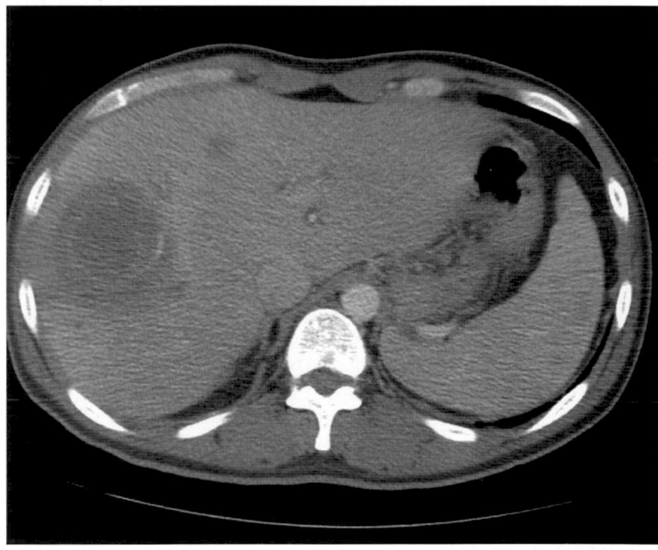

FIGURE 89.7 Computed tomography of a patient with amebic liver abscess who presented with fever, right upper quadrant pain and pleuritic pain.

tenderness, are distinguishable from amebic and pyogenic abscesses by CT (multiple clustered fluid collections without surrounding stranding or enhancement).

Thus, the primary consideration in the differential diagnosis of amebic liver abscess is the distinction between pyogenic abscess and amebic abscess. The two cannot be distinguished clinically. Amebic liver abscesses are often large, single abscesses of the right lobe, whereas pyogenic abscesses more often multiple, but the overlap is significant [23]. Pyogenic liver abscess is much more common than amebic liver abscess in developed countries, has positive blood cultures in half the patients and patients tend to be older than 50 years, present with jaundice and abnormalities of the gallbladder and interhepatic ducts on imaging. Empiric antibiotics can be tried, but if the patient is progressing and the diagnosis is unclear despite blood cultures, serology and stool studies, many patients undergo aspiration for diagnosis. Upon aspiration, amebic abscesses are described as "anchovy paste", chocolate-colored fluid consisting predominantly of necrotic hepatocytes. Gram stain is negative, unlike most cases of pyogenic liver abscess. Trophozoites are rarely seen from aspirates, as these are usually found at the junction of the abscess and viable liver, which usually requires an open drainage procedure [24, 25].

The differential diagnosis of amebic dysentery includes any other dysenteric infection, thus bacterial stool culture should be performed to identify *Shigella, Campylobacter, Salmonella*, enteroinvasive *Escherichia coli*, and enterohemorrhagic *E. coli*. Non-infectious causes of abdominal pain and bloody diarrhea include IBD, ischemic colitis, diverticulitis, and arterio-venous malformation. Occasionally, patients with ongoing intestinal symptoms undergo colonoscopy with biopsy and the diagnosis is made by the pathologist, where clues include patchy areas of ulceration and periodic acid-Schiff staining trophozoites (not to be confused with macrophages). IBD has been confused pathologically with amebic colitis; thus, in a patient with possible exposure to *E. histolytica*, the diagnosis of IBD should be confirmed with the pathologist, as steroids can worsen amebiasis.

TREATMENT

AMEBIC COLITIS

Since the 1960s, the mainstay of therapy for amebic colitis has been the nitroimidazoles, in particular metronidazole and tinidazole. Powell and coworkers performed the first clinical trial of metronidazole in patients with acute amebic dysentery which demonstrated the superiority of 800 mg tid given for 10 days [26]. Lower doses were less effective, but subsequent studies have demonstrated that the 800 mg po tid regimen can be shortened to 5 days [27, 28]. Newer studies have successfully used nitroimidazoles with longer half-lives including tinidazole [29], secnidazole [30] and ornidazole for even shorter durations. Tinidazole has had the most experience, is better tolerated than metronidazole and can be administered for only 3 days [31, 32]. The common side effects of metronidazole include nausea, headache, anorexia and a metallic taste; less common ones include a disulfuram-like reaction to alcohol, vomiting and peripheral neuropathy. The nitroimidazoles are rapidly absorbed after oral administration and are not effective against luminal trophozoites and exhibit a 40–60% rate of parasite persistence in the intestine after therapy with these agents [12, 33]. Therefore, a course of treatment should be followed with a course of a luminal agent. A potential new agent for intestinal amebiasis is nitazoxanide. This drug, administered at 500 mg po bid for three days, was associated with resolution of *E. histolytica/E. dispar*-associated diarrhea in 80–90% of patients (vs. 40–50% in patients receiving placebo) along with microscopic improvement [34]. The tetracyclines have also been used but they are not as effective as metronidazole [35].

AMEBIC LIVER ABSCESS

The initial amebic colitis trials with metronidazole also included groups of "not severely ill patients" with amebic liver abscess. Liver abscess was found to be, in general, more responsive than colitis. We recommend the standard high dose of metronidazole for 10 days or tinidazole for 5 days [36] as the lower-dose or single-dose groups had slower recoveries or more failures [37].

SEVERE DISEASE

The metronidazole trials to date have been in "not severely ill patients". In a severely ill patient who cannot take oral medications, such as those with fulminant amebic colitis, it is logical to assume that intravenous metronidazole would be effective in these patients; however, data is limited to a case series from Japan that showed promise [38].

In patients with either colitis or liver abscess failing or progressing on metronidazole, a potential alternative or additional therapy is emetine. It is derived from ipecac, has been used since the 1920s and is as potent as the nitroimidazoles *in vitro*. The drug is cardiotoxic and congestive failure and deaths have been reported. Electrocardiogram monitoring is recommended. The drug is given intramuscularly. The synthetic derivative dehydroemetine is less cardiotoxic and is recommended over emetine if available. Procurement is difficult. In the USA, it is available from the Centers for Disease Control and Prevention (CDC) Drug Service for metronidazole-refractory amebiasis (1600 Clifton Road, MS/D09 Atlanta, GA 30333; Tel: (404) 639-3670; Fax: (404) 639-3717).

When patients fail medical treatment and undergo open surgery for acute abdomen, gastrointestinal bleeding or toxic megacolon [39], mortality is extremely high and broad-spectrum antibiotics should be added for bacterial spillage into the peritoneum.

Chloroquine has also been used for amebic liver abscess and has shown similar cure rates to metronidazole, although improvement was slower [40]. It is reported to have little effect on intestinal disease and little *in vitro* activity [41]. Extended courses have been recommended for liver abscess because relapses have historically been common, but these probably reflect the drug's ineffectiveness against intestinal parasites; 20 days should be adequate if followed by a course of a luminal agent. For severe liver abscess progressing on metronidazole/tinidazole beyond 72 hours, switching to chloroquine and dehydroemetine can be considered [42]; however, procurement of the dehydroemetine is difficult and should not delay consideration of drainage.

DRAINAGE

The role for liver abscess drainage is when antibiotics are failing in order to prevent impending rupture. Any liver abscess rupture is a high-mortality event (6–30%), particularly if into the pericardium [43], and requires open surgery. Given the high mortality, the question of when to prophylactically drain an abscess arises. Criteria that would prompt consideration of drainage include an abscess >10 cm in diameter, a left lobe abscess to prevent rupture into the pericardium or any abscess close to a serosal surface (Fig. 89.8). Aspiration is also indicated for abscesses that are not promptly responding to drugs alone and for abscesses of uncertain cause. The majority of amebic liver abscesses that are relatively small (<10 cm) usually respond to drug therapy alone. Many studies indicate that routine drainage of amebic liver abscess confers no clinical benefit over antibiotics alone [44] and a meta-analysis concluded therapeutic aspiration could not be supported or refuted because of lack of evidence [45]. One study showed that failure to respond by 72 hours in terms of prolonged fever, leukocytosis and hepatomegaly identified a group at high risk for abscess rupture [46]. We therefore feel that ongoing pain while on appropriate therapy for 72 h is a reasonable criteria for drainage, especially with large left lobe abscesses, as these are associated with a greater frequency of complications [25]. Percutaneous aspiration under ultrasound guidance has shown good results compared with open drainage or needle aspiration [47]. Serial liver scans and sonograms have shown that most liver abscesses completely heal 4–8 months after chemotherapy. The resolution time may be longer for large abscesses; however, patients usually remain asymptomatic in these cases.

ASYMPTOMATIC INTESTINAL COLONIZATION

The WHO recommends against treatment of asymptomatic patients when only a microscopic diagnosis by stool examination is available (i.e. *E. histolytica/E. dispar/E. moshkovskii*) [1]. If *E. histolytica* is confirmed by specific testing (fecal antigen test, serology) or is suspected (e.g. close contact with a case of invasive amebiasis or during an outbreak of amebiasis) then treatment is appropriate. There are at least three classes of luminal agents that have shown efficacy in clinical trials for asymptomatic intestinal colonization: dichloracetanilide derivatives, oral aminoglycosides and 5-hydroxyquinolines. The specific agents include diloxanide furoate, paromomycin and iodoquinol/diiodohydroxyquin. All have a large, worldwide experience and poor gastrointestinal absorption, which allows high luminal concentrations but renders them less effective in invasive disease. One of these

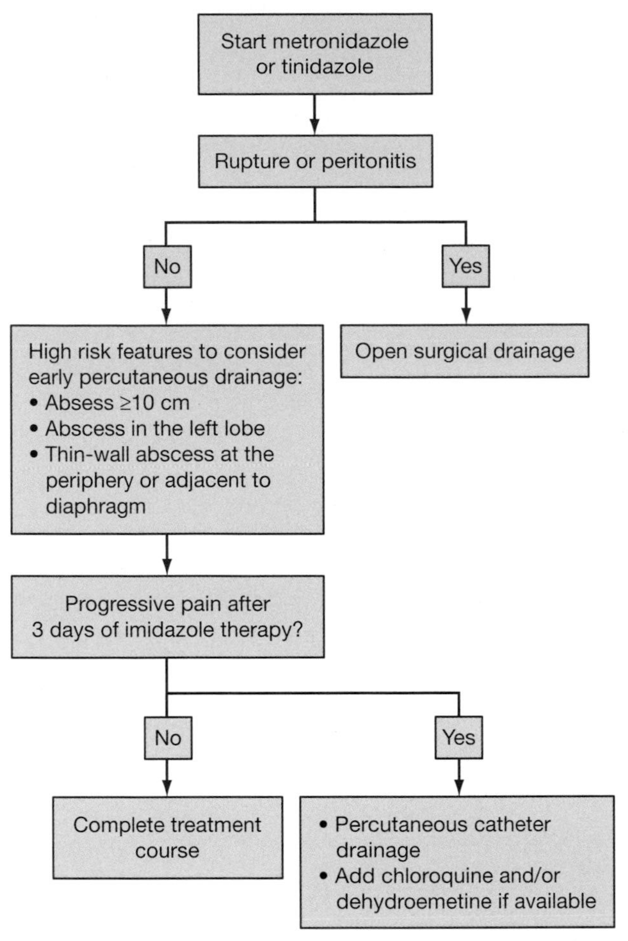

FIGURE 89.8 Algorithmic approach to the management of amebic liver abscess.

BOX 89.1 Anti-amebic drugs for children and pregnant women

Children

Most anti-amebic drugs mentioned have pediatric dosing regimens (Table 89-1). Tinidazole is only approved in the USA in children over 3 years old and nitazoxanide in children over 1 year old.

Pregnancy

Of the drugs mentioned for asymptomatic infection, paromomycin has been used safely in pregnancy [54] and would be the drug of choice. For invasive intestinal disease, there is continued controversy over the use of metronidazole in pregnancy with reports of facial defects and central nervous system tumors in children born to mothers taking metronidazole in the first trimester [55] but large analyses have simultaneously found no increased risk above controls [56]. A caveat is that the dose used for *E. histolytica* infection is higher than that used in most analyses. Some would recommend a trial of paromomycin for mild invasive intestinal disease [57]. For severe colitis or liver abscess, we feel that the risk of metronidazole to the fetus is less than that of the disease to the mother, particularly in second or third trimester. One could consider trying chloroquine for liver abscess, as this drug has been used safely (at lower doses) in pregnant women for malaria prophylaxis.

TABLE 89-1 Antimicrobial Therapy for *Entamoeba histolytica* Infection

Clinical syndrome	Drugs of choice	Adult dose (pediatric dose)	Reference	Evidence base
Asymptomatic or post-treatment intestinal cure	Paromomycin	25–35 mg/kg/d po ÷ tid × 7 d	[48]	**3**
	Diloxanide	500 mg po tid (20 mg/kg/d ÷ tid) × 10 d	[51]	**4**
	Iodoquinol	650 mg po tid (30–40 mg/kg/d ÷ tid) × 20 d		
Intestinal amebiasis	Metronidazole	750 mg po tid (35–50 mg/kg/d ÷ tid) × 5–10 d	[26]	**3**
	Tinidazole	2 g po qd (50 mg/kg qd) × 3–5 d	[58]	**3**
	Nitazoxanide	500 mg po bid × 3 d	[34]	**1**
Amebic liver abscess	Metronidazole	750 mg po tid (35–50 mg/kg/d ÷ tid) × 10 d	[40]	**3**
			[26]	**3**
	Tinidazole	2 g po qd (50 mg/kg qd) × 5d	[59]	**2**
			[36]	**2**
	Nitazoxanide	500 mg po bid × 3 d (age adjusted dosing)	[34]	**2**
Severe disease failing oral metronidazole/ tinidazole	Metronidazole	1500 mg IV qd (7.5–30 mg/kg/day)	[38]	4
	Dehydroemetine	1–1.5 mg/kg/d IM or SC for 5 d	[60]	2
	Chloroquine (liver abscess only)	600 mg po qd × 2 days, then 300 mg po qd × 14 d	[40]	3

IM, intramuscularly; IV, intravenously; SC, subcutaneously.

courses should always be given after a treatment course for invasive intestinal or extra-intestinal disease to reduce the rate of relapse.

Paromomycin has also been effective in a number of trials. We consider it our drug of choice for luminal infection because it is widely available and demonstrated better efficacy than diloxanide [48]. Many of these have also shown cure rates for mild invasive disease [49, 50]. Side effects with oral therapy are generally mild, but include diarrhea and other gastrointestinal disturbances and less commonly, headache and dizziness. Therapy should be given with meals and for a full seven days, as failures have occurred with shorter courses.

Diloxanide furoate is a relative of chloramphenicol used since the 1950s. The CDC experience with the drug from 1977 to 1990 documented a parasitologic cure rate in 86% of patients with asymptomatic *E. histolytica/E. dispar* infection [51]. The drug is well-tolerated, with only 14% of patients reporting mild side effects—mainly flatulence or other gastrointestinal symptoms. In the USA, the drug is only available through compounding pharmacies. Iodoquinol (diiodohydroxyquionoline) has been widely used for asymptomatic intestinal colonization because it is effective and inexpensive. A large study in India found it to be 85% effective in non-dysenteric *E. histolytica/E. dispar* patients [52]. However, it requires a 20-day course and there have been case reports of loss of vision [53], we would thus consider it a second-line agent. Common side effects include constipation and enlargement of the thyroid gland (the drug contains 64% iodine) (see **Box 89.1**).

REFERENCES

1. WHO/PAHO/UNESO. A consultation of experts on amebiasis. Epidemiol Bull Pan Amer Health Org 1997;18:13.
2. Ali IK, Hossain MB, Roy S, et al. *Entamoeba moshkovskii* infections in children, Bangladesh. Emerg Infect Dis 2003;9:580–4.
3. Caballero-Salcedo A, Viveros-Rogel M, Salvatierra B, et al. Seroepidemiology of amebiasis in Mexico. Am J Trop Med Hyg 1994;50:412–9.
4. Haque R, Mondal D, Duggal P, et al. *Entamoeba histolytica* infection in children and protection from subsequent amebiasis. Infect Immun 2006;74:904–9.
5. Acuna-Soto R, Maguire JH, Wirth DF. Gender distribution in asymptomatic and invasive amebiasis. Am J Gastroenterol 2000;95:1277–83.
6. Blessmann J, Van Linh P, Nu PA, et al. Epidemiology of amebiasis in a region of high incidence of amebic liver abscess in central Vietnam. Am J Trop Med Hyg 2002;66:578–83.
7. Stauffer W, Abd-Alla M, Ravdin JI. Prevalence and incidence of Entamoeba histolytica infection in South Africa and Egypt. Arch Med Res 2006; 37:266–9.
8. Freedman DO, Weld LH, Kozarsky PE, et al. Spectrum of disease and relation to place of exposure among ill returned travelers. N Engl J Med 2006;354:119–30.
9. Geltman PL, Cochran J, Hedgecock C. Intestinal parasites among African refugees resettled in Massachusetts and the impact of an overseas pre-departure treatment program. Am J Trop Med Hyg 2003;69:657–62.
10. Allason-Jones E, Mindel A, Sargeaunt P, Katz D. *Entamoeba histolytica* as a commensal intestinal parasite in homosexual men. New Engl J Med 1986; 315:353–6.
11. Hung CC, Ji DD, Sun H-Y, et al. Increased risk for *Entamoeba histolytica* infection and invasive Amebiasis in HIV seropositive men who have sex with men in Taiwan. PLoS Negl Trop Dis 2008;2:e175.
12. Irusen EM, Jackson TF, Simjee AE. Asymptomatic intestinal colonization by pathogenic *Entamoeba histolytica* in amebic liver abscess: prevalence, response to therapy, and pathogenic potential. Clin Infect Dis 1992;14:889–93.
13. Walker EL, Sellards AW. Experimental entamoebic dysentery. Philippine J Sci 1913;8:253–330.
14. Guo X, Houpt E, Petri WA, Jr. Crosstalk at the initial encounter: interplay between host defense and ameba survival strategies. Curr Opin Immunol 2007;19:376–84.
15. Haque R, Mondal D, Karim A, et al. Prospective case-control study of the association between common enteric protozoal parasites and diarrhea in Bangladesh. Clin Infect Dis 2009;48:1191–7.
16. Gotohda N, Itano S, Okada Y, et al. Acute appendicitis caused by amebiasis. J Gastroenterol 2000;35:861–3.
17. Haque R, Huston CD, Hughes M, et al. Amebiasis. N Engl J Med 2003; 348:1565–73.
18. Katzenstein D, Rickerson V, Braude A. New concepts of amebic liver abscess derived from hepatic imaging, serodiagnosis, and hepatic enzymes in 67 consecutive cases in San Diego. Medicine (Baltimore) 1982;61:237–46.
19. Ibarra-Pérez C. Thoracic complications of amebic abscess of the liver: report of 501 cases. Chest 1981;79:672–7.
20. Viriyavejakul P, Riganti M. Undiagnosed amebic brain abscess. Southeast Asian J Trop Med Public Health 2009;40:1183–7.
21. Hejase MJ, Bihrle R, Castillo G, Coogan CL. Amebiasis of the penis. Urology 1996;48:151–4.
22. Hiatt RA, Markell EK, Ng E. How many stool examinations are necessary to detect pathogenic intestinal protozoa? Am J Trop Med Hyg 1995;53:36–9.
23. Lodhi S, Sarwari AR, Muzammil M, et al. Features distinguishing amoebic from pyogenic liver abscess: a review of 577 adult cases. Trop Med Int Health 2004;9:718–23.
24. Nordestgaard AG, Stapleford L, Worthen N, et al. Contemporary management of amebic liver abscess. Am Surg 1992;58:315–20.
25. vanSonnenberg E, Mueller PR, Schiffman HR, et al. Intrahepatic amebic abscesses: indications for and results of percutaneous catheter drainage. Radiology 1985;156:631–5.
26. Powell SJ, MacLeod I, Wilmot AJ, Elsdon-Dew R. Metronidazole in amoebic dysentery and amoebic liver abscess. Lancet 1966;2:1329–31.
27. Powell SJ, Wilmot AJ, Elsdon-Dew R. Further trials of metronidazole in amoebic dysentery and amoebic liver abscess. Ann Trop Med Parasitol 1967; 61:511–4.
28. Powell SJ, Wilmot AJ, Elsdon-Dew R. Single and low dosage regimens of metronidazole in amoebic dysentery and amoebic liver abscess. Ann Trop Med Parasitol 1969;63:139–42.
29. Garcia EG. Treatment of symptomatic intestinal amoebiasis with tinidazole. Drugs 1978;1:16–8.
30. Soedin K, Syukran OK, Fadillah A, Sidabutar P. Comparison between the efficacy of a single dose of secnidazole with a 5-day course of tetracycline and clioquinol in the treatment of acute intestinal amoebiasis. Pharmatherapeutica 1985;4:251–4.
31. Bassily S, Farid Z, el-Masry NA, Mikhail EM. Treatment of intestinal *E. histolytica* and G. lamblia with metronidazole, tinidazole and ornidazole: a comparative study. J Trop Med Hyg 1987;90: 9–12.
32. Gonzales ML, Dans LF, Martinez EG. Antiamoebic drugs for treating amoebic colitis. Cochrane Database Syst Rev 2009;CD006085.
33. Spillmann R, Ayala SC, Sanchez CE. Double-blind test of metronidazole and tinidazole in the treatment of asymptomatic *Entamoeba histolytica* and *Entamoeba* hartmanni carriers. Am J Trop Med Hyg 1976;25:549–51.
34. Rossignol JF, Kabil SM, El-Gohary Y, Younis AM. Nitazoxanide in the treatment of amoebiasis. Trans R Soc Trop Med Hyg 2007;101:1025–31.
35. Masters DK, Hopkins AD. Therapeutic trial of four amoebicide regimes in rural Zaire. J Trop Med Hyg 1979;82:99–101.
36. Hatchuel W. Tinidazole for the treatment of amoebic liver abscess. S Afr Med J 1975;49:1879–81.
37. Lasserre R, Jaroonvesama N, Kurathong S, Soh CT. Single-day drug treatment of amebic liver abscess. Am J Trop Med Hyg 1983;32:723–6.
38. Kimura M, Nakamura T, Nawa Y. Experience with intravenous metronidazole to treat moderate-to-severe amebiasis in Japan. Am J Trop Med Hyg 2007; 77:381–5.
39. Takahashi T, Gamboa-Domínguez A, Gomez-Mendez TJ, et al. Fulminant amebic colitis: analysis of 55 cases. Dis Colon Rectum 1997;40:1362–7.
40. Cohen HG, Reynolds TB. Comparison of metronidazole and chloroquine for the treatment of amoebic liver abscess. A controlled trial. Gastroenterology 1975;69:35–41.
41. Neal RA. Experimental amoebiasis and the development of anti-amoebic compounds. Parasitology 1983;86:175–91.
42. Badalamenti S, Jameson JE, Reddy KR. Amebiasis. Curr Treat Options Gastroenterol 1999;2:97–103.
43. Adams EB, MacLeod IN. Invasive amebiasis. II. Amebic liver abscess and its complications. Medicine 1977;56:325–34.
44. Van Allan RJ, Katz MD, Johnson MB, et al. Uncomplicated amebic liver abscess: prospective evaluation of percutaneous therapeutic aspiration. Radiology 1992;183:827–30.
45. Chavez-Tapia NC, Hernandez-Calleros J, Tellez-Avila FI, et al. Image-guided percutaneous procedure plus metronidazole versus metronidazole alone for uncomplicated amoebic liver abscess. Cochrane Database Syst Rev 2009; CD004886.
46. Thompson JE, Jr, Forlenza S, Verma R. Amebic liver abscess: a therapeutic approach. Rev Infect Dis 1985;7:171–9.
47. Singh JP, Kashyap A. A comparative evaluation of percutaneous catheter drainage for resistant amebic liver abscesses. Am J Surg 1989;158:58–62.
48. Blessmann J, Tannich E. Treatment of asymptomatic intestinal *Entamoeba histolytica* infection. N Engl J Med 2002;347:1384.
49. Simon M, Shookhoff HB, Terner H, et al. Paromomycin in the treatment of intestinal amebiasis; a short course of therapy. Am J Gastroenterol 1967; 48:504–11.

50. Sullam PM, Slutkin G, Gottlieb AB, Mills J. Paromomycin therapy of endemic amebiasis in homosexual men. Sex Transm Dis 1986;13:151–5.
51. McAuley JB, Herwaldt BL, Stokes SL, et al. Diloxanide furoate for treating asymptomatic *Entamoeba histolytica* cyst passers: 14 years' experience in the United States. Clin Infect Dis 1992;15:464–8.
52. Kaur J, Mathur TN. Comparative drug trials in symptomatic and asymptomatic non-dysenteric amoebic colitis. Indian J Med Res 1972;60:1547–53.
53. Fleisher DI, Hepler RS, Landau JW. Blindness during diiodohydroxyquin (Diodoquin) therapy: a case report. Pediatrics 1974;54:106–8.
54. Kreutner AK, Del Bene VE, Amstey MS. Giardiasis in pregnancy. Am J Obstet Gynecol 1981;140:895–901.
55. Thapa PB, Whitlock JA, Brockman Worrell KG, et al. Prenatal exposure to metronidazole and risk of childhood cancer: a retrospective cohort study of children younger than 5 years. Cancer 1998;83:1461–8.
56. Caro-Patón T, Carvajal A, Martin de Diego I, et al. Is metronidazole teratogenic? A meta-analysis. Br J Clin Pharmacol 1997;44:179–82.
57. McAuley JB, Juranek DD. Paromomycin in the treatment of mild-to-moderate intestinal amebiasis. Clin Infect Dis 1992;15:551–2.
58. Swami B, Lavakusulu D, Devi CS. Tinidazole and metronidazole in the treatment of intestinal amoebiasis. Curr Med Res Opin 1977;5:152–6.
59. Islam N, Hasan K. Tinidazole and metronidazole in hepatic amoebiasis. Drugs 1978;15(suppl. 1):26–9.
60. Jain NK, Madan A, et al. Hepatopulmonary amoebiasis. Efficacy of various treatment regimens containing dehydroemetine and/or metronidazole. J Assoc Physicians India 1990;38:269–71.

90 Giardiasis

Rodney D Adam

Key features

- Giardiasis is a small intestinal infection that presents with subacute diarrhea, malabsorption and weight loss
- Asymptomatic infections are common, especially in children in highly endemic regions
- Transmission may occur by ingestion of contaminated water or from direct fecal–oral transmission
- The diagnosis is established by stool microscopy or stool antigen tests
- Nitroimidazoles are the mainstay of treatment
- Symptoms of irritable bowel syndrome may occur after resolution of infection

INTRODUCTION

Giardiasis is a small intestinal infection resulting from infection with the flagellated protozoan parasite *Giardia lamblia* (syn. *G. intestinalis, G. duodenalis*), likely first reported by Van Leeuwenhoek in 1681 [1].

EPIDEMIOLOGY

Giardia lamblia is constituted by seven different molecular types (genotypes A through G), each with some degree of host specificity. It is likely some of these genotypes will eventually be considered distinct species. Genotypes A and B are found in humans, and occasionally in a variety of other mammals. Conversely, genotypes C through G are found in a variety of other mammals [2]. They have a moderate degree of host specificity and have never been identified from human infections. Therefore, it is likely that most human infections result (directly or indirectly) from human-to-human transmission. However, there are clearly exceptions. Beavers have been implicated as a source of water-borne human outbreaks in a couple of reports. However, some controversy remains regarding the potential of household pets, especially dogs, as sources for human infection. Most studies have shown the predominant or exclusive presence of genotypes C and D in dogs. However, some studies have identified genotypes A and B in dogs, fueling the controversy of whether dogs are a potential source of human giardiasis.

The most commonly identified risk factors relate to water-borne transmission, including backpacking, recreational water use, or having a shallow well for drinking water. Occasional large outbreaks due to contaminated water have been identified, including a recent outbreak of over 3000 symptomatic cases in a Norwegian city. The seasonality of infections in the US with increased occurrence in the summer and early fall probably reflect the increased use of recreational water facilities.

The increased incidence in children who attend daycare facilities reflects direct fecal–oral transmission, while the increased incidence in homosexual men most likely results from oral–anal sexual contact. HIV infection has not been reported as a significant risk factor. Although less common than water-borne transmission, food-borne transmission has also been documented. Hypogammaglobulinemia has been associated with an increased risk of giardiasis [3]. Isolated IgA deficiency may also be a risk factor, but remains controversial. Impaired gastric acid secretion also increases the risk for acquisition of giardiasis.

Within the US, northern states have a higher incidence of giardiasis than the southern states, with case rates peaking at 30 per 100,000 population in Vermont (US average = 7) [4], perhaps due to more prolonged cyst survival in cool moist climates. The above rates markedly underestimate the incidence, but stool prevalence rates of 2–5% are primarily from symptomatic patients and are overestimates.

Although there is little evidence for acquired resistance to infection, there appears to be partial resistance to symptomatic infection. Evidence includes a water-borne outbreak of giardiasis in a ski resort in the Rocky Mountains of the US, where local residents had a lower risk of symptoms. Similarly, very high rates of symptomatic disease (50–100%) have been reported in Finnish travelers to St. Petersburg, Russia, in the 1960s. In contrast, children in highly endemic regions such as Peru or Palestine are frequently asymptomatic; for example, in a shanty town near Lima, Peru, where the quality of available drinking water is poor, children are universally infected by the age of 2 years and are rapidly re-infected after treatment [5]. In these otherwise asymptomatic children, there is some evidence for growth retardation. However, because of malnutrition and other infection, it has been difficult to determine whether there is a causal relationship between giardiasis and growth retardation in these children. These observations suggest at least two very different patterns of transmission and disease. Populations with high rates of water contamination and continuing endemic transmission typically have high prevalence rates, but few attributable symptoms. Conversely, in populations with generally safe water, transmission is irregular and prevalence is low. However, when infections do occur, they are frequently symptomatic.

NATURAL HISTORY, PATHOGENESIS, AND PATHOLOGY

The life cycle of *G. lamblia* consists of two forms, the trophozoite and the cyst. The cyst is oval in shape and approximately 8 by 12 µm in size and contains four nuclei that can be visualized microscopically. The cyst is environmentally resistant, and as few as 10 cysts can initiate infection after ingestion. After passage through the stomach, the cyst excysts to produce two binucleate trophozoites that are pear-shaped and approximately 10–12 µm in length by 5–7 µm in width. The trophozoites move by the beating of four pairs of flagellae and attach to the wall of the small intestine by their concave ventral sucking disk (see Fig. 90.1). When the trophozoites detach from the intestinal wall, an imprint displays the site of their attachment. The trophozoites

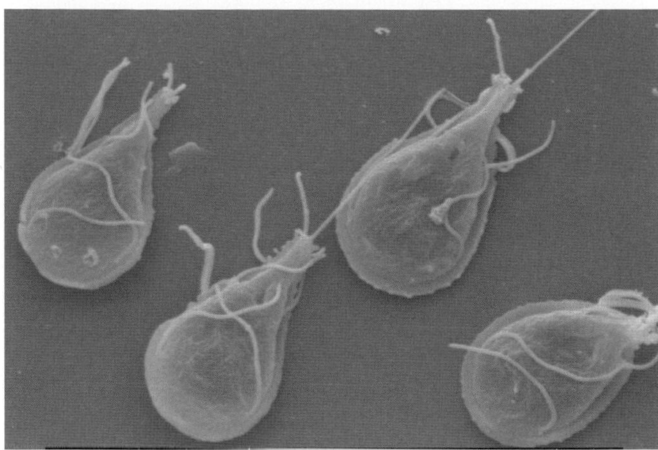

FIGURE 90.1 A scanning electron micrograph of *Giardia lamblia* trophozoites demonstrates the convex dorsal surface. Several of the eight flagella can be seen.

replicate by binary fission and some of these trophozoites encyst after exposure to bile or as a result of cholesterol starvation, and are passed in the feces to continue the cycle of infection [6].

The course of naturally acquired giardiasis is highly variable, ranging from transient colonization to prolonged infection and from asymptomatic to severe diarrhea and weight loss. As noted above, partial immunity may account for some of those differences. In addition, there is some evidence for differences in pathogenicity among different isolates. In human volunteer studies, all 10 volunteers became infected with the GS isolate (genotype B) and five developed symptoms. On the other hand, none of five volunteers were infected with ISR (genotype A1). Genotype A2 differs about 1–2% from genotype A1 in DNA sequence, while genotype B differs by nearly 20% from both, suggesting that it may properly be considered a different species. Interestingly, some studies correlating symptoms with genotype have found that genotype B infections are more frequently symptomatic, while others have found that symptoms are more associated with genotype A2. Genotype A1 has seldom been identified in these studies.

Patients with symptomatic disease have villous shortening which can range from mild to severe, both from one patient to another and even within the same patient. Chronic inflammatory changes are frequently found.

There is no evidence for toxin-mediated diarrhea and mucosal invasion has not been convincingly shown. Therefore, much of the recent interest has focused on an immunopathogenic mechanism for the diarrhea. Animal models [7] and human observations [8] have shown epithelial cell dysfunction and impairment of the barrier function, likely involving intraepithelial lymphocytes.

The surfaces of trophozoites are coated with a cysteine-rich variant-specific surface protein (VSP) that evokes a significant immune response [9]. However, the organism can switch expression from one to another member of this large gene family, and this antigenic variation may contribute to the chronicity of the infection.

CLINICAL FEATURES

For patients who develop symptomatic disease, there is typically a 1- to 2-week incubation period after exposure, followed by diarrhea that may be self-limited but frequently lasts 6 weeks or longer in the absence of treatment. Table 90-1 shows the approximate frequency of symptoms reported from a number of studies of symptomatic giardiasis [10–15]. Patients typically have diarrhea or loose stools marked by loose greasy stools with a foul odor. The daily stool volume is typically normal and one to several stools daily is usual. The diarrhea

TABLE 90-1 Symptoms of Giardiasis*

Symptom	Average frequency (%)
Diarrhea	95
Abdominal cramps	70
Weakness or malaise	70
Nausea	60
Weight loss	50
Anorexia (decreased appetite)	50
Abdominal distention (bloating/distension)	50
Flatulence	50
Vomiting	30
Fever	20

*The table includes the approximate frequency of the signs and symptoms reported in six studies of symptomatic giardiasis [10–15]. It is important to note that there is substantial variability of symptoms among studies.

is frequently accompanied by abdominal pain, bloating, flatulence, and malabsorption with weight loss (Table 90-1). Fatigue is commonly found. Fever is uncommon, and when present, it is found early and resolves with a few days. Bloody diarrhea and systemic toxicity are not seen with giardiasis and should raise the suspicion for invasive bacterial infections or amebiasis.

The physical examination is typically normal or demonstrates nonspecific abnormalities. Mild abdominal tenderness may be present, but severe tenderness should suggest an alternative diagnosis. Likewise, significant fluid loss is uncommon with giardiasis, so evidence of dehydration on examination or by laboratory testing should prompt a search for alternative diagnoses.

PATIENT EVALUATION, DIAGNOSIS AND DIFFERENTIAL DIAGNOSIS

Giardiasis should be suspected in patients who present with subacute or chronic diarrhea, especially when the diarrhea is accompanied by weight loss. The onset of giardiasis can be relatively indolent, and frequently patients do not present for evaluation early, therefore giardiasis should be considered seriously in patients with at least 5 to 7 days of diarrhea. In contrast, most diarrhea caused by viral and bacterial pathogens resolves within 3 to 5 days [16]. In addition, the incubation period for giardiasis is typically 1 to 2 weeks, which distinguishes it from many other infectious etiologies. The differential diagnosis includes those illnesses that present with subacute or chronic diarrhea of a small intestinal source. The fluid and electrolyte loss caused by some small intestinal pathogens is distinctly uncommon with giardiasis. Thus, the list of pathogens that could produce diarrhea mimicking giardiasis is short, but could include atypical presentations of *Campylobacter* or *Salmonella* infections. Both celiac disease and tropical sprue present with chronic diarrhea that may be accompanied by weight loss. Giardiasis typically has a more readily defined onset of symptoms than celiac disease or tropical sprue. Celiac disease may be a more common cause of diarrhea in the US, but is much less common in many developing regions, so a travel and exposure history is important. Whipple's disease is rare, but can present with chronic diarrhea and weight loss. Extraintestinal manifestations are common with Whipple's, but are not seen with giardiasis, with the exception of the occasional urticarial rash that has been reported. Lactose intolerance is a common cause of chronic diarrhea, but does not cause weight loss and resolves with elimination of lactose from the diet. Irritable bowel syndrome frequently presents with chronic diarrhea, but does not cause weight loss. As noted below, it is particularly common after an episode of giardiasis. Chronic diarrhea is commonly found in advanced HIV infection with or without an identifiable pathogen. Conversely, HIV-infected patients are at increased risk for a variety of enteric pathogens, but there is not a notable increase in frequency or severity of giardiasis in these patients. *Campylobacter* or *Salmonella* spp. can occasionally cause prolonged diarrhea, so these pathogens should be considered.

The initial diagnostic test when giardiasis is considered is a microscopic examination of a concentrated fecal specimen for cysts or trophozoites. Cysts are much more commonly found than trophozoites, and can be identified equally well from fresh or preserved specimens. In contrast, freshly collected specimens are required for the identification of trophozoites. When trophozoites are found, they correlate highly with symptomatic infection. Three separate specimens should be evaluated for optimal sensitivity. Alternatively, there are several commercial *Giardia* cyst antigen tests available, all of which detect cyst antigens in fecal samples, either by immunoassay or by immunofluorescence or chromatographic detection (Table 90-2). These are more sensitive than conventional microscopy, such that a single test can suffice. The sensitivity of the immunoassay tests is in the 93–100% range and the fluorescent antibody test near 100%, but with the caveat that there is not an adequate gold standard for a validation of the diagnosis, so these numbers should be taken with caution. The specificity of the tests is in the 98–99% range, so there should be few false-positive results in populations with a high prevalence. One limitation of these antigen-based tests is that they detect cysts, but not trophozoites. However, the enzyme imunoassay is less labor-intensive and does not require the availability of a fluorescent microscope. The use of PCR testing has been reported, but is not yet commercially available.

For some patients with giardiasis, fecal examinations are repeatedly negative but *Giardia* trophozoites can be detected in the duodenum by endoscopy or by the string test. The string test involves the patient swallowing a capsule on the end of a string, pulling it out after 4 hours to overnight, and then examining the end microscopically for the presence of trophozoites. An alternative approach is to perform an upper endoscopy with a biopsy and sampling of duodenal contents (see Fig. 90.2 for a histologic specimen of the small intestine showing a flattened villous and a mononuclear inflammatory response), which adds the potential of identifying other entities such as tropical or celiac sprue.

There are no serologic tests that are useful for the diagnosis of giardiasis.

In clinical practice, it is very common to empirically treat for giardiasis in patients who have a clinical presentation consistent with giardiasis, especially in resource-poor areas.

TREATMENT

Drugs from several different classes have excellent efficacy for treatment of giardiasis (Table 90-3) [17,18]. The nitroimidazoles are the most commonly used drugs in the US, and perhaps worldwide, primarily metronidazole and tinidazole. These two drugs are essentially 100% absorbed by the oral route. Initial concerns regarding metronidazole in pregnancy have been allayed, at least for the second and third trimesters, by extensive experience with treating bacterial vaginosis. Nausea and a metallic taste are common and potentially treatment-limiting side effects. These drugs also have a disulfiram-like activity after ethanol ingestion, so alcohol use during treatment is prohibited. Single-dose and short courses of therapy with metronidazole have had high failure rates, so treatment should be continued for 5 to 10 days, while tinidazole demonstrates excellent efficacy with single-dose therapy, which may make it the preferred agent in many settings. Secnidazole and ornidazole are other nitroimidazoles that have excellent efficacy with single-dose treatment courses, but are not available in the US.

Albendazole is an antihelminthic agent that inhibits tubulin and has activity against giardiasis. In addition, its broad antihelminthic activity may be an advantage in settings with a high prevalence of intestinal helminth infections. However, single-dose therapy has demonstrated poor efficacy for the treatment of giardiasis, so treatment courses of 5 days are used. Some studies have shown reduced efficacy in comparison with nitroimidazoles. Albendazole has been associated with embryopathy, so it should be avoided at least during the first trimester of pregnancy.

Quinacrine has excellent efficacy and at one time was the drug of choice in the US, but has been largely replaced by the nitroimidazoles, partly because of nausea and vomiting and occasional reports of psychosis.

Nitazoxanide has activity for *Giardia* and *Cryptosporidium* as well as other microbes and has been approved for use in the US. Nitazoxanide has been studied in children using 3-day courses, yielding response rates of about 70–80%, and has been well tolerated.

Furazolidone became popular for treating giardiasis in children because it is tolerated better than quinacrine and is available in liquid suspension. In clinical studies, it has yielded cure rates of 80–94%. However, compliance is more difficult than with some drugs, since it is administered four times daily for 7 to 10 days.

Paromomycin has been evaluated in a few earlier studies, demonstrating an efficacy of about 55–90% [17]. It is commonly recommended for treatment of giardiasis during pregnancy, at least during the first trimester, because of its perceived safety in that setting.

Persistent symptoms after treatment of giardiasis are common and usually do not represent continued infection. After a large outbreak of giardiasis in Norway, as many as 40% of patients had prolonged

TABLE 90-2 Commercially Available Tests for Fecal Diagnosis of Giardiasis

Manufacturer	Test name	Ag detected	Method
Meridian	ImmunoCard STAT Giardia/Cryptosporidium	Not stated	Immuno-chromatographic assay
Meridian	Merifluor Giardia/Cryptosporidium	Not stated	Direct fluorescent Ab
Tech-lab	Pt5012-Giardia II	CWP1	ELISA
Biosite	Triage Parasite Panel for Giardia, Entamoeba histolytica and Cryptosporidium		Enzyme immunoassay
BD	ColorPAC Giardia/Crypto	CWP1	
Remel	X/pect Giardia or Giardia/Crypto	Not stated	Rapid immunoassay

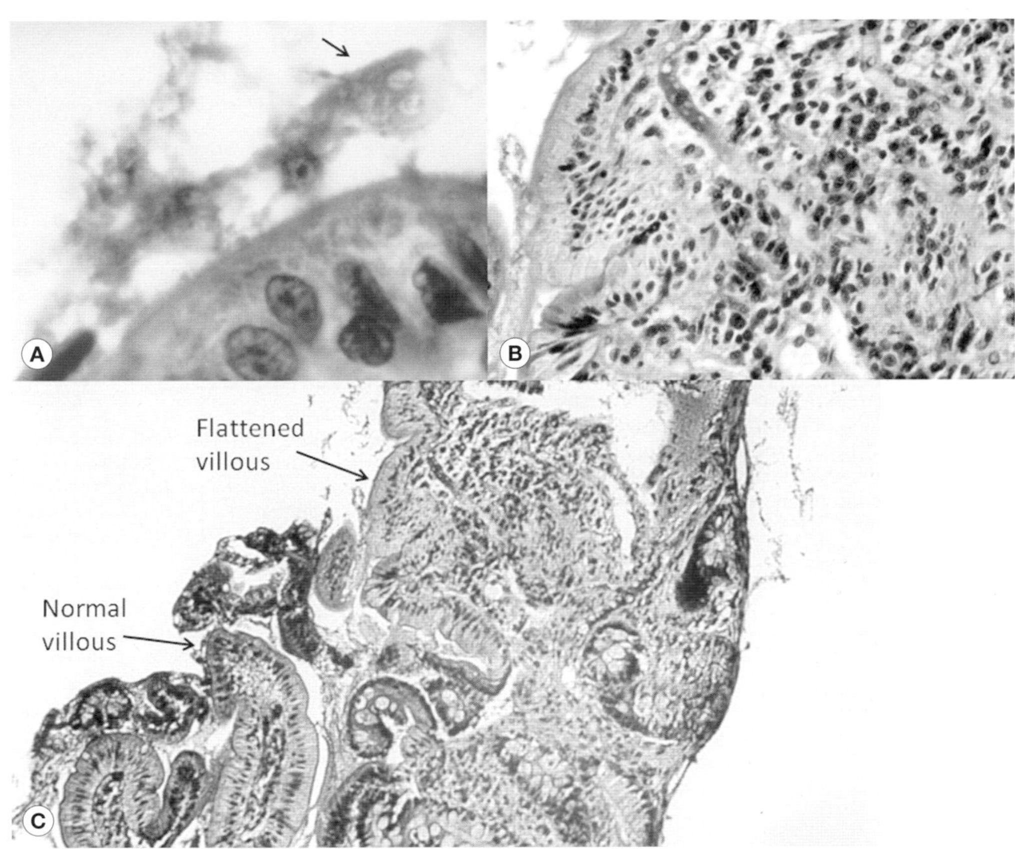

FIGURE 90.2 A jejunal biopsy specimen from a patient with giardiasis. **A.** A trophozoite is demonstrated in the lumen. **B.** A diffuse mononuclear inflammatory response is demonstrated. **C.** A flattened villous and a normal villous are shown in the same biopsy specimen.

TABLE 90-3 Treatment of Giardiasis*

Drug	FDA approved/ Commerically available	FDA approved indication for the treatment of giardiasis	Oral bioavailability (%)	Half-life	Dose (adult and maximum pediatric dose)	Duration of treatment	Treatment efficacy (%)
Metronidazole	Yes/Yes	No	100	6–10 h	5 mg/kg tid (250 mg)	5 to 10 days	90–100
Tinidazole	Yes/Yes	Yes	100	12 h	Adults: 50 mg/kg (2 g) Pediatric patients older than 3 years of age: 50 mg/kg (up to 2 g) with food	Single dose	90–100
Albendazole	Yes/Yes	No	1–5	8–12 h	15 mg/kg qid (400 mg)	5 days	90–100
Paromomycin	Yes/Yes	No	0	NA	10 mg/kg tid (500 mg)	5 to 10 days	55–90
Furazolidone	No/No	No		10 min	2 mg/kg qid (100 mg)	7 to 10 days	80–94
Nitazoxanide	Yes/Yes	Yes	Parent drug not detected	1.3–1.8 h	Adults: 500 mg bid Ages 1–3: 100 mg bid Ages 4–11: 200 mg bid	3 days	70–80
Quinacrine	No	No	Good	5–14 days	2 mg/kg tid (100 mg)	5 to 7 days	80–100

*These agents have all been studied in controlled (and usually randomized) studies [17,18]. The treatment efficacy reflects the success found with the majority of studies. Quinacrine is no longer generally available in the US, but can be obtained from a compounding pharmacy. NA, not applicable.

fatigue and abdominal symptoms without evidence of ongoing infection [19] or benefit from *Giardia*-specific treatment. Persistent gastrointestinal symptoms are common after treatment of several other intestinal pathogens as well [20]. Therefore, if someone has persistent or recurrent symptoms after treatment for giardiasis, the presence or absence of giardiasis should be confirmed by fecal examination. A negative test in someone with persistent diarrhea but no weight loss suggests post-infectious irritable bowel or perhaps lactose intolerance. However, with a negative fecal examination in the setting of weight loss, upper endoscopy should be considered, to identify other diagnoses such as gluten enteropathy.

For patients with documented relapse after treatment, re-treatment is usually effective. Drug resistance has been proposed as a possible reason for treatment failure; however, because of culture difficulties, few susceptibility studies have been performed. In addition, relapses may be more common in the setting of immunoglobulin deficiency, so immunoglobulin levels should be determined. Patients who fail re-treatment with a standard course of a nitroimidazole usually respond to subsequent treatment with metronidazole in addition to either albendazole or quinacrine.

PREVENTION

The majority of cases of giardiasis occur through the ingestion of contaminated water, so backpackers and travelers to regions with inadequately purified water should purify the water by filtration with a 1–2-µm (or smaller) pore size or by heating the water to 70 °C for 10 minutes or boiling. Halogenation will also inactivate cysts but must be prolonged. Contaminated hands are the source of *Giardia* in the setting of daycare or food, therefore hand washing should be employed.

REFERENCES

1. Adam RD. Biology of *Giardia lamblia*. Clin Microbiol Rev 2001;14:447–75.
2. Caccio SM, Ryan U. Molecular epidemiology of giardiasis. Mol Biochem Parasitol 2008;160:75–80.
3. Oksenhendler E, Gerard L, Fieschi C, et al. Infections in 252 patients with common variable immunodeficiency. Clin Infect Dis 2008;46:1547–54.
4. Yoder JS, Beach MJ; Centers for Disase Control and Prevention (CDC). Giardiasis surveillance – United States, 2003–2005. MMWR Surveill Summ 2007;56:11–18.
5. Gilman RH, Marquis GS, Miranda E, et al. Rapid reinfection by Giardia lamblia after treatment in a hyperendemic Third World community. Lancet 1988;1:343–5.
6. Carranza PG, Lujan HD. New insights regarding the biology of *Giardia lamblia*. Microbes Infect 2010;12:71–80.
7. Buret AG. Mechanisms of epithelial dysfunction in giardiasis. Gut 2007;56:316–17.
8. Troeger H, Epple HJ, Schneider T, et al. Effect of chronic *Giardia lamblia* infection on epithelial transport and barrier function in human duodenum. Gut 2007;56:328–35.
9. Nash TE. Surface antigenic variation in *Giardia lamblia*. Mol Microbiol 2002;45:585–90.
10. Brodsky RE, Spencer HC Jr, Schultz MG. Giardiasis in American travelers to the Soviet Union. J Infect Dis 1974;130:319–23.
11. Kent GP, Greenspan JR, Herndon JL, et al. Epidemic giardiasis caused by a contaminated public water supply. Am J Public Health 1988;78:139–43.
12. Moore GT, Cross WM, McGuire D, et al. Epidemic giardiasis at a ski resort. N Engl J Med 1969;281:402–7.
13. Osterholm MT, Forfang JC, Ristinen TL, et al. An outbreak of foodborne giardiasis. N Engl J Med 1981;304:24–8.
14. Shaw PK, Brodsky RE, Lyman DO, et al. A communitywide outbreak of giardiasis with evidence of transmission by a municipal water supply. Ann Intern Med 1977;87:426–32.
15. Walzer PD, Wolfe MS, Schultz MG. Giardiasis in travelers. J Infect Dis 1971;124:235–7.
16. Pawlowski SW, Warren CA, Guerrant R. Diagnosis and treatment of acute or persistent diarrhea.Gastroenterology 2009;136:1874–86.
17. Gardner TB, Hill DR. Treatment of giardiasis. Clin Microbiol Rev 2001;14:114–28.
18. Rossignol JF. Cryptosporidium and Giardia: treatment options and prospects for new drugs. Exp Parasitol 2010;124:45–53.
19. Robertson LJ, Hanevik K, Escobedo AA, et al. Giardiasis – who do the symptoms sometimes never stop? Trends Parasitol 2010;26:75–82.
20. Spiller R, Garsed K. Postinfectious irritable bowel syndrome. Gastroenterology 2009;136:1979–88.

Cryptosporidiosis 91

Lihua Xiao, Jeffrey K Griffiths

Key features

- Cryptosporidiosis is an intestinal infection caused by intracellular protozoan *Cryptosporidium* species
- Cryptosporidiosis is a cosmopolitan cause of acute and chronic diarrhea, clinically indistinguishable from many other enteric pathogens, and one of the leading causes of diarrhea globally
- Specific diagnosis requires additional laboratory testing of stool specimens, such as acid-fast staining, compared with other parasites
- Cryptosporidiosis is a common intestinal infection in AIDS patients causing malabsorption and chronic diarrhea; it can infect the biliary system and respiratory tract. Resolution of the infection requires intact cell-mediated immunity, which in persons with HIV/AIDS often means that highly active anti-retroviral therapy (HAART) must be initiated
- Cryptosporidiosis is a frequent cause of mortality in persons with AIDS and sometimes malnutrition or other forms of immunosuppression, with death from wasting or dehydration. Testing for this parasite should always be considered in immunocompromised people with diarrhea
- Most human disease is caused by the human-adapted species *Cryptosporidium hominis*, but substantial disease is caused by zoonotic *Cryptosporidium parvum* (often found in young cattle and other herbivores) and occasionally parasite species adapted to other mammals and birds
- No highly effective therapy exists and the form of the parasite involved in transmission is highly resistant to water chlorination. Nitazoxanide is modestly effective in immunocompetent persons. Thus, the prevention of infection is critical especially for persons with HIV/AIDS
- *Cryptosporidium* can be killed by heating contaminated food or water. Filtration and ultraviolet light disinfection render drinking water safe for consumption

INTRODUCTION

Human cryptosporidiosis was first reported in 1976. It is a classic diarrheal "emerging disease" because it has a very low infectious dose, is most severe in immunocompromised populations, is highly resistant to anti-parasitic therapy, has human and nonhuman reservoirs, and can cause major epidemics when public health measures break down. Cryptosporidiosis is most common in developing countries, but remains a significant pathogen of children and the elderly in industrialized nations, with waterborne, foodborne, person-to-person and zoonotic transmission pathways [1, 2]. It is a common cause of wasting and lethal diarrhea in HIV-infected persons and acute and persistent diarrhea in children.

EPIDEMIOLOGY

Cryptosporidium spp. are amongst the most common diarrheal pathogens worldwide. In developing countries ~20% of diarrheic children have cryptosporidiosis [3, 4], contrasting with 1–5% in North America and Europe. Infection usually occurs before 2 years in the former [3–5] and before 5 years in the latter [6–8]. Prevalence is higher in rural areas [4, 6] and during rainy seasons [3–5]; seropositivity increases with age, suggesting continued exposure. Malnutrition [3, 5], HIV/AIDS [9] and other immunocompromising conditions significantly increase the risk, severity and persistence of cryptosporidiosis. It is an AIDS-defining opportunistic infection and frequently afflicts malnourished children with persistent diarrhea. Cryptosporidiosis-affected children may have impaired growth and cognitive function [2], and have multiple symptomatic episodes before they acquire partial protective immunity [10].

Water, residential surfaces and food may be contaminated by *Cryptosporidium*-containing feces, and serve as sources of infection, as well as person-to-person transmission where hygienic standards are low [10, 11]. In industrialized countries transmission is less frequent, likely because of public health interventions relating to clean food, water treatment and sanitation. Transmission have also been linked to international travel, contact with animals or children with diarrhea, recreational water exposure and multiple sexual partners or anal intercourse [7, 9–12].

NATURAL HISTORY, PATHOGENESIS, AND PATHOLOGY

Replication of *Cryptosporidium* only occurs in the gastrointestinal tract of vertebrates. The incubation period ranges from 4 to 10 days after oocyst ingestion (Fig. 91.1) [2, 13]. Excretion of infectious oocysts in feces begins approximately when symptoms begin and may persist for months. The infectious dose is low (10–1000 oocysts); in animal models a single oocyst can cause infection. Unlike many other coccidian parasites, the oocysts of Cryptosporium spp. are immediately infectious when they are passed in stool. Internal autoinfection is common and likely to be responsible for the chronic nature of the disease in immunocompromised people. *Cryptosporidium hominis* and *C. parvum* cause ~ 75% and 20% of human disease respectively [11, 14]. *Cryptosporidium hominis* is more virulent in humans than other species and only infects humans, whereas *C. parvum* infects many ruminants, such as cattle and sheep (Fig. 91.1) [14]. *Cryptosporidium meleagridis*, an avian species, is the third most commonly identified human pathogen.

The natural history is quite variable (Table 91-1). Transient infection may be asymptomatic or symptomatic with diarrhea, which is most

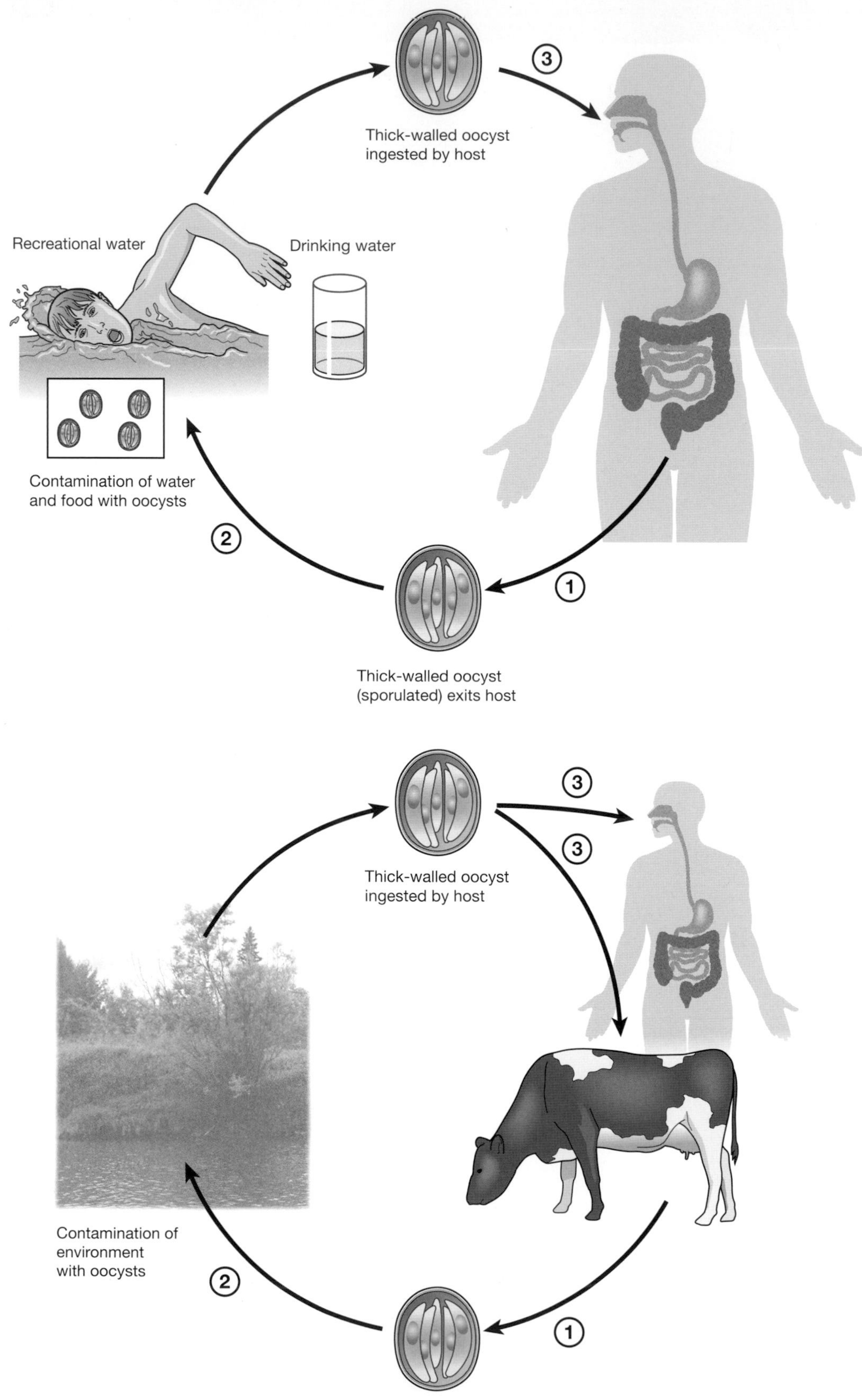

FIGURE 91.1 Life cycle of *Cryptosporidium hominis* (upper panel) and *Cryptosporidium parvum* (lower panel). Sporulated oocysts are excreted by the infected host through feces (1). Transmission of *C. parvum* and *C. hominis* occurs mainly through contact with contaminated water (e.g. drinking or recreational water), food and infected persons (for *C. hominis* and *C. parvum*) or animals (for *C. parvum* only). Zoonotic and anthroponotic transmission of *C. parvum* and anthroponotic transmission of *C. hominis* occur through exposure to infected individuals or water, food, and fomites contaminated by feces of infected animals/persons (2). Humans (for *C. hominis* and *C. parvum*) and animals (for *C. parvum*) become infected after ingestion (and possibly inhalation) of oocysts (3). Sporozoites released by oocysts go through several rounds of multiplications in the small intestine and colon and sporulated oocysts are generated and excreted by infected persons or animals. Oocysts are infective upon excretion, thus permitting direct and immediate fecal-oral transmission *[reproduced with permission from Laboratory Identification of Parasites of Public Health Concern (DPDx): http://www.dpd.cdc.gov/dpdx/].*

TABLE 91-1 Clinical Features of Cryptosporidiosis in Different Groups of Patients

	Immunocompetent persons in industrialized nations*	**Immunocompromised persons†**	**Immunocompetent children in developing countries§**
Length and severity of illness	Self-limiting illness (mean 12–13 days, median 9–11 days)	Severe, chronic or intractable illness with increased mortality	Asymptomatic (77%), acute (77% ill children with <7 days of diarrhea; median 2 days) or chronic illness (9% ill children with >14 days of diarrhea)
Clinical features	Diarrhea (98–100%)	Diarrhea	Diarrhea
	Watery (81–93%) Median maximal No. of stool/day (5–12)	Chronic (36%) Cholera-like (33%) Transient (15%) Relapsing (15%)	Watery (91–96%)
	Abdominal pain (60–96%)	Abdominal pain (60–89%)	Vomiting (57–71%)
	Vomiting (48–65%)	Vomiting (21–37%)	Fever (6–37%)
	Nausea (35–70%)	Nausea (50–56%)	Effects on fitness and nutrition
	Fatigue (87%)	Weight loss (37–74%)	Malnutrition Weight loss Stunt growth Impaired cognitive function
	Anorexia (51–81%)	Anorexia (55–74%)	
	Fever (36–59%)	Fever (44–53%)	
	Muscle or joint aches (53%)	Muscle or joint aches (56–66%)	
		Biliary involvement (23–29%)	
		Sclerosing cholangitis (26%)	
		Pancreatitis (3–33%)	
		Respiratory involvement	
		Cough (8–44%)	

*[20, 29–31]
†[22, 31–34]
§[5, 35, 36]
Adapted from Chalmers RM, Davies AP. Minireview: Clinical cryptosporidiosis. Exp Parasitol 2009;124:138–46.

severe in young children. Asymptomatic infections are seen after prior symptomatic infections. Disease resolution depends upon intact cell-mediated immunity and the antibody response appears to be nearly irrelevant [15]. Persistent infection can also be relatively asymptomatic or quite severe with malabsorption and weight loss. A cholera-like, severely dehydrating, rapidly fatal syndrome in persons with AIDS has been described. While persistent infection occurs in persons with inflammatory bowel disease, immunosuppression, or renal disease, the greatest burden is in pediatric persistent diarrhea and in persons with HIV/AIDS.

Cryptosporidium parasites infect the colonic mucosa and, less commonly, the small intestine and stomach. Replicating parasites may, however, infect the entire gut from oropharynx to anus. Histologically, mononuclear cell infiltration in the lamina propia, mucosal cell apoptosis and mucosal inflammation with villus blunting, and cryptitis are seen which can lead to a loss of barrier function and malabsorption (Fig. 91.2). Illness severity correlates with the extent of infection and host immunity. In persons with HIV, infection of the crypts suggests more severe disease, as does infection of the proximal small bowel with villus flattening [2, 16–18]. Diarrhea with chloride secretion and impaired glucose absorption is mediated by Substance P, a gastrointestinal tract neuropeptide [19].

This parasite (Fig. 91.3) uniquely occupies an intracellular but extracytoplasmic site. This may account for its resistance to therapeutic drugs which are effective against similar parasites (such as malaria, *Toxoplasma* or *Babesia*) which are intracellular but intracytoplasmic. It has been theorized that drugs that enter the host cell cytoplasm may not be able to cross the membrane between the cytoplasm and the parasite.

Immune competence is an important determinant in the severity and duration of intestinal disease in humans. Cryptosporidiosis is a self-limiting illness of 7–14 days duration in immunocompetent individuals but it can be a life threatening illness in the severely immunocompromised (such as people with AIDS), hypogammaglobulinemia or those receiving immunosuppressive drugs for cancer or to prevent rejection in transplantation.

CLINICAL FEATURES

Enteric cryptosporidiosis has no unique clinical signs or symptoms and it resembles many other forms of diarrheal disease. First infections are usually symptomatic with watery diarrhea, vomiting, nausea, abdominal cramps and fatigue. Blood or leukocytes are rarely seen in stool specimens. Low grade fever and cough also occur. In developing countries where repeated exposure is common, most infected children are asymptomatic. Those with symptoms are generally sick for less than seven days (median of two days). Weight loss and dehydration are common. Cryptosporidiosis is more common in malnourished children and those with persistent diarrhea. Both asymptomatic and symptomatic cryptosporidiosis appear to cause malnutrition,

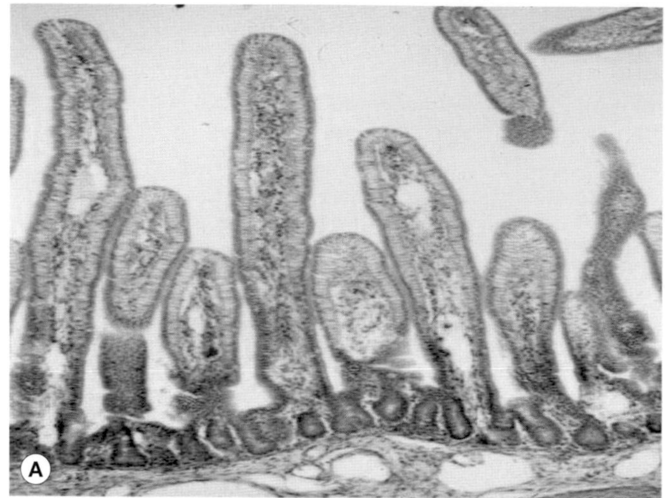

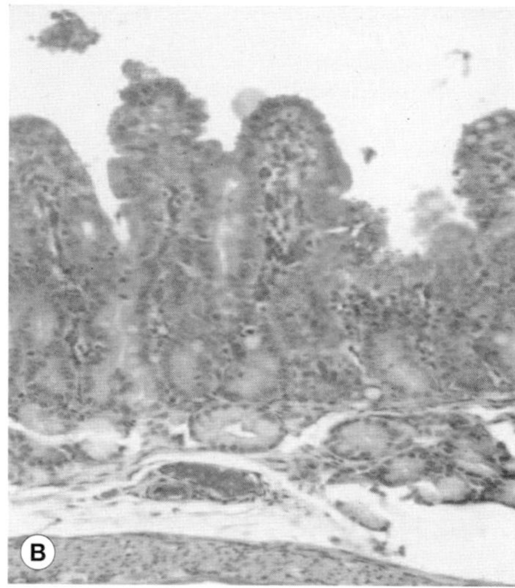

FIGURE 91.2 Normal (A) and experimentally-infected (B) piglet intestine demonstrating the blunted villi and cryptitis seen with *Cryptosporidium* infection *(courtesy of Dr Saul Tzipori)*.

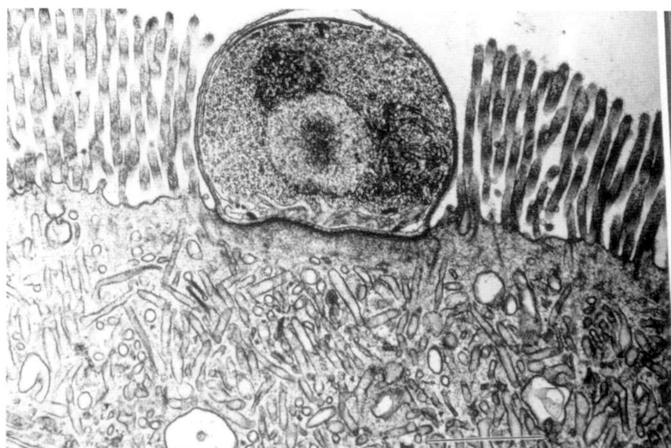

FIGURE 91.3 Electron micrograph of a developing *Cryptosporidium* parasite. It is located on the apical surface of the intestinal cell; host cell membranes can be seen enveloping the globular parasite. At the base of the parasite, an electron-thick membrane can be seen separating the intracellular parasite from the host cell cytoplasm *(courtesy of Dr Saul Tzipori)*.

stunted growth and impaired cognitive function [2]. Immunocompetent persons with cryptosporidiosis in industrialized nations usually have clinical symptoms of explosive, watery diarrhea [12, 20, 21] which may last for a median of 9–11 days. Hospitalization may occur in 7–22% of patients [12, 21]. Because very few persons with mild diarrhea are tested for cryptosporidiosis, this apparent disease difference may be somewhat biased because the patients had especially severe disease or were part of an epidemic where diagnostic testing was done.

Some patients have joint pain, eye pains, recurrent headache, dizziness and fatigue, which are more common with *C. hominis* than with *C. parvum* [20]. *Cryptosporidium* can trigger inflammatory bowel diseases and irritable bowel syndrome [2].

Persistent infection in immunocompromised persons may progress from asymptomatic to symptomatic as immune status declines. Biliary tract involvement may lead to clinical cholangitis [16] and respiratory disease, to mild hypoxia and shortness of breath [13, 16]. Respiratory infection has been considered a rare HIV/AIDS complication, but recent data suggest it may be common in normal children with enteric infection, suggesting that respiratory transmission may occur. In persons with HIV/AIDS, cryptosporidiosis causes increased mortality and shortened survival [22]. In people with the cholera-like form of the disease characterized by massive fluid loss, severe abdominal pain, malabsorption, anorexia and significant weight loss, survival may only be for days or several weeks. To summarize, variations in immune status and the extent and sites of infection contribute to differences in disease severity and survival [17, 18], as may the species of the parasite [11].

PATIENT EVALUATION, DIAGNOSIS, AND DIFFERENTIAL DIAGNOSIS

The medical focus with mild diarrheal disease is generally on detecting and preventing dehydration rather than on making a specific diagnosis. Cryptosporidiosis is usually mild and thus under-diagnosed as with most cryptosporidiosis no diagnostic testing is performed. Suspicion for *Cryptosporidium* is increased when the patient has persistent or chronic diarrhea, is malnourished, has an immunosuppressive condition or another risk factor (Box 91.1). One important clue is that the incubation period is longer (~1 week) than it is for viral or bacterial diseases (1–3 days) yet shorter than for giardiasis (~2 weeks). The differential diagnoses for routine cryptosporidiosis includes many hundreds of viral and bacterial pathogens which have a similar presentation. *Giardia, Isospora* and *Cyclospora* infections may also mimic cryptosporidiosis.

Because cryptosporidiosis is a frequent cause of AIDS-related acute and chronic diarrhea, clinicians must have a low threshold for ordering these special tests in persons with known, or suspected, HIV. Many clinicians incorrectly believe that *Cryptosporidium* is detected via classical "ova and parasites" testing. The differential diagnosis of diarrhea in persons with AIDS includes not only common bacterial pathogens, but also *Cryptosporidium*, species of microsporidia, *Isospora belli, Mycobacterium avium* complex and cytomegalovirus. In sub-Saharan Africa, the vast majority of chronic diarrhea in persons with HIV is caused by either *Cryptosporidium* or microsporidia [2]. Tests for *Cryptosporidium* should always be ordered when the cause for diarrhea is unclear.

Enteric cryptosporidiosis is diagnosed by examining stool specimens, or by biopsy and examination of histologic sections of infected intestine, biliary system or respiratory tract. *Cryptosporidium* oocysts are ~5μm in size. Fecal oocysts are detected using acid-fast staining, antigen detection via ELISA, PCR; or a direct immunofluorescent antibody (DFA) assay [23]. Oocysts can also be detected via direct wet-mounted feces microscopy (see Fig. 91.4). Detection of oocysts is easier if the number being excreted is high. In some laboratories, oocysts are concentrated using the modified ethyl acetate concentration method with detection of stained fecal concentrates by microscopy. Modified acid-fast staining is frequently used in developing countries because of its low cost, ease of use, the ability to use a standard microscope and simultaneous detection of other pathogens relevant to persons with HIV/AIDS, such as *Isospora, Cyclospora* and *Mycobacteria* species. In experienced hands, modified acid-fast staining and microscopy will detect ~85% of the cases of cryptosporidiosis detected via PCR. In industrialized nations, antigen detection and DFA are increasingly prevalent. Oocysts are intermittently shed in stools. If *Cryptosporidium* infection is suspected and initial stool specimen is negative, multiple specimens at intervals of 2–3 days should be examined [23]. Yeasts are morphologically similar to *Cryptosporidium* spp. but do not stain or stain the same color as the counterstain. Many commercial or hospital laboratories do not routinely provide acid fast staining when physicians request ova and parasite examinations, *Cryptosporidium* testing is only done with a specific request.

BOX 91.1

Diarrhea ± vomiting

Increased Suspicion:

Persistent or chronic diarrhea
Immunosuppression, HIV/AIDS
Malnutrition

Travel

Residence in Developing Country

Zoonotic Exposure

Ongoing epidemic outbreak

No bacterial pathogen found with prior culture

Negative 'Ova and Parasites' exam

Failure to respond to empiric treatment

Diagnose with:

1. Acid-fast staining (inexpensive, high sensitivity for most clinical cases, especially with experienced microscopists)
2. PCR (expensive research tool, but detects cased with low levels of parasite excretion and allows genetic characterization)
3. Anitgen-detection ELISA/ICT kit (used in some industrialized country hospitals)
4. Immunofluorescent antibody (highly sensitive research technique)

AIDS patients with *Cryptosporidium* sclerosing cholangitis usually have elevated serum alkaline phosphatase levels and right upper quadrant pain if there is also biliary involvement [16]. Diagnosis is by endoscopic retrograde cholangiopancreatography (ERCP) and biopsy. Ultrasonography or computed tomography may reveal biliary involvement but do not provide an etiological diagnosis. Respiratory involvement is characterized by hypoxia and the presence of diffuse infiltrates on chest radiography. It can be diagnosed by detecting oocysts via acid-fast staining, DFA or PCR in sputa, or via biopsy. Bronchoscopy may be necessary to differentiate it from *Pneumocystis* pneumonia.

TREATMENT AND PREVENTION

Oral or intravenous rehydration, antimotility agents and nutritional support are used for the symptomatic treatment of diarrhea (see Box 91.2) [24]. Almost no drugs have been shown to be even modestly effective in controlled clinical trials [10, 24–26]. Nitazoxanide (NTZ) is the only Food and Drugs Administration (FDA)-approved drug for cryptosporidiosis. NTZ can shorten clinical disease by a day or so on average and reduce parasite loads in immunocompetent patients [25]. Unfortunately, NTZ is not consistently effective for immunodeficient persons [16] (Table 91-2). An open-label study did find that a sustained positive clinical response was observed in 59% of 365 patients with HIV/AIDS who received high doses (500–1500 mg of NTZ twice daily) for prolonged periods (median of 62 days) [27], although it was unclear whether study patients were on anti-retroviral therapy. However, a recent controlled trial of high-dose, prolonged (28 days) NTZ therapy in HIV infected children found no significant benefit. Mortality did not differ between control and NTZ treatment arms and was 28% at 28 days. Our personal advice is that NTZ can be considered for mildly immunocompromised HIV/AIDS patients, for persons in whom cancer chemotherapy is being temporarily deferred because of cryptosporidiosis, or when trying to limit infection during HAART initiation [26]. Paromomycin and macrolides, such as azithromycin, have led to anecdotal success, though not in controlled trials [24, 26], and, when no other options exist, they could be tried in combination with NTZ as a salvage attempt. No studies of NTZ in combination

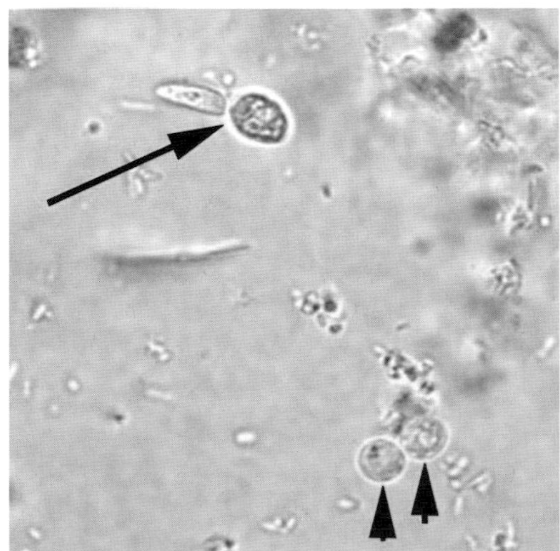

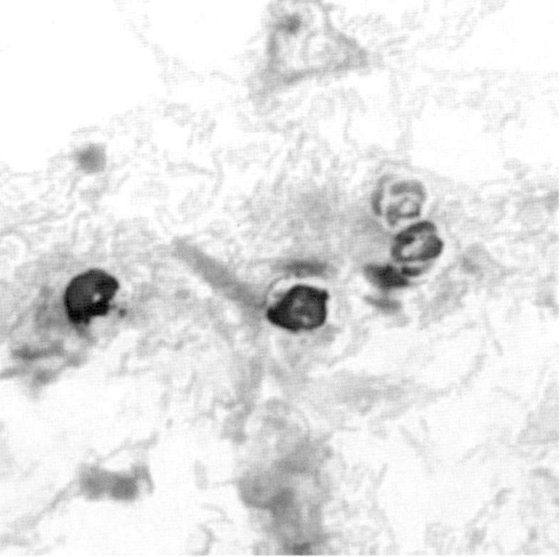

FIGURE 91.4 *Cryptosporidium* oocysts as seen in direct wet-mount microscopy (left) and as stained with the modified acid-fast method. The *Cryptosporidium* oocysts are marked with pink arrows in the image on the left and a budding yeast is marked with the brown arrow. In the image on the right, sporozoites can be seen within the two stained oocysts on the right *(courtesy of the Centers for Diseases Control Public Health Image Library).*

BOX 91.2

Confirmed Cryptosporidiosis →

Evaluate for HIV/AIDS

Evaluate nutritional status and hydration

Reverse dehydration and keep hydrated during evaluation process

If malnourished (e.g. from persistent diarrhea), begin aggressive nutritional rehabilitation which improves cell-mediated immunity. Treat any co-infections

Consider anti-*Cryptosporidium* therapy with drugs such as nitazoxanide, paromomycin, azithromycin if symptoms are severe or not improving with supportive therapy. No clinical studies have shown any consistent benefits with these drugs for persons with HIV/AIDS but there are anecdotal reports of success.

If the person has HIV/AIDS , focus on hydration and aggressive nutritional support.

Treat any co-infections.

Begin anti-retroviral therapy which will, if successful, reverse the underlying immunosuppression and may allow the person to resolve the infection. This may take weeks.

with other agents have been published, and thus we emphasize that HAART is the critical therapy for persons with HIV/AIDS.

The most effective *Cryptosporidium* treatment and prophylaxis for AIDS patients is HAART to restore cell-mediated immunity [24, 25, 28]. It is believed that this is related to $CD4^+$ cell replenishment in treated persons and perhaps the anti-parasitic activities of HAART protease inhibitors [25, 28]. Some protease inhibitors (indinavir, nelfinavir and ritonavir) demonstrate anti-cryptosporidial activity [24]. Relapse of cryptosporidiosis is common in AIDS patients who have stopped taking HAART [10]. Because malnutrition may occur because of cryptosporidiosis, or contribute to its persistence, most experienced clinicians aggressively treat malnutrition. Nutritional support may help restore cellular immunity in the severely malnourished and, in persons with HIV/AIDS, allow survival when HAART is being initiated.

Cholecystectomy may be used in the treatment of cryptosporidial acalculous cholecystitis and ERCP with sphincterotomy and/or stent placement can ameliorate sclerosing cholangitis [24]. The therapy of respiratory cryptosporidiosis has not been systematically explored. In our opinion, both biliary and respiratory disease in the immunocompromised is best treated by HAART or temporarily stopping the use of chemotherapy if the person has cancer.

PREVENTION

To prevent fecal-oral transmission, strict attention to personal hygiene, especially hand-washing, is emphasized. Cooking kills *Cryptosporidium* in food. Oocysts are killed by pasteurization (72 °C for 5 seconds), heating to 60 °C for 30 minutes, or freezing at -7 °C for 1 hour. No safe and effective disinfectant has been identified for decontaminating produce.

Preventing *Cryptosporidum* contamination of drinking water requires modern water filtration and purification systems that are not available in lower income countries. Concentrations of chlorine (1–2 mg/l) used to disinfect drinking water are not effective against

TABLE 91-2 Efficacy of Nitazoxanide in Double-Blind Placebo-Controlled Studies

Patient population	Study location	Dose	Oocyst clearance		Resolution of diarrhea		Reference
			Placebo	*Treatment*	*Placebo*	*Treatment*	
HIV+ persons							
Adults	Mexico	500 or 1000 mg twice daily for 14 days	5/21 (24%)	22/49 (45%)	10/20 (50%)	21/34 (62%)	[37]
Malnourished children	Zambia	100 mg twice daily for 3 days	5/24 (21%)	5/25 (20%)	6/24 (25%)	2/25 (8%)	[38]
Adults with $CD4^+$ <50	Thailand	100 mg twice daily for 8 weeks	0/20 (0%)*	2/22 (9%)*	1/20 (5%)*	7/22 (32%)*	[25]
Children aged 1–11 years old	Zambia	200 mg (if 1–3 years old) or 400 mg twice daily (4–11 years) for 28 days	9/26 (35%)	7/26 (27%)	8/26 (35%) in "well" group	11/26 (42%) in "well" group	[39]
HIV– persons							
Malnourished children	Zambia	100 mg twice daily for 3 days	3/22 (14%)	13/25 (52%)	5/22 (23%)	14/25 (56%)	[38]
Adults and children	Egypt	100 (1–3-year-old), 200 (4–11-year-old) or 500 mg (>11–year-old) twice daily for 3 days	11/50 (22%)	39/49 (67%)	20/49 (41%)	39/49 (80%)	[40]
Adults and children	Egypt	500 mg twice daily for 3 days	10/27 (37%)	26/28 (93%) for tablets; 28/31 (90%) for suspension	11/27 (41%)	27/28 (96%) for tablets; 27/31 (87%) for suspension	[41]

*Based on partial data presented in Pantenburg B, Cabada MM, White AC, Jr. Treatment of cryptosporidiosis. Expert Rev Anti Infect Ther 2009;7:385–91.

Cryptosporidium. Oocycts exposed to full strength bleach can still infect mice. Personal use filters that have an absolute pore size of 1 micron or smaller are effective.

Cryptosporidiosis can be avoided in the highly immunocompromised by education and careful avoidance behaviors to include drinking only filtered or boiled water, ingesting only cooked food, thorough hand-washing, avoiding bathing or swimming in water used by other people or animals and avoiding contact with people or animals (especially calves and lambs) with diarrhea. Companion dogs and cats should be examined and cleared of infection by a veterinarian.

REFERENCES

1. Mor SM, DeMaria A Jr, Griffiths JK, Naumova EN. Cryptosporidiosis in the elderly population of the United States. Clin Infect Dis 2009;48:698–705.
2. Chalmers RM, Davies AP. Minireview: Clinical cryptosporidiosis. Exp Parasitol 2009;124:138–46.
3. Mor SM, Tzipori S. Cryptosporidiosis in children in sub-saharan Africa: a lingering challenge. Clin Infect Dis 2008;47:915–21.
4. Snelling WJ, Xiao L, Ortega-Pierres G, et al. Cryptosporidiosis in developing countries. J Infect Dev Ctries 2007;1:242–56.
5. Bhattacharya MK, Teka T, Faruque AS, Fuchs GJ. Cryptosporidium infection in children in urban Bangladesh. J Trop Pediatr 1997;43:282–6.
6. Snel SJ, Baker MG, Venugopal K. The epidemiology of cryptosporidiosis in New Zealand, 1997–2006. N Z Med J 2009;122:47–61.
7. Nichols GL, Chalmers RM, Sopwith W, et al. Cryptosporidiosis: A report on the surveillance and epidemiology of Cryptosporidium infection in England and Wales. Drinking Water Directorate Contract Number DWI 70/2/201. Drinking Water Inspectorate, UK. 2006;142.
8. Yoder JS, Beach MJ. Cryptosporidiosis surveillance—United States, 2003–2005, MMWR Surveill Summ 2007;56:1–10.
9. Hunter PR, Nichols G. Epidemiology and clinical features of cryptosporidium infection in immunocompromised patients. Clin Microbiol Rev 2002;15: 145–54.
10. Cama VA, Bern C, Roberts J, et al. Cryptosporidium species and subtypes and clinical manifestations in children, Peru. Emerg Infect Dis 2008;14: 1567–74.
11. Cama VA, Ross JM, Crawford S, et al. Differences in clinical manifestations among Cryptosporidium species and subtypes in HIV-infected persons. J Infect Dis 2007;196:684–91.
12. Robertson B, Sinclair MI, Forbes AB, et al. Case-control studies of sporadic cryptosporidiosis in Melbourne and Adelaide, Australia. Epidemiol Infect 2002;128:419–31.
13. Greenberg PD, Koch J, Cello JP. Diagnosis of *Cryptosporidium parvum* in patients with severe diarrhea and AIDS. Digestive Dis Sci 1996;41:2286–90.
14. Xiao L. Molecular epidemiology of cryptosporidiosis: An update. Exp Parasitol 2010;124:80–9.
15. Pantenburg B, Dann SM, Wang HC, et al. Intestinal immune response to human Cryptosporidium sp. infection. Infect Immun 2008;76:23–9.
16. De Angelis C, Mangone M, Bianchi M, et al. An update on AIDS-related cholangiopathy. Minerva Gastroenterol Dietol 2009;55:79–82.
17. Clayton F, Heller T, Kotler DP. Variation in the enteric distribution of cryptosporidia in acquired immunodeficiency syndrome. Am J Clin Pathol 1994; 102:420–5.
18. Lumadue JA, Manabe YC, Moore RD, et al. A clinicopathologic analysis of AIDS-related cryptosporidiosis. AIDS 1998;12:2459–66.
19. Hernandez J, Lackner A, Aye P, et al. Substance P is responsible for physiologic alternations such as increased chloride ion secretion and glucose-malabsorption in Cryptosporidiosis. Immunol Infect 2007;75:11137–423.
20. Hunter PR, Hughes S, Woodhouse S, et al. Health sequelae of human cryptosporidiosis in immunocompetent patients. Clin Infect Dis 2004;39: 504–10.
21. Goh S, Reacher M, Casemore DP, et al. Sporadic cryptosporidiosis, North Cumbria, England, 1996–2000. Emerg Infect Dis 2004;10:1007–15.
22. Manabe YC, Clark DP, Moore RD, et al. Cryptosporidiosis in patients with AIDS - correlates of disease and survival. Clin Infect Dis 1998;27:536–42.
23. Smith HV. Diagnostics. In: Fayer R, Xiao L, eds. Cryptosporidium and Cryptosporidiosis, 2nd edn. Boca Raton: CRC Press; 2008:173.
24. Rossignol JF. Cryptosporidium and Giardia: Treatment options and prospects for new drugs. Exp Parasitol 2010;124:45–3.
25. Pantenburg B, Cabada MM, White AC, Jr. Treatment of cryptosporidiosis. Expert Rev Anti Infect Ther 2009;7:385–91.
26. Abubakar I, Aliyu SH, Arumugam C. et al. Treatment of cryptosporidiosis in immunocompromised individuals: systematic review and meta-analysis. Br J Clin Pharmacol 2007;63:387–93.
27. Rossignol JF. Nitazoxanide in the treatment of acquired immune deficiency syndrome-related cryptosporidiosis: results of the United States compassionate use program in 365 patients. Aliment Pharmacol Ther 2006;24:887–94.
28. Bachur TP, Vale JM, Coelho IC, et al. Enteric parasitic infections in HIV/AIDS patients before and after the highly active antiretroviral therapy. Braz J Infect Dis 2008;12:115–22.
29. Anon. Cryptosporidiosis in England and Wales: prevalence and clinical and epidemiological features. Public Health Laboratory Service Study Group. BMJ 1990;300:774–7.
30. MacKenzie WR, Hoxie NJ, Proctor ME, et al. A massive outbreak in Milwaukee of cryptosporidium infection transmitted through the public water supply. N Engl J Med 1994;331:161–7.
31. Frisby HR, Addiss DG, Reiser WJ, et al. Clinical and epidemiologic features of a massive waterborne outbreak of cryptosporidiosis in persons with HIV infection. JAIDS 1997;16:367–73.
32. McGowan I, Hawkins AS, Weller IV. The natural history of cryptosporidial diarrhoea in HIV-infected patients. AIDS 1993;7:349–54.
33. Hashmey R, Smith NH, Cron S, et al. Cryptosporidiosis in Houston, Texas. A report of 95 cases. Medicine 1997;76:118–39.
34. Vakil NB, Schwartz SM, Buggy BP, et al. Biliary cryptosporidiosis in HIV-infected people after the waterborne outbreak of cryptosporidiosis in Milwaukee. N Engl J Med 1996;334:19–23.
35. Khan WA, Rogers KA, Karim MM, et al. Cryptosporidiosis among Bangladeshi children with diarrhea: a prospective, matched, case-control study of clinical features, epidemiology and systemic antibody responses. Am J Trop Med Hyg 2004;71:412–9.
36. Guerrant DI, Moore SR, Lima AA, et al. Association of early childhood diarrhea and cryptosporidiosis with impaired physical fitness and cognitive function four-seven years later in a poor urban community in northeast Brazil. Am J Trop Med Hyg 1999;61:707–13.
37. Rossignol JF, Hidalgo H, Feregrino M, et al. A double-'blind' placebo-controlled study of nitazoxanide in the treatment of cryptosporidial diarrhoea in AIDS patients in Mexico. Trans R Soc Trop Med Hyg 1998;92:663–6.
38. Amadi B, Mwiya M, Musuku J, et al. Effect of nitazoxanide on morbidity and mortality in Zambian children with cryptosporidiosis: a randomised controlled trial. Lancet 2002;360:1375–80.
39. Amadi B, Mwiya M, Sianongo S, et al. High dose prolonged treatment with nitazoxanide is not effective for cryptosporidiosis in HIV positive Zambian children: a randomised controlled trial. BMC Infect Dis 2009;9:195.
40. Rossignol JF, Ayoub A, Ayers MS. Treatment of diarrhea caused by Cryptosporidium parvum: a prospective randomized, double-blind, placebo-controlled study of Nitazoxanide. J Infect Dis 2001;184:103–6.
41. Rossignol JF, Kabil SM, el-Gohary Y, Younis AM. Effect of nitazoxanide in diarrhea and enteritis caused by Cryptosporidium species. Clin Gastroenterol Hepatol 2006;4:320–4.

92 Cyclosporiasis

David R Shlim, Bradley A Connor

Key features

- A prolonged protozoal infection characterized by initial severe diarrhea, which evolves into an illness with prominent fatigue and anorexia, along with intermittent nausea, and diarrhea
- The organism has now been described in at least two dozen countries. In countries where local transmission has been studied, the risk is distinctly seasonal
- Outbreaks have occurred in North America due to imported food
- Microscopic diagnosis of the oocysts excreted in stool is enhanced by doing a concentration procedure followed by modified acid-fast staining
- The only effective treatment is trimethoprim–sulfamethoxazole

INTRODUCTION

Cyclosporiasis is an intestinal infection with the coccidian organism *Cyclospora cayetanensis*. Infection is associated with diarrhea, fatigue, anorexia, and a prolonged course in the absence of treatment. *Cyclospora* was definitively identified in 1993 [1], after being independently discovered by four different researchers dating back to 1979 [2,3].

EPIDEMIOLOGY

Since it was first noted in 1979, *Cyclospora* has been identified in an increasing number of countries throughout the world, including Papua New Guinea, Haiti, Nepal, Peru, the US, Mexico, Puerto Rico, India, Guatemala, Morocco, Pakistan, South Africa, the Dominican Republic, Malaysia, Thailand, Cambodia, the Solomon Islands, Vietnam, Indonesia, Kenya, and Tanzania. Infection is distinctly seasonal in most environments, for reasons that have not been determined. The organism has been known to be transmitted in both food and water. There is evidence that halogens, such as chlorine, may not disinfect *Cyclospora* oocysts in water [4]. Large outbreaks of cyclosporiasis in the US in the mid-1990s were traced to Guatemalan raspberries, and later imported fresh salad greens and fresh basil [5]. A recent review details the epidemiology of *Cyclospora*, summarizes reported food- and water-borne outbreaks, and lists case reports in both returning travelers and those without a travel history [6].

NATURAL HISTORY, PATHOGENESIS, AND PATHOLOGY

The seasonality of *Cyclospora* is one of its most striking features. In Nepal, the organism is present from May (just before the rainy season) until October (just after the rainy season) [3]. The peak risk is in June and July. In Peru, the *Cyclospora* season extends from January to July, with a peak from April to June. In Guatemala, the main season of risk is May to September. The organism exists in both a sporulated and unsporulated form. Although there are reasons to believe that only the sporulated form is likely to be infectious, human volunteers did not become infected when fed high inoculums of either sporulated or unsporulated oocysts [7]. The route of infection is presumed to be fecal–oral. However, person-to-person transmission has not been clearly documented, suggesting that there is some necessary but unknown environmental factor. No nonhuman hosts have been identified.

The organism infects the upper intestine, causing flattening of the villi, crypt hyperplasia, inflammation and malabsorption. The complete asexual and sexual life cycle has been identified in cytoplasmic vacuoles in enterocytes located at the tips of intestinal villi on the small intestine of infected humans. *Cyclospora* oocysts are excreted in stool, but are not likely to be immediately infectious. Sporozoites have been found intracellularly in extracytoplasmic parasitophorous vacuoles at the luminal surface of the enterocyte in duodenal biopsies. Asymptomatic excretion of *Cyclospora* has not been found among travelers in Nepal, but has been reported among children in Peru. Untreated infections last from 2 to 12 weeks, with an average of 6 weeks [3].

CLINICAL FEATURES

The incubation period is 2–7 days. The onset of illness is often abrupt, with severe watery diarrhea, nausea, and vomiting. Abdominal pain, including cramps, epigastric discomfort, and distention, is present in most patients with acute cyclosporiasis. Fever can occur in 30% of cases in the initial 3 days of illness. After 2 to 3 days, the severity of illness decreases and the illness goes into a more chronic phase. Anorexia and fatigue are the two most prominent and consistent symptoms, and patients with a good appetite almost never have cyclosporiasis. The symptoms of anorexia and fatigue are fairly consistent, while nausea and diarrhea can come and go. Weight loss almost always occurs in untreated cases. Diarrhea is not prominent late in the disease, in which the hallmark symptoms are profound fatigue and anorexia.

PATIENT EVALUATION, DIAGNOSIS, AND DIFFERENTIAL DIAGNOSIS

The history of illness should include any foreign travel that may have put the patient at risk for cyclosporiasis. However, sporadic cases occur in the US without a history of foreign travel owing to local acquisition

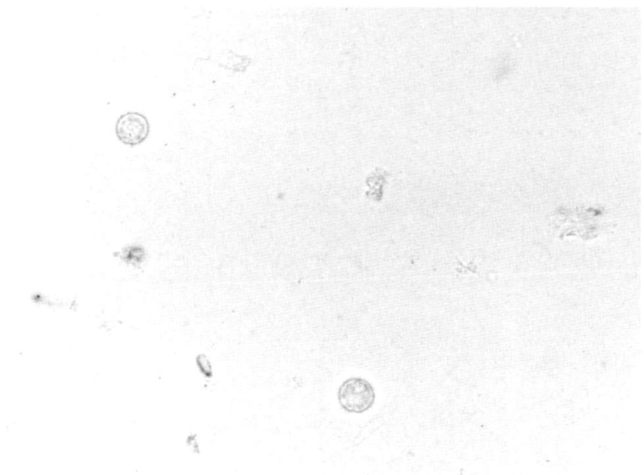

FIGURE 92.1 Unstained *Cyclospora* oocysts in a concentrated stool preparation. An experienced microscopist can easily learn to recognize unstained oocysts.

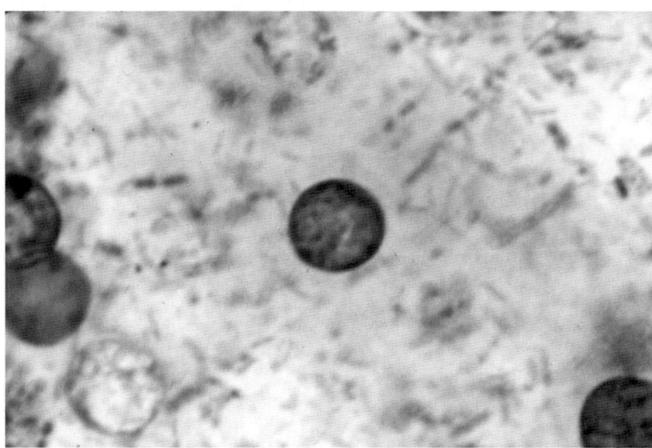

FIGURE 92.2 *Cyclospora* oocysts stained with a modified acid-fast stain in a concentrated stool preparation. Note the variable staining, from nearly white to dark red.

from endemic foci and ingestion of contaminated imported foods. Fatigue and anorexia should be specifically inquired about. A history of sudden onset of moderately severe diarrhea that becomes less severe and more chronic after several days should increase the suspicion of cyclosporiasis. Many patients with *Cyclospora* have already taken an antibiotic, such as ciprofloxacin. Because the initial phase of cyclosporiasis closely resembles a bacterial infection, and gets better spontaneously within a few days, it often appears as if the initial course of empiric antibiotics was beneficial, although the patient fails to return to his or her usual state of health. Tests for malabsorption, such as the d-xylose absorption test, although rarely necessary, are abnormal in cyclosporiasis.

The differential diagnosis, at the beginning of the illness, would include pathogenic enteric bacteria or viruses. However, as the illness progresses, the differential would include other intestinal protozoa, including *Giardia lamblia*. A rare cause of illness in travelers, *Cystoisospora belli*, can produce a prolonged diarrhea after travel, and is sensitive to trimethoprim–sulfamethoxazole. Fatigue and weight loss can be caused by *Entamoeba histolytica*, but anorexia is not as prominent. *Dientamoeba fragilis* can cause prolonged, low-grade intestinal symptoms, but without anorexia or weight loss. Fatigue and weight loss can be due to tropical sprue, which is a rare cause of prolonged diarrhea in travelers. Celiac sprue occasionally manifests during foreign travel.

The diagnosis is confirmed by stool examination. Although organisms can be detected in unstained stool by an experienced microscopist (Fig. 92.1), the organism is most easily detected using a concentration technique such as formalin–ethyl acetate centrifugation, and then staining with a modified acid-fast stain (Fig. 92.2). Individuals with acute and severe disease can shed few organisms, so concentration techniques are essential. Concentration of the stool has been shown to increase the diagnostic yield by over 40% [8]. Once identified on acid-fast staining, *C. cayetanensis*, which measures 8 to 10 μm, must be distinguished form *Cryptosporidium* spp., which measure only 4 to 5 μm. Ultraviolet fluorescence microscopy can be useful as *C. cayetanensis* is autofluorescent while *Cryptosporidium* spp. are not. *Cyclospora* oocysts stain variably with modified Ziehl-Neelsen acid-fast stain. Some oocysts stain dark red, others stain pale pink and some do not take up stain at all. Safranin stains oocysts uniformly when the fecal smear and stain are heated by microwave treatment. Other stains used in parasite detection, such as Giemsa and trichrome, do not stain *Cyclospora* oocysts. The organism is consistently shed in the stools of infected patients until the illness ends. *C. cayetanensis* does not cause an inflammatory diarrhea and fecal leukocytes are not usually seen.

Reliable, commercially available serologic assays to determine human exposure to *Cyclospora* are not available.

TREATMENT

Trimethoprim–sulfamethoxazole (TMP-SMX) is the only proven effective treatment of cyclosporiasis. In a randomized placebo controlled trial, a dose of sulfamethoxazole 800 mg and trimethoprim 160 mg given twice daily for 7 days was 94% curative [9]. The few patients who were not cured with 7 days of therapy were cured by a total of 10 days of treatment. In patients who are diagnosed early during the acute phase when diarrhea is prominent, the response to TMP-SMX is fairly rapid, within 1–2 days. In later-stage illness, people start to feel better quite rapidly, but since they have usually been ill for a while before treatment, they do not feel better all at once. The recommended adult dose and regimen is sulfamethoxazole 800 mg and trimethoprim 160 mg given twice daily for 7 days. The treatment dose for children is sulfamethoxazole 20 mg/kg and trimethoprim 4 mg/kg every 12 hours for 7 days.

Cyclosporiasis has been described among HIV-positive patients in Haiti. The symptoms were not more severe than in immunocompetent patients. Infection was easily treated with TMP-SMX, but relapse or re-infection was common. A dose of TMP-SMX three times per week prevented subsequent *Cyclospora* infection in HIV-positive patients during 7 months of surveillance [10].

In an evaluation of alternate regimens for patients who cannot tolerate sulfa-based treatments, 10 of 11 (90%) HIV-positive patients in Haiti given ciprofloxacin 500 mg twice daily for 7 days were asymptomatic on day 8 and 64% (7 of 11) had negative stool specimens. The standard regimen of TMP-SMX usually eliminates parasites by day 8, even in HIV-infected patients. Anecdotal use of ciprofloxacin in immunocompetent patients with *Cyclospora* in other settings, however, has not been effective. In a case report, nitazoxanide, 500 mg twice daily for 7 days, resulted in improved symptoms and clearing of *Cyclospora* oocysts from the stool in a patient with severe sulfa allergies [11]. Nitazoxanide was tried in an informal study at the CIWEC Clinic in Kathmandu, and did not appear efficacious. A wide variety of antimicrobials have been tried against *Cyclospora* without success, including albendazole, trimethoprim (used alone), azithromycin, nalidixic acid, tinidazole, metronidazole, quinacrine, tetracycline, doxycycline, and diloxanide furoate. Thus, currently, only ciprofloxacin and nitazoxanide have any published evidence that they might be effective against *Cyclospora* in individuals who cannot take TMP-SMX.

REFERENCES

1. Ortega YR, Sterling CF, Gilman RH, et al. Cyclospora species: a new protozoan pathogen of humans. N Engl J Med 1993;328:1308–12.
2. Ashford RW. An undescribed coccidian in man. Ann Trop Med Parasitol 1979;73:497–500.
3. Shlim DR, Cohen MT, Eaton M, et al. An alga-like organism associated with an outbreak of prolonged diarrhea among foreigners in Nepal. Am J Trop Med Hyg 1991;45:383–9.
4. Rabold JG, Shlim DR, Rajah R, et al. Cyclospora outbreak associated with chlorinated drinking water. Lancet 1994;344:1360–1.
5. Herwaldt BL. *Cyclospora cayetanensis*: a review, focusing on the outbreaks of cyclosporiasis in the 1990s. Clin Infect Dis 2000;31:1040–57.
6. Ortega YR, Sanchez R. Update on *Cyclospora cayetanensis*, a food-borne and waterborne parasite. Clin Microbiol Rev 2010;23:218–34.
7. Alfano-Sobsey EM, Eberhard ML, Seed JR, et al. Human challenge pilot study with *Cyclospora cayetanensis*. Emerg Infect Dis 2004;10:726–8.
8. Shlim DR. Cyclospora cayetanensis. Clin Lab Med 2002;22:927–36.
9. Hoge CW, Shlim DR, Ghimere M, et al. Placebo-controlled trial of co-trimoxazole for the treatment of Cyclospora infections among travelers and foreign residents in Nepal. Lancet 1995;345:691–3.
10. Verdier R, Fitzgerald DW, Johnson WD, Pape JW. Trimethoprim-sulfamethoxazole compared with ciprofloxacin for treatment and prophylaxis of *Isospora belli* and *Cyclospora cayetanensis* infection in HIV-infected patients. Ann Intern Med 2000;132:885–8.
11. Zimmer SM, Schuetz AN, Franco-Paredes C. Efficacy of nitazoxanide for cyclosporiasis in patients with sulfa allergy. Clin Infect Dis 2007;44:466–7.

Cystoisospora belli (syn. *Isospora belli*) 93

Rebecca Dillingham, Eric R Houpt

Key features

- A cause of persistent diarrhea found in tropical areas in immunocompromised patients
- Treatable with trimethoprim-sulfamethoxazole (TMP-SMX)

INTRODUCTION

Isospora belli was first identified in US troops abroad during World War I but was not studied further until 1970 when Brandborg and colleagues identified it in tissue sections from patients with malabsorptive enteritis [1]. The Centers for Disease Control and Prevention (CDC) recently revised the genus to *Cystoisospora belli* based on its morphologic and lifecycle characteristics. *Isospora* remains the designation for species infecting passerine birds [2]. Not all published work makes this distinction and, for now, *Cystoisospora belli* and *Isospora belli* can remain synonymous for the clinician.

EPIDEMIOLOGY

Humans are the only known hosts for *C. belli*, although other *Cystoisospora*/*Isospora* species are found throughout the animal kingdom. *Cystoisospora belli* has been reported throughout the tropics and subtropics. Even in endemic areas, infection is most common in those with profound immunocompromise. A hospital-based study from Ethiopia evaluated causes of diarrhea and found infection only in HIV-infected persons at a rate of 7% [3]. Outside of endemic areas, disease is occasionally seen in patients with a history of travel to these areas or immunocompromise, including instances after organ transplantation.

NATURAL HISTORY, PATHOGENESIS AND PATHOLOGY

Acquisition of *Cystoisospora* is thought to be caused by ingestion of food or water contaminated with mature oocysts from human feces. In studies of HIV-infected patients with diarrhea in Haiti, sub-Saharan Africa and south Asia, *C. belli* was identified in 3–26% of stool specimens examined [4, 5]. A community-based study of children in Guinea-Bissau found a low incidence (11 cases/168.7 child years at risk) but a strong association with diarrhea—as strong as any enteropathogen studied [6]. When observed histopathologically, *C. belli* can be found invading beyond the epithelium into the lamina propria [1]. Infiltration of eosinophils into the lamina propria and peripheral eosinophilia can be seen [7].

CLINICAL FEATURES

Cystoisospora belli generally produces an asymptomatic or self-limited diarrheal illness in otherwise healthy persons. Symptoms are nonspecific, with watery diarrhea and abdominal pain, cramps, nausea and low-grade fever usually lasting less than 1 month. In immunocompromised patients, diarrhea may be prolonged and more severe. In one study of HIV-infected patients, the median duration of diarrhea was 5.8 months [4]. Rarely, dissemination of infection to mesenteric and tracheobronchial lymph nodes, liver, gallbladder or spleen has been reported [2, 8].

PATIENT EVALUATION, DIAGNOSIS AND DIFFERENTIAL DIAGNOSIS

Cystoisosporiasis should be considered in residents of, or travelers to, tropical areas who experience persistent diarrhea. There are no characteristic physical findings or laboratory abnormalities, although peripheral eosinophilia is sometimes noted, as are Charcot-Leyden crystals in the stool [7]. Fecal leukocytes usually are not seen [4]. *Cystoisospora* infection is confirmed by stool microscopy (Fig. 93.1). The oocysts can be seen with saline wet mount, but are commonly visualized after modified acid-fast staining and are clearly distinguishable because of their large and elliptical size (10–30 μm). Other techniques, including lactophenol cotton blue staining, the auramine-rhodamine technique, Giemsa staining and the heated safranin-methylene blue technique have also been used. Shedding of oocysts may be intermittent and detection may require up to three stool examinations [9]. No serologic tests for *Cystoisospora* are commercially available. PCR assays for use on stool samples have been developed in research labs [10].

TREATMENT

Cystoisosporiasis can be treated successfully in patients with or without immunocompromise, though relapse or re-infection occurs in the latter. The regimen of choice for adults in both groups is one double-strength tablet of trimethoprim-sulfamethoxazole (TMP/SMX; 160 mg/800 mg) orally 2–4 times daily for 10 days (the higher

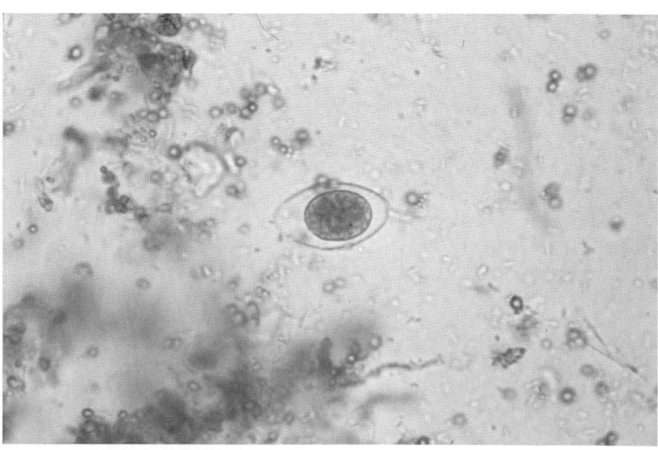

FIGURE 93.1 *Cystoisospora belli* in iodine-stained stool specimen from patient with diarrhea *(image courtesy of Herman Zaiman collection)*.

TABLE 93-1 Antimicrobial therapy for *Cystoisospora belli* infection

Scenario	Drug	Adult dose	Reference
Treatment (recommended for immunocompetent and immunocompromised patients)	Trimethoprim/sulfamethoxazole	160 mg/800 mg po bid × 7–10 d	[11, 12]
	Ciprofloxacin	500 mg po bid × 7 d	[11]
	Pyrimethamine	75 mg po qd × 3–4 w (+ leucovorin 5–25 mg/day)	[13]
Maintenance (recommended for immunocompromised patients)	Trimethoprim/sulfamethoxazole	160 mg/800 mg po tiw	[12]
	Sulfadoxine/pyrimethamine	500 mg/25 mg po weekly	[12]
	Pyrimethamine	25 mg po qd (+ leucovorin 5–25 mg/day)	[13]

dose may be needed for immunocompromised patients). In Haiti, this treatment resulted in complete symptomatic relief for most patients within 2–3 days and for all patients within 7 days [4, 11]. In Haiti, 47% of HIV-infected individuals who did not receive prophylaxis after treatment for cystoisosporiasis relapsed [4]; therefore, maintenance therapy is recommended for immunocompromised individuals with one of two regimens—one double-strength TMP-SMX tablet three times a week or one Fansidar tablet (pyrimethamine 25 mg plus sulfadoxine 500 mg) once a week [12]. For treatment of patients who are intolerant of sulfonamide-containing medications, alternative regimens include: ciprofloxacin 500 mg twice daily for 7 days or oral pyrimethamine 50–75 mg/day in individual doses (plus leucovorin 10–25 mg/day) [11, 13]. In cases of severe extraintestinal disease or during intestinal malabsorption, treatment with intravenous TMP/SMX has been used [14]. The presence of cystoisosporiasis should not delay the initiation of anti-retroviral therapy in HIV-infected patients requiring therapy [6] (Table 93-1).

REFERENCES

1. Brandborg LL, Goldberg SB, Breidenbach WC. Human coccidiosis–a possible cause of malabsorption. N Engl J Med 1970;283:1306–13.
2. Restrepo C, Macher AM, Radany EH. Disseminated extraintestinal isosporiasis in a patient with acquired immune deficiency syndrome. Am J Clin Pathol 1987;87:536–42.
3. Assefa S, Erko B, Medhin G, et al. Intestinal parasitic infections in relation to HIV/AIDS status, diarrhea and CD4 T-cell count. BMC Infect Dis 2009;9:155.
4. DeHovitz JA, Pape JW, Boncy M, Johnson WD, Jr. Clinical manifestations and therapy of *Isospora belli* infection in patients with the acquired immunodeficiency syndrome. N Engl J Med 1986;315:87–90.
5. Dwivedi KK, Prasad G, Saini S, et al. Enteric opportunistic parasites among HIV infected individuals: associated risk factors and immune status. Jpn J Infect Dis 2007;60:76–81.
6. Dillingham RA, Pinkerton R, Leger P, et al. High early mortality in patients with chronic acquired immunodeficiency syndrome diarrhea initiating antiretroviral therapy in Haiti: a case-control study. Am J Trop Med Hyg 2009;80:1060–4.
7. Lindsay DS, Dubey JP, Blagburn BL. Biology of Isospora spp. from humans, nonhuman primates, and domestic animals. Clin Microbiol Rev 1997;10: 19–34.
8. Benator DA, French AL, Beaudet LM,et al. Isospora belli infection associated with acalculous cholecystitis in a patient with AIDS. Ann Intern Med 1994;121:663–4.
9. Valentiner-Branth P, Steinsland H, Fischer TK, et al. Cohort study of Guinean children: incidence, pathogenicity, conferred protection, and attributable risk for enteropathogens during the first 2 years of life. J Clin Microbiol 2003; 41:4238–45.
10. ten Hove RJ, van Lieshout L, Brienen EA, et al. Real-time polymerase chain reaction for detection of *Isospora belli* in stool samples. Diagn Microbiol Infect Dis 2008;61:280–3.
11. Verdier RI, Fitzgerald DW, Johnson WD, Jr, Pape JW. Trimethoprim-sulfamethoxazole compared with ciprofloxacin for treatment and prophylaxis of *Isospora belli* and *Cyclospora cayetanensis* infection in HIV-infected patients. A randomized, controlled trial. Ann Intern Med 2000;132:885–8.
12. Pape JW, Verdier RI, Johnson WD, Jr. Treatment and prophylaxis of *Isospora belli* infection in patients with the acquired immunodeficiency syndrome. N Engl J Med 1989;320:1044–7.
13. Weiss LM, Perlman DC, Sherman J, et al. *Isospora belli* infection: treatment with pyrimethamine. Ann Intern Med 1988;109:474–5.
14. Bialek R, Overkamp D, Rettig I, Knobloch J. Case report: Nitazoxanide treatment failure in chronic isosporiasis. Am J Trop Med Hyg 2001;65:94–5.

Miscellaneous Intestinal Protozoa 94

Lynne S Garcia

Key features

- The less common intestinal protozoa *Balantidium coli, Dientamoeba fragilis, Entamoeba polecki*, and *Blastocystis hominis* are considered pathogenic and are often associated with symptoms
- *Dientamoeba fragilis* can be difficult to identify, even on a permanent stained smear; laboratories using skilled microscopists and permanent stained smears often report seeing more *D. fragilis* than *Giardia lamblia* (*intestinalis, duodenalis*)
- *Blastocystis hominis* remains one of the most common protozoans found in human fecal specimens and may be present more often than either *D. fragilis* or *G. lamblia*
- As the various strains or subspecies of *B. hominis* look very similar (some of which are pathogenic and some are non-pathogenic), this explains the ongoing controversy regarding the pathogenicity of "*B. hominis*"—a controversy that may eventually be resolved at the molecular level
- *Entamoeba polecki* can often be confused with other organisms in the genus *Entamoeba*; these amebae are probably often misidentified or missed during routine diagnostic testing

This chapter discusses the less common intestinal amebae, flagellates and ciliates that parasitize humans (Table 94-1). Most change their form and function from the active, feeding trophozoites to the resting, more resistant cyst form, which is primarily responsible for transmission, These protozoa are most often transmitted through food, water or other materials that are contaminated with fecal material; prevalence is often correlated with socioeconomic conditions. Most produce nonspecific intestinal symptoms, thus diagnosis requires microscopic identification of the organisms present. Fecal immunoassays and molecular methods are becoming available for these protozoa; however, their use remains somewhat limited.

The microscopic examination of the stool specimen, normally called the ova and parasite examination (O&P), consists of three separate techniques: the direct wet smear (on very soft or liquid fresh stool only), the concentration (wet mount of concentrate sediment is examined) and the permanent stained smear (the most important part of the O&P for the identification of intestinal protozoa). Microscopic identification is based on specific characteristics of the trophozoites and cysts, most of which are best seen in the permanent stained fecal smear [1, 2]. Key characteristics of the trophozoites include the type of motility (not commonly seen), cytoplasm inclusions and the number and morphology of the nuclei. Distinguishing features of the cysts include the size and shape, number and morphology of the nuclei, type of cytoplasmic inclusions (chromatoidal bars) and the presence and size of vacuoles.

94.1 Balantidiasis

INTRODUCTION

Balantidiasis is an intestinal infection caused by *Balantidium coli*, a pathogenic ciliated protozoan [2, 3].

EPIDEMIOLOGY

Balantidium coli is widely distributed in domestic pigs, which serve as the main reservoir for human infection. Transmission is fecal–oral (e.g. through contaminated food or water). Human infection occurs worldwide but has mostly been reported from Southeast Asia, the Western Pacific islands and rural South America. Pig farmers or abattoir workers are at particular risk. Sporadic reports exist of epidemics in institutionalized groups in developed countries. Transmission from nonhuman primates and rats may also occur.

NATURAL HISTORY, PATHOGENESIS, AND PATHOLOGY

Cysts can remain viable for weeks in moist feces and contaminated soil. After ingestion, excystation occurs in the bowel and the trophozoites live in the large intestine, where they remain asymptomatic in the lumen or invade the intestinal mucosa, producing abscesses beneath the surface or ulcers (Fig. 94.1).

CLINICAL FEATURES

Balantidium infection takes three forms: asymptomatic infection; chronic non-bloody diarrhea, often with halitosis; and severe invasive disease with dysentery similar to amebiasis. The diarrhea may persist for weeks to months prior to the development of dysentery.

TABLE 94-1 Miscellaneous Intestinal Protozoa

Organism	Pathogenicity	Organism stage		
		Trophozoite	*Cyst*	*Other*
Amebae				
Entamoeba polecki	+	+	+	
Flagellates				
Dientamoeba fragilis	+	+	–	
Ciliates				
Balantidium coli	+	+	+	
Other (may be reclassified)				
Blastocystis hominis	+	–	–	Multiple forms

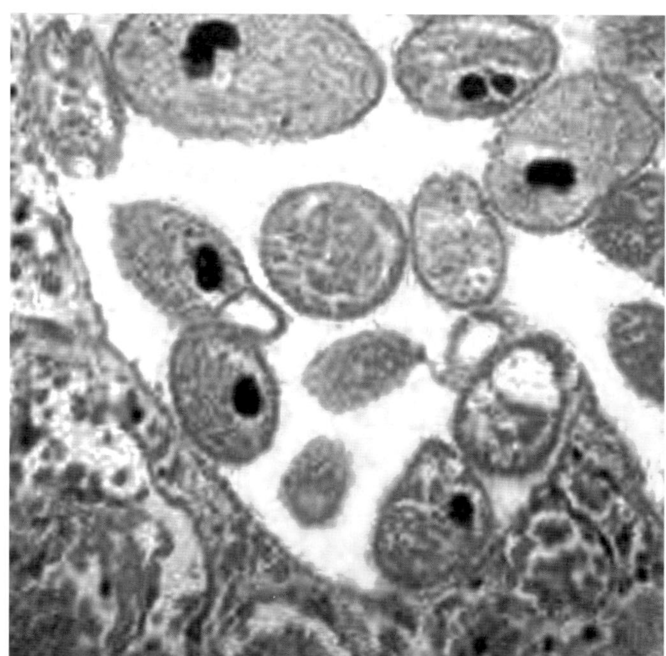

FIGURE 94.1 *Balantidium coli*. Tissue section of a colon biopsy specimen showing necrosis and organisms within an ulcerated area.

There may be tremendous fluid loss, with a type of diarrhea similar to that seen in cholera or in some coccidial or microsporidial infections. Rarely, extra-intestinal disease has been reported involving the lung, appendix, liver, peritoneum and genitourinary tracts, particularly in immunocompromised persons.

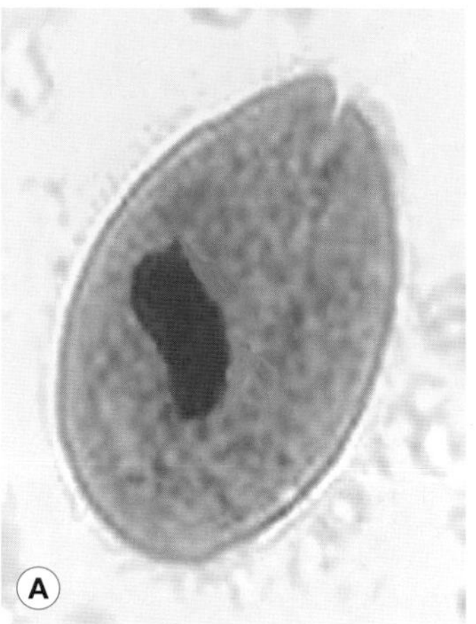

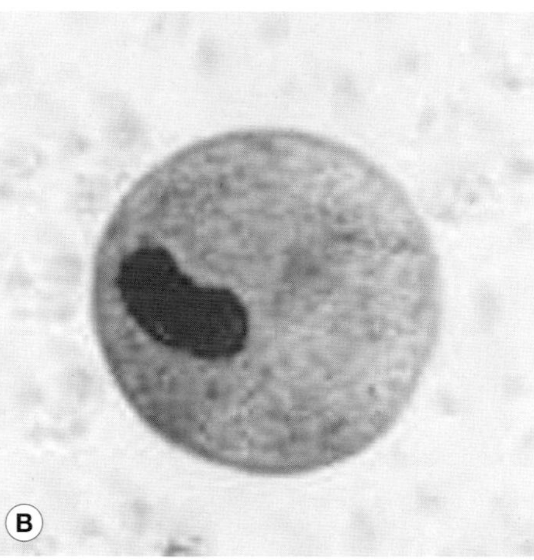

FIGURE 94.2 *Balantidium coli*. **(A)** trophozoite from a fecal specimen (note the large macronucleus); **(B)** cyst from a fecal specimen (note the large macronucleus). Organisms in wet preparations may be easier to see; occasionally in stained preparations that are stained too dark, the organisms may resemble large debris.

DIAGNOSIS

Wet preparation examinations of fresh and concentrated fecal material (O&P examination) will demonstrate the organisms (Fig. 94.2). Organism recognition and identification on a permanent stained smear is difficult; these ciliates are so large that they tend to stain very darkly, thus obscuring any internal morphology.

TREATMENT

Treatment generally involves tetracycline, 500 mg four times a day for 10 days, or doxycycline. Metronidazole 750 mg po tid for 5 days [4] or iodoquinol, 650 mg, three times a day for 20 days have also been used.

94.2 *Dientamoeba fragilis*

INTRODUCTION

Dientamoeba fragilis is an ameboflagellate closely related to *Histomonas* and *Trichomonas* spp. (Fig. 94.3) [2,5,6].

EPIDEMIOLOGY

Dientamoeba fragilis is found worldwide and past surveys provide incidence rates of 1.4–19%. Much higher incidence figures have been reported for mental institution inmates, missionaries and Native Americans in Arizona. In some laboratories in countries such as Canada and the Netherlands, *D. fragilis* is the most common protozoa found on stool ova and parasite examination. The life cycle and mode of transmission of *D. fragilis* have not been confirmed, although transmission via helminth eggs such as those of *Ascaris* and *Enterobius* spp. has been postulated. The cyst stage has not been confirmed to date.

NATURAL HISTORY, PATHOGENESIS, AND PATHOLOGY

Dientamoeba fragilis is assumed to be noninvasive and thus elicit symptoms by epithelial irritation. The significance of two genetically distinct forms of *D. fragilis* may, ultimately, serve to clarify the issues of virulence and clinical perceptions regarding pathogenicity. In some cases, the organism has been found in the biliary tree.

CLINICAL FEATURES

Although its pathogenic status is still not well defined, *D. fragilis* has been associated with diarrhea and a number of other symptoms, including intermittent diarrhea, abdominal pain, nausea, anorexia, malaise, fatigue, poor weight gain, and unexplained eosinophilia. The most common symptoms in patients infected with this parasite appear to be intermittent diarrhea and fatigue. A number of studies have even incriminated *D. fragilis* as a cause of irritable bowel syndrome and allergic colitis.

DIAGNOSIS

Diagnosis of *D. fragilis* infections depends on proper stool collection (a minimum of three fecal specimens, one collected every other day) and processing techniques. Although the survival time for this parasite has been reported as 24–48 h, the survival time in terms of morphology is limited, and stool specimens must be examined immediately or preserved in a suitable fixative soon after defecation. It is very important that permanently-stained smears of stool material be examined with the oil immersion objective (100 ×, total magnification 1000×). These organisms have been recovered in formed stool; therefore, a permanent stained smear must be prepared for every stool sample submitted for a parasite examination (O&P). Organisms seen in direct wet mounts may appear as refractile, round forms; the nuclear structure cannot be seen without examination of the permanent stained smear. Although the organisms can be isolated in culture, this approach is not a routine procedure in most clinical laboratories.

TREATMENT

We recommend treatment in individuals with persistent symptoms and *D. fragilis* infection, particularly if *D. fragilis* is the only pathogen found. No clinical trials have been performed to evaluate therapies against *D. fragilis*. Clinical improvement has been observed in adults receiving tetracycline, diiodohydroxyquin, metronidazole and paromomycin. We favor paromomycin at a dosage of 500 mg three times a day for 7 days because this is the shortest course and appears effective.

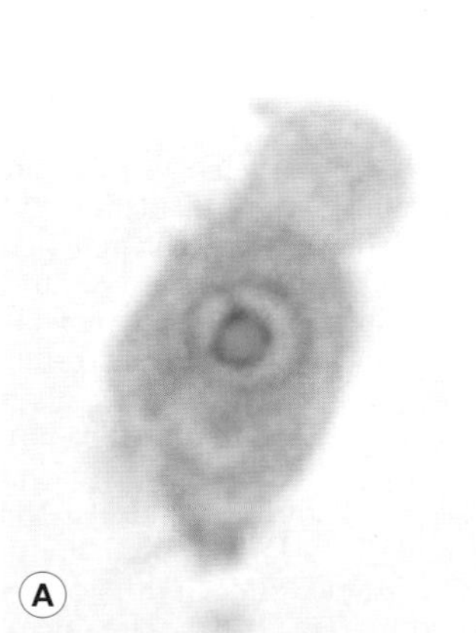

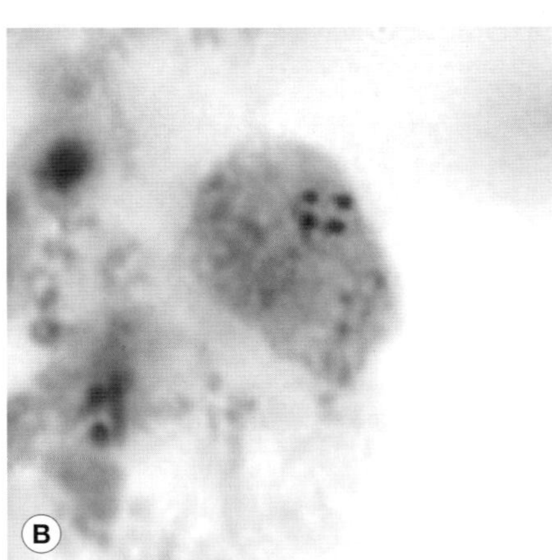

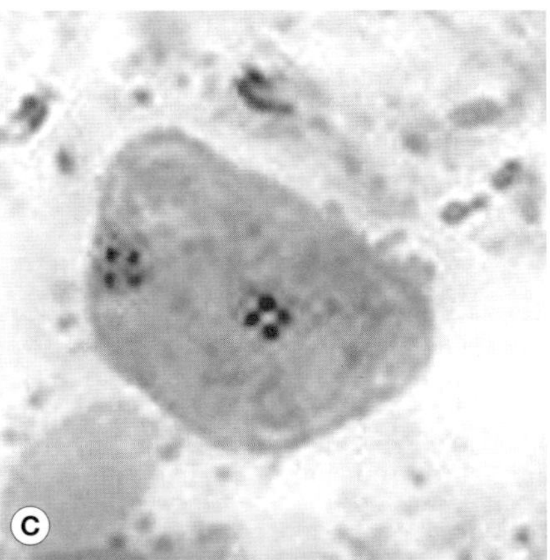

FIGURE 94.3 *Dientamoeba fragilis*. **(A)** trophozoite from stool (one nucleus, note the nuclear chromatin is getting ready to fragment); **(B)** trophozoite (one nucleus, nuclear chromatin has already fragmented); **(C)** trophozoite (two nuclei with fragmented chromatin). No known cyst form.

94.3 *Entamoeba polecki*

INTRODUCTION

Entamoeba polecki is an infrequently pathogenic ameba commonly found in the intestines of pigs and monkeys [2,7,8].

EPIDEMIOLOGY

The organism is found worldwide and highly prevalent in certain areas of the world such as Papua New Guinea. Transmission is likely human-human or from pigs, monkeys or domestic animals.

CLINICAL FEATURES

Although the majority of cases diagnosed with *E. polecki* infection have been asymptomatic, several cases have been documented in which the patients were symptomatic. Symptoms included anorexia, diarrhea, mucoid stools, abdominal pain, malaise and eosinophilia.

DIAGNOSIS

Differentiation of this organism from either *E. histolytica/E. dispar/ E. moshkovskii* or *E. coli* is rarely accomplished on the basis of a wet preparation examination and is difficult even with the permanent stained smear (Fig. 94.4). The nuclear morphology of the trophozoite is almost a composite of those of *E. histolytica/E. dispar, E. moshkovskii* and *E. coli*. Without some of the cyst stages for comparison, it would be very difficult to identify this organism to the species level on the basis of the trophozoite alone. The cyst normally has only a single nucleus, chromatoidal material like that seen in *E. histolytica* and, frequently, an inclusion body. This mass tends to be round or oval and is not sharply defined on the edges. The material, which is not glycogen, remains on the permanent stained smear and stains less intensely than nuclear material or chromatoidal bars.

TREATMENT

As for *E. histolytica*, metronidazole 750 mg three times a day for 10 days, often followed by diloxanide furoate, 500 mg three times a day for 10 days, has been used to eradicate the organism.

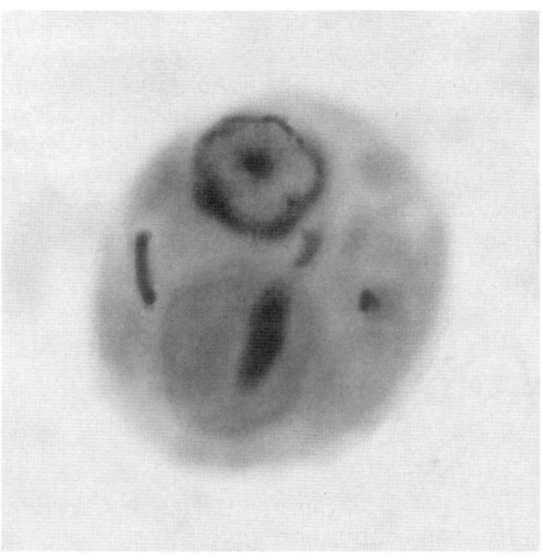

FIGURE 94.4 *Entamoeba polecki*. Uninucleate cyst in stool. Note the prominent inclusion, chromatoidal bars and single nucleus (morphology of the nucleus is a composite of all the *Entamoeba* species nuclei).

94.4 *Blastocystis hominis*

INTRODUCTION

Recently, this organism has been removed from the protozoa and reclassified in a separate group, the Stramenopila, and there are multiple subtypes at the protein or DNA level [10–12]. Analysis of 10 stocks of *B. hominis* isolated from human stools revealed two distinct subtypes, which may partially explain why some patients are asymptomatic and some have clinical symptoms.

EPIDEMIOLOGY

Blastocystis hominis is found worldwide with a prevalence in some studies as high as 58% and generally exceeds that of other organisms; even 15% of stool submitted in the USA for O&P examination may be positive. Fecal-oral transmission is postulated. Studies suggest the existence of numerous zoonotic isolates with frequent animal-to-human and human-to-animal transmission and of a large potential reservoir in animals for infections in humans. The pathogenicity of *B. hominis* has long been controversial. Several case-control analyses show no increase in prevalence in patients with diarrhea, with high carriage rates in asymptomatic individuals. Many patients infected with *Blastocystis* also carry other pathogens; endoscopic studies have not found intestinal pathology, thus causality can be difficult to discern.

CLINICAL MANIFESTATIONS

In some studies, *Blastocystis* has been associated with diarrhea, cramps, nausea, fever, vomiting and abdominal pain. An association with irritable bowel syndrome and intestinal obstruction has also been reported. One case of *Blastocystis* arthritis has also been reported.

DIAGNOSIS

Routine stool examinations are very effective in recovering and identifying *B. hominis*, although the permanent stained smear is the procedure of choice. The examination of wet preparations may not easily reveal the organism; morphology can be difficult to see at the lower magnifications. If the fresh stool is rinsed in water before fixation (for the concentration method), *B. hominis* organisms, other than the cysts, will be destroyed, thus possibly yielding a false-negative report. The organisms should be quantitated on the report form, i.e. as rare, few, moderate or many. The classic form that is usually seen in the human stool specimen varies tremendously in size, from 6–40 µm, and is characterized by a large central body, which may be involved with carbohydrate and lipid storage (visually appearing like a large vacuole) (Fig. 94.5). The more amebic form is occasionally seen in diarrheal fluid but may be extremely difficult to recognize. Generally, *B. hominis* will be identified on the basis of the more typical round form with the central body.

Quantitation of *Blastocystis* in stool (>5 organisms per oil immersion field) has been proposed to inform whether *Blastocystis* is a pathogen, but this also remains controversial and poorly studied. ELISA and fluorescent-antibody tests have been developed for detection of serum antibody to *B. hominis* infections.

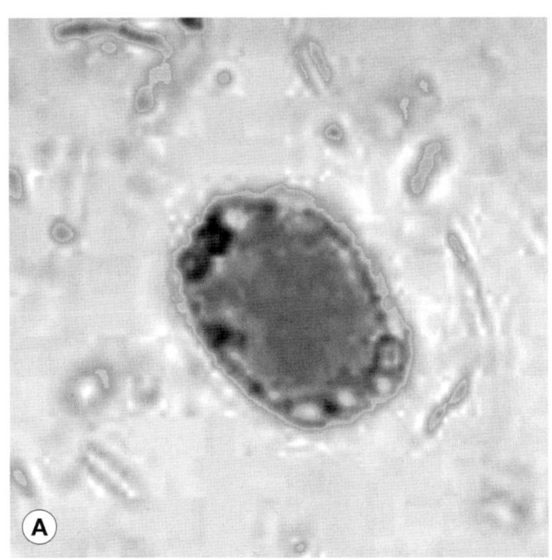

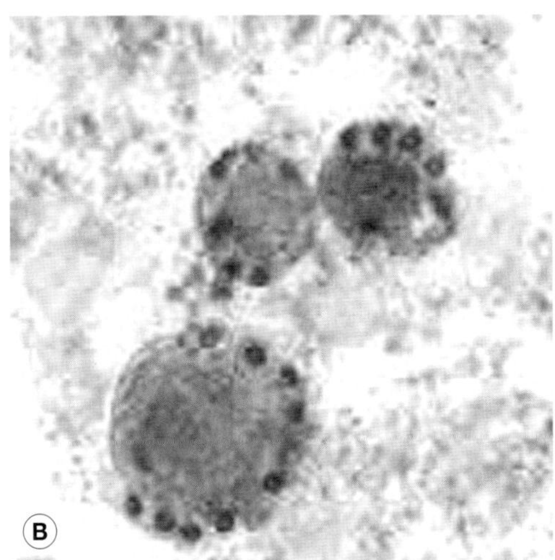

FIGURE 94.5 *Blastocystis hominis*. Central body forms from stool. Note the small nuclei around the periphery; also note the organism on the left **(A)** is dividing.

TREATMENT

Routine treatment of asymptomatic *Blastocystis* infection is not recommended. It reasonable to treat symptomatic *Blastocystis* infection if no other pathogens are found, particularly if repeat stool studies confirm the parasite. Treatment is most commonly attempted with metronidazole at the amebiasis dose of 750 mg TID for 5–10 days. Successful treatment with nitazoxanide and trimethoprim-sulfamethoxazole has also been reported. Parasitologic and clinical cure rates are relatively low at ~70%.

94.5 Non-pathogenic Intestinal Protozoa

A number of non-pathogenic amebae and flagellates are often found during the routine O&P stool examination, including *E. coli, Endolimax nana, Iodamoeba bütschlii, Chilomastix mesnili* and *Pentatrichomonas* (formerly trichomonsa) *hominis* (Tables 94-2 and 94-3). Although these are non-pathogens, this finding indicates the patient has come in contact with something contaminated with fecal material containing infective cysts. If the patient is symptomatic, it is important to perform additional testing to detect possible pathogens that might also be present.

TABLE 94-2 Trophozoites of Miscellaneous Intestinal Protozoa

Parasite	Size* µm (normal range)	Motility	Stained nucleus (number)	Peripheral chromatin flagella; or cilia	Cytoplasm	Inclusions
Entamoeba polecki	8–15 (10–12)	Same as *E. coli*	Difficult to see in unstained preparations (1); intermediate between *E. histolytica* and *E. coli*	Fine and large granules; even or uneven arrangement; karyosome usually central	Finely granular	Bacteria
Dientamoeba fragilis	Shaped like amebae 5–15 (9–12)	Usually nonprogressive	Usually not visible in unstained preparations; 40% one nucleus; 60% two nuclei; karyosome composed of cluster of 4–8 granules	Internal flagella not visible, even in stained preparations	Tremendous variability in size and shape; finely granular; usually vacuolated	Bacteria, yeasts, other debris
Balantidium coli	Ovoid with tapering anterior end; 50–100 (40–70) longby 40–50 wide	Rotary, boring, may be rapid	One large kidney-shaped macronucleus; one small, round micronucleus (very difficult to see even in stained preparation)	Cilia may be seen in unstained or stained preparations	Cytoplasm may be vacuolated	Small debris

*These measurements refer to wet preparation measurements. After permanent staining (including dehydration), some trophozoite measurements may be 1–1.5 microns less. In general, shrinkage is more obvious and greater with the cyst forms.

TABLE 94-3 Cysts of Miscellaneous Intestinal Protozoa

Parasite	Size* µm (normal range)	Shape	Stained nucleus (number); karyosome	Peripheral chromatin; flagella; or cilia	Cytoplasm	Inclusions
Entamoeba polecki	5–11	Usually spherical	Mature cyst (1), rarely more; morphology similar to that seen in trophozoite	Similar to trophozoite	Granular	Many chromatoidal bars with pointed ends; half of cysts contain spherical or ovoid "inclusion mass"
*Blastocystis hominis***	6–40; tremendous size variation in a single specimen	Usually round	Large central body (looks like large vacuole) surrounded by small, multiple nuclei	No peripheral chromatin	Large vacuole (central body area)	More amebic form seen in diarrheal fluid, but is extremely difficult to identify; may be confused with yeast cells
Dientamoeba fragilis	No cyst form					
Balantidium coli	50–70 (50–55)	Spherical or oval	One large, kidney-shaped macronucleus; one small, round micronucleus (very difficult to see even in stained preparation)	Cilia more difficult to see in the cyst form	Vacuoles very small	Small debris, no inclusions

*These sizes refer to the wet preparation measurements. When organisms are stained/dehydrated, often the measurements from the permanent stained smear may be 1–1.5 micron smaller in size.
***Blastocystis hominis* is now classified in the Stramenopila kingdom (no longer in the Protozoa kingdom) [12].

REFERENCES

1. Beaver PC, Jung RC, Cupp EW. Clinical Parasitology, 9th edn. Philadelphia: Lea & Febiger; 1984.
2. Garcia LS. Diagnostic Medical Parasitology, 5th edn. Washington: ASM Press; 2007.
3. Schuster FL, Ramirez-Avila L. Current world status of *Balantidium coli*. Clin Microbiol Rev 2008;21:626–38.
4. Garcia-Laverde A, de Bonilla L.Clinical trials with metronidazole in human balantidiasis. Am J Trop Med Hyg 1975;24:781–3.
5. Johnson EH, Windsor JJ, Clark CG. Emerging from obscurity: biological, clinical and diagnostic aspects of *Dientamoeba fragilis*. Clin Microbiol Rev 2004;17:563–70.
6. Stark DJ, Beebe N, Marriott D, et al. Dientamoebiasis: clinical importance and recent advances. Trends Parasitol 2006;22:92–6.
7. Gay JD, Abell TL, Thompson JH, et al. *Entamoeba polecki* infection in Southeast Asian refugees: Multiple cases of a rarely reported parasite. Mayo Clin Proc 1985;60:523.
8. Salaki JS, Shirey JL, Strickland GT. Successful treatment of symptomatic *Entamoeba polecki* infection. Am J Trop Med Hyg 1979;28:190.
9. Verweij JJ, Polderman AM, Clark CG. Genetic variation among human isolates of uninucleated cyst-producing *Entamoeba* species. J Clin Microbiol 2001; 39:1644–6.
10. Sohail MR, Fischer PR. *Blastocystis hominis* and travelers. Travel Med Infect Dis 2005;3:33–8.
11. Tan TC, Suresh KG, Smith HV. Phenotypic and genotypic characterization of *Blastocystis hominis* isolates implicates subtype 3 as a subtype with pathogenic potential. Parasitol Res 2008;104:85–93.
12. Cox FEG. Taxonomy and classification of human parasitic protozoa and helminths. In: Versalovic J, Carroll KC, Funke G, et al. (eds). Manual of Clinical Microbiology, 10th ed, Section VIII Parasitology. ASM Press, Washington, DC, 2011:2041–6.

Trichomoniasis 95

Michael F Rein

Key features

- Trichomoniasis (synonym: "trich") is a common sexually transmitted disease caused by a protozoan parasite that infects the urogenital tract of men and women
- The vagina is the most common site of infection in women
- Most women present with vaginal discharge, often yellow or green, often frothy; vulvovaginal irritation; and external dysuria
- The urethra is the most common site of infection in men
- Most men with trichomoniasis do not have signs or symptoms; however, some men may temporarily have an irritation inside the penis, mild discharge, or slight burning after urination or ejaculation

INTRODUCTION

Trichomoniasis is a common, worldwide, urogenital infection with *Trichomonas vaginalis* [1]. The protozoan was first described in purulent genital secretions by Donné in 1836. Trichomoniasis is a frequent cause of symptomatic vaginitis and a less common cause of nongonococcal urethritis (NGU).

EPIDEMIOLOGY

Trichomoniasis is sexually transmitted by penile–vaginal coitus. The organism is not acquired by fellatio, cunnilingus, or insertive or receptive anal intercourse. Because it is sexually transmitted, it is common in populations at higher risk for other sexually transmitted infections (STIs). Its presence in an individual is a marker for high-risk behaviors, and coincident STIs should be sought. Sexual partners, even if asymptomatic, should be treated simultaneously. The presence of trichomoniasis increases the risk of acquisition of HIV infection [2]. Women who deliver while infected rarely transmit the infection to the neonate, in whom it may present vaginally or, rarely, in the respiratory tract.

For many years, it has been estimated that there are 3–5 million new cases annually in the US and an overall prevalence among women of about 3% [3]. The incidence and prevalence appear higher among African-American women and, not surprisingly, among commercial sex-workers. Infection is detected in about three-quarters of the male sexual partners of infected women [4], and re-infection is common [5]. Nonvenereal acquisition by adults is very rare. Cure rates are demonstrably improved if sexual partners are treated simultaneously. Some estimates suggest that the incidence of trichomoniasis in the US may have gradually decreased over the last 40 years. This may be due to the large amount of metronidazole and other imidazoles used in the same population for the treatment of bacterial vaginosis.

Although usually carried asymptomatically by men, *T. vaginalis* may cause between 7% and 22% of cases of NGU in some populations [6]. Some studies suggest that male circumcision may reduce the likelihood of transmission [7].

NATURAL HISTORY, PATHOGENESIS, AND PATHOLOGY

Infected vaginal discharge contains 10^1 to 10^5 organisms/mL, with symptomatic women generally manifesting the larger numbers. *T. vaginalis* damages squamous epithelial cells through direct contact, and the process results in microulcerations and microscopic hemorrhages of the vaginal walls and exocervix. Columnar epithelium is not affected, and thus trichomoniasis presents with vaginitis but not with endocervicitis. The simultaneous presence of an endocervical discharge should alert the clinician to the possibility of coincident infection with *Neisseria gonorrhoeae* or *Chlamydia trachomatis*. Invasion of tissue does not occur.

T. vaginalis is isolated from the urethra in most infected women. Organisms can cause ulcerations beneath the prepuce [6].

The immune response to trichomonal infection remains incompletely defined. Infection elicits an outpouring of polymorphonuclear neutrophils (PMNs), which are easily visualized on wet mount and serve as an aid in differential diagnosis. The presence of many PMNs may actually contribute to pathogenesis. A low-grade humoral response is detected in serum and vaginal secretion, but immunity to re-infection is not produced.

CLINICAL FEATURES

HISTORY

In various series, 50% to 90% of women with trichomoniasis have symptoms. Individual symptoms are relatively nonspecific. Many women with trichomoniasis have other STIs, and it is sometimes difficult to attribute specific clinical features to trichomoniasis alone. Vaginal discharge is recognized by 50% to 75% of infected women, but the discharge is considered malodorous by only 10%. One-quarter to one-half of infected women suffer vulvar irritation or pruritus, and up to 50% suffer dyspareunia. Dysuria may be internal or external.

Lower abdominal discomfort is described by only 10% of women, and its presence, particularly if accompanied by an adnexal tenderness on bimanual examination, should suggest the possibility of coincident salpingitis from other pathogens.

Some women report that symptoms began or were exacerbated immediately following the menstrual period. In experimentally induced infection, incubation periods ranged from 3 to 28 days.

Most infected men come to treatment as sexual contacts of infected women. *T. vaginalis* causes a minority of cases of nongonococcal urethritis, presenting as some combination of dysuria and urethral discharge, and resembling NGU of more common etiologies. Trichomonal urethritis is usually recognized when the condition fails to respond to standard antibacterial therapies [6,8]. Rarely, epididymitis is encountered, and the organism has been identified in the prostate [6].

PHYSICAL EXAMINATION

The vulva is erythematous in less than one-third of patients. On speculum examination, excessive discharge is noted in 50% to 75% of infected women. A yellow vaginal discharge suggests trichomoniasis, but the classically yellow or green, frothy discharge is seen in only a minority of patients. Indeed, bubbles are present in only 8% to 50% of infected women in various series, and since bubbles are also observed in bacterial vaginosis, their presence is nonspecific [9].

Vaginal wall erythema, occasionally with edema, is observed in 20% to 75% of cases, and punctate hemorrhages are observed on the vaginal walls or the exocervix (strawberry cervix) in about 2% of women during routine physical examination, but the characteristic hemorrhages are visualized in 45% by colposcopy.

In my experience, mild adnexal tenderness is occasionally elicited on bimanual examination. This may be due to pelvic adenitis induced by the infection, but its presence should raise concerns for coincident salpingitis.

COMPLICATIONS

Trichomoniasis is generally a benign disease. Gestational trichomoniasis has been associated with premature rupture of the fetal membranes and preterm delivery [10]. Unfortunately, two studies suggest that treating trichomoniasis in pregnancy is actually associated with an increased frequency of these complications [11,12]. Symptomatic infections require treatment, but some specialists recommend postponing treatment of asymptomatic trichomoniasis in pregnancy until after the 37th week of gestation [13].

Trichomoniasis, with its brisk inflammatory response and microulcerations of the genital epithelium, may increase the risk of acquiring HIV [2]. In addition, treatment of trichomoniasis reduces the concentration of HIV in vaginal secretions about fourfold, theoretically reducing the risk of transmitting the HIV [14].

A possible association of trichomoniasis with pelvic inflammatory disease and cervical cancer is sometimes hypothesized, but observations may be confounded by frequent past or present co-infection with other sexually transmitted agents, such as chlamydia or human papillomavirus, more strongly associated with upper tract disease and genital malignancy.

TABLE 95-1 Typical Features of Trichomoniasis and Differentials

	Trichomoniasis	Vulvovaginal candidiasis	Bacterial vaginosis
Symptoms			
Vulvar irritation	4+	4+	0–1+
Dysuria	20%	External	0
Odor	0–2+	0	1+–4+
Signs			
Labial erythema	1+–4+	1–4+	0
Satellite lesions	0	Frequent	0
Discharge			
Consistency	Frothy (25%)	Minimal to curdy	Homogeneous, often frothy
Color	Yellow-green (25%)	White	Gray, white
Adherence to vaginal walls	0	Often	Usually
Whiff test	60–90%	0	70–90%
Alkalinity	≥4.7 (70–90%)	≤4.5	≥4.7 (90%)
Bimanual examination			
Adnexal tenderness	Occasional	0	0
Vaginal wall tenderness	0–2+	0–2+	0
Wet mount			
Epithelial cells	Normal	Normal	Clue cells (90%)
PMN/ epithelial cell	≥1	Variable	≤1
Bacteria	Rods or coccobacilli	Rods	Coccobacilli and motile rods
Pathogens	Trichomonads (70%)	Yeasts and pseudohyphae (50%)	Nonspecific

PMN, polymorphonuclear neutrophils.

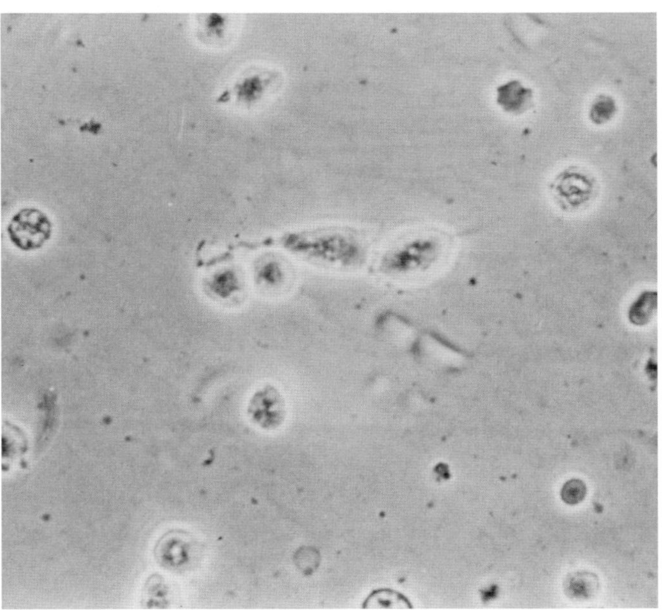

FIGURE 95.1 Trichomoniasis. Wet mount of vaginal discharge showing several round polymorphonuclear neutrophils and two ovoid trichomonads. Anterior flagella are visible. (Phase contrast, ×1000.)

PATIENT EVALUATION, DIAGNOSIS, AND DIFFERENTIAL DIAGNOSIS

Clinicians often manage symptomatic women who present with some combination of vaginal discharge, vulvar irritation, and odor. The clinical and laboratory features that assist in differentiating trichomoniasis from bacterial vaginosis and candidiasis are presented in Table 95-1. A history of contact with a new partner supports the diagnosis of sexually transmitted vaginitis. Odor without much irritation is more consistent with bacterial vaginosis than with trichomoniasis, in which irritation is more prominent. After completing the physical examination, it is useful to determine the pH of vaginal secretions. This is conveniently accomplished by inserting a strip of indicator paper into the vaginal discharge pooled in the lower lip of the speculum. Normal vaginal pH of 4.7 or less is maintained in most patients with vulvovaginal candidiasis. Vaginal pH is elevated above 4.7 in most women with trichomoniasis, but an elevated pH is also found in most women with bacterial vaginosis and is not specific. The pH of vaginal material may be artifactually elevated if contaminated with cervical discharge or semen. After the pH has been determined, several drops of 10% to 20% potassium hydroxide should be added to the discharge in the speculum. The clinician then seeks the elaboration of a pungent, fishy, amine-like odor. This positive result of the whiff test is manifested by 75% of women with trichomoniasis but also by most women with bacterial vaginosis. The whiff test is not positive in vulvovaginal candidiasis. Such point-of-care testing is particularly useful in resource-poor venues [15].

Definitive diagnosis is based on demonstrating the parasite (Fig. 95.1). A swab of vaginal material can be agitated in about 1 mL of saline and a drop transferred to a microscope slide to which a coverslip is then applied. This wet mount is observed at 400× with the substage condenser racked down and the substage diaphragm closed. Its sensitivity for trichomoniasis is only about 60%. *T. vaginalis* culture systems are commercially available but expensive. Diagnosis in men is difficult and depends on newer molecular techniques [16]. The Pap smear can detect trichomonal infection, but the Gram stain is useless.

TREATMENT

Decades of experience and old studies confirm the value of oral 5′-nitroimidazoles for treating men and women. Metronidazole or tinidazole are preferred in the US, but in other parts of the world, ornidazole and nimorazole are used as well. High-dose vaginal suppositories are available in some areas, but low-dose metronidazole vaginal preparations designed for bacterial vaginosis are inadequate for trichomoniasis. Male partners should be treated simultaneously even if asymptomatic. Treatment of trichomoniasis can be effectively accomplished with metronidazole 2 g orally in a single dose, tinidazole 2 g orally in a single dose, or metronidazole 500 mg orally twice daily for 7 days. Metronidazole can be used in pregnancy (Category B), but tinidazole (Category C) should not [13,17]. The optimal management of patient allergy or trichomonal resistance to the imidazoles remains incompletely defined.

REFERENCES

1. Van der Pol B. *Trichomonas vaginalis* infection: the most prevalent nonviral sexually transmitted infection received the least public health attention. Clin Infect Dis 2007;44:13–22.
2. McClelland RS, Sangare L, Hassan WM, et al. Infection with *Trichomonas vaginalis* increases the risk of HIV-1 acquisition. J Infect Dis 2007;195:698–702.
3. Sutton M, Sternberg M, Koumans EH, et al. The prevalence of *Trichomonas vaginalis* infections among reproductive-age women in the United States. Clin Infect Dis 2007;45:1139–26.
4. Sena AC, Miller WC, Hobbs MM, et al. *Trichomonas vaginalis* infection in male sexual partners: implications for diagnosis, treatment, and prevention. Clin Infect Dis 2007;44:13–22.
5. Van der Pol B, Williams JA, Orr DP, et al. Prevalence, incidence, natural history, and response to treatment of *Trichomonas vaginalis* infection among adolescent women. J Infect Dis 2005;192:2039–44.
6. Krieger JN: Trichomoniasis in men: old issues and new data. Sex Transm Dis 1995;22:83–96.
7. Gray RH, Kigozi G, Serwadda D, et al. The effects of male circumcision on female partners' genital tract symptoms and vaginal infections in a randomized trial in Rakai, Uganda. Am J Obstet Gynecol 2009;200:42.e1–e7.
8. Centers for Disease Control and Prevention. Sexually transmitted diseases treatment guidelines, 2006. MMWR Recomm Rep 2006;55:36–7.
9. Wolner-Hanssen P, Krieger JN, Stevens CE, et al. Clinical manifestations of vaginal trichomoniasis. JAMA 1989;264:571–6.
10. Cotch MF, Pastorek JG 2nd, Nugent RP, et al. *Trichomonas vaginalis* associated with low birth weight and preterm delivery. The Vaginal Infections and Prematurity Study Group. Sex Transm Dis 1997;24:353–60.
11. Rigg MA, Klebanoff MA. Treatment of vaginal infections to prevent preterm birth: a meta-analysis. Clin Obstet Gynecol 2004;47:796–807.
12. Hay P, Czeizel AE. Asymptomatic trichomonas and candida colonization in pregnancy outcome. Best Pract Clin Obstet Gynecol 2007;21:403–9.
13. Centers for Disease Control and Prevention. Sexually transmitted disease treatment guidelines, 2010. MMWR 2010;59(RR-12):58–61.
14. Wang CC, McClelland RS, Reilly M, et al. The effect of treatment of vaginal infections on shedding of human immunodeficiency virus type 1. J Infect Dis 2001;183:1017–22.
15. Madhivanan P, Krupp K, Hardin J, et al. Simple and inexpensive point-of-care tests improve diagnosis of vaginal infections in resource-constrained settings. Trop Med Int Health 2009;14:703–8.
16. Hobbs MM, Lapple DM, Lawing LF, et al. Methods for detection of *Trichomonas vaginalis* in the male partners of infected women: implications for control of trichomoniasis. J Clin Microbiol 2006;44:3994–9.
17. Okun N, Gronau KA, Hannah ME. Antibiotics for bacterial vaginosis or *Trichomonas vaginalis* in pregnancy: a systematic review. Obstet Gynecol 2005;105:857–68.

SECTION

B

INFECTIONS OF THE BLOOD AND RETICULOENDOTHELIAL SYSTEM

96 Malaria

Terrie Taylor, Tsiri Agbenyega

Key features

- The clinical presentation of uncomplicated malaria is a nonspecific, undifferentiated febrile illness. It is not possible to confirm or exclude the diagnosis of malaria based on clinical presentation alone
- Malaria infection in non-immune individuals is a medical emergency
- Malaria infection is not synonymous with malaria illness, particularly in malaria-endemic areas where older children and adults have acquired immunity to malaria disease and are commonly found with asymptomatic parasitemias
- The diagnosis of malaria should be parasitologically confirmed by the microscopic visualization of parasites on a peripheral blood smear or detecting parasite antigen with a rapid diagnostic test (RDT)
- Repeating smears every 12 hours for 36–48 hours if initial smears are negative is warranted in non-immune individuals who are at risk. It not necessary to time smears with elevations in temperature to make a parasitologic diagnosis
- Patients who are unable to take anti-malarial medication by mouth require parenteral therapy – a loading dose is essential
- When possible, decisions regarding the use of anti-malarial medications should be based on parasitologic evidence (blood film or malaria RDT)

INTRODUCTION

Malaria is an ancient and enduring scourge of mankind with a rich and fascinating history [1]. About 3 billion people – nearly half of the world's population – are at risk of malaria infection and illness. Every year, this leads to about 250 million malaria cases and nearly 1 million malaria deaths. Malaria has shaped the human genome, complicated major military campaigns, eluded pharmacologic attacks, adversely affected international economic indicators and frustrated generations of clinicians, scientists and policy makers.

Malaria is an acute and chronic disease caused by obligate intracellular protozoa of the genus *Plasmodium*. Historically, four species of malaria parasites were considered capable of infecting humans: *Plasmodium falciparum, Plasmodium vivax, Plasmodium ovale* and *Plasmodium malariae;* however, recently, a fifth – *Plasmodium knowlesi* – has been recognized as a significant human pathogen [2]. The majority (56%) of malaria infections are in sub-Saharan Africa, followed by Southeast Asia (27%), the Eastern Mediterranean (12%) and South America (3%) [3]. The parasites are transmitted to humans by female *Anopheles* mosquitos. The clinical presentation is highly variable but is generally characterized by an undifferentiated febrile illness with headache, chills and rigors, anemia and splenomegaly. *Plasmodium falciparum* is the species most commonly associated with severe and complicated disease.

Plasmodium vivax is the dominant species found outside of Africa; its distribution (the Middle East, Asia, the Western Pacific and Central and South America) complements that of *P. ovale* (primarily West Africa). *Plasmodium malariae* has a worldwide distribution, generally in isolated pockets, and, to date, *P. knowlesi* is restricted to South and Southeast Asia, primarily in areas harboring macaque monkeys (Fig. 96.1).

In sub-Saharan Africa, nearly all of the malaria-associated morbidity and mortality is caused by *P. falciparum*. Individuals of all ages remain susceptible to infection, but immunity to severe disease develops over time, the result of repeated exposure to bites from infected anopheline mosquitoes. Anti-disease immunity is related to transmission intensity, but its specific characteristics and determinants are not well understood. Non-immune individuals – typically young children in sub-Saharan Africa, but tourists and soldiers in other malaria-endemic areas are included in this category – are at risk of developing severe and complicated malaria. Semi-immune people can be infected (i.e. parasitemic) but asymptomatic; when semi-immune people do develop a malaria illness, it is generally marked by fever and malaise and rarely becomes life-threatening.

There is a broad geographic overlap between the distributions of HIV and malaria, especially falciparum malaria. Co-infection is associated with a transient increase in HIV RNA [4]. HIV-infected individuals, particularly those with CD4 counts <200 cells/μl, are more susceptible to malaria infection and have higher parasitemias [5]. Data on whether HIV serostatus has any impact on malaria disease severity are conflicting.

Contemporary efforts to address the multiple challenges of malaria control, prevention and, perhaps, elimination (reduction to zero of malaria infection in a defined geographic area) or eradication (permanent extinction of malaria transmission throughout the world) include using combination chemotherapy *exclusively* (to slow the development and spread of drug resistant parasites), attempting to develop a malaria vaccine and scaling-up interventions which are known to be effective (e.g. long-lasting insecticide-treated bed nets, indoor residual spraying of insecticide).

EPIDEMIOLOGY

TRANSMISSION

The epidemiology of malaria is fundamentally determined by the dynamics and intensity of parasite transmission. Vector abundance and longevity are major contributors to transmission rates and these are strongly influenced by temperature, rainfall and humidity. The most direct measure of transmission intensity is the entomologic inoculation rate (EIR) – the number of infectious female anopheline bites per person per year. In general, EIRs of <10/year are considered "low transmission", 10–49/year "intermediate transmission" and

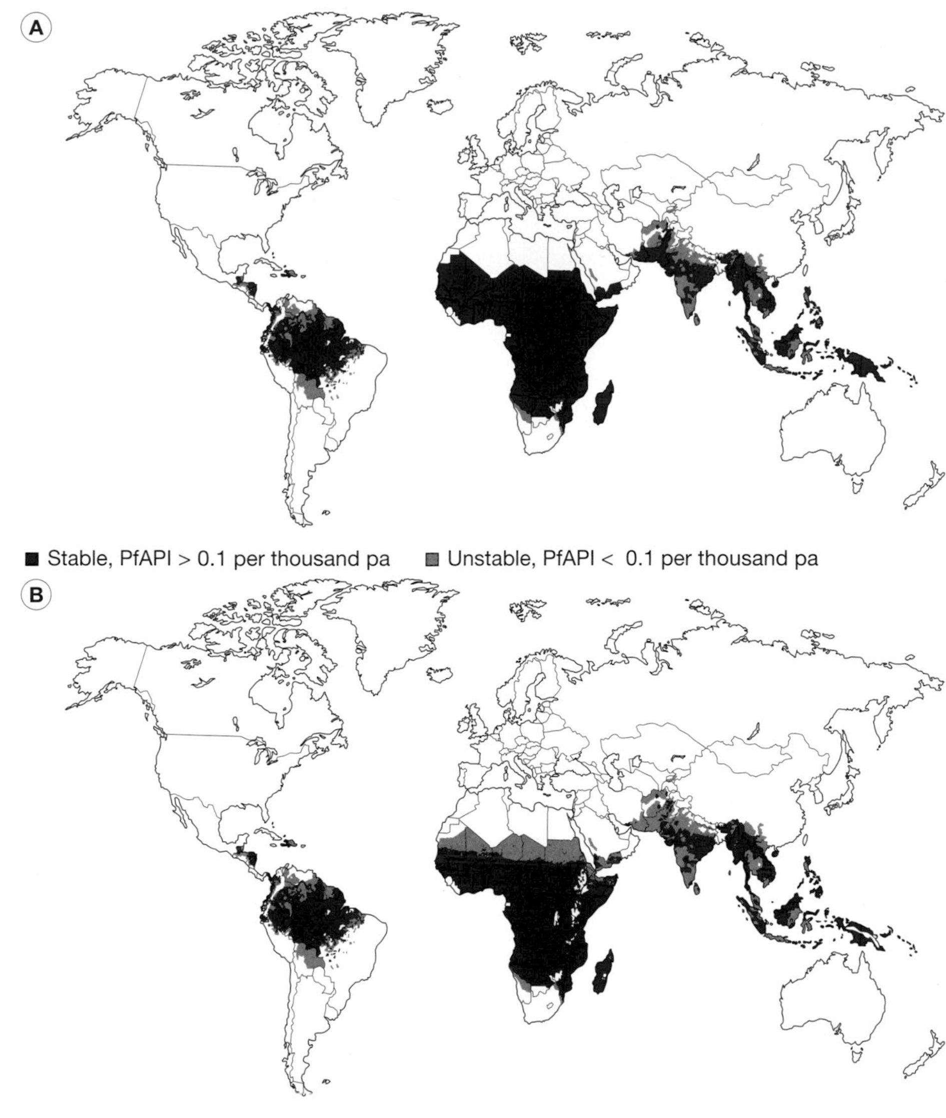

FIGURE 96.1 *P. falciparum* malaria risk defined by annual parasite incidence (top) and temperature and aridity (bottom). Areas were defined as stable (dark blue areas, where *Pf*API ≥0.1 per thousand pa), unstable (light blue, where *Pf*API <0.1 per thousand pa), or no risk (no color). The few areas for which no *Pf*API data could be obtained, mainly found in India, are not colored. The borders of the 87 countries defined as *P. falciparum* endemic are shown. The aridity mask excluded risk in a step-wise fashion, reflected mainly in the larger areas of unstable (light blue) areas compared to the top panel, particularly in the Sahel and southwest Asia (southern Iran and Pakistan). *Reproduced from Guerra CA, Gikandi PW, Tatem AJ, et al. The limits and intensity of Plasmodium falciparum transmission: implications for malaria control and elimination worldwide. PLoS Med 2008;5(2):e38.*

≥ 50/year "high transmission". For clinicians working in settings where data on EIRs are not readily available, surrogate measures include the spleen rate and parasite prevalence rates in children (Box 96.1). Transmission dynamics are regarded as stable when transmission is constant throughout the year, or predictably seasonal. Unstable transmission (characteristic of epidemics) occurs when there are changes in the environment (e.g. sudden, heavy rains) or in the population (e.g. migration).

Malaria transmission is also influenced by climate. The optimal conditions occur when the temperature is between 20°C and 30°C and the mean relative humidity is at least 60%. Sporogony does not occur at temperatures below 16°C or higher than 33°C. Water temperatures regulate the duration of the aquatic cycle of the mosquito vector. A high relative humidity increases mosquito longevity and therefore increases the probability that an infected mosquito will survive long enough to become infective.

The proximity of human habitation to breeding sites directly influences vector-human contact and, therefore, transmission. The stability of breeding sites is influenced by water supply, soil and vegetation. Irrigation schemes, dams and other man-made changes affecting land use can radically alter stable patterns of malaria transmission.

ACQUIRED IMMUNITY

The incidence and prevalence of malaria *illness* is determined largely by acquired immunity. The burden of disease and death is borne by non-immune individuals. In areas of stable transmission (e.g. most of sub-Saharan Africa), young children are the non-immune individuals at risk of life-threatening malaria. Older children and adults are "semi-immune"; their malaria infections may be asymptomatic or they may develop uncomplicated malaria illnesses.

Attributing a cause-and-effect relationship between parasites and the often nonspecific symptoms of an uncomplicated malaria illness in semi-immune patients is difficult and bedevils the diagnosis of a "malaria illness" in this group (see *"Interpreting the results of malaria diagnostic tests"* below).

Where transmission is unstable, there is little acquired immunity and individuals from all age groups can develop severe disease. Whether

BOX 96.1 Useful Malaria Vocabulary

- **Pre-patent period:** the time from inoculation of sporozoites from mosquitoes until asexual erythrocytic stage parasites are detected by microscopy in the bloodstream. This measure can be influenced by the parasite detection technique (PCR > rapid diagnostic tests > microscopy).
- **Incubation period:** the time from inoculation of sporozoites from mosquitoes until an individual develops clinical signs or symptoms of malaria – this is always longer than the pre-patent period, but the time difference is determined by immune status. Non-immune individuals develop symptoms with low parasitemias, so the incubation period is shorter than in semi-immune individuals, who may be able to tolerate significant parasitemias without becoming symptomatic.
- **Recurrence:** repeat intra-erythrocytic infection causing malaria-associated symptoms.
  - **Relapse:** a recurrent infection caused by a new brood of blood-stage parasites emerging from hypnozoites in the liver (*P. vivax, P. ovale*).
  - **Recrudescence:** a recurrent infection caused by the growth of an undetectable blood stage infection (generally the result of drug resistance, unusual pharmacokinetics or an incomplete dose). It can also occur in immunocompromised individuals, most famously with *P. malariae*.
  - **Re-infection:** a recurrent infection caused by new exposure to infective mosquitoes, best differentiated from recrudescence by molecular methods.
- **Endemicities:** this traditional measure has been based on different indicators over the years, and is most useful as a general description of the relationship between parasite transmission and malaria disease in a given setting (Table 96-6).
- **Stable malaria** is present when natural transmission occurs over many years and there is a predictable incidence of illness and prevalence of infection. Transmission is generally high and epidemics are unlikely.
- **Unstable malaria** occurs in settings where transmission rates vary from year to year and population immunity is low. Epidemics are more likely in this setting.
- **Autochthonous (indigenous) malaria** is contracted locally. Secondary cases are those derived from imported cases and are referred to as **introduced malaria**.
- **Induced malaria** is acquired by blood transfusion, shared needles, intentional inoculation, or laboratory accident.
- **Cryptic malaria** cases are those that occur in isolation and are not associated with secondary cases.
- **Imported malaria** infections are associated with individuals returning from malaria-endemic areas. Increased international air travel has escalated the incidence of **imported malaria** (and other infectious diseases) to non-endemic areas. Tourists often travel during the incubation period and do not become ill until after they return home.
- **Entomologic inoculation rate:** sporozoite positive mosquito bites per unit time.
- **Annual parasite incidence (API):** number of new parasite confirmed cases per 1000 population.
- **Spleen rate:** proportion of individuals in a stated age range with enlarged spleens.

acquired immunity can wax and wane with transmission intensity remains to be seen [6], but this will become increasingly important as malaria control efforts increase and expand.

INNATE IMMUNITY

On a population level, several genetic polymorphisms and mutations conferring risk or protection have been identified; most involve mutations in the alpha or beta chain of hemoglobin (hemoglobinopathies), such as sickle cell anemia and trait, the thalassemias, hemoglobin C, red blood cell enzyme deficiencies, such as glucose 6 phosphate deficiency (G6PD), or mutations affecting the red cell exoskeleton, such as ovalocytosis. Individuals with sickle cell trait (HbAS) are less likely to develop severe malaria once infected than are individuals who are homozygous (HbAA). Practically speaking, information on genetic polymorphisms is rarely available quickly enough to be useful during an acute illness; it may be potentially useful when considering risks associated with travel to malaria-endemic areas and it provides some insight into mechanisms of disease pathogenesis, susceptibility and protection.

NATURAL HISTORY, PATHOGENESIS, AND PATHOLOGY

Malaria is usually transmitted during the bite of an infected female *Anopheles* mosquito or, more rarely, through the direct inoculation of infected red blood cells (i.e. congenital malaria, transfusion malaria and malaria from contaminated needles).

LIFECYCLE

Infection begins when sporozoites in mosquito saliva enter the bloodstream and, within 30 minutes, have invaded hepatocytes (Fig 96.2). The duration of the asexual replication phase inside the hepatocytes varies from 11–12 days in *P. falciparum*, *P. vivax* and *P. ovale*, to 35 days in *P. malariae* (Table 96-1). The nucleus undergoes repeated division, resulting in the formation of thousands of uninucleate *merozoites*, each measuring 0.7–1.8 μm in diameter. The nucleus of the liver cell is displaced, but there is no inflammatory reaction in the surrounding liver tissue, and the host is asymptomatic.

In *P. falciparum* and *P. malariae* infections, the liver tissue schizonts/meronts rupture at about the same time and none persists in the liver. In contrast, *P. vivax* and *P. ovale* have two types of exoerythrocytic forms: a primary type develops and ruptures within 6–9 days; the secondary type – the hypnozoite – may remain dormant in the liver for weeks, months, or up to 5 years before developing, and causing *relapses* of erythrocytic infection unless the patient is treated with primaquine – a drug that targets this lifecycle stage. The pre-patent period for *P. knowlesi* in humans has not yet been determined. Most infected hepatocytes rupture when the schizont forms mature and the merozoites that are released into the circulation quickly attach to, and invade, red blood cells.

Plasmodium falciparum and *P. knowlesi* are capable of invading erythrocytes of any age, but *P. vivax* and *P. ovale* selectively invade reticulocytes. Serial cycles of asexual replication take place in erythrocytes and, again, the duration varies with the species, ranging from 24 hours in *P. knowlesi* to 48 hours in *P. falciparum*, *P. vivax* and *P. ovale*, and 72 hours in *P. malariae* (Table 96-1).

The youngest stages in the blood are small, rounded trophozoites, known as *ring forms*. As they grow, they become more irregular and ameboid. During development, the parasites consume hemoglobin leaving an iron-containing compound known as hematin or hemozoin as the product of digestion; it is visible in the cytoplasm of the parasite as dark granules. The schizont/meront stage begins when the

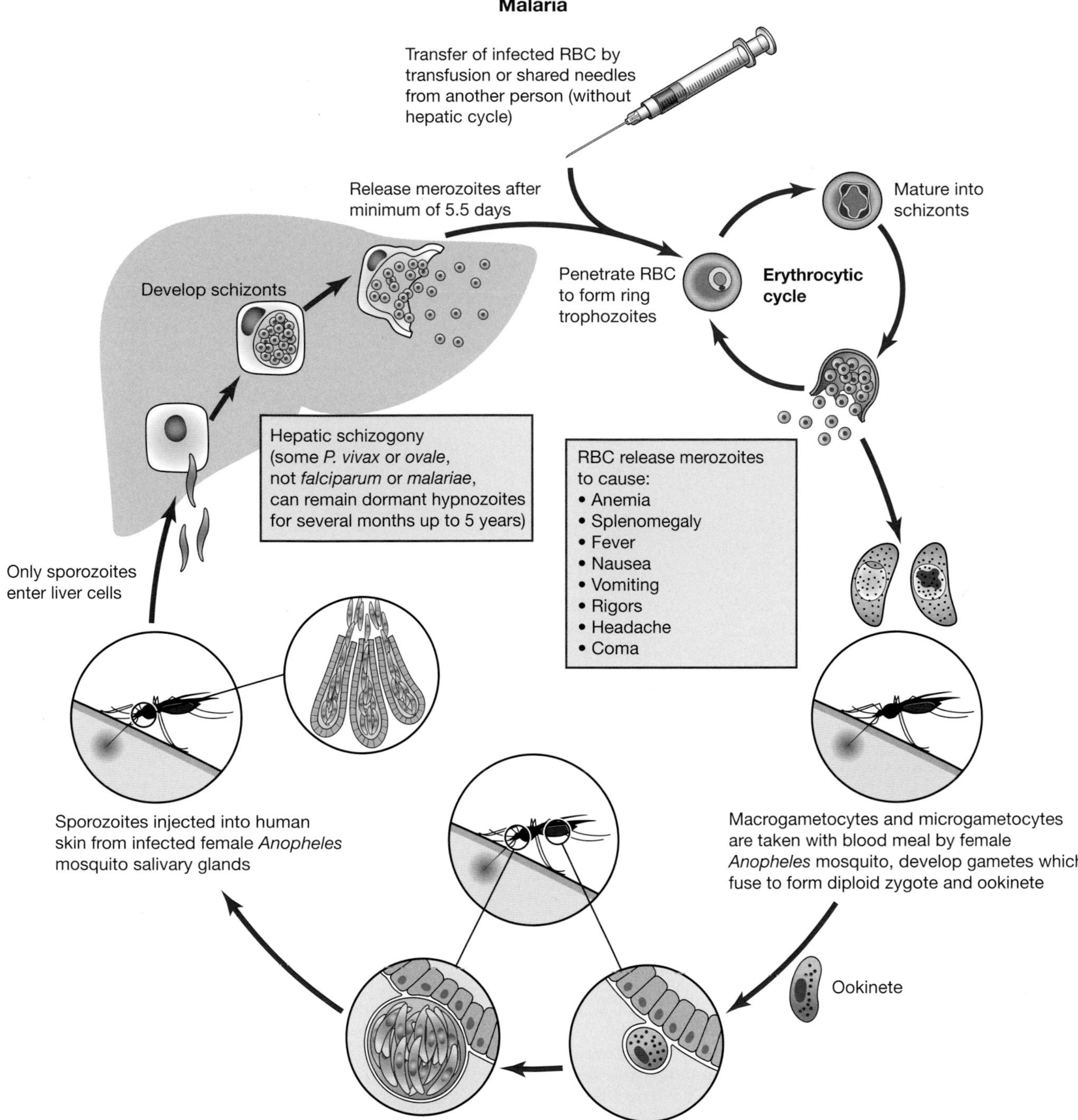

FIGURE 96.2 Malaria lifecycle.

parasite undergoes nuclear division and culminates in segmentation to form *merozoites.*

In response to a variety of stimuli, some parasites undergo gametocytogenesis. When male and female gametes are ingested by a female anopheline taking a blood meal from a human host, the sexual replication phase of the malaria parasite ensues, starting in the mosquito mid-gut and ending in the salivary glands. The erythrocytic lifecycle continues until it is abrogated by effective chemotherapy or reined in by the host's acquired immunity.

The life cycle of *P. falciparum* differs from the other four human malaria parasites in one important respect: during the latter half of the intra-erythrocytic cycle, mature falciparum-infected red blood cells (schizonts) effectively disappear from the peripheral blood. These late-stage parasites are very active metabolically, consuming up to 75 times more glucose than earlier ring stages and generating lactate as an end product. At this stage, the red cell surface is studded with "knobs" (proteins of parasite origin) and these mediate the cytoadherence of parasitized red cells to receptors on the luminal surface of endothelial cells. This leads to sequestration of the parasitized red cells in various organs (brain, gut, subcutaneous fat, cardiac muscle), particularly in capillaries and post-capillary venules, in such large numbers that blood flow is impaired [7] (Fig. 96.3).

The "natural history" of malaria infection and illness is difficult to capture. In its early stages, a malaria illness is indistinguishable from other common causes of fever. In endemic areas, and for returning travelers, if malaria infections are identified as such and treated

TABLE 96-1 Parasite Characteristics

Characteristic	*P. falciparum*	*P. vivax*	*P. malariae*	*P. ovale*	*P. knowlesi*
Geographic distribution	Widespread	Widespread, but rare in West Africa	West Africa, Philippines, Indonesia, Papua New Guinea	Infrequent, localized areas	South Asia
Clinical disease	Can be severe	Generally mild, occasionally severe	Generally mild*	Generally mild	Generally mild, but can be severe
Pre-patent period (days)	11–12	11–12	33	11–12	Unknown
Incubation period (days)	13–14	13–14	35	13–14	Unknown
Exoerythrocytic (liver) cycle (days)	5.5–7	6–8	9	12	16
Intra-erythrocytic cycle (hrs)	43–52	48	72	48	24
Sequestration-cytoadherence	Yes	No	No	No	No
Earliest appearance of gametocytes (days)	10	3	Unknown	Unknown	Unknown
Hypnozoite stage (i.e. potential for relapse from liver stage)	No	Yes	No	Yes	No
Age of red blood cell infected by the parasite	All ages	Reticulocytes	Reticulocytes	Older red cells	All ages
Peripheral parasitemia	High; multiply infected cells common	Low	Low	Low	May be high
Morphology (light microscope)					
Rings					
Trophozoites					
Schizonts	Rarely seen in peripheral blood, 16–20 merozoites	20–24 merozoites – generally more than 12	4–16 merozoites – usually <12	6–12 merozoites – usually <12	8–16 merozoites – usually <12
Gametocytes					

*Severe malaria in a patient thought to have *P. malariae* should raise the suspicion of *P. knowlesi*.

promptly with effective drugs, clinical progression is rare. If the initial symptoms are not attributed to malaria, "tertiary care" may not be sought until complications (commonly coma and convulsions) develop. Volunteers who are "challenged" with the bites of infected mosquitoes for research studies are provided with effective therapy at the first sign of infection and their natural history is truncated at that point. The mean incubation period (Box 96.1) is 8.9 days (range 7–14); the most commonly reported symptoms are fatigue, myalgias, arthralgias, headache, chills and nausea. The mean pre-patent period (Box 96.1) is slightly longer (10.5 days, range 9–14) and the appearance of peripheral parasitemia is associated with a mild, transient pancytopenia in most patients.

PATHOGENESIS

Pathophysiologic changes in malaria are caused by a number of different parasite-derived stimuli involving many different organ systems. Blood-stage parasites are the main source of these various stimuli; exoerythrocytic stages, gametocytes and sporozoites do not induce pathophysiologic changes. Malaria pathogenesis and pathology are linked inextricably to stages in the lifecycle (Fig. 96.2).

Fever

Schizont rupture is the likely source of the fevers associated with malaria, although the specific pyrogens have yet to be identified. The fevers are rarely as periodic as the erythrocytic cycles themselves, probably because parasite population dynamics within a host are not synchronous.

Anemia

Malarial anemia results largely from the hemolysis of infected red blood cells at the time of schizont rupture, accelerated immune-mediated destruction of uninfected red blood cells, bone marrow suppression and dyserythropoiesis, despite appropriate concentrations of erythropoietin. Severe intravascular hemolysis, also known as blackwater fever and manifesting as hemoglobinuria, can precipitate acute renal failure.

Hypoglycemia

Because of its deleterious effects on the central nervous system (CNS), and because of the necessity for treatment with exogenous glucose, this is the most important of the biochemical aberrations described to date [8]. Hypoglycemia (usually defined as blood glucose concentrations <40 mg/dL or 2.2 mmol/L) can develop, prior to any antimalarial treatment, in up to 20% of children with severe *P. falciparum* malaria. Plasma insulin levels are low and gluconeogenic precursors and adrenal hormones are present in high concentrations in the blood, so parasite consumption of glucose and/or inadequate hepatic gluconeogenesis are the most likely etiologies for pretreatment of hypoglycemia. It is not possible to detect hypoglycemia on clinical

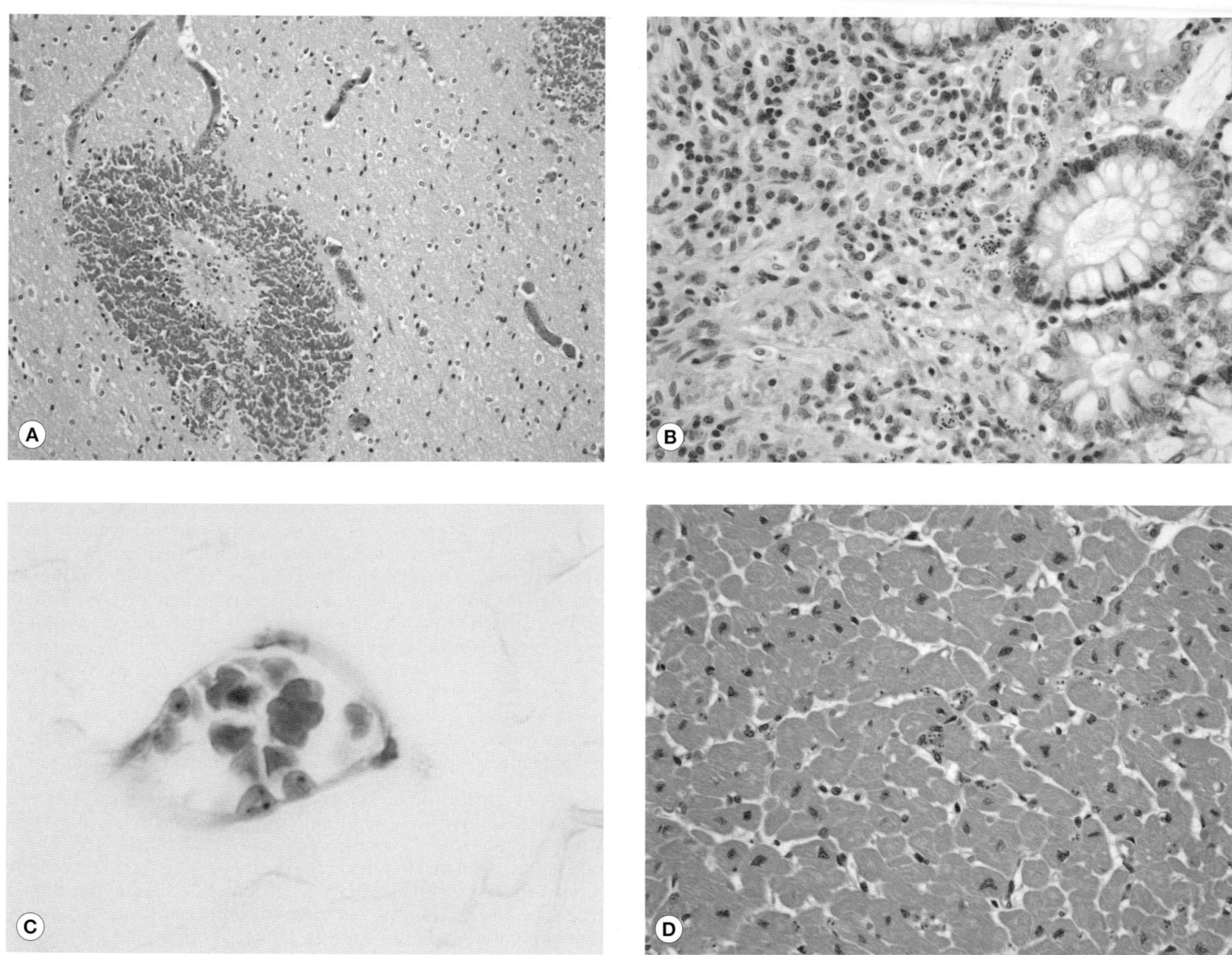

FIGURE 96.3 Four human tissue autopsy samples demonstrating sequestration and other pathologies in cerebral malaria. **(A)** The brain: several of the classic features can be seen including a ring hemorrhage surrounding a blood vessel which contains a fibrin plug; distended congested blood vessels throughout the section; and sequestered parasites (hematoxylin and eosin [H&E], 200×). **(B)** The colon has many parasites sequestered in tissues, similar to the entire glandular gastrointestinal tract, which are most prominent in the small capillaries of the lamina propria. In this section, the presence of later stage trophozoites and schizonts can be readily appreciated (H&E, 400×). **(C)** The adipose tissue of the skin can variably contain sequestered parasites within the rich vessel network (H&E, 1000×). Many other organs, including the heart **(D)**, show variable amounts of sequestered parasites (H&E, 400×). *(Courtesy of Dr Danny A Milner).*

grounds in these patients, so in situations where the blood glucose cannot be measured in comatose parasitemic patients, immediate treatment with 50% dextrose is recommended. Unconscious patients who present with pretreatment hypoglycemia have a worse prognosis than those who do not, and the risk of a poor outcome is inversely associated with blood glucose concentrations, even those above the traditional cutoff of 2.2 mmol/L (40 mg/dL) [8]. Anti-malarial treatment can precipitate hypoglycemia. Rapid infusions of quinine (>10 mg/kg/hr) can stimulate pancreatic insulin secretion; pregnant women appear to be especially susceptible to this complication of treatment.

Metabolic acidosis

Acidosis is now recognized as an important marker of severity in falciparum malaria infections. "Acidotic breathing" alone was associated with a 19% mortality rate in Kenyan children. In this population, the mortality rate in children with impaired consciousness uncomplicated by acidotic breathing was 12%; in children with acidotic breathing and impaired consciousness, the mortality rate was 32% [8] (Fig. 96.4). Elevated plasma and cerebrospinal fluid (CSF) lactate levels are also associated with a poor outcome but few studies have examined both pH and lactate, so although they are likely to be highly correlated, the precise relationship is not known. Acidosis and hypoglycemia are strongly associated, suggesting parasite and/or host metabolism may be contributing to both. Full-blown circulatory shock is rarely a feature of severe and complicated malaria, so grossly impaired perfusion is unlikely to be a cause of the metabolic acidosis of malaria. This acidosis generally improves rapidly once intravenous (IV) treatment with an effective anti-malarial drug and maintenance fluids is started. The transient nature of the acidosis is consistent with the possibility that seizures are a contributing factor. Convulsions are common in malaria, and seizures alone can cause an acute lactic acidosis. Acidosis persists longer in those patients who die and is also associated with a slower respiratory rate; this suggests that the usual centrally-mediated respiratory response to metabolic acidosis may be compromised in these patients.

Acute respiratory distress (ARDS)

Non-cardiogenic pulmonary edema is a common feature of complicated malaria in adults, but only rarely develops in children. The specific cause of this syndrome in malaria patients has yet to be identified [9].

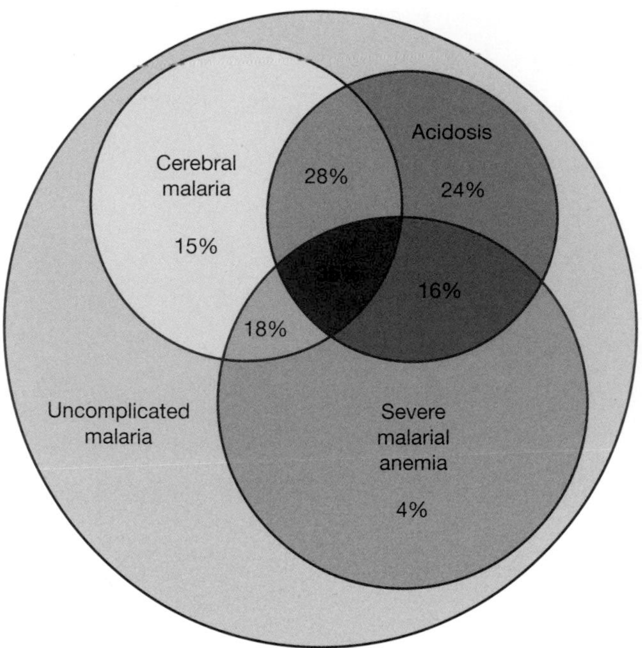

FIGURE 96.4 Venn diagram of complicated malaria syndromes. The percentage values represent the mortality rates in Kenyan children with the various syndromes. *(Adapted from Marsh K, Forster D, Waruiru C, et al. Indicators of life-threatening malaria in African children. N Engl J Med 1995;332: 1399–404).*

Renal abnormalities

Nonspecific mildly elevated urea nitrogen and creatinine levels, proteinuria and abnormal urinary sediment are common in malaria. Acute renal failure is a common complication of severe malaria, particularly in adults. As in cerebral malaria, the insult often resolves and most patients do not require long-term dialysis [10].

Neurologic changes and coma

The clinical syndrome of cerebral malaria is associated with the sequestration of erythrocytes harboring late-stage *P. falciparum* parasites (trophozoites and schizonts) in the cerebral microcirculation. Putative mechanisms include obstruction leading to hypoperfusion with anoxic damage, endothelial cell activation and blood–brain barrier compromise, and platelet activation with microthrombus formation (Fig. 96.3). Alternatively, a cytokine cascade leading to a systemic inflammatory response-type scenario, initiated by the interaction of parasitized red cells and host immune cells has been postulated; this mechanism would be independent of sequestration and could be invoked for the other four species of malaria parasite involved in human disease [11].

CLINICAL FEATURES

PRODROMAL SYMPTOMS

Some patients have vague prodromal symptoms, such as malaise, myalgia, low back pain, headache, anorexia and mild fever, before parasitemia can be detected by the usual microscopic techniques. These manifestations may persist for 2–3 days before an acute paroxysm begins. The incubation period, or time from exposure to onset of symptoms, can be prolonged by partial immunity and/or by chemoprophylaxis.

PERIODICITY

In primary attacks, several days are required before the periodicity predicted by the lengths of various parasite lifecycles is established. Often, in patients with "asynchronous" infections, this periodicity is never clinically apparent. After 5–7 days, *P. vivax, P. malariae* and *P. ovale* infections can become synchronous and cause periodic febrile paroxysms. In *P. vivax* and *P. falciparum* malaria, schizonts mature and rupture with tertian periodicity, i.e. every 48 hours; *P. vivax* malaria has been referred to as *benign tertian malaria* and *P. falciparum* malaria as *malignant tertian malaria. Plasmodium malariae* schizonts rupture at 72-hour intervals, causing a quartan periodicity. The typical paroxysm has an abrupt onset with a feeling of coldness and a chill. The patient's teeth may chatter prompting the need for warmth or cover. Within 30–60 minutes, the patient feels hot and has profuse sweating, usually accompanied by a headache, malaise and myalgia. Temperatures of 40–41 °C (104–106 °F) are usual in primary falciparum infections, but peak fevers in infections with the other three species of plasmodia are usually lower, i.e. 39–40 °C (102–104 °F). The hot stage lasts from 2–6 hours. The sweating stage, in which the patient's temperature falls rapidly, lasts 2–3 hours. The entire paroxysm averages 9–10 hours. In between paroxysms, the patient may feel well.

UNCOMPLICATED MALARIA

Uncomplicated malaria illness is by far the most common clinical manifestation of a malaria infection and fever, or history of fever, is the most common symptom. There are no pathognomonic signs by which "uncomplicated malaria" can be distinguished from common viral causes of fever (Box 96.2). The presence of malaria parasitemia increases the odds of a causal connection, especially in non-immune individuals, where peripheral parasitemia is nearly always associated with symptoms. Many semi-immune individuals (generally long-term residents of malaria-endemic areas) can harbor parasites without becoming symptomatic and, in these individuals, peripheral blood parasitemia may well be "incidental" to the symptoms [12]. In practical terms, symptomatic, parasitemic individuals who are alert enough to take oral medications are considered to have "uncomplicated malaria".

Important aspects of the clinical history include travel itinerary, malaria precautions (chemoprophylaxis, use of bed nets and repellents) and recent prior treatment with anti-malarial drugs. The physical exam is useful for identifying *other* potential etiologies. In endemic areas, the presence of hepato- or splenomegaly tilt the differential diagnosis toward malaria, as does thrombocytopenia. For non-immune travelers, the presence of fever, splenomegaly, hyperbilirubinemia and thrombocytopenia make malaria more likely [13].

Common presenting signs are generalized constitutional symptoms including fever, chills, dizziness, backache, myalgia, malaise and fatigue (frequently summarized as "total body pain" by endemic-area adults). Gastrointestinal symptoms (i.e. anorexia, nausea, vomiting, abdominal pain and diarrhea) can be prominent, causing confusion with gastroenteritis. Patients may have nonproductive cough and dyspnea, consistent with acute respiratory infections. Young children and semi-immune adults may present with only fever and headache.

LABORATORY FINDINGS

Anemia, leukopenia and thrombocytopenia are usual. The reticulocyte count is normal or depressed, despite the hemolysis, and becomes elevated usually 5–7 days after the parasitemia has cleared. Urinalysis reveals albuminuria and urobilinogen; increased conjugated bilirubin is present in many patients. Some patients are jaundiced and concomitant abnormalities in liver function tests may cause diagnostic confusion with viral hepatitis. Serum alanine aminotransferase (ALT) and aspartate transaminase (AST), are usually elevated. Both the direct and the indirect bilirubin can be elevated. Prothrombin times can be prolonged. Hyponatremia is not uncommon; in some patients, the clinical picture is consistent with inappropriate secretion of antidiuretic hormone (ADH), but this is not a universal finding. Increases in serum creatinine and blood urea nitrogen may be transient, or they may presage acute renal failure. Hypoglycemia frequently complicates falciparum malaria and can occur both before treatment and as a result of quinine therapy.

The five human malaria parasites have similar clinical presentations for uncomplicated disease and are best distinguished from each other

BOX 96.2 Differential Diagnosis of Uncomplicated Malaria*

	Symptoms	Physical exam	Lab tests	Geography
Malaria	Fever Nonspecific myalgias, arthalgia, malaise Nausea, vomiting	Hepatomegaly Splenomegaly	Malaria smear positive Thrombocytopenia Hyperbilirubinemia	Primarily tropical areas
Viral syndromes (flu, pneumonia, early gastroenteritis)	Fever Nonspecific myalgias, arthalgia, malaise Nausea, vomiting	Lymphadenopathy	Low white cell count, lymphocyte predominant	Worldwide, frequently seen in local epidemics
Bacterial pneumonia	Fever Productive cough	Tachypnea Increased respiratory effort (inter- and subcostal recession, use of accessory muscles) Crepitations (rales) Decreased oxygen saturation (<90%)	Leukocytosis	Worldwide
Meningitis (bacterial or viral)	Fever Altered mental status	Neck stiffness	Concomitant parasitemia uncommon in bacterial meningitis WBCs in CSF (> 5–10/μl, or >10 times higher than the predicted CSF WBC count†)	
Dengue	Retro-orbital pain Pain/tenderness of the extraocular eye muscles, particularly on extreme lateral gaze	Skin rash develops in at least 50% by day 2–3	Leukopenia Thrombocytopenia	Less common in sub-Saharan Africa
Leptospirosis	Fever, headache, dry cough, shaking, chills, nausea, vomiting, diarrhea, muscle pain, abdominal pain	Muscle tenderness (myositis), conjunctivitis, hepatosplenomegaly	Elevated creatine kinase, abnormal urine sediment, proteinuria, normal to elevated WBC counts	Worldwide distribution, association with fresh-water exposure
Typhus	High fever, dry cough, low back pain, headache, nausea, vomiting, abdominal pain, diarrhea, nausea, chills, delirium, photophobia, myalgia	Rash begins on the chest and spreads to the rest of the body (except the palms of the hands and soles of the feet). The early rash is a light rose color and fades when pressed. Later, the rash becomes dull and red and does not fade. People with severe typhus may also develop small areas of bleeding into the skin (petechiae)	Anemia Thrombocytopenia Two-to-five-fold elevation of liver enzymes	Worldwide distribution, murine typhus (*Rickettsia typhi*) seen in areas of poor hygiene and cold tempertures. Epidemic typhus (*Rickettsia prowzekii*) associated with exposure to rat fleas or rat feces
Viral hemorrhagic fevers	Fever, bleeding diathesis, malaise, fatigue, myalgias, headache, vomiting, diarrhea, hypotension, shock	Flushing of the face and chest, frank bleeding, ecchymoses, renal failure, edema	Cytopenias seen early in illness with elevated WBC seen in late disease, coagulation abnormalities	Worldwide distribution and caused by several families of RNA viruses

*Individual patients may have more than one diagnosis.
†Predicted CSF WBC count/μl = CSF RBC count × (peripheral blood WBC count ÷ peripheral blood RBC count).
CSF, cerebrospinal fluid; RBC, red blood cell; WBC, white blood cell.

by geography (Fig. 96.1), by parasite density (parasitemias >2% are more commonly seen in *P. falciparum* and *P. knowlesi*) and by parasite morphology – best appreciated on thin blood films (Table 96.1). Low-grade infections of *P. malariae* can persist for years and individuals with *P. vivax* and *P. ovale* may have pre-patent periods of a year or more.

Non-immune individuals with *P. falciparum* infections may deteriorate very rapidly; prompt and effective treatment in this high-risk group is important and should be provided on an emergent basis. When feasible, patients should be monitored closely to detect early signs of clinical deterioration. A high index of suspicion is warranted for travelers and others who have been in malaria-endemic areas.

TABLE 96-2 Features of Complicated Malaria

Physical findings	Laboratory investigations
• Impaired consciousness/ unrousable coma (Blantyre Coma Score ≤2) (children > adults) • Prostration (unable to walk or sit up) • Failure to feed • Convulsions (more than 2 in 24 hours) (children > adults) • Acidotic breathing (children > adults) • Shock (systolic blood pressure <70 mmHg in adults, <50 mmHg in children) • Clinical jaundice + evidence of another organ dysfunction (adults > children) • Abnormal spontaneous bleeding • Pulmonary edema (radiologic evidence) (adults > children)	• Hypoglycemia (<2.2 mmol/L or 40 mg/dl) (children > adults) • Metabolic acidosis (plasma bicarbonate <15 mmol/L) (children > adults) • Severe anemia (hemoglobin <5 g/dl, PCV < 15%) (children > adults) • Hemoglobinuria • Hyperparasitemia (>2%, or 100,000/μl in low transmission setting, >5%, or 250,000/μl in high transmission settings) • Hyperlactatemia (>5 mmol/L) • Renal impairment (creatinine> 265 μmol/L) (adults > children)

PCV, packed cell volume.

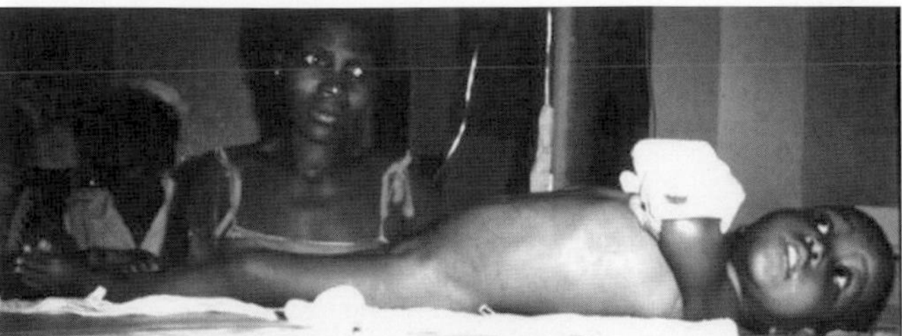

FIGURE 96.5 Child in coma with eyes wide open.

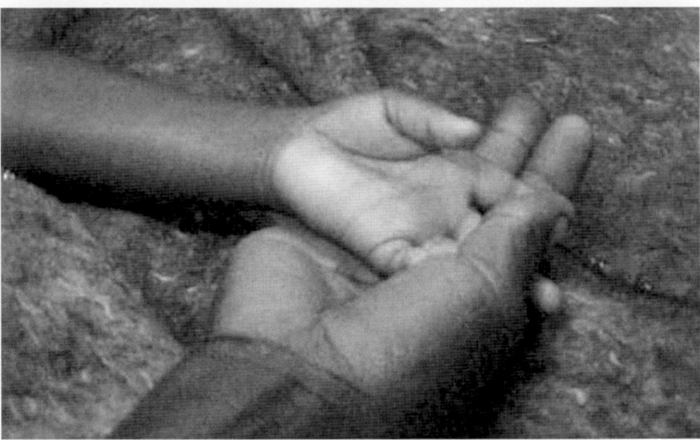

FIGURE 96.6 Pallor.

Serial examination of the peripheral blood (every 12 hours) may aid in the identification of low density parasitemias; thrombocytopenia is another helpful clue in oligo-parasitemic or initially aparasitemic patients.

COMPLICATED MALARIA

Long considered to be unique to falciparum malaria, several of the features of complicated malaria (Table 96-2) have now been described in patients with *P. vivax* and *P. knowlesi* infections. In addition to the complications described in Table 96-2, splenic rupture is a rare complication of *P. vivax* infections, and nephrotic syndrome is occasionally seen in patients after a *P. malariae* illness.

In a parasitemic patient, the presence of any of the clinical or laboratory features of complicated malaria represents a medical emergency; these patients should be provided with the best available medical care.

The clinical presentation of complicated malaria is different in adults than it is in children (Table 96-2). Cerebral malaria alone is more characteristic of pediatric severe malaria, whereas multi-organ system involvement is seen frequently in adults with complicated malaria illnesses.

Cerebral malaria is a highly variable clinical syndrome consisting of *P. falciparum* parasitemia of any density and coma (Blantyre Coma Score ≤2 in children/Glasgow Coma Score ≤9 in adults, unrelated to hypoglycemia, meningitis or a postictal state). Children with cerebral malaria frequently demonstrate symptoms suggesting widespread involvement of the CNS, including generalized tonic-clonic convulsions, focal seizures, posturing (opisthotonos, decerebrate rigidity, decorticate rigidity), conjugate gaze deviations and respiratory rhythm abnormalities (including Cheyne-Stokes respirations). Convulsions (focal and generalized) are very common, particularly in children. Intracranial pressure is often elevated in children with cerebral malaria and deaths consistent with various herniation syndromes have been described. An unusual feature of pediatric malarial comas is that the eyes are frequently wide open (Fig. 96.5) – this can be confusing for parents and caregivers. Among patients who survive, the recovery is relatively rapid; most children who survive an episode of cerebral malaria have regained full consciousness within 48 hours. The rapid evolution and reversibility of the dramatic neurologic features of cerebral malaria are among the most intriguing aspects of the disease.

The clinical history is generally notable for a sudden deterioration in the patient's clinical status – the transition from uncomplicated to complicated malaria can be as brief as a single seizure.

With point-of-care bedside tests for malaria parasitemia, blood glucose, hemoglobin or hematocrit and lactate combined with a careful physical examination, nearly all patients with complicated malaria can be identified quickly and without sophisticated laboratory support.

Important elements of the physical examination include inspection for prostration (the inability to sit unaided or, in infants who cannot yet sit, to look for the mother's breast and feed) and deep breathing, assessing the Blantyre [14] or Glasgow Coma Score (Box 96.3), inspecting nail beds and conjunctivae for pallor (Fig. 96.6), cardiac and pulmonary auscultation for signs of high output cardiac failure (i.e. a systolic murmur, a gallop rhythm, widened pulse pressure, enlarging liver), measuring blood pressure and checking capillary refill (Box 96.4) (to identify patients in shock), and palpating the abdomen to identify hepato- and splenomegaly and urinary retention. Acute renal failure will become evident over time on the basis of urinary output and can be confirmed by measures of serum creatinine. In order to identify hyperparasitemia, the capacity to stain blood films and count parasites is required.

Among patients meeting the standard clinical case definition of cerebral malaria [15], a careful ocular funduscopic exam is very useful for distinguishing patients with "true" cerebral malaria from patients with incidental parasitemias and a non-malarial cause of coma (see *"Complicated Malaria"* below).

METABOLIC ACIDOSIS

Capillary blood pH <7.3, plasma bicarbonate <15 mmol/L or plasma lactate concentrations >5 mmol/L are all associated with severe disease and with poor outcomes. Acidosis, manifested clinically as

BOX 96.3 Coma Scales for Adults and Children

	Glasgow Coma Scale (GCS; adults)		Blantyre Coma Score (BCS; children)	
Motor Response (to painful stimuli: pressure on nail bed, sternum, supraorbital ridge)	Obeys commands	6		
	Localizes	5	Localizes	2
	Flexion/withdraws	4	Withdraws	1
	Abormal flexion (decorticate)	3		
	Extension (decerebrate)	2	Extension (decerebrate)	0
	No response	1	No response	0
Verbal Response (to painful stimuli or speech)	Oriented, converses normally	5	Normal cry, appropriate speech	2
	Confused, disoriented	4		
	Utters inappropriate words	3		
	Incomprehensible sounds	2	Abnormal cry	1
	Makes no sounds	1	Makes no sounds	0
Eyes	Opens eyes spontaneously	4		
	Opens eyes in response to voice	3		
	Opens eyes in response to pain	2	Follows moving objects	1
	Does not open eyes	1	Unable to follow moving objects	0

BOX 96.4 Assessing Capillary Refill

1. Observe the color of the nail bed.
2. Press on the nail bed of any digit until it blanches completely.
3. Release pressure.
4. Count ("one-one thousand, two-one thousand) until the nail bed completely regains its normal color.
5. Normal capillary refill is <2 seconds; prolonged capillary refill times suggest that the patient is in shock.

Self-calibration by the examining clinician is helpful.

abnormally deep breathing is a poor prognostic feature in parasitemic children with or without neurologic compromise.

SEVERE ANEMIA

Life-threatening anemia can develop rapidly; children who have adjusted to a low hemoglobin or hematocrit can rapidly decompensate when challenged by a febrile illness such as malaria. Decisions regarding blood transfusion are difficult, particularly in malaria-endemic areas where HIV infection is common. Decisions to transfuse are generally made on the basis of hemodynamic grounds (signs of high-output heart failure include hypotension, poor capillary refill, systolic murmurs and hepatosplenomegaly), level of consciousness and evidence of acidosis. Estimates of parasite density are helpful in predicting the need for blood transfusion (see below, *"Treatment"*). Anemic children who are clinically stable may be treated conservatively, but close observation is recommended.

RESPIRATORY FAILURE

Respiratory failure associated with ARDS can develop rapidly; clinically it is indistinguishable from the ARDS that develops as a result of septicemia, toxic inhalants or other causes. Patients become hypoxemic and may require mechanically-assisted ventilation. Aggressive management of malaria-associated ARDS should be used wherever available.

ALGID MALARIA

The majority of patients with severe malaria remain well perfused, but a small proportion develop algid malaria – defined as low blood pressure, cold and clammy extremities, hypoglycemia and acidosis. In most cases, this represents septic shock and pathogens are cultured from the blood. The judicious administration of antibiotics, fluids and inotropes is recommended for this small group of patients. The sudden onset of hypotension in a patient with vivax malaria should prompt consideration of splenic rupture or subcapsular bleeding.

ACUTE RENAL FAILURE

Mild proteinura, azotemia and oliguria occur frequently in otherwise uncomplicated *P. falciparum* infections. Acute renal failure is another complication that is far more common among adults than among children; it is also more common in patients with hemoglobinuria ("blackwater fever"). Acute renal failure can also result from acute tubular necrosis, a sequelae of reduced renal perfusion. Anuria is a poor prognostic sign and hemoperfusion, renal or peritoneal dialysis are often necessary. Few data exist to describe the proportion of patients on dialysis who recover renal function but, as in cerebral malaria, renal abnormalities are reversible and patients appropriately supported through the critical period often enjoy a full recovery.

POST-MALARIA NEUROLOGIC SYNDROME

This is a rare transient neurologic syndrome, reported most commonly in non-immune travelers after a successfully treated episode of severe falciparum malaria. The onset is generally within 1–2 weeks of recovery, but can be as long as 2 months after. The clinical features range from confusion and tremors, to aphasia, seizures, ataxia, psychosis and impaired consciousness. There may be a lymphocytic pleocytosis in the CSF; imaging studies may or may not show nonspecific white matter changes. The symptoms are generally self-limiting; steroids have been used with good results in some patients [16].

MALARIA IN PREGNANCY

The effects of malaria infection in pregnancy are visited on the expectant mother via peripheral parasitemia and on the fetus/newborn via parasite sequestration in the intervillous spaces of the placenta.

In general, pregnant woman are more susceptible to malaria infection than their non-pregnant counterparts; this is most noticeable in areas of low transmission, where few adults have acquired anti-disease immunity. Susceptibility to infection decreases with each succeeding pregnancy.

The placenta provides a new site for sequestration, a phenomenon unique to infections with *P. falciparum*, and, as with peripheral parasitemia, semi-immune women are less likely to have placental sequestration than non-immune women, and the placentae of multigravidae are less likely to contain evidence of parasite sequestration than those of primigravidae. The receptor on the syncytiotrophoblast lining the intervillous spaces of the placenta is chondroitin sulfate A, and binding is mediated by a specific variant surface antigen, var2csa [17].

Clinical manifestations in the mother are determined by the extent of acquired immunity. In sub-Saharan Africa, where most studies have been carried out, mild febrile illnesses and anemia are the most common features. In relatively non-immune pregnant women, severe and complicated malaria, often characterized by hypoglycemia and pulmonary edema, can occur. Pregnancy-induced immune suppression generally results in more severe disease, especially in the group at highest risk, primigravid, non-immune women. Parasitemia rates are at their highest during the second trimester, and the period of increased risk can extend into the post-partum period for 1–2 months [18].

Adverse maternal and perinatal outcomes of malaria in pregnancy include anemia, miscarriage, fetal growth restriction (small for gestational age), low birth weight (<2500 g at birth), pre-term births and congenital infection. Again, the likelihood of these outcomes is related to maternal gravidity and degree of acquired anti-malarial immunity.

TRANSFUSION MALARIA

Any of the five species of human malaria can be transmitted directly from an infected blood donor, accidental infection by a contaminated needle, or from infected intravenous drug users sharing needles. The incubation period following infection is as short as a few days for *P. falciparum*, but can be up to 40 days or longer for *P. malariae* [19].

PATIENT EVALUATION, DIAGNOSIS AND DIFFERENTIAL DIAGNOSIS

UNCOMPLICATED MALARIA

At the individual patient level, accurate diagnosis and treatment of uncomplicated malaria enhances the chances of a prompt cure and minimizes the likelihood of disease progression. At the population level, the appropriate management of uncomplicated malaria, particularly large numbers of patients with uncomplicated malaria, as is common in endemic areas, will diminish the reservoir of infected individuals while minimizing the development and spread of drug-resistant parasites.

To minimize the unnecessary or inappropriate use of anti-malarial drugs, parasitologic confirmation of clinically suspected cases is now recommended by the World Health Organization (WHO) [20]. Malaria parasites can be identified in a sample of peripheral blood via light microscopy or using rapid diagnostic tests (RDTs), which are based on the detection of parasite enzymes or antigens. When it is performed well, light microscopy is sensitive and specific and allows for the recognition of various malaria parasite species. There is a large initial cost for acquiring equipment and training technicians, and ongoing quality assurance and quality control are expensive, but the day-to-day operational costs are low, especially when high throughput is required. The "gold standard" approach uses Giemsa stain and oil-immersion microscopy.

RDTs are antigen-based dipstick, cassette or card tests in which a colored line indicates that plasmodial antigens have been detected. They are relatively simple to perform and interpret and they do not require electricity, but not all tests can distinguish between species, and some cannot distinguish new infections from recently and effectively-treated infections (Box 96.5). The choice of a specific RDT

BOX 96.5 Microscopy versus Malaria Rapid Diagnostic Tests (RDTs)

	Thin film microscopy	Thick film microscopy	RDTs
Speciation	Yes	Possible	Yes
Quantification	Yes	Optimal	RDTs give qualitative "yes" or "no" results but intensity of the parasite line correlates to antigen present
Can use to follow response to treatment	Yes	Yes	No; HRP2- based tests specific for *P. falciparum* can remain positive for days after successful treatment.
Electricity required	Yes	Yes	No
Training and skill required	Extensive training; acquired skill		Limited training; can be used in remote settings
Sensitivity	Vary by skill of microscopist		Vary among tests
Cost	May be less expensive in busy settings		$0.50–$1 per test
Storage			Temperature ranges; humidity a problem unless individually foil-wrapped
Detects other pathogens in blood	White cell count, platelet count, *Borrelia*, *Trypanosoma*, *Babesia* spp.		No
Malaria parasites detected	All species Species differentiation on the basis of different morphologies	All species	*P. falciparum* only and *P. falciparum*/*P. vivax* combinations
Mixed infections	Yes	Yes	Usually no
False-positives	Artifact	Artifact	Antigenemia can persist after parasitemia has cleared
False-negatives	Low parasite density		Prozone effect Low parasite density

HRP2, histidine-rich protein 2.

depends on its intended use. For example, does it need to distinguish between a recent malaria infection and a current infection? Should it be able to distinguish between falciparum and non-falciparum species? Will treatment decisions be based on the results, or is it being employed for epidemiologic purposes?

The choice of which malaria RDT to use in a given situation is complex and depends on availability, cost, quality of the test and performance characteristics. The WHO sponsors independent RDT product testing in collaboration with the Foundation for Innovative New Diagnostics (FIND), the Special Program for Research and Training in Tropical Diseases (TDR) and the WHO Global Malaria Program (GMP). Testing is performed at the US Centers for Disease Control and Prevention (CDC). Summary results of the most recent round are available online [21]. These comparisons help to inform procurement decisions for national malaria control programs and to guide United Nations (UN) procurement policies.

In resource-constrained endemic areas, parasitologic diagnosis is not always available – even when it is available, quality and accuracy are a continuing challenge. When parasitologic diagnoses are not available, algorithms devised on the basis of the prevalence of parasitemia in various age groups [22] help to balance the risk of under-treating those at risk of progressing to severe disease against the risks of unnecessary drug use in the semi-immune population, excessive costs and drug pressure, which could accelerate the development of drug resistant parasites.

Serial parasitologic assessments after the start of treatment are helpful for documenting response to treatment; if these are paired with an assessment of anemia (either hemoglobin concentration or hematocrit), it may be possible to anticipate the need for blood transfusion (see below for guidelines).

BLOOD FILMS

The gold standard of malaria diagnosis remains the blood film. For detecting parasites, a thick blood film is superior as it concentrates the red cells by a factor of 20–40. Identifying species on thick films may be difficult because the red cells have lysed and the morphologic features of the parasites have been altered. Species identifications are made more easily using thin blood films. Thick and thin films can be prepared on the same slide, although they are processed differently (thin films must be fixed in methanol before they are stained). Quantitating parasitemias, even semiquantitatively (0, + - ++++) is useful for predicting whether the illness is likely to be caused by malaria, for anticipating the need for blood transfusion and for following response to anti-malarial treatment.

Parasites can be counted as a percentage of red cells on a thin film, or against white blood cells on a thick film, and if the total red cell or white cell counts are known, the parasite densities can be calculated. Blood can be stained with Giemsa, Leishman, Field or Wright's stains.

The most important initial distinction is to determine whether malaria parasites are present: for this, a thick film is most efficient. Species identification is best done on thin films (Table 96-1). The golden brown malaria pigment (hemozoin) in monocytes or leukocytes suggests a current or recent malaria infection, even in the absence of a patent parasitemia.

INTERPRETING THE RESULTS OF MALARIA DIAGNOSTIC TESTS

In practice, clinicians in malaria-endemic areas with little diagnostic capacity prescribe anti-malarial drugs to symptomatic individuals whenever parasites are detected; however, the clinical challenge is to decide if *additional* treatment (e.g. antibiotics) is needed. In semi-immune individuals, asymptomatic or "incidental" parasitemia is common, and the presence of peripheral parasitemia can be misleading. In these individuals, it would be prudent to consider other etiologies for the symptoms, particularly in patients with lower density parasitemias (Box 96.2). Anti-malarial treatment is warranted if parasites are detected, but additional treatment may also be required.

A second dilemma is the febrile individual with a *negative* malaria test. Withholding anti-malarial drugs in situations where malaria infection is a real possibility is difficult for clinicians. The dangers of missing a malaria diagnosis and thus delaying treatment are well known. This apprehension, accompanied by a degree of skepticism regarding the reliability of the parasitologic diagnosis (especially via microscopy), is used to justify a "better safe than sorry" approach to the use of anti-malarial drugs. In malaria-endemic areas, patients themselves, along with parents and other caregivers, have come to expect malaria chemotherapy for many febrile illnesses. Clinical evidence for other non-malaria diagnoses should be sought (Box 96.2) to support the decision to withhold anti-malarials in patients who are not infected with plasmodia.

The absence of parasites in the peripheral blood should prompt the clinician to consider other etiologies of the patient's symptoms. In non-immune patients at risk for malaria infection, several parasitologic assessments carried out at 12-hour intervals during a 36–48 hour period are recommended before concluding that the individual is free of infection. Intra-erythrocytic falciparum parasites are typically in circulation for the first 24–36 hours of the 48-hour lifecycle, and the intra-erythrocytic parasites for the other four infecting species are always present in the peripheral blood, so it is not necessary to "time" blood collections to any particular symptoms (e.g. fever, rigor, diaphoresis). The WHO recommends withholding anti-malarial treatment in the face of negative (often repeatedly negative) tests; in practice, as noted above, this can be difficult, given the well-known dangers of untreated malaria and the challenges of obtaining a reliable parasitologic diagnosis.

COMPLICATED MALARIA

Parasitemic individuals with any of the clinical or laboratory features described in Table 96-2 are likely to have complicated malaria, but the possibility of a "false-positive" assessment should be considered, particularly (but not exclusively) in the semi-immune population. The mortality rate of untreated severe malaria is probably over 75%; with good management, the mortality rate of cerebral malaria is roughly 15–20%.

Concomitant meningitis should be excluded via lumbar puncture; if a lumbar puncture is contraindicated on clinical grounds, the patient should be provided with the appropriate antibiotic coverage (penicillin + gentamicin, or ceftriaxone).

Co-infections with blood-borne bacteria are common and should be sought when the capacity exists [23, 24]. Septic shock should be considered in the differential diagnosis and empiric antibiotic therapy administered if there are signs of acidosis or impaired perfusion.

An autopsy-based study of pediatric cerebral malaria demonstrated that the standard clinical case definition of cerebral malaria was incorrect in approximately 25% of cases – non-malarial causes of death were identified and those patients had no evidence of parasite sequestration in the cerebral microcirculation. In contrast, 75% of cases in this series did have cerebral sequestration of parasitized erythrocytes and no other causes of death were identified at autopsy [25]. The best clinical indicator of "true" cerebral malaria was the presence of at least one of the three features of a recently described malaria retinopathy: vessel color changes, macular or extra-macular whitening, and white-centered hemorrhages [26] (Fig 96.7). With autopsy findings as the gold standard, the specificity of retinal findings is 93%, the sensitivity is 97% and the positive and negative predictive values are 97% and 93% respectively.

Malarial retinopathy is best appreciated in eyes that have been fully dilated with mydriatics (a combination of tropicamide and phenylephrine eye drops will dilate the eyes within 15–20 minutes) and examined with a hand-held direct ophthalmoscope (which provides magnification) and an indirect ophthalmoscope (which provides a three-dimensional perspective, as well as a wider field of view). These examinations are routine for trained ophthalmologists, but non-ophthalmologist clinicians can learn to recognize these features, too. Ninety percent of retinopathy-positive patients can be identified on

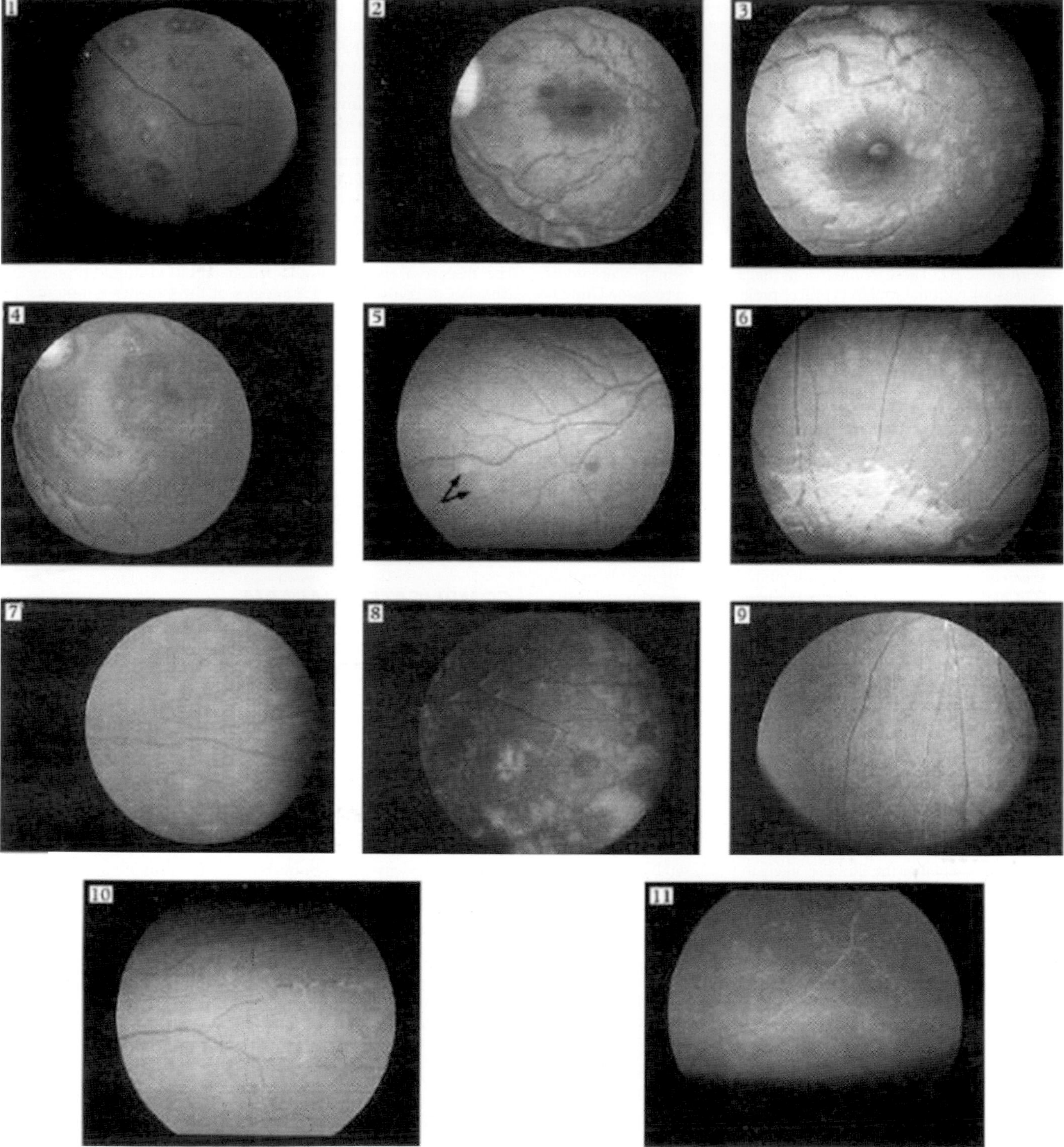

FIGURE 96.7 Malaria retinopathy. Examples of clinical ocular fundus findings in African children with *P. falciparum* malaria. 1, Retinal hemorrhages, some with white centers. 2. Grade 2 macular whitening, less than 1/3 of the disc area of whitening. 3. Grade 2 macular whitening, between 1/3 and 1 disc area of whitening. 4. Grade 3 macular whitening, greater than 1 disc area of whitening. 5. Grade 1 extramacular whitening, note 2 foci of whitening. 6. Grade 2 extramacular whitening; scattered white spots in the upper half of the photograph represent the density of whitening for the 2+ grade. 7. Grade 3 extramacular whitening; this definite mosaic represents the minimum whitening for the 3+ grade. 8. Grade 3 extramacular whitening; confluence of whitening. 9. Abnormal vessels; orange delineation of vessels. 10. Abnormal vessels; segmental whitening. 11. Abnormal vessels, extensive delineation of capillaries with some irregular delineation of terminal portion of larger vessels. *(From Lewallen S, Harding SP, Ajewole J, et al. A review of the spectrum of clinical ocular fundus findings in P. falciparum malaria in African children with a proposed classification and grading system. Trans Roy Soc Trop Med Hyg 1999;93:619–22.).*

the basis of observations of the optic disc, the macula and the area in between [27].

Severe pneumonia was a common cause of death in parasitemic children who satisfied the clinical case definition of cerebral malaria in the autopsy study described above. Pneumonia may be suspected on the basis of the history and physical examination, and should definitely be considered when oxygen saturations are <90%. Given the frequency of this particular co-morbidity, empiric antibiotic therapy based on the clinical assessment is reasonable [28].

If pediatric patients have a history of aspirin intake, or if there is hepatomegaly in the face of recurrent hypoglycemia, Reyes Syndrome should be included in the differential diagnosis.

TREATMENT

CLEARING THE PARASITE

For patients who are able to swallow, oral medications (Table 96-3) are recommended [20]. Prior treatment is common, and should be taken into consideration when deciding how to treat individual patients; quinine use following mefloquine may be arrhythmogenic, for instance.

Although chloroquine is no longer recommended by the WHO as the primary treatment of *P. falciparum* infections, it remains the most commonly used drug in a few parts of the world including Haiti, the Dominican Republic, most regions of the Middle East, and Central America, west of the Panama Canal. Even in settings where chloroquine-resistance is widespread, the drug, an effective analgesic and antipyretic, has considerable popularity.

Chloroquine is recommended for the blood-stage infections of *P. malariae, P. ovale* and most *P. vivax* infections. Chloroquine-resistant vivax malaria has been reported from Indonesia and Papua New Guinea, and those infections should be treated with artemisinin combination therapies, atovaquone-proguanil, mefloquine or quinine followed by doxycyline or tetracycline.

Primaquine is required for radical cures of the liver stage parasites in *P. vivax* and *P. ovale*. In most situations, a daily dose (0.25–0.5 mg/kg) of primaquine for two weeks is sufficient. Patients should be screened for G6PD-deficiency prior to administration of primaquine. In settings where laboratory testing is not available, a test dose of primaquine followed by careful observation and repeated measures of hemoglobin or hematocrit may be necessary.

In general, though, monotherapy for falciparum malaria has been supplanted by drug combinations (co-formulated or co-packaged) of artemisinin-based compounds (rapidly parasiticidal, but with short half-lives) and partner drugs (more slowly acting, but with longer half-lives). The artemisinins typically clear 90% of the parasites within 24–36 hours and the partner drug clears the rest. Most regimens (Table 96-3) require twice daily administration of the drug combination over three days. The WHO currently recommends five different combinations; specific choices depend on prevailing parasite drug sensitivities, procurement opportunities and cost [20].

For patients who are unable to swallow, parenteral drug treatment is required; both options are contemporary formulations of traditional, plant-based remedies. Quinine (and its stereoisomer, quinidine) come from the bark of the cinchona tree and the artemisinins are derived from *Artemesia annua,* known colloquially as "sweet wormwood".

The cinchona alkaloids have been the mainstay of treatment for complicated malaria since they were introduced to Europe from Peru in the 17th century. Quinine is used more commonly, but quinidine is as effective, albeit more likely to engender cardiac dysrhythmias. Although the IV route is preferred, intramuscular administration is effective – the drug, as formulated (at 300 mg base/ml) is fairly acidic, though and should be diluted 4–6-fold prior to intramuscular injection. Large-volume injections should be divided between two large muscle masses (preferably the anterior thighs).

Irrespective of the alkaloid selected, a loading dose is required in order to achieve a therapeutic drug concentration quickly. More care is required to administer quinine and quinidine than the artemisinins. Quinine and quinidine, when infused too rapidly, stimulate the pancreatic secretion of insulin and hypoglycemia may ensue.

Intravenous quinine was enshrined as the treatment for severe malaria well before pharmacokinetic studies were possible; current regimens have evolved on the basis of experience and some computer modeling. Regimens for intramuscular quinine and the intravascular/intramuscular formulations of the artemisinin derivatives are based on sound pharmacokinetics (Table 96-4).

Randomized clinical trials comparing IV quinine with IV artesunate have established the superiority of IV artesunate in adults and children [29, 30].

Patients with complicated malaria should receive parenteral antimalarials for at least 24 hours; after that, a full course of an effective oral drug can be administered, beginning as soon as the patient can swallow (Table 96-4).

PREGNANT PATIENTS

For pregnant women living in malaria-endemic areas, the WHO recommends Intermittent Preventive Treatment during pregnancy (IPTp) [20] with two doses of sulfadoxine-pyrimethamine (SP) administered at monthly intervals after the onset of fetal movements. IPTp should be extended into the third trimester for HIV-infected pregnant women who are not taking cotrimoxazole prophylaxis.

Chemotherapy for pregnant women who develop malaria illnesses during pregnancy is similar to that recommended for non-pregnant patients with the following caveats:

- few pharmacokinetic studies have been carried out in pregnant women;
- chloroquine is well tolerated;
- the recommended doses of quinine and quinidine are safe;
- mefloquine may be associated with an increased risk of stillbirth [31], but can be used when no other treatment options are available;
- tetracycline, doxycycline, primaquine and halofantrine are contraindicated in pregnancy, and neither primaquine or the tetracyclines should be used while breastfeeding;
- primaquine is contraindicated during pregnancy, given the uncertain G6PD status of the fetus.

There are very few data on the safety of the artemisinin drugs during pregnancy; in general, they are not recommended during the first trimester and amodiaquine use during pregnancy is eschewed because of the risk of agranulocytosis.

TREATING THE PATIENT

Supportive care

Dedicated nursing care is important in the management of these patients. Vital signs, urine output and an appropriate coma score should be monitored as frequently as possible. The most common causes of a drop in coma score following the initiation of therapy are convulsions, hypoglycemia and anemia. Blood glucose, lactate, parasitemia and hemoglobin/hematocrit can be monitored every 4–6 hours on fingerprick samples of blood. Patients not on ventilatory support should be nursed in the lateral decubitus position to minimize the chance of aspiration. IV fluids containing 5% dextrose are important initially, but nasogastric tube feeding can be started within 18–24 hours of admission if the patient is unable to eat.

Fever

There is no consensus on how best to treat malarial fevers. Aggressive fever management may decrease the risk of convulsions and subsequent neurologic damage but parasite sequestration is less effective at higher temperatures. Acetaminophen/paracetamol and ibuprofen are all effective antipyretics in malaria patients.

TABLE 96-3 Oral Anti-Malarial Drugs

Parasite	Treatment regimens	Clinical caveats
P. falciparum	WHO-recommended artemisinin-based combination therapy (ACT): • Artemether + lumefantrine (AL) Given at 0, 8, 24, 36, 48 and 60 hours: 5–15 kg: 1 tablet 16–25 kg: 2 tablets 26–35 kg: 3 tablets >35 kg: 4 tablets (adult dose) • Artesunate + amodiaquine (AS + AQ) 4 mg/kg/day AS and 10 mg/kg/day AQ daily for 3 days • Artesunate + mefloquine (AS + MQ) 4 mg/kg/day AS daily for 3 days. MQ can be taken as 15 mg/kg on day 1 and 10 mg/kg on day 2, or as 8.3 mg/kg/daily for 3 days • Artesunate + sulfadoxine-pyrimethamine (AS + SP) 4 mg/kg AS daily for 3 days; 25 mg/1.25 mg/kg SP on Day 1 • Dihydroartemisinin + piperaquine (DHA + PPQ) 4 mg/kg AS plus 18 mg/kg PPQ daily for 3 days	Generally very well-tolerated
	Other options: • Chloroquine (if known to be chloroquine sensitive) Adults: 600 mg base (=1000 mg salt) p.o., followed by 300 mg base (=500 mg salt) p.o. at 6, 24 and 24 hours Children: 10 mg base/kg p.o., followed by 5 mg base/kg p.o. at 6, 24 and 48 hours • Oral quinine sulfate plus doxycycline, tetracycline or clindamycin	Chloroquine can cause significant pruritus in dark-skinned individuals Overdoses (>2 g) can be fatal; adrenaline and diazepam are antidotes Bitter taste Bitter taste Frequent dosing needed because of a short half-life Cinchonism: tinnitus, nausea, headaches, dizziness and disturbed vision Overdosing leads to cardiotoxicity, more so with quinidine
	• Quinine sulfate: 542 mg base (= 650 mg salt) p.o. three times a day for 3 days (7 days for infections acquired in Southeast Asia) • Doxycycline: 100 mg p.o. twice a day for 7 days • Tetracycline: 250 mg p.o. four times a day for 7 days • Clindamycin: 20 mg base/kg/day, p.o., divided three times a day for 7 days	Rapid IV or IM administration can precipitate hypoglycemia Doxycycline and tetracycline are not recommended during pregnancy or in children under the age of 8 years. Clindamycin is recommended for these two groups Doxycycline should be taken with food to minimize the risk of esophageal erosions Both drugs may cause photosensitivity and disrupt normal flora enough to precipitate vaginal yeast infections
	• Atovaquone-proguanil Adult tablet: 250 mg atovaquone, 100 mg proguanil Pediatric tablet: 62.5 mg atovaquone, 25 mg proguanil 5–8 kg: two 25-mg pediatric tablets daily for 3 days 9–10 kg: three 25-mg pediatric tablets daily for 3 days 11–20 kg: one adult 100-mg tablet daily for 3 days 21–30 kg: two adult 100-mg tablets daily for 3 days 31–40 kg: three adult 100-mg tablets daily for 3 days >40 kg: four adult 100-mg tablets daily for 3 days • Mefloquine Adults: 684 mg base (= 750 mg salt) p.o., followed by 456 mg base (= 500 mg salt) p.o., 6–12 hours later Children: 13.7 mg base/kg (= 15 mg salt/kg) p.o., followed by 9.1 mg base/kg (= 10 mg salt/kg) p.o., 6–12 hours later	Atovaquone targets an element of the parasite electron transport chain and is thus well-tolerated by the host Proguanil interferes with folate metabolism and has been associated with aphthous oral ulcers Side effects include vomiting, dizziness, and exacerbation of cardiac conduction abnormalities Not recommended for individuals with a history of psychiatric disorders May disrupt sleep or cause vivid dreams
	Treatment failure within 14 days Second-line treatment: • a different ACT, known to be effective in the region • AS + tetracycline, doxycycline or clindamycin, for 7 days • quinine + tetracycline, doxycycline or clindamycin, for 7 days See above for details re dosage regimens	
	Treatment failure after 14 days Repeat the original ACT unless it contained MQ; in that case, use a different ACT	

TABLE 96-3 Oral Anti-Malarial Drugs—cont'd

Parasite	Treatment regimens	Clinical caveats
P. vivax, P. ovale	Chloroquine See above for details re dosage regimen	
	Radical cure (liver stages) • 14-day course of primaquine Adult: 15 mg daily for 14 days. In Oceania and Southeast Asia, the dose of primaquine should be 30 mg daily for 14 days Children: 0.25 mg base/kg body weight, taken with food once daily for 14 days. In Oceania and Southeast Asia, the dose of primaquine should be 0.5 mg/kg body weight. In mild/moderate G6PD deficiency: Adult: 45–60 mg weekly for 8 weeks Children: 0.75 mg base/kg body weight should be given once a week for 8 weeks. In severe G6PD deficiency, primaquine is contraindicated and should not be used	Primaquine is contraindicated in individuals with G6PD deficiency and during pregnancy Malaria infection as a result of blood transfusion or organ transplantation does not require radical cure Primaquine is a gametocytocidal drug
Chloroquine resistant *P. vivax* (Papua New Guinea, Indonesia)	Artemisinin-based combination therapy: • DHA + PPQ • AL • AS + AQ followed by primaquine Quinine + doxycycline or tetracycline, followed by primaquine Atovaquone-proguanil followed by primaquine Mefloquine followed by primaquine See above for details re dosage regimens	AS + SP is not effective in many locales
P. malariae, P. knowlesi	Chloroquine See above for details re dosage regimen	Effective against gametocytes

G6PD, glucose 6 phosphate deficiency; IM, intramuscular; IV, intravenous; WHO, World Health Organization.

TABLE 96-4 Parenteral Anti-Malarial Drugs

Parasite	Treatment regimens	Clinical caveats
P. falciparum	**For all regimens:** • Continue parenteral treatment for at least 24 hours • When the patient is able to swallow, administer a treatment dose of a locally-effective drug (ACT, oral quinine + doxycycline or clindamycin, atovaquone-proguanil, mefloquine)	
	Artesunate 2.4 mg/kg IV at 0, 12 and 24 hours, then daily until oral medication can be given	Well-tolerated Effective against a broad range of lifecycle stages (early ring stages up to schizonts and gametocytes)
	Quinine dihydrochloride: IV Loading dose: 12.5 mg base/kg (= 20 mg salt/kg), IV, over 4 hours Maintenance dose: 20–30 mg/kg salt/day (divided into 2–3 daily doses, every 8–12 hours) Quinine should be used with caution in patients on mefloquine prophylaxis **Quinine dihydrochloride: IM** Loading dose: 6.25 mg base/kg (= 10 mg/kg salt), IM (dilute quinine to 60 mg/ml), repeat after 4 hours Maintenance doses: 6.25 mg base/kg (=10 mg/kg salt), IM, every 8–12 hours **Quinidine gluconate** Loading dose: 24 mg salt/kg loading dose, IV, over 4 hours Maintenance dose: 12 mg salt/kg, IV over 4 hours, every 8 hours, for at least 24 hours or until oral medication can be given	Cardiotoxic Can induce hypoglycemia Most effective against late rings and early trophozoites
	Artemether Loading dose: 3.2 mg/kg body weight IM Maintenance dose: 1.6 mg/kg IM per day until oral medication can be given	Well-tolerated Effective against a broad range of lifecycle stages (early ring stages up to schizonts and gametocytes)

IM, intramuscular; IV, intravenous.

Convulsions

Fits are a very common complication of malaria illnesses. Febrile convulsions are distinguished by a fairly rapid recovery of consciousness but, in patients with cerebral malaria, the coma is often initiated with a convulsion. Multiple fits are common, as are clinically "silent" fits, evident only electroencephalographically. In practice, decisions regarding the use of anti-epileptic drugs are made on the basis of a thoughtful and detailed clinical exam focusing on the eyes (looking for evidence of nystagmus, hippus [also known as pupillary athetosis – spasmodic, rhythmic (<0.04 Hz), but irregular dilating and contracting pupillary movements involving the sphincter and dilator muscles] and absence of the light reflex), the respiratory rate and rhythm (shallow, irregular respirations may be a "seizure equivalent"), the mouth and fingers (infrequent fine twitching movements of the tongue, a single finger, or the corner of the mouth can also be seizure equivalents). Occasionally, seizures emerge when hypoglycemia is corrected. Often a trial of a rapidly acting anticonvulsant (i.e. paraldehyde or diazepam) can help to identify subtle convulsions.

Standard anticonvulsant protocols are difficult to develop because of the heterogeneity of the patient population, but commonly used drugs include the benzodiazpines (IV, per rectum [PR] or sublingual), paraldehyde (IM), phenobarbital (IV) and phenytoin (IV). There is little experience with levetiracetam in malaria to date, but it may prove to be useful. A study of prophylactic phenobarbital, administered on admission to children with cerebral malaria, was deleterious [32]; as a result, clinicians are advised to treat clinically-evident seizures and to watch for subtle evidence for subclinical events.

Anemia

The evidence base for treating severe malarial anemia is scanty. "Transfusion triggers" are difficult to develop because the rate at which an anemia develops is as important as the absolute value of the hemoglobin concentration but, in general, transfusions begin to be considered when the hemoglobin drops below 5 gm/dL [packed cell volume (PCV) = 15%]. Clinical clues include signs of hemodynamic instability (passive congestion of the liver, systolic flow murmurs, extra heart sounds, rales, tachycardia) and cerebral hypoperfusion. The clinical decision regarding transfusion should take into account the peripheral parasitemia, as well as the hemoglobin concentration (or hematocrit): the higher the parasitemia, the lower the hemoglobin or hematocrit are likely to drop. The usual practice is to transfuse whole blood (20 ml/kg) or packed cells (10 ml/kg), irrespective of the degree of the anemia or the intensity of the parasitemia. About 5% of pediatric patients require a second transfusion.

Hypoglycemia

Patients with severe malaria can develop hypoglycemia if quinine is infused too rapidly; when it develops as part of the disease process, it worsens the prognosis for the patient. If hypoglycemia is identified, the patient should be given 50% dextrose (1 ml/kg) IV, and the glucose should be re-checked soon thereafter and then regularly until they regain consciousness.

Acidosis

Acidosis in severe malaria is manifested as deep, Kussmaul-like respirations [33] and can occur with, or without, associated hyperlactatemia. It is frequently a sign of hypovolemia [34]. A large trial in children with a variety of febrile illnesses (57% had malaria) and "compensated shock" compared bolus therapy (normal saline and albumin) with conservative management with no boluses and found that outcomes were significantly better in those who received no additional fluid bolus [35]. When justified, blood transfusions are helpful in this situation; when blood is not indicated, cautious fluid repletion, beginning with normal saline (10 ml/kg) may be helpful. Acidosis may also be a sign of sepsis so collecting a blood culture and starting empiric antibiotic therapy may be justified.

Pulmonary edema/ARDS

This complication is more common in adults, and can develop several days after admission and the initiation of anti-malarial treatment. Prompt intubation and assisted ventilation are the only recognized treatments; clinical trials of this specific malaria complication have not been carried out, so treatment recommendations are based on extrapolations from other conditions [35].

Renal failure

This complication is also more common in adults with severe malaria than in children. Untreated, the mortality rate is over 70%. Patients should receive adequate renal replacement therapy – hemofiltration is superior to peritoneal dialysis in terms of mortality and cost-effectiveness [36]. The role of hemodialysis has not been assessed in a randomized trial, but is likely to be superior to peritoneal dialysis in patients who are hemodynamically stable [37].

Treating the process

Many trials of adjuvant therapies targeting putative pathogenic processes have been conducted. Only a few, even when subjected to meta-analysis, have been adequately powered, and none has demonstrated a positive impact on outcome (Table 96-5).

CONCLUSION

Malaria remains a major cause of morbidity and mortality in endemic areas, and is the largest single cause of fever in travelers returning from malaria-endemic regions. Prompt recognition and treatment of malaria disease is helpful in terms of preventing disease progression, and prompt recognition and treatment of non-malarial disease (even in parasitemic individuals) is equally important.

Patients with severe and complicated malaria can be managed well in resource-poor settings with careful attention to IV fluid support, blood transfusions, convulsions, blood glucose and the airway.

PLASMODIUM OVALE

Plasmodium ovale was first described in the blood of a soldier returning from East Africa in 1922 [38]. Although *P. ovale* has been reported from all continents, it is only in tropical Africa and New Guinea that it is relatively common. In West Africa, a blood film *P. ovale* parasite positive rate between 0.7% and 10% has been found [39]. *Plasmodium ovale* is a common cause of morbidity in the endemic communities with the highest incidence of febrile episodes among children aged 0–7 years old, but clinical attacks can be seen in all age groups. *Plasmodium ovale* can be seen in up to 15% of returning travelers. As febrile episodes are often treated empirically in endemic areas and the confirmation of low-density *P. ovale* infections by microscopy is demanding, the true incidence of *P. ovale* malaria is likely underestimated. *Plasmodium ovale* in African immigrants can present months after arrival in a new region.

Characterization of *P. ovale* from Southeast Asia based on the small subunit rRNA gene and parts of the cysteine protease, ookinete surface protein and cytochrome b genes, indicate that *P. ovale* can be divided into at least two types – classic and variant – which do not differ morphologically [40]. Variant *P. ovale* is associated with a higher parasite density in humans. A recent study of 55 *P. ovale* isolates from around the world showed that variant and classic *P. ovale* co-exist and do not recombine [41].

Plasmodium ovale causes a relatively mild form of malaria that is very rarely severe (ARDS) or fatal (death caused by splenic rupture reported). The most frequent symptoms are fever with temperatures higher than 38.5°C (seen in half the cases), body aches, chills, nausea, abdominal pain, diarrhea and nonproductive cough. Mild heptomegaly and splenomegaly, thrombocytopenia lower than 100,000/mm^3, elevation in hepatic enzymes (AST/ALT) and mild

TABLE 96-5 Trials of Adjuvant Therapy in Complicated Malaria

Therapeutic Intervention	Pathogenic Target	Impact	Recommendation	Reference
Dexamethasone	Cerebral edema	No effect/deleterious effect	Not recommended currently	[87, 88]
Intravenous immune globulin	Reverse sequestration	Sequential trial, halted because superiority was unlikely	Not recommended	[89]
Phenobarbital	Seizure prophylaxis	Adverse effect when administered to all patients with cerebral malaria	Not recommended for use on *all* patients, but should be considered in those with a documented history of seizures	[32]
Mannitol	Cerebral edema	No effect on outcome	Not recommended currently	[90, 91]
Erythropoietin	Neuroprotection, anti-cytokine	In progress	Await outcome of study	[92]
Desferrioxamine	Inhibit parasite growth, protect against free radical-mediated damage	No impact on outcome	Not recommended	[93, 94]
Dichloroacetate	Lactic acidosis	Positive impact on lactic acidosis, unknown effect on mortality	Not used routinely	[95]
Anti-tumor necrosis factor antibody	Cytokine cascade	Positive impact on fever, but no effect on outcome	Not recommended	[96]
L-arginine	Improve endothelial cell function, generate nitric oxide	In progress	Await outcome of study	[97]
N-acetylcysteine	Antioxidant	No effect noted on multiple outcome indicators	Not recommended	[98]
Activated charcoal	Immune modulation	Prevents CM in mice, does not interfere with artesunate kinetics in healthy volunteers	Await outcome of study	[99]
Crystalloids vs. colloids	Intravascular volume depletion and acidosis	Intravenous fluid boluses were found to be deleterious	Fluid boluses in moderately dehydrated patients are not recommended	[35]
Pentoxifylline	Inhibition of TNF	Trend toward improved survival in earlier studies, not substantiated subsequently	Not recommended	[100–104]
Levamisole	Inhibit sequestration	Trial underway	Await outcome of study	[29, 30]
Exchange blood transfusion	Enhance parasite clearance	Improved parasite clearance times, no impact on outcome	Worth a try only in settings where intravascular volume can be monitored	[105, 106]

Source for trials currently underway: http://www.controlled-trials.com (accessed 13 Mar 2011).
CM, cerebral malaria; TNF, tumor necrosis factor.

TABLE 96-6 Endemicity

Criterion	Hypoendemic	Mesoendemic	Hyperendemic	Holoendemic	Reference
Spleen rate: 2–9 years	0–10%	11–50%	>50%	>75%	[83]
Parasite prevalence: 2–9 years	0–10%	11–50%	>50%	>75%	
Stability	*Unstable*		*Stable*		[84]
Types of epidemic	True	Exaggerated seasonal			[85]
Entomological Inoculation Rate (EIR)	<0.25	0.25–10	11–140	>140	[86]

The degree of endemic malaria is determined by examination of a statistically significant sample of a population and is assessed and classified as in the Table.

hyperbilirubinemia are seen in about 50% of patients. The hemoglobin count tends to be normal. The undifferentiated febrile clinical presentation cannot be distinguished from other malarias.

Plasmodium ovale is considered a relapsing malaria [42]. However, the relapse frequency and relapse interval of *P. ovale* is poorly described. Recently, the existence of a true hypnozoite in *P. ovale* malaria has been questioned [43]. The existence of *P. ovale* hypnozoites has never been proven by biologic experiments. On one hand, indirect evidence of the existence of hypnozoites, i.e. reports on the occurrence of true relapses undoubtedly caused by this parasite is rare; true *P. ovale* relapses have been reported only occasionally. On the other hand, *P. ovale* cases reported without any preventive medication where relapses did not occur outnumber reported relapses caused by this parasite. If true hypnozoites exist then the relapse frequency must be very low.

DIAGNOSIS

There tends to be lower initial parasitemias (<500 parasites per µl) with *P. ovale* malaria, making the diagnosis by routine microscopy insensitive. *Plasmodium ovale* and *P. vivax* can be difficult to distinguish morphologically by oil immersion microscopy. Mixed infections, especially in endemic areas, are common. In endemic regions where *P. falciparum* and/or *P. vivax* predominate, *P. ovale* is frequently overlooked. For more accurate diagnosis and estimates of the burden of *P. ovale* infections, more sensitive diagnostic methods are needed [44].

Plasmodium ovale malaria is currently problematic to diagnose in travelers, with early attempts complicated by the lack of specific clinical features, the rarity of biologic changes and the poor sensitivity of diagnostic tools to detect low parasitaemia. Thus, the diagnosis is commonly delayed or missed.

Molecular diagnosis and differentiation of the two subspecies can be accomplished with PCR protocols in reference laboratories [45], but the genetic polymorphisms of the two subspecies require appropriate protocols [46].

Rapid diagnostic tests (RDTs) have not been developed to detect *P. ovale*, and the performance of currently-available RDTs varies greatly in their capability to detect *P. ovale* parasites. Sensitivity varies between 0% and 80%, with parasite density a key factor [47–50]. A negative RDT test result cannot exclude the diagnosis of *P. ovale* malaria.

TREATMENT

Chloroquine at 25 mg/kg divided over three days is the treatment of choice if a mono-infection with *P. ovale* is confirmed. Artemisinin combination treatments (ACTs) are effective and could be used in settings of diagnostic uncertainty. Currently, a radical cure dose of 30 mg primaqine base (0.5 mg/kg) by mouth daily for 14 days is recommended to eliminate hypnozoites; however, note the controversy in this regard above. Use of lower dose primaquine has been associated with therapeutic failures and recurrent *P. ovale* malaria [51].

PLASMODIUM MALARIAE

Plasmodium malariae was first described by Golgi in 1886 when he noted the relationship between the 72-hour lifecycle of the parasite in the blood of patients and the corresponding appearance of fever and chills (the paroxysm) [52]. Fever caused by *P. malariae* was historically known as "quartan malaria" because of the appearance of fever every fourth day (assuming the first day of fever is day 1). *Plasmodium malariae* has been reported from all continents but is only relatively common in tropical Africa and the Southwest Pacific. The prevalence of *P. malariae* varies from less than 1% to as high as 30–40% in focal areas of West Africa and Indonesia based on standard light microscopy detection of parasites on thick films. In the endemic communities, *P. malariae* is a common cause of morbidity with the highest incidence of febrile episodes among children less then 10 years old. As febrile episodes are often treated empirically and the confirmation of low-density *P. malariae* infections by microscopy is difficult, the true incidence of *P. malariae* malaria is underestimated.

Plasmodium malariae is unique in that without treatment, blood stage parasites persist for extremely long periods of time – likely the lifetime of the host. The persistent, low-density parasitemia in otherwise healthy individuals may produce distinctive clinical features, or individuals may be so asymptomatic that they qualify as blood donors. This is why *P. malariae* causes about 25% [53] of transfusion related cases of malaria although it accounts for only 1–2% of imported cases of malaria [54].

Likewise, asymptomatic persons can re-introduce *P. malariae* into previously malaria-free areas [55]. Years later, when carriers are immunosuppressed with drugs [56] or stressed by surgery [57], the parasites can recrudesce and they become symptomatic with typical symptoms of malaria.

The most important and unique feature of prolonged *P. malariae* parasitemia is an irreversible, immune-mediated, nephrotic syndrome first noted in West Africa in the 1960s [58, 59]. Nephrotic syndrome caused by *P. malariae* can also present outside of malaria endemic areas years after the last exposure [60].

CLINICAL PRESENTATION

Plasmodium malariae is a relatively mild form of malaria, although the initial paroxysms can be similar to those seen with *P. falciparum* and *P. vivax*. The undifferentiated febrile presentation is indistinguishable from other malarias. Deaths associated with *P. malariae* are not from acute infection but rather caused by end-stage renal disease [61].

The nephrotic syndrome associated with chronic *P. malariae* is caused by an immune complex, basement membrane nephropathy and presents no differently from nephrotic syndrome associated with other causes. Usually, there is a several-month history of progressively worsening lower extremity edema, frothy urine, hypertension and multiple abnormal laboratory findings including proteinuria, hypoalbuminemia, hyperlipidemia, high serum creatinine and anemia. Renal biopsy is usually required to confirm the diagnosis and properly guide management [61]. *Plasmodium malariae* as the true cause of the nephrotic syndrome may be very difficult to diagnose because the patients may have exceedingly low parasitemias and negative rapid diagnostic test (RDT) results. Parasitologic confirmation in this syndrome requires exhaustive, expert, microscopic review of smears and carefully directed molecular methods [60].

DIAGNOSIS

The preferred diagnostic method to confirm *P. malariae* remains traditional Giemsa-stained thick and thin peripheral blood smears. In the growing parasite, pigment increases rapidly with many jet-black granules. The trophozoite assumes variable shapes but often stretches across the width of the red blood cell to appear as a "band form" (see Fig. 96.3), which is often considered diagnostic, although this band form can be seen with other species, especially *P. knowlesi* and *P. inui*. Red blood cells infected with trophozoites of *P. malariae* parasites are not enlarged and do not contain prominent stippling, which distinguishes them from *P. vivax* and *P. ovale* [62].

When considering the microscopic diagnosis of *P. malariae*, three considerations should be kept in mind:

- there tends to be lower initial and maximal parasitemias with *P. malariae* than with other species because the number of merozoites per red blood cell replication cycle is lower (6–14), the three-day versus two-day developmental cycle produces slower growth, and *P. malariae*'s preference for older red blood cells limits the number of cells that can be infected [62];

- in endemic regions where *P. falciparum* and/or *P. vivax* predominate, mixed infections are the rule and *P. malariae* is frequently overlooked unless more sensitive diagnostic methods, such as molecular diagnostic tests, are used [63];
- even careful microscopic examination may not be sufficient to morphologically distinguish *P. knowlesi* – an emerging cause of severe and potentially fatal malaria in Southeast Asia – from *P. malariae* on the peripheral smear [64]. Molecular methods may be needed to confirm the diagnosis of *P. malariae* where the two parasite distributions overlap.

RDTs for malaria are not developed to specifically diagnose *P. malariae*, and the detection of parasites relies on various pan-*Plasmodium* capture reagents not specifically optimized for *P. malariae*. The performance of currently available RDTs varies greatly (0–100%) in their capability to detect *P. malariae* parasites. Clinical studies are usually designed to evaluate the sensitivity and specificity of RDTs for *P. falciparum* and *P. vivax*, and small numbers of *P. malariae* are encountered and reported. Whether the poor sensitivity is because of the very low parasitemias (and presumably low antigen levels) in patients or because of the lack of cross-reaction with the capture reagents is not known. A negative RDT test result cannot exclude the diagnosis of *P. malariae* malaria.

Molecular testing is not commercially available or standardized, and results may vary based on regional differences in target gene sequences; caution should be used when relying solely on molecular results to make clinical decisions. As also seen in *P. ovale*, the targets of *P. malariae* molecular probes may exhibit geographic variation suggesting subspecies of *P. malariae* [65] and an additional reason why PCR reactions could yield a false-negative result.

TREATMENT

The treatment of choice for the typical, uncomplicated febrile illness associated with *P. malariae* mono-infection is chloroquine at 25 mg/kg total dose divided over three days. Artemisinin combination treatments (ACTs), as well as other anti-malarial drugs, are effective and could be used in settings of diagnostic uncertainty.

Clinicians should be aware of the possibility of occasional recurrent parasitemias with clinical symptoms following treatment with a standard course of chloroquine [66]. These cases likely represent delayed parasite clearance rather than true resistance. There is a 16–59 day range in the length of the pre-patent period in experimental mosquito transmitted *P. malariae* [62] and it is thought that some parasites could emerge from the liver days or weeks after treatment is initiated when drug levels are inadequate to prevent parasitemia [67]. On such occasions, either re-treatment with a full treatment course of chloroquine or another standard anti-malarial treatment regimen would be satisfactory.

Treating the underlying *P. malariae* in fully established nephrotic syndrome does not improve renal function, as segmental sclerosis and hyalinization of the nephron are irreversible. These patients often become hemodialysis dependent. To prevent end-stage renal disease, *P. malariae* must be considered, diagnosed and effectively treated as soon as renal symptoms develop [61].

PLASMODIUM KNOWLESI

Plasmodium knowlesi is primarily a parasite infecting macaque monkeys. Sporadic human infections, generally linked to macaque exposures, were the rule [68], (aside from a brief flirtation with *P. knowlesi* as malaria therapy for syphilis in the 1930s [69]), until a 2004 outbreak of "hyperparasitemic *P. malariae*" in the Kapit division of Malaysian Borneo was confirmed as *P. knowlesi* using molecular methods [70]. *Plasmodium knowlesi* is now established as a common cause of malaria on the Malaysian Peninsula in particular, and in Southeast Asia in general, especially in populations living in close proximity to the simian reservoir [81].

The most common clinical syndrome is a febrile illness, indistinguishable from uncomplicated falciparum malaria, but a small proportion of patients (<10%) progress to severe and complicated disease, in which respiratory distress (ARDS) and renal failure feature more prominently than in severe falciparum malaria [68, 71–74]. In contrast to falciparum malaria, coma is a relatively rare complication of infection with *P. knowlesi*. Surprisingly, the salient findings in the one case of fatal *P. knowlesi* malaria that was autopsied are similar to fatal falciparum malaria: there was selective accumulation of parasitized red cells in the brain, heart and kidneys, the brain was slate gray in color and there were petechial hemorrhages scattered through the cerebrum and cerebellum [75]. *Plasmodium knowlesi* is a quotidian parasite, undergoing asexual replication every 24 hours, which may explain the relatively high incidence of severe anemia [73]. Thrombocytopenia, often profound, is nearly a constant feature in *P. knowlesi* infections, but no clinically evident coagulopathies have been reported [71–74]. The disease in children is fairly similar to that in adults, but there is one striking contrast in pediatric infections with *P. knowlesi* compared with *P. falciparum*: pediatric *P. knowlesi* infection is restricted to school-age children, whereas falciparum malaria affects all ages [72].

Microscopically, *P. knowlesi* resembles *P. falciparum* young ring stages and *P. malariae* in the mature trophozoite blood stages, therefore a high index of suspicion and judicious use of molecular methods are required to establish the diagnosis definitively [76]. Median parasitemias are typically approximately 1400 parasites per microliter (interquartile range 6–250,000) [71]. To date, there is no evidence that *P. knowlesi* is a relapsing malaria and, thus far, treatment with a wide variety of anti-malarial drugs (quinine, artesunate, various artemisinin combination therapies [ACTs], mefloquine, with and without primaquine) have been successful [71–74].

Plasmodium knowlesi malaria has been called the "fifth human malaria", but there is, as yet, no definitive evidence for cyclical transmission by mosquitoes from human to human. Without this evidence, it remains a simian malaria with occasional zoonotic human infections [77]. Analysis of archival blood films suggests that *P. knowlesi* has infected humans for many years in Malaysian Borneo [78] and recent epidemiologic studies suggest that macaque monkeys are the reservoir host [79]. The recent upsurge in clinical episodes may be related to changes in human exposure to monkeys, deforestation and a decline in *P. vivax* infections [80].

DIAGNOSIS

Plasmodium knowlesi infections are limited to areas where humans (local residents or travelers) are near the reservoir hosts: long-tailed (*Macaca fascularis*) and pig-tailed macaques (*Macaca nemestrina*). Microscopic identification of a malaria infection is the first step, but because of the morphologic similarities between *P. falciparum, P. malariae* and *P. knowlesi*, the definitive diagnosis of *P. knowlesi* rests on molecular detection using a nested PCR technique [14]. Combinations of rapid diagnostic tests (RDTs) can be used to increase diagnostic certainty, but there is no RDT specifically for *P. knowlesi* at this time.

TREATMENT

This parasite has been subjected to less drug pressure than any other malaria parasite infecting humans and has been fully susceptible to a broad range of anti-malarial drugs administered according to standard oral and parenteral regimens (chloroquine, quinine, artemether-lumefantrine, artesunate [71–74]). Primaquine has been used as presumptive anti-relapse treatment, but there is no evidence of a hypnozoite stage, so it may not be necessary [74].

REFERENCES

1. Carter R, Mendis KN. Evolutionary and historical aspects of the burden of malaria. Clin Microbiol Rev 2002;15:564–94.
2. Cox-Singh J, Davis TM, Lee KS, et al. *Plasmodium knowlesi* malaria in humans is widely distributed and potentially life threatening. Clin Infect Dis 2008; 46:165–71.
3. Hay SI, Guerra CA, Gething PW, et al. A world malarial map: *Plasmodium falciparum* endemicity in 2007. PLoS Med 2009;6:e1000048.
4. Kublin JG, Patnaik P, Jere CS, et al. Effect of *Plasmodium falciparum* malaria on concentration of HIV-1-RNA in the blood of adults in rural Malawi: a prospective cohort study. Lancet 2005;365:233–40.
5. Laufer MK, van Oosterhout JJ, Thesing PC, et al. Impact of HIV-associated immunosuppression on malaria infection and disease in Malawi. J Infect Dis 2006:193:872–8.
6. O'Meara WP, Bejon P, Mwangi TW, et al. Effect of a fall in malaria transmission on morbidity and mortality in Kilifi, Kenya. Lancet 2008;372: 1555–62.
7. Pongponratn E, Riganti M, Punpoowong B, Aikawa M. Microvascular sequestration of parasitized erythrocytes in human falciparum malaria: a pathological study. Am J Trop Med Hyg 1991;44:168–75.
8. Willcox ML, Forster M, Dicko MI, et al. Blood glucose and prognosis in children with presumed severe malaria: is there a threshold for 'hypoglycaemia'? Trop Med Int Health 2010;15:232–40.
9. Haldar K, Murphy SC, Milner DA, Taylor TE. Malaria: mechanisms of erythrocytic infection and pathological correlates of severe disease. Annu Rev Pathol 2007;2:217–49.
10. Elsheikha HM, Sheashaa HA. Epidemiology, pathophysiology, management and outcome of renal dysfunction associated with plasmodia infection. Parasitol Res 2007;101:1183–90.
11. Idro R, Jenkins NE, Newton CR. Pathogenesis, clinical features, and neurological outcome of cerebral malaria. Lancet Neurol 2005;4:827–40.
12. Reyburn H, Mbatia R, Drakeley C, et al. Overdiagnosis of malaria in patients with severe febrile illness in Tanzania: a prospective study. BMJ 2004;329: 1212.
13. Taylor SM, Molyneux ME, Simel D, et al. Does this patient have malaria? JAMA 2010;304:2048–56.
14. Molyneux ME, Taylor TE, Wirima JJ, Borgstein A. Clinical features and prognostic indicators in paediatric cerebral malaria: a study of 131 comatose Malawian children. Q J Med 1989:71:441–59.
15. World Health Organization. Severe falciparum malaria. Trans Roy Soc Trop Med Hyg 2000;94(suppl. 1):S1–90.
16. Markley JD. Post-malaria neurological syndrome: a case report and review of the literature. J Travel Med 2009;16:424–30.
17. Fried M, Duffy PE. Adherence of *Plasmodium falciparum* to chondroitin sulfate A in the human placenta. Science 1996;272:1502–4.
18. Diagne N, Roger C, Sokhan CS, et al. Increased susceptibility to malaria during the early postpartum period. N Engl J Med 2000;343:598–603.
19. Kitchen AD, Chiodini PL. Malaria and blood transfusion. Vox Sang 2006; 90:77–84.
20. World Health Organization guidelines for the treatment of malaria. Geneva: World Health Organization; 2010. Available at: http://whqlibdoc.who.int/publications/2010/9789241547925_eng.pdf (accessed 6 November 2011).
21. Malaria rapid diagnostic test performand – results of WHO product testing of malaria RDTs: Round 3 (2010–2011). Available at: http://apps.who.int/tdr/svc/publications/tdr-research-publications/rdt_round3.
22. Smith T, Schellenberg JA, Hayes R. Attributable fraction estimates and case definitions for malaria in endemic areas. Stat Med 1994;13:2345–58.
23. Berkley J, Mwarumba S, Bramham K, Lowe B. Bacteraemia complicating severe malaria in children. Trans R Soc Trop Med Hyg 1999;93:283–6.
24. Bronzan RN, Taylor TE, Mwenechanya J, et al. Bacteremia in Malawian children with severe malaria: prevalence, etiology, HIV coinfection, and outcome. J Infect Dis 2007;195:895–904.
25. Taylor TE, Fu WJ, Carr RA, et al. Differentiating the pathologies of cerebral malaria by postmortem parasite counts. Nat Med 2004;10:143–5.
26. Beare NA, Taylor TE, Harding SP, et al. Malarial retinopathy: a newly established diagnostic sign in severe malaria. Am J Trop Med Hyg 2006;75: 790–7.
27. Beare NA, Lewallen S, Taylor TE, Molyneux ME. Redefining cerebral malaria by including malaria retinopathy. Future Microbiol 2011;6:349–55.
28. Bassat Q, Machevo S, O'Callaghan-Gordo C, et al. Distinguishing malaria from severe pneumonia among hospitalized children who fulfilled integrated management of childhood illness criteria for both diseases: a hospital-based study in Mozambique. Am J Trop Med Hyg 2011;85:626–34.
29. Dondorp A, Nosten F, Stepniewska K, Day N, White, South East Asian Quinine Artesunate Malaria Trial (SEAQUAMAT) group. Artesunate versus quinine for treatment of severe falciparum malaria: a randomised trial. Lancet 2005;366:717–25.
30. Dondorp AM, Fanella CF, Hendriksen KDE, et al. Artesunate versus quinine in the treatment of severe falciparum malaria in African children (AQUAMAT); an open-label, randomized trial. Lancet 2010;376:1647.
31. Nosten F, Vincenti M, Simpson J, et al. The effects of mefloquine treatment in pregnancy. Clin Infect Dis 1999;28:808–15.
32. Crawley J, Waruiru C, Mithwani S, et al. Effect of phenobarbital on seizure frequency and mortality in childhood cerebral malaria: a randomised, controlled intervention study. Lancet 2000;355:701.
33. Marsh K, Forster D, Waruiru C, et al. Indicators of life-threatening malaria in African children. N Engl J Med 1995;332:1399–404.
34. Molyneux EM, Maitland K. Intravenous fluids – getting the balance right. N Engl J Med 2005;353:941–4.
35. Maitland K, Kiguli S, Opoka RO, et al; the FEAST Trial Group. Mortality after fluid bolus in african children with severe infection. N Engl J Med 2011; 364:2483–95.
36. Day N, Dondorp AM. The management of patients with severe malaria. Am J Trop Med Hyg 2007;77(suppl. 6):29–35.
37. Phu NH, Hien TT, Mai NT, et al. Hemofiltration and peritoneal dialysis in infection-associated acute renal failure in Vietnam. N Engl J Med 2002; 247:895–902.
38. Stephens JWW. A new malaria parasite of man. Ann Trop Med 1922;16: 383–8.
39. Petersen E, Hogh B, Marbiah NT, et al. A longitudinal study of antibodies to the *Plasmodium falciparum* antigen Pf155/RESA and immunity to malaria infection in adult Liberians. Trans R Soc Trop Med Hyg 1990;84: 339–45.
40. Win TT, Jalloh A, Tantular IS, et al. Molecular analysis of *Plasmodium ovale* variants. Emerg Infect Dis 2004;10:1235–40.
41. Sutherland CJ, Tanomsing N, Nolder D, et al. Two nonrecombining sympatric forms of the human malaria parasite *Plasmodium ovale* occur globally. J Infect Dis 2010;201:1544–50.
42. Collins WE, Jeffery GM. *Plasmodium ovale*: parasite and disease. Clin Microbiol Rev 2005;18:570–81.
43. Richter J, Franken G, Mehlhorn H, et al. What is the evidence for the existence of *Plasmodium ovale* hypnozoites? Parasitol Res 2010;107:1285–90.
44. Mueller I, Zimmerman PA, Reeder JC. *Plasmodium malariae* and *Plasmodium ovale* – the "bashful" malaria parasites. Trends Parasitol 2007;23:278–83.
45. Oguike MC, Betson M, Burke M, et al. *Plasmodium ovale curtisi* and *Plasmodium ovale wallikeri* circulate simultaneously in African communities. Int J Parasitol 2011;41:677–83.
46. Calderaro A, Piccolo G, Perandin F, et al. Genetic polymorphisms influence *Plasmodium ovale* PCR detection accuracy. J Clin Microbiol 2007;45: 1624–7.
47. Win TT, Tantular IS, Pusarawati S, et al. Detection of Plasmodium ovale by the ICT malaria P.f/P.v. immunochromatographic test. Acta Trop 2001;80: 283–4.
48. Bigaillon C, Fontan E, Cavallo JD, et al. Ineffectiveness of the Binax NOW malaria test for diagnosis of *Plasmodium ovale* malaria. J Clin Microbiol 2005;43:1011.
49. Marx A, Pewsner D, Egger M, et al. Meta-analysis: accuracy of rapid tests for malaria in travelers returning from endemic areas. Ann Intern Med 2005; 142:836–46.
50. Grobusch MP, Hanscheid T, Zoller T, et al. Rapid immunochromatographic malarial antigen detection unreliable for detecting *Plasmodium malariae* and *Plasmodium ovale*. Eur J Clin Microbiol Infect Dis 2002;21:818–20.
51. Bottieau E, van Gompel A, Peetermans WE. Failure of primaquine therapy for the treatment of *Plasmodium ovale* malaria. Clin Infect Dis 2005;41: 1544–5.
52. Golgi C. Malarial infection. Arch Sci Med 1886;10:109–35.
53. Mungai M, Tegtmeier G, Chamberland M, Parise M. Transfusion-transmitted malaria in the United States from 1963 through 1999. N Engl J Med 2001; 344:1973–8.
54. Mali S, Steele S, Slutsker L, Arguin PM; Centers for Disease Control and Prevention (CDC). Malaria surveillance–United States, 2008. MMWR Surveill Summ 2010;59:1–15.
55. Tikasingh E, Edwards C, Hamilton PJ, et al. A malaria outbreak due to *Plasmodium malariae* on the Island of Grenada. Am J Trop Med Hyg 1980;29: 715–9.
56. Vinetz JM, Li J, McCutchan TF, Kaslow DC. *Plasmodium malariae* infection in an asymptomatic 74-year-old Greek woman with splenomegaly. N Engl J Med 1998;338:367–71.

57. Chadee DD, Tilluckdharry CC, Maharaj P, Sinanan C. Reactivation of *Plasmodium malariae* infection in a Trinidadian man after neurosurgery. N Engl J Med 2000;342:1924.
58. Gilles HM, Hendrickse RG. Possible aetiological role of *Plasmodium malariae* in "nephrotic syndrome" in Nigerian children. Lancet 1960;i:806–7.
59. Abdurrahman MB, Greenwood BM, Narayana P, et al. Immunological aspects of nephrotic syndrome in Northern Nigeria. Arch Dis Child 1981; 56:199–202.
60. Hedelius R, Fletcher JJ, Glass WF, II, et al. Nephrotic syndrome and unrecognized *Plasmodium malariae* infection in a US Navy sailor 14 years after departing Nigeria. J Travel Med 2011;18:288–91.
61. Eiam-Ong S. Malarial nephropathy. Semin Nephrol 2003;23:21–33.
62. Collins WE, Jeffery GM. *Plasmodium malariae*: parasite and disease. Clin Microbiol Rev 2007;20:579–92.
63. Mueller I, Zimmerman PA, Reeder JC. *Plasmodium malariae* and *Plasmodium malariae* – the "bashful" malaria parasites. Trends Parasitol 2007;23:278–83.
64. Singh B, Kim Sung L, Matusop A, et al. A large focus of naturally acquired *Plasmodium knowlesi* infections in human beings. Lancet 2004;363:1017–24.
65. Liu Q, Zhu S, Mizuno S, et al. Sequence variation in the small-subunit rRNA gene of *Plasmodium malariae* and prevalence of isolates with the variant sequence in Sichuan, China. J Clin Microbiol 1998;36:3378–81.
66. Maguire JD, Baird JK. The "non-falciparum" malarias: the roles of epidemiology, parasite biology, clinical syndromes, complications and diagnostic rigour in guiding therapeutic strategies. Ann Trop Med Parasitol 2010;104:283–301.
67. Müller-Stöver I, Verweij JJ, Hoppenheit B, et al. *Plasmodium malariae* infection in spite of previous anti-malarial medication. Parasitol Res 2008;102: 547–50.
68. Maguire JD, Baire JK. The "non-falciparum" malarias: the role of epidemiology, parasite biology, clinical syndromes, complications and diagnostic rigour in guiding therapeutic strategies. Ann Trop Med Parasitol 2010;104:283–301.
69. Nicol WE. Malaria in general paresis of the insane. BMJ 1935;2:760.
70. Singh B, Kim Sung L, Matusop A, et al. A large focus of naturally acquired *Plasmodium knowlesi* infections in human beings. Lancet 2004;363;1017–24.
71. Daneshvar C, Davis TME, Cox-Singh J, et al. Clinical and laboratory features of human *Plasmodium knowlesi* infection. Clin Inf Dis 2011;52:1356–62.
72. Barber BE, William T, Jikal M, et al. *Plasmodium knowlesi* in children. EID 2011;17:814–20.
73. William T, Menon J, Rajahram G, et al. Severe *Plasmodium knowlesi* malaria in a tertiary care hospital, Sabah, Malayasia. EID 2011;17:1248–55.
74. Kantele A, Jokiranta TS. Review of cases with the emerging fifth human malaria parasite, *Plasmodium knowlesi*. Clin Inf Dis 2011;52:1256–362.
75. Cox-Singh J, Hiu J, Lucas SB, et al. Severe malaria – a case of fatal *Plasmodium knowlesi* infection with *post-mortem* findings: a case report. Mal J 2010; 9:10.
76. Lee K-S, Cox-Singh J, Singh B. Morphological features and differential counts of *Plasmodium knowlesi* parasites in naturally acquired human infections. Mal J 2009;8:73
77. Collins WE, Barnwell JW. *Plasmodium knowlesi*: Finally being recognized. J Inf Dis 2009;199.1107–8.
78. Lee K-S, Cox-Singh J, Brooke G, et al. *Plasmodium knowlesi* from archival blood films: further evidence that human infections are widely distributed and not newly emergent in Malaysian Borneo. Int J Parasitol 2009;39: 1125–8.
79. Lee K-S, Divis PCS, Zakaria SK, et al. *Plasmodium knowlesi*: reservoir hosts and tracking the emergence in humans and macaques. PLoS Pathogens 2011;7: e1002015.
80. Cox-Singh J, Singh B. Knowlesi malaria: newly emergent and of public health importance? Trends Parasitol 2008;24:406–10.
81. Cox-Singh J, David TME, Lee K-S, et al. *Plasmodium knowlesi* malaria in humans is widely distributed and potentially life-threatening. Clin Inf Dis 2008;46:165–71.
82. White NJ. Malaria. In: Cook GC, Zumla A, eds. Manson's Tropical Diseases, 22nd edn. Saunders; 2009:1201–300.
83. World Health Organization. Report of the Malaria Conference in Equatorial Africa (WHO Technical Report Series, No. 38). Geneva: World Health Organization; 1951.
84. World Health Organization. 2005.
85. World Health Organization. Prevention and control of malaria epidemics. Third meeting of the Technical Support Network, 10–11 December 2001 (WHO/CDS/RBM/2002.40). Geneva: World Health Organization; 2002.
86. Beier JC, Killeen GF, Githure JI. Short report: entomologic inoculation rates and *Plasmodium falciparum* malaria prevalence in Africa. Am J Trop Med Hyg 1999;61:109–13.
87. Warrell DA, Looareesuwan S, Warrell MJ, et al. Dexamethasone proves deleterious in cerebral malaria. A double-blind trial in 100 comatose patients. N Engl J Med 1982;306(6):313–19.
88. Hoffman SL, Rustama D, Punjabi NH, et al. High-dose dexamethasone in quinine-treated patients with cerebral malaria: a double-blind, placebo-controlled trial. J Infect Dis 1988;158:325–31.
89. Taylor TE, Molyneux ME, Wirima JJ, et al. Intravenous immunoglobulin in the treatment of paediatric cerebral malaria. Clin Exp Immunol 1992; 90:357–62.
90. Namutangula B, Ndeezi G, Byarugaba JS, Tumwine JK. Mannitol as adjunct therapy for childhood cerebral malaria in Uganda: a randomized clinical trial. Malar J 2007;6:138.
91. Mohanty S, et al. Brain swelling and mannitol treatment in adult cerebral malaria: a randomized trial. Clin Inf Dis 2011;53(4):349–55.
92. Picot, S (study in progress).
93. Gordeuk V, Thuma P, Brittenham G, et al. Effect of iron chelation therapy on recovery from deep coma in children with cerebral malaria. N Engl J Med 1992;327(21):1473–7.
94. Thuma PE, Mabeza GF, Biemba G, et al. Effect of iron chelation therapy on mortality in Zambian children with cerebral malaria. Trans R Soc Trop Med Hyg 1998;92:214–18.
95. Agbenyega T, Planche T, Bedu-Addo G, et al. Population kinetics, efficacy, and safety of dichloroacetate for lactic acidosis due to severe malaria in children. J Clin Pharmacol 2003;43(4):386–96.
96. van Hensbroek MB, Palmer A, Onyiorah E, et al. The effect of a monoclonal antibody to tumor necrosis factor on survival from childhood cerebral malaria. J Infect Dis 1996;174:1091–7.
97. Anstey, N (study in progress).
98. Charunwatthana P, Abul Faiz M, Ruangveerayut R, et al. N-acetylcysteine as adjunctive treatment in severe malaria: a randomized, double-blinded placebo-controlled clinical trial. Crit Care Med 2009;37(2):516–22.
99. De Souza JB, Okomo U, Alexander ND, et al. Oral activated charcoal prevents experimental cerebral malaria in mice and in a randomized controlled clinical trial in man did not interfere with the pharmacokinetics of parenteral artesunate. PLoS One 2010;5:e9687.
100. Di Perri G, Di Perri IG, Monteiro GB, et al. Pentoxifylline as a supportive agent in the treatment of cerebral malaria in children. J Infect Dis 1995; 171(5):1317–22.
101. Hemmer CJ, Hort G, Chiwakata CB, et al. Supportive pentoxifylline in falciparum malaria: no effect on tumor necrosis factor alpha levels or clinical outcome: a prospective, randomized, placebo controlled study. Am J Trop Med Hyg 1997;56:397–403.
102. Looareesuwan S, Wilairatana P, Vannaphan S, et al. Pentoxifylline as an ancillary treatment for severe falciparum malaria in Thailand. Am J Trop Med Hyg 1998;58:348–53.
103. Das BK, Mishra S, Padhi PK, et al. Pentoxifylline adjuvant improves prognosis of human cerebral malaria in adults. Trop Med Int Health 2003; 8:680–4.
104. Lell B, Köhler C, Wamola B, et al. Pentoxifylline as an adjunct therapy with cerebral malaria. Malaria J 2010;9:368.
105. van Genderen PJ, Hesselink DA, Bezemer JM, et al. Efficacy and safety of exchange transfusion as an adjunct therapy for severe Plasmodium falciparum malaria in nonimmune travelers: a 10-year single-center experience with a standardized treatment protocol. Transfusion 2010;50(4):787–94.
106. Riddle MS, Jackson JL, Sanders JW, Blazes DL. Exchange transfusion as an adjunct therapy in severe Plasmodium falciparum malaria: a meta-analysis. Clin Infect Dis 2002;34:1192–8.

97 African Trypanosomiasis

Sanjeev Krishna, August Stich

Key features

- Synonyms: human African trypanosomiasis, sleeping sickness, encephalitis lethargica
- Infection caused by protozoa genus *Trypanosoma* and transmitted by tsetse fly
- Hematologic stage (I) associated with systemic illness
- Neurologic stage (II) associated with progressive disease, disability, and death if untreated
- May be difficult to diagnose
- Treatments are associated with significant toxicity

INTRODUCTION

The description of sleeping sickness preceded by centuries the discovery of its cause. John Atkin (1685–1757) described "a sleepy distemper" reminiscent of second stage trypanosomiasis off the coast of Guinea in 1721, and Thomas Masterman Winterbottom (1766–1859) published an account of lethargy in Sierra Leone that was sometimes associated with "small glandular tumors in the neck" in West African slaves. However, it was only after Pasteur's (1822–1895) demonstration that microorganisms can cause disease that trypanosomes began to be identified in the blood of animals in the middle of the nineteenth century.

David Livingstone (1813–1873) had already written (1858) of a *nagana,* a disease of horses ("which follows the bite of the tsetse") when Captain David Bruce (1855–1931) identified trypanosomes in large mammals in Ubombo, Zululand (in 1895). Bruce experimented with tsetse flies and dogs to demonstrate transmission of trypanosomes.

The first human infection was described by Robert Forde (1861–1948) together with Everett Dutton (1877–1905). They identified trypanosomes in a sailor returning from The Gambia to Liverpool and classified them as a new species, *Trypanosoma gambiense,* in 1902.

Aldo Castellani (1878–1971) went to Entebbe to assist with an epidemic of sleeping sickness that was devastating communities there and first reported trypanosomes in the cerebrospinal fluid (CSF) of patients in 1903, albeit in somewhat controversial circumstances. In 1910, John Stephens (1865–1946) and Harold Fentham (1875–1937) described in detail a morphologically different parasite – "with a nucleus at the posterior (non-flagellar) end" – from another patient who had been seen in Liverpool and named it *T. rhodesiense* as the patient had returned from a prospecting expedition in northeastern Rhodesia. This parasite was more virulent in laboratory models than *T. gambiense.* A year later, Allan Kinghorn (1880–1953) and Warrington Yorke (1883–1943) showed that *Glossina morsitans* can transmit *T. rhodesiense* to monkeys.

Although arsenic had been used by Livingstone to treat a mare with *nagana,* and Forde used it (Fowler's solution) to treat his patient from The Gambia, it fell upon Ernst Friedham (1899–1989) to carry out the first drug trials of arsenic derivatives in the 1940s and to select melarsoprol, which was licensed in 1949.

The control of trypanosomiasis in endemic areas crucially depends upon public health measures that were developed during the major epidemics in the last century, including one in the Congo (1896–1906, killing 500,000) and Uganda then as well as in the 1970s. Eugene Jamot (1879–1937) in the 1920s evolved the concept of a mobile team for case finding, which has proved to be so important for control in recent years.

Scientific studies of trypanosomes have resulted in the discovery of antigenic variation, GPI anchors, polycistronic transcription, RNA splicing, mitochondrial RNA editing, and several unusual metabolic pathways, but, as yet, precious few new agents for treatment. Perhaps the recent publication of the full sequence of the genome of the kinetoplastids, including *Trypanosoma* spp., will help to rectify this anomaly [1].

Human African trypanosomiasis (HAT) is an acute (caused by *T. b. rhodesiense*) or chronic (caused by *T. b. gambiense*) protozoal infection that invariably progresses to a fatal outcome unless treated (see Table 97-1 for forms of HAT). Other human trypanosomiases include infections in the Americas by *T. cruzi* that causes Chagas disease and occasional infections with *T. evansi* (in India), and *T. congolense* and *T. b. brucei* (in Africa). *T. b. brucei* is almost exclusively an animal subspecies that causes economically important disease in ungulates. In Malawi, a more chronic version of *T. b. rhodesiense* has been described, possibly with a distinct immunopathogenetic mechanism.

Stage I hemolymphatic infection is when there is no evidence of central nervous system (CNS) involvement (no clinical signs and ≤5 lymphocytes/mm^3 in the CSF). Stage II meningoencephalitic infection is when the parasite has penetrated into the CNS as evidenced by a lymphocytic pleocytosis (>5 lymphocytes/mm^3 in CSF) associated with or without CNS symptoms and signs. An "intermediate stage" of infection has also been described and used in some countries to guide therapy, defined as infection with trypanosomes in patients who have between 6 and 20 lymphocytes/mm^3 in the CSF. The clinical relevance of this "intermediate stage" and its consequences for treatment are still unclear [2].

EPIDEMIOLOGY

Within the subkingdom Protozoa and Order kinetoplastida, the genus *Trypanosoma* belongs to the family Trypanosomatidae and subgenus *Trypanozoon.* Despite early descriptions of morphologic differences between *T. rhodesiense* and *T. gambiense,* it is accepted that the three species in this subgenus, *T. brucei, T. evansi,* and *T. equiperdum,* are morphologically indistinguishable. *T. brucei* itself is now divided into three subspecies: the two human pathogens *T. b. gambiense* and *T. b. rhodesiense* and the animal pathogen *T. b. brucei.* It is their epidemiology, molecular biology, and clinical behavior that establishes the

TABLE 97-1 Forms of HAT

East African sleeping sickness	West African sleeping sickness
Trypanosoma brucei rhodesiense	*Trypanosoma brucei gambiense*
Zoonosis; wild (antelopes, e.g. bushbuck) and occasionally domestic animals as reservoir and source of case clusters; epidemic outbreaks, mainly in East Africa (Tanzania, Zambia, Malawi)	Mainly anthroponosis with evidence for several other mammal species; severe public health problem in some West and Central African countries (DRC, Sudan, Angola, CAR)
Transmitted by savannah tsetse flies (Morsitans group)	Transmitted by riverine tsetse flies (Palpalis group)
Acute onset, chancre frequent, rapid progression; death frequently in stage I (cardiac failure)	Febrile disease, slow progression; death usually in stage II after many months or years
Parasites usually in high number and easily detectable, serological tests unreliable	Parasitemia scanty, serology reliable in later stages

strongest distinctions between subspecies. *T. brucei* is transmitted by tsetse flies and develops in their midgut and salivary glands (hence "salivarian" trypanosomes) [3].

In nature, *T. b. brucei* can infect all domestic animals, camels, some antelopes and carnivores; *T. b. rhodesiense* infects humans, domestic livestock, and some wild antelopes, and *T. b. gambiense* infects humans, pigs, and sheep and only occasionally other orders. *T. b. rhodesiense* and *T. b. brucei* are easily grown in rodents, whereas *T. b. gambiense* requires immunosuppressed rodents, multimammate, or thicket rats to yield reasonable rates of isolation after subinoculation.

Trypanosomes are flagellated, extracellular protozoa (Fig. 97.1) that are slender and long (12–42 µm) in the bloodstream. They have a single, tubular mitochondrion located near the flagellum, which contains circular DNAs within concatenated structures called the kinetoplast. Short "stumpy" forms are taken up by tsetse when they feed, and in the midgut they develop into procyclic forms and multiply by binary fission. After about 2 weeks in the gut, trypanosomes migrate to the salivary glands as epimastigotes, where they develop into metacyclic forms that can infect the next host. There are many coordinated changes in the metabolism and antigenicity of the parasite as it develops its morphologic program in each host. In contrast to *Leishmania* spp and *T. cruzi*, there is no evidence for intracellular stages of *T. brucei.*

VECTOR

African trypanosomes are transmitted by different species of tsetse fly (*Glossina* spp) found in microfoci between the latitudes 14°N and 29°S (Fig. 97.2) [4]. The genus of these biologically unique insects comprises 31 distinct species and subspecies. Only few are potential vectors of HAT, the most important being *G. morsitans* (Fig. 97.3) and *G. palpalis*. Their distinctive behavior, ecology (warm temperatures), and chosen habitat (shade, and humidity for resting and larviposition) explain many epidemiologic features of sleeping sickness. Tsetse flies can live for many months in the wild, but give birth to only about eight larvae per lifetime. Both sexes feed on blood, inflicting a painful bite. A relatively small proportion of flies in the field (<1%) are competent to transmit infection, with a higher proportion found in epidemics (<5%).

NATURAL HISTORY, PATHOGENESIS, AND PATHOLOGY

Normal human plasma has a trypanolytic factor that does not allow animal trypanosomes (including *T. b. brucei* and *T. evansi*) to survive. This protective factor, serum resistance antigen, is made of apolipoprotein L1, apolipoprotein A-I, and haptoglobin-related protein, which together are found in the densest subfraction of high-density lipoprotein (HDL3) and in another lipid-poor complex of IgMs. This mechanism has helped to explain how a human case of *T. evansi* developed, as the patient was deficient in apolipoprotein L1. Normal

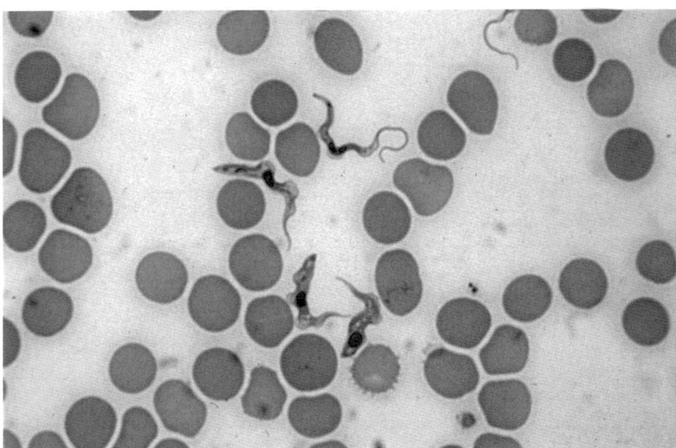

FIGURE 97.1 Trypanosomes in peripheral blood (Giemsa stain).

human serum or recombinant apoLI inserts anionic pores in the lysosomal membrane of parasites, causing lysis through osmotic swelling [5].

Apart from serum resistance antigen, which acts to protect against innate host defense, parasites have also evolved a dense surface coat of glycoprotein (variant surface glycoprotein or VSG), which is shed when the host's immune system develops anti-VSG IgM and IgG antibody responses. Approximately 10^7 molecules of single VSG are expressed at any one time, being replaced with an antigenically distinct version in a smaller, proliferating subset of parasites (about 2%) that multiply to replace the ones that have already been recognized. As the host immune response attempts to catch up by generating new VSG antibodies, the parasites produce new surface coats. New VSGs are generated through programmed DNA rearranging from a non-expressed context to an expression-linked, telomerically located region. Whilst this elaborate antigenic switching mechanism is well understood in molecular terms, it has not yielded a solution to the problem it creates for making a vaccine against this organism.

POLYCLONAL ACTIVATION OF B CELLS

A further consequence of antigenic variation is chronic stimulation of the host's immune system with hypergammaglobulinemia, penetration of trypanosomes into privileged sites such as the CNS, and stimulation of the cytokine and mediator networks, exhausting defense mechanisms. Much of the IgM and IgG antibody is directed to non-VSG antigens, with production of rheumatoid factor-like reactivity, anti-DNA antibodies and heterophile antibodies, some of which can be confusing if identified in screening tests. Cross-reactivity with numerous other serologic tests is common and can be misleading.

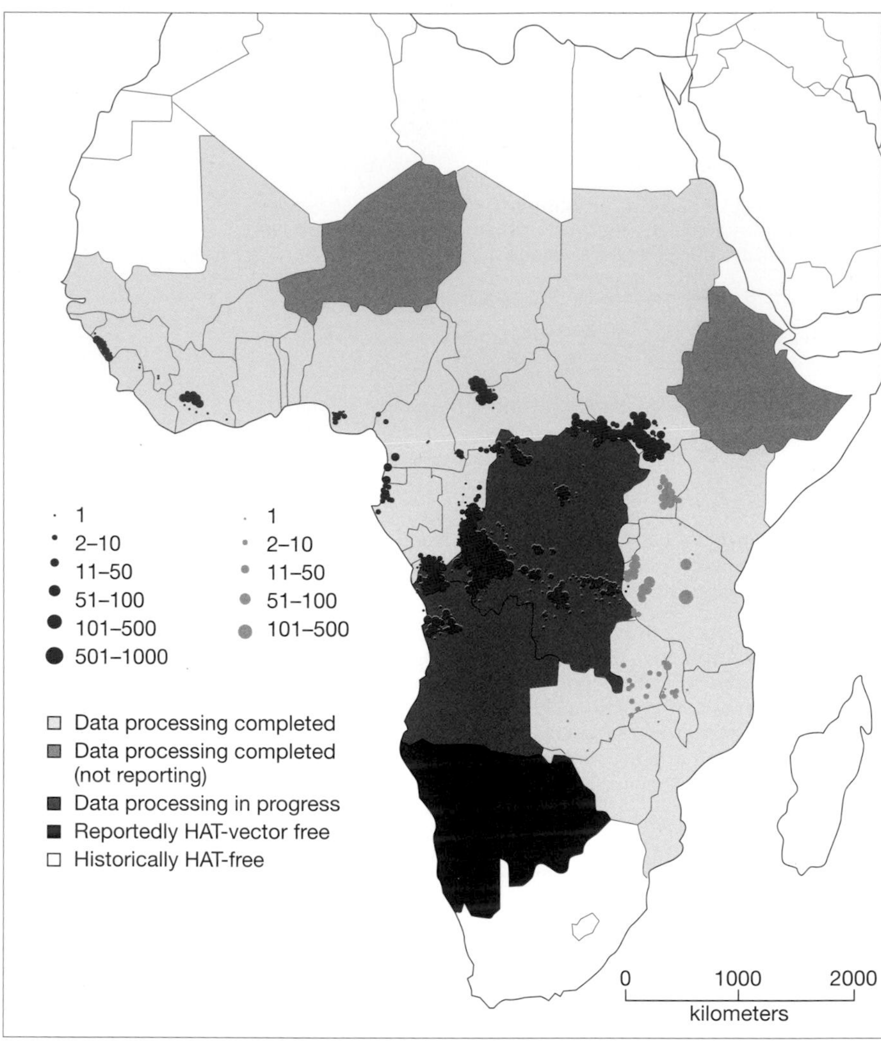

FIGURE 97.2 Map of distribution of human African trypanosomiasis

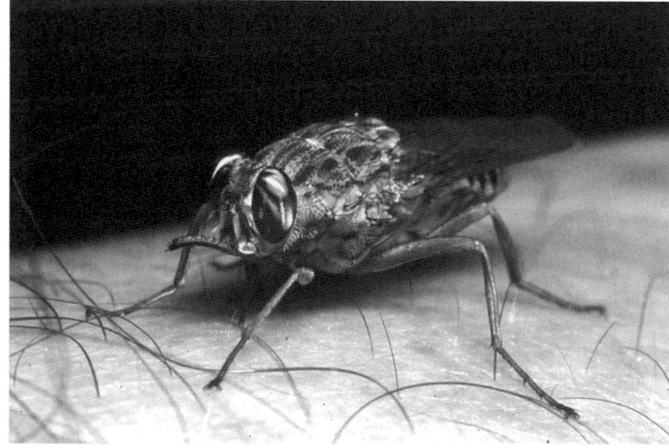

FIGURE 97.3 *Glossina morsitans.*

CLINICAL FEATURES

There is no unique clinical picture of HAT, and the disease in all its stages offers a sometimes wide range of differential diagnoses. The infection often has an insidious onset, but *T. brucei*, whether the East or West African subspecies, will invariably kill if the patient is not treated in time. The natural course of HAT can be divided into different and distinct stages. Their determination by various laboratory investigations is important for the clinical management of the patient.

THE TRYPANOSOMAL CHANCRE

Tsetse bites can be quite painful. In the case of an infection, a local reaction called trypanosomal chancre (Fig. 97.4) can develop at the site where the fly has injected parasites with its saliva. A small raised papule develops after about 5 days. It increases rapidly in size, surrounded by an intense erythematous tissue reaction with local edema and regional lymphadenopathy. Although some chancres have a very angry appearance, they are usually not very painful unless they become ulcerated and superinfected. They heal without treatment after several weeks, leaving a permanent, hyperpigmented spot. Trypanosomal chancres occur in more than half the cases of *T. b. rhodesiense*. In *T. b. gambiense*, they are much less common and often go undetected in endemic populations. Inexperienced clinicians might misdiagnose chancres as cutaneous manifestations of bacterial diseases, such as superinfected insect bites, eschar or cutaneous anthrax.

HEMOLYMPHATIC STAGE (HAT STAGE I)

In *T. b. rhodesiense* infection, this hemolymphatic stage is very dramatic and pronounced, clinically often resembling severe *Plasmodium falciparum* malaria or septicemia. Patients may die within the first weeks after the onset of symptoms, mostly through cardiac involvement (myocarditis). In the early stage of *T. b. gambiense* infection,

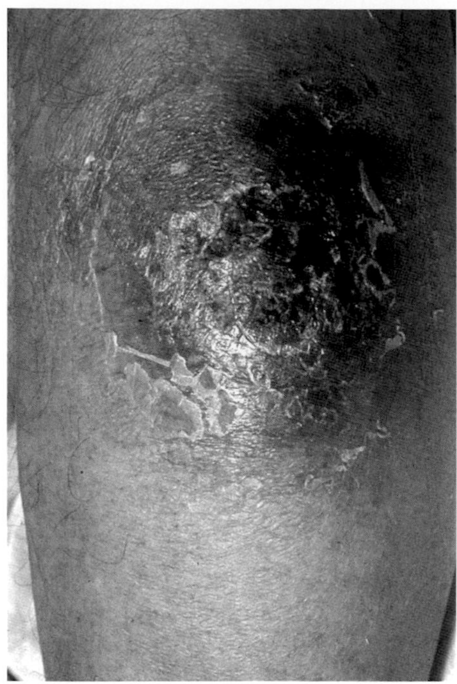

FIGURE 97.4 Trypanosomal chancre on the leg.

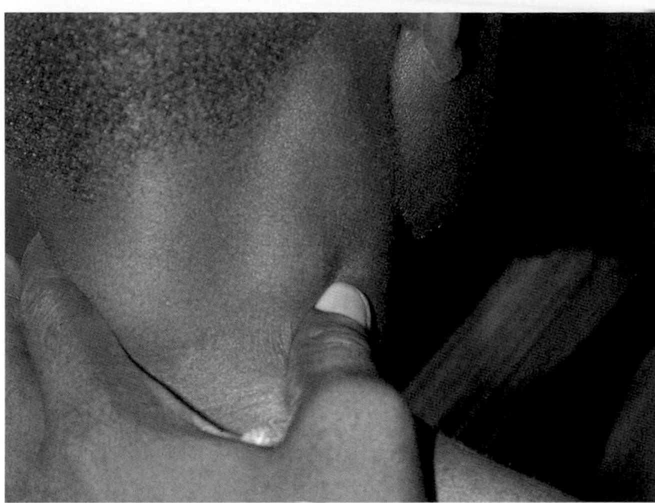

FIGURE 97.5 Winterbottom's sign.

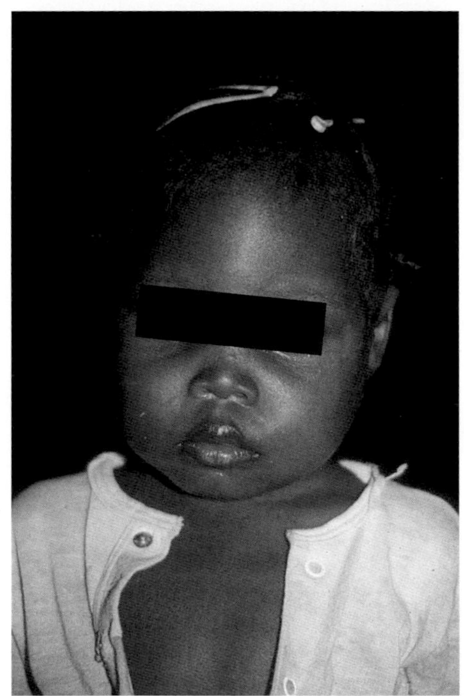

FIGURE 97.6 "Puffy face" syndrome.

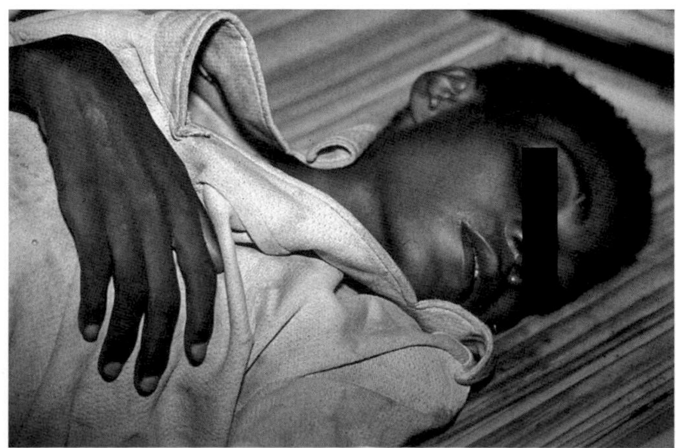

FIGURE 97.7 Patient with late-stage trypanosomiasis.

symptoms are usually infrequent and mild. Laboratory findings indicate raised levels of markers of inflammation (CRP, ESR), normal to low WBC counts, anemia, and often a marked thrombocytopenia, depending on the severity of the clinical condition [6].

After the initial phase, febrile episodes become less severe as the disease progresses. Fever is often undulating, reflecting the lyses of waves of parasites in the bloodstream. A reliable sign, particularly in *T. b. gambiense* infection, is the enlargement of lymph nodes in the posterior triangle of the neck (Winterbottom's sign, Fig. 97.5). Other typical signs are a fugitive patchy or circinate rash, a myxedematous infiltration of connective tissue ("puffy face syndrome", Fig. 97.6), and an inconspicuous periostitis of the tibia with delayed hyperesthesia (Kérandel's sign).

MENINGOENCEPHALITIC STAGE (HAT STAGE II)

Within weeks in *T. b. rhodesiense* and months (sometimes years) in *T. b. gambiense* infection, cerebral involvement will invariably follow the early stages of HAT. Trypanosomes cross the blood–brain barrier and enter the CSF by mechanisms that are still not clearly understood.

The onset of stage II is insidious and may not be determined clinically. As the disease progresses, patients complain of increasing headache and some may detect a marked change in behavior and personality. Neurologic symptoms, which follow gradually, can be focal or generalized, depending on the site of cellular damage in the CNS. Radiologic changes include bilateral, hyperintense signals at MRI T2-signal prolongation, predominantly involving the periventricular and frontal white matter as well as affecting capsules, basal ganglia and cerebellum. The pathohistologic correlate is a perivascular infiltration of inflammatory cells ("cuffing") and glial proliferation, resembling cerebral endarteritis. Neuronal elements may be less affected [7].

Convulsions in late-stage trypanosomiasis are common, usually indicating a poor prognosis. Periods of confusion and agitation slowly evolve towards a stage of distinct perplexity (Fig. 97.7) when patients lose interest in their surroundings and their own situation. Inflammatory reactions in the hypothalamic structures lead to a dysfunction in circadian rhythms and sleep regulatory systems. Sleep patterns become fragmented and finally result in a somnolent and comatose

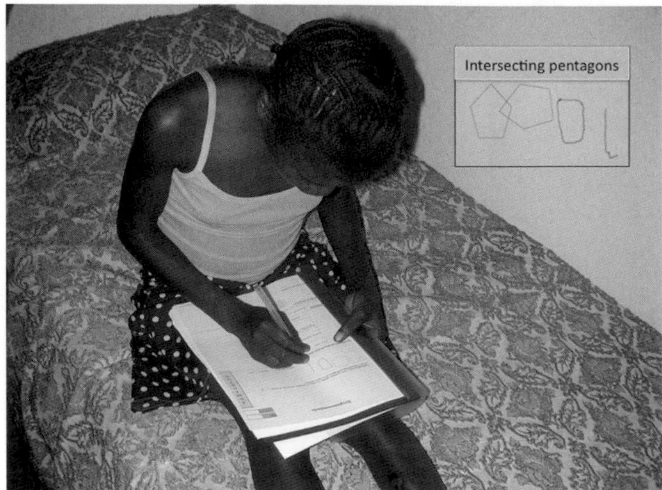

FIGURE 97.8 Patient with late-stage trypanosomiasis asked to copy a figure (intersecting pentagons) shown in inset.

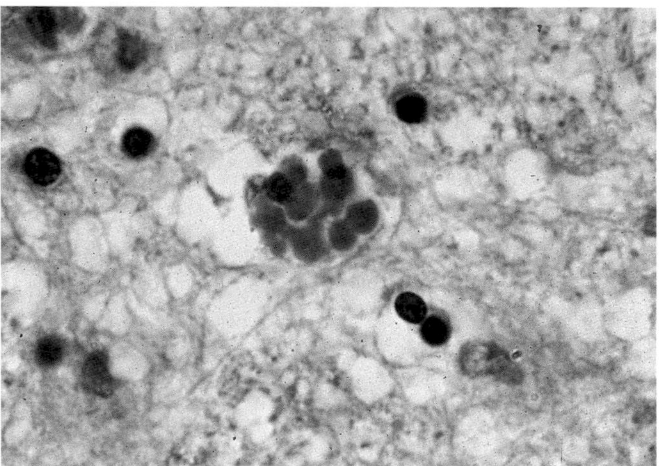

FIGURE 97.9 Morular cell of Mott (H&E stain) in cerebrospinal fluid of patient with stage II disease.

state. Other evidence of CNS involvement includes inability to execute relatively simple tasks (Fig. 97.8). In some cases, morular cells of Mott, activated plasma cells with eosinophilic inclusions containing IgM antibodies, can be seen in the CSF (Fig. 97.9). Progressive wasting and dehydration follows the inability to eat and drink.

In children, HAT seems to progress even more rapidly. Parents often notice insomnia and behavioral changes, and stage II is usually already reached when the diagnosis is established.

PATIENT EVALUATION, DIAGNOSIS, AND DIFFERENTIAL DIAGNOSIS

Few infections demand a confirmed diagnosis as much as African trypanosomiasis, because the treatments available can be fatally toxic. Clinical suspicion is triggered when a patient returns from an area endemic for trypanosomiasis. A distinction should be made between the two forms: For *T. b. rhodesiense* infections, the appearance of a chancre and the presence of high fever should raise suspicion and trigger a vigorous search for parasites in the blood film. *T. b. gambiense* infections can present, sometimes months or years after exposure, with symptoms that may be relatively nonspecific, even sometimes mimicking psychoses. Again, detection of parasites is critical to management, and these can be sought in aspirate from a chancre, in blood, lymph fluid in glands, or in the CSF. In endemic areas, active case finding relies on serologic screening tests for *T. b. gambiense* that identify individuals at high risk of being infected [8]. In some circumstances when serologic tests are strongly positive, there are appropriate clinical findings, and especially when there is evidence of advanced (stage II) disease, treatment can be given empirically. For infection with *T. b. rhodesiense*, serologic tests are unhelpful, but parasites are much easier to detect because they are commonly present in greater abundance in the bloodstream.

T. b. gambiense can cause disease even though it may be present in numbers well below the limits for detection (for example, <10 parasites/mL) by any method that examines body fluids. Repeated examinations for parasites, or, if possible, subinoculation into a susceptible species, may help in detection.

ASPIRATION OF CHANCRE OR LYMPH NODE

Chancres mark the portal of entry of trypanosomes and are more common in *T. b. rhodesiense*, where half the patients may manifest this sign, whereas they are less common in *T. b. gambiense* infections, particularly in patients in endemic areas. If present, they are a good source of parasites. Fluid from enlarged lymph nodes, frequently posterior cervical nodes that form Winterbottom's sign, can be aspirated and visualized immediately (×400) with direct microscopy or, if available, dark-field illumination. Fresh preparations contain motile trypanosomes that catch the eye by jostling their neighboring cells.

BLOOD FILMS

Thick blood films, stained with Field's or Giemsa's stains identical to the ones used for malaria diagnosis, can sometimes show trypanosomes, although concentration techniques are required routinely to identify parasites in a *T. b. gambiense* infection. Morphology may be poor in thick films, but the longer time required to examine thin films that preserve morphology may outweigh their value in screening for this infection. In contrast, blood film examinations are much more useful in *T. b. rhodesiense* infections.

CONCENTRATION METHODS

Many approaches to concentrate parasites before visualization have been successfully developed. Probably the most robust one relies on a mini anion exchange column that allows trypanosomes through its cellulose matrix when 300 μL of blood is added to it (compared to ~10 μL of blood volume examined on a thick film). The kit is not commercially available and is used only by specialized laboratories. Another method has been adapted from malaria diagnosis, the quantitative buffy coat (QBC) method. A similar approach uses capillary tube centrifugation (CTC). These approaches can be combined with better visualization techniques such as fluorescence labeling to improve parasite recognition and together with field-adapted, relatively cheap fluorescence microscopes with light-emitting diodes as source illumination are being developed by the Foundation for Innovative New Diagnostics (FIND), which aims to improve diagnostic approaches for African trypanosomiasis.

NUCLEIC ACID AMPLIFICATION TECHNIQUES

Genus, species and subspecies specific primers are well described and available for use in epidemiologic studies of African trypanosomiasis, but conventional PCR currently lacks sensitivity to detect parasites in low abundance in the clinic. Newer approaches including the use of isothermal PCR techniques that demand much less in the way of equipment are being investigated by FIND, but until now molecular diagnostic tests are still inferior to conventional parasite detection.

SEROLOGIC ASSAYS

A card agglutination test (CATT) has been used for many years to screen for antibodies against *T. b. gambiense* using a mixture of abundant parasite antigens. This is a rapid, field-adapted test that detects antibodies by their ability to agglutinate antigen, but does not confirm the infection. Rather, a positive result should stimulate the search for parasites. The CATT can be obtained from the Department of Parasitology, Prince Leopold Institute of Tropical Medicine, Nationalestraat 155 B – 2000 Antwerp, Belgium (www.itg.be).

TREATMENT

Treatment of HAT is difficult and dangerous for the patient in all stages. Hospitalization is usually necessary. Patient management requires not only the availability and correct administration of drugs with numerous side effects, but also good general medical skills and nursing care to deal with treatment reactions and concomitant pathologies, as most patients with late stage trypanosomiasis are severely ill and malnourished [9]. However, sleeping sickness is a disease of rural, remote places where the healthcare system is rudimentary. The active foci of sleeping sickness are usually in far-away and insecure places, which are difficult to access. Many treatment centers work under emergency conditions with extremely restricted resources.

However, if managed properly, HAT can be cured, especially when the diagnosis is made at an early stage of the disease.

Still, HAT treatment is not standardized. Trypanosomiasis treatment regimens vary considerably between countries and treatment centers, as many country programs have traditionally developed their own treatment protocols. Results from different centers are comparable to only a very limited extent. Few properly conducted and sufficiently powered clinical trials are available to evaluate duration, dosage, possible combinations of drugs, and co-administration of auxiliary treatments. Sufficient infrastructure for carrying out clinical research exists in only a handful of places.

MANAGEMENT OF HAT STAGE I

The treatment of HAT depends on the trypanosome subspecies and the stage of the disease (Tables 97-2 & 97-3).

Pentamidine

Since its introduction in 1937, pentamidine has become the drug of choice for *gambiense* HAT stage I, achieving cure rates as high as 98%. But in *T. rhodesiense* HAT there are frequent failures. Lower rates of cellular pentamidine uptake in *T. b. rhodesiense* may explain these differences. Some cures of stage II infections have also been reported, but CSF drug levels are usually not sufficiently high to guarantee a reliable trypanosomicidal effect in the CNS.

Pentamidine is usually given by deep intramuscular injection, which sometimes can be managed on an outpatient basis. If hospital care and reasonable monitoring conditions are available, an intravenous infusion, given in normal saline over 2 hours, might be used instead. The main advantage of pentamidine over other drugs is the short treatment course and ease of administration. Adverse effects are related to the route of administration or its dose and are usually reversible.

In clinical medicine, pentamidine is also used as second-line therapy for visceral leishmaniasis and especially in the prophylaxis and treatment of opportunistic *Pneumocystis jiroveci* pneumonia in AIDS. Since the start of the HIV pandemic, the cost of pentamidine was increased more than tenfold by producers, making it unaffordable for health institutions in low-income countries. After an intervention led by the World Health organization (WHO), a limited amount of pentamidine is now made available for use in HAT through a public–private partnership..

Suramin

In the early twentieth century, the development of the complex sulphated naphthylamine suramin ("Bayer 205"), resulting from German research on the trypanosomicidal activity of various dyes and heavy metals, was a major breakthrough in the field of tropical medicine. For the first time, African trypanosomiasis, at least in its early stages, became treatable without causing major harm. Suramin, under the trade name of Germanin® soon became a figurehead of German research in tropical medicine. That German politicians tried to use suramin to regain access to Africa to reverse the loss of the German colonies after World War I is another sad chapter on how tropical medicine was instrumentalized for political ambitions.

Suramin is still the drug of choice to treat stage I HAT caused by *T. b. rhodesiense*. Like pentamidine, it does not reach therapeutic levels in CSF. Suramin is injected intravenously after dilution in distilled water.

Adverse effects, especially pyrexia and nephrotoxicity, depend on nutritional status, concomitant illnesses (especially onchocerciasis) and the patient's clinical condition. Although life-threatening reactions like anaphylactic shock have been described, serious adverse effects are rare.

MANAGEMENT OF HAT STAGE II

Melarsoprol

Until the systematic introduction of the arsenical compound melarsoprol in 1949, late stage trypanosomiasis was virtually untreatable. Since then, it has remained the most widely used stage II antitrypanosomal drug for both *T. b. gambiense* and *rhodesiense* infections and has thus saved many lives. However, melarsoprol displays a high rate of dangerous adverse effects [10]. In addition, there is increasing evidence of frequent relapses and resistance in some parts of Congo, Angola, Sudan and Uganda.

TABLE 97-2 Drugs for the Treatment of HAT

	Stage 1 ***hemolymphatic stage (no evidence of CNS involvement)***	**Stage 2** ***meningoencephalitic stage (pathological CSF findings)***
Trypanosoma brucei rhodesiense	Suramin	Melarsoprol
Trypanosoma brucei gambiense	Pentamidine	Eflornithine (+ nifurtimox) alt.: melarsoprol

TABLE 97-3 Treatment Protocols for Antitrypanosomal Drugs

Suramin	Test dose 5 mg/kg, afterwards 20 mg/kg (max. 1 g/day) on day 1, 3, 7, 14, 21
Pentamidine	4 mg/kg every second day (max. 200 mg/day) for 7–10 days
Melarsoprol	2.2 mg/kg daily for 10 days (dosage regimen only evaluated for *T. b. gambiense*)
Eflornithine	100 mg/kg every 6 hours for 14 days
NECT (nifurtimox–eflornithine combination therapy)	Nifurtimox 5 mg/kg three times daily for 10 days Eflornithine 200 mg/kg twice daily for 7 days

Melarsoprol clears trypanosomes rapidly from the blood, lymph and CSF. It is given by slow intravenous injection; extravascular leakage must be avoided because of possible tissue necrosis. The most important adverse effect is an acute encephalopathy, usually appearing around day 5 to 8 of the treatment course in 5–14% of all patients. Severe headache, convulsions, rapid neurologic deterioration, or deepening of coma are the indicators of a reaction which is immune-mediated by release of parasite antigens in the first days of treatment. MRI changes associated with this reaction are of a diffuse hemorrhagic encephalopathy and cerebral edema. The overall case fatality under treatment ranges between 2% and 12%, depending on the stage of disease and the quality of medical and nursing care. Simultaneous administration of glucocorticosteroids (prednisolone 1 mg/kg body weight; maximum 40 mg daily) might reduce mortality, especially in cases with high CSF pleocytosis [11].

Eflornithine (DFMO)

Initially developed as antitumor agent, eflornithine (alpha-difluoromethylornithine) was introduced in 1980 as an antitrypanosomal drug, in the hope that it might replace melarsoprol for treatment of stage II trypanosomiasis. However, exorbitant costs and limited availability have restricted its use mostly to melarsoprol-refractory cases of *gambiense* sleeping sickness. *T. b. rhodesiense* is much less sensitive due to a much higher turnover rate of the target enzyme ornithine decarboxylase, and, therefore, cannot be treated with eflornithine.

Eflornithine can be taken orally, but intravenous administration is preferred as it achieves a much higher bioavailability and success rate. The infusion should be administered slowly over a period of at least 30 minutes. Continuous 24-hour administration is preferable if facilities allow.

The range of adverse reactions to eflornithine is wide, as with other cytotoxic drugs in cancer treatment. Their occurrence and intensity increase with the duration of treatment and the severity of the patient's general condition.

In the late 1990s, eflornithine was no longer produced for use against HAT, despite pleas from WHO. The discovery of its therapeutic effect in cosmetic creams against facial hair helped to restimulate a production line and thus had a beneficial "spin-off effect" for HAT. In 2001, agreements were signed between WHO and two major drug-producing companies (Bayer HealthCare and Sanofi-Aventis) which led to a "public–private partnership" (PPP) and helped to assure a sufficient supply of eflornithine and other drugs essential for the treatment of HAT. In 2006, the agreement was prolonged until 2011, and there are already promising signs for its continuation.

Nifurtimox

Ten years after its introduction for the treatment of American trypanosomiasis in 1967, nifurtimox was found to be effective in the treatment of *gambiense* sleeping sickness. It has a place as second-line treatment in melarsoprol-refractory cases and especially as a partner in combination therapies. Nifurtimox is generally not well tolerated, with gastrointestinal (nausea, epigastric pain) and neurologic (polyneuropathies, ataxia) symptoms being the most pronounced, but adverse effects are usually not severe. They are dose-related and rapidly reversible after discontinuation of the drug.

Combination Treatments in HAT

Melarsoprol, eflornithine and nifurtimox interfere with trypanothione synthesis and activity at different stages. There is also experimental evidence that combinations of suramin and stage II drugs might be beneficial. Therefore, by reducing the overall dosage of each individual component, drug combinations could perhaps reduce the frequency of serious side effects, and the development of resistance. Based on this concept, important progress was made in 2009 by a multicenter trial, testing a combination of nifurtimox and eflornithine. NECT (nifurtimox– eflornithine combination therapy) has the potential to develop into the preferred first-line treatment for stage II *gambiense* HAT in the future [12].

PREVENTION

Individual Protection

Pentamidine or suramin chemoprophylaxis is of historical interest, and can no longer be recommended. Insect repellents are only of limited use, as tsetse flies are visually attracted to their prey. Long-sleeved, bright clothing is the best defence against attacking tsetse flies. Infested strips of land are often well known to the local population and should be avoided as far as possible. Even in foci of disease, less than 1 % of the flies are infective, so HAT among tourists and occasional visitors to endemic areas is rare, although it continues to be reported in returned travelers. Recently, *rhodesiense* HAT has been reported in visitors to game parks in Tanzania and Zambia.

Control in Endemic Areas

In the past, tremendous efforts were undertaken to control the threat posed by sleeping sickness to human lives and economic development in rural Africa. Control programs are based on a combination of treatment of patients, mass screening, and vector control, usually by trapping. The most important strategy is active case finding. This requires mobile teams which regularly visit villages in endemic areas. Mostly based on the results of CATT screening, patients, preferably in the early stage of the disease, are identified and treated. Gradually, the parasite reservoir is depleted. As *Glossina* is a relatively incompetent vector and susceptible to control measures such as insecticide application or trapping, the combination of various approaches can lead to a complete break of the transmission cycle. This was achieved in the past in many places, and some recent successes have been accomplished, usually through the work of committed non-governmental organizations (Sudan, Angola, CAR). However, the resurgence of sleeping sickness in areas ridden by war and civil unrest in the last 25 years, in combination with the decreasing availability of drugs and the general loss of interest in health in Africa, gives rise to the fear that HAT will still continue to be a severe public health problem in the future.

REFERENCES

1. Barrett MP, Boykin DW, Brun R, Tidwell RR. Human African trypanosomiasis: pharmacological re-engagement with a neglected disease. Br J Pharmacol 2007;152:1155–71.
2. Brun R, Blum J, Chappuis F, Burri C. Human African trypanosomiasis. Lancet 2010;375:148–59.
3. Brun R, Balmer O. New developments in human African trypanosomiasis. Curr Opin Infect Dis 2006;19:415–20.
4. Simarro PP, Cecchi G, Paone M, et al. The atlas of human African trypanosomiasis: a contribution to global mapping of neglected tropical diseases. Int J Health Geogr 2010;9:57.
5. Pays E, Vanhollebeke B. Human innate immunity against African trypanosomes. Curr Opin Immunol 2009;21:493–8.
6. Stich A, Abel PM, Krishna S. Human African trypanosomiasis. BMJ 2002;325:203–6.
7. Kager PA, Schipper HG, Stam J, Majoie CB. Magnetic resonance imaging findings in human African trypanosomiasis: a four year follow-up study in a patient and review of the literature. Am J Trop Med Hyg 2009;80: 947–52.
8. Magnus E, Vervoort T, van Meirvenne N. A card-agglutination test with stained trypanosomes (C.A.T.T.) for the serological diagnosis of *T. b. gambiense* trypanosomiasis. Ann Soc Belg Med Trop 1978;58:169–76.
9. Burri C, Stich A, Brun R. Current chemotherapy of human African trypanosomiasis. In: Maudlin I, Holmes PH, Miles MA, eds. Trypanosomiasis. Wallingford, UK: CABI Publishing; 2004.
10. Burri C, Nkunku S, Merolle A, et al. Efficacy of new, concise schedule for melarsoprol in treatment of sleeping sickness caused by *Trypanosoma brucei gambiense*: a randomised trial. Lancet 2000;355:1419–25.
11. Pepin J, Milord F, Guern C, et al. Trial of prednisolone for prevention of melarsoprol-induced encephalopathy in *gambiense* sleeping sickness. Lancet 1989;i:1246–50.
12. Priotto G, Kasparian S, Mutombo W, et al. Nifurtimox-eflornithine combination therapy for second-stage African *Trypanosoma brucei gambiense* trypanosomiasis: a multicentre, randomised, phase III, non-inferiority trial. Lancet 2009;374:56–64.

American Trypanosomiasis (Chagas disease) 98

Rogelio López-Vélez, Francesca F Norman, Caryn Bern

Key features

- Caused by *Trypanosoma cruzi*, a flagellate protozoan parasite of the order Kinetoplastida, family Trypanosomatidae
- Endemic in the Americas from Mexico to northern Argentina and Chile. Twenty-eight million people are at risk; it is estimated that 8–10 million people are currently infected. Forty-one thousand and two hundred new infections and 12,500 deaths are estimated to occur annually
- The southern half of the USA has enzootic vector-borne transmission and rare autochthonous human cases
- Owing to migration now seen in North America, Europe (particularly Spain), Australia and Japan, acute Chagas disease has rarely been reported in travelers returning from endemic countries
- Transmitted by hematophagous triatomine vectors (Hemiptera, Reduviidae, Triatominae), more than 100 species of mammal act as reservoirs
- *Trypanosoma cruzi* can also be transmitted congenitally, by blood transfusion or organ donation, and via contaminated food or drink
- Factors that may affect pathogenesis include parasite burden, the severity of the initial infection, host immune response and human genetic factors. Tissue inflammation may be caused directly by the parasite and secondary to the host's immune response
- The natural history includes the acute phase lasting 2–3 months and the chronic phase, which lasts the lifetime of the host. An estimated 20–30% of people who initially have the indeterminate (asymptomatic) form progress over a period of years to clinically-evident cardiac and/or gastrointestinal disease
- Severe and fatal cases of *T. cruzi* infection following organ, tissue, or cell transplantation, and HIV co-infection can occur
- Diagnosis of acute and early congenital *T. cruzi* infection requires demonstration of the parasite in blood by microscopy, PCR or hemoculture. Diagnosis of chronic infection relies on serologic tests (e.g. ELISA) to detect IgG antibodies to *T. cruzi*
- Indication for anti-parasitic therapy depends on the phase of the disease and the clinical status and age of the patient. There are currently only two available drugs: benznidazole and nifurtimox
- Prevention and control relies on residual application of long-lasting insecticides in human dwellings and peridomestic structures, and serologic screening of blood donors, pregnant women and the newborns of women found to be infected
- Chagas disease has now emerged in North America and Europe. Physicians in non-endemic countries should therefore be aware of the existence, or even the potential transmission, of this parasitic disease during their routine clinical practice

INTRODUCTION

Chagas disease is a zoonotic protozoan infection transmitted by hematophagous triatomine bugs (Hemiptera, Reduviidae, Triatominae), a subfamily of the reduviid bugs (http://www.cdc.gov/parasites/chagas/gen_info/vectors/index.html). In 1909, Carlos Chagas, a Brazilian scientist, discovered the etiologic agent (the flagellate protozoan parasite *Trypanosoma cruzi*), described the clinical picture of acute disease and documented the vector and reservoir hosts.

In Latin America, Chagas disease affects millions and is one of the leading causes of cardiomyopathy with a high morbidity and mortality rates [1].

Thanks to efforts undertaken to control the vector and secure blood supply, the incidence and prevalence have decreased considerably since the 1990s. However, imported Chagas disease is increasingly recognized as an emerging problem in the USA and Europe as a result of immigration from Latin America. Most immigrants were infected during childhood and may now be at an age when the first manifestations of cardiomyopathy would be expected to appear. Clinicians in non-endemic areas may, therefore, face migrants with symptomatic or asymptomatic *T. cruzi* infection, as well as acute infections transmitted congenitally, through organ donation or blood transfusions. Chagas disease is considered a neglected tropical disease, characterized by an urgent need for new tools for screening, treatment and test of cure.

EPIDEMIOLOGY

VECTOR-BORNE TRANSMISSION, VECTORS AND NON-HUMAN RESERVOIR HOSTS

Trypanosoma cruzi is carried in the gut of the triatomine bug; transmission occurs when infected bug feces are inoculated through the bite wound or intact mucous membranes [2]. Vector-borne transmission occurs exclusively in the Americas and remains the predominant mechanism for new human infections.

Triatomines of both sexes must take blood meals to develop through their nymphal stages to adults; females require a blood meal to lay eggs. Thus, nymphs and adults of either sex may be infected with *T. cruzi*, but infection rates increase with increasing vector stage and age. There are at least 130 triatomine species in the Americas, many of which have been documented to carry *T. cruzi*. However, a handful of highly domiciliated vector species are of disproportionate importance in the human epidemiology of disease [3]. These include: *Triatoma infestans* in the Southern Cone (Argentina, Bolivia, Chile, Paraguay, southern Peru, Uruguay and southern Brazil); *Rhodnius prolixus* and *Triatoma dimidiata* in northern South America and Central America; and *Panstrongylus megistus* and *Triatoma brasiliensis* in Brazil. Most domestic species feed nocturnally and are able to complete their blood meal without waking the host. The major Latin American vectors defecate during, or immediately after taking, a blood meal, increasing the likelihood of infecting the host. Some triatomine species can infest both domestic and sylvatic sites and may play a bridging role.

More than 100 species of mammals have been reported to carry natural infections with *T. cruzi*. Sylvatic transmission cycles are maintained by wild mammals and triatomine species; the vectors often colonize nests of rodent or marsupial reservoir hosts. Wild triatomine adults may fly into human dwellings, attracted by light, and cause sporadic human infections. Domestic transmission cycles occur where vectors are adapted to living in human houses and nearby animal enclosures. The peridomestic environment provides abundant hosts that act as blood meal sources and poor quality housing provides crevices and other diurnal hiding places for triatomines. In endemic communities, a high proportion of houses may be infested, and a house and its immediate surroundings may support large colonies of bugs. Dogs, cats and guinea pigs act as important domestic *T. cruzi* reservoir hosts, while opossums, rodents, armadillos and raccoons are important sylvatic hosts.

NON-VECTORIAL TRYPANOSOMA CRUZI TRANSMISSION

Trypanosoma cruzi can also be transmitted congenitally, by blood transfusion or organ donation, and via contaminated food or drink. An estimated 5–6% (range 1–10%) of infants of infected mothers are born with congenital *T. cruzi* infection [4]. Congenital transmission can occur from women who were infected congenitally, perpetuating the disease in the absence of the vector. Factors reported to increase risk include higher maternal parasitemia level, less robust maternal anti-*T. cruzi* immune responses, HIV and, in an animal model, parasite strain. Transfusional transmission of *T. cruzi* was first hypothesized in 1936 and the first documented occurrence was published in 1952. The risk of *T. cruzi* transmission per infected unit transfused is estimated to be 10–25% [5]. Platelet transfusions are thought to pose a higher risk than those of other components, such as packed red cells. Uninfected recipients who receive an organ from a *T. cruzi*-infected donor may develop acute *T. cruzi* infection. However, transmission is not universal and varies depending on the organ transplanted and degree of immunosuppression [6]. In a series of 16 uninfected recipients of kidneys from infected donors, only 3 (19%) acquired *T. cruzi* infection; cardiac transplantation is thought to pose a much higher risk. Eighteen instances of transmission by organ transplantation have been documented in the literature to date (12 kidney, 1 kidney and pancreas, 3 liver, 2 heart transplants) [6]. Recently, increasing attention has focused on the oral route of *T. cruzi* transmission, with several outbreaks attributed to contaminated fruit or sugar cane juice reported from Brazil and Venezuela [7, 8].

GEOGRAPHIC DISTRIBUTION AND DISEASE BURDEN

Historically, Chagas disease primarily affected rural Latin America [2, 9]. In settings with endemic vector-borne transmission, *T. cruzi* infection is usually acquired in childhood. Because the infection is lifelong, the seroprevalence in an area with sustained vector-borne transmission rises with age and may reach high levels in adulthood, reflecting cumulative incidence. The country with the highest estimated prevalence of *T. cruzi* infection is Bolivia, where many endemic rural communities have adult infection prevalences >20%, followed by Argentina, El Salvador and Honduras. However, vector-borne transmission occurred historically throughout the Americas from the southern USA to Chile and Argentina in the south [2]. Because cardiac and gastrointestinal manifestations usually begin in early adulthood and progress over a period of years (to decades), the prevalence of symptomatic clinical disease increases with increasing age.

Several Chagas disease control initiatives have made major advances in decreasing house infestation and ensuring *T. cruzi* screening of blood supplies [9, 10]. As a consequence, the estimated global prevalence of Chagas disease has fallen from 18 million in 1991 to 8–10 million in 2005. At the same time, migration has brought infected individuals to cities both within and outside of Latin America. The estimated disease burden outside of Latin America includes as many as 67,000 *T. cruzi*-infected immigrants in Spain and tens of thousands in Italy, France and Switzerland [11]. Immigrants with Chagas disease are also known to be living in Japan, Australia and Canada (Fig. 98.1).

The USA is a special case in that the southern half of the USA contains established enzootic cycles of *T. cruzi*, involving several triatomine vector species and mammalian hosts, such as rodents, raccoons, opossums and domestic dogs. A total of seven vector-borne *T. cruzi* infections are documented to have occurred in the USA since the 1950s, but most are presumed to go undetected [12]. Nevertheless, the number of autochthonous *T. cruzi* infections is dwarfed by the estimated 300,000 infected immigrants from endemic areas of Latin America [13].

CONTROL AND PREVENTION

Application of long-lasting insecticides in human dwellings and peridomestic structures is effective against domestic triatomine vectors, but must be followed by monitoring for re-infestation [9]. Between 1991 and 2004, four sub-regional control programs were established. The major aims were to control transmission by domestic vectors through house spraying programs and to prevent blood-borne *T. cruzi* transmission by establishing blood donation screening. Programs to address congenital *T. cruzi* infection were subsequently added in several countries.

The Southern Cone Initiative, the first program to be established, has resulted in the certification of elimination of transmission by *T. infestans* in Chile (1999), Uruguay (1997) and Brazil (2006), plus several departments/provinces of Argentina and Paraguay [10]. The success of the Southern Cone Initiative inspired the subsequent establishment of initiatives in Central America, the Amazon and Andean countries. *Trypanosoma cruzi* transmission by *R. prolixus* was certified as interrupted throughout Guatemala in 2008.

Serologic screening of blood components for *T. cruzi* is now compulsory in all but one of the endemic countries in the region, and the prevalence of infection in screened donors has decreased substantially [14]. Nevertheless, Chagas disease screening coverage by country was estimated to vary from 25% to 100% in 2002, and the risk of transmission through blood transfusion, though much decreased, has not been eliminated. The residual risk in Latin America where screening has been implemented is estimated to be 1 : 200,000 units.

Congenital Chagas disease screening programs usually rely on prenatal serologic screening followed by microscopic examination of concentrated cord blood from infants of seropositive mothers [4]. Conventional IgG serology is recommended after nine months of age for infants with negative screening tests at birth. These programs have been challenged by suboptimal sensitivity of cord blood screening and high loss to follow-up later in infancy.

Surveys of sentinel populations, usually children younger than five years of age or new military recruits, are used to monitor the impact of control initiatives: steep declines in *T. cruzi* infection prevalence have been documented in many Latin American countries. However, focal vector-borne transmission continues in most endemic countries of Latin America and the success of the Southern Cone Initiative is now challenged by re-infestation from residual vector colonies and

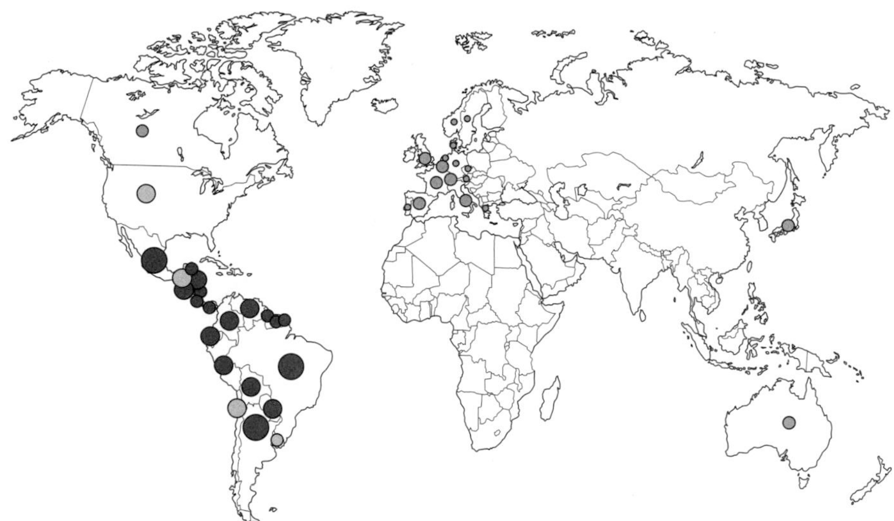

FIGURE 98.1 Distribution of cases of *Trypanosoma cruzi* infection, based on official estimates and status of vector transmission worldwide, 2006–2009. *(From WHO, Global Health Observatory. http://gamapserver.who.int/mapLibrary/Files/Maps/Global_chagas_2009.png).*

the development of insecticide resistance, especially in the Gran Chaco—a heavily infested ecologic zone shared by Argentina, Bolivia and Paraguay.

NATURAL HISTORY AND PATHOGENESIS

LIFE CYCLE

Trypanosoma cruzi is a flagellate protozoan parasite of the order Kinetoplastida, family Trypanosomatidae, which passes part of the life cycle in the triatomine vector and part in the human or nonhuman mammalian host. In the mammalian host, infective trypomastigotes circulate in the bloodstream and intracellular dividing amastigotes occur in tissues. Dividing epimastigotes and infective metacyclic trypomastigotes are found in the vector. Triatomine vectors are infected by ingestion of circulating trypomastigotes in a blood meal. In the triatomine midgut, trypomastigotes transform into epimastigotes which replicate by binary fission. Daughter epimastigotes migrate to the vector hindgut and differentiate into metacyclic trypomastigotes. Infective metacyclic trypomastigotes are excreted during defecation and enter the mammalian host by penetrating the bite wound or other breaks in the skin, or through intact mucous membranes. Trypomastigotes circulate in blood, invade cells and differentiate into amastigotes which replicate and then transform into trypomastigotes. Infected cells rupture and disseminate trypomastigotes into the circulation to invade adjacent cells and other tissues at distant sites via the bloodstream and lymphatics, with special affinity for muscle and ganglion cells. A blood meal with ingestion of trypomastigotes by the vector completes the cycle (Fig. 98.2) [2].

PATHOGENESIS AND PATHOLOGY

Both parasite and host factors are thought to influence the development of clinical manifestations and severity of disease following *T. cruzi* infection. The pathogenesis of Chagas disease is not completely understood, but possible factors that may alter chronic severity include the parasite burden and severity of the initial infection, re-infections, the host immune response and human genetic factors. Distinct evolutionary lineages of the parasite (*T. cruzi* Discrete Typing Units [DTUs] I–VI) have been identified [15]. Specific *T. cruzi* DTUs may be associated with different geographical distributions, transmission cycles and susceptibility to trypanocidal drugs. The occurrence of the digestive form of Chagas disease principally in areas south of the Amazon basin is believed to be as a result of differences in parasite strains [16]. Multiple DTUs with different tissue tropism may coexist in the same patient and the type detected in blood may not be the same as that found in tissue lesions. Recent data suggest that specific parasite DTUs may be more frequently associated with cardiac involvement [17]. Parasite molecules such as cruzipain and trans-sialidases regulate adhesion and invasion of host cells and/or immune evasion; variations in expression of these molecules may influence the virulence of *T. cruzi*.

Tissue damage appears to be caused both by direct parasite effects and secondary to the host's immune response. Cross-reactivity between *T. cruzi* antigens and auto-antigens, and an imbalance between $CD4^+$ and $CD8^+$ T lymphocyte responses leading to excessive production of inflammatory cytokines may have roles in immune-mediated tissue damage [2, 18].

During the acute phase of infection (usually corresponding to the first 2–3 months after infection), all types of nucleated cells may be infected and inflammatory changes are especially marked close to ruptured infected cells. Lesions reveal localized inflammatory reactions, acute diffuse myocarditis with myocyte necrosis, interstitial edema and inflammatory cell infiltrates [19]. Inflammatory lesions may also be found in the smooth muscle of the esophagus and colon, and the central and peripheral nervous systems.

In nearly all infected individuals, an effective host immune response, involving T helper-1, $CD4^+$ and $CD8^+$ lymphocytes and the production of interferon-γ, tumor necrosis factor-α and interleukin-12, develops within 60 days of infection which controls the parasitemia. However, in the absence of effective treatment, tissue infection persists for the life of the host. In the indeterminate form of the chronic phase, isolated inflammatory foci may be found in tissues.

The parasite is difficult to detect in the chronic phase, but there is now a consensus that parasite persistence is required for development of disease. A positive correlation between parasite DNA in tissue lesions and disease progression and severity has been shown [20].

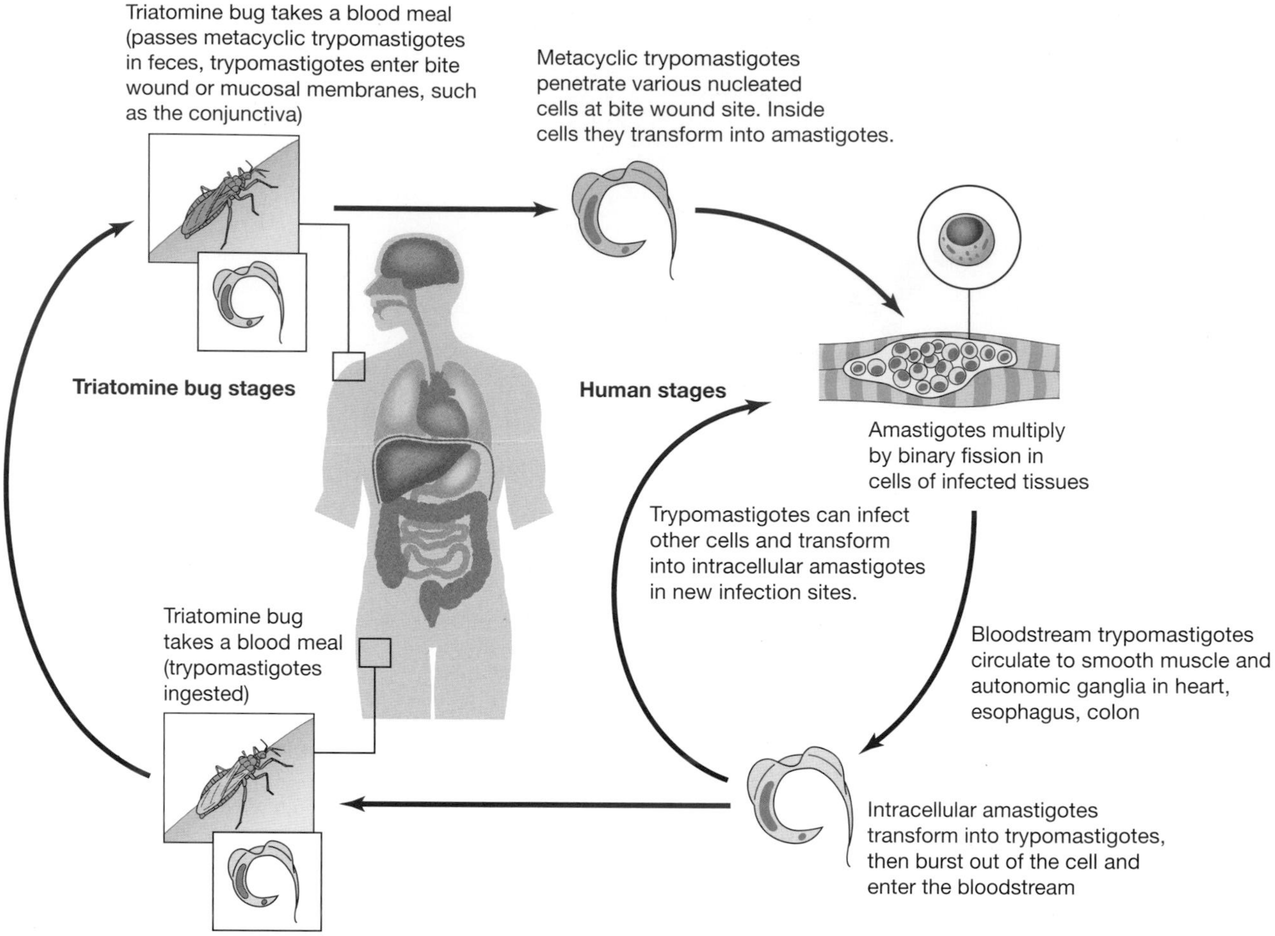

Triatomine bug takes a blood meal (passes metacyclic trypomastigotes in feces, trypomastigotes enter bite wound or mucosal membranes, such as the conjunctiva)

Metacyclic trypomastigotes penetrate various nucleated cells at bite wound site. Inside cells they transform into amastigotes.

Triatomine bug stages

Human stages

Amastigotes multiply by binary fission in cells of infected tissues

Trypomastigotes can infect other cells and transform into intracellular amastigotes in new infection sites.

Triatomine bug takes a blood meal (trypomastigotes ingested)

Bloodstream trypomastigotes circulate to smooth muscle and autonomic ganglia in heart, esophagus, colon

Intracellular amastigotes transform into trypomastigotes, then burst out of the cell and enter the bloodstream

FIGURE 98.2 Life cycle of *Trypanosoma cruzi*.

However, the pathogenesis of cardiomyopathy includes components of immunologically-mediated damage to heart tissue; autoantibodies that cross-react with heart tissue may contribute to the pathology. A low-level, ongoing myocarditis of all chambers leads to diffuse myocardial fibrosis, scarring of the conduction system and reduction in cardiac fibers, often leading to dilated cardiomyopathy, sometimes accompanied by an apical aneurysm.

Gastrointestinal involvement in chronic Chagas disease is thought to be produced by destruction of autonomic ganglia in the gut walls, with unmasking as a result of age-related attrition of the remaining nerve cells and eventually leading to megaesophagus and/or megacolon [21].

CLINICAL MANIFESTATIONS

ACUTE TRYPANOSOMA CRUZI *INFECTION*

Following vector-borne *T. cruzi* exposure, the incubation period is 1–2 weeks, after which the acute phase of infection begins [2]. The acute phase lasts 8–12 weeks and is characterized by circulating trypomastigotes detectable by microscopy of fresh blood or buffy coat smears. Most patients are asymptomatic or have mild, nonspecific symptoms, such as fever, lymphadenopathy and/or hepatosplenomegaly, and do not come to clinical attention during the acute phase. In some patients, acute infection is associated with inflammation and swelling at the site of inoculation, known as a chagoma. Chagomas typically occur on the face or extremities, and parasites may be demonstrable in an aspirate of the lesion. Inoculation via the conjunctiva leads to the characteristic unilateral swelling of the upper and lower eyelid known as the Romaña sign (Fig. 98.3). Severe acute disease occurs in less than 1% of patients; manifestations include acute myocarditis, pericardial effusion, and/or meningoencephalitis. Acute Chagas disease carries an estimated risk of mortality in the range of 1 in 200 to 1 in 400 cases [2]. Orally-transmitted *T. cruzi* infection appears to be associated with more severe acute morbidity and higher mortality than vector-borne infection. For example, 75% of 103 infected individuals in a 2007 outbreak in a Caracas school linked to contaminated fruit juice were symptomatic, 59% had electrocardiography (ECG) abnormalities, 20% were hospitalized and there was one death from acute myocarditis [8].

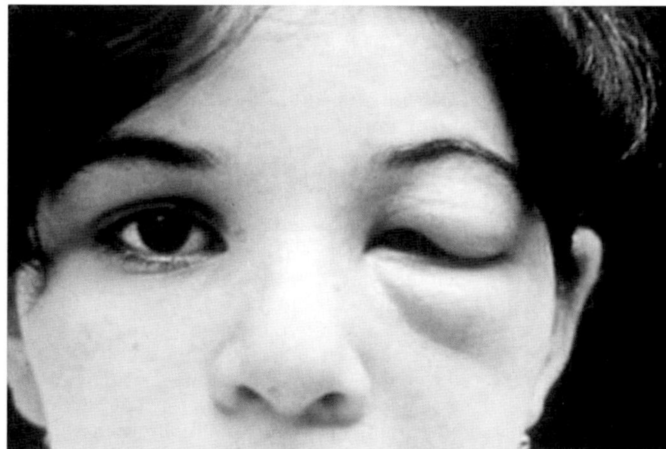

FIGURE 98.3 Acute Chagas disease in a child. The eye sign of Romaña is present. This is frequently seen in acute cases and is presumed to mark the point of entry of the parasite. *(From Special Programme for Reseach & Training in Tropical Diseases, World Health Organization).*

CHRONIC TRYPANOSOMA CRUZI *INFECTION*

Eight to 12 weeks after infection, parasitemia levels become undetectable by microscopy and, in the absence of effective anti-trypanosomal treatment, the individual passes into the chronic phase of *T. cruzi* infection. Despite the absence of microscopically-detectable parasites in the peripheral blood, persons with chronic *T. cruzi* infection can transmit the parasite to the vector and directly to other humans through blood components, organ donation and congenitally. Persons with chronic *T. cruzi* infection, but without signs or symptoms of Chagas disease, are considered to have the indeterminate or aysmptomatic form. An estimated 20–30% of people who initially have the indeterminate form of Chagas disease progress over a period of years (to decades) to clinically-evident cardiac and/or gastrointestinal disease [2].

CHAGAS CARDIOMYOPATHY

Chagas cardiomyopathy is characterized by chronic inflammation affecting all chambers of the heart, conduction system damage and often an apical aneurysm [22]. The first manifestations usually consist of right bundle branch block, left anterior fascicular block and/or segmental left ventricular wall motion abnormalities (Table 98-1) [2, 23]. Later manifestations include: complex ventricular extrasystoles and non-sustained and sustained ventricular tachycardia; sinus node dysfunction leading to severe bradycardia; a high degree of atrioventricular block; an apical aneurysm, usually in the left ventricle; emboli as a result of thrombus formation in the dilated left ventricle or aneurysm; and progressive dilated cardiomyopathy with congestive heart failure. Signs of impaired left ventricular function, New York Heart Association functional class III or IV, cardiomegaly on chest x-ray and/or non-sustained ventricular tachycardia on 24-hour ambulatory ECG monitoring indicate poor prognosis and high risk of mortality in the short-term [24].

TABLE 98-1 Interpretation of Electrocardiogram (ECG) Findings in a Patient with Chagas disease

ECG findings characteristic of and common in Chagas disease
Right bundle branch block
Incomplete right bundle branch block with QRS 0.10-0.11 (in adults)*
Left anterior fascicular block
1° atrioventricular block
2° atrioventricular block
Complete atrioventricular block
Bradycardia and other manifestations of sinus node dysfunction
Ventricular extrasystoles, often frequent, multifocal and/or paired
Non-sustained or sustained ventricular tachycardia
ECG findings less common but clinically significant in Chagas disease
Atrial fibrillation or flutter
Left bundle branch block
Low QRS voltage
Q waves
Nonspecific ECG findings
Nonspecific ST-T wave changes
Minor increase in PR interval
rsR′ not meeting duration criteria for right bundle branch block

*Criteria based on the Minnesota Code Manual of Electrocardiographic Findings with modifications from Maguire JH, Mott KE, Souza JA, et al. Electrocardiographic classification and abbreviated lead system for population-based studies of Chagas' disease. Bull Pan Am Health Organ 1982;16:47–58. Different criteria may be required for ECGs in children.

CHAGAS DIGESTIVE DISEASE

Gastrointestinal involvement is less common than Chagas heart disease. This form is more frequently seen in patients infected in the countries of the Southern Cone, and is rare in northern South America, Central America and Mexico. The effects on the esophagus span a spectrum from asymptomatic motility disorders through mild achalasia to severe megaesophagus. Symptoms include dysphagia, odynophagia, esophageal reflux, weight loss, aspiration, cough and regurgitation. As in idiopathic achalasia, the risk of esophageal carcinoma is elevated. Megacolon (Fig. 98.4) is characterized by prolonged

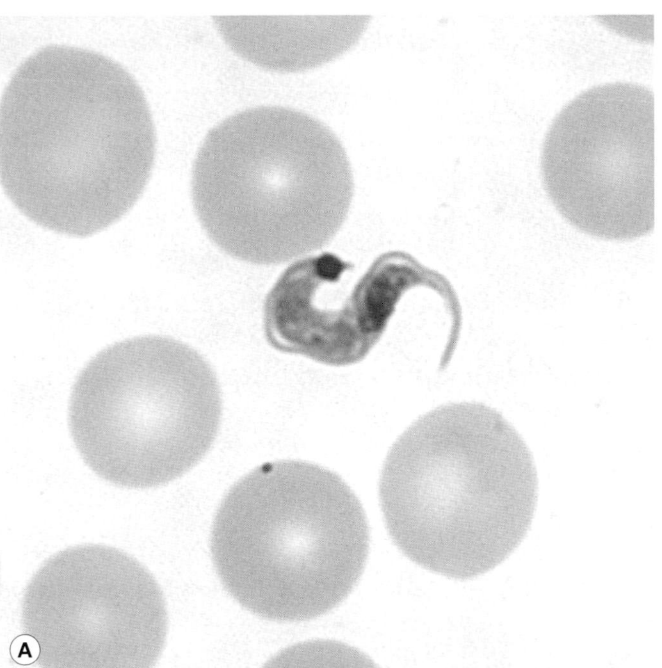

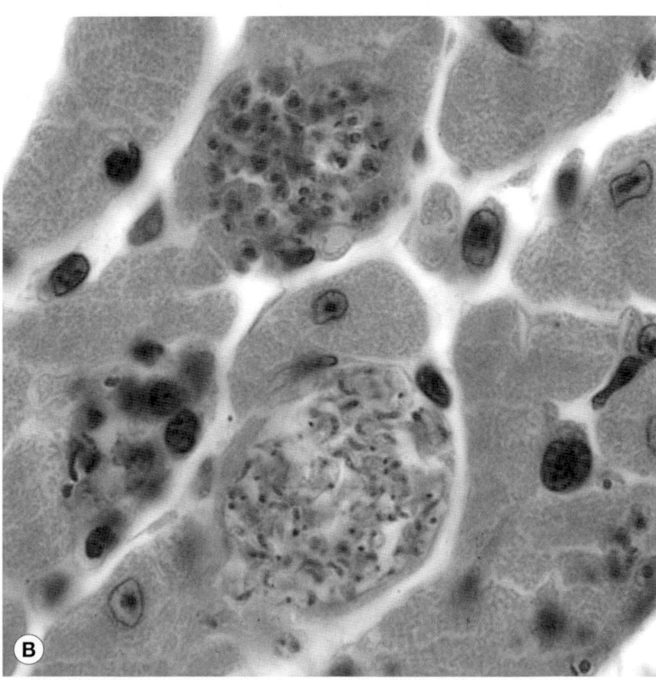

FIGURE 98.4 (A) The trypomastigote form of *Trypanosoma cruzi* in a Giemsa-stained peripheral blood smear from a patient with acute Chagas disease. **(B)** Several nests of *T. cruzi* amastigotes in a hematoxylin and eosin stained slide of heart muscle tissue. The parasites in the nest at the bottom of the image are in the process of transformation to trypomastigotes *(Fom Division of Parasitic Diseases and Malaria, Centers for Disease Control and Prevention).*

constipation and may give rise to fecaloma, volvulus and bowel ischemia.

CONGENITAL TRYPANOSOMA CRUZI *INFECTION*

Most infected newborns are asymptomatic or have subtle findings, but a minority presents with severe life-threatening disease [4]. The manifestations of symptomatic congenital Chagas disease can include low birth weight, prematurity, low Apgar scores, hepatosplenomegaly, anemia and thrombocytopenia. Severely affected neonates may have myocarditis, meningoencephalitis, gastrointestinal megasyndromes, anasarca, pneumonitis and/or respiratory distress. In published studies from the 1990s and earlier, mortality among infected infants was significantly higher than in uninfected infants, ranging from <5% to 20%. However, even severe congenital Chagas disease may not be recognized, as signs are often non-specific or the diagnosis is not considered. More recent cohort studies have shown lower rates of severe congenital Chagas disease and some investigators hypothesize that disease severity has decreased as a result of better vector control and decreasing maternal parasite exposure.

TRYPANOSOMA CRUZI *INFECTION IN THE IMMUNOCOMPROMISED HOST*

Acute *Trypanosoma cruzi* infection in organ transplantation recipients

Acute *T. cruzi* infection in organ recipients has several features that differ from acute *T. cruzi* infection in immunocompetent hosts [6]. The incubation period can be prolonged over several months to more than one year. A relatively severe clinical spectrum has been reported, with manifestations that include fever, malaise, anorexia, hepatosplenomegaly, acute myocarditis and decreased cardiac function; 2 of the 18 reported patients presented with fulminant myocarditis and congestive heart failure.

Reactivation of chronic *Trypanosoma cruzi* infection in organ recipients

Patients with chronic *T. cruzi* infection are considered candidates for organ transplants. Indeed, in a large cohort of heart transplant patients, survival of patients who received the transplant because of chronic Chagas cardiomyopathy was better than among those with idiopathic or ischemic cardiomyopathy, and *T. cruzi* reactivation was a rare cause of death [25]. The cumulative risk of reactivation among patients who received a heart transplant for Chagas cardiomyopathy ranged from 29% to 50% in published cohort studies. Reactivation was diagnosed at times varying from 38 days to more than 7 years after transplantation. In addition to fever and acute Chagas myocarditis in the transplanted heart, common manifestations of reactivation disease include inflammatory panniculitis and skin nodules [26]. Central nervous system (CNS) involvement has been reported, but is a much less frequent manifestation of reactivation among transplant recipients than in AIDS patients. Reactivation should be considered in the differential diagnosis of febrile episodes and apparent rejection crises. When reactivation is suspected, serial monitoring by peripheral blood buffy coat examination and PCR is recommended (see below *"Utility of PCR for Diagnosis or Monitoring"* and Box 98.1).

BOX 98.1 Management of *Trypanosoma cruzi*-infected Blood Donors in the USA

In December 2006, the USA Food and Drug Administration (FDA) approved an ELISA assay to screen for antibodies to *T. cruzi* in donated blood. A second *T. cruzi* ELISA was approved for blood bank screening in April 2010. No confirmatory test has been approved by the FDA but, to date, most blood banks have used the radioimmune precipitation assay (RIPA). The FDA has not issued formal guidance for appropriate use of the tests and screening of blood donations remains voluntary. In data collated by the American Association of Blood Banks (AABB) through to 18 April 2011, 1406 confirmed seropositive donations have been detected in 43 states, with the largest numbers found in California, Florida and Texas (http://www.aabb.org/programs/biovigilance/Pages/chagas.aspx).

The management of a blood donor with reported positive results by blood bank screening assays should begin with confirmation by at least two serologic tests conducted by a diagnostic laboratory. Options for *T. cruzi* serologic testing in the USA are relatively limited. Three ELISA kits based on parasite lysate or recombinant antigens (Ortho ELISA (Raritan, NJ, USA), Wiener Chagatest 3.0 (Riobamba, Rosario, Argentina), Hemagen (Columbia, MD, USA)) are currently FDA-cleared for diagnostic application. Of these three tests, the Ortho and Wiener ELISAs demonstrated high sensitivity and specificity in published evaluations [50, 51]. The Centers for Disease Control (CDC) offers consultation to clinicians in the USA regarding patients with suspected Chagas disease and, when determined to be appropriate, serologic testing. The CDC routinely tests each specimen by two conventional serologic assays and, when necessary, uses a third test to resolve discordant results. The CDC also provides information concerning patient evaluation and treatment, and acts as a reference laboratory for *Trypanosoma cruzi* PCR (Parasitic Diseases Public Inquiries: Tel.: 404-718-4745; email parasites@cdc.gov; for emergencies after business hours, on weekends and federal holidays, CDC Emergency Operations Center: Tel.: 770-488-7100; website: http://www.cdc.gov/parasites/chagas/index.html).

Patients with confirmed infection should be counseled not to donate blood in future and testing should be offered to family members with likely exposure to vectorial transmission and children of *T. cruzi*-infected women. The evaluation of a *T. cruzi*-infected individual should include a complete medical history and physical examination, including a detailed review of cardiac and gastrointestinal systems, and a 12-lead electrocardiogram (ECG) with 30-second rhythm strip. If the findings of this basic evaluation suggest the presence of cardiomyopathy, a comprehensive cardiac examination, including 24-hour ambulatory ECG monitoring, ECG and exercise testing, is recommended. If gastrointestinal symptoms are present, barium contrast studies should be performed.

Anti-trypanosomal treatment is recommended for all cases of acute and congenital Chagas disease, reactivated infection and *T.cruzi*-infected individuals aged ≤18 years old. In adults aged 19–50 years without advanced heart disease, etiologic treatment may slow development and progression of cardiomyopathy and should generally be offered (Infectious Diseases Society of America strength of recommendation B, quality of evidence II). Treatment is considered optional for those older than 50 years. Individualized treatment decisions for adults should balance the potential benefit, prolonged course and frequent side effects of the drugs. In the USA, the CDC is currently the only source of anti-trypanosomal drugs (contact information above).

TABLE 98-2 Differential Diagnosis of *Trypanosoma cruzi* Infection

	Clinical manifestations	Differential diagnosis
Acute *T. cruzi* infection	Asymptomatic Fever Myocarditis, pericardial effusion, meningoencephalitis, hepatosplenomegaly, lymphadenopathy Chagoma (inflammation at site of inoculation) Romaña sign (unilateral bipalpebral swelling)	Parasitic infections: toxoplasmosis, schistosomiasis, leishmaniasis, malaria Viral infections: CMV, EBV, HIV Bacterial infections: brucellosis, typhoid fever, infective endocarditis Localized signs of portal of entry (Chagoma, Romaña sign): local allergic reaction to insect bite, lesions secondary to trauma
Chronic *T. cruzi* infection cardiac disease	Arrhythmias, dilated cardiomyopathy/heart failure, cardiac aneurysm formation +/– thrombotic events	Other causes of dilated cardiomyopathy: ischemic heart disease, viral infections (coxsackie, CMV, HIV, EBV, echovirus infections), bacterial infections (post-streptococcal rheumatic fever, rickettsial disease, Lyme disease), fungal infections (histoplasmosis), other parasitic infections, deposition diseases (amyloidosis, hemochromatosis), cardiomyopathy secondary to drugs and toxins (chemotherapeutic agents, anti-retrovirals, ethanol, cocaine), nutritional deficiencies, rheumatologic diseases (SLE, scleroderma), granulomatous disorders (sarcoidosis), endocrinologic disorders (thyroid disease, diabetes mellitus), familial causes
Gastrointestinal (GI) disease	Upper GI tract: motility disorders/achalasia, megaesophagus, increased risk of esophageal carcinoma Lower GI tract: megacolon	Upper GI: primary idiopathic achalasia, malignancy (pseudoachalasia), amyloidosis, sarcoidosis, neurofibromatosis and eosinophilic gastroenteritis Lower GI (constipation): malignancy, metabolic disorders, amyloidosis, systemic sclerosis
Congenital *T. cruzi* infection	Low birth weight, hepatosplenomegaly, anemia/thrombocytopenia, meningoencephalitis, pneumonitis/respiratory distress	Toxoplasmosis, rubella, CMV, syphilis, HIV
T. cruzi infection in the immunocompromised host		
Acute infection in organ transplant recipients	Fever, hepatosplenomegaly, myocarditis (fulminant), congestive heart failure	Acute rejection Infections occurring in post-transplant patients
Reactivation of infection in organ recipients	Fever, myocarditis, inflammatory panniculitis/skin nodules (CNS disease)	Acute rejection Infections occurring in post-transplant patients
Reactivation of infection in HIV/AIDS patients	Meningoencephalitis, space-occupying CNS lesions, (myocarditis, skin lesions, parasitic invasion of GI tract)	Toxoplasmosis, lymphoma, progressive multifocal leucoencephalopathy, cryptococcosis, tuberculosis

CMV, cytomegalovirus; CNS, central nervous system; EBV, Epstein-Barr virus; SLE, systemic lupus erthyematosus.

Reactivation Chagas disease in HIV/AIDS patients

Reactivation of *T. cruzi* infection in HIV/AIDS patients can cause severe clinical disease with high risk of mortality [27, 28]. However, reactivation is not universal, even in those with low $CD4^+$ lymphocyte counts. The only published prospective cohort study followed 53 HIV-*T. cruzi* co-infected patients in Brazil for 1–190 months; 11 (21%) had *T. cruzi* reactivation diagnosed based on symptoms and/or microscopically-detectable parasitemia [28]. Even in the absence of clinical reactivation, parasitemia levels are higher among HIV-co-infected patients compared with HIV-negative patients. Symptomatic *T. cruzi* reactivation in AIDS patients is most commonly reported to cause meningoencephalitis and/or *T. cruzi* brain abscesses; the presentation may be confused with CNS toxoplasmosis and should be considered in the differential diagnosis of mass lesions on imaging or CNS syndromes in AIDS patients. The second most commonly reported sign is acute myocarditis, sometimes superimposed on pre-existing chronic Chagas cardiomyopathy. Patients may present with new arrhythmias, pericardial effusion, acute cardiac decompensation or accelerated progression of chronic heart disease. Less common manifestations of reactivation in HIV/AIDS patients include skin lesions, erythema nodosum and parasitic invasion of the peritoneum, stomach or intestine.

DIFFERENTIAL DIAGNOSIS

In the acute phase, the differential diagnosis includes many parasitic, viral and bacterial infections (Table 98-2). Localized signs of a portal of entry must be differentiated from a local allergic reaction to an insect bite, or lesions secondary to trauma.

Chronic cardiac involvement caused by Chagas disease should be differentiated from other causes of dilated cardiomyopathy, such as ischemic heart disease, many infectious causes, deposition diseases, cardiomyopathy secondary to drugs and toxins, nutritional deficiencies, rheumatologic diseases, granulomatous disorders, endocrinologic disorders and familial causes. The differential diagnosis of esophageal motility abnormalities includes primary idiopathic achalasia, malignancy (pseudoachalasia), amyloidosis, sarcoidosis, neurofibromatosis and eosinophilic gastroenteritis. Chronic constipation can result from malignancy, metabolic disorders, amyloidosis and systemic sclerosis.

TABLE 98-3 Summary of Diagnostic Testing for Chagas disease

Setting	Microscopy	PCR	Anti-*T. cruzi* IgG serology
Acute infection	Useful	Very useful	Takes several weeks to become positive
Early congenital infection	Useful	Very useful	Only useful after ~9 months
Chronic infection	Not useful	Not useful	Best test
Reactivation	Useful	Quantitative PCR useful	Not useful
Monitoring in organ recipient or accidental exposure	Useful	Very useful	Useful but seroconversion may be delayed or never occur

Congenital Chagas disease must be differentiated from congenital toxoplasmosis, rubella, cytomegalovirus, syphilis and HIV.

The differential diagnosis of CNS lesions in immunosuppressed hosts (especially HIV-infected patients) includes toxoplasmosis, lymphoma, progressive multifocal leucoencephalopathy, cryptococcosis and tuberculosis. In the setting of non-HIV-related immunosuppression (typically transplant patients), the differential diagnosis of myocarditis, menigoencephalitis or cutaneous lesions is extensive and includes the wide range of infections which may be found in transplant recipients. *Trypanosoma cruzi* infection in a transplant patient may also mimic acute organ rejection.

DIAGNOSIS

Appropriate diagnostic testing for *T. cruzi* infection varies depending on the phase of the disease and the status of the patient (Table 98-3).

DIAGNOSIS OF ACUTE TRYPANOSOMA CRUZI *INFECTION*

Because the parasitemia level is high during the acute phase, motile trypomastigotes can be detected by microscopy of fresh preparations of anti-coagulated blood or buffy coat [3]. Parasites may also be visualized by microscopy of blood smears stained by Giemsa or other standard stains. Even without treatment, the parasitemia level decreases within 90 days of infection and is undetectable by microscopy in the chronic phase. PCR is a sensitive diagnostic tool in the acute phase of Chagas disease and to monitor for acute *T. cruzi* infection in the recipient of an infected organ, or after accidental exposure [6].

DIAGNOSIS OF CONGENITAL TRYPANOSOMA CRUZI *INFECTION*

In the first months of life, congenital Chagas disease is an acute *T. cruzi* infection and similar diagnostic methods are employed [4]. Concentration methods give better sensitivity than direct examination of whole blood. The most widely used technique in Latin American health facilities is the microhematocrit method. In this technique, cord or neonatal blood is collected and sealed in 4–6 heparinized microhematocrit tubes, centrifuged and the buffy coat layer examined by microscopy. Repeated sampling on several occasions during the first months of life increases sensitivity, but may not be acceptable to the parents of a neonate. Hemoculture can increase sensitivity, but the technique is not widely available, and results are not available for 30–60 days. Molecular techniques have higher sensitivity and detect congenital infections earlier in life compared with the microhematocrit method [29]. Transient detection of parasite DNA has occasionally been reported in specimens from infants who subsequently are found to be uninfected [4]. For this reason, positive PCR results on two samples drawn on separate occasions are sometimes required for confirmation of congenital infection. PCR is increasingly used for the early diagnosis of congenital Chagas disease in Latin America and is the method of choice in industrialized countries. For infants not diagnosed at birth, conventional IgG serology (as outlined below for chronic *T. cruzi* infection) is recommended after nine months of age, when transferred maternal antibody has disappeared and the congenital infection has passed into the chronic phase.

DIAGNOSIS OF CHRONIC TRYPANOSOMA CRUZI *INFECTION*

Diagnosis of chronic infection relies on tests to detect IgG antibodies to *T. cruzi*, most commonly the ELISA and immunofluorescent antibody assay (IFA). No single serologic assay has sufficient sensitivity and specificity to be relied on alone; two tests based on different antigens (e.g. whole parasite lysate and recombinant antigens) and/or techniques (e.g. ELISA, IFA, immunoblot) are used in parallel to increase the accuracy of the diagnosis [3]. Published data suggest that the sensitivity of serologic assays varies by geographical location, possibly because of *T. cruzi* strain differences and resulting antibody responses [30, 31]. Inevitably, a proportion of individuals tested by two assays will have discordant serologic results and need further testing to resolve their infection status. The status of some individuals remains difficult to resolve, even after a third test, because there is no true gold standard assay for chronic *T. cruzi* infection [32]. Assays such as the radioimmune precipitation assay (RIPA) and trypomastigote excreted-secreted antigen immunoblot (TESA-blot) are promoted as reference tests but even these do not have perfect sensitivity and specificity, and may not be capable of resolving the diagnosis.

UTILITY OF PCR FOR DIAGNOSIS OR MONITORING

Molecular techniques currently provide the most sensitive tools to diagnose acute phase and early congenital Chagas disease and to monitor for acute *T. cruzi* infection in the recipient of an infected organ or after accidental exposure (Table 98-3). PCR assays usually show positive results days to weeks before circulating trypomastigotes are visible by microscopy of peripheral blood [29]. In chronic *T. cruzi* infection, PCR is used as a research tool, but is not generally a useful diagnostic test. Although PCR results will be positive for a proportion of patients, the sensitivity is highly variable depending on characteristics of the population tested, as well as the PCR primers and methods used. Quantitative PCR assays (e.g. real-time PCR) are useful for monitoring for reactivation in immunosuppressed patients with chronic *T. cruzi* infection, such as an organ recipient or HIV-co-infected patient. In these patients, a positive result on conventional PCR does not prove reactivation, but quantitative PCR assays showing rising parasite numbers over time provide the earliest and most sensitive indicator of reactivation [33]. The Centers for Disease Control (CDC) currently performs several conventional and real-time PCR assays with primers targeting kinetoplast and nuclear DNA (Box 98.1) [34–36].

PATIENT EVALUATION

The initial evaluation of a patient diagnosed with *T. cruzi* infection should begin with the complete medical history and physical examination. Details on family history, potential exposure to the vector and history of blood transfusion in endemic areas should be recorded. A detailed review of systems should focus on cardiovascular and gastrointestinal symptoms (Table 98-4). Screening should be offered to other family members, including children of seropositive mothers,

TABLE 98-4 Symptoms Suggestive of Chagas disease that Should Be Covered in the Review of Systems

Cardiac symptoms
Arrhythmias and conduction system disease
Palpitations
Syncope
Presyncope or dizziness
Congestive heart failure
Dyspnea
Decreased exercise tolerance
Peripheral edema
Other
Thromboembolic phenomena (transient ischemic attack or stroke)
Atypical chest pain
Gastrointestinal symptoms
Esophagus
Requires longer time to eat than others (early sign)
Dysphagia for both liquids and solids (solids usually worse)
Progression of dysphagia
Regurgitation and aspiration
Odynophagia
Weight loss
Colon
Prolonged constipation
Acute abdominal pain (volvulus or ischemia)
Abrupt worsening of symptoms

and the patient should be advised regarding possible transmission routes (such as blood and organ donation). An HIV test and/or evaluation for other causes of immunosuppression should be considered, as management of Chagas disease in these patients merits special attention.

Every patient should have a resting 12-lead ECG with a 30-second rhythm strip; other tests should be ordered if warranted by signs and symptoms elicited during the history and examination. In the strict sense, the indeterminate form is defined by positive anti-*T. cruzi* serology in an asymptomatic person with a normal physical examination, a normal 12-lead ECG and normal radiologic examination of the chest, esophagus and colon. However, patients with a normal ECG and no cardiovascular and gastrointestinal symptoms have a favorable prognosis and yearly follow-up may be sufficient without having to perform any additional tests [2, 37].

Patients with cardiovascular symptoms and/or ECG abnormalities suggestive of Chagas cardiac disease (Tables 98-1 and 98-4) should undergo further evaluation, including two-dimensional (2-D) ECG, exercise testing and 24-hour ambulatory ECG monitoring. The need for additional cardiac studies should be assessed on an individual basis. A barium swallow or enema should be performed in patients with upper or lower gastrointestinal symptoms respectively. Esophageal manometry may be of use for patients with suggestive symptoms in whom the barium swallow is inconclusive. Patients with mega-esophagus may be at increased risk for esophageal cancer and an upper gastrointestinal endoscopy may be indicated, especially in patients with new, or progressive, symptoms. An increased risk of colorectal cancer has not been found in patients with megacolon.

Additional procedures may have a role in patient evaluation in the future. Segmental cardiac wall motion abnormalities detected by 2-D ECG and areas of myocardial fibrosis demonstrated by delayed-enhancement magnetic resonance imaging (MRI) have been found in patients with normal ECGs; research studies suggest that minor abnormalities of ventricular contractility may be predictive of future deterioration in function [38–40]. Diastolic dysfunction and elevated blood levels of brain natriuretic peptide (BNP) appear to correlate with prognosis in patients with cardiomyopathy owing to a variety of etiologies, including Chagas disease [41]. 2-D echo and 24-hour ambulatory ECG monitoring results are used to assess risk in some prognostic scores for Chagas disease [24].

MANAGEMENT

Currently, the only available anti-trypanosomal drugs with proven efficacy in humans are benznidazole and nifurtimox. Both drugs have a high rate of adverse effects, especially in adults, and require prolonged treatment courses (usually 60–90 days). Tolerance and compliance are therefore suboptimal. There are currently no pediatric formulations. Although the cure rate in acute and early congenital infection is high and has been accepted as standard of care since these drugs were introduced in the 1970s, their use in the chronic phase has been more controversial, because of the lack of a reliable test of cure and the variable natural history of the disease. Adverse effects of benznidazole and nifurtimox with recommendations for management are outlined in Table 98-5. Benznidazole and nifurtimox are not approved by the USA Food and Drugs Administration (FDA), but both can be obtained free of charge from the CDC and used under investigational protocols (Box 98.1). Questions about drug access outside the USA can be addressed to the World Health Organization (www.who.int/neglected_diseases/diseases/chagas/en/index.html).

SPECIFIC ANTI-PARASITIC DRUGS

Nifurtimox, a nitrofuran compound, acts through production of nitrogenated free radicals (e.g. superoxide, hydrogen peroxide) for which parasites have much lower detoxification capacity than vertebrates [42]. Benznidazole, a nitroimidazole derivative, is thought to act through the mechanism of reductive stress by covalent binding of nitroreduction intermediates to parasite molecules [42]. Both drugs are rapidly absorbed from the gastrointestinal tract (plasma levels peak at 1 hour after a single oral dose); the average biological half-life is 12 hours. Nifurtimox is rapidly and extensively metabolized in the liver using cytochrome P-450 and P-450 reductase. Interindividual variability suggests that metabolism of nifurtimox may be under genetic control. Elimination of both drugs is predominantly renal. Hepatic or renal function impairment increase blood concentrations of the medication, increasing the risk of side effects. Concurrent alcohol intake may enhance the occurrence of side effects. In tissue other than the liver (testicles, ovaries, adrenal glands, colon, esophagus), the reducing activity is variable. Both drugs are mutagenic and have been reported to increase the risk of lymphomas in experimental animals but no increase in incidence of human lymphoma has been reported among treated populations. The drugs are known to be teratogenic in experimental animals and their use in pregnant women is contraindicated. Risk for significant infant exposure to drugs through breast milk seems small and below the level of exposure of infants with Chagas disease receiving nifurtimox treatment. This potential degree of exposure may not justify discontinuation of breastfeeding [43].

Recent trials have all used benznidazole and this drug is usually better tolerated than nifurtimox; for these reasons benznidazole is viewed by most experts as the first line treatment. Nevertheless, individual tolerance varies—if one drug must be discontinued, the other can be used as an alternative. Nifurtimox is indicated for a patient in the acute phase with documented benznidazole treatment failure.

Evidence base for anti-trypanosomal drug therapy

In symptomatic acute *T. cruzi* infection, treatment reduces severity and shortens the clinical course. The parasitologic cure rate in acute and early congenital infection ranges from 60% to 100% in published reports [2].

The degree of efficacy in chronic *T. cruzi* infection is still uncertain, in part because of a lack of a reliable test of cure. Results by conventional

TABLE 98-5 Specific Antiparasitic Treatment for *Trypanosoma cruzi*: Dosage, Regimens and Toxicity

Drug and dosage regimen*	Toxicity†,§
Benznidazole (Rochagan® or Radanil®) Released in 1971 by Roche but production is being transferred to Lafepe in Pernambuco (Brazil). Available in 100-mg tablets. Standard dosage regimen: 5-10 mg/kg/day (7.5 mg/kg/day) p.o. in 2 doses for 30–60 days in adults and children >12 years or >40 kg; 10 mg/kg/day p.o. in 2 doses for 30–60 days in children <12 years or <40 kg	**Dermatologic adverse effects** in 25–30%. The rash rarely progresses to exfoliative dermatitis. The dermatitis is usually mild-to-moderate and manageable with topical or low-dose systemic corticosteroids. The drug should be discontinued immediately in case of severe or exfoliative dermatitis or dermatitis associated with fever and lymphadenopathy **Gastrointestinal tract complaints** in 10–40%. Anorexia, nausea, vomiting, and occasionally abdominal pain and diarrhea. (Taken with meals to minimize gastrointestinal irritation) **Dose-dependent peripheral neuropathy** in 30%. Paresthesias, acute polyneuritis. It occurs most commonly late in the treatment course and the drug should be discontinued. It is nearly always reversible but may take months to resolve **Bone marrow suppression** is rare and should prompt immediate treatment interruption **Additional adverse effects** include anorexia and weight loss, nausea and/or vomiting, myalgias and arthralgias, insomnia and dysgeusia **Monitoring**: laboratory testing (complete blood cell count and levels of hepatic enzymes, bilirubin, serum creatinine and blood urea nitrogen) before beginning treatment and repeated every 2–3 weeks during the treatment course. Patients should be monitored for dermatitis beginning 10 days after initiation of treatment. Alcohol should be avoided
Nifurtimox (Lampit®) Released in 1967 by Bayer, but suspended the production in Argentina in 1997. In 2000, production was resumed at the company's plant in Ilopango (El Salvador). Available in 30-mg and 120-mg tablets. Standard dosage regimen: 8–10 mg/kg/day p.o. in 3–4 doses for 90–120 days in adults; 12.5–15 mg/kg/day in 3–4 doses for 90–120 days in children aged 11–16 years; 15–20 mg/kg/day p.o. in 3–4 doses for 90–120 days in children 1–10 years	**Gastrointestinal tract complaints** in 30–70%. Anorexia, nausea, vomiting, and occasionally abdominal pain and diarrhea **Central nervous system toxicity**. Irritability, insomnia, disorientation and, less often, tremors. Less common but more serious are paresthesias, polyneuropathy and peripheral neuritis. The peripheral neuropathy is dose-dependent, appears late in the treatment course and should prompt interruption **Additional adverse effects** include skin disorders, headache, dizziness or vertigo, nervous excitation, myalgias and arthralgias **Monitoring**: laboratory testing (complete blood cell count and levels of hepatic enzymes, bilirubin, serum creatinine and blood urea nitrogen) before beginning treatment and repeated at 4–6 weeks and at the end of treatment¶. Patients should be weighed and monitored for symptoms and signs of peripheral neuropathy every 2 weeks, especially during the second and third months of treatment. Alcohol should be avoided

*Neither drug is commercialized in Western countries but can be obtained under investigational/foreign drug protocols.
†Children have fewer adverse effects than adults and tolerate higher doses.
§Contraindicated in pregnancy or severe hepatic or renal dysfunction.
¶Treatment must be discontinued with the appearance of peripheral neuropathy, leucopoenia (white blood cell count <2.500 cells/μl) or severe rash not responding to oral steroids. Mild rash may be managed initially with oral antihistamines or steroids and by decreasing the dose or stopping the anti-trypanosomal drugs temporarily. A threefold increase in aspartate transaminase serum levels is an indication for decreasing or stopping the anti-trypanosomal drugs temporarily (reversible temporary secondary effect).

serology remain positive for years (to decades) after successful treatment and experimental tests of cure have not been rigorously validated. In the second half of the 1990s, two double-blinded, randomized, placebo-controlled trials of benznidazole treatment in children with chronic *T. cruzi* infection demonstrated cure rates of 60–85%, as measured by conversion to negative serology four years post-treatment and, in one trial, by xenodiagnoses [44, 45]. Each trial used a different, experimental serologic test to assess cure. Based on these trials, treatment of children up to 12 years of age with chronic *T. cruzi* infection became the standard of care by the late 1990s.

The evidence base for anti-trypanosomal treatment of adults with longstanding chronic *T. cruzi* infection remains suboptimal, but, since 2000, there has been an increasing trend to offer treatment to these patients. This trend is based on the growing consensus that persistence of parasites, coupled with an unbalanced immune response in some individuals, leads to the sustained inflammatory responses that underlie the characteristic lesions of chronic Chagas disease. In contrast to long-held views, this new paradigm indicates that elimination of *T. cruzi* may be a prerequisite to arrest the evolution of Chagas disease and avert its irreversible long-term consequences, and implies that Chagas disease must be treated primarily as an infectious and not an autoimmune condition. In a non-randomized, non-blinded trial that included 566 adults followed for a mean of 9.8 years, benznidazole treatment was associated with decreased development and progression of Chagas cardiomyopathy [46]. Based on these, and other data, most experts now recommend that treatment be offered to adults with chronic *T. cruzi* infection in the absence of advanced cardiomyopathy. In a systematic review of 696 studies and meta-analysis of 9 studies on the treatment of chronic Chagas disease with benznidazole compared with placebo or no treatment [47], benznidazole increased the probability of response to therapy 18-fold. However, up to 18% of patients discontinued treatment because of toxicity. A multicenter, randomized, double-blinded, placebo-controlled trial of benznidazole 5 mg/kg/day for 60 days in patients with mild-to-moderate Chagas cardiomyopathy is currently under way (BENEFIT study). Data from this study are expected in 2012–2013 and should help clarify treatment decisions for this group of patients.

INDICATIONS FOR ANTI-TRYPANOSOMAL THERAPY

Recommendations for anti-trypanosomal therapy vary according to phase and form of Chagas disease and by patient age (Table 98-6).

Treatment of acute and early congenital infection

All acute and congenital infections should be treated. The earlier treatment is begun, the better the response obtained. There is currently no pediatric formulation of benznidazole or nifurtimox, and preparation of the drugs for infants and young children should be performed by a compounding pharmacy. A dispersible tablet containing a pediatric dose of benznidazole is under development.

TABLE 98-6 Recommendations for Anti-trypanosomal Drug Therapy in Chagas Disease

Recommendation by clinical and demographic group	Grade†
Recommended	
• Acute infection	AII
• Early congenital infection	AII
• Children aged <12 years with chronic infection	AI
• Children aged 13–18 years with chronic infection	AIII
• Reactivated infection in patient with HIV/AIDS or other immunosuppression	AII§
Offered	
• Adults aged 19–50 years with indeterminate form or mild-moderate cardiomyopathy	BII
• Women of reproductive age	BIII
Optional	
• Adults >50 years old without advanced cardiomyopathy	CIII
Generally not offered	
• Patients with advanced cardiomyopathy	DIII
• Patients with megaesophagus with significant impairment of swallowing (await surgical correction)	DIII
Contraindicated	
• Pregnancy	EIII
• Severe renal or hepatic insufficiency	EIII

Adapted from Bern C, Montgomery SP, Herwaldt BL, et al. Evaluation and treatment of Chagas disease in the United States: a systematic review. JAMA 2007;298: 2171–81. Drugs and dosage regimens outlined in Table 98-5.

†Infectious Diseases Society of America quality of evidence standards. Strength of recommendation graded A–E. A: both strong evidence for efficacy and substantial clinical benefit support recommendation for use; should always be offered. B: moderate evidence for efficacy or strong evidence for efficacy but only limited benefit, support recommendation for use. Should generally be offered. C: evidence for efficacy is insufficient to support a recommendation for or against use; or evidence for efficacy might not outweigh adverse consequences or cost of treatment under consideration. Optional. D: moderate evidence for lack of efficacy or for adverse outcome supports recommendation against use. Should generally not be offered. E: good evidence for lack of efficacy or for adverse outcome supports recommendation against use. Should never be offered. Quality of evidence supporting the recommendation graded as I–III. I: evidence from at least one properly designed, randomized clinical trial. II: evidence from at least one well-designed clinical trial without randomization, from cohort or case-controlled analytic studies (preferably from more than one center), or from multiple time-series studies; or dramatic results from uncontrolled experiments. III: evidence from opinions of respected authorities based on clinical experience, descriptive studies, or reports of expert committees.

§Follows standard dosing recommendations but may need to be prolonged to 90 days for benznidazole or 120 days for nifurtimox. Drug toxicity may be increased.

Management of accidental exposures

Management of accidental exposures remains controversial. Some experts advocate presumptive prophylaxis of all moderate-to-high risk accidental exposures with a short course of benznidazole (7–10 mg/kg/day for 10 days). However, the efficacy of short-course therapy has not been established, and presumptive treatment may suppress parasitemia and mask indicators of inadequately treated infection. Laboratory monitoring, preferably by PCR, as well as serology, at regular intervals (e.g. weekly for four weeks, then monthly for four months) is therefore generally recommended, and treatment is usually only offered if infection is documented.

Treatment of chronic infection

Treatment is indicated for all children up to age 18 years with chronic *T. cruzi* infection. For adults between 19 and 50 years who do not have advanced cardiomyopathy, treatment should generally be offered, bearing in mind the less certain efficacy and the higher frequency of side effects in adults compared with children. For adults older than 50 years, treatment is considered optional and should reflect a careful assessment of the potential risks and benefits. Characteristic early signs (e.g. right bundle branch block) may indicate a higher risk of future cardiac progression and may alter the risk-benefit equation toward treatment. On the other hand, a patient over 50 years of age with longstanding infection and no cardiac signs or symptoms may have a low risk of developing significant disease during the rest of their lifetime.

Treatment of immunocompromised patients

Reactivation carries a high risk of morbidity and mortality even with adequate anti-parasitic treatment. Treatment consists of the standard daily dosage regimen, but the course may need to be prolonged based on the clinical and parasitologic response.

In patients with pre-existing *T. cruzi* infection who undergo organ transplantation, presumptive anti-trypanosomal treatment is unlikely to be curative and is not recommended in the absence of evidence of reactivation. Monitoring for *T. cruzi* reactivation is recommended with the same schedule used for rejection monitoring, for example 1, 3, 6, 9 and 12 months after transplantation, plus one month after steroid treatment for rejection and when fever or other symptoms occur. Laboratory testing should include microscopy and/or PCR of serial peripheral blood or buffy coat specimens, plus PCR and histologic examination of endomyocardial biopsy specimens collected for routine rejection monitoring.

In HIV-*T. cruzi* co-infected patients, standard dosing regimens are used for treatment of reactivation, but a more prolonged course (90–120 days) may be needed. The usefulness of suppressive treatment (secondary prophylaxis) after treatment has not been established. Secondary prophylaxis with benznidazole 5 mg/kg/day p.o. in two doses administered three days per week has been used empirically but data on efficacy are lacking. Early effective anti-retroviral therapy is essential in HIV-*T. cruzi* co-infected patients. Benznidazole is mainly metabolized in the liver by the cytochrome P-450 system and some anti-retroviral drugs could increase or decrease efficacy and toxicity of benznidazole. Moreover, some anti-retrovirals can add toxicity to benznidazole: fosamprenavir and abacavir produce cutaneous toxicity, zidovudine produces bone marrow suppression and didanosine, stavudine and efavirenz are toxic to the nervous system. There are no published reports of immune reconstitution syndrome (IRIS) in HIV-*T. cruzi* co-infected patients.

DOCUMENTATION OF RESPONSE AFTER SPECIFIC TREATMENT

For monitoring response to treatment of acute, early congenital or reactivated *T cruzi* infection, direct examination of blood or buffy coat, hemoculture and PCR have high sensitivity. In the chronic phase, negative seroconversion by conventional assays occurs after successful treatment, but takes years (to decades), making this an impractical test of cure. There is currently no standard test recommended for the assessment of response to treatment in chronic *T. cruzi* infection. Changes in *T. cruzi*–specific T cell and antibody responses measured by the frequency of peripheral interferon gamma-producing T cells specific for *T. cruzi* have been advocated as a surrogate marker of treatment efficacy, but would require further validation and adaptation to a more practical format [48].

NOVEL ANTI-TRYPANOSOMAL DRUG CANDIDATES

New drugs with high efficacy and with a better side effect profile are urgently needed, especially for the treatment of chronic infection [49]. Triazole derivatives combine potent inhibition of *T. cruzi* ergosterol biosynthesis and pharmacokinetic properties (long terminal elimination half-life and large distribution volume), and currently represent the most promising candidates. Posaconazole reduces parasitism and inflammation in the heart in experimental acute and chronic murine infection. E-1224 (Eisai Pharmaceuticals, Woodcliff Lake, NJ, USA), a water soluble pro-drug of ravuconazole, has *in vitro* and *in vivo* activity against *T. cruzi;* a phase II clinical trial is underway in adults with asymptomatic chronic infection. Other promising drug candidates include Tak-187 (a triazole) and inhibitors of protein or purine synthesis, trypanothione metabolism, cysteine protease, phospholipids (miltefosine) or pyrophosphate metabolism (residronate). In the future, drug combinations may improve efficacy and prevent development of resistance. *In vitro* synergy has been shown for azole derivatives with benznidazole and nifurtimox, and for posaconazole with amiodarone or dronedarone.

MANAGEMENT OF CARDIAC DISEASE

(Table 98-7)

Congestive heart failure treatment

In the absence of randomized controlled trials, treatment of patients with Chagas heart failure has been extrapolated from guidelines developed for the management of heart failure from other causes [2, 23]. Increased doses of diuretics are justified in the advanced stages of disease because of the predominance of systemic congestive manifestations over signs of pulmonary congestion. Angiotensin-converting enzyme inhibitors (captopril, enalapril) can reduce myocarditis and fibrosis in *T. cruzi* infection in animal models. Calcium channel antagonists (verapamil) may act early in the course of *T. cruzi* infection to prevent ventricular dilatation and myocardial dysfunction in animal models. Palliative procedures, such as dynamic cardiomyoplasty and partial left ventriculectomy, are contraindicated because of unsatisfactory results.

TABLE 98-7 Management of Cardiac Disease in *Trypanosoma cruzi* Infected Patients

Grade of cardiopathy	Risk of death	Selected treatment
No	Low	APD
Mild with NSVT and no LVSD	Intermediate	APD + amiodarone
Mild with LVSD and no NSVT	Intermediate	APD + ACE-inhibitor + β-blocker + diuretic (for selected patients)
Moderate	High	Amiodarone + ACE-inhibitor + β-blocker + diuretic (for selected patients) + consider implantable cardioverter defibrilator
Severe (NHYA class III or IV)	Very high	Amiodarone + ACE-inhibitor + β-blocker (if tolerated) + diuretic-spironolactone + digitalis + consider implantable cardioverter defibrillator + consider cardiac transplant

Adapted from Rassi A Jr, Rassi A, Marin-Neto JA. Chagas disease. Lancet 2010;375: 1388–402.
ACE: angiotensin-converting enzyme; APD: anti-parasitic drugs (benznidazole or nifurtimox); LVSD: left ventricular systolic dysfunction, measured by echocardiography or cardiomegaly by chest radiography or both; NSVT: non-sustained ventricular tachycardia, detected by 24-h Holter monitoring; NYHA: New York Heart Association.

Anti-arrhythmic treatment

Almost all of the widely used anti-arrhythmic agents have been used in patients with Chagas disease. The potential role of β-blockers, possibly in combination with amiodarone, to reduce mortality remains to be established. Observational data suggest that amiodarone may improve survival in cardiomyopathy patients at high risk of death from malignant arrhythmias. Thus, amiodarone is usually recommended as the treatment of choice for all patients with sustained ventricular tachycardia, and for those with non-sustained ventricular tachycardia and myocardial dysfunction. The β-blockers have been classically avoided in chagasic patients because of conduction defects, but, in some studies, β-blockers have been associated with improved survival. Because of the high occurrence of thromboembolic phenomena, oral anti-coagulants are recommended for patients with atrial fibrillation, previous embolism, apical aneurysm and mural thrombus. Recommendations for permanent cardiac pacing are sinus node dysfunction, atrial fibrillation with AV block, second and third degree AV block and trifascicular block, among others. Implantable cardioverter-defibrillators are the first line therapeutic option for primary and secondary prevention of terminating life-threatening arrhythmias in patients with depressed LV function. Radiofrequency catheter ablation could be an option in patients with recurrent ventricular tachycardia. Infrared laser has been experimentally tested with promising results. Cardiac resynchronization has become an established treatment for patients with moderate-to-severe heart failure, wide QRS complex, optimized heart failure treatment and evidence of ventricular dysynchrony, and it is also a promising therapy for patients with refractory heart failure.

Cell therapy

Heart transplantation is currently the only available option for patients with heart failure who have failed optimal medical management. The potential benefit of transplantation of bone marrow cells for treatment of Chagas heart failure is being assessed in a multicenter, randomized, controlled trial sponsored by the Brazilian Health Ministry.

MANAGEMENT OF DIGESTIVE DISEASE

There are no data to suggest that anti-parasitic treatment affects progression of gastrointestinal tract disease. Patients with megaesophagus with significant dysphagia will not be able to take oral drugs.

Treatment of megaesophagus is similar to that for idiopathic achalasia [21]. Sublingual nitrates and nifedipine induce lower esophageal-sphincter relaxation and could be used before meals. Endoscopic botulin toxin injection in the sphincteric region is rarely used because of its transitory efficacy. The same is true for endoscopic pneumatic balloon dilatation, which is reserved for selected cases. Non-advanced megaesophagus is best treated by laparoscopic Heller's myotomy and fundoplication, a more definitive form of treatment. In advanced cases, different techniques of esophageal resection have been used with variable results.

The early stage of colonic dysfunction can be treated with a fiber-rich diet and abundant fluid intake, as well as laxatives and intermittent enemas. Fecal impaction can occur as the disease progresses, requiring manual emptying under general anesthesia. Patients with megacolon who fail to respond to conservative measures, and those with frequent fecaloma or sigmoid volvulus, need to undergo surgical organ resection.

REFERENCES

1. Bocchi EA, Guimaraes G, Tarasoutshi F, et al. Cardiomyopathy, adult valve disease and heart failure in South America. Heart 2009;95:181–9.
2. Rassi A Jr, Rassi A, Marin-Neto JA. Chagas disease. Lancet 2010;375: 1388–402.
3. World Health Organization Expert Committee. Control of Chagas Disease. Brasilia, Brazil: World Health Organization; 2002. Report No.: WHO technical report series number 905.
4. Oliveira I, Torrico F, Munoz J, Gascon J. Congenital transmission of Chagas disease: a clinical approach. Expert Rev Anti Infect Ther 2010;8:945–56.
5. Wendel S. Transfusion-transmitted Chagas' disease. Curr Opin Hematol 1998; 5:406–11.
6. Chin-Hong PV, Schwartz BS, Bern C, et al. Screening and treatment of Chagas disease in organ transplant recipients in the United States: Recommendations from the Chagas in Transplant Working Group. Am J Transplant 2011;11: 672–80.
7. Nobrega AA, Garcia MH, Tatto E, et al. Oral transmission of Chagas disease by consumption of acai palm fruit, Brazil. Emerg Infect Dis 2009;15:653–5.
8. de Noya B, Diaz-Bello Z, Colmenares C, et al. Large urban outbreak of orally acquired acute Chagas disease at a school in Caracas, Venezuela. J Infect Dis 2010;201:1308–15.
9. Dias JC, Silveira AC, Schofield CJ. The impact of Chagas disease control in Latin America: a review. Mem Inst Oswaldo Cruz 2002;97:603–12.
10. Dias JC. Elimination of Chagas disease transmission: perspectives. Mem Inst Oswaldo Cruz 2009;104(suppl. 1):41–5.
11. Gascon J, Bern C, Pinazo MJ. Chagas disease in Spain, the United States and other non-endemic countries. Acta Trop 2010;115:22–7.
12. Bern C, Kjos S, Yabsley M, Montgomery SP. *Trypanosoma cruzi* and Chagas Disease in the United States. Clin Microbiol Rev 2011;24:655–81.
13. Bern C, Montgomery SP. An estimate of the burden of Chagas disease in the United States. Clin Infect Dis 2009;49:e52–4.
14. Schmunis GA, Cruz JR. Safety of the blood supply in Latin America. Clin Microbiol Rev 2005;18:12–29.
15. Zingales B, Andrade SG, Briones MR, et al. A new consensus for *Trypanosoma cruzi* intraspecific nomenclature: second revision meeting recommends TcI to TcVI. Mem Inst Oswaldo Cruz 2009;104:1051–4.
16. Miles MA, Feliciangeli MD, de Arias AR. American trypanosomiasis (Chagas' disease) and the role of molecular epidemiology in guiding control strategies. BMJ 2003;326:1444–8.
17. Burgos JM, Diez M, Vigliano C, et al. Molecular identification of *Trypanosoma cruzi* discrete typing units in end-stage chronic Chagas heart disease and reactivation after heart transplantation. Clin Infect Dis 2010;51:485–95.
18. Lescure FX, Le Loup G, Freilij H, et al. Chagas disease: changes in knowledge and management. Lancet Infect Dis 2010;10:556–70.
19. Coura JR, Borges-Pereira J. Chagas disease: 100 years after its discovery. A systemic review. Acta Trop 2010;115:5–13.
20. Schijman AG, Vigliano CA, Viotti RJ, et al. *Trypanosoma cruzi* DNA in cardiac lesions of Argentinean patients with end-stage chronic chagas heart disease. Am J Trop Med Hyg 2004;70:210–20.
21. de Oliveira RB, Troncon LE, Dantas RO, Menghelli UG. Gastrointestinal manifestations of Chagas' disease. Am J Gastroenterol 1998;93:884–9.
22. Marin-Neto JA, Cunha-Neto E, Maciel BC, Simoes MV. Pathogenesis of chronic Chagas heart disease. Circulation 2007;115:1109–23.
23. Rassi A Jr, Rassi A, Little WC. Chagas' heart disease. Clin Cardiol 2000;23:883–9.
24. Rassi A Jr, Rassi A, Rassi SG. Predictors of mortality in chronic Chagas disease: a systematic review of observational studies. Circulation 2007; 115:1101–8.
25. Bocchi EA, Fiorelli A. The paradox of survival results after heart transplantation for cardiomyopathy caused by *Trypanosoma cruzi*. First Guidelines Group for Heart Transplantation of the Brazilian Society of Cardiology. Ann Thorac Surg 2001;71:1833–8.
26. Riarte A, Luna C, Sabatiello R, et al. Chagas' disease in patients with kidney transplants: 7 years of experience 1989–1996. Clin Infect Dis 1999;29: 561–7.
27. Diazgranados CA, Saavedra-Trujillo CH, Mantilla M, et al. Chagasic encephalitis in HIV patients: common presentation of an evolving epidemiological and clinical association. Lancet Infect Dis 2009;9:324–30.
28. Sartori AM, Ibrahim KY, Nunes Westphalen EV, et al. Manifestations of Chagas disease (American trypanosomiasis) in patients with HIV/AIDS. Ann Trop Med Parasitol 2007;101:31–50.
29. Duffy T, Bisio M, Altcheh J, et al. Accurate real-time PCR strategy for monitoring bloodstream parasitic loads in Chagas disease patients. PLoS Negl Trop Dis 2009;3:e419.
30. Sosa-Estani S, Gamboa-Leon MR, Del Cid-Lemus J, et al. Use of a rapid test on umbilical cord blood to screen for *Trypanosoma cruzi* infection in pregnant women in Argentina, Bolivia, Honduras, and Mexico. Am J Trop Med Hyg 2008;79:755–9.
31. Verani J, Seitz A, Gilman R, et al. Geographic variation in the sensitivity of recombinant antigen-based rapid tests for chronic *Trypanosoma cruzi* infection. Am J Trop Med Hyg 2009;80:410–5.
32. Tarleton RL, Reithinger R, Urbina JA, et al. The challenges of Chagas Disease—grim outlook or glimmer of hope. PLoS Med 2007;4:e332.
33. Diez M, Favaloro L, Bertolotti A, et al. Usefulness of PCR strategies for early diagnosis of Chagas' disease reactivation and treatment follow-up in heart transplantation. Am J Transplant 2007;7:1633–40.
34. Piron M, Fisa R, Casamitjana N, et al. Development of a real-time PCR assay for *Trypanosoma cruzi* detection in blood samples. Acta Trop 2007;103: 195–200.
35. Schijman AG, Altcheh J, Burgos JM, et al. Aetiological treatment of congenital Chagas' disease diagnosed and monitored by the polymerase chain reaction. J Antimicrob Chemother 2003;52:441–9.
36. Schijman AG, Bisio M, Orellana L, et al. International study to evaluate PCR methods for detection of *Trypanosoma cruzi* DNA in blood samples from Chagas disease patients. PLoS Negl Trop Dis 2011;5:e931.
37. Bern C, Montgomery SP, Herwaldt BL, et al. Evaluation and treatment of Chagas disease in the United States: a systematic review. JAMA 2007;298: 2171–81.
38. Pazin-Filho A, Romano MM, Almeida-Filho OC, et al. Minor segmental wall motion abnormalities detected in patients with Chagas' disease have adverse prognostic implications. Braz J Med Biol Res 2006;39:483–7.
39. Rochitte CE, Oliveira PF, Andrade JM, et al. Myocardial delayed enhancement by magnetic resonance imaging in patients with Chagas' disease: a marker of disease severity. J Am Coll Cardiol 2005;46:1553–8.
40. Viotti RJ, Vigliano C, Laucella S, et al. Value of echocardiography for diagnosis and prognosis of chronic Chagas disease cardiomyopathy without heart failure. Heart 2004;90:655–60.
41. Garcia-Alvarez A, Sitges M, Pinazo MJ, et al. Chagas cardiomyopathy: the potential of diastolic dysfunction and brain natriuretic peptide in the early identification of cardiac damage. PLoS Negl Trop Dis 2010;4.
42. Urbina JA, Docampo R. Specific chemotherapy of Chagas disease: controversies and advances. Trends Parasitol 2003;19:495–501.
43. Garcia-Bournissen F, Altcheh J, Panchaud A, Ito S. Is use of nifurtimox for the treatment of Chagas disease compatible with breast feeding? A population pharmacokinetics analysis. Arch Dis Child 2010;95:224–8.
44. Andrade AL, Zicker F, de Oliveira RM, et al. Randomised trial of efficacy of benznidazole in treatment of early *Trypanosoma cruzi* infection. Lancet 1996; 348:1407–13.
45. Sosa Estani S, Segura EL, Ruiz AM, et al. Efficacy of chemotherapy with benznidazole in children in the indeterminate phase of Chagas' disease. Am J Trop Med Hyg 1998;59:526–9.
46. Viotti R, Vigliano C, Lococo B, et al. Long-term cardiac outcomes of treating chronic Chagas disease with benznidazole versus no treatment: a nonrandomized trial. Ann Intern Med 2006;144:724–34.

47. Perez-Molina JA, Perez-Ayala A, Moreno S, et al. Use of benznidazole to treat chronic Chagas' disease: a systematic review with a meta-analysis. J Antimicrob Chemother 2009;64:1139–47.
48. Laucella SA, Mazliah DP, Bertocchi G, et al. Changes in *Trypanosoma cruzi*-specific immune responses after treatment: surrogate markers of treatment efficacy. Clin Infect Dis 2009;49:1675–84.
49. Urbina JA. Specific chemotherapy of Chagas disease: Relevance, current limitations and new approaches. Acta Trop 2010;115:55–68.
50. Gorlin J, Rossmann S, Robertson G, et al. Evaluation of a new *Trypanosoma cruzi* antibody assay for blood donor screening. Transfusion 2008;48:53–40.
51. Ramirez JD, Guhl F, Umezawa ES, et al. Evaluation of adult chronic Chagas' heart disease diagnosis by molecular and serological methods. J Clin Microbiol 2009;47:3945–51.

Leishmaniasis 99

Alan J Magill

99.1 Leishmaniasis: General Principles

DEFINITION

Protozoan parasites of the genus *Leishmania*, transmitted by sandflies of the genera *Phlebotomus* (Old World leishmaniasis) and *Lutzomyia* (New World leishmaniasis) cause a diverse group of cutaneous and visceral clinical syndromes that can be referred to as the leishmaniases.

LIFE CYCLE

The *Leishmania* life cycle is shown in Figure 99.1. Promastigotes in the female sandfly are introduced into the skin of a vertebrate host during a blood meal. The promastigotes invade reticulo-endothelial cells, transform into amastigotes (round- or oval-shaped structures) measuring 2–5 μm in diameter found within reticuloendothelial cells (Fig. 99.2). Amastigotes multiply within phagolysosomes, and invade other reticuloendothelial cells [1]. In Wright's- or Giemsa-stained preparations, the pale blue cytoplasm is surrounded by a plasma membrane and contains a large, dark purple nucleus and a small, purple, rod-shaped structure – the kinetoplast. The kinetoplast is a complex body and appears as an electron-dense granular band with a distinct fibrillar pattern, lying within an extension of the mitochondrion. Sandflies feeding on infected individuals ingest parasitized cells, and the amastigotes transform into promastigotes, which multiply in the gut and migrate to the proboscis, completing the cycle.

TAXONOMY

The taxonomy of *Leishmania* can be confusing, and there is no single, generally agreed-on classification. One clinically useful taxonomic classification is presented in Table 99-1. Although minor differences in size and morphology of amastigotes are reported, the species that infect humans cannot be reliably distinguished morphologically. Reference isolates are assigned to species and subspecies based on their geographic origin, the clinical syndrome they produce, developmental biology in sand flies and ecologic characteristics. Traditionally, promastigotes derived from *in vitro* culture are analyzed by protein electrophoresis and the pattern of isoenzymes obtained is compared

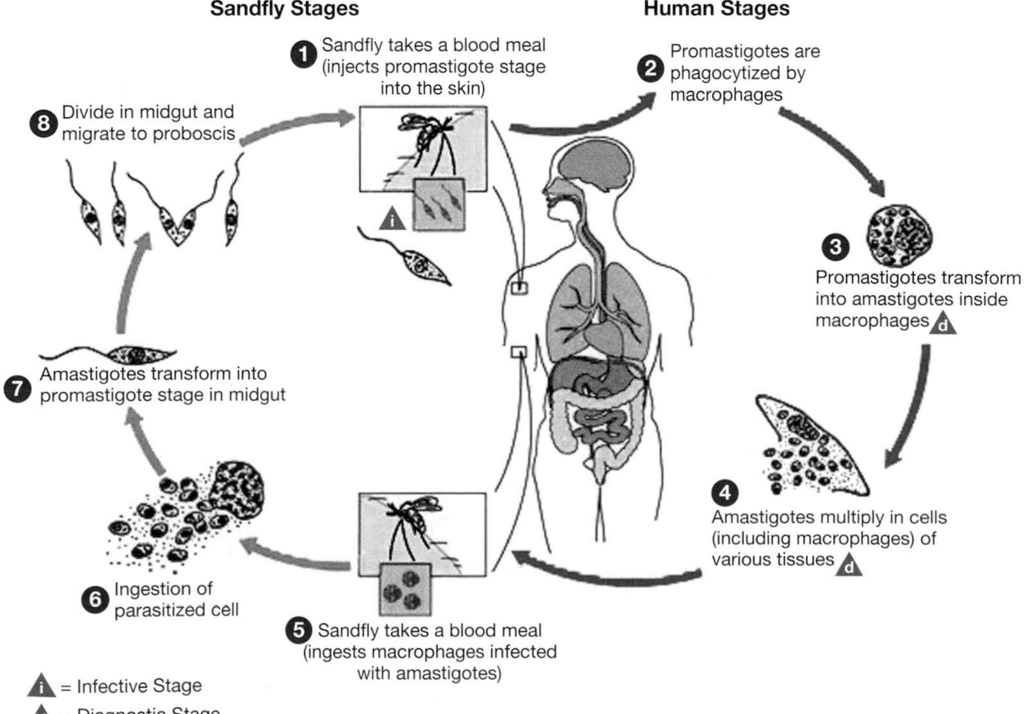

FIGURE 99.1 Life cycle of *Leishmaniasis. (Adapted from http://dpd.cdc.gov/dpdx/HTML/Leishmaniasis.htm)*

TABLE 99-1 *Leishmania* found in humans

Subgenus	*L. (Leishmania)*	*L. (Leishmania)*	*L. (Viannia)*	*L. (Viannia)*
Old World	*L. donovani* *L. infantum*	*L. major* *L. tropica* *L. killick*[a] *L. aethiopica* *L. infantum*		
New World	*L. infantum*	*L. infantum* *L. infantum* *L. mexicana* *L. pifanoi*[a] *L. venezuelensis* *L. garnhami*[a] *L. amazonensis*	*L. braziliensis* *L. guyanensis* *L. panamensis* *L. shawi* *L. naiffi* *L. lainsoni* *L. lindenbergi* *L. peruviana* *L. colombiensis*[b]	*L. braziliensis* *L. panamensis*
Principal tropism	Viscerotropic	Dermotropic	Dermotropic	Mucotropic

[a]Species status is under discussion.
[b]Taxonomic position is under discussion.

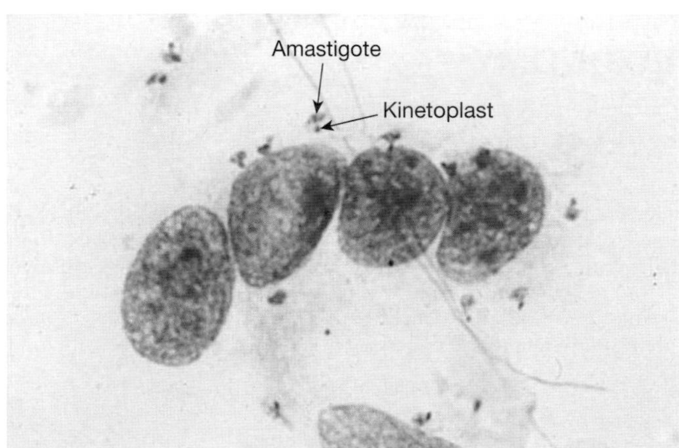

FIGURE 99.2 Amastigotes from cutaneous leishmaniasis.

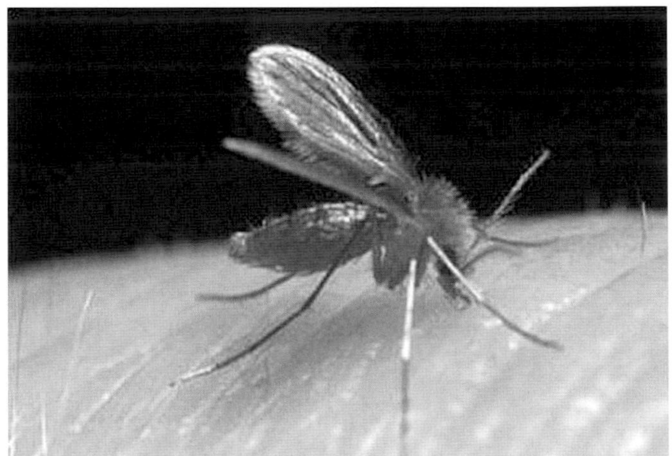

FIGURE 99.3 A sandfly: *Phlebotomus longipes.*

with reference standards. Molecular methods to characterize nuclear and kinetoplast DNA from cutaneous lesions, liver and spleen, and bone marrow specimens and cultured isolates are available and widely used.

CLINICAL CLASSIFICATION

A simplified clinical classification separates the leishmaniases into three major syndromes: (1) visceral leishmaniasis, (2) cutaneous leishmaniasis, and (3) mucosal leishmaniasis. (Table 99-2) Visceral leishmaniasis is characterized classically by fever, wasting, pancytopenia, hepatosplenomegaly (especially splenomegaly), and hypergammaglobulinemia. "Incomplete", or atypical, syndromes, in which one or more of these clinical features are missing, are common. Visceral leishmaniasis is usually caused by parasites of the *Leishmania donovani* complex. The typical clinical presentation of cutaneous leishmaniasis is a localized, nonhealing ulcerative skin lesion. Less common cutaneous leishmaniasis presentations include nodular, psoriaform and verrucous forms. Other, less common, cutaneous syndromes include diffuse cutaneous leishmaniasis, post-Kala-azar dermal leishmaniasis (PKDL) and leishmaniasis recidivans. In the New World, mucosal leishmaniasis is most often associated with *Leishmania (Viannia) braziliensis* and characterized by a primary cutaneous lesion that may be followed months to years later by destructive nasopharyngeal lesions ("espundia"). In the Old World, mucosal leishmaniasis-like syndromes associated with *Leishmania major* have rarely been reported.

Another clinically useful classification is to describe clinical syndromes in terms of the parasite burden. For example, polyparasitic syndromes, such as visceral leishmaniasis and diffuse cutaneous leishmaniasis, are characterized by very large numbers of parasites in the host. Oligoparasitic syndromes, such as mucosal and cutaneous leishmaniasis and leishmaniasis recidivans, have relatively fewer parasites. This has implications for the clinician in choosing the best technique for diagnosis and determining optimal treatment.

TRANSMISSION AND EPIDEMIOLOGY

The phlebotomine sandflies that transmit *Leishmania* parasites are small (1.5–2.5 mm), hairy flies that are recognized by their characteristic hopping movement and the position of their wings, which are held in a nearly erect V configuration over the body (Fig. 99.3). Sandflies are generally inactive in daylight, seeking shelter in dark, moist places. They breed in dark, damp places rich in organic matter, for example leaf litter in tropical rain forests, rubble and loose earth, caves and rock holes [2]. Female sandflies feed on a variety of warm- and

TABLE 99-2 Leishmania infecting humans

Clinical syndrome	*Leishmania* species	Geographic distribution
Visceral Leishmaniasis		
Classic Indian sub-continent Kala-azar	*L. donovani*	Bangladesh, India, Nepal,
East African visceral leishmaniasis	*L. donovani* *L. infantum*	Sudan, Ethiopia, Kenya, Uganda, Eritrea
Visceral leishmanisis and viscerotropic leishmaniasis (rare)	*L. tropica*	Sub-Saharan Africa, East Africa India, Israel, Kenya, Saudi Arabia
Infantile visceral leishmaniasis	*L. infantum*	Mediterranean littoral Central Asia, China, Middle East
American visceral leishmaniasis	*L. chagasi* *L. amazonensis*	South and Central America
Typical Cutaneous Leishmaniasis (CL)*		
Old World		
Dry or urban Oriental sore	*L. tropica*	Mediterranean littoral, Middle East, Southwest Asia
Moist or rural Oriental sore	*L. major*	Central Asia, Middle East, southwest Asia, sub-Saharan Africa
Nodular CL	*L. aethiopica*	Ethiopia, Kenya
Nodular CL	*L. infantum*	Central Asia, Iran, Mediterranean littoral
New World		
Leishmania (Leishmania)		
	L. chagasi/infantum L. mexicana ("chiclero ulcer") L. venezuelensis L. amazonensis	Honduras, Costa Rica Central America, Mexico, Texas Venezuela Amazon basin
Leishmania (Viannia)		
	L. braziliensis L. guyanensis ("Pian bois") L. panamensis L. peruviana ("uta") L. shawi, L. naiffi, L. lainsoni, L. lindenbergi L. amazonensis	Brazil, Bolivia, Colombia, Ecuador, Paraguay, Peru, Venezuela Brazil, Colombia, French Guiana, Guyana, Surinam Costa Rica, Colombia, Panama Peru, Argentina South America South America
Disseminated CL	L. amazonensis	Brazil
Mucosal Leishmaniasis		
	L. (V.) braziliensis "Espundia" L. panamensis (rare) L. guyanensis (rare) L. major, L. aethiopica (rare)	Argentina, Brazil, Bolivia, Ecuador, Paraguay, Peru Colombia, Costa Rica, Panama Guyana, Surinam, northern Amazon Basin Sudan
Diffuse Cutaneous Leishmaniasis (DCL)		
	L. aethiopica *L. pifanoi* *L. mexicana* *L. amazonensis*	Ethiopia, Kenya, Namibia, Yemen Venezuela Dominican Republic, Mexico, Texas Amazon basin
Post–Kala-azar Dermal Leishmaniasis (PKDL)		
	L. donovani	Bangladesh, India, Nepal, Ethiopia, Kenya, Sudan
Leishmaniasis Recidivans		
	L. tropica	Middle East, North Africa

*Typical CL refers to the classic chronic ulcerative disease. Atypical CL refers to nodular and sporotrichoid presentations and less common atypical forms, e.g., plaques, verrucous, and psoriaform lesions.

cold-blooded hosts, including humans, cats, dogs, rodents, cattle, bats, birds, and lizards. They can acquire *Leishmania* with their first blood meal and are capable of disease transmission 7–10 days later. They then remain infective throughout adult life, which is usually only a few weeks. *Leishmania*-infected sandflies have abnormal feeding behavior, with increased probing while attempting to take a blood meal. This behavior may facilitate transmission to the vertebrate host.

Sandfly saliva contains maxadilan, a potent vasodilatory peptide. The presence, and relative abundance, of maxadilan has been correlated with the course of human infection. For example, sandflies of the *Lutzomyia longipalpis* complex transmit *Leishmania chagasi* in the New World. Visceral leishmaniasis caused by *L. chagasi* is common in Brazil but rare in Costa Rica, whereas non-ulcerative cutaneous leishmaniasis caused by *L. chagasi* is found in Costa Rica but not in Brazil. Costa Rican sandfly saliva has a negligible content of salivary maxadilan, induces very little erythema but enhances cutaneous proliferation, whereas Brazilian sandfly saliva has more maxadilan, induces moderate-to-marked erythema, but does not exacerbate cutaneous infections [3]. Substances in sandfly saliva are at least partly responsible for the tropism observed in *Leishmania* isolates.

Transmission of *Leishmania* is either zoonotic (mammalian reservoir, often canine or rodent reservoirs) or anthroponotic (human reservoir). Zoonotic transmission can occur in completely wild (sylvatic) or peri-domestic situations. Two important human diseases – Indian sub-continent visceral leishmaniasis caused by *L. donovani* and urban cutaneous leishmaniasis caused by *Leishmania tropica* – are characterized by anthroponotic transmission [4]. The epidemiology of various forms of leishmaniasis is discussed in Chapters 99.2, 99.3 and 99.4 below.

Globally, there are an estimated 1.5–2.0 million new cases and 70,000 deaths annually, and about 350 million are at risk of infection. Cutaneous leishmaniasis is endemic in more than 70 countries of the tropics and neo-tropics, with 90% of cases reported from Afghanistan, Algeria, Brazil, Pakistan, Peru, Saudi Arabia, and Syria [5]. Cutaneous leishmaniasis is under-reported in most areas and active surveillance reveals a 5–10-fold higher number of actual cases.

Although most parasite transmission is by the bite of infected sand flies, several other routes of transmission include blood transfusion [6], needle-sharing in drugs users [7], congenital transmission [8], sexual contact [9] and laboratory accidents [10].

IMMUNOLOGY

The protective immune response to leishmaniasis is primarily cell-mediated. High titers of antibodies detected in visceral leishmaniasis appear to play no part in defense against the parasite. In contrast, a positive leishmanin skin test correlates with resistance to leishmaniasis. It is negative during active visceral leishmaniasis, becoming positive after recovery. In addition, some patients with subclinical, self-curing visceral leishmaniasis have had positive leishmanin skin tests associated with well-developed tuberculoid granulomas demonstrated in liver biopsies. Cell-mediated immunity (CMI) is not entirely beneficial, as it also causes tissue destruction. The onset of ulceration correlates with the development of a positive leishmanin skin test in cutaneous leishmaniasis. In mucosal leishmaniasis, the reaction to the leishmanin skin test is much larger in individuals with more severe mucosal damage.

SPECTRUM OF CLINICAL DISEASE

In all forms of leishmaniasis, there is a spectrum of clinical disease [11]. In cutaneous leishmaniasis, the spectrum varies from a progressive nonhealing lesions associated with anergy (diffuse cutaneous leishmaniasis) to the exaggerated hypersensitivity seen in mucosal leishmaniasis and leishmaniasis recidivans, in which severe tissue damage is mediated by the immune response. In visceral leishmaniasis, many infections are subclinical and self-healing, although malnutrition or an immunosuppressive process can reactivate latent infection. In those who develop the syndrome of visceral leishmaniasis, delayed hypersensitivity specifically to leishmanial antigens and nonspecifically to tuberculin and other unrelated antigens is suppressed; there is proliferation of reticuloendothelial cells and an exaggerated humoral immune response with the production of polyclonal, nonprotective immunoglobulins.

DIAGNOSTIC TESTING

Parasitologic diagnosis refers to the demonstration of amastigotes in tissues or clinical specimens, visualizing promastigotes in *in vitro* cultures or the detection of parasite genetic material. Immunologic diagnosis refers to the detection of an antibody or delayed-type hypersensitivity (DTH) response in the host to *Leishmania* antigens.

It is important to note there is not a single diagnostic test that is optimal in all clinical settings. It is always preferable to perform more than one parasitologic assay when possible. For example, smears, cultures, and PCR can be employed in the confirmation of parasites from a bone marrow or splenic aspirate.

IN VITRO *CULTURE*

Promastigotes can be grown in a variety of media at 22–25°C. A biphasic medium, for example Nicolle's modification of Novy and MacNeal's medium (NNN) is often used [12]. Schneider's *Drosophila* medium supplemented with fetal bovine serum is often more effective in primary isolation from New World cutaneous lesions. When animal or human specimens are being cultured, penicillin and streptomycin should be added with the inoculum to prevent bacterial overgrowth. 5-Fluorocytosine can be used to inhibit fungal contamination, but amphotericin B should not be added as it may inhibit growth of *Leishmania*. Promastigotes are generally found 2–7 days after inoculation of amastigotes into Schneider's medium and after 7–21 days in NNN medium.

THE LEISHMANIN SKIN TEST

Injection of killed promastigotes (Montenegro test) or preparations made from killed promastigotes will induce a DTH reaction in individuals with prior exposure to *Leishmania*. In most leishmanin skin test (LST) preparations currently in use, cultured promastigotes are washed in 0.5% phenol saline, diluted to 1×10^6/ml, and 0.1 ml is injected intradermally. Another method is to disrupt a promastigote pellet via sonication or microfluidization. The resulting material is filtered to remove particulates and the crude, soluble solution is standardized by protein content. The injection site is examined 48 hours later and induration of ≥5 mm is considered a positive test. A positive LST denotes present or past infection with *Leishmania*. The LST is generally positive when the lesions of cutaneous and mucosal leishmaniasis are present, but negative in active visceral leishmaniasis. Although *Leishmania* share common antigens with mycobacteria and trypanosomes, the LST is not positive in pulmonary tuberculosis, leprosy, African trypanosomiasis, or Chagas' disease. Occasional false-positive reactions have been noted in patients with glandular tuberculosis and systemic fungal infections, but rigorous studies have not been done.

Although there are many different LST preparations in use worldwide, there are no licensed or available LSTs for use in the USA (as of 2012). Sensitivity, specificity and appropriate dose-ranging studies in different geographic settings with standardized products have not been performed. It is not advisable to assume that performance characteristics obtained in one area are applicable to another. For example, a study in Brazil comparing LSTs made from New World antigens to LSTs made from Old World antigens showed markedly different results in individuals with confirmed cutaneous and visceral leishmaniasis. The Old World LST, containing *L. major*, detected only 19% of prior cutaneous leishmaniasis cases, whereas the New World LST, containing a mixture of New World parasites, detected 100% of the prior cutaneous leishmaniasis cases [13]. In addition, a soluble antigen from New World *L. chagasi* detected 96% of cases of prior visceral leishmaniasis, whereas an Old World LST, made from *Leishmania infantum*, detected 71% of cases.

PRINCIPLES OF TREATMENT

DEFINITION OF CURE

Cure or response to treatment is defined as clinical or parasitologic. Clinical cure is the resolution of the signs and symptoms of disease within a defined time period. For example, resolution of fever and improved sense of wellbeing in the first week or so of treatment for visceral leishmaniasis accompanied by resolution of anemia and splenomegaly with weight gain in the following weeks is a satisfactory clinical response to treatment. Final clinical cure is achieved with no recurrence of symptoms (no relapse) at 6 months. The complete epithelialization of an ulcer without recurrence at 6 months in cutaneous leishmaniasis is a common definition of clinical cure. Achievement of clinical cure is the patient care goal.

Parasitologic cure refers to the eradication of *Leishmania* parasites which occurs infrequently with the leishmaniases. Infection is usually life-long. Parasitologic response is often defined as the decrease or absence of parasites by smear or culture within a defined time period following treatment. For example, a splenic aspiration may be 3+ prior to therapy and smear-negative at the end of therapy, indicating a parasitologic response. Parasitologic response endpoints are utilized in research studies to assess response to treatment but are not commonly used or recommended in routine clinical care.

PERSISTENCE OF VIABLE PARASITES

Successful chemotherapy leading to clinical cure does not eradicate parasites from the host. For example, viable parasites can be obtained from healed scars of New World cutaneous leishmaniasis years following successful therapy leading to clinical cure [14]. As in tuberculosis, reactivation of overt disease following immunosuppression results from old foci of infection that were controlled by an immune response [15]. Recurrent disease in patients with AIDS–*Leishmania* co-infections supports the fact that an intact immune system is required for sustained clinical cure.

VARIABILITY OF TREATMENT REGIMENS

Leishmania are a diverse group of protozoan parasites found in many different geographic regions of the tropical and subtropical world. Each parasite "species" exists within a unique zoonotic or anthroponotic cycle. Some of these parasites infect humans and lead to a wide variety of systemic, cutaneous and mucosal clinical syndromes. Each geographic region has a unique combination of parasite strains, sandfly vectors, mammalian reservoirs and human hosts of different genetic backgrounds. A treatment regimen that is efficacious in one area may not be efficacious in another. For example, what works best for visceral leishmaniasis in India may not be optimal for East Africa [16]. Therefore, it is not possible, or desirable, to recommend a single treatment regimen that would be safe and effective for all forms of the disease in all geographic regions.

99.2 *Visceral Leishmaniasis (Kala-azar)*

DEFINITION

Visceral leishmaniasis is a systemic illness caused by parasites of the *Leishmania donovani* complex and characterized by irregular fever, enlargement of the spleen and liver, weight loss, pancytopenia and hypergammaglobulinemia. The disease is also known as Kala-azar (Hindi for black sickness).

ETIOLOGY

Visceral leishmaniasis is most often caused by species of the *L. donovani* complex: (1) *Leishmania donovani sensu sticto* in the Indian subcontinent; (2) *Leishamania donovani sensu lato* in East Africa; and, (3) *Leishmania infantum* found around the Mediterranean littoral, in the Middle East, Africa, China and in the Americas. New World visceral leishmaniasis was thought to be caused by a different parasite, *Leishmania chagasi*, but *L. chagasi* and *L. infantum* are very similar (if not identical) and it is likely the organism was imported to the New World by the dogs of the conquistadors and early settlers [17]. There are no clinically useful morphologic or serologic methods for distinguishing the species, but there are differences between *L. donovani* and *L. infantum* infections in epidemiology, clinical features and responses to treatment that suggest distinct species are involved. Organisms with biochemical characteristics of *Leishmania tropica* have occasionally been isolated from bone marrow cultures of patients with visceral leishmaniasis and "viscerotropic leishmaniasis" in Kenya, the Middle East, and India.

DISTRIBUTION AND INCIDENCE

Mediterranean or infantile Kala-azar caused by *L. infantum* is found in Portugal, Spain, France, Italy, Greece, Yugoslavia, North Africa, the Mediterranean islands, Lebanon, Iraq, Iran, Saudi Arabia, Yemen, southern Russia, central Asia, and northern China (Fig. 99.4). Indian Kala-azar occurs in the eastern part of India (Assam, Bengal, Bihar, Uttar Pradesh, Madras, Sikkim), Nepal and Bangladesh. African Kala-azar is common in Kenya, Ethiopia, and the Sudan, but sporadic cases occur in Chad, Upper Volta, the Central African Republic, Uganda, the Democratic Republic of Congo, Zambia, and Somalia. American Kala-azar occurs in north-eastern Brazil, Paraguay, Argentina, Venezuela, Colombia, Guatemala, El Salvador, Honduras, and Mexico (Fig. 99.5). Reliable or current incidence figures are not available but, in 1992, the worldwide incidence of visceral leishmaniasis was estimated to be at least 100,000 per year [18].

TRANSMISSION AND EPIDEMIOLOGY

Leishmania donovani is transmitted by phlebotomine sandflies of the genera *Phlebotomus* in the Old World and *Lutzomyia* in the New World. Regional epidemiology depends on the interaction of sandflies, reservoir hosts and susceptible humans. Visceral leishmaniasis is associated with poor nutrition and desperate poverty. Population movements of non-immune individuals into endemic areas can result in epidemics.

RESERVOIR HOSTS

Humans

In India, where the domestic sandfly vector *Phlebotomus argentipes* feeds solely on humans, people appear to be the only reservoir.

Domestic Dogs

Dogs are the main reservoir for *L. infantum*-associated disease. Non-HIV-associated disease in this area usually occurs in infants and young children. Young dogs and certain breeds (foxhounds and beagles) are especially susceptible to infection with *L. infantum* and develop overt disease that is often fatal.

Wild Canines

In southern France and central Italy, foxes with unapparent infection are the reservoir and visceral leishmaniasis is primarily a rural disease

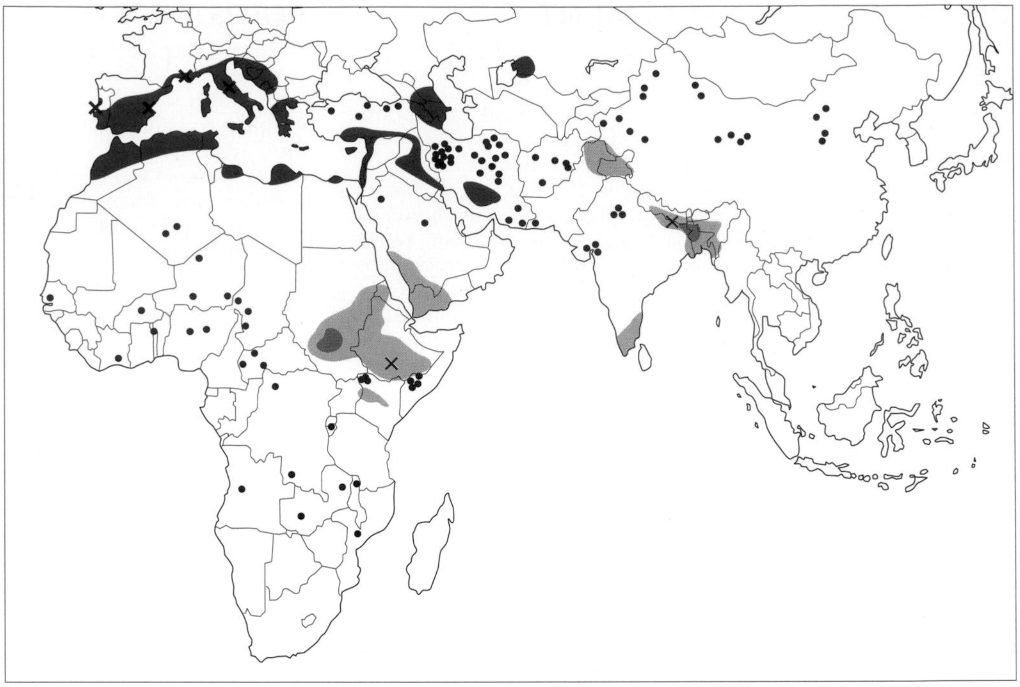

90% of VL in 5 countries: Bangladesh, India, Nepal, Sudan, & Brazil

- ■ *L. infantum*
- ■ *L. donovani*
- ■■ Endemic zones
- ■ Hyperendemic zones
- × Increasing leishmaniasis - HIV co-infection
- ✖ Decreasing leishmaniasis - HIV co-infection
- • Sporadic cases

FIGURE 99.4 Geographic distribution of Old World visceralizing leishmania *(adapted with permission from Magill AJ. Epidemiology of the leishmaniases. Dermatol Clin 1995;13:505–23.)*

L. infantum

- • Sporadic cases
- ■ Endemic zones
- ■ Hyperendemic zones

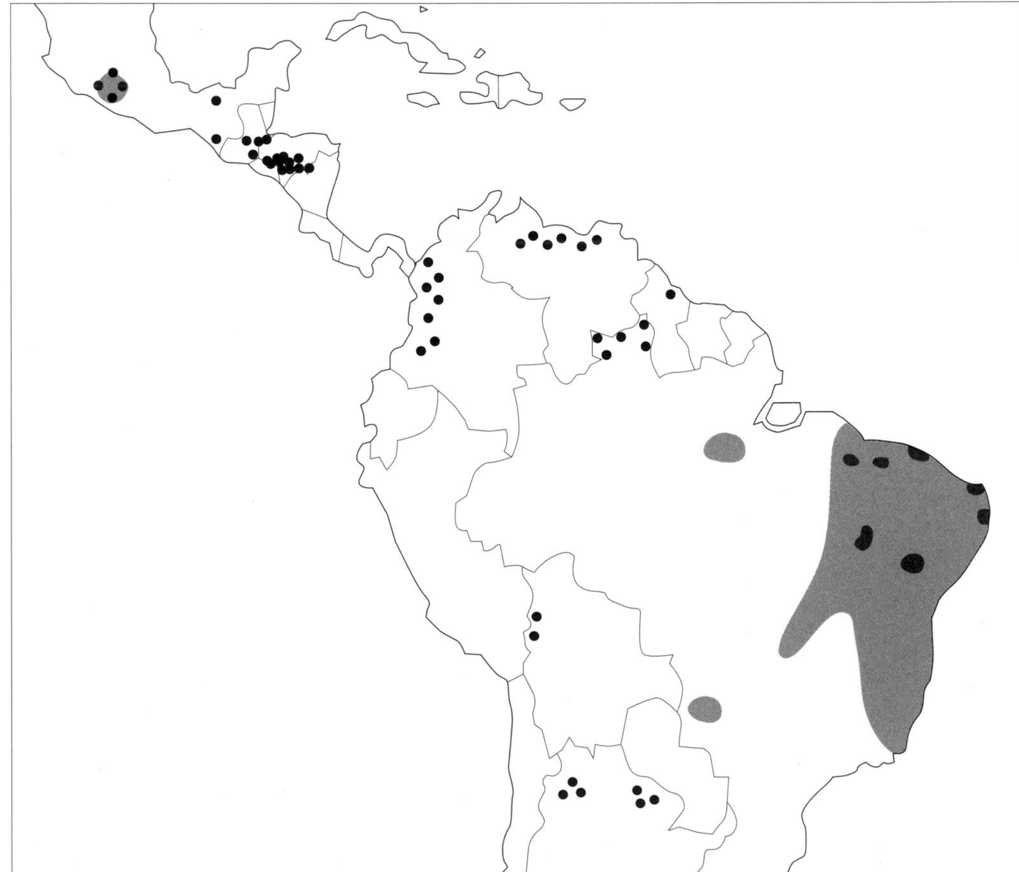

FIGURE 99.5 Geographic distribution of New World visceralizing leishmania *(adapted with permission from Magill AJ. Epidemiology of the leishmaniases. Dermatol Clin 1995;13:505–23.)*

affecting older children and adults. Foxes are also reservoirs in Brazil and jackals are probably an important source of the sporadic, mainly rural, cases that occur in the Middle East and central Asia.

Multiple Hosts, Rodents

The epidemiology of visceral leishmaniasis in Africa is incompletely understood. In Kenya, where *Phlebotomus martini* is the probable vector, epidemics of visceral leishmaniasis occurred in the 1950s and 1970s, suggesting a human reservoir, but domestic dogs have occasionally been found infected with *L. donovani*. In the Sudan, between the epidemics in the 1950s and the current, ongoing, one, visceral leishmaniasis usually occurs sporadically in nomads who occupy temporary villages in the dry season near patches of scrub that harbor the vector *Plebotomus orientalis*. *Leishmania donovani* has been isolated from rodents in the Sudan; rodents may be important in maintaining enzootic foci in interepidemic periods. Parasite isolates from East Africa are more closely related biochemically to *L. donovani*.

PATHOGENESIS

Following inoculation by the sandfly, promastigotes enter reticuloendothelial cells and multiply. Parasites spread to local lymph nodes and then, hematogenously within macrophages, to the liver, spleen, and bone marrow, resulting in a spectrum of outcomes from asymptomatic infection to oligosymptomatic disease with spontaneous resolution or disseminated infection and the clinical syndrome of visceral leishmaniasis. Patients with progressive disease develop marked splenomegaly as a result of hyperplasia of reticuloendothelial cells filled with parasites. In acute cases, the spleen is smooth and friable, but in the more usual chronic cases it is firm. Splenic infarcts are common. The liver is usually enlarged and contains numerous amastigote-laden Kupffer cells with little, or no, surrounding cellular reaction. In subclinical cases, non-caseating granulomas with few parasites are scattered throughout the liver. Lymph nodes may be enlarged and contain macrophages filled with amastigotes, usually with few surrounding lymphocytes. Tonsillar lymphoid tissue may also contain *Leishmania*. In subclinical cases or in lymphatic leishmaniasis, there is a granulomatous and giant cell reaction closely resembling tuberculosis but without caseation. In the gastrointestinal tract, there is proliferation of reticuloendothelial cells in the duodenum and jejunum, infiltration of the submucosa with parasitized cells and, sometimes, villous atrophy with hyperplasia of crypt cells. Small ulcerations may occur in which parasites can be demonstrated. The bone marrow usually contains numerous parasite-laden macrophages. The skin may contain *Leishmania* and, in fatal cases, all levels beneath the epidermis are often heavily infiltrated, with masses of parasitized cells concentrated around the sweat glands and arterioles. Parasites have also been identified in heart muscle and the adrenal glands. The kidneys may show an interstitial nephritis or a mild proliferative glomerulonephritis and may contain immune complexes. Renal amyloidosis is an uncommon late complication.

CLINICAL MANIFESTATIONS

SYMPTOMS

The incubation period is generally 2–6 months, although disease occasionally occurs many years after the patient has left an endemic area. The patient usually does not recall a primary skin lesion. The onset of the disease in naïve adults (migrants, soldiers, and visitors to an endemic area) is frequently acute with high fever, chills, and malaise [19]. This syndrome, initially described early in the 20th century in India, is often mistaken for malaria; however, early clinicians commented that visceral leishmaniasis patients did not appear as "toxic" as malaria patients. In endemic areas, the disease progression is described as more gradual, with intermittent fever, progressive enlargement of the spleen and liver, and vague abdominal discomfort. The initial acute illness may not be recognized. Other common symptoms include weight loss, epistaxis, diarrhea, and nonproductive cough.

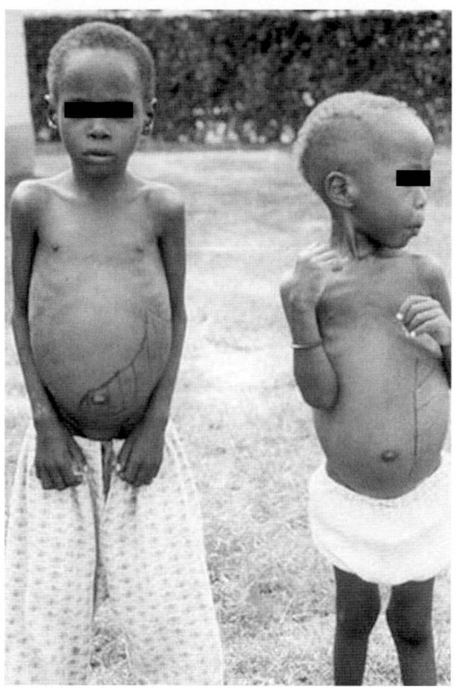

FIGURE 99.6 Overt Kala-azar.

SIGNS

The patient is often weak and emaciated. The abdomen is usually distended by a markedly enlarged spleen and a moderately enlarged liver (Fig. 99.6). In acute visceral leishmaniasis, the spleen may not be palpably enlarged. Femoral and inguinal lymphadenopathy is often noted, especially in African visceral leishmaniasis, and generalized lymphadenopathy is a feature of lymphatic leishmaniasis. Trophic changes of the hair (thinning, dryness, hypopigmentation, and loss of curl) and of the skin on the lower legs are common. Heart murmurs are often present and edema of the legs, jaundice, petechiae, and purpura may sometimes be noted. Mucosal lesions are occasionally seen in patients with visceral leishmaniasis in the Sudan and rarely in patients from East Africa and India. Oral lesions appear as nodules or ulcers of the gum, palate, tongue, or lip. Lesions of the nasal mucosa may cause perforation of the septum. Nasopharyngeal and laryngeal lesions present with mucosal swelling and hoarseness. These lesions may be associated with active visceral infections or with post-Kala-azar dermal leishmaniasis (PKDL). They respond to therapy and may be caused by an exaggerated, nonhealing immune response. Uncommon presenting syndromes, which precede the development of overt visceral leishmaniasis, include bacteremia, acute hepatitis and Guillain-Barré syndrome. Only after the classic signs and symptoms of visceral leishmaniasis develop are these unusual (or uncommonly recognized) manifestations of visceral leishmaniasis associated with *Leishmania* infection. In addition, uncommon systemic manifestations associated with overt visceral leishmaniasis include retinal hemorrhages, massive hepatic necrosis, pancytopenia without splenomegaly, cholecystitis and distal extremity paresthesias. Lymphatic leishmaniasis also occurs not infrequently. Both generalized and regional adenopathy with, and without, systemic symptoms may occur. *Leishmania* infection is an uncommon, treatable cause of secondary hematophagocytic syndrome, especially in children [20]. This syndrome is oligoparasitic and parasitologic confirmation can be difficult [21].

LABORATORY ABNORMALITIES

Hematologic

Hemoglobin concentrations of 5–9 g/dl, white blood cell (WBC) counts of 2000–4000/mm^3 and platelet counts of 50,000–200,000/mm^3 are typical, although much lower counts are sometimes seen in advanced disease [22]. The anemia is multifactorial. Erthrocyte survival time is shortened owing to hypersplenism and possibly to autoimmune mechanisms. Bone marrow depression is indicated by a reticulocytosis lower than expected for the degree of anemia. Coexistent iron deficiency may be present. The Coombs test is usually positive, with both C3 and IgG present on red blood cells, but does not correlate with the severity of the anemia. The neutrophil survival time is shortened and the WBC differential demonstrates neutropenia, relative lymphocytosis, and an almost complete absence of eosinophils. Agranulocytosis is rare.

Other

Liver transaminases (alanine transaminase [ALT] more than aspartate transaminase [AST]) are mildly elevated in the majority of patients, but elevations of serum bilirubin are uncommon. The prothrombin time is usually 2–4 seconds longer than that in controls, and serum albumin is generally less than 3 g/dl. A polyclonal hypergammaglobulinemia of 5–10 g/dl, most of which is IgG, is usual. In some reports, albuminuria is common, but in others the urinalysis is normal, as are tests of renal function.

COMPLICATIONS

Bacterial pneumonia may be present on admission or may develop during treatment. Pulmonary tuberculosis and HIV are common co-infections, and it should be suspected in any patient responding poorly to specific anti-*Leishmania* therapy. Cancrum oris, a necrotizing oral infection, occurs late in the course when neutropenia is severe. Hepatic cirrhosis is an uncommon sequela of visceral leishmaniasis and portal hypertension may cause persistent splenomegaly, despite successful treatment of Kala-azar. Post-Kala-azar anterior uveitis can occur after treatment for visceral leishmaniasis. Patients present with deteriorating visual acuity – slit lamp examination shows irregular nodules in the iris. Other rare ocular complications reported are retinal hemorrhages, keratitis, central retinal vein thrombosis, papillitis, and iritis. Disseminated intravascular coagulation, immune complex-mediated glomerulonephritis and renal amyloidosis presenting with a nephrotic syndrome are also rarely seen. Death in patients with visceral leishmaniasis is often associated with, and perhaps caused by, concurrent infections, for example tuberculosis, dysentery, measles, and bacterial pneumonias. Deaths caused by cardiac failure in severely anemic persons also occur.

SUBCLINICAL OR OLIGOSYMPTOMATIC INFECTIONS

In areas endemic for visceral leishmaniasis, many inhabitants develop a positive skin test without a history of overt clinical disease – such individuals appear to be resistant to naturally occurring and experimental infection with *L. donovani*. The difference between true asymptomatic infection and oligosymptomatic disease is difficult to establish in most endemic areas because the etiology of nonspecific illness is rarely diagnosed and does not warrant evaluation in the context of the culture and healthcare infrastructure. For example, in a prospective study in Brazil, 28 out of 86 children with antibodies to *L. donovani* developed classic visceral leishmaniasis within a few weeks to 15 months after seroconversion. Twenty others remained asymptomatic during observation for up to 5 years and 38 had a prolonged "subclinical" illness, manifested by mild constitutional symptoms and intermittent hepatomegaly that resolved without anti-leishmanial treatment after an average of 35 months [23]. Other reports of nonspecific, chronic illness, associated with "viscerotropic" *Leishmania* infection have come from Italy [24] and Saudi Arabia [25, 26]. One patient presented more than 2 years after the last possible exposure. These relatively mild, nonspecific illnesses are characterized by cough, malaise, chronic fatigue, abdominal pain, and intermittent fevers and diarrhea and have been parasitologically confirmed from bone marrow or lymph node aspirates and are likely more common than currently appreciated. Therefore, "viscerotropic" leishmaniasis should be considered in individuals with unexplained constitutional complaints in endemic areas or in travelers with a history of exposure.

INFECTIONS IN IMMUNOCOMPROMISED HOSTS

Prior to the routine use of modern anti-retroviral therapy for HIV infection, *Leishmania* was a significant opportunistic infection in patients with AIDS. Co-infection with *Leishmania* and HIV is a recognized problem in the Southern Mediterranean and has been reported in 20 other countries [27]. As the incidence of HIV infection increases in India, Brazil, and East Africa, the numbers of people at risk of co-infection will also increase dramatically.

Clinical signs and symptoms of visceral leishmaniasis usually occur as a late-stage manifestation in patients with AIDS. CD4 T lymphocyte counts, when reported, are usually less than 50 mm^3 and are almost always less than 200 mm^3. In general, patients with overt disease associated with visceral leishmaniasis have very high parasite burdens but seem to tolerate the parasite co-infection reasonably well. Many clinicians believe that *Leishmania* does not cause severe symptoms in these patients but rather is just one more of the many opportunistic infections that plague patients with severely depressed CD4 counts. Numerous viscerotropic, dermotropic and novel *L. infantum* zymodemes have been isolated from co-infected patients in Europe.

The clinical presentation of visceral leishmaniasis in AIDS patients is similar to the presentation in non-HIV-infected hosts. Fever, splenomegaly and pancytopenia are common. Involvement of the gastrointestinal tract is more common in AIDS patients. Abundant parasite-laden macrophages are found in the submucosa from the esophagus to the rectum. Co-infected patients may have atypical presentations that include a variety of pulmonary syndromes, for example pleural effusion and pulmonary nodules. Afebrile patients with minimal splenomegaly have also been reported.

The principles of diagnosis in HIV-co-infected patients are not different. The parasite burden tends to be higher and serologic tests may be negative; therefore, classic parasitologic methods are preferable. Fever or hepatosplenomegaly in an HIV-infected patient who has resided in, or visited, an area endemic for visceral leishmaniasis should prompt an examination of the bone marrow with both smears, cultures, and PCR for *Leishmania*.

Visceral leishmaniasis may also occur as an opportunistic infection in immunocompromised patients associated with solid organ (renal, heart) transplantation [28], persons receiving immunosuppressive therapy [29, 30] and chronic corticosteroid use [31]. Unexplained fever, splenomegaly and cytopenias in an immunocompromised patient with an appropriate exposure history should prompt consideration of leishmaniasis. Standard parasitologic diagnostic methods are usually sufficient. The problem is almost always a failure to consider the diagnosis.

POST-KALA-AZAR DERMAL LEISHMANIASIS (PKDL)

PKDL is a cutaneous syndrome seen following the treatment of visceral leishmaniasis, usually with pentavalent antimony [32, 33]. The syndrome consists of macules and papules first occurring around the mouth and spreading to the rest of the face and, to a lesser extent, on the extensor surfaces of the arms, the trunk and, occasionally, the legs. Initially, they appear as small hypopigmented patches, which enlarge and may progress to nodules that sometimes resemble leprosy.

PKDL occurs in up to 20% of patients with visceral leishmaniasis in India, with skin lesions usually appearing 2–10 years after successful treatment of visceral leishmaniasis. PKDL has been reported in over 50% of Sudanese visceral leishmaniasis patients treated and the lesions often appear within a few months of treatment. In the Sudan, onset of PKDL was reported to occur at a mean of 56 days (range: 0–180 days) (Fig. 99.7).

Histologically, there is a spectrum of cellular response, varying from numerous parasites with few inflammatory cells to a granulomatous reaction containing few parasites. Parasites isolated from patients

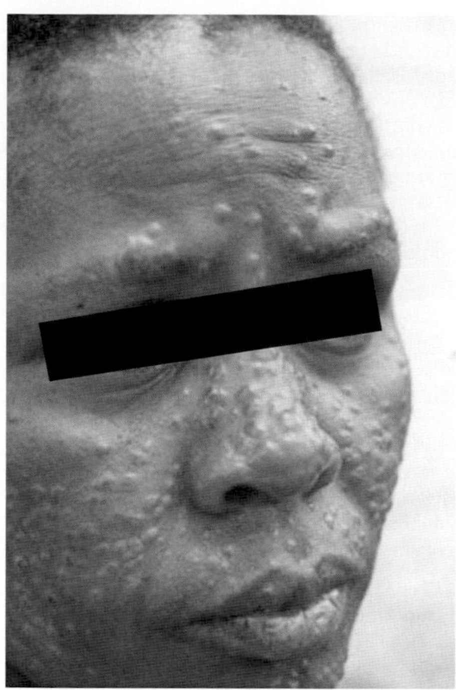

FIGURE 99.7 Nodular lesions of post-Kala-azar dermal leishmaniasis in a Kenyan woman.

with PKDL are serologically and biochemically identical to *L. donovani* isolated from patients with visceral leishmaniasis. Because the lesions of PKDL may persist for up to 20 years, such patients may act as a chronic reservoir of infection.

DIAGNOSIS

CLINICAL DIAGNOSIS

A clinical diagnosis of visceral leishmaniasis can be made with varying degrees of certainty depending on the local epidemiologic factors and clinical presentation The positive predictive value of a clinical diagnosis of late-stage visceral leishmaniasis, with classic signs and symptoms, in an endemic area is likely to be very high. Although a confirmatory parasitologic diagnosis is preferable prior to starting treatment, in settings where safely performing an invasive procedure is difficult, a presumptive diagnosis can be made when clinical improvement in response to appropriate therapy is seen within a week or so. A clinical diagnosis early in the course of infection when the classic features of disease are not yet established is much less certain.

DEMONSTRATION OF PARASITES

Specimens can be obtained from the bone marrow, liver, spleen, or enlarged lymph nodes. Splenic aspiration has the highest sensitivity. In experienced hands, the procedure is safe and well tolerated; however, deaths have occurred after splenic aspiration, presumably owing to splenic laceration – careful observation after the procedure is mandatory [34, 35]. Contraindications to splenic aspiration are a soft spleen in acute disease, a prothrombin time ≥5 seconds compared with the normal control, or a platelet count below 40,000/mm^3. The procedure uses a 21-gauge needle attached to a 5-ml syringe, which is inserted just under the skin over the middle of the spleen or via an intercostal approach if the spleen is minimally enlarged. As suction is applied, the needle is rapidly inserted into the spleen and withdrawn, with the needle remaining in the spleen only a fraction of a second. The small amount of splenic tissue and blood in the needle is expressed into culture medium and onto slides for thin smears. Splenic smears stained with Giemsa or Leishman's stain demonstrate amastigotes in >95% of cases. Splenic smears are often quantitated by the method of Chulay and Bryceson to assist in response to therapy [36].

Bone marrow aspiration is preferred in many areas because of concern about the hazards of splenic aspiration and unfamiliarity with the technique. Bone marrow smears usually contain relatively fewer amastigotes, and parasites are found in only 50–85% of cases compared with splenic aspirates. Amastigotes are also frequently found in aspirates or biopsies of liver specimens or lymph nodes. Buffy coat smears can demonstrate amastigotes in Indian and Kenyan Kala-azar, but it is unusual to make the diagnosis by this method.

The confirmation of visceral leishmaniasis is usually not difficult, as it is a polyparasitic syndrome; however, the parasite burden in early disease in non-immunes or in those with hemophagocytic syndrome can be very light and more sensitive techniques such as culture and PCR are needed [37]. PCR amplification of *Leishmania* DNA from liver and bone marrow are routinely reported.

The early macules and hypopigmented lesions of PKDL have few parasites but papular or nodular lesions of PKDL usually have abundant parasites and can easily be seen on smears or grown in culture.

SEROLOGIC TESTS

High-titer anti-leishmanial antibodies are present in visceral leishmaniasis and can be detected by ELISA, immunofluorescence, and direct agglutination. Sensitivity and specificity vary based on the antigens used in the assay and the infecting parasites. Whole promastigotes, crude promastigote lysates and recombinant antigens are in use. In general, current serologic tests for visceral leishmaniasis have sensitivities >90% but with lower specificities. False-positive results, especially with lower titers, can be seen in malaria, trypanosomiasis, tuberculosis, enteric fever, and schistosomiasis. In addition, antibodies may persist for many months following treatment for visceral leishmaniasis.

The ELISA test using whole, soluble promastigote or recombinant antigens appears as sensitive and specific as the indirect fluorescent antibody test (IFA) and, because of economy and technical practicality, it is especially useful for large-scale epidemiologic studies. Both the IFA and ELISA can be performed on sera eluted from filter papers impregnated with 50 µl of capillary blood.

The IFA is positive in more than 95% of patients with visceral leishmaniasis, generally with titers above 1:256. Whole, culture-derived promastigotes are fixed in wells of a special glass slide. Serum at different dilutions is applied to the wells. Antibodies in the serum that bind to surface antigens on the promastigotes are then detected by an antibody to the Ig molecule conjugated to a fluorescent marker. A microscopist reports a titer (the reciprocal of the dilution) that corresponds to a certain percentage of parasites that fluoresce. IFA testing is somewhat subjective and requires rigorous technique and relatively expensive equipment.

The direct agglutination test (DAT) is based on direct agglutination of *L. donovani* promastigotes that react specifically with anti-leishmania antibodies in the serum specimen resulting in agglutination of the promastigotes. Serial, twofold dilutions (starting 1:100) from the serum samples, are made in a V-shaped microtiter plate. The antigen is added and the plates are read the next day. Agglutination is visible as a blue/purple mat in the wells of the microtiter plate. The freeze-dried antigen is available from the Royal Tropical Institute (KIT) Biomedical Research in Amsterdam, The Netherlands (http://www.kit.nl/-/INS/52859/Royal-Tropical-Institute) and can be stored at ambient temperature for at least 2 years. After reconstitution of the antigen in saline and storage at 4 °C, the antigen can be used at least for a week. DAT test sensitivity and specificity estimates were 94.8% (95% confidence interval 92.7–96.4%) and 85.9% (72.3–93.4%), respectively, in a meta-analysis [38].

The recombinant protein rK39 is used as the capture antigen in ELISA tests and in point-of-care, dipstick-type, rapid diagnostic tests to detect antibodies in the serum of patients with visceral leishmaniasis. In the same meta-analysis, the rK39 test sensitivity and specificity were very similar to the DAT at 93.9% (87.7–97.1%) and 90.6% (66.8–97.9%) respectively [38]. Sensitivity is higher and more homogeneous in the studies carried out in South Asia and the specificity varies depending on the choice of controls. Quantitative titers to rK39 determined by ELISA also decrease following successful chemotherapy and tend to rise in cases of relapse, making it useful for the recognition of treatment failures. In the rapid assays, the rK39 antigen is striped onto nitrocellulose paper and a drop of whole blood is placed onto a sample pad with immunolabeled gold. Human IgG binds to the labeled gold and migrates up the strip. If antibodies to rK39 are present in the serum, they bind to the rK389 antigen stripe giving a visual positive test result. A Food and Drug Administration (FDA)-cleared rK39 assay is commercially available (Kalazar Detect™, Inbios International Inc., Seattle, WA, USA; http://www.inbios.com/rapid-tests/kalazar-detect). The rK39 test is not useful in screening asymptomatic individuals for infection but should be used in individuals with a compatible clinical syndrome.

LEISHMANIN SKIN TEST (LST)

The Leishmanin skin test (LST) test is almost uniformly negative in active visceral leishmaniasis but becomes positive in 90% of patients 6 weeks to 1 year after recovery. Tuberculin sensitivity is usually similarly depressed during active Kala-azar, indicating a broad defect in cell-mediated immunity (CMI).

DIFFERENTIAL DIAGNOSIS

The differential diagnosis of late-stage visceral leishmaniasis is limited. Hematologic and lymphatic malignancies, disseminated histoplasmosis and hepatosplenic schistomiasis have rarely been reported to mimic late-stage visceral leishmaniasis. Early disease has a much broader differential that includes malaria, African trypanosomiasis, brucellosis, enteric fevers, bacterial endocarditis, generalized histoplasmosis, chronic myelocytic leukemia, Hodgkin disease and other lymphomas, sarcoidosis, hepatic cirrhosis, and tuberculosis. Tropical splenomegaly syndrome is especially difficult to differentiate, although high titers of antimalarial antibodies and a characteristic histologic appearance of the liver suggest this disease. Patients with multiple myeloma and Waldenström's macroglobulinemia have monoclonal hypergammaglobulinemia.

TREATMENT

NONSPECIFIC OR SUPPORTIVE CARE

Patients should receive a nutritious diet, as patients are often malnourished. Antimicrobial agents are given when concurrent pneumonia, tuberculosis or other bacterial infections are suspected. Patients with chronic disease generally tolerate anemia well, but blood transfusion may be needed if associated with respiratory distress or the hemoglobin level falls below 6 g/dl. Coexistent iron or vitamin deficiency my also require specific treatment.

SPECIFIC ANTI-LEISHMANIAL THERAPY

Pentavalent antimony compounds (SbV) have historically been the drugs of choice for the treatment of visceral leishmaniasis worldwide since their introduction in the mid-1930s. However, reports of primary treatment failures with SbV in India became more prevalent in the mid-1990s leading to trials of amphotericin B compounds as initial therapy for both Mediterranean and Indian visceral leishmaniasis. Currently, many favor the use of liposomal amphotericin B as first-line therapy for visceral leishmaniasis. SbV remains efficacious when given at appropriate doses in East Africa and the Americas.

PENTAVALENT ANTIMONIALS (SbV)

There are two widely available commercial SbV formulations: sodium stibogluconate (SSG; Pentostam®, GlaxoSmithKline, UK) largely used in English-speaking countries and meglumine antimoniate (Glucantime®, Sanofi-Aventis, Suzano, Brazil) commonly used in Latin America and French-speaking parts of Africa and Europe. There are numerous local and regional manufacturers around the world of SSG and other SbV formulations. It is not known how these different preparations compare with each other in terms of safety and efficacy, as no comparative trials have ever been performed. However, it is unwise to assume one preparation will perform the same as another or have the same safety and tolerability profile. Deaths have been associated with the use of generic SbV and every batch of generic SSG should be subject to rigorous quality control prior to use [39].

SbV can be administered intravenously or intramuscularly. There is variation in the total antimony (Sb) content, the proportion of SbV to trivalent Sb (trivalent Sb is much more toxic than SbV), and the physical and chemical characteristics of different lots of SbV from the same manufacturer and between preparations from different manufacturers. Many investigators believe these lot variations are responsible for the different safety and efficacy profiles observed in treated patients. Several cardiac deaths in India were associated with use of a SbV preparation with high osmolarity [40]. In addition, SbV dissociates or polymerizes over time, so storage conditions and shelf-life are important considerations. Storage at 4 °C in the dark is optimal.

In the USA, Pentostam® is available from the Centers for Disease Control and Prevention (CDC) under an investigational new drug (IND) application. The recommended treatment regimen for visceral leishmaniasis is 20 mg of SbV/kg/day given intravenously for 28 days. Undiluted intravenous injections are not recommended. The daily dose can be given as 1:10 dilution with 5% D/W to reduce the incidence of local thrombosis through a steel butterfly needle placed and removed daily. In endemic areas, the intramuscular route of administration is more common although the large-volume injections are moderately painful.

SbV drugs are safe, although with a poorly tolerated side effect profile. Nausea, anorexia, abdominal pain, malaise, headache, arthralgias, myalgias, and lethargy are frequent, beginning about 7–10 days into therapy [41]. These side effects are more noticeable in cutaneous leishmaniasis and mucosal leishmaniasis patients, as they do not have systemic symptoms associated with their disease. In general, visceral leishmaniasis patients seem to tolerate SbV better than cutaneous leishmaniasis or mucosal leishmaniasis patients. In particular, large joint arthralgias can be quite problematic. Fortunately, these symptoms resolve shortly after therapy is complete.

Shortly after beginning therapy, patients treated with SbV preparations develop elevations in serum amylase and serum lipase, lipase greater than amylase, which peak at 7–14 days [42]. Although most are asymptomatic, many develop some degree of anorexia, nausea and mid-epigastric pain consistent with pancreatitis. Lipase and amylase levels return to normal despite continuing the drug.

Deaths attributed to pancreatic necrosis have been reported in patients receiving SbV; therefore, monitoring of serum amylase and lipase in patients is recommended. When patients develop symptoms or signs of pancreatitis, it is recommended that SSG be temporarily halted for a few days. Serum amylase and lipase rapidly return to normal and the regimen can then usually be completed without another interruption. Even in asymptomatic patients, it is reasonable to temporarily interrupt therapy for significant elevations of serum amylase or lipase.

Anemia, neutropenia, and thrombocytopenia associated with hypoplasia of the bone marrow have all been seen during SbV therapy and are occasionally severe enough to interrupt therapy. Abnormalities reverse on discontinuation of the drug. Again, baseline values prior to treatment and monitoring during therapy are recommended if feasible. Transient increases in serum transaminases are also seen in the majority of patients during treatment. AST levels rise three- to fourfold above the upper limit of normal between days 7 and 14 but decline despite continued therapy. Renal tubular acidosis and acute renal failure associated with SbV have been reported. SSG causes lymphopenia that has been associated with occasional cases of herpes zoster occurring during the course of treatment.

Electrocardiographic (ECG) abnormalities, including nonspecific ST- and T-wave changes and T-wave flattening or inversion, occur in more than half of patients receiving SSG; the frequency of these changes is proportional to the total daily dose and the duration of therapy [43]. Torsades de pointes with prolonged QT intervals and syncopal episodes have also been reported. An ECG should be obtained prior to therapy and repeated weekly for standard doses; if doses above 20 mg/kg/day are considered, more frequent ECG monitoring should be considered. Treatment should be suspended if the corrected QT interval (the measured QT interval divided by the square root of the RR interval) becomes prolonged beyond 0.50 seconds. T-wave flattening or inversion, the most common ECG abnormality during antimony administration, is not an indication to stop treatment [44].

AMPHOTERICIN B

Amphotricin B deoxycholate was successfully introduced to treat cases of visceral leishmaniasis that failed to respond to SbV in the 1990s, especially in India. The regimen is 1 mg/kg administered by slow intravenous infusion over 4–6 hours every 2 days, until a total dose of about 20 mg/kg has been given. Although some initiate treatment with an incremental escalation of doses in an attempt to decrease the infusion-related side effects of amphotericin B, a clinical trial of 120 Indian patients with visceral leishmaniasis showed no difference in infusion-related side effects between those receiving the incremental dose and those receiving 1 mg/kg from day 1 [45]. The widespread use of amphotericin B deoxycholate has been hindered because of the well-known infusion-related side effects of fever, chills and thrombophlebitis, long-term problems of renal insufficiency, anemia and hypokalemia, and poor tolerability (anorexia, nausea). Also, amphotericin B deoxycholate should be used with caution in those previously receiving SbV. Sudden cardiac death has been reported following the first dose of amphotericin B deoxycholate in these patients. It is thought that the ECG abnormalities associated with SbV therapy predispose to cardiac events [46]. It seems prudent to recommend that a baseline ECG be obtained and a rest period be observed until the ECG normalizes, usually within 10 days of the end of SbV therapy, and any electrolyte abnormalities be corrected before starting amphotericin B deoxycholate.

The desire to develop less toxic and more effective preparations of amphotericin B to treat systemic mycoses led to the introduction of lipid-associated amphotericin B preparations in the mid-1990s. Liposomal amphotericin B (LAMB) (AmBisome®, Astellas Pharma US, Inc., USA) was approved in 1997 by the FDA for the treatment of visceral leishmaniasis [47, 48].

LAMB has been shown in a series of trials to be a very effective and safe drug for the treatment of visceral leishmaniasis acquired in Brazil, India, Kenya, and the Mediterranean [16, 49–51]. The current FDA-approved regimen for immunocompetent patients, based on data from the Mediterranean and Brazil, is 3 mg/kg daily on days 1–5, a sixth dose on day 14 and a seventh dose on day 21 (total dose with this regimen is 21 mg/kg). Overall success rate with this dose regimen is practically 100%. Lower-dose regimens have been effective in trials from Brazil, India, and Kenya. A dose of 3–4 mg/kg daily on days 1–5 with a sixth dose on day 10 is probably adequate for visceral leishmaniasis acquired in the Mediterranean and Brazil, and a dose of 2–3 mg/kg daily on days 1–5 and a sixth dose on day 10 for visceral leishmaniasis acquired in East Africa and India. Culminating a series of investigations spanning a decade, Indian investigators have shown that a single 10 mg/kg dose of LAMB was >95% efficacious [51]. Lower-dose regimens may have a somewhat lower efficacy than the near 100% reported with the higher-dose regimen, but the cost savings and decreased potential for infusion-related side effects may make a lower-dose regimen optimal for some geographic regions. The current FDA-approved regimen for immunosuppressed patients is a higher-dose regimen of 4 mg/kg daily on days 1–5, 10, 17, 24, 31 and 38 (total dose of 40 mg/kg). Even with the higher total dose, relapse is common in immunocompromised patients. For the rare cases of visceral leishmaniasis treated in the non-endemic areas, LAMB is the recommended drug and should be used unless contraindicated.

PAROMOMYCIN

Paromomycin is an aminoglycoside with broad anti-parasitic activity. Parenteral paromomycin used as monotherapy has been shown to be effective in Indian visceral leishmaniasis at a dose of 15 mg/kg paromomycin sulfate (11 mg base) given intramuscularly for 21 days for a cure rate of 93–95% [52]. The efficacy was shown to be 85% in East Africa at an increased dose of 20 mg/kg (15 mg base) per day for 21 days [53]. There is no experience with this drug in *L. infantum* foci (Mediterranean, South America). Mild pain at the injection site is the commonest adverse event (55%). Reversible ototoxicity occurs in 2% of patients. Occasional elevated hepatic enzyme concentrations and rare renal toxicity and tetany have been reported.

MILTEFOSINE

Miltefosine was originally developed as an oral anticancer drug but was later shown to have anti-leishmanial activity. Miltefosine commonly induces gastrointestinal side-effects such as anorexia, nausea, vomiting (38%), and diarrhea (20%). Most episodes are brief and resolve as treatment is continued. Occasionally, the side effects can be severe and require interruption of treatment. Skin allergy, elevated hepatic transaminase concentrations and, rarely, renal insufficiency may be observed. Miltefosine should be taken after meals and, if multiple doses are to be taken, they should be divided. Miltefosine is potentially teratogenic and should not be used by pregnant women or women with child-bearing potential for whom adequate contraception cannot be assured for the duration of treatment and for 3 months afterwards. Miltfosine is given at a dose of 2.5 mg/kg per day for 28 days to children aged 2–11 years and for people aged 12 years and above at a dose of 50 mg/day for those weighing <25 kg, 100 mg/day for 25–50 kg body weight and 150 mg/day for >50 kg body weight for 28 days, has shown a 95% cure rate in immunocompetent patients in India [54, 55] and about 90% in Ethiopia [56].

COMBINATION TREATMENT

The use of long-duration monotherapy in unsupervised settings is concerning for the risk of developing resistance to established or newly introduced drugs, especially in anthroponotic foci. The current World Health Organization (WHO) policy is to limit the use of monotherapy to liposomal LAMB [57].

Combination treatment has the potential advantages of shortening the duration of treatment, reducing the overall dose of medicines and reducing the probability of selection of drug-resistant parasites which will improve compliance, reduce drug toxicities, lower costs and prolong the effective life of the available medicines.

Several trials of combinations have been conducted, with favorable results. A combination of paromomycin and antimonials resulted in a higher cure rate in visceral leishmaniasis patients in Bihar, India than antimonials alone, to which lack of response was common. In East Africa, the combination of sodium stibogluconate at 20 mg/kg SbV + plus paromomycin given at 15 mg/kg (11-mg base) for 17 days showed an efficacy of 93%. The safety and efficacy of the combination treatment and sodium stibogluconate alone were similar. Furthermore, there were no differences in the efficacy of the combination treatment in Ethiopia, Kenya, and the Sudan, suggesting that this regimen could be used across the region. In several phase 3 studies in India, three separate combinations showed 98–99% cure rates. The treatment included two sequential administrations, with either liposomal amphotericin B (5 mg/kg, single infusion) plus 7 days' miltefosine (dosage as above) or liposomal amphotericin B (5 mg/kg, single infusion) plus 10 days' paromomycin (11-mg/kg base), and co-adminstration of 10 days' miltefosine plus 10 days' paromomycin (dose as above). No safety issues were recorded.

TREATMENT OF RELAPSES

Relapse usually occurs within 6 months of the end of treatment, often within a few months. Persistent splenomegaly and thrombocytopenia are useful prognostic indicators. Co-infection with tuberculosis and HIV should be considered in those who fail to respond or relapse. Successful treatment of coexisting tuberculosis usually results in response of the visceral leishmaniasis. Patients who fail to respond or relapse after initial therapy should be treated with a different drug regimen. For example, if a visceral leishmaniasis patient fails to respond to liposomal amphotericin B, then a trial of SbV could begin. Additional doses, or higher doses, of the same regimen could be tried, but only under close supervision.

SPLENECTOMY

Splenectomy is rarely indicated in patients with visceral leishmaniasis. The more common dilemma is inadvertent splenectomy because of failure to consider the diagnosis of visceral leishmaniasis [58]. Patients with a protracted clinical course and frequent relapses who are resistant to treatment and develop severe cytopenias with massive splenomegaly may require splenectomy. The use of elective splenectomy is effective for restoring the hematologic parameters and reduces the need for blood transfusions, but it does not avoid relapsing visceral leishmaniasis. There is usually a prompt rise in hemoglobin levels and WBC and platelet counts after splenectomy, but additional chemotherapy is necessary, or cure is unlikely [59]. Splenectomized patients are at increased risk of overwhelming sepsis because of penumococci and other encapsulated bacteria and should receive anti-pneumococcal vaccination before splenectomy. Because malaria is often fatal in splenectomized individuals, life-long anti-malarial prophylaxis is essential in countries where malaria occurs.

POST-KALA-AZAR DERMAL LEISHMANIASIS (PKDL)

Treatment of PKDL depends on the severity of the condition in individual patients. In Bangladesh, India, and Nepal either an extended regimen of amphotericin B deoxycholate at 1 mg/kg per day by infusion (20 days on, 20 days off), up to 60–80 doses over 4 months or miltefosine orally at 50 mg three times daily for 60 days or twice daily for 90 days for 12 weeks is recommended. Disappearance of the lesion is considered clinical cure. In East Africa, PKDL is not routinely treated, as the majority of cases (85%) heal spontaneously within a year. Only patients with severe or disfiguring disease, those with lesions that have remained for longer than 6 months, those with concomitant anterior uveitis and young children with oral lesions that interfere with feeding are treated. Treatment with either SSG at 20 mg/kg SbV+ per day for up to 2 months or a 20-day course of liposomal amphotericin B at 2.5 mg/kg per day is recommended. Clinical cure is defined as flattening of lesions and improvement of dyschromia, although pigmentary changes may persist indefinitely.

HIV CO-INFECTION

Response to initial treatment with pentavalent antimony is only 50%, whereas response to liposomal amphotericin B is near 100%. However, relapse is common after both drugs. The optimal induction therapeutic regimen, including choice of drug, dose and duration for different infecting parasites is not known. Optimal intermittent maintenance regimens are likewise unknown. Currently, immune system reconstitution through highly active anti-retrovial therapy (HAART) is the optimal therapy, where feasible. It is reasonable to recommend an initial course of induction therapy using LAMB to decrease the parasite burden closely followed by HAART to raise the CD4 cell count.

PREGNANCY

Treatment of pregnant women is always a risk–benefit assessment. The possibility of a fatal outcome of leishmaniasis for the mother, the fetus and the newborn is much greater than the risk for adverse drug effects. When untreated, spontaneous abortion, small-for-birth date and congenital leishmaniasis have been described [60]. SbV and miltefosine should not be used in pregnancy [57, 61]. Miltefosine is potentially embryotoxic and teratogenic and should not be used during pregnancy. Women of child-bearing age should be tested for pregnancy before treatment and use effective contraception for 3 months after treatment.

Amphotericin B deoxycholate and LAMB are the best therapeutic options for visceral leishmaniasis. No abortions or vertical transmission have been reported in mothers treated with liposomal amphotericin B [61, 62].

PROGNOSIS

Infection with *L. donovani* comprises a spectrum of diseases, and spontaneous cure of inapparent infection is more common than was formerly realized. In contrast, the established syndrome of visceral leishmaniasis is almost always fatal in the absence of specific chemotherapy.

Response to treatment should be monitored by daily assessment of sense of wellbeing, appetite, temperature and weekly assessment of hemoglobin, platelet and neutrophil counts, body weight and spleen size. Repeat splenic or bone marrow aspirates to document parasitologic improvement are not routinely indicated in the face of clinical improvement. In most patients, the fever disappears within days, appetite returns and the patient feels better. The hemoglobin level rises and the spleen becomes smaller within 2 weeks, although return to baseline size may not occur until months after therapy. When fever persists and the general condition does not improve during treatment, concomitant tuberculosis or HIV infection should be suspected. Within 6–12 months, the spleen usually becomes non-palpable, and elevated immunoglobulin levels and serologic tests become normal. Persistent splenomegaly after otherwise successful treatment may be caused by portal hypertension.

Follow-up examination is important for the early detection and treatment of relapses. Relapse is suggested by an increase in spleen size, a fall in hemoglobin levels, and a decrease in eosinophil counts to fewer than 50/mm^3 and should be confirmed by the demonstration of parasites. Relapses are most common during the first 2–6 months after finishing treatment but, occasionally, they occur several years later, particularly in patients who become immunocompromised by disease or medication.

PREVENTION AND CONTROL

TREATMENT OF CASES

In epidemics of visceral leishmaniasis in which humans are the reservoir (India and, perhaps, parts of East Africa), aggressive case-management may help interrupt the epidemic.

POST-KALA-AZAR DERMAL LEISHMANIASIS (PKDL)

Patients with PKDL can actively transmit *Leishmania* parasites and may represent a persistent human reservoir responsible for ongoing transmission as these patients seldom receive treatment [63].

RESERVOIR CONTROL

Zoonotic visceral leishmaniasis (ZVL) caused by *Leishmania infantum* is an important disease of humans and dogs. Transmission among dogs can be maintained by non-sandfly routes, such as congenital and sexual transmission, as well as between dogs by sandfly transmission. Dogs are the only confirmed primary reservoir of infection. Review of intervention studies examining the effectiveness of current control methods highlights the lack of randomized controlled trials of both dog culling and residual insecticide spraying. Topical insecticides (deltamethrin-impregnated collars and pour-ons) have been shown to provide a high level of individual protection to treated dogs, but further community-level studies are needed [64].

VECTOR CONTROL

In India, during the early part of the 20th century, houses known to be microfoci were burned. During the malaria eradication campaigns, visceral leishmaniasis virtually disappeared from India but when spraying of dichlorodiphenyltrichloroethane (DDT) was stopped, the incidence of visceral leishmaniasis increased to high levels.

VACCINES

A variety of vaccine preparations, including killed promastigotes with, and without, adjuvants, parasite fractions, recombinant antigens, and genetically-engineered "avirulent" live parasites have been evaluated without success or are in clinical trials. None are licensed or commercially available at this time [65].

99.3 Cutaneous Leishmaniasis of the Old World

DEFINITION

Cutaneous leishmaniasis of the Old World is characterized by chronic slow-to-heal ulcerative and nodular skin lesions. Uncommon syndromes in the Old World include diffuse cutaneous leishmaniasis, mucocutaneous leishmaniasis and leishmaniasis recidivans. Local names for this disease include Oriental sore, Baghdad boil, Delhi boil, Biskra button, and Aleppo evil.

ETIOLOGY

Most Old World cutaneous leishmaniasis is caused by infections with *Leishmania tropica* and *Leishmania major* and less commonly with *Leishmania aethiopica, Leishmania infantum*, and *Leishmania killicki* that are often geographically focal diseases.

DISTRIBUTION AND EPIDEMIOLOGY

The geographic distribution of Old World CL is shown in Figure 99.8. Old World CL usually occurs in semi-arid or desert ecologic zones. In established transmission foci, cutaneous leishmaniasis is a childhood disease with increasing prevalence with age to about the mid-teenage years. Adults have acquired immunity and are seldom affected. In newly emerging foci, all individuals are non-immune and significant epidemics with very high attack rates are common [66].

LEISHMANIA MAJOR

Leishmaniasis major is a zoonotic infection of desert rodents with humans infected as incidental hosts. The great gerbil (*Rhombomys opimus)* lives in dry desert areas of central Asia, in southern Russia, throughout Iran and Pakistan, and in parts of Iraq and north-western India and China. These gerbils may have an infection rate as high as 30%, with cutaneous lesions on relatively hairless parts of the body – chiefly the head, ears and base of the tail. Other rodents in these areas play a secondary role in maintaining the infection. In North Africa, Saudi Arabia, and Israel, the fat desert gerbil *(Psammomys obesus)* and other rodents (*Meriones* spp.) are important reservoir hosts. Inhabitants of villages near gerbil burrows may have infection prevalence rates of 100% and others who enter the ecosystem, for example travelers, hunters, and military personnel, may also experience high attack rates. The peak incidence of infection occurs from June to October, with lesions appearing in October to March. Most children in endemic areas acquire a sore between 2 and 3 years of age, rarely reaching maturity without a scar. Cutaneous leishmaniasis caused by *L. major* is also found sporadically in a wide area of sub-Saharan Africa where the Nile rat *(Arvicanthis niloticus)* is a major reservoir host, although infection has been demonstrated in other rodents.

LEISHMANIA TROPICA

Leishmania tropica is a very heterogeneous species complex with strains that can be distinguished on ecologic, biochemical and serologic

- ■ *L. infantum*
- ▨ *L. major*
- □ *L. donovani*
- ⊞○ *L. tropica*
- ■ *L. aethiopica*
- □ *L. archibaldi*
- × Increasing leishmaniasis - HIV co-infection
- × Decreasing leishmaniasis - HIV co-infection
- ★ Isolated lymphadenopathy reported
- ▪ Mucous forms reported
- • Diffuse cutaneous forms reported
- \+ Post-kala-azar forms reported

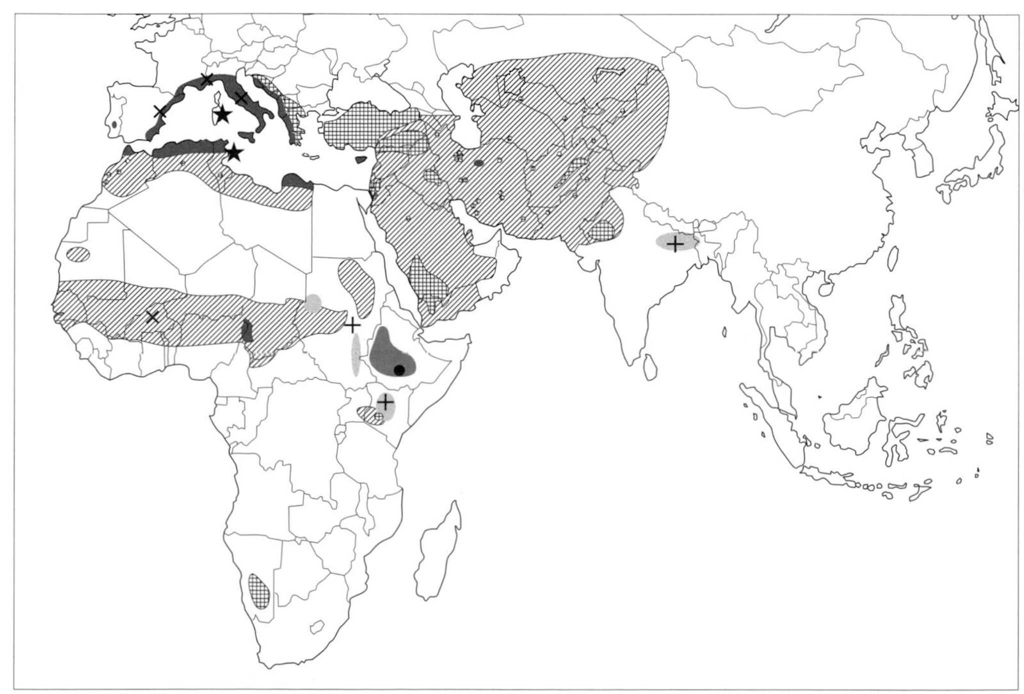

FIGURE 99.8 Geographic distribution of Old World cutaneous leishmania *(Reproduced with permission from Magill AJ. Epidemiology of the leishmaniases. Dermatol Clin 1995;13: 505–23.)*

grounds. Zoonotic *L. tropica* is a parasite of dogs and rodents and is associated with rural disease. Anthroponotic *L. tropica* is a parasite of humans and occurs in urban environments. The infection was formerly common in many large cities of the Middle East (Baghdad, Teheran, Aleppo, and Damascus) leading to it being known as "urban" cutaneous leishmaniasis. It is also found in southern Italy, Greece, Pakistan, and north-western India. With residual insecticide spraying for malaria control, there was a marked decrease in the sandfly populations and concomitant decline in the incidence of urban cutaneous leishmaniasis. However, a major epidemic of anthroponotic cutaneous leishmaniasis caused by *L. tropica* has occurred in war-ravaged Kabul, Afghanistan, with thousands of cases identified [67].

LEISHMANIA AETHIOPICA

Leishmania aethiopica is a zoonotic parasite found in stable, low endemicity foci in mountain valleys of the Rift Valley of Ethiopia and Kenya. The mammalian reservoir is the rock hyrax *(Procavia habessinica)* and the tree hyrax *(Heterohyrax brucei)*, with the high-altitude sandfly vectors *Phlebotomus longipes* (Ethiopia) and *Phlebotomus pedifer* (Kenya). Human cases are closely associated with proximity to hyrax colonies and often occur when homesteads encroach on the zoonotic cycle on deforested mountain slopes [68].

LEISHMANIA INFANTUM

Leishmania infantum, the usual cause of Mediterranean visceral leishmaniasis, has been isolated from indurated, nodular cutaneous lesions, as well as in countries throughout the Mediterranan littoral, Iran, the Caucasus, and foci in the New World [69]. Isoenzyme analysis shows that "dermotropic" *L. infantum* strains are more commonly found in cutaneous lesions and have also been isolated from visceral sites in AIDS patients.

PATHOGENESIS

The development of clinical disease following infection depends on the parasite strain and inoculum, the genetically determined host innate and acquired immune responses, prior exposures and sandfly factors to include components of the saliva [66]. The host inflammatory responses mediate disease expression resulting in asymptomatic infection to predominantly self-healing ulcerative cutaneous leishmaniasis or chronic, nonhealing diffuse cutaneous leishmaniasis, mucosal leishmaniasis or leishmaniasis recidivans. In general, disease resolution is mediated by cell-mediated immune responses (CMI). In self-healing cutaneous leishmaniasis, delayed-type hypersensitivity is usually present and tends to correlate to ulcer size and number, as determined by skin test reactivity [70]. In leishmaniasis recidivans, there is healing in the center of the lesion but failure to heal peripherally, where a granulomatous reaction without caseation is seen. Parasites are scanty and the histologic changes are similar to those of lupus vulgaris. In diffuse cutaneous leishmaniasis, there is a defect in the CMI response and numerous macrophages filled with amastigotes are seen with no cellular reaction or only a few surrounding lymphocytes.

CLINICAL MANIFESTATIONS

The incubation period of cutaneous leishmaniasis is generally 2–8 weeks but, in exceptional cases, the incubation period may be as long as 3 years. The first sign of cutaneous leishmaniasis is often an unnoticed area of erythema at the site of the sandfly bite that slowly becomes an inflammatory papule. It may persist as a flattened plaque or may progress to a nodule after a few days or weeks, with the surface becoming covered with fine, papery scales (Fig. 99.9), which are white and dry at first, but later become moist and adherent, uncovering a shallow ulcer as they fall off. As the ulcer enlarges, it oozes serous fluid and may become covered with a thick crust. A raised, indurated area with a characteristic dusky discoloration surrounds the edge of the ulcer. Satellite lesions are common and may ultimately merge with the parent lesion. Over many weeks to months the typical features of ulcerative cutaneous leishmaniasis emerge [71].

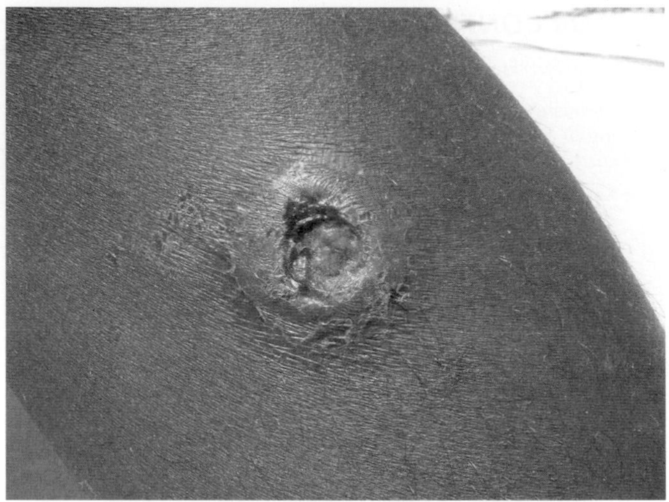

FIGURE 99.9 Cutaneous leishmania caused by *Leishmania major*.

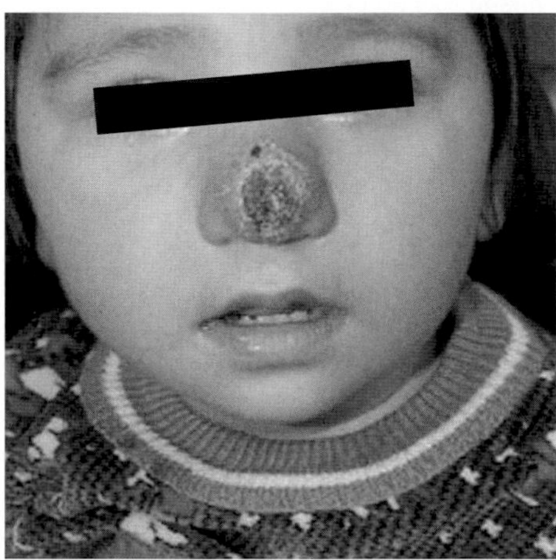

FIGURE 99.10 *Leishmania tropica*.

Different forms of cutaneous leishmaniasis vary in some of their clinical features. The lesions of rural disease caused by *L. major* tend to be larger, multiple and can be accompanied by marked inflammation and crusting. They mature rapidly and heal relatively quickly, lasting a few months. The lesions of urban disease caused by *L. tropica* tend to be smaller, single, develop more slowly and persist for a year or more (Fig. 99.10).

Cutaneous leishmaniasis lesions caused by *L. aethiopica* are the least inflamed and most chronic; however, most lesions usually eventually heal spontaneously within 2–5 years. *Leishmania aethiopica* gives rise principally to localized cutaneous nodular lesions; less frequently, it gives rise to oronasal leishmaniasis, which may distort the nostrils and lips, and a small percentage of infected individuals develop nonhealing diffuse cutaneous leishmaniasis. Most lesions evolve slowly and may spread locally. Ulceration is late or absent.

The clinical appearance of the lesions reflects the degree of the host's immune response and may vary from small papules to non-ulcerated plaques to large ulcers with well-defined, raised, indurated margins. When multiple lesions are present, they are usually similar in appearance and enlarge and heal together. After a few months to more than a year, healing begins with central granulation tissue that spreads peripherally. The resultant depressed white or pink scar is often cosmetically disfiguring, especially when on the face. *Leishmania major* infections may be associated with severe scarring, which can cause disability if located at critical sites, for example the wrist or elbow, and substantial stigma for affected individuals.

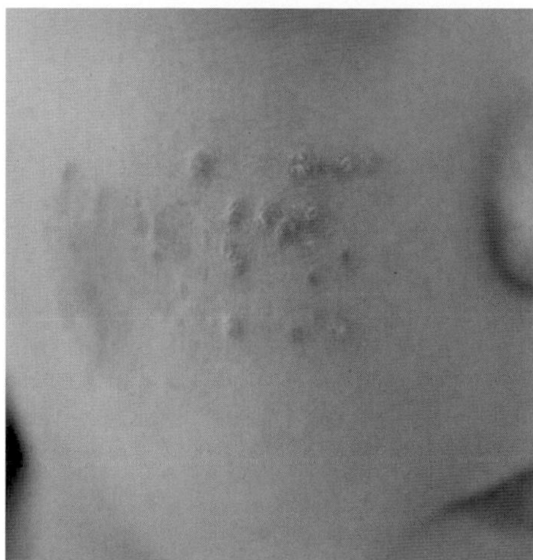

FIGURE 99.11 Leishmaniasis recidivans.

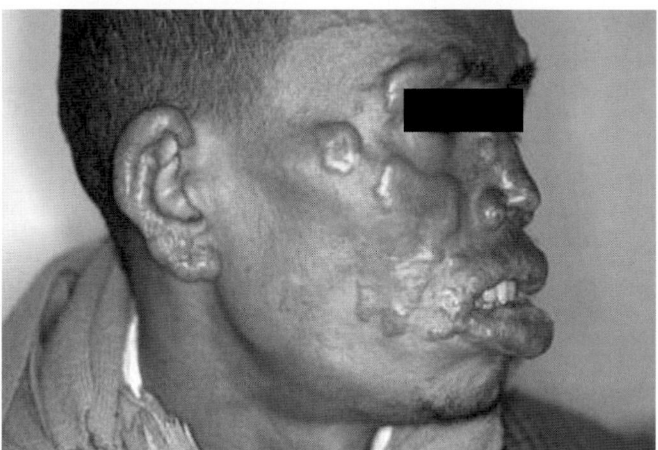

FIGURE 99.12 A male outpatient [Armauer Hansen Research Institute (AHRI), Addis Ababa) with diffuse cutaneous leishmaniasis. The condition is similar to, and often misdiagnosed as, leprosy. *(Reproduced with permission from the World Health Organization/TDR (WHO/TDR/Crump http://apps.who.int/tdr/publications/tdr-image-library?idNumber=03061505).)*

Lesions usually occur on exposed parts of the body, for example face, hands, feet, arms, and legs, but rarely on the trunk and never on the palms or soles or hairy scalp. Uncommon sites of ulcers include the ears, tongue, and eyelids. Fever has occasionally preceded the appearance of multiple nodules. Lymphatic spread may occur in *L. major* infections, with subcutaneous nodules in a linear distribution and regional lymphadenopathy. When the primary lesion is on the hand, this may resemble sporotrichosis. Secondary bacterial infection, defined as purulence or abscess, of an ulcer is unusual; however, bacterial colonization of ulcer surfaces is common.

LEISHMANIASIS RECIDIVANS

Leishmaniasis recidivans is a rare chronic form of cutaneous leishmaniasis caused by *L. tropica,* which is found primarily in Iran, Iraq, and North Africa. This clinical manifestation usually begins on the face (95%), slowly progresses, healing in the center and advancing at the periphery, and is characterized by the development of recrudescing lupoid papules or nodules that form mostly around, or in, the site of primary healed lesions (Fig. 99.11). Leishmaniasis recidivans lesions spread slowly, may persist for 20–40 years and rarely respond to treatment, thus becoming destructive and disfiguring over the years. Patients often relate a history of seasonal variation in the activity of the lesions. They usually became worse in the summer and improve in the winter. Patients express little discomfort about their lesions [72].

Also known as lupoid leishmaniasis, the scarcity of amastigotes in the lesions in direct smears and tissue specimens easily leads to misdiagnosis of lupus vulgaris (cutaneous tuberculosis), both clinically and histologically. The dense scar tissue in the center of the lesion contains small granulomas, whereas the nodules and papules at the periphery resemble the "apple jelly" nodules of lupus vulgaris.

DIFFUSE CUTANEOUS LEISHMANIASIS

Diffuse cutaneous leishmaniasis is an uncommon result of infection with *L. aethiopica* in Ethiopia and Kenya. Diffuse cutaneous leishmaniasis usually begins as a single, nodular, non-ulcerating lesion (often on the face), which enlarges and is followed by multiple, widely disseminated cutaneous macules, papules, nodules or plaques, or by diffuse infiltration of the skin (especially on extensor surfaces of the limbs and on the face) resulting in lesions scattered over the entire body (especially on the face and nose, limbs and buttocks), where thickening of the eyebrows and earlobes may resemble lepromatous leprosy [73] (Fig. 99.12). The lesions do not ulcerate and may coalesce to form plaques. Mucosal involvement is confined to the borders of the nostrils and lips. This disease does not heal spontaneously and relapses are frequent after treatment. The nodules of diffuse cutaneous leishmaniasis are often described as soft and fleshy, whereas the nodules of lepromatous leprosy are often more indurated. Although parasites are rarely recovered from blood and bone marrow, visceral disease does not develop. The leishmanin skin test (LST) is persistently negative unless, and until, recovery occurs.

DIAGNOSIS

DEMONSTRATION OF THE ORGANISM

Typical ulcerative lesions should be thoroughly cleaned and exudative crusts debrided to a clean ulcer base. Using a No. 10 scalpel blade, one can scrape the clean surface to obtain material about the size of a rice grain: place on glass slides for staining and microscopic diagnosis; place in culture media; and place in 95% ethanol for DNA or RNA extraction for PCR testing. Tissue juice aspirated from the margin of lesions can also be cultured. Cultures generally become positive within 2–7 days in Schneider's medium, but may take longer (up to 21 days) to grow in Novy and MacNeal's medium (NNN) medium.

In nodular lesions amastigotes can sometimes be identified in slit skin smears prepared as for diagnosing leprosy. The margin of the lesion is squeezed between the thumb and forefinger until bloodless; a scalpel blade is used to make a small incision; the cut edge of the incision is scraped with the blade; and the tissue juice on the blade is spread on a clean glass slide and stained with Giemsa stain. Alternatively, a small biopsy specimen may be removed from the edge of the lesion and an impression smear made by pressing the cut surface lightly against a slide. A portion of the biopsy specimen is macerated and cultured in NNN or Schneider's medium and the remainder fixed for pathologic examination. Varying numbers of organisms can be identified in histologic sections according to the immune status of the individual.

Leishmania amastigotes have a kinetoplast and must be differentiated from yeast cells and the intracellular forms of *Histoplasma capsulatum* and *Toxoplasma gondii* that do not have kinetoplasts. In leishmaniasis recidivans, organisms are rarely seen in biopsy specimens or on smear but can more often be isolated by culture or PCR. The LST is strongly positive in typical ulcerative CL.

SKIN TEST

The LST becomes positive within 3 months of the onset of skin lesions and remains positive for life. Skin test-positive individuals may have skin lesions for which the etiology is not leishmaniasis.

SEROLOGIC TESTS

Low titers of anti-leishmanial antibodies are detected in many patients with cutaneous leishmaniasis, but these tests are generally of little diagnostic help.

DIFFERENTIAL DIAGNOSIS

On clinical grounds, the lesions of cutaneous leishmaniasis must be distinguished from diphtheritic or veldt sores, tropical ulcer, tertiary syphilis, yaws, lupus vulgaris, blastomycosis, basal cell carcinoma, squamous cell carcinoma and other causes of chronic nodules and ulcers. Although the LST is sometimes helpful, definitive diagnosis depends on demonstration or isolation of the organism.

TREATMENT

TYPICAL OLD WORLD CUTANEOUS LEISHMANIASIS

The majority of Old World cutaneous leishmaniasis lesions, especially rural zoonotic cutaneous leishmaniasis caused by *L. major*, are self-healing, requiring a few months to heal completely. Urban anthroponotic cutaneous leishmaniasis caused by *L. tropica* can take many months or a few years to heal. In general, systemic treatment is less commonly employed in Old World disease compared with New World disease. There is a paucity of evidence-based data from high-quality clinical trials in Old World cutaneous leishmaniasis [74].

LOCAL THERAPY

Local treatments include thermotherapy, cryotherapy, topical paromomycin ointments, intralesional administration of SbV and combinations of all of the above.

Local heat therapy is useful in treating small lesions. One or two applications of localized heat (50 °C for 30 s) with the ThermoMed® device was as effective as intralesional SbV (70% cure rate) in *L. tropica* acquired in Afghanistan [75] and more effective (70% cure rate) than systemic SbV+ in *L. major* acquired in Iraq [76]. The device is expensive but works on a battery – a significant advantage for field use. Local anesthesia must be applied to the lesion prior to using the device. A blister is seen 1–2 days after thermotherapy, but appears to be well-tolerated. Application of a topical antibiotic ointment and wound care decreases the incidence of secondary wound infections.

Cryotherapy is achieved with application of liquid nitrogen every 3–7 days for 1–5 sessions. Each weekly administration is usually two application cycles of 10–15 seconds of freezing time, with a thawing interval of 20 seconds. Freezing should reach up to a few millimeters of healthy skin surrounding the lesion. Liquid nitrogen application requires specific devices and a skilled healthcare provider. Post-cryotherapy care includes daily cleansing with an antiseptic solution and topical application of antibiotic ointment.

Topical paromomycin creams at various doses, regimens and formulations have been used for decades. A topical formulation of 15% paromomycin with 12% methylbenzethonium chloride in soft white paraffin (Leshcutan®, Teva, Israel) gives variable responses in *L. major* ranging from 30–75%, and little-to-no efficacy in *L. tropica*. Because this preparation causes significant local reactions consisting of pruritus, paresthesias and vesicle formation in about 25% of patients, other, better-tolerated preparations have been developed. A 10% paromomycin/10% urea formulation used twice daily for 14 days was no better than placebo in controlled trials in Iran and Tunisia. A longer regimen (up to 12 weeks) of 12–15% paromomycin/10% urea applied daily cured 23 out of 27 patients at the Hospital for Tropical Diseases in London in a mean of 6.7 weeks and was reported as nontoxic. None of the topical agents are effective against cutaneous leishmaniasis caused by *L. tropica*. A third-generation formulation of 15% paromomycin and 0.5% gentamicin was shown to be superior to placebo in *L. major* acquired in Tunisia and was safe and well-tolerated [77]. Although the next generation of paromomycin-based topicals appears quite promising, the best formulation and optimal dose regimen are not yet determined. It is likely that the optimal dose regimens will have to be determined for each major geographic area.

Intralesional SbV, defined as local infiltration of 0.3–0.8 mL of SbV, has been used extensively for Old World cutaneous leishmaniasis with some success and merits consideration, especially for early, non-ulcerated lesions. Each lesion is injected individually, dividing the dose into four quadrants if possible. The reported number of injections and the daily dose used vary widely, but efficacy is similar to intramuscular administration. Intralesional SbV can be very painful depending on the location injected but avoids systemic toxicity and reduces costs.

Combinations of intralesional SbV co-administered with cryotherapy have been shown to be superior to either one alone [78].

SYSTEMIC CHEMOTHERAPY

Systemic treatment is indicated for large, or multiple, lesions and to patients with lesions in functionally or cosmetically important areas, for example the wrist, feet, and ankles, or face when local treatments are not indicated. SbV can be given intramuscularly or intravenously at 20 mg Sb/kg/day for 10–20 days. Cutaneous leishmaniasis caused by *L. tropica* and *L. aethiopica* usually requires a longer treatment duration, while cutaneous leishmaniasis caused by *L. major* may be adequately treated with the shorter 10-day regimen. The true efficacy of SbV in Old World cutaneous leishmaniasis in most locations has never been established and is thought by many to be minimally effective [57].

Oral fluconazole at 200 mg daily for 6 weeks was shown to shorten the time to healing in *L. major* infections in Saudi Arabia compared with placebo [79]. A more recent randomized controlled trial in patients with *L. major* in Iran showed that a higher fluconazole dose of 400 mg was superior to the 200 mg dose in shortening the time to healing [80]. The optimal dose of fluconazole remains to be determined.

LEISHMANIASIS RECIDIVANS

The World Health Organization (WHO)-recommended treatment for leishmaniasis recidivans is 15–20 mg SbV+/kg per day intramuscularly or intravenously for 15 days plus oral allopurinol 20 mg/kg for 30 days, to treat leishmaniasis recidivans caused by *L. tropica* [57].

DIFFUSE CUTANEOUS LEISHMANIASIS

Diffuse cutaneous leishmaniasis in Ethiopia and Kenya responds poorly to treatment with SbV. The WHO currently recommends 20 mg SbV+/kg per day intramuscularly or intravenously plus paromomycin, 15 mg (11-mg base)/kg per day intramuscularly for 60 days or longer to treat diffuse cutaneous leishmaniasis [57]. Whatever the regimen used, treatment should be prolonged for several weeks beyond clinical cure.

PREVENTION AND CONTROL

VECTOR CONTROL

Reducing the vector population can decrease the incidence of cutaneous leishmaniasis. Improved general sanitation and removal of refuse and rubble in which sandflies breed reduces the incidence of urban cutaneous leishmaniasis. Residual spraying with dichlorodiphenyltrichloroethane (DDT) for malaria control had eliminated cutaneous leishmaniasis in many areas, although it has returned with the cessation of spraying.

RESERVOIR CONTROL

In the central Asian republics of the former Soviet Union, cutaneous leishmaniasis incidence has been reduced by deep plowing of fields to destroy burrows and eliminate gerbils from the area.

IMMUNIZATION

Intracutaneous vaccination with live, attenuated *L. major* promastigotes was used for many years in Russia, Israel, Iran, Iraq and Jordan. ("leishmanization"), and a lesion is allowed to develop and run its natural course. This results in a single scar in a cosmetically-acceptable location, and the immunity that develops is comparable to that following a natural infection. There is a small risk of developing a cutaneous leishmaniasis lesion requiring treatment or the development of leishmaniasis recidivans at the site of immunization.

99.4 Cutaneous Leishmaniasis of the New World

DEFINITION

Cutaneous leishmaniasis of the New World is a zoonosis caused by parasites of the species complexes *Leishmania mexicana* and *Leishmania braziliensis* (Fig. 99.4 and Table 99-1). Mucosal leishmaniasis, also known as "espundia", is characterized by destructive oral, nasal or pharyngeal lesions and is usually associated with *L. braziliensis* infection. Local names for New World cutaneous leishmaniasis include uta (Peru), chiclero ulcer or bay sore (Mexico), dicera de Baurid (Brazil), and pian bois or forest yaws (Guyana). Collectively, these diseases are also referred to as American cutaneous leishmaniasis.

ETIOLOGY

New World cutaneous leishmaniasis parasites are divided into two complexes, the *L. (Leishmania)* complex and *L. (Viannia)* complex that are known to infect humans (Fig. 99.4). Members of the *L. (Leishmania)* complex develop in the midgut and foregut of their sandfly vectors, whereas members of the *L. (Viannia)* complex develop in the hindgut, as well as the midgut and foregut. *L. infantum* has also been isolated from lesions of CL on rare occasions.

DISTRIBUTION AND EPIDEMIOLOGY

The geographic distribution of New World cutaneous leishmaniasis is shown in Fig. 99.13. New World cutaneous leishmaniasis is an uncommon disease in returning travelers from endemic areas but should be considered when evaluating an ulcerative lesion in persons with an exposure or travel history. Those conducting field studies are at highest risk, but casual tourists with brief exposures also become infected. Sylvatic or wild transmission cycles are adapting to peridomestic environments with domestic animal reservoirs associated with increasing urbanization. In addition, people moving into endemic areas for natural products extraction (oil and gas, timber, road building, etc.), armed conflicts and increasingly adventurous travel and ecotourism lead to new infections and epidemics of cutaneous leishmaniasis in non-immune people [81].

LEISHMANIA MEXICANA

The parasite causing chiclero ulcer is common throughout southern Mexico, Belize, and Guatemala, and causes the rare cases of cutaneous leishmaniasis acquired in the southern USA. It is transmitted among forest rodents by *Lutzomyia olmeca*, which is not highly attracted to humans. However, the prolonged exposure of "chicleros", who live for many months in the forest collecting chewing gum latex from chicle trees, explains the high incidence of infection in these workers, i.e. 30% during the first year of employment. Timber cutters, road builders and agricultural workers are also commonly infected. In south Texas, the southern plains wood rat, *Neotoma micropus*, is the reservoir and *Lutzomyia anthophora* the primary vector of the enzootic cycle [82].

LEISHMANIA AMAZONENSIS

This parasite occurs in the Amazon region of Brazil and neighboring countries. It is primarily a disease of forest rodents, but marsupials and foxes can be secondary hosts. Infection rates of 20% occur in some rodent species in Brazil, but human disease is uncommon because the vector *Lutzomyia flaviscutellata* is nocturnal, is not very anthropophilic and lives in swampy areas of the forest seldom frequented by people.

LEISHMANIA VENEZUELENSIS

This parasite has been isolated only from humans with cutaneous leishmaniasis and diffuse cutaneous leishmaniasis in Venezuela. *Lu. olmeca bicolor* is the probable vector. The mammalian host has not yet been discovered.

LEISHMANIA (VIANNIA) BRAZILIENSIS

Leishmania braziliensis, which primarily causes infection of forest rodents, causes cutaneous leishmaniasis and mucosal leishmaniasis in humans. Human infection occurs in all endemic countries of the Americas except Guyana, Surinam and the USA. *Leishmania braziliensis* likely causes a spectrum of illness across its geographic range and is associated with multiple sandfly vectors. Disease is common among persons living in farming communities in newly cleared forest areas, and in road construction and mining workers [83].

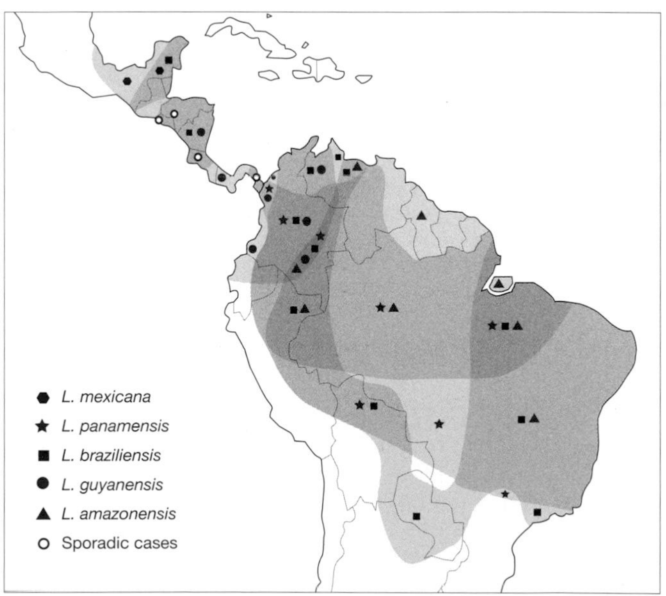

FIGURE 99.13 Geographic distribution of New World cutaneous Leishmania. *Leishmania braziliensis* is found from Mexico to Argentina. *Leishmania peruviana* is found on the Western slopes of the Peruvian Andes. *Leishmania guyanensis* is found north of the Amazon river in Brazil, Guyana, Surinam, French Guiana, Venezuela, Colombia and Ecuador. *Leishmania panamensis* is found in Honduras, Nicaragua, Costa Rica, Panama, Colombia, Ecuador and Venezuela. *Leishmania amazonensis* is found in Brazil. *Leishmania mexicana* is found in Texas, Mexico, Belize, Guatemala, the Dominican Republic, Honduras, Costa Rica, Panama, Colombia and Venezuela. *Leishmania venezuelensis* is found in Venezuela. Symbols and shading mark the distribution overlaps between species. *(reproduced with permission from Magill AJ. Epidemiology of the leishmaniases. Dermatol Clin 1995;13:505–23.)*

LEISHMANIA (VIANNIA) PANAMENSIS

This parasite is found from Guatemala in the north through Central America and Colombia and Ecuador in the south. The principal reservoir is the tree sloth, *Choloepus hoffmanni*. Other sloths, procyonids, and forest primates are secondary hosts. The major vector, *Lutzomyia trapidoi*, usually lives in the forest canopy in close contact with the known reservoirs. However, at certain times of the year, when rainfall is moderate, it can be found close to the ground where it can bite humans. Human disease is common in rural agricultural workers, especially in the first year after settlement before deforestation is complete, and in military personnel participating in jungle warfare training.

LEISHMANIA (VIANNIA) GUYANENSIS

Pian bois or forest yaws, the human disease caused by *Leishmania guyanensis* occurs in the Guyanas and northern Brazil. Because the principal vector, *Lutzomyia umbratilis*, has a high infection rate (up to 7%) and readily bites humans in the daytime when disturbed from its resting sites on tree trunks. Disease is common among forest workers. The major reservoir of *L. guyanensis* is the two-toed forest sloth.

LEISHMANIA (VIANNIA) PERUVIANA

Leishmania peruviana is found in high Andean valleys between 800 and 3000 meters above sea level in Peru. Dogs with unapparent infection are the principal reservoir hosts for transmission. Human disease (uta) is contracted in, and around, the home and, in some villages, 90% of people are infected or scarred.

INFECTIONS CAUSED BY OTHER LEISHMANIA *SPECIES*

Parasites have been cultured from lesions of cutaneous leishmaniasis in various parts of South America that have isoenzyme patterns and growth characteristics in culture and laboratory animals that are different from those of known species of *Leishmania*. *Leishmania infantum* causes non-ulcerative nodular cutaneous leishmaniasis in Honduras and Costa Rica.

DIFFUSE CUTANEOUS LEISHMANIASIS

A diffuse form of cutaneous leishmaniasis is rarely seen in Bolivia, Brazil, Colombia, Costa Rica, Dominican Republic, Ecuador, Guatemala, Mexico, Peru, Venezuela, or the USA. Diffuse cutaneous leishmaniasis in the New World is usually associated with *L. mexicana* and *L. amazonensis* infections.

CLINICAL MANIFESTATIONS

CUTANEOUS DISEASE

The lesions of New World cutaneous leishmaniasis are generally similar to those of Old World disease. A few weeks to several months after infection, an erythematous, often pruritic, papule develops at the site of inoculation. The initial papule may become scaly or gradually enlarge, developing a raised indurated margin with central ulceration. Verrucous and acneiform lesions are uncommon, but nodular lesions are seen in about 10%. Ulcerative lesions are usually painless unless secondarily infected. The natural history varies depending on the infecting species, location of the lesion and host immunity. *Leishmania mexicana* infections generally have one or a few lesions that heal spontaneously within six months. In Guatemala, 22 out of 25 lesions caused by *L. mexicana* (88%) completely re-epithelialized by a median lesion age of 14 weeks (range: 6–44 weeks) and 17 (68%) were classified as cured six months later [84]. However, lesions on the ear occur in 40% of patients and are chronic, lasting many years. Simple cutaneous lesions caused by parasites of the *L. braziliensis* complex generally require 6–18 months for spontaneous healing but sometimes persist much longer. In addition, enlargement of the lymph nodes draining the bite site commonly accompanies, or precedes, the ulcer in *L. braziliensis* infections [85, 86]. Multiple skin lesions owing to metastatic spread along lymphatics are common with *L. guyanensis* infections, and subcutaneous lymphatic nodules resembling sporotrichosis are often seen in *L. panamensis* infections.

Trauma to uninvolved skin can lead to the formation of lesions caused by *Leishmania* (Koebner phenomenon) [87]. Persons living in endemic areas note the ulcers of cutaneous leishmania develop along machete cuts or other such blunt and sharp trauma. Postoperative granulomas caused by *Leishmania* have also been reported as postsurgical complications.

MUCOSAL DISEASE

One to five percent of persons infected with *L. braziliensis* develop mucosal leishmaniasis. Mucosal leishmaniasis is more commonly seen in Bolivia, Brazil and Peru, and is much less common in northern South America and Central America [88]. The lesions of ML may appear concurrently with the primary cutaneous ulcer but more often several months to many years after healing of the initial cutaneous lesion. The nasal mucosa is the first site involved. Initially, patients may complain of nasal stuffiness, difficulty in breathing through their nose and occasional bleeding as their first symptoms associated with erythema and edema of the involved nasal mucosa. This proceeds to septum ulceration covered with a mucopurulent exudate. There is often mutilating destruction of the nasal septum (Fig. 99.14), palate, lips, pharynx and larynx in severe mucosal leishmaniasis. The lesions are chronic and progressive and death can be caused by aspiration or inanition. Mucosal leishmaniasis can also less commonly be seen with *L. panamensis* and *L. guyanensis* infections. Hoarseness should prompt evaluation of the vocal cords for laryngeal involvement. Mucosal leishmaniasis does not spontaneously resolve, is more difficult to treat especially in patients with severe or extensive disease and secondary bacterial infections are common.

There is currently no way to predict the development of mucosal leishmaniasis in a person with primary cutaneous leishmaniasis. However, risk factors for the development of mucosal leishmaniasis are male gender, older age, severe malnutrition and lesion duration of over four months [89]. In addition, a genetic component for the risk of developing mucosal leishmaniasis has long been suspected to include association between human leukocyte antigen (HLA) loci and

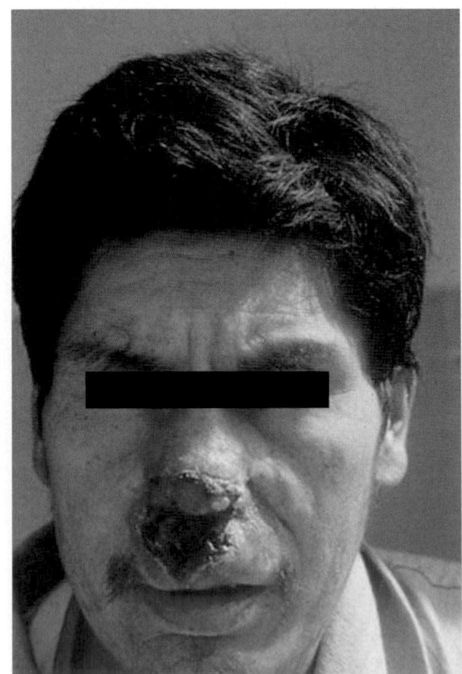

FIGURE 99.14 Mucosal leishmaniasis.

the presence of mucosal leishmaniasis and polymorphisms in the tumor necrosis factor alpha (TNF-α) and beta (TNF-β) genes associated with high circulating levels of TNF-α.

DIFFUSE CUTANEOUS LEISHMANIASIS

The initial lesion is usually a macule, papule, or nodule (rarely an ulcer). Because of an immunologic defect in the host, the parasite spreads locally and hematogenously to cause generalized nodular lesions consisting of heavily parasitized macrophages. The nasal mucosa and laryngopharynx are sometimes involved, but visceral lesions do not occur.

DIAGNOSIS

DEMONSTRATION OF THE ORGANISM

As in other forms of leishmaniasis, definitive diagnosis requires demonstration of the parasite. The methods are the same as those for diagnosis of cutaneous leishmaniasis of the Old World (see Chapter 99.3). Studies in Guatemala and Colombia show that yields of parasites are similar whether the material is collected from the edge of the lesion or from the ulcer base provided appropriate debridement is performed. It is important to completely debride the crusted exudative material from the ulcer before trying to scrape or aspirate. Wet-to-dry gauze pads are often required for adequate debridement. This can be quite painful for the patient and local anesthesia with injectable 1% lidocaine with epinephrine is recommended, if available. Use of topical anesthetics such as lidocaine and prilocaine have also proven useful. The sensitivity of culture can also be improved by 20–25% if 3–5 cultures per ulcerative lesion are obtained [90, 91]. In practice, if the only goal is to demonstrate parasites prior to instituting therapy, then several smears can be made and examined before resorting to culture. Organisms are generally more numerous in smears and biopsy specimens of cutaneous leishmaniasis caused by *L. mexicana* but are often scanty in *L. braziliensis* infection of both the skin and mucous membranes, especially in long-standing disease. Cultures of tissue juice aspirated from the indurated margin of a skin lesion or of biopsy specimens of skin or mucosal lesions are more likely to confirm *L. braziliensis* infection.

Although assay performance is laboratory-dependent and the general availability is poor, the use of PCR to amplify *Leishmania* DNA targets is now very common in endemic areas.

SKIN TEST

The leishmanin skin test (LST) is positive in almost all patients with active cutaneous leishmaniasis and mucosal leishmaniasis, although it may be negative during the first few months. Treatment is occasionally justified despite the failure to demonstrate parasites in persons with typical lesions and a positive skin test, especially in those with espundia. In diffuse cutaneous leishmaniasis, the skin test is uniformly negative.

SEROLOGIC TESTS

Standard serologic tests are not useful for diagnosis of New World cutaneous leishmaniasis or mucosal leishmaniasis. Assays using crude antigen preparations are positive at low titer in only 70–80% of cases and are especially likely to be negative early in the course of the disease, when a diagnosis is most desired.

DIFFERENTIAL DIAGNOSIS

New World cutaneous leishmaniasis must be distinguished from sporotrichosis, blastomycosis, yaws, syphilis, cutaneous tuberculosis, *Mycobacterium marinum* infection, and dermatologic cancers. Diseases that may resemble espundia include paracoccidioidomycosis, histoplasmosis, tuberculosis, syphilis, malignant tumors and lethal midline granuloma. Nodular diffuse cutaneous leishmaniasis must be differentiated from lepromatous leprosy.

TREATMENT

TYPICAL NEW WORLD CUTANEOUS LEISHMANIASIS

Systemic chemotherapy is generally indicated in New World cutaneous leishmaniasis in contrast to Old World cutaneous leishmaniasis. New World cutaneous leishmaniasis tends to be more severe and to last longer than cutaneous leishmaniasis of the Old World. Indications for systemic treatment include the multiplicity of lesions, the chronicity of untreated disease or progression of mucosal disease in the absence of chemotherapy. The therapeutic decision is a risk:benefit ratio of the intervention for each patient; no single treatment approach fits all clinical presentations. Experience with local therapy for New World cutaneous leishmaniasis is limited as local therapy was long considered unsuitable for the treatment of New World cutaneous leishmaniasis, especially in those patients infected with *L. braziliensis* or *L. panamensis* because of the potential risk of mucosal leishmaniasis and the belief that systemic treatment could prevent metastasis and mucosal leishmaniasis. However, systemic treatment does not guarantee prevention of later mucosal leishmaniasis and it is now considered acceptable to use local therapy in selected cases of New World cutaneous leishmaniasis.

Pentavalent antimonials

A randomized controlled trial in patients with *L. panamensis* infections showed that treatment with sodium stibogluconate (SSG) at a dosage of 20 mg of Sb/kg/day for 20 days gave a significantly higher cure rate than did a dosage of 10 mg of Sb/kg/day for 20 days [92]. This dosage and duration are also recommended for other forms of simple New World cutaneous leishmaniasis. Lower doses and shorter regimens may be effective in certain geographic regions. Toxicity of SSG is discussed in Chapter 99.2. If toxicity does occur at the higher doses, the drug should be withheld for a few days until side effects resolve and treatment can then usually be resumed at the same dose.

Amphotericin B

In patients unresponsive to SbV, amphotericin B deoxycholate is usually effective. One mg/kg doses are administered by slow intravenous infusion on alternate days. Prolonged treatment to a total of 2–3 g is generally required. LAMB is increasingly being used as the drug of choice to treat cutaneous leishmaniasis in higher income countries with generally good results, although there are case reports of failure [93].

Pentamidine

Pentamidine was as effective as pentavalent antimonials for curing cutaneous leishmaniasis caused by *L. panamensis* or *L. guyanensis* in Brazil, Colombia, French Guiana and Suriname. Recent trials in Colombia have shown that 2 mg/kg given intramuscularly (IM) every other day for seven doses or 3 mg/kg given IM every other day for four doses cured 72 out of 75 (96%) evaluable patients [94]. The injections were well tolerated and no significant side effects were noted. It is, however, less efficient than antimonials against disease caused by *L. braziliensis*

Ketoconazole

Ketoconazole gave a 70% cure rate in patients with cutaneous leishmaniasis caused by *L. panamensis* in Guatemala; however, it is less effective for *L. braziliensis*, curing only seven out of 23 (30%) infections [95]. Because it can be given orally, ketoconazole may thus have a role in some patients for whom parenteral therapy is not possible.

Miltefosine

Current World Health Organization (WHO) recommendations include miltefosine at 2.5 mg/kg day orally for 28 days for cutaneous leishmaniasis caused by *L. mexicana, L. guyanensis* and *L. panamemsis* [57]. Miltefosine is also 75% effective against CL caused by *L. braziliensis* acquired in Bahia Brazil [96], 70% effective in Colombia, 70% in Bolivia [97], but only 53% effective in Guatemala [98]. The response of *L. braziliensis* to miltefosine may vary depending on the geographic area.

Local agents

Intralesional injections of SbV, accepted therapy for disease in the Old World, have not seen wide use in the Americas. There are no large comparative trials on which to base recommendations.

Topical application of paromomycin formulations has been evaluated in Ecuador and Colombia. In Ecuador, an open, non-randomized trial of 15% paromomycin with 12% methylbenzethonium chloride in white paraffin cured 90% of 52 patients [99]. In Colombia, another open, non-randomized trial of 15% paromomycin with 5% methylbenzethonium chloride combined with parenteral Glucantime at 20 mg/kg daily for 7 days cured 18 out of 20 (90%) patients [100]. The true efficacy remains to be determined in controlled trials, but topical paromomycin formulations may have a role in combination with SbV to decrease the number of injections required for cure.

MUCOSAL LEISHMANIASIS

Current WHO recommendations for the treatment of mucosal leishmaniasis include SbV at 20 mg/kg per day intramuscularly or intravenously for 30 days, SbV plus oral pentoxifylline at 400 mg/8 h for 30 days [101], amphotericin B deoxycholate at 0.7–1 mg/kg by infusion every other day up to 25–45 doses, or liposomal amphotericin B: 2–3 mg/kg daily by infusion up to a total dose of 40–60 mg/kg. Miltefosine at 2.5–3.3 mg/kg per day orally for 28 days has been shown to be efficacious in an open label study in Bolivia [102]. The cure rate for the 36 patients who had "mild" disease (i.e. affecting nasal skin and nasal mucosa) was 83%. The cure rate for the 36 patients who had more extensive disease (involving the palate, pharynx and larynx) was 58%. Reportedly, patients refused to be randomized to parenteral agents because they preferred the oral agent. The cure rate for an almost contemporary group receiving amphotericin B (45 mg/kg over 90 days) was 50%.

In patients with advanced mucosal leishmaniasis, adequate nutrition must be ensured and destructive or obstructive lesions may require ventilatory support or treatment, as in aspiration pneumonia. Plastic surgery may be required after parasitologic cure in patients with extensive tissue destruction from espundia.

DIFFUSE CUTANEOUS LEISHMANIASIS

In contrast to Ethiopian diffuse cutaneous leishmaniasis, Venezuelan diffuse cutaneous leishmaniasis often improves after initial treatment with SbV, although relapse is invariable and patients who relapse often do not respond to additional SbV treatment.

Miltefosine produces a dramatic clinical and parasitologic response in patients with diffuse cutaneous leishmaniasis and improvement continued during drug administration, but patients relapse and develop new lesions when treatment is stopped [103]. Continuous use or intermittent treatments may be useful.

PROGNOSIS

Cutaneous lesions usually heal (complete epithelialization) within 1–2 months after initiation of treatment with SbV, although large ulcers may require longer. In a study of ulcerative cutaneous leishmaniasis caused by *L. braziliensis*, 32% of lesions had re-epithelialized at the end of a 3-week treatment course, 60% at 6 weeks, and 90% at 13 weeks. Mucosal disease caused by *L. braziliensis*, which may appear many years after the primary cutaneous lesion has resolved, is progressive unless treated. The risk of espundia may be reduced in persons whose primary cutaneous lesions are adequately treated. Diffuse cutaneous leishmaniasis is characteristically a relapsing or chronically progressive disease.

PREVENTION AND CONTROL

Vaccines and chemoprophylactic drugs are not available. Because of the forest location of vectors and reservoirs, control of American cutaneous leishmaniasis and mucosal leishmaniasis is not possible. The only exception is uta, which, because of its domiciliary nature, can be mimimized by spraying houses with insecticides. Insect repellents, long-sleeved shirts and fine-mesh bed-netting may reduce the risk of infection for individual travelers. Permethrin-impregnated clothing is also effective. In a study of Colombian military personnel in an endemic area for 6.6 weeks and followed for an additional 12 weeks, 4 out of 143 (3%) soldiers wearing permethrin-impregnated uniforms acquired disease, whereas 18 out of 143 (18%) soldiers who did not wear impregnated uniforms acquired disease [104].

REFERENCES

1. Kaye P, Scott P. Leishmaniasis: complexity at the host-pathogen interface. Nat Rev Microbiol 2011;9:604–15.
2. Killick-Kendrick R. Phlebotomine vectors of the leishmaniases: a review. Med Vet Entomol 1990;4:1–24.
3. Warburg A, Saraiva E, Lanzaro GC, et al. Saliva of *Lutzomyia longipalpis* sibling species differs in its composition and capacity to enhance leishmaniasis. Philos Trans R Soc Lond B Biol Sci 1994;345:223–30.
4. Magill AJ. Epidemiology of the leishmaniases. Dermatol Clin 1995;13: 505–23.
5. Desjeux P. Leishmaniasis. Nat Rev Microbiol 2004;2:692.
6. Cardo LJ. Leishmania: risk to the blood supply. Transfusion 2006;46: 1641–5.
7. Pineda JA, Martin-Sanchez J, Macias J, Morillas F. Leishmania spp infection in injecting drug users. Lancet 2002;360:950–1.
8. Meinecke CK, Schottelius J, Oskam L, Fleischer B. Congenital transmission of visceral leishmaniasis (Kala Azar) from an asymptomatic mother to her child. Pediatrics. 1999;104:e65.
9. Symmers WS. Leishmaniasis acquired by contagion: a case of marital infection in Britain. Lancet 1960;1:127–32.
10. Herwaldt BL, Juranek DD. Laboratory-acquired malaria, leishmaniasis, trypanosomiasis, and toxoplasmosis. Am J Trop Med Hyg 1993;48:313–23.
11. Pearson RD, Sousa AQ. Clinical spectrum of Leishmaniasis. Clin Infect Dis 1996;22:1–13.
12. Schuster FL, Sullivan JJ. Cultivation of clinically significant hemoflagellates. Clin Microbiol Rev 2002;15:374–89.
13. Abramson MA, Dietze R, Frucht DM, et al. Comparison of New and Old World leishmanins in an endemic region of Brazil. Clin Infect Dis 1995; 20:1292–7.
14. Mendonca MG, de Brito ME, Rodrigues EH, et al. Persistence of leishmania parasites in scars after clinical cure of American cutaneous leishmaniasis: is there a sterile cure? J Infect Dis 2004;189:1018–23.
15. Dereure J, Duong Thanh H, Lavabre-Bertrand T, et al. Visceral leishmaniasis. Persistence of parasites in lymph nodes after clinical cure. J Infect. 2003; 47:77–81.
16. Berman JD, Badaro R, Thakur CP, et al. Efficacy and safety of liposomal amphotericin B (AmBisome) for visceral leishmaniasis in endemic developing countries. Bull World Health Organ 1998;76:25–32.
17. Kuhls K, Alam MZ, Cupolillo E, et al. Comparative microsatellite typing of new world leishmania infantum reveals low heterogeneity among populations and its recent old world origin. PLoS Negl Trop Dis 2011;5:e1155.
18. Desjeux P. Human leishmaniases: epidemiology and public health aspects. World Health Stat Q 1992;45:267–75.
19. Most H, Lavietes PH. Kala azar in American military personnel; report of 30 cases. Medicine (Baltimore) 1947;26:221–84.
20. Gagnaire MH, Galambrun C, Stephan JL. Hemophagocytic syndrome: A misleading complication of visceral leishmaniasis in children – a series of 12 cases. Pediatrics 2000;106:E58.
21. Levy L, Nasereddin A, Rav-Acha M, et al. Prolonged fever, hepatosplenomegaly, and pancytopenia in a 46-year-old woman. PLoS Med 2009;6:e1000053.
22. Varma N, Naseem S. Hematologic changes in visceral leishmaniasis/kala azar. Indian J Hematol Blood Transfus 2010;26:78–82.
23. Badaro R, Jones TC, Carvalho EM, et al. New perspectives on a subclinical form of visceral leishmaniasis. J Infect Dis 1986;154:1003–11.

24. Pampiglione S, Manson-Bahr PE, Giungi F, et al. Studies on Mediterranean leishmaniasis. 2. Asymptomatic cases of visceral leishmaniasis. Trans R Soc Trop Med Hyg 1974;68:447–53.
25. Magill AJ, Grogl M, Gasser RA Jr, et al. Visceral infection caused by *Leishmania tropica* in veterans of Operation Desert Storm. N Engl J Med 1993;328: 1383–7.
26. Magill AJ, Grogl M, Johnson SC, Gasser RA Jr. Visceral infection due to *Leishmania tropica* in a veteran of Operation Desert Storm who presented 2 years after leaving Saudi Arabia. Clin Infect Dis 1994;19:805–6.
27. Alvar J, Aparicio P, Aseffa A, et al. The relationship between leishmaniasis and AIDS: the second 10 years. Clin Microbiol Rev 2008;21:334–59.
28. Antinori S, Cascio A, Parravicini C, et al. Leishmaniasis among organ transplant recipients. Lancet Infect Dis 2008;8:191–9.
29. Kopterides P, Mourtzoukou EG, Skopelitis E, et al. Aspects of the association between leishmaniasis and malignant disorders. Trans R Soc Trop Med Hyg 2007;101:1181–9.
30. De Leonardis F, Govoni M, Lo Monaco A, Trotta F. Visceral leishmaniasis and anti-TNF-alpha therapy: case report and review of the literature. Clin Exp Rheumatol 2009;27:503–6.
31. Tuon FF, Sabbaga Amato V, Floeter-Winter LM, et al. Cutaneous leishmaniasis reactivation 2 years after treatment caused by systemic corticosteroids – first report. Int J Dermatol 2007;46:628–30.
32. Zijlstra EE, Musa AM, Khalil EA, et al. Post-kala-azar dermal leishmaniasis. Lancet Infect Dis 2003;3:87–98.
33. Ramesh V, Singh R, Salotra P. Short communication: post-kala-azar dermal leishmaniasis–an appraisal. Trop Med Int Health 2007;12:848–51.
34. Kager PA. Splenic aspiration in visceral leishmaniasis. Rev Soc Bras Med Trop 1992;25:217–23.
35. Kager PA, Rees PH, Manguyu FM, et al. Splenic aspiration; experience in Kenya. Trop Geogr Med 1983;35:125–31.
36. Chulay JD, Bryceson AD. Quantitation of amastigotes of *Leishmania donovani* in smears of splenic aspirates from patients with visceral leishmaniasis. Am J Trop Med Hyg 1983;32:475–9.
37. Myles O, Wortmann GW, Cummings JF, et al. Visceral leishmaniasis: clinical observations in 4 US army soldiers deployed to Afghanistan or Iraq, 2002–2004. Arch Intern Med 2007;167:1899–901.
38. Chappuis F, Rijal S, Soto A, et al. A meta-analysis of the diagnostic performance of the direct agglutination test and rK39 dipstick for visceral leishmaniasis. BMJ 2006;333:723.
39. Rijal S, Chappuis F, Singh R, et al. Sodium stibogluconate cardiotoxicity and safety of generics. Trans R Soc Trop Med Hyg 2003;97:597–8.
40. Sundar S, Sinha PR, Agrawal NK, et al. A cluster of cases of severe cardiotoxicity among kala-azar patients treated with a high-osmolarity lot of sodium antimony gluconate. Am J Trop Med Hyg 1998;59:139–43.
41. Aronson NE, Wortmann GW, Johnson SC, et al. Safety and efficacy of intravenous sodium stibogluconate in the treatment of leishmaniasis: recent U.S. military experience. Clin Infect Dis 1998;27:1457–64.
42. Gasser RA, Jr, Magill AJ, Oster CN, et al. Pancreatitis induced by pentavalent antimonial agents during treatment of leishmaniasis. Clin Infect Dis 1994;18:83–90.
43. Chulay JD, Spencer HC, Mugambi M. Electrocardiographic changes during treatment of leishmaniasis with pentavalent antimony (sodium stibogluconate). Am J Trop Med Hyg 1985;34:702–9.
44. Sundar S, Chakravarty J. Antimony toxicity. Int J Environ Res Public Health 2010;7:4267–77.
45. Thakur CP, Sinha GP, Barat D, Singh RK. Are incremental doses of amphotericin B required for the treatment of visceral leishmaniasis? Ann Trop Med Parasitol 1994;88:365–70.
46. Maheshwari A, Seth A, Kaur S, et al. Cumulative cardiac toxicity of sodium stibogluconate and amphotericin B in treatment of kala-azar. Pediatr Infect Dis J 2011;30:180–1.
47. Meyerhoff A. U.S. Food and Drug Administration approval of AmBisome (liposomal amphotericin B) for treatment of visceral leishmaniasis. Clin Infect Dis 1999;28:42–8.
48. Berman JD. U.S Food and Drug Administration approval of AmBisome (liposomal amphotericin B) for treatment of visceral leishmaniasis. Clin Infect Dis 1999;28:49–51.
49. Davidson RN, Di Martino L, Gradoni L, et al. Liposomal amphotericin B (AmBisome) in Mediterranean visceral leishmaniasis: a multi-centre trial. Q J Med 1994;87:75–81.
50. Sundar S, Chakravarty J. Liposomal amphotericin B and leishmaniasis: dose and response. J Glob Infect Dis 2010;2:159–66.
51. Sundar S, Chakravarty J, Agarwal D, et al. Single-dose liposomal amphotericin B for visceral leishmaniasis in India. N Engl J Med 2010;362:504–12.
52. Sundar S, Jha TK, Thakur CP, et al. Injectable paromomycin for Visceral leishmaniasis in India. N Engl J Med 2007;356:2571–81.
53. Hailu A, Musa A, Wasunna M, et al. Geographical variation in the response of visceral leishmaniasis to paromomycin in East Africa: a multicentre, open-label, randomized trial. PLoS Negl Trop Dis 2010;4:e709.
54. Sundar S, Jha TK, Thakur CP, et al. Oral miltefosine for Indian visceral leishmaniasis. N Engl J Med 2002;347:1739–46.
55. Bhattacharya SK, Sinha PK, Sundar S, et al. Phase 4 trial of miltefosine for the treatment of Indian visceral leishmaniasis. J Infect Dis 2007;196:591–8.
56. Ritmeijer K, Dejenie A, Assefa Y, et al. A comparison of miltefosine and sodium stibogluconate for treatment of visceral leishmaniasis in an Ethiopian population with high prevalence of HIV infection. Clin Infect Dis 2006;43:357–64.
57. Control of the leishmaniases: Report of a meeting of the WHO Expert Committee on the Control of Leishmaniases 22–6 March 2010. Geneva: World Health Organization; 2010.
58. Jones L, Davies SN, Newland AC, Jenkins GC. A narrow escape from splenectomy. Br Med J (Clin Res Ed) 1985;290:687–8.
59. Troya J, Casquero A, Muniz G, et al. The role of splenectomy in HIV-infected patients with relapsing visceral leishmaniasis. Parasitology 2007;134:621–4.
60. Pagliano P, Carannante N, Rossi M, et al. Visceral leishmaniasis in pregnancy: a case series and a systematic review of the literature. J Antimicrob Chemother 2005;55:229–33.
61. Mueller M, Balasegaram M, Koummuki Y, et al. A comparison of liposomal amphotericin B with sodium stibogluconate for the treatment of visceral leishmaniasis in pregnancy in Sudan. J Antimicrob Chemother 2006; 58:811–5.
62. Topno RK, Pandey K, Das VN, et al. Visceral leishmaniasis in pregnancy – the role of amphotericin B. Ann Trop Med Parasitol 2008;102:267–70.
63. Addy M, Nandy A. Ten years of kala-azar in west Bengal, Part I. Did post-kala-azar dermal leishmaniasis initiate the outbreak in 24-Parganas? Bull World Health Organ 1992;70:341–6.
64. Quinnell RJ, Courtenay O. Transmission, reservoir hosts and control of zoonotic visceral leishmaniasis. Parasitology 2009;136:1915–34.
65. Modabber F. Leishmaniasis vaccines: past, present and future. Int J Antimicrob Agents 2010;36(suppl. 1):S58–61.
66. Reithinger R, Dujardin JC, Louzir H, et al. Cutaneous leishmaniasis. Lancet Infect Dis 2007;7:581–96.
67. Reithinger R, Mohsen M, Aadil K, et al. Anthroponotic cutaneous leishmaniasis, Kabul, Afghanistan. Emerg Infect Dis 2003;9:727–9.
68. Lemma A, Foster WA, Gemetchu T, et al. Studies on leishmaniasis in Ethiopia. I. Preliminary investigations into the epidemiology of cutaneous leishmaniasis in the highlands. Ann Trop Med Parasitol 1969;63:455–72.
69. del Giudice P, Marty P, Lacour JP, et al. Cutaneous leishmaniasis due to *Leishmania infantum*. Case reports and literature review. Arch Dermatol 1998;134:193–8.
70. Antonelli LR, Dutra WO, Almeida RP, et al. Activated inflammatory T cells correlate with lesion size in human cutaneous leishmaniasis. Immunol Lett 2005;101:226–30.
71. Ridley DS, Ridley MJ. The evolution of the lesion in cutaneous leishmaniasis. J Pathol 1983;141:83–96.
72. Sharifi I, Fekri AR, Aflatoonian MR, et al. Leishmaniasis recidivans among school children in Bam, South-east Iran, 1994–2006. Int J Dermatol 2010;49:557–61.
73. Bryceson AD. Diffuse cutaneous leishmaniasis in Ethiopia. I. The clinical and histological features of the disease. Trans R Soc Trop Med Hyg 1969;63: 708–37.
74. Gonzalez U, Pinart M, Reveiz L, Alvar J. Interventions for Old World cutaneous leishmaniasis. Cochrane Database Syst Rev 2008:CD005067.
75. Reithinger R, Mohsen M, Wahid M, et al. Efficacy of thermotherapy to treat cutaneous leishmaniasis caused by *Leishmania tropica* in Kabul, Afghanistan: a randomized, controlled trial. Clin Infect Dis 2005;40:1148–55.
76. Aronson NE, Wortmann GW, Byrne WR, et al. A randomized controlled trial of local heat therapy versus intravenous sodium stibogluconate for the treatment of cutaneous *Leishmania major* infection. PLoS Negl Trop Dis 2010; 4:e628.
77. Ben Salah A, Buffet PA, Morizot G, et al. WR279,396, a third generation aminoglycoside ointment for the treatment of *Leishmania major* cutaneous leishmaniasis: a phase 2, randomized, double blind, placebo controlled study. PLoS Negl Trop Dis 2009;3:e432.
78. Asilian A, Sadeghinia A, Faghihi G, Momeni A. Comparative study of the efficacy of combined cryotherapy and intralesional meglumine antimoniate (Glucantime) vs. cryotherapy and intralesional meglumine antimoniate (Glucantime) alone for the treatment of cutaneous leishmaniasis. Int J Dermatol 2004;43:281–3.
79. Alrajhi AA, Ibrahim EA, De Vol EB, et al. Fluconazole for the treatment of cutaneous leishmaniasis caused by *Leishmania major*. N Engl J Med 2002;346: 891–5.

80. Emad M, Hayati F, Fallahzadeh MK, Namazi MR. Superior efficacy of oral fluconazole 400 mg daily versus oral fluconazole 200 mg daily in the treatment of cutaneous leishmania major infection: a randomized clinical trial. J Am Acad Dermatol 2011;64:606–8.
81. Grimaldi G Jr, Tesh RB. Leishmaniases of the New World: current concepts and implications for future research. Clin Microbiol Rev 1993;6:230–50.
82. McHugh CP, Melby PC, LaFon SG. Leishmaniasis in Texas: epidemiology and clinical aspects of human cases. Am J Trop Med Hyg 1996;55:547–55.
83. Jones TC, Johnson WD Jr, Barretto AC, et al. Epidemiology of American cutaneous leishmaniasis due to *Leishmania braziliensis braziliensis*. J Infect Dis 1987;156:73–83.
84. Herwaldt BL, Arana BA, Navin TR. The natural history of cutaneous leishmaniasis in Guatemala. J Infect Dis 1992;165:518–27.
85. Barral A, Guerreiro J, Bomfim G, et al. Lymphadenopathy as the first sign of human cutaneous infection by *Leishmania braziliensis*. Am J Trop Med Hyg 1995;53:256–9.
86. Barral A, Barral-Netto M, Almeida R, et al. Lymphadenopathy associated with *Leishmania braziliensis* cutaneous infection. Am J Trop Med Hyg 1992; 47:587–92.
87. Wortmann GW, Aronson NE, Miller RS, et al. Cutaneous leishmaniasis following local trauma: a clinical pearl. Clin Infect Dis 2000;31:199–201.
88. Marsden PD. Mucosal leishmaniasis ("espundia" Escomel, 1911). Trans R Soc Trop Med Hyg 1986;80:859–76.
89. Machado-Coelho GL, Caiaffa WT, Genaro O, et al. Risk factors for mucosal manifestation of American cutaneous leishmaniasis. Trans R Soc Trop Med Hyg 2005;99:55–61.
90. Navin TR, Arana FE, de Merida AM, et al. Cutaneous leishmaniasis in Guatemala: comparison of diagnostic methods. Am J Trop Med Hyg 1990; 42:36–42.
91. Weigle KA, de Davalos M, Heredia P, et al. Diagnosis of cutaneous and mucocutaneous leishmaniasis in Colombia: a comparison of seven methods. Am J Trop Med Hyg 1987;36:489–96.
92. Ballou WR, McClain JB, Gordon DM, et al. Safety and efficacy of high-dose sodium stibogluconate therapy of American cutaneous leishmaniasis. Lancet 1987;2:13–6.
93. Wortmann G, Zapor M, Ressner R, et al. Lipsosomal amphotericin B for treatment of cutaneous leishmaniasis. Am J Trop Med Hyg 2010;83: 1028–33.
94. Soto J, Buffet P, Grogl M, Berman J. Successful treatment of Colombian cutaneous leishmaniasis with four injections of pentamidine. Am J Trop Med Hyg 1994;50:107–11.
95. Navin TR, Arana BA, Arana FE, et al. Placebo-controlled clinical trial of sodium stibogluconate (Pentostam) versus ketoconazole for treating cutaneous leishmaniasis in Guatemala. J Infect Dis 1992;165:528–34.
96. Machado PR, Ampuero J, Guimaraes LH, et al. Miltefosine in the treatment of cutaneous leishmaniasis caused by *Leishmania braziliensis* in Brazil: a randomized and controlled trial. PLoS Negl Trop Dis 2010;4:e912.
97. Soto J, Rea J, Valderrama M, et al. Efficacy of extended (six weeks) treatment with miltefosine for mucosal leishmaniasis in Bolivia. Am J Trop Med Hyg 2009;81:387–9.
98. Soto J, Arana BA, Toledo J, et al. Miltefosine for new world cutaneous leishmaniasis. Clin Infect Dis 2004;38:1266–72.
99. Krause G, Kroeger A. Topical treatment of American cutaneous leishmaniasis with paramomycin and methylbenzethonium chloride: a clinical study under field conditions in Ecuador. Trans R Soc Trop Med Hyg 1994; 88:92–4.
100. Soto J, Hernandez N, Mejia H, et al. Successful treatment of New World cutaneous leishmaniasis with a combination of topical paromomycin/ methylbenzethonium chloride and injectable meglumine antimonate. Clin Infect Dis 1995;20:47–51.
101. Machado PR, Lessa H, Lessa M, et al. Oral pentoxifylline combined with pentavalent antimony: a randomized trial for mucosal leishmaniasis. Clin Infect Dis 2007;44:788–93.
102. Soto J, Toledo J, Valda L, et al. Treatment of Bolivian mucosal leishmaniasis with miltefosine. Clin Infect Dis 2007;44:350–6.
103. Zerpa O, Ulrich M, Blanco B, et al. Diffuse cutaneous leishmaniasis responds to miltefosine but then relapses. Br J Dermatol 2007;156:1328–35.
104. Soto J, Medina F, Dember N, Berman J. Efficacy of permethrin-impregnated uniforms in the prevention of malaria and leishmaniasis in Colombian soldiers. Clin Infect Dis 1995;21:599–602.

Babesiosis 100

Edouard Vannier, Peter J Krause

Key features

- Babesiosis is an emerging infectious disease caused by intra-erythrocytic protozoan parasites. Frequent symptoms include fever, fatigue, chills, sweats and headache
- Babesiosis typically is transmitted by *Ixodes* ticks, occasionally through blood transfusion and, rarely, transplacentally
- Healthy people over 50 years of age and immunocompromised individuals, including those who are asplenic, have a malignancy or HIV infection, are at increased risk of severe disease and death
- Definitive diagnosis is made by visualizing parasites on peripheral blood smears or amplifying *Babesia* DNA by PCR. Detection of anti-*Babesia* antibody in serum indicates active or past infection
- Standard therapy is a single 7–10-day course of atovaquone and azithromycin or clindamycin and quinine. Partial or complete exchange transfusion is recommended for severe cases. Highly immunocompromised individuals with persistent infection should be treated for at least 6 weeks, including 2 weeks after the parasite is no longer detected on blood smear

INTRODUCTION

Babesiosis is a tick-borne infectious disease caused by intra-erythrocytic protozoan parasites of the genus *Babesia*. Wild and domestic animals are reservoir hosts for more than 100 *Babesia* species. Humans are infected by a few of these species. The parasite is named in honor of the Romanian pathologist Viktor Babes who investigated the cause of febrile hemoglobinuria in cattle and visualized the microorganism in their red blood cells. Described since biblical times as an important disease of livestock, babesiosis was first recognized as a human disease in 1956. Thousands of cases have subsequently been reported, primarily in the USA where babesiosis is classified as an emerging infectious disease.

EPIDEMIOLOGY

GEOGRAPHIC DISTRIBUTION

USA

The first confirmed human case was identified in 1969 on Nantucket Island and was caused by *Babesia microti*, a parasite of small rodents. *Babesia microti* is the most common cause of human babesiosis and is now endemic in the northeast (from Maine to Delaware) and in the upper mid-west (Minnesota and Wisconsin). The number of cases and the geographical range of babesiosis have steadily increased over the last two decades. In 2009, more than 700 cases were reported to public health departments in endemic states, although this number is certainly an underestimate. Babesiosis became a nationally notifiable disease in January 2011. Factors thought to account for the emergence of babesiosis include an increase in deer that are a critical host in the lifecycle of the vector tick (*Ixodes scapularis*), spread of *B. microti*-infected ticks to new areas and a heightened awareness of the disease by physicians and the general public [1]. Several cases caused by *Babesia duncani* have been reported on the west coast. A few cases caused by *Babesia divergens*-like organisms have been reported from Kentucky, Missouri, and Washington State [1].

Europe

About 30 cases have been attributed to *B. divergens*, a parasite of cattle [2]. Most have been reported from the UK, Ireland and France, particularly from regions with extensive cattle farming. Isolated cases have been reported from Croatia (index case), Finland, Georgia (ex-USSR), Spain, Portugal and Sweden. A single autochthonous case of *B. microti* infection has been documented in Germany. Four cases infected with *Babesia venatorum* (EU1), a species closely related to *B. odocoilei* that infect white-tailed deer in the USA, have been reported from Italy, Austria and Germany [2].

Asia, Africa and South America

Two cases in Taiwan and one in Japan were infected with *B. microti*-like organisms [1]. A case in South Korea has been attributed to *Babesia* KO1, a species closely related to those found in sheep. In the few cases reported from Africa, China, and India, the *Babesia* spp. were not fully characterized. Asymptomatic infection has been reported from Mexico and Colombia.

MODE OF TRANSMISSION

Babesia microti is typically transmitted during the blood meal of infected *Ixodes scapularis* nymphal ticks. Transmission occurs from May through to September, with most cases presenting from June to August. Most infected individuals do not recall a tick bite. The tick species that transmit *B. duncani* and *B. divergens*-like organisms remain unknown. In Europe, *Ixodes ricinus* is the main vector for transmission of *B. divergens* and *B. venatorum*.

Babesia microti is the most commonly reported microorganism transmitted through blood transfusion in the USA [3–5]. More than 150 cases have been reported, primarily following packed red blood cell transfusion, but many cases are thought to go unreported or unrecognized [3]. Transfusion-transmitted *B. duncani* infection has been documented on three occasions [5]. Transfusion-transmitted babesiosis can occur anywhere and at any time of the year, but most cases are reported in endemic areas during autumn and winter. The incubation period varies from 1 to 9 weeks but in one case was 6 months. Of the 11 deaths attributed to transfusion-transmitted babesiosis and reported to the US Food and Drugs Administration (FDA) between 1998 and 2008, ten occurred between 2005 and 2008 [4, 5]. Recent increases in the number of transfusion-transmitted babesiosis cases and associated mortality are a major concern of the transfusion medicine community.

Babesiosis has rarely been transmitted transplacentally. Three such cases have been reported, all caused by *B. microti*.

CLINICAL MANIFESTATIONS

BABESIA MICROTI *INFECTION*

Symptoms of *B. microti* infection vary in number and intensity. Three patterns of infection have been described: i) asymptomatic infection; ii) mild-to-moderate viral-like illness; and, iii) severe illness that may be fulminant and culminate in prolonged illness or death.

As many as a quarter of adults and half of children do not have symptoms [6]. Asymptomatic infection may persist for weeks to months following resolution of symptoms, even after standard antibiotic therapy has been administered [7]. The infection is also asymptomatic during the incubation period that typically lasts from 1 to 4 weeks following tick bite.

Babesiosis is a viral-like illness that consists of a gradual onset of malaise and fatigue followed by fever as high as 40.6 °C (105 °F) and one or more of the following: chills, sweats, headache, myalgia, anorexia, non-productive cough, arthralgia and nausea [1, 6]. Less commonly noted are emotional lability and depression, hyperesthesia, sore throat, abdominal pain, conjunctival injection, photophobia and weight loss. Fever is the most common finding on physical examination. Rash is seldom noted, although ecchymoses and petechiae have been described. Mild splenomegaly, hepatomegaly, or both, occasionally occur. Slight pharyngeal erythema, jaundice, hematuria, and retinopathy with splinter hemorrhages and retinal infarcts have been reported. Severe infection requires hospital admission and often occurs in people over 50 years of age and in people immunocompromised by asplenia, malignancy, HIV infection or immunosuppressive drugs [1, 8]. The most common complications consist of pulmonary edema [acute respiratory distress syndrome (ARDS)], disseminated intravascular coagulopathy (DIC), congestive heart failure and renal failure [9]. Splenic infarcts and splenic rupture have been noted. Highly immunocompromised hosts may experience a persistent or relapsing illness [8]. Outcome is fatal in 6–9% of all hospitalized cases and up to 28% of cases in immunocompromised hosts.

OTHER BABESIA *INFECTIONS*

Patients infected with *B. divergens* present with a fulminant illness and nearly all reported cases have occurred in splenectomized individuals [2]. Symptoms include high fever, shaking chills, intense sweats, headache, myalgia and lumbar and abdominal pain. Hemoglobinuria and jaundice are almost always present. Several decades ago most cases were fatal but, with the advent of exchange transfusion combined with effective antibiotic therapy, death is rare. Cases of *B. duncani* infection have been few and have ranged in severity from asymptomatic to fatal. Similarly, *B. venatorum* infection has ranged from mild to severe.

DIAGNOSIS

The diagnosis of babesiosis should be considered in any person who resides in, or has traveled to, an endemic area and who presents with symptoms of babesiosis during the summer or early autumn.

The definitive diagnosis of babesiosis is made by microscopic analysis of Giemsa-stained thick or thin blood smears, although parasites can be visualized using Wright's stain (Fig. 100.1, Table 100-1) [1]. *Babesia* typically appear as ring forms that may be mistakenly identified as *Plasmodium falciparum*. Trophozoites divide by binary fission, yielding two to four merozoites that remain in close proximity. The four merozoites are distributed as a "Maltese cross", but this pattern is seldom noted.

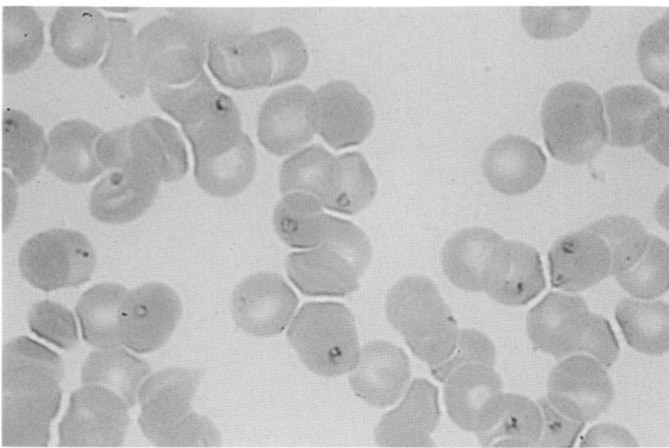

FIGURE 100.1 Ring forms of *Babesia microti* on a Giemsa-stained human blood film (magnification x1000).

TABLE 100-1 Diagnosis of Babesiosis

Epidemiology
• Residence in, or travel to, an area endemic for babesiosis • *Ixodes* tick bite within 1 to 4 weeks • Blood transfusion within 1 to 9 weeks
Symptoms
• Fever, fatigue, chills, sweats, headache, myalgia, anorexia, non-productive cough, arthralgia and nausea • Less common: emotional lability and depression, hyperesthesia, sore throat, abdominal pain, conjunctival injection, photophobia and weight loss
Signs on physical examination
• Fever • Splenomegaly, hepatomegaly, pallor
Common laboratory diagnostic procedures
• Visualization of *Babesia* parasites on peripheral blood smears • Amplification of *Babesia* DNA in blood using PCR • Presence of serum *Babesia* IgM antibody or a fourfold rise in *Babesia* IgG antibody

When parasites are too few to be detected on blood smears, as often occurs in the early phase of infection and after resolution of symptoms, infection is best detected by PCR [1]. Amplification and sequence analysis of the entire18S rRNA gene allows for molecular classification of *Babesia* species.

Supportive laboratory findings include moderate-to-severe hemolytic anemia, thrombocytopenia, an elevated reticulocyte count and an elevated erythrocyte sedimentation rate. The leukocyte count is normal-to-slightly decreased, with a "left shift." In severe cases, elevated serum bilirubin and liver enzyme concentrations, elevated serum blood urea nitrogen and creatinine concentrations, and hematuria and proteinuria are noted.

Immunofluorescence assay (IFA) serology is useful in confirming the diagnosis. IgM antibody titers ≥1:64 and IgG antibody titers of ≥1:1024 signify active, or recent, infection. IgG titers typically decrease to ≤1:64 within 12 months. Thin blood smears, PCR and serology tests are available at most large commercial laboratories in endemic areas. Certain university medical center laboratories and the Centers for Disease Control and Prevention (CDC) serve as reference laboratories.

TREATMENT

BABESIA MICROTI *INFECTION*

Patients are occasionally diagnosed with *Babesia* infection after they have become asymptomatic following acute illness. No controlled trials are available to guide optimal therapy for such patients, but a regimen of atovaquone and azithromycin for 7–10 days has been suggested for people who experience asymptomatic parasitemia for 3 months or longer in order to minimize the risks of clinical relapse and transfusion-transmitted babesiosis. Mild-to-moderate viral-like illness is best treated with the combination of atovaquone and azithromycin for 7–10 days (Table 100-2). Severe infection should be treated with the combination of clindamycin and quinine, although quinine is often associated with transient hearing impairment or gastrointestinal upset. In the first antibiotic treatment trial for human babesiosis [10], the combination of atovaquone and azithromycin was compared with clindamycin and quinine – the first successful therapeutic regimen used for the treatment of babesiosis. These combinations were equally effective in clearing symptoms and parasitemia. Adverse effects were reported in 15% of patients who received atovaquone and azithromycin compared with 72% of those who received clindamycin and quinine. Drug reactions were so severe that the regimen was discontinued or the dosage decreased in about a third of those taking clindamycin and quinine, but in only 2% of those taking atovaquone and azithromycin. Partial, or complete, exchange blood transfusion is recommended in case of intense parasitemia (>10%), severe anemia, pulmonary edema, or renal or hepatic compromise [1]. For highly immunocompromised people who suffer persistent infection, antimicrobial therapy should be administered for at least 6 weeks, including 2 weeks during which the parasite is no longer detected on blood smear [8].

TABLE 100-2 Treatment of Babesiosis

Treatment	Dose	Frequency
Atovaquone and azithromycin		
Atovaquone	Adult: 750 mg	Every 12 hours
	Child: 20 mg/kg (maximum 750 mg/dose)	Every 12 hours
Azithromycin	Adult: 500–1000 mg	On day 1
	250 mg	On subsequent days
	Child: 10 mg/kg (maximum 500 mg/dose)	On day 1
	5 mg/kg (maximum 250 mg/dose)	On subsequent days
Clindamycin and quinine		
Clindamycin	Adult: 600 mg	Every 8 hours
	Child: 7–10 mg/kg (maximum 600 mg/dose)	Every 6–8 hours
	Intravenous administration	
	Adult: 300–600 mg	Every 6 hours
	Child: 7–10 mg/kg (maximum 600 mg/dose)	Every 6–8 hours
Quinine	Adult: 650 mg	Every 6–8 hours
	Child: 8 mg/kg (maximum 650 mg/dose)	Every 8 hours

All antibiotics are administered by mouth, unless otherwise specified. All doses are administered for 7–10 days except for persistent or relapsing infection (see text). For immunocompromised patients, successful treatment regimens have included higher doses of azithromycin (600–1000 mg per day) in combination with atovaquone.

Exchange transfusion

Partial, or complete, exchange transfusion should be considered for the treatment of severe cases, including those who experience parasitemia >10%, severe anemia, pulmonary edema, or renal or hepatic compromise.

OTHER BABESIA *INFECTIONS*

Babesia divergens infections are treated with exchange transfusion in combination with clindamycin and quinine [2]. The combination of pentamidine and trimethoprim-sulfamethoxazole was successfully used to treat a mild case of *B. divergens* infection. Infections with *B. duncani* and *B. venatorum* are treated with clindamycin and quinine, along with exchange transfusion and hemodialysis, when necessary.

PREVENTION

Areas where ticks, deer and mice are known to thrive should be avoided during the primary transmission season, especially by people who are immunocompromised. Clothing that covers the lower part of the body and that is sprayed or impregnated with diethyltoluamide, dimethyl phthalate or permethrin (Permanone) is recommended. A search for ticks on people and pets should be carried out and the ticks removed with the use of tweezers when possible. Application of acaricide to deer decreases the risk of tick-borne disease in people by reducing tick numbers. In the USA, the indefinite deferral of prospective blood donors who report past *Babesia* infection is the only measure currently employed to protect the blood supply. The results of an interim analysis of the first laboratory-based strategy for screening blood donors who are infected with *Babesia* suggests that the combined use of *Babesia microti* IFA and qPCR is effective in reducing the incidence of transfusion-transmitted babesiosis. Treatment of blood products with pathogen reduction methods is being developed [4–5]. No vaccine for human babesiosis is available.

ACKNOWLEDGEMENTS

This work was supported by a generous gift from The Gordon and Llura Gund Foundation and grants from the National Institutes of Health (R01 AG019781 [EV] and R21 AI088079 [PJK]).

REFERENCES

1. Vannier E, Gewurz BE, Krause PJ. Human babesiosis. Infect Dis Clin North Am 2008;22:469–88.
2. Hunfeld KP, Hildebrandt A, Gray JS. Babesiosis: Recent insights into an ancient disease. Int J Parasitol 2008;38:1219–37.
3. Herwaldt BL, Linden JV, Bosserman E, et al. Transfusion-associated babesiosis in the United States: a description of cases. Ann Intern Med 2011;155: 509–19.
4. Gubernot DM, Nakhasi HL, Mied P, et al. Transfusion-transmitted babesiosis in the United States: Summary of a workshop. Transfusion 2009;49:2759–71.
5. Leiby DA. Transfusion-transmitted *Babesia* spp.: bull's-eye on *Babesia microti*. Clin Microbiol Rev 2011;24:14–28.
6. Krause PJ, McKay K, Gadbaw J, et al. Increasing health burden of human babesiosis in endemic sites. Am J Trop Med Hyg 2003;68:431–6.
7. Krause PJ, Spielman A, Telford SR, III, et al. Persistent parasitemia after acute babesiosis. N Engl J Med 1998;339:160–5.
8. Krause PJ, Gewurz BE, Hill D, et al. Persistent and relapsing babesiosis in immunocompromised patients. Clin Infect Dis 2008;46:370–6.
9. Hatcher JC, Greenberg PD, Antique J, Jimenez-Lucho VE. Severe babesiosis in Long Island: review of 34 cases and their complications. Clin Infect Dis 2001;32:1117–25.
10. Krause PJ, Lepore T, Sikand VK, et al. Atovaquone and azithromycin for the treatment of babesiosis. N Engl J Med 2000;343:1454–8.

SECTION

C

TISSUE INFECTION

101 Toxoplasmosis

Luc Paris

Key features

- *Toxoplasma gondii* is a common intracellular protozoan parasite with a worldwide distribution
- Although *T. gondii* usually causes asymptomatic infections, 10–20% of patients with acute infection may develop cervical lymphadenopathy and/or a flu-like illness. The clinical course is usually benign and self-limited with symptoms usually resolving within a few weeks-to-months
- Atypical strains of *T. gondii* are responsible for a severe infectious syndrome with pulmonary involvement seen in travelers living in, or returning from, South America, particularly the Amazon area
- Ocular *Toxoplasma* infection, an important cause of retinochoroiditis in the USA, can be the result of congenital infection or infection after birth. In congenital infection, patients are often asymptomatic until the second or third decade of life, when lesions develop in the eye
- Congenital toxoplasmosis results from an acute primary infection acquired by the mother during pregnancy. The incidence and severity of congenital toxoplasmosis vary with the trimester during which infection was acquired
- Immunodeficient patients often have central nervous system (CNS) disease but may have retinochoroiditis, pneumonitis or other systemic disease. In patients with AIDS, toxoplasmic encephalitis is the most common cause of intracerebral mass lesions
- The diagnosis of *T. gondii* is based on serologic methods in immunocompetent individuals and parasitologic methods in immunocompromised individuals
- Treatment is not needed for a healthy person who is not pregnant. Treatment is usually recommended for pregnant women, persons who are immunocompromised, or persons with ocular disease or severe illness
- The drug of choice for treatment of symptomatic toxoplasmosis is pyrimethamine plus a sulfa drug, usually sulfadiazine. Trimethoprim-sulfamethoxazole may be used in many settings and may be preferred because of its wide availability

INTRODUCTION

Toxoplasmosis is caused by an intracellular protozoan parasite, *Toxoplasma gondii*, which can infect humans and virtually all warm-blooded animals worldwide. *Toxoplasma gondii* was discovered in 1908 simultaneously by Nicolle and Manceaux in Tunisia and Splendore, Brazil, and toxoplasmosis became recognized as a human disease in 1939–1940 [1]. The complete lifecycle of the parasite was described at the end of the 1960s [2]. Our understanding of this parasitic disease has evolved recently with the availability of new genomic data. Classically, *Toxoplasma* was considered to be benign in immunocompetent persons but potentially severe in immunocompromised patients and for the fetus. Today, we know that the clinical spectrum and severity of disease depends on both the host and the pathogen's genetic background, the immune status of the host and the host-parasite interaction. Toxoplasmosis is a possible etiology for a severe infectious syndrome in travelers living in, or returning from, tropical countries.

EPIDEMIOLOGY

THE PARASITE AND ITS LIFE CYCLE

(Fig. 101.1)

Human infection is acquired by ingesting food or water contaminated with oocysts shed in the feces of wild and domestic cats, or tissue cysts in uncooked meat. The oocyst is ovoid, measures 9 × 13 μm and can remain viable for more than a year in moist soil. After sporulation (ranging from two days to three weeks, depending on the ambient temperature) takes place, the oocyst is infectious. Millions of initially non-infectious (unsporulated) oocysts are shed in the cat's feces. Although oocysts are usually only shed for 1–2 weeks, large numbers may be shed.

Virtually all warm-blooded animals, especially birds and rodents, can be intermediate hosts in nature and become infected after ingesting soil, water or plant material contaminated with oocysts. Oocysts transform into tachyzoites shortly after ingestion and multiply rapidly during the acute infection. These rapidly dividing tachyzoites localize in neural and muscle tissue and are responsible for acute illness (Fig. 101.2). They destroy their host cells, enter adjacent cells, and give rise to focal necrosis with a vigorous local inflammatory reaction. Tachyzoites divide every 5–12 hours and can cause significant cell destruction before effective immunity is acquired. After 3–6 weeks, the infection persists with only slowly-dividing bradyzoites inside tissue cysts. Neither chemotherapy nor host immunity can affect the parasite once this transformation occurs. The long-lived bradyzoites persist in a viable state inside cysts during the remainder of the hosts' life without signs of host reaction; they are responsible for latency and reactivation.

Cysts ranging in size from 5–50 μm in diameter appear primarily in the brain, the retina and in skeletal and cardiac muscles (Fig. 101.3). Cysts are usually spherical in the brain but more elongated in cardiac and skeletal muscles. Cats become infected after consuming intermediate hosts harboring tissue cysts and may also become infected directly by ingestion of sporulated oocysts. Animals bred for human consumption and wild game may also become infected with tissue cysts after ingestion of sporulated oocysts in the environment. A very specific phenomenon with *T. gondii* is the transmission of infection from one intermediate host to another by carnivorism, without need for passage through a definitive host.

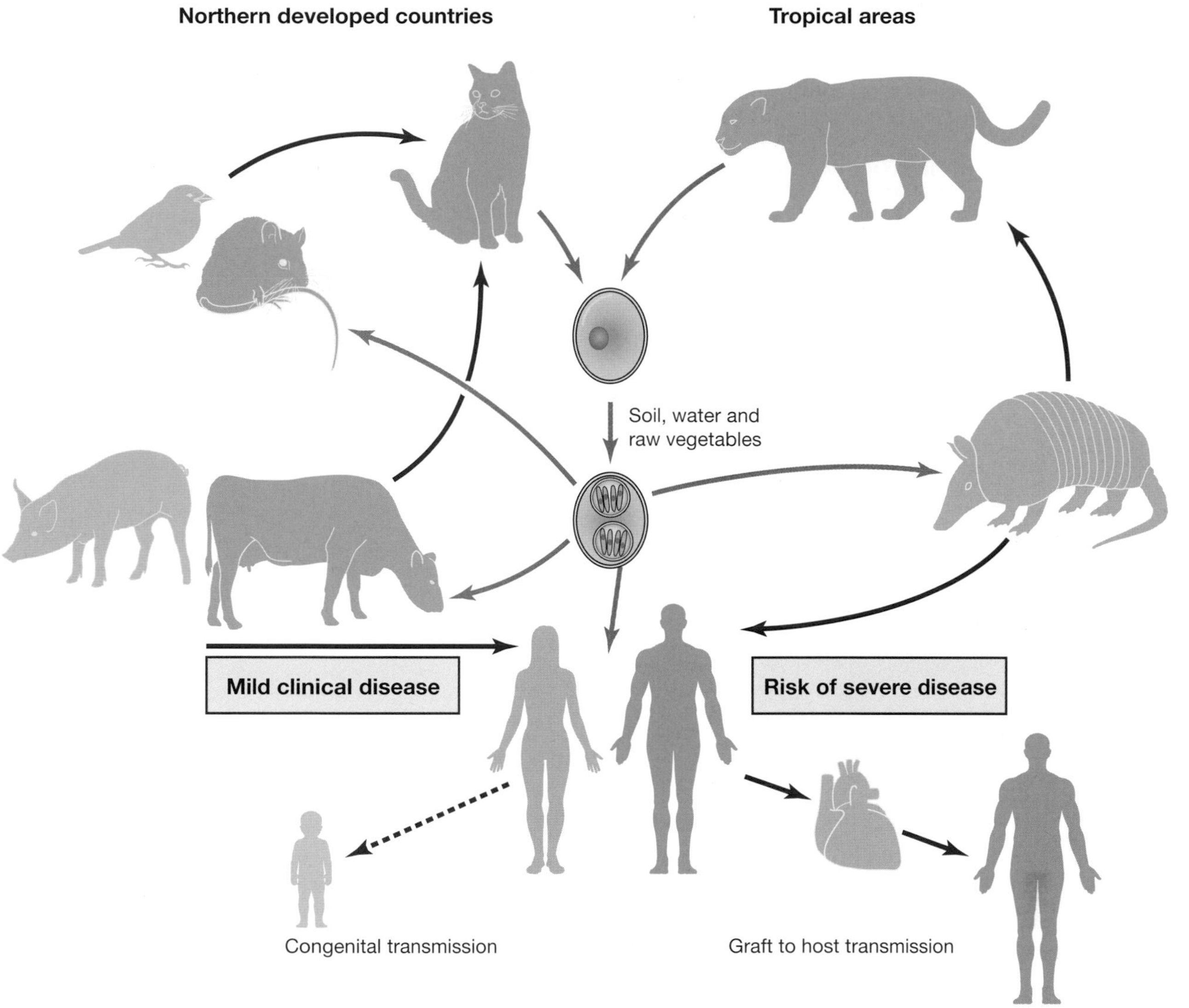

Northern developed countries

Tropical areas

Soil, water and raw vegetables

Mild clinical disease

Risk of severe disease

Congenital transmission

Graft to host transmission

FIGURE 101.1 Life cycle of *Toxoplasma gondii.* Dashed arrow indicate transmission by tachyzoites; dark blue arrows indicate transmission by cysts (bradyzoites); and light blue arrows indicate transmission by oocysts.

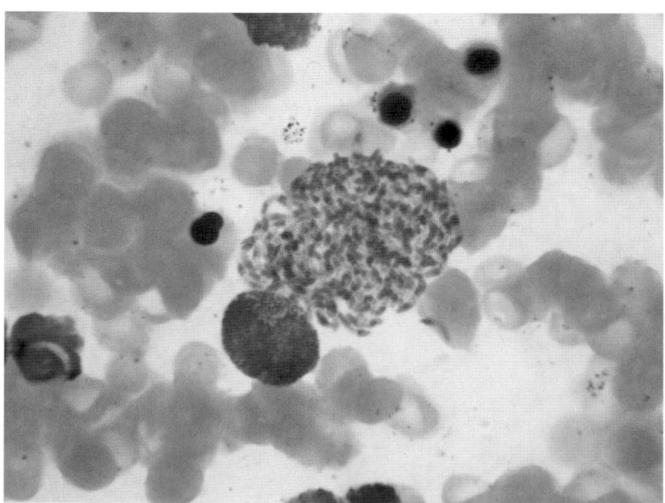

FIGURE 101.2 Numerous intracellular *Toxoplasma gondii* in bone marrow. Coloration RAL 1555 ×1000. *(From personal collection, Luc Paris, Laboratoire de Parasitologie-Mycologie, Groupe Hospitalier Pitié-Salpêtrère, Paris, France).*

TRANSMISSION

Humans become infected by ingesting tissue cysts when eating raw or undercooked meat (lamb, beef or pork) of animals harboring tissue cysts, and by ingestion of oocysts in soil-contaminated food (raw vegetables) or drinking water—believed to be the major source of infection in tropical areas. Transmission can also occur when changing the litter box of a pet cat, by blood transfusion or organ transplantation, and transplacentally from mother to fetus, leading to congenital infections.

A transplanted solid organ from a donor seropositive for toxoplasmosis can transmit *T. gondii* to a seronegative recipient. Heart transplant recipients are particularly at risk for this mode of acquisition, and additional cases have been described with other organs (kidney, lung, liver). Although *T. gondii* has been isolated from the peripheral blood of acutely symptomatic patients, transmission by transfusion is rare.

Transplacental infection occurs in approximately 30% of women if they are first infected during pregnancy and thus have no pre-existing immunity. The risk of transmission to the uterus is lowest in the time just after conception (<1%) and increases to virtually 100% if the mother is infected just before delivery. Additionally, transplacental transmission during chronic infection has been observed in immunosuppressed women.

Although uncommon, occupational exposure and transmission via needlestick can occur when working with live *Toxoplasma*-infected materials in the laboratory.

DISTRIBUTION AND PREVALENCE (Fig. 101.4)

Toxoplasma is distributed worldwide, but the incidence in humans varies widely [3]. Prevalence depends on local eating habits, environmental conditions, and the presence of definitive hosts. Prevalence also increases with age. The overall prevalence in Western Europe is 30–50%. Since the initial studies of the 1950s and 1960s, a trend towards lower seroprevalence has been observed in many European countries. In France, the prevalence declined from more than 80% in the 1960s to 54.3% in 1995, and to 43.8% in 2003. This has been attributed to improved hygiene, new habits of food consumption (e.g. freezing of meat) and better awareness in the general population regarding the risks of consuming undercooked meat. The same phenomenon has been described in the USA, where the seroprevalence declined from 14.1% in the 1988–1994 National Health and Nutrition Examination Survey (NHANES) to 9% in the 1999–2004 NHANES.

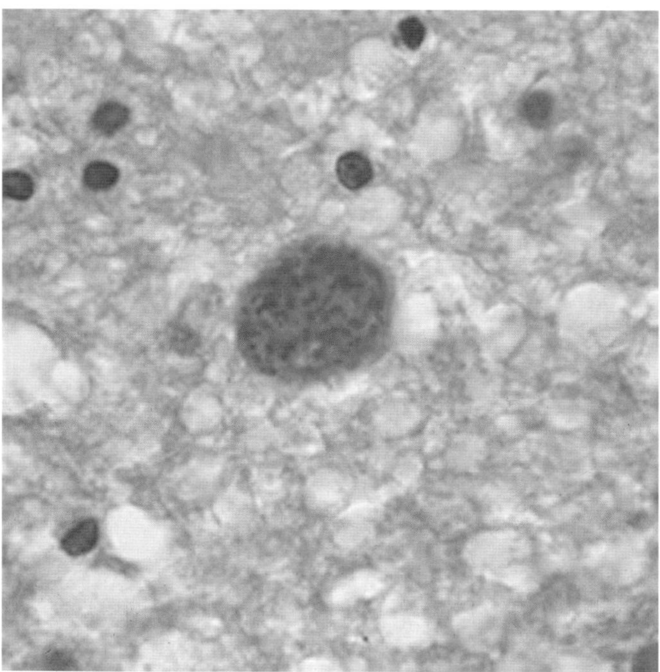

FIGURE 101.3 Cysts in the brain.

In developing and tropical countries, prevalence depends on environmental conditions and climate. It is higher in urban than in rural areas, and higher in wet compared with dry climates. Foci of high prevalence (>80%) exist in Latin America, parts of Eastern/Central Europe, the Middle East, parts of Southeast Asia and Africa. Regional seroprevalence variation relates to the dietary practices of individual subpopulations. A trend toward lower seroprevalence has also been observed in Africa: in Gabon, the prevalence in Franceville was 56% in 2007 compared with 71% 15 years earlier. Prevalence is generally higher in South America (e.g. 53% in Southern Brazil) or in Africa (e.g. 46% in Tanzania and 40.8% in Lagos, Nigeria) than in India (20.3% in Bangalore) or in the Far East (<10% in Korea or China). Globally, toxoplasmosis seroprevalence is continuingly evolving, subject to regional socioeconomic parameters and population habits.

GENETIC DIVERSITY OF TOXOPLAMA GONDII

Early studies of parasite genotypes revealed a clonal population structure comprising three lineages, named types I, II and III [4]. These archetypal lineages were isolated in Europe and North America from humans and domestic animals. Types I and III are common worldwide; type II predominates in Western Europe and the USA, but has not been described in South America to date. Further studies performed on strains isolated in other geographic areas [5] or from wild animals have revealed a greater genetic diversity. There is a relationship between this genetic diversity and the clinical expression of the infection, as shown in South America where several cases of severe toxoplasmosis, some fatal, were described in immunocompetent patients. Initial observations were in patients returning from French Guiana, in whom recombinant or atypical (unrelated to any of the archetypal lineages) strains were implicated [6, 7] . These recombinant and atypical strains are not well adapted to human hosts, perhaps explaining the greater severity of human infection. As more data become available from America and Africa, a new classification is emerging with several haplogroups described in Brazil and in Africa [8].

PATHOPHYSIOLOGY

The primary route of infection is via oral ingestion into the gastrointestinal tract and progression through lymphatics to widespread dissemination. Asexual multiplication of the parasite occurs within the

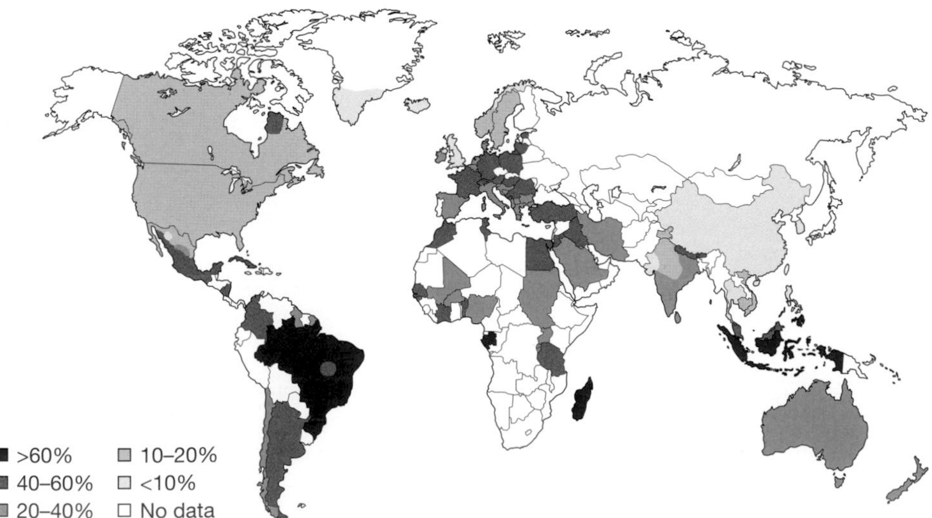

FIGURE 101.4 Global status of *Toxoplasma gondii* seroprevalence *(adapted from Pappas G, Roussos N, Falagas, ME. Toxoplasmosis snapshots: global status of Toxoplasma gondii seroprevalence and implications for pregnancy and congenital toxoplasmosis. Int J Parasitol 2009;39:1385–94.).*

intestinal epithelial cells following ingestion of infective cysts. This early infection period is associated with peripheral parasitemia with *T. gondii* tachyzoites circulating freely, or within mononuclear phagocytic cells, until the development of an effective immune response. Differentiation of tachyzoites into bradyzoites correlates with the onset of protective immunity and begins after a few days. In the setting of T cell immune deficiency, bradyzoites can reactivate into tachyzoites. The genetic background of the host may have influence the risk of reactivation. This is well known in HIV-infected patients for whom the risk of reactivated toxoplasmosis is higher or lower depending on the host's human leukocyte antigen (HLA) haplotype. The absence of effective T cell immunity in the fetus explains the gravity of congenital toxoplasmosis.

CLINICAL MANIFESTATIONS

Although infection with *T. gondii* in developed countries is asymptomatic in 80% of newly infected patients, there are several distinct clinical syndromes.

ACUTE POSTNATAL-ACQUIRED TOXOPLASMOSIS IN IMMUNOCOMPETENT PATIENTS

In the 20% of patients with symptoms at presentation, the disease is generally mild. The incubation period is 1–2 weeks. The most frequent symptoms are fever, asthenia and a single, enlarged cervical lymph node, but regional and generalized lymphadenopathy can occur. The lymph nodes are nontender and do not suppurate. Macular or urticarial rash, arthralgia, myalgia and hepatitis are less common findings. The clinical presentation may resemble a mild influenza-like episode. Symptoms usually resolve spontaneously within a few weeks or months. Ocular involvement is also possible—more frequently reported in South America (particularly Brazil) —but not specifically associated with recent primary infection or with a wild toxoplasmosis cycle. In Europe and North America the great majority of these classical mild cases are supposedly caused by infection with a type II strain. Clinically, the patient presents with a mononucleosis syndrome and the diagnosis is made by serology.

There have been fewer than 100 cases of severe primary toxoplasmosis caused by an atypical or recombinant strain of *T. gondii* in immunocompetent patients reported. The majority of these patients were infected in French Guiana, but cases have also been reported from other areas. In some European cases, the source of infection has been determined to be undercooked horse meat imported from South America [9]. Clinically, the patient presents with a marked, nonspecific infectious syndrome with visceral involvement. Fever higher than 39 °C and prolonged more than 10 days is prominent. In two-thirds of cases there is weight-loss of >5% body weight, generalized lymphadenopathy, elevated liver enzyme levels and pulmonary involvement. Fifty percent of the patients have severe headache and a third have diarrhea, hepatosplenomegaly or chorioretinitis. Other reported complications include Guillain-Barré syndrome, pericarditis, myositis and cutaneous rash. Prognosis is poorer with lung involvement, which occurs generally 10–15 days after the onset of fever and may require hospitalization. For a third of the patients there is an acute respiratory distress syndrome. The main differential diagnosis in South America is histoplasmosis. Without treatment, this severe presentation can be fatal. The diagnosis can be confirmed by classical serology, but direct parasitologic diagnosis is also possible in many cases. An outbreak of severe acute primary toxoplasmosis in a Surinamese village was described with 11 cases; all the patients were infected by the same atypical strain. There were five disseminated acute toxoplasmosis—all hospitalized—with one death; four less severe cases (without hospitalization) and two lethal cases of congenital toxoplasmosis. Different clinical outcomes may be explained by different genetic background in hosts or by the size or type of parasite inoculum [10]. It is important to consider the diagnosis of acute toxoplasmosis in patients who live in, or have recently travelled to, South America—especially the Amazon region—and who present with a severe infectious syndrome with pulmonary involvement.

TOXOPLASMOSIS IN IMMUNOCOMPROMISED HOSTS

In immunocompromised patients, toxoplasmosis is a severe disease. Most cases are reactivation of chronic infection resulting from impaired of T cell immunity. High-risk groups include HIV-infected patients with a CD4 cells count <100/mm^3, patients treated with immunosuppressive agents and bone marrow transplant patients. Such patients, if seronegative, are also at risk for newly acquired infection. Although classically a localized and a disseminated form have been described, in reality the presentation is often less distinct. Initial diagnosis will often focus on a clinically localized finding, whereas further evaluation will reveal disseminated infection. The most common clinical presentation is multifocal necrotizing encephalitis. Patients present with headache and a focal deficit with fever in 50% of cases [11]. Other common neurologic presentations include generalized seizures, with or without encephalitis. Compute tomography (CT) and magnetic resonance imaging (MRI) of the head typically show multiple, low-density lesions at corticomedullary junction or in the basal ganglia that enhance following administration of intravenous contrast (Fig. 101.5). Meningeal signs are uncommon. Mononuclear cerebrospinal fluid (CSF) pleocytosis and mildly elevated protein in the CSF are common.

Another common clinical presentation is pneumonia (which can resemble pneumocystosis) but any organ can be involved because

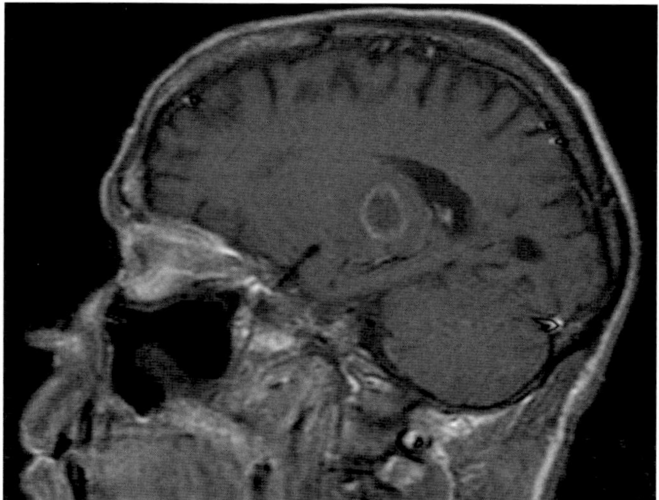

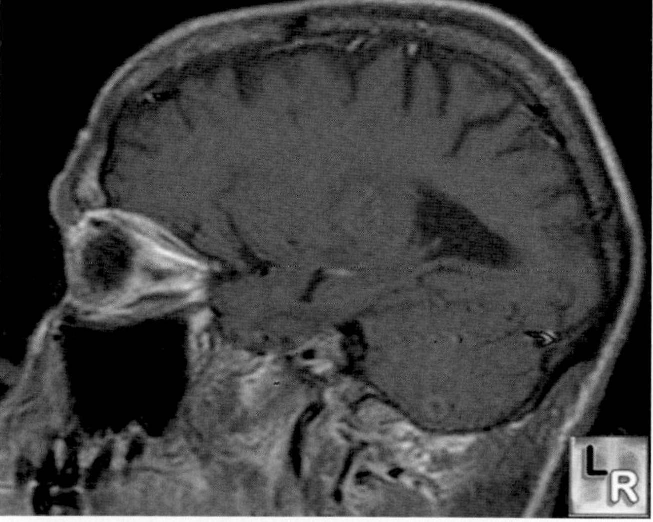

FIGURE 101.5 MRI toxoplasma encepahalitis.

T. gondii infects all nucleated cell types. Forty percent of AIDS patients with ocular localization will also have a brain abscess. Disseminated toxoplasmosis usually presents with high and prolonged fever with altered mental status, arthralgia, rash and focal clinical (CNS abscess, pneumonia) or laboratory (elevated liver enzymes, hemophagocytosis) findings. There is a higher rate of cerebral involvement in AIDS patients than in those whose immunosuppression is not HIV related; for these patients, pulmonary involvement is more frequent. In tropical areas, the rate of toxoplasma reactivation is dependent on the local prevalence of infection in the community.

Although host factors are much more involved than parasite factors in immunocompromised patients' susceptibility to toxoplasmosis [12], the genetic makeup of the particular *T. gondii* strain involved may be associated with atypical presentations. Ghosn et al. [13] reported one case of inguinal lymphadenopathy in a HIV patient with undetectable viral load and CD4 cell count of >500/mm^3. This patient was likely infected by *T. gondii* in the West Indies several years before. An atypical strain was isolated from the lymph node and the patient required treatment with trimethoprim-sulfamethoxazole followed by secondary prophylaxis.

Severe generalized toxoplasmosis with high fatality rates occurs when recipient negative persons receive donor positive organs. Universal prophylaxis with trimethoprim-sulfamethoxazole (TMP-SMX) is effective in preventing post-transplant toxoplasmosis [14]

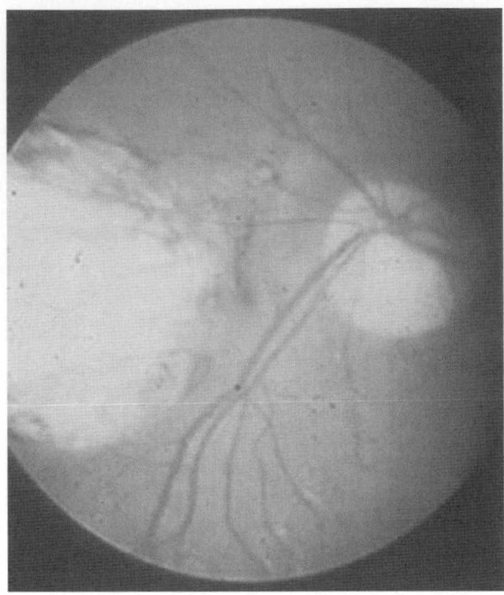

FIGURE 101.6 Active ocular toxoplasmosis.

MANAGEMENT OF ACUTE TOXOPLASMOSIS DURING PREGNANCY

Primary infection of the mother with consequent infection of the placenta is the mechanism for congenital transmission. The placenta allows transmission to the fetus in 30–50% of infections acquired in pregnancy. The rate of transplacental infection and severity of disease in the fetus vary with the time of infection in relation to gestation. When maternal infection occurs in the first trimester, the risk of fetal infection is only about 10% but disease is severe. When maternal infection occurs in the third trimester, the risk of fetal infection rises to 65% and approaches 100% at term; however, neonatal infection in these cases is usually asymptomatic.

Suspected or confirmed toxoplasmosis during pregnancy leads to complex and ongoing management challenges [15]. With appropriate monitoring and management of seroconversion, the great majority (70–80%) of congenital infection is asymptomatic. In settings where such prenatal monitoring is unavailable, congenital infection rates are much higher.

One strategy is to place pregnant women suspected of having toxoplasmosis on spiramycin 1 g, three or four times daily to prevent fetal infection, if this has not yet occurred, while waiting for the results of serologic testing. If a recent infection with toxoplasmosis is confirmed, an amniocentesis is performed and PCR testing of amniotic fluid is done. If positive, one option would be to terminate the pregnancy, depending on the parent's wishes. If the PCR is negative, infection did not occur and spiramycin could be continued through delivery. In resource-limited, lower-income counties, the sophisticated reference laboratories for serologic testing and antenatal diagnostic procedures are not available.

CONGENITAL TOXOPLASMOSIS

Severe congenital toxoplasmosis presents at birth with intracranial calcifications, hydrocephalus and chorioretinitis. The diagnosis is more difficult in mild or asymptomatic forms. Sequelae may develop just after delivery, or later. Physicians must consider congenital toxoplasmosis when a newborn exhibits ocular abnormalities (chorioretinitis, blindness, strabismus, cataracts or nystagmus), epilepsy, mental retardation, microcephaly, intracranial calcifications, diarrhea, hypothermia or anemia. The main determinant of the severity of congenital toxoplasmosis remains the stage of pregnancy at the time of infection. In non-archetypal (i.e. not types I, II or III) strains, primary infection of the mother does not appear to have any unique consequences for the mother, although the few reported cases have been associated with severe congenital disease in the newborn [16]. Presence of such atypical strains of *T. gondii* could explain a reported case of re-infection with congenital transmission in a mother who had been exposed to toxoplasmosis before conception, suggesting that acquired immunity against archetypal strains may not protect against reinfection by atypical strains [9].

OCULAR TOXOPLASMOSIS

Ocular toxoplasmosis is the main cause of posterior uveitis worldwide [17]. Previously considered a late sequelae of congenital toxoplasmosis, it is now believed the majority of ocular disease in immunocompetent patients is postnatally-acquired infection [18, 19]. Ocular involvement is not specifically associated with recent primary infection, but can be delayed several months (or even years) after primary infection [20]. In all cases, the main clinical presentation of chorioretinitis is a focally necrotic retinal lesion with fuzzy outlines (Fig. 101.6). It is accompanied by a whitish vitreous exudate that sometimes obscures the lesion [21]. A new lesion can occasionally arise from the edge of an old one. This chorioretinitis may be associated with edema of the retina and optic nerve, optic neuritis, iridocyclitis and, in rare instances, panuveitis. In congenital toxoplasmosis, the ocular lesions are more likely bilateral versus unilateral in postnatally acquired cases. Ocular toxoplasmosis is characterized by recurrent episodes of chorioretinitis that can be associated with severe morbidity if the disease extends to structures critical for vision or if there is a retinal detachment. The timing of recurrences is unpredictable, but the individual risk is estimated to be as high as 50%. The genetic diversity of *T. gondii* may partially explain this phenomenon. A high prevalence of ocular toxoplasmosis has been reported in South America [22] and Africa [23]. In the UK, the risk of ocular toxoplasmosis is 100 times higher in black people born in West Africa than in subjects born in Britain [23]. In Brazil, the incidence of ocular toxoplasmosis is 17.7% compared with 0.6% in Alabama (USA). Similarly, in Brazil, the ocular sequelae of congenital toxoplasmosis are more frequent, more recurrent and more severe than in Europe [24]. As discussed previously, there is considerable genetic diversity in tropical areas with many atypical strains of *T. gondii* circulating; in Brazil there is no archetypal strain II that predominates in USA. Type II strain in France can be responsible for ocular toxoplasmosis in both immunocompetent and immunocompromised patients [25]. Cumulatively, these data suggest that some strains probably have a tropism for eye tissues but that there are also host factors involved in the occurrence of ocular toxoplasmosis.

TABLE 101-1 Interpretation of Toxoplasma Antibody Tests

IgG result	IgM result	Report/interpretation for humans*
Negative	Negative	No serological evidence of infection with *Toxoplasma*
Negative	Equivocal	Possible early acute infection or false-positive IgM reaction. Obtain a new specimen for IgG and IgM testing. If results for the second specimen remain the same, the patient is probably not infected with *Toxoplasma*
Negative	Positive	Possible acute infection or false-positive IgM result. Obtain a new specimen for IgG and IgM testing. If results for the second specimen remain the same, the IgM reaction is probably a false-positive.
Equivocal	Negative	Indeterminate: obtain a new specimen for testing or retest this specimen for IgG in a different assay.
Equivocal	Equivocal	Indeterminate: obtain a new specimen for both IgG and IgM testing.
Equivocal	Positive	Possible acute infection with *Toxoplasma*. Obtain a new specimen for IgG and IgM testing. If results for the second specimen remain the same or if the IgG becomes positive, both specimens should be sent to a reference laboratory with experience in diagnosis of toxoplasmosis for further testing.
Positive	Negative	Infected with *Toxoplasma* for more than 1 year.
Positive	Equivocal	Infected with *Toxoplasma* for probably more than 1 year or false-positive IgM reaction. Obtain a new specimen for IgM testing. If results with the second specimen remain the same, both specimens should be sent to a reference laboratory with experience in the diagnosis of toxoplasmosis for further testing.
Positive	Positive	Possible recent infection within the last 12 months, or false-positive IgM reaction. Send the specimen to a reference laboratory with laboratory with experience in the diagnosis of toxoplasmosis for further testing.

*except infants
Adapted from CDC: http://www.dpd.cdc.gov/dpdx/HTML/Toxoplasmosis.htm.

DIAGNOSIS

LABORATORY DIAGNOSIS

The differential diagnosis of the various syndromes of toxoplasmosis is broad and laboratory confirmation is recommended in all suspected cases, and is essential in the immuncompromised or in those with severe syndromes. The diagnosis of toxoplasmosis is confirmed by direct detection of parasites in patient specimens or by serology.

DIRECT DETECTION AND IDENTIFICATION OF THE PARASITE

Toxoplasma tachyzoites or cysts can be demonstrated on tissue imprints, biologic fluids (blood, bronchoalveolar lavage, CSF, amniotic fluid) or biopsies (CNS, lymph node, bone marrow) that are fixed and stained appropriately. The diagnosis of acute infection requires the visualization of tachyzoites. The tachyzoites of toxoplasmosis must be distinguished from other intracellular parasites such as *Histoplasma*, *Leishmania*, *Sarcocystis* and *Trypanosoma cruzi*. Isolation of parasites from blood or other body fluids by intraperitoneal inoculation in mice is very useful in isolating the strain. The mice should be tested for the presence of *Toxoplasma* organisms in the peritoneal fluid 6–10 days post-inoculation; if no organisms are found, serology can be performed on the animals 4–6 weeks post-inoculation. There are no accepted cell culture techniques for diagnosis because of a lack of sensitivity. The detection of *T. gondii* DNA by real-time PCR has superseded the classical methods. Several studies confirm that rep529 is the more sensitive DNA target for the diagnosis [26, 27]. Sensitivity using this technique is 95% for antenatal diagnosis in amniotic fluid and for disseminated toxoplasmosis in blood. In localized toxoplasmosis, the sensitivity is similar if PCR is performed on an appropriate sample (BAL (broncho alveolar lavage), cerebral biopsy) but is less sensitive in blood. In AIDS patients with cerebral abscesses, PCR on CSF is positive in only 30–60% of cases.

SEROLOGIC TESTING

Serologic diagnosis is the routine method of diagnosis for most patients and is based on the detection of *T. gondii*-specific IgG and IgM antibodies. The historic gold standard is the dye test developed by Sabin and Feldman in 1948 for the detection of IgG [28]. In 1968, Remington developed an indirect immunofluorescence (IIF) test for IgM detection [29]. The dye test is only available in a specialized reference laboratories and the IIF test requires specific material, therefore, today, the great majority of laboratories use ELISA or electrochemiluminescence immunoassay (ECLIA). Agglutination and indirect hemagglutination tests are easy to perform. Results of IgG studies are generally expressed as international units per milliliter (IU/mL), whereas IgM levels are reported as an index or as serial dilutions. The modern gold standard for IgM is the immuno-sorbent agglutination assay (ISAgA). The interpretation of toxoplasma antibody tests can be complex (Table 101-1).

The determination of the avidity of anti-toxoplasma IgG antibodies by their ability to stay bound to the antigen when exposed to chaotropic salt solutions, can be useful to distinguish early versus later infection. Anti-toxoplama antibodies formed in the few months following infection are less tightly bound (lower avidity) than antibodies found much later in the infection (higher avidity). Avidity assays may be useful in the differential diagnosis of lymphadenopathy and dating infection in pregnant women [30]. The Food and Drug Administration (FDA)-cleared VIDAS TOXO IgG Avidity assay (bioMérieux Inc., Hazelwood, MO, USA) helps determine whether a pregnant woman or a person with swollen lymph nodes testing positive for toxoplasmosis developed the infection within the past 4 months.

DIAGNOSIS OF ACUTE POSTNATAL-ACQUIRED TOXOPLASMOSIS IN IMMUNOCOMPETENT PATIENTS

Acute infection is assessed by seroconversion from a negative to a positive serology. It is the appearance of IgG that defines seroconversion; the presence of IgM alone can be nonspecific or related to cross-reactions. If no negative baseline sample exists, a fourfold rise in IgG titers, combined with a positive IgM, drawn at 2–3 week intervals and run in parallel is highly suggestive of an acute infection. Modern IgM immunosorbent assays are very sensitive and specific but the persistence of these IgM antibodies means that their presence is not, by itself, sufficient to diagnose an acute infection. In such cases, a high IgG avidity index may exclude an acute infection. The lack of standardization between assays may lead to discrepant results; no conclusions can be drawn comparing two results obtained from two different laboratories using different reagents. Routine serology tests are sufficient for diagnosis of "Guyanese toxoplasmosis" strains; serologic response to these strains is generally brisk, with very high IgG titers and a long persistence of specific IgM and IgA.

The differential diagnosis of acute toxoplasmosis is broad and includes infectious mononucleosis caused by Epstein-Barr and cytomegalovirs viruses, acute HIV infection, cat-scratch disease, tuberculosis, lymphoma, Hodgkin's disease and sarcoidosis.

DIAGNOSIS OF TOXOPLASMOSIS IN IMMUNOCOMPROMISED HOSTS

Positive serology indicates only that the diagnosis is possible. A negative serology excludes the diagnosis, except in case of primary infection; for these patients, the appearance of an IgM and IgG response can be delayed. The diagnosis is confirmed by demonstration of the parasite in biopsies or biologic fluids by PCR. In the case of cerebral lesions, a therapeutic trial is frequently initiated, with biopsy performed only if there is no clinical improvement after one week of treatment. Brain biopsy without a therapeutic trial is indicated in immunocompromised patients with a negative specific IgG serologic test, non-enhancing single lesions and those on routine prophylaxis with TMP/SMX because these abnormalities are unlikely to be caused by *Toxoplasma*.

The most common clinical presentation of *T. gondii* infection among patients with AIDS is focal encephalitis with headache, confusion, or motor weakness and fever [31]. Physical examination might demonstrate focal neurologic abnormalities and, in the absence of treatment, disease progression results in seizures, stupor and coma.

Retinochoroiditis, pneumonia and evidence of other multifocal organ system involvement can be observed after dissemination of infection but are rare manifestations in this patient population. A CT scan or MRI of the brain will typically show multiple contrast-enhancing lesions, often with associated edema [32]. However, toxoplasmosis also can manifest as single lesions in the brain.

The differential diagnosis of CNS toxoplasmosis in immunocompromised individuals mimics other causes of enhancing mass lesions such as lymphoma, metastatic carcinoma, tuberculoma, and brain abscess.

DIAGNOSIS OF CONGENITAL TOXOPLASMOSIS

The gold standard for the antenatal diagnosis of congenital toxoplasmosis is PCR performed on amniotic fluid. If there are no abnormalities on fetal ultrasound, the mother is treated until delivery. If severe abnormalities are detected on ultrasound, medical interruption of the pregnancy might be considered based on the parents' choice and local laws. If an antenatal diagnosis is negative or was not performed, neonatal diagnosis is done via child/mother comparison via the immunoblot method and inoculation of placental tissue into mouse peritoneum. After one week of life, the presence of IgA or IgM in the child serum confirms the diagnosis. IgG passively transferred from mother to child should disappear by 10–12 months.

The differential diagnosis of congenital toxoplasmosis includes congental infections with cytomegalovirus, herpes simplex, rubella, *Listeria*, syphilis, *T. cruzi* and erythroblastosis fetalis.

DIAGNOSIS OF OCULAR TOXOPLASMOSIS

The current gold standard for diagnosis of ocular toxoplasmosis is a thorough an ophthalmologic examination. In patients with atypical lesions, laboratory methods may confirm the diagnosis [33]. The most reliable method is aspiration of aqueous humor that can be tested for local specific antibody production or for *T. gondii* DNA by PCR. The ratio of local specific intraocular antibody production compared with serum antibody (Goldmann-Witmer coefficient) is calculated as (anti-*Toxoplasma* IgG in aqueous humor/total IgG in aqueous humor)/(anti-*Toxoplasma* IgG in serum/total IgG in serum). A value of 2 is considered evidence of intraocular Ab synthesis. Immunoblotting can also be utilized.

The differential diagnosis of acute toxoplasmic encephalitis includes uveitis caused by syphilis, tuberculosis, leprosy and sacrcoidosis.

TREATMENT

Most drugs used for the treatment of toxoplasmosis are active only against the tachyzoite forms of the parasite and treatment does not eradicate the infection. Atovaquone has limited *in vitro* activity against the cyst forms.

Specific treatment is not indicated for a healthy person with mild symptoms who is not pregnant, as they usually resolve within a few weeks. Treatment is usually recommended for severe illness in the immunocompetent, infection acquired infection during pregnancy, clinical manifestations compatible with toxoplasmosis in immunosuppressed patients, congenital infection (whether the infant is symptomatic or not), or persons with active ocular disease or severe illness. The treatment of toxoplasmosis in immunocompromised patients is a medical emergency. Primary prophylaxis is used in severely immunosuppressed patients. Current treatment recommendations are found in Table 101-2.

Standard therapy for most indications is a combination of oral pyrimethamine and a sulfonamide. A 200-mg loading dose of pyrimethamine given in divided doses is followed by a daily dose of 1 mg/kg in adults and every 1–3 days for children.

The new gold standard in tropical countries should be TMP/SMX. Maintenance therapy is given until effective immune reconstitution occurs. Primary prophylaxis is necessary for patients with CD4 T cell depletion of less than 200 cells/mm^3. The regimen is the same for primary or secondary prophylaxis, with one tablet (160 trimethoprim/800 mg sulfamethozole) daily.

Treatment recommendations in pregnancy vary; in some countries treatment by pyrimethamine-sulfonamide is systematically given in cases of seroconversion after the first trimester of the pregnancy. In others locations, spiramycin is given until the result of amniocentesis is known and pyrimethamine-sulfonamide used only if the antenatal diagnosis is positive. There is also variability in the duration of the pyrimethamine-sulfonamide regimen used (only one month or until delivery). Changes in antibody titers are not useful for monitoring responses to therapy.

Patients with *Toxoplasma* encephalitis should be monitored routinely for adverse events and clinical and radiologic improvement. Common pyrimethamine toxicities include rash, nausea and bone marrow suppression (neutropenia, anemia and thrombocytopenia) that can often be reversed by increasing the dose of leucovorin to 50–100 mg/day administered in divided doses. Common sulfadiazine toxicities include rash, fever, leukopenia, hepatitis, nausea, vomiting, diarrhea and crystalluria. Common clindamycin toxicities include fever, rash, nausea, diarrhea (including pseudomembranous colitis or diarrhea related to *Clostridium difficile* toxin) and hepatotoxicity. Common TMP-SMX toxicities include rash, fever, leukopenia, thrombocytopenia and hepatotoxicity. Drug interactions between anticonvulsants and anti-retroviral agents should be evaluated carefully and doses adjusted according to established guidelines. Several cases of neurologic disease have been attributed to immune reconstitution and toxoplasmosis, but more data are needed to verify that such cases are immune reconstitution syndrome related to *T. gondii* [34].

CONCLUSION

Since its recognition as a human pathogen in 1939, understanding of *Toxoplasma* has evolved dramatically. Since the end of the 1990s, description of *T. gondii's* genetic composition has led to a better understanding of its biological diversity and pathologic variability. We

TABLE 101-2 Current Treatment Recommendations for Toxoplasmosis

Clinical syndrome	Recommended drug regimen	Comments	Alternate drug regimen	Comments	References
Acquired postnatal toxoplasmosis in immunocompetent individuals					
Asymptomatic infection or mild illness	No treatment	Exception is pregnant women Mild illness resolves spontaneously	Spiramycin 1–2 grams twice daily (adult) and 25 mg/kg twice daily (children) weighing less than 20 kg. Administer for 2–4 weeks	Spiramycin is not a FDA approved drug	[35]
Severe illness (visceral involvement or severe or persistent symptoms)	Adults: 200 mg of pyrimethamine given for one day as a loading dose followed by 50–75 mg per day plus 1–1.5 g sulfadiazine four times per day. Treatment may be indicated for 2–4 weeks	To avoid the hematologic toxicity of pyrimethamine, folinic acid (Leucovorin) is administered in a dose of 5–10 mg daily for adults and 1 mg daily for children.	If sulfa allergic or intolerant then use pyrimethamine plus clindamycin at 600 mg orally or intravenously four times daily		
Immuncocompromised patients					
Encephalitis in HIV infected patients with AIDS	Adults: 200 loading mg of pyrimethamine given for one day followed by 50–75 mg per day plus sulfadiazine at 100–150 mg/kg (e.g. 4–6 g/day for an adult in 1–1.5 g four times per day plus folinic acid (leucovorin) 5–10 mg with each dose of pyrimethamine) Children: pyrimethamine 1 mg/kg plus sulfadiazine 100–150 mg/kg given in four divided daily doses To avoid the hematologic toxicity of this regimen, folinic acid is administered in a dose of 25 mg daily for adults and 1 mg daily for children	Pyrimethamine penetrates the brain parenchyma efficiently, even in the absence of inflammation Adjunctive corticosteroids (e.g. dexamethasone) should be administered to patients with TE when clinically indicated only for treatment of a mass effect associated with focal lesions or associated edema Anticonvulsants should be administered to patients with TE who have a history of seizures, but should not be administered as prophylactics to all patients Anticonvulsants, if administered, should be continued at least through the period of acute therapy. Acute therapy for TE should be continued for at least six weeks, if there is clinical and radiologic improvement. Longer courses might be appropriate if clinical or radiologic disease is extensive or response is incomplete at six weeks. Because of the potential immunosuppressive effects of corticosteroids, they should be discontinued as soon as clinically feasible. Patients receiving corticosteroids should be monitored closely for the development of other OIs, including CMV retinitis and TB disease	The preferred alternative regimen for patients who are unable to tolerate or who fail to respond to first-line therapy is pyrimethamine plus clindamycin plus leucovorin TMP/SMX is 10/50 mg/kg/day given BID, or 15/75 mg/kg/day Atovaquone at 750 mg four times a day plus pyrimethomine	Add folinic acid if mental status is altered and until clinical improvement is seen (generally 3–5 days) If the patient is comatose, treatment is initially given intravenously at the same dose TMP-SMX was reported in a small (77 patients) randomized trial to be effective and better tolerated than pyrimethamine-sulfadiazine Great inter-individual variability in drug atovaquone absorption	[36, 37]

TABLE 101-2 Current Treatment Recommendations for Toxoplasmosis—cont'd

Clinical syndrome	Recommended drug regimen	Comments	Alternate drug regimen	Comments	References
Maintenance therapy in the immunocompromised	Pyrimethamine 25–50 mg daily plus sulfadiazine 2–4 grams daily plus leucovorin 5 mg/kg daily	Suppressive treatment should be continued for duration of immunosuppression Regimen also protects against *Pneumocystis jiroveci* pneumonia All HIV positive patients with positive *Toxoplasma* serology and CD4 T lymphocyte counts less than 200/mcl If CD4 counts are above 200/mcl and viral load is controlled, maintenance therapy can be stopped	Clindamycin 300–450 mg three times daily TMP/SMX Dapsone at 50 mg daily plus pyrimethamine 50 mg/week and leucovorin 10 mg/week 750 mg atovaquone twice daily	Alternative regimens used for those who are sulfa intolerant	
Pregnant women	Spiramycin is traditionally used during the first and second trimesters in pregnant women who seroconverted during the first trimester of pregnancy The dose is 3–4 grams daily in divided doses. pyrimethamine/sulfadiazine and leucovorin (for late-second and third trimesters) for women with acute *T. gondii* infection diagnosed at a reference laboratory during gestation	Pyrimethamine is teratogenic and should not be used in the first trimester			
Congential toxoplasmosis in the neonate	Pyrimethamine plus a sulfonamide, given to the neonate for 3–12 months depending of the severity of the disease and local recommendations Sulfadiazine can be replaced by sulfadoxine with an intake every 10 days	No uniform or consensus recommendations			
Ocular toxoplasmosis	Combination pyrimethamine-sulfonamide (same regimen as used in immunocompromised) and corticosteroids	Maintenance therapy with TMP/SMX should be given if a lesion is considered vision-threatening or for mono-ocular patients Long-term maintenance treatment reduces the rate of recurrence The best regimen is not determined but should be one tablet (80 mg/400 mg) per day if adequately tolerated	Many other drug combinations are cited in the literature, principally pyrimethamine plus a macrolide, but there is no randomized study evaluating these regimens against the TMP/SMX		[38]

CMV, cytomegalovirus; FDA, Food and Drugs Administration; OI, opportunistic infection; TB, tuberculosis; TE, toxoplasmosis encephalitis.

know today that the disease, once considered to be benign, is potentially severe in immunocompetent patients. Acute toxoplasmosis must be considered in the differential diagnosis of a patient living in, or returning from, tropical areas—particularly the Amazon region of South America—who presents with a severe infectious syndrome with pulmonary involvement.

REFERENCES

1. Weiss LM, Dubey JP. Toxoplasmosis: A history of clinical observations. Int J Parasitol 2009;39:895–901.
2. Dubey JP. History of the discovery of the life cycle of *Toxoplasma gondii*. Int J Parasitol 2009;39:877–82.
3. Pappas G, Roussos N, Falagas, ME. Toxoplasmosis snapshots: global status of *Toxoplasma gondii* seroprevalence and implications for pregnancy and congenital toxoplasmosis. Int J Parasitol 2009;39:1385–94.
4. Howe DK, Sibley LD. *Toxoplasma gondii* comprises three clonal lineages: correlation of parasite genotype with human disease. J Infect Dis 1995;172:1561–6.
5. Lehmann T, Graham DH, Dahl ER, et al. Variation in the structure of *Toxoplasma gondii* and the roles of selfing, drift, and epistatic selection in maintaining linkage disequilibria. Infect Genet Evol 2004;4:107–14.
6. Bossi P, Caumes E, Paris L, et al. *Toxoplasma gondii*-associated Guillain-Barre syndrome in an immunocompetent patient. J Clin Microbiol 1998;36:3724–5.
7. Darde ML, Villena I, Pinon JM, Beguinot I. Severe toxoplasmosis caused by a *Toxoplasma gondii* strain with a new isoenzyme type acquired in French Guyana. J Clin Microbiol 1998;36:324.
8. Al-Kappany YM, Rajendran C, Abu-Elwafa SA, et al. Genetic diversity of *Toxoplasma gondii* isolates in Egyptian feral cats reveals new genotypes. J Parasitol 2010;96:1112–14.
9. Elbez-Rubinstein A, Ajzenberg, D Darde ML, et al. Congenital toxoplasmosis and reinfection during pregnancy: case report, strain characterization, experimental model of reinfection, and review. J Infect Dis 2009;199:280–5.
10. Demar M, Ajzenberg D, Maubon D, et al. Fatal outbreak of human toxoplasmosis along the Maroni River: epidemiological, clinical, and parasitological aspects. Clin Infect Dis 2007;45:e88–95.
11. Luft BJ, Remington JS. Toxoplasmic encephalitis in AIDS. Clin Infect Dis 1992;15:211–22.
12. Ajzenberg D, Year H, Marty P, et al. Genotype of 88 *Toxoplasma gondii* isolates associated with toxoplasmosis in immunocompromised patients and correlation with clinical findings. J Infect Dis 2009;199:1155–67.
13. Ghosn J, Paris L, Ajzenberg D, et al. Atypical toxoplasmic manifestation after discontinuation of maintenance therapy in a human immunodeficiency virus type 1-infected patient with immune recovery. Clin Infect Dis 2003;37:e112–14.
14 Martina MN, Cervera C, Esforzado N, et al. *Toxoplasma gondii* primary infection in renal transplant recipients. Two case reports and literature review. Transpl Int 2011;24:e6–12.
15. Montoya JG, Remington JS. Management of *Toxoplasma gondii* infection during pregnancy. Clin Infect Dis 2008;47:554–66.
16. Ajzenberg D, Cogne N, Paris L, et al. Genotype of 86 *Toxoplasma gondii* isolates associated with human congenital toxoplasmosis, and correlation with clinical findings. J Infect Dis 2002;186:684–9.
17. Commodaro AG, Belfort RN, Rizzo LV, et al. Ocular toxoplasmosis: an update and review of the literature. Mem Inst Oswaldo Cruz 2009;104:345–50.
18. Balasundaram MB, Andavar R, Palaniswamy M, Venkatapathy N. Outbreak of acquired ocular toxoplasmosis involving 248 patients. Arch Ophthalmol 2010;128:28–32.
19. Montoya JG, Remington JS. Toxoplasmic chorioretinitis in the setting of acute acquired toxoplasmosis. Clin Infect Dis 1996;23:277–82.
20. Silveira, C, Belfort R, Jr, Muccioli C, et al. A follow-up study of Toxoplasma gondii infection in southern Brazil. Am J Ophthalmol 2001;131:351–4.
21. Delair E, Latkany P, Noble AG, et al. Clinical manifestations of ocular toxoplasmosis. Ocul Immunol Inflamm 2011;19:91–102
22. Glasner PD, Silveira C, Kruszon-Moran D, et al. An unusually high prevalence of ocular toxoplasmosis in southern Brazil. Am J Ophthalmol 1992;114:136–44.
23. Gilbert RE, Stanford MR, Jackson H, et al. Incidence of acute symptomatic toxoplasma retinochoroiditis in south London according to country of birth. BMJ 1994;310:1037–40.
24. Gilbert RE, Freeman K, Lago EG, et al. Ocular sequelae of congenital toxoplasmosis in Brazil compared with Europe. PLoS Negl Trop Dis 2008;2:e277.
25. Fekkar A, Ajzenberg D, Bodaghi B, et al. Direct genotyping of *Toxoplasma gondii* in ocular fluid samples from 20 patients with ocular toxoplasmosis: predominance of type II in France. J Clin Microbiol 2011;49:1543–7.
26. Mesquita RT, Ziegler AP, Hiramoto RM, et al. Real-time quantitative PCR in cerebral toxoplasmosis diagnosis of Brazilian human immunodeficiency virus-infected patients. J Med Microbiol 2010;59:641–7.
27. Sterkers Y, Varlet-Marie E, Cassaing S, et al. Multicentric comparative analytical performance study for molecular detection of low amounts of *Toxoplasma gondii* from simulated specimens. J Clin Microbiol 2010;48:3216–22.
28. Sabin AB, Feldman HA. Dyes as microchemical indicators of a new immunity phenomenon affecting a protozoon parasite (toxoplasma). Science 1948;108:660–3.
29. Remington JS, Miller MJ, Brownlee I. IgM antibodies in acute toxoplasmosis. II. Prevalence and significance in acquired cases. J Lab Clin Med 1968;71:855–66.
30. Fricker-Hidalgo H, Saddoux C, Suchel-Jambon AS, et al. New Vidas assay for Toxoplasma-specific IgG avidity: evaluation on 603 sera. Diagn Microbiol Infect Dis 2006;56:167–72.
31. Luft BJ, Brooks RG, Conley FK. Toxoplasmic encephalitis in patients with acquired immune deficiency syndrome. JAMA 1984;252:913–17.
32. Kupfer MC, Zee CS, Colletti PM, et al. MRI evaluation of AIDS-related encephalopathy: toxoplasmosis vs. lymphoma. Magn Reson Imaging 1990;8:51–7.
33. Fekkar A, Bodaghi B, Touafek F, et al. Comparison of immunoblotting, calculation of the Goldmann-Witmer coefficient, and real-time PCR using aqueous humor samples for diagnosis of ocular toxoplasmosis. J Clin Microbiol 2008;46:1965–7.
34. Martin-Blondel G, Alvarez M, Delobel P, et al. Toxoplasmic encephalitis IRIS in HIV-infected patients: a case series and review of the literature. J Neurol Neurosurg Psychiatry 2011;82:691 3.
35. Georgiev VS. Management of toxoplasmosis. Drugs 1994;48:179.
36. Beraud G, Pierre-Francois S, Foltzer A, et al. Cotrimoxazole for treatment of cerebral toxoplasmosis: an observational cohort study during 1994-2006. Am J Trop Med Hyg 2009;80:583–7.
37. Torre D, Casari S, Speranza F, et al. Randomized trial of trimethoprim-sulfamethoxazole versus pyrimethamine-sulfadiazine for therapy of toxoplasmic encephalitis in patients with AIDS. Italian Collaborative Study Group. Antimicrob Agents Chemother 1998;42:1346–9.
38. Silveira C, Belfort R, Jr, Muccioli C, et al. The effect of long-term intermittent trimethoprim/sulfamethoxazole treatment on recurrences of toxoplasmic retinochoroiditis. Am J Ophthalmol 2002;134:41–6.

102 Pathogenic and Opportunistic Free-living Ameba Infections

Govinda S Visvesvara

Key features

- *Naegleria fowleri* causes an acute and fulminating primary amebic meningoencephalitis (PAM) in children and young adults with a history of recent aquatic activities and leads to death within a week
- *Acanthamoeba* spp. cause chronic but fatal granulomatous amebic encephalitis (GAE) and disseminated infections of the skin and other organs in immunocompromised people; they can also cause *Acanthamoeba* keratitis, most frequently in association with soft or hard contact lenses
- *Balamuthia mandrillaris* causes a chronic but fatal granulomatous amebic encephalitis in both immunocompromised and immunocompetent people

DEFINITION

Acanthamoeba spp., *Balamuthia mandrillaris* and *Naegleria fowleri* are pathogenic and opportunistic free-living amebae (POFLA) that primarily cause central nervous system (CNS) infections in humans and other animals. *Acanthamoeba* spp. and *B. mandrillaris* cause a chronic infection called granulomatous amebic encephalitis (GAE) lasting from 2 weeks to 2 years. GAE is often associated with dissemination to the skin, lungs, kidney, thyroid and liver. Cases of GAE occur at any time of the year without relation to seasonality. *Acanthamoeba* can also cause keratitis. *N. fowleri* causes an acute and fulminating infection called primary amebic meningoencephalitis (PAM) leading to death within 7–10 days. PAM usually occurs during the summer months when the ambient temperature is high [1–3]. Recently, *Sappinia pedata* (previously identified as *S. diploidea*), a saprophytic ameba normally isolated from soil contaminated with fecal material of lizards, elk and bison, was identified in a brain biopsy specimen of a previously healthy 38-year-old man who developed meningoencephalitis, suggesting that other POFLA besides *Acanthamoeba*, *Balamuthia* and *Naegleria* spp. may also cause human disease [2,4,5].

HISTORY AND ETIOLOGY

The concept that POFLA, particularly *Acanthamoeba* spp., may cause human disease was developed by C. G. Culbertson in 1958 when he isolated an ameba from a control monkey kidney cell culture used during the development of polio vaccine. This ameba, now called *Acanthamoeba culbertsoni*, produced meningoencephalitis in cortisone-treated monkeys and mice upon intranasal instillation [1–3]. The first documented human cases were reported by Fowler and Carter in 1965 [6].

The life cycle of *Acanthamoeba* spp. consists of two stages: a trophozoite stage and a resistant cyst. The trophozoite measures 15–45 μm and is uninucleate with a centrally placed, large, densely staining nucleolus (see Fig. 102.2). The free-living trophozoite feeds on bacteria and environmental organic debris. Cysts measure 10–25 μm and are uninucleate and double-walled: the outer wall (the ectocyst) is wrinkled and contains protein; the inner wall (the endocyst) is usually stellate, polygonal, oval or spherical and contains cellulose. Pores covered by opercula are present at the point of contact between the ectocyst and the endocyst [1–3]. Both trophozoite and cyst stages are presumed to be capable of causing human infection.

B. mandrillaris, previously called leptomyxid ameba, also has two stages in its life cycle. The trophozoite is irregular in shape, uninucleate, and measures from 12 to 60 μm. The nucleus contains a large centrally placed nucleolus. Occasionally, in infected human tissues, trophic stages containing a large nucleus with two or three nucleoli seen (which helps differentiate it from *Acanthamoeba*). Cysts are also uninucleate, more or less spherical, range in size from 12 to 30 μm, and appear to be double-walled with a wavy ectocyst and a spherical endocyst under light microscopy. Ultrastructurally, the cysts are tripartite with an outer thin, irregular ectocyst, an inner thick endocyst, and a middle amorphous fibrillar mesocyst [2].

N. fowleri has three stages in its life cycle: a trophozoite, a cyst and a flagellated form. It is thus also described as an ameboflagellate. *Naegleria* differentiates into this pear-shaped biflagellate stage in response to sudden changes in the ionic concentration of the environment. The trophozoite measures 10–25 μm and is uninucleate; the nucleus is spherical and contains a large, centrally placed, dense nucleolus. Cysts are round, measure 7–14 μm and contain a single nucleus with a central dense nucleolus; the dense cyst walls are plugged with one or more flat pores [1,2]. *Acanthamoeba* spp. and *N. fowleri*, but not *B. mandrillaris*, can be cultivated on non-nutrient agar plates coated with suitable Gram-negative bacteria such as *Escherichia coli* or *Enterobacter aerogenes*. The amebae will feed on the bacteria, multiply and differentiate into cysts within a few days. All three amebae can be grown axenically without bacteria as well as on mammalian cell cultures [1–3].

EPIDEMIOLOGY

The POFLA are ubiquitous and occur worldwide. *Acanthamoeba* and *Naegleria fowleri* have been isolated from a wide range of aquatic and environmental niches as well as from dust in the air and even the nasal passages and throats of healthy individuals. *B. mandrillaris* has also been isolated from the soil. *Acanthamoeba* spp. can harbor pathogenic microorganisms such as *Legionella* spp., *Mycobacteria*, *Francisella tularensis*, *E. coli* O157, *Burkholderia*, *Parachlamydia* and mimiviruses and hence may be of additional public health importance [1–3].

PRIMARY AMEBIC MENINGOENCEPHALITIS (PAM)

PAM has a worldwide distribution [1,2], occurring in active healthy children and young adults with a history of recent contact with fresh water. The ameba enters through the nasal passages, penetrates the cribriform plate, reaches the subarachnoid space, then invades the brain parenchyma. The incubation period of PAM varies from 2 to 15 days. PAM is characterized clinically by the sudden onset of bifrontal or bitemporal headaches, fever, nausea, vomiting and stiff neck. Nuchal rigidity usually occurs with positive Kernig's and Brudzinski's signs. Other signs and symptoms include abnormalities in taste or smell, cerebellar ataxia, and photophobia. Signs of increased intracranial pressure, lethargy, and confusion ensue, leading to generalized seizures, coma and death within a week to 10 days.

DIAGNOSTIC MICROBIOLOGY

The CSF is characterized by pleocytosis, with predominance of polymorphonuclear leukocytes but with an absence of bacteria. The CSF pressure is elevated (100–600 mmHg). Glucose concentration may be slightly reduced or normal, but the protein content is elevated, ranging from 100 mg/100 mL to 1000 mg/100 mL. Differentiation of PAM from acute pyogenic or bacterial meningoencephalitis is made by recognizing motile amebae in direct wet mount examination of the CSF. Smears of CSF should also be stained with Giemsa or trichrome in order to detect the characteristic *Naegleria* nuclear morphology [1,2]. Neuroimaging can be nonspecific but can include edema, basilar meningeal enhancement, and obliteration of the cisterns around the midbrain and the subarachnoid space [7]. Many cases have been diagnosed postmortem based on examination of hematoxylin and eosin (H&E)-stained sections, immunohistochemical tests and PCR assay. Recently, a real-time multiplex PCR has been developed which identifies *N. fowleri* DNA in the CSF within 5 hours, thus greatly facilitating rapid and accurate diagnosis [8].

Little information exists on the antibody response to *N. fowleri* infection, probably because most patients die before serum antibodies become detectable. However, in one patient who survived PAM, an antibody titer of 1:4096 to *N. fowleri* was demonstrated by immunofluorescence in serum samples obtained at 7, 10 and 42 days of hospitalization [2]. Low levels of antibodies to *N. fowleri* and other *Naegleria* species in sera of hospitalized patients and in apparently healthy people have been reported. Apparently, normal human serum, but not heat-inactivated serum, stimulates production of protein kinases in *N. fowleri*, which may be effective in destroying complement and protecting amebae from the membrane-attack complex of the complement cascade [2].

PATHOLOGIC FEATURES

At autopsy, the cerebral hemispheres are swollen and edematous. The olfactory bulbs and the orbitofrontal cortices are necrotic and hemorrhagic. The arachnoid membrane is severely congested with scant purulent exudate. Amebic trophozoites, but not cysts, are usually seen within the Virchow–Robin spaces with minimal or no inflammatory reaction (Fig. 102.1) [1,2].

MANAGEMENT

The few patients who have survived this infection have done so primarily because of early diagnosis and aggressive treatment with intrathecal and/or intravenous amphoterecin B, miconazole and oral rifampin [2,9]. Amphotericin B and azithromycin were found to be synergistic *in vitro* and in a mouse model [10].

PREVENTION

The trophic and the cyst forms of *N. fowleri* are susceptible to chlorine and are killed at 2 mg/L. It is therefore important for swimming pools to be maintained properly with adequate chlorination at all times [1,2]. Warning signs should be posted in geographic areas with warm, freshwater bodies of water, particularly during the summer months.

GRANULOMATOUS AMEBIC ENCEPHALITIS (GAE)

GAE caused by *Acanthamoeba* spp. usually occurs in chronically ill, debilitated individuals, in immunosuppressed patients including those who have AIDS, or in those who have received broad-spectrum

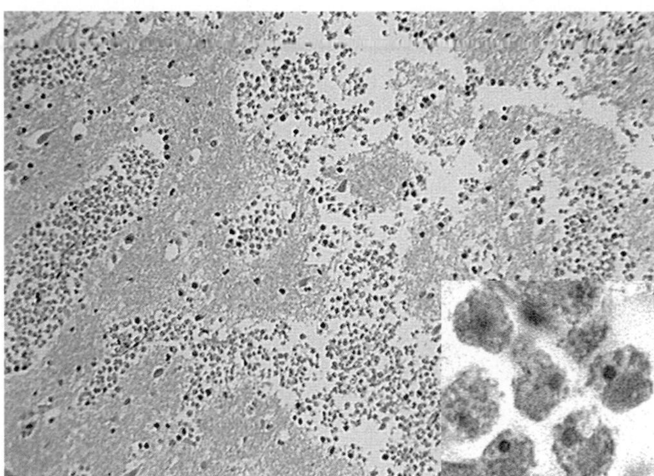

FIGURE 102.1 Central nervous system section of a primary amebic meningoencephalitis (PAM) case, demonstrating numerous trophozoites of *Naegleria fowleri* (H&E; ×400). Note the absence of cysts. Inset: trophozoites showing large nucleus with densely staining nucleolus (×1000).

antibiotics or chemotherapeutic medications [1–3]. *B. mandrillaris* causes infection in both immunodeficient and immunocompetent individuals [2]. GAE is an insidious disease and has a long and protracted clinical course. Clinical signs can progress from personality changes, headache, low-grade fever, nausea and vomiting, to lethargy, diplopia, hemiparesis, seizures, depressed levels of consciousness and coma. Third and sixth cranial nerve palsies may be seen in some patients. GAE may mimic bacterial leptomeningitis, tuberculous or viral meningitis, or single or multiple space-occupying lesions. Pneumonitis may also occur.

DIAGNOSTIC MICROBIOLOGY

CSF in patients with GAE reveals a lymphocytic pleocytosis with mildly elevated protein and normal levels of glucose. Neuroimaging studies can reveal single or multiple heterogeneous, hypodense, non-enhancing, space-occupying lesions involving the basal ganglia, cerebral cortex, subcortical white matter, cerebellum and pons, suggesting abscess, tumor or intracerebral hematoma. Brain and skin biopsies are important diagnostic procedures. Molecular techniques such as PCR and real-time PCR have also been used recently to identify *Acanthamoeba* in the CSF, brain and corneal tissue as well as in tear fluid. *Acanthamoeba* spp. can be easily cultured from infected tissue on bacterially seeded agar plates [1–3]. *B. mandrillaris* can be isolated from the CNS by inoculating monkey kidney cell culture with brain tissue [2].

PATHOLOGIC FEATURES

The cerebral hemispheres are edematous. Encephalomalacia with multifocal areas of cortical softening and hemorrhagic necrosis may be seen. Multifocal necrotic lesions often accompanied by *Acanthamoeba* trophozoites and cysts (Fig. 102.2) may also be seen in the posterior fossa structures, midbrain, thalamus, brainstem and cerebellum. Occasionally, angiitis may be seen with perivascular cuffing by inflammatory cells, chiefly lymphocytes, a few plasma cells and macrophages. In patients with AIDS, ulcerations of the skin with acute and chronic inflammation and trophozoites and cysts may be seen. The kidneys, prostate gland, adrenal glands, lungs and liver may also be involved, suggesting hematogenous dissemination. Recently, two clusters of transmission of *B. mandrillaris* infection through solid organ transplantation were reported, further suggesting that the route of invasion to the brain is via the bloodstream [11]. Histopathologically, *Balamuthia* can be differentiated from *Acanthamoeba* since the nucleus of *Balamuthia* sometimes contains

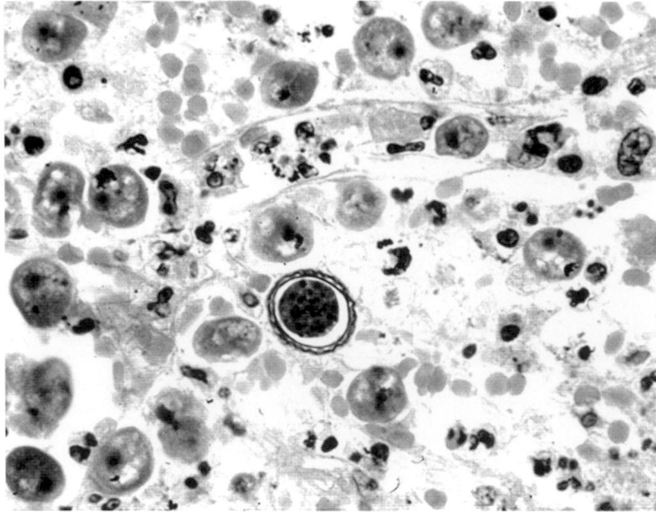

FIGURE 102.2 Central nervous system section of a granulomatous amebic encephalitis (GAE) case due to *Acanthamoeba*, demonstrating many trophozoites and a cyst (Masson's trichrome; ×1000).

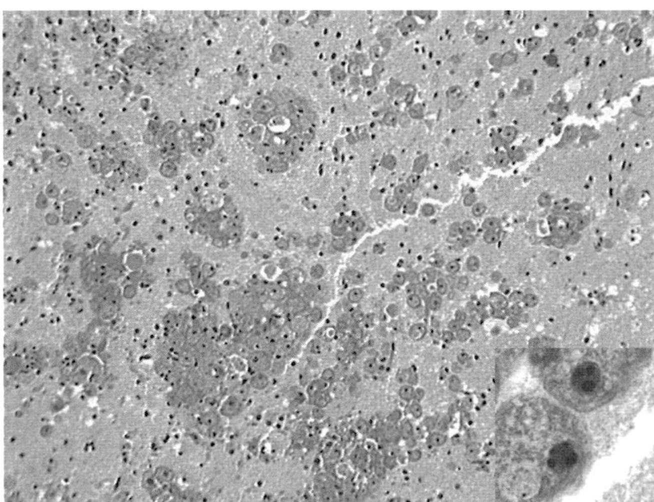

FIGURE 102.3 Central nervous system section of a granulomatous amebic encephalitis (GAE) case due to *Balamuthia mandrillaris*, showing numerous trophozoites of *B. mandrillaris* (H&E; ×100). Inset: more than one nucleolus can be seen within the nucleus of the trophozoite (×1000).

multiple nucleoli (Fig. 102.3). Immunohistochemical analysis using rabbit anti-*Acanthamoeba* spp. or anti-*B. mandrillaris* sera can also differentiate the two amebae [1–3].

MANAGEMENT

There is no effective treatment for GAE and therefore the prognosis is poor. Diagnosis of GAE is often made postmortem. A few patients diagnosed pre-mortem and a few with cutaneous infections without CNS involvement have been successfully treated with a combination of antimicrobials including pentamidine isethionate, sulfadiazine, flucytosine, fluconazole or itraconazole, and miltefosine [12,13].

Although the majority of patients with *Balamuthia* GAE have died, a few patients have survived the infection. Notably, two transplant recipients have survived after treatment with a combination of pentamidine isethionate, sulfadiazine, a macrolide (azithromycin or clarithromycin), fluconazole, 5-fluorocytosine and miltefosine [2,8,11,14]. Two Peruvian patients with cutaneous lesions recovered after prolonged therapy with albendazole and itraconazole [2].

Prevention

Since *Acanthamoeba* spp. can grow and colonize hot water tanks, jacuzzis, filters used in HVAC units, and in-line filters used for purifying portable water supplies and eye wash stations, periodic inspection and cleaning of these systems is recommended.

ACANTHAMOEBA KERATITIS (AK)

AK is a sight-threatening inflammation of the cornea caused by amebae introduced by ocular trauma or by contact lens wear and the use of nonsterile homemade saline solution that has been contaminated. *Acanthamoeba* present in the environment or the contaminated lens solution adhere to corneal epithelial cells and secrete proteolytic and collagenolytic enzymes that contribute to the pathogenesis of AK. According to recent studies, the initial process of invasion occurs when a 136-kDa mannose-binding protein (MBP), a lectin expressed on the surface of *Acanthamoeba*, adheres to mannose glycoproteins on the surface of the epithelial cells and destroys them [15]. *Acanthamoeba* trophozoites may also produce "food cups" with which they directly ingest epithelial cells. The hallmark of AK is severe ocular pain, photophobia, a central or paracentral 360° stromal ring infiltrate, and a recurrent breakdown of corneal epithelium, with a waxing and waning clinical course. The lesion is refractory to the usual antibacterial, antiviral and antimycotic medications with which it is often presumptively treated. If proper treatment is not provided, AK may lead to a vascularized scar within a thin cornea, causing impaired vision or perforation of the cornea and loss of the eye [2,3,15].

The first case of AK in the US was reported in 1975 in a farmer from south Texas with ocular trauma of the right eye. Subsequently, contact lens use (particularly soft hydrogel lenses) and the use of nonsterile homemade saline solutions have been identified as additional risk factors for AK. Recently, an epidemiologic survey conducted by the Centers for Disease Control and Prevention (CDC) of a multistate outbreak of *Acanthamoeba* keratitis revealed that the national increase in the number of *Acanthamoeba* keratitis cases was associated with the use of Advanced Medical Optics Complete® MoisturePlus™ multipurpose contact lens solution, leading to an international recall by the manufacturer [16].

DIAGNOSTIC MICROBIOLOGY

Accurate diagnosis of AK requires deep corneal scrapings and biopsy. Unfixed specimens should be cultured on bacterially seeded agar plates (as above). Smears should also be prepared and stained with Giemsa–Wright, Hemacolor, or with Wheatly's or Masson's trichrome stain which help differentiate trophozoites of *Acanthamoeba* spp from host corneal cells. Confocal microscopy has also been used recently to diagnose AK [2,3].

MANAGEMENT

Unlike with GAE, successful treatment of AK is feasible, using aggressive topical application of polyhexamethylene biguanide or chlorhexidine gluconate in combination with propamidine isethionate (Brolene) and neomycin. Debridement of the cornea, penetrating keratoplasty and corneal grafting has also been performed with good results in some patients. Recurrence of AK has been reported after corneal transplantation because of persistence of *Acanthamoeba* cysts in the corneal stroma [15].

Prevention

Eye-care professionals need to educate patients about the proper care and use of contact lenses. Contact lenses and contact lens paraphernalia, particularly the solutions, should be kept meticulously clean. Contact lens wearers should follow the directions and recommendations of the manufacturers and eye-care professionals. Contact lens use should be avoided during swimming or other water sports.

DISCLAIMER

The findings and conclusions in this report are those of the authors and do not necessarily represent the views of the Centers for Disease Control and Prevention.

REFERENCES

1. Martinez AJ, Visvesvara GS. Free-living, amphizoic and opportunistic amebas. Brain Pathol 1997;7:583–98.
2. Visvesvara GS, Moura H, Schuster FL. Pathogenic and opportunistic free-living amoebae: *Acanthamoeba* spp., *Balamuthia mandrillaris, Naegleria fowleri*, and *Sappinia diploidea*. FEMS Immunol Microbiol 2007;50:1–26.
3. Marciano-Cabral F, Cabral G. *Acanthamoeba* spp. as agents of disease in humans. Clin Microbiol 2003;16:273–307.
4. Gelman BB, Popov V, Cahlijub G, et al. Neuropathological and ultrastructural features of amebic encephalitis caused by *Sappinia diploidea*. J Neuropathol Exp Neurol 2003;62:990–8.
5. Qvarnstrom Y, da Silva AJ, Schuster FL, et al. Molecular confirmation of *Sappinia pedata* as causative agent of amebic encephalitis. J Infect Dis 2009; 199:1139–42.
6. Fowler M, Carter RF. Acute pyogenic meningitis probably due to *Acanthamoeba* sp.: a preliminary report. Br Med J 1965;2:740–3.
7. Singh P, Kochhar R, Vashishta RK, et al. Amebic meningoencephalitis: spectrum of imaging findings. Am J Neuroradiol 2006;27:1217–21.
8. Qvarnstrom Y, Visvesvara GS, Sriram R, Da Silva AJ. A multiplex real-time PCR assay for simultaneous detection of *Acanthamoeba* spp., *Balamuthia mandrillaris* and *Naegleria fowleri*. J Clin Microbiol 2006;44:3589–95.
9. Seidel JS, Harmatz P, Visvesvara GS, et al. Successful treatment of primary amebic meningoencephalitis. N Engl J Med 1982;306:346–8.
10. Soltow SM, Brenner GM. Synergistic activities of azithromycin and amphotericin B against *Naegleria fowleri* in vitro and in a mouse model of primary amebic meningoencephalitis. Antimicrob Agents Chemother 2007;51:23–7.
11. Centers for Disease Control 2010. *Balamuthia mandrillaris* transmitted through organ transplantation – Mississippi, 2009. MMWR Morb Mortal Wkly Rep 2010;59:1165–70
12. Slater CA, Sickel JZ, Visvesvara GS, et al. Successful treatment of disseminated *Acanthamoeba* infection in an immunocompromised patient. N Engl J Med 1994;331:85–7.
13. Aichelberg AC, Walochnik J, Assadian O, et al. Successful treatment of disseminated *Acanthamoeba* infection and granulomatous amoebic encephalitis in an immunocompromised patient with military tuberculosis and tuberculous meningitis with miltefosine, an alkylphosphocholine. Emerg Infect Dis 2008;14:1743–6.
14. Deetz TR, Sawyer MH, Billman G, et al. Successful treatment of *Balamuthia* amoebic encephalitis: presentation of two cases. Clin Infect Dis 2003;37: 1304–12.
15. Dart JKG, Saw VPJ, Kilvington S. *Acanthamoeba* keratitis: diagnosis and treatment update. Am J Ophthalmol 2009;148:487–99.
16. Verani J, Lorick S, Yoder JS, et al. National outbreak of *Acanthamoeba* keratitis associated with use of a contact lens solution, United States. Emerg Infect Dis 2009;15:1236–42.

103 Sarcocystosis

Benjamin M Rosenthal

Key features

- *Sarcocystis* parasites are a rare cause of eosinophilic enteritis, subcutaneous nodules, and eosinophilic myositis
- Humans are definitive hosts for *Sarcocystis hominis* and *Sarcocysti suihominis*, the agents responsible for intestinal sarcocystosis. Ingesting sarcocysts found in uncooked or undercooked beef or pork may cause mild enteritis, but most infections are thought to be asymptomatic
- Humans may also become dead-end (intermediate) hosts for nonhuman *Sarcocystis* spp. after the accidental ingestion of oocysts. This ingestion leads to muscular sarcocystosis, a clinical spectrum ranging from asymptomatic muscle cysts to a severe, acute, eosinophilic myositis associated with systemic symptoms with peripheral eosinophilia
- Most human cases have been described from Southeast Asia, but *Sarcocystis* parasites have a worldwide distribution, especially where livestock is raised, and human infections in other areas have been described but may be under-recognized

TRANSMISSION AND EPIDEMIOLOGY

Humans are the definitive hosts when they consume undercooked pork or beef containing tissue cysts (sarcocysts) (Fig. 103.1) of the two recognized human species, *Sarcocystis hominis* and *Sarcocystis suihominis*, and they develop intestinal sarcocystosis – a transient infection restricted to the gastro-intestinal tract.

The vast majority of over 100 different parasite species are found in other mammals. In nature, carnivores acquire infection by consuming prey whose tissues harbor encysted parasites. The carnivores excrete the parasite oocysts which are then consumed by herbivores ingesting contaminated vegetation or water. Humans are accidental intermediate hosts for several other *Sarcocystis* species.

Sarcocystis parasites have a worldwide distribution. Our understanding of the epidemiology of human sarcocystosis relies on sporadic case reports and occasional outbreaks, mostly described from Southeast Asia, especially Malaysia and Thailand. Limited seroprevalence studies and stool surveys confirm widespread distribution and exposures, and suggest human infections are likely under-recognized [2]. Incidental findings at autopsy suggest widespread infection in endemic areas. One series of 100 consecutive, routine autopsies from Malaysia documented evidence of sarcocystosis in 21% of muscle tissue examinations [3].

PATHOGENESIS

Sarcocystis parasites are obligatory, two-host, intracellular, intestinal, coccidian parasites. *Sarcocystis hominis* and *S. suihominis* use humans as definitive hosts and are responsible for intestinal sarcocystosis in the human host. Humans may also become dead-end hosts for non-human *Sarcocystis* spp. after the accidental ingestion of oocysts.

Both sporulated oocysts (containing two sporocysts) and individual sporocysts can be passed in stool. Sporocysts contain four sporozoites and a refractile residual body. Sporocysts ingested by the intermediate host (cattle for *S. hominis* and pigs for *S. suihominis*) rupture, releasing sporozoites. Sporozoites enter endothelial cells of blood vessels and undergo schizogony, resulting in first-generation schizonts. Merozoites derived from the first generation invade small capillaries and blood vessels, becoming second-generation schizonts. The second-generation merozoites invade skeletal and heart myocytes, as well as neurons, and develop into metrocysts and undergo a series of internal mitotic divisions (endodyogeny). When filled with bradyzoites, the metrocyst becomes a sarcocyst (Fig. 103.2A) that will be infectious when eventually consumed by the definitive host. There is no evidence that rupture of sarcocysts in the intermediate host can initiate new rounds of replication in the intermediate host.

Much of our understanding of the pathogenesis of intestinal infection in humans comes from experiments infecting human volunteers with sarcocysts (although, arguably, unnaturally large numbers were ingested). Several days after exposure, and for several days thereafter, infected persons will excrete oocysts and infective sporocysts in the stool. Although people can experience lengthy, indeed lifelong infection with sarcocysts, the identity and natural history of those parasites remain unknown. Excellent, illustrated reviews of zoonotic sarcocystosis are available [4–6].

CLINICAL MANIFESTATIONS

Human disease can manifest as either an enteric infection or as a muscular infection (Table 103-1) Older reviews of sarcocystis infections in man are available [7, 8].

ENTERIC INFECTION

Most individuals with intestinal sarcocystosis remain asymptomatic and naturally occurring gastrointestinal illness is rare, or rarely recognized. Symptoms induced by experimental challenge include nausea, abdominal discomfort and self-limited diarrhea, with symptom severity dependent on the amount of meat consumed [5]. Onset of diarrhea is generally rapid (in some subjects 3–6 hours post-ingestion), normally within 48 hours of ingestion. Illness is typically brief and self-limited, usually resolving within 36 hours of onset. A segmental, eosinophilic, necrotizing enteritis attributed to sexual forms of *Sarcocystis* has been reported; however, causation in these cases was not definitely established [9]. The intensity of symptoms may be related to the infectious dose of sarcocysts ingested, rather than the infecting species of *Sarcocystis*.

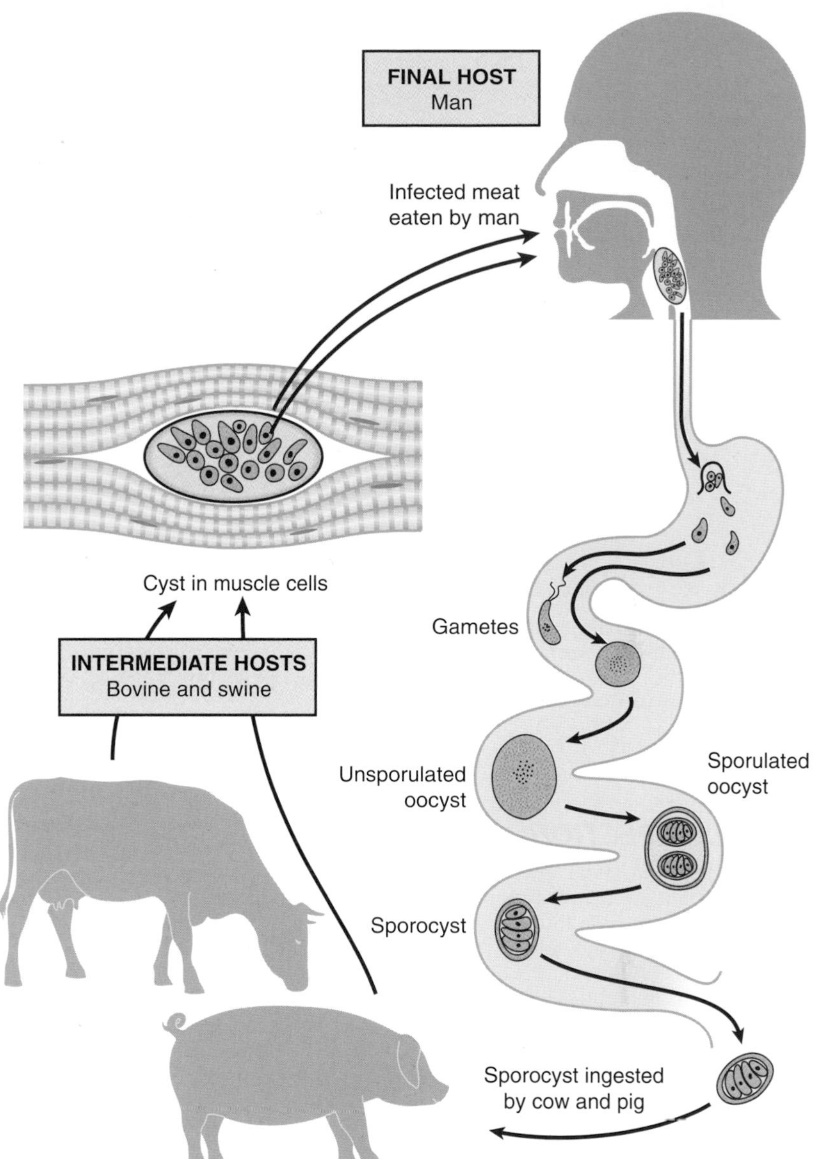

FIGURE 103.1 Schematic representation of the lifecycle of *Sarcocystis hominis* and *Sarcocystis suihominis*. *(reproduced with permission from Murrell KD, Fayer R, Dubey JP. Parasitic Organisms. Advances in Meat Research. West Port, CT: AVI Publishing Co.; 1986.)*

TABLE 103-1 Parasite Development and Disease Manifestations in Humans

Characteristic	Muscular infection	Intestinal infection
Source of infection	Water or food contaminated with feces from unknown carnivore or omnivore	Raw or undercooked meat
Infective stage	Oocyst or free sporocysts	Sarcocyst containing bradyzoites
Developmental stages	Intravascular schizonts (not seen); intramuscular sarcocysts	Sexual stages in lamina propria; oocysts excreted in feces
Time from ingestion of infective stage to symptoms	Weeks to months, lasting months to years	3–6 h, lasting 36 h
Symptoms	Musculoskeletal pain, fever, rash, cardiomyopathy, bronchospasm, subcutaneous swelling	Nausea, loss of appetite, vomiting, stomachache, bloat, diarrhea, dyspnea, and tachycardia
Diagnosis	Biopsy specimen containing sarcocyst; antibodies to bradyzoites	Oocysts or sporocysts in feces, beginning 5–12 days after ingestion
Therapy (none approved)	Co-trimoxazole, furazolidone, albendazole, anticoccidials, pyrimethamine, anti-inflammatories	None

Reproduced with permission from Fayer R. Sarcocystis *spp. in human infections. Clin Microbiol Rev 2004;17:894–902.*

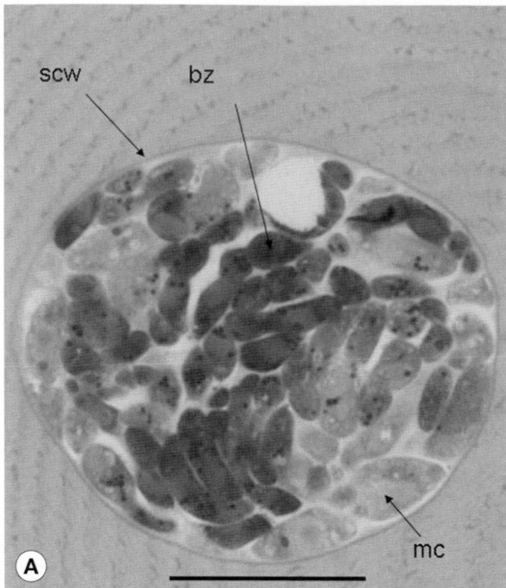

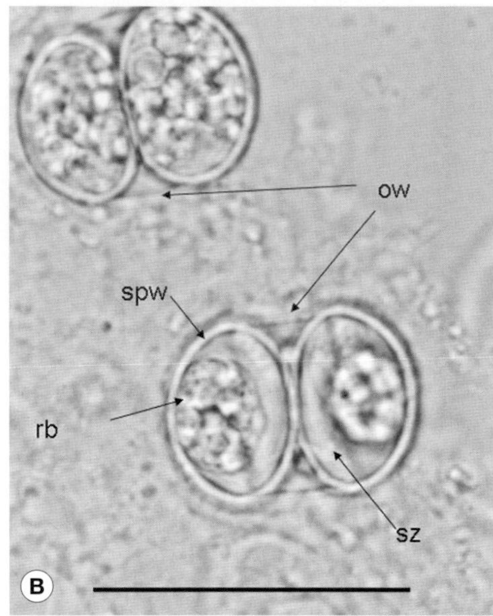

FIGURE 103.2 Photomicrographs of *Sarcocystis muris.* **(A)** Developing sarcocyst in muscle tissue. Immature metrocytes (mc) and mature bradyzoites (bz) are enclosed by the sarcocyst wall (scw). **(B)** Two sporulated oocysts. Sporozoites (sz) and residuum bodie (rb) are enclosed by the prominent sporocysts wall (spw) which, in turn, are paired within the oocyst wall (ow). In many instances, unpaired sporocysts will be recovered owing to rupture of the oocysts wall. The scale bar denotes 20 microns.

MUSCLE INFECTION

As with gastrointestinal involvement, muscular sarcocystosis is usually, but not always, asymptomatic. When humans ingest sporocysts, and thus become intermediate hosts, the release of meronts to the endothelium and subsequent merozoite invasion of striated muscle can correlate with vasculitic and/or musculoskeletal symptomatology. In an outbreak of eosinophilic myositis in a 15-man U.S. military unit operating in Malaysia, an acute illness consisting of fever, myalgias, bronchospasm, fleeting pruritic rashes, transient lymphadenopathy, and subcutaneous nodules associated with eosinophilia, elevated erythrocyte sedimentation rate, and elevated levels of hepatic enzymes and muscle creatinine kinase were reported in 7 out of the 10 exposed personnel [10]. One patient had serious, chronic sequelae; the other team members had milder, self-limited illnesses. Muscle tissue biopsy of the index case showed an unidentified *Sarcocystis* species.

When cases are symptomatic, painful muscle swellings, measuring 1–3 cm in diameter and initially associated with erythema of the overlying skin, occur episodically, and last from 2 days to 4 weeks. Sometimes, lesions are accompanied by fever, diffuse myalgia, muscle tenderness, weakness, eosinophila, and bronchospasm. A discharging sinus, painful swelling with erythema, an ill-defined mass, and chronic pain with ulceration have been reported from New Zealand [11].

DIAGNOSIS

Sporulated sporocysts, each containing four sporozoites, and oocysts containing two sporocysts enclosed by a protective wall, can be visualized microscopically in freshly voided stool specimens with the aid of flotation procedures (Fig. 103.2B). *Sarcocystis* oocysts resemble *Isospora* oocysts – they are acid-fast and contain two sporocysts. Generally, parasite species cannot be differentiated microscopically for clinical practice; however, variation in the 18S rDNA provides a basis to discriminate among excreted parasites [12]. Oocysts measure 15 x 20 μm and sporocysts measure 12 x 6 μm. Owing to the fragile nature of the oocyst wall, individual sporocysts may also be detected in stool. Infection can also be confirmed by visualizing trophozoites or bradyzoites in biopsy tissue.

Definitive diagnosis of sarcocystis myositis is by muscle biopsy. Other muscle cyst-forming organisms, such as *Toxoplasma gondii* and *Trypanosoma cruzi*, must be excluded. Sarcocysts are septate and the cell wall is distinct ultrastructurally. Bradyzoites of *Sarcocystis* and *T. gondii* are periodic acid–Schiff positive, but *T. cruzi* is not. Intact sarcocysts can measure up to 100 μm in diameter and 325 μm in length, but are more often in the 20–60 μm range and are not generally accompanied by an inflammatory reaction in the surrounding tissue. However, if pain is a major complaint, then mild inflammatory reactions are often seen [11].

In the absence of muscle biopsy, eosinophila in the presence of a compatible clinical syndrome and epidemiologic exposure support a probable diagnosis, especially if other diagnoses can be excluded. Serology is difficult to obtain and of uncertain value. Seroprevalence of 10–20% has been described in adults in rural areas of Laos and Tibet [13].

TREATMENT

Because *Sarcocystis* organisms in muscle and intestine are fully formed, terminal stages in the host and parasites will not spread to new cells – treatment directed towards the muscle and enteric infection is unsatisfactory. Although various treatments have been used for symptomatic muscular infection (see Table 103-1) none can be recommended and there is no specific treatment for *Sarcocystis* infection described. Treatment is symptomatic and palliative – corticosteroids should palliate episodic allergic inflammatory reactions following cyst rupture or to alleviate more chronic, systemic symptoms. Because the intracystic bradyzoites are not capable of infecting new cells in the host, there is no risk of recrudescence.

PREVENTION

Muscle involvement can be prevented by avoiding food and water that are potentially contaminated with feces of predatory carnivores. Enteric infection can be prevented by avoiding ingestion of raw or undercooked beef and pork. Sporocysts are hardy, resisting treatment with bleach, chlorhexidine, and the iodophore Betadyne [14]. Most frozen (–20°C) or well-cooked meats are safe, however.

PUBLIC HEALTH BURDEN

The public health burden of human sarcocystosis remains unknown. Although veterinary data implicate immune suppression as a clinical risk factor for sarcocystosis, and although pregnancy and AIDS markedly exacerbate toxoplasmosis (caused by a closely related zoonotic parasite), less is currently known about how vulnerability to sarcocystosis may vary among individuals [15].

Intensive transmission should be limited to those who routinely consume uncooked meat and live where untreated human wastes routinely expose livestock to renewed exposure [9]. Indeed, epidemics have been documented where such circumstances prevail. However, the population at risk for such infections has never been defined with certainty. Prevalent *S. hominis* in European cattle [16], but not in American cattle [17], suggest that geographic variation in risk may occur, even among developed countries.

REFERENCES

1. Murrell KD, Fayer R, Dubey JP. Parasitic Organisms. Advances in Meat Research. West Port, CT: AVI Publishing Co.; 1986.
2. Wilairatana P, Radomyos P, Radomyos B, et al. Intestinal sarcocystosis in Thai laborers. Southeast Asian J Trop Med Public Health 1996;27:43–6.
3. Wong KT, Pathmanathan R. High prevalence of human skeletal muscle sarcocystosis in southeast Asia. Trans R Soc Trop Med Hyg 1992;86:631–2.
4. Dubey JP, Fayer R. Sarcocystosis. Br Vet J 1983;139:371–7.
5. Fayer R. *Sarcocystis* spp. in human infections. Clin Microbiol Rev 2004;17: 894–902.
6. Dubey JP, Speer CA, Fayer R. Sarcocystosis of animals and man. Boca Raton: CRC Press; 1989.
7. Jeffrey HC. Sarcosporidiosis in man. Trans R Soc Trop Med Hyg 1974;68:17–29.
8. Beaver PC, Gadgil K, Morera P. *Sarcocystis* in man: a review and report of five cases. Am J Trop Med Hyg 1979;28:819–44.
9. Bunyaratvej S, Unpunyo P, Pongtippan A. The *Sarcocystis*-cyst containing beef and pork as the sources of natural intestinal sarcocystosis in Thai people. J Med Assoc Thai 2007;90:2128–35.
10. Arness MK, Brown JD, Dubey JP, et al. An outbreak of acute eosinophilic myositis attributed to human *Sarcocystis* parasitism. Am J Trop Med Hyg 1999;61:548–53.
11. Mehrotra R, Bisht D, Singh PA, et al. Diagnosis of human *Sarcocystis* infection from biopsies of the skeletal muscle. Pathology 1996;28:281–2.
12. Xiang Z, Chen X, Yang L, et al. Non-invasive methods for identifying oocysts of *Sarcocystis* spp. from definitive hosts. Parasitol Int 2009;58:293–6.
13. Giboda M, Ditrich O, Scholz T, et al. Current status of food-borne parasitic zoonoses in Laos. Southeast Asian J Trop Med Public Health 1991;22 (suppl.):56–61.
14. Dubey JP, Saville WJ, Sreekumar C, et al. Effects of high temperature and disinfectants on the viability of *Sarcocystis* neurona sporocysts. J Parasitol 2002;88:1252–4.
15. Velásquez JN, Di Risio C, Etchart CB, et al. Systemic sarcocystosis in a patient with acquired immune deficiency syndrome. Hum Pathol 2008;39:1263–7.
16. Vangeel L, Houf K, Chiers K, et al. Molecular-based identification of *Sarcocystis hominis* in Belgian minced beef. J Food Prot 2007;70:1523–6.
17. Pritt B, Trainer T, Simmons-Arnold L, et al. Detection of *Sarcocystis* parasites in retail beef: a regional survey combining histological and genetic detection methods. J Food Prot 2008;71:2144–7.

104 Microsporidiosis

Louis M Weiss

Key features

- Microsporidia are a diverse group of obligate intracellular eukaryotic parasites most closely related to fungi
- Microsporidia form characteristic spores that are diagnostic for the phylum. Spores possess a unique organelle—the polar tubule or polar filament—which is coiled inside the spore
- Spores of species associated with human infection measure 1–4 μm
- While Microsporidia can infect immunocompetent hosts, they are more commonly seen in the setting of cell-mediated immune dysfunction
- The most common manifestations of infection are diarrhea and keratoconjunctivitis; however, Microsporidia can infect virtually any organ, causing a variety of symptoms, including disseminated disease, hepatitis, myositis, kidney and urogenital infection, ascites, cholangitis, and asymptomatic carriage
- Examination of stool or urine specimens using special stains is a practical method for the diagnosis of microsporidiosis. Definitive species diagnosis requires transmission electron microscopy visualization of spore ultrastructure or molecular methods (PCR)
- Albendazole is the drug of choice to treat gastroenteritis caused by *Encephalitozoon intestinalis* and to treat disseminated microsporidiosis with or without local manifestations (*Encephalitozoon hellem, Encephalitozoon cuniculi, E. intestinalis, Pleistophora* sp., *Trachipleistophora* sp., *Brachiola vesicularum*)
- Fumagillin is the drug of choice to treat gastroenteritis and disseminated infection caused by *Enterocytozoon bieneusi*, but is associated with thrombocytopenia
- The treatment of choice for ocular microsporidiosis (*E. hellem, E. cuniculi, Vittaforma corneae*) is oral albendazole plus topical fumagillin. Corneal infections with *V. corneae* often do not respond to chemotherapy and may require keratoplasty

INTRODUCTION

First recognized by Nageli in 1857 as the cause of disease in silkworms, microsporidia were not suspected as being a cause of human disease until 1959, when they were found in a child with encephalitis. Conclusive evidence of Microsporidia as pathogens dates to 1973, when a 4-month-old athymic boy died with severe diarrhea and malabsorption caused by *Nosema* (now *Anncaliia*) *connori* (Fig. 104.1). Interest and knowledge of microsporidia as parasites of man have expanded dramatically since they were first described as a cause of persistent diarrhea and systemic disease in persons with AIDS [1].

Microsporidia are obligate intracellular parasites which are classified in a separate phylum—the Microsporidia—consisting of approximately 170 genera and more than 1200 species [2, 3]. They are classified based on their ultrastructural features, including size and morphology of the spores, number of coils of the polar tube, developmental lifecycle and host–parasite relationship [4]. Molecular data, based primarily on small subunit RNA genes, have also been used to define taxonomic relationships and for the diagnosis of these pathogens. Although traditionally believed to be "primitive" protozoa, molecular phylogenetic analysis has suggested that the Microsporidia are instead related to the Fungi [5, 6]. The genome size of the Microsporidia varies from 2.3 to 19.5 Mb with that of the Encephalitizoonidae being less than 3.0 Mb, making them among the smallest eukaryotic nuclear genomes so far identified.

EPIDEMIOLOGY

The Microsporidia infect virtually all animal phyla, including other protists. They have a worldwide distribution and are important agricultural parasites in insects, fish, and mammals. They have been found in every tissue and organ, and spores are common in environmental sources [2]. Many human infections are likely zoonotic and/or transmitted by water [7]. Domestic and wild animals may be naturally infected with *E. cuniculi, E. intestinalis*, and *Enterocytozoon bieneusi*. Birds, especially parrots (parakeets, love birds, budgies), are naturally infected with *E. hellem*. *Enterocytozoon bieneusi* and *V. corneae* have

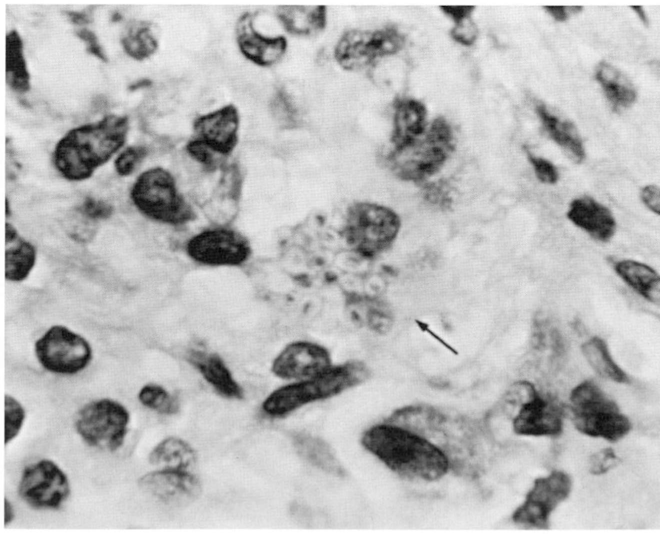

FIGURE 104.1 *Anncaliia (Nosema) connori* (arrow) in a human infant (×1260) *(courtesy of Drs Daniel Connor and Ann Cali, and the Armed Forces Institute of Pathology, Photograph Neg. No. 71–5882).*

been identified in surface waters, and spores of *Nosema* sp. (likely *Anncaliia algerae*) have been identified in ditchwater. Human-to-human transmission is likely although not proven.

Prevalence of microsporidiosis varies from not detected to over 80% depending on the geographic region, method of diagnosis and demographic characteristics of the population being studied. Microsporidiosis is increasingly recognized in non-HIV-infected populations, such as travelers, children, the elderly and organ transplant recipients. Most infections in immunocompetant and naïve hosts are likely self-limited or asymptomatic. Current understanding suggests that Microsporidia are as common in humans as they are in other mammals, and are associated with travel or residence in developing nations [8]. Microsporidal keratitis is increasingly recognized in endemic areas and is likely associated with exposure to soil, muddy water and minor trauma, with higher incidence during the rainy season [9].

NATURAL HISTORY, PATHOGENESIS, AND PATHOLOGY

The Microsporidia are single-cell, intracellular parasites containing a nucleus with a nuclear envelope, an intracytoplasmic membrane system, chromosome separation on mitotic spindles, a vesicular Golgi and a mitochondrial "remnant". The infectious spore is characteristic of the phylum: it is unicellular with an environmentally-resistant spore wall, one or two nuclei and an extrusion apparatus consisting of a single polar tube with an anterior attachment complex. During germination, the polar tube rapidly everts forming a hollow tube that both transports and inoculates the sporoplasm into the host cell [2].

Most microsporidial infections occur when infectious spores are ingested or inhaled. *Enterocytozoon bieneusi*, the most frequently encountered intestinal microsporidia in patients with AIDS, primarily causes intestinal infections with less frequent extra-intestinal infections. Like *E. bieneusi*, *Encephalitozoon intestinalis* may infect enterocytes and cause chronic diarrhea. However, through the infection of macrophages, *E. intestinalis* can disseminate to different organs, especially the kidneys, from which spores are shed in the urine.

The lifecycle of microsporidia begins when the spores germinate, resulting in the extrusion of its polar tubule and infects a host epithelial cell or is phagocytosed by a host cell. The spore injects the infective sporoplasm into the eukaryotic host cell or into a parasitophorous vacuole through the polar tubule. Inside the cell, the sporoplasm undergoes extensive multiplication either by merogony (binary fission) or schizogony (multiple fission). This development can occur either in direct contact with the host cell cytoplasm (e.g. *E. bieneusi*) or inside a parasitophorous vacuole (e.g. *E. intestinalis*). Either free in the cytoplasm or inside a parasitophorous vacuole, microsporidia develop by sporogony to mature spores. During sporogony, a thick wall is formed around the spore, which provides resistance to adverse environmental conditions. When the spores increase in number and completely fill the host cell cytoplasm, the cell membrane is disrupted and releases the spores to the surroundings. These free mature spores can infect new cells, thus continuing the cycle.

Within their hosts, most species infect the digestive tract, but reproductive, respiratory, muscular, excretory and nervous system infections are well documented [2]. Microsporidiosis in humans is most often identified in the setting of immune deficiencies (especially in patients with AIDS) [7]. A strong humoral response occurs during infection and includes antibodies that react with the spore wall and polar tube. The immunosuppressed states associated with microsporidiosis (e.g. AIDS and transplantation) are characterized by defects in cell-mediated immunity. Spontaneous cure of microsporidiosis can be induced by immune reconstitution with combination anti-retroviral treatment (cART) [10].

CLINICAL FEATURES

Microsporidian genera associated with human disease and their site of infection are described in Table 104-1. Human microsporidiosis represents an important and emerging opportunistic disease, occurring mainly, but not exclusively, in severely immunocompromised patients with AIDS. Additionally, cases of microsporidiosis in immunocompromised persons not infected with HIV, as well as in immunocompetent persons, also have been reported. Microsporidia is likely a common enteric pathogen causing self-limited disease and asymptomatic carriage. The clinical manifestations of microsporidiosis are very diverse, varying according to the causal species, with chronic or persistent diarrhea being the most common presenting syndrome. Microsporidiosis can also present as keratoconjunctivitis, disseminated disease, hepatitis, myositis, kidney and urogenital infection, ascites and/or cholangitis.

The genus *Microsporidium* is used to designate Microsporidia of uncertain taxonomic status. No one genus is uniquely associated with a specific clinical syndrome; rather, there is considerable overlap in clinical disease across species.

INFECTIONS IN IMMUNE COMPETENT PATIENTS

Chronic diarrhea and ocular infections are the most common presentations in immunocompetent hosts. *Enterocytozoon bieneusi* has been identified as a cause of self-limited diarrhea in immunocompetent patients and travelers, and has been found in up to 10% of African children with diarrhea. *Encephalitozoon intestinalis* was found in 8% of the stools of patients in a survey for the etiology of diarrhea in Mexico and has been seen in travelers with chronic diarrhea (Fig. 104-2). Cerebral infections owing to *Encephalitozoon* sp. were identified serologically in a 3-year-old boy with seizures and hepatomegaly and a 9-year-old Japanese boy with headache, vomiting, spastic convulsions and recurrent fever. An unidentified Microsporidia responsive to albendazole was described causing multiple cerebral lesions in a 33- year-old man in Japan. *Pleistophora spp.* have been identified in the skeletal muscle of an HIV-negative patient with myositis.

Ocular infections with ulcer or deep cornea stroma infection associated with eye pain have been reported in immune-competent patients [11]. In 1973 and 1981, two cases were documented in immune

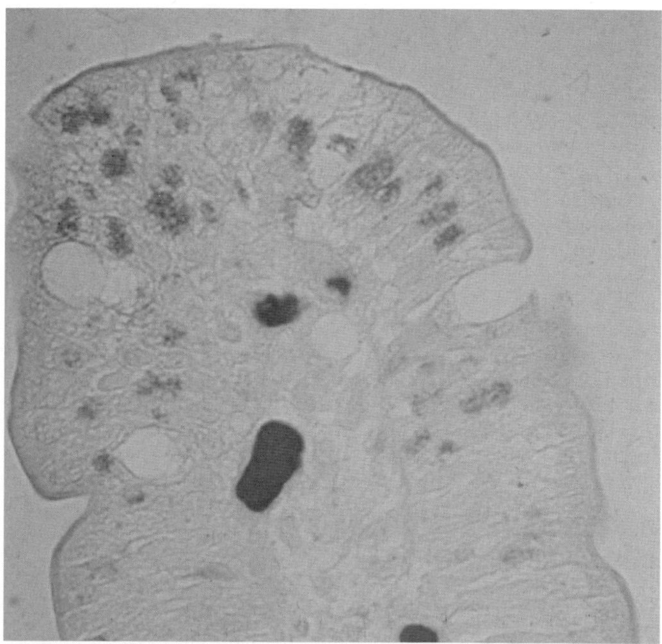

FIGURE 104.2 *Encephalitozoon intestinalis* gastrointestinal tract infection. As can be seen in this tissue section stained with a modified trichrome stain, this organism is present on the apical and basal surface as well as in the lamina propria. This is consistent with a disseminating infection *(courtesy of Drs Donald P. Kotler and Jan M. Orensten).*

TABLE 104-1 Microsporida Identified as Pathogenic in Humans

Microsporidian genus and species	Clinical manifestation (syndromes in bold described in immunocompetent hosts)
Genus Encephalitozoon	
*Encephalitozoon intestinalis (*syn. *Septata intestinalis)*	**Chronic diarrhea**, intestinal perforation, keratoconjunctivitis, cholangitis, nephritis, osteomyelitis of the mandible and upper respiratory infections
Encephalitozoon cuniculi	**Chronic diarrhea, encephalitis (with seizures)**, peritonitis, urethritis, cellulitis, prostatitis, sinusitis, keratoconjunctivitis, cholangitis, cystitis, hepatitis, nephritis and disseminated infection with fever
Encephalitozoon hellem	Keratoconjunctivitis, sinusitis, pneumonitis, nephritis, cystitis, urethritis, prostatits, diarrhea and disseminated infection
Genus Enterocytozoon	
Enterocytozoon bieneusi	**Chronic diarrhea**, acalculous cholecystitis, wasting syndrome, sinusitis, rhinitis and can invade cholangioepithelium leading to sclerosing cholangitis, cholangiopathy and cholecystitis
Genus Trachipleistophora	
Trachipleistophora anthropophthera	Disseminated infection, keratoconjunctivits, encephalitis
Trachipleistophora hominis	Myositis, stromal keratitis, (probably disseminated infection)
Genus Pleisitophora	
Pleistophora ronneafiei and *Pleistophora* sp.	**Myositis**
***Genus Anncaliia* (syn. *Brachiola*)**	
A. vesicularum	Myositis
A. connori	Disseminated infection
A. algerae	Keratoconjunctivits, myositis, cellulitis
Genus Nosema/Vittaforma	
Nosema ocularum	**Keratoconjunctivitis**
Vittaforma (Nosema) corneae	**Keratoconjunctivitis**, urinary tract infections
Genus Microsporidium	
Microsporidium africanus	**Corneal ulcer**
Microsporidium ceylonensis	**Corneal ulcer**

competent patients from Botswana (*Microsporidium africanus*) and Sri Lanka (*M. ceylonesis)*. Other cases of keratitis have since been identified to be caused by *Nosema ocularum* and *N. corneum* (now *V. cornea*). Treatment of these infections has often required surgery (keratoplasty and/or corneal transplant). *Encephalitozoon* spp. and *Trachipleistophora anthropophthera* corneal infections have been described in contact lens-wearers. These infections have responded to topical therapy. In a report from India on 40 immune competent patients, epidemic keratoconjuctivits has been associated with Microsporidia [12]. Many of these resolved without specific treatment.

INFECTIONS IN PATIENTS WITH IMMUNE DEFICIENCIES

While the majority of reported infections have been in patients with AIDS (and CD4 counts less than 100 cells/mm^3), infections have been seen in organ transplantation patients, patients with various hematologic malignancies and those being treated with immunosuppressive medications (especially antibodies to tumor necrosis factor [TNF]-α). Gastrointestinal infection usually involves chronic diarrhea of 3–10 bowel movements per day, anorexia, weight loss and bloating without associated fever. It is usually caused by *E. bieneusi* and, occasionally, *E. intestinalis;* however, other microsporida have also been demonstrated in cases of diarrheal disease (e.g. *Anncaliia connori, Vittaforma spp., E. hellem, E. cuniculi*). In patients undergoing liver and bone marrow transplantation, clinical manifestations have included watery, non-bloody diarrhea; nausea; and diffuse abdominal pain. Kotler and Orenstein found that 39% of patients with HIV and diarrhea, presenting to a gastroenterology clinic had microsporidosis and that the presence of Microsporidia was associated with wasting, a mean CD4 count of 28 cells/mm^3 and an abnormal D-xylose test result, whereas only 2.6% of HIV-infected patients without diarrhea had microsporidiosis [13]. Coyle and colleagues, using PCR employing primers to the small subunit rRNA gene of *E. bieneusi*, also found a significant association between the presence of diarrhea and Microsporidia in patients with AIDS [11].

Ocular infection in immune compromised hosts has been restricted to the superficial epithelium of the cornea and conjunctiva (i.e. superficial keratoconjunctivitis) (Fig. 104.3). This keratitis rarely progresses to corneal ulceration. Most patients present with bilateral coarse punctate epithelial keratopathy and conjunctival inflammation resulting in redness, foreign body sensation, photophobia and changes in visual acuity [14]. Biopsy specimens examined with transmission electron microscopy (TEM) have revealed numerous microsporidian

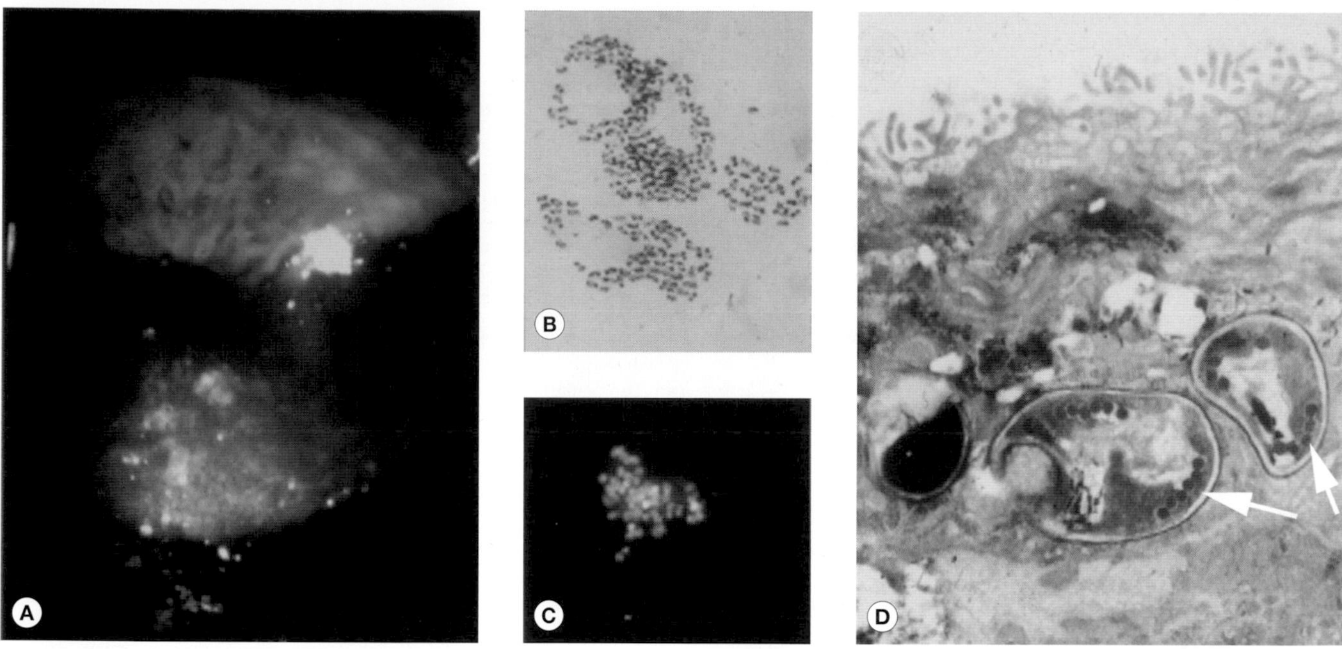

FIGURE 104.3 *Encephalitozoon hellem* keratoconjunctivitis. **(A)** Slit lamp examination demonstrating punctuate keratoconjunctivitis, **(B)** conjunctival scraping stained with Giemsa demonstrating organisms with typical morphology of microsporidia, **(C)** conjunctival scraping stained with calcofluor white demonstrating fluorescent spores, **(D)** TEM of *Encephalitozoon hellem* in conjunctival tissue from a patient with keratoconjunctivitis. The characteristic coiled polar tube is present in cross section (arrows).

spores within the corneal and conjunctival epithelium. Of the reports in the literature of microsporidian keratitis caused by Encephalitozoonidae, all but three have been attributed to *E. hellem*, including three cases originally classified as *E. cuniculi*. *Trachipleistophora* spp. has also been associated with keratoconjunctivitis in patients with AIDS and *Anncaliia algerae* in a patient with hematological malignancy. Ocular disease is usually associated with disseminated disease and examination of urine sediments for can confirm microsporidian spores. Physical examination reveals conjunctival hyperemia with superficial punctate keratopathy. Slit lamp examination usually demonstrates punctate epithelial opacities, granular epithelial cells (with irregular flourescein uptake), conjunctival injection, superficial corneal infiltrates and an inflamed anterior chamber.

Several species of Microsporidia have been described as causing myositis in patients with immune deficiencies, often with associated disseminated infections. These cases have presented with myalgias, weakness, elevated serum creatinine phosphokinase and aldolase levels, and abnormal electromyography consistent with an inflammatory myopathy. *Trachipleistophora hominis* has been described in several patients with AIDS as a cause of disseminated disease with an associated myositis. *Trachipleistophora anthropophthera* was described in several patients with AIDS having encephalitis associated with myositis. *Anncaliia* (*Brachiola*) *vesicularum* and *Pleistophora ronneafiei* have been reported as isolated cases of myositis. Myositis was documented to be caused by *A. algerae* in a patient with rheumatoid arthritis treated with steroids and monoclonal antibody to TNF-α (Fig. 104.4). Systemic infection with *V. corneae* has been reported in a patient with AIDS. In a child with leukemia, skin infection with involvement of the cellular elements of the dermis caused by *A. algerae* has been reported.

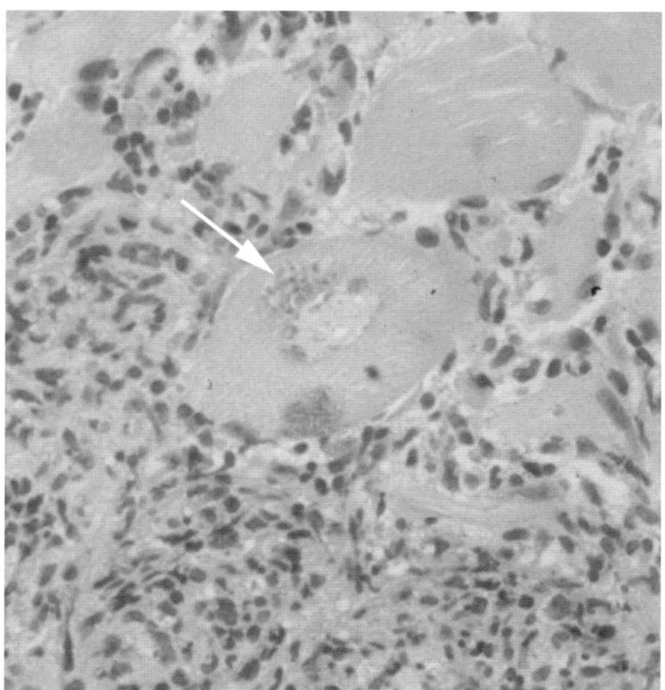

FIGURE 104.4 *Anncaliia (Bracheola) algerae* myositis. The organisms are found in muscle fibers (arrow) with inflammatory cells in the surrounding supporting tissue.

PATIENT EVALUATION, DIAGNOSIS, AND DIFFERENTIAL DIAGNOSIS

A confirmed diagnosis of microspordiosis requires parasitologic confirmation of the parasite in a clinical specimen with an appropriate laboratory test. There are several methods useful for diagnosing suspected microsporidiosis.

Examination of stool specimens by light microscopy using modified trichrome stain (chromotrope 2R) (Fig. 104.5), Uvitex 2B or calcofluor white is the standard method for diagnosing gastrointestinal microsporidiosis. Overall, the sensitivity of Uvitex 2B and calcofluor white is slightly higher than that of modified trichrome stain; however, the specificity of the chemofluorescent stains is lower. Microscopy does not allow identification of microsporidia to the species level.

TABLE 104-2 Treatment Options for Microspordiosis

Organism	Preferred therapy	Dose and duration	Other options/issues
All disseminated (systemic) Microsporidian Infections except *Enterocytozoon bieneusi*	Albendazole*	400 mg twice daily × 4 weeks	• If patient has AIDS, initiate or optimize cART regimens with goal of immune reconstitution to CD4 >100 cells/μL. In patients with AIDS and low CD4 counts, immune reconstitution with optimized cART should be considered the intervention of choice along with the concurrent initiation of albendazole. Continue albendazole treatment until CD4 >200 cells/μL • Fluid support in patients with diarrhea resulting in severe dehydration • Nutritional supplement for patients with severe malnutrition and wasting • The pediatric dose of albendazole is 10mg/kg/day not to exceed the adult dose of 800 mg per day. • Duration of treatment for microsporididosis is not well established. Relapse may occur on discontinuation of albendazole. Prolonged treatment may be required
Gastrointestinal infections caused by *Enterocytozon bieneusi*	Oral fumagillin	20 mg three times daily or 60 mg once daily	• Fumagillin is not available in the USA. Use requires IND to import to the US. Consult with Sanofi-Adventis, France • There is no known pediatric dose adjustment for oral fumagillin • Thrombocytopenia is a known drug-related adverse reaction • Oral albendazole results in modest clinical improvement in about 50% of patients in some studies and no improvement in others
Ocular infections	Fumagillin solution (Fumidil B 3mg/mL in saline or fumagillin 70 μg/ml)	Two drops every 2 hours for 4 days; then 2 drops 4 times daily	• Treatment for ocular infection should be continued indefinitely • Chronic maintenance therapy may be discontinued if patients: (1) remain asymptomatic with regards to signs and symptoms of microsporidiosis; and (2) sustained CD4+ T-lymphocyte counts >200 cells/μL for ≥6 months on ART • Pediatric dose is topical therapy as per the adult dose • Ocular infection frequently accompanied by disseminated infection, may also require oral albendazole

*Although albendazole is a Food and Drug Administration-approved drug, there is no approved indication for microsporididosis.
Adapted from Wittner M, Weiss LM. The Microsporidia and Microsporidiosis. Washington, DC: ASM Press; 1999:xvii,1:1–553.
cART, combined anti-retroviral therapy; IND, investigational new drug application.

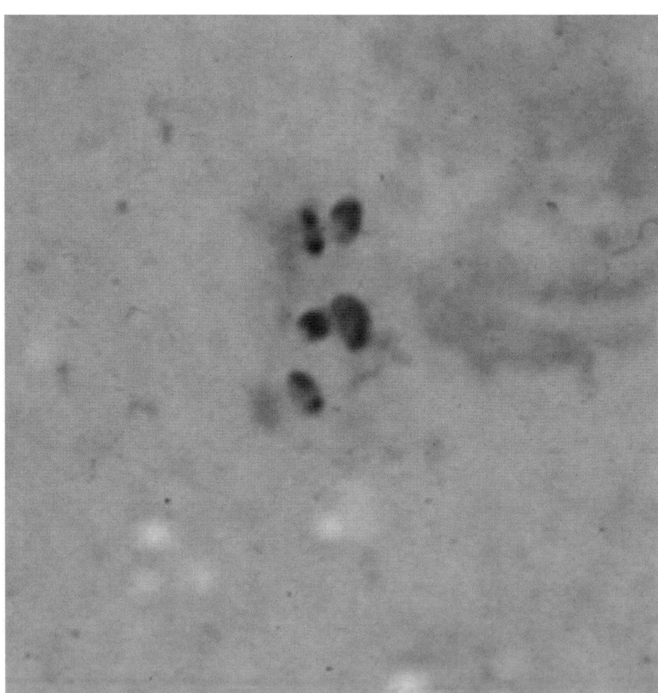

FIGURE 104.5 *Enterocytozoon bieneusi* in a fecal specimen, visualized with modified trichrome stain (chromotrope 2R).

The most widely used staining technique is the Chromotrope 2R method or its modifications. This technique stains the spore and the spore wall a bright pinkish red. Often, a belt-like stripe, which also stains pinkish red, is seen in the middle of the spore. However, this technique is lengthy and time consuming, requiring about 90 min. The "Quick-Hot Gram Chromotrope technique" cuts down the staining time to less than 10 minutes and provides a good differentiation from the lightly stained background fecal materials so that the spores stand out for easy visualization [15]. The spores stain dark violet and the belt-like stripe is enhanced. In some cases, dark staining Gram-positive granules are also clearly seen. Chemofluorescent agents, such as Calcofluor white, are also useful in the quick identification of spores in fecal smears. The spores measure 0.8–1.4 μm in the case of *E. bieneusi* and 1.5–4 μm in *B. algerae*, *Encephalitozoon* spp., *V. corneae*, and *Nosema* spp. If stool examination is negative in the setting of chronic diarrhea (more than two months' duration), endoscopy should be performed. In patients with enteric microsporidiosis undergoing endoscopy, the small intestine has provided the highest diagnostic yield, but organisms have also been seen in colonic biopsy material.

Definitive species diagnosis of microsporidiosis currently requires TEM visualization of spore ultrastructure (Fig. 104.3D) and developmental stages or molecular methods (PCR). TEM is expensive, time-consuming and not feasible for routine diagnosis. Species-specific rRNA primers for PCR have been described and are available in reference laboratories [e.g. Centers for Disease Control and Prevention (CDC)]. Thus, molecular diagnosis with species-specific PCR primers is commonly believed to be the gold standard for identification of microsporidian species [16].

As renal involvement with shedding of spores in the urine is common in all of the species of Microsporidia that disseminate, urine specimens should be obtained whenever the diagnosis of microsporidiosis is considered. This has therapeutic implications, as the Microsporidia that disseminate (e.g. *Encephalitozoon*) are usually sensitive to albendazole, whereas those that do not disseminate (e.g. *E. bieneusi*) are resistant. In tissue sections (Figs 104.2 and 104.5), touch preparations or corneal scrapings (Figs 104.3B, C), Microsporidia are discernible with hematoxylin-eosin, Giemsa, tissue Gram or chromotrope 2R stains. Histologically, microsporidian spores are easily discernible with a modified tissue chromotrope 2R or tissue Gram stain (Brown-Hopp or Brown-Brenn) in sections prepared from fixed tissue using routine procedures.

TREATMENT (Table 104-1)

Microsporidiosis is primarily an opportunistic infection in the immunocompromised host.

Studies have demonstrated that immune reconstitution can result in clinical response in patients with microsporidiosis secondary to immune dysfunction. Immune reconstitution with cART in patients with AIDS or reversal of iatrogenic immunosuppression, when possible, is an important management principle [2].

Immune reconstitution syndrome (IRIS) has been reported in a patient with microsporidiosis treated with anti-retroviral therapy [17]; however, based on clinical experience, IRIS reactions are not common in this setting. Aspartyl protease inhibitors of HIV have been shown to inhibit replication of *E. intestinalis* in tissue culture.

Albendazole is a benzimidazole effective against many helminths and protozoa that inhibits microtubule assembly. Albendazole was initially shown effective in severely immunosuppressed (<50 CD4 cells/ml) patients with AIDS with systemic disease, disseminated infection with *E. intestinalis* and chronic diarrhea. Treatment with albendazole 400 mg twice daily resulted in a dramatic and rapid clinical resolution of diarrhea and transient elimination of the organism from feces and urine [18]. In a subsequent small, randomized, double-blind, controlled trial, albendazole at 400 mg twice daily for three weeks led to rapid clinical improvement and elimination of the pathogen [19]. Prevention of relapse is best accomplished by immune reconstitution but albendazole at 400mg twice daily was shown to significantly delay relapse [19]. Treatment with albendazole for intestinal disease caused by *E. bieneusi* in patients with AIDS has not proven effective. Albendazole at 400 mg twice daily for one month in patients with chronic diarrhea, weight loss and malabsorption did not clear infection, although there was a statistically significant decrease in bowel movements from seven per day to four per day [20].

Albendazole has also been used for the treatment of clinical syndromes caused by microsporidia other than *E. intestinalis* although clinical trial data is lacking. Clinical and radiographic improvement was seen in a case of chronic sinusitis caused by *E. hellem* treated with albendazole 400 mg bid. Marked clinical improvement with albendazole occurred in a patient with disseminated infection caused by *E. cuniculi* involving the conjunctiva, sinuses, kidneys and lungs. Resolution of myositis was noted in patients infected with a *Nosema*-like microsporidian and in a case of disseminated infection with myositis caused by *T. hominis* treated with albendazole. Albendazole as a systemic agent is indicated if the organism is demonstrated in the urine or in nasal smears of patients with keratoconjunctivitis.

Albendazole is recommended for the treatment of acute microsporidial infections in immunocompetant non-immune children in endemic areas and also returning travelers. In a randomized, open study in Costa Rica, albendazole at 15 mg/kg/day twice a day for seven days was effective in improving clinical symptoms and decreasing duration of illness from 10 days to 5 days in children ages 6–36 months [21].The data in returning adult travelers are less robust but if microsporidial spores are detected in a patent with persistent diarrhea, a trial of albendazole would be indicated [22].

Fumagillin, an antibiotic derived from the fungus *Aspergillus fumigatus*, have *in vitro* and *in vivo* activity against *E. cuniculi*, *E. hellem*, *E. intestinalis*, *E. bieneusi*, *Nucleospora* (*Ent.*) *salmonis*, and *V. corneae*. Fumagillin has been demonstrated in a dose-escalation trial, case reports and a randomized clinical trial to be effective for the treatment of human infection with *E. bieneusi* at a dose of 60 mg/day (20 mg three times daily) for 2 weeks [23]. The main limiting toxicity of treatment was thrombocytopenia beginning about a week after initiation of treatment and reaching a nadir three days after the end of treatment. Thrombocytopenia was reversible in 1–2 weeks on stopping fumagillin treatment. Complete blood counts should be monitored every other day and the drug discontinued if platelet counts fall below 75,000 per cubic millimeter. Oral fumagillin at 20 mg/kg 3 or 4 times daily for 7–10 days is also recommended in transplant-associated microsporidiosis caused by *E. bienusi*, although the optimal dose regimen has not been defined [24].

Solutions of the soluble salt, Fumidil B (fumagillin bicylohexylammonium), applied topically have been demonstrated to be nontoxic to the cornea and treatment of ocular microsporidiosis can be accomplished using a 3-mg/ml solution of Fumidil B in saline (fumagillin 70 μg/ml) [11]. Treatment should probably be continued indefinitely, as recurrence has been reported upon stopping the drops.

The efficacy of imidazole compounds on microsporidiosis is variable. Other medications used without success in the treatment of gastrointestinal microsporidiosis are azithromycin, metronidazole, paromomycin, sulfamethoxazole and quinacrine.

Microsporidal keratitis with and without systemic involvement is a specialized clinical manifestation that requires management in conjunction with an ophthalmologist. Topical flouroquinolones as monotherapy or in combination with topical fumagillin, topical steroids and systemic albendazole may all be appropriate depending on the extent of infection [25].

For a review of drugs used in microsporidiosis in humans and animals see Costa and Weiss [26]. Neither oral nor topical fumagillin is an approved drug by the United States Food and Drug Administration (FDA) and are not easily available in the USA.

PREVENTION

As the Microsporida that infect humans are likely food- or water-borne pathogens, standard sanitary measures that prevent contamination of food and water with the urine and feces of animals should decrease the chance for infection. Hand-washing and general hygienic habits probably reduce the chance for contamination of the conjunctiva and cornea in contact lens wearers. The presence of infective spores in various bodily fluids suggests that universal precautions in healthcare settings and general attention to hand-washing and other personal hygiene measures should be useful in preventing primary infections. Immune compromised patients may wish to consider using bottled or filtered water in some settings. No prophylactic anti-parasitic agents have been identified for these organisms.

REFERENCES

1. Desportes I, Le Charpentier Y, Galian A, et al. Occurrence of a new microsporidan: *Enterocytozoon bieneusi* n.g., n. sp., in the enterocytes of a human patient with AIDS. J Protozool 1985;32:250–4.
2. Wittner M, Weiss LM. The Microsporidia and Microsporidiosis. Washington, DC: ASM Press; 1999:xvii,1:1–553.
3. Didier ES. Microsporidiosis: an emerging and opportunistic infection in humans and animals. Acta Trop 2005;94:61–76.
4. Sprague V, Becnel JJ, Hazard EI. Taxonomy of the phylum Microspora. Crit Rev Microbiol 1992;18:285.
5. Weiss LM, Vossbrinck CR. Microsporidiosis: molecular and diagnostic aspects. Adv Parasitol 1998;40:351–95.
6. Lee SC, Corradi N, Byrnes EJ, 3rd, et al. Microsporidia evolved from ancestral sexual fungi. Curr Biol 2008;18:1675–9.
7. Weber R, Bryan RT, Schwartz DA, Owen RL. Human microsporidial infections. Clin Microbiol 1994;7:426.

8. Didier ES, Stovall ME, Green LC, et al. Epidemiology of microsporidiosis: sources and modes of transmission. Vet Parasitol 2004;126:145–66.
9. Sharma S, Das S, Joseph J, et al. Microsporidial keratitis: need for increased awareness. Surv Ophthalmol 2011;56:1–22.
10. Khan I, Moretto M, Weiss LM. Immune response against *Encephalitozoon cuniculi* infection. Microbes Infect 2001;3:401–5.
11. Coyle CM, Wittner M, Kotler DP, et al. Prevalence of microsporidiosis *(Enterocytozoon bieneusi* and *Encephalitozoon [Septata] intestinalis)* in AIDS related diarrhea as determined by the polymerase chain reaction to microsporidian small subunit ribosomal RNA. Clin Infect Dis 1996;23:1002.
12. Das S, Sharma S, Sahu SK, et al. New microbial spectrum of epidemic keratoconjunctivitis: clinical and laboratory aspects of an outbreak. Br J Ophthalmol 2008;92:861–2.
13. Kotler DP, Orenstein JM. Prevalence of intestinal microsporidiosis in HIV infected individuals referred for gastroenterological evaluation. Am J Gastroenterol 1994;89:1998.
14. Rastrelli PD, Didier ES, Yee RW. Microsporidial keratitis. Ophthalmol Clin North Am 1994;7:617.
15. Moura H, Schwartz DA, Bornay-Llinares F, et al. A new and improved "quick-hot Gram-chromotrope" technique that differentially stains microsporidian spores in clinical samples, including paraffin-embedded tissue sections. Arch Pathol Lab Med 1997;121:888–93.
16. Weiss LM, Vossbrinck CR. Microsporidiosis: molecular and diagnostic aspects. Adv Parasitol 1998;40:351–95.
17. Sriaroon C, Mayer CA, Chen L, et al. Diffuse intra-abdominal granulomatous seeding as a manifestation of immune reconstitution inflammatory syndrome associated with microsporidiosis in a patient with HIV. STDS 2008;22:611–12.
18. Molina JM, Oksenhendler E, Beauvais B, et al. Disseminated microsporidiosis due to *Septata intestinalis* in patients with AIDS: Clinical features and response to albendazole therapy. J Infect Dis 1995;171:245.
19. Molina JM, Chastang C, Goguel J, et al. Albendazole for treatment and prophylaxis of microsporidiosis due to *Encephalitozoon intestinalis* in patients with AIDS: a randomized double-blind controlled trial. J Infect Dis 1998;177:1373–7.
20. Dieterich DT, Lew EA, Kotler DP, et al. Treatment with albendazole for intestinal disease due to *Enterocytozoon bieneusi* in patients with AIDS. J Infect Dis 1994;169:178–83.
21. Tremoulet AH, Avila-Aguero ML, París MM, et al. Albendazole therapy for Microsporidium diarrhea in immunocompetent Costa Rican children. Pediatr Infect Dis J 2004;23:915–18.
22. Wichro E, Hoelzl D, Krause R, et al. Microsporidiosis in travel-associated chronic diarrhea in immune-competent patients. Am J Trop Med Hyg 2005;73:285–7.
23. Molina JM, Tourneur M, Sarfati C, et al. Fumagillin treatment of intestinal microsporidiosis. N Engl J Med 2002;346:1963–9.
24. Lanternier F, Boutboul D, Menotti J, et al. Microsporidiosis in solid organ transplant recipients: two Enterocytozoon bieneusi cases and review. Transpl Infect Dis 2009;11:83–8.
25. Loh RS, Chan CM, Ti SE, et al. Emerging prevalence of microsporidial keratitis in Singapore: epidemiology, clinical features, and management. Ophthalmology 2009;116:2348–53.
26. Costa SF, Weiss LM. Drug treatment of microsporidiosis. Drug Resist Update 2000;3:384–99.

Miscellaneous Tissue Protozoa 105

Edward T Ryan

Protozoal organisms may be seen during histologic examination of tissue samples in a number of infectious processes other than toxoplasmosis, Chagas' disease, sarcocystosis and microsporidiosis. Leishmanial organisms infect monocytic and macrophage cell lines, and leishmaniasis is most commonly categorized as cutaneous, mucocutaneous or visceral (see Chapter 99). In immunocompetent individuals with leishmaniasis, the most commonly involved tissues include bone marrow, spleen, liver, lymph nodes, skin, and mucous membranes of the nasopharyngeal area. In immunocompromised individuals, there may also be involvement of gastrointestinal tissues and mesenteric lymph nodes [1, 2]. Histologic examination of these tissues will disclose intra-marcophage protozoal *Leishmania* species parasites, often *Leishmania donovani*. Gastrointestinal involvement is most commonly encountered in individuals with severe immunocompromising states, including advanced HIV infection or AIDS (most commonly in individuals with a CD4 count of <200/mm^3). Immunocompromised individuals with gastrointestinal leishmaniasis may present with diarrhea, dysphagia, abdominal discomfort, and weight loss. Endoscopy may disclose normal-appearing superficial mucosa in almost half of cases [1]; however, histologic examination will disclose infiltration of the lamina propria and submucosal tissue with leishmanial-laden macrophages and monocytes. In rare cases, involvement of the peritoneum and pleural cavities has also been described [3].

Similarly, cryptosporidiosis is most commonly considered an intracellular protozoal infection of the intestinal mucosal epithelial surface (see Chapter 91). However, tissue involvement may extend beyond the intestinal epithelial surface in individuals who are severely immunocompromised, including individuals with AIDS, severe combined immunodeficiency syndrome, severe hypogammaglobulinemia, or lymphoma. Such extension usually involves the biliary system and may include bile duct wall thickening, acalculus cholecystitis, sclerosing cholangitis, and ampullary stenosis [4]. There have also been rare reports involving severely immunocompromised individuals with cryptosporidial involvement extending into the respiratory epithelium lining the trachea, bronchi, and bronchioles [5, 6].

REFERENCES

1. Laguna F, García-Samaniego J, Soriano V, et al. Gastrointestinal leishmaniasis in human immunodeficiency virus-infected patients: report of five cases and review. Clin Infect Dis 1994;19:48–53.
2. Stenzinger A, Nemeth J, Klauschen F, et al. Visceral leishmaniasis in a patient with AIDS: early pathological diagnosis using conventional histology, PCR and electron microscopy is the key for adequate treatment. Virchows Arch 2012;460:357–60.
3. Muñoz-Rodríguez FJ, Padró S, Pastor P, et al. Pleural and peritoneal leishmaniasis in an AIDS patient. Eur J Clin Microbiol Infect Dis 1997;16:246–8.
4. Seaman DL, Chahal P, Sanderson SO, et al. Biliary cryptosporidiosis in a patient without HIV infection: endosonographic, cholangiographic, and histologic features (with video). Gastrointest Endosc 2009;70:590–2.
5. Moore JA, Frenkel JK. Respiratory and enteric cryptosporidiosis in humans. Arch Pathol Lab Med 1991;115:1160.
6. Travis WD, Schmidt K, MacLowry JD, et al. Respiratory cryptosporidiosis in a patient with malignant lymphoma. Report of a case and review of the literature. Arch Pathol Lab Med 1990;114:519.

PART

6

HELMINTHIC INFECTIONS

106 General Principles

G Thomas Strickland, David R Hill

DEFINITIONS

Helminth is derived from the Greek word *helmins* and means worm. As usually interpreted, the word denotes several groups of parasitic worms. In contrast to unicellular protozoa, the helminths are large, multicellular organisms with complex tissues and organs.

CLASSIFICATION

There are three groups of helminths that parasitize humans: annelids (segmented worms); nematodes (roundworms); and, platyhelminths (flatworms).

ANNELIDA

Hirudinea (leeches) is the only class of annelids of medical importance.

NEMATODA

Members of this phylum are nonsegmented roundworms. They are characterized by longitudinally oriented muscles. They are bilaterally symmetrical and have a complete digestive tract; the sexes are usually distinct. The word nematode is derived from the Greek *nema* for thread and *eidos* for form.

It is useful to divide nematodes into groups according to the body organ of humans in which they reside.

Adults That Reside in the Gut

This group includes the following species: *Ascaris lumbricoides, Ancylostoma duodenale* and *Necator americanus, Trichuris trichiura, Enterobius vermicularis, Strongyloides stercoralis, Capillaria philippinensis* and *Trichostrongylus orientalis* (Chapters 107–109).

Adults That Reside in the Blood, Lymphatic, or Subcutaneous Tissues

This group includes the following species: *Wuchereria bancrofti, Brugia malayi, Brugia timori, Loa loa, Onchocerca volvulus, Mansonella ozzardi, Mansonella perstans,* and *Mansonella streptocerca,* and *Dracunculus medinensis* (Chapters 110–113).

Larval Stages that Cause Human Pathologic Conditions in Various Tissues

These, with the exception of *Trichinella spiralis* (Chapter 115), are nonhuman parasites that are unable to develop to adults in humans, an aberrant host. In general, these nematodes follow the same migration pattern as in their definitive host, except that it is interrupted.

Infections That Are Usually Limited to the Skin and Subcutaneous Tissues

Creeping eruption is primarily caused by the dog and cat hookworms [i.e. *Ancylostoma braziliense, Ancylostoma caninum,* (Chapter 109)]. Skin penetration by human hookworms and *Strongyloides* (Chapter 109) sometimes causes similar findings.

Infections Primarily Involving the Muscles

The larvae of *Trichinella spiralis* can migrate through many tissues, including the heart and brain, before encysting in muscle.

Infections Causing a Visceral Larva Migrans Syndrome

The larval stages of the dog and cat ascarids, *Toxocara canis* and *Toxocara cati* (Chapter 116), cause lesions in multiple organs, principally the liver, brain, lungs, and eye.

Angiostrongylus costaricensis (Chapter 119) and marine ascarids (e.g. the anisakids and eustrongylids) primarily cause abdominal lesions.

Angiostrongylus cantonensis, the rat lungworm, causes eosinophilic meningitis (Chapter 118). *Gnathostoma spinigerum,* a stomach worm of domestic and wild cats and dogs, can cause a creeping eruption, an abdominopulmonary hypereosinophilia syndrome, and an eosinophilic myeloencephalitis (Chapter 117).

The dog heartworm, *Dirofilaria immitis,* sometimes causes pulmonary nodules in humans following bites from infectious mosquitoes (Chapter 113). A pulmonary hypereosinophilia syndrome can be caused by migrating human ascarids, hookworm, and *Strongyloides* larvae and microfilariae of *W. bancrofti, B. malayi.*

PLATYHELMINTHES

Flatworms are usually dorsoventrally flattened, bilaterally symmetrical and have three body layers lacking a body cavity. They include the trematodes and cestodes. The word is derived from the Greek *platys,* meaning broad, and *helmins,* meaning worm.

TREMATODA

This class includes the flukes that are parasitic to humans and animals. They are usually hermaphroditic and a digestive canal is present in adult stages. Trematode eggs are excreted in the stool, urine, or sputum of the definitive host. All flukes require a mollusk as their first intermediate host. The larval stage that escapes from the mollusk may then enter a second intermediate host (fish, crustacean), encyst on vegetation, or penetrate directly into the skin of the definitive host. Infection generally results from the ingestion of insufficiently cooked fish, crustaceans, and vegetation.

The important trematodes of humans belong to the following genera: (1) adults that live in the venous system—*Schistosoma* (Chapter 122); (2) adults that live in the intestines—*Fasciolopsis, Echinostoma, Heterophyes, Gastrodiscoides,* and *Metagonimus* (Chapter 123); (3) adults that live in the biliary system—*Clonorchis, Opisthorchis, Fasciola,* and *Dicrocoelium* (Chapter 124); and (4) adults that live in the bronchi—*Paragonimus* (Chapter 125).

CESTODA

This comprises the true tapeworms, which have a head (scolex) and segments (proglottids). Adults are all parasitic and hermaphroditic and live in the intestinal lumen of vertebrate hosts. Those that can infect humans include *Diphyllobothrium latum* and *Diphyllobothrium pacificum, Taenia saginata* and *Taenia solium, Hymenolepis nana* and *Hymenolepis diminuta* and *Dipylidium caninum*. Their invasive larval stages (hydatid, cysticercus, sparganum, coenurus) can be found in various organs and tissues of humans and other intermediate hosts (Chapters 127–131).

ANATOMY AND PHYSIOLOGY

Helminths are complicated multicellular organisms. Those infecting humans range in length from 0.3 mm (e.g. *T. canis* and *A. braziliense* larvae) to 12 m (e.g. adult *T. saginata*). They are round (nematodes) or flat (flukes and tapeworms). They all have an outer coating—the cuticle—which provides protection and is involved in active transport of water, electrolytes, and other substances.

Almost all helminths are unable to multiply in their host. The reproductive organs make up a large portion of the body cavities. The nematodes are sexually distinct, with separate males and females. The trematodes and cestodescan have separate male and female sexes (schistosomes) or male and female reproductive organs in the same worm or proglottid segment (other flukes and the tapeworms). The trematodes reproduce by self-fertilization or by cross-fertilization, and sperm can be transferred between adjacent mature proglottids of the tapeworms.

TRANSMISSION

Parasitic worms infect humans in almost all regions of the world, but there is a particular abundance in the tropics of parasite species and infected individuals. Many parasites require special conditions of temperature and humidity for survival and multiplication. Others require particular vertebrate or invertebrate hosts, for example fish, snails, crustaceans, or insects, for the completion of their lifecycles. The intermediate hosts, particularly insect vectors, are also more abundant in warm climates.

ORAL TRANSMISSION

The distribution of intestinal nematodes whose eggs are passed in human feces is affected by climatic conditions (e.g. rainfall, temperature, and humidity), as well as sanitary practices. There can be pollution of soil, water supplies, and foods (particularly vegetables), resulting in a high prevalence of fecally transmitted nematodes.

Eating habits account for the transmission of other helminths. Ingestion of undercooked or raw meat (*T. spiralis, Taenia* species) or fish (anisakid larvae, *D. latum,* and *Clonorchis sinensis* and *Opisthorchis* species) infected with larval stages of the parasite transmits some helminths. Other helminthic infections follow the ingestion of larvae-contaminated water (*D. medinensis*), raw snails (*Angiostrongylus* species), raw or undercooked crabs (*Paragonimus westermani*), and aquatic plants (*Fasciola hepatica* and *Fasciolopsis buski*).

People are infected with *Toxocara canis* and *Echinococcus granulosus* following the ingestion of substances contaminated with dog feces containing the helminth eggs.

TRANSMISSION BY SKIN PENETRATION

Larval stages of hookworm and *S. stercoralis* in the soil cause infection when they penetrate intact skin. The larvae of dog and cat hookworms can penetrate unbroken skin, but cannot develop fully in humans, and cause a creeping eruption. Cercariae of *Schistosoma* species penetrate the skin of those exposed to contaminated water. Species not capable of developing in humans cause a rash called swimmer's itch.

TRANSMISSION BY BITE OF A VECTOR

The filarial parasites develop within the biologic vector, which is also an intermediate host. These can be mosquitoes (*W. bancrofti* or *B. malaya*), black flies (*O. volvulus*), or *Chrysops* flies (*Loa loa*).

MAGNITUDE OF THE HEALTH PROBLEM

TROPICS AND SUBTROPICS

Because many people are infected with more than one species of helminth, there are more different species of helminths infecting people than there are people in the world. The numbers infected with hookworms, *Ascaris, Trichuris,* pinworm, schistosomes, onchocerca and filariae are each in the many millions, although they have often been "neglected" in tropical disease control priorities. A common trinity of intestinal helminthiasis, termed the soil-transmitted helminths, includes ascariasis, hookworm infection, and trichuriasis.

The magnitude of disease caused by helminths is related to the intensity of infection. Individuals with light infections have few, or no, abnormal findings, whereas those with heavy and prolonged infections often have clinical symptoms and signs and can develop complications. This is well documented in schistosomiasis, hookworm disease, onchocerciasis, and filariasis.

TEMPERATE CLIMATES

Prior to the middle of the twentieth century, the helminthiases were a significant cause of morbidity in the USA. Infections with the intestinal nematodes were particularly common in the Southeast. However, improvements in sanitation have decreased the incidence, except cosmopolitan parasites such as pinworm.

MIGRANTS AND TRAVELERS

Helminths can be found in migrants to high-income countries and in those who have lived for prolonged periods in tropical regions. The usual intestinal nematodes, as well as the liver flukes (*C. sinensis* and *Opisthorchis viverrini*), the lung fluke *(P. westermani)* and *Schistosoma mekongi* and *Schistosoma japonicum,* are sometimes found in migrants from Southeast Asia. Those from Mexico and Central America may have intestinal nematodes. Epilepsy caused by cerebral cysticercosis is seen in migrants from Latin America. Migrants from Africa can have intestinal nematodes, *S. mansoni* and *S. haematobium, T. saginata, W. bancrofti,* and *O. volvulus.*

CHEMOTHERAPY

Treatment of helminths involves mass drug treatment of populations and treatment of individuals. Mass drug treatment can be given to decrease the burden of infection and disease in a population, for example, ivermectin treatment of filiarial infections in Africa or albendazole for soil-transmitted helminths. Treatment of an individual has the aim of decreasing the intensity of worm infection or curing infection. Therapy of specific helminths will be covered in subsequent chapters.

SECTION

A

INTESTINAL NEMATODE INFECTIONS

107 Nematodes Limited to the Intestinal Tract (*Enterobius vermicularis, Trichuris trichiura, Capillaria philippinensis* and *Trichostrongylus* spp.)

Donald AP Bundy, Edward S Cooper, Simon Brooker

Key features

- These worms exhibit marked clinical differences; however, they are all confined to the gut as larvae and adults
- Enterobiasis (pinworm infection) occurs in children and their families worldwide; it is usually asymptomatic but can produce pruritus ani and vulvovaginitis
- Trichuriasis (whipworm) is a Neglected Tropical Disease affecting 800 million people in the tropics, with physical and developmental consequences in mild cases, and colitis and dysentery in heavy infection
- Capillariasis is a rare zoonosis in East Asia, now emerging in the Middle East, which can progress to severe malabsorption and diarrhea due to autoinfection
- Trichostrongyliasis is usually an asymptomatic zoonosis of Asia and the Middle East
- Treatment of these infections requires multiple dosing – see [14] for systematic review

ENTEROBIASIS

The pinworm *Enterobius vermicularis* was described by Linnaeus in 1758, and is found worldwide.

EPIDEMIOLOGY

Enterobiasis occurs in tropical and temperate regions and in rural and urban populations. It is among the most common helminthic infections in the US and Western Europe, where it is found in children of all socioeconomic classes. The prevalence is greatest among young school-aged children, where personal hygiene and exposure to infected peers are contributing factors [1]. Transmission is common within families. Anyone who handles infected children's clothing or bedding is at risk.

NATURAL HISTORY, PATHOGENESIS AND PATHOLOGY

Infection follows ingestion of eggs from soiled hands or contaminated food. Eggs hatch in the upper small intestine, releasing larvae that migrate to the ileum, molting twice to become adults and mating in the lower small intestine. Adult females settle in the cecum, appendix, or adjacent areas of the ascending colon and live up to 13 weeks, with oviposition occurring as early as 5 weeks, after which the gravid female leaves the colon and migrates out of the anus to lay eggs. Approximately 11,000 eggs are produced by each gravid female. The eggs are ovoid and asymmetrically flattened. The shell has a thick outer albuminous layer which has a role in adherence to skin. The eggs contain larvae that must undergo further maturation to become infective. Atmospheric oxygen acts as a stimulus to development; at body temperature, eggs are infective within 6 hours. They begin to lose infectivity after 1 or 2 days under warm, dry conditions, but can survive for 2 weeks at lower temperature and higher humidity; the maximum reported survival is 19 weeks.

E. vermicularis rarely causes intestinal pathology. Worms are occasionally found in the appendix after surgical excision (Fig. 107.1A), but only occasionally cause acute appendicitis [2]. On rare occasions, adult worms reach the peritoneum by traversing the female genital tract or migrating through a perforation in the bowel caused by appendicitis, diverticulitis, or intestinal malignancy. Granulomatous reactions to dead worms or eggs have been found in the vaginal wall, cervix, endometrium, salpinx, ovary and peritoneum, and can be confused with tuberculosis or metastatic neoplasms. On rare occasions, pinworms have been found in the conjunctival sac and the external auditory canal, where eggs presumably were delivered by soiled fingers.

CLINICAL FEATURES

Cutaneous irritation in the perianal region is the most prominent clinical feature. Local symptoms vary from a mild tickling sensation to pain [3]. Symptoms tend to be most troublesome at night and can produce sleep disturbances and restlessness. *Pruritus ani* results in scratching and trauma to the skin, and can lead to secondary bacterial infection. The eosinophil count in persons with *E. vermicularis* infection is usually normal.

E. vermicularis is a well-recognized cause of vulvovaginitis in prepubertal girls. It has also been incriminated as a potential cause of secondary enuresis and urinary tract infection. Peritoneal granulomas secondary to migrating *E. vermicularis* have been associated with abdominal pain in adult women. More commonly, peritoneal nodules are found incidentally at the time of laparotomy (Fig. 107.1B).

PATIENT EVALUATION, DIAGNOSIS, AND DIFFERENTIAL DIAGNOSIS

The diagnosis of enterobiasis depends on identifying adult worms or ova. Adult female worms are small, whitish, and pin-shaped (Fig. 107.2). They are occasionally seen in the perianal or vaginal area.

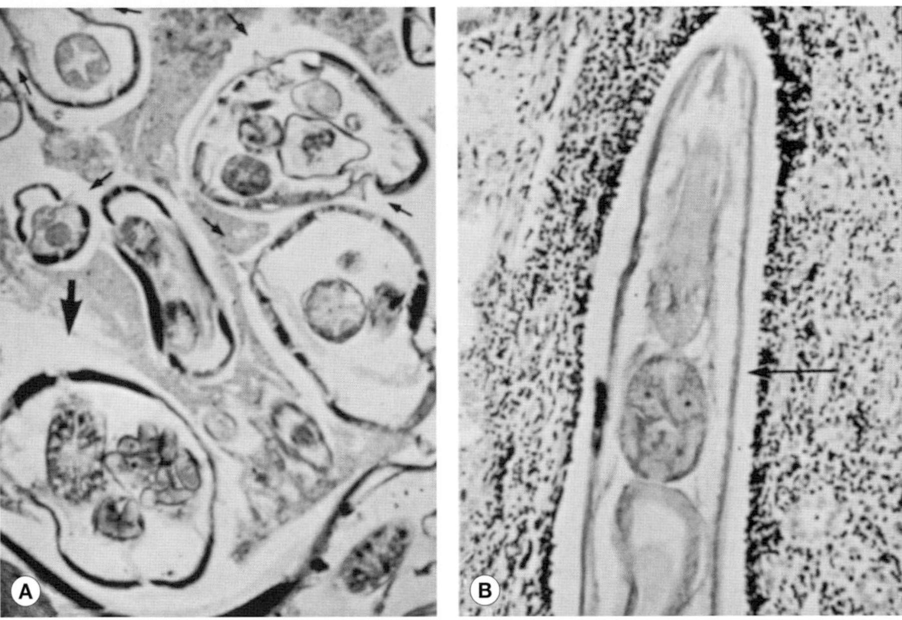

FIGURE 107.1 *Enterobius vermicularis* in appendix. **(A)** Cross-section of adult pinworms in lumen shows bilateral crests (*narrow arrows*); one worm contains eggs (*wide arrow*). **(B)** Longitudinal section of adult worm in lymphatic nodule shows prominent esophageal bulb (*arrow*). *(Courtesy of the Louisiana State University School of Medicine, New Orleans.)*

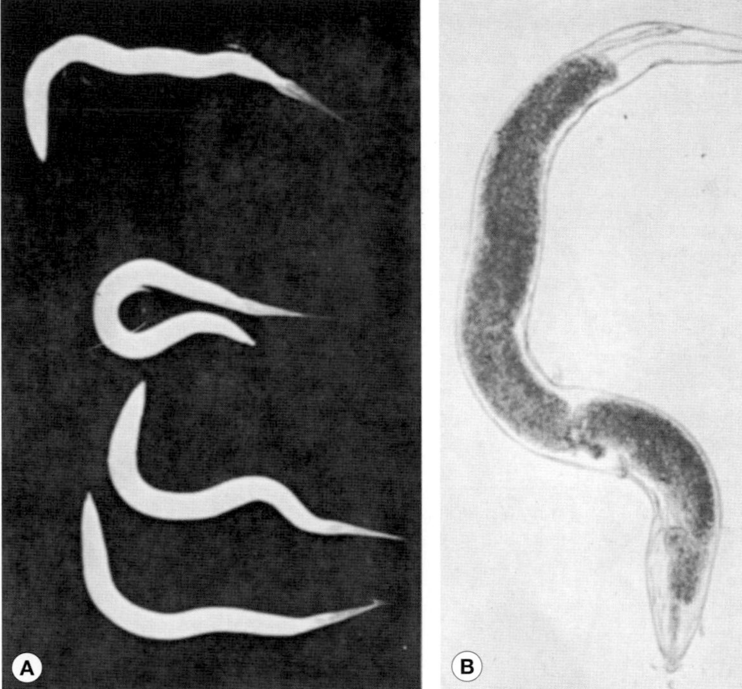

FIGURE 107.2 *Enterobius vermicularis* adult female worms. **(A)** Note shapes and the clear, attenuated, and pointed posterior end. **(B)** Note cephalic alae, bulb behind esophagus, vulva, egg mass, anus, and pointed posterior end. *(Courtesy of the Louisiana State University School of Medicine, New Orleans.)*

The most successful diagnostic approach uses a strip of transparent tape, which is held with the adhesive side out, affixed to a tongue depressor. Before the person defecates or bathes on arising in the morning, the buttocks are spread and the tape is pressed against the anal or perianal skin. The strip is transferred to a microscope slide, adhesive side down. Debris can be cleared by adding a drop of toluene. Eggs are prominent at low power. Examination of a single smear detects approximately 50% of infections, and 90% are detected with three swabs. Six negative swabs on separate days are necessary to exclude the diagnosis.

Routine stool examination is positive in only 10–15% of infected persons. Rarely, eggs are found incidentally in Papanicolaou-stained vaginal smears or in urine sediment.

TREATMENT

E. vermicularis is susceptible to several anthelmintic drugs, with cure rates of >90%. Mebendazole (100 mg orally) or pyrantel embonate (10 mg/kg) is given in a single dose and repeated once or twice 2 to 4 weeks later. Albendazole is given as a single dose (400 mg for adults and children >2 years; 100 mg for children <2 years), and repeated after 7 days. Piperazine 50 mg/kg is taken on each of seven successive days and repeated after 2 to 4 weeks. Because family members are usually infected, treatment for the entire family is recommended. Benzimidazoles should not be given during the first trimester of pregnancy.

Hygiene measures, including hand washing, particularly after bowel movements, are important. Simple laundering of clothes and linen is adequate to disinfect them.

TRICHURIASIS

Trichuris trichiura (whipworm) was thought to be benign; however, it is now recognized that intense infection is associated with colitis and dysentery, and that moderate infection can impair development in childhood [4]. It is estimated that 800 million people are infected. The name *whipworm* derives from the morphology of the 3- to 5-cm adult.

EPIDEMIOLOGY

Trichuris is distributed worldwide, where fecal contamination of moist soils allows maturation of eggs. Infection often occurs concurrently with ascariasis and has similar population dynamics (see Chapter 108). Recent analyses utilizing geographical information systems, remote sensing and spatial statistics have helped to better define the environment limits of transmission, enabling the development of risk maps [5]. In many areas where latrines have been installed, the incidence of soil-transmitted nematodes is still high because of the practice of using untreated feces as fertilizer (night soil). As with other helminths, the intensity of infection in communities is uneven. In a community where the average worm burden is 100 worms, most individuals will have considerably fewer but some harbor several thousand [6]. These individuals appear to be predisposed to intense infection for immunologic or ecologic reasons, and tend to reacquire infections of above average intensity after successful treatment. There is now evidence of genetic variation in susceptibility within communities [7]. Intensity of infection is age-related, with the most intense infections typically occurring in children of school age [8]. Treatment of this age group has been advocated as a cost-effective approach to community-wide control because it will reduce transmission to the rest of the population.

NATURAL HISTORY, PATHOGENESIS AND PATHOLOGY

T. trichiura infects humans as its primary host, but numerous members of the genus *Trichuris* infect domestic animals. *T. suis* is a morphologically identical parasite that rarely and abortively infects humans, and *T. vulpis* of dogs has been reported occasionally in humans. The life cycle of *T. trichiura* (Fig. 107.3) begins with ingestion of the embryonated egg. Larvae emerge in the cecum, where they penetrate the crypts of Lieberkühn and migrate within the mucosal epithelium. On molting to the adult, the posterior end is projected out of the epithelium, leaving the threadlike anterior portion embedded in a

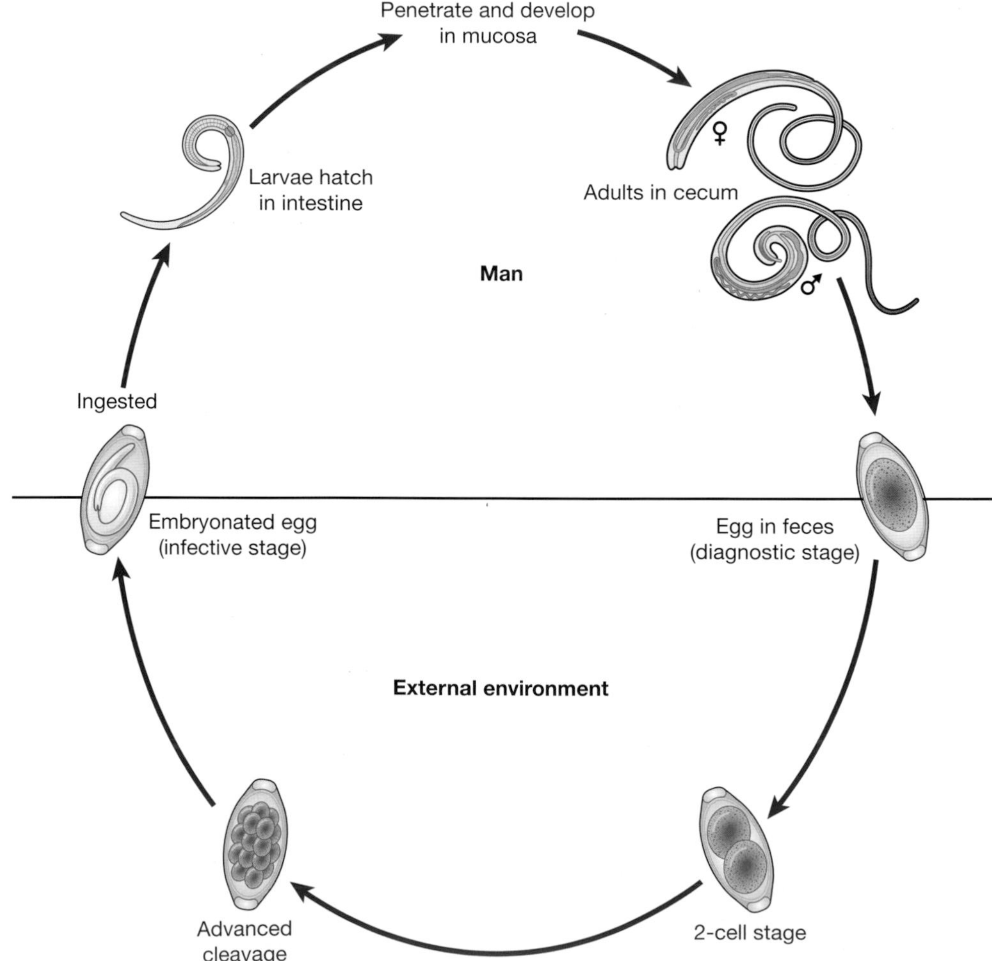

FIGURE 107.3 Life cycle of *Trichuris trichiura*. *(From Melvin DM, Brooke MM, Sadun EH: Common Intestinal Helminths of Man. Atlanta, Centers for Disease Control. DHEW Publication No. [CDC] 75–8286, 1964.)*

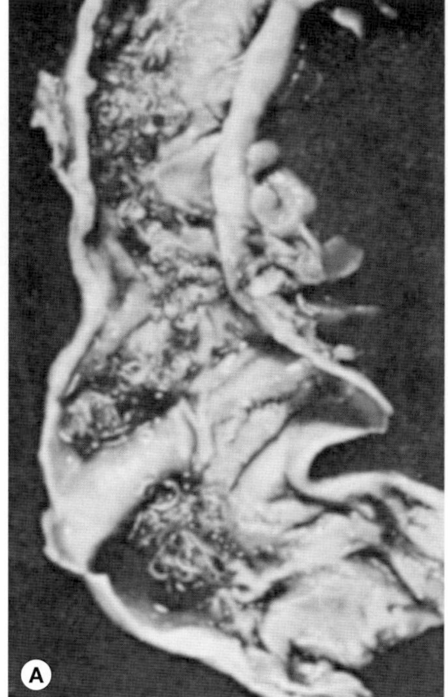
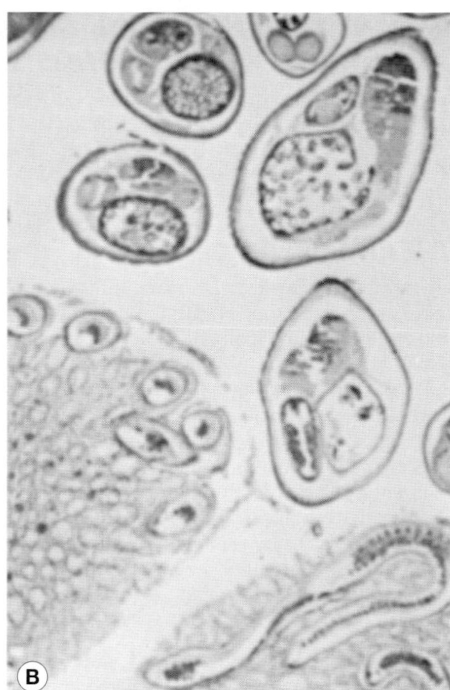

FIGURE 107.4 (A) Masses of *Trichuris trichiura* (whipworms) in colon of a child. **(B)** Section of large intestine showing adult whipworms (natural infection of *T. vulpis* in dog). Thin anterior portions of worms are embedded and threaded in the mucosa; broader posterior parts of worms, containing eggs, are in lumen. *(Courtesy of the Louisiana State University School of Medicine, New Orleans.)*

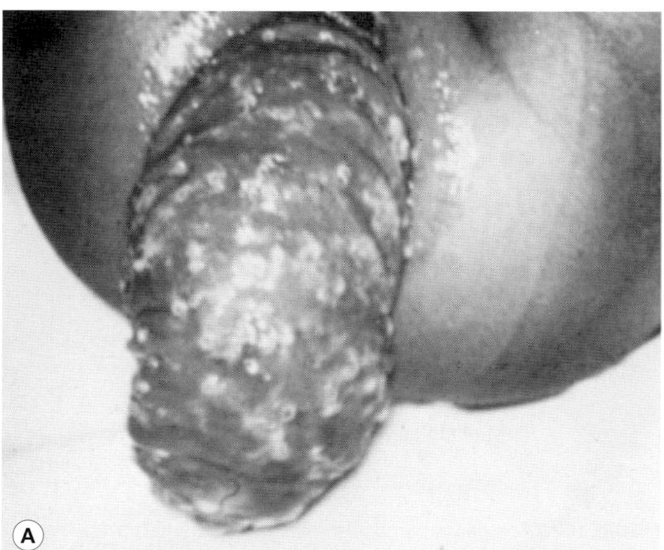
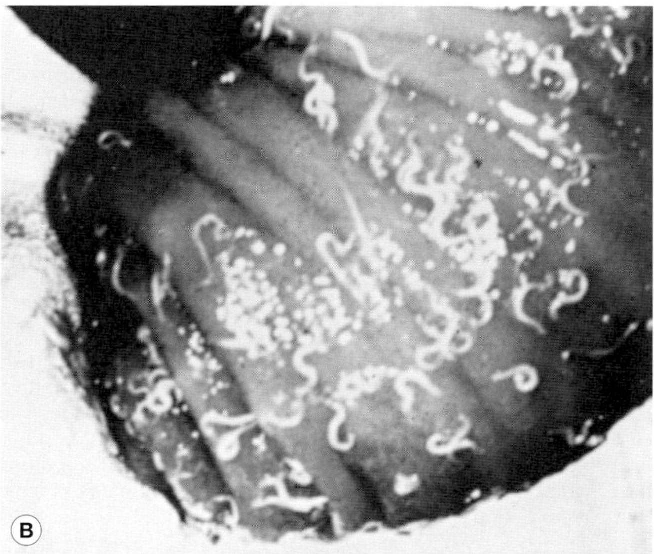

FIGURE 107.5 (A) Prolapse of rectum in a heavy infection with *Trichuris trichiura*. **(B)** Adult *T. trichiura* attached to prolapsed bowel. *(Courtesy of Drs P C Beaver and R V Platou, Tulane University School of Medicine, New Orleans.)*

syncytium created from epithelial cells. The mature female produces 2000 to 6000 eggs per day. Eggs are passed in feces, where they must mature in soil for a period that varies with temperature but is at least 10 to 14 days. About 3 months is necessary for a patent infection to be produced from the ingestion of eggs. Adult worms can persist for years.

Infection results in a well-defined humoral immune response (Th2-mediated), and IgE-mediated local anaphylaxis; cell-mediated inflammatory responses are conspicuously absent [9]. Local eosinophilic infiltration is present in the submucosa, and in heavy infection the bowel wall may be edematous and friable [10]. Under these circumstances, the mucosa can bleed easily, but worms do not suck blood. Blood loss from inflamed mucosa can be important in people with marginal iron intake [11]. Heavy infection (Fig. 107.4) can manifest abdominal pain and chronic diarrhea, and rectal prolapse (Fig. 107.5).

The clinical picture of trichuriasis has been divided into two descriptions: the classic dysenteric form (trichuris dysentery syndrome, massive infantile trichuriasis) and the more recently recognized milder form, chronic *Trichuris* colitis with growth retardation [4]. Although the latter is not sharply demarcated from the former, affected children are more likely to be brought to medical attention because of short stature rather than because of chronic diarrhea. Finger clubbing and rectal prolapse with chronic diarrhea in children are considered pathognomonic of trichuriasis in endemic areas. Recent studies suggest that infection can impair not only physical growth but also cognitive ability [12,13]. This could lead to education compromise.

PATIENT EVALUATION, DIAGNOSIS, AND DIFFERENTIAL DIAGNOSIS

Characteristic barrel-shaped eggs (50 × 20 μm) with polar hyaline plugs in a stool specimen are diagnostic (Fig. 107.7).

In severe cases, the clinical picture can resemble hookworm, acute appendicitis, or amebic dysentery.

TREATMENT

Therapy of trichuriasis is more difficult than that of other soil-transmitted nematodes [14]. A 3-day course of either mebendazole 100 mg twice daily or albendazole 400 mg once a day is usually curative in heavy infections [15]. Ivermectin, 200 μg/kg orally for 3 days, is an alternative therapy. However, compliance with a 3-day course is lower than with single-dose treatment. A single dose of mebendazole 500 mg or albendazole 400 mg may be effective in mild to moderate infections and is appropriate for community treatment. Oxantel pamoate and combination therapy with mebendazole and ivermectin show better efficacy against heavy infections, but optimal treatment doses have yet to be established. Although high priority should be given to the treatment of pregnant women, these drugs should not be administered during the first trimester.

INTESTINAL CAPILLARIASIS

Capillaria philippinensis is related to *Trichuris trichiura*. It is capable of autoinfection and therefore can cause pathology of the small intestine after a relatively light exposure.

EPIDEMIOLOGY

Most cases have been recognized in the Philippines, where the infection was first noted in the 1960s [16]. Endemic areas are recognized in several provinces where both sporadic cases and outbreaks occur. A few cases have been reported from Thailand, Japan and Taiwan, and may be expected in other areas of Asia where freshwater fish are eaten without cooking [17]. There are case reports from Egypt and Iran [18].

NATURAL HISTORY, PATHOGENESIS AND PATHOLOGY

Infection is spread by ingestion of several species of freshwater fish that have infectious larvae within muscle. The natural reservoir host has not been identified, but fish-eating water birds are probable. The custom of eating raw fish probably determines transmission. Outbreaks have occurred when fecal contamination of freshwater lagoons has allowed eggs from infected patients to be disseminated in large numbers to a local source of fish.

After ingestion of infected fish, larvae can invade the small bowel, causing a chronic malabsorption-diarrhea syndrome characterized by induration and villous atrophy which is most prominent in the jejunum (Fig. 107.6). Adult worms invade the mucosa and lamina propria. Although inflammation is not prominent around parasites, chronic inflammation is noted within the lamina propria. The small intestine can contain thousands of parasites because of the ability of the adult females to produce infectious larvae. The chronic, usually watery, diarrhea leads to electrolyte and protein abnormalities. Muscle wasting and myocardial degeneration ensue terminally. Death has been attributed to hypokalemic or metabolic cardiomyopathy or to secondary infection of debilitated patients.

PATIENT EVALUATION, DIAGNOSIS AND DIFFERENTIAL DIAGNOSIS

The diagnosis is made by finding characteristic eggs in the stool (Fig. 107.7); larvae may also be seen. Repeated examinations may have to be made because shedding of diagnostic stages may be infrequent or sporadic.

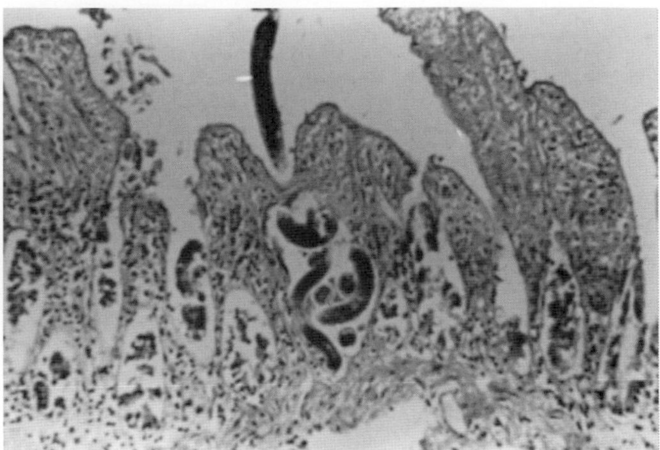

FIGURE 107.6 *Capillaria philippinensis*. Three transverse sections of larval *C. philippinensis* embedded in intestinal glands (×100). *(Courtesy of Armed Forces Institute of Pathology, Photograph Neg. No. 69–1065.)*

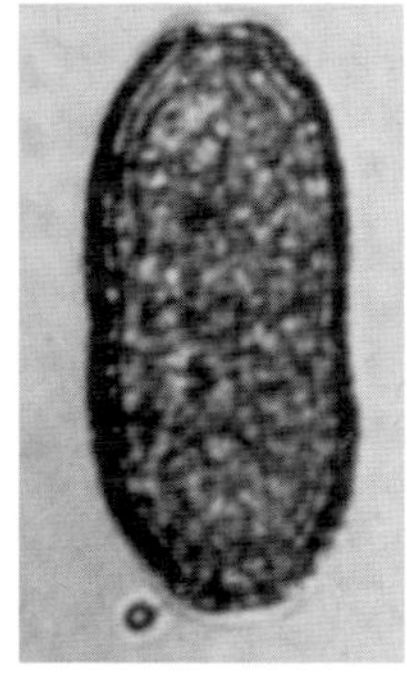

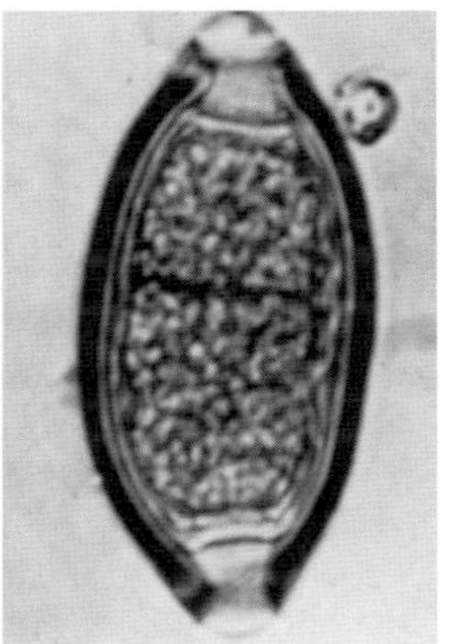

	CAPILLARIA PHILIPPINENSIS	TRICHURIS TRICHIURA
Size:	45 X 21 μm	52 X 26 μm
Shape:	peanut	ellipse
Plugs:	bipolar not protuberant	bipolar protuberant
Shell:	pitted	smooth

FIGURE 107.7 Comparison of *Capillaria philippinensis* and *Trichuris trichiura* eggs. *(From Whalen GE, et al.: Lancet 1:13, 1969.)*

TREATMENT

Because autoinfection can lead to clinical deterioration, infection with *Capillaria* should be promptly treated with mebendazole 100 mg twice daily or 200 mg once daily for 20 days. Albendazole is also effective at 400 mg daily in two divided doses for 10 days [16]. Failure to complete the course usually results in relapse. Supportive fluid, electrolyte and nutritional therapy may also be necessary. Cooking of fish prevents infection.

TRICHOSTRONGYLIASIS

Trichostrongyliasis is caused by any of several *Trichostrongylus* species infecting herbivores. Humans become infected when they ingest food or water contaminated by the feces of infected animals or humans. *Trichostrongylus* adults reside in the duodenum or the upper jejunum with their heads embedded in the mucosa.

EPIDEMIOLOGY

Trichostrongylus species have been reported from many areas of the world. Human infections appear to be most prevalent in the Middle East and Asia. The most thorough investigations have been carried out in Iran, where nine *Trichostrongylus* species have been identified in humans. In general, *T. colubriformis* is the species usually encountered in the Near and Middle East, whereas *T. orientalis* is the principal species in Asia. *Trichostrongylus* species and related genera are common parasites of herbivorous animals, including cattle, sheep, donkeys, goats, deer, and rabbits. The use of sheep or cow manure as fertilizer contributes to spread of infection in farming communities. Humans are often incidental hosts and vary in their susceptibility to different *Trichostrongylus* species. The prevalence of human infection can be 1% or 2% in endemic areas. The use of night soil in Asia creates conditions favorable to the spread of *T. orientalis,* which appears to be spread primarily from humans to humans.

NATURAL HISTORY, PATHOGENESIS, AND PATHOLOGY

Under favorable conditions of humidity and temperature, ova hatch in the environment within 24 to 36 hours. They are resistant to cold and desiccation. The hatched larvae pass through three free-living stages, reaching the infective stage in 60 hours or more. Eggs and larvae flourish in areas with shade, high humidity, and vegetation. Infection usually follows ingestion of larvae in contaminated food or water, although larvae can enter through unbroken skin. Unlike *Strongyloides stercoralis* and the hookworms, *Trichostrongylus* species do not need to migrate through the lungs for completion of the life cycle.

Little is known about the pathology of human trichostrongyliasis [19]. The usual site of infection is the duodenum or the upper jejunum. Adult worms are thought to suck blood at times and to damage the mucosa of the small intestine at or near their sites of attachment. Most human infections are mild and asymptomatic, but epigastric pain, diarrhea and flatulence can occur. Rarely, anemia and emaciation are associated with heavy infections. Eosinophilia is present in a minority and sometimes exceeds 25%.

PATIENT EVALUATION, DIAGNOSIS AND DIFFERENTIAL DIAGNOSIS

The diagnosis of trichostrongyliasis depends on the identification of ova in the stool. Concentration techniques are necessary. Care should be taken to differentiate *Trichostrongylus* eggs, which are larger and more pointed on one or both ends, from those of the hookworms. The diagnosis is occasionally made by finding *Trichostrongylus* larvae in duodenal aspirates. Identification of species requires examination of adult worms.

TREATMENT

Mebendazole 100 mg twice daily for 3 days or a single dose of albendazole 400 mg is effective. Pyrantel pamoate 11 mg/kg once (maximal dose 1 g) can be used as an alternative. Although thiabendazole 25 mg/kg twice daily (maximal daily dose of 3 g) for 2 days is effective, thiabendazole-resistant *Trichostrongylus* strains have been identified, and the drug is associated with side effects. Prevention of infection involves sanitary disposal of human excreta and prevention of fecal contamination of the topsoil by infected animals. Potentially contaminated vegetables should be thoroughly cooked and water boiled before ingestion.

REFERENCES

1. Wang LC, Hwang KP, Chen ER. *Enterobius vermicularis* infection in schoolchildren: a large-scale survey 6 years after a population-based control. Epidemiol Infect 2010;138:28–36.
2. Ramezani MA, Dehghani MR. Relationship between *Enterobius vermicularis* and the incidence of acute appendicitis. Southeast Asian J Trop Med Public Health 2007;38:20–3.
3. Otu-Bassey IB, Ejezie GC, Epoke J, Useh MF. Enterobiasis and its relationship with anal itching and enuresis among school-age children in Calabar, Nigeria. Ann Trop Med Parasitol 2005;99:611–16.
4. Bundy DAP, Cooper ES. *Trichuris* and trichuriasis in humans. Adv Parasitol 1989;28:107–73.
5. Brooker S, Clements ACA, Bundy DAP. Global epidemiology, ecology and control of soil-transmitted helminth infections. Adv Parasitol 2006;62: 221–61.
6. Bundy DA. Epidemiological aspects of *Trichuris* and trichuriasis in Caribbean communities. Trans R Soc Trop Med Hyg 1986;80:706–18.
7. Williams-Blangero S, Vandeberg JL, Subedi J, et al. Two quantitative trait loci influence whipworm (*Trichuris trichiura*) infection in a Nepalese population. J Infect Dis 2008;197:1198–203.
8. Bundy DA, Cooper ES, Thompson DE, et al. Age-related prevalence and intensity of *Trichuris trichiura* infection in a St Lucian community. Trans R Soc Trop Med Hyg 1987;81:85–94.
9. Bradley JE, Jackson JA. Immunity, immunoregulation and the ecology of trichuriasis and ascariasis. Parasite Immunol 2004;26:429–41.
10. Cooper ES, Spencer JM, Whyte-Alleng CAM, et al. Immediate hypersensitivity in the colon of children with *Trichuris* dysentery. Lancet 1991;338:1104–7.
11. Ramdath DD, Simeon DT, Wong MS, Grantham-McGregor SM. Iron status of schoolchildren with varying intensities of *Trichuris trichiura* infection. Parasitology 1995;110:347–51.
12. Taylor-Robinson DC, Jones AP, Garner P. Deworming drugs for treating soil-transmitted intestinal worms in children: effects on growth and school performance. Cochrane Database Syst Rev 2007;(4):CD000371.
13. Bundy DAP, Kremer M, Bleakley H, et al. Deworming and development: asking the right questions, asking the questions right. PLoS Negl Trop Dis 2009;3:e362.
14. Keiser J, Utzinger J. Efficacy of current drugs against soil-transmitted helminth infections: systematic review and meta-analysis. JAMA 2008;299:1937–48.
15. Steinmann P, Utzinger J, Du ZW, et al. Efficacy of single dose and triple-dose albendazole and mebendazole against soil-transmitted helminth infections and *Taenia* spp.: single-blind randomized controlled trial. Trop Med Int Health 2009;14S:194.
16. Cross JH, Basaca-Sevilla V. Albendazole in the treatment of intestinal capillariasis. Southeast Asian J Trop Med Public Health 1987;18:507–10.
17. Saichua P, Nithikathkul C, Kaewpitoon N. Human intestinal capillariasis in Thailand. World J Gastroenterol 2008;14:506–10.
18. Ahmed L, el-Dib NA, el-Boraey Y, Ibrahim M. *Capillaria philippinensis*: an emerging parasite causing severe diarrhoea in Egypt. J Egypt Soc Parasitol 1999;29:483–93.
19. Boreham RE, McCowan MJ, Ryan AE, et al. Human trichostrongyliasis in Queensland. Pathology 1995;27:182–5.

108 Intestinal Nematodes: Ascariasis

Donald A P Bundy, Nilanthi de Silva, Simon Brooker

Key features

- Ascariasis is the most prevalent human helminth and Neglected Tropical Disease, with an estimated more than 1 billion infections worldwide; it is also among the most common chronic infections of humans
- Morbidity and transmission are related to the worm burden, which has a non-normal distribution such that most people have few worms, and a few have many
- Most infections have insidious effects on growth and development, including cognitive development, but large worm burdens can result in intestinal obstruction, particularly in young children
- Intense infection is most common in school-age children who are the targets for school-based community control efforts
- *Ascaris* is easy to treat with one of several effective drugs in a single dose – see [11] for a systematic review

INTRODUCTION

Ascaris lumbricoides, the largest of the intestinal nematodes, is also the most prevalent, with more than 1 billion people infected worldwide [1]. This is partly because the female worm produces a prodigious number of eggs that are relatively resistant to drying or to extremes of temperature. The adult worms usually remain in the small intestine; passage of the larvae through the lungs is accompanied by pneumonitis, which is usually subclinical. Recent research indicates that moderate to heavy worm burdens can adversely affect cognitive development in schoolchildren and that even light worm burdens can impact the health of younger children [2–4]. A large burden of worms can cause a fatal intestinal obstruction [5]. Much of the morbidity associated with infection can be decreased by periodic chemotherapy.

Ascariasis is one of the seven common Neglected Tropical Diseases that can be controlled by regular but infrequent community chemotherapy. The others are blinding trachoma, hookworm and whipworm infection, lymphatic filariasis, schistosomiasis and onchocerciasis.

A. lumbricoides has no important animal reservoir, although the morphologically similar *A. suum* may occasionally infect humans and *A. lumbricoides* may infect pigs.

EPIDEMIOLOGY

The prevalence of infection varies geographically, it is highest in the warm and humid equatorial regions [6]. Approximately 71% of all infections have been estimated to occur in Asia (especially in China, India, and Southeast Asia), 14% in sub-Saharan Africa, and 12% in Latin America and the Caribbean [1]. There can be small localized areas of high transmission. Only cold, arid climates are free of infection; absence of infection in temperate areas is probably due to historical improvements in hygiene and sanitation, rather than non-permissive environmental conditions. Analyses employing geographic information systems, remote sensing and spatial statistics show that the prevalence of *A. lumbricoides* is strongly related to estimates of land surface temperature (LST), such that prevalence is generally <5% in areas where maximum LST exceeds 36–37°C [6]. Within environmentally determined, distributional limits, there exists considerable local random spatial variation, due presumably to differences in personal hygiene, sanitation and socioeconomic status. Infection is equally common in urban and rural settings.

Even in areas of high prevalence, the intensity of infection is not uniform. A small proportion usually harbors the majority of worms, and this subset of heavily infected people is concentrated in children <10 years [7]. Age-intensity profiles are typically convex, with maximum intensity at 5–10 years of age, and rapidly decline to a low level throughout adulthood. There is no epidemiological difference by sex. In addition, both individuals and families are predisposed to high or low intensity of infection, such that the size of the worm burden reacquired after successful treatment is positively associated with the intensity of infection before treatment [7]. Factors that determine predisposition probably include differences in exposure and variations in individual susceptibility, some of which has been attributed to genetics.

NATURAL HISTORY, PATHOGENESIS AND PATHOLOGY

Adult females reside in the human distal small intestine and produce up to 200,000 eggs per day that are deposited in the intestinal lumen and excreted in feces (Fig. 108.1). Under suitable environmental conditions of warm, moist, shaded soils, the embryo molts; the infectious stage is a second-stage larva. Infection is by ingestion or possibly by inhalation of contaminated dust. Larvae hatch in the jejunum, penetrate the intestinal wall, and migrate by way of hepatic venules to the right side of the heart and the pulmonary circulation, where they break into the alveolar spaces and undergo two further molts. From the alveoli, the 1.5-mm-long larvae ascend to the trachea and are swallowed, undergo a last molt in the intestine, and develop to adults. Larvae migrating through the lungs can induce pulmonary hypersensitivity in sensitized hosts, which can be manifested as asthma. Eosinophilic inflammation and granulomatous reaction can be seen in the lungs, as well as hypersecretion of mucus, bronchiolar inflammation, and serous exudate. The intestinal phase of the infection is generally asymptomatic, but moderately heavy infections can affect the health, growth, and physical fitness of children. *Ascaris* produces disturbances in the absorption of several nutrients including lactose, nitrogen, and vitamin A, each of which could contribute to growth faltering [3,4]. Heavy worm burdens can cause more serious complications; the most frequently reported, especially in children <10 years

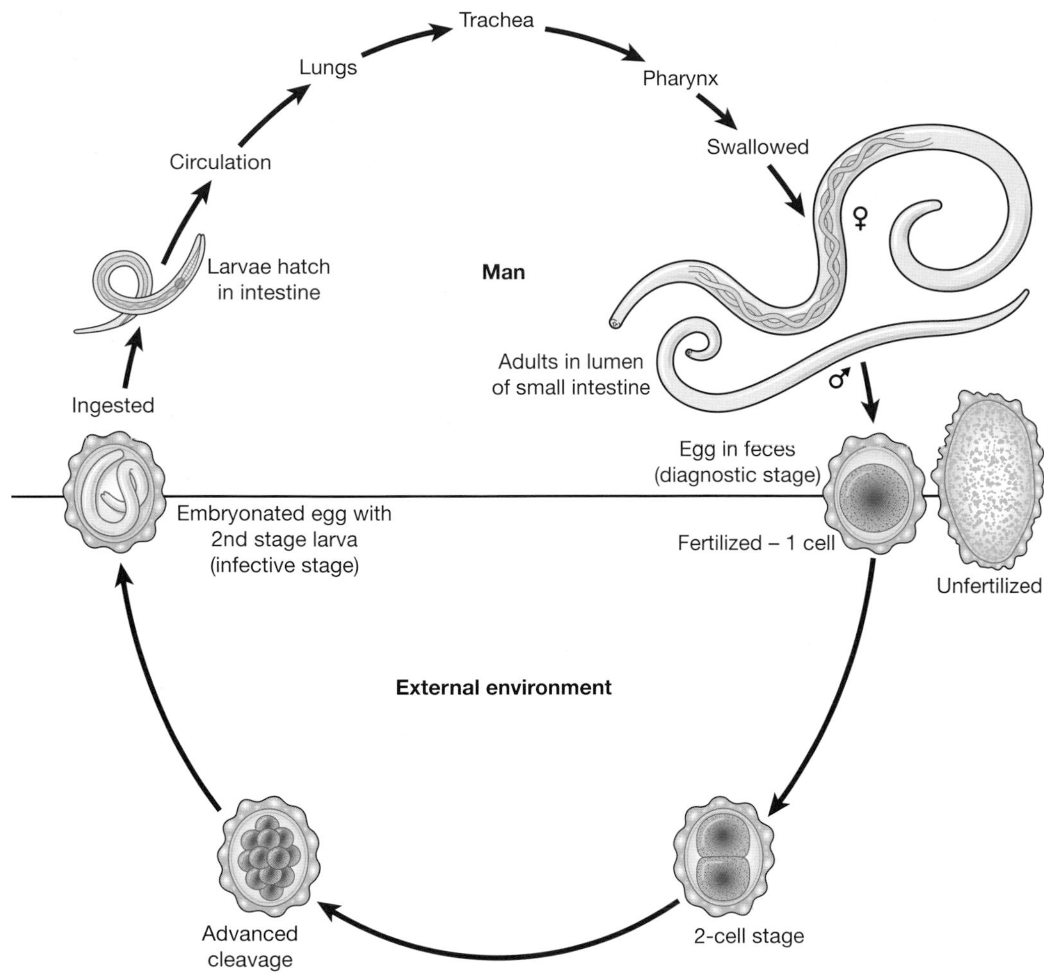

FIGURE 108.1 Life cycle of *Ascaris lumbricoides*. *(From Melvin DM, Brooke MM, Sadun EH: Common Intestinal Helminths of Man. Atlanta, Centers for Disease Control, DHEW Publication No. [CDC] 75–8286, 1964.)*

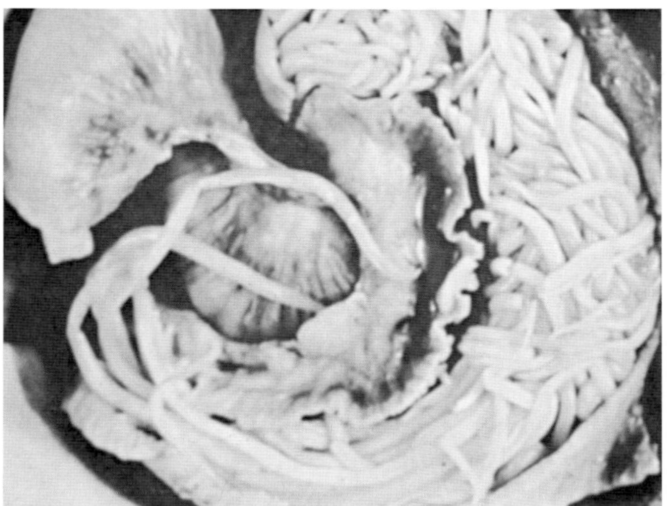

FIGURE 108.2 Terminal part of ileum opened, showing obstructing bolus of ascarids. *(Courtesy of Drs D W Aiken and F N Dickman. From JAMA 164:1317, 1957.)*

old, is obstruction of the terminal ileum by a bolus of worms (Fig. 108.2).

It can take from 10 to 12 weeks from ingestion of eggs to the production of eggs. The number of adult worms per infected person can vary widely in an infected population; egg production per female worm decreases as the worm burden increases, and thus egg counts may not linearly reflect intensity of infection. Adults live for approximately a year.

IMMUNE RESPONSE

The human immune response is associated with elevated immunoglobulin (Ig)E, tissue eosinophilia and mastocytosis, and a strong localized T helper cell type 2 (Th2) response. Although cross-sectional studies of communities often show features consistent with development of immunity to *Ascaris*, examination of antibody responses to *A. lumbricoides* has not shown humoral immunity to have a role in limiting infection. Antibodies to both adult and larval *Ascaris* antigens simply reflect the intensity of infection. It is likely that infection with *Ascaris* modulates allergic responses to non-parasite allergens, and affects allergic sensitization and expression of allergic diseases such as asthma [8,9]. It is also possible that immunomodulation in chronic infections could affect HIV-1 disease progression. A recent placebo-controlled, randomized clinical trial conducted among adult Kenyans co-infected with HIV-1 and *A. lumbricoides* found that treatment with albendazole resulted in significantly increased CD4 counts during 3 months of follow-up [10].

CLINICAL FEATURES

PULMONARY MIGRATION

Ascaris larvae usually cause few symptoms along their migratory path, but in sensitized hosts, pulmonary manifestations can start within 1 week after ingestion of eggs. Symptoms are likely to occur where transmission is seasonal or sporadic, e.g., in Saudi Arabia. Other allergic manifestations to migrating larvae, such as urticaria, are more common at the end of the pulmonary phase. Fever, cough, wheezing and dyspnea can be accompanied by sputum production, sometimes with small amounts of blood; chest pain and cyanosis are noted in the most severe cases. Chest film examination can show unilateral or bilateral abnormalities, ranging from nodular densities to diffuse interstitial patterns. The illness usually is limited to several weeks, but can persist as long as larvae pass through the lungs. Leukocytosis and marked eosinophilia can occur, fulfilling the clinical picture of Löffler's syndrome. Rarely, severe pulmonary inflammation has progressed to death.

INTESTINAL INFECTIONS

The intestinal phase of the infection is generally asymptomatic, but even moderately heavy infections can affect the health, growth, and physical fitness of children.

The more serious complications of ascariasis result from migration of adult worms. Migrating worms can reach the upper gastrointestinal (GI) tract and be vomited or passed per rectum. Worms can intertwine and form a bolus, which can cause partial or complete intestinal obstruction, with abdominal pain, vomiting, and occasionally a palpable abdominal mass (Fig. 108.2). Rarely, such a mass causes a volvulus or leads to perforation of the small intestine. More frequently, the migrating worms enter ducts or diverticula, where they can perforate or cause obstruction. The common bile duct is the most often obstructed, leading to biliary colic or cholangitis (Fig. 108.3). A worm that ascends higher in the biliary tree can result in liver abscess or can penetrate the bile duct and lead to bile peritonitis. When the pancreatic duct is obstructed it can lead to pancreatitis. Appendicitis can be triggered by *Ascaris* obstructing the appendix (Fig. 108.4).

Heavy worm burdens can cause more serious complications; the most frequently reported, especially in children <10 years old, is obstruction of the terminal ileum by a bolus of worms [5] (Fig. 108.2). Rarely, the section of intestine containing the bolus of worms may act as a fixed point resulting in a volvulus. Ileocecal intussusception as well as solitary intestinal perforation has been attributed to *Ascaris*, but the causative role of *Ascaris* in these cases is not always clear.

PATIENT EVALUATION, DIAGNOSIS AND DIFFERENTIAL DIAGNOSIS

The diagnosis of ascariasis is made by stool examination. Characteristic eggs (55 to 75 μm by 35 to 50 μm) can be seen on direct or concentrated stool specimens. Unfertilized eggs can be more difficult to identify because of their atypical size and appearance. Decorticate eggs lacking the outer mamillated covering are sometimes produced, and these may be confused with the eggs of other nematodes; the thick hyaline shell is typical of *Ascaris*. Infections consisting of only male worms produce no eggs; if such infections are symptomatic, the worms may sometimes be detected radiologically as linear filling defects outlined by contrast media (Fig. 108.5). Intestinal worms may sometimes ingest barium and be seen as thin, curved linear densities. In cases of suspected biliary ascariasis or pancreatitis, duodenoscopy with retrograde cholangiopancreatography can be useful both in establishing a diagnosis and in providing a nonsurgical means of removing the worms. Ultrasonography is also useful in the diagnosis of biliary ascariasis but is of less value in pancreatitis.

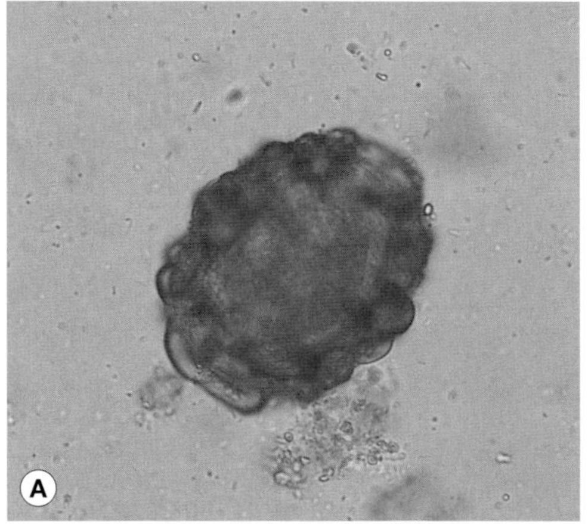

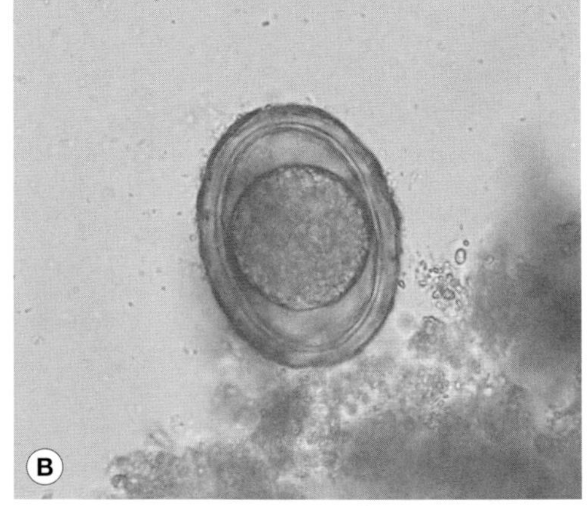

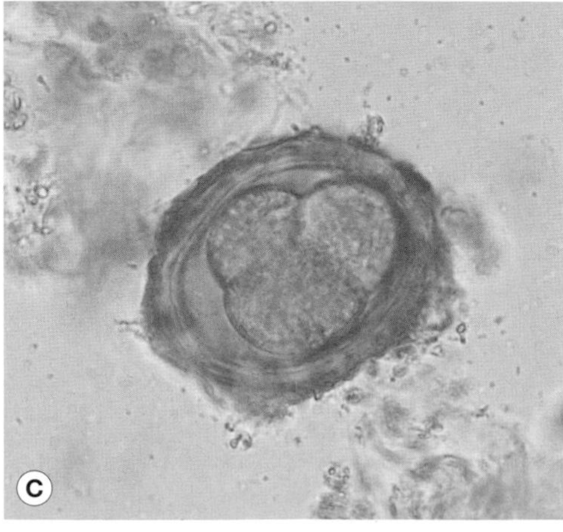

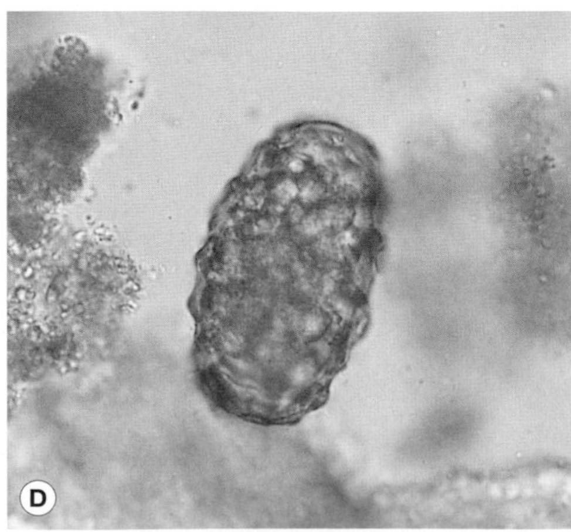

FIGURE 108.3 *Ascaris lumbricoides* eggs in saline smears (×400 magnification) showing **(A)** mammilated outer cortex **(B)** fertilized decorticated egg **(C)** embryonated egg **(D)** unfertilized egg.

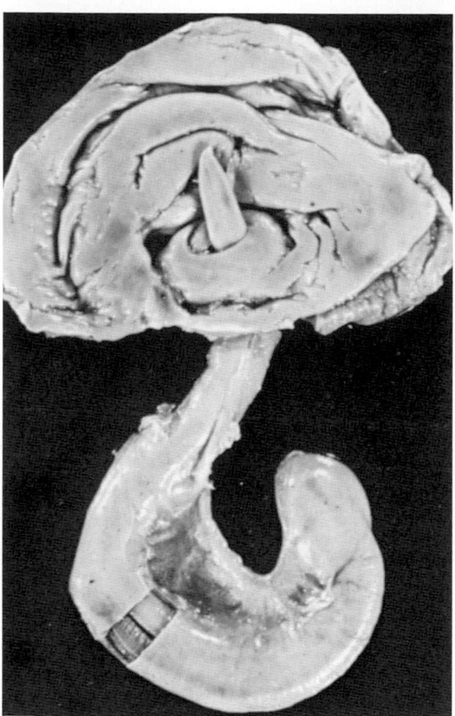

FIGURE 108.4 Adult *A. lumbricoides* in appendix. *(Courtesy of the Louisiana State University School of Medicine, New Orleans.)*

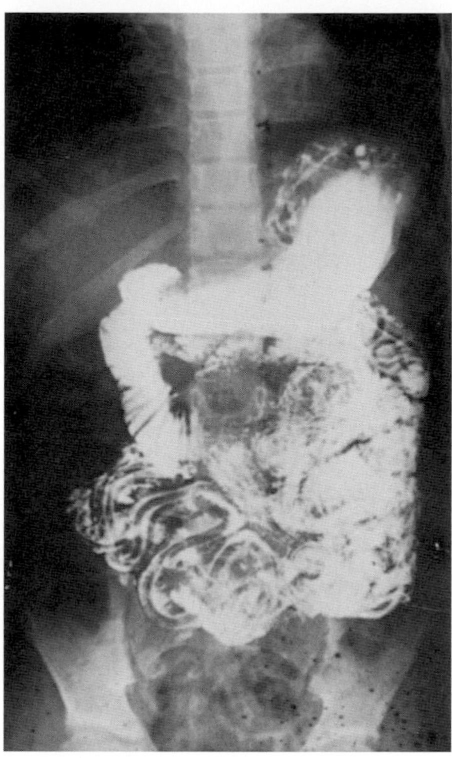

FIGURE 108.5 Adult *A. lumbricoides* visualized in small intestine by x-ray following barium. Ascarids may be detected at times without barium, by air contrast, but are less distinct. *(Courtesy of Louisiana State University School of Medicine and the Charity Hospital of New Orleans.)*

TREATMENT

CHEMOTHERAPY

There are several effective drugs for treatment of ascariasis, with cure rates of >90% commonly achieved [11]. Mebendazole given at a dosage of 100 mg twice daily for 3 days or as a single dose of 500 mg, or albendazole at a single dose of 400 mg, are highly effective. Levamisole (either 80 mg or 2.5 mg/kg) is similarly efficacious. Transient GI discomfort and headache have been reported with these drugs. Pyrantel pamoate (10 mg/kg up to a maximum of 1 g) can be given as a single dose. Adverse effects include occasional GI disturbances, headaches, dizziness, rash and fever. Treatment with benzimidazoles should not be administered during the first trimester of pregnancy.

SUPPORTIVE THERAPY

Intestinal obstruction may necessitate surgery. However, patients who are clinically stable and well hydrated can often be successfully managed conservatively with nasogastric suction, intravenous hydration, and antispasmodics followed by anthelminthics given by nasogastric tube once the obstruction has subsided. In these cases, treatment is given after the obstruction is relieved to avoid paralyzing the worms in the ileum, which could precipitate complete obstruction. Obstruction of the bile or pancreatic ducts must be relieved endoscopically or surgically, but conservative therapy may be appropriate in simple biliary colic.

PREVENTION

Without improvements in sanitation, re-infection following treatment is common, especially as the eggs can remain viable in the environment for years. Chemotherapy targeted at school-age children delivered through schools is a feasible and effective approach to worm control, reducing rates of anemia and improving growth, especially weight [12,13]. By targeting school-age children for repeated chemotherapy, the worm burden in the community can be reduced, thus alleviating morbidity and reducing transmission.

REFERENCES

1. de Silva NR, Brooker S, Hotez P, et al. Soil-transmitted helminths: updating the global picture. Trends Parasitol 2003;19:547–51.
2. O'Lorcain P, Holland CV. The public health importance of *Ascaris lumbricoides*. Parasitology 2000;121:S51–71.
3. Hall A, Hewitt G, Tuffrey V, de Silva N. A review and meta-analysis of the impact of intestinal worms on child growth and nutrition. Matern Child Nutr 2008;4(Suppl 1):118–236.
4. Taylor-Robinson DC, Jones AP, Garner P. Deworming drugs for treating soil-transmitted intestinal worms in children: effects on growth and school performance. Cochrane Database Syst Rev 2007;(4):CD000371.
5. de Silva NR, Guyatt HL, Bundy DAP. Morbidity and mortality due to *Ascaris*-induced intestinal obstruction. Trans R Soc Trop Med Hyg 1997;91:31–6.
6. Brooker S, Clements ACA, Bundy DAP. Global epidemiology, ecology and control of soil-transmitted helminth infections. Adv Parasitol 2006;62:221–61.
7. Bundy DAP, Medley G. Immuno-epidemiology of human geohelminthiasis: ecological and immunological determinants of worm burden. Parasitology 1992;104(Suppl):S105–19.
8. Cooper PJ. Interactions between helminth parasites and allergy. Curr Opin Allergy Clin Immunol 2009;9:29–37.
9. Leonardi-Bee J, Pritchard D, Britton J. Asthma and current intestinal parasite infection: systematic review and meta-analysis. Am J Respir Crit Care Med 2005;174:514–23.
10. Walson JL, Otieno PA, Mbuchi M, et al. Albendazole treatment of HIV-1 and helminth co-infection: a randomized, double blind, placebo-controlled trial. AIDS 2008;22:1601–9.
11. Keiser J, Utzinger J. Efficacy of current drugs against soil-transmitted helminth infections: systematic review and meta-analysis. JAMA 2008;299:1937–48.
12. Bundy DAP, Shaeffer S, Jukes M, et al. School-based health and nutrition programs. In: Jamison D, Breman J, Measham A, et al., eds. Disease Control Priorities in Developing Countries, 2nd edn. New York: The World Bank and Oxford University Press; 2006:1091.
13. Bundy DAP, Kremer M, Bleakley H, et al. Deworming and development: asking the right questions, asking the questions right. PLoS Negl Trop Dis 2009;3:e362.

109 Hookworm and *Strongyloides* Infections

Peter J Hotez, Robert H Gilman

Key features

- Hookworm and *Strongyloides* are intestinal nematodes that penetrate exposed skin, usually of the feet, hands, buttocks, and legs, to establish infection
- Hookworm infection leads to intestinal blood loss and iron-deficiency anemia, especially in Africa, Asia, and Latin America. Infection results in developmental and cognitive delays in children, as well as reductions in future wage earning
- Hookworm is common in pregnant women in low-income countries, resulting in poor birth outcome
- Deworming with benzimidazole anthelminthics is the major therapeutic approach to reduce the number of hookworms in the intestine and improve anemia. For severe anemia, especially for pregnant women, additional iron supplementation may be necessary
- *Strongyloides stercoralis* infection leads to diarrhea, and can cause chronic infection lasting decades without treatment
- Infection is difficult to diagnose because of the paucity of larvae detected in feces
- Hyperinfection with *Strongyloides* is linked to exogenous steroid use or other immune dysregulation and is associated with high mortality
- Deworming with ivermectin is the major therapeutic approach for *Strongyloides*. In hyperinfection, prolonged treatments are sometimes required, along with management of secondary bacteremias and bacterial meningitis

HOOKWORM INFECTIONS

INTRODUCTION

Human hookworm infection is a global cause of anemia and malnutrition [1]. Approximately 85% of cases are caused by *Necator americanus*, followed by *Ancylostoma duodenale*; *Ancylostoma ceylanicum*, which infects a number of animals, is occasionally found in humans in restricted geographic areas; *Ancylostoma braziliense* is a cause of cutaneous larva migrans, and *Ancylostoma caninum* is a rare cause of eosinophilic enteritis. The hallmark of hookworm disease resulting from moderate and heavy infections is iron-deficiency anemia (IDA) due to parasite blood feeding and chronic blood loss [1]. Because hookworms are responsible for a significant proportion of IDA in low- and middle-income countries, some global disease burden estimates indicate that hookworm infection is one of the most important parasitic diseases. During the first few decades of the twentieth century hookworm infection was common in the rural southeastern US, but it has been eliminated as a public health problem following urbanization and economic development.

EPIDEMIOLOGY

Approximately 600 million people are infected worldwide, with the largest number of cases in sub-Saharan Africa, Asia, and tropical regions of the Americas [2]. Hookworm infection is soil-transmitted and acquired most commonly when infective larvae in the soil penetrate exposed human skin anywhere on the body. Environmental factors favoring hookworm transmission are extreme rural poverty and poor sanitation, appropriate soil conditions, including sandy or loamy soils that facilitate the migration of hookworm larvae, high temperatures, and adequate moisture, rainfall and shade. In most endemic areas, similar to other soil-transmitted helminthiases, the prevalence of hookworm infection rises sharply in the first few years of life and then reaches a plateau. However, unlike ascariasis and trichuriasis, the intensity of hookworm infection often continues to rise in adulthood. These observations partly explain the high intensity of hookworm infection found among women of reproductive age and among some elderly populations [3].

NATURAL HISTORY, PATHOGENESIS, AND PATHOLOGY

Hookworm ova are passed in the feces and develop in the soil (Fig. 109.1). Under optimal conditions, each egg liberates a rhabditiform larva, which gradually doubles in size, and molts twice to become a slender, non-feeding, infective third-stage larva (L3). L3 larvae live in the top one-half inch of soil, with their ends projecting upward from the surface. When contact is made with human skin, the larvae penetrate the skin (including feet, hands, buttocks, and legs) by releasing proteases and other hydrolytic enzymes. *A. duodenale* L3 larvae are also orally infective. Larval migration in the skin is associated with immediate hypersensitivity. Following skin penetration, the larvae gain access to the venous circulation and are carried to the lungs, where they migrate through the respiratory tree to the pharynx. Larvae are swallowed, pass through the esophagus and stomach, and arrive in the small intestine before molting to become adults. Eosinophilia typically begins shortly after larvae first enter the gut. Eggs appear in the stool 5 weeks or more after invasion of the skin by infective larvae.

Almost all of the pathology is caused by the adult stages, which are small, cylindrical, creamy-white nematodes roughly 1 cm in length (Figs 109.1 & 109.2). At the site of parasite attachment in the gut, hookworms lacerate capillaries in the mucosa or arterioles in the submucosa and bleeding ensues following secretion of hookworm anticoagulants (Figs 109.2 & 109.3). Hookworms ingest host blood, lyse the red cells, and then degrade host hemoglobin through an ordered cascade of hemoglobin-digesting proteases. It has been estimated that, through this mechanism, 25 adult *N. americanus* hookworms will cause the loss of 1 mL of blood per day, which contains

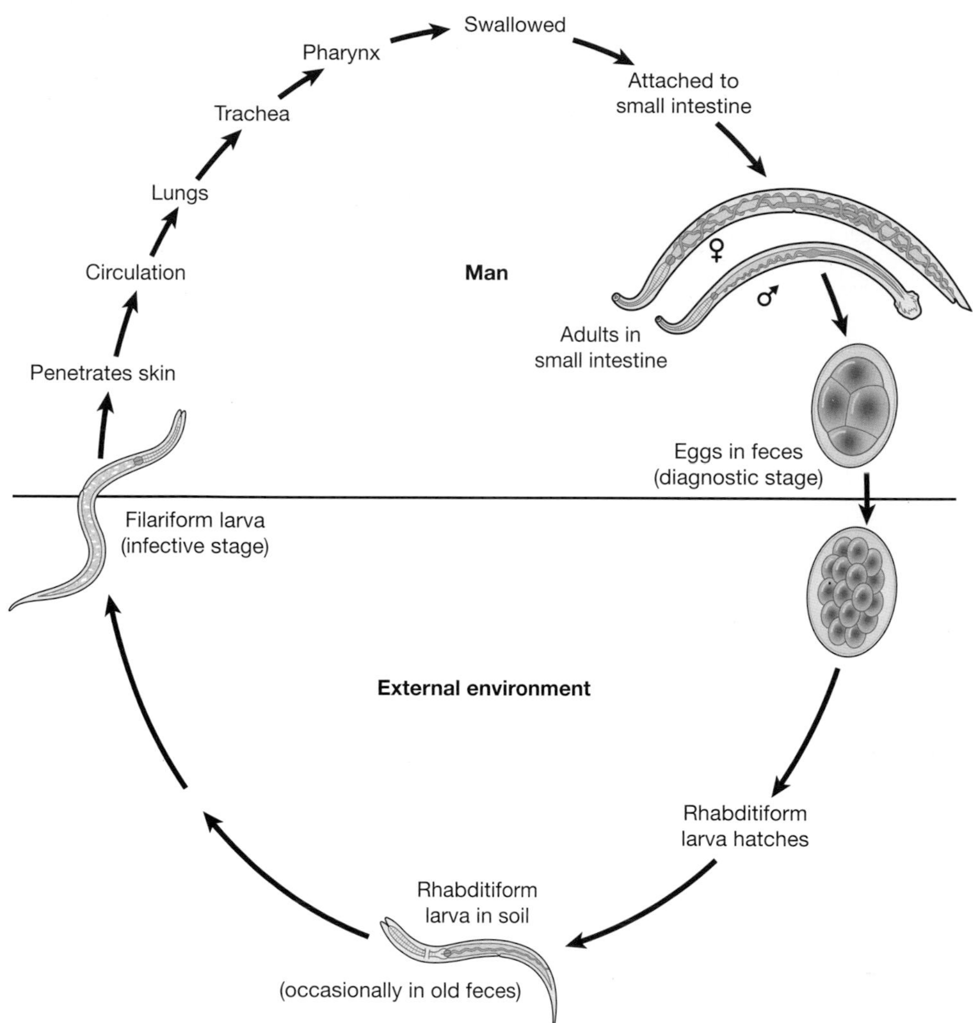

FIGURE 109.1 Life cycle of hookworm. *(Redrawn from Melvin DM, Brooke MM, Sadun EH: Common Intestinal Helminths of Man. Atlanta, Centers for Disease Control, DHEW Publication No. [CDC] 75–8286, 1964.)*

roughly 0.5 mg of iron. This amount is equivalent to the daily iron intake of a child [4].

CLINICAL FEATURES

The clinical features of hookworm infection correspond to the life cycle of the organism and the intensity of infection [1].

Ground Itch and Cutaneous Larva Migrans

Associated with the penetration of the skin by L3 larvae, there is intense itching, and, in some instances, erythematous, pruritic papules at the site of penetration. Cutaneous larva migrans is a related condition caused by skin penetration of animal hookworms, classically *A. braziliense*, and results in raised, reddened, serpiginous tracks that mark the migration of the worm. They are the most frequent on the lower extremities, followed by the buttocks and anogenital area, although both the trunk and upper extremities may also be affected.

Pulmonary Manifestations

As larvae pass through the lungs, patients may complain of cough and wheezing. In a small percentage of patients, eosinophilic infiltrates appear on chest film.

Gastrointestinal Manifestations

Epigastric pain and tenderness occur early in the intestinal phase. Abdominal pain can be severe enough to suggest peptic ulcer disease.

Iron Deficiency Anemia (IDA)

The hallmark of chronic hookworm disease is IDA, which manifests as a microcytic and hypochromic anemia. The development of IDA depends on the number and species of infecting hookworm, the iron reserves and requirements of the host, and the availability of iron in the diet. Lassitude, weakness, apathy, and depression are characteristic of anemia. On physical examination, the mucous membranes, conjunctivae, and skin appear pale. Iron deficiency has also been associated with koilonychia and angular stomatitis. A yellowish-green hue (chlorosis) that results in a sallow complexion can be seen in heavy infections. Anemia is often accompanied by eosinophilia, and, in severe cases, protein loss and hypoalbuminemia occur. In children, chronic hookworm infection and disease lead to deficits in growth and physical fitness as well as reductions in intelligence and cognition. These changes can lead to reduced school performance and attendance. IDA from chronic hookworm infection in pregnancy is associated with increased maternal morbidity as well as low birthweight and prematurity. Severe cases of hookworm anemia and hypoalbuminemia are accompanied by cardiovascular changes.

PATIENT EVALUATION, DIAGNOSIS, AND DIFFRENTIAL DIAGNOSIS

Hookworm disease should be considered in any patient from an endemic area who presents with anemia, eosinophilia, or both. The diagnosis is confirmed by identifying hookworm ova in the stool (Fig. 109.1). The eggs of *N. americanus* and *A. duodenale* are almost

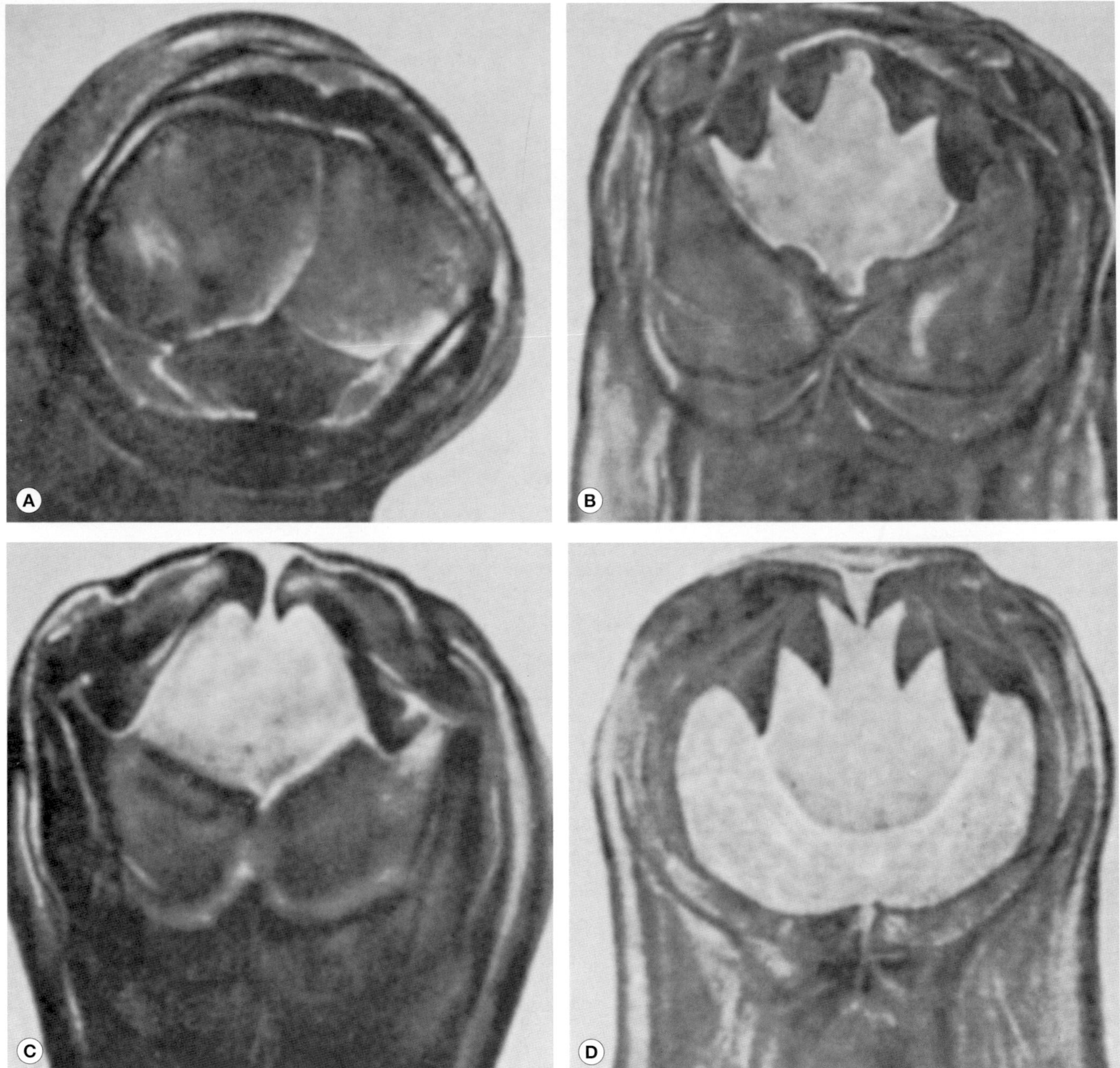

FIGURE 109.2 (A) Mouthparts of *Necator americanus*. Note two pairs of chitinized cutting plates characteristic of this species. **(B)** Mouthparts of *Ancylostoma duodenale*. Note two large pairs of teeth, each of the medial pair bearing a small accessory process. **(C)** Mouthparts of *A. braziliense*. Note two pairs of teeth, a large outer pair and a small inner pair without accessory processes. **(D)** Mouthparts of *A. caninum*. Note three well-developed pairs of teeth.

indistinguishable, and both are eliminated in feces in two- to eight-celled stages of cleavage. A clear space is present between the cells and the shell (Fig. 109.1). Direct fecal examination in saline or an iodine solution is suitable for detection of clinically significant infections. This technique identifies persons with more than 1200 eggs per gram of stool. Zinc sulfate flotation or formalin–ether concentration techniques can be used to identify persons with lighter infections. For purposes of epidemiologic studies, it is sometimes necessary to perform quantitative fecal egg counts, which roughly correlate with the number of hookworms in the intestine. The Kato–Katz quantitative method is used widely, but the method requires immediate evaluation as the technique can selectively destroy hookworm eggs over time, leaving only *Ascaris*, *Trichuris*, and schistosome eggs in areas of co-endemicity.

TREATMENT

The therapy of hookworm infection disease is treatment with an oral anthelminthic agent. In resource-poor countries where hookworm infection is endemic, the drugs are usually administered as part of mass treatment programs, either as part of child health days or through school-based deworming programs on an annual or more frequent basis [5]. For hookworm infection, deworming produces benefits in physical and intellectual development and hemoglobin levels. For decades, single doses of either of two benzimidazole agents, albendazole or mebendazole, were considered first-line treatments. However, in a systematic review and meta-analysis, the cure rate of single-dose oral albendazole (400 mg) was 72% and the cure rate of single-dose mebendazole (500 mg) was only 15% [6]. Therefore,

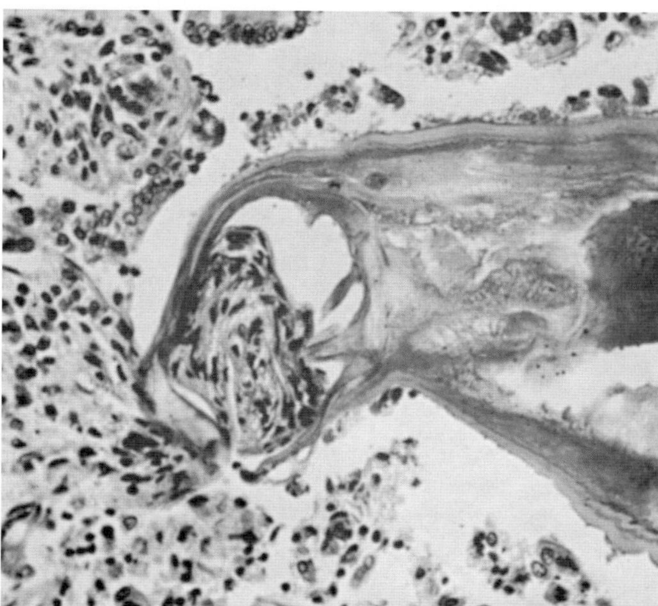

FIGURE 109.3 Longitudinal section through hookworm attached to intestinal mucosa. *(Courtesy of Dr Pedro Morera, Facultad de Microbiologia, Universidad de Costa Rica.)*

when used as a single dose in mass drug administration, albendazole may be the only acceptable agent. Outside of resource-poor settings, mebendazole when administered in a dose of 100 mg orally twice daily for three successive days may be as effective as albendazole, as well as pyrantel pamoate administered as a dose of 11 mg/kg (max. 1 g) for 3 days.

Because of the teratogenicity and embryotoxicity of albendazole and other benzimidazoles when used in high doses in laboratory animals, two special circumstances warrant caution. In children greater than 1 year but less than 2 years of age, albendazole should be administered at one-half of the recommended dose (200 mg), weighing the effect of chronic hookworm infection on development and growth, with the theoretical risks of treatment. Similarly, in women in their second and third trimesters of pregnancy, treatment has had proven benefits in terms of reduced maternal and perinatal morbidity and mortality [3]. No anthelminthic treatment should be administered during the first trimester, but subsequently the risks of treatment need to be weighed against the high risk of hookworm infection on pregnancy outcome. During pregnancy, treating anemia of hookworm disease with both anthelminthic drugs and iron therapy is superior to either treatment alone An experimental vaccine to prevent hookworm infection and re-infection is under development [7,8].

STRONGYLOIDES INFECTIONS

INTRODUCTION

Strongyloidiasis, threadworm infection, results from infection by *Strongyloides stercoralis,* the female of which is usually embedded in the mucosa of the small intestine. *S. stercoralis* is unusual among helminths in its ability to multiply within the host and maintain persisting infection for years. Recognized since 1876, when Normand described the larvae in stools of French soldiers in Southeast Asia with Cochin-China diarrhea, *S. stercoralis* has a complex life cycle of entering the skin, migrating through the lungs, and residing in the small bowel (Fig. 109.4).The capacity of *S. stercoralis* to overwhelm immunocompromised hosts with hyperinfection is well recognized. There is a link between strongyloidiasis and co-infection with human T-cell lymphotrophic virus type 1 (HTLV-1) [9, 10]. Although almost all *Strongyloides* infections are with *S. stercoralis,* the primate parasite *S. fulleborni* is recognized in humans in Africa and in Papua New Guinea, where it is a cause of "swollen belly syndrome" particularly among infants and young children.

EPIDEMIOLOGY

Strongyloidiasis has a patchy, widespread distribution through warm, wet tropical and subtropical areas. In temperate regions, it is encountered in institutions where sanitary facilities are poor or in moist conditions such as mines or tunnels. Some have conservatively estimated that 30 to 100 million people are infected. The difficulties in diagnosing strongyloidiasis have contributed to our limited understanding of the global prevalence and disease burden [9, 10]. *Strongyloides* infections are endemic in tropical Asia, Africa, and Latin America, as well as in rural Appalachia in the US and in parts of southern and eastern Europe. Although infection is widespread, the prevalence is typically low (<10%). Prevalence is reportedly elevated in older HTLV-1-affected patients in regions where this virus is endemic (e.g. Japan, Caribbean).

Immigrants, travelers, or military veterans from endemic areas, e.g., southern Asia, can have prolonged infections. The latter are usually older males, veterans who have lived in endemic tropical areas, and those with underlying malignant, metabolic, pulmonary or renal disease. They have mild to moderate chronically relapsing symptoms. Because infection can be maintained for 40 years or more, and because effective therapy has been available only since 1967, many persons, e.g. military personnel who were in the South Pacific in World War II, the Korean War, or the Vietnam War, may remain infected and at risk for episodic symptoms of chronic infection or overwhelming hyperinfection, especially if they receive corticosteroid therapy.

NATURAL HISTORY, PATHOGENESIS, AND PATHOLOGY

The life cycle of *S. stercoralis* is complex (Fig. 109.4). Like other intestinal nematodes, it can involve host and soil stages. However, unlike most other helminths, the life cycle can also occur completely in the soil (free-living cycle) or completely in the host (internal or external autoinfection). Autoinfection is the basis of both persistence of infection, as well as overwhelming hyperinfection syndrome in patients receiving corticosteroids.

Human infection begins with exposure of the skin to L3 larvae that reside in fecally contaminated, moist soil (Fig. 109.4). These larvae have slender bodies, and notched tails that distinguish them from hookworm larvae. The L3 migrate through the lungs and ascend the airways to the trachea and epiglottis before being swallowed to complete their life cycle in the small intestine. There, after two molts, adult females (2.2 mm long) emerge, penetrate and reside in the superficial mucosa of the duodenum and jejunum. The evidence for the existence of male worms is controversial. In the intestine, adult female worms, eggs, and larvae are found in the superficial submucosa and in the mucosal crypts, causing mechanical trauma, mucous discharge and microscopic ulceration but usually minimal inflammation. Progressive involvement may lead to edema, flattened villi, malabsorption, and even ulceration, enteritis and secondary bacterial invasion.

Nearly 1 month after infection, the adult female lays oval, thin-shelled, embryonated eggs that closely resemble hookworm eggs but are usually not seen because they rapidly hatch in the intestinal mucosa to produce first-stage, noninfectious rhabditiform larvae (Fig. 109.5). It is this rhabditiform larval stage that is characteristically found in the stool or the upper small bowel. Under favorable soil conditions, rhabditiform larvae transform into infective L3 within 24 hours after fecal passage, a process that may also occur in the perianal region after defecation. L3 larvae can also survive for several weeks under moist conditions, and develop into adult male and female worms (Fig. 109.4).

Alternatively, autoinfection can occur by rapid transformation of rhabditiform larvae to infectious L3 in the gut lumen, where they penetrate the intestinal mucosa (*internal autoinfection*) to proceed via

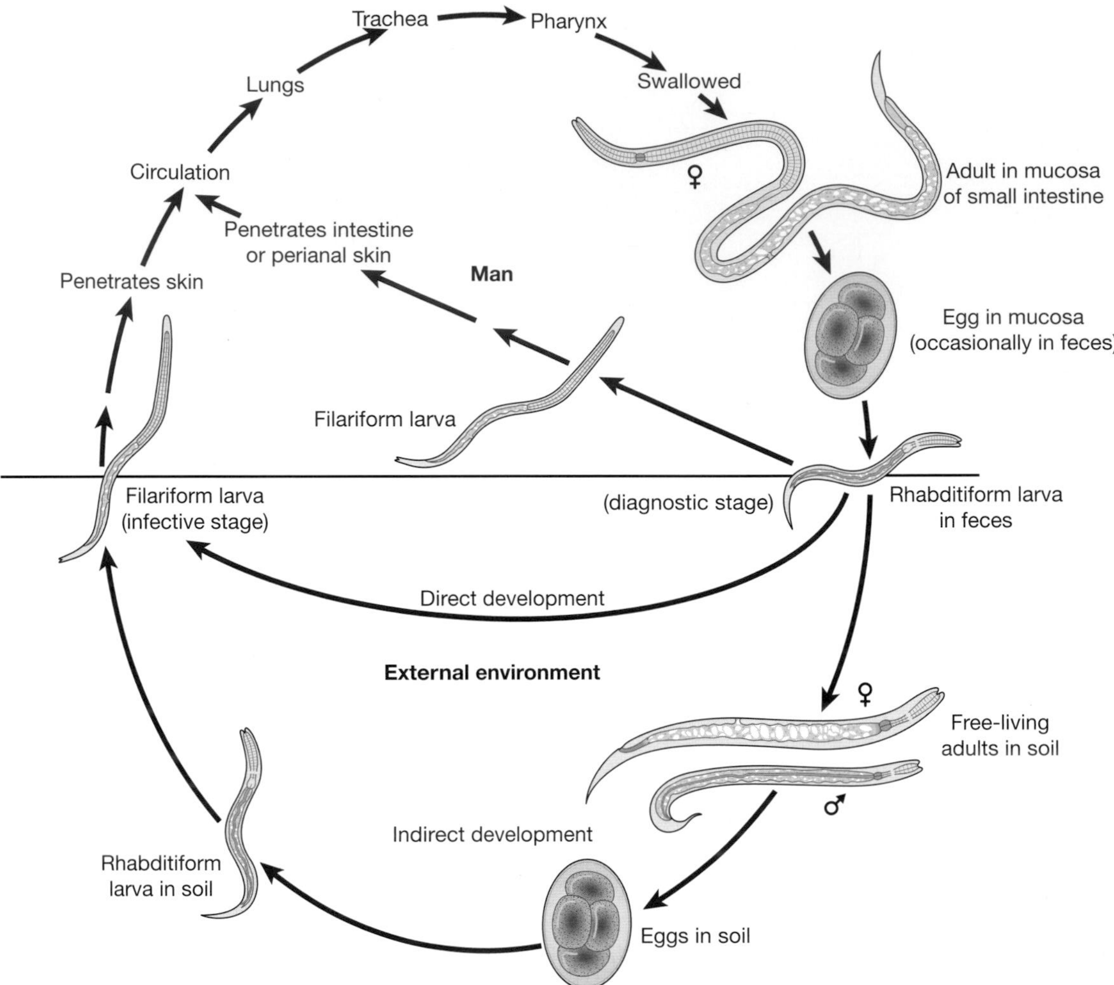

FIGURE 109.4 Life cycle of *Strongyloides stercoralis*. *(Redrawn from Melvin DM, Brooke MM, Sadun EH: Common Intestinal Helminths of Man. Atlanta, Centers for Disease Control, DHEW Publication No. [CDC] 75–8286, 1964.)*

the lungs to maintain infection (Fig.109.4). Under selected conditions, the autoinfective process may become dysregulated, leading to large number of L3 penetrating the gut, cycling through the lungs and re-entering the intestine. This process can lead to hyperinfection, associated secondary bacteremias and bacterial meningitis. Among conditions associated with hyperinfection are immunosuppressive drug therapies, especially corticosteroids. Other conditions are hematologic malignancies, solid organ transplantations, and autoimmune disorders, although in many of these conditions corticosteroids are used during treatment. Infection with HTLV-1 (as well as co-infections with tuberculosis, leprosy, syphilis) is another risk factor; however, the basis for this has not been established. In some patients with hyperinfection, the migrating larvae can develop to adult worms in ectopic sites, e.g. the lung and central nervous system. This condition is known as disseminated strongyloidiasis. In cases of external autoinfection, the L3 may also develop in the colorectal area and penetrate the perianal skin with resultant pruritic creeping eruption or *larva currens* and *external autoinfection*.

CLINICAL FEATURES

The clinical manifestations of *S. stercoralis* infection are acute infection, chronic persisting infection, and the hyperinfection syndrome. The latter two syndromes are the best characterized [9, 10].

Acute Infection

Although an estimated one-third or more of individuals are asymptomatic, a pruritic maculopapular rash or rapidly migrating linear urticaria called *larva currens*, which is usually seen on the buttocks area with external autoinfection, can occur. Cough, shortness of breath, wheezing, fever, transient pulmonary infiltrates, and eosinophilia are infrequent, but may be encountered with the migration of larvae through the lungs. When adult worms develop and penetrate the mucosa in the small bowel, nonspecific aching or epigastric abdominal pain and diarrhea can develop. With heavy infections, vomiting, malabsorption, steatorrhea, weight loss, edema, or a paralytic ileus with edema in the small bowel wall are recognized.

Chronic, Persisting Infection

This condition probably occurs as a result of internal autoinfection and is best described in military veterans or in former prisoners of war who have returned from endemic tropical areas in Asia or in the South Pacific. The classically recognized triad of symptoms is larva currens, abdominal pain, and diarrhea. An endemic focus also occurs in southeastern Kentucky and elsewhere in Appalachia, where most patients are usually white, male, older than 50 years, and from lower socioeconomic backgrounds. Viral HTLV-1 infection is an important risk factor for chronic, persisting infection.

Hyperinfection Syndrome

Gastrointestinal signs and symptoms are common but nonspecific and include crampy abdominal pain, bloating, watery diarrhea and constipation. Patients can develop an ileus and small bowel obstruction, with diffuse tenderness and hypoactive bowel sounds. Pulmonary manifestations are variable, and larva currens is common. Of

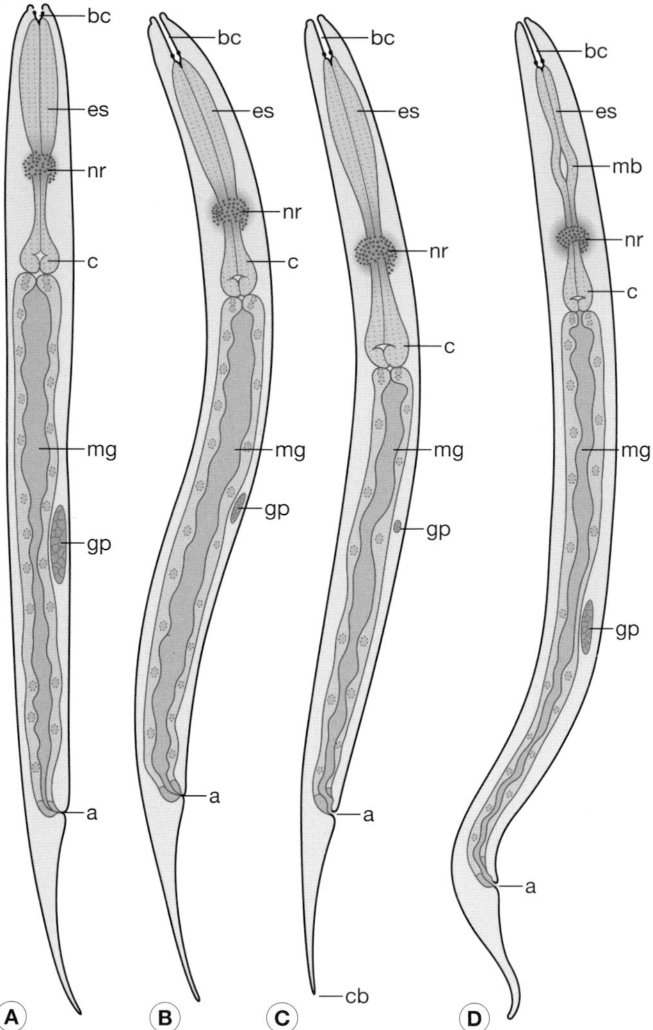

FIGURE 109.5 Figures of typical rhabditiform larval stages of: **(A)** *Strongyloides*; **(B)** hookworm; **(C)** *Trichostrongylus*; and **(D)** *Rhabditis* (ca. ×400). Explanation of labels: *a*, anus; *bc*, buccal chamber; *c*, cardiac bulb of esophagus; *cb*, beadlike swelling of caudal tip; *es*, esophagus; *gp*, genital primordia; *mb*, midesophageal bulb; *mg*, midgut; *nr*, nerve ring. *(Redrawn from Beaver PC, Jung RC, Cupp EW: Clinical Parasitology, 9th ed. Philadelphia, Lea & Febiger, 1984.)*

special concern is the high mortality, often with bacterial infection secondary to extensive larval spread from the intestine. Sepsis, meningitis, peritonitis and endocarditis are commonly documented, often with the microbiological recovery of Gram-negative enteric bacteria [9, 10].

PATIENT EVALUATION, DIAGNOSIS, AND DIFFRENTIAL DIAGNOSIS

Any individual from a strongyloidiasis-endemic area who is diagnosed with HTLV-1 infection or who is expected to undergo corticosteroid therapy (including doses as low as 1 mg of dexamethasone daily) should be screened for strongyloidiasis. The important aspects of diagnosing *Strongyloides* infections include a high index of suspicion in patients with histories of exposure and characteristic skin and intestinal symptoms. Second, an experienced person may have to diligently search in fecal specimens to find the characteristic rhabditiform larvae (Fig. 109.5). Several researchers have made efforts to improve the likelihood of finding *Strongyloides* larvae by amplifying the indirect life cycle *in vitro*. They have placed feces on nutrient agar and looked for tracks of bacteria from migrating larvae, used the Baermann funnel gauze concentration method, or used Harada Mori cultures on vertical strips of damp filter paper (where the larvae migrate down). Although previous serologic tests were complicated by lack of sensitivity and specificity, an improved immunofluorescence antibody assay using *Strongyloides* antigen has been described. Improved ELISA also gives high specificity and sensitivity, particularly if combined with Western blot. All immunodiagnostic methods are complicated by cross-reactivity with other nematode helminth infections. Sensitivity may decrease in co-infection with HTLV-1. *S. stercoralis* antigen is not widely available for routine diagnostic use.

TREATMENT

Because of the potential for chronic symptomatic infection, autoinfection over many years, and the hyperinfection syndrome, all individuals who are infected with *S. stercoralis* should be treated. The first-line treatment for acute or chronic infection is ivermectin, at a recommended dose of 200 μg/kg per day orally, on two successive days. The safety of ivermectin in young children (<15 kg) and in pregnancy has not been established. Albendazole at 400 mg orally twice a day for 7 days is an alternative. Albendazole should be taken with a fatty meal to promote absorption; ivermectin should be taken on an empty stomach and with water. Patients with HTLV-1 should be treated until their stools are negative for larvae or until they become seronegative. Treatment of immunocompromised patients suspected of having a life-threatening, hyperinfection syndrome should be continued until the clinical signs resolve. Because the autoinfective life cycle requires at least 2 weeks, some investigators recommend that treatment and screening should continue at least until fecal cultures have been negative for this period of time. A veterinary parental formulation has been used in patients who are unable to take or reliably absorb oral medications. In disseminated strongyloidiasis, combination therapy with albendazole and ivermectin has been suggested, although there are no carefully controlled clinical trials to support this. In patients with hyperinfection, co-infection with enteric bacteria is common, as well as bacteremia and bacterial meningitis; patients may require co-administration of oral or parenteral antibiotics. Patients with *Strongyloides* hyperinfection are infectious and may require isolation. Following treatment for hyperinfection, some clinicians choose to keep patients on chronic suppressive therapy with anthelminthic agents.

REFERENCES

1. Hotez PJ, Brooker S, Bethony JM, et al. Hookworm infection. N Engl J Med 2004;351:799–807.
Review of the major features of human hookworm infection.
2. Bethony J, Brooker S, Albonico M, et al. The soil-transmitted helminth infections. Lancet 2006;367:1521–32.
3. Brooker S, Hotez PJ, Bundy DAP. Hookworm-related anaemia among pregnant women: a systematic review. PLoS Negl Trop Dis 2008;2:e291.
4. Crompton DW. The public health importance of hookworm parasitology. Parasitology 2000;121(Suppl):S39–50.
5. Hotez PJ. Mass drug administration and the integrated control of the world's high prevalence neglected tropical diseases. Clin Pharmacol Ther 2009;85:649–64.
6. Keiser J, Utzinger J. Efficacy of current drugs against soil-transmitted helminth infections: systematic review and meta-analysis. JAMA 2008;299:1937–48.
Up-to-date meta-analysis of the major drugs used to treat intestinal helminthiases.
7. Diemert D, Bethony J, Hotez PJ. Hookworm vaccines. Clin Infect Dis 2008;46:282–8.
8. Hotez PJ, Bethony JM, Diemart DJ, et al. Developing vaccines to combat hookworm infection and intestinal schistosomiasis. Nat Rev Microbiol 2010;8(11):814–26.
9. Keiser PB, Nutman TB. *Strongyloides stercoralis* in the immunocompromised population. Clin Microbiol Rev 2004;17:208–17.
Up-to-date review of hyperinfection and disseminated infection, with treatment and patient management recommendations.
10. Ramanathan R, Nutman T. *Strongyloides stercoralis* infection in the immunocompromised host. Curr Infect Dis Rep 2008;10:105–10.

SECTION

B

FILARIAL INFECTIONS

110 Lymphatic Filariasis

LeAnne M Fox, Christopher L King

Key features

- Filariasis is a mosquito-transmitted nematode infection where the burden of infection correlates with exposure to infected mosquitos
- There is widespread chronic infection in 72 countries, with 1.3 billion people at risk and 120 million infected
- Adult parasites (up to 10 cm in length) live in the host lymphatics for many years and can lead to lymphatic dysfunction
- Clinical disease ranges from acute filarial lymphangitis (AFL) and acute dermatolymphangioadenitis (ADLA) to intermittent or chronic lymphedema in the extremities and/or hydroceles in men. The majority of infected individuals are asymptomatic
- Risk of infection is very low in travelers who are in endemic countries for less than a year
- Individuals first exposed or infected with lymphatic filariasis as adults are more likely to have clinical disease and eosinophilia

INTRODUCTION

Lymphatic filariasis is caused by infection with three species of parasite, *Wuchereria bancrofti*, *Brugia malayi* and *Brugia timori*. This mosquito-transmitted infection occurs throughout the tropics, but is highly heterogeneous in its distribution, infecting a high proportion of people in some communities and few in others [1]. The parasites can persist for years in humans and, consequently, the burden of disease occurs in adults.

The nematodes live in human lymphatics resulting in lymphatic damage and dysfunction that leads to recurrent swelling and disfigurement of the limbs (elephantiasis), genitalia (hydroceles) in men and sometimes breasts in women. Occasionally, infected individuals may develop a retrograde lymphadenitis and lymphangitis. The disfigurement resulting from lymphatic filariasis can have substantial economic and psychosocial consequences, particularly among individuals whose livelihoods depend on physical labor.

Descriptions of elephantiasis are found in early Indian, Egyptian and Persian writings, and epidemiologic association of elephantiasis with hydrocele, chylocele and chyluria were established by the middle of the 19th century. Their common etiology, however, remained a mystery until discoveries were made of microfilariae in hydrocele fluid (Demarquay, 1863), chylous urine (Wucherer, 1868) and blood (Lewis, 1872), and of the adult worm in a lymphatic abscess (Bancroft, 1877). Patrick Manson first described uptake of microfilariae by *Culex* mosquitoes and their maturation to infective forms (1875–89). This was the first description of the mosquito as a vector for any of the parasitic diseases and paved the way to his discovery of malaria transmission. Manson also made the association of endemic microfilaremia with elephantiasis and other lymphatic diseases.

EPIDEMIOLOGY

Currently, there are an estimated 1.34 billion people living in endemic areas in 72 countries with 120 million people infected. More than 90% of infections are caused by *W. bancrofti* for which humans are the only natural host.

Lymphatic filariasis is endemic in Africa, Asia, the Indian subcontinent, the western Pacific Islands, focal areas of Latin America, and the Caribbean – particularly Haiti and the Dominican Republic (Fig. 110.1). Approximately 65% of those at risk reside in south and South-east Asia, 30% in sub-Saharan Africa and the remainder in other parts of the tropical world [2]. In the Americas, endemic foci persist on the island of Hispaniola and in coastal areas of Guyana and north-eastern Brazil. Infection with *Brugia malayi* is limited to Asia (India, Malaysia) and several western Pacific island groups (Indonesia and the Philippines). There are fewer than 10–20 million persons in these areas who are infected with *B. malayi*. Unlike *W. bancrofti*, *B. malayi* has feline and primate reservoirs. *Brugia timori* is only found on the islands of south-eastern Indonesia. Both China and the Republic of Korea were considered endemic until recently, but have declared elimination of lymphatic filariasis as a public health problem in 2007 and 2008, respectively [2].

The distribution of lymphatic filariasis is highly focal within an endemic area. This is as a result of the different feeding and breeding behaviors of the mosquito vectors that are capable of transmitting lymphatic filariasis. For example, *W. bancrofti* is transmitted in much of rural Africa by *Anopheles* species [3], whereas in many urban areas of the world, including India and in the Western Hemisphere, *W. bancrofti* is transmitted by *Culex* mosquitoes [4]. Other vectors include *Aedes* species in some Pacific islands and *Mansonia*, which transmits *B. malayi* [5]. Lymphatic filariasis may be less efficiently transmitted than other vector-borne parasitic infections and therefore less commonly infects travelers with short-term exposure [6]. The microfilariae of *W. bancrofti* and *B. malayi* have a nocturnal periodicity where a few microfilaria appear in the circulation beginning around 18.00 h, but with the large majority in the peripheral circulation between 22.00 h and 02.00 h, coinciding with the time when most mosquito vectors take their blood meal [7]. In contrast, there is no clear-cut periodic cycle for *Aedes*-transmitted microfilariae in the South Pacific.

Infection, detected by microfilaria in the blood, is gradually acquired until the third or fourth decade of life. In areas of intense transmission, initial infection, detected as the presence of circulating filarial antigen, commonly occurs between the ages of 2 and 4 years and the prevalence of microfilaremia increases rapidly between the ages of 5 and 10 years [8, 9]. The proportion of age group infection and frequency of disease varies in different endemic areas. The chronic manifestations, such as lymphedema and hydrocele (in males), occur

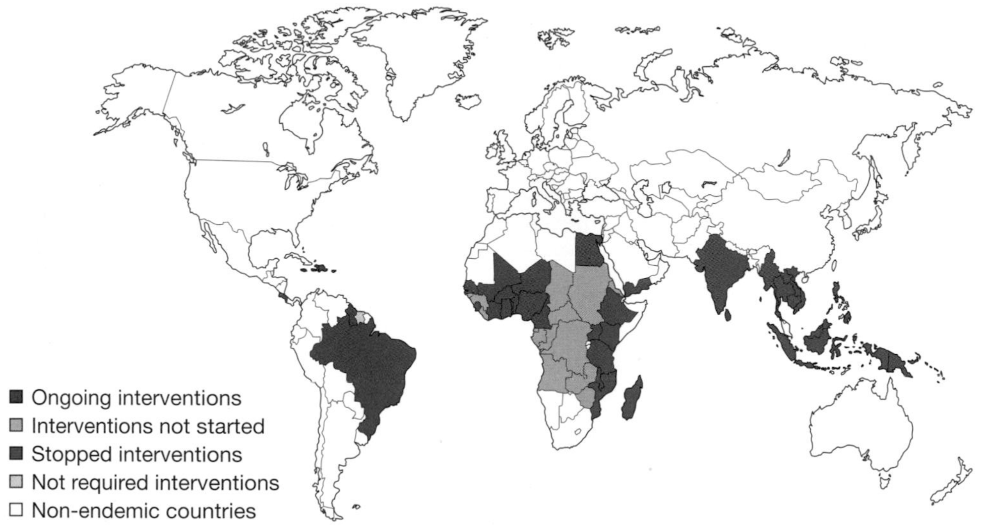

FIGURE 110.1 Global distribution of lymphatic filariasis and status of mass drug administration as of 2009.

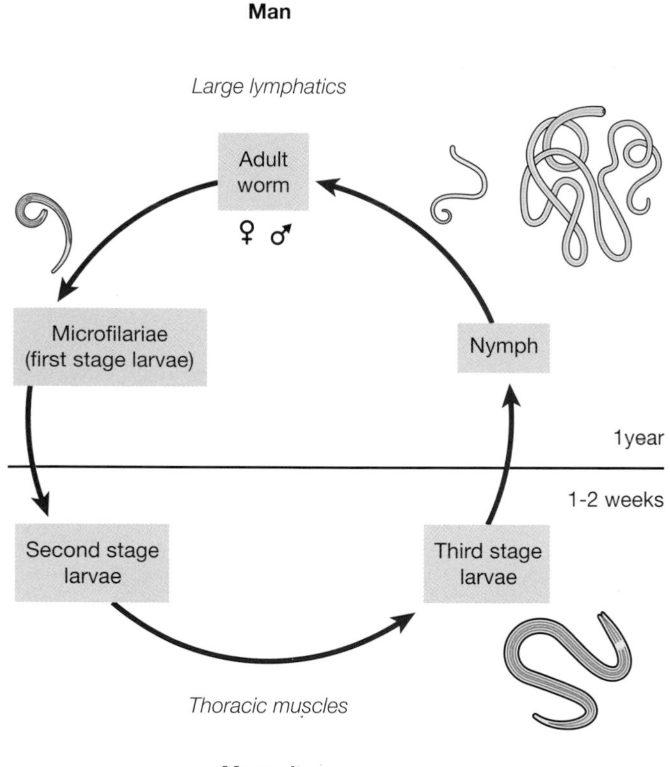

FIGURE 110.2 Life Cycle of lymphatic filariasis.

infrequently in people younger than 10 years and generally increase with age [8]. The role of gender in susceptibility to infection and disease is poorly understood. Hydrocele is the most common clinical manifestation of *W. bancrofti*, whereas chronic lymphedema has been more common in women. Occupation and socioeconomic status are important risk factors as filariasis affects primarily persons of the lowest socioeconomic levels. Host genetics may be important in susceptibility and development of lymphatic filariasis, but more research is needed.

NATURAL HISTORY, PATHOGENESIS, AND PATHOLOGY

Wuchereria bancrofti, *B. malayi* and *B. timori* have five morphologically distinct stages of their lifecycle (Fig. 110.2). The first stage larvae or microfilariae are released from fecund adult female worms that release up to 10,000 microfilariae per day, which circulate in the blood. Microfilariae are approximately 250 μm long and 10 μm wide and have an acellular sheath. Microfilariae of *W. bancrofti* and *B. malayi* differ morphologically based on the pattern of nuclei in the caudal and cephalic regions. Microfilariae are most abundant in the circulation at night (nocturnal periodicity), and during the day the microfilariae sequester in the deep vascular beds. This periodicity is thought to prolong the survival of microfilariae (~9 months) and result in high levels of microfilaria in some individuals (e.g. >10,000/ml).

Microfilariae are ingested by mosquitos and exsheath following the blood meal, penetrate the mosquito gut wall and migrate to the mosquito's thoracic muscle where they grow and undergo two molts to infective third-stage larvae (L3) in 10–14 days. L3 larvae migrate to the mouthparts of the mosquitos where they are deposited in the dermis during feeding. The L3 actively enter the feeding site, migrate to the local lymphatics where they quickly molt to L4 stage larvae and then migrate centrally in the lymphatic systems to develop into sexually-mature, adult worms at 6–9 months. Adult worms are long, thread-like organisms, hence the name filariae, with female worms ranging from 40–100 mm and males 20–40 mm in length. A striking feature of adult worms is the ability to cause massive dilation of the surrounding and proximal lymphatics, indicating release and/or stimulation of potent lymphangiogenic factors by adult worms. This lymphatic dilation leads to lymphatic valvular dysfunction and the inability to remove interstitial fluid and lymphedema. Death of adult worms and associated inflammation (acute filarial lymphangitis) can accelerate the process of lymphatic dysfunction. Although treatment can reverse some of the dysfunction, there is often persisting damage, putting an individual at risk for bacterial super-infections. The type, and extent of, overt clinical disease is related to where adult worms accumulate. Large numbers of adults appear to accumulate in lymphatics draining the lower extremities (inguinal and obturator lymphatics), axillary nodes in the upper extremities and, for *W. bancrofti* in men, in the lymphatics draining the spermatic cord, epididymis and tunica vaginalis surrounding the testis.

An important characteristic of *W. bancrofti* and *Brugia* species is the presence of an obligate intracellular bacterial endosymbiont, *Wolbachia*. *Wolbachia* parasites support essential biochemical pathways necessary for the parasite survival especially for embryogenesis and molting that is critical for transition from one parasite stage to another [10, 11].

CLINICAL FEATURES

The clinical expression of lymphatic filariasis varies from subclinical infection to pronounced chronic manifestations. The three species of parasite cause similar signs and symptoms, although urogenital disease and chyluria do not occur with *Brugia* infection.

SUBCLINICAL INFECTION

Most infected persons are asymptomatic, despite circulating microfilariae or filarial antigen in the peripheral blood [12]. Although they may be clinically asymptomatic, infected individuals have underlying lymphatic damage [13, 14]. Microscopic hematuria or proteinuria are also found in infected persons [15].

ACUTE MANIFESTATIONS

Infected persons may exhibit acute manifestations, particularly acute filarial lymphangitis (AFL) and acute dermatolymphangioadenitis (ADLA). AFL involves acute inflammation of a lymphatic vessel that progresses distally along the vessel and is thought to be caused by the death of the adult worm [16]. Patients usually give a history of pain, erythema and tenderness in the affected lymph node region for hours or a day prior to the onset of lymphangitis. Localized inflammatory nodules in breast, scrotum or subcutaneous tissues have also been reported.

ADLA is a separate and clinically distinct syndrome that is caused by bacterial infection of the small collecting lymphatic vessels in areas of lymphatic dysfunction [16, 17]. Unlike true filarial lymphangitis, this syndrome develops in a reticular rather than a linear pattern and is more commonly associated with severe pain, fever and chills. There is often a history of injury to the skin, such as trauma, insect bites or interdigital fungal infections. ADLA is often diagnosed as cellulitis and symptoms can last 3–15 days.

The adenolymphangitis of brugian filariasis (both *B. malayi* and *B. timori*) is more distinct, more dramatic and more destructive. In brugian filariasis, a single local abscess can form along the lymphatic tract, most often in the inguinal area, but sometimes in the axillae. These can suppurate and form sterile abscesses that often leak lymph before healing with a characteristic scar (Fig. 110.3).

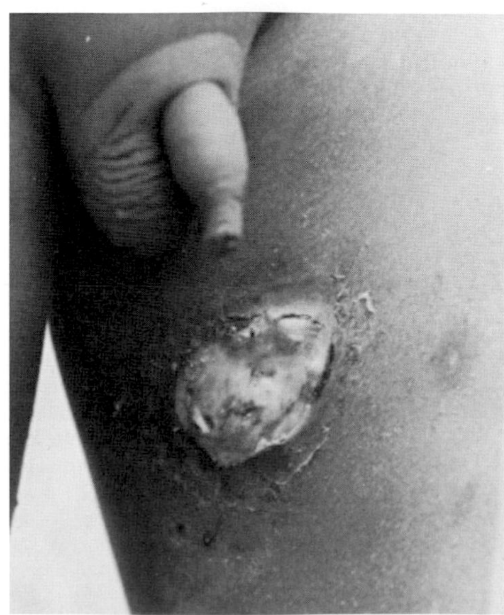

FIGURE 110.3 Clean-based ulcer resulting from the rupture of a filarial abscess *(courtesy of Dr David Dennis)*.

CHRONIC MANIFESTATIONS

It is estimated that of the 120 million persons infected worldwide, approximately one-third, or 40 million, have some form of clinically-overt disease; 25 million with hydrocele and 15 million with lymphedema or elephantiasis.

GENITAL MANIFESTATIONS

In many endemic areas, the most common chronic manifestation of lymphatic filariasis caused by *W. bancrofti* is hydrocele. Other forms of genital disease including epididymitis, orchitis, funiculitis, lymphedema of the scrotum and vulvar lymphedema have also been noted [18, 19]. (Figs 110.4 and 110.5). The pathogenesis of filarial hydrocele is thought to be as a result of lymphatic damage caused by living adult *W. bancrofti*. In filariasis-endemic areas, clinically-apparent hydrocele may actually be chylocele, resulting from rupture of dilated intrascrotal lymphatic vessels and leakage of lymph into the cavity of the testicular tunica vaginalis [20]. Hydroceles can become quite large (over 30 cm in diameter) and inguinal lymph nodes may be enlarged.

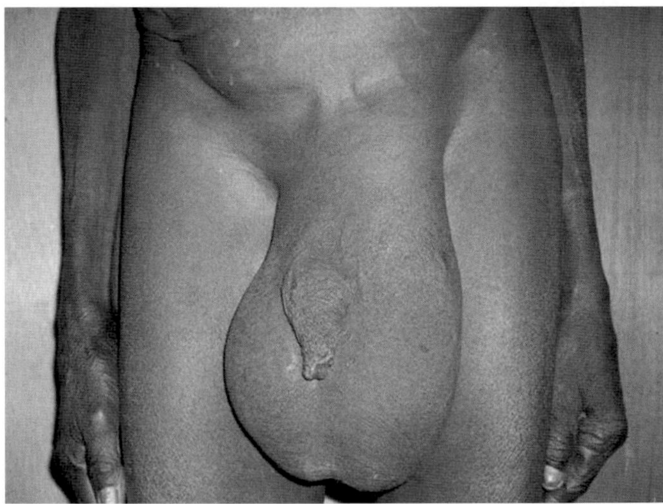

FIGURE 110.4 Man from the Democratic Republic of the Congo with bilateral filarial hydrocele progressing to "hanging-groin" *(courtesy of Dr Tony Ukety)*.

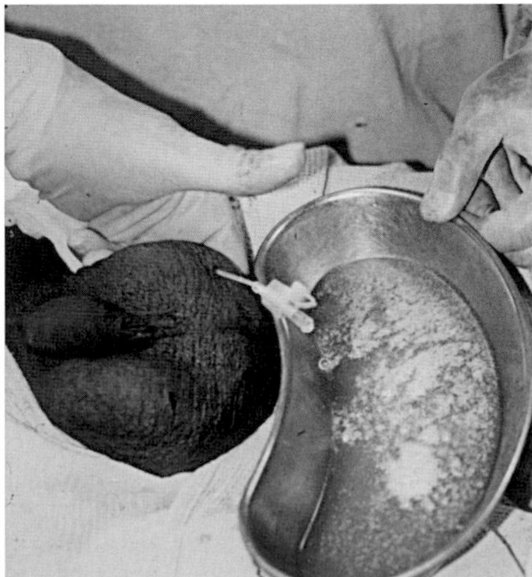

FIGURE 110.5 Hydrocele is the most common manifestation of clinical filariasis in males, necessitating mandatory genital examination in all patients. Straw-colored hydrocele fluid is non-inflammatory and generally without microfilariae. Therapeutic drainage is discouraged, as fluid rapidly re-accumulates.

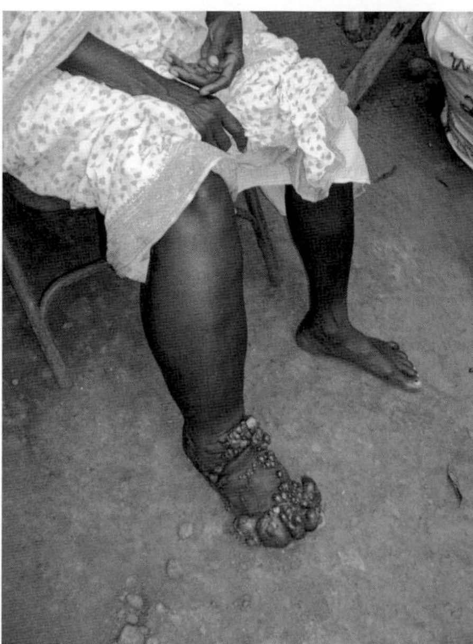

FIGURE 110.6 Filarial elephantiasis showing nodular and verrucous changes of the skin *(courtesy of Mr Jonathan Rout, Church's Auxiliary for Social Action, Bhubaneswar, India).*

Men with lymphedema of the scrotum can have rupture of dilated lymphatic vessels in the scrotal wall with oozing of lymph to the exterior. Genital manifestations of lymphatic filariasis occur only with *W. bancrofti* infection.

LYMPHEDEMA AND ELEPHANTIASIS

Lymphedema is a common chronic manifestation of lymphatic filariasis and occurs in the legs, scrotum, penis, breast and arms. Disease is more prevalent in the lower extremities, where assymetrical involvement is common. In bancroftian filariasis, lymphedema may involve the entire limb, whereas in brugian filariasis, the swelling is restricted to the distal extremities below the knee or elbow.

Grading systems, describe the severity of lymphedema. The World Health Organization (WHO) classification consists of four grades:

Grade I: pitting edema that is reversible upon elevation of the extremity;
Grade II: non-pitting edema that is not reversible upon elevation of the extremity;
Grade III: non-pitting edema that is not reversible with elevation associated with thickened skin or skin folds;
Grade IV: non-pitting edema with fibrotic and papillomatous skin lesions and the presence of skin folds (elephantiasis) (Fig. 110.6) [21].

Another grading (staging) system has been proposed containing seven categories and providing a more refined description of lymphedema stage based on depth of skin folds and types of papillomatous lesions [22].

Reversible episodes of lymphedema of the extremities progress to elephantiasis in the distribution of the affected lymphatics over a period of years. Factors involved include: repeated attacks of ADLA [20]; the intensity of filarial transmission within a population [23]; and the presence of *Wolbachia* [10]. ADLA episodes originate from breaks in the epidermis and contribute to lymph stasis, secondary bacterial infection and fibrosis.

In *Brugia* infection, insidious onset of chronic lymphedema or elephantiasis is less common than in bancroftian filariasis. Sclerotic, cordlike lymphatics and enlarged firm nodes of the arms and legs are usual.

CHYLURIA

Chyluria, resulting from rupture of dilated retroperitoneal lymphatic structures into the renal pelvis, is a rare, but serious, manifestation of lymphatic filariasis. As a result of loss of chyle, which contains dietary lipids, proteins and vitamins, weight loss and malnutrition can ensue. The condition is painless. The frequency of chyluria in filariasis endemic areas has not been established, but it is lower than lymphedema or hydrocele [24].

TROPICAL PULMONARY EOSINOPHILIA

Tropical pulmonary eosinophilia (TPE) is a distinct clinical entity that results from *W. bancrofti* or *B. malayi* infection [25]. Most cases have been reported in long-term residents from India, although there are cases from Pakistan, Sri Lanka, Brazil, Guyana and Southeast Asia. Men aged 20–40 years old are most commonly affected with a male/female ratio of 4:1. The pathogenesis of TPE is postulated to result from an exaggerated allergic type hypersensitivity response to microfilariae as they migrate through the pulmonary blood vessels. TPE is characterized by a paroxysmal, nonproductive cough (which is more severe at night), wheezing, low-grade fever, adenopathy, generalized malaise and weight loss, accompanied by pronounced peripheral blood eosinophilia (>3000 cells/mm^3), elevated serum IgE (>10,000 ng/ml), and elevated antifilarial antibody titers. Typically, peripheral microfilaremia is absent in patients with TPE. Chest radiographs can be normal or show diffuse small (1–3 mm in diameter) interstitial or reticulonodular infiltrates with increased bronchovascular markings. Pulmonary function tests show restrictive abnormalities, although obstructive defects can be seen. Treatment with diethylcarbamazine provides symptomatic improvement with decreases in eosinophilia and serum IgE. In advanced, untreated cases, the disease can progress to chronic restrictive lung disease with diffuse interstitial fibrosis. [26]

LYMPHATIC FILARIASIS IN EXPATRIATES AND TRAVELERS

AFL has been well documented in travelers to endemic areas. Two-to-six months after exposure, acute inflammation develops in a lymphatic vessel and its associated lymph nodes, most frequently in the leg, scrotal area or arm. Characteristically, the inflammation progresses distally along the lymphatic vessel, which becomes indurated, tender and erythematous, and resolves spontaneously within 3–7 days. Because biopsies reveal intense inflammation and nonliving adult worms, acute filarial lymphangitis is thought to be caused by the death of the adult worm [20]. The risk of developing chronic manifestations of lymphatic filariasis for the traveler is very low, as the parasite is inefficiently transmitted to humans by infected mosquitoes [6].

PATIENT EVALUATION, DIAGNOSIS, AND DIFFERENTIAL DIAGNOSIS

PATIENT EVALUATION

The diagnosis of lymphatic filariasis depends on the appropriate epidemiologic history, clinical findings and laboratory tests. Acquisition of filarial infection requires prolonged exposure, generally greater than three months, in a filariasis endemic area. While most infected individuals are clinically asymptomatic, a clinical diagnosis can be made in those with acute episodic adenolymphangitis, hydrocele or irreversible lymphedema. Eosinophilia is inconsistent in individuals with long-standing exposure and infection. In children, filarial lymphadenopathy is seen commonly [8, 27]. Adult worms can be detected by ultrasonography of the inguinal, crural and axillary lymph nodes, and vessels of infected children [14].

DIAGNOSIS

A definitive diagnosis requires detection of the parasite, parasite antigen or parasite DNA. The standard for diagnosis is microscopic detection of microfilariae on a thick blood film with Giemsa or hematoxylin staining (Fig. 110.7), but filtration of 1–5 ml of blood through

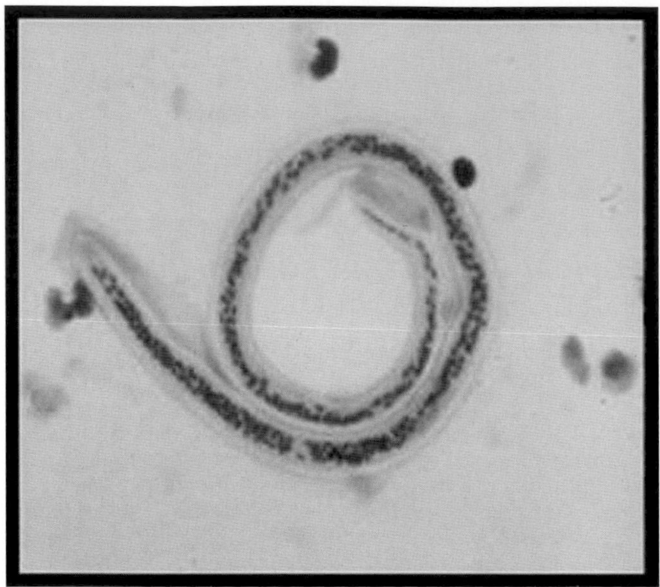

FIGURE 110.7 Microfilaria of *W. bancrofti* on a thick blood film stained with hematoxylin *(courtesy of Dr Mark L. Eberhard, Division of Parasitic Diseases and Malaria, Centers for Disease Control and Prevention, Atlanta, GA, USA).*

a 3–5-µm nucleopore filter or centrifugation of fluid fixed in 2% formalin (Knott's concentration technique) are more sensitive methods [28]. Diagnostic sampling must take into account the periodicity of microfilaria. For example, microfilaria of *W. bancrofti* circulate at highest concentration at night; therefore, blood specimens should be collected between 22.00 h and 02.00 h. Microfilaria can be found in blood, hydrocele fluid and, occasionally, in other fluids, such as urine. Microfilariae of the three species are distinguished morphologically.

Other tests may be helpful in individuals who do not have microfilaremia. Assays that detect circulating *W. bancrofti* antigen, primarily from the adult worm, are available and allow diagnosis of both microfilaremic and amicrofilaremic infections, even in the daytime blood of those with nocturnally-periodic microfilariae. Two assays for circulating antigens exist, an ELISA [29] and a rapid-format immunchromatographic card test [30]. Both assays have high sensitivity and specificity, but are not currently Food and Drugs Administration (FDA)-approved for diagnosis of filariasis in the USA. There are currently no tests for circulating antigens in brugian filariasis.

Antibody-based assays have suffered from poor specificity as they cannot distinguish among the filarial parasites that infect humans. Improvements have been made with the detection of antifilarial IgG4, which cross-reacts less with other nonfilarial helminthes [31]. Elevated antifilarial IgG4 levels indicate active filarial infection. Species-specific recombinant antigens have also been developed for brugian and bancroftian filariasis [32]. In addition, a rapid dipstick has been developed for the detection of *B. malayi* infection in endemic areas [33].

PCR-based assays to detect *W. bancrofti* and *B. malayi* in blood may be available in research laboratories [34, 35].

Adult worms localized in lymphatic vessels or lymph nodes have been found in pathologic specimens [27]. Examination of superficial lymphatics of the extremities and female breast or the intrascrotal lymphatics in men using high-frequency ultrasound in conjunction with Doppler techniques has demonstrated motile adult worms within dilated lymphatics, termed the filaria dance sign [36–39]. Filarial worms have been visualized in the intrascrotal lymphatics in up to 85% of infected men [38]. Ultrasonography has also been used to visualize the adult worms of children [40, 14]. Radionuclide lymphoscintigraphic imaging of the extremities has demonstrated lymphatic dilatation and dysfunction in both asymptomatic persons and those with lymphedema [13].

DIFFERENTIAL DIAGNOSIS

The differential diagnosis varies based on the clinical presentation. Bacterial infection, thrombophlebitis or trauma can be mistaken for acute filarial adenolymphangitis. Filarial lymphangitis is retrograde, which helps differentiate it from bacterial lymphangitis. Tuberculosis, leprosy, sarcoidosis and other systemic granulomatous diseases may be confused with filarial disease. Chronic lymphedema can be caused by malignancy, postoperative changes, congenital malformations or a hereditary form of lymphostasis (Milroy's disease), as well as renal or cardiac failure. Physical examination cannot distinguish a filarial from a nonfilarial cause of lymphedema or elephantiasis. A foreign body reaction to silica dust introduced into traumatized legs, termed podoconiosis, accounts for elephantiasis in some parts of the world.

Patients with filarial lymphedema are often amicrofilaremic, so that diagnosis depends on the epidemiologic and clinical history as well as the physical examination and can be supported by positive serology. In cases of orchitis and epididymitis, sexually transmitted infections must be considered. For tropical pulmonary eosinophilia, a failure to respond to DEC treatment should suggest an alternative diagnosis.

TREATMENT

Diethylcarbamazine (DEC, 6 mg/kg per day for 12 days for a total dose of 72 mg/kg or single-dose DEC at 6 mg/kg) is the recommended treatment for active lymphatic filariasis (antigen and/or microfilaremia positive, adults worms by ultrasound). DEC is active against both the microfilaria and adult worms, although treatment may not kill all adult worms. Infected individuals, particularly those with parasitemia, are at increased risk for adverse reactions from DEC treatment. Reactions are associated with the rapid killing of adult worms, which can lead to scrotal pain in men or acute lymphangioadenitis with nodules containing dying worms. Rapid killing of microfilariae induces systemic inflammation, most likely from release *Wolbachia* antigens. To reduce this risk of side effects, an escalating dose of DEC can be used. Alternatively, individuals can be pretreated with 1–3 days of oral steroids, depending on the intensity of infection as most severe reactions occur within the first 48 hours.

The mechanism of action of DEC is still not completely understood, but it results in the sequestration of microfilariae and their eventual destruction by the immune system, and is dependent on inducible nitric oxide synthase and cyclooxygenase. It is important to exclude co-infections with onchocerciasis and loiasis. Co-infections are most likely to occur in areas of west and central Africa, but not in Asia or the Pacific regions. Treatment with DEC can cause rapid death of *Onchocerciasis volvulus* microfilaria in the skin (or eye), resulting in severe skin and eye reactions. High levels of circulating microfilaria from *Loa loa* have been associated with severe systemic reactions and even death with DEC treatment.

Other drugs are effective against *W. bancrofti* and *Brugia* species. Albendazole inhibits the polymerization of worm β-tubulin and microtubule formation. A single dose of 400 mg decreases *W. bancrofti* microfilaraemia for 6–12 months and when it is used in combination with diethylcarbamazine (or ivermectin), the numbers of microfilaria are reduced for a longer length of time than after a single dose of DEC. A combined dose of DEC (6 mg/kg daily) plus 400 mg daily of albendazole is likely to kill adult worms more rapidly than DEC alone and the combination could shorten the duration of DEC therapy, although this has not been tested.

Ivermectin is highly active against microfilaria, and contributes to sterilization of adult worms, but does not kill them. It acts by hyperpolarization of glutamate-sensitive channels and was shown to block the contractile activity of the excretory/secretory vesicle [41]. As a result, molecules that may modulate the immune response are not released, leaving the microfilaria susceptible to host killing near release from adult worms rather than in the peripheral circulation or skin in onchocerciasis. There are less adverse reactions in subjects co-infected with onchocerciasis.

As *Wolbachia* are essential for *W. bancrofti* and *Brugia* spp. treatment with a course lasting 4, 6 or 8 weeks of a doxycycline, 200 mg daily, results in long-term sterility and eventual death of >90% of adult worms [42]. This slow death of worms is an advantage as it leads to fewer side effects compared with more rapidly-acting drugs like DEC. Shorter courses of doxycycline do not kill most adult worms, except in a recent study showing that three weeks of doxycycline followed by a single dose of DEC (6 mg/kg) had similar efficacy [43] to 4 weeks or more of doxycycline. There is evidence that anti-*Wolbachia* therapy leads to improvements in lymphatic pathologic features and decreased severity of lymphoedema and hydrocele [44]. The disadvantages of doxycycline are that it is contraindicated in children <9 years of age and in pregnant or breastfeeding women. Therefore, a four-week course of doxycycline could be considered in the appropriate patient. More potent drugs are needed to kill adult worms. Flubendazole, which is related to albendazole, is highly effective in killing adult worms; however, in its current formulation, it cannot be absorbed from the gut and is under further development.

PREVENTION AND CONTROL

There is no specific recommendation for prevention of *W. bancrofti* and *Brugia* spp. infection for the traveler or short-term residents other than bed nets and/or topical mosquito repellants, as transmission is inefficient and infections require many months, or even years, to acquire. In 2000, a global program to eliminate lymphatic filariasis (GPELF) by 2020 was launched. The main goal of GPELF is to break the cycle of transmission of disease between mosquitoes and human beings, mainly through mass drug distribution of diethylcarbamazine or ivermectin combined with albendazole. This program has distributed over 2.4 billion doses of drugs in more than 60 countries endemic for lymphatic filariasis. The increased use of bed nets as part of a worldwide malaria control program will also have a substantial impact on transmission of lymphatic filariasis as the two infections are often co-endemic and often share the same mosquito vectors. Hopefully, in several decades, lymphatic filariasis will be a disease of historical interest; however, there remain tremendous challenges to attain this goal.

REFERENCES

1. Taylor MJ, Hoerauf A, Bockarie M. Lymphatic filariasis and onchocerciasis. Lancet 2010;376:1175–85.
2. World Health Organization. Global Programme to Eliminate Lymphatic Filariasis (GPELF) Progress Report 2000–2009 and Strategic Plan 2010–2020. Geneva: World Health Organization; 2010:6–8.
3. Merelo-Lobo AR, McCall PJ, Perez MA, et al. Identification of the vectors of lymphatic filariasis in the Lower Shire Valley, southern Malawi. Trans R Soc Trop Med Hyg 2003;97:299–301.
4. Ramaiah KD, Das PK. Seasonality of adult *Culex quinquefasciatus* and transmission of bancroftian filariasis in Pondicherry, south India. Acta Trop 1992;50:275–83.
5. Chang MS. Operational issues in the control of the vectors of Brugia. Ann Trop Med Parasitol 2002;96:S71–S76.
6. Lipner EM, Law MA, Barnett E, et al. Filariasis in travelers presenting to the GeoSentinel Surveillance Network. PloS Negl Trop Dis 2007;1:e88.
7. O'Conner FW. Filarial periodicity with observations and on the mechanisms of migration of the microfilariae and from parent worm to the blood stream. PR Public Health Trop Med 1931;6:263.
8. Witt C, Ottesen EA. Lymphatic filariasis: An infection of childhood. Bull World Health Org 2001;6:582–606.
9. Malhotra I, Ouma JH, Wamachi A, et al. Influence of maternal filariasis on childhood infection and immunity to Wuchereria bancrofti in Kenya. Infect Immun 2003;71:5231–7.
10. Hise AG, Gillette-Ferguson I, Pearlman E. The role of endosymbiotic *Wolbachia* bacteria in filarial disease. Cell Microbiol 2004;6:97–104.
11. Rajan TV. Relationship of anti-microbial activity of tetracycline to their ability to block the L3 and L4 molt of the human filarial parasite *Brugia malayi*. Am J Trop Med Hyg 2004;71(1):24–8.
12. Ottesen EA. Infection and disease in lymphatic filariasis—an immunological perspective. Parasitology 1992;104:571.
13. Shenoy RK, Suma TK, Kumaraswami V, et al. Lymphoscintigraphic evidence of lymph vessel dilation in the limbs of children with *Brugia malayi* infection. J Commun Dis 2008;40:91–100.
14. Fox LM, Furness BW, Haser JK, et al. Ultrasonographic examination of Haitian children with lymphatic filariasis: a longitudinal assessment in the context of antifilarial drug treatment. Am J Trop Med Hyg 2005;72:642–8.
15. Dreyer G, Ottesen EA, Galdino E, et al. Renal abnormalities in microfilaremic patients with Bancroftian filariasis. Am J Trop Med Hyg 1992;46:745–51.
16. Dreyer G, Medeiros Z, Netto MJ, et al. Acute attacks in the extremities of persons living in an area endemic for bancroftian filariasis: Differentiation of two syndromes. Trans Roy Soc Trop Med Hyg 1999;93:413–17.
17. Olszewski WL, Jamal S, Manokaran G, et al. Bacteriologic studies of blood, tissue fluid, lymph, and lymph nodes in patients with acute dermatolymphangioadenitis (DLA) in course of 'filarial' lymphedema. Acta Trop 1999; 73:217–24.
18. Aguiar-Santos AM, Leal-Cruz M, Netto MJ, et al. Lymph scrotum: an unusual urological presentation of lymphatic filariasis. A case series study. Rev Inst Med Trop Sao Paulo 2009;51:179–83.
19. Adesiyun AG, Samaila MO. Huge filarial elephantiasis vulvae in a Nigerian woman with subfertility. Arch gynecol Obstet 2008;278:597–600.
20. Dreyer G, Noroes J, Figueredo-Silva J, et al. Pathogenesis of lymphatic disease in bancroftian filariasis: A clinical perspective. Parasitol Today 2000;16: 544–8.
21. World Health Organization. Informal consultation on evaluation of morbidity in lymphatic filariasis. WHO/TDR/FK/92.31. Geneva: World Health Organization; 1992.
22. Dreyer G, Addiss DG, Dreyer P, Norões J. Basic lymphoedema management: Treatment and prevention of problems associated with lymphatic filariasis. Hollis: Hollis Publishing Co.; 2002.
23. Kazura JW, Bockarie M, Alexander N, et al. Transmission intensity and its relationship to infection and disease due to *Wuchereria bancrofti* in Papua New Guinea. J Infect Dis 1997;176:242–6.
24. Dreyer G, Mattos D, Noroes J. Chyluria. Rev Assoc Med Bras 2007;53:460–4.
25. Ottesen EA, Nutman TB. Tropical pulmonary eosinophilia. Annu Rev Med 1992;43:417–24.
26. Rom WN, Vijayan VK, Cornelius MJ, et al. Persistent lower respiratory tract inflammation associated with interstitial lung disease in patients with tropical pulmonary eosinophilia following conventional treatment with diethylcarbamazine. Am Rev Respir Dis 1990;142:1088–92.
27. Figueredo-Silva J, Dreyer G. Bancroftian filariasis in children and adolescents: clinical–pathological observations in 22 cases from an endemic area. Ann Trop Med Parasitol 2005;99:759–69.
28. Eberhard ML, Lammie PJ. Laboratory diagnosis of filariasis. Clin Lab Med 1991;11:977–1010.
29. More SJ, Copeman DB. A highly specific and sensitive monoclonal antibody-based ELISA for the detection of circulating antigen in bancroftian filariasis. Trop Med Parasitol 1990;41:403–6.
30. Weil GJ, Lammie PJ, Weiss N. The ICT Filariasis Test: a rapid-format antigen test for diagnosis of bancroftian filariasis. Parasitol Today 1997;13:401–4.
31. Lal RB, Ottesen EA. Enhanced diagnostic specificity in human filariasis by IgG4 antibody assessment. J Infect Dis. 1988;158:1034–7.
32. Lammie PJ, Weil G, Rahmah N, et al. Recombinant antigen-based antibody assays for the diagnosis and surveillance of lymphatic filariasis—a multicenter trial. Filaria J 2004;3:9.
33. Rahmah N, Taniawati S, Shenoy RK, et al. Specificity and sensitivity of a rapid dipstick test (Brugia Rapid) in the detection of Brugia malayi infection. Trans R Soc Trop Med Hyg 2001;95:601–4.
34. Kanjanavas P, Tan-ariya P, Khawak P, et al. Detection of lymphatic *Wuchereria bancrofti* in carriers and long-term storage of blood samples using semi-nested PCR. Mol Cell Probes 2005;19:169–72.
35. Kluber S, Supali T, Williams SA, et al. Rapid PCR-based detection of *Brugia malayi* DNA from blood spots by DNA detection test strips. Trans R Soc Trop Med Hyg 2001;95:169–70.
36. Amaral F, Dreyer G, Figueredo-Silva J, et al. Live adult worms detected by ultrasonography in human bancroftian filariasis. Am J Trop Med Hyg 1994;50:753–7.
37. Dreyer G, Brandao AC, Amaral F, et al. Detection of ultrasound of living adult *Wuchereria bancrofti* in the female breast. Mem Inst Oswaldo Cruz 1996;91(1):95–6.
38. Dreyer G, Santos A, Noroes J, et al. Ultrasonographic detection of living adult *Wuchereria bancrofti* using a 3.5-MHz transducer. Am J Trop Med Hyg 1998;59:399–403.
39. Mand S, Marfo-Debrekyei Y, Dittrich M, et al. Animated documentation of the filaria dance sign (FDS) in bancroftian filariasis. Filaria J 2003;2:3.

40. Dreyer G, Noroes J, Addiss D, et al. Bancroftian filariasis in a paediatric population: An ultrasonographic study. Trans Roy Soc Trop Med Hyg 1999;93:633–6.
41. Moreno Y, Nabhan JF, Solomon J, et al. Ivermectin disrupts the function of the excretory–secretory apparatus in microfilariae of *Brugia malayi*. Proc Natl Acad Sci USA 2010;107:20120–5.
42. Taylor MJ, Makunde WH, McGarry HF, et al. Macrofilaricidal activity after doxycycline treatment of *Wuchereria bancrofti*: a double-blind, randomised placebo-controlled trial. Lancet 2005;365:2116–21.
43. Supali T, Djuardi Y, Pfarr KM, et al. Doxycycline treatment of *Brugia malayi*-infected persons reduces microfilaremia and adverse reactions after diethylcarbamazine and albendazole treatment. Clin Infect Dis 2008;46:1385–93.
44. Debrah AY, Mand S, Specht S, et al. Doxycycline reduces plasma VEGF-C/sVEGFR-3 and improves pathology in lymphatic fi lariasis. PLoS Pathog 2006;2:e92.

Loiasis 111

Amy D Klion

Key features

- Loiasis, infection with the filarial nematode *Loa loa*, is endemic in Central and West Africa
- Characteristic clinical manifestations include episodic angioedema (Calabar swellings) and subconjunctival migration of adult worms (eyeworm)
- Microfilariae are found in the peripheral blood during the day
- Treatment with diethylcarbamazine (DEC) is curative in most cases, but is associated with severe side effects in patients with high levels of circulating microfilariae
- Weekly DEC is effective in preventing loiasis in travelers to endemic regions

INTRODUCTION

Infection with the filarial nematode *Loa loa* was first described by Mongin in 1770, when he extracted an adult worm from the eye of an African slave [1]. The clinical manifestations were not fully described, however, until 1781 by Guyot. Adult worms migrate through the subcutaneous tissues causing intermittent "Calabar swellings" and sometimes migrate beneath the conjunctiva (hence the popular name *eye worm*). Although many infected people are asymptomatic despite large numbers of circulating microfilariae in the blood, administration of microfilaricidal agents, including diethylcarbamazine and ivermectin, can cause severe, sometimes fatal, treatment-associated reactions. This has created challenges for the Global Programme to Eliminate Lymphatic Filariasis.

EPIDEMIOLOGY

It has been estimated that *Loa loa* infects 3 to 13 million people in Central and West Africa with a distribution that mirrors the distribution of the *Chrysops* fly vectors, which breed in wet mud on the edge of shaded streams beneath the high-canopied rain forest. The endemic areas of Africa are illustrated in Figure 111.1. Isolated cases have also been reported in Uganda, Malawi, Zambia and Ethiopia, and in the region from Ghana to Guinea.

Infection rates are usually higher in adults, particularly males, than in children, probably because of increased exposure to biting flies. Non-human primates harbor a form of *Loa*, but there is no evidence that they act as reservoir hosts for human *Loa loa*, and infection of humans by the simian strain has not been demonstrated.

NATURAL HISTORY, PATHOGENESIS AND PATHOLOGY

Loa loa is transmitted by large tabanid flies of the genus *Chrysops*, known in Africa as red flies (Fig. 111.2). The species *C. silacea* and *C. dimidiata* are the most important. Microfilariae are ingested by the vector during a blood meal and develop over the course of 10 to 12 days into infective filariform (L3) larvae. Many larvae (up to 100) can develop in a single fly. When the fly bites a new host, larvae are injected and develop into adult worms over the course of 6 to 12 months. Adult *Loa* are thin transparent worms that migrate through the subcutaneous tissues at rates of up to 1 cm/min. Females measure 50–70 × 0.5 mm, and males 30–35 × 0.3–0.4 mm. The cuticle of the middle region in both sexes has numerous small bosses that aid in identifying portions of worms removed at biopsy. Adult worms can survive for up to 17 years. Following sexual mating, microfilariae are released into the bloodstream, where they exhibit diurnal periodicity [2]. Peak microfilarial levels in the blood range from undetectable to more than 100,000 parasites/mL and are remarkably stable in an individual person over time. Of note, *Loa loa* does not harbor the

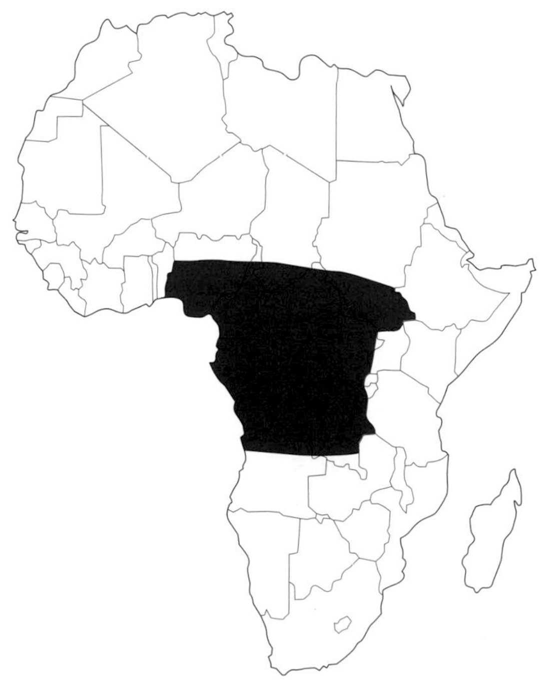

FIGURE 111.1 Geographic distribution of loiasis. Endemic areas are shaded. Please note that the prevalence of infection within an endemic area is typically focal.

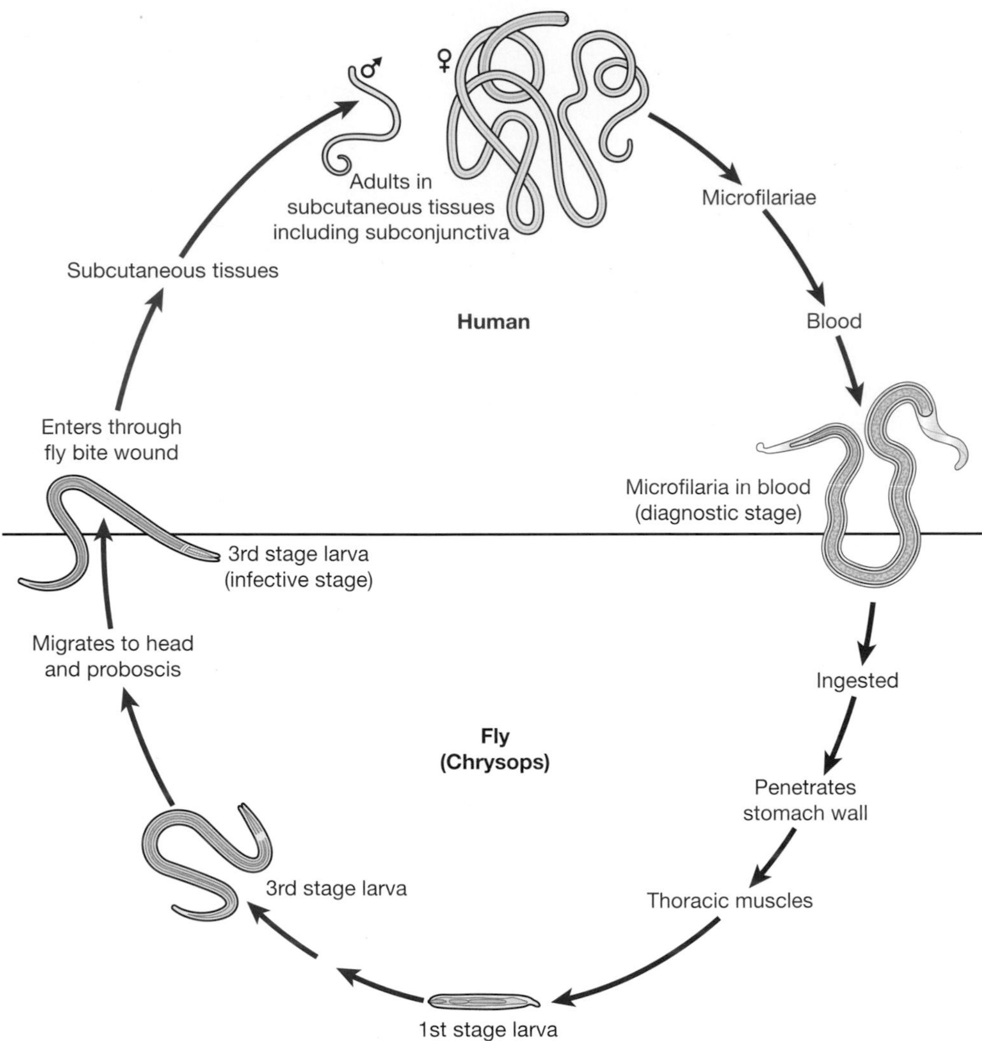

FIGURE 111.2 *Loa loa* life cycle

bacterial endosymbiont *Wolbachia*, found in most other filarial pathogens of humans [3].

CLINICAL FEATURES

The clinical spectrum of loiasis is broad, ranging from asymptomatic infection to life-threatening complications of encephalitis, cardiomyopathy and renal failure. With the exception of eye worm and renal abnormalities (see below), clinical signs and symptoms are more common in visitors to *Loa*-endemic areas than in people native to these areas and reflect a heightened immune response to the parasite. Conversely, microfilariae are detectable in the peripheral blood of most endemic individuals with loiasis but are rare in infected visitors [4].

CALABAR SWELLINGS

Recurrent episodes of localized angioedema, or Calabar swellings (Fig. 111.3), are one of the characteristic manifestations of loiasis. Although their precise etiology is unproved, Calabar swellings are thought to be a hypersensitivity response to antigenic material released by a migrating, developing or adult worm. They are most common on the face and extremities. Typically, an area of pain or itching develops, followed within hours by the development of a 10- to 20-cm area of nonpitting edema. The edema lasts from a few days to several weeks and is usually painless, except when the location of the swelling causes restriction of joint movement or nerve compression. Peripheral nerve compression is most common in the region of the carpal tunnel and may be transiently exacerbated by diethylcarbamazine (DEC) treatment.

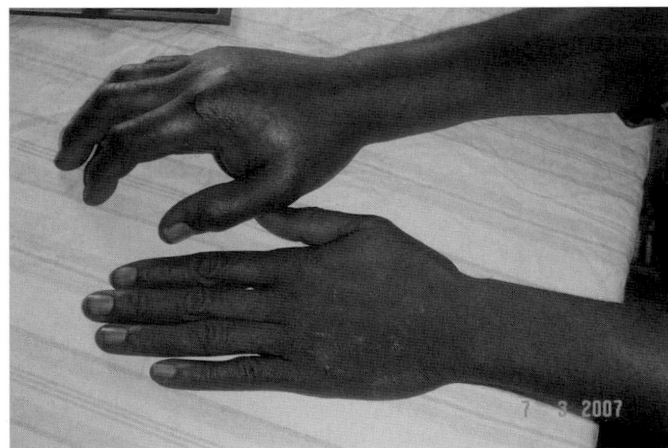

FIGURE 111.3 Calabar swelling. *(Courtesy of Joseph Kamgno.)*

EYE WORM

Subconjunctival migration of the adult eye worm (Fig. 111.4), is generally accompanied by transient swelling of the lid and intense

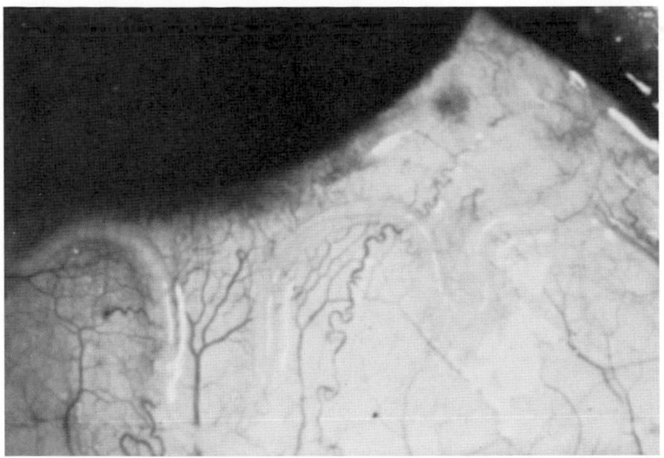

FIGURE 111.4 Subconjunctival migration of an adult *Loa loa* worm.

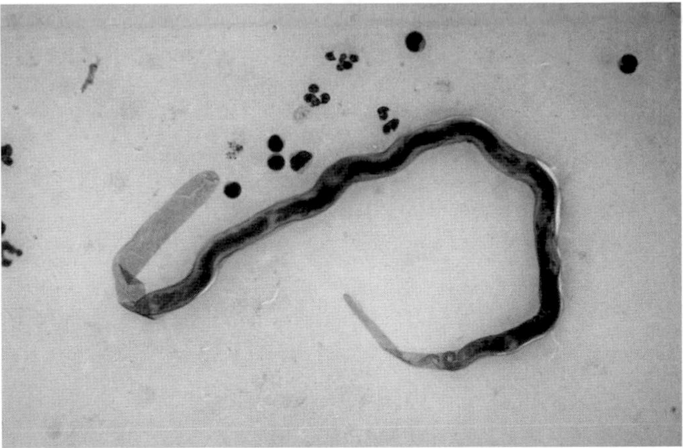

FIGURE 111.5 *Loa loa* microfilaria in a thick blood smear of peripheral blood stained with Delafield's hematoxylin (180×), showing the sheath (clear halo) and nuclei extending to the tip of the tail. *(Courtesy of W Meyers, Armed Forces Institute of Pathology.)*

conjunctivitis. Although most episodes resolve spontaneously and completely, rare cases of retinal artery occlusion and macular retinopathy due to aberrant migration of the adult parasite have been reported.

OTHER SYMPTOMS

Nonspecific systemic symptoms including pruritus, urticaria, myalgia, arthralgia, fatigue and malaise are common. Eosinophilia is marked in most infected individuals.

COMPLICATIONS

Central Nervous System

The most serious complication of *Loa loa* infection is meningoencephalitis, which occurs predominantly in patients with high numbers of circulating microfilariae, particularly in the setting of treatment with DEC or ivermectin.

The severity of central nervous system involvement ranges from mild headache and meningismus to coma and death. Occasionally, microfilariae are found in the cerebrospinal fluid, and, in fatal cases, degenerating microfilariae have been seen in necrotizing granulomas in the brain.

Renal

Hematuria and proteinuria are commonly seen in loiasis and may be due to immune complex glomerulonephritis or mechanical trauma resulting from the filtration of large numbers of microfilariae. The urinary sediment is usually unremarkable, except for the occasional detection of microfilariae. Transient worsening may occur following DEC treatment; most cases resolve completely with treatment, and progression to chronic renal insufficiency is unusual.

Endomyocardial Fibrosis

Loiasis has been implicated in the etiology of some cases of endomyocardial fibrosis (EMF) in equatorial Africa based on the higher prevalence of EMF in *Loa*-endemic areas than in other regions in Africa and high levels of antifilarial antibodies detected in some individuals with EMF. Although clinical resolution of biopsy-proven EMF with antifilarial therapy has been documented in one patient with concomitant loiasis, the relationship between these two clinical entities remains unclear.

Other Complications

Transient pulmonary infiltrates and pleural effusion have been reported. Other uncommon manifestations of loiasis include arthritis, lymphangitis and hydrocele.

PATIENT EVALUATION, DIAGNOSIS AND DIFFERENTIAL DIAGNOSIS

Loiasis should be considered in an individual with a compatible travel history and unexplained eosinophilia, Calabar swellings, or an adult worm migrating under the skin or across the eye. Sometimes, the diagnosis is suggested by dead, calcified worms seen on a roentgenogram. Most people have a history of prolonged exposure in an endemic area, although cases have been reported after 1–2 weeks in a highly endemic area.

DEFINITIVE DIAGNOSIS

Demonstration of *Loa loa* microfilariae in the blood or identification of an adult *Loa loa* worm removed from the subcutaneous tissue is diagnostic. Microfilariae can be distinguished from microfilariae of *Wuchereria bancrofti* and *Mansonella perstans*, other filarial pathogens whose geographic distribution overlaps that of *Loa loa*, by their diurnal periodicity, their size (approximately 290 × 7.5 μm), the presence of a sheath and three or more nuclei extending to the tip of the tail (Fig. 111.5). Blood should be drawn between 10 am and 2 pm (with adjustment made for recent [<2 weeks] travel from a different time zone) to coincide with peak levels of microfilariae. Although microfilariae can be seen in thick blood smears stained with Giemsa or Wright's stain, concentration techniques, including Knott's concentration, saponin lysis, and filtration of anticoagulated blood through a 5-μm Nuclepore filter, are useful in patients with low numbers of circulating microfilariae. Species-specific PCR-based diagnostics are more sensitive than blood filtration, but are available only in research settings [5].

PRESUMPTIVE DIAGNOSIS

Immunodiagnostic tests are available commercially and at some academic centers and may be useful in confirming the diagnosis of filariasis in travelers from endemic areas who have characteristic clinical symptoms or unexplained eosinophilia but no detectable microfilariae in blood [6]. Currently available tests do not distinguish between the human filariae, including lymphatic filariasis and onchocerciasis, which have overlapping geographic distributions with loiasis. The high prevalence of antifilarial antibodies in native populations of *Loa*-endemic areas limits the utility of serologic tests in this group.

DIFFERENTIAL DIAGNOSIS

In the absence of definitive, parasitologic evidence of infection, the diagnosis of loiasis can be difficult. Angioedema mimicking Calabar

TABLE 111-1 Treatment of Loiasis

Indication	Treatment	Dose	Comments	Evidence
Treatment of choice	DEC	3 mg/kg three times daily for 21 days	Severe side effects in patients with high mf levels	Multiple anecdotal reports and small case series
Pre-treatment for patients with high mf levels	Cytapheresis	N/A	Requires special settings	Case series
	Albendazole	200 mg twice daily for 21 days		Double-blind trial
Refractory disease	Albendazole	200 mg twice daily for 21 days		Case series
Prophylaxis	DEC	300 mg weekly		Double-blind trial

DEC, diethylcarbamazine; mf, microfilariae.

swellings can be associated with C1 esterase deficiency, other helminth infections such as gnathostomiasis and trichinosis, and allergic diseases. Subconjunctival migration of an adult worm is highly suggestive of loiasis, although other etiologies, including *Dirofilaria repens* and *Thelazia californiensis*, have been described.

TREATMENT

In patients with few or no circulating microfilariae, DEC at a dose of 8 to 10 mg/kg/day for 21 days is the drug of choice (**Table 111-1**). The drug is not directly toxic to the parasites but works in conjunction with the host immune responses to kill microfilariae and adult worms. DEC is curative in most cases, although multiple courses of therapy are often necessary, and relapses have been documented as late as 8 years after treatment [7].

Mild side effects of DEC treatment, including Calabar swellings, urticaria, arthralgias, fever and right upper quadrant tenderness, are common during the first few days of therapy and generally respond to antihistamines or a short course of corticosteroids. DEC should not be used in patients with concomitant onchocerciasis, because of the risk of severe cutaneous and ocular reactions in these individuals. Serious complications of DEC treatment, including meningoencephalitis and renal failure, are most common in patients with high numbers of circulating microfilariae (>2500/mL) and are thought to be due to the massive release of antigens from dying microfilariae [8]. Although advocated in the past, neither a gradual increase in DEC dose nor pretreatment with corticosteroids is completely effective in preventing encephalitis in such patients. Consequently, if therapy is indicated in a patient with high numbers of circulating microfilariae, cytapheresis should be used to reduce the microfilarial load prior to the initiation of DEC and corticosteroid therapy [9].

Albendazole, at a dose of 200 mg twice daily for 3 weeks, reduced *Loa* microfilaremia by approximately 80% over the course of several months without adverse effects [10]. Shorter courses of higher-dose albendazole appear to be less effective [11]. Albendazole is thought to have an effect on adult parasites by inhibiting microtubular function and glucose uptake. Albendazole has been used successfully in DEC-refractory *Loa loa* infection.

Ivermectin, the treatment of choice for onchocerciasis, has activity against *Loa loa* microfilariae, but little, if any, effect on adult worms. Consequently, since ivermectin is not curative and causes similar side effects to those seen with DEC in patients with high microfilarial loads [12], it should not be used for the treatment of loiasis. Doxycycline is not effective in loiasis due to the absence of the bacterial endosymbiont *Wolbachia*.

Elimination of insect vectors using larvicides has been hampered by the inaccessibility of vector breeding sites. Clearance of forest around dwellings, screening houses, and use of protective clothing can effectively reduce personal exposure to *Chrysops* in endemic areas. DEC at a dose of 300 mg weekly is effective in preventing loiasis in long-term travelers to endemic areas [13].

REFERENCES

1. Mongin. Observation on a worm found under conjunctiva in Maribou, Saint Domingue Island. J Med Chir Pharm Paris 1770;32:338–9.
2. Duke BOL. Behavioural aspects of the life cycle of Loa. In: Canning ED, Wright CA, eds. Behavioural Aspects of Parasite Transmission. London: Academic Press; 1972:97–108.
3. Büttner DW, Wanji S, Bazzocchi C, et al. Obligatory symbiotic *Wolbachia* endobacteria are absent from *Loa loa*. Filaria J 2003;2:10.
4. Klion AD, Massougbodji A, Sadeler B-C, et al. Loiasis in endemic and non-endemic populations: immunologically mediated differences in clinical presentation. J Infect Dis 1881;163:1318–25.
5. Nutman TB, Zimmerman PA, Kubofcik J, et al. ELISA-based detection of PCR products: a universally applicable approach to the diagnosis of filarial and other infections. Parasitol Today 1994;10:239–43.
6. Burbelo PD, Ramanathan R, Klion AD, et al. Rapid, novel, specific, high-throughput assay for diagnosis of *Loa loa* infection. J Clin Microbiol 2008; 46:2298–304.
   Diagnosis of loiasis can be difficult, especially in the absence of microfilariae in the blood. The authors describe a novel antibody assay for specific diagnosis of Loa loa infection.
7. Klion AD, Ottesen EA, Nutman TB. Effectiveness of diethylcarbamazine in treating loiasis acquired by expatriate visitors to endemic regions: long term follow-up. J Infect Dis 1994;169:604–10.
8. Carme B, Boulesteix J, Boutes H, et al. Five cases of encephalitis during treatment of loiasis with diethylcarbamazine. Am J Trop Med Hyg 1991; 44:684–90.
9. Chandenier J, Pillier-Loriette C, Datry A, et al. Value of cytapheresis in the treatment of loaiasis with high blood microfilaria levels. Results in 7 cases. Bull Soc Pathol Exot Filiales 1987;80:624–33.
10. Klion AD, Massougbodji A, Horton J, et al. Albendazole in human loiasis: results of a double-blind, placebo-controlled trial. J Infect Dis 1993;168: 202–6.
11. Tsague-Dongmo L, Kamgno J, Pion SDS, et al. Effects of a 3-day regimen of albendazole (800 mg daily) on *Loa loa* microfilaremia. Ann Trop Med Parasitol 2002;96:707–15.
12. Gardon J, Gardon-Wendel N, Demanga-Ngangue, et al. Serious reaction after mass treatment of onchocerciasis with ivermectin in an area endemic for *Loa loa* infection. Lancet. 1997;350:18–22.
    Severe post-treatment reactions have been recognized as a complication of DEC treatment of loiasis for decades. This study demonstrates similar post-treatment reactions during mass administration of ivermectin for onchocerciasis control.
13. Nutman TB, Miller KD, Mulligan M, et al. Diethylcarbamazine prophylaxis for human loiasis. Results of a double-blind study. N Engl J Med 1988;319: 752–6.

Onchocerciasis 112

Philip J Cooper, Thomas B Nutman

Key features

- Onchocerciasis (also known as river blindness and enfermedad de Robles) is caused by the filarial nematode *Onchocerca volvulus*
- The parasite is transmitted by *Simulium* black flies
- Infection with *O. volvulus* can cause visual impairment and blindness, including anterior segment disease: sclerosing keratitis and iridocyclitis, and posterior segment disease: optic atrophy and chorioretinopathy
- It is the world's second leading infectious cause of blindness
- Infection with *O. volvulus* can also cause debilitating skin disease, including localized onchodermatitis ("sowda") and chronic papular onchodermatitis
- Ivermectin is the treatment of choice
- Control of onchocerciasis consists of semi-annual or annual treatment of populations

INTRODUCTION

Onchocerciasis was first described in 1875 by John O'Neill, a British naval surgeon, among inhabitants of the West African coast suffering from a pruritic skin disease known as "craw-craw". Onchocerciasis remains today a leading cause of debilitating skin and ocular disease in endemic regions in Africa, the Arabian Peninsula, and parts of Latin America. Forty percent of disability-adjusted life years attributed to the disease are due to visual impairment, and 60% to the severe itching with skin disease. Infection has been associated with increased mortality independent of its effects on sight, and poses a major hurdle to economic wellbeing in highly endemic areas of Africa. However, control programs using repeated community treatments with ivermectin can prevent public health consequences of the disease and eliminate the infection in endemic regions in the Americas and possibly in Africa.

EPIDEMIOLOGY

Onchocerciasis is found in 36 countries, where an estimated 37 million people are infected, and some 500,000 suffer significant visual loss of which about one-half are blind [1, 2]. An estimated 85.6 million people are thought to be at risk of infection worldwide [1]. Onchocerciasis is most prevalent in sub-Saharan Africa (Fig. 112.1A) and is a major public health problem along rivers where the black fly vectors breed, from Senegal, Guinea, and Sierra Leone in the West to southern Sudan and the Ethiopian Highlands in the East. In the Americas, isolated foci remain in Mexico, Guatemala, Colombia, Ecuador, Venezuela, and Brazil [3] (Fig. 112.1B). The infection is also found in Yemen [4]. Blinding disease in highly endemic communities in the savanna of West Africa heretofore has affected up to 30% of the population. Onchocerciasis foci have been classified epidemiologically into hyperendemic, mesoendemic, and hypoendemic, according to disease prevalence: >60%, 30–60%, and <30%, respectively. In highly endemic areas, *O. volvulus* infection is acquired early in life and over 90% of inhabitants may be infected by the age of 20 years. In communities with a low prevalence of infection, there is often little evidence of clinical disease. Onchocerciasis accounts for approximately 1 in 500 medical conditions diagnosed in returned travelers, and the risk of infection will be higher among travelers to rural areas of Africa where the parasite is endemic [5].

NATURAL HISTORY, PATHOGENESIS AND PATHOLOGY

Infectious *O. volvulus* L3 larvae are transmitted by black flies (Fig. 112.2) and develop into adults that are found in subcutaneous fibrous nodules or onchocercomata (Fig. 112.3). Male adults migrate between nodules where they fertilize sedentary females. Females release thousands of larvae or microfilariae into the surrounding tissues where they can be ingested by feeding black flies to complete the life cycle (see Fig. 112.4). The period from an infective bite to the detection of microfilariae in skin is generally between 10 and 20 months. Individuals infected with *O. volvulus* can suffer disease affecting the skin, lymph nodes, and eyes. Pathology in these tissues is caused by inflammatory reactions that follow the death of microfilariae. It can be caused by the secretion of toxic products by granulocytes, the deposition of immune complexes in the tissues, or by inflammatory mechanisms induced by release of *Wolbachia* (bacteria infecting the filariae)-derived products. Most clinical manifestations associated with *O. volvulus* infection are related to the chronic effects of repeated episodes of inflammation. Clinical disease can also follow short periods of exposure such as among visitors to or expatriates living in endemic areas.

Skin disease is caused by skin-dwelling microfilariae that secrete enzymes such as collagenase during their migration, causing long-term damage to dermal collagen and elastin. Loss of skin elasticity and early aging characterize chronic disease. Microfilariae are seen histologically at the dermo-epidermal junction (Fig. 112.5A) and "live" intact microfilariae are generally observed free of inflammatory cells. The inflammatory changes take place in the upper dermis and include edema and fibrosis. Acute papules show intraepidermal microabscess formation with dead or degenerating microfilariae surrounded by eosinophils and neutrophils (Fig. 112.5B). There can be loss of melanin from basal cells, loss of elastic fibres in the dermis, and atrophy of the dermis. The dermatitis correlates with where microfilariae predominate, particularly around the buttocks and pelvic girdle where the inguinal and femoral nodes show evidence of lymphadenitis and fibrosis. Lichenified onchodermatitis (LOD) (also known as localized onchocerciasis or "sowda") (Fig. 112.6C) is

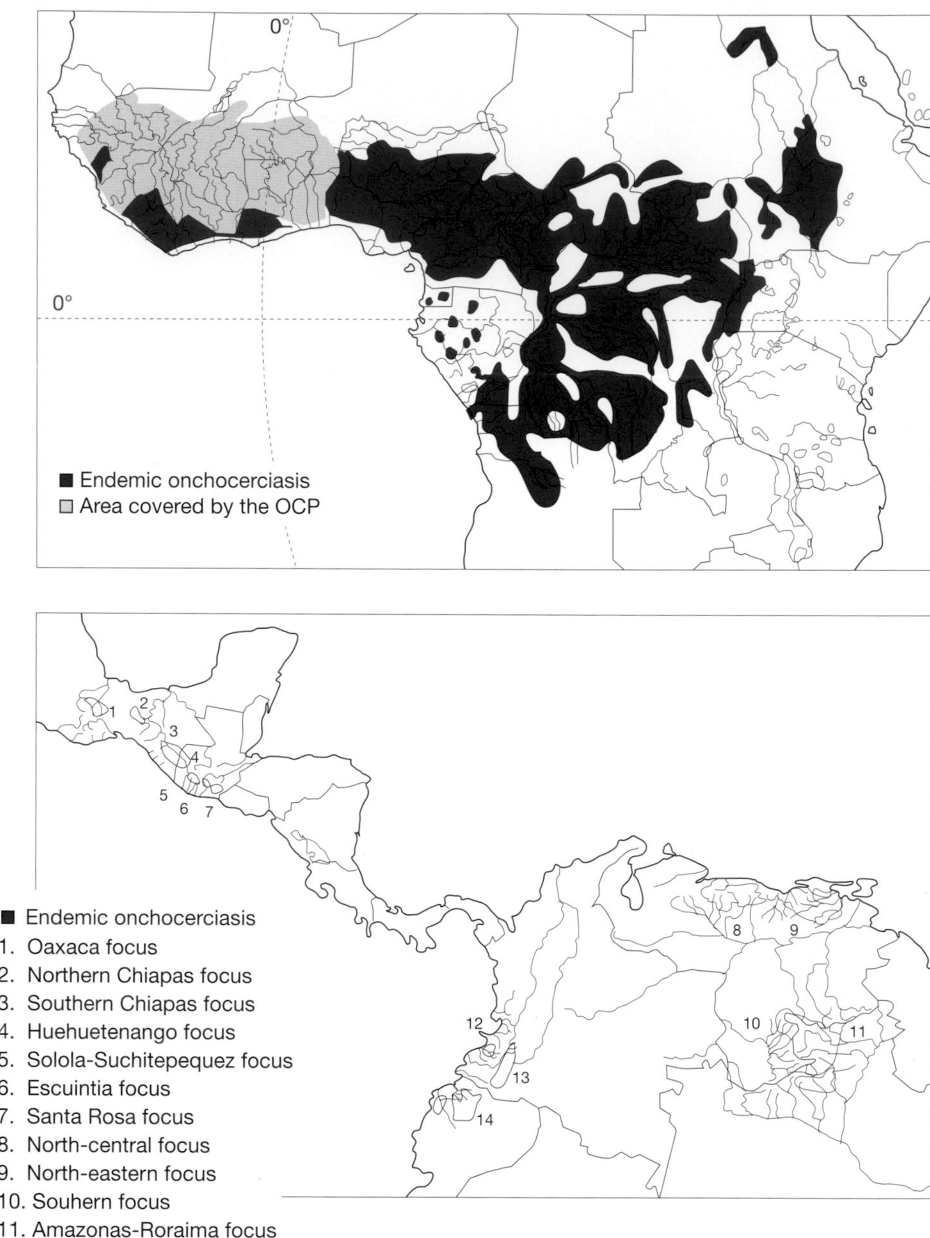

FIGURE 112.1 Maps showing the distribution of onchocerciasis: Africa and Central and South America. *(By permission of the World Health Organization.)*

characterized by enlarged, soft, regional lymph nodes associated with localized skin changes that histologically show a hyperreactive inflammatory cell infiltrate with sclerosis and edema but few microfilariae. Scarring in lymph nodes may lead to regional lymphedema, hanging groin (Fig. 112.6F), or elephantiasis.

Individuals with higher microfilarial burdens are more likely to develop severe ocular disease. Ocular lesions are caused by the invasion and local death of microfilariae. Microfilariae can enter the eye through the bulbar conjunctiva, along the sheaths of the scleral vessels and nerves, or by embolization in the choroidal or ciliary capillaries. Punctate keratitis (Fig. 112.7A) is observed clinically in the corneal stroma and clears without scarring. Punctate opacities are focal accumulations of lymphocytes and eosinophils around degenerating microfilariae with local edema. Sclerosing keratitis (Fig. 112.7B) is a progressive fibrovascular pannus and inflammatory infiltrate composed mainly of lymphocytes and eosinophils which starts at the level of Bowman's membrane. Mild, chronic uveitis is common with heavy microfilarial invasion of the anterior chamber. Lesions of the posterior chamber include optic atrophy and chorioretinopathy. The extent of chorioretinal changes is highly variable and the retinal pigment epithelium can show migration, clumping, atrophy, or focal hyperplasia. Chronic nongranulomatous chorioretinitis consists of an infiltrate of lymphocytes, plasma cells and eosinophils with secondary degenerative changes in the overlying retinal pigment epithelium and neuroretina. Loss of the photoreceptors and outer layers of the retina can be due to inflammatory damage to the retinal pigment epithelium and choriocapillaris. This is followed by consecutive loss of the inner neuroretina, ganglion cells, and nerve fibres. Profound chorioretinal atrophy can develop with loss of almost all the retina and choroid. Optic atrophy is common in the more advanced stages of ocular onchocerciasis (Fig. 112.7E,F).

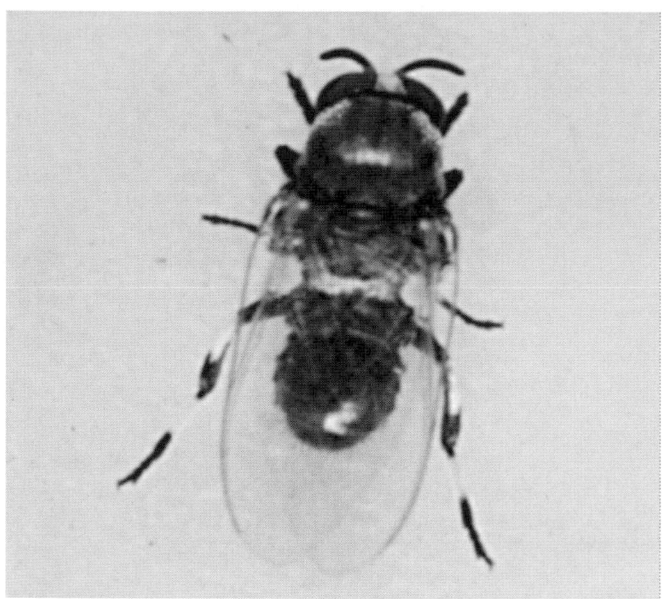

FIGURE 112.2 One of the black flies in the *Simulium damnosum* complex. The length of the fly is about 3.5 mm (×14.8). *(Courtesy of the Armed Forces Institute of Pathology, Photograph Neg. No. 72-4519E.)*

CLINICAL FEATURES

SKIN DISEASE

The earliest and most troublesome symptom of onchocercal skin involvement is itching [6]. The skin changes have been classified as acute papular onchodermatitis (APOD), chronic papular onchodermatitis (CPOD), lichenified onchodermatitis (LOD), atrophy, and depigmentation [6]. More than one skin disease type can coexist in an individual. APOD consists of small pruritic papules (Fig. 112.6A). Because of pruritus, there can be excoriations, secondary infection, and ulceration. APOD is the typical presentation in individuals with short exposure histories, and in such individuals, microfilariae may not be detectable.

CPOD consists of flat-topped papules that vary in size and height above the skin surface (Fig. 112.6B). Some lesions can be macular. Itching can occur, and individuals with CPOD may also have acute lesions. LOD or "sowda" typically affects young adults and is characterized by pruritic, hyperpigmented and hyperkeratotic plaques (Fig. 112.6C). The distribution is asymmetric, involving one limb, and is associated with regional lymphadenopathy. In later stages, the skin can be grossly lichenified. Itching is intense in the acute stage; this condition can coexist with APOD or CPOD. Atrophy of the skin is relatively common in areas of high endemicity (Fig. 112.6D). Atrophic skin adopts many of the characteristics of aging, such as loss of elasticity, and the skin appears excessively wrinkled. Hairs may be lost and sweating reduced. Onchocercal depigmentation or "leopard skin" is associated with patches of complete pigment loss and generally affects the lower leg anteriorly (Fig. 112.6E). A rare manifestation is "hanging groin" or "adenolymphocele" that is observed only in heavy and longstanding infections, and consists of a pouch of lymphedematous tissue in which hang atrophic inguinal or femoral nodes (Fig. 112.6F). Inflammatory damage to the lymph nodes and lymphatics may, over the long term, lead to elephantiasis of the limbs or genitalia.

NODULES

Onchocercomata are subcutaneous fibrous nodules containing adult worms, found in the region of the iliac crest, the trochanter, the sacrum, the upper thorax and head (Fig. 112.8). Nodules are often absent among patients with short exposure histories but may become detectable later in the course of the infection.

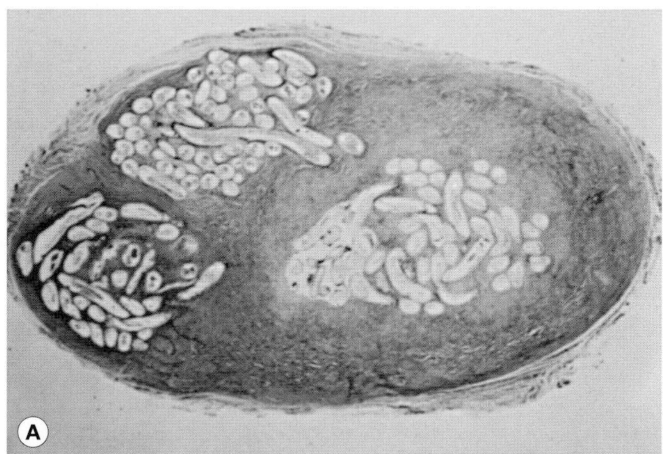

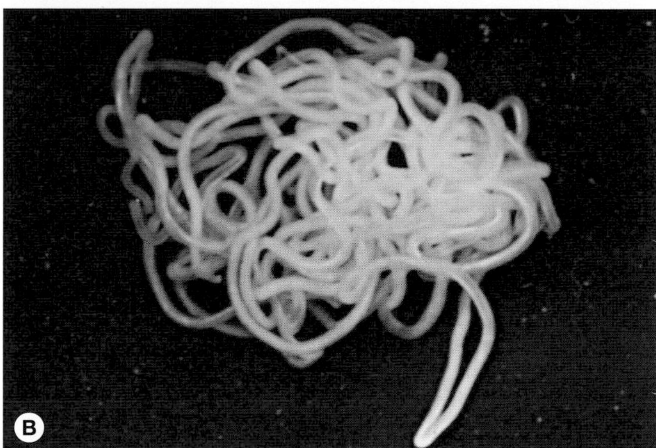

FIGURE 112.3 Adult worms of *O. volvulus*. **(A)** Microscopic section through an onchocercal nodule (1.3 × 0.7 cm), showing several coiled adult worms (mostly gravid females). The worms are surrounded and incarcerated by hyalinized scar (Russell-Movat, ×8.2). *(Courtesy of the Armed Forces Institute of Pathology, Photograph Neg. No. 69-3639).* **(B)** Entangled adult worms, after collagenase digestion of an onchocercal nodule. The cluster measures about 1.1 × 0.9 cm. The individual worms are up to 0.5 mm across and 50 cm long (×6.9). *(Courtesy of the Armed Forces Institute of Pathology, Photograph Neg. No. 80-12068.)*

LYMPH NODES

Lymph node changes are commonly seen where they drain areas of onchodermatitis. Usually the nodes are only slightly enlarged, firm, and nontender. Acute regional lymphadenopathy can accompany acute papular eruptions and lymphedema, but lymph node pathology is usually clinically silent.

EYE DISEASE

Punctate keratitis (fluffy or snowflake opacities) consists of opacities of the superficial corneal stroma (Fig. 112.7A). They can be seen by the naked eye or visualized using a slit lamp. Up to 100 or more opacities measuring 0.5 mm in diameter may be observed, and these lesions heal without scarring. Punctate keratitis can be asymptomatic or accompanied by conjunctival injection, chemosis, limbitis and epiphora. Longstanding and heavy infections can result in massive invasion of the cornea, leading to the development of sclerosing keratitis, a slowly progressive scarring of the cornea (Fig. 112.7B). Severe anterior uveitis (iridocyclitis) can occur with the development of posterior synechiae and pear-shaped deformity of the pupil, a loss of the iris pigment frill and a pumice-stone appearance of the iris [7]. Extensive synechiae can cause seclusio- and occlusio-pupillae, secondary cataracts, and secondary glaucoma [7].

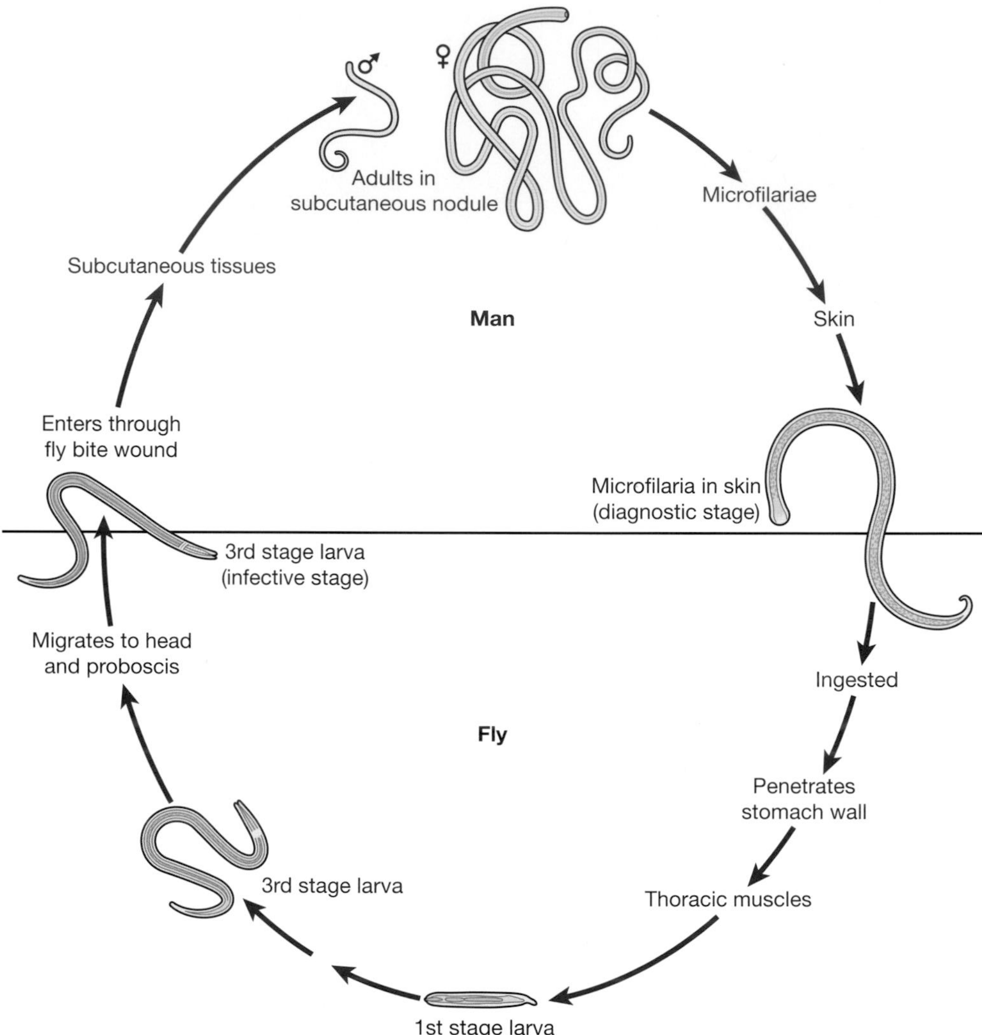

FIGURE 112.4 Life cycle of *O. volvulus*. *(Based on Melvin DM, Brooke MM, Healy GR. et al. Common Blood and Tissue Parasites: Life Cycle Charts. Atlanta: Centers for Disease Control, 1961.)*

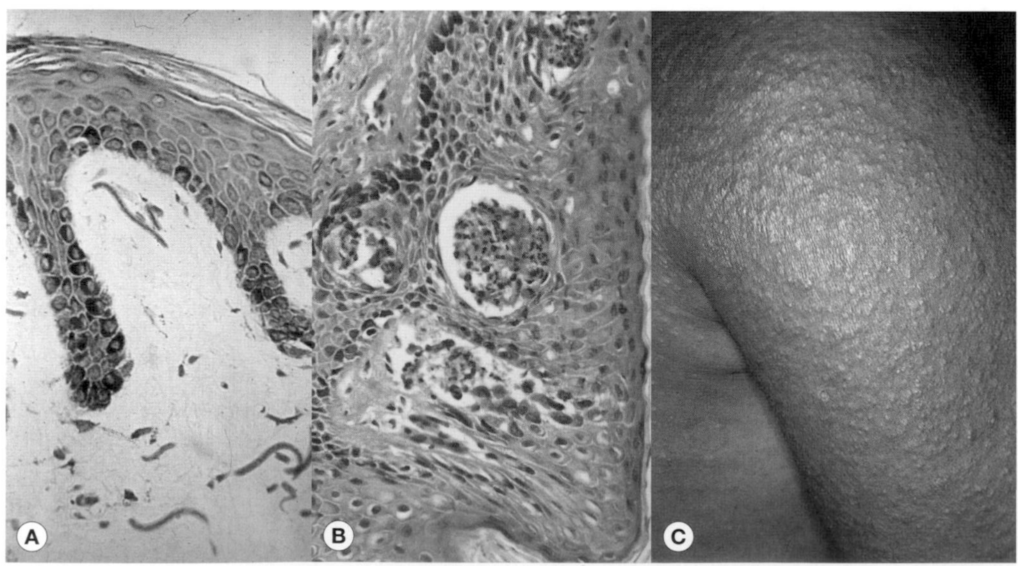

FIGURE 112.5 Effects of diethylcarbamazine (DEC) on *O. volvulus* microfilariae. **(A)** *O. volvulus* microfilariae are found at the dermo-epidermal junction, eliciting minimal host inflammatory response. **(B)** After DEC treatment, intraepidermal microabscesses can form in the epidermis, characterized by dead and degenerating microfilariae surrounded by eosinophils and neutrophils. **(C)** Edema and papular dermatitis developing after DEC treatment.

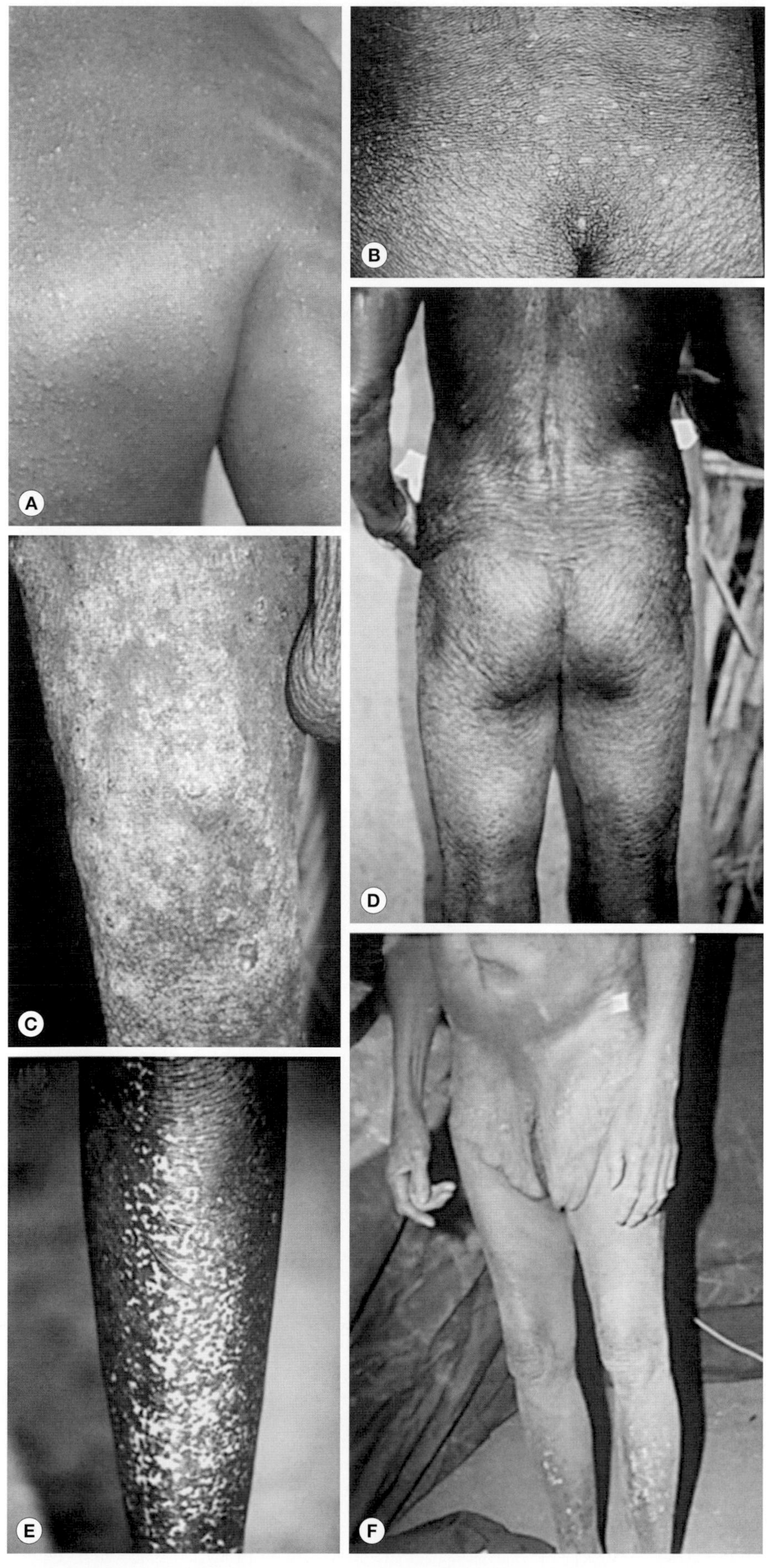

FIGURE 112.6 Skin changes in onchocerciasis. **(A)** Acute papular onchodermatitis. **(B)** Chronic papular onchodermatitis. **(C)** Lichenified onchodermatitis. **(D)** Onchocercal atrophy confined to the buttocks. **(E)** Depigmentation or "leopard skin". **(F)** Hanging groin, with redundant folds of atrophic skin. *(Courtesy of Dr. M. Murdoch.)*

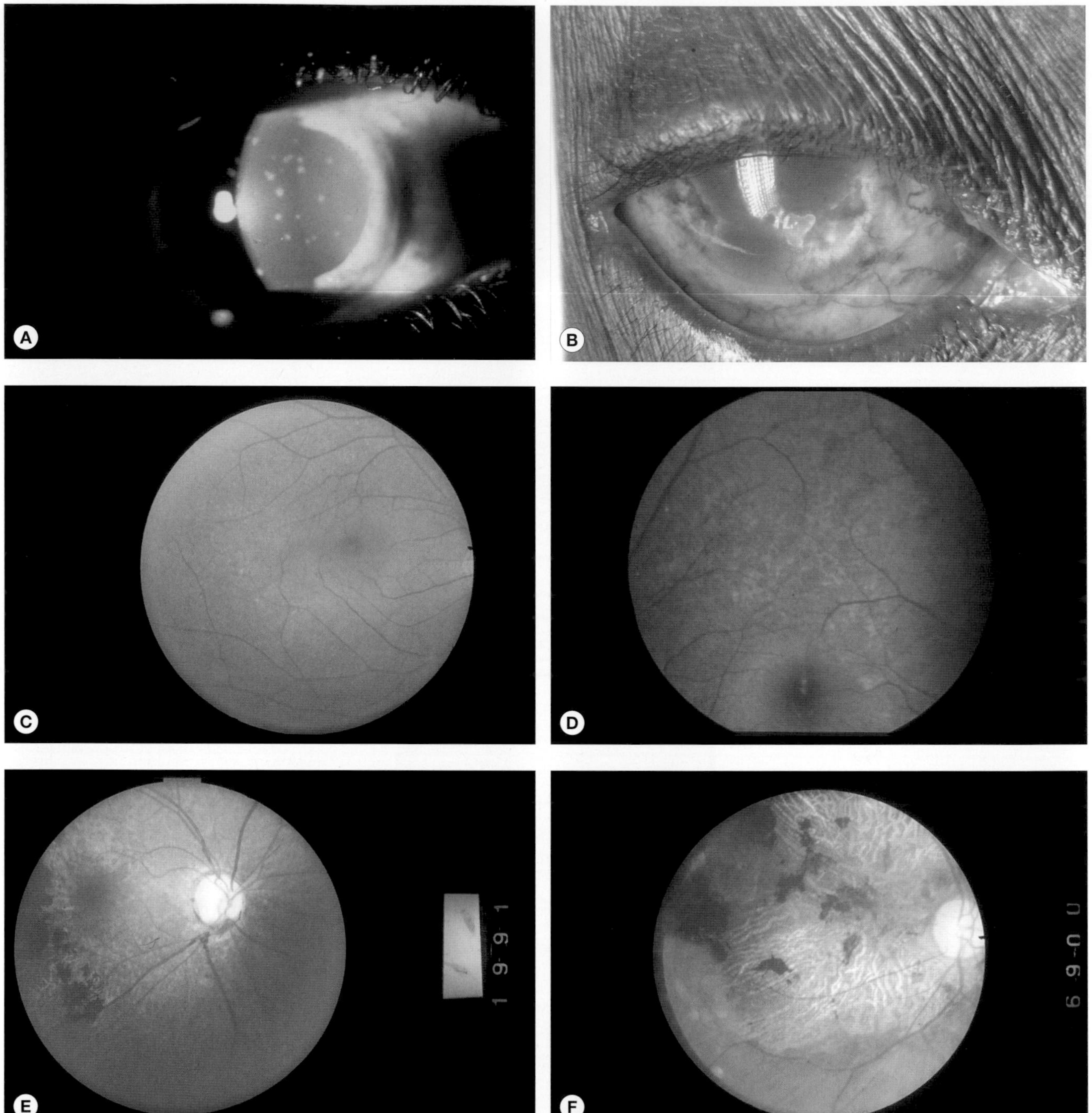

FIGURE 112.7 Ocular changes in onchocerciasis. **(A)** Punctate opacities in the cornea. **(B)** Sclerosing keratitis. *(Courtesy of Dr I Murdoch.)* **(C)** Early mottling of retina temporal to the macula (arrow). **(D)** Mottling of retina temporal to macula *(Courtesy of Dr R Proaño.)* **(E)** Post-neuritic optic atrophy with peripapillary pigmentation and temporal chorioretinal scar. **(F)** Post-neuritic optic atrophy and geographic atrophy of the retinal pigment epithelium with choriocapillary atrophy. *(Courtesy of Dr. I. Murdoch.)*

Chorioretinitis or chorioretinopathy is slowly progressive, taking many years before visual loss is evident. It is characterized by retinal pigment epithelial atrophy and chorioretinal scarring [7]. Chorioretinopathy in onchocerciasis is first seen as a loss of pigment lateral to the macula (Fig. 112.7C,D) or nasal to the optic disc at the level of the retinal pigment epithelium (RPE). Pigment loss appears as a grey-yellow mottling. RPE loss progresses in an arc around the macula and eventually may become confluent, producing areas of geographic atrophy (Fig. 112.7F). Extensive atrophy can be accompanied by choriocapillary atrophy (the choroidal vessels become exposed) and subretinal fibrosis. The macula is often preserved until late in the course of disease. Mild forms of RPE atrophy may be detected only by fluorescein angiography. Fundal changes are usually symmetric. Post-neuritic optic atrophy reflects previous episodes of active inflammation of the optic nerve [7] (Fig. 112.7E). Onchocercal optic atrophy can also follow extensive destruction of the retina (Fig. 112.7F). Both forms are generally accompanied by inflammatory changes such as peripapillary hyperpigmentation and sheathing of the central retinal vessels.

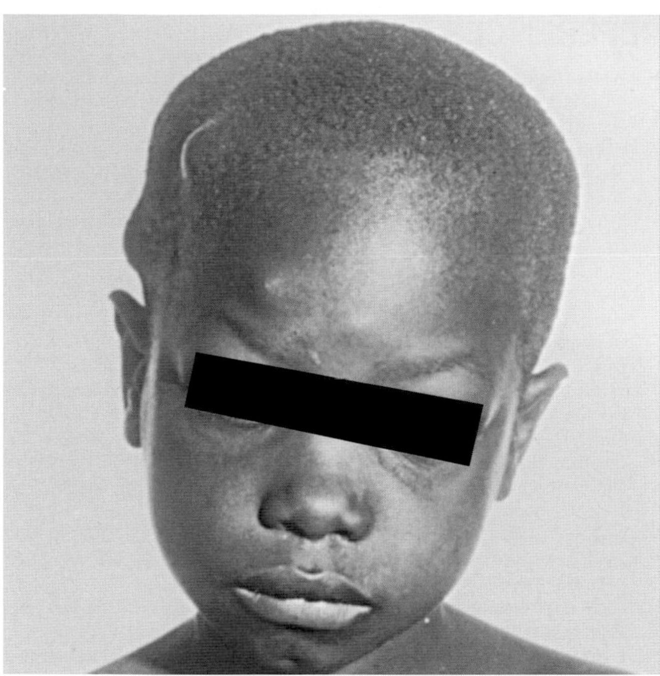

FIGURE 112.8 Young boy from the Democratic Republic of the Congo with three onchocercal nodules of his forehead and skull. *(Courtesy of the Armed Forces Institute of Pathology, Photograph Neg. No. 69-3619.)*

BOX 112.1 Pediatric Considerations – Patient Evaluation

- Children who have not been in endemic areas for long periods have a very low chance of infection
- Infected children generally present with acute manifestations such as APOD, punctate keratitis, or a palpable subcutaneous nodule

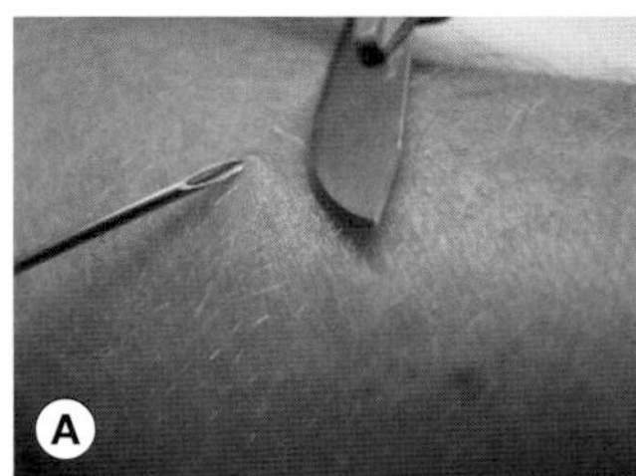

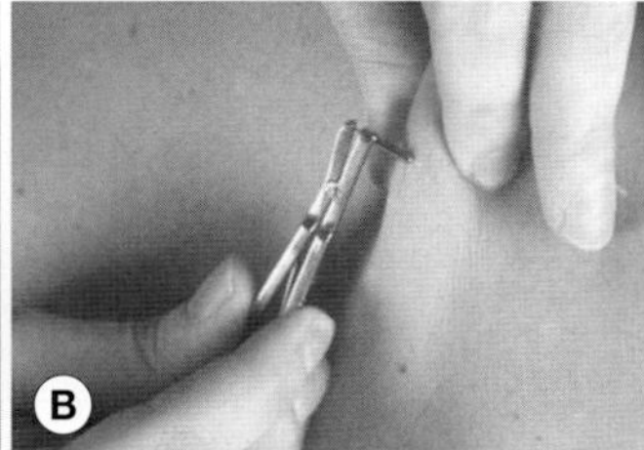

FIGURE 112.9 Sampling of skin for diagnosis of *O. volvulus* infection. **(A)** Skin snips being removed with needle and scalpel. Note the small tent of skin that is lifted up by the needle. **(B)** Skin snip using a corneoscleral punch.

OTHER COMPLICATIONS

Chronic infections are associated with low body weight and diffuse musculoskeletal pain. A form of dwarfism, Nakalanga dwarfism, has been attributed to pituitary involvement in this disease in the Mabira forest of Uganda [8]. An association with epilepsy has also been reported [8, 9]. Other conditions are reproductive abnormalities with secondary amenorrhea, spontaneous abortion, and infertility.

PATIENT EVALUATION, DIAGNOSIS AND DIFFERENTIAL DIAGNOSIS

The chance of acquiring *O. volvulus* infection increases with greater exposure time in endemic regions (Box 112.1). Some patients may be diagnosed through investigation of eosinophilia. A presumptive diagnosis can be made based on a history of exposure in an endemic area, the presence of subcutaneous nodules, or typical skin and/or ocular signs. Early onchodermatitis is rarely diagnosed correctly and must be distinguished from atopic dermatitis, food allergies, contact dermatitis, insect bites and scabies. Chronic skin lesions can be mistaken for severe chronic eczema, malnutrition and presbydermia. "Leopard skin" must be distinguished from other causes of hypochromia, including vitiligo and leprosy.

Definitive diagnosis depends on the identification of microfilariae in skin snips or of the adult worms from excised or aspirated nodules [10]. Ocular microfilariae can be detected by slit lamp examination. The chances of detection are increased if patients are asked to sit with their head between their legs for up to 10 minutes prior to examination. Microfilariae in the anterior chamber are seen as small wriggling worms. Live microfilariae in the cornea are transparent and coiled up. Skin snips can be obtained using a corneoscleral punch (Fig. 112.9A) or by elevating a crease of skin with the point of a needle (Fig. 112.9B) and obtaining a small circular disc-shaped slice of epidermis and superficial dermis using a scalpel blade. The skin snip is then incubated on a glass slide in saline and examined using a dissecting microscope (or magnifying glass) to detect emergent microfilariae [10].

Assays to detect specific antibodies to *Onchocerca* [11–14] and PCR [15] to detect onchocercal DNA in skin snips are now in use in specialized laboratories and are highly sensitive and specific. Although current serologic assays have limited ability to discriminate past exposures from current infections, the detection of *O. volvulus* DNA in microscopically negative skin snips is useful in individuals with light infections.

Individuals with no evidence of *O. volvulus* microfilariae in the skin or eyes can be challenged using the Mazzotti test. The patient is given a single oral dose of 25–50 mg of diethylcarbamazine (DEC). Patients should have a complete ocular examination before considering the performance of this test because DEC may cause irreversible damage to the posterior segment of the eye. Infected individuals develop intense pruritus between 30 minutes and 24 hours after the test, which can be accompanied by erythema, edema and papular dermatitis (Fig. 112.5C). The presence of *M. streptocerca* may cause false-positive reactions.

TREATMENT

Ivermectin is the most important drug for the treatment of onchocerciasis. It is well tolerated, highly efficacious, and rapidly reduces microfilarial numbers in the skin [16]. The drug is administered as a single dose of 150 μg/kg. Because ivermectin has limited effects on adult worms, treatment must be repeated at annual or semi-annual intervals for the duration of the lives of adult worms to suppress dermal microfilarial levels [17]. Ivermectin significantly reduces the itching of reactive onchocercal skin disease (APOD, CPOD and LOD), but because microfilariae can re-invade the skin within 6 months of treatment, annual treatments may not be sufficient to control pruritus, and treatments every 3 months may be necessary for the first 1–2 years. Contraindications for ivermectin treatment are conditions associated with an impaired blood–brain barrier because penetration into the CNS can cause lethargy, ataxia, tremors and death. The drug is not approved for use in children weighing less than 15 kg (Box 112.2), pregnant women, and mothers nursing infants during the first week of life. Ivermectin has no significant drug interactions.

Ivermectin has a marked beneficial effect on anterior segment disease [7, 18]. A single dose of ivermectin is associated with a reduction in the prevalence of punctate corneal opacities and microfilariae

BOX 112.2 Pediatric Considerations – Treatment

- Ivermectin is not approved for use in children weighing less than 15 kg
- Doxycycline is contraindicated in children aged below 9 years and in pregnant women

in the anterior chamber (MfAC). Repeated treatments result in an improvement in the early lesions of iridocyclitis and sclerosing keratitis. There is evidence that ivermectin may also have a useful effect even in relatively advanced cases of iridocyclitis. The benefits of ivermectin on posterior segment disease are less clear, with the drug shown to be beneficial against the development of optic atrophy but not chorioretinal diseases [7, 18]. Control programs using ivermectin are expected to have a major impact on the development of the lesions of ocular onchocerciasis, and should prevent much of the visual loss and blindness associated with this infection [7, 18].

There are few side effects and it is generally well tolerated. A mild clinical reaction (Mazzotti-like reaction) occurs in 10–20% of patients receiving a first dose of ivermectin; a more severe reaction may be seen. Most reactions occur on the second day after treatment, although severe reactions can commence within 12 hours. During subsequent treatments, the frequency and severity of adverse reactions is reduced. Reactions are characterized by worsening of rash in previously affected areas. Edema can affect one limb or the face and is associated with enlarged tender regional lymph nodes. A systemic reaction may be observed, characterized by fever, arthralgia, musculoskeletal pain, and severe postural hypotension. Patients with LOD tend to have more severe reactions following treatment. Mild reactions require only symptomatic treatment (e.g. antihistamines and antipyretics). Severe reactions may require intramuscular or intravenous steroids. Extreme caution should be exercised in those with a possible exposure history to loiasis – the death of *Loa loa* microfilariae can cause severe, or even fatal, encephalitis [19]. It is recommended that the presence of heavy infections with *Loa loa* should be excluded using thin blood films [19].

Because a *Wolbachia* endosymbiotic bacteria is present in *O. volvulus* and is required for the survival of *Onchocerca*, doxycycline at a daily dose of 200 mg for 6 weeks inhibits *O. volvulus* fertility and kills approximately 50% of adult worms when given with a single standard dose of ivermectin [20–22]. Such treatment regimens have even been used in small community-based treatment programs. This approach (doxycycline plus ivermectin) provides a macrofilaricidal treatment option for individuals who do not live in endemic areas and are thus unlikely to get re-infected.

CONTROL

The initial objective of onchocerciasis control strategies was to reduce community microfilarial burdens to levels that were associated with negligible morbidity. Elimination of onchocerciasis is now considered a realistic objective not only in small foci in parts of Latin America (e.g. Ecuador) [3, 23, 24] but also in many regions of Africa [25]. Currently, the focus of control strategies is through semi-annual (in Latin America) [3] or annual distribution (in Africa) [26] of ivermectin that has been provided gratis by the manufacturer (Merck & Co) for as long as it is needed. The highly successful Onchocerciasis Control Programme (OCP) in West Africa that relied on vector control measures was phased out in 2002 [26], and control presently relies on ivermectin as the primary control measure [26]. Concerns for both suboptimal microfilaricidal responses to ivermectin or possible resistance [27] have surfaced such that measures that would be adjunctive to annual ivermectin distribution are being sought.

REFERENCES

1. World Health Organization (WHO). Onchocerciasis and its Control. Report of a WHO Expert Committee on Onchocerciasis Control. WHO Technical Report Series 852. Geneva: WHO; 1995.
2. World Health Organization (WHO). Working to Overcome the Global Impact of Neglected Tropical Diseases. WHO/HTM/NTD/2010.1. Geneva: WHO; 2010.
3. [Anonymous]. Report from the Inter-American Conference on Onchocerciasis, November 2007. Wkly Epidemiol Rec 2008;83:256–60.
4. [Anonymous]. African Programme for Onchocerciasis Control – report on task force meeting, July 2008. Wkly Epidemiol Rec 2008;83:307–12.
5. Lipner EM, Law MA, Barnett E, et al. For the GeoSentinel Surveillance. Filariasis in travelers presenting to the GeoSentinel Surveillance Network. PLoS Negl Trop Dis 2007;1:e88.
6. World Health Organization (WHO). The Importance of Onchocercal Skin Disease. TDR/ONCHO/95.1. Geneva: WHO; 1995.
7. Abiose A. Onchocercal eye disease and the impact of Mectizan treatment. Ann Trop Med Parasitol 1998;92:S11–12.
8. Duke BO. Onchocerciasis, epilepsy and hyposexual dwarfism. Trans R Soc Trop Med Hyg 1998;92:236.
9. Pion SD, Kaiser C, Boutros-Toni F, et al. Epilepsy in onchocerciasis endemic areas: systematic review and meta-analysis of population-based surveys. PLoS Negl Trop Dis 2009;3:e461.
10. Eberhard ML, Lammie PJ. Laboratory diagnosis of filariasis. Clin Lab Med 1991;11:977–1010.
11. Burbelo PD, Leahy HP, Iadorola MJ, Nutman TB. A four antigen mixture for rapid assessment of *Onchocerca volvulus* infection. PLoS Negl Trop Dis 2009;3:e438.
12. Lobos E, Weiss N, Karam M, et al. An immunogenic *Onchocerca volvulus* antigen: a specific and early marker of infection. Science 1991;251:1603–5.
13. Ramachandran, CP. Improved immunodiagnostic tests to monitor onchocerciasis control programmes – a multicenter effort. Parasitol Today 1993;9:77–9.
14. Weil GJ, Steel C, Liftis F, et al. A rapid-format antibody card test for diagnosis of onchocerciasis. J Infect Dis 2000;182:1796–9.
15. Zimmerman PA, Guderian RH, Aruajo E, et al. 1994. Polymerase chain reaction-based diagnosis of *Onchocerca volvulus* infection: improved detection of patients with onchocerciasis. J Infect Dis 1994;169:686–9.
16. Greene BM, Taylor HR, Cupp EW, et al. Comparison of ivermectin and diethylcarbamazine in the treatment of onchocerciasis. N Engl J Med 1985; 313:133–8.
17. Basanez MG, Pion SD, Boakes E, et al. Effect of single-dose ivermectin on *Onchocerca volvulus*: a systematic review and meta-analysis. Lancet Infect Dis 2008;8:310–22.
18. World Health Organization (WHO). The effect of repeated ivermectin treatment on ocular onchocerciasis. Report of an informal consultation. TDR/TDE/ONCHO 1993;4–5.
19. Gardon J, Gardon-Wendel N, Demanga N, et al. Serious reactions after mass treatment of onchocerciasis with ivermectin in an area endemic for *Loa loa* infection. Lancet 1997;350:18–22.
20. Hoerauf A, Volkmann L, Hamelmann C, et al. Endosymbiotic bacteria in worms as targets for a novel chemotherapy in filariasis. Lancet 2000;355: 1242–3.
21. Hoerauf A, Specht S, Buttner M, et al. *Wolbachia* endobacteria depletion by doxycycline as antifilarial therapy has macrofilaricidal activity in onchocerciasis: a randomized placebo-controlled study. Med Microbiol Immunol 2008;197:295–311.
22. Hoerauf A, Specht S, Marfo-Debrekyei Y, et al. Efficacy of 5-week doxycycline treatment on adult *Onchocerca volvulus*. Parasitol Res 2009;104:437–47. *Doxycycline is the first effective and well-tolerated macrofilaricidal drug.*
23. Thylefors B, Alleman M. Towards the elimination of onchocerciasis. Ann Trop Med Parasitol 2006;100:733–46.
24. Osei-Atweneboana MY, Eng JK, Boakye DA, et al. Prevalence and intensity of *Onchocerca volvulus* infection and efficacy of ivermectin in endemic communities in Ghana: a two-phase epidemiological study. Lancet 2007;369:2021–9.
25. Cupp EW, Sauerbrey M, Richards F. Elimination of human onchocerciasis: history of progress and current feasibility using ivermectin (Mectizan) monotherapy. Acta Trop 2011 (in press). *Useful review of the use of ivermectin in control programs and potential for elimination of infection using ivermectin alone in Latin American and Africa.*
26. Vieira JC, Cooper PJ, Lovato R, et al. Impact of long-term treatment with ivermectin for onchocerciasis in Ecuador: potential for elimination of infection. BMC Med 2007;5:9.
27. Taylor MJ, Awadzi K, Basanez MG, et al. Onchocerciasis control: vision for the future from a Ghanian perspective. Parasit Vectors 2009;2:7.

Miscellaneous Filariae 113

Amy D Klion

Key features

- *Mansonella* species that infect humans include *M. perstans*, *M.ozzardi*, and *M. streptocerca*
- *Mansonella* species vary considerably in their geographic distribution and the location of adult and larval parasites in the host
- Despite high prevalences of infection in endemic areas, clinical manifestations of *Mansonella* infections are uncommon
- *Dirofilaria* infection is a zoonosis spread by mosquitoes that is worldwide in distribution
- The most common presentation of *Dirofilaria immitis* (dog heartworm) infection in humans is an asymptomatic coin lesion seen on chest radiography
- Responses of *Mansonella* and *Dirofilaria* parasites to antifilarial treatment vary by species

MANSONELLA PERSTANS INFECTION

INTRODUCTION

Microfilariae of the filarial parasite *Mansonella perstans* (synonyms: *Dipetalonema perstans, Acanthocheilonema perstans, Tetrapetalonema perstans*) were first described in the blood of an African by Manson in 1891; in 1898, the adult parasite was extracted from the mesentery of an Amerindian in Guyana [1]. Generally believed to cause little pathology and, until recently, refractory to antifilarial chemotherapy, *M. perstans* has been understudied.

EPIDEMIOLOGY

M. perstans is endemic throughout much of tropical Africa, especially in the region from Senegal east to Uganda and south to Zimbabwe, and in South America along the Atlantic coast from Panama to Argentina. Minor foci have also been identified in Algeria and Tunisia. Although the total number of people infected with *M. perstans* is unknown, the prevalence of microfilaremia may reach 100% in highly endemic areas [2]. Infection of travelers is rare [3]. Nonhuman primates (gorillas and chimpanzees) can harbor infection with *M. perstans*, but do not appear to be a major reservoir of infection.

NATURAL HISTORY, PATHOGENESIS, AND PATHOLOGY

M. perstans is transmitted by biting midges of the genus *Culicoides*, of which the species C. *milnei* and C. *grahamii* are the most important. The infected larvae penetrate the skin and develop over the course of 9 to 12 months into adult worms (males 35–45 mm × 50–70 μm; females 60–80 mm × 100–150 μm) that inhabit the pleural, peritoneal and pericardial cavities, as well as the mesentery, perirenal and retroperitoneal tissues [4]. Microfilariae of *M. perstans*, which are small (3.5–4.5 μm × 100–200 μm) and unsheathed with a round terminal nucleus at the tip of the tail (Fig. 113.1), circulate in the blood without periodicity. Some isolates of *M. perstans* harbor the bacterial endosymbiont *Wolbachia*, found in most other filarial pathogens of humans [5].

CLINICAL FEATURES

Although most patients with *M. perstans* infection are asymptomatic, clinical manifestations include transient subcutaneous swellings similar to the Calabar swellings of loiasis, urticaria, pruritus, arthralgias, abdominal pain, and fatigue. Serositis, including pleuritis and pericarditis, meningoencephalitis, neuropsychiatric disturbances, hepatitis, granulomatous nodules in the conjunctiva, retinal lesions and periorbital inflammation surrounding dead adult worms (*bung-eye* or *bulge-eye*) have also been described. Eosinophilia and elevated serum IgE levels are common [6].

PATIENT EVALUATION, DIAGNOSIS, AND DIFFERENTIAL DIAGNOSIS

The diagnosis of *M. perstans* infection is most often made when microfilariae are detected incidentally in the peripheral blood. Infection should also be considered in individuals with a history of prolonged residence in an endemic area who present with unexplained eosinophilia and/or any of the clinical signs and symptoms described above. Microfilariae can be seen in thick blood smears stained with Giemsa or Wright's stain; concentration techniques are useful in patients with low numbers of circulating microfilariae. Species-specific PCR-based diagnostics are more sensitive than blood filtration, but are available only in research settings. Rarely, adult worms are recovered intact or appear in histologic sections.

TREATMENT

M. perstans infection is relatively refractory to most antifilarial therapies, including diethylcarbamazine (DEC), ivermectin and albendazole [7]. The current recommended therapy, DEC at a dose of 8–10 mg/kg/day for 21 days, is rarely curative, and multiple courses of therapy are often needed. Mebendazole (100–200 mg daily for 14–21 days) alone or in combination with DEC (400 mg daily for 21 days) appears to be more effective than DEC alone, clearing *M. perstans* microfilaremia in up to 37% of subjects in one study [7]. In a more recent randomized trial, doxycycline (200 mg daily for 6 weeks), which has activity against the intracellular endosymbiont *Wolbachia*, was 100% effective in clearing *M. perstans* microfilariae from the blood of infected subjects in Mali for up to 36 months [8].

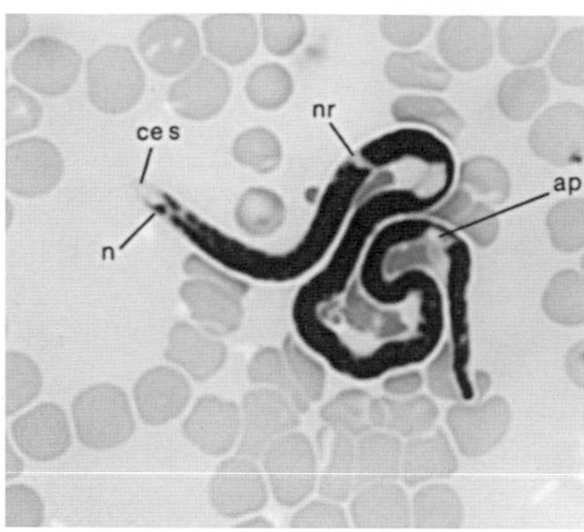

FIGURE 113.1 Thin blood film, *Mansonella perstans* microfilaria (Giemsa stain, ×890); cephalic space (ces), nucleus (n), nerve ring (nr), anal pore (ap). *(Courtesy of the Armed Forces Institute of Pathology, Photograph Neg. No. 74.5605.)*

MANSONELLA OZZARDI INFECTION

INTRODUCTION

In 1897, Manson first described microfilariae in the blood of Amerindians in Guyana [9]. He named the species *Filaria ozzardi* after Ozzard, who obtained the specimens. In 1929, Faust named the new genus *Mansonella*.

EPIDEMIOLOGY

M. ozzardi is restricted to Central America, South America (Colombia, Venezuela, Guyana, Suriname, Brazil, Argentina, Bolivia) and the Caribbean islands (Puerto Rico, Antigua, Guadeloupe, Nevis, Dominican Republic, Haiti, Martinique, St Kitts, St Lucia, St Vincent, and Trinidad). Although the total number of people infected with *M. ozzardi* is unknown, the prevalence of microfilaremia may reach 70% in highly endemic villages. Infection of travelers is uncommon [3]. Humans are the only major reservoir of infection.

NATURAL HISTORY, PATHOGENESIS, AND PATHOLOGY

M. ozzardi is transmitted by biting midges of the genus *Culicoides* as well as by the black fly, *Simulium amazonicum*. Infective larvae penetrate the skin and develop over the course of months to years into adult worms that are often found in the thoracic and peritoneal cavities, and have also been described in the lymphatics. *M. ozzardi* adult females measure 65–81 mm × 210–250 μm. Only a fragment of a male worm (38 mm × 200 μm) from humans has been described. Microfilariae can be found in the skin and blood, where they circulate without periodicity [10]. *M. ozzardi* microfilariae are small (3–5 μm × 170–240 μm) and sheathless and are characterized by a cephalic space 2 to 6 μm long with two or three overlapping nuclei and a caudal space 3 to 8 μm long with oval terminal nuclei (Fig. 113.2). *M. ozzardi* harbors the bacterial endosymbiont *Wolbachia* [11].

CLINICAL FEATURES

Although most patients with *M. ozzardi* infection are asymptomatic [12], clinical manifestations include urticaria, pruritic skin eruptions, edema, lymphadenopathy, articular pains, fever, headache, vertigo, and pulmonary symptoms. Peripheral eosinophilia is common.

PATIENT EVALUATION, DIAGNOSIS, AND DIFFERENTIAL DIAGNOSIS

M. ozzardi infection should be considered in individuals with a compatible travel history who present with unexplained eosinophilia and/or any of the clinical signs and symptoms described above. Definitive diagnosis can be made by demonstration of microfilariae in the blood (see Chapter 111) or in skin snips (see Chapter 112). Currently available serologic tests are not species-specific and do not differentiate between exposure and infection. PCR-based diagnostics are available only in research settings.

TREATMENT

Although diethylcarbamazine (DEC) and albendazole appear ineffective in the treatment [13], resolution of clinical symptoms and reduction of microfilarial levels have been reported in a single patient treated with ivermectin [14]. More recently, a placebo-controlled, double-blind study of 40 patients in Trinidad demonstrated an 82% reduction in *M. ozzardi* microfilarial levels after 4 years of annual ivermectin (6 mg/year) [15]. The efficacy of doxycycline in treating infections with other *Wolbachia*-containing filarial parasites has been well documented but has not been explored in *M. ozzardi* infection.

STREPTOCERCIASIS

INTRODUCTION

In 1922, Macfie and Corson described microfilariae in the skin of Ghanaians that were morphologically distinct from *Onchocerca volvulus* [16]. Adult male and female worms were not demonstrated in humans until 1972 and 1975, respectively [17]. The clinical significance of streptocerciasis is likely underestimated due to overlap in symptomatology and geographic distribution with onchocerciasis.

EPIDEMIOLOGY

Although streptocerciasis was believed to be limited to the tropical rain forests of western and central Africa, including northern Angola, Cameroon, Central African Republic, People's Republic of Congo, Equatorial Guinea, Nigeria, and the Democratic Republic of Congo, a focus was identified in western Uganda [18]. Prevalence rates vary widely, but can reach 90% focally. Infection of travelers is uncommon [3]. Although natural infection of nonhuman primates occurs, their importance as reservoirs of streptocerciasis remains unknown.

NATURAL HISTORY, PATHOGENESIS, AND PATHOLOGY

M. streptocerca is transmitted by the biting midge, *Culicoides grahamii*. The infective larvae penetrate the skin and develop over the course of months to years into adult worms that live in the dermis of the upper trunk and shoulder girdle. *M. streptocerca* adult worms measure approximately 27 mm × 85 μm (females) and 17 mm × 50 μm (males). Dermal microfilariae are small (2.5–5 μm × 180–240 μm), unsheathed and characterized by a sharp curving of the posterior end that frequently gives them a shepherd's crook configuration (Fig. 113.3). The cephalic space is 3 to 5 μm long with four oval nuclei in single file followed by seven to ten smaller rounder nuclei. There are no published data on the presence of *Wolbachia* in *M. streptocerca*.

CLINICAL FEATURES

The clinical manifestations of streptocerciasis appear to be restricted to the skin and lymph nodes [19]. Although infection is often asymptomatic, the most common complaint is chronic pruritus, most pronounced over the shoulder girdle and thorax. Characteristic findings include dermal thickening, non-anesthetic hypopigmented macules, and axillary or inguinal adenopathy. Occasionally, papules may be present. Peripheral blood eosinophilia is common.

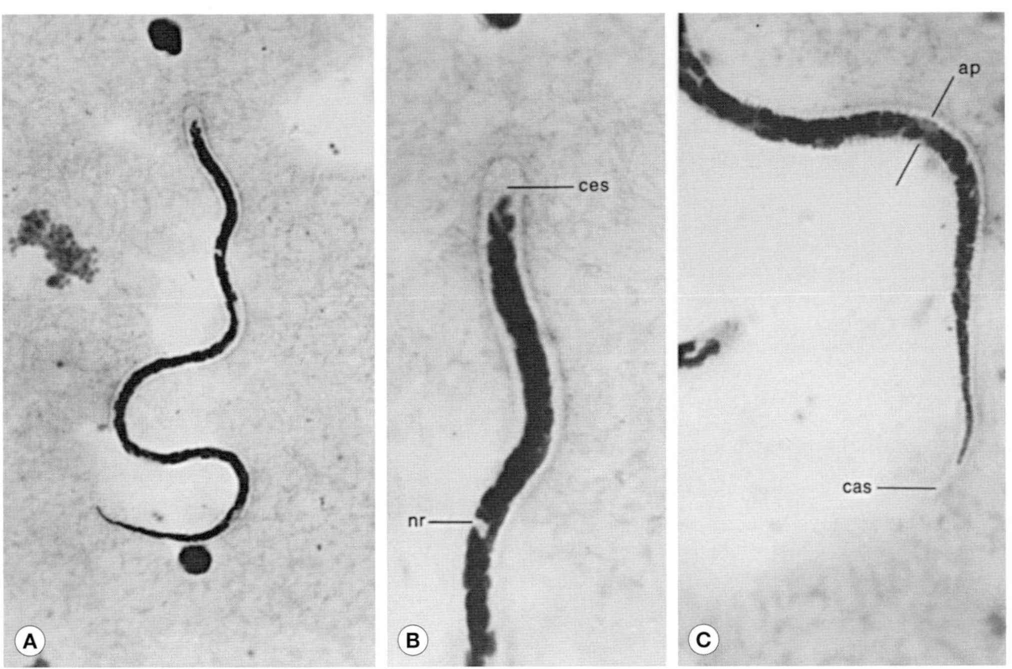

FIGURE 113.2 Thick blood film, *Mansonella ozzardi* microfilaria (Giemsa stain). **(A)** ×820. *(Courtesy of the Armed Forces Institute of Pathology, Photograph Neg. No.74-19692.)* **(B)** Anterior end, cephalic space (ces), nerve ring (nr), ×1620. **(C)** Posterior end, anal pore (ap), caudal space (cas), ×1620.

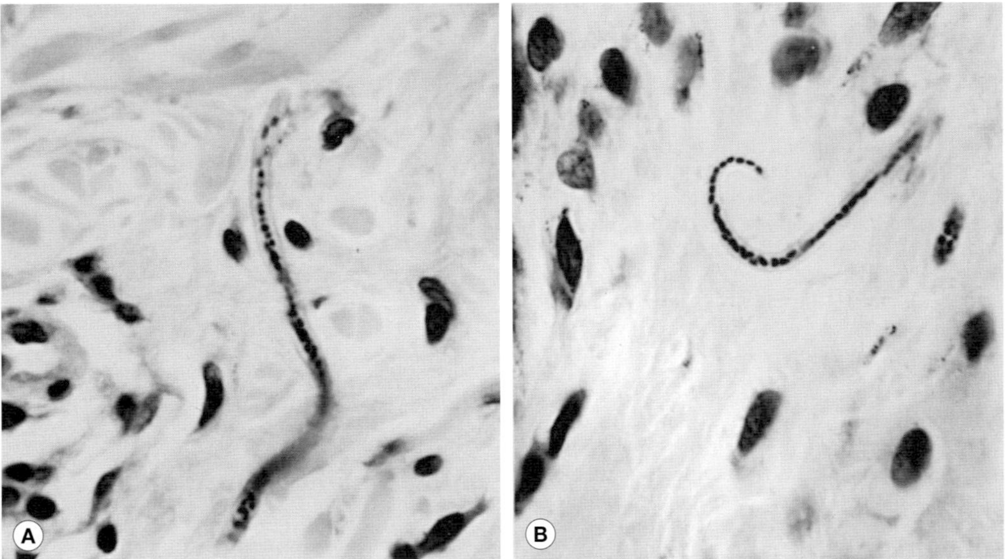

FIGURE 113.3 Diagnostic features of microfilariae of *Mansonella streptocerca* in sections of skin. The microfilariae are extravascular in the dermal collagen. **(A)** Anterior end, showing cephalic space and nuclei (×1080). *(Courtesy of the Armed Forces Institute of Pathology, Photograph Neg. No.71-10075.)* **(B)** Posterior end with "shepherd's crook" configuration and nuclei that reach nearly to the tip (×1080). *(Courtesy of the Armed Forces Institute of Pathology, Photograph Neg. No.71-10074.)*

PATIENT EVALUATION, DIAGNOSIS, AND DIFFERENTIAL DIAGNOSIS

M. streptocerca infection should be considered in individuals with a compatible exposure history who present with pruritus, a macular hypopigmented rash, or bilateral inguinal or axillary adenopathy. Diagnosis is made by morphologic identification of microfilariae from skin snips or biopsies (see Chapter 112). PCR has been described and is more sensitive than standard techniques [20]. As in other *Mansonella* infections, serology is not helpful in making a diagnosis. Skin histopathology may be necessary to distinguish *M. streptocerca* macular lesions from those of early leprosy.

TREATMENT

DEC (6 mg/kg/day) for 14 to 21 days is effective in killing both microfilariae and adult worms, but can be accompanied by an exacerbation of clinical symptoms, including pruritus, papular eruptions (Fig. 113.4), urticaria, arthralgias, myalgias, fever, headache, nausea, and vomiting. These effects generally subside within 24 to 48 hours

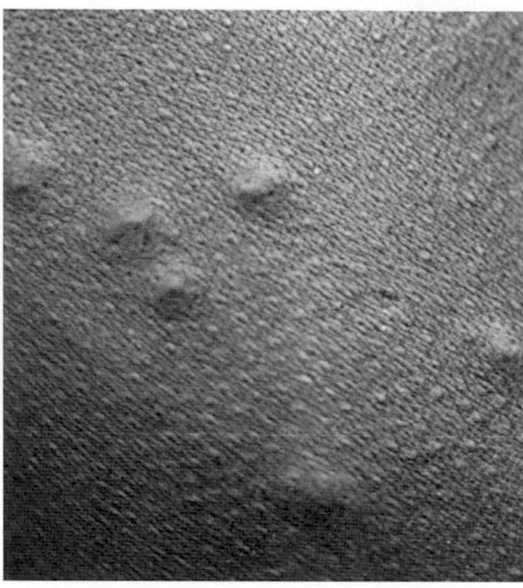

FIGURE 113.4 Multiple papules on the chest of a Congolese man with streptocerciasis. Papules developed within 18 hours after ingestion of 50 mg of diethylcarbamazine. *(Courtesy of the Armed Forces Institute of Pathology, Photograph Neg. No.77-5005.)*

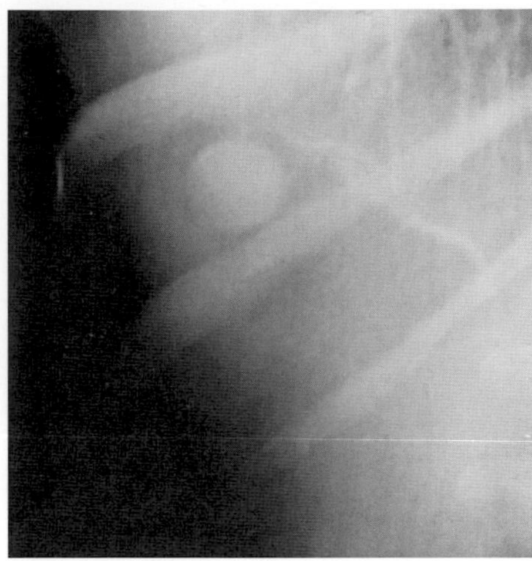

FIGURE 113.5 Roentgenogram of "coin lesion" 2.5 by 2.0 cm, in right lung. *(Courtesy of the Armed Forces Institute of Pathology, Photograph Neg. No.72-10156.)*

and can be managed symptomatically with antihistamines and anti-inflammatory agents. Ivermectin (150 μg/kg as a single dose) has been shown to reduce *M. streptocerca* microfilarial levels [21], although there have been no studies examining the clinical effects of this treatment. The use of doxycycline has not been explored.

DIROFILARIASIS

INTRODUCTION

Dirofilariasis, infection caused by filarial nematodes of the genus *Dirofilaria*, is the most common zoonotic filariasis. Human dirofilariasis was first described in 1885. Unlike other filarial infections of humans, which are restricted to the tropics and subtropics, dirofilariasis has a worldwide distribution. Two distinct clinical forms are recognized: pulmonary dirofilariasis, caused by the dog heartworm, *Dirofilaria immitis*, and subcutaneous dirofilariasis caused by a variety of species, including *D. tenuis* and *D. repens*.

EPIDEMIOLOGY

The true incidence and geographic distribution of human dirofilariasis are unknown [22]. In general, human infection is determined by the prevalence of infection in the natural host and the extent to which humans are exposed to the mosquito vectors. Pulmonary dirofilariasis has a cosmopolitan distribution with cases reported from North and South America, Australia, Japan, and Europe. Subcutaneous dirofilariasis has been reported worldwide.

NATURAL HISTORY, PATHOGENESIS, AND PATHOLOGY

Dirofilaria are zoonotic filarial parasites that are transmitted to their natural hosts by mosquito vectors. The location of the adult worms and microfilariae varies depending on the species. All *Dirofilaria* examined to date harbor the bacterial endosymbiont *Wolbachia* [22].

Pulmonary Dirofilariasis

Although *D. immitis* infects the cat, fox, wolf, coyote, sea lion, and other mammals, the dog is by far the most important reservoir host. Coiled masses of adult worms inhabit the right ventricle and produce microfilariae, which are taken up by the mosquito vector in a blood meal. In human infection, parasites likely develop partially in the right ventricle before dying and being swept into small pulmonary arteries. Neither mature adult worms nor microfilaria have been found in humans.

Subcutaneous Dirofilariasis

Most subconjunctival dirofilarial infections in humans in North America are due to *D. tenuis*, a raccoon parasite, and in Europe, Africa, and Asia, due to *D. repens*, a dog and cat parasite. Rare cases of subconjunctival disease due to *D. immitis* have been reported in Asia and Australia. Other species that have been identified as causes of subcutaneous infections in humans include *D. striata*, a parasite of wildcats, and *D. ursi*, a parasite of bears. Humans are not a definitive host for these parasites, and although occasionally gravid worms have been identified, microfilariae have not been detected.

CLINICAL FEATURES

Pulmonary Dirofilariasis

Most cases of pulmonary dirofilariasis present as asymptomatic coin lesions on routine chest radiography (Fig. 113.5). Lesions are most often solitary, 1–3 cm in diameter, sharply defined and located in the periphery of the lung. When symptoms do occur, they are cough, hemoptysis, fever, chills, and malaise.

Subcutaneous Dirofilariasis

The most dramatic presentation of subcutaneous dirofilariasis is the presence of a moving adult worm in the conjunctiva (Fig. 113.6). This is often accompanied by swelling of the eyelid and face and a burning sensation. Occasionally, worms are found in the retina or within the eye and present as eye pain and blurred vision. Subcutaneous lesions in other parts of the body present as small (0.5–1.5 cm), painless nodules that develop over days to weeks. The nodule may or may not be painful, erythematous, and accompanied by a feeling of movement. Systemic signs are unusual. The most common locations are the eyelid, scrotum, breast, arm, and leg, although any part of the body can be involved.

PATIENT EVALUATION, DIAGNOSIS, AND DIFFERENTIAL DIAGNOSIS

Pulmonary dirofilariasis should be considered in patients presenting with a coin lesion on radiography without risk factors for or other clinical findings suggestive of malignancy. Rarely, subcutaneous dirofilariasis can mimic a localized tumor [23,24]. Unfortunately, definitive diagnosis can only be made by identification of the worm in a

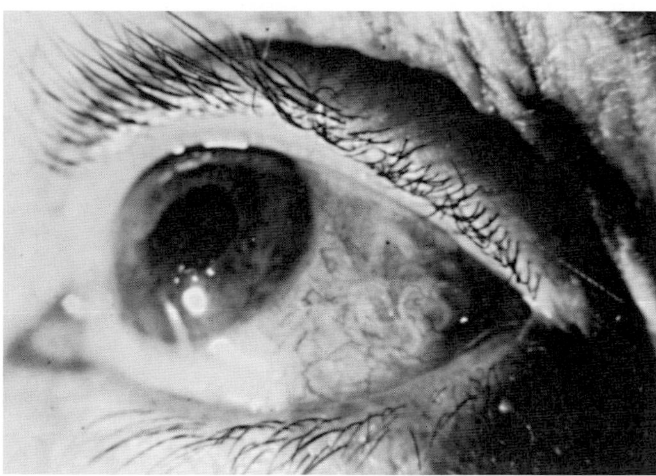

FIGURE 113.6 Female *Dirofilaria tenuis* in conjunctiva of left eye. *(Courtesy of the Armed Forces Institute of Pathology, Photograph Neg. No.74-6351-1.)*

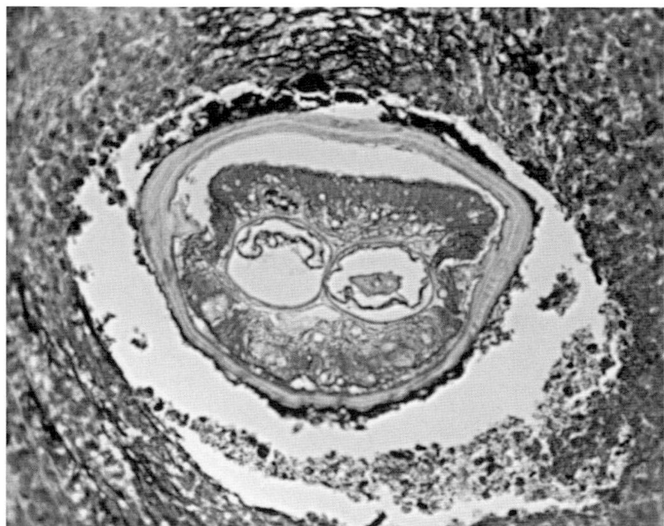

FIGURE 113.7 Transverse section of immature female *Dirofilaria immitis* in lung (Movat stain, ×275). *(Courtesy of the Armed Forces Institute of Pathology, Photograph Neg. No.71-1045.)*

biopsy or autopsy specimen. Filarial serology may be positive or negative, is not species-specific, and is rarely helpful in establishing a diagnosis.

Histopathology typically reveals a central zone of necrosis surrounded by granulomatous inflammation and a fibrous wall. A single, coiled, usually necrotic and sometimes calcified, worm is found in the lumen of an artery within the area of necrosis (pulmonary dirofilariasis) or in a subcutaneous abscess (Fig. 113.7). Dirofilaria have a number of morphologic features that help in their identification in tissue sections, including their relatively large size (100 to 350 μm in diameter), a thick cuticle, and abundant musculature. Species-specific PCR has also been used to identify and differentiate between *Dirofilaria* species in tissues [25].

TREATMENT

The only known treatment is surgical removal of the worm, as has often occurred during the diagnostic workup. Removal of the worm is not essential, however, except in cases where ongoing inflammation is likely to cause permanent damage (ex. a worm inside the anterior chamber of the eye). Most worms die without treatment and are absorbed without clinical sequelae.

REFERENCES

1. Manson P. Parental form of *Filaria perstans*. Br Med J 1899;1:429.
2. Wanji S, Tendongfor N, Esum M, et al. Epidemiology of concomitant infections due to *Loa loa, Mansonella perstans*, and *Onchocerca volvulus* in rain forest villages of Cameroon. Med Microbiol Immunol 2003;192:15–21.
3. Lipner EM, Law MA, Barnett E, et al. Filariasis in travelers presenting to the GeoSentinel Surveillance Network. PLoS Negl Trop Dis 2007;1:e88.
4. Baird JK, Neafie RC, Lanoie L, Connor DH. Adult *Mansonella perstans* in the abdominal cavity in nine Africans. Am J Trop Med Hyg 1987;37:578–84.
5. Keiser PB, Coulibaly Y, Kubofcik J, et al. Molecular identification of *Wolbachia* from the filarial nematode *Mansonella perstans*. Mol Biochem Parasitol 2008;160:123–8.
6. Fux CA, Chappuis B, Holzer B, et al. *Mansonella perstans* causing symptomatic hypereosinophilia in a missionary family. Travel Med Infect Dis 2006;4:275–80.
7. Bregnani ER, Rovellini AA, Mbaidoum N, Magnini MG. Comparison of different anthelminthic drug regimens against *Mansonella perstans* filariasis. Trans R Soc Trop Med Hyg 2006;100:458–63.
8. Coulibaly YI, Dembele B, Diallo AA, et al. A randomized trial of doxycycline for *Mansonella perstans* infection. N Engl J Med 2009;361:1448–58.
   Mansonella perstans *infection is refractory to standard antifilarial therapies. Based on the premise that* M. perstans *contains the intracellular symbiont* Wolbachia, *this study demonstrates that doxycycline is effective in lowering* M. perstans *microfilaremia, providing the first example of effective therapy for this infection.*
9. Manson P. On certain new species of nematode haematozoa occurring in America. Br Med J 1897;1930:1837–8.
10. Nathan MB, Bartholomew CF, Tikasingh ES. The detection of *Mansonella ozzardi* microfilariae in the skin and blood with a note on the absence of periodicity. Trans R Soc Trop Med Hyg 1978;72:420–2.
11. Casiraghi M, Favia G, Cancrini G, et al. Molecular identification of *Wolbachia* from the filarial nematode *Mansonella ozzardi*. Parasitol Res 2001;87:417–20.
12. Bartoloni A, Cancrini G, Bartalesi F, et al. *Mansonella ozzardi* infection in Bolivia: prevalence and clinical associations in the Chaco region. Am J Trop Med Hyg 1999;61:830–3.
13. Bartholomew CF, Nathan MB, Tikasingh ES. The failure of diethylcarbamazine in the treatment of *Mansonella ozzardi* infections. Trans R Soc Trop Med Hyg 1978;72:423–4.
14. Nutman TB, Nash TE, Ottesen EA. Ivermectin in the successful treatment of a patient with *Mansonella ozzardi* infection. J Infect Dis 1987;156:662–5.
15. Gonzalez AA, Chadee DD, Rawlins SC. Ivermectin treatment of mansonellosis in Trinidad. West Indian Med J 1999;48:231–4.
16. Macfie JWS, Corson JF. A new species of filarial larva found in the skin of natives in the Gold Coast. Ann Trop Med Parasitol 1922;16:465–71.
17. Neafie RC, Connor DH, Meyers WM. *Dipetalonema streptocerca* (Macfie and Corson, 1922): description of the adult female. Am J Trop Med Hyg 1975;24:264–7.
18. Fischer P, Bamuhiiga J, Buttner DW. Occurrence and diagnosis of *Mansonella streptocerca* in Uganda. Acta Trop 1997;63:43.
19. Meyers WM, Connor DH, Harman LE, et al. Human streptocerciasis. A clinicopathologic study of 40 Africans (Zairians) including identification of the adult filaria. Am J Trop Med Hyg 1972;21:528–45.
20. Fischer P, Buttner DW, Bamuhiiga J, Williams SA. Detection of the filarial parasite *Mansonella streptocerca* in skin biopsies by a nested polymerase chain reaction-based assay. Am J Trop Med Hyg 1998;58:816–20.
21. Fischer P, Tukesiga E, Buttner DW. Long-term suppression of *Mansonella streptocerca* microfilariae after treatment with ivermectin. J Infect Dis 1999;180:1403–5.
22. Simon F, Morchon R, Gonzalez-Miguel J, et al. What is new about animal and human dirofilariosis? Trends Parasitol 2009;25:404–9.
   The authors provide an excellent recent review of both human and animal dirofilariasis, addressing epidemiology, the host–parasite relationship, and the role of the intracellular endosymbiont Wolbachia *in pathogenesis and treatment.*
23. Fleck R, Kurz W, Quade B, et al. Human dirofilariasis due to *Dirofilaria repens* mimicking a scrotal tumor. Urology 2009;73:209.e1–e3.
24. Perret-Court A, Coulibaly B, Ranque S, et al. Intradural dirofilariasis mimicking a Langerhans cell histiocytosis tumor. Pediatr Blood Cancer 2009;53:485–7.
25. Favia G, Lanfrancotti A, Della Torre A, et al. Polymerase chain reaction-identification of *Dirofilaria repens* and *Dirofilaria immitis*. Parasitology 1996;113:567–71.

SECTION

C

OTHER TISSUE NEMATODE INFECTIONS

114 Dracunculiasis

Ernesto Ruiz-Tiben

Key features

- Human dracunculiasis manifests as an ulcer on the skin, with the nematode *Dracunculus medinensis* protruding through the lesion
- It is an incapacitating disease of poor residents in rural areas without access to safe drinking water. It severely affects agricultural productivity and school attendance
- Infection occurs after ingestion of freshwater copepods that contain the larval worm. Acute manifestations begin about 1 year after infection with the formation of a skin blister, accompanied by redness and irritation (burning sensation), and usually preceded by fever and allergic symptoms, including intense generalized itching
- The intense skin irritation prompts the patient to seek relief by immersing the lesion in water. After the blister breaks, an ulcer-like lesion develops with the anterior end of the parasite exposed, allowing the adult female worm to discharge larvae into the water
- Lesions occur on the lower extremities, including the ankle or foot in about 90% of cases, but the parasite can exit from anywhere on the body
- Other manifestations are due to abscess formation if the worm is broken during the process of manual extraction or when they die before exiting the body and calcify. Chronic manifestations of arthritis, synovitis, and muscle and tendon contractures with resultant ankylosis of the limb are rare
- Synonyms: Guinea worm disease, dracontiasis, dracunculosis

INTRODUCTION

Dracunculiasis is caused by the nematode *Dracunculus medinensis,* and is a disabling disease of poor rural residents in parts of six countries in Africa [1, 2]. This infection manifests by 2–3-foot (~1 m)-long worms that emerge directly through a lesion on the skin; it has an enormous adverse impact on agricultural production and school attendance. The infection is close to being eradicated. *D. medinensis* has been known since ancient Egyptian times. The life cycle of the parasite was first fully described by Alexei Fedechenko in 1870 [3].

EPIDEMIOLOGY

During the nineteenth and twentieth centuries, dracunculiasis was common in much of southern Asia, and in North, West and East Africa. When the Dracunculiasis Eradication Program was getting underway in 1986, an estimated 3.5 million cases occurred annually in India, Pakistan, and 16 African countries [4]. Transmission of dracunculiasis in Yemen was confirmed during 1994, and the World Health Organization (WHO) declared the Central African Republic to have indigenous transmission in 1996, making it the twentieth endemic country [5]. By 2008, only 4619 cases were reported from six remaining endemic countries: Ethiopia and Sudan in East Africa, and Ghana, Mali, Niger, and Nigeria in West Africa (Fig. 114.1) [1,2]. Because of the global campaign, Asia became free of the disease in 1997.

People become infected when they drink water containing tiny freshwater copepods called "Cyclops" or "water fleas", which act as intermediate hosts and harbor infective larvae [6]. When the ingested

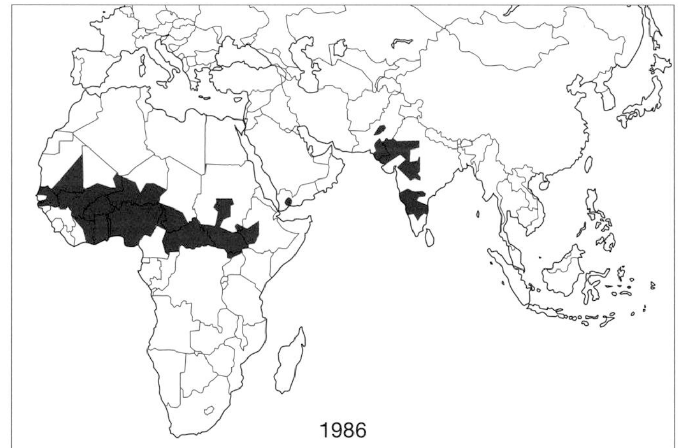

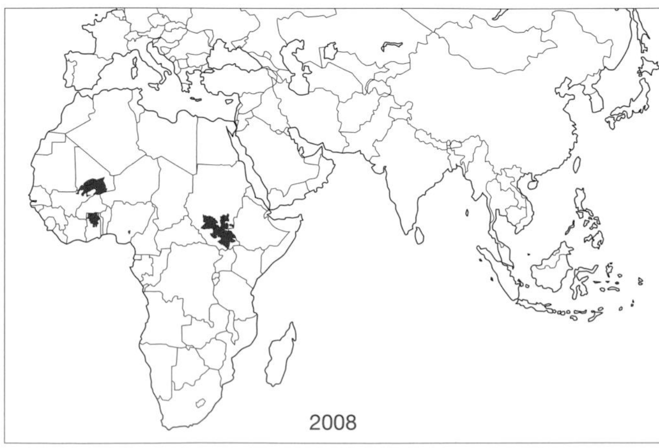

FIGURE 114.1 Extent of areas in Africa affected by dracunculiasis in 1986 and in 2008.

copepods are killed by the digestive juices in the stomach, the larvae are released and move to the small intestine, where they penetrate the intestinal wall and migrate to the connective tissues of the thorax [6]. Male and female larvae mature and mate 60–90 days after infection. Over the next 10–14 months, gravid female worms mature, reaching lengths of 70–100 cm (2–3 feet), and slowly migrate to the surface of the body (Fig. 114.2), where they become visible through ulceration. On contact with fresh water, powerful contractions cause a loop of the worm's uterus to break and discharge a swarm of motile larvae. Contraction of the worm and discharge of larvae may be repeated if the lesion is again submerged in water, until the entire brood of larvae is discharged. Motile free-swimming larvae are ingested whole by copepods and mature in the body cavity in about 2 weeks. Stagnant sources of drinking water such as ponds, cisterns, pools in dried-up river beds, and shallow unprotected hand-dug wells commonly harbor copepods, and are the usual sites where infection is transmitted.

Seasonality varies according to location. In the remaining countries with endemic transmission in the Sahel area of Africa (e.g. Mali, Niger, northern Nigeria, Southern Sudan, and Ethiopia), transmission usually peaks during the rainy season at mid-year (May–September). This is because stagnant surface sources of water are more common during the 5–6-month-long rainy season. In currently endemic countries near the Gulf of Guinea (e.g. Ghana and southern Nigeria), the disease peaks during the dry season, from October to March, when mostly stagnant sources of drinking water remain, in contrast to abundant surface water sources during the rest of the year. The seasonal emergence of the worm often coincides with harvest or planting seasons, and thus significantly affects agricultural productivity and also school attendance. Sudan, the country with the highest incidence of dracunculiasis, in 2008 reported 47% of 3618 cases of dracunculiasis among young adults (ages 16–35); 47% of the cases were male (Makoy SYL, personal communication).

NATURAL HISTORY, PATHOGENESIS, PATHOLOGY, AND CLINICAL FEATURES

Infected people remain asymptomatic for approximately a year after infection, until the mature female worm approaches the skin and forms a painful papule in the dermis. This papule can become a blister within 24 hours or may enlarge for several days before blistering (Fig. 114.3). The blister is accompanied by redness and induration, and is usually preceded by systemic symptoms of low-grade fever and allergic symptoms (erythema, urticarial rash, intense pruritus,

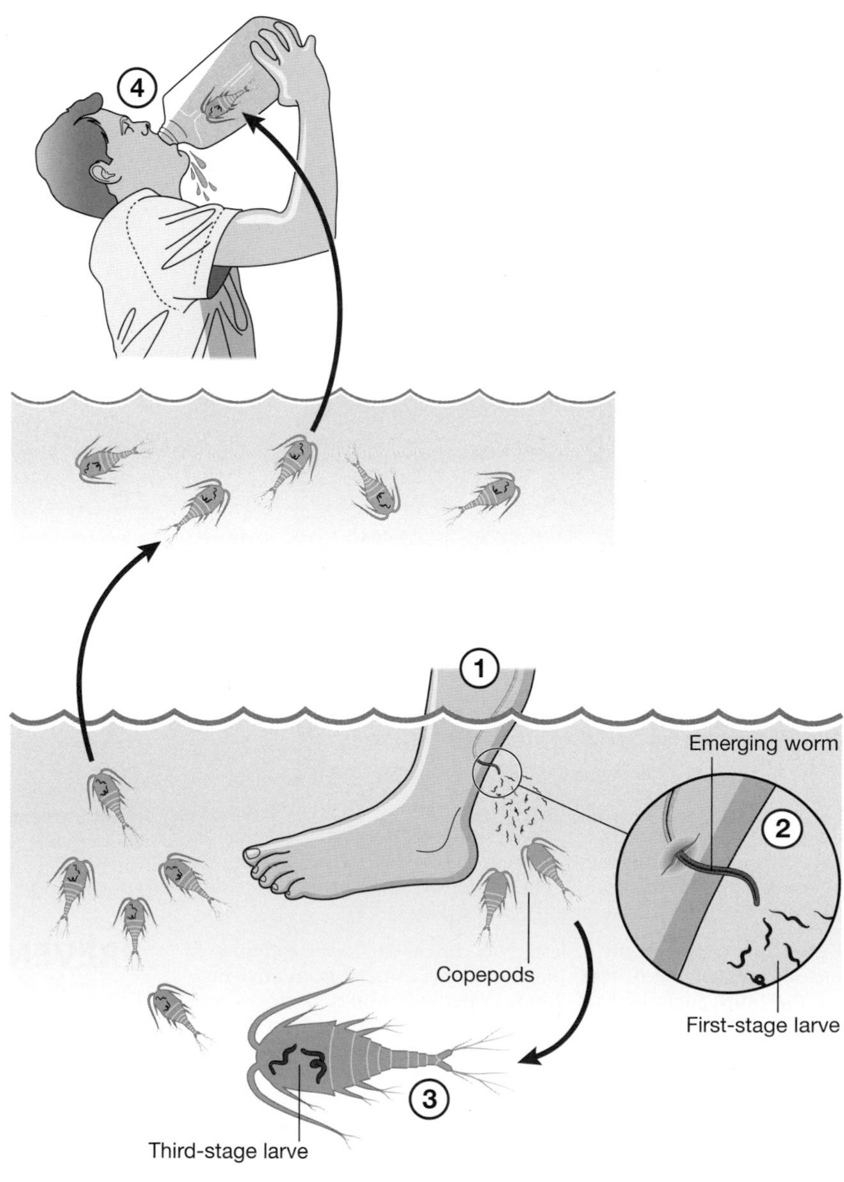

FIGURE 114.2 Life cycle of *Dracunculus medinensis*. *(Courtesy of Encyclopedia Britannica, Inc., © 1996.)*

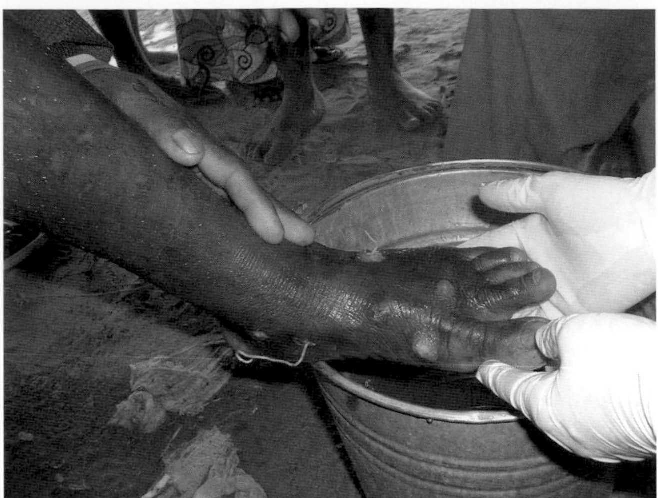

FIGURE 114.3 Blisters caused by *Dracunculus medinensis* and rupture of blisters resulting in skin lesions with protruding Guinea worms. *(Courtesy of Elizabeth Long, The Carter Center.)*

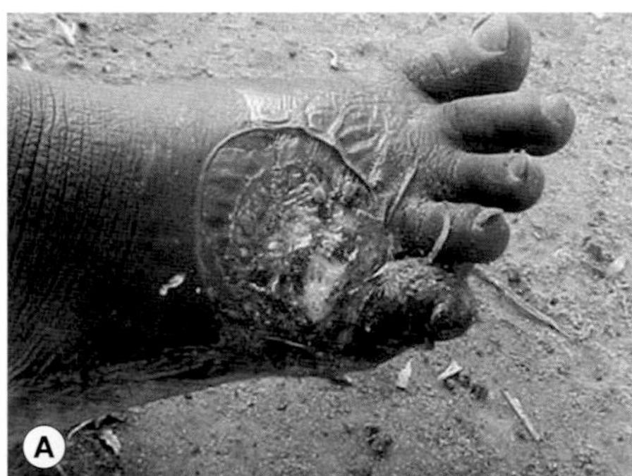

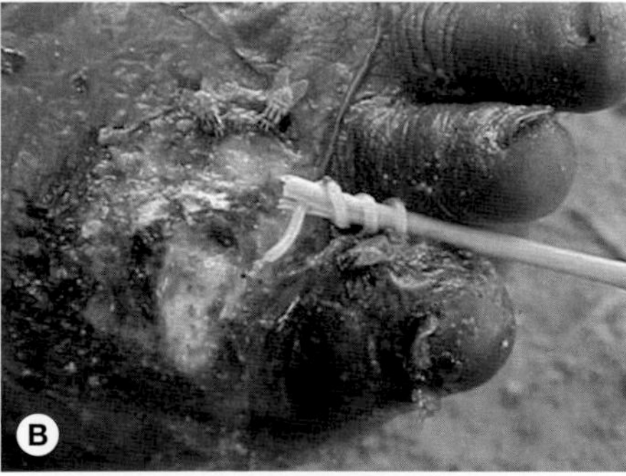

FIGURE 114.4 Pyogenic organisms invade the superficial lesion and worm tract, aggravating the condition. *(Courtesy of The Carter Center.)*

dizziness, nausea, vomiting). The lesion produces intense irritation and burning, inducing the patient to seek relief by immersing the affected limb in water, where the blister breaks, allowing the adult worm to discharge larvae into the water (Fig. 114.4).

Eighty to ninety percent of lesions occur on the lower extremities, including the ankle or foot, but the worms can exit from anywhere on the body, including the head, upper extremities, buttocks and genitalia. More than one worm may emerge from a given patient either simultaneously or sequentially over a period of weeks or months. As the worm emerges through the skin lesion, the affected person pulls it out slowly and carefully (because of inflammation and pain), usually by winding a few centimeters of the worm each day on a small stick. This very painful process may last many weeks.

Pain and other symptoms may lessen with the rupture of the blister, but, at this time, pyogenic organisms invariably invade the superficial lesion and worm tract and aggravate the condition (Fig. 114.4). If the worm breaks during extraction and the remaining part retracts into the tissue, an intense inflammatory reaction occurs, with pain, swelling, and cellulitis along the worm tract, and usually the formation of an abscess. The reported period of incapacitation ranges from 2 to 16 weeks (average 8.5 weeks) [7–14] and more than half of a village's population may be affected at the same time. In addition to the blisters and skin lesions, the secondary bacterial infections usually exacerbate local inflammation and often lead to sepsis, abscesses, septic arthritis, contracture of muscles near joints, or even tetanus [15].

Chronic manifestations are due to inflammation of the joints, with signs and symptoms of arthritis, synovitis [16], and muscle and tendon contractures with resultant ankylosis of the limb [17]. Migration of the worms to the retroperitoneum and from the retroperitoneum to the subcutaneous tissue in the leg sometimes results in aberrant (ectopic) locations such as the pancreas, lung, periorbital tissues, testis, pericardium [18], and the spinal cord, producing compression [19] as well as focal abscess formation.

PATIENT EVALUATION, DIAGNOSIS, AND DIFFERENTIAL DIAGNOSIS

There are no serodiagnostic tests available to detect a patient with an incubating Guinea worm. Diagnosis is based on the clinical history and findings with an appropriate exposure. The blister fluid is bacteriologically sterile and initially contains polymorphonuclear leukocytes and later lymphocytes, eosinophils and macrophages. Larvae are always present in the fluid and white blood cells adhere to them [6]. With time, the blister and worm track can become secondarily infected.

Because differentiation between human and zoonotic species of *Dracunculus* (which rarely affect humans) requires morphologic examination of adult male worms (which are rarely available), efforts are underway to map the genome of the Guinea worm's DNA in order to ascertain the infecting parasite's species more precisely. Although there are several known zoonotic species of *Dracunculus*, only *medinensis* is specific to humans. A molecular tool is now available to differentiate between *D. medinensis* and other tissue-dwelling nematodes, including other *Dracunculus* species that may on rare occasions infect humans [20]. Work on determining the genome of *D. medinensis* is ongoing at the Centers for Disease Control and Prevention (Eberhard ML, personal communication).

TREATMENT

There is no curative drug or vaccine against dracunculiasis. Infected people do not develop immunity. Applying wet compresses to the lesion may relieve pain during the worm's emergence. Placing an occlusive bandage on the wound keeps it clean and may help prevent the patient from contaminating sources of drinking water. Oral analgesics and anti-inflammatory medicines can be administered to alleviate pain and inflammation. Topical antiseptics or antibiotic ointment may minimize the risk of secondary bacterial infections, reduce inflammation, and may permit removal of the worm by gentle traction over a number of days. Systemic antibiotics may be used in established infections. Patients usually recover completely, but repeated infections may occur.

PREVENTION

Prevention of dracunculiasis includes education of the at-risk population about the disease and avoidance measures, filtration of drinking water to remove copepods, and prevention of infected people from entering water intended for drinking. Developing safe sources for drinking water is also a key feature of control [21]. The global eradication program has achieved great success towards its goal, with only six remaining endemic countries [1, 2].

REFERENCES

1. Hopkins DR, Ruiz-Tiben E, Eberhard ML, Roy S. Progress towards global eradication of dracunculiasis, January 2008-June 2009. MMWR Morb Mortal Wkly Rep 2009;58:1123–5.
   This paper provides an update on the status of the global campaign to eradicate dracunculiasis as of mid-2009. Annual cases of dracunculiasis have decreased from 3.5 million to fewer than 10,000 since the World Health Assembly mandated eradication in 1986. The number of indigenous dracunculiasis cases continued to decline and fell below 5000 for the first time in 2008. In 2009, the continued success of the eradication campaign is threatened most by program disruptions from sporadic insecurity, violence and unrest, particularly in Southern Sudan.
2. World Health Organization. Dracunculiasis eradication: global surveillance summary 2008. Wkly Epidemiol Rec 2009;84:162–71.
   This report summarizes the status of the global campaign to eradicate dracunculiasis as of the end of 2008, when only 4619 cases were reported from six countries (Ethiopia, Ghana, Mali, Niger, Nigeria, and Sudan) a reduction of 52% from the 9585 cases reported in 2007. The status of national campaigns is discussed country by country.
3. Fedchenko AP. Concerning the structure and reproduction of the guinea worm (Filaria medinensis L.). Proceedings of the Imperial Society of the Friends of Natural Sciences, Anthropology, and Ethnography. Vol 8 (in Russian), 1870, Reprinted in: Am J Trop Med Hyg 1971:20:511–23.
4. Watts SJ. Dracunculiasis in Africa: its geographical extent, incidence, and at-risk population. Am J Trop Med Hyg 1987;37:119–25.
5. World Health Organization. Dracunculiasis: global surveillance summary: 1996. Wkly Epidemiol Rec 1997;72:133–9.
6. Muller R. Dracunculus and dracunculiasis. Adv Parasitol 1971;6:73–151.
7. Belcher DW, Wurapa FK, Ward WB, et al. Guinea worm in southern Ghana: its epidemiology and impact on agricultural productivity. Am J Trop Med Hyg 1975;24:243–9.
8. Khan HD, Aminuddin M, Shah CH. Epidemiology and socio-economic implications of dracunculiasis in eleven rural communities of District Bannu (Pakistan). J Pakistani Med Assoc 1986;36:233–9.
9. Smith GS, Blum D, Huttley SRA. Disability from dracunculiasis: effect on mobility. Ann Trop Med Parasitol 1989;83:151–8.
10. Watts SJ. Guinea worm: an in depth study of what happens to mothers, families, and communities. Soc Sci Med 1989;29:1043–9.
11. Adeyeba OA, Kale OO. Epidemiology of dracunculiasis and its socio-economic impact in a village in south-west Nigeria. West Afr J Med 1991;10:208–15.
12. Ilegbodu VA, Ilegbodu AE, Wise RA, et al. Clinical manifestations, disability, and use of folk medicine in dracunculiasis in Nigeria. J Trop Med Hyg 1991;94:35–41.
13. Chippaux JP, Benzou A, Agbede K. Social and economic impact of dracunculiasis: a longitudinal study carried out in two villages in Benin. Bull World Health Organ 1992;70:73–8.
14. Rhode JE, Sharma BL, Patto H, et al. Surgical extraction of Guinea worm: disability reduction and contribution to disease control. Am J Trop Med Hyg 1993;48:71–6.
15. Adeyeba OA. Secondary infections in dracunculiasis: Bacteria and morbidity. Int J Zoonoses 1985;12:147.
16. Robineau M, Sereni D. Arthrite aiguë du genou avec presence intra-articulaire de microfilaires de *D. medinensis*. Évolutions clinique et immunologique compares. A propos d'un cas. Bull Soc Pathol Exot Filiales 1978;71:85–9.
17. el Garf A. Parasitic rheumatism: rheumatic manifestations associated with calcified guinea worm. J Rheumtol 1985;12:976–9.
18. Kinare SG, Parulkar GB, Sen PK. Constrictive pericarditis resulting from dracunculosis. Br Med J 1962;1:845.
19. Odaibo SK, Agowun IA, Oshagbemi K. Paraplegia complicating dracontiasis. J R Coll Surg 1986;31:376–8.
20. Bimi L, Freeman AR, Eberhard ML, et al. Differentiating *Dracunculus medinensis* from *D. insignis*, by the sequence analysis of the 18S rRNA gene. Ann Trop Med Parasitol 2005;99:511–17.
21. Barry M. The tail end of guinea worm – global eradication without a drug or a vaccine. N Engl J Med 2007;356:2561–4.

115 Trichinellosis

Fabrizio Bruschi, K Darwin Murrell

Key features

- Trichinellosis (also called trichinosis) is the name for a parasite infection caused by the nematode *Trichinella*
- It is acquired by humans from eating the muscles of wild or domestic animals harboring the larval stage of the parasite
- The severity of disease is usually proportional to the number of larvae ingested, and the disease is characterized by fever, gastrointestinal symptoms, myositis, swollen eyelids, and eosinophilia
- The diagnosis is made by muscle biopsy and a highly specific serologic test (e.g. Western blot)
- Treatment involves symptom management, corticosteroid use, and anthelmintics (albendazole or mebendazole)

INTRODUCTION

Trichinellosis has been a zoonotic disease for thousands of years, acquired by humans from eating insufficiently cooked infected meat. *Trichinella* was first described in 1835 by James Paget, when studying muscle tissue from a cadaver. The eight species of *Trichinella* responsible for infection occur in many wild and domestic animals distributed throughout the Arctic, temperate and tropical zones [1]. Virtually all mammals are susceptible to infection although only humans appear to be prone to developing clinical disease. While diminishing in developed countries, outbreaks continue to be reported in developing regions, especially Southeast Asia, Latin America, and Africa [2].

EPIDEMIOLOGY

Trichinellosis is an important food-borne zoonosis because of the economic burden associated with maintaining systems to prevent it entering the human food chain, particularly from domestic swine (meat inspection). The prevalence of swine infection due to *T. spiralis* has greatly diminished because of the widespread adoption of modern pig-rearing systems. However, outbreaks due to infected horse meat and game animals, often involving other species (especially *T. britovi, T. murrelli,* and *T. nativa)* frequently occur. Such outbreaks have occurred recently in China, Thailand, Laos, Vietnam, Mexico, Argentina, and Bolivia (Table 115-1). More than 100 species of mammals are susceptible. The infective encysted larvae (trichina) may remain viable in the host's musculature for several years (depending upon host species). Their ability to survive long periods in decaying and putrefying muscle increases the probability of successful transmission in nature.

A feature of *Trichinella* epidemiology is the existence of two normally separate ecologic systems, the sylvatic and the domestic. The two biotopes may become linked through man's activities, resulting in the exposure of humans to *Trichinella* species normally confined to wild animals. Only *T. spiralis* is highly infective to pigs; consequently, commercial pig production needs to have stringent barriers to exposure to wild animals, especially commensal rats, and uncooked meat scraps [1].

NATURAL HISTORY, PATHOGENESIS, AND PATHOLOGY

When humans consume raw or rare flesh infected with first-stage *Trichinella* larvae (which may be encysted or not, depending on the species) (Fig. 115.1), the larvae are freed from the muscles by digestion in the stomach. The larvae, resistant to gastric juice, pass into the small intestine, burrow beneath the columnar epithelium and lie just above the lamina propria. There, they undergo four molts and develop into adult worms, male and female, which mate. After fertilization, the females begin to discharge live (newborn) early first-stage larvae, the production of which can continue for 4 to 16 weeks or more, depending on host species, until the adult worms are finally expelled from the intestine; the longevity of adult worms in the human intestine is not known.

Newborn larvae make their way into the lamina propria, to a draining lymph node or blood vessel, and are carried to the arterial circulation via the thoracic duct. Larvae arrive at striated skeletal muscle cells, where, after invasion, they induce changes that culminate in a new cell phenotype termed the nurse cell; the nurse cell can develop a collagenous capsule around the larvae (in the case of the encapsulated *Trichinella*). After 21 days, the larvae are fully infective. In humans, calcification of the cyst may begin within 6 months to a year, a process that eventually leads to death of the encysted larvae.

CLINICAL FEATURES

The degree of illness is usually related to infection level, particularly the number of larvae per gram of muscle: in light subclinical infections, up to ten larvae; in moderate infections, 50 to 500 larvae; and in severe, life-threatening infections, 1000 or more larvae. The species of *Trichinella* may also be an important variable. Most human infections with *Trichinella* have been attributed to *T. spiralis*; infections with *T. nelsoni* and *T. britovi* appear to be less clinically severe [3].

The symptoms of trichinellosis can be separated into an early intestinal phase, a later phase associated with inflammatory and allergic responses caused by muscle invasion, and a convalescent phase. The incubation period ranges from 5 to 51 days; the course of infection is more severe. During this period, gastrointestinal symptoms occur. The incubation period ends when the acute infection phase begins and is characterized by the fever, myalgia, periorbital edema, and eosinophilia (i.e., the so-called trichinotic syndrome or general trichinosis syndrome). Acute infection lasts 1 to 8 weeks, and it may have a mild, moderate, or severe course, depending on the fever severity and length, the intensity of symptoms, the time taken to recover from disease, and the presence of complications.

TABLE 115-1 Recent Trichinellosis Cases

Country	Period	Number of cases	Sources
United States	1996–2005	61	Pork; game
Canada	2005	9	Bear
Argentina	1990–2002	6919	Pork; game
Bulgaria	1993–2000	5683	Pork; game
Croatia	1997–2000	1047	Pork
Serbia	1995–2001	3925	Pork
Germany	1996–2007	99	Pork; game
Russia	1998–2002	864	Game; pork
Israel	2002	30	Pork
Turkey	2004	418	Pork
China	1964–2004	23,004	Pork; dog; game
Thailand	1994–2007	136	Pork
Laos	2005	625	Pork

Adapted from Bruschi F, Murrell KD. Trichinellosis. In: Guerrant RL, Walker DH, Weller PF, eds. Tropical Infectious Diseases: Principles, Pathogens and Practice, 3rd edn. Philadelphia: Churchill Livingstone Elsevier; 2011.

INTESTINAL OR ENTERAL PHASE

The initial consequences of infection occur within the first week after ingestion of larval worms in inadequately cooked meat (Table 115–2). The symptoms, reflecting mucosal irritation as adult worms develop in the small intestine, include nausea, abdominal cramps, loss of appetite, vomiting, low-grade fever, and either mild diarrhea or constipation. Frontal headaches, dizziness, and weakness can also occur, especially in light to moderate infections. Severe diarrhea, persisting for weeks, can be seen in heavy infections. Infected Inuit Indians in North America experience an unusually high frequency of diarrhea and a low frequency of myalgia. This may reflect chronic exposure and the development of intestinal immunity [4].

MUSCLE INVASION OR PARENTERAL PHASE

This stage, beginning as early as 9 to 10 days after exposure, is associated with penetration of the newborn larvae into muscle cells, initiating an inflammatory response of neutrophils, eosinophils, lymphocytes, and macrophages. It especially occurs in the extraocular muscles; masseters; muscles of the larynx, tongue, diaphragm, and neck; intercostals; and muscular attachments to tendons and joints. The fibers become edematous and enlarged. This process reaches its peak at about 5 to 6 weeks of infection and diminishes when the larvae are encapsulated.

Early symptoms are swelling of the eyelids and facial edema. After this, muscle swelling, tenderness, pain on movement, and fever can develop. Headache, fainting, urticaria, splinter hemorrhages, conjunctivitis, loss of appetite, hoarseness, dysphagia, dyspnea, and edema of the legs can also occur. Fever can be delayed until several weeks after infection, but temperature may eventually reach 104 °F for a week or more in heavy infections.

Pain is noticed at about the time facial edema appears. It is most severe between the second and fourth weeks of infection but may persist for a longer period and can be intense enough to make chewing, talking, and swallowing difficult. Respiratory symptoms, including dyspnea, result from involvement of respiratory muscles, and myocarditis, sometimes fatal, may result from larval invasion of the heart, but immunopathologic processes could also play a role.

Neurologic Complications

Neurologic symptoms can accompany migration of the larvae through central nervous system tissue; resulting in intracerebral hemorrhage and meningitis. Patients can exhibit dizziness, ataxia, hysteria, psychotic disturbances, seizures, monoparesis, and eventually coma in severe infections. Larvae cannot successfully encyst in the nervous system.

CONVALESCENT PHASE

Beginning in the second month after infection, myalgia, along with fever and itching, decreases. At this time, evidence of congestive heart failure may appear, especially if the patient becomes active too soon. Larvae remain alive in the cysts for one or more years, depending on the species, even after the cyst wall becomes calcified. These larvae release antigens that lead to a persistent low to moderate eosinophilia and stimulate specific circulating antibody. Fatal outcome is infrequent in trichinellosis, normally occurring only in massive infections, and is most frequently associated with myocarditis, encephalitis, and pneumonitis. In the period 2002–2007, of 66 cases of trichinellosis reported in the US, no fatalities were reported [5].

PATIENT EVALUATION, DIAGNOSIS, AND DIFFERENTIAL DIAGNOSIS

An algorithm for identification of trichinellosis cases (see Table 115-3), as well as one for chronic trichinellosis and sequelae, has been developed by Dupouy-Camet and Bruschi [6]. Diagnosis can be made by direct or indirect demonstration of infection. Eosinophilia, leukocytosis, elevated levels of muscle enzymes, and increased immunoglobulin levels, especially total IgE, are the most characteristic laboratory findings of this disease. Specific immunodiagnostic tests are now available.

DIRECT DEMONSTRATION OF WORMS

Enteral Phase

Adult *Trichinella* can sometimes be recovered from the intestinal mucosa at autopsy and could, theoretically, be recovered from a living patient by duodenal aspiration or biopsy.

Parenteral Phase

The muscle stage offers the best chance for direct demonstration of worms. The larvae can be found on examination of a biopsy of a superficial skeletal muscle. A specimen measuring approximately 1 cm^3 should be taken, preferably from either the deltoid or gastrocnemius muscle. A portion of the specimen is fixed and examined histologically. The remainder is processed either by: 1) compression between glass slides, followed by microscopic examination; and/or 2) digestion in 1% pepsin and 1% hydrochloric acid, followed by microscopic examination of a filtrate or washed sediment of the digested specimen.

INDIRECT DEMONSTRATION

A nondiagnostic biopsy does not exclude the possibility of infection. Circulating antibody can be detected even in lightly infected patients 3 to 4 weeks after infection and as early as 2 weeks in heavily infected individuals. The fluorescent antibody test and ELISA are the most useful serologic tests. ELISA using larval E/S (excretory/secretory) antigens is sensitive and can also detect a rise and fall in titer [7]. ELISA should be confirmed by Western blot, which should show reactivity against the TSL-1 antigen family (40–70 kDa) in the reduced form [7].

DIFFERENTIAL DIAGNOSIS

Trichinellosis can mimic a wide variety of diseases. Mild cases can be misdiagnosed as influenza or other viral fevers unless the clinician

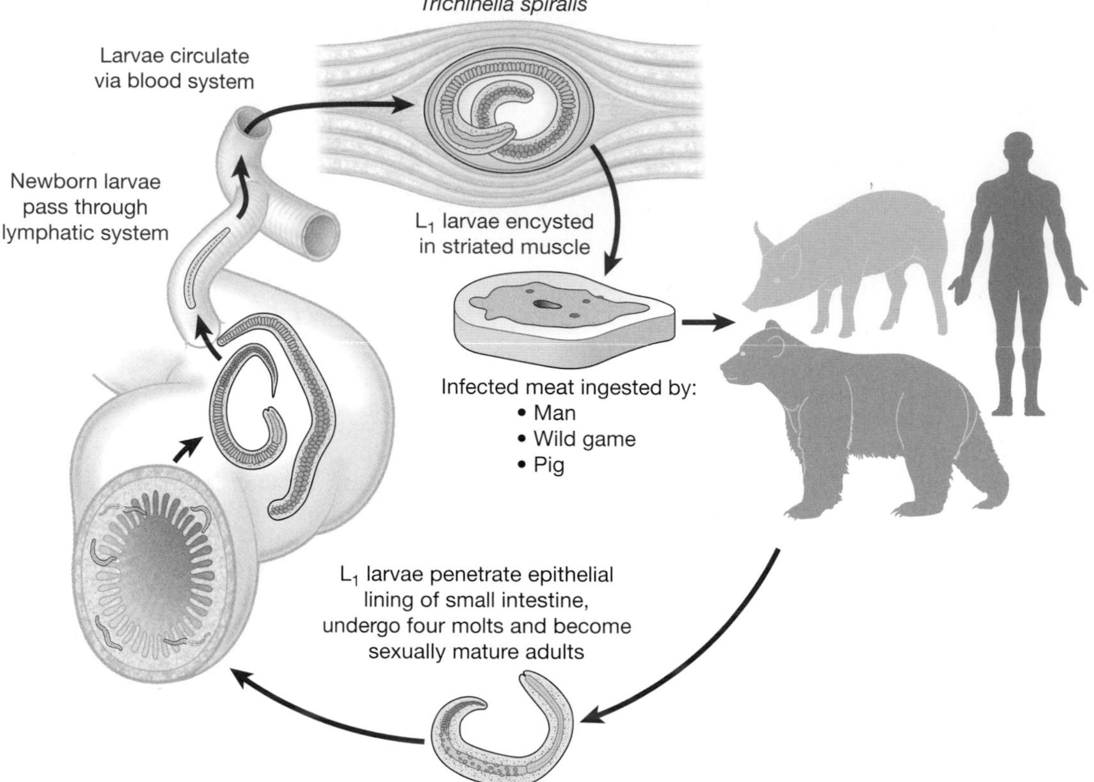

FIGURE 115.1 Life cycle of *Trichinella spiralis* showing stages and locations of development.

TABLE 115-2 Clinical Phases of Trichinellosis

Days after infection	Developmental phase	Symptoms and signs (heavy infections)
2 to 7	Intestinal	Gastrointestinal signs, i.e. nausea, abdominal pain, headache
9 to 28	Muscle	Muscular pain, facial edema, fever, chills, eosinophilia, tachycardia, coma, respiratory difficulties
14+	Encystment or chronic	Mental apathy, neurotoxic symptoms, possible myocarditis, anemia, muscular swelling

TABLE 115-3 Signs and Symptoms Useful in Assessing the Probability of Being Infected With *Trichinella*

Group A	Group B	Group C	Group D
Fever	Diarrhea	Eosinophilia (> 1 G/l and/or increased IgE levels)	Positive serology (with a highly specific test)
Eyelid and/or facial edema	Neurological signs	Increased levels of muscular enzymes	Seroconversion
Myalgia	Cardiological signs		Positive muscular biopsy
	Conjunctivitis		
	Subungual hemorrhages		
	Cutaneous rash		

The diagnosis is:
Very unlikely: one A or one B or one C
Suspected: one A or two B and one C
Probable: three A and one C
Highly probable: three A and two C
Confirmed: three A, two C, and one D; any of groups A or B and one C and one D

Reproduced with permission from Dupouy-Camet J, Bruschi F. Management and diagnosis of human trichinellosis. In: Dupou12y-Camet J, Murrell KD, eds. FAO/WHO/OIE Guidelines for the Surveillance, Management, Prevention and Control of Trichinellosis. Paris: OIE; 2007:37–69.

recognizes a history of recent ingestion of pork or game, febrile myalgia, periorbital edema, and rising eosinophilia (to 50% or higher), and confirms the diagnosis by either serologic tests or muscle biopsy. Similar symptoms among others who dined on the same occasion reflect a common source of infection and further substantiate the diagnosis.

TREATMENT

It is difficult to differentiate the efficacy of drug therapy from natural recovery of infection in mild to moderate cases. Symptomatic treatment [6] includes analgesic and antipyretic drugs, bed rest, and corticosteroids (prednisolone at 50 mg/day), especially in severe infections to prevent shock-like symptoms. Antiparasitic treatment [6] is with mebendazole (in adults, usually at a daily dose of 5 mg/kg [in some countries up to 20–25 mg/kg/day] in two doses for a period of 10 to 15 days) or albendazole (administered at a dose of 15 mg/kg/day in two doses for 10 to 15 days, in adults). For severe infection, treatment may be repeated after 5 days.

Factors such as the *Trichinella* species, intensity of infection (worm burden), duration of infection, and the host's response characteristics, especially immunocompetence and/or premunition, should help dictate treatment. Unfortunately, only a limited number of prospective, controlled clinical trials of treatment for trichinellosis have been carried out, which has led to uncertainties in the treatment choice [6].

REFERENCES

1. Pozio E, Murrell KD. Systematics and epidemiology of *Trichinella*. Adv Parasitol 2006;63:367–439.
   This reference represents the landmark for people involved in the study of taxonomy of the genus Trichinella.
2. Bruschi F, Murrell KD. Trichinellosis. In: Guerrant RL, Walker DH, Weller PF, eds. Tropical Infectious Diseases: Principles, Pathogens and Practice, 3rd edn. Philadelphia: Churchill Livingstone Elsevier; 2011.
3. Bruschi F, Murrell KD. New aspects of human trichinellosis: the impact of new *Trichinella* species. Postgrad Med J 2002;78:15–22.
4. Murrell KD, Bruschi F. Clinical trichinellosis. Prog Clin Parasitol 1994;4:116–50.
5. Kennedy ED, Hall RL, Montgomery SP, et al. Trichinellosis surveillance – United States, 2002-2007. MMWR Surveill Summ 2009;58:1–7.
6. Dupouy-Camet J, Bruschi F. Management and diagnosis of human trichinellosis. In: Dupouy-Camet J, Murrell KD, eds. FAO/WHO/OIE Guidelines for the Surveillance, Management, Prevention and Control of Trichinellosis. Paris: OIE; 2007:37–69.
   This reference is one of the most complete and updated reviews on human trichinellosis.
7. Gamble HR, Pozio E, Bruschi F, et al. International Commission on Trichinellosis: recommendations on the use of serological tests for the detection of *Trichinella* infection in animals and man. Parasite 2004;11:3–13.

116 Toxocariasis

Dana M Woodhall

Key features

- Toxocariasis is a zoonotic infection that occurs worldwide and predominately affects children
- Humans become infected by ingesting eggs in contaminated soil or, rarely, by consuming undercooked meat of an animal infected with *Toxocara* larvae
- Two main clinical presentations are ocular toxocariasis and visceral toxocariasis. In visceral toxocariasis, body organs, such as the liver, are affected
- Diagnosis of toxocariasis is made by clinical presentation and testing for antibody to the *Toxocara* parasite
- Anthelmintics, corticosteroids and supportive treatment are the mainstays of treatment

INTRODUCTION

Toxocariasis is caused by the dog and cat roundworms *Toxocara canis* or *Toxocara cati*. In 1950, Wilder was the first person to detect the nematode larvae in a series of enucleated eyes. In 1952, *Toxocara* larvae were identified and documented in humans by Beaver and colleagues who described a series of patients presenting with eosinophilia and systemic disease [1]. Today, toxocariasis is recognized as a zoonotic infection that occurs anywhere dogs or cats are present, and causes a spectrum of disease in humans, ranging from asymptomatic infection to the development of visceral, ocular or covert toxocariasis. Diagnosing *Toxocara* infection remains a challenge as no standardized clinical definition of disease exists and presenting symptoms can be vague.

EPIDEMIOLOGY

The geographic distribution of toxocariasis is worldwide. In the USA, the overall seroprevalence for antibodies to *Toxocara* is 14%; in other countries, studies have demonstrated seroprevalence ranges from 4–86%; however, a positive serologic test does not necessarily indicate active clinical disease [2]. Higher seropositivity has been noted in non-Hispanic blacks and linked to low socioeconomic status, increased blood lead levels and dog or cat ownership. The true prevalence of active clinical disease remains unknown.

Playgrounds and sandboxes are common sources of *Toxocara*, as animals frequently defecate there. An older study demonstrated contamination rates in soil as high as 40% [3]. Children comprise the majority of patients diagnosed with toxocariasis as they often visit contaminated areas and put their fingers, toys, or other objects into their mouths. A few studies have cited a male predominance for seropositivity, possibly associated with greater risk activities, such as an increased likelihood to accidentally ingest dirt. Other associations with *Toxocara* infection include geophagia and residing in warmer climates.

NATURAL HISTORY, PATHOGENESIS, AND PATHOLOGY

Dogs and cats are the definitive hosts of *T. canis* and *T. cati*. In addition to the ingestion of *Toxocara* eggs from the environment, infection in puppies and kittens can also occur prenatally or early postnatally through lactogenic transmission. In puppies only, transplacental transmission can occur. In dogs and cats, the *Toxocara* lifecycle is completed when *Toxocara* larvae develop into egg-laying adult worms in the intestine.

Adult *Toxocara* worms in dog and cat intestines produce eggs that are shed in the feces. Once in the external environment, *Toxocara* eggs require 2–4 weeks at temperatures of >10°C to embryonate and become infective. Transmission of *Toxocara* to humans occurs through ingestion of embryonated eggs directly from the soil or from contaminated fomites or hands (Fig. 116.1). Transmission may also occur following ingestion of undercooked meat from an animal infected with *Toxocara* larvae. Humans and other animals are paratenic hosts for *Toxocara*, as the larvae do not undergo further development into adult worms.

In humans, after embryonated eggs are swallowed, the shell is partially digested in the intestine and the larva escapes. Larvae enter the vascular system and may burrow into tissues, causing hemorrhage, necrosis, and secondary inflammation. Larvae have been found in every tissue and organ system, including the liver, lungs, heart, and brain. Granulomas, 1–2 mm in diameter, usually form around the larvae. These have a preponderance of eosinophils. Later, fibrosis and possible calcification occur. Despite a vigorous immunologic response, *Toxocara* larvae can survive for years and continue to cause clinical disease [4].

CLINICAL FEATURES

The development of clinical disease depends on the parasite load, the host's immune response and migration path of the larvae. In many cases, infection is asymptomatic; however, two syndromes, visceral toxocariasis and ocular toxocariasis, are well defined. It is uncommon for patients to present with manifestations of both visceral and ocular toxocariasis.

VISCERAL TOXOCARIASIS (VISCERAL LARVA MIGRANS)

Visceral toxocariasis, usually diagnosed in very young children (mean age 2–4 years), is a marked inflammatory immune response to numerous larvae migrating to the liver or other tissues. Signs and symptoms may include fever, abdominal pain, or hepatomegaly. Symptoms may also include wheezing or coughing; pulmonary infiltration is evident in a third of patients. A potential association between infection with *Toxocara* and asthma or neurologic manifestations, such as

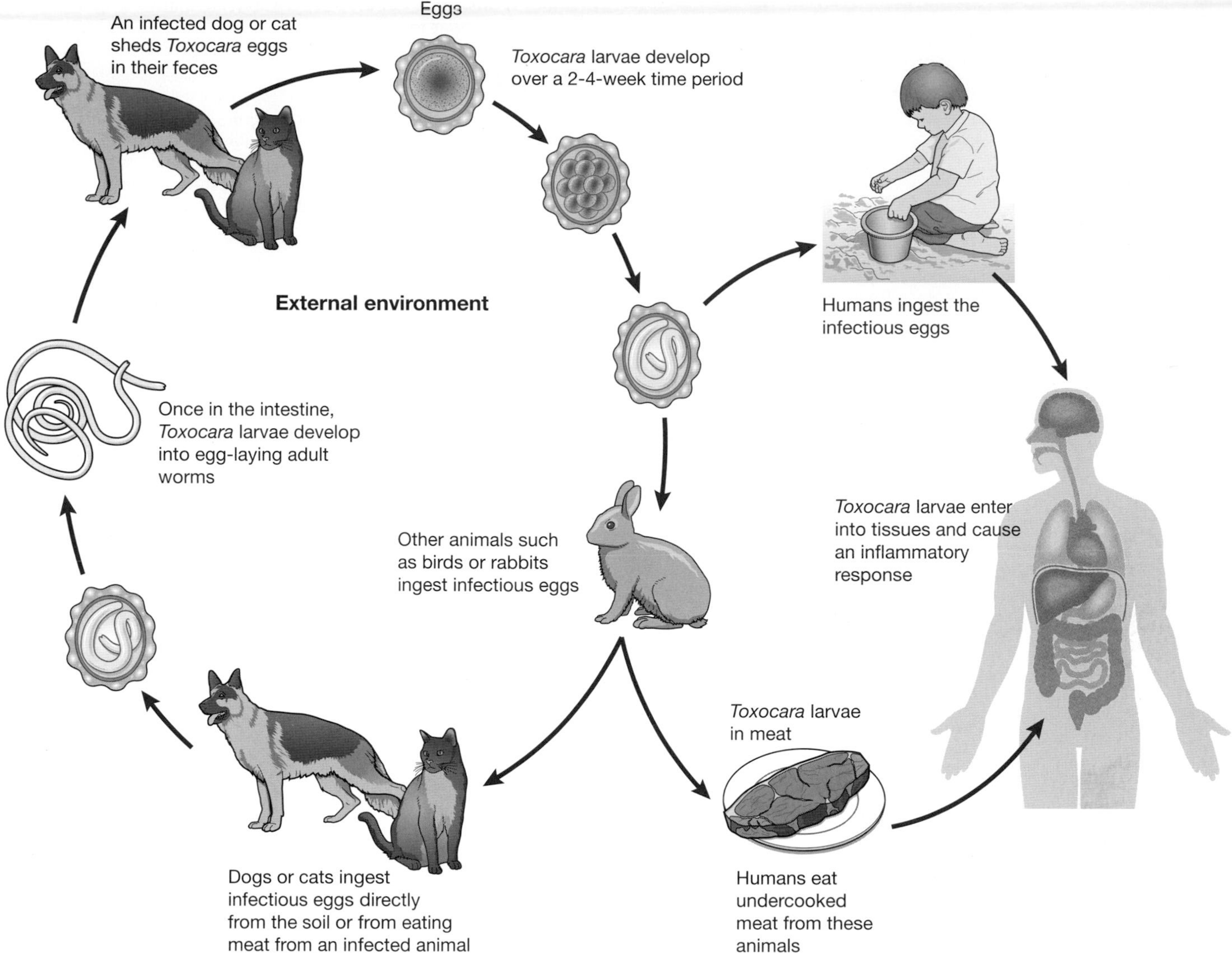

FIGURE 116.1 *Toxocara* lifecycle.

seizures, has been described [5, 6]. Rare fatal cases have resulted from larval migration to the myocardium or the central nervous system (CNS) [1].

OCULAR TOXOCARIASIS (OCULAR LARVA MIGRANS)

Ocular involvement is more common in older children and adults (mean age 7–17 years). Ocular toxocariasis is caused by migration of *Toxocara* larvae to the eye resulting in inflammation and scarring which can lead to permanent vision loss [7]. Ocular disease is usually unilateral and typically affects the posterior segment of the eye. Presenting symptoms can include eye redness, eye pain, strabismus, photophobia or vision changes. Specific signs, such as subretinal granulomatous mass, endophthalmitis or posterior pole granuloma can be evident on ophthalmologic exam.

COVERT OR COMMON TOXOCARIASIS

The term "covert" or "common" toxocariasis is used to describe signs and symptoms that are mild and nonspecific but together form a recognizable symptom complex consistent with toxocariasis. Such symptoms can include abdominal pain, anorexia, sleep and behavior disturbances, wheezing, and fever.

PATIENT EVALUATION, DIAGNOSIS, AND DIFFERENTIAL DIAGNOSIS

The diagnosis of visceral toxocariasis should be considered in persons with a persistently elevated eosinophil count. Identification of larvae in biopsy tissue permits definitive diagnosis of *Toxocara* infection (Fig. 116.2); other larval nematodes can be differentiated based on characteristic morphologic features. However, biopsy is often unrewarding because, unless the infection is massive, specimens may not yield larvae.

A history of geophagia or association with dogs or cats is helpful. The clinical and laboratory findings (other than serologic tests) are nonspecific and do not help to differentiate visceral toxocariasis from other conditions associated with eosinophilia. Because the parasite does not mature beyond the larval stage in human tissues, adult worms do not develop in the intestine and diagnosis by egg detection in feces is not possible.

Loss of vision in a child may not be recognized immediately. Disuse of the affected eye commonly leads to strabismus and the parents may note that a squint has developed. In other individuals, routine examination may reveal poor or absent sight in one eye; ophthalmologic exam can demonstrate vitritis, retinal scarring, granuloma formation,

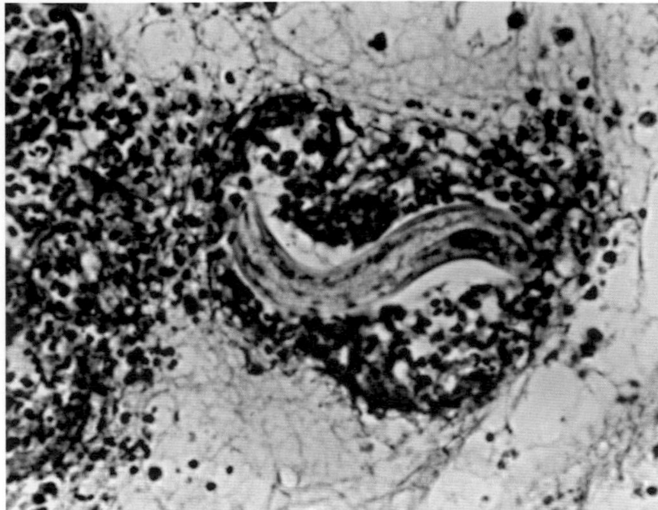

FIGURE 116.2 A portion of a *Toxocara canis* larva is surrounded by inflammatory cells in a preretinal mass. *(× 220; Courtesy of the Armed Forces Institute of Pathology, Photograph Neg. No. 29856329081.)*

or retinal detachment. *Toxocara* larva is rarely identified on ophthalmologic exam.

LABORATORY FINDINGS

Eosinophilia is common in active visceral toxocariasis, but its duration is inconsistent and is probably related to the quantity and recentness of the infecting dose and the frequency of re-infection. In ocular toxocariasis, peripheral eosinophilia is often absent.

SEROLOGIC TESTS

ELISA, using excretory-secretory antigens from infective-stage larvae, is the diagnostic test of choice. In patients whose clinical signs and history suggest visceral toxocariasis, a positive *Toxocara* ELISA is strong presumptive evidence of *Toxocara* infection. A rising or falling titer with a twofold difference in a recently ill patient is consistent with visceral toxocariasis. Because *Toxocara* antibody titers can remain elevated for years after initial infection, a measurable titer is not proof of a causative relationship between *T. canis* or *T. cati* and the current illness. Surveys have shown that as many as 1–10% of asymptomatic children have ELISA titers of 1:32 or more. In patients with ocular lesions compatible with toxocariasis, positive ELISA titers support the diagnosis but do not rule out other eye pathology. Toxocaral ELISA testing is available at the Centers for Disease Control and Prevention (CDC) and several other clinical laboratories in the USA.

DIFFERENTIAL DIAGNOSIS

Visceral toxocariasis must be differentiated from infections caused by other tissue-migrating helminths (other ascarids, hookworm, filiaria, *Strongyloides stercoralis*, and *Trichinella spiralis*) and hypereosinophilic syndromes. Hepatic capillariasis can be confused with toxocariasis involving the liver when patients present with hepatomegaly, eosinophilia, and abnormal liver function test results. Differentiation between the two diseases is through liver biopsy which may demonstrate eggs of *Capillaria* species within a hepatic granuloma. Retinoblastoma, ocular tumors, developmental anomalies, exudative retinitis (Coats disease), tuberculosis, trauma, and other childhood uveitides should be considered as possible alternative diagnoses in patients with ocular toxocariasis.

TREATMENT

Asymptomatic toxocariasis does not require anthelmintic therapy. Although there are isolated reports of ocular disease occurring years after exposure to *Toxocara*, available data suggest that asymptomatic individuals have spontaneous resolution of their eosinophilia and seroreactivity without adverse sequelae.

Treatment of patients with symptoms of visceral toxocariasis is primarily supportive. Anthelmintics, albendazole (400 mg PO BID), or mebendazole (100–200mg PO BID), have been used for treatment in adults and children although the optimum duration of treatment remains unknown. A 5-day course is considered sufficient, although some practitioners treat for up to 20 days for severe infections. Severe pulmonary, myocardial, or CNS involvement may warrant corticosteroid therapy.

Treatment of acute ocular toxocariasis is directed toward suppressing the inflammatory response. Systemic and intraocular corticosteroids (prednisone 30–60 mg PO each day for 2–4 weeks; triamcinolone acetonide 40 mg sub-tenon weekly for 2 weeks; or topical prednisolone acetate) are commonly utilized [8]. The benefit of concurrent use of anthelminthic drugs in managing ocular toxocariasis remains unclear. A single study showed improved visual acuity in persons treated with albendazole and corticosteroids, however, there was no comparison group [9]. Relapse and progression of ocular disease are common and often lead to permanent structural damage. Intraocular fibrous adhesions, retinal traction and detachment, and chronic vitreal inflammation are most effectively managed by surgical intervention. Surgical procedures may include pars plana vitrectomy or scleral buckling.

Implementation of simple prevention strategies can lead to a reduction in the number of cases of human toxocariasis. Good hygiene practices such as hand-washing and teaching children not to eat dirt will minimize human exposure to infectious eggs. Excluding pets from play areas and prompt disposal of pet feces will decrease environmental contamination. Routine veterinarian care for pets, including deworming, will reduce *Toxocara* infection in dogs and cats. Healthcare providers should educate patients about toxocariasis to increase public awareness of this preventable disease.

REFERENCES

1. Despommier D. Toxocariasis: clinical aspects, epidemiology, medical ecology, and molecular aspects. Clin Microbiol Rev 2003;16:265–72.
2. Won KY, Kruszon-Moran D, Schantz PM, Jones JL. National seroprevalence and risk factors for Zoonotic Toxocara spp. infection. Am J Trop Med Hyg 2008; 79:552–7.
3. Dubin S, Segall S, Martindale J. Contamination of soil in two city parks with canine nematode ova including *Toxocara canis*: a preliminary study. Am J Public Health 1975;65:1242–5.
4. Glickman LT, Schantz PM. Epidemiology and pathogenesis of zoonotic toxocariasis. Epidemiol Rev 1981;3:230–50.
5. Buijs, J, Borsboom G, van Gemund JJ. Toxocara seroprevalence in 5-year old elementary schoolchildren: relation with allergic asthma. Am J Epidemiol 1994;140:839–47.
6. Critchley EM, Vakil SD, Hutchinson, DN. Toxoplasma, Toxocara, and epilepsy. Epilepsia 1982;23:315–23.
7. Stewart JM, Cubillan LD, Cunningham ET. Prevalence, clinical features, and causes of vision loss among patients with ocular toxocariasis. Retina 2005; 25:1005–13.
8. Taylor MR. The epidemiology of ocular toxocariasis. J Helminthol 2001;75: 109–18.
9. Barisani-Asenbauer T, Maca SM, Hauff W, et al. Treatment of ocular toxocariasis with albendazole. J Ocul Pharmacol Ther 2001;17:287:94.

Gnathostomiasis 117

Paron Dekumyoy, Dorn Watthanakulpanich

Key features

- Human gnathostomiasis, is also called Tau-cheed (Thailand), Yangtze River edema and Shanghai's rheumatism (China), Rangoon tumor (Myanmar), Woodbury bug (Australia), Chokofishi (Japan), and nodular migratory eosinophilic panniculitis or traveling cutaneous inflammation (Ecuador)
- *Gnathostoma* species cause subcutaneous migratory swellings, piercing sensations and, less commonly, ocular and central nervous system disease
- Gnathostomiasis is a food-borne parasitic zoonosis. Consumption of intermediate/paratenic hosts, usually raw fish, shrimp, crab, frog, or chicken, is the source of infection
- Treatment is surgical when the worm can be accessed or medical with albendazole and/or ivermectin

INTRODUCTION

Parasites of the genus *Gnathostoma* are nematode infections of cats and other carnivores. Five species that affect humans are reported: *Gnathostoma spinigerum* (the most common; Richard Owen, 1836); *Gnathostoma hispidum* (Fedtschenko, 1872); *Gnathostoma doloresi* (Tubangui, 1925); *Gnathostoma nipponicum* (Yamaguti, 1941); and *Gnathostoma binucleatum* (Almeyda-Artigas, 1991). Gnathostomiases have similar manifestations, including subcutaneous migratory swellings.

EPIDEMIOLOGY

Gnathostomiases, especially *G. spinigerum*, have become more common. Since 1889, patients infected with *G. spinigerum* have been reported in Thailand (Fig. 117.1) and *G. binucleatum* is currently in Mexico and other neighboring Latin American countries. *Gnathostoma hispidum*, *G. doleresi*, and *G. nipponicum* have been reported in Japan and China [1]. A few gnathostomiasis cases have been reported from non-endemic countries, for example *G. spinigerum* infection in Zambia, South Africa and Brazil, and *G. hispidum* infection in Spain. It is likely that gnathostomiasis is under-reported in many Asian countries.

Definitive hosts for gnathostomiasis are dogs, cats, pigs, wild pigs, weasels, and other mammals [1, 2]. Several species of amphibians, reptiles, avians, and mammals act as intermediate hosts of both *G. spinigerum* and *G. binucleatum*. In Thailand, 48 species of vertebrates (including 20 species of freshwater fish) can serve as second intermediate and/or paratenic hosts. In Mexico, 25 species of fish and seven species of fish-eating birds are recorded as intermediate hosts.

Human gnathostomiases are found more frequently in adults than children, and in more females than males, with the exception of Vietnam where males are more frequently infected [3, 4]. Occupation, dietary habits and social aspects affect the probability of infection. Patients as young as 3 days old have been reported, suggesting prenatal or perinatal transmission [5, 6].

NATURAL HISTORY, PATHOGENESIS, AND PATHOLOGY

Adult nematodes coil in the stomach muscles of the definitive host. Eggs are passed in feces and, when exposed to water, release larvae. These larvae are ingested by freshwater copepods that are ingested, in turn, by an intermediate host, where larvae invade and lodge in muscle. Humans acquire the parasite by consuming the second- or third-stage larvae from infected intermediate hosts or paratenic hosts. In humans, larvae cannot develop into adult worms and will penetrate the stomach wall and migrate randomly within the human host. These larvae measure 2.5–12.5 mm. The incubation period, or the time between ingestion of a worm and the first appearance of cutaneous manifestations, is usually from 3 to 4 weeks, although it can be as long as several years. Untreated, the worm can live in humans for several years; therefore, a long, asymptomatic interval can be followed by a sudden recurrence of symptoms [7].

Infection results in nonspecific symptoms, such as fever, mild malaise, urticaria, and epigastric pain, followed by external (cutaneous) or internal (visceral) larva migrans. The migrating worm produces several toxins (acetylcholine, hyaluronidase, proteolytic enzyme, and hemolytic substance). The pathologic picture of swelling and track-like necrosis demonstrates an intense cellular infiltration with neutrophils, mononuclear cells, plasma cells, and large numbers of eosinophils. Allergic changes are seen with hyper-eosinophilia. The parasite can migrate to the ocular system and central nervous system (CNS) causing localized inflammation and destruction.

CLINICAL FEATURES

The most common manifestation is intermittent, migratory swelling in the skin and subcutaneous tissues. If the swelling is subcutaneous, there are usually signs of inflammation, redness, and pain. The swelling is hard and non-pitting and lasts for 1–4 weeks before it disappears. Re-appearance of swelling can occur after an asymptomatic interval of 1 week to several months in a new location not far from the previous one (Figs 117.2 and 117.3).

Patients can initially suffer from epigastric pain, nausea, or vomiting which are likely caused by penetration of the gastric wall by the ingested larvae. Other features can be fever, liver tenderness, and pleuro-pulmonary involvement. Frequent coughing, hemoptysis, chest pain, dyspnea, pneumothorax, hematuria with or without renal pain, and granuloma formation in the peritoneal cavity can occur. With CNS invasion, eosinophilic meningitis or meningoencephalitis, subarachnoid, intracerebral or intraventricular hemorrhage, radiculopathy, paralysis, seizures, altered conciousness, coma and death can

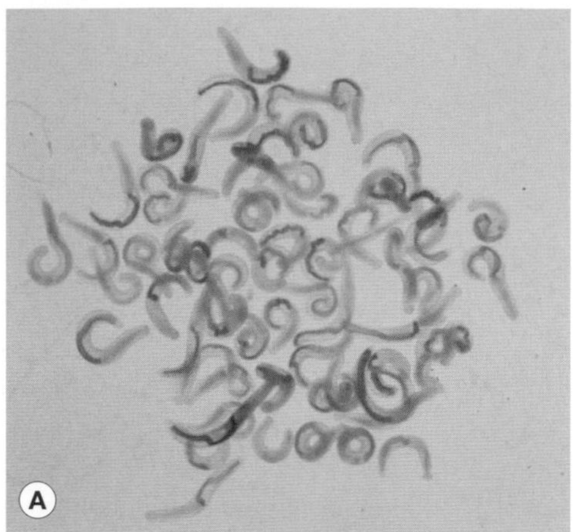

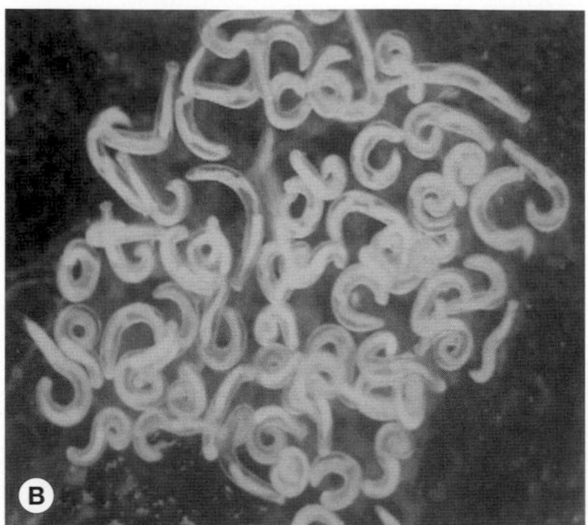

FIGURE 117.1 *Gnathostoma spinigerum* advanced third-stage larvae from livers of freshwater eels. A specific characteristic is the head-bulb and body; its body length is in a range of 2.5–6 mm.

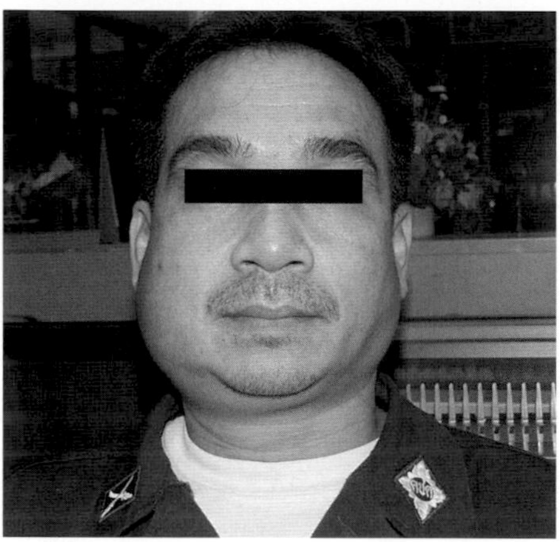

FIGURE 117.2 Cutaneous infection with *Gnathostoma spinigerum* with migrating intermittent edema at the right mandibular area.

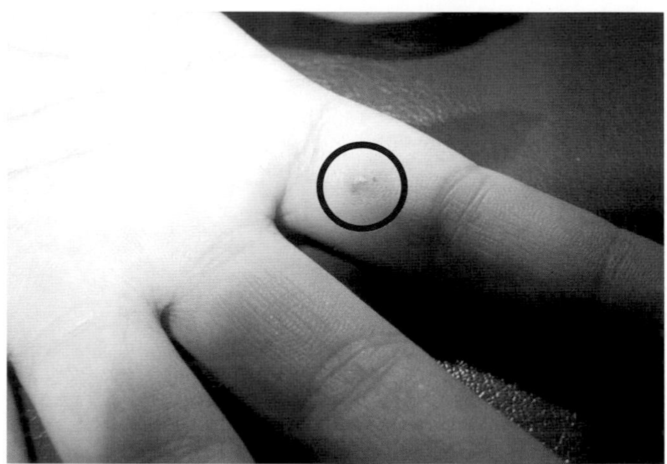

FIGURE 117.3 Cutaneous infection with *Gnathostoma spinigerum* with involvement of the left index finger.

occur [1, 6]. With ocular invasion, probably by migration of the worm along the optic nerves, there can be decreased visual acuity and blindness.

With *G. binucleatum*, clinical features are similar to *G. spinigerum* with the additional invasion of peripheral extremities, face, head, and possibly cardiac tissue [8].

Physical examination findings depend on the area of the body into which the worms migrate and vary between *Gnathostoma* species. In cases of *G. spinigerum* and *G. binucleatum* infection, the disease can persist in subcutaneous tissue with relapses over several years, while in cases of *G. hispidum*, *G. nipponicum*, and *G. doloresi* infection, surface skin lesions spontaneously disappear within 3 months even without treatment. A peripheral blood leukocytosis with hyper-eosinophilia occurs in acute cases. The degree of eosinophilia (sometimes as high as 90%) does not correlate with clinical severity. In cerebral gnathostomiasis, the cerebrospinal fluid (CSF) is usually bloody or xanthochromic and has a pleocytosis [9].

PATIENT EVALUATION, DIAGNOSIS, AND DIFFERENTIAL DIAGNOSIS

The initial evaluation should be focused on characteristic clinical findings, travel or residence in a gnathostomiasis endemic area, and dietary history suggesting ingestion of intermediate or paratenic hosts. An increased eosinophil count in peripheral blood or CSF can be present; however, the eosinophil count may also not be elevated, which may lead to a delay in diagnosis. In one clinical series, 47% had eosinophilia [7].

The differential diagnosis for cerebral, visceral and cutaneous gnathostomiases includes intracerebral tuberculosis, syphilis, lymphoma, eosinophilic meningitis, or meningoencephalitis, intracranial haemorrhage, localized angioedema, and helminth infections of loiasis, spirurina larvae, and baylisascariasis (roundworms of raccoons). Computerized tomography (CT), magnetic resonance imaging (MRI), and ultrasound can assist in the detection of gnathostomiasis, but serologic tests should accompany imaging studies. Antibody detection using serum and/or CSF can be used to identify a specific IgG to a 24-kDa antigen from *G. spinigerum* larvae. This test is highly sensitive and specific [10]. *Gnathostoma spinigerum* cDNA recombinant antigens have also been developed for antibody detection – two matrix metalloproteinase-like proteins. The sensitivity and specificity of these tests have yet to be established.

TREATMENT

Definitive therapy is surgical removal of the worms. Extraction of superficial cutaneous *Gnathostoma* can be performed by needles or scratching [1], and surgical extraction for intravitreal gnathostomiasis. Albendazole (400 mg twice a day for 21–28 days) demonstrated a

90–94% cure rate for cutaneous gnathostomiasis [11, 12]. In albendazole- and/or ivermectin-treated patients, gnathostomes may be stimulated to move to the skin surface [13, 14]. Patients on a month of albendazole can experience nausea, headache, and vomiting, and should be monitored for liver toxicity. Ivermectin at 0.2 mg/kg single dose has been shown to be effective in killing third-stage larvae of *G. spinigerum*, with cure rates of 76%, while repeated ivermectin used in relapsed cases demonstrates cure rates of nearly 100% [15]. In one study, ivermectin at 0.2 mg/kg body weight for 2 consecutive days demonstrated a cure rate of 100% with mild side effects [16]. A combination of supportive, symptomatic and anti-inflammatory treatments can also be used. In CNS gnathostomiasis, corticosteroids may have an additional role in reducing CNS inflammation and intensive neurologic care is important in critical cases; however, recurrence of symptoms is possible. Therefore, post-treatment, long-term follow-up of antibody levels and eosinophilia may be helpful to observe decreases over time. Following antibody levels for at least 1 year is recommended.

REFERENCES

1. Waikagul J, Diaz Camacho SP. Gnathostomiasis. In: Murrell KD, Fried B, eds. Food-Borne Parasitic Zoonoses. New York: Springer; 2007:235–261.
2. Rojekittikhun W, Chaiyasith T, Nuamtanong S, Komalamisra C. *Gnathostoma* infection in fish caught for local consumption in Nakhon Nayok province, Thailand, I. Prevalence and fish species. Southeast Asian J Trop Med Public Health 2004;35:523–30.
3. Xuan LT, Hoa PTL, Dekumyoy P, et al. *Gnathostoma* infection in South Vietnam. Southeast Asian J Trop Med Public Health 2004;35(suppl. 1): 97–9.
4. Bussaratid V, Dekumyoy P, Desakorn V et al. Predictive factors for *Gnathostoma* seropositivity in patients visiting gnathostomiasis clinic at hospital for tropical diseases, Thailand in 2000-2005. Southeast Asian J Trop Med Pub Health 2010;41:1316–21.
5. Miyazaki I. *Gnathostoma* and gnathostomiasis in Japan. Prog Med Parasitol Japan 1966;3:531.
6. Daengsvang S. *Gnathostoma spinigerum* and human gnathostomiasis : a brief review. The 25th Anniversary of the Faculty of Tropical Medicine, Bangkok, Thailand 1986;124–47.
7. Moore DA, McCroddan J, Dekumyoy P, Chiodini PL. Gnathostomiasis: an emerging imported disease. Emerg Infect Dis 2003;9:647–50.
8. Lazo RF. *Gnathostoma* and Gnathostomiasis in Ecuador. Southeast Asian J Trop Med Public Health 2004;35(suppl.1):92–96.
9. Punyagupta S, Bunnag T, Juttijudata P. Eosinophilic meningitis in Thailand: clinical and epidemiological characteristics of 162 patients with myeloencephalitis probably caused by *Gnathostoma spinigerum*. J Neurol Sci 1990; 96:241–56.
10. Tapchaisri P, Nopparatana C, Chaicumpa W, Setasuban P. Specific antigen of *Gnathostoma spinigerum* for immunodiagnosis of human gnathostomiasis. Int J Parasitol 1991;21:315–19.
11. Kraivichian P, Kulkumthorn M, Yingyoud P, et al. Albendazole for the treatment of human gnathostomiasis. Tran R Soc Trop Med Hyg 1992;86: 418–21.
12. Suntharasamai P, Riganti M, Chittamas S, Desakorn V. Albendazole stimulates outward migration of *Gnathostoma spinigerum* to the dermis in man. Southeast Asian J Trop Med Health 1992; 23:716–22.
13. Boongird P, Phnapradit P, Siridej N, et al. Neurological manifestation of gnathostomiasis. J Neurol Sci 1977 31:279–91.
14. Kraivichian K, Nuchprayoon S, Siriyasatien P, et al. Resolution of eosinophilia after treatment of cutaneous gnathostomiasis. J Med Assoc Thai 2005;88(suppl. S4):163–66.
15. Kraivichian K, Nuchprayoon S, Sitichalernchai P, et al. Treatment of cutaneous gnathostomiasis with ivermectin. Am J Trop Med Hyg 2004;71:623–28.
16. Nontasut P, Claesson BA, Dekumyoy P, et al. Double-dose ivermectin vs albendazole for the treatment of gnathostomiasis. Southeast Asian J Trop Med Public Health 2005;36:650–52.

118 Eosinophilic Meningitis (*Angiostrongylus cantonensis*, *Parastrongylus cantonensis*)

Yupaporn Wattanagoon, John H Cross[†]

Key features

- *Angiostrongylus* is the most common parasitic cause of eosinophilic meningitis
- The most common mode of transmission is raw snail consumption. Many patients have been infected by eating uncooked paratenic hosts, such as freshwater prawns, crabs, frogs and monitor lizards. Contaminated vegetables and fruits may also transmit the infection
- Ocular involvement occurs in about 1% of patients
- Pathologic changes include infiltration of lymphocytes, eosinophils and plasma cells in meninges. Granuloma formation may be found surrounding dead parasites
- Treatment is often symptomatic. Corticosteroids can improve symptoms. Albendazole and mebendazole with or without corticosteroids have limited clinical experience

INTRODUCTION

The first discovery of the worm, *Angiostrongylus cantonensis* in the pulmonary arteries and hearts of domestic rats in Canton, China was reported by Chen in 1935. However, the first case of human infection was documented in 1945 in Taiwan. Since then, there have been reports of outbreaks or sporadic infection of this parasite in many parts of the world. It is estimated that 150 million people are at risk.

EPIDEMIOLOGY

Nearly 3000 cases of *Angiostrongylus cantonensis* have been reported worldwide since 1945 [1]. However, these figures only include reports from publications in international journals; the incidence of angiostrogyliasis meningitis is likely under-reported. Endemic areas are in Asia, the Pacific Islands and Australia. Outbreaks of sporadic cases of eosinophilic meningitis have been reported in travelers returning from endemic areas. In Thailand, where most cases have been reported, the estimated incidence has ranged from 0.19–2.25 per 100,000 population during the years 1996–2000. The majority of the cases are young adults, but children are also affected. In most reports, males are affected more frequently than females.

NATURAL HISTORY, PATHOGENESIS AND PATHOLOGY

Humans become infected after ingestion of third-stage larvae of *A. cantonensis* when eating undercooked intermediate hosts, such as snails or slugs. Many paratenic hosts have been implicated as sources of infection, including prawns, crabs, frogs and monitor lizards. Unclean vegetables, fruits and drinking water are occasionally sources of infection. After ingestion, larvae are released in the intestine and invade the intestinal wall entering into the circulation, passing through liver, heart, lungs and, finally, moving to the brain. In humans, the larvae will molt into fourth-stage larvae but will not develop further and usually die in the brain after 1–2 months. Occasionally, larvae may invade the orbits causing ocular disease. Pathologic changes involve an inflammatory response to the presence or movement of larvae in the brain. Lymphocytes, plasma cells and eosinophils infiltrate the meninges or around the cerebral vessels, forming a granuloma around the dead parasites. Migration of worms makes parasitic tracks with hemorrhage and microcavities. Hemosiderin, eosinophils, glial scars and Charcot-Leyden crystals can be seen in the track. Living worms have been detected in pulmonary vessels of patients from Taiwan, Australia, Jamaica and Thailand during necropsy [2–5].

CLINICAL FEATURES

Clinical manifestations are associated with worm migration and inflammatory response to the worm. Disease severity and incubation period depend on the number of larva ingested. The disease is generally benign and self-limiting with some patients only experiencing a mild headache that spontaneously subsides, but, occasionally, there is severe illness with long-lasting neurologic sequelae. The incubation period ranges from one day to many weeks. Some patients develop gastrointestinal symptoms when the ingested larvae are released and invade the intestinal wall causing abdominal discomfort, nausea and vomiting. For patients with neurologic involvement, most patients develop signs and symptoms of meningitis, but occasionally develop encephalitis. The most common signs and symptoms of patients with eosinophilic meningitis or meningoencephalitis are headache, nausea, vomiting, fever, blurred vision, diplopia, paraesthesia, urinary retention, altered consciousness or coma, and focal neurologic deficit [6, 7] (Fig. 118.1). Headache is usually gradual. Fever is low grade; however, high grade fever is more common in children. Neck stiffness, positive Brudzinsky or Kernig's sign, papilloedema, cranial nerve palsy and sensory impairment may be detected. Patients usually recover spontaneously within a few weeks. Drug treatment can shorten the duration of headache and reduce the number of lumbar punctures required. Case mortality rate is very low; death is more common in children.

About 1% of angiostrongyliasis patients have ocular involvement [8]. Many of these cases have been reported from Thailand, Indonesia, Japan, Taiwan, India, Sri Lanka and Australia [8–15]. Ocular angiostrongyliasis is usually found in association with meningitis. The parasite can be seen in the anterior or posterior chamber without causing inflammation. In such cases, patients usually complain of seeing something moving in the eye without visual loss. Cases in which the larval migration causes an inflammatory or granulomatous reaction in the retina, vitreous or anterior or posterior chamber may present with loss of vision, eye pain and redness (Figs 118.2 and 118.3). Signs of iritis, vitreous haziness, ophthalmitis or retinal detachment can be detected. Patients who present with visual impairment may not regain normal visual acuity after recovery.

[†]Deceased

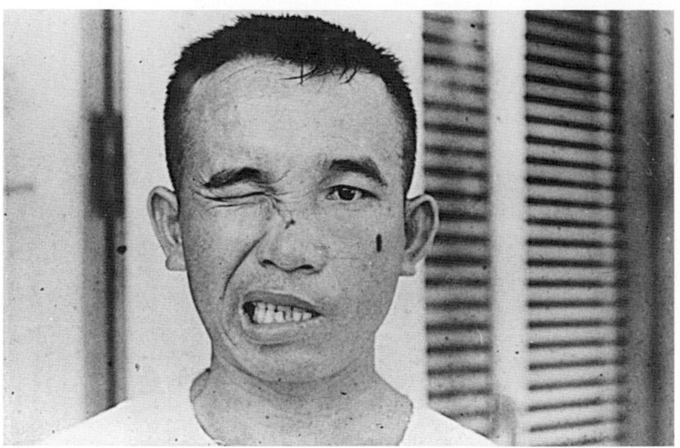

FIGURE 118.1 Unilateral facial paralysis of the lower motor neuron type in a patient with *Angiostrongylus* meningitis. *(Courtesy of Professor Thanongsak Bunnag, Thailand).*

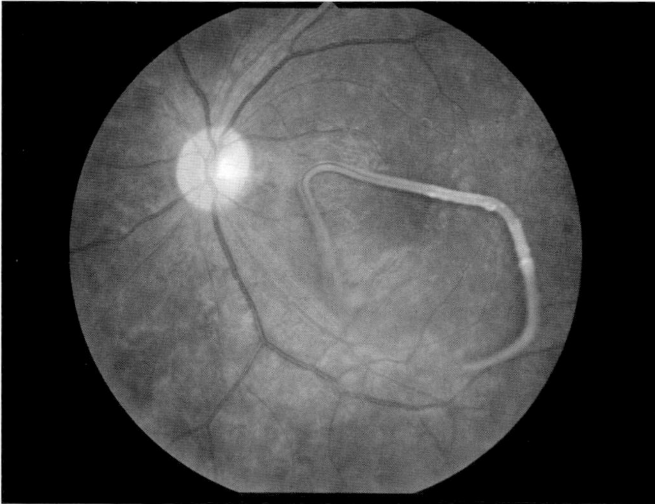

FIGURE 118.2 Ocular angiostrongyliasis. An intravitreal *Angiostrongylus* nematode killed with laser photocoagulation before surgical removal. *(Courtesy of Dr Suthasinee Sinawat, Department of Ophthalmology, Khon Kaen University, Khon Kaen, Thailand).*

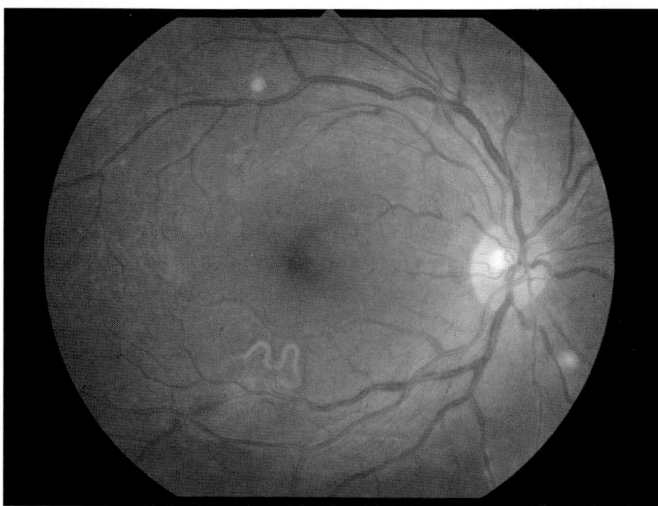

FIGURE 118.3 Ocular angiostrongyliasis. A subretinal *Angiostrongylus* nematode in the inferotemporal quadrant. *(Courtesy of Dr Suthasinee Sinawat, Department of Ophthalmology, Khon Kaen University, Khon Kaen, Thailand).*

PATIENT EVALUATION, DIAGNOSIS AND DIFFERENTIAL DIAGNOSIS

In the appropriate epidemiologic setting, patients who present with symptoms and signs of meningitis should be evaluated for *Angiostrongylus*. Severe cases present with meningoencephalitis or have cranial nerve involvement; presentation in children tends to be more severe than in adults. Careful examination of the eyes should be done. Laboratory criteria for diagnosis of eosinophilic meningitis include cerebrospinal fluid (CSF) eosinophils of more than 10 cells/ml or 10% of CSF white blood cells (WBC). Angiostrongyliasis patients usually have a high CSF pressure above 200 mmH_2O, and the CSF usually contains between 500 and 2000 leukocytes/mm^3 with more than 20% eosinophils, normal glucose and slightly raised protein. Complete blood examination reveals eosinophilia in the majority of cases.

Patients with focal neurodeficit or encephalitis should receive a computed tomography (CT) or magnetic resonance imaging (MRI) scan to exclude other conditions. MRI findings of *Angiostrongylus* meningitis can be normal or show meningeal enhancement without focal lesion or abnormal micronodular enhanced lesions [16]. Small parasitic tracks may be detected by MRI. Brain edema may be seen in severe cases.

The definitive diagnosis of *Angiostrongylus* meningitis is based on detection of the parasite in the CSF sample or in the eye. When no parasite is obtained, serologic diagnosis can be performed by detection of *Angiostrongylus* antibodies or antigen in serum or CSF by ELISA or immunoblot technique.

DIFFERENTIAL DIAGNOSIS

Eosinophilic meningitis can be caused by other parasitic infections, such as gnathostomiasis, paragonimiasis, cysticercosis, schistosomiasis, toxocariasis, baylisascariasis or trichinellosis (Fig. 118.4). In Thailand, gnathostomiasis is an important differential and should be suspected if the patient has a previous history of migratory swellings and they have hemorrhagic or xanthochromic spinal fluid and eosinophilic pleocytosis. Serologic diagnosis can be performed to differentiate these two infections.

TREATMENT

Most patients spontaneously recover within a few weeks after receiving supportive treatment to alleviate headache. Acetaminophen and repeated lumbar punctures may be clinically indicated.

There have been a few clinical trials of treatment; most of those have included eosinophilic meningitis, but not always specifically documented *Angiostrongylus* infection (Box 118-1). Oral prednisolone (60 mg/day divided into three doses) for two weeks significantly

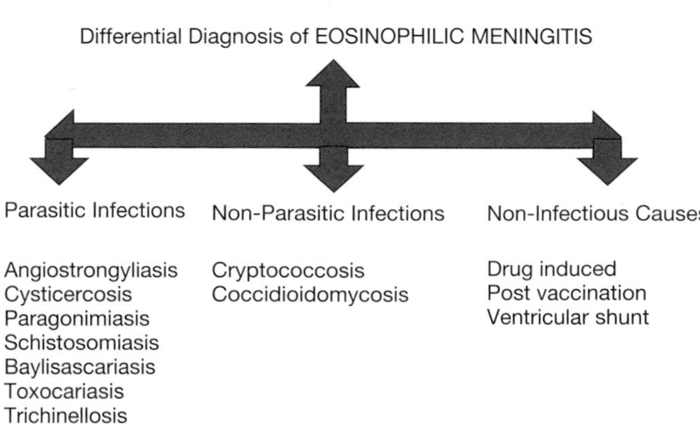

FIGURE 118.4 Differential diagnosis of eosinophilic meningitis.

shortened the duration of headache and the number of repeated lumbar punctures when compared with placebo in patients with eosinophilic meningitis presumably from angiostrongyliasis [17]. In 26 eosinophilic meningitis patients using a combination of corticosteriod (prednisolone 60 mg/day divided into three doses) and albendazole (15 mg/kg/day divided into two doses) for two weeks, treated patients had a similar duration of headache compared with patients receiving prednisolone only [18]. Forty-one patients treated with a combination of prednisolone and mebendazole (10 mg/kg/day) for two weeks had a similar duration of headache compared with the previous study with prednisolone treatment [19]. Treatment of eosinophilic meningitis with prednisolone and albendazole was no different in relieving headache than treatment with prednisolone alone [20]. A small trial comparing the efficacy of albendazole (15 mg/kg/day divided into two doses) and placebo demonstrated a decreased duration of headache in the albendazole treated group [21] (Box 118.1).

BOX 118.1 Summary of Clinical Trials for Eosinophilic Meningitis Due to Angiostrongyliasis

Drug trial	Study design	No. of patients	Results
Prednisolone vs. placebo [17]	RCT	110	Significantly shortened duration of headache, decreased number of lumbar punctures in prednisolone group
Prednisolone + albendazole [18]	Pilot prospective	41	Duration of headache comparable with prednisolone-alone arm of the RCT
Prednisolone + mebendazole [19]	Pilot prospective	26	Duration of headache comparable with prednisolone-alone arm of the RCT
Albendazole vs. placebo [21]	RCT	66	Trend to shorter duration of headache in albendazole group
Prednisolone + albendazole vs. prednisolone alone [20]	RCT	104	No difference in headache resolution

RCT, randomized controlled trial.

REFERENCES

1. Wang QP, Lai DH, Zhu XQ, et al. Human angiostrongyliasis. Lancet Infect Dis 2008;8:621–30.
2. Hung TP, Chen ER. Angiostrongyliasis (*Angiostrongylus cantonensis*). In: Vinken P, Bruyn G, Klawans H, eds. Handbook of Clinical Neurology. New York: Elsevier; 1988;8:545–62.
3. Cooke-Yarborough C, Kornberg A, Hogg G, et al. A fatal case of angiostrongyliasis in an 11-month-old infant. Med J Aust 1999;170:541–3.
4. Lindo JF, Escoffery CT, Reid B, et al. Fatal autochthonous eosinophilic meningitis in a Jamaican child caused by *Angiostrongylus cantonensis*. Am J Trop Med Hyg 2004;70:425–8.
5. Sonakul D. Pathological findings in four cases of human angiostrongyliasis. Southeast Asian J of Trop Med Public Health 1978;9:220–7.
6. Punyagupta S, Juttisudata P, Bunnag T. Eosinophilic meningitis in Thailand. Clinical studies of 484 typical cases probably caused by *Angiostrongylus cantonensis*. Am J Trop Med Hyg 1975;24:921–31.
7. Hwang KP, Chen ER. Clinical studies on *Angiostrongyliasis cantonensis* among children in Taiwan. Southeast Asian J Trop Med Public Health 1991; 22(Suppl):194–9.
8. Sawanyawisuth K, Kitthaweesin K, Limpawattana P, et al. Intraocular angiostrongyliasis: clinical findings, treatments and outcomes. Trans Roy Soc Trop Med Hyg 2007;101:497–501.
9. Kanchanaranya C, Punyagupta S. Case of ocular angiostrongyliasis associated with eosinophilic meningitis. Am J Ophthalmol 1971;71:931–4.
10. Sunardi W, Lokollo DM, Margono SS. Ocular angiostrongyliasis in Semarang Central Java. Am J Trop Med Hyg 1977;26:72–4.
11. Nelson RG, Warren RC, Scotti A, et al. Ocular Angiostrongyliasis in Japan: A Case Report. Am J Trop Med Hyg 1988;38:130–2.
12. Toma H, Matsumura S, Oshiro C, et al. Ocular angiostrongyliasis without meningitis symptoms in Okinawa, Japan. J Parasitol 2002;88:211–13.
13. Maholtra S, Mehta DK, Arora R, et al. Ocular angiostrongyliasis in a child—first case report from India. J Trop Pediatr 2006;52:223–5.
14. Ihalamulla RL, Fernando SD, Weerasena KH, et al. A further case of Parastrongyliasis (=Angiostrongyliasis) from the eye of a patient in Sri Lanka. Ceylon Med Sci 2007;50:15–17.
15. Sinawat S, Sanguansak T, Angkawinijwong T, et al. Ocular angiostrongyliasis: clinical study of three cases. Eye 2008;22:1446–8.
16. Jin E, Ma D, Liang Y, et al. MRI findings of eosinophilic meningoencephalitis due to *Angiostrongylus cantonenesis*. Clin Radiol 2005;60:242–50.
17. Chotmongkol V, Sawanyawisuth K, Thavornpithak Y. Corticosteroid treatment of eosinophilic meningitis. Clin Infect Dis 2000;31:660–2.
18. Chotmongkol V, Wongjitrat C, Sawadpanit K, Sawanyawisuth K. Treatment of eosinophilic meningitis with combination of albendazole and corticosteroid. Southeast Asian J of Trop Med Public Health 2004;35:172–4.
19. Chotmongkol V, Sawadpanit K, Sawanyawisuth K, et al. Treatment of eosinophilic meningitis with combination of predinisolone and mebendazole. Am J Trop Med Hyg 2006; 74:1122–4.
20. Chotmongkol V, Kittimongkolma S, Niwattayakul K, et al. Comparison of prednisolone plus albendazole with prednisolone alone for treatment of patients with eosinophilic meningitis. Am J Trop Med Hyg 2009;81:443–5.
21. Jitpimolmard S, Sawanyawisuth K, Morakote N, et al. Albendazole therapy for eosinophilic meningitis caused by *Angiostrongylus cantonensis*. Parasitol Res 2007;100:1193–6.

Abdominal Angiostrongyliasis 119

Pedro Morera

Key features

- Characterized by granulomatous inflammation with eosinophilic infiltration of the intestinal wall
- The lifecycle involves rodents (definitive hosts) and mollusks (intermediate hosts)
- Human infection mostly occurs in Central and South America, from southern Mexico to Argentina
- Children are more frequently infected and the male-to-female ratio for infection is 2:1
- Prevention involves avoiding ingesting slugs and raw food and water that may be contaminated with slugs or slug secretions
- Synonyms include: *Angiostrongylus costaricensis, Morerastrongylus costaricensis* [1], and eosinophilic granuloma
- There is no specific anti-parasitic therapy; surgical treatment may be necessary

INTRODUCTION

Abdominal angiostrongylosis, caused by *Angiostrongylus costaricensis* is characterized by a granulomatous inflammatory reaction with heavy eosinophilic infiltration of the intestinal wall, especially in the ileocecal region. The disease has been observed in Costa Rica since 1952; since 1971, it has been reported from most countries of the Americas, especially Central and South America. In addition, cotton rats naturally infected with the parasite have been found in the USA.

EPIDEMIOLOGY

The disease has been reported from the USA to Argentina, including some Caribbean islands. One human case has been reported from Africa. In Costa Rica, its distribution is universal, from sea level to an altitude of 2000 meters. With the first recognition of *A. costaricensis* until the mid-1980s, 20–60 cases were reported annually. Secondary to better identification of the disease by medical personnel, the annual incidence increased to 600 cases per year (20 cases per 100,000 inhabitants). Improvements in sanitation and mollusk control since 2000 have decreased the number of cases to about 185 cases/year over the last 10 years.

NATURAL HISTORY, PATHOGENESIS, AND PATHOLOGY

Angiostrongylus costaricensis is a filariform nematode normally living within the mesenteric arteries of the definitive host—a rodent. The female is 33 mm long with vulva and anus located near the caudal end; the male is 20 mm long with a copulatory bursa and two spicules approximately 300 μm in length [2]. Eggs are released within the mesenteric arteries and carried by the blood into the intestinal wall, where they embryonate (Fig. 119.1). First-stage larvae hatch and migrate through the intestinal wall. They are excreted in the rat's feces and reach the soil, where they are eaten by the intermediate host—usually slugs. Two molts take place in the mollusk and, after 18 days, the infective third-stage larva matures. The definitive host, usually the cotton rat, becomes infected by eating the mollusk. The prepatent period lasts 24 days [3].

In Costa Rica, the cotton rat, *Sigmodon hispidus*, is the most important host, but at least 12 different species of rat and one coati have been found to be naturally infected. Marmosets and two rodents have been found infected with *A. costaricensis* in eastern Peru and southern Brazil, respectively [4].

Although several mollusks are naturally infected with *A. costaricensis*, veronicellid slugs are considered the main intermediate hosts. Humans become infected when they ingest slugs or food items contaminated with small mollusks or their secretions, for example small slugs hidden in salad greens could be finely chopped and inadvertently eaten raw. Several cases have followed ingestion of mollusks by infants. Most human infections are probably caused by ingestion of the infective larvae shed in the mollusk's secretions (Fig. 119.1). Slugs have been found in ripe fruits that have fallen to the ground. Characteristic mucous trails left by the mollusks can be observed throughout endemic areas. The propensity for small children to put things in their mouths could explain why they have the highest infection rates.

At least two species of veronicellid slugs in Costa Rica (*Saranisula plebeia* and *Diplosolenodes occidentalis*) and several species in Brazil (*Phyllocaulis variegatus* and *Sarasinula linguaeformis*, among other species) are naturally infected with *A. costaricensis*. Fifty percent of 6025 slugs from 20 Costa Rican localities, from sea level to an altitude of 2000 meters, were found to be infected and more than 16,000 infected larvae were counted in a single specimen.

In most cases, lesions caused by *A. costaricensis* are located in the ileocecal region. They also occur in the hepatic flexure and descending colon, regional lymph nodes, liver, and testicles. Two major pathogenic mechanisms are present: (i) the adult worms living within the mesenteric arteries (Fig. 119.2) damage the endothelium, inducing thrombosis and, consequently, necrosis of the tissues perfused by the vessels; and (ii) eggs, embryos, and larvae, as well as excretion-secretion products, cause inflammatory reactions. These features, as well as the patient's susceptibility and the number and localization of parasites, determine the pathophysiology of the infection.

INTESTINAL LESIONS

Gross pathology shows a hardened and thickened intestinal wall with yellowish foci in the serosal surface of the intestine. The intestinal lumen is reduced, sometimes causing partial or complete obstruction. Necrotic areas can perforate. In many cases, cecal lesions are detected during an appendectomy. Histopathology demonstrates

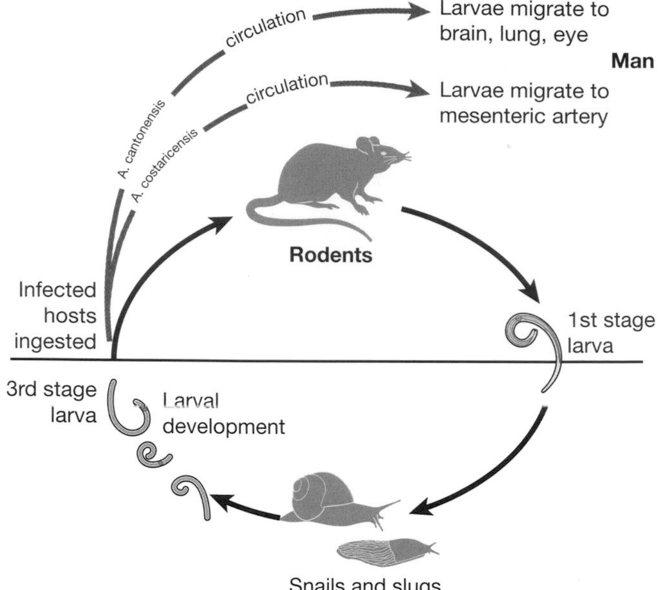

FIGURE 119.1 Life cycle of *Angiostrongylus cantonensis* and *A. costaricensis*.

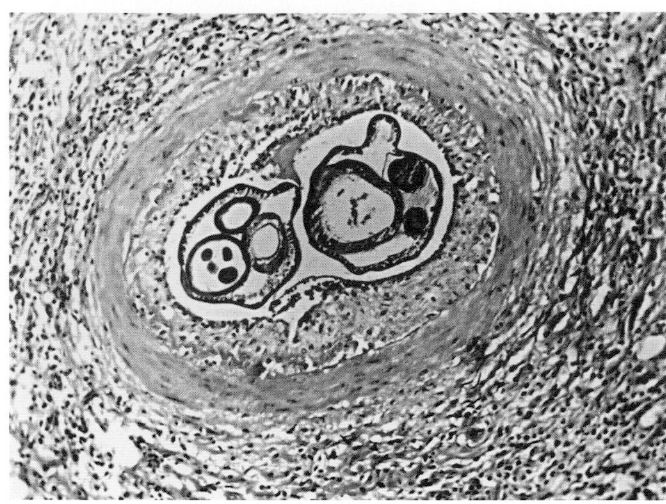

FIGURE 119.2 Adults of *Angiostrongylus costaricensis* within a mesenteric artery. The intima is swollen and the endothelium is damaged.

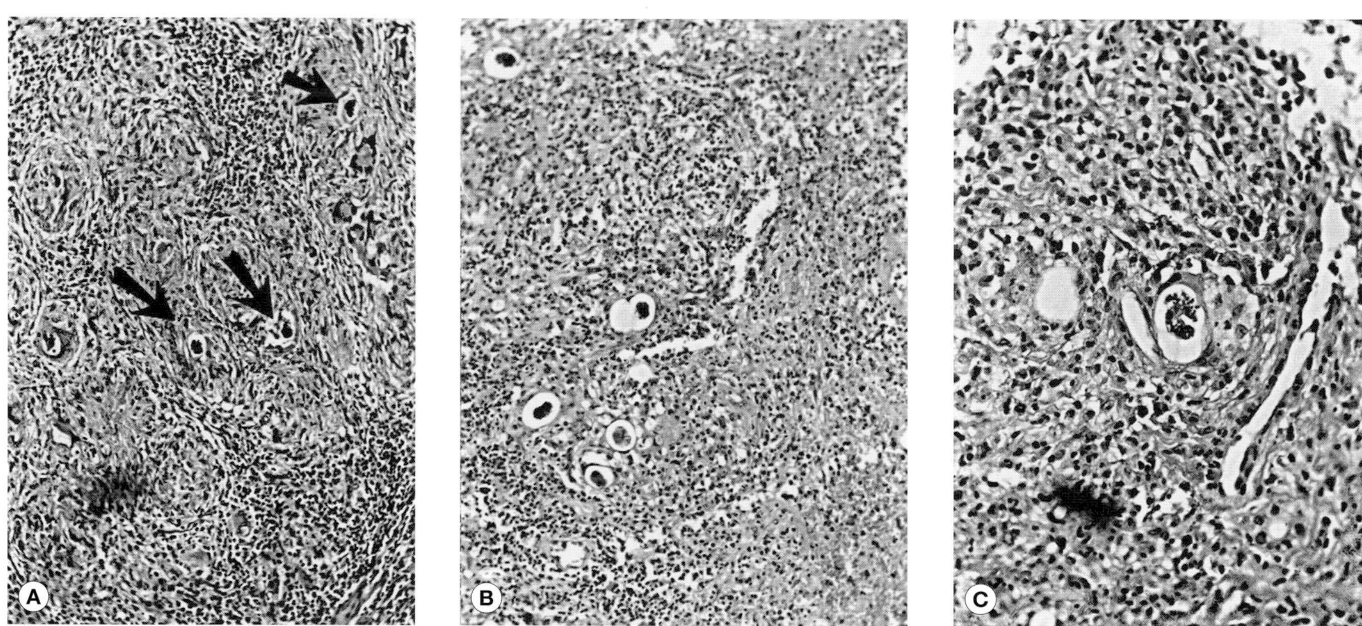

FIGURE 119.3 *Angiostrongylus costaricensis* ova in tissues. **(A)** Section of the intestine showing several granulomas and giant cells. Eggs (arrows) are scattered in the tissue. **(B)** Eggs in the cecal wall surrounded by inflammatory cells (eosinophils). **(C)** Embryonated eggs in the liver.

granulomatous inflammatory reactions (Fig. 119.3A) with heavy eosinophilic infiltration, especially in the intestinal mucosa and submucosa; the serosa and muscular layers are often involved to a lesser degree. Eggs (Fig. 119.3B), embryos, and larvae are in small cavities lined by endothelium. Unfertilized eggs usually degenerate and are difficult to recognize. These structures, as well as the excretion-secretion antigens, are easily identified by immunochemical techniques. Large areas of necrosis are caused by arterial thrombosis.

EXTRAINTESTINAL LESIONS

Eggs and embryos are present in the mesenteric lymph nodes, which show reticuloendothelial hyperplasia and eosinophilic infiltration. Hepatic lesions caused by *A. costaricensis* are similar to those caused by *Toxocara canis* (Chapter 116). However the finding of eggs (Fig. 119.3C), larvae and even adult worms in the hepatic parenchyma establishes the diagnosis. In excised testicles, worms have been observed obstructing the arteries of the spermatic cord and there can be extensive parenchymal hemorrhagic necrosis.

CLINICAL FEATURES

Abdominal angiostrongylasis predominantly affects children. Among 116 patients studied in a pediatric hospital, 50% were school age, 40% were preschool age and 10% were infants; two-thirds were male [5]. When worms are located in the ileocecal region, most patients complain of pain in the right iliac fossa and the right flank. Palpation in this area often causes pain. Rectal examination is also painful in about one-half of the patients and most patients present with fever of 38–38.5°C, rarely accompanied by chills. In chronic cases, a mild fever may persist for several weeks. Anorexia, vomiting, and constipation are also present in about half the patients.

An important finding is the palpation of a tumor-like mass in the right lower quadrant that can be confused with a malignancy. Although a few patients have no hematologic abnormalities, leukocytosis and eosinophilia are usually present. White blood cell counts usually range between 15,000 and 50,000/mm^3 and eosinophilia from 20–50%. The leukocytosis has been as high as 169,000/mm^3, with a 91% eosinophilia.

EXTRAINTESTINAL FINDINGS

Sometimes the patient complaints of pain in the right upper quadrant. In these cases, the liver is almost always enlarged and tender to palpation. At laparoscopy, small yellowish spots (granulomas) are seen on the surface of the liver. Most patients have hepatic involvement along with intestinal angiostrongyliasis. When the testicle is involved, the patient experiences acute pain, accompanied by redness and then purple discoloration. Eosinophilia and leukocytosis are also conspicuous. All patients with testicular necrosis have been misdiagnosed as having testicular torsion—the correct diagnosis being made only following surgery.

PATIENT EVALUATION, DIAGNOSIS, AND DIFFERENTIAL DIAGNOSIS

The clinical diagnosis is based on characteristic features. The symptoms and findings can be confused with those of appendicitis—the appendix is frequently involved, with the diagnosis made at surgery. Radiologic or other imaging can demonstrate suggestive findings usually localized in the terminal ileum, cecum, appendix, and ascending colon. Studies using contrast medium show incomplete filling and irritability of the involved areas. The lumen is reduced by the thickening of the intestinal wall and often resembles colon carcinoma (Fig. 119.4). Laboratory diagnosis can involve both ELISA and PCR [6]. A latex agglutination test has high sensitivity and specificity and can be performed in small laboratories. Eggs and larvae do not appear in the stools.

TREATMENT

Surgery is sometimes required for abdominal angiostrongyliasis. However, as knowledge of this often self-limiting disease increases, more cases have been followed without surgery. Two drugs—diethycarbamazine and thiabendazole—have been used, but there are no clinical trials demonstrating efficacy [7]. *In vitro* and *in vivo* trials in experimentally infected rats demonstrate that parasites can be excited, rather than killed, by the drugs, causing erratic migrations and worsening of the lesions. Thus, chemotherapy is not recommended until experimental studies demonstrate a more efficacious drug.

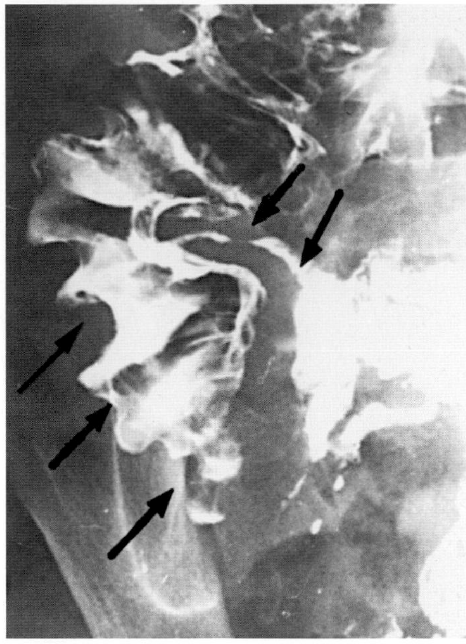

FIGURE 119.4 Radiograph after barium enema showing filling defects in the ileocecal region and ascending colon. The external wall of the colon shows festooned aspect of mucosa.

REFERENCES

1. Chabaud A. Description de *Stefankostrongylus dubosti* n.sp. parasite du Potamogale et essai de clasification des Nematodes Angiostrongylinae. Ann Parasit Hum Comp 1972;47:735–44.
2. Morera, P, Céspedes R. *Angiostrongylus costaricensis* n. sp. (Nematoda: Metastrongylidae) a new lungworm occurring in man in Costa Rica. Rev Biol Trop 1971;18:173–85.
3. Morera P. Life history and redescription of *Angiostrongylus costaricensis* Morera and Céspedes, 1971. Am J Trop Med Hyg 1973;22:613–21.
4. Graeff-Teixetra C, Thomé JW, Pinto SCC, et al. *Phyllocaulis variegatus* an intermediate host of *Angiostrongylus costaricensis* in South Brazil. Mem Inst Osvaldo Cruz (Rio de Janeiro) 1989;84:65–8.
5. Loria-Cortes R, Lobo-Sibaja HF. Clinical abdominal angiostrongyliasis. A study of 116 children with intestinal eosinophilic granuloma caused by *Angiostrongylus costaricensis*. Am J Trop Med Hyg 1980;29:538.
6. Arámburu da Silva AC, Graeff-Teixeira C, Zaha A. Diagnosis of abdominal angiostrongyliasis by PCR from sera of patients. Rev Inst Med Trop (São Paulo) 2003;45:295–7.
7. Morera P, Perez F, Mora F, et al. Visceral larva migrans-like syndrome caused by *Angiostrongylus costaricensis*. Am J Trop Med Hyg 1982;31:67.

120 Cutaneous Larva Migrans

Susan P Montgomery

Key features

- Cutaneous larva migrans (CLM) is a creeping eruption caused by the migration of larval nematodes in the epidermis. Most infections are associated with *Ancylostoma braziliense*, a hookworm of both dogs and cats
- Diagnosis is made clinically; serologic testing is not widely available
- Symptoms and signs are one or more erythematous, serpiginous tracks in the epidermis, pruritus, erythema and mild swelling. Allergic reactions and folliculitis can occur
- CLM is often associated with travel to tropical or near tropical areas where environmental conditions favor larval development. The burden of disease in resident populations of the developing world is undefined
- CLM can be prevented by avoiding contact with potentially contaminated soil or sand. Although infection with zoonotic hookworm larvae is self-limiting, treatment can shorten the duration of clinical disease

INTRODUCTION

Cutaneous larva migrans (CLM) is a dermatologic condition caused by the migration of animal nematode larvae, most commonly the larvae of the dog and cat hookworm *Ancylostoma braziliense*. Other common dog and cat hookworms, *A. caninum*, *A. ceylanicum* and *Uncinaria stenocephala*, have been associated with disease [1].

Creeping eruption, the clinical manifestation of CLM, was first reported to be associated with *A. braziliense* larvae by Kirby-Smith et al. in 1926 [2]. Although other parasites can cause similar symptoms, the specific clinical and epidemiological features of disease caused by migrating *A. braziliense* larvae distinguish the etiology of this disease, often referred to as hookworm-related CLM. CLM is most often reported in returning travelers who have had soil and/or sand exposures in regions where *A. braziliense* is endemic in resident dog and cat populations [1,3]. The global burden of disease remains undefined [4].

EPIDEMIOLOGY

Dog and cat hookworms occur throughout the world, although hookworm species have differing geographic ranges (Table 120-1). *A. braziliense* is found in warmer climates along the Atlantic but not Pacific coasts of the Americas from the southeastern US, throughout the Caribbean, and into South America. From animal studies, *A. braziliense* has also been reported in parts of Africa, Australia, and Southeast Asia. *A. caninum* is found wherever dogs are present in warmer climates but the distribution of *U. stenocephala* is restricted to colder climates [1].

CLM is most frequently reported among travelers to tropical or near tropical parts of the world; traveler infections likely represent only a small proportion of the true global burden of disease. Among travelers, the frequency of reported CLM is associated with reason for travel, e.g. tourist or business; the geographic area visited; and age [3,5]. Infection is associated with increased likelihood of unprotected skin exposure among vacationing tourists and younger age groups. In less developed areas of the world, dogs and cats are often free-ranging and have high rates of infection with hookworm, and soil and sand contamination is widespread [4–6]. In a survey of a rural population in Brazil, the prevalence of CLM during the rainy season was 14.9% among children less than 5 years old and 0.7% among adults aged 20 years and older [7]. The prevalence in resident populations is poorly defined as CLM typically is not considered a public health priority.

Patients usually report skin exposure to soil or sand, and lesions will be located on the body area in contact with soil while sitting or standing, especially the feet, buttocks and thighs. Rarely, infection has been linked to exposure to contaminated clothing or plant material [1,6]. The most common symptom is pruritus; pain has also been reported, as well as stinging sensations at the time of larval penetration through the skin [5,6,8].

NATURAL HISTORY, PATHOGENESIS, AND PATHOLOGY

Animal hookworm eggs are shed in the feces of the animal host and develop into infective filariform larvae in the soil, where they can survive for several weeks under appropriate environmental conditions. When human skin comes in contact with contaminated soil or sand, larvae attempt to penetrate the skin, but the larvae of most species of animal hookworm cannot penetrate beyond the dermis [1]. The larvae of *A. braziliense* will migrate in the epidermis for several weeks before dying, after which lesions resolve spontaneously. *A. caninum* and *A. ceylanicum* larvae can penetrate more deeply and have been associated with other clinical syndromes, including eosinophilic enteritis. Rarely, eosinophilic pneumonitis has been reported in patients with CLM, possibly due to larval penetration involving the lungs. Allergic reactions can occur in multiply exposed individuals with extreme inflammatory response at the location of the track [1,6,8].

CLINICAL FEATURES

Signs and symptoms appear shortly after the larvae penetrate the skin, typically within a few days of infection although delay of onset for up to several months has been reported. In reported outbreaks of CLM, the median time to onset ranged from 10 to 15 days [6,8]. The

TABLE 120-1 Epidemiology and Clinical Characteristics of Parasites Associated With Cutaneous Disease Including Cutaneous Larva Migrans

	Host species	Geographic distribution	Clinical characteristics
Ancylostoma braziliense	Cat, dog	Atlantic coast of SE United States, Caribbean, South America south to Uruguay; Africa; Australia; Asia	Linear tracks which are often raised and pruritic; moves 1–2 cm/day; may persist up to 3 months
Ancylostoma caninum	Dog	Tropical to temperate climates worldwide	Linear tracks are rare, more often associated with folliculitis; occasional myositis or eosinophilic enteritis; persists up to 1 month
Uncinaria stenocephala	Cat, dog	Colder climates of North America, South America, Europe, Asia, Australia, and New Zealand	Relationship with cutaneous larva migrans is unclear; may cause transient linear tracks
Ancylostoma duodenale, Necator americanus	Human	Tropical to temperate climates worldwide	Transient papular rash at sites of penetration, usually lasts less than 1 week. Urticarial rash can develop as larvae migrate in lungs
Gnathostoma spinigerum	Cat, dog	Asia and South Asia, especially Thailand and Japan; Central America and Mexico; Africa	Intermittent pruritic, erythematous and painful swellings in subcutaneous tissues; lesions last 1–2 weeks but infection can persist for years
Strongyloides stercoralis	Human	Tropical to temperate climates worldwide	Urticarial rashes, less commonly transient linear tracks with pruritus; lesions perianal with autoinfection; migrate several cm/day; lesions resolve within 7–14 days

first symptom is typically intense pruritus followed by a raised, erythematous track that starts near the site of penetration. The track, typically about 3 mm wide and up to 20 mm long, can move in the skin at a rate of several millimeters per day; the larva itself is usually migrating somewhere ahead of the track. Usually, only one or a few tracks are present but there may be multiple tracks in more intense infections. Vesiculobullous lesions and edema can accompany the track; folliculitis is uncommon and may be related to the infecting species of hookworm. Eosinophilia is not consistently present and is likely when larvae have penetrated to deeper tissues or a greater inflammatory reaction is present [6,8].

PATIENT EVALUATION, DIAGNOSIS, AND DIFFERENTIAL DIAGNOSIS

Cutaneous larva migrans is a clinical diagnosis based on the presence of characteristic pruritus and an erythematous raised track that moves randomly in the dermis, as well as a history of skin exposure to contaminated soil or sand in endemic areas. Serologic testing to confirm infection is not available; skin biopsy is not useful since the location of the migrating larva cannot be predicted by the visible track. Clinical features and travel history can also help to define differential diagnoses, including other parasitic infections such as human hookworm, gnathostomiasis, strongyloidiasis, or noninfectious conditions such as cutaneous pili migrans. Myiasis and scabies can mimic CLM [1,6,8].

TREATMENT

CLM can be prevented by wearing shoes, sitting or lying on protective mats while at the beach, and taking other protective measures to avoid contact with contaminated soil or sand. Regular deworming of cats and dogs and prompt disposal of animal waste in the environment help to control sources of infective larvae [1]. CLM is self-limiting; larvae migrating in the skin usually will die after 5–6 weeks, although delayed onset and persistent clinical disease have been reported. Treatment may be necessary to resolve severe symptoms and address secondary bacterial infections. Cryotherapy is not recommended, as the larvae migrate randomly in advance of the visible tracks and may not be in the treated area. Topical therapy with anthelminthics has been shown to be effective but needs repeated applications over large areas of skin. Oral treatment with albendazole (400 mg/day orally for 3–7 days) or ivermectin (200 μg/kg orally single dose) eliminates the symptoms and kills the migrating larvae; in more severe cases of folliculitis, additional doses may be necessary. Rarely, relapse can occur but usually is resolved by repeated treatment [6,8,9].

Pediatric treatment: In children over 15 kg, a single dose of ivermectin 200 μg/kg orally is effective. Children under the age of 2 years should receive albendazole 200 mg orally for 3 days. Topical preparations of either drug have been suggested as alternative treatments in children.

REFERENCES

1. Bowman DD, Montgomery SP, Zajac AM, et al. Hookworms of dogs and cats as agents of cutaneous larva migrans. Trends Parasitol 2010;26:162–7.
2. Kirby-Smith J, Dove W, White G. Creeping eruption. Arch Dermatol Syphilol 1926;13:137–73.
3. Lederman ER, Weld LH, Elyazar IR, et al. Dermatologic conditions of the ill returned traveler: an analysis from the GeoSentinel Surveillance Network. Int J Infect Dis 2008;12:593–602.
4. Feldmeier H, Heukelbach J. Epidermal parasitic skin diseases: a neglected category of poverty-associated plagues. Bull World Health Organ 2009;87:152–9.
5. Blackwell V, Vega-Lopez F. Cutaneous larva migrans: clinical features and management of 44 cases presenting in the returning traveler. Br J Dermatol 2001;145:434–7.
6. Heukelbach J, Feldmeier H. Epidemiological and clinical characteristics of hookworm-related cutaneous larva migrans. Lancet Infect Dis 2008;8:302–9.
7. Heukelbach J, Jackson A, Ariza L, Feldmeier H. Prevalence and risk factors of hookworm-related cutaneous larva migrans in a rural community in Brazil. Ann Trop Med Parasitol 2008;102:53–61.
8. Hochedez P, Caumes E. Hookworm-related cutaneous larva migrans. J Travel Med 2007;14:326–33.
9. Caumes E. Treatment of cutaneous larva migrans and *Toxocara* infection. Fundam Clin Pharmacol 2003;17:213–16.

121 Anisakidosis

Davidson H Hamer

Key features

- Humans are accidental hosts to the intermediate larva of marine nematodes, especially *Anisakis simplex* and *Pseudoterranova decipiens*
- Infection results from consumption of raw or undertreated marine fish or squid
- The greatest burden of disease is in Japan but increased awareness of anisakidosis and adventurous eating habits have resulted in a greater worldwide distribution of disease
- Major clinical syndromes include gastric, intestinal, extraintestinal, and allergic anisakidosis
- Endoscopy can be used for both diagnosis and treatment of gastric anisakidosis
- Prolonged freezing, flash freezing at low temperatures, and adequately cooking marine fish are effective for prevention

INTRODUCTION

Humans are accidental hosts to the intermediate larval stage of several species of zoonotic intestinal nematodes, which are acquired by the consumption of raw or undercooked marine fish or squid. Anisakidosis was first recognized more than 50 years ago in a patient in the Netherlands who presented with an eosinophilic intestinal lesion associated with severe abdominal pain. During the last two decades, these nematodes have been increasingly identified as causes of gastric, intestinal, and allergic syndromes in humans who have occupational exposure or frequently consume seafood.

Most human infections are caused by *Anisakis simplex* (also known as the herring worm) and *Pseudoterranova decipiens* (cod or seal worm) [1,2]. Other less common members of the family Anisakidae are the *A. simplex* complex (e.g. *A. pegreffi*) and the *Pseudoterranova* complex, as well as *A. physeteris*, *Contracaecum* spp. and *Thynnascaris* spp. The term anisakidosis refers to disease caused by any member of the family Anisakidae, whereas anisakiasis is caused by worms of the genus *Anisakis* and pseudoterranovosis by the genus *Pseudoterranova*.

EPIDEMIOLOGY

The annual incidence is greatest in Japan, where the consumption of raw fish is common. Of the approximately 20,000 reported cases worldwide, more than 90% occur in Japan [3]. Most other cases have been described in Korea and Europe, especially the Netherlands, Germany, France, Spain and Italy. During the last two decades, there have been increasing reports from the US, Canada, Brazil, Chile, Egypt and New Zealand. The increase in prevalence of anisakidosis can be attributed to improved endoscopic diagnosis, increased consumption of raw or lightly cooked seafood, and larger populations of the definitive hosts [4]. While there have been approximately 60 cases reported in the US, anisakidosis is most likely greatly underdiagnosed and underreported.

Anisakidosis is associated with consuming raw, marinated, or incompletely cooked fish. In Japan, infections occur more frequently in coastal populations and in men aged 20 to 50 years. Fish served in sushi bars tend to be less contaminated or even free of *Anisakis* as sushi chefs are experts in identifying larval infestation. The risk of infection is greater with less-expensive marine fish such as cod, herring, mackerel and squid that are more frequently consumed at home or in local restaurants. The main fish species responsible for anisakiasis in Japan are mackerel and squid. In the Netherlands, herring is mainly responsible; in the US, Pacific salmon; and in Spain, pickled anchovies. Pseudoterranovosis rarely occurs in Japan and Europe. By contrast, it is more frequent in the US and Canada where *P. decipiens* is mainly transmitted by the Atlantic or Pacific cod, Pacific halibut, and red snapper.

Limited data from seafood markets suggest that substantial proportions of fish are infected with third-stage larvae (L3) of *A. simplex*. In Spain, greater infection rates in fish from the Atlantic Ocean are present than in those from the Mediterranean Sea. A substantial proportion of cod harvested in the Atlantic Ocean is infected with *P. decipiens* (Fig. 121.1).

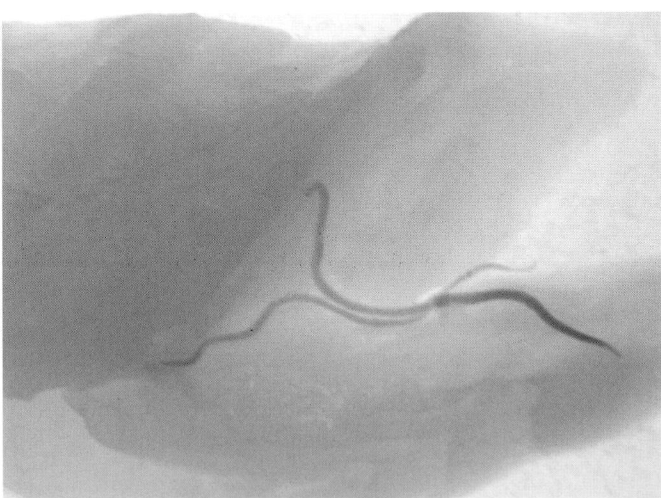

FIGURE 121.1 *Pseudoterranova decipiens* larvae embedded in the flesh of Atlantic cod.

NATURAL HISTORY, PATHOGENESIS, AND PATHOLOGY

The adult worm is found in the stomachs or intestines of marine mammals such as whales, dolphins, sea lions, and seals [5]. Eggs hatch in seawater to form free-living larvae (L2) that infect intermediate hosts, usually crustaceans, e.g. krills (Fig. 121.2). Within the first intermediate host, the parasite matures into L3 larvae which are subsequently ingested by marine fish or squid, which serve as transport (second intermediate) hosts. The third-stage larvae migrate into the viscera, peritoneal cavity and musculature of this host. Ingestion of uncooked fish or squid by a marine mammal (final host) or humans (accidental hosts) leads to infection. The nematode larvae develop into fourth-stage larvae and then adults in the marine mammal final host.

Primary hosts for *Anisakis* are dolphins, porpoises, and whales. Primary hosts for *P. decipiens* are seals, walruses, and sea lions.

After ingestion of raw or undercooked saltwater fish by humans, the larvae embed themselves in the gastric or intestinal mucosa and then die. The burrowing or dead larva precipitates an intense hypersensitivity reaction characterized by a granulomatous, eosinophilic tissue infiltrate. A Th2 immune response has been demonstrated in humans, with mucosal and submucosal inflammatory infiltrate composed of eosinophils and lymphocytes.

CLINICAL FEATURES

There are four major clinical syndromes in humans: gastric, intestinal, ectopic (or extra-gastrointestinal), and allergic [3]. Infection with *P.*

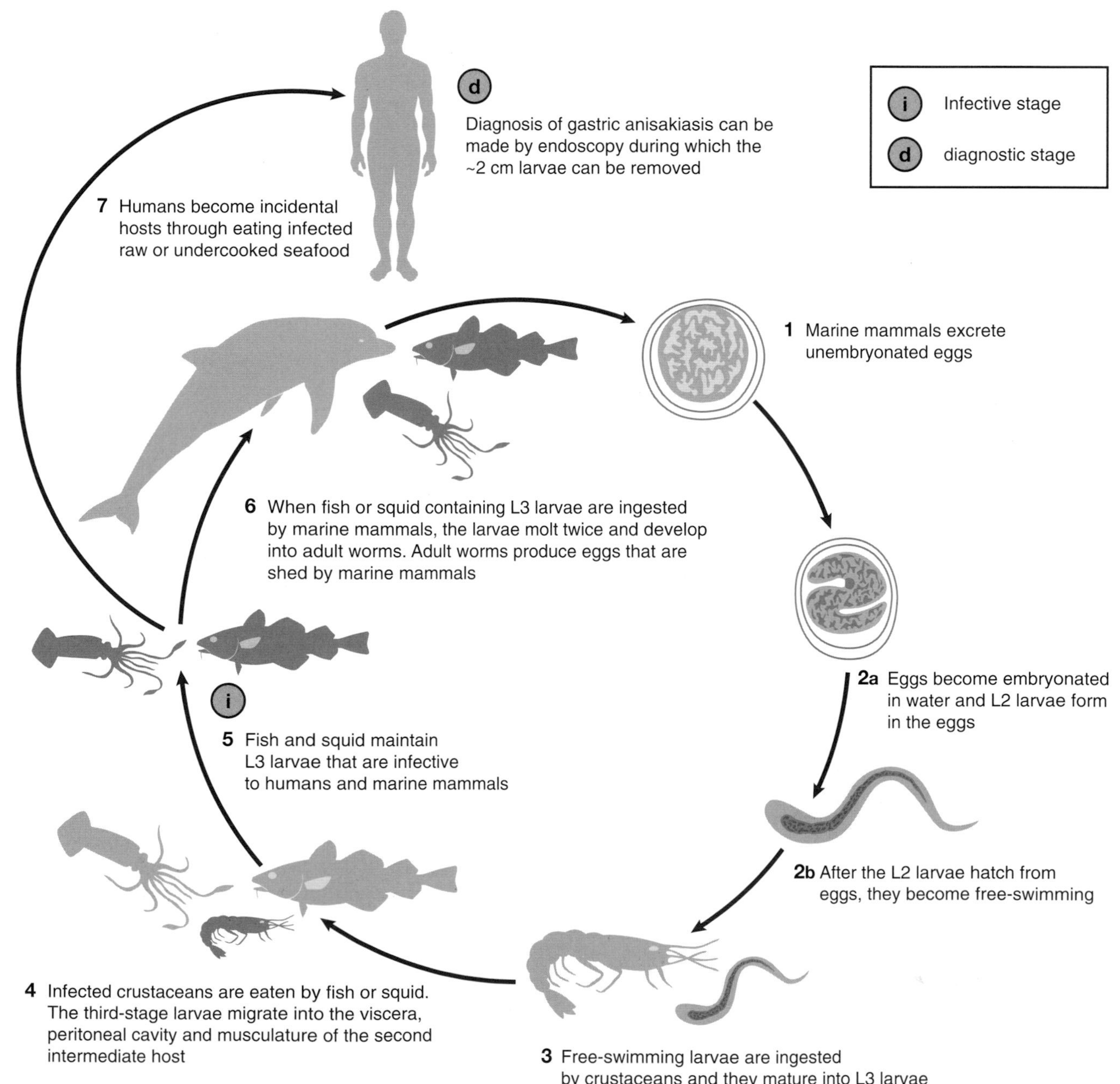

FIGURE 121.2 Life cycle of anisakids.

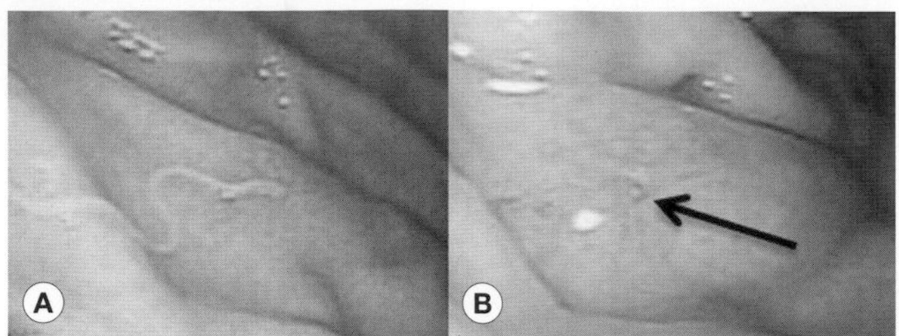

FIGURE 121.3 Third-stage larva of *Anisakis simplex* burrowing into the gastric mucosa. Surrounding erythema and edema of the mucosa are evident. *(Endoscopic view courtesy of Drs Tomohiro Kato and Itaru O-I, Department of Medicine, Daini Hospital, Tokyo Women's Medical University.)*

decipiens usually involves only the stomach and tends to be milder than disease due to *Anisakis* spp., which may cause symptomatic gastric or intestinal infections. Asymptomatic infections with *Pseudoterranova* spp. may come to medical attention when the patient coughs up a live or dead worm. This usually occurs within 48 hours of the ingestion of infected fish and may be preceded by a sensation of feeling a worm crawling in the upper esophagus or pharynx, termed "tingling throat syndrome".

Gastric anisakiasis is heralded by the abrupt (generally 1–12 hours after ingestion of raw fish) onset of severe epigastric pain, nausea, vomiting, and low-grade fever (Fig. 121.3). There is frequently leukocytosis with intense eosinophilia. Untreated gastric disease may lead to chronic, ulcer-like symptoms and can be more difficult to diagnose.

Intestinal anisakiasis is characterized by intermittent or constant abdominal pain that may be severe enough to result in peritoneal signs or a partial bowel obstruction. Symptoms may not appear until 5 to 7 days or longer after ingestion of the anisakid larvae. Intestinal infections predominantly occur in the terminal ileum; colonic or jejunal involvement is less common. Rare complications include small bowel obstruction, ileal stenosis, intussusception, intestinal perforation, and pneumoperitoneum.

Ectopic, extra-gastrointestinal and intraperitoneal anisakiasis are less common complications which result from an anisakid larva penetrating the full thickness of the stomach or intestine. This can lead to larval migration within the peritoneal cavity and, less commonly, the pleural cavity, mesentery, liver, pancreas, ovary, and subcutaneous tissue.

Anisakidosis may be associated with a strong allergic response [6]. Generally within 1 to 2 hours after the ingestion of infected fish, allergic reactions develop with manifestations ranging from urticaria and isolated angioedema to anaphylaxis. Allergic reactions are accompanied by high levels of IgE including specific anti-*A. simplex* IgE. High levels of fish consumption and occupational exposure (e.g. fish processing) are associated with increased risk of allergy to *A. simplex*.

PATIENT EVALUATION, DIAGNOSIS, AND DIFFERENTIAL DIAGNOSIS

A history of recent consumption of raw or inadequately prepared fish or squid followed by the acute onset of epigastric or right lower quadrant abdominal pain provide important diagnostic clues. Gastroscopic or surgical removal and examination of the larva provides a definitive diagnosis of gastric anisakidosis. Besides directly visualizing the worm embedded in the gastric mucosa, endoscopy can reveal erythema, edema, erosions, a tumor-like nodule, or thickened gastric folds, which can suggest a diagnosis of lymphoma or gastric cancer. Gastric anisakidosis can be misdiagnosed as a peptic ulcer, gastritis, or gastric carcinoma. As a result of the vague symptoms associated with intestinal infections, the differential diagnosis is broad and includes appendicitis, ileitis, diverticulitis, eosinophilic gastroenteritis, cholecystitis, colonic tumor, and inflammatory bowel disease. Extraintestinal infections may be confused with acute peritonitis, tuberculous peritonitis, and pancreatic cancer.

Detection of anti-*A. simplex* IgE by ELISA, latex agglutination, or other immunoassays can be used for the serodiagnosis of anisakiasis, but is not commercially available [6,7]. The diagnosis of allergy to *A. simplex* should be based on the following: a compatible history of allergic reactions after consumption or exposure to fish; positive skin-prick test; elevated specific anti-*A. simplex* IgE; and a lack of reaction to fish proteins. Multiplex PCR methods have been developed for identification of specific marine nematodes species in fish, but these are not available for human use.

TREATMENT

Endoscopic extraction is the preferred treatment of gastric anisakidosis unless the larva is spontaneously regurgitated. Surgical removal of the larvae may be necessary for intestinal or extraintestinal infections, especially if complications such as intestinal obstruction, appendicitis, or peritonitis occur. If the diagnosis of intestinal anisakidosis can be established without the need for an invasive procedure, then conservative, supportive therapy will often lead to clinical resolution. Limited evidence suggests that albendazole (400 to 800 mg daily for 6 to 21 days) is effective [8].

PREVENTION

The best protection against anisakidosis is to avoid consumption of raw or inadequately cooked, marinated, or salted marine fish or squid. The risk of human infection can also be reduced by visual examination of fish, extraction of visible parasites, and removal of heavily parasitized fish from the market. Eviscerating fish as soon as possible after catch may decrease the number of larvae in the fish flesh by preventing migration from the intestinal tract into the edible musculature. Additional protective measures include thorough cooking, freezing at −20°C (−4°F) for 7 days, or blast freezing to −35°C (−31°F) for 15 hours or longer.

REFERENCES

1. Audicana MT, Kennedy MW. *Anisakis simplex*: from obscure infectious worm to inducer of immune hypersensitivity. Clin Microbiol Rev 2008;21:360–79.
   This review presents a comprehensive summary of the immunopathogenesis of anisakiasis.
2. McClelland G. The trouble with sealworms (*Pseudoterranova decipiens* species complex, Nematoda): a review. Parasitology 2002;124:S183–203.
3. Hochberg N, Hamer DH. Anisakidosis: perils of the deep. Clin Infect Dis 2010;51:806–12.
   This is a recently published comprehensive review of the epidemiology, clinical manifestations, treatment and prevention of anisakidosis.
4. Chai JY, Murrell KD, Lymbery AJ. Fish-borne parasitic zoonoses: Status and issues. Int J Parasitol 2005;35:1233–54.
5. Ishikura H, Kikuchi K, Nagasawa K, et al. Anisakidae and anisakidosis. Prog Clin Parasitol 1993;3:43–102.
6. Audicana MT, Ansotegui IJ, de Corres LF, Kennedy MW. Anisakis simplex: dangerous – dead and alive? Trends Parasitol 2002;18:20–5.
   This brief review provides an excellent overview of anisakiasis with an emphasis on the role of this parasite as a cause of food allergy in Spain and methods for diagnosis of allergy to A. simplex.
7. López-Serrano MC, Gomez AA, Daschner A, et al. Gastroallergic anisakiasis: findings in 22 patients. J Gastroenterol Hepatol 2000;15:503–6.
8. Pacios E, Arias-Diaz J, Zuloaga J, et al. Albendazole for the treatment of anisakiasis ileus. Clin Infect Dis 2005;41:1825–6.

SECTION

D

TREMATODE INFECTIONS

122 Schistosomiasis

Bruno Gryseels, G Thomas Strickland

Key features

- Schistosomiasis is caused by several species of blood flukes, with the three most important being *Schistosoma mansoni*, *Schistosoma haematobium* and *Schistosoma japonicum*
- Infection is focally widespread in most of Africa, Southeast Asia and large parts of South America. Two hundred million people are estimated to be infected; 85% of them live in sub-Saharan Africa. In countries where praziquantel therapy has been widely used, the burden of schistosomiasis is a fraction of what it was 30 years ago
- The lifecycle requires a snail intermediate host that is specific to each parasite species
- Schistosome ova that are deposited in surface water with stools or urine release primary larvae (miracidiae) that infect the snails and develop into free living secondary larvae (cercariae). Humans are infected when cercariae penetrate the skin during exposure to water
- In endemic areas, large proportions of the population can be infected, especially children. Many infections result only in vague, nonspecific or hidden morbidity
- The disease has both acute and chronic phases. Acute schistosomiasis (Katayama fever) occurs a few weeks after exposure and is caused by the body's reaction to developing larvae (schistosomula) migrating through the body. Chronic schistosomiasis occurs after years of infection and is primarily caused by cellular immunity and fibrosis as a reaction to ova retained in the tissues. Ectopic lesions may cause neurologic, pulmonary or genital schistosomiasis
- *Schistosoma mansoni* and *S. japonicum* primarily cause intestinal and hepatic pathology; *S. haematobium* primarily damages the urinary tract
- Diagnosis is based on microscopic detection of ova, serology or imaging
- Praziquantel provides safe, inexpensive and effective oral therapy. Extensive mass drug administration programs have, over the past 20 years, reduced morbidity and transmission in many countries

INTRODUCTION

Schistosomiasis is caused by trematodes (fluke worms) of the genus *Schistosoma* (Phylum Platyhelminthes, Class Trematoda) that live in blood vessels [1–3]. Humans become infected when infectious motile cercariae penetrate the skin during freshwater contact. Three main species infect humans. *Schistosoma mansoni* (Africa, Arabia and South America) and *S. japonicum* (China and the Philippines) causes intestinal and hepatosplenic schistosomiasis. *Schistosoma haematobium* causes urinary tract schistosomiasis in Africa and Arabia. *Schistosoma intercalatum* is only of local importance in some pockets in West and Central Africa, *Schistosoma mekongi* in the Mekong delta and *Schistosoma malayensis* in Malaysia [1–4]. Each schistosome species is transmitted by specific freshwater snails: *Biomphalaria* genus for *S. mansoni*, *Bulinus* for *S. haematobium* and *Oncomelania* (which are amphibious) for *S. japonicum* [5, 6].

The number of people with schistosomiasis is estimated by the World Health Organization (WHO) at more than 200 million in 74 countries, with over 700 million people at risk [7–9]. The actual figures may be lower, as the numbers of infections and people at risk are dwindling quickly in major historical foci, such as Egypt, Brazil and China [3]. Today, over 85% of cases occur in sub-Saharan Africa [8]. The WHO has classified schistosomiasis as one of the "Neglected Tropical Diseases" (NTD), a group of parasitic and infectious diseases that create considerable havoc among low-income and deprived populations in developing countries but that receive less attention than global threats such as HIV/AIDS, tuberculosis and malaria [9].

Transmission of schistosomes requires a tropical climate, the presence of suitable snail hosts, human settlement, contamination by excreta of the surface waters and human contact with these waters [1–3]. Notwithstanding these uniform conditions, the epidemiology of schistosomiasis varies greatly between continents, countries, regions and even neighboring villages. Snail populations, cercarial densities and human water contact show strong temporal and spatial variations, depending upon local ecology. The distribution of worms in local populations is often extensive, with prevalence commonly between 30% and 100%, but the severity of infection and disease can be very uneven. Typically, the highest prevalence and intensities of infection are found in children between the ages of 8 and 15 years, whereas adults usually have fewer exposures and develop acquired resistance to infection.

Severe disease is usually associated with heavy worm burdens, but may develop after only several years of silent, or mildly symptomatic, infection. Since the advent of safe schistosomicides, especially praziquantel, it has become possible to interrupt the insidious disease cycle, even in the face of continued transmission and re-infection [8, 10]. Therefore, modern control strategies focus primarily on the regular treatment of people at risk, especially school-aged children, or through mass drug administration (MDA) programs.

HISTORY

The evolutionary pathway of *S. japonicum* probably lies in the Yangtze River Valley, *S. mansoni* probably originated in the Nile River basin, and *S. haematobium* in the African Great Lake area [1–3, 11]. Calcified schistosome eggs and, more recently, specific antigens have been detected in Egyptian, Sudanese and Chinese mummies dating from several millennia BC. There are no comparable paleo-epidemiological traces in South America, where *S. mansoni* was imported with the slave trade in the 16th and 17th centuries.

In 1851, the young German pathologist Theodore Bilharz first identified *S. haematobium* as the etiologic agent of Egyptian endemic hematuria during an autopsy in Cairo. He also described the underlying pathology of the urinary system and bilharziasis, or bilharzia, is still used to denominate schistosomal disease. Association of chronic liver disease, characterized by hepatomegaly and splenomegaly, was not reported until Symmer described the typical "clay pipe stem fibrosis" in Egypt in 1904. The complete lifecycle of the parasite and the role of the snail intermediate host were described in 1913 by Miyairi and confirmed experimentally by Leiper in 1915. McDonough introduced the first effective chemotherapy using tartar emetic in 1918.

Schistosomiasis attracted little research attention in the USA until US troops became exposed to infection with *S. japonicum* on the island of Leyte, during the re-invasion of the Philippines in 1944. In the late 1950s, a mouse model of *S. mansoni* infection with hepatosplenomegaly, portal hypertension and esophageal varices was developed and the pathology was shown to be caused by schistosome ova trapped in the presinusoidal venules of the liver. In the 1960s, the immunologic complexities of the host's granulomatous response to the schistosome egg and the mechanisms of concomitant protective immunity began to be defined. It was determined in the 1970s that chronic disease often takes decades to develop and is associated with heavy worm burdens [12]. Until the 1980s, schistosomiasis could only be treated with toxic drugs, such as tartar emetic and, later, niridazole. The large-scale use of intravenous tartar emetic in Egypt between 1950 and 1980 is thought to have caused a massive iatrogenic spread of hepatitis C, considerably aggravating, and probably also obfuscating, schistosomal liver disease [13]. Most control programs in that period relied on the chemical destruction of the vector snails with copper sulphate or niclosamide (Bayluscid®), which was expensive, technically demanding and toxic to fish [1, 3].

In the 1970s, hycanthone, metrifonate and oxamniquine were developed, but these still had disadvantages, for example single-species activity, side effects or the need for repeated administration. The development of praziquantel in 1979, in a then unique public-private partnership between the WHO and the pharmaceutical industry, heralded a breakthrough for the treatment and control of schistosomiasis [1, 14]. It is highly effective and safe against all species in a single dose. More recently, less expensive generic brands, drug donations and renewed international support for neglected diseases control enabled the introduction of MDA, often combined with other anthelminthics, for the control of schistosomal morbidity. In 2001, the World Health Assembly officially recommended this strategy for all regions where schistosomiasis still constitutes a serious public health problem, along with integrated case management in primary healthcare, health education, safe water supply and improved sanitation [15].

BIOLOGY

SPECIES

The genus *Schistosoma* belongs to the class of Trematoda (flukes), phylum of Platyhelminthes (flatworms). They differ from other human flukes by: (i) having separate sexes; (ii) living in blood vessels; (iii) having non-operculated eggs; and (iv) lacking an encysted metacercarial stage. Humans are definitive hosts for *S. japonicum*, *S. mansoni*, *S. haematobium*, *S. mekongi*, *S. malayensis* and *S. intercalatum* [1].

Dozens of other schistosome species infect animals, some of which are occasionally found in humans, including *S. mattheei*, *S. bovis*, *S. curassoni*, *S. rodhaini*, *S. margrebowiei*, *S. spindale* and *S. incognitum*. Recent genetic studies confirmed that some of these species may form productive and pathogenic hybrids with human schistosomes [16]. The infective larvae or cercariae of other nonhuman schistosomes and related trematodes, mostly parasites of birds or small mammals, can attack or penetrate human skin causing dermatitis, but die without migration or maturation. These exposures also occur in temperate climates and cause "swimmers' itch" during summers in North America and Europe [17].

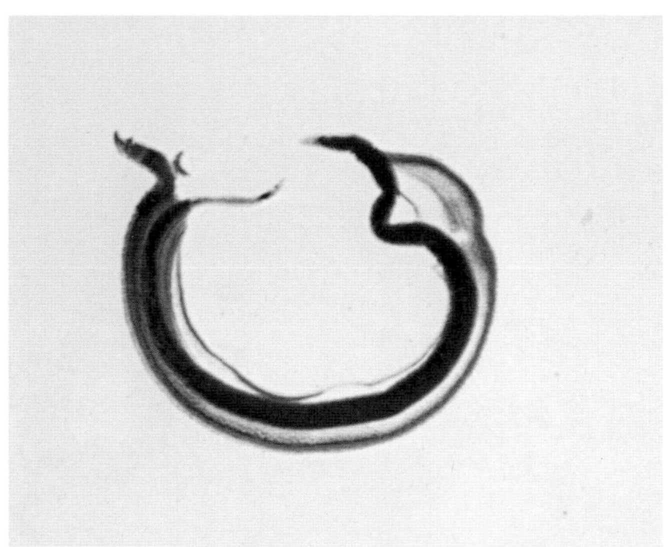

FIGURE 122.1 Morphology of adult male and female *Schistosoma mansoni*. *(Courtesy of the Armed Forces Institute of Pathology, Photograph Neg. No. 56-3334).*

MORPHOLOGY AND METABOLISM (Fig. 122.1)

Adult schistosomes are white-greyish worms with a cylindrical body, tend to be 10–20 mm long and 0.3–0.6 mm thick. The tegument of adult schistosomes consists of a double layer, of which the outer one is continuously shed and renewed. The male tegumental surface may be tuberculated or smooth, depending on the species; the surface of the female worm is smooth in all species. The adult male worm is shorter, thicker and flatter than the longer, slender female. With his flattened body, the male worm forms a groove or "gynecophoric channel", in which the female positions herself for most of her life. Copulation takes place permanently as the male and female genital orifices superpose in the gynecophoric channel.

Schistosomes feed on nutrients and cells in the blood, and metabolize globulins and hemoglobin through anaerobic glycolysis into pigment-like debris. As the gut terminates blindly, the debris is regurgitated into the host's bloodstream. The pigment may be deposited in the Kupffer cells and macrophages of the liver and other organs, showing as typical pigmentation in histologic stains.

REPRODUCTION AND TRANSMISSION (Fig. 122.2)

Adult schistosome pairs live within the perivesical (*S. haematobium*) or mesenteric (other species) venous plexus. Studies in migrants show that live eggs, and thus adult worms, can still be found for more than 30 years after last exposure [18]. The average lifespan of adult schistosomes is estimated at 3–5 years, but may be shorter in areas with high levels of transmission and worm turn-over [19].

The favored location of the adult worms and, consequently, egg deposition and ensuing pathology, varies according to species. *Schistosoma haematobium* is concentrated near the bladder and around the ureters, *S. mansoni* in the inferior mesenteric vessels of the large intestine and *S. japonicum* in the superior mesenteric vessels of the large and small intestine.

The females produce large, oval or round ova of 100–170 µm in length with a typical terminal or lateral spine at a daily rate of hundreds (African species) to several thousands (Oriental species) with often clustered ova of 70–100 µm in length. The spines are formed during the release of the eggs from the ovipore and may serve as an anchor against the blood flow – helping eggs to start their journey through the vascular wall and into the tissues.

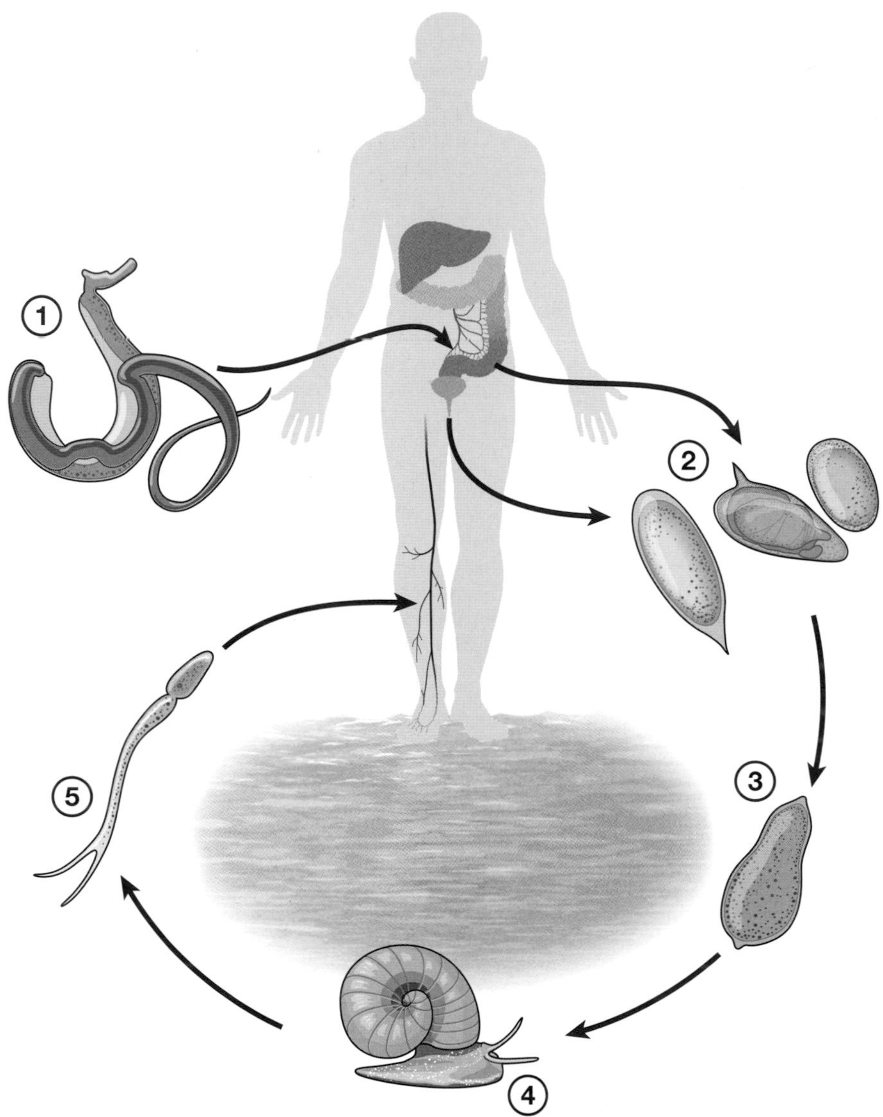

FIGURE 122.2 Transmission cycle of schistosomes. *(Reproduced with permission from Gryseels B, Polman K, Clerinx J, Kestens L. Human schistosomiasis. Lancet 2006; 368:1106–18.)*

Each ovum contains one ciliated larva, called a miracidium, which matures over 6–10 days. The miracidium secretes proteolytic enzymes that help the eggs to penetrate through the vascular wall and into surrounding tissues into the lumen of the bladder (*S. haematobium*) or the intestine (other species). About 50% of the eggs are eventually excreted with the urine or the feces, where they may stay viable for seven days (African species) or up to several months (Oriental species), depending on the temperature and humidity in the environment. The other ova are dislodged and partly destroyed in the liver or spleen, but many remain stuck in the tissues of the bladder or ureters, the intestinal wall, or the liver or spleen (depending on species) where immune responses lead to most of the host's pathology.

The excreted ova release the miracidium upon contact with water of the right temperature (20–30°C), which then swims freely and swiftly around in search of its snail intermediate host. They are propelled by flagellating cilia and guided by positive phototaxis and chemotaxis (attracted by light and snail substances) and negative geotaxis (moving away from the bottom mud). In addition to this typical movement and cilia, the miricidia have pulsating flame and gland cells. They can remain infective for 6–12 hours and penetrate the snail intermediate host's soft parts by aid of lytic substances.

After snail penetration, the miracidium loses its cilia and transforms into a non-motile sac-like embryo: the mother sporocyst. Over the next 10–15 days, germinal cells in the mother sporocyst differentiate into motile daughter sporocysts. The daughter sporocysts migrate to, and grow in, the hepatic and gonadal tissue of the snail, where they metamorphose within 2–4 weeks into bifurcated, mobile larvae called cercariae. The entire non-sexual reproduction stage in the snail takes 4–6 weeks, but cercariae may be shed for up three months at a rate of dozens (*S. japonicum*) to thousands (*S. mansoni*, *S. haematobium*) per day. While snail life expectancy is reduced by schistosome infection because of damage to hepatic and gonadal tissue, one snail infected by one miracidium can shed thousands of cercariae every day for months and may produce up to 100,000 cercariae in its lifetime.

The cercariae are unisexual, highly mobile larvae measuring 400–600 μm in length. They feature a pear-shaped head with two embryonic suckers and a long slender tail ending in a typical short fork. Cercarial shedding is stimulated by direct sunlight and temperatures between 24–30°C, leading to peak transmission rates between 11.00 h and 15.00 h and, in subtropical regions, during summer months. *Schistosoma japonicum* cercariae may also be shed at night.

Cercariae may survive up to 48–72 hours, though infectivity starts to decrease after 12 hours. Activity in water varies with the species: *S. mansoni* and *S. haematobium* cercariae move vertically, alternating between active movements toward the surface and slow sinking; *S. japonicum* cercariae tend to remain at rest in the water surface film unless disturbed. When cercariae meet a suitable definitive host, they attach themselves to its skin by their ventral or oral suckers, assisted by mucoid secretions. Vertical, vibratory movements and lytic secretions lead to penetration of the skin, usually complete within 3–5 minutes. Only some of the cercariae will develop further after penetration, depending on the physiologic and immunologic reactions of the host.

The cercariae lose their tail and undergo an intensive outer membrane modification to become schistosomula which are tolerant to a saline environment and, even more strikingly, to at least part of the hosts' immune responses. They remain in subcutaneous tissue for about 48 hours before beginning the 3–6 day migration through the bloodstream to the heart and then the lungs, where they are able to stretch the capillaries between the arterioles and venules. Within 5–10 days they reach the small vessels of the liver where they mature within another 3–4 weeks into adult male or female worms, mate and migrate against the blood flow to their perivesicular or mesenteric destination where the cycle starts all over again. Egg deposition and excretion thus starts 6–8 weeks after infection.

THE SNAIL INTERMEDIATE HOSTS AND OTHER RESERVOIR HOSTS

The snail intermediate hosts of *S. mansoni* and *S. haematobium* are red-brownish in color and are non-operculate, i.e. they have no cover or lid on the shells. The major intermediate hosts for *S. haematobium* and *S. intercalatum* are *Bulinidae*, with conic shells with a left-twisted spiral. The genus *Biomphalaria* serves as the intermediate host for *S. mansoni* and is characterized by its disk- or lens-shaped shells [1, 5, 6]. The snail intermediate hosts of *S. japonicum*, members of *Oncomelania hupensis* species, are operculate with conical or turriculate shells.

Other freshwater mollusks serve as intermediate hosts for incomplete avian schistosome infections (causing cercarial dermatitis) but may be difficult to distinguish from the intermediate hosts of human schistosomes, requiring the use of rigid determination keys or genetic analysis.

The aquatic snails important to the transmission of *S. mansoni* and *S. haematobium* live in lightly-shaded, slow-flowing shallow waters. *Biomphalaria*, and particularly *Bulinus*, can survive protracted droughts, hiding in moist mud until the next rains come and rivers swell again. The amphibious *Oncomelania* intermediate host of *S. japonicum* spends part of its time out of water, preferring moist soil in marshy habitats, at the edge of slow-flowing streams, or irrigation canals. It can survive dry periods, as well as long and cold winters. The population dynamics of the snails, and consequently the transmission dynamics of the parasite populations, may differ greatly from one area, one season or one year to another. The infective dynamics of the intermediate host are such that usually less than 0.5% is infected with schistosomes at any one time. As only a very small proportion of the total snail population can be sampled, it may be difficult to find any infected snails or cercariae even in highly endemic areas [20].

There is no identified functional reservoir host for *S. haematobium*. *Schistosoma mansoni* infects rodents and baboons living in some endemic areas and they can maintain the transmission cycle. However, humans are by far the main reservoir of infection. In contrast, *S. japonicum* is a zoonotic parasite that naturally infects dogs, cats, cattle, water buffaloes, pigs, horses, sheep, goats and rodents; some of these, i.e. cattle and water buffaloes, are as important for transmission as humans [6, 20].

IMMUNOLOGY

PROTECTIVE IMMUNITY

Epidemiologic and clinical observations show that people living in endemic areas develop acquired immunity, but only after several years of exposure [21]. Indeed, prevalence and intensities of infection decline after the age of 10–15 years. Cross-sectional data are, however, difficult to relate with exposure, as the worm burdens in adults were built up slowly over many years [21]. The availability of praziquantel has also allowed testing and confirming of this hypothesis by measuring re-infection rates after population-based treatment. After confirmed chemotherapeutic cure, egg counts usually rise much quicker to initial levels in children than in adults, with minimal correlation to exposures to contaminated water. This partial immunity is mediated by IgE against larval and adult worm antigens, which stimulate eosinophils to release cytotoxins targeting schistosomulae [22]. Efforts to develop a protective vaccine are ongoing but are unlikely to result in a commercially-available product in the near future [3, 22, 23].

MORBID IMMUNITY

The main pathology in schistosomiasis is actually caused by cellular immune responses against eggs retained in the tissues, rather than the adult worms [12, 24]. The enzymes and metabolites released by the ova that are trapped in the tissues provoke granulomatous reactions by eosinophils, monocytes and lymphocytes orchestrated by CD4+ T cells. In the early stages of infection, cytokine responses are predominantly of the TH1 type featuring interferon-γ. As egg production proceeds, they shift to a TH2 profile with high levels of IgE, interleukin (IL)-4 and eosinophilia. In long-standing chronic infection, this TH2 profile modulates to production of IL-10, IL-13 and IgG_4, which leads to the regression of the granulomas and their replacement by collagen. In most infected persons, however, anti-inflammatory IL-10, and possibly transforming growth factor (TGF)-β, induced by regulatory T cells, prevents excessive TH1 or TH2 polarization and, hence, severe disease manifestations in the late stages of the disease.

IMMUNE RESPONSES AND CO-INFECTIONS

Various bidirectional interactions between immune responses to schistosomiasis and HIV/AIDS have been described, but their clinical significance remains undetermined [3, 25]. Treatment of concomitant schistosomiasis appears to have little effect on HIV viral load or results, at most, in a lower HIV RNA increase in patients with a delayed intervention. Reduced CD4+ T cell counts may increase the susceptibility to schistosome infections and serodiagnostic reliabilities may be affected in concomitant infections.

There have been experimental animal and human studies reporting that chronic schistosomiasis, by downregulating the TH1 and upregulating the TH2 immune responses, could cause viral infections, notably hepatitis B and C, to become chronic and more severe [26]. The situation is complicated as parenteral treatment of schistosomiasis has caused the spread of some blood-borne viral infections [13], but the clinical importance of the immunosuppressive effects of schistosomiasis on hepatitis B and C is less than the pathophysiology caused by having multiple infections.

EPIDEMIOLOGY

GEOGRAPHIC DISTRIBUTION (Fig. 122.3)

The distribution of the different species depends primarily on the ecology of the snail hosts. The introduction and sustained transmission of *Schistosoma* infections requires suitable snail hosts, a tropical climate for at least 4–6 months a year, human settlement, fecal or urinary contamination of the surface waters harboring the snails and human contact with these waters. The geographic distribution of schistosomiasis is, thus, largely confined to an area between 36° north and 34° south latitude, where freshwater temperatures average 25–30 °C and socioeconomic conditions impose regular contact with snail-infested water [1, 3, 4]. In addition, within populations and age groups, schistosomes are not evenly distributed – a small number of individuals carry most of the parasite burden [27].

The epidemiology of schistosomiasis is highly focal and can vary strongly from one area, village or hamlet to another [1, 3, 4]. While *S. haematobium* mostly occurs in warm plains, *S. mansoni* can be transmitted in a variety of ecotypes, from savannah to rain forest and highland areas of up to 2500 m. Transmission of both species takes place in the great lakes of Central and East Africa; in many other small

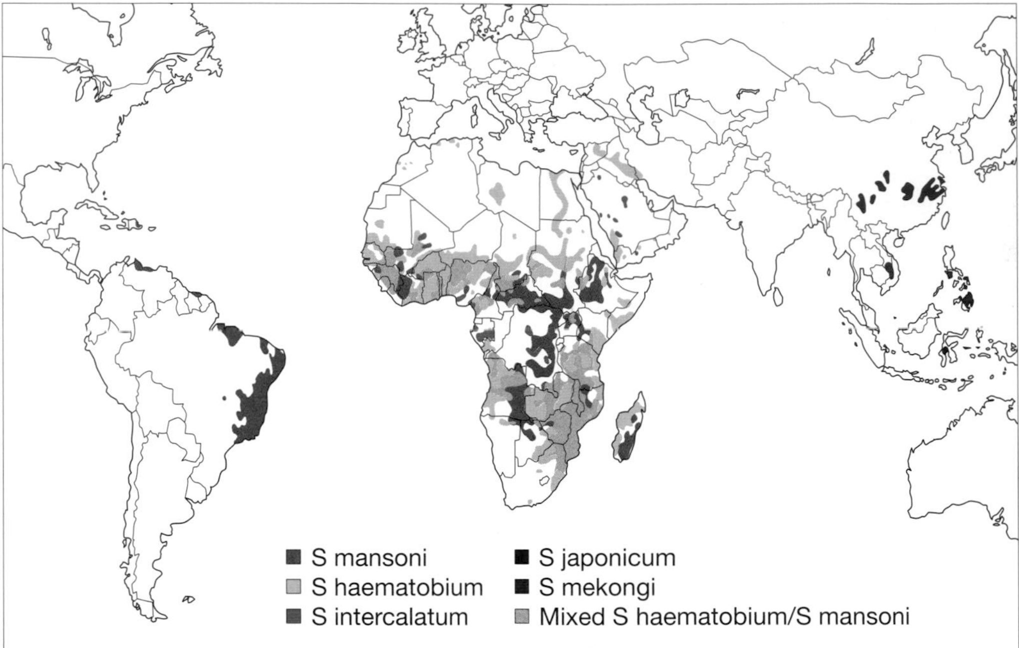

FIGURE 122.3 World distribution map of schistosomiasis *(Reproduced with permission from Gryseels B, Polman K, Clerinx J, Kestens L. Human schistosomiasis. Lancet 2006;368: 1106–18.).*

and large, natural and artificial lakes throughout the continent; in surface irrigation and drainage systems; and in innumerable natural streams and ponds. Transmission of *S. japonicum* takes place in hot southern areas in China, as well as in the mountains of Sichuan and the central lakes, where winters are severe but summers are hot and long enough to allow intense seasonal transmission.

The main foci of *S. mansoni* are in sub-Saharan Africa, including Madagascar; Lower and Middle Egypt; the Arabian peninsula; northeast Brazil; Surinam; Venezuela; and parts of the Caribbean. *Schistosoma haematobium* occurs in large parts of sub-Saharan Africa, Madagascar, Middle and Upper Egypt, the Maghreb and the Arabian peninsula. *Schistosoma japonicum* is found along the central lakes and the Yangtze River in China, including the mountain areas of Sichuan and Yunnan; and Mindanao, Leyte and other small sites in the Philippines. It is not clear whether transmission still occurs in some small historical pockets in Indonesia. The distribution of *S. mekongi* is limited to the central Mekong basin in Laos and Cambodia, and of *S. intercalatum* to pockets in West and Central Africa.

Schistosomiasis is typically an infection of traditional rural areas, but it has also spread to many human settlements around artificial dams and irrigated lands [1–3, 28]. Examples are Lake Nasser and several newly reclaimed areas in Egypt; Lake Volta in West Africa; dams on the Senegal River in Mali, Mauritania and Senegal; hundreds of small village dams throughout Africa; the irrigated sugar estates in Brazil; canal systems in China, and, possibly in the future, the Three Gorges Dam area. Despite mandatory and elaborate risk assessments, food production and socioeconomic development take precedence over future health concerns. Urban schistosomiasis is becoming an increasing problem throughout Africa, South America and Asia. In many shantytowns, snail populations thrive in local canals, drains or small irrigated plots. As sanitation and water supply are often poor, migratory and other exchanges with rural endemic areas easily leads to the establishment of permanent transmission within city boundaries.

COMMUNITY EPIDEMIOLOGY

Our understanding of the epidemiology of schistosomiasis is based on indirect measures of worm burdens, i.e. the presence and number of eggs excreted by individuals in a known volume of excreta [1, 3, 27]. These are useful at the community and group level, but much less accurate in individuals owing to significant day-to-day and individual variations of egg excretion. Worm burdens have been directly counted in only a few autopsy studies, and further approximated in mathematical models or using circulating antigen levels. Other methodologic handicaps include difficulty measuring snail densities and infection rates, cercarial of miracidial densities, human water contact or acquired resistance [20].

The overall prevalence of infection in communities living under endemic conditions is usually between 30% and 100% [1]. However, particularly in areas with low intensities of transmission and infections, many light infections go undetected on routine screening, and the true prevalence may be 2–3 times higher than that observed [29]. In addition, many adults who are microscopically negative for ova have probably had earlier infections, as demonstrated by the persistence of specific antibodies.

Depending on the intensity of transmission and local habits, infections can be detected in toddlers from the age of 6 months onwards – sometimes even earlier [30]. In almost all foci, prevalence and intensities of infection, as measured by egg excretion, rise strongly from the age of 5–7 years to a peak in the age group between the age of 8 and15 years, and then decline substantially in adults [1, 3]. The peak age usually falls a few years earlier in heavily infected communities. Boys are usually more heavily infected than girls as they play more often and intensively in water. In adults, gender differences depend on occupational activities.

While these observations can be partly explained by water contact patterns, many epidemiologic, clinical and immunologic studies indicate that people living in endemic areas develop some form of acquired resistance after years of exposure [1, 22]. However, similar age-related infection rates are also observed in communities only recently exposed to transmission through migration or newly established transmission. As acquired immunity cannot be invoked in such cases, it might represent age-related innate resistance, possibly influenced by hormonal changes [21].

CLINICAL DISEASE AND PATHOLOGIC CORRELATES

The pathogenesis of schistosomiasis is largely based upon the host reaction against the different parasite stages, rather than their presence. The adult worms living in the bloodstream are seldom associated with clinical illness. They rarely cause vascular obstruction in ectopic areas, for example cerebral or spinal arteries. Early clinical manifestations associated with migratory schistosomulae include

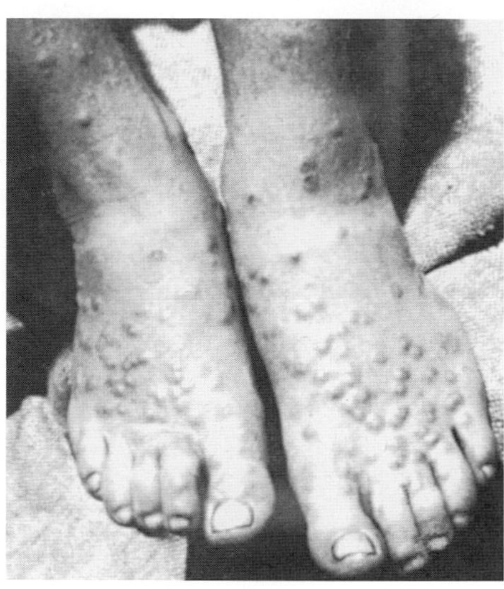

FIGURE 122.4 Swimmers' itch. *(Courtesy of Dr A J Bearup, School of Public Health and Tropical Medicine, University of Sydney, NSW, Australia).*

cercarial dermatitis and acute systemic schistosomiasis (Katayama fever). Chronic schistosomiasis is largely associated with the granulomatous and fibrotic responses to *Schistosoma* ova during mature, chronic infections [12]. Severity of clinical disease and susceptibility to praziquantel varies between geographic areas, suggesting *Schistosoma* subspecies, or strain differences, between and within countries and continents; apparently, immunogenetic traits among populations affect the epidemiology and pathophysiology of schistosomiasis as well [3].

CERCARIAL DERMATITIS (Fig. 122.4)

Non-sensitized and sensitized individuals respond with marked differences to the penetration of the skin by cercariae. Initial exposures produce only mild, transient reactions that can be unnoticed or cause only a mild prickling sensation as the water evaporates and the parasites penetrate the skin. Macules usually appear within 12 hours on the exposed skin in non-sensitized persons and rapidly disappear. However, in previously sensitized persons they are followed by pruritic papules, erythema and, in more severe cases, vesicles, edema and pruritus. Cercarial dermatitis most commonly occurs with *S. mansoni* and *S. haematobium* and is unusual with *S. japonicum*. A similar "swimmers' itch" is also frequently caused by cercariae of animal and bird trematodes in tropical areas or during summer in temperate climate zones, including Europe and North America [1, 17]. Pathologically, these focal lesions show edema and heavy dermal and epidermal eosinophil and mononuclear cell infiltrates resulting from subcutaneous cercarial death. Cercarial dermatitis resolves in 7–10 days without permanent tissue damage or scarring.

ACUTE SCHISTOSOMIASIS (KATAYAMA FEVER)

Acute schistosomiasis, or "Katayama fever" by its historical Japanese name, is a systemic hypersensitivity reaction against the migrating schistosomulae and/or the onset of egg production, occurring within a few weeks to months after a primary infection [31, 32]. It can be caused by all schistosome species. Usually, the onset is sudden with fever, fatigue, myalgia, malaise, nonproductive cough, marked peripheral eosinophilia, elevated IgE and patchy infiltrates on chest x-ray. Early symptoms are mostly caused by allergic reactions to the migratory schistosomulae as they congregate in the pulmonary microvasculature en route to the liver. A few weeks later, abdominal symptoms may develop because of the migration and positioning of the mature worms and the start of ovideposition in the tissues. Most patients recover spontaneously after 2–10 weeks, but some develop a persistent and serious illness with weight loss, dyspnea, diarrhea, diffuse abdominal pain, toxemia, hepatosplenomegaly and generalized rash. Intense infections occasionally are fatal.

Acute schistosomiasis caused by *S. mansoni* and *S. haematobium* is rarely reported within chronically exposed populations. It is not an infrequent diagnosis in tourists, travelers and others accidentally exposed to transmission. Most cases in Western travel clinics are imported from sub-Saharan Africa, often in family or group clusters [31, 33]. Exposures frequently occur in Lakes Malawi, Victoria and Volta, the Zambesi and Niger deltas, the Dogon country of Mali, and lake resorts in South Africa. The infective water contacts range from bathing and swimming to scuba diving, water skiing and rafting. Serious neurologic complications can occur as a result of ectopic worms or eggs in the spinal cord.

Katayama fever caused by *S. japonicum* infections can present as serious, sometimes fatal, serum sickness-like disease which possibly results from the early release of large quantities of egg antigens that cross-react with antibodies to schistosomula, resulting in immune complexes that cause hypertrophy of lymphoreticular tissue [1–3, 32. This prototypic Katayama syndrome is characterized by fever, hepatosplenomegaly and cachexia which may evolve directly to severe hepatosplenic fibrosis and portal hypertension. Unlike African schistosomiasis, it is not restricted to primary infection, but also occurs in people living in endemic areas and in those with a history of previous infections. In China, true "rebound epidemics" have been reported in endemic communities exposed to floods.

CHRONIC PATHOLOGY AND ILLNESS

In chronically established infections most pathology is caused by cellular and fibrotic immune reactions against eggs that are trapped in the tissues during their perivesical or peri-intestinal migration, or after embolization to the liver, spleen, lungs or cerebrospinal system [12, 34, 35]. The ova secrete proteolytic enzymes that sensitize local lymphocytes which in turn mobilize macrophages, lymphocytes, eosinophils and fibroblasts that encapsulate the egg with a typical granuloma. Early, acute granulomas are usually composed of eosinophils and neutrophils, as well as mononuclear cells. Macrophages, lymphocytes, fibroblasts and multinucleated giant cells dominate the chronic granuloma. The acute granuloma is large and diffuse, whereas the more chronic granuloma is smaller and better circumscribed (Fig. 122.5).

The egg granuloma is thought to be protective, as well as pathogenic. In healthy hosts it reduces, or confines, tissue necrosis. Granuloma formation is largely a product of TH2 cytokines. As cell-mediated immunity reactions are downregulated over time, the granulomas are reduced in size and gradually replaced by collagen depositions. In some, but not all patients, this balance is disturbed and the collagen deposition leads to fibrosis. Depending on the tissue egg load, a great number of microlesions may merge into the typical fibrotic streaks that cause most of the irreversible pathology in all forms of schistosomiasis. The severity of chronic diseases is thus related to the intensity of infection on one hand, and individual immune responses on the other. Severe forms are mostly seen in individuals with previously high parasite loads, and probably some form of immunogenetic predisposition [3, 24].

While in such cases schistosomiasis is a serious and sometimes life-threatening disease, many infections remain asymptomatic or cause only mild, vague or intermittent symptoms of malaise, drowsiness, abdominal discomfort and mucus or blood-specked diarrhea [1–3]. In endemic areas, it is common to detect many infected persons without, at first sight, noticeable consequences. Often, however, treatment is followed by spontaneous, widespread reports of improved wellbeing, fitness and appetite. Also in tourists or migrants, infection is regularly a chance finding, sometimes decades after exposure.

URINARY SCHISTOSOMIASIS

The eggs of *S. haematobium* provoke granulomatous inflammation, ulceration and pseudopolyposis of the mucosa and submucosa of the bladder and the ureters [3, 36]. Obstructive uropathy occurs when such lesions are located in the ureter or in the bladder near the ureteral inlet. Bladder and ureteral obstruction may result in urine stasis,

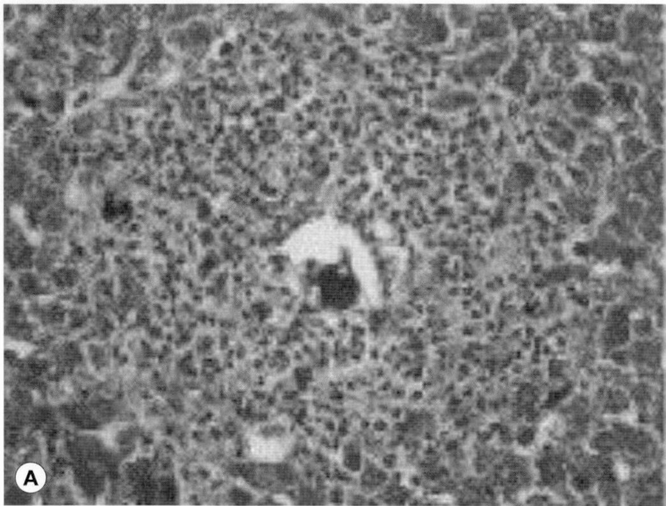

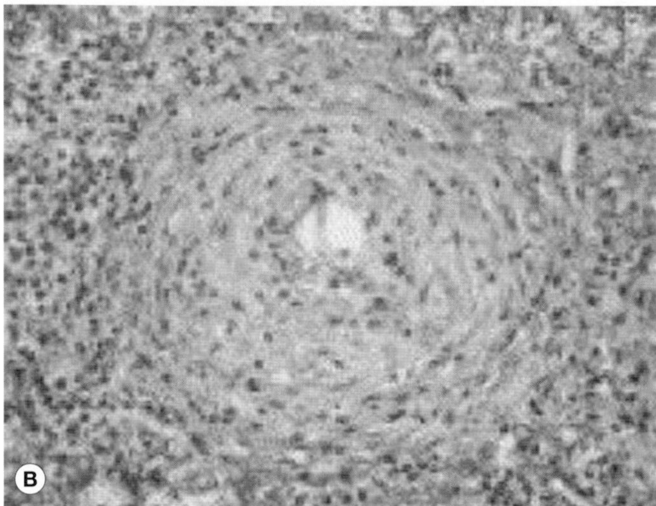

FIGURE 122.5 Histopathology in schistosomiasis: early **(A)** and late **(B)** egg granulomas in the liver. *(Reproduced with permission from Gryseels B, Polman K, Clerinx J, Kestens L. Human schistosomiasis. Lancet 2006;368:1106–18.)*

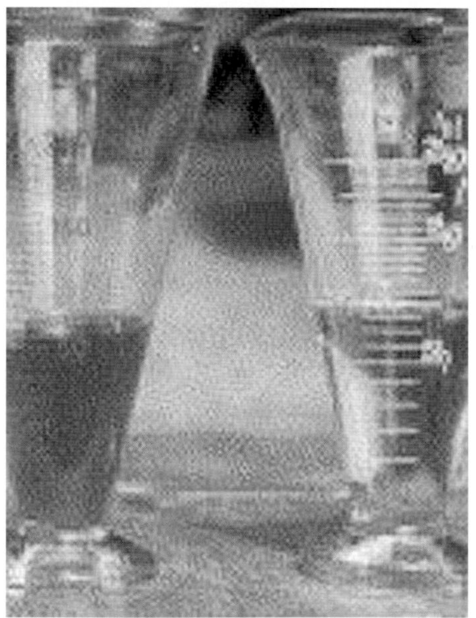

FIGURE 122.6 Urinary schistosomiasis: macroscopic hematuria, the "red flag" of urinary schistosomiasis in children. *(Reproduced with permission from Gryseels B, Polman K, Clerinx J, Kestens L. Human schistosomiasis. Lancet 2006;368:1106–18.)*

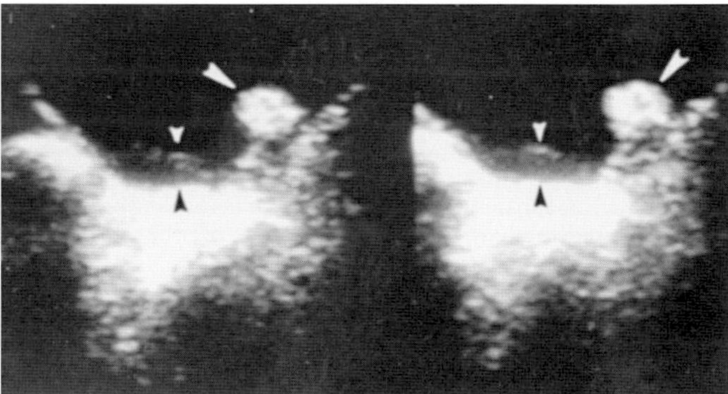

FIGURE 122.7 Urinary schistosomiasis. Ultrasonographic view of bladder. Thickening and irregularity of the bladder wall (small arrows) and a large polyp (large arrows) are present.

disruption of the normal bacteriostatic mechanisms of the bladder mucosa and urinary tract infection. Although rarer following the widespread use of antischistosomal chemotherapy, abdominal radiographs may show calcium deposits around extensive deposits of calcified *Schistosoma* eggs in the bladder wall.

Common early symptoms of urinary schistosomiasis include dysuria, urinary frequency and urgency, proteinuria and, particularly, hematuria. In endemic areas, the latter is the "red flag of schistosomiasis" in children between the age of 5 and 10 years old, sometimes mistakenly considered as the onset of menstruation in girls, or even as a similar coming of age in boys (Fig. 122.6). Typically, blood is first seen in the terminal urine; in more severe cases, the urine can be dark-colored and bacterial super-infection is a common complication. These symptoms mostly wane as the child becomes older. In non-treated populations exposed to *S. haematobium*, microhematuria can be present in 40–100% of infected children [39]. Bladder pathology and upper urinary tract lesions can be detected by ultrasound or radiology in many infected people (Figs 122.7 and 122.8). Many cases with serious morphologic lesions show a surprisingly preserved renal function.

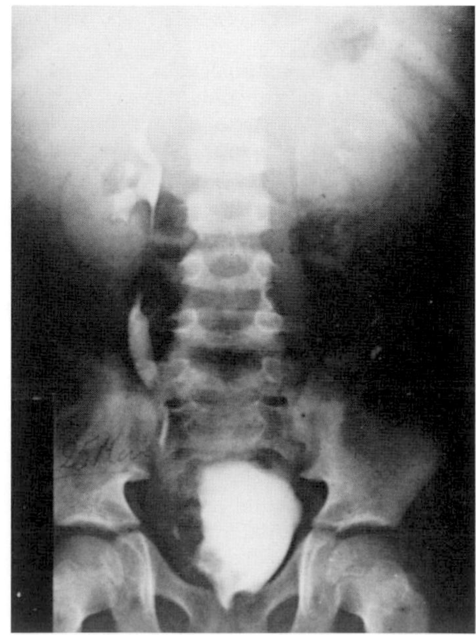

FIGURE 122.8 Urinary schistosomiasis. Intravenous pyelogram showing a large bladder filling defect caused by granulomatous polyp formation. Early right hydronephrosis and hydroureter are also present. *(Courtesy of U.S. Naval Medical Research Unit No.3, Cairo, Egypt).*

Lesions can reverse spontaneously with age and usually heal well after antischistosomal therapy. Chronic infection may lead to obstructive uropathy, renal failure and bladder cancer.

Obstructive Uropathy (Figs 122.7 and 122.8)

Fibrosis of the bladder and lower ureters with hydroureter and hydronephrosis occurs in the lower third of the ureter or in the bladder. It may remain clinically silent for years, while being easily visualized in pyelograms or ultrasound, and is usually reversible with chemotherapy. Hydronephrosis is initially caused by compression; the parenchyma can eventually be destroyed leading to renal failure. Secondary chronic bacteriuria and pyelonephritis, sometimes complicated by septicemia, may be the presenting manifestation and can be fatal.

Bladder Cancer

Chronic urinary schistosomiasis is epidemiologically associated with high incidences of squamous cell bladder carcinoma in Egypt and, less clearly, in some other African foci [3, 37]. In Egypt, the incidence of bladder cancer has decreased over the past 2–3 decades along with the prevalence of urinary schistosomiasis following praziquantel MDA. In addition to causing chronic inflammation of the bladder wall, the schistosomal lesions may enhance the exposure of the bladder epithelium to carcinogenic substrates. Apart from gross hematuria, bladder cancer often presents with frequency, urgency, dysuria, weight loss and metastasis to the inguinal, femoral and retroperitoneal lymph nodes.

INTESTINAL SCHISTOSOMIASIS

The eggs of *S. mansoni*, *S. japonicum* and other species migrate through the intestinal wall where they provoke mucosal granulomatous inflammation, pseudopolyposis, micro-ulcerations and superficial bleeding. Most lesions are situated in the large bowel and the rectum; small bowel pathology is rare [38].

Most common symptoms attributed to intestinal schistosomiasis are chronic or intermittent abdominal pain and discomfort, loss of appetite and mucous diarrhea with or without blood, although occult blood in the stool is very common [1–3, 39]. Physical examination may be normal or show moderate abdominal distention, diffuse mild abdominal tenderness and hyperactive bowel sounds.

Intestinal polyposis, ulcers, fistula and strictures have been attributed to *S. mansoni*. In such cases, diffuse, protein-losing enteropathy may occur, with chronic mucohemorrhagic diarrhea, weight loss and anemia. Physical examination reveals a distended abdomen with diffuse tenderness or localized tenderness over the transverse and descending colon. Severe, long-standing granulomatous or polypous lesions may result in partial or complete bowel obstruction and, in rare cases, appendicitis or perforation. Intense dysenteric syndromes are exceptional, but in some cases fatal. *Schistosoma japonicum* and *S. mansoni* have both been associated with colon cancer, but the evidence for causation is weak.

The reported frequency of intestinal disease in people living in endemic areas infected with *S. mansoni* or *S. japonicum* is usually 10–50% [39]. In general, intestinal morbidity is strongly correlated with intensities of infection, both at the population and at the individual level.

HEPATOSPLENIC SCHISTOSOMIASIS

(Figs 122.9 and 122.10)

Hepatic schistosomiasis can be caused by *S. mansoni*, *S. japonicum* and *S. mekongi*. The pathologic impact of *S. intercalatum* is restricted to mild intestinal disease. Hepatic and hepatosplenic schistosomiasis can be caused by either early inflammatory or late fibrotic hepatic disease, with quite different underlying pathology and prognoses [1–3].

Inflammatory Hepatic Schistosomiasis

This is an early reaction to ova trapped in the hepatic presinusoidal periportal spaces where many granulomas are produced (Fig. 122.5A).

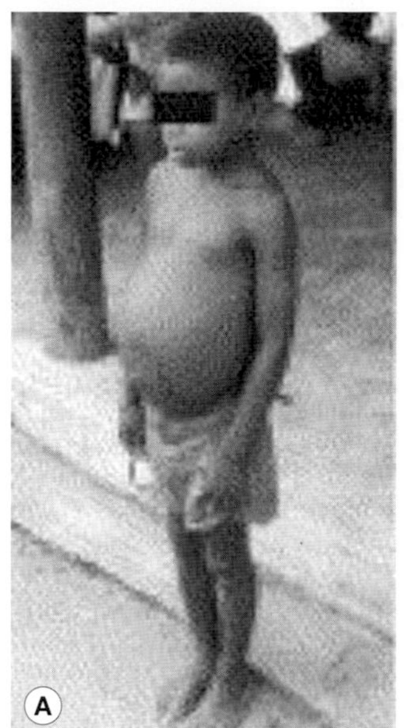

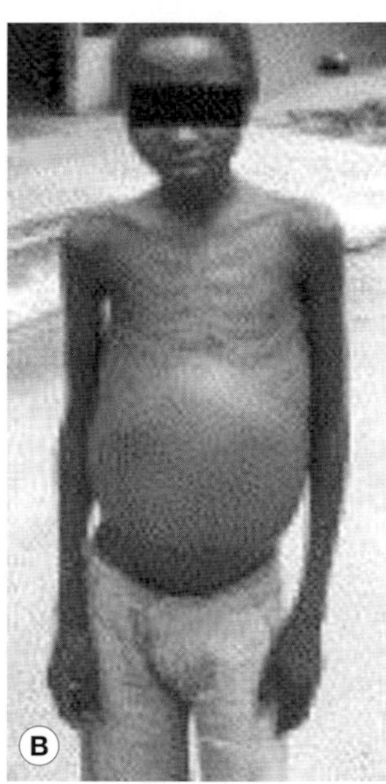

FIGURE 122.9 Early **(A)** and late **(B)** hepatosplenic schistosomiasis mansoni. *(Reproduced with permission from Gryseels B, Polman K, Clerinx J, Kestens L. Human schistosomiasis. Lancet 2006;368:1106–18.)*

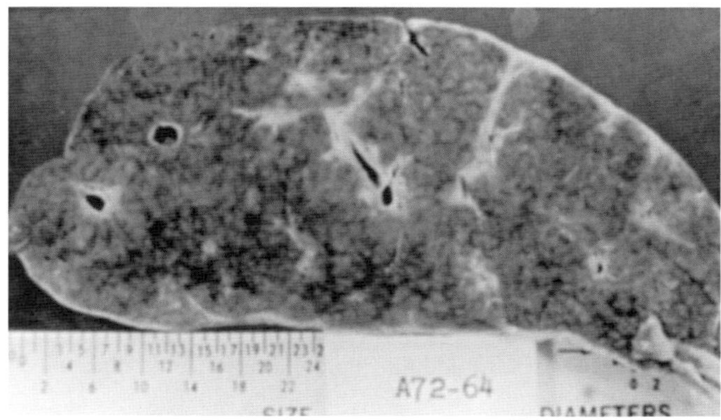

FIGURE 122.10 Cut surface of the liver showing Symmer's clay pipe stem fibrosis in a patient infected with *Schistosoma mansoni*. *(Courtesy of U. S. Naval Medical Research Unit No. 3, Cairo, Egypt).*

It is the main cause of schistosomal hepatomegaly in children and adolescents, often associated with hyperplastic splenomegaly and strongly correlated with the intensity of infection. Typical features include sharp-edged enlargement of the left lobe of the liver and nodular splenomegaly. In most cases, the organomegaly is mild but sometimes the liver and spleen may extend below the umbilicus and into the pelvis (Fig. 122.9A). Usually, liver cell function is normal and jaundice is absent. In young children, clinical differentiation from malaria may be difficult. In heavily endemic areas, this type of hepatomegaly, with or without splenomegaly, is present in 30% or more of infected children and adolescents, but much less in adults. The frequency and severity correlate with intensities of infection, but are also subject to methodologic variations, immunogenetic predisposition and other confounding factors [39].

Fibrotic or Chronic Hepatic Schistosomiasis

This complication develops years later in the course of infection and in a minority of those infected. It is believed to be a consequence of long-standing intense infection, as well as dysfunctional or overpolarized immune responses which fail to downregulate granulomatous and fibrotic reactions [24]. Diffuse collagen deposits in the periportal spaces occur (Fig. 122.5B) and confluence of the resulting fibrotic streaks leads to the pathognomic "Symmer's pipe stem fibrosis", in which the elongated periportal fibrotic lesions resemble clay pipe stems (Fig. 122.10). Physical occlusion of the portal veins leads to portal hypertension, increased splenic vein pressure and tortuosity and splenomegaly. Portal hypertension results in collateralization of the abdominal venous circulation, which may show externally as a "caput medusa", and leads internally to portocaval shunting and gastrointestinal varices. This condition also facilitates the distribution of *Schistosoma* eggs into the general circulation and the occurrence of ectopic lesions in the lungs, spinal cord (Fig. 122.11) or the brain. End-stage hepatosplenic schistosomiasis can be marked by ascites (Fig. 122.9B).

The extent of exposure, immunogenetic predisposition, concomitant infections and nutritional deficiencies all contribute to the severity of the disease. The liver is not necessarily enlarged, but is usually hard and nodular on palpation. In contrast to cirrhosis, the parenchyma, hepatocellular functions and its biologic parameters remain largely unaffected. Fibrotic hepatic schistosomiasis is mainly seen in young and middle-aged adults, although it can occur in heavily infected adolescents. In *S. mansoni* infections, this takes at least 5–15 years to develop, by which time ova may not be present or detectable. In *S. japonicum*, the progression may be more rapid, in some cases with little, or no, interval between acute and chronic disease.

Bleeding from gastro-esophageal varices is the most serious, and often fatal, complication of fibrotic hepatic schistosomiasis. In *S. mansoni* infections, it tends to recur and become more severe over time; in *S. japonicum*, bleeding is often sudden and massive. Repeated or occult bleeding may lead to anemia, hypoalbuminemia, cachexia and growth retardation. Ascites can be caused by a combination of hypoalbuminemia and portal hypertension, or concomitant infection with hepatitis B or C.

Advanced liver fibrosis caused by schistosomiasis used to be a frequent and severe health problem in large parts of Egypt, Brazil, China, the Philippines and other countries. Over the past few decades, chemotherapy and general socioeconomic development have led to a dramatic reduction of such morbidity worldwide. Symptomatic liver fibrosis has always been less frequent in sub-Saharan Africa, except for some East-African foci, for example West Nile in Uganda, Machakos in Kenya and Gezirah in Sudan [39]. These varying continental and regional morbidity patterns may be partially explained by ethnic and genetic factors, in addition to the intensities of exposure to infection.

OTHER COMPLICATIONS AND ECTOPIC SCHISTOSOMIASIS

Pulmonary Schistosomiasis

This syndrome is a complication of portocaval shunting caused by portal hypertension in chronic *S. mansoni* infection which allows ova to pass into the peri-alveolar capillary beds [1, 3, 40]. The ensuing granulomas cause obliterative arteritis which leads to fibrosis resulting in pulmonary hypertension, increased right heart pressure, pulmonary artery and right atrial dilatation, and right ventricular hypertrophy. Schistosomal cor pulmonale has been mostly described in Brazil and Egypt, but appears to have become much less frequent over the last decades.

Schistosomal Glomerulonephritis

Immune complexes can be deposited in the renal glomeruli during *S. mansoni* infections [41]. Schistosomal glomerulonephritis used to be found quite commonly in renal biopsies from patients with *S. mansoni* infection in Brazil, but this finding was usually asymptomatic or clinically insignificant. Nephrotic syndrome is seen occasionally in patients with *S. mansoni* or *S. haematobium* infections, sometimes associated with chronic *Salmonella* bacteremia or bacteriuria.

Genital Schistosomiasis

Schistosoma haematobium and *S. mansoni* ova that are trapped in the reproductive organs remain mostly occult in endemic areas, but are a regular finding in travelers. Hypertrophic and ulcerative lesions of the vulva, vagina and cervix may facilitate the transmission of sexually transmitted infections, including HIV. Lesions of the ovaries and the fallopian tubes can lead to infertility. In males, the epididymis, testicles, spermatic cord and prostate may be affected; hemospermia is a common symptom [42].

Neuroschistosomiasis

This severe complication is caused by inflammation around ectopic worms or eggs in the cerebral or spinal venous plexus, which can evolve to irreversible fibrotic scars if left untreated [1–3, 43]. Ectopic *S. mansoni* and *S. haematobium* infections mainly cause spinal cord pathology with transverse myelitis, which is also a potential complication of acute schistosomiasis in travelers [31, 33]. Symptoms vary with the location and the degree of the myelitis, and may include paraplegia and loss of bladder and/or anal sphincter control. Sometimes, the patient may have pain or loss of sensation; rarely there will be a rash around the body affecting the dermatome at the level of the spinal cord lesion.

Schistosoma japonicum, possibly because of the larger number and smaller size, or the clustering of the eggs, is associated with cerebral granulomatous lesions that can be either diffuse or focal, possibly depending on whether eggs have been randomly embolized from a distance or locally-released by ectopic worm pairs. Depending on type and location, the resulting syndrome may have an epileptic, paralytic or meningo-encephalitic character. The acute phase, which occurs months after exposure, may be accompanied by fever, urticaria, eosinophilia and angioneurotic edema suggesting an allergic encephalopathy. There may be delirium, confusion, personality changes, incontinence, coma, nuchal rigidity, pyramidal track signs and cerebellar symptoms. The acute phase may merge into a chronic phase, which could be asymptomatic or mimic intracranial neoplasm. Epileptic syndromes often include Jacksonian or grand mal seizures, stemming from lesions in the parietal lobe. Other neurologic signs and symptoms are headaches, speech difficulties, visual disturbances, papilledema and cerebellar symptoms [43].

Other Sites

Ectopic schistosomal lesions in the skin can present as maculopapules or wart-like protuberances, the latter particularly in the genital area [2]. Schistosomal granulomas in the peritoneum may be mistaken for endometriosis, miliary tuberculosis or cancer metastasis. Granulomas around stray eggs have also been documented in the pancreas, gallbladder, stomach, heart, kidney and adrenal glands, with or without recognized clinical manifestations.

ASSOCIATION OF SCHISTOSOMIASIS AND OTHER INFECTIONS

Chronic *Salmonella* Co-Infections

Schistosomiasis has been associated with the presence of several co-infections, especially chronic persistent *Salmonella* bacteremia [1]. Possible explanations include immunologic tolerance caused by schistosomiasis and the physical attachment and proliferation of *Salmonella* bacteria on, or in, adult worms. The syndrome was seen mainly in males between the age of 15–30 years, but has become rare. It is characterized by a long history of indolent febrile disease, bacteremia with one or more *Salmonella* species and chronic active schistosomiasis. It differs from enteric fever caused by *S. typhi* by negative stool cultures, a petechial rash on the lower extremities rather than on the abdomen, and the absence of systemic complications, for example prostration, delirium or localized infections.

Co-Infections with Hepatitis B and C

Chronic *S. mansoni* infected patients co-infected with hepatitis B or C are prone to have clinically more severe infections. Prior parenteral treatment for schistosomiasis may also have substantially increased the risk for hepatitis infections in some areas, especially Egypt [13,

26]. Patients with co-infections more often develop jaundice, intractable ascites and hepatic failure. In fact, patients with chronic schistosomiasis who have elevations in serum alanine transaminase (ALT) or aspartate transaminase (AST) have a high probability of having concomitant hepatitis B and/or C infections. Proper precautions should be taken in the management of the patient and the handling of blood samples.

INDIRECT PATHOLOGY AND MORBIDITY

Before the advent of modern treatment and control, *S. japonicum* infection was believed to be related to reduced stature, weight, weight-for-height, skin-fold thickness, muscle mass and other anthropometric measures, especially during childhood and adolescence. These clinical and epidemiologic observations, although historical and not always rigorously documented, indicate an independent effect of the infection on nutrition, growth and development. This impact on physical development was widespread and is thought to have substantially reduced economic productivity in China at one time, when schistosomiasis was considered "the plague of gods" and its control received high political priority [2].

However, early studies to establish an association between general wellbeing, anthropometric indices, nutritional status and physical or cognitive performance, and the presence or intensity of *S. mansoni* or *S. haematobium* infection were largely inconclusive or contradictory [39]. Possibly, they were obscured by the frequent comorbidities from malarial, intestinal helminths, protozoa, bacterial and viral infections. As severe disease from *Schistosoma* infections has waned in many areas, subtle or "indirect" morbidity has become the target of more focused research efforts and is providing a rationale for sustained control strategies. Significant associations have now been demonstrated for anemia, nutritional status, cognitive and physiologic capacities [44].

GLOBAL BURDEN OF DISEASE (GBD)

Schistosomiasis is highly prevalent but the associated morbidity is low and variable. The GBD of schistosomiasis, as expressed in Disability-Adjusted Life Years (DALY), depends on the number of people infected on one hand, and the mortality and disability attributed to it on the other [45]. The total number of cases in the world is estimated by the WHO at 200 million, a figure that is consistently quoted in the literature but may need to be revised downward in view of recent trends [2, 7–9]. The GBD estimates report up to 15,000 lives lost to schistosomiasis annually, and applies a "disability weight" of 0.06. The total number of DALYs lost to schistosomiasis is estimated at 1.75–2.0 million, of which 85% are in sub-Saharan Africa. This is a fraction of the GBD of AIDS, malaria or tuberculosis, and puts it in the same league as lymphatic filariasis, leishmaniasis and trypanosomiasis. Schistosomiasis would account for 0.1% of the GBD in the world and 0.4% of the GBD in sub-Saharan Africa.

These figures have been contested by many schistosomiasis experts when advocating for global control efforts [8, 44, 46, 47]. Upgrades of as much as a 40-fold increase of schistosomiasis mortality in sub-Saharan Africa, and a 4–30-fold upgrade of the disability weight have been proposed. These revised data have not been empirically validated, however, and remain inconsistent with total mortality and GBD data. This does not reduce the need, however, to bring treatment and control to affected populations.

DIAGNOSIS

MEDICAL HISTORY AND EXAMINATION

Within endemic areas, schistosomiasis must be suspected in all patients presenting any symptom, however vague, that can be related to the infection. In travelers and migrants, a careful residence or travel history can help establish the diagnosis of schistosomiasis [31, 33]. In several sub-Saharan areas, both *S. mansoni* and *S. haematobium*, and even *S. intercalatum*, can be contracted. The patient who has lived in, or visited, endemic areas must be asked about skin contact with freshwater of any kind, even if considered locally as safe or snail-free. Contacts of any type or duration can lead to infection. The patient may, or may not, report itching or rash shortly after the water contact. Visual inspection may help diagnose "swimmers' itch" after recent exposure.

A medical history may reveal intermittent symptoms since the potential exposure, including flu-like syndromes in the weeks or months thereafter. Malaise, fatigue, muscle pains, appetite loss, intermittent diarrhea, vague abdominal pain and red or dark urine are potential warning signs – partly depending on the suspected species. A neurologic history and examination is performed to exclude early cerebrospinal involvement. Abdominal palpation may reveal hepatomegaly or splenomegaly of varying degrees and abdominal tenderness or distention, but also may be entirely negative.

LABORATORY FINDINGS

Rapid tests can include a visual inspection or a hematuria dip-stick test of the urine for *S. haematobium*, or occult blood in the stools for *S. mansoni* and *S. japonicum*; these are very useful tools for rapid diagnosis and community screening in the endemic areas [1–3, 39]. In tourists and migrants, the most important hematologic indicator is eosinophilia, which is usually elevated in acute schistosomiasis but may be negative in chronic cases. Other hematologic or biochemical parameters, including liver function tests, are often within normal limits but abnormal values can indicate chronic complications, for example anemia or renal failure, or comorbidities, such as hepatitis. Mild anemia is not unusual in infected persons living in endemic areas and the serum alkaline phosphatase level may be elevated. If the ALT or AST levels are elevated, a concomitant hepatitis B and/or C infection should be suspected. Recently, DNA detection in serum was shown to be very sensitive and specific for the early diagnosis of schistosomiasis [48].

SCHISTOSOMA *OVA IDENTIFICATION BY MICROSCOPY* (Fig. 122.11)

The microscopic demonstration and identification of eggs in excreta remains the gold standard for the diagnosis of active schistosomiasis, but has low sensitivity in light infections [29]. In rare cases, incidental exposure may lead to infection with only male or female worms, in which case there is no ova production. If eggs are found, their size and shape allows easy detection and identification under low magnification. Direct microscopic examinations of wet-mounted slides are not reliable, as they contain only a few milligrams of feces or milliliters of urine. Concentration methods and repeated examinations in different urine or stool specimens on different days may be required to confirm the presence of active infections. Stools may be concentrated with general techniques, for example Ritchie's formol-ether method, or more specific ones, such as conical flask sedimentation in glycerine water, sieving or miracidial hatching. Urine may be centrifuged, sedimented or passed through paper or nylon filters with a variety of devices [1, 49, 50]. Sensitivity increases considerably with the weight or volume of the sample examined. The excretion of *S. haematobium* eggs in the urine is not uniform over a day, and samples collected between 10.00 h and 14.00 h are more likely to be positive. Also, physical exercise before sampling increases the chance of finding eggs in the urine. The microscopic examination of crushed rectal snips, obtained during proctoscopy or sigmoidoscopy, is remarkably sensitive for *S. mansoni* and *S. japonicum*, as well as *S. haematobium* infection. Rectal biopsies can be performed during proctoscopy or sigmoidoscopy by taking 1–3 small mucosal samples from inflamed or granulomatous lesions, or from random areas of normal-appearing mucosa. The mucosal sample is pressed between a cover slip and a glass slide until it becomes transparent. If ova are present, they can be seen under low power microscopy. Also, bladder biopsies obtained during cystoscopy can be directly examined for eggs. The biopsies can be partly fixed in formalin for histologic staining and examination, which may reveal eggs, as well as inflammation and typical granulomas.

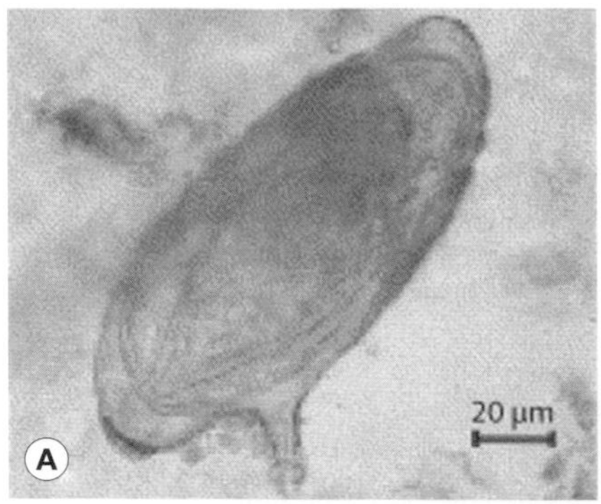

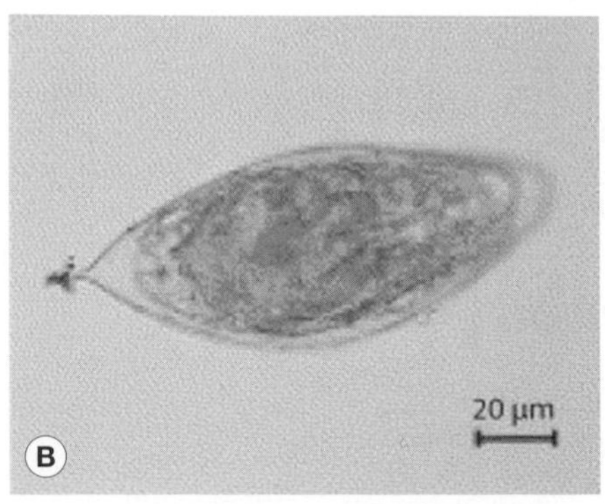

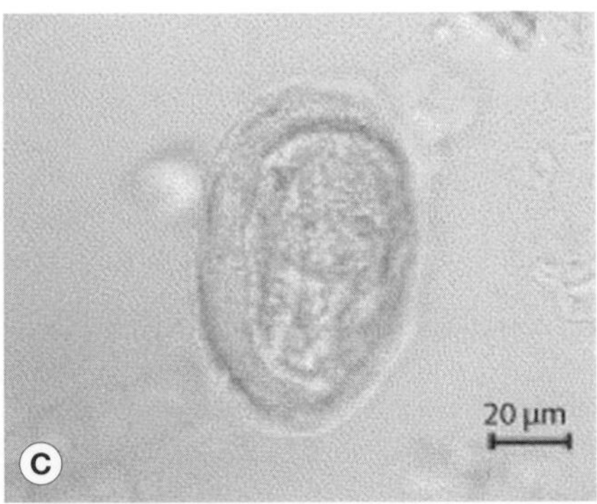

FIGURE 122.11 Schistosome eggs under the microscope. **(A)** *S. mansoni* (from lateral spine); **(B)** *S. haematobium* (from terminal spine); **(C)** *S. japonicum* (from small lateral spine). *(Reproduced with permission from Gryseels B, Polman K, Clerinx J, Kestens L. Human schistosomiasis. Lancet 2006;368:1106–18.)*

Egg counts in calibrated samples provide a quantitative assessment of the infection. Quantitative egg counts after standardized urine filtration or in calibrated fecal thick smears (Kato-Katz method) are especially useful for epidemiologic surveys and control, as they correlate reasonably well with worm burdens and morbidity. For the Kato-Katz method, a 50 mg sample of feces is pressed through a 105-mesh steel sieve and fitted in the hole of a punched template, which rests on a glass microscope slide. This calibrated sample of filtered feces is then covered with a cellophane cover-slip impregnated with glycerin, inverted and pressed onto a bed of filter paper. The slide is left for 24–48 hours while the fecal matter clears. Then, all eggs on the slide are counted under a microscope. Multiplying by 20 gives the number of eggs per gram of feces (EPG). Limitations of the test are that formed stools are desirable, light infections tend to be missed when examining small amounts of feces, and the microscopist must be reliable. The most common quantitative technique for urine is filtrating 10 ml with a syringe through a paper, nucleopore or nytrel filter, which is then examined under a microscope and the number of eggs counted. This method provides a measure of eggs per 10 ml of urine [49, 50].

In clinical settings and in field surveys requiring accuracy, 3–5 repeated examinations with Kato-Katz or 10 ml urine filtration may be needed. It may be important to verify the ova's viability, particularly to determine whether drug treatment has been successful. Dead *Schistosoma* ova in the tissues can be excreted in the urine and stool for months after adult worms are dead. Eggs passed more than one week after treatment are usually not viable. Microscopic examination of viable eggs will reveal clear, transparent structures with moving organelles (flame cells) of the miracidium. Dead eggs are often deformed, dark or half-empty, and show no internal movement. Alternatively, ova may be hatched to demonstrate their viability by diluting a small amount of urine or stool sediment in distilled water at room temperature and exposing it to light for 15–20 minutes. Ideally, it is put in a covered, darkened flask with a narrow top, which is left exposed to the light. Examination with a hand-held lens will reveal swimming miracidia.

SEROLOGY

Antibody-Based Serum Assays

Many serologic methods have been developed for the indirect diagnosis of schistosomiasis [49–52]. These are quite sensitive but can not distinguish a past infection from a present active one. Some tests also may cross-react with other helminths and they are not easily applicable in the field. Serologic assays are important, however, for diagnosis in travelers, migrants and other occasionally-exposed people. They can also provide important circumstantial evidence when complications of schistosomiasis are suspected, especially neuroschistosomiasis, even when urine and stools are microscopically negative. Most routine techniques detect IgG, IgM or IgE against soluble worm antigen (SWA) or crude egg antigen (CEA) by enzyme immune assays (EIA). Seroconversion takes place usually within 4–8 weeks after infection, but, rarely, antibodies might not be detected for 4–5 months after infection. Most assays remain positive for at least two years after cure, and often much longer.

Circulating Schistosome Antigens

Circulating anodic antigen (CAA) and circulating cathodic antigen (CCA) can be detected and quantified in serum or urine with labeled monoclonal antibodies in different formats, including reagent strips [50, 52, 53]. These are *Schistosoma* gut glycoproteins regurgitated with the metabolized blood particles into the circulation of the human host. Antigen detection in serum is not sensitive in light infections, however, and therefore not very useful for clinical applications. These assays are primarily used in epidemiologic and therapeutic studies. Urine-based assays are more sensitive, but less specific.

CHEMICAL TESTING

Using reagent strips to test for blood in urine and simple questionnaires for visible hematuria are inexpensive, easy and effective tools for the screening and rapid assessment of urinary schistosomiasis [1–3, 29, 49, 50]. Indirect diagnostic methods for intestinal or hepatic schistosomiasis, for example examining the stool for mucus and blood, are reasonably sensitive, but less specific.

ENDOSCOPY AND CYSTOSCOPY

Endoscopy can visualize esophageal varices; sigmoidoscopy and colonoscopy allow visualizing of typical schistosomiasis lesions and provide access to biopsy specimens for tissue egg identification [1, 54]. The endoscopist can visualize small petechiae in otherwise normal rectal mucosa, dull patches with a sandpaper-like appearance, superficial erosions, stellate superficial ulcerations, hyperemic, easy bleeding areas, and granulomatous or polyp disease; the latter can be removed during the procedure. Laparoscopy can reveal granulomatous inflammation or periportal fibrosis. Needle biopsies of the liver may not sample the hard fibrotic lesions; wedge biopsies may be needed, for instance, to differentiate periportal fibrosis from post-infectious or alcoholic cirrhosis. Cystoscopy may reveal hemorrhagic inflammation, granulomatosis, polyposis, fibrosis or calcification of the bladder, and allow biopsy sampling.

IMAGING (Figs 122.7, 122.8, 122.12)

X-Rays and Scans

Intravenous pyelography and ultrasonography allow visualization of renal, ureteral and bladder pathology quite easily and plain x-rays may show calcified tissues and lesions, including renal or bladder stones (Figs 122.7 and 122.8) [55]. In hepatic schistosomiasis, contrast radiology can demonstrate portal vein distension or

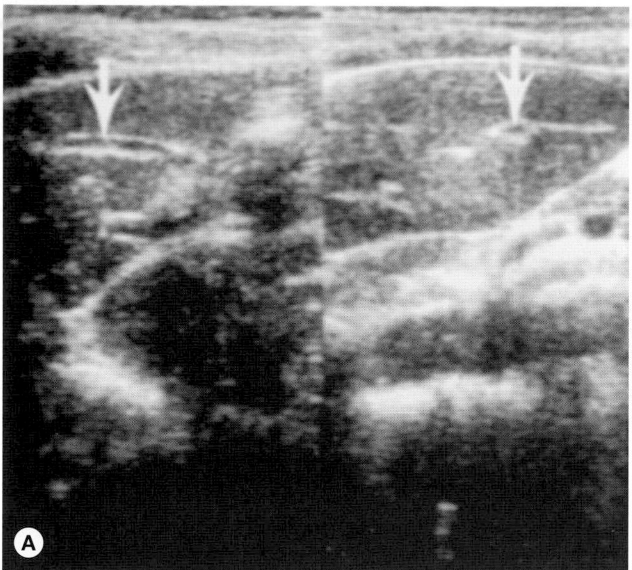

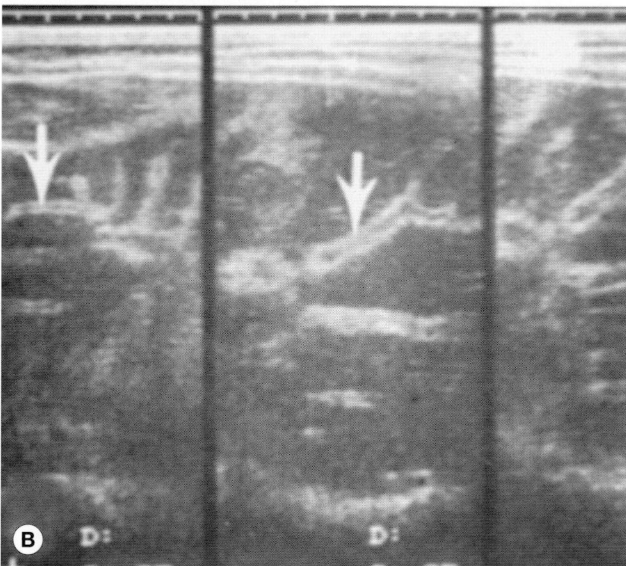

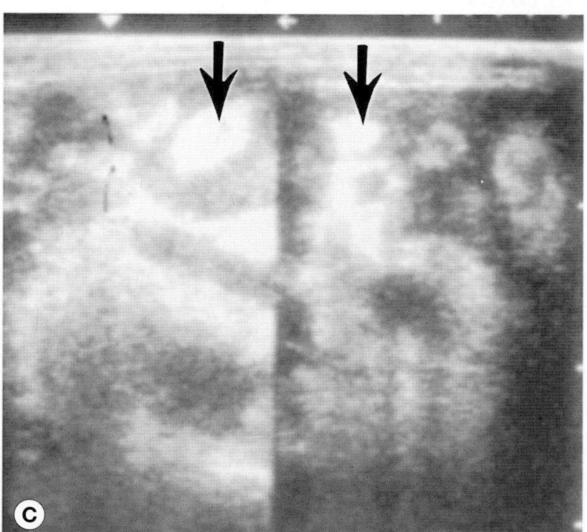

FIGURE 122.12 Minimal **(A)**, moderate **(B)** and extensive **(C)** periportal fibrosis of the liver demonstrated by ultrasonography. The arrows point to typical lesions.

gastro-esophageal varices. Computerized tomography, myelography and magnetic resonance can be useful for detailed imaging, especially for neuroschistosomiasis.

Ultrasound

Over the past three decades, ultrasonography has provided marked improvement in the diagnosis and study of schistosomiasis pathology [56, 57]. Sonography is an excellent noninvasive technique to demonstrate the pathognomonic periportal fibrosis and can estimate the degree of portal hypertension by measuring the distension of the portal vein (Fig. 122.12). Standardized protocols have been developed in order to classify hepatic fibrosis and urinary tract lesions. These protocols require specific expertise and experience, and results may be subject to considerable inter- and intra-observer variation.

TREATMENT

Once active infection is confirmed by detection of ova, or a clinical diagnosis of schistosomiasis is made, specific chemotherapy is indicated.

CHEMOTHERAPEUTIC AGENTS

Praziquantel, the drug of choice, is effective against all schistosome species, as well as other flukes (e.g. *Clonorchis sinensis* and *Paragonimus westermani*) and cestodes (e.g. *Taenia saginata, Taenia solium, Diphyllobothrium latum* and *Hymenolepis nana*) [2, 3, 54, 58]. Praziquantel is mostly marketed as scored 600-mg tablets. The drug acts within an hour after ingestion by provoking tetanic contraction of the adult worms and damaging their tegument, but the precise molecular mechanisms remain unknown. The antigens revealed induce humoral and cellular immune responses, enhancing the direct drug action. Side effects are mild and include nausea, vomiting, malaise and abdominal pain. In heavy infections, acute colic with bloody diarrhea may occur, probably provoked by massive worm shifts and antigen releases induced by praziquantel.

The original brand of praziquantel, Biltricide® (Bayer), has lost most market share to about 30 generic brands. Consequently, the price falling from $2.00–4.00 to less than $0.20 per treatment has made the drug widely available for control purposes [58]. On the downside of this development, large pharmaceutical companies have given up investments to find new schistosomicides [14].

The quality of generic praziquantel may vary and counterfeit praziquantel has been reported in Sudan [59]. The toxicity, mutagenicity and embryotoxicity of praziquantel are very low in animal models and, after 30 years of widespread application, no significant safety problems have been documented in humans. It is therefore no longer recommended to withhold treatment from young children and pregnant women [60].

The standard single dose of 40 mg/kg of body weight for treating *S. mansoni, S. haematobium* or *S. intercalatum* may be subcurative [1–3, 54]. Higher regimens are not always well-tolerated, however, and should be given in split doses, several hours apart. For population-based treatment, in which the reduction of egg loads and morbidity is the main objective, 40 mg/kg remains recommended [10]. People with high egg counts may be given two doses of 30 mg/kg, 3–6 hours apart. This higher split-dose is also routinely recommended for treatment of *S. japonicum, S. mekongi* and *S. malayensis* infections.

Praziquantel does not act on ova or on immature worms. Viable, tissue-dwelling eggs may be excreted for several weeks after successful treatment and schistosomulae or young adult worms may survive treatment and become viable adult worms. The optimal course, therefore, if cure is the goal, is to repeat the microscopic examination of the stool and/or urine for ova 4–6 weeks after treatment. After a single dose of 40 mg/kg, intensities of infection, as measured by egg counts or antigen levels, are almost invariably reduced by 90–95%. Parasitologic cure is usually achieved in 70–95% of treated patients, but these percentages may be considerably lower in populations with high initial egg counts and exposed to intense transmission and re-infection [61]. For individual case-management, or when there is no risk of re-infection, 60–120 mg/kg in split doses may be given. Repeat treatment 6–12 weeks later can be used to cure prepatent infections, particularly if eosinophilia, high antibody titers or symptoms persist. Definitive parasitologic cure in people leaving endemic areas is proven by the disappearance of viable eggs from the excreta for at least six months after treatment. In some cases, egg release is interrupted but starts again a few weeks later. Adult worms may be incapacitated temporarily by chemotherapy and resume mating and activity later. A few remaining schistosomes may cause little or no harm, but if complete eradication of all worms is envisaged, a conclusive laboratory evaluation may have to consist of thorough examination of excreta on three consecutive days, serologic reconversion, clearing of eosinophilia and, possibly, examination of a rectal or vesical biopsy. For population-based treatment in endemic areas, aiming more at morbidity rather than infection control, pursuing complete cure in all those treated is impractical and not pertinent.

The cure rate (percentage of infected people converting to negative stools or urine) can vary according to the sensitivity of method used, the timing of the follow-up, and the intensity of transmission. The optimal time of follow-up is 4–6 weeks after treatment. However, in areas and periods of intense transmission, residual surviving of worms in those with high worm burdens, maturation of prepatent infections and rapid re-infection may result in seemingly low cure rates [61]. A better measure of success is the reduction of mean egg counts as an indicator of the risk for severe morbidity, and the impact on the long-term resolution of pathology as measured by ultrasound, hematuria reagent strips testing for blood, or clinical evaluation [62, 63].

Most schistosome-induced pathology resolves after praziquantel treatment. Clinical, radiologic and sonographic studies have demonstrated regression over weeks-to-months of intestinal and vesical lesions, reactive hepatomegaly, and even severe upper urinary tract lesions and liver fibrosis. Thus, the prognosis is usually good, except in advanced cases with parenchymal hydronephrosis or renal failure in urinary schistosomiasis, or severe liver fibrosis with established portal hypertension with recurrent bleeding from esophageal varices and ascites in hepatosplenic schistosomiasis.

Resistance against praziquantel was feared in some high transmission foci, but the low local cure rates were shown to be caused by intense continuing transmission [61]. Tolerant *S. mansoni* strains were reported in Egypt, but have not been independently confirmed. If existent, they have not spread further in spite of intense drug pressure. To date, true drug resistance to praziquantel in human populations has not been convincingly documented.

Recently, derivatives of artemisinin, a drug for the treatment of malaria, were shown to be effective against the immature stages of *S. japonicum*, *S. mansoni* and, possibly, *S. haematobium* [64]. They could, in principle, be used to treat acute schistosomiasis or as a prophylactic agent. In a clinical trial in China, repeated administration throughout the transmission season greatly reduced parasite burden of *S. japonicum* and prevented early manifestations of infection. Trials in Africa, as a stand-alone drug or in combination with praziquantel, showed prophylactic but no curative potential. However, their preventive application is not recommended, as artemisinin should be preserved for treatment of drug-resistant malaria.

TREATMENT OF ACUTE SCHISTOSOMIASIS AND COMPLICATIONS

Topical steroid creams and oral antihistamines can provide symptomatic relief for cercarial dermatitis. Katayama fever is primarily treated with corticosteroids, for example prednisone 40 mg daily for 5–14 days, to suppress the hypersensitivity reaction. This treatment should be followed by praziquantel to eliminate the adult worms [31, 32, 54].

Neuroschistosomiasis requires specialized care, again with corticosteroids and, if necessary, anticonvulsants prior to praziquantel treatment [43, 54]. Caution is required in the rare case of concurrent neurocysticercosis, on which praziquantel is also active but may provoke epileptic seizures owing to the destruction of the cerebral cysts.

Bleeding from esophageal varices may be treated symptomatically with β-blockers, endoscopic sclerotherapy, splenectomy, or splenorenal or portocaval shunts. In advanced urinary schistosomiasis, destructed and non-functional kidneys may have to be removed [54].

CONTROL AND PREVENTION

Until late in the 20th century, schistosomiasis was a high-priority public health problem among the populations in Egypt, the Maghreb, Brazil, China and the Philippines [1–3, 11, 26]. Large-scale national control programs, based on the chemical or physical destruction of the snail intermediate hosts, case-finding and general improvement in hygiene, involved large teams of malacologists, epidemiologists, clinicians and laboratory technicians in specialized programs. Apart from a few research or pilot projects, most of the lower-income endemic countries, especially in sub-Saharan Africa, remained devoid of such efforts and often lacked the means to diagnose and treat clinical cases.

SNAIL CONTROL

Attempts to exterminate the snail populations with chemicals (molluscicides) are expensive, logistically demanding and often inconclusive. An efficient application requires considerable human and material resources, as well as detailed epidemiologic and malacologic surveillance. Snail populations can be reduced but rarely exterminated, requiring molluscicide treatment to be repeated regularly and for a long period. The toxicity of molluscicides to fish and other aquatic organisms causes ecologic concerns. Focal application in specific "hot spots" where schistososome-infected snails reside and human infections are occurring may be useful in preventing local infections. In general, however, chemical snail control has been all but abandoned as a standard control strategy. Snail control can also be pursued in some cases by thorough and regular weeding, hydraulic engineering and alternative irrigation practices, but such measures are tedious and expensive. The introduction of competitor snails, natural predators such as ducks or fish, or plant molluscicides, is not effective in practice.

MASS DRUG ADMINISTRATION (MDA) PROGRAMS

The introduction of praziquantel heralded a shift in control strategies to interventions aimed at the definitive human host, rather than at the intermediate snail host. This strategy of "morbidity control" has a more immediate impact on infection and disease and requires much less expertise. It was officially adopted by the WHO in 2002 and has become the standard approach in most endemic countries [1–3, 6, 8, 10, 58]. Its main objective is to reduce community-wide infection rates and intensities of infection in order to prevent schistosomal morbidity (by reducing ova retained in the host's body) and, over time, transmission of infection (by reducing ova passed from the host into the environment). Various chemotherapy strategies can be applied, including indiscriminate mass treatment, treatment of particular risk groups, especially school-aged children, and active case-finding followed by treatment (Fig. 122.13). Thirty years of experience have shown that population-based treatment is feasible and safe, and effectively reduces prevalence and intensity of infection, as well as morbidity. Its impact on transmission is more difficult to measure, and a limited number of residual eggs passing into the environment can maintain considerable transmission potential. However, in most areas where MDA has been applied over a number of years, transmission appears to have waned. Still, regular surveillance and/or regular re-treatment must be envisaged.

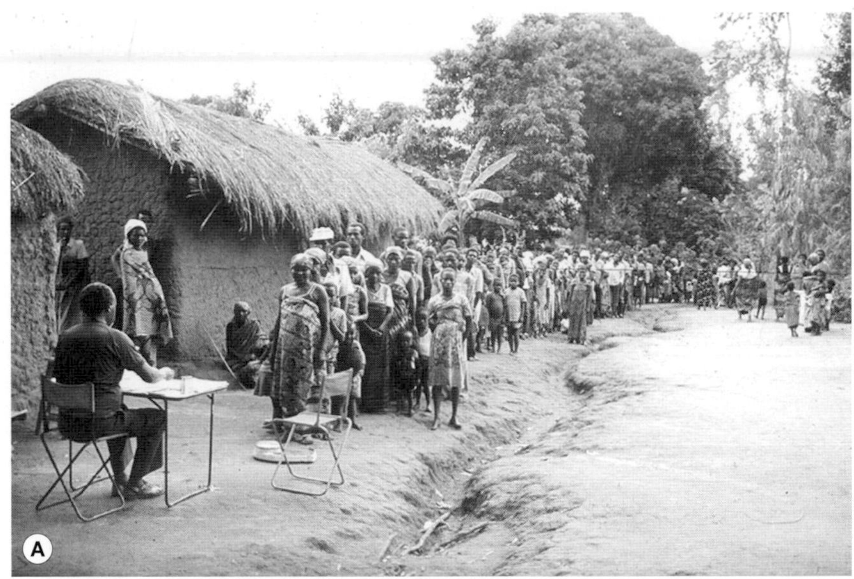

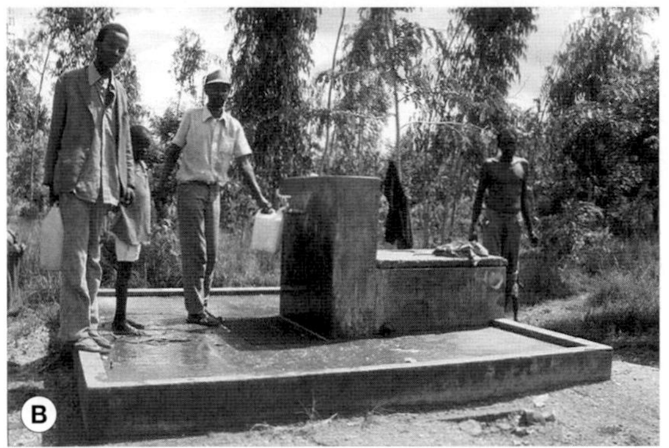

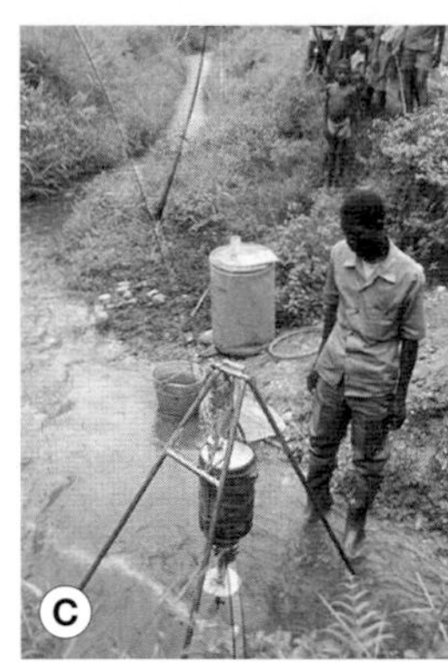

FIGURE 122.13 Schistosomiasis control in the field **(A)** Mass treatment with praziquantel in the community. **(B)** Safe water suppy, **(C)** Snail control with molluscicides. *(Reproduced with permission from Bruno Gryseels; Infectious Disease Clinics of North America; vol 26; Issue 2; 383-397; Elsevier Inc ©2012).*

INTEGRATED CONTROL METHODS

Schistosomiasis can be eliminated by behavioral changes, safe water supply and sanitary engineering. This happened in Japan in the 1950s, far before modern drugs were developed [65]. In low-income countries, the prevention of schistosomiasis necessitates more than providing safe drinking water. Sites free of exposure to infective cercariae for washing, bathing, laundering, swimming and crop irrigation are also required. Moreover, these must be adapted to local attitudes and circumstances, and long-term maintenance is a frequently problematic necessity. Specific educational programs can enhance the knowledge and perception of schistosomiasis, but is often insufficient in reducing exposure in the absence of adequate alternatives for water contact.

In several countries with sufficient resources and the political will to implement and sustain population-based therapy, the public health impact of schistosomiasis has decreased dramatically over the past decades. These middle-income nations are usually characterized by general socioeconomic progress and substantial improvements in water supply, sanitation and healthcare. While residual transmission pockets may remain difficult to extinguish, general prevalence and intensities of infection are kept low by regular MDA. It is estimated that the number of remaining infections in Brazil and China, and possibly even Egypt, has been reduced to less than one million. Even more strikingly, severe morbidity in these countries has all but disappeared; cases of advanced hepatosplenic disease with hematemesis, advanced hydronephrosis or schistosomiasis-associated bladder cancer, once common, have become anecdotal. In Morocco, Tunisia, Iraq and Puerto Rico the infection has been eliminated.

CONTROL IN SUB-SAHARAN AFRICA

Early pilot projects with population-based chemotherapy in sub-Saharan Africa showed promising results in the short-term, but the re-treatment schedules and vertical structures employed were not sustainable once foreign assistance was withdrawn [2, 8, 20]. Quick wins were as quickly lost to rapid re-infection, while regular health services were left deprived and demotivated for further action. National resources and capacities are limited, while decision makers are faced with many priorities. Some programs that were built up more gradually, by improving passive or active case finding through regular healthcare structures, have had less impressive short-term results but appeared to be more sustainable. However, as the disease continues to spread to new development areas and city slums, efforts to control schistosomiasis remain a public health priority in large parts of the continent.

GLOBAL TARGET TO CONTROL SCHISTOSOMIASIS

Renewed efforts have been launched to control schistosomiasis in resource-poor countries following a call by the WHO to international agencies, charities and pharmaceutical companies to provide praziquantel and other anthelminthic drugs at low, or no, cost [9, 10, 15]. The joint "Global Target" is to annually treat at least 75% of all school-aged children at risk of infection using a standardized strategy based on local epidemiologic characteristics of schistosomal infections. Active MDA programs are being launched in an increasing number of sub-Saharan African countries [47]. An important new asset is the integration of schistosomiasis control with MDA for

TABLE 122-1 Other Schistosome Species Causing Human Intestinal Disease

	Schistosoma intercalatum	*Schistosoma mekongi*	*Schistosoma mattheei*
Distribution	African disease only. Endemic in parts of Cameroon, Gabon, Democratic Republic of Congo and other areas of Central and West Africa; although occasionally co-existent with *S. mansoni* and *S. haematobium*, usually found as the sole species in known transmission foci	Lower Mekong River basin in Laos and Cambodia	South Africa. Natural infection of sheep, cattle, horses and antelope that occasionally infects humans. Always found in association with *S. mansoni* or *S. haematobium*
Clinical manifestations	Anorexia, nausea, abdominal pain, diarrhea with blood and mucus; rectal and genital lesions; hepatomegaly and rectal bleeding pain in left iliac fossa with tenesmus	Similar to *S. japonicum*; acute schistosomiasis in non-immune travelers; generalized weakness, diarrhea and abdominal distress; hepatomegaly and splenomegaly. CNS and cardiopulmonary complications not described	Relatively mild intestinal disease, mucoid diarrhea; diffuse intermittent abdominal pain and cramping, malaise, hepatomegaly
Diagnosis	Eggs are similar to *S. haematobium* in shape and in possessing a terminal spine but are usually longer (140–240 μm), often have a central bulge and are shed in stool, not urine; terminal spine is characteristically bent; eggs are Ziehl-Neelsen (acid-fast) positive	Eggs in stool and rectal biopsy. The eggs are similar to *S. japonicum* but are generally smaller (50–80 μm by 40–65 μm); they also contain a small, inconspicuous spine. Elevated alkaline phosphatase	Eggs resemble *S. intercalatum* and measure 120–180 μm in length and have a terminal spine; eggs present in stool or occasionally urine
Treatment	Praziquantel at 40 mg/kg body weight in single dose	Praziquantel at 60 mg/kg single dose or 2 × 30 mg/kg in divided doses	Praziquantel at 40 mg/kg single dose

CNS, central nervous system.

other neglected parasitic diseases, for example lymphatic filariasis, onchocerciasis and intestinal helminths, as well as provision of vitamins and nutritional supplements [66]. To increase sustainability, these campaigns are carried out wherever possible through community health workers or regular health services rather than vertical mobile teams. However, many health systems may still be too weak and overburdened to sustain these programs, or to execute them with the necessary epidemiologic vigor [67]. The over-reliance on drugs may also reduce efforts for the implementation of the other, more structural, elements of the WHO resolution, for example accessible care for clinical cases, safe water supply, improved sanitation and behavioral changes [68]. The massive, and sometimes uncontrolled, use of praziquantel brings along a risk for the development of drug resistance, while there are no alternative antischistosomal drugs in the pipeline [69]. Thus, while further progress towards the elimination of schistosomiasis as a public health problem can be expected, the global efforts need to be accompanied with national and local expertise and vigilance.

Although a vaccine to prevent schistosomiasis is unlikely to be available during the next decades, one that would reduce infection rates may improve a multifaceted approach to control schistosomal morbidity and transmission. A combination of chemotherapy, reduction of water contact and contamination, and possibly snail control and vaccination, could lead to the elimination of schistosomiasis in much of the world. However, the ultimate challenge in the eradication of schistosomiasis is to improve living standards and alleviate poverty, which is the underlying cause of this and many other health problems in the tropics.

OTHER HUMAN SCHISTOSOME INFECTIONS

Characteristics of three other *Schistosoma* species causing human disease are outlined in Table 122-1.

REFERENCES

1. Jordan P, Webbe G, Sturrock FS. Human Schistosomiasis. Wallingford: CAB International; 1993.
2. Ross AG, Bartley PB, Sleigh AC, et al. Schistosomiasis. N Engl J Med 2002; 346:1212–20.
3. Gryseels B, Polman K, Clerinx J, Kestens L. Human schistosomiasis. Lancet 2006;368:1106–18.
4. Doumenge JP, Mott KE. Global distribution of schistosomiasis: CEGET/WHO Atlas. World Health Stat Q 1984;37:186–99.
5. Brown DS. Freshwater snails of Africa and their medical importance, 2nd edn. London: Taylor and Francis; 1994.
6. Ross AGP, Sleigh AC, Li Y, et al. Schistosomiasis in the People's Republic of China: Prospects and challenges for the 21st century. Clin Microbiol Rev 2001;14:270–95.
7. Chitsulo L, Engels D, Montresor A, Savioli L. The global status of schistosomiasis and its control. Acta Trop 2000;77:41–51.
8. World Health Organization Expert Committee. Prevention and Control of Schistosomiasis and Soil-Transmitted Helminthiasis. Technical report series. Geneva: World Health Organization; 2002.
9. World Health Organization. Schistosomiasis. Available at: http://www.who.int/mediacentre/factsheets/fs115/en/index.html (accessed 14 November 2011).
10. World Health Organization. Preventive chemotherapy in human helminthiasis. Geneva: World Health Organization; 2006.
11. Jordan P. From Katayama to the Dakhla Oasis: the beginning of epidemiology and control of bilharzia. Acta Tropica 2000;77: 9–40.
12. Warren KS. The pathology, pathobiology and pathogenesis of schistosomiasis. Nature 1978;273:609–12.
13. Frank C, Mohamed MK, Strickland GT, et al. The role of parenteral antischistosomal therapy in the spread of hepatitis C virus in Egypt. Lancet 2000;355: 887–91.
14. Reich R, Govindaraj R. Dilemmas in drug development for tropical diseases. Experiences with praziquantel. Health Policy 1998;44:1–18.
15. World Health Organization. Fifty-fourth World Health Assembly. Resolution WHA54.19. Schistosomiasis and soil-transmitted helminths. Geneva: World Health Organization; 2001.

16. Huyse T, Webster BL, Geldof S, et al. Bidirectional introgressive hybridization between a cattle and human schistosome species. PloS Pathogens 2009;5: e1000571.
17. Horak P, Kolarova L. Molluscan and vertebrate immune responses to bird schistosomes. Parasite Immunol 2005;27:247–55.
18. Harris ARC, Russell RJ, Charters AD. A review of schistosomiasis in immigrants in Western Australia, demonstrating the unusual longevity of *Schistosoma mansoni*. Trans Roy Soc Trop Med Hyg 1984;78;385–8.
19. Fulford AJC, Butterworth AE, Ouma JH, Sturrock RF. A statistical approach to schistosome population dynamics and estimation of the life-span of *Schistosoma mansoni* in man. Parasitology 1995;110:307–16.
20. Gryseels B. Uncertainties in the epidemiology and control of schistosomiasis. Am J Trop Med Hyg 1996;55(suppl. 5):103–8.
21. Gryseels B. Human resistance to schistosoma infections: Age or experience? Parasitol Today 1994;10:380–84.
22. Capron A, Riveau G, Capron M, Trottein F. Schistosomes: the road from host-parasite interactions to vaccines in clinical trials. Trends Parasitol 2005;21: 143–9.
23. Siddiqui AA, Siddiqui BA, Ganley-Leal L. *Schistosomiasis* vaccines. Hum Vaccin 2011;7:11.
24. Wilson MS, Mentink-Kane MM, Pesce JT, et al. Immunopathology of schistosomiasis. Immun Cell Biol 2007;85:148–54.
25. Secor WE. Interactions between schistosomiasis and infection with HIV-1. Parasite Immun 2006;28:597–603.
26. Strickland GT. Liver disease in Egypt: hepatitis C superseded schistosomiasis as a result of iatrogenic and biological factors. Hepatology 2006;43: 915–22.
27. Gryseels B, De Vlas SJ. Worm burdens in schistosome infections. Parasitol Today 1996;12:115–9.
28. Steinmann P, Keiser J, Bos R, et al. Schistosomiasis and water resources development: systematic review, meta-analysis, and estimates of people at risk. Lancet Infect Dis 2006;6:411–25
29. De Vlas SJ, Gryseels B. Underestimation of *Schistosoma mansoni* prevalences. Parasitol Today 1992;8:274–7.
30. Stothard JR, Sousa-Figuereido JC, Betson M, et al. *Schistosoma mansoni* infections in young children: when are schistosome antigens in urine, eggs in stool and antibodies to eggs first detectable? PLoS Negl Trop Dis 2011;5:e938.
31. Clerinx J, Van Gompel A. Schistosomiasis in travellers and migrants. Travel Med Infect Dis 2011;9:6–24.
32. Ross AG, Vickers D, Olds GR, et al. Katayama syndrome. Lancet Infect Dis 2007;7:218–24.
33. Jelinek T, Nothdurft HD, Loscher T. Schistosomiasis in travelers and expatriates. J Travel Med 1996;13:160–4.
34. Cheever AW, Hoffmann KF, Wynn TA. Immunopathology of schistosomiasis mansoni in mice and men. Immunol Today 2000;21:465–6.
35. Abath FGC, Morais CNL, Montenegro CEL, et al. Immunopathogenic mechanisms in schistosomiasis: what can be learnt from human studies? Trends in Parasitology 2006;22:85–91.
36. Chen MG, Mott KE. Progress in assessment of morbidity due to *Schistosoma haematobium* infection: a review of recent literature. Trop Dis Bull 1989; 86:R1–36.
37. Vennervald BJ, Polman K. Helminths and malignancy. Parasite Immunol 2009;31:686–96.
38. Cheever AW. A quantitative post-mortem study of schistosomiasis mansoni in man. Am J Trop Med Hyg 1968;17:38–64.
39. Gryseels B. The relevance of schistosomiasis for public health. Trop Med Parasitol 1989;40:134–42.
40. Schwartz E. Pulmonary schistosomiasis. Clin Chest Med 2002;23:433–43.
41. Barsoum R, Harrington JT, Mathew CM, et al. The changing face of schistosomal glomerulopathy. Kidney Int 2004;66:2472–84.
42. Feldmeier H, Leutscher P, Poggensee G, Harms G. Male genital schistosomiasis and haemospermia. Trop Med Int Health 1999;4:791–3.
43. Carod-Artal FJ. Neuroschistosomiasis. Expert Rev Anti Infect Ther 2010:8: 1307–18.
44. King CH, Dickman K, Tisch DJ. Regauging the cost of chronic helminthic infection: meta-analysis of disability-related outcomes in endemic schistosomiasis. Lancet 2005;365:1561–9.
45. Mathers CD, Ezzati M, Lopez AD. Measuring the burden of neglected tropical diseases: The global burden of disease framework. PLoS Negl Trop Dis 2007;1:e114.
46. van der Werf MJ, De Vlas SJ, Brooker S, et al. Quantification of clinical morbidity associated with schistosome infection in sub-Saharan Africa. Acta Trop 2003;86:125–39.
47. World Health Organization. Working to overcome the global impact of neglected tropical diseases. Geneva: World Health Organization; 2011.
48. Clerinx J, Bottieau E, Wichmann D, et al. Acute schistosomiasis in a cluster of travelers from Rwanda: Diagnostic contribution of schistosome DNA detection in serum compared to parasitology and serology. J Travel Med 2011; 18:367–72.
49. Feldmeier H, Poggensee G. Diagnostic techniques in schistosomiasis control. A review. Acta Trop 1993;52:205–20.
50. Rabello A. Diagnosing schistosomiasis. Mem Inst Oswaldo Cruz 1997; 92:669–76.
51. Tsang VC, Wilkins PP. Immunodiagnosis of schistosomiasis. Immunol Invest 1997;26:175–88.
52. Deelder AM, Qian ZL, Kremsner PG, et al. Quantitative diagnosis of Schistosoma infections by measurement of circulating antigens in serum and urine. Trop Geogr Med 1994;46:233–8.
53. van Dam GJ, Wichers JH, Ferreira TMF, et al. Diagnosis of schistosomiasis by reagent strip test for detection of circulating cathodic antigen. J Clin Microb 2004;42:5458–61.
54. Olds GR, Dasarathy S. Schistosomiasis. Curr Treat Options Infect Dis 2000; 2:88–99.
55. Palmer PES, Reeder CC. International Registry of Tropical Imaging. Radiology Department, Uniformed Services University USA. 2005. Available at: http://tmcr.usuhs.mil (accessed 14 November 2011).
56. Hatz CF. The use of ultrasound in schistosomiasis. Adv Parasitol 2001; 48:225–84.
57. Richter J, Hatz C, Haussinger D. Ultrasound in tropical and parasitic diseases. Lancet 2003;362:900–2.
58. Fenwick A, Savioli L, Engels D, et al. Drugs for the control of parasitic diseases: current status and development in schistosomiasis. Trends Parasitol 2003; 19:509–15.
59. Sulaiman SM, Mamadou T, Engels D, et al. Counterfeit praziquantel. Lancet 2001;358:666–7.
60. World Health Organization. Report of the WHO informal consultation on the use of praziquantel during pregnancy/lactation and albendazole/mebendazole in children under 24 months. Geneva: World Health Organization; 2002.
61. Gryseels B, Mbaye A, De Vlas SJ, et al. Are poor responses to praziquantel for the treatment of *Schistosoma mansoni* infections in Senegal due to resistance? An overview of the evidence. Trop Med Int Health 2001;6:864–73.
62. Richter J. The impact of chemotherapy on morbidity due to schistosomiasis. Acta Trop 2003;86:161–83.
63. Magnussen P. Treatment and re-treatment strategies for schistosomiasis control in different epidemiological settings: a review of 10 years' experiences. Acta Trop 2003;86:243–54.
64. Utzinger J, Xiao SH, Tanner M, Keiser J. Artemisinins for schistosomiasis and beyond. Curr Opin Investig Drugs 2007;8:105–116.
65. Minai M, Hosaka Y, Ohta N. Historical view of schistosomiasis japonica in Japan: implementation and evaluation of disease-control strategies in Yamanashi Prefecture. Paras Int 2003;52:321–6.
66. Molyneux DH, Hotez PJ, Fenwick A. "Rapid-impact interventions": how a policy of integrated control for Africa's neglected tropical diseases could benefit the poor. PLoS Med 2005;2:e336.
67. Cavalli A, Bamba SI, Traore MN, et al. Interactions between global health initiatives and country health systems: the case of a neglected tropical diseases control program in Mali. PLoS Neglected Trop Dis 2010;4:e798.
68. Mahmoud A, Zerhounic E. Neglected Tropical Diseases: moving beyond mass drug treatment to understanding the science. Health Affairs 2009;28: 1726–33.
69. Geerts S, Gryseels B. Drug resistance in human helminths: current situation and lessons from livestock. Clin Microbiol Rev 2000;13:207–22.

123 Intestinal Fluke Infections

Yupaporn Wattanagoon, Danai Bunnag

Key features

- Intestinal flukes are primarily distributed in Asia, although *Heterophyidae* species are also seen in North Africa and the Middle East
- Humans acquire infection by eating raw contaminated water plants, for example *Fasciolopsis buski*, by ingesting raw freshwater fish, for example *Heterophyidae*, or through uncooked snails, snakes, or frogs
- Most infections are asymptomatic; diarrhea and abdominal pain are common complaints in symptomatic patients
- Malabsorption and protein-losing enteropathy can be seen in severe *F. buski* infection, particularly in children
- Therapy of intestinal flukes is with praziquantel

INTRODUCTION

Intestinal flukes vary in size from large to minute. There are over 70 species that infect humans. The majority of infections are caused by flukes from the families *Fasciolidae, Echinostomatidae*, and *Heterophyidae* (Table 123-1). A smaller number are caused by the *Gastrodiscidae, Plagiorchiidae, Microphallidae*, and *Diplostomatidae* families (Table 123-1). Many species have been discovered incidentally by identification of adult worms in stool after anthelminthic treatment [1]. The source of infection varies according to the intermediate host, for example infected freshwater fish, aquatic plants, snails, or tadpoles.

EPIDEMIOLOGY

More than 50 million people are infected by intestinal flukes [2]. Most cases have been reported from Southeast Asia, the Far East, the Middle East, and Africa. On a few occasions, cases have been reported from Europe, North America, or Australia. Intestinal flukes have been reported from:

- *Fasciolopsis buski:* India, Thailand, Loa People's Democratic Republic (PDR), Cambodia, Indonesia, Taiwan, China, Japan, Malaysia, and the Philippines;
- *Echinostomatidae* species: north-eastern Thailand (about 50% prevalence), the Philippines, Indonesia, and Taiwan;
- *Heterophyidae* species, usually *Heterophyes heterophyes* and *Metagonimus yokogawai*: Nile delta of Egypt, Iran, Tunisia, Turkey, Southeast Asia and the Far East, such as Japan, Korea, Taiwan, mainland China, the Philippines, and Indonesia;
- *Gastrodiscidae* species (*G. hominis*): common in Asia especially in India (Assam, Bihar, and Orissa). Cases also reported from Vietnam, Thailand, Myanmar, China, the Philippines, Kazakhstan, and Guyana. Reservoir hosts are pigs, deer mice (*Tragulus*

TABLE 123-1 List of Various Species of Intestinal Flukes that Infect Humans and Their Habitats

Intestinal Fluke Family	Intestinal Fluke Species	Habitats
Fasciolidae	*F. buski*	Small intestine
Echinostomatidae	*E. ilocanum* *E. malayanum* *E. revolutum* *E. lindoense* *E. recurvatum* *E. jassyense (E. melis)* *E. macrorchis* *E. cinetorchis* *Hypoderaeum conoideum* *Echinochasmus perfoliatus* *Paraphostomum sufrartyfex* *Himasthla meuhlensi*	Small intestine
Heterophyidae	*H. heterophyes* *H. yokogawai* *H. taichui* *Metagonimus yokogawai* *Metagonimus minutus* *Centrocestus formosanus* *Haplorchis pumilio* *Diorchitrema formosanum* *D. amplicaecale* *Pygidiopsis summa* *Stellantchasmus falcatus* *Procerovum calderoni*	Small intestine
Gastrodiscoidiae	*G. hominis*	Cecum and ascending colon
Lecithodendriae	*P. bonnei* *P. molenkempi*	Small intestine
Microphallidae	*Spelotrema brevicaeca*	Small intestine
Plagiorchiidae	*P. philippinensis* *P. javensis* *P. muris*	Small intestine
Alariasis	*Alaria americana*	Small intestine
Neodiplostomumiasis	*Neodiplostomum seoulense*	Small intestine

Data from [8, 17, 18].

napu), and rats. It has been proposed that sylvanic cycles persist [3];
- *Lecithodendriidae* species (*Phaneropsolus bonnei* and *Prosthodendrium molenkempi*): endemic in Southeast Asia, especially Thailand, Lao PDR, and Indonesia [4].

NATURAL HISTORY, PATHOLOGY AND PATHOGENESIS

The lifecycles of most intestinal flukes are similar except for the intermediate hosts. Adult flukes reside in the intestines of the definitive hosts and release eggs that are passed in stool. When the embryonated eggs reach water, they release miracidia which penetrate the snail intermediate host and develop into sporocysts, radiae and then cercariae. Cercariae leave the snails and, depending on the species of fluke, encyst as metacercariae on aquatic plants, in fish, freshwater snails, snakes, or frogs (Table 123-2). Humans, or other definitive hosts, become infected after eating metacercariae in uncooked infected or contaminated second intermediate hosts. Metacercariae excyst in the duodenum, attach to the intestinal wall and develop into adult worms that produce eggs and complete the lifecycle.

When flukes attach to the intestinal wall they can cause inflammation with cellular infiltration, ulceration and increased mucus secretion. Heavy infection can lead to local necrosis, erosion and hemorrhage. Intestinal obstruction can occur with heavy worm burden. Malabsorption and protein-losing enteropathy can occur in severe cases of *F. buski* infection. Occasionally, ova or adult worms of minute intestinal flukes (e.g. *Heterophidiae*) can enter blood vessels and travel to ectopic sites, such as the heart or brain.

CLINICAL FEATURES

Most cases are asymptomatic and are discovered after anthelminthic treatment for other conditions. Symptomatic cases report mild gastrointestinal symptoms such as abdominal pain, colic, flatulence, and diarrhea, which can be watery or foul-smelling with mucus and blood. Severe infection with *F. buski* in children can present with chronic diarrhea and protein losing enteropathy. Rarely, intestinal perforation occurs, which can be fatal [5].

TABLE 123-2 List of Reported Definitive and Reservoir Hosts and, First and Second Intermediate Hosts of Various Intestinal Flukes

Intestinal fluke family	Intestinal fluke species	Definitive host	First intermediate host	Second intermediate host
Fasciolidae	*Fasiolopsis buski*	Pigs and humans	Planorbid snail *Segmentina hemisphaerula*, *Hippeutis cantori*, *Gyraulus* species *Segmentina* (*Trochorbis*)	Water caltrop, water chestnut, water bamboo water morning glory water lily shoots, watercress and other edible aquatic vegetation
Echinostomatidae	*Echinostoma ilocanum*	Birds, mammals, sometimes humans	Planorbid snails *Gyraulus convexiusculus* *Hippeutis umbilicus* *Gyraulus prashdi*	Freshwater snails (*Pila, Viviparus, Lymnaea*), fish, tadpoles or vegetation
	Echinostoma malayanum	Rats, dogs	Freshwater snails *Indoplanorbis exustus* *Lymnaea leuteola*	*I. exustus, L. (Radix) rubiginosa*, *G. convexiusculus* and in tadpoles, *V. javanicus* and *Pila scutata*
	Echinostoma revolutum	Ducks, geese and rats	Freshwater snails *I. exustus*, *L. (Radix) rubiginosa* *Physa* species (*Segmentina* species and *Helisoma* species)	Mollusks, tadpole and clams (*Corbicula producta*)
	Hypoderaeum conoideum	Ducks, other fowl, rats and humans		*I. exustus, L. (Radix) rubiginosa* and tadpoles
Heterophyidae	*Heterophyes heterophyes*	Dogs, cats, foxes, birds, and other fish-eating mammals	Freshwater snails *Perinella conica Cerithedea cingulata* (syn. *Tymphonotonus microptera*	Brackish or freshwater fish in mullet and minnow species *Mugil cephalus, M. capito, Tilapia nilotica, Aphanius fasciatus Gambusia affinis* and *Acanthogobius* species
	Metagonimus yokogawai	Dogs, cats, pigs and pelicans	Snail: *Semisulcospira libertina* and related species	Freshwater fish, particularly Cyprinidae: trout (*Plectoglossus altivelis* and *Odontobulis obscurus*) and salmon (*Salmo perryi* and *Tribolodon hakonensis*)
Lecithodendriae	*Planeropsolus bonnei* *Planeropsolus molenkempi*	Monkeys (*Nycticebus coucang, Macaca iris, Macaca mulatta* and *Macaca fuscicularis)* Insectivorous bats *(Scotophilus kuhlii* and *Taphozons melanopogon)* Rats *(Rattus rattus)*	Snails (*Bithynia* species)	Dragonflies and damselflies

Physical examination shows no abnormality in asymptomatic or mild cases. In severe cases, protein malnutrition, anemia and edema of the face and extremities can be detected caused by chronic protein and blood loss and B12 malabsorption [6]. There are occasional reports of infection at ectopic sites from some species, for example *Alaria Americana*, that has caused lesions in the vitreous and the retina [7], and has disseminated throughout the body [8].

PATIENT EVALUATION, DIAGNOSIS, AND DIFFERENTIAL DIAGNOSIS

Routine laboratory tests are usually normal in mild cases. Anemia and eosinophilia can be seen in severe cases of *F. buski*. Low serum albumin and B_{12} level has occurred with protein-losing enteropathy.

Confirmatory diagnosis is made by:

1. Identification of adult worms, with specific species confirmation based on the worm characteristics.
2. Identification of ova in fecal samples: It can be difficult to diagnose worm species because the ova of these parasites are similar to others in the same family or the liver fluke species, for example *F. buski* is similar to *Fasciola hepatica* or *Fasciola gigantica* ova, and minute intestinal flukes ova, for example *H. heterophyes*, *Prostodendrium molenkampi*, *Phaneropsolus bonnei*, *M. yokogawai* ova are similar to *O. viverrini*, *O. felineus*, and *C. sinensis* ova.
   The sensitivity of the above methods can be enhanced by using the methiolate iodine-formaline (MIF) technique [9].
3. PCR: PCR distinguishes intestinal flukes based on their DNA sequences. Using PCR–restriction fragment length polymorphism (PCR-RFLP) and simple sequence repeat anchored PCR, differentiation among various species of *Metagonimus* genus [10, 11] and six species of *Heterophyidae* genus has been possible [12].
4. Serology: similar to most intestinal parasitic infections, serology is not routinely performed. However, in patients infected with multiple pathogens, it can be useful for confirmation, for example *F. buski* and *F. gigantica* [13].

Other intestinal parasites or liver flukes can give similar symptoms of abdominal pain, flatulence, and diarrhea. Severe cases may be similar to intestinal schistosomiasis but without liver or splenic enlargement. Risk factors based on endemic area, eating habits, or travel history should be carefully elicited. Co-infection with other intestinal can be common in endemic areas.

TREATMENT

Praziquantel is the anthelminthic of choice. One field trial of treatment for *F. buski* demonstrated that praziquantel 15 mg/kg orally in a single dose at bedtime gave a 100% cure rate and was similar to the higher dose praziquantel (25 or 40 mg/kg), but with fewer side effects [14]. The Medical Letter recommends 75 mg/kg in three divided doses [15].

There have been no controlled trials of praziquantel for other intestinal flukes. However praziquantel at 15, 25, or 40 mg/kg in a single oral dose has been used successfully [16].

PREVENTION

Important methods to prevent infection are proper cleaning of raw water plants and cooking of vegetables, freshwater fish, or other intermediate hosts before consumption. Improved sanitation and hygiene will help to prevent fecal contamination of freshwater.

REFERENCES

1. Radomyos P, Bunnag D, Harinasuta T. Worms recovered in stools following praziquantel treatment. Drug Res 1984;34:118688.
2. World Health Organization. WHO Study Group: Control of Foodborne Trematode Infections. World Health Organ Techn Rep Ser No. 849. Geneva: World Health Organization; 1995.
3. Surinthrangkul B, Gonthian S, Pradatsundarasar A. *Gastrodiscoides hominis* from man in Thailand. J Med Assoc Thai 1965;48:96.
4. Manning GS, Lertprasert P. Studies on the life cycle of *Planeropsolus bonnei* and *Prosthodendrium molenkempi* in Thailand. Ann Trop Med Parasitol 1973;67:361.
5. Bhattacharjee HK, Yadav D, Bagga D. Fasciolopsiasis presenting as intestinal perforation: a case report. Trop Gastroenetrol 2009;30:40–1.
6. Chai JY, Shin JH, Lee SH, Rim HJ. Foodborne intestinal flukes in Southeast Asia. Korean J Parasitol 2009;47(suppl.):S69–102.
7. McDonald HR, Kazacos KR, Schatz H, Johnson RN. Two cases of intraocular infection with *Alaria* mesocercaria (Trematoda). Am J Ophthalmol 1994; 117:447–55.
8. Freeman RS, Stuart PF, Cullen JB, et al: Fatal human infection with mesocercariae of the trematode *Alaria americana*. Am J Trop Med Hyg 1976;25:803–7.
9. Wang LC. Improvement in the identification of intestinal parasites by a concentrated merthiolate-iodine-formaldehyde technique. J Parasitol 1998; 84:457–8.
10. Yang HJ, Guk SM, Han ET, Chai JY. Molecular differentiation of three species of Metagonimus by simple sequence repeat anchored polymerase chain reaction (SSR-PCR) amplification. J Parasitol 2000;86:1170–2.
11. Yu JR, Chai JY. Metagonimus. In: Liu D, ed. Molecular Detection of Foodborne Pathogens. Boca Raton, FL: CRC Press; 2010.
12. Dzikowski R, Levy MG, Poore MF, et al. Use of rDNA polymorphism for identification of Heterophyidae infecting freshwater fishes. Dis Aquat Organ 2004;59:35–41.
13. Quang TD, Duong TH, Richard-Lenoble D, et al. Emergence in humans of fascioliasis (from *Fasciola gigantica*) and intestinal distomatosis (from *Fasciolopsis buski*) in Laos. Sante 2008;18:119–24.
14. Bunnag D, Radomyos P, Harinasuta T. Field trial of the treatment of fasciolopsiasis with praziquantel. Southeast Asian J Trop Med Public Health 1983;14:216–19.
15. Medical Letter. Drugs for parasitic infections. Treatment Guidelines from the Medical Letter 2010(suppl.):e1–e20.
16. Pungpak S, Radomyos P, Radomyos BE, Schelp FP, et al. Treatment of *Opisthorchis viverrini* and intestinal fluke infections with Praziquantel. Southeast Asian J Trop Med Public Health 1998;29:246–9.
17. Hong SJ, Cho TK, Hong SJ, et al. Fifteen human cases of *Fibricola seoulensis*. Korean J Parasitol 1984;22:61–9.
18. Hong ST, Shoop WL. *Neodiplostomum seoulense*, the amended name for *Fibricola seoulensis*. Korean J Parasitol 1995;33:399.

Liver Fluke Infections 124

Yupaporn Wattanagoon, Danai Bunnag

Key features

- The major flukes causing liver infection are *Opisthorchis* spp., *Clonorchis sinensis*, and *Fasciola* spp. Less common causes are *Dicrocoelium* and *Eurytrema*
- *Clonorchis* is limited to East and Southeast Asia, *O. viverrini* to Southeast Asia and *O. felineus* is widely distributed in eastern Europe. *Fasciola* spp. occurs in many countries of the world
- *Opisthorchis* and *Clonorchis* are acquired through ingestion of raw or undercooked cyprinid fish (e.g. carp) containing infective metacercariae and *Fasciola* after eating freshwater plants with encysted metacercariae. Herbivorous animals are the usual hosts of *Fasciola* spp.
- *Clonorchis* and *Opisthorchis* reside in the biliary tree; acute symptoms are more common with *O. felineus*. Chronic infection with these species is strongly associated with cholangiocarcinoma
- Symptoms with *Fasciola* occur during migration of the fluke through liver parenchyma or during ectopic migration
- Detection of characteristic ova in stool is the usual mode of diagnosis. Serology can also be useful
- Treatment of *Opisthorchis* and *Clonorchis* is usually with praziquantel, whereas *Fasciola* is treated with triclabendazole

124.1 Opisthorchiasis and Clonorchiasis

INTRODUCTION

Opisthorchiasis and clonorchiasis are caused by liver flukes in the genus *Opisthorchiadae* and *Clonorchiadae*. The three most common species causing disease in humans are *Opisthorchis viverrini, O. felineus,* and *Clonorchis sinensis*.

EPIDEMIOLOGY

Opisthorchis viverrini is endemic in Southeast Asia – mainly Thailand, Lao People's Democratic Republic, the southern part of Vietnam, and Cambodia. The prevalence in north-eastern Thailand was as high as 90% during the 1980s and remains around 20%, despite control measures. *Opisthorchis felineus* is endemic in Russia and Eastern Europe, and *C. sinensis* is common in Korea, China, and northern Vietnam. In endemic areas, children as young as 1 year old have been infected with *O. viverrini*.

NATURAL HISTORY, PATHOGENESIS, AND PATHOLOGY

Humans are an incidental host of *O. viverrini, O. felineus,* and *Clonorchis sinensis*. Consumption of raw or undercooked cyprinid fish (e.g. carp) containing metacercaria – the infective stage of these flukes – results in infection. The metacercaria, released in the intestine, move through the Ampula of Vater into the common bile duct to the gallbladder and the peripheral bile ducts in the liver, and develop into adult worms (Fig. 124.1). Adult worms release eggs that are passed in the feces. Once in freshwater, the eggs hatch and release miracidia that are taken up by snails in which parasite amplification occurs. Cercariae emerge from snails and infect susceptible fresh water fish, encysting as metacercariae.

The presence of adult worms in the bile duct causes chronic irritation; the worms also release toxic metabolic substances. The immune response leads to infiltration with eosinophils and mononuclear cells in periductal areas; secondary bacterial infections can occur. There is bile duct epithelial cell desquamation, epithelial cell hyperplasia and glandular proliferation (Fig. 124.2). Intrahepatic bile ducts become dilated with distal clubbing and cystic changes. The gallbladder can be dilated and contain whitish bile [1], and its wall can demonstrate hypertrophic epithelial cells. Severity of pathology depends on both intensity and duration of infection. The chronic changes combined with endogenous and exogenous carcinogens, notably nitrosamines, induce mutagenic changes in the bile duct epithelium and can lead to cholangiocarcinoma.

CLINICAL FEATURES

Acute symptoms are more common with *C. sinensis* and *O. felineus* infection and are rare with *O. viverrini*. High fever, arthralgia, myalgia, lymph node enlargement, eosinophilia and, occasionally, facial edema can occur after 2–3 weeks of infection during worm migration and development [2]. As the worms are not yet mature, ova will not be detected in the feces at this stage. Illness usually

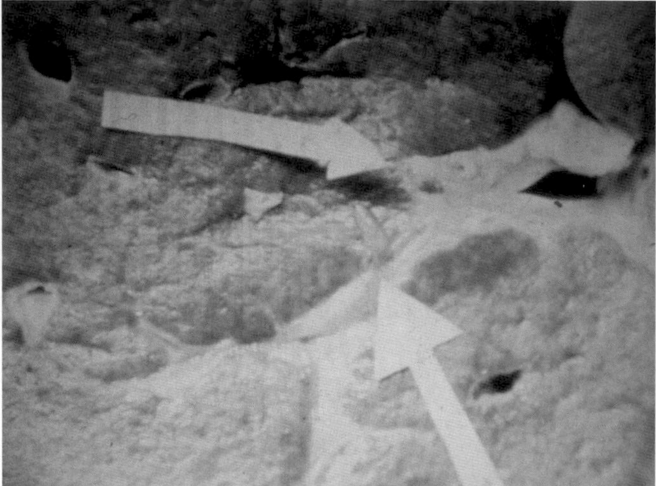

FIGURE 124.1 Adult *Opisthorchis viverrini* in the intrahepatic bile ducts in a gross specimen from a patient with cholangicarcinoma. *(Courtesy of Asst. Professor Mario Riganti, Faculty of Tropical Medicine, Mahidol University.)*

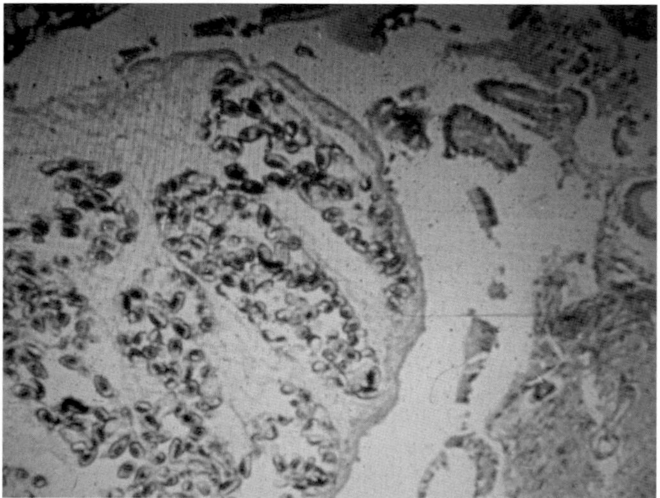

FIGURE 124.2 Microscopic pathology of intrahepatic ducts, epithelial desquamation, hyperplasia and proliferation with presence of an adult fluke inside the bile duct lumen. *(Courtesy of Asst. Professor Mario Riganti, Faculty of Tropical Medicine, Mahidol University.)*

lasts for 1–2 weeks. Allergic hepatitis is occasionally observed, especially in severe cases.

Chronic infections are usually asymptomatic. Most infections are detected by routine stool examination. In symptomatic cases, nonspecific symptoms, such as lassitude, anorexia, flatulence, abdominal discomfort, poor appetite, and occasional loose stools are complaints. A peculiar hot sensation over the right upper abdomen is a characteristic symptom found in *O. viverrini* infection. Low-grade fever and hepatomegaly can be found on examination [3].

Complications such as relapsing cholangitis or abscess caused by secondary bacterial infections are common in advanced infection. Patients present with fever, jaundice, and abdominal pain with hepatomegaly and an enlarged gallbladder. Cholangiocarcinoma is highly associated with opisthorchis and clonorchis infection [4], especially when combined with consumption of a diet high in nitrosamines. Animal studies have documented that hamsters infected with *O. viverrini* developed cholangiocarcinoma when fed a high nitrosamine diet [5].

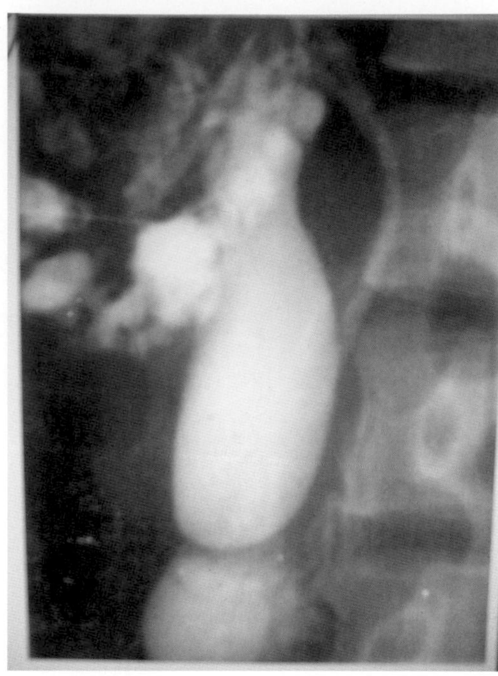

FIGURE 124.3 Dilated intrahepatic bile ducts and gall bladder seen on cholangiogram. *(Courtesy of Dr Tula Dhiensiri.)*

PATIENT EVALUATION AND DIFFERENTIAL DIAGNOSIS

As patients with early or mild infection can be asymptomatic, diagnosis usually relies on routine stool examination. People in endemic areas who eat uncooked fish and have nonspecific abdominal symptoms should have yearly stool examinations for *Opisthorchis* or *Clornorchis* ova. However, these ova can be difficult to differentiate from flukes present in the small intestine [6]. Patients with intestinal fluke infection usually have chronic watery diarrhea.

Acute opisthorchiasis or clonorchiasis are differentiated from acute fascioliasis, acute schistosomiasis and other tissue parasites by exposure history and epidemiology.

In late-stage disease, patients can present with obstructive jaundice, cholangitis, or cholangiocarcinoma; other causes of obstructive jaundice, such as biliary tract stones, should be investigated.

DIAGNOSIS

Stool examination for *Opisthorchis* or *Clonorchis* ova is the standard for diagnosis. Other specimens that can be used for ova detection are duodenal fluid or bile collected via endoscopic retrograde cholangiopancreatography (ERCP) or during surgery.

Serology can be used for diagnosis of acute infection, but is not helpful in chronic infection or re-infection in endemic areas, as a positive antibody will persist after treatment. Detection of co-proantigen can be used as a "test of cure" after treatment.

PCR can detect *Opisthorchis* DNA in fecal samples and distinguish it from intestinal flukes with high sensitivity and specificity. It is also useful for epidemiologic surveys [7].

Ultrasonography of the liver and gallbladder in early infections usually shows an enlarged non-functioning gall bladder with sludge. Later stage infections can show dilatation of intrahepatic bile ducts or a mass. A liver mass with intralesional bile duct dilatation is suggestive of cholangiocarcinoma. Cholangiography was performed before the availability of computed tomography (CT) or magnetic resonance imaging (MRI). Dilated intrahepatic bile ducts with distal clubbing may be visualized (Fig. 124.3), as well as occasional filling defects owing to the presence of adult flukes (Fig. 124.4). CT or MRI is useful for staging of cholangiocarcinoma.

TREATMENT

OPISTHORCHIS VIVERRINI

Praziquantel is the drug of choice. At a dose of 25 mg/kg body weight orally three times over 1–2 days, the cure rate was 100% [8]. A single dose of 40 mg/kg at bedtime gave a 91–95% cure, while a dose of 50 mg/kg gave 97% cure rate but with a higher rate of adverse events [9, 10]. Therefore, praziquantel, 40 mg/kg, is recommended for mass treatment.

Albendazole at 400 mg twice daily for 3–7 days yielded only a 40–63% cure rate [11].

CLONORCHIS SINENSIS

Praziquantel is effective for clonorchiasis. Twenty-five mg/kg, three times per day for 1 day yields an 85% cure rate, while the same dose given for 2 days cures up to 100%. A single dose of 40 mg/kg yielded only a 25% cure rate [12].

Patients with secondary cholangitis should be treated with antimicrobials. Cholangiocarcinoma, if detected early, can be resected. However if detected late, palliative treatment by drainage of bile can help to relieve symptoms of obstructive jaundice. The prognosis is poor for these patients as chemotherapy or radiation therapy are usually not effective for cholangiocarcinoma.

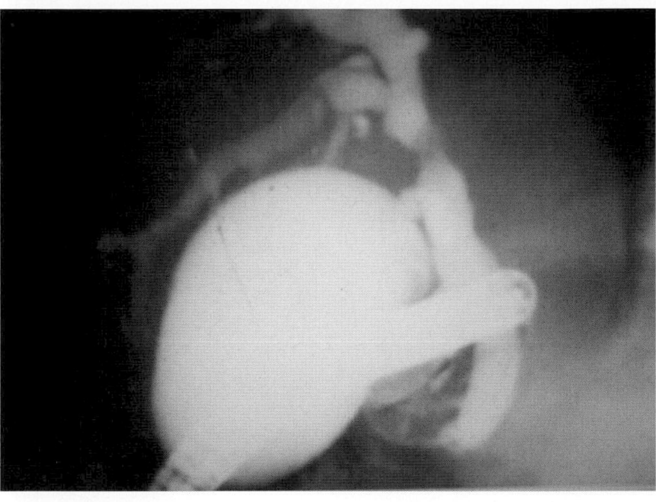

FIGURE 124.4 Cholangiogram with dilated bile ducts with filling defect due to the presence of an adult fluke in the lumen. *(Courtesy of Dr Tula Dhiensiri.)*

PREVENTION AND CONTROL

Thorough cooking of fish is the best way to prevent infection. This should be enforced through continuous health education in endemic areas. Control measures through mass treatment programs and improving sanitation can reduce the prevalence.

124.2 Fascioliasis

INTRODUCTION

Fascioliasis is infection by sheep liver flukes, *Fasciola* spp. The two species that infect humans are *Fasciola hepatica* and *Fasciola gigantica* (Fig. 124.5) Other herbivorous animals such as cattle, goats, water buffalo, horses, camels, hogs, rabbits, and deer can be infected with *Fasciola* spp.

EPIDEMIOLOGY

Human fascioliasis has been reported worldwide. Endemic areas are South America, the Middle East, Asia, Africa, Europe, and the USA.

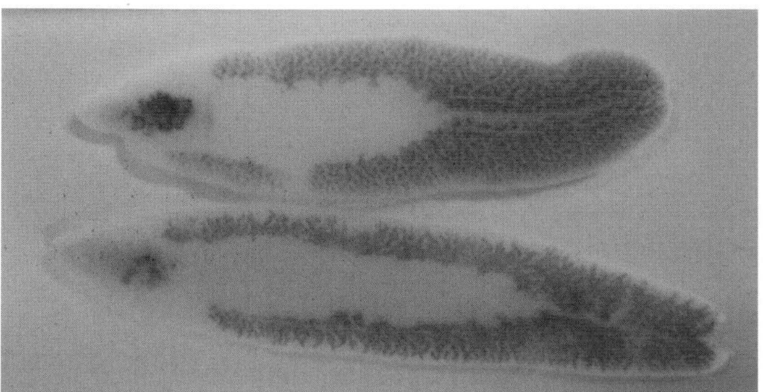

FIGURE 124.5 *Fasciola* spp. *Fasciola hepatica* and *Fasciola gigantiga* adult flukes.

NATURAL HISTORY, PATHOGENESIS, AND PATHOLOGY

Humans acquire *Fasciola* after ingestion of aquatic plants, such as fresh watercress, that are contaminated with *Fasciola metacercaria*. The metacercaria excyst in the duodenum and penetrate through the intestinal wall into the peritoneal cavity. They enter the liver through Glisson's capsule, moving through the liver parenchyma to their final habitat – the bile ducts – where they attain maturity and begin laying eggs. The immature parasites can wander, causing ectopic foci in organs such as the heart, lung, brain, and subcutaneous tissues.

The pathologic changes in human fascioliasis are related to the stages of infection. In the early stage of immature worm migration (migratory phase), the young flukes create migratory tracts in the liver parenchyma, producing subcapsular hemorrhages and hepatic necrosis with cellular infiltration of eosinophils and lymphocytes, leading to hepatic abscesses and, finally, fibrosis. Common bile duct obstruction rarely occurs. Once reaching the large bile duct, adult flukes cause hyperplasia, desquamation and cystic dilatation of bile ducts. Ectopic fascioliasis is common.

CLINICAL FEATURES

Human fascioliasis is usually mild. Clinical symptoms can be described in relation to the phases of infection.

MIGRATORY PHASE

Symptoms occur when young flukes migrate through the liver capsule and parenchyma before reaching the bile ducts. They include dyspepsia, anorexia, nausea, vomiting, pain in the right

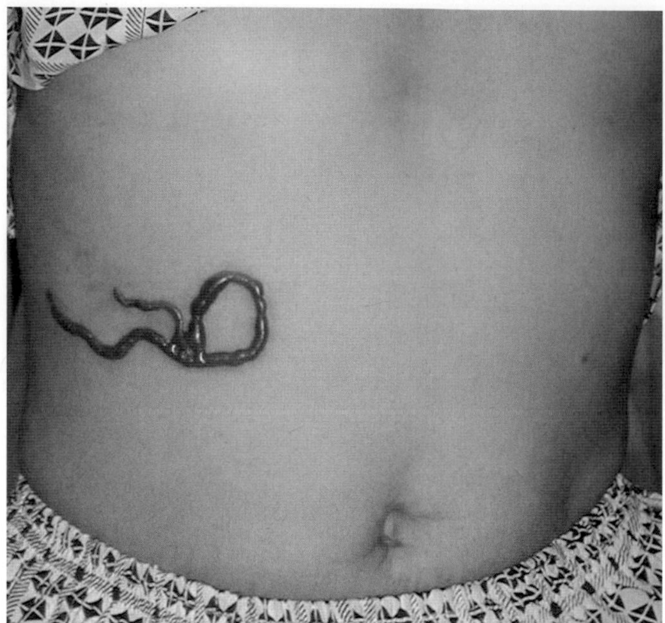

FIGURE 124.6 Ectopic fascioliasis. Cutaneous serpiginous hemorrhagic vesicular parasitic tract over the abdominal wall caused by *Fasciola gigantica*. *(Courtesy of Dr Nguyen Thien Hung, Medic Medical Centre, Ho Chi Minh City, Vietnam.)*

hypochondrium, and hepatomegaly. Urticaria and eosinophilia are common.

BILIARY TRACT INFECTION

Once the flukes reside in the bile ducts, most patients have no clinical symptoms. On rare occasions, bile duct occlusion can occur leading to signs and symptoms of obstructive jaundice or pancreatitis. In highly endemic areas, growth stunting in children occurs [13].

Ectopic Fascioliasis

Clinical symptoms and signs depend on the site of infection. Parasitic tracts, nodules or abnormal masses can be found in subcutaneous tissues (Fig. 124.6), the intestinal wall, lung, heart, or brain, and can be accompanied by hemorrhage, for example intracranial hemorrahge.

Pharyngeal Form

The pharyngeal form is caused by consumption of young flukes in infected livers of goats or sheep. The flukes attach to the mucosa of laryngopharyngeal tissue causing localized edema of the pharynx or larynx leading to dysphagia and dyspnea. Patients can die from asphyxia if not recognized.

PATIENT EVALUATION, DIAGNOSIS, AND DIFFERENTIAL DIAGNOSIS

The standard method of diagnosis is detection of *Fasciola* ova in fecal samples. Ova should be differentiated from *Fasciolopsis buski* ova, which is a large intestinal fluke. Eggs can also be found in bile or duodenal aspirate.

Serologic diagnosis is useful for diagnosis of acute phase and ectopic fascioliasis as stool examination will be negative in these patients. Detection of antibody by ELISA or immunoblots using *F. gigantica* excretory secretory antigen have high sensitivity and specificity.

Recovery of adult worms from surgical or autopsy specimens, or stool collection after treatment, can help to confirm the diagnosis.

Radiologic examinations including ultrasonography and CT of the liver are helpful, especially during the hepatic or migratory phase. Subcapsular hypodense areas and intrahepatic hypoechoic nodular lesions with poorly defined contours may be found on ultrasonogram. CT can show multiple hypodense nodules and tunnel-like, branching hypodense tracts representing the migratory tracts of young flukes [14]. During the biliary phase, adult fasciola may appear as a leaf-like echogenic object without acoustic shadow in the gallbladder or common bile ducts [15]. Filling defects owing to the presence of adult fasciola in the bile duct can also be demonstrated during endoscopic retrograde cholangiopancreatography (ERCP).

TREATMENT

Following reports of the failure of praziquantel in fascioliasis, triclabendazole, nitazoxanide, and artesunate have been tried. Praziquantel at 25mg/ kg three times daily for 1–2 days was only partially effective in treating fascioliasis. Triclabendazole 10 mg/kg single dose, or two doses for 1 day, is effective, with cure rates of 79% and 92% respectively. A randomized placebo-controlled trial of nitazoxanide 500 mg twice daily for 7 days gave a 60% cure rate. Children aged 4–11 years old were given a dose of 200 mg twice daily and children aged 2–3 years old received 100 mg twice daily for 7 days; this resulted in a 40% cure rate [16]. A randomized, controlled trial compared triclabendazole 10 mg/kg for two doses at 12-h intervals and artesunate 4 mg/kg once a day for 10 days for the treatment of acute fascioliasis in Vietnam. Artesunate-treated patients were significantly more likely to be free of abdominal pain, but were less likely to be symptom-free 3 months after treatment (76% vs. 92%) [17].

Surgical resection or ERCP removal of adult flukes can be done in cases with biliary tract obstruction.

PREVENTION AND CONTROL

Proper cooking or cleaning of aquatic plants before consumption will prevent accidental *Fasciola* infection. In endemic areas, adequate mass chemotherapy of infected animals and proper sanitary protection of pastures are important control measures.

124.3 Dicroceliasis and Eurytremiasis

INTRODUCTION

Dicroceliasis and eurytremiasis are caused by the liver flukes *Dicrocoelium dendriticum* and *Eurytrema pancreaticum*. Herbivorous animals such as sheep, goats, and cattle are the natural host. Humans are accidental hosts.

EPIDEMIOLOGY

Dicroceliasis is common in animals in Europe, northern Africa and parts of the Far East, and is less common in North and South America. Only a few human cases have been reported, mainly from Europe.

Eurytrema pancreaticum has been reported from autopsy findings in China and Japan [18]. Animal infections have been reported in cattle, water buffalo, sheep, and goats in Asia and occasionally in camels and monkeys in northern China, Brazil, Venezuela, and Madagascar.

NATURAL HISTORY, PATHOGENESIS, AND PATHOLOGY

Humans acquire dicroceliasis by accidental ingestion of food contaminated with infected ants of the species, *Formica fusa,* which is the second intermediate host. Acquisition of eurytremiasis follows accidental ingestion of food contaminated with infected grasshoppers or crickets – the second intermediate host. In both infections, metacercaria excyst in the duodenum and migrate through the ampula of Vater. For dicroceliasis, they move retrograde to the bile ducts where they develop into adult worms. In eurytremiasis, they move retrograde to the pancreatic duct and, rarely, the bile ducts, where they develop into adult worms. Pathologic changes are similar to those of *Opisthorchis* infections.

CLINICAL FEATURES

There have been only rare documented cases of re-infection. In dicroceliasis, dyspepsia, abdominal pain, flatulence, and watery diarrhea have been reported [19]. In eurytremiasis, symptoms include abdominal distress, dyspepsia, vomiting, and diarrhea. Occasionally jaundice and an enlarged tender liver have been documented.

DIAGNOSIS

Demonstration of ova of each species in fecal specimens is diagnostic. Spurious infection should be suspected if patients have a history of raw sheep liver consumption. Patients should be put on a liver-free diet for 3 days and a repeat stool examination performed.

TREATMENT

No therapeutic trials have been conducted. Praziquantel 25 mg/kg three times a day for 1 day or triclabendazole 10 mg/kg single dose after a meal have both been used successfully in single case treatment of dicroceliasis [19]. Most cases of eurytremiasis have been successfully treated with praziquantel 25 mg/kg three times a day for 1 day.

REFERENCES

1. Riganti M, Pungpak S, Punpoowong B, et al. Human pathology of *Opisthorchis viverrini* infection: A comparison of adults and children. Southeast Asian J Trop Med Public Health 1989;20:95–100.
2. Xu Z, Zhong H, Cao W. Acute clonorchiasis: Report 2 cases. Chin Med J 1970;92:423–6.
3. Pungpak S, Riganti M, Bunnag D, Harinasuta T. Clinical features in severe *Opisthorchiasis viverrini*. Southeast Asian J Trop Med Public Health 1985; 16:405–9.
4. Haswell-Elkins MR, Mairiang E, Mairiang P, et al. Cross-sectional study of *Opisthorchis viverrini* infection and cholangiocarcinoma in communities within a high risk area in northeast Thailand. Int J Cancer 1994;59:505–9.
5. Thamvit W, Bhramarapravati N, Sahaphong S, et al. Effects of Dimethylnitrosamine on induction of Cholangiocarcinoma in *O. viverrini* infected Syrian golden hamsters. Cancer Res 1978;38:4634–39.
6. Radomyos P, Bunnag D, Harinasuta T. Worms recovered in stools following helminthic infections. Southeast Asian J Trop Med Public Health 1984;15:44.
7. Lovis L, Mark TK, Phongluxa K, et al. PCR Diagnosis of *Opisthorchis viverrini* and *Haplorchis taichui* infections in an endemic Lao community: a comparison of diagnostic methods for parasitilogical field surveys. J Clin Microbiol 2009;47:1517–23.
8. Bunnag D, Harinasuta T. Studies on the chemotherapy of human opisthorchiasis in Thailand. I. Clinical trial of praziquantel. Southeast Asian J Trop Med Public Health 1980;11:528–31.
9. Bunnag D, Harinasuta T. Studies on the chemotherapy of human opisthorchiasis. III Minimum effective dose of Praziquantel. Southeast Asian J Trop Med Public Health 1981;12:413–17.
10 Pungpak S, Bunnag D, Harinasuta T. Studies on the chemotherapy of human opisthorchiasis: Effective dose of praziquantel in heavy infection. Southeast Asian J Trop Med Public Health 1985;16:248–52.
11. Pungpak S, Bunnag D, Harinasuta T. Albendazole in the treatment of opisthorchiasis and concomitant intestinal helminthic infections. Southeast Asian J Trop Med Public Health 1984;15:44–50.
12. Rim HJ, Lyu KS. Chemotherapeutic effect of praziquantel (EMBAY 8440) in the treatment of clonorchiasis sinensis. Korea Univ Med J 1979;16:459–70.
13. Stork MG, Venables GS, Jennings SMF, et al. An investigation of endemic fascioliasis in Peruvian village children. J Trop Med Hyg 1973;76:231–5.
14. Kabaalioglu A, Ceken K, Alimoglu E, et al. Hepatobiliary fascioliasis: Sonographic and CT findings in 87 patient during the initial phase and long termfollow-up. Am J Roentgenol 2007;189:824–8.
15. Richter J, Freise S, Mull R, Millán JC. Fascioliasis: sonographic abnormalities of the biliary tract and evolution after treatment with triclabendazole. Trop Med Int Health 1999;4(11):774–81.
16. Kaiser J, Utzinger J. Chemotherapy for major food borne trematodes: a review. Expert Opin Pharmacother 2004;5:1711–26.
17. Tran TH, Ng TT, Nguyen HM, et al. A randomized controlled pilot study of artesunate versus triclabendazole for human fascioliasis in Central Vietnam. Am J Trop Med Hyg 2003;78:388–92.
18. Ishii Y, Koga M, Fujino T, et al. Human infection with the pancreatic fluke *Eurytrema pancreaticum*. Am J Trop Med Hyg 1983;32:1019–22.
19. Ceniz ZT, Yilmaz H, Dulger AC, Cicek M. Human infection with dicrocelium dendriticum in Turkey. Ann Saudi Med 2010;30:159–61.

125 Paragonimiasis

Yupaporn Wattanagoon, Danai Bunnag

Key features

- More than ten species of *Paragonimus* are infective to humans; *Paragonimus westermani* is the most commonly reported
- Infection is acquired by ingestion of raw freshwater crabs or crayfish containing metacercaria
- Ectopic manifestations are common
- Paragonimiasis should be differentiated from pulmonary tuberculosis, especially when presenting with hemoptysis
- Treatment is usually successful with praziquantel

INTRODUCTION

Paragonimiasis is the infection caused by lung flukes of the genus Paragonimus. More than ten species of Paragonimus are infective to humans; the most commonly reported is *P. westermani*. The disease is acquired through eating raw, or undercooked, freshwater crabs (Fig. 125.1) or crayfish containing the infective metacercaria stage of the fluke.

EPIDEMIOLOGY

There are more than 22 million people infected globally [1] and about 200 million people at risk. Paragonimiasis is prevalent in Asia – especially Southeast Asia, Africa, and Central and South America. *Paragonimus westermani*, or oriental lung fluke infection, is common in Asia – especially in China, the Philippines, Thailand, and Vietnam, whereas *Paragonimus mexicanus* causes infection in Central and South America, and *Paragonimus africanus* and *Paragonimus uterobilateralis* are the major causes of infection in Africa. Human infection with *Paragonimus kellicotti* has been reported in the USA.

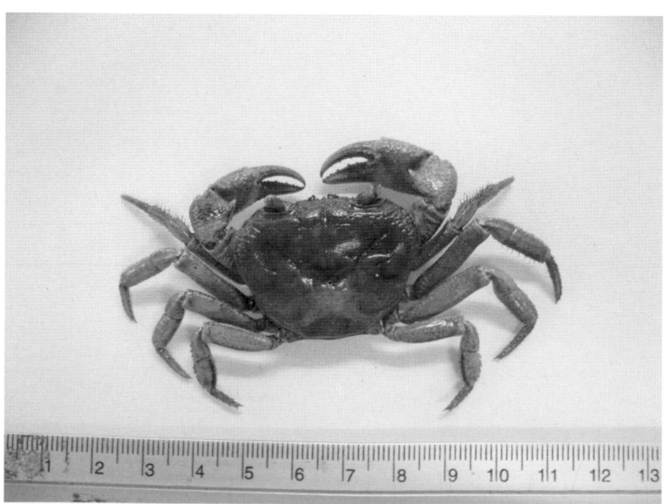

FIGURE 125.1 Potamon crab: an intermediate host for paragonimiasis.

NATURAL HISTORY, PATHOLOGY, AND PATHOGENESIS

The wide variation in pathologic findings depends on the number of infecting worms, duration of infection and tissues affected. Toxic and allergic factors may be involved.

Infection with *P. westermani* is acquired though ingestion of metacerariae in undercooked, or raw, crab or crayfish. Ingestion of different snails or crustaceans can lead to infection with other *Paragonimus* species. The metacercariae excyst, penetrate the intestinal wall, enter the abdominal cavity and then cross the diaphragm into the lung, where they mature into adult worms over a period of approximately 2 months. Adults worms produce eggs that gain access to the tracheobronchial tree through fistulas from the parasitic lung cyst. Eggs are coughed up and shed into the environment through sputum or after swallowing and passage in the feces. Once in freshwater, the eggs hatch releasing miracidia that infect snail hosts where parasite amplification and development occurs. Cercariae are released from the snail and infect crustacean hosts. In some cases, infection can be from a paratenic host, such as wild boars [2].

PULMONARY LESIONS

Migration of larval flukes in the lungs (and frequently in other tissues) induces local necrosis, hemorrhage and inflammatory exudate, which is followed by fibrous encapsulation into a worm cyst. In the lungs, initial lesions are usually located a few centimeters beneath the pleural surface, near bronchioles or bronchi. Pathology includes bronchopneumonia, interstitial pneumonia, bronchitis, bronchiectasis, atelectasis, fibrosis, pleural thickening, pleural effusion, angiitis obliterans, and periphlebitis.

Macroscopically, the worm cysts are 1–4 cm, distended, grayish-white nodules. In cross section they have irregular outlines and cavities, within which are 1–2 worms and, uncommonly, 3, 4 or 0. The total number of cysts in the lungs is usually <20, with the larger proportion located in the right lung.

Microscopically, the cyst wall consists of granulation tissue with fibroblasts, lymphoid cells, mononuclear cells, plasma cells, and eosinophils. Within the cavity are numerous Charcot-Leyden crystals, *Paragonimus* eggs, and necrotic material. In the vicinity of the cysts are tunnels, burrows, egg tubercles, and calcified eggs.

ECTOPIC LESIONS

Young, or even mature, flukes can migrate from the lungs and reach almost any organ, including the breast, psoas muscle, testes, scrotum, spermatic cord, liver, gut wall, other abdominal viscera, uterine and vaginal wall, spinal cord, and brain. In the ectopic site, the flukes reach sexual maturity. Cysts, granulomas, or abscess can then form around the flukes or their eggs. Some immature flukes migrate from the lungs through the jugular or carotid foramen at the base of the skull to reach the temporal and occipital lobes of the brain, where they produce necrosis and eosinophilic granulomatous reactions. In China, migratory subcutaneous swellings are common with *Pagumogonimus skrjabini* infection, and ova have been found at the centers of small eosinophilic granulomas in the pericardium, meninges, and liver.

CLINICAL MANIFESTATIONS

In light infections, the majority of patients are asymptomatic. Even in heavy infections, most patients have few symptoms and appear well, despite severe pathology. The disease can be classified into acute and chronic stages involving pulmonary or extrapulmonary sites.

ACUTE STAGE

This stage corresponds to the period of invasion and migration of young flukes. Although this stage often passes undiagnosed, findings can include diarrhea, abdominal pain, urticaria, and eosinophilia, followed by fever, chest pain, cough, dyspnea, malaise, and night sweats. The symptoms usually spontaneously resolve after 1–2 months.

CHRONIC STAGE

Pulmonary Paragonimiasis

The incubation period is about 6 months (range: 1–27 months). Cough, sputum and chest discomfort increase gradually and are similar to those in chronic bronchitis. The cough is spasmodic, usually occurs on walking or after exertion, and is productive. Sputum is characteristically gelatinous, tenacious and rusty-brown. Hemoptysis is common and can be aggravated by strenuous exertion. Pleuritic chest pain is also common. About half of the patients complain of breathlessness on exertion and some complain of wheezing. Mild fever may be present.

Physical signs in the chest are not distinct; digital clubbing can be seen. Secondary bronchopneumonia and lung abscess are complications. Pleural involvement includes unilateral or bilateral pleural effusion or, in rare instances, pseudochylothorax. In endemic areas, co-infection of pulmonary paragonimiasis and tuberculosis is not uncommon.

EXTRAPULMONARY PARAGONIMIASIS

Cerebral and spinal paragonimiasis

In endemic areas of Asia, 25% of hospitalized cases are as a result of brain invasion. Eighty percent of these patients are <10 years old and most are males. Cerebral disease is particularly prevalent in rural South Korea, where it is the most common cause of cerebral tumor. As many as 10 round or oval cysts, measuring a few millimeters to 10 cm in diameter, are found in the temporal and occipital lobes, near the jugular foramen.

In the acute phase, manifestations can resemble meningoencephalitis. Patients suffer headache, vomiting, fever, and visual disturbances. With progression, patients can have papilledema, bitemporal hemianopsia, facial palsy, hemiplegia, paraplegia, Jacksonian seizures, and coma. Death during the acute phase is not uncommon. In nonfatal cases, spontaneous remission occurs in 1–2 months, but recurrence may follow. Pleocytosis of the cerebrospinal fluid (CSF) with a high eosinophil count is usually seen. Cysts can be demonstrated by computed tomography or angiography.

Rarely, spinal cord involvement presents as paraplegia or monoplegia, with weakness of the extremities and disturbance in sensation.

Abdominal paragonimiasis

Findings can include abdominal pain and tenderness, bloody diarrhea, nausea, vomiting, palpable nodules, and abscess formation in the liver, spleen, or abdominal cavity. These may simulate a bacterial infection. In some instances, cysts rupture into the intestinal lumen releasing *Paragonimus* eggs that can be recovered in the feces.

Migratory subcutaneous paragonimiasis

Migratory subcutaneous nodules occur in 20–60% of patients with *P. skrjabini* and 10% of those with *P. westermani* infections. They are firm, tender, slightly mobile, a few millimeters to 10 cm in diameter and are often mildly irritating. The most common sites are the lower abdomen, inguinal region, and thigh.

In China, *P. skrjabini* is unable to develop to maturity in the lungs. Instead of findings of hemoptysis and ova in the sputum, the striking feature is trematode larva migrans associated with migratory subcutaneous nodules accompanied by marked eosinophilic leukocytosis and necrotic liver lesions. In many cases, the nodules contain juvenile flukes. Brain involvement with subarachnoid hemorrhage occurs.

PATIENT EVALUATION, DIAGNOSIS, AND DIFFERENTIAL DIAGNOSIS

A presumptive diagnosis can be made in a patient who has a history of chronic bronchitis, blood-streaked sputum and occasional hemoptysis, and who lives in an endemic area and has eaten raw crustaceans.

Laboratory tests show an eosinophilic leukocytosis. Chest radiographs in the early stage show ill-defined opacities. Later radiographic findings include cavitary lesions, lung infiltration (nodular, patchy or linear type) (Fig. 125.2), calcified foci, pleural thickening, pleural effusions, and hilar enlargement [3]. Pleural fluid can be serous, serosanguinous, or chylus. It is characteristically an exudate with a high amount of protein (6–7 g/dl), very low glucose level (<10 mg/dl), high lactate dehydrogenase (1000 u/dl), elevated percentage of eosinophils (12–75%), and low pH (<7.1) [4]. Occasionally, the fluid may be chylous [5].

Confirmation is made by finding characteristic eggs in sputum, stool, pleural effusion, or CSF, or adult flukes in subcutaneous nodules, in other surgical specimens or, rarely, in sputum.

Serologic diagnosis can be used for detection of antibody of *Paragonimus* spp. via complement fixation, ELISA and immunoblot – they give high sensitivity and specificity [6]. Antigen detection using monoclonal antibody is useful for detecting active infection [7]. Immunodiagnosis is particularly useful for diagnosis of extrapulmonary disease when paragonimus ova cannot be detected in sputum or stool

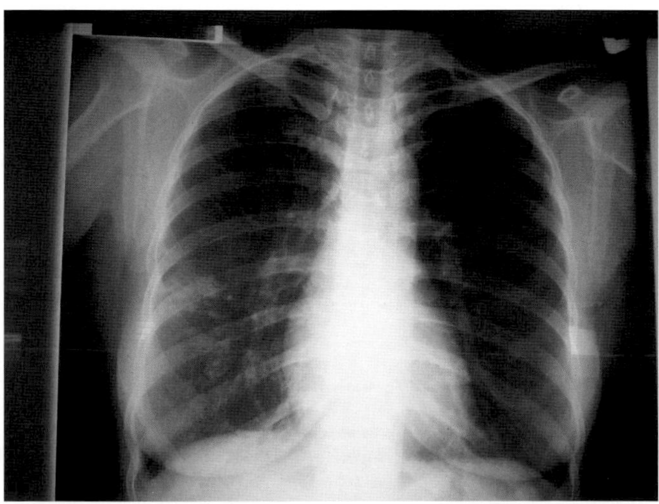

FIGURE 125.2 Demonstrating infiltration of right lung in a patient with paragonimiasis. *(Courtesy of Asst. Professor Udomsak Silachamroon, Faculty of Tropical Medicine, Mahidol University.)*

samples. Most treated patients become seronegative after about 6–12 months.

The differential diagnosis of pulmonary paragonimiasis includes pulmonary tuberculosis, lung abscess, chronic bronchitis or bronchiectasis, and primary and metastatic pulmonary carcinoma. In many areas where tuberculosis is common, the eating of raw freshwater crabs or pork is also common. Patients presenting with chronic cough or hemoptysis with acid-fast bacilli-negative sputum should be investigated for paragonimiasis as the prevalence of paragonimiasis may be as high as 50% and patients can be cured with antihelminthic drugs within a few days. Cerebral and spinal paragonimiasis must be differentiated from abscess, tuberculoma and other helminthic infections, including fascioliasis, schistosomiasis, cysticercosis, hydatid disease, angiostrongyliasis, and gnathostomiasis.

Abdominal symptoms mimic many acute conditions, including appendicitis and amebic liver abscess. Subcutaneous paragonimiasis can be confused with gnathostomiasis, sparganosis, onchocerciasis, and cysticercosis.

TREATMENT

The drug of choice is praziquantel 25 mg/kg three times per day after meals for 3 days. The cure rate is almost 100% [8–10]; only a few patients with heavy infections require a second course of treatment. Symptoms improve rapidly and disappear within a few months. Eggs clear from the sputum in a few weeks, whereas the radiologic pulmonary lesions can take months to clear. The dosage in cerebral paragonimiasis is often higher and must be adjusted according to the clinical response. Because convulsions and coma have been observed, treatment should proceed in the hospital with corticosteroids administered to prevent brain edema. A randomized, controlled trial in small numbers of patients showed that triclabendazole 5 mg/kg/day for 3 days or 10 mg/kg bid for 1 day orally gives the same cure rate as praziquantel but has a faster egg reduction rate [11]. The drug is not available as widely as praziquantel. Bithionol in a dose of 30–50 mg/kg/d on alternate days for 10–15 days is also effective, although the drug has treatment-limiting side effects [12]. Surgical resection of ectopic paragonimiasis, such as subcutaneous nodules or masses can cure extrapulmonary paragonimiasis.

Pulmonary paragonimiasis is rarely fatal; even without treatment, flukes die or disappear within 10–20 years. Pleural effusions can be protracted and recur even after treatment. Most cases of cerebral disease are associated with chronic morbidity as a result of epilepsy and other neurologic sequelae. Five percent of the patients die as a result of hemorrhage – usually in the first 2 years of the disease.

PREVENTION AND CONTROL

Health education, especially for young school-children, is needed to change the dietary customs of eating raw, or undercooked, crab or crayfish. Mass treatment with bithionol in some endemic areas in Korea proved effective in reducing the prevalence of paragonimiasis. Mollusciciding is impractical.

REFERENCES

1. Haswell-Elkins MR, Ekkins DB. Lung and liver flukes. In: Leslie C, Albert B, Max S, eds. Toplley and Wilson's Microbiology and Microbial infections, Vol.5, 9th edn. New York: Oxford University Press; 1998:507–20.
2. Miyazaki I, Habe S. A newly recognized mode of human infection with the lung fluke *Paragonimus westermani*. J Parasitol 1976;62:646–8.
3. Vanijanonda S, Bunnag D, Harinasuta T. Radiological findings in pulmonary paragonimiasis heterotremus. Southeast Asian J Trop Med Pub Health 1984; 15:122.
4. Romeo DP, Pollock JJ. Pulmonary paragonimiasis: diagnostic value of pleural fluid analysis. South Med J 1986;79:241–3.
5. Thewjitcharoen Y, Poopitaya S. Paragonimiasis presenting with unilateral pseudochylothorax: case report and literature review. Scand J Infect Dis 2006; 38:386–8.
6. Slemenda SB, Maddison SE, Jong EC, Moore DD. Diagnosis of paragonimiasis by immunoblot. Am J Trop Med Hyg 1988;39:469–71.
7. Zhang Z, Zhang Y, Shi Z, et al. Diagnosis of active *Paragonimus westermani* infections with a monoclonal antibody-based antigen detection assay. Am J Trop Med Hyg 1993;49:329–34.
8. Udonsi JK. Clinical field trials of praziquantel in pulmonary paragonimiasis due to *Paragonimus uterobilateralis* in endemic populations of the Igwun Basin, Nigeria. Trop Med Parasitol 1989;40:65–8.
9. Nawa Y. Re-emergence of Paragonimiasis. Intern Med 2000;39:353–4.
10. Johnson RJ, Jong EC, Dunning SB, et al. Paragonimiasis: diagnosis and the use of praziquantel in treatment. Rev Infect Dis 1985;7:200–6.
11. Calvopiña M, Guderian RH, Paredes W, et al. Treatment of human pulmonary paragonimiasis with triclabendazole: clinical tolerance and drug efficacy. Trans R Soc Trop Med Hyg 1998;92:566–9.
12. Kim JS. Treatment of *Paragonimus westermani* infections with bithionol. Am J Trop Med Hyg 1970;19:940.

SECTION

E

CESTODE INFECTIONS

126 Tapeworm Infections

Joseph D Mega, Gerson Galdos-Cardenas, Robert H Gilman

Key features

- There are three main *Taenia* species: *Taenia saginata*, *Taenia solium*, and *Taenia asiatica*. *Taenia solium* is also infectious in its larval form, causing human cysticercosis (see Chapter 127). *Taenia* infection occurs after ingestion of undercooked beef (*T. saginata*) or pork (*T. solium*) that are infected with larval cysticerci. Most intestinal infections are asymptomatic
- The broad tapeworm, *Diphyllobothrium latum*, is acquired after eating raw or poorly cooked fish. Most *D. latum* infections are asymptomatic
- Both *Taenia* and *D. latum* infections can be prevented by adequate cooking or freezing of beef, pork, or fish
- The dwarf tapeworm *Hymenolepis nana* is acquired after ingestion of eggs in conditions of poor hygiene, usually by children. With large worm burdens it can cause nonspecific gastrointestinal symptoms
- Infection with the dog tapeworm, *Dipylidium caninum*, occurs occasionally when a person accidentally swallows an infected flea
- All of the tapeworms can be treated with praziquantel or niclosamide

126.1 Taeniasis

INTRODUCTION

Human infection with *Taenia* species is one of the most common parasitic infections. These tapeworms cause extensive human morbidity and major production losses to domestic food animals. Human infection with *Taenia* has been documented since antiquity; the first lifecycles for any tapeworm were demonstrated with *Taenia* almost 150 years ago [1]. The highest incidence is seen in areas where undercooked pork and beef are consumed. Humans can serve as the definitive host for all *Taenia* species, as well as an accidental intermediate host of *T. solium* through ingestion of tapeworm eggs. This can lead to human cysticercosis, the most common helminthic parasite affecting the central nervous system (CNS) [2]. While the majority of taeniasis is caused by *T. saginata*, the three species of *Taenia* should be distinguished in order to evaluate a patient's risk of developing neurocysticercosis (see Chapter 127).

EPIDEMIOLOGY

INFECTION

Taeniasis incidence and prevalence are highest where cattle and swine have access to human fecal contamination and where raw or undercooked beef or pork is consumed. *Taenia solium* occurs most frequently in areas of poor sanitation where free-roaming pigs can become massively infected with cysticerci. Urban sewage used to fertilize cattle pastures is a risk factor for *T. saginata* infection if it is not properly sanitized [3].

Because meat consumption is the main route of transmission of taeniasis, infection is uncommon prior to the age at which people begin to eat meat. In rural Mexico, *T. solium* infection has been reported with similar frequency in all age groups older than two years. However, individuals who neither consume nor raise pork may still be at risk for cysticercosis if they ingest *T. solium* eggs. This mode of transmission was reported in orthodox Jews in New York City who acquired infection from contaminated food prepared by domestic helpers from endemic countries [4].

GEOGRAPHY

Both *T. saginata* and *T. solium* have a global distribution. It is estimated that 50 million people worldwide are infected with *T. saginata* and 5 million with *T. solium* [5]. The prevalence of taeniasis can vary greatly within, and between, countries.

Taenia saginata is most prevalent in East Africa, the Middle East, parts of Central and South America, central and Southeast Asia and eastern Europe. High prevalence has been demonstrated in Bali, East Africa and Tibetan populations in China [6]. The highest prevalence in Europe is in Slovakia and Turkey; however, levels for the region as a whole are low and range from less than 1% to 10% [3, 7]. Prevalence in Mexico has ranged from less than 1% to 6.5% [8, 9]. In the USA, most cases of *T. saginata* are introduced by migrants from Latin America. A survey along the Texas-Mexico border showed prevalence of 3% [10]. Most diagnostic tests used in surveys of taeniasis do not distinguish between species, which may confound *T. saginata* prevalence estimates in areas where *T. solium* is also present.

Taenia solium's cosmopolitan distribution is limited to areas of the world where pork is consumed. This makes rates of infection extremely low in Muslim countries, particularly the Middle East. *Taenia solium* is endemic in most of Latin America, with the highest seroprevalences seen in Peru, Honduras, Ecuador, Guatemala, Bolivia, Venezuela, Brazil, and Mexico [11, 12]. Other high prevalence regions include India, China, Southeast Asia, Slavic countries, and sub-Saharan Africa. Some villages in Uganda report up to 45% of pigs to be infected with *T. solium* [11]. Western Europe and North America have few infections.

Taenia asiatica is limited to Asia. Prevalence is particularly high in regions where people routinely eat undercooked pork with viscera. Taiwan, Korea, North Sumatra, Indonesia, Vietnam, and several provinces in China have a prevalence as high as 21% [13, 14].

NATURAL HISTORY, PATHOGENESIS, AND PATHOLOGY

Adult tapeworms have segmentally arranged hermaphroditic sexual units called proglottids, which mature as they progress distally from the neck of the tapeworm. The most distal (gravid) proglottids are periodically released and can pass, intact, in human feces or rupture, scattering thousands of eggs that remain infectious for months.

Taenia saginata worms are 4–12 meters in length and can contain 1000–2000 proglottids. The morphology of the proglottid helps to distinguish the different species. *Taenia saginata's* gravid proglottid has 12 or more primary uterine branches. *Taenia solium* worms are shorter (between 1.5 and 8 meters) and usually contain less than 1000 proglottids – the proglottid has an identifiable uterine pore and less than 12 primary uterine branches. *Taenia asiatica* is slightly smaller in size (4–8 meters in length, 300–1000 proglottids) but is otherwise indistinguishable from *T. saginata*. The two species are distinct based on molecular phylogenetic work [15].

Taenia lifecycles are unique, in that mammals serve as both definitive and intermediate hosts. The typical *Taenia* lifecycle involves two mammalian hosts: a carnivorous or omnivorous definitive host and a herbivorous intermediate host. Infection with the larval-stage worm in the musculature, visceral organs or CNS of the intermediate host follows ingestion of parasite proglottids or eggs. The definitive host acquires the larvae from consuming infected meat or viscera. The adult-stage worm then develops in the intestinal lumen of the definitive host and sheds gravid proglottids or eggs in the feces [1].

Humans acquire *T. saginata* through consumption of measly beef infected with the larval form, called a cysticercus. Once larvae are ingested, the scolex within the cysticercus evaginates through the cyst wall and, using its four suckers, the scolex attaches to the jejunal wall. Worms can migrate frequently.

The scolices of the three *Taenia* species are morphologically unique. *Taenia saginata* lacks a crown or rostellum with hooks. The scolex of *T. solium* is about 1 mm wide and possesses four suckers and a distinctive rostellum armed with a double row of large and small hooklets. *Taenia asiatica* exhibits a rostellum, but lacks hooks [16].

Maturation into adult worms takes 10–12 weeks and results in the shedding of terminal proglottids (10–15 per day) and free eggs in the stool. Adult worms can live as long as 25 years; however, average infections are shorter.

Taenia solium is acquired through the consumption of measly pork. Upon ingestion of cysticerci (*Cysticercus cellulosae*) undergo the same process as *T. saginata*. Maturation in the gut takes 5–12 weeks and worms can persist for years. Groups of 3–5 gravid proglottids can be shed in the stool on a daily basis.

The lifecycle of *T. asiatica* within its definitive host is identical to that of *T. saginata*; however, it begins with consumption of measly pork viscera, especially liver.

Although cattle serve as the primary intermediate host for *T. saginata*, the parasite can infect other domesticated bovine, including water buffalo and yak. Reindeer are a host in northern latitudes [3].

Pigs become infected with *T. solium* by ingesting gravid proglottids or eggs found in contaminated environments, where *T. solium* eggs remain viable for many months [12]. Dogs can become infected, presenting as an alternate intermediate host that may maintain infection in areas of Asia where dog consumption occurs [13].

Taenia asiatica is typically found only in pigs. Oncospheres from *T. asiatica* have a predilection for viscera and preferentially migrate to, and encyst in, the liver. After four weeks, the viscera becomes infectious. Cysticercosis attributable to *T. asiatica* does not occur.

Infection is most often caused by a single *Taenia* worm, but infections with multiple tapeworms may occur, in which case the size of the tapeworms is inversely proportional to the numbers that are present [17, 18]. Worms obtain nourishment through the movement of host nutrients across the parasite's body surface (tegument) [6].

CLINICAL FEATURES

Taeniasis should be suspected in patients who live in, or have traveled to, endemic areas where consumption of raw or undercooked beef or pork is common.

Most adult *Taenia* carriers are asymptomatic. In the case of *T. saginata*, carriers often first become aware of infection when they experience the sensation of motile segments migrating through the perianal area or in their underwear. *Taenia saginata* proglottids are passed on an almost daily basis in the stool. *Taenia solium* proglottids are not motile and less frequently passed in the stool. Thus, the presence of motile segments helps to rule out *T. solium*.

Symptomatic patients with tapeworms complain of mild abdominal discomfort, cramps, colicky pain, nausea, vomiting, fatigue, anorexia and weight loss [6]. Rare acute complications can occur, more commonly with *T. saginata*, as a result of proglottids migrating to unusual anatomic sites. Intestinal perforation [19], intestinal obstruction [20], pancreatitis, cholangitis and cholecystitis as a result of aberrant proglottid migration have all been reported [21–23].

A history of taeniasis with *T. solium* increases an individual's risk of the more serious condition cysticercosis (see Chapter 127).

PATIENT EVALUATION, DIAGNOSIS, AND DIFFERENTIAL DIAGNOSIS

T. saginata infections can be tentatively diagnosed from a patient's history, particularly if migrating proglottids were in the perianal area or underwear. When proglottids are observed, the differential diagnosis is limited to *Taenia* species and *D. caninum*, a common tapeworm of dogs. As the treatment for these two infections is similar, examination of proglottids from stool is mostly to rule out a patient's risk of cysticercosis. In patients with nonspecific gastrointestinal (GI) symptoms, the differential diagnosis includes other intestinal parasites and primary GI disorders.

MICROSCOPY

If a patient provides gravid proglottides, species identification should be attempted by counting the number of uterine branches using light microscopy. Specimens should be collected in saline or water and can be fixed in formalin, dehydrated in glycerol and then flattened between two microscope slides. India ink can be injected into the lateral genital pore to enhance visibility of the uterine branches. Twelve branches or less is diagnostic of *T. solium* and 12 or more may be either *T. saginata* or *T. asiatica*, depending on geographic location.

If only mature, non-gravid proglottids are available, a stained segment of *T. solium* will show a three-lobed ovary; *T. saginata* exhibits a vaginal sphincter. Cleansing the intestine with a purge immediately before treatment may improve recovery of parasite material for species identification [24].

Taenia eggs are periodically absent from feces during infection. When present, the eggs of all *Taenia* species appear identical [24, 25]. *Taenia* eggs consist of a mature six-hooked (hexacanth) embryo, termed an oncosphere (Figs 126.1 and 126.2).

IMMUNOLOGIC TESTS

Parasite specific co-proantigens (CoAg) are amenable to immunologic detection. A CoAg ELISA detecting worm somatic or excretory-secretory products is at least twofold more sensitive at identifying human carriers compared with traditional stool examination [25]. A microplate ELISA and dipstick test demonstrate a sensitivity of about 95% with false-negative tests at <1% [26]. These tests are also useful in assessing treatment, as CoAgs disappear from feces within one week of successful treatment [27]; however, they are unable to differentiate between species.

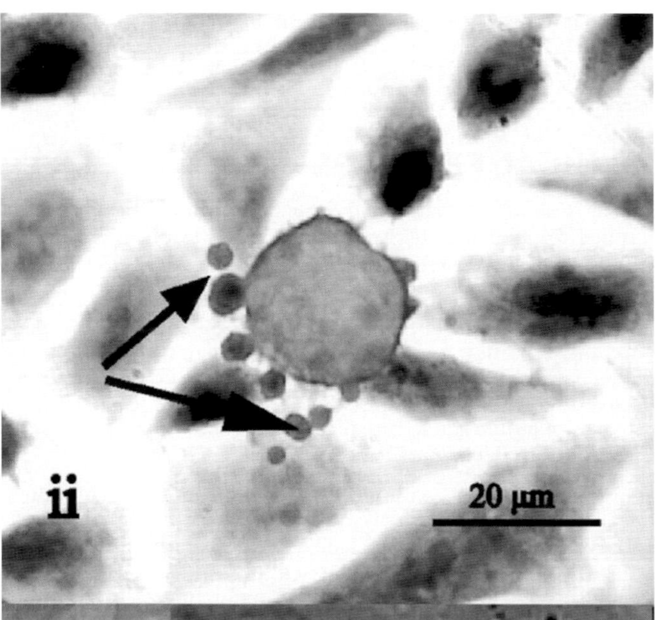

FIGURE 126.1 Secretory vesicles of *Taenia solium* oncosphere.

Copro-PCR for detection of DNA in human stool can make species-specific diagnoses prior to treatment [28–30].

Species-specific stool tests capable of identifying taeniasis and cysticercosis using a single fecal sample detect a *T. solium* oncosphere-specific protein Tso31 by PCR. In a field trial in Peru, this test was 100% sensitive and specific for identifying *T. solium*, and did not cross-react with other parasites [31].

TREATMENT

All three forms of human taeniasis can be eliminated (85–98% efficacy) with a single oral dose of niclosamide (2 g PO) or praziquantel (5–10 mg/kg PO) [6]. Praziquantel presents a small risk that asymptomatic viable brain cysts of *T. solium* will be activated during treatment, resulting in neurologic sequelae of seizures and headache [32]. For this reason, some consider niclosamide the drug of choice because it is not systemically absorbed. Despite being included on the World Health Organization's (WHO) list of essential drugs, its use has been discontinued in the USA [33].

During treatment of *T. solium*, autoinfection or dissemination with parasite eggs can occur. Medications that induce vomiting should be avoided, as retrograde peristalsis may allow gravid proglottids to be digested with egg hatching, penetration of larvae and development of cysticercosis. Adverse effects from praziquantel are abdominal discomfort, diarrhea, headache, dizziness, and drowsiness [34].

Some clinicians recommend a bowel purge within two hours of treatment. This will help to prevent release of eggs from disintegrating gravid proglottids. However, no documented cases of cysticercosis have occurred by this mechanism. If successful, a purge will also improve the likelihood of recovering an intact tapeworm within 6–12 hours, aiding in species identification. Finally, if the scolex of the tapeworm is not expelled, the worm can regenerate

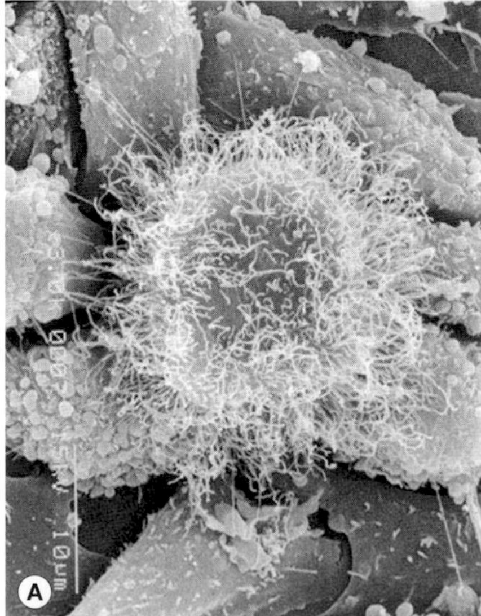

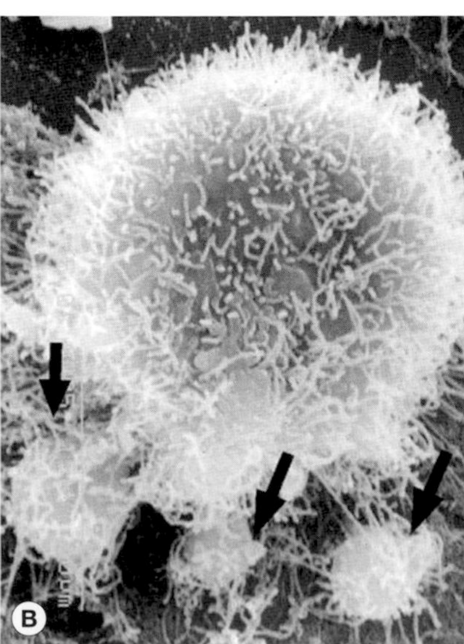

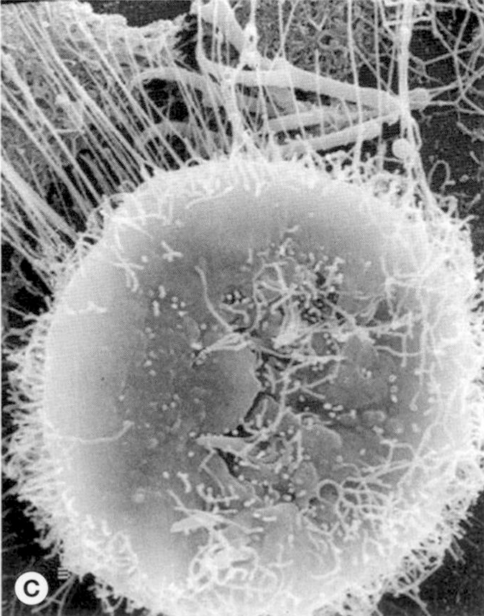

FIGURE 126.2 Scanning electron micrographs of *T. solium* oncospheres adhering to fixed monolayer CHO-K1 cells. **(A)** *T. solium* oncospheres attached to the surface of CHO cells by elongated microvilli. **(A)** Secretory vesicles (arrows) that are present outside the oncosphere membrane. Microvilli are on the surface membrane of the oncosphere and secretory vesicles. **(C)** Elongate microvilli that are attached to the surface of CHO cells. Hooks are present outside the oncosphere.

within two months [12]. Electrolyte-polyethyleneglycol solution is more effective than castor oil in producing intact scolices and proglottids and is the preferred purgative [18].

Other anthelminth drugs used to treat roundworm infections (e.g. albendazole) are not as effective. Nitazoxanide cured *T. saginata* unresponsive to niclosamide, praziquantel or both, and should be considered in resistant cases of taeniasis [35].

PREVENTION AND CONTROL

Infections with *Taenia* can be prevented by adequate cooking or freezing of beef and pork or, in the case of *T. asiatica*, pig liver. Freezing meat kills cysticerci of all species when the internal temperature drops below -5°C (23°F) for at least 4 days or around –20°C for at least 12 hours. Cooked meat or viscera are safe to eat when it loses its pink color (>70°C), or is "well done".

126.2 Diphyllobothriasis

INTRODUCTION

The broad-tapeworm, *Diphyllobothrium latum*, is the main species of *Diphyllobothrium* [36]. This tapeworm is acquired by ingestion of larval stages (plerocercoid) present in raw or insufficiently cooked fish. Worldwide, other species can infect humans such as *Diphyllobothrium nihonkaiense* in coastal Japan and *Diphyllobothrium klebanovskii* along the Amur River drainage in far-eastern Siberia. Species of parasites primarily infecting fish eating birds such as gulls (*Diphyllobothrium dendriticum*), and gulls and dogs in Alaska (*Diphyllobothrium dalliae*) can also infect humans [37].

EPIDEMIOLOGY

There is an association of *Diphyllobothrium* tapeworms and cold-water regions such as Scandinavia and North America [38]. Diphyllobothriasis is associated with consumption of raw or poorly cooked fish, including raw salted or marinated fish fillets commonly eaten in Europe and South America and "sushi" and "sashimi" in Japan [39]. *Diphyllobothrium latum* is found in salmonid species and in the musculature of several fish species in North America (pike, yellow perch, walleye and sauger), Europe and northern Asia (pike, perch, ruffe and burbot).

In North America, diphyllobothriasis was a reportable disease in the USA until 1982; most cases occurred in the Great Lakes region, central Canada (Manitoba) and Alaska. Between 1977 and 1981, the Centers for Disease Control and Prevention (CDC) estimated about 125–200 cases occurred in the USA [40]. Decreasing trends of human diphyllobothriasis have been observed in historically endemic countries of Western Europe (Finland, Poland, Romania, Sweden, Norway, Estonia, Latvia and Lithuania) and in North America over the last 20 years [41]. This decline is thought to be as a result of increased awareness of the disease, stricter monitoring of food fish, a change of eating habits and higher standards of public hygiene.

Reports of diphyllobothriasis have increased in areas around Swiss, Italian and French lakes, where raw or undercooked perch is consumed. In the last six years, sporadic cases have been reported in some countries previously considered to be disease free (Austria, Czech Republic, Belgium, the Netherlands, and Spain), presumably linked to the consumption of raw imported fish [40].

South America, Chile, Peru, Argentina, Brazi, and Ecuador have reported human infections caused by *Diphyllobothrium pacificum* and *D. latum* [42–44]. Diphyllobothriasis is frequently reported along the coast of the Sea of Japan, where the majority of human infections are caused by *D. nihonkaiense.* Since 1970, an average of 100 cases per year has been reported in Japan [45]. Prevalences of 1.0–3.3% have been reported in Okhotsk (Russia) and up to 45 human cases from Korea. Rare clinical cases attributed to different species of *Diphyllobothrium* have been reported in the Middle East. There are no reliable reports from Africa and Australia [46].

NATURAL HISTORY, PATHOGENESIS, AND PATHOLOGY

Unembryonated eggs are released into the stool; a single worm can produce up to 1 million eggs per day. The motile first-stage larva hatches in the water, and can infect many species of first intermediate hosts (copepods) [47]. The larva penetrates the intestinal wall of the copepod and develops into the procercoid. After ingestion of infected copepods by the second intermediate hosts (freshwater, anadromous or marine fish), the procercoid enters their tissues and develops into the plerocercoid stage. Plerocercoids develop rapidly into adults in the definitive hosts' intestine, yielding their first eggs 2–6 weeks later [48]. Most *Diphyllobothrium* species have a low specificity at the adult stage, implying that humans can become infected with parasites of carnivore mammals or even fish-eating birds [40].

Diphyllobothrium tapeworms can grow up to 2–15 meters in length (3000–4000 segments). Parasites can live up to 20 years and their growth rate may be as high as 22 cm/day.

Diphyllobothrium are characterized by a scolex with a paired slit-like attachment groove (bothrium) on the dorsal and ventral surfaces. A proliferative zone (neck) is usually present posterior to the scolex. The remaining body (strobila) is composed of a high number of proglottids, each containing one set of genital organs of both sexes [40].

CLINICAL FEATURES

Eggs are passed in stools approximately 15–45 days after ingestion of larvae. The presence of the tapeworm can be noted because of the expulsion of segments with the stools. Adult parasites can survive for decades [40].

Although most *Diphyllobothrium* species are large and can have a mechanical effect on the host, many infections are asymptomatic. Diarrhea, discomfort and abdominal pain are observed in about 20%. Other symptoms such as fatigue, constipation, pernicious anemia, headache, and allergic reactions may also be present. Tapeworms usually attach in the ileum. Rarely, the worms attach in a bile duct. Massive infections, although uncommon, can result in intestinal obstruction, and migrating segments can cause cholecystitis or cholangitis [49].

When prolonged or heavy *D. latum* infection is present, megaloblastic anemia can occur and is characterized by macrocytic red cells and often associated with low platelet or white blood cell counts. Approximately 80% of the B_{12} intake is absorbed by the worm making B_{12} unavailable to the host. Although about 40% of *D. latum*-infected individuals show low B_{12} levels, only 2% or less develop clinical anemia. *Diphyllobothrium*-associated pernicious anemia is now rarely reported [50].

Symptoms with *D. nihonkaiense* infection are generally mild [51].

PATIENT EVALUATION, DIAGNOSIS, AND DIFFERENTIAL DIAGNOSIS

Human broad tapeworm diagnosis is based on finding eggs of an ovoid shape with an operculum on a narrowed pole. In most cases, identification at the species level is difficult as *Diphyllobothrium* species can only be differentiated on the basis of the shape and size of the scolex, which is usually absent in clinical samples [40]. At present, molecular methods represent the most reliable tool to identify clinical samples of *Diphyllobothrium* at the species level. However, these are available only at research laboratories.

TREATMENT

A single oral dose of 25 mg/kg praziquantel is highly effective against human *D. latum* infections. Lower doses of 10 mg/kg are effective against human infections with *D. pacificum* [40]. Oral administration of a single dose of praziquantel at 5–10 mg/kg has been reported to be effective and safe for *D. nihonkaiense* infections, but a single administration of a 25–50-mg/kg dose is usually used [52]. An alternative drug is niclosamide (a single dose of 1 g in children older than 6 years and 2 g in adults).

Intraduodenal gastrographin (used for contrast-enhanced intestinal radiographs) can be efficacious in the treatment of large cestodes. However, this method is cumbersome in practice. It will lead to the discharge of a complete, living worm with the scolex and is suitable for species identification [40].

Infections with *Diphyllobothrium* tapeworms can be prevented by eating well-cooked fish or deep-frozen fish (at least −10°C for 24 h) or by placing the fish in a concentration of brine (12% NaCl) [46].

126.3 Hymenolepiasis

INTRODUCTION

Humans are infected mainly by two species of tapeworms of the genus *Hymenolepis*:

- *Hymenolepis nana*: dwarf tapeworm (1–5 cm long), the most common tapeworm infection of humans;
- *Hymenolepis diminuta*: considerably larger (20–90 cm long); a rodent tapeworm that rarely infects humans [53].

EPIDEMIOLOGY

Hymenolepis nana has a worldwide distribution with estimates of 50–75 million carriers. There is a high prevalence in Central America. *Hymenolepis nana* infection is observed in households with poor hygiene and overcrowding, and can have a prevalence of 5–25% in children [54]. In the southeastern USA, as many as 1% of young school-children are infected.

Hymenolepis diminuta has a cosmopolitan distribution with prevalence up to 1% in parts of India. Children are most likely to contract infection after contact/play with stored grain or cereals.

NATURAL HISTORY, PATHOGENESIS, AND PATHOLOGY

Humans are the natural host for *H. nana*, which has a direct lifecycle (no intermediate host is needed); animal hosts of other *Hymenolepis* species utilize insect intermediate hosts. Infective eggs containing a hexacanth embryo or oncosphere are released to the intestine after disintegration of the proglottid [55]. The cysticercoid develops directly in the intestinal villi. After several days, it emerges and develops into a tapeworm in a few weeks. Autoinfection within the gut can possibly occur. *Hymenolepis nana* can also infect rodents and be transmitted via beetles or fleas [56].

Accidental ingestion of cysticercoid infected beetles, fleas or other insects in various grain products can rarely cause human infection with *H. diminuta* [47].

CLINICAL FEATURES

The presence of an adult tapeworm occurs 3–4 weeks after direct egg/oncosphere infection. Abdominal discomfort, irritability, diarrhea and possibly malabsorption can be caused by large burdens of *H. nana* tapeworms (>300) in children. However, clinical signs in adults are rare; only in heavy infection have diarrhea and abdominal discomfort been noted. Diarrhea results from damage to the mucosal surface. Infection in adults, but not in young children, is generally self-limited [57].

The prepatent period of *H. diminuta* in humans is about three weeks and infection is mild. Diarrhea, nausea, and anorexia have occurred but these symptoms are not unusual.

PATIENT EVALUATION, DIAGNOSIS, AND DIFFERENTIAL DIAGNOSIS

Diagnosis is made by the identification of ova in stool samples. Egg counts in stool of over 10,000 eggs per gram are considered heavy infection.

TREATMENT

Praziquantel (25 mg/kg in adults and children), niclosamide (>90% efficacy) and nitazoxanide (75–93% efficacy) are effective. A carrier's family/household members should also be treated. Treatment is successful if eggs are not observed in stool samples one month post-treatment [58]. Prevention includes improved environmental and personal hygiene.

126.4 Dipylidiasis

INTRODUCTION

Dipylidium caninum is the most common cestode of domestic dogs. It can also infect cats. It is a small-to-medium-sized (10–50 cm) tapeworm, pink in color, with double-pored, barrel-shaped segments [59]. It can infect humans when a person accidentally swallows an infected flea (*Ctenocephalides canis* or *Ctenocephalide felis*) [54].

EPIDEMIOLOGY

Humans, usually young children (0.5–5 years old) probably acquire infection after accidental ingestion of fleas or lice during contact with pets [60]. Prevalence in dogs ranges from 1–60% in studies performed in South and Central America. In Europe, prevalence in wild foxes has ranged from 1–50% in several countries, including Spain, France, England, and Greece [60].

NATURAL HISTORY, PATHOGENESIS, AND PATHOLOGY

Infection is transmitted to dogs (or cats) by ingesting fleas or body lice *(Trichodectes* spp.*)* that are infected with the larval cysticercoid stage of the tapeworm. More than 20–30 tapeworms of different lengths may reside in the dog small intestine with each worm containing 60–175 proglottids. Egg packets can be expelled by the contraction of the proglottid or by disintegration of the proglottids in the perianal region. Each onchosphere has six hooklets [55, 56].

CLINICAL FEATURES

Close contact between young children and dogs and cats is responsible for this mainly asymptomatic infection. However, proglottids can cause anal irritation, loss of appetite, abdominal pain or diarrhea [57].

PATIENT EVALUATION, DIAGNOSIS, AND DIFFERENTIAL DIAGNOSIS

Infection is usually asymptomatic and its detection occurs by the discovery of small white motile rice-like segments in underwear or diapers. Microscopic confirmation can be made by the presence of characteristic egg packets/sacs containing numerous hooked oncospheres [47].

TREATMENT

Praziquantel and niclosamide are effective treatments. Regular treatment of pet dogs or cats with anthelmintics and antiflea collars is preventive [58].

REFERENCES

1. Hoberg EP. Taenia tapeworms: their biology, evolution and socioeconomic significance. Microbes Infect 2002;4:859–66.
2. Verastegui M, Gilman R, Aeana Y, et al. *Taenia solium* oncosphere adhesion to intestinal epithelial and Chinese hamster ovary cells in vitro. Infect Immunity 2007;75:5158.
3. Cabaret J, Geerts S, Madeline M, et al. The use of urban sewage sludge on pastures: the cysticercosis threat. Vet Res 2002;33:575–97.
4. Schantz PM, Moore AC, Munoz JL, et al. Neurocysticercosis in an Orthodox Jewish community in New York City. N Engl J Med 1992;327:692–5.
5. Schantz PM. *Taenia solium* cysticercosis/taeniasis is a potentially eradicable disease: developing a strategy for action and obstacles to overcome. In: García HH, Martínez M, eds. Teniasis/Cisticercosis por *T. solium*. Lima: ICN; 1996: 227–30.
6. Craig P, Ito A. Intestinal cestodes. Curr Opin Infect Dis 2007;20:524–32.
7. Dornu P, Praet N. *Taenia saginata* in Europe. Vet Parasitol 2007;149:22–4,
8. Flisser A, Sarti E, Lightowlers M, Schantz P. Neurocysticercosis: regional status, epidemiology, impact and control measures in the Americas. Acta Tropica 2003;87:43–51.
9. Flisser A, Rodriguez-Canul R, Willingham AL, III. Control of the taeniosis/cysticercosis complex: Future developments. Vet Parasitol 2006;139:283–92.
10. Behravesh BC, Mayberry LF, Bristol JR, et al. Population-based survey of taeniasis along the United States-Mexico border. Ann Trop Med Parasitol 2008;102:325–33.
11. Pawlowski Z, Allan J, Sarti E. Control of *Taenia solium* taeniasis/cysticercosis: From research towards implementation. Int J Parasitol 2005;35:1221–32.
12. Willingham AL, III, Engels D. Control of *Taenia solium* Cysticercosis/Taeniosis. Adv Parasitol 2006;61;509–66.
13. Ito A, Nakao M, Wandra T. Human taeniasis and cysticercosis in Asia. Lancet 2003;362:1918–20.
14. Fan PC, Chung WC. Sociocultural factors and local customs related to taeniasis in East Asia. Kaohsiung J Med Sci 1997;13:647–52.
15. Hoberg EP. Phylogeny of Taenia: species definitions and origins of human parasites. Parasitol Int 2006;50(suppl.):S23–30.
16. Flisser A, Viniegra A, Aguilar-Vega L, et al. Portrait of human tapeworms. J Parasitol 2004;90:914–6.
17. Read CP. The "crowding effect" in tapeworm infections. J Parasitol 2000: 86(2):206–8.
18. Jeri C, Gilman RH, Lescano AG, et al. Species identification after treatment for taeniasis. Lancet 2004;363:949–50.
19. Jongwutiwes S, Putaporntip C, Chantachum N, Sampatanukul P. Jejunal perforation caused by morphologically abnormal *Taenia saginata* infection. J Infect 2004;49:324–8.
20. Karanikas ID, Sakellaridis TE, Alexiou CP, et al. Taenia saginata: a rare cause of bowel obstruction. Trans R Soc Trop Med Hyg 2007;101:527–8.
21. Plane P, Ronceray J, Dubin P. Acute pancreatitis from obstruction of Wirsung's canal by *Taenia saginata*. J Chir (Paris) 1980;117:193–4.
22. Bordon LM. Intestinal obstruction due to *Taenia saginata* infection: a case report, J Trop Med Hyg 1992;95:352–3.
23. Negre A. Rupture into the free peritoneum of a liver abscess caused by the presence of *Taenia saginata* in the right lobe. Mem Acad Chir (Paris) 1957; 83:493–5.
24. Garcia HH, Gonzalez AE, Evans CAW, Gilman RH. *Taenia solium* cysticercosis. Lancet 2003;362:547–56
25. Allan JC, Craig PS. Coproantigens in taeniasis and echinococcosis. Parasitol Int 2006;55(suppl.):S75–80.
26. Allan JC, Velasquez Tohom M, Torres Alvarez R, et al. Field trial of diagnosis of Taenia solium taeniasis by coproantigen enzyme linked immunosorbent assay. Am J Trop Med Hyg 1996;54:352–6.
27. Allan JC, Avila G, Garcia-Noval J, et al. Immunodiagnosis of taeniasis by coproantigen detection. Parasitology 1990;101:473–7.
28. Mayta H, Talley A, Gilman RH, et al. Differentiating *Taenia solium* and *Taenia saginata* infections by simple hematoxylin-eosin staining and PCR-restriction enzyme analysis. J Clin Microbiol 2000;38:133–7.
29. Gonzalez LM, Montero E, Sciutto E, et al. Differential diagnosis of *Taenia saginata* and *Taenia solium* infections: from DNA probes to polymerase chain reaction. Trans R Soc Trop Med Hyg 2002;96:S243–50.
30. Yamasaki H, Allan JC, Sato MO, et al. DNA differential diagnosis of taeniasis and cysticercosis by multiflex PCR. J Clin Microbiol 2004;42:548–53.
31. Mayta H, Gilman RH, Prendergast E, et al. Nested PCR for specific diagnosis of *Taenia solium* taeniasis. J Clin Microbiol 2008;46(1):286–9.
32. Flisser A, Madrazo I, Placarte A, et al. Neurological symptoms in occult neurocysticercosis after single taenicidal dose of praziquantel. Lancet 1993;243:748.
33. Pawlowski ZS. Role of chemotherapy of taeniasis in prevention of neurocysticercosis. Parasitol Int 2006;55(suppl. 1):S105–9.
34. Loukas A, Hotez PJ. Chemotherapy of helminth infections. In: Brunton LL, Lazo JS, Parker KL, eds. Goodman & Gilman's The Pharmacological Basis of Therapeutics; 2006. Available at: http://www.accessmedicine.com (accessed 8 November 2011).
35. Lateef M, Zargar SA, Khan AR, et al. Successful treatment of niclosamide- and praziquantel-resistant beef tapeworm infection with nitazoxanide. Int J Infect Dis 2008;12:80–2.
36. Adams AM, Rausch RL. Diphyllobothriasis. In: Connor DH, Chandler FW, Schwartz DA, et al, eds. Pathology of Infectious Diseases, vol. 2. Stamford; McGraw-Hill Professional; 1997;1377–90.
37. Schmidt GD. CRC handbook of tapeworm identification. Boca Raton: CRC Press; 1986.
38. Dick T. Diphyllobothriasis: the *Diphyllobothrium latum* human infection conundrum and reconciliation with a worldwide zoonosis. In: Murrell KD, Fried B, eds. Food-borne Parasitic Zoonoses: Fish and Plant-borne Parasites (World Class Parasites), vol. 11. London: Springer; 2008:151–84.
39. Lee KW, Suhk HC, Pai KS, et al. *Diphyllobothrium latum* infection after eating domestic salmon flesh. Korean J Parasitol 2001;39:319–21.
40. Scholtz T, Garcia HH, Kuchta R, Wicht B. Update on the human broad tapeworm (genus *Diphyllobothrium*), including clinical relevance. Clin Microbiol Rev 2009;22:146–60.
41. Scholz T, Garcia HH, Kuchta R, Wicht B. Update on the human broad tapeworm (Genus *Diphyllobothrium*), including clinical relevance. Clin Microbiol Rev 2009;22:146–60.
42. Atias A, Cattan PE. Primer caso humano de infeccion por *Diphyllobothrium pacificum* en Chile. Rev Med (Chile) 1976;104:216–7 [in Spanish].
43. Eduardo MBP, Sampaio JLM, Goncalves EMN, et al. *Diphyllobothrium* spp.: um parasita emergence em São Paulo, asociado ao consumo de peixe cru – sulis e sashimis. Bol Epidemiol Paulista 2005;2:1–5.
44. Skeříková A, Brabec J, Kuchta R, et al. Is the human-infecting *Diphyllobothrium pacificum* a valid species or just a South American population of the Holarctic fish broad tapeworm, *D. latum*? Am J Trop Med Hyg 2006;75:307–10.
45. Awakura A. The infection of *Diphyllobothrium nihonkaiense* plerocercoid in salmonids of Japan. Jpn Soc Syst Parasitol Circular 1992;10:1–4 [in Japanese].
46. Alkhalife IS, Hassan RR, Abdel-Hameed AA, Al-Khayal LA. Diphyllobothriasis in Saudi Arabia. Saudi Med J 2006;27:1901–4.
47. Raether W, Hanel H, Epidemiology, clinical manifestations and diagnosis of zoonotic cestode infections: an update. Parasitol Res 2003;91:412–38.

48. Andersen K, Gibson DI. A key to three species of larval *Diphyllobothrium* Cobbold, 1858 (Cestoda: Pseudophyllidea) occurring in European and North American freshwater fishes. Syst Parasitol 1989;13:3–9.
49. Marty AM, Neafie RC. Diphyllobothriasis and sparganosis. In: Meyers WM, ed. Pathology of Infectious Diseases, vol. 1. Helminthiases. Washington: Armed Forces Institute of Pathology; 2000:165–83.
50. Donoso SM, Raposo L, Reyes H, et al. Severe megaloblastic anaemia secondary to infection by *Diphyllobothrium latum*. Rev Med Chile 1986;114:1171–4.
51. Wicht B, de Marval F, Peduzzi R. *Diphyllobothrium nihonkaiense* (Yamane et al., 1986) in Switzerland: first molecular evidence and case reports. Parasitol Int 2007;56:195–9.
52. Ohnishi K, Kato Y. Single low-dose treatment with praziquantel for *Diphyllobothrium nihonkaiense* infections. Intern Med 2003;42:41–3.
53. Neafie RC, Marty AM. Unusual infections in humans. Clin Microbiol Rev 1993;6:34–56.
54. Andreassen J. Intestinal tapeworms. In: Cox FEG, Kreier JP, Wakelin D, eds. Topley and Wilson's Microbiology and Microbial Infection, 9th edn, vol 5. London: Arnold; 1998:521–37.
55. Schantz PM. Tapeworms (cestodiasis). Gastroenterol Clin North Am 1996; 25:637–53.
56. Thompson RCA, McManus DP. Aetiology: parasites and life cycles. In: Eckert J, Thompson RC, Bucklar H, et al., eds. Manual on Echinococcosis in Humans and Animals a Public Health Problem of Global Concern. Geneva: World Organization for Animal Health; 2001:1–19.
57. Despommier DD, Gwadz RW, Hotez PJ, eds. Parasitic diseases, 3rd edn. New York, Berlin: Springer; 1994.
58. Mehlhorn H, ed. Encyclopedic Reference of Parasitology, Vol. 1: Biology-Structure-Function; Vol. 2: Diseases-Treatment-Therapy, 2nd edn. Berlin, Heidelberg: Springer; 2001.
59. Brandstetter W, Auer H. *Dipylidium caninum*, a rare parasite in man. Wien Klin Wochenschr 1994;106:115–6 [article in German].
60. Neira OP, Jofré ML, Muñoz SN. *Dipylidium caninum* infection in a 2 year old infant: case report and literature review. Rev Chilena Infectol 2008;25: 465–71.

Larval Cestode Infections (Cysticercosis) 127

Hector H Garcia, Robert H Gilman

Key features

- Neurocysticercosis (NCC) is the invasion of the human central nervous system (CNS) by larvae of the pork tapeworm *Taenia solium*; it is a major cause of seizures and other neurologic morbidity worldwide
- Parenchymal brain disease can follow a benign course and is usually associated with seizures
- Extraparenchymal (intraventricular or subarachnoid) disease is progressive, has a poor prognosis and usually presents with hydrocephalus or intracranial hypertension
- Diagnosis of NCC is based on brain imaging—computed tomography (CT) and magnetic resonance imaging (MRI)—and supported by specific serology (western blot with purified antigens). Antigen detection assays may be of help in monitoring the course of disease
- Management should be individualized and includes symptomatic treatment (analgesics, anti-epileptic drugs, anti-inflammatory drugs) and anti-parasitic therapy with albendazole or praziquantel. The use of anti-parasitic therapy is of benefit in most cases, but there are specific contraindications

INTRODUCTION

Cysticercosis is the infection of human tissues with larvae of the pork tapeworm, *Taenia solium*. Endemic in most of the world, this parasitic disease is a major cause of seizures and other neurologic morbidity.

EPIDEMIOLOGY

Neurocysticercosis is estimated to be the most common parasitic infection of the brain and the most common cause of adult-onset epilepsy worldwide. Cysticercosis is endemic on all continents except Australasia and is common in non-Muslim developing countries, including much of South and Central America, Asia and Africa. Prevalence varies depending on the prevalence and type of animal husbandry, hygiene and dietary practices. In endemic countries, approximately 30% of seizure disorders are caused by neurocysticercosis [1]. Industrialized porcine production, meat inspection and sewage disposal has helped to prevent propagation of the parasite lifecycle in high income countries, but immigration from, and travel to, endemic regions leads to sporadic cases of cysticercosis. For example, cysticercosis accounts for as many as 2% of neurologic/neurosurgical admissions in southern California and immigrant tapeworm carriers (Latin American cooks) caused an outbreak of cysticercosis in Orthodox Jews in New York City [2].

NATURAL HISTORY, PATHOGENESIS AND PATHOLOGY

The natural history of cysticercosis is poorly defined because most infections are asymptomatic and many of those who are symptomatic have a long prepatent period. Symptomatic cysticercosis is a serious disease that can be progressive and have fatal consequences. In general, numerous intracranial cysticerci are associated with more severe disease that is less likely to respond to treatment. The location of cysticerci is also important: patients with <20 cysticerci with a parenchymal location and the absence of hydrocephalus have a better prognosis than those who have basal or ventricular lesions, especially if associated with hydrocephalus.

Cysticercosis is contracted when humans ingest material contaminated by human feces containing tapeworm eggs, not from eating infected pork containing cysticerci; this would lead to gut infection with the tapeworm. When humans ingest tapeworm eggs, they act as the intermediate, dead-end host and develop cysticerci within their tissues in the same way as pigs (Fig. 127.1). Strict vegetarians and people who have never eaten pork can develop cysticercosis if they ingest fecally-contaminated food items. Humans harboring an

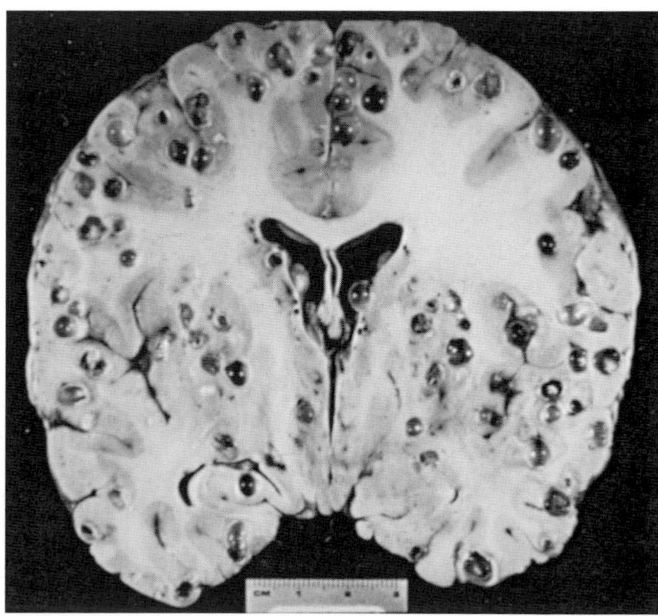

FIGURE 127.1 Sagital section of brain of a 13-year-old girl who died from a massive infection with cerebral cysticercosis. *(Courtesy of Dr D C Gajdusek of the National Intstitutes of Health, and Dr S C Bauserman of the Armed Forces Institute of Pathology; Papua New Guinea Med J 21:329, 1978.)*

intestinal tapeworm can infect themselves (anus–hand–mouth) or others, directly or through unhygienic food preparation. Internal autoinfection has been suggested, but is not common. Most patients with cysticercosis do not harbor an adult tapeworm in their intestines at the time of the diagnosis and most people infected with a tapeworm do not develop symptomatic cysticercosis. It is not known what proportion of tapeworm carriers will develop cysticercosis over time.

Living cysticerci actively evade and suppress immune recognition, especially within immunologically privileged sites, such as the brain and the eyes. Histopathology of live cysts from human tissues shows minimal host inflammation. Only rarely do living cysticerci induce symptoms—usually by causing obstruction to the flow of cerebrospinal fluid (CSF) by pressure on adjacent tissues. Symptoms most commonly result from inflammation owing to the host's immune response to dying cysticerci. This explains the usual delay between infection and cyst establishment (which occurs within three months of infection), and the development of symptoms several years later. English soldiers returning from India and remaining in the UK, a non-endemic area, developed seizures caused by cysticercosis after a median of 3–5 years [3].

Inflammation around the cysticerci can be asymptomatic or lead to acute symptoms that can be fatal. Lymphocytes and plasma cells usually outnumber giant multinuclear cells and foamy macrophages. Eosinophils are conspicuous. Adjacent necrosis and perivascular infiltration of mononuclear lymphoid cells can lead to granuloma, fibrous scar or calcification. In the same patient, cysticerci at different sites may be viable or at various stages of degeneration.

In the CNS, two forms of cysticerci are found. Cysticerci located in the brain parenchyma or floating freely in the ventricles are spherical or ovoid, 5–10-mm structures, each of which contains a scolex (Fig. 127.1). A second, uncommon form called racemose cysticerci are large, lobulated vesicular structures that lack a scolex and are usually found in the basal cisternal spaces resembling a bunch of grapes. Racemose cysticerci are not usually present in pediatric cases. They may be a degenerative form or a response to a different anatomic location.

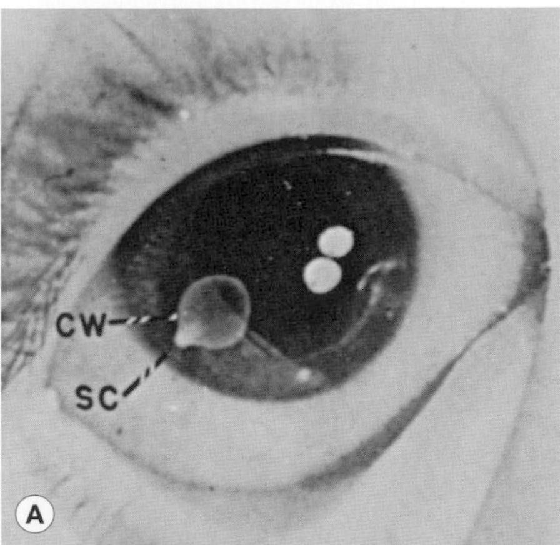

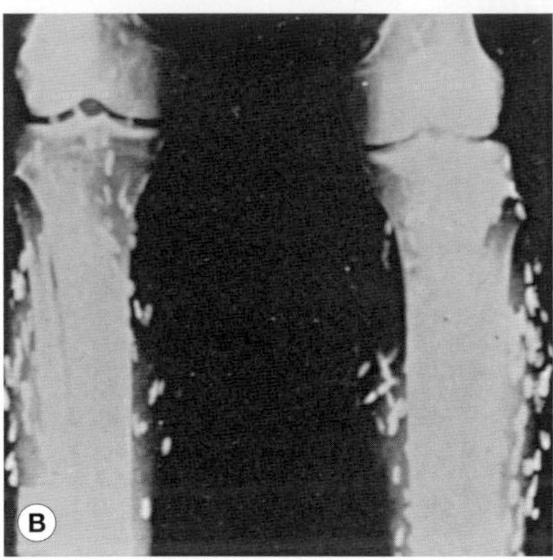

FIGURE 127.2 A Cysticercosis in human eye showing scolex (SC) and cyst wall (CW). *(Courtesy of Dr A Trejos, Costa Rica.)*. **B** *(Courtesy of Dr M. Campagna.)*

CLINICAL MANIFESTATIONS

Although cysticerci can infect any tissue, most clinically relevant lesions affect the brain and spinal cord (neurocysticercosis), or the eye (Fig. 127.2A). Clinical features of cysticercosis vary widely, depending on the number, size and location of the larvae, as well as on the stage of evolution and inflammatory response.

NEUROCYSTICERCOSIS

The clinical expression of neurocysticercosis corresponds to whether the parasites are intraparenchymal (within the brain hemispheres or cerebellum) or extraparenchymal (intraventricular or subarachnoid lesions).

The most frequent symptom of intraparenchymal cysticercosis is seizures. Focal seizures with secondary generalization are most common, but any type of epilepsy can occur. Single or multiple cysticerci within the brain parenchyma can be inflamed and surrounded by focal encephalitis and edema.

Extraparenchymal NCC is associated with intracranial pressure with or without hydrocephalus. When the subarachnoid space at the base of the brain is affected, basal arachnoiditis is often particularly severe, causing cranial nerve palsies and potentially fatal raised intracranial pressure. Intraventricular or basal cysticercosis is a frequent cause of obstructive hydrocephalus in endemic regions. Intermittent, positional headache may represent a free-floating cysticerci in the fourth ventricle (Brun's syndrome). Meningeal inflammation around subarachnoid cysts can cause vasculitis and cerebral infarcts, usually when the base of the brain is affected [4].

The encephalitic form occurs predominantly in children and young females and consists of massive infection of the brain (Fig. 127.1). Lesions are in the same phase of development, and cause an immune reaction leading to severe brain edema. These patients have intracranial hypertension, seizures that are difficult to control and a reduced level of consciousness. Rare clinical forms include dementia or other psychiatric symptoms (often in association with hydrocephalus), or chronic meningitis.

Spinal cysticercosis, although uncommon, is associated with increased pressure either directly from the cysticercus or secondary to the inflammatory reaction. Spinal cysticercosis is more frequently subarachnoid and only rarely intramedullary. Cervical spinal cysticercosis is usually associated with racemose cysticercosis of the posterior fossa.

OPHTHALMIC CYSTICERCOSIS

Cysticerci infecting the eye are retinal or subretinal, but may float freely in the vitreous or aqueous humors (see Fig. 127.2). Light entering the eye during ophthalmoscopy may induce movement and even envagination of a living parasite. Inflammation around degenerating cysticerci usually threatens vision by causing chorioretinitis, retinal detachment or vasculitis.

MUSCULAR AND SUBCUTANEOUS CYSTICERCOSIS

Some patients have characteristic subcutaneous cysticerci palpable as pea-like nodules. These are usually asymptomatic, although transient local pain and tenderness can occur as cysticerci degenerate. The frequency of subcutaneous nodules varies considerably by geographic area, with <5% of patients in South America and >20% of patients in

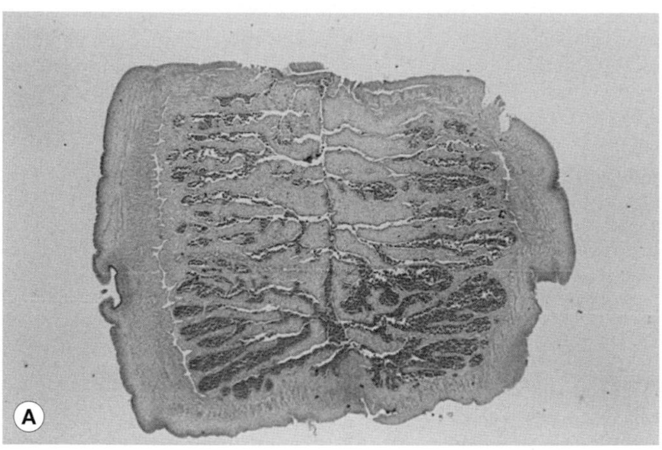

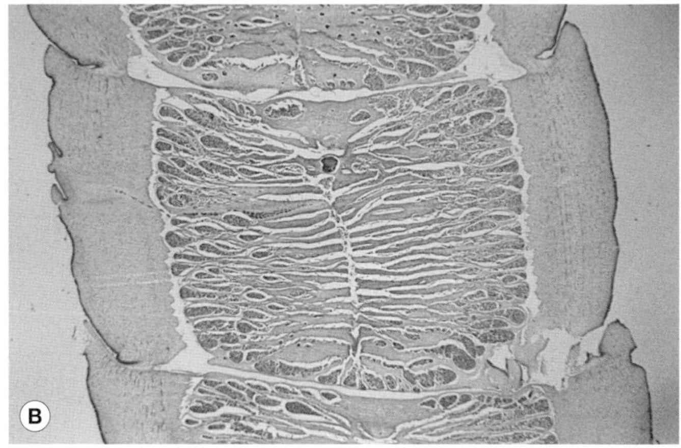

FIGURE 127.3 Proglottid segments of *Taenia solium* **(A)** and *Taenia saginata* **(B)**. T. solium **(A)** has fewer uterine branches than *T. saginata* **(B)**.

Asia having subcutaneous nodules. These lesions are easy to sample by biopsy and can thus provide proof of disease.

Large numbers of cysticerci can infect muscles and rare cases of massive muscular pseudohypertrophy have been reported (Fig. 127.2B). These patients can also have many cysticerci in multiple other localizations.

PATIENT EVALUATION, DIAGNOSIS AND DIFFERENTIAL DIAGNOSIS

NCC should be suspected in patients presenting with neurologic symptoms and a history of living in, or traveling in, endemic regions, particularly if they have late onset seizures or raised intracranial pressure. Given the variability of clinical manifestations, the diagnosis is based on neuroimaging findings and supported by serology.

HISTORY OF TAENIASIS

Patients should be asked whether they have passed tapeworm segments, even decades previously, and stool specimens should be examined for tapeworm eggs to rule out concurrent intestinal tapeworm infections. While in most cases, the infective tapeworm dies long before the symptoms of NCC develop, it may still be found in approximately 10% of NCC patients. Younger individuals, or those with many viable brain parasites, have a higher risk of concurrent taeniasis. The diagnostic yield of standard co-proparasitologic examination is low and the finding of *Taenia* spp. eggs does not differentiate intestinal *Taenia saginata* from *Taenia solium* infections as eggs are morphologically identical. Treatment with an anthelminthic agent causes the worm to be passed in the feces, allowing definitive identification of the tapeworm species (see Fig. 127.3). A tapeworm co-proantigen detection ELISA assay has much better sensitivity, although it is not widely available [5, 6].

IMAGING

CNS imaging using either CT or MRI is the key tool for the diagnosis of NCC. Living cysticerci are visible as 5–10-mm hypodense lesions that do not enhance with intravenous contrast (Fig. 127.3). Degenerating cysticerci, which are more likely to be associated with symptoms, are surrounded by edema with ring or nodular enhancement after administration of intravenous contrast. End-stage calcified cysticerci are seen as hyperdense lesions. MRI provides more detailed images of living and degenerating cysticerci (Fig. 127.4). MRI frequently demonstrates cysticerci that may not be seen on CT, especially small lesions or those located in the posterior fossa. MRI is better than CT in defining edema and other inflammatory images, but its sensitivity to detect calcifications is lower. Plain radiographs of the thighs or other muscles may reveal calcifications along the fascial planes formed by degenerated cysticerci (see Fig. 127.2B).

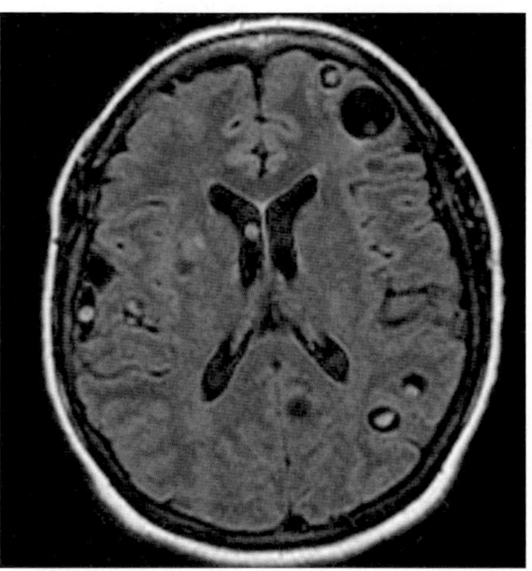

FIGURE 127.4 MRI scan of the brain of a patient with multiple cysticerci. The Scolex of the larval parasite can be seen within several cysticera. There is also an intraventricular parasite in the frontal horn. *(Courtesy of Dr T. Nash).*

SEROLOGY AND CEREBROSPINAL FLUID (CSF) EXAMINATION

Several different types of serologic tests have been used to diagnose cysticercosis. The enzyme-linked immunoelectrotransfer blot (EITB, western blot) is the assay of choice. It has >98% sensitivity and specificity, although it has only 0–80% sensitivity for a single ring-enhancing lesion. This test uses a group of purified glycoprotein antigens in an immunoblot to detect infection-specific antibodies in serum or CSF. One of its advantages is its equal sensitivity in serum or CSF, so a lumbar puncture is not required. Despite the reliability of this assay, results must be interpreted with caution in patients from endemic areas, where some healthy urban populations and >10% of rural villagers in pig-raising areas can be seropositive [7]. Patients with clinical symptoms tend to have more specific bands than those who are asymptomatic, and patients with strong reactions to several antibody bands have more intracranial lesions than those with fewer bands. The cysticercosis EITB has largely superseded less sensitive ELISA assays.

CSF findings may be normal and, even when abnormal, there are no characteristic features. Moderate CSF pleocytosis and elevated protein concentration can be noted. Eosinophils are found in approximately one quarter of patients with cysticercosis. Antigen detection ELISA assays, developed in the late 1980s, have been recently revisited. They have poor sensitivity in intraparenchymal NCC but can provide a useful monitoring tool for follow-up of patients with extraparenchymal disease [8, 9].

BIOPSY

A search should be made for subcutaneous cysticerci, excision or biopsy of which confirms the diagnosis of cysticercosis. The gross biopsy specimen is a white, fluid-filled, semi-opaque bladder typically 5–10 mm in diameter, but rarely up to 70 mm. The bladder contains a solid, 2-mm long larval tapeworm scolex. Microscopic examination reveals four suckers and a double row of hooks on the scolex by which an ingested scolex attaches to the human intestinal wall.

DIFFERENTIAL DIAGNOSIS

The heterogeneous clinical features of cysticercosis make diagnosis difficult, but the combination of imaging and reliable serology greatly facilitates diagnosis. A single ring-enhancing intracranial lesion may present a difficult differential diagnosis, because 20–50% of patients with these lesions can have a negative EITB. Other possible causes are tuberculosis (more common), neoplasm or brain abscess caused by bacteria, fungi or *Toxoplasma gondii*. In some cases, differentiating a tuberculoma from a cysticercal granuloma is difficult, often necessitating empiric therapy for tuberculosis [10]. The differential diagnosis of cystic images other than cysticercosis are subarachnoid or porencephalic cysts, hydatid cysts and cystic astrocytomas. Intracranial calcifications can also be caused by tuberculosis, toxoplasmosis, tuberous sclerosis and cytomegalovirus. Cysticerci outside the CNS are easier to identify, but subcutaneous cysticerci may be mistaken for subcutaneous lipomas.

TREATMENT

Treatment of neurocysticercosis involves symptomatic and anti-parasitic therapies. Symptomatic treatment is a key part of management. It includes analgesics, anticonvulsants, anti-inflammatories (mostly steroids) and management of intracranial hypertension when present. Anticonvulsant drugs should be administered as for any other cause of epilepsy. Raised intracranial pressure, with or without associated arachnoiditis, usually responds to oral corticosteroids that may be required long-term in cases of persistent intracranial inflammation. Insertion of a ventriculoperitoneal shunt for hydrocephalus can be beneficial in the short-term, but shunt blockage is common when the CSF protein concentration is elevated. Concomitant use of corticosteroids in patients with ventriculoperitoneal shunts has been reported to improve prognosis.

Anti-parasitic treatment of cysticercosis involves killing living brain parasites by using albendazole (15 mg/kg/day in two doses, orally for 8–15 days) or praziquantel (50–75mg/kg/day in three doses, orally for 15 days). Treatment of patients with viable or degenerating cysts with anti-parasitic therapy seems to be associated with better seizure evolution [4, 11, 12].

Albendazole is currently the drug of choice because of slightly greater efficacy, better availability and lower cost. A short course of three doses of 75–100 mg/kg of praziquantel in the same day (every two hours) has been reported to be efficacious in patients with one or two cysts. Between the second and the fifth days of anti-cysticercal therapy, patients usually have an exacerbation of neurologic symptoms attributed to local inflammation as a result of the death of the larvae. For this reason, albendazole or praziquantel should be given under hospital conditions, usually with corticosteroids to control edema and intracranial hypertension. Co-administration of corticosteroids reduces the blood levels of praziquantel; however, this is not thought to be clinically relevant.

PERILESIONAL EDEMA AROUND CALCIFIED CYSTICERCI

In approximately 50% of patients with seizures associated only with calcified lesions (without viable parasites), an area of pericalcification edema appears on MRI taken a few days after a seizure. This resolves spontaneously in the following weeks and should not be interpreted as representing survival of parasites, but most likely represents an inflammatory reaction around parasite debris and/or edema associated with seizure activity [13, 14].

PEDIATRIC CYSTICERCOSIS

Pediatric cases are usually found in older children or young teenagers with recent onset seizures and a single degenerating cyst. Rarely, massive infections present with headache and intracranial hypertension. Diagnostic and therapeutic considerations are similar to those for adults.

ASYMPTOMATIC NEUROCYSTICERCOSIS

In most cases, viable cysticerci living within the human brain are asymptomatic, but they may occasionally be discovered by imaging studies performed for other reasons. If the cysticerci are not causing symptoms and are not associated with radiologic evidence of inflammation, the parasites may be assumed to be alive and successfully evading immune-mediated inflammation. There are no data on the benefits of anti-parasitic treatment of asymptomatic cysticercosis. In such cases, cestocidal treatment would kill the parasites and allow prophylactic or therapeutic administration of corticosteroids if treatment caused symptoms. However, cysticerci infecting the brain often resolve without symptoms; thus, an alternative choice is not to treat, but to advise patients to seek medical help if neurologic symptoms develop.

OPHTHALMIC CYSTICERCOSIS

The inflammation associated with a degenerating intraocular cysticercus may result in permanent loss of vision. Reports of successful treatment with cestocidal drugs, cryotherapy and photocoagulation await further confirmatory studies. Ocular cysticercosis is usually treated surgically. Excision of a living cysticercus before the onset of significant intraocular inflammation has a good prognosis.

MUSCULAR AND SUBCUTANEOUS CYSTICERCOSIS

Asymptomatic subcutaneous or intramuscular cysticerci do not require treatment, but imaging studies should be performed to preclude the presence of neurologic infection. Cysticerci causing symptoms through local pressure may be excised or treated with cestocidal drugs. Transient symptomatic inflammation around degenerating cysticerci is ameliorated by corticosteroid or nonsteroidal anti-inflammatory drugs.

PREVENTION AND CONTROL

Transmission of cysticercosis depends on the presence of tapeworm carriers. Human infection with intestinal tapeworms is prevented by freezing or adequate cooking of cysticercotic (measly) pork. In contrast, human cysticercosis results from fecal-oral contamination with material containing *T. solium* eggs, and basic hygiene and sanitation prevent this disease [15, 16].

REFERENCES

1. Garcia HH, Del Brutto OH. Neurocysticercosis: updated concepts about an old disease. Lancet Neurol 2005;4:653–61.
2. Schantz PM, Moore AC, Muñoz JL, et al. Neurocysticercosis in an orthodox Jewish community in New York City. N Engl J Med 1992;327:692–5.
3. Flisser A. Taeniasis and cysticercosis due to *Taenia solium*. Prog Clin Parasitol 1994;4:77–116.
4. Proano JV, Madrazo I, Avelar F, et al. Medical treatment for neurocysticercosis characterized by giant subarachnoid cysts. N Engl J Med 2001;345:879–85.
5. Allan JC, Wilkins PP, Tsang VC, Craig PS. Immunodiagnostic tools for taeniasis. Acta Trop 2003;87:87–93.

6. Jeri C, Gilman RH, Lescano AG, et al. Species identification after treatment for human taeniasis. Lancet 2004;363:949–50.
7. Tsang VC, Brand JA, Boyer AE. An enzyme-linked immunoelectrotransfer blot assay and glycoprotein antigens for diagnosing human cysticercosis (*Taenia solium*). J Infect Dis 1989;159:50–9.
8. Dorny P, Brandt J, Geerts S. Immunodiagnostic approaches for detecting *Taenia solium*. Trends Parasitol 2004;20:259–60.
9. Rodriguez S, Dorny P, Tsang VC, et al. Detection of *Taenia solium* antigens and anti-*T. solium* antibodies in paired serum and cerebrospinal fluid samples from patients with intraparenchymal or extraparenchymal neurocysticercosis. J Infect Dis 2009;199:1345–52.
10. Rajshekhar V, Chandy MJ. Validation of diagnostic criteria for solitary cerebral cysticercus granuloma in patients presenting with seizures. Acta Neurol Scand 1997;96:76–81.
11. Del Brutto OH, Roos KL, Coffey CS, Garcia HH. Meta-analysis. Cysticidal drugs for neurocysticercosis: albendazole and praziquantel. Ann Intern Med 2006;145:43–51.
12. Sotelo J, Del Brutto OH, Penagos P, et al. Comparison of therapeutic regimen of anticysticercal drugs for parenchymal brain cysticercosis. J Neurol 1990; 237:69–72.
13. Nash TE, Del Brutto OH, Butman JA, et al. Calcific neurocysticercosis and epileptogenesis. Neurology 2004;62:1934–8.
14. Nash TE, Pretell EJ, Lescano AG, et al. Perilesional brain oedema and seizure activity in patients with calcified neurocysticercosis: a prospective cohort and nested case-control study. Lancet Neurol 2008;7:1099–105.
15. Schantz PM, Cruz M, Sartie E, Pawlowski ZS. Potential eradicability of taeniasis and cysticercosis. Bull Pan Am Health Organ 1993;27:397–403.
16. Roman G, Sotelo J, Del Brutto OH, et al. A proposal to declare neurocysticercosis an international reportable disease. Bull World Health Organ 2000;78: 399–406.

128 Cystic Echinococcosis

Pedro L Moro, Peter M Schantz

Key features

- Zoonotic parasitic disease principally transmitted between dogs and domestic livestock, particularly sheep
- Human cystic echinococcosis occurs in parts of the world where sheep are raised and dogs are used to herd livestock
- The liver is the most common site of the echinococcal or hydatid cyst followed by lungs; cysts occur less frequently in the spleen, kidneys, heart, bone, and central nervous system
- New sensitive and specific diagnostic methods and effective therapeutic approaches against cystic hydatid disease (CHD) have been developed in the last 10 years
- Treatment options include surgery, chemotherapy with anthelminthic agents, or puncture-aspiration-injection-re-aspiration (PAIR), the latter being restricted to the treatment of liver cysts
- Despite some progress in the control of echinococcosis, this zoonosis continues to be a major public health problem in several countries and in several others it constitutes an emerging and re-emerging disease

INTRODUCTION

Cystic echinococcosis is the infection of humans and mammals by the larval stage of the zoonotic cestode *Echinococcus granulosus* [1]. It is also known as cystic hydatid disease (CHD).

EPIDEMIOLOGY

Echinococcal infection is widely prevalent in regions of the world where dogs are used to care for large flocks of sheep. It is widely distributed in South America, the areas bordering the Mediterranean Sea, southern and central Russia, central Asia, China, Australia, and Africa [1–3]. In South America, echinococcosis is endemic in Argentina, Bolivia, Chile, southern Brazil, Peru, and Uruguay [4].

Studies using portable ultrasonography and chest radiography in endemic areas of Peru showed that 6% of the population had hydatid cysts [2, 5]. The infection rates were 32% in dogs and 89% in sheep in the same area [2]. In north-west Turkana, Kenya, ultrasonography demonstrated 5.6% of the tribe had hepatic hydatid cysts [6].

Autochthonous cases of human hydatid disease are rare in the USA; however, foci of endemic transmission in the sheep–dog cycle have been detected in recent years in Arizona and New Mexico [7]. Cystic echinococcosis has re-emerged in certain areas where it was once believed to be controlled, such as in Bulgaria and Wales [8]. Populations at most risk use dogs to herd sheep but also keep them as house pets. The Turkana of Kenya, who have the highest infection rate in the world, live very closely with dogs (Fig. 128.1A). In endemic regions, the practice of feeding raw infected viscera of slaughtered livestock to dogs facilitates transmission of *E. granulosus.*

NATURAL HISTORY, PATHOGENESIS, AND PATHOLOGY

The adult tapeworm of *E. granulosus* parasitizes a wide variety of canids (e.g. domestic dogs, foxes, wolves, and dingoes), which serve as final, definitive hosts. These adult worms are small, ranging in size 2–12 mm in length, with 3–6 segments. They typically localize in the lower duodenum and jejunum of the definitive host. Embryophores (eggs) containing infective embryos are expelled in large numbers in the feces of the final host. Intermediate hosts are usually farm animals (e.g. sheep, cattle, swine or horses), that acquire infection by ingestion of infectious eggs in the pasture (Fig. 128.2). The embryo or oncosphere is released by the action of gastric and intestinal enzymes, penetrates the intestinal wall and is transported by the blood stream to the liver or other organs. Once the oncosphere reaches its final location, it develops into an echinococcal cyst (metacestode). The echinococcal cyst is a fluid-filled, spherical, unilocular cyst that consists of an inner germinal layer of cells supported by an acellular, laminated membrane of variable thickness. Each cyst is surrounded by a host-produced layer of granulomatous adventitial reaction. Small vesicles called brood capsules bud internally from the germinal layer and produce multiple protoscolices by asexual division.

In humans, who are accidental hosts, the slowly growing hydatid cysts can attain a volume of several liters and contain many thousands of protoscolices. With time, internal septations and daughter cysts can form, disrupting the unilocular pattern typical of the young echinococcal cysts.

CLINICAL FEATURES

Signs and symptoms of hydatid disease depend on the organ involved and the size of the cyst. The onset of symptoms varies from months to several years and results from pressure exerted by the growing cyst. Cysts grow at varying rates.

Cysts occur more frequently in the liver (52–77%; Fig. 128.1A, B), followed by the lungs (9–44%; Fig. 128.3) and other locations (13–19%). Most infections have a single cyst.

LIVER CYSTS

Liver cysts occur more frequently in the right lobe—most individuals with hepatic hydatid cysts are asymptomatic [9]. Physical examination may reveal abdominal distention (Fig. 128.1A) and a palpable mass in the upper right quadrant of the abdomen, with or without hepatomegaly. When the cyst has reached large dimensions, complications usually occur. Cysts sometimes become infected with bacteria and can clinically resemble a liver abscess. Acute signs and symptoms follow rupture of a cyst, which can occur spontaneously, secondary to a traumatic event or during surgery. Rupture may occur into a bile

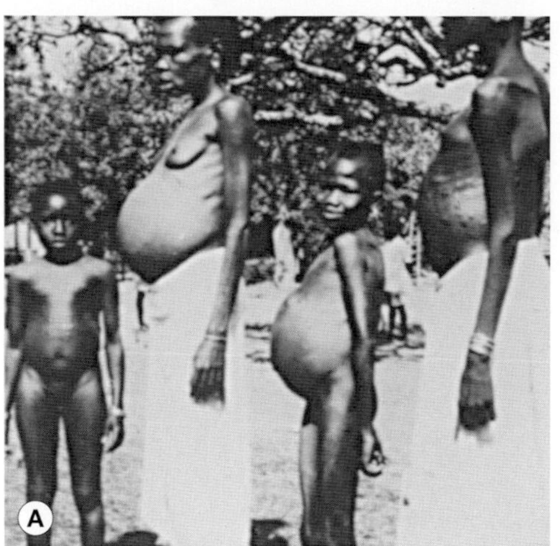

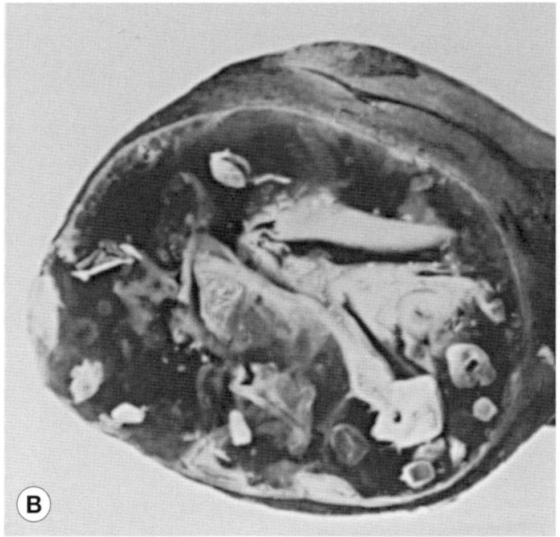

FIGURE 128.1 Cystic hydatid disease. **(A)** Abdominal distention from hydatid cysts in Turkana, Kenya *(reproduced from Muller R. Worms and Disease. London: William Heinemann Medical Books; 1975.).* **(B)** Unilocular hydatid cyst in human liver containing hydatid sand consisting of daughter cysts and free scoleces in the cyst fluid. *(Courtesy of the Armed Forces Institute of Pathology, Photograph Neg. No. N-31977).*

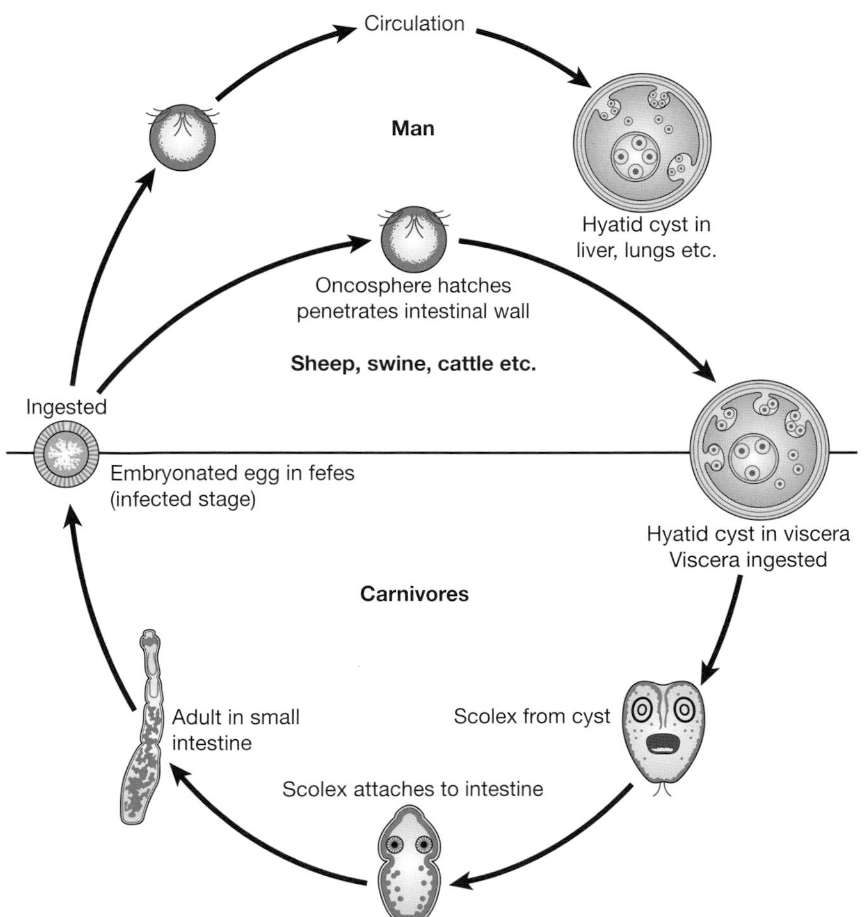

FIGURE 128.2 Life cycle of *Echinococcus granulosus* *(modified from Melvin DM. Common Blood and Tissue Parasites of Man. Life Cycle Charts. Atlanta: Centers for Disease Control; 1979.).*

duct, resulting in obstructive jaundice and colic-like pain followed by bacterial overgrowth. Rupture into the peritoneal cavity usually leads to secondary formation of numerous peritoneal cysts from released protoscolices and, on rare occasions, to peritonitis. Rupture and leakage of cyst fluid may also lead to an erythematous rash or to anaphylaxis.

LUNG CYSTS

Non-complicated lung cysts rarely produce symptoms and are usually found incidentally after a routine chest radiograph (Fig. 128.3)[10]. In patients who are symptomatic, chest pain with fever, cough, dyspnea and hemoptysis are often the presenting symptoms; the illness can be confused with pulmonary tuberculosis. Complete or

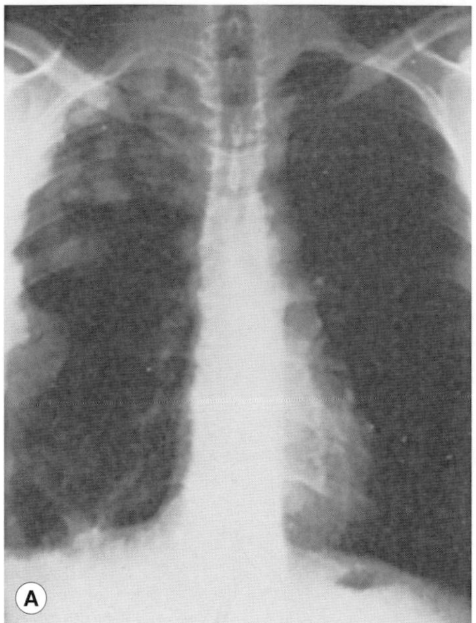

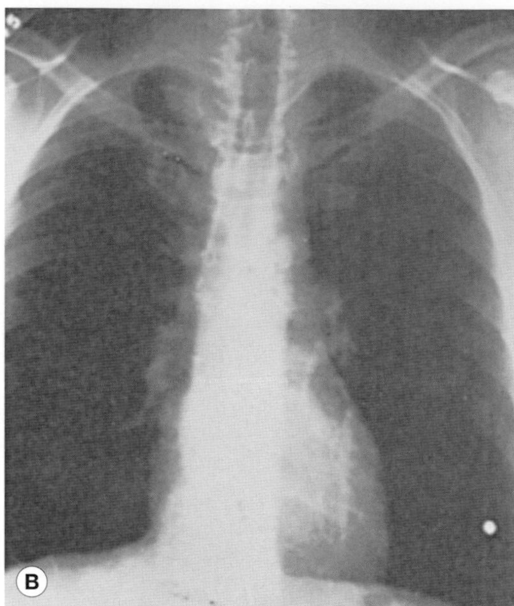

FIGURE 128.3 Echinococcosis. **(A)** Chest radiograph of a young Italian carpenter with multiple cysts in the right upper lung fields and a large cyst on the right lateral chest wall. **(B)** Chest radiograph almost 4 years later following a prolonged course of mebendazole therapy. No lesions are present on the radiograph.

partial rupture of a cyst often leads to expectoration of hydatid fluid and/or membranes, followed by bacterial overgrowth and a lung abscess. Physical examination may reveal dullness with absence of breath sounds. Rupture into the lung may cause pneumothorax and empyema, allergic reactions (e.g. pruritus, urticaria) and, rarely, anaphylactic shock. Rupture into the pleural space with secondary formation of hydatid occurs rarely.

OTHER SITES

Hydatid cysts have been reported in almost any organ. The spleen is the next most common abdominal organ affected, accounting for 3–5% of all abdominal cysts. Heart or intracerebral cysts each have been reported in 1–1.5% of patients.

PATIENT EVALUATION, DIAGNOSIS, AND DIFFERENTIAL DIAGNOSIS

The presence of an enlarged liver and/or palpable mass in the right upper quadrant of the abdomen, or a cannon ball-appearing lesion on chest radiographs suggests the clinical diagnosis of hydatid disease. A patient coming from an endemic area who gives a history of expectoration of a salty-tasting fluid with hemoptysis has a high probability of having a pulmonary hydatid cyst.

Hepatic hydatid cysts can be confused with any space-occupying lesion, including congenital liver cysts, choledochal cysts, amebic or bacterial liver abscess, and primary and secondary hepatic tumors. Symptoms caused by lung cysts may be similar to those of pulmonary tuberculosis. Congenital cysts, bronchogenic cysts, and lung abscesses may also be confused with pulmonary hydatid cysts.

Abdominal ultrasonography and computed tomography (CT) are the methods of choice for detecting abdominal cysts (Fig. 128.4) [11]. In 1995, the World Health Organization-informal Working Group on Echinococcosis (WHO-IWGE) developed a standardized classification that could be applied in all settings to allow for a natural grouping of the cysts into three relevant groups: active cystic echinococcosis (CE) 1 and 2, transitional (CE3) and inactive (CE4 and 5). The WHO-IWGE classification differs from the previous Gharbi's classification introduced in 1981 by adding a "cystic lesion" (CL) stage (undifferentiated). CE3 transitional cysts are differentiated into CE3a (with detached endocyst) and CE3b (predominantly solid with daughter vesicles). CE1 and CE3a are early stages and CE4 and CE5 late stages.

A posteroanterior chest radiograph is the method of choice for diagnosis of lung cysts (Fig. 128.3).

A wide variety of serologic assays have been developed with varying sensitivities and specificities (Chapter 152). However, a considerable number of patients, particularly those with lung cysts, may not develop a detectable immune response [12]. Parasitologic examination of expectorated or aspirated fluid may reveal protoscolices and/or hooklets (Fig. 128.5).

TREATMENT

Treatment indications for cystic echinococcoses are complex and should be based on cyst characteristics, available medical/surgical expertise and equipment, and adherence of patients to long-term monitoring. No clinical trial has compared different treatment modalities; therefore, there is no single best treatment option for cystic echinococcosis.

"WATCH AND WAIT"

Ultrasound surveys have revealed the presence of cysts which have consolidated and calcified and have become inactive. If such lesions do not compromise organ functions or cause symptoms then a "Watch and wait" approach may be taken leaving the cysts untreated. Careful ultrasound monitoring should be done in these situations [13].

CHEMOTHERAPY

Benzimidazole therapy can cure, or partially improve, two-thirds of cysts [14]. The efficacy of benzimidazoles depend on a variety of factors such as the size, type and location of the cysts. For example, bone cysts respond very poorly to benzimidazoles as a result of poor diffusion of the drug to the site of the parasitic lesion.

Benzimidazoles are also indicated in patients with multiple cysts in one or more organs or with peritoneal hydatidosis. Perioperative use

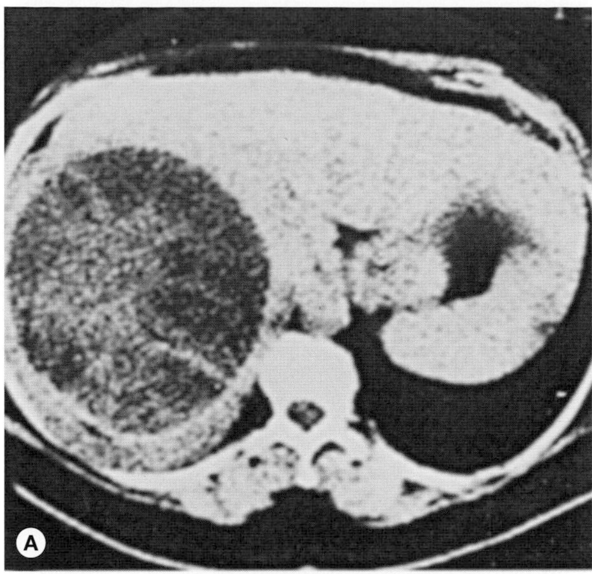

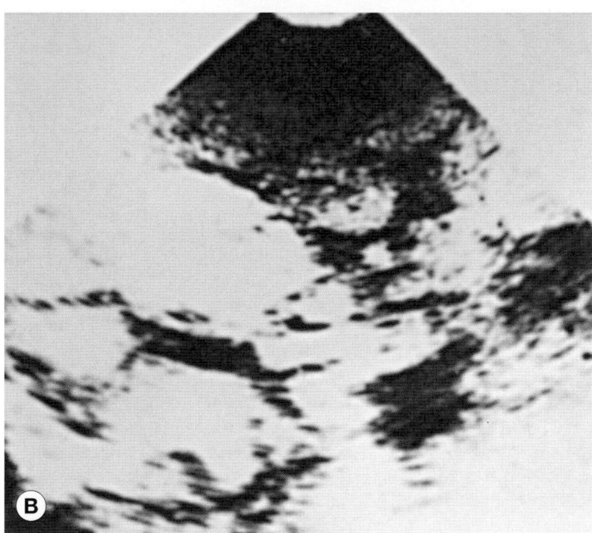

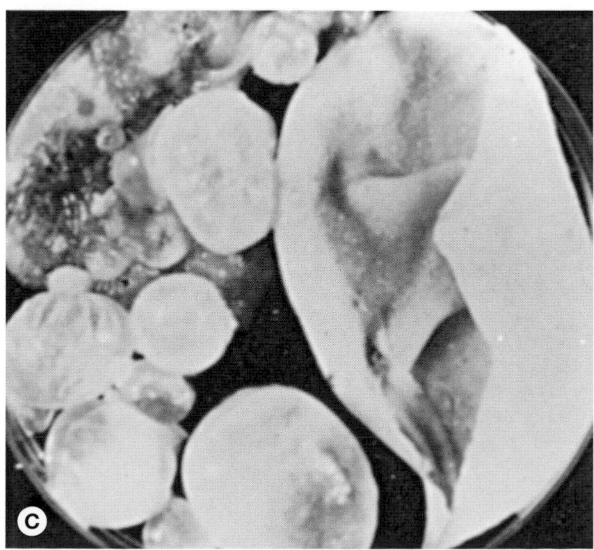

FIGURE 128.4 Cystic hydatid disease. **(A)** CT scan showing septate densities within the 12-cm cyst. **(B)** Sonogram of the same cyst showing the septate densities. **(C)** Daughter cysts removed from the same cyst *(Courtesy of the Armed Forces Institute of Pathology)*.

of benzimidazoles can reduce the risk of secondary echinococcosis following surgery. Albendazole should also be used in prophylaxis before and after puncture-aspiration-injection-re-aspiration (PAIR).

Both albendazole (10–15 mg/kg/day) and mebendazole (40–50 mg/kg/day) have demonstrated efficacy against cystic echinococcosis [15–17]. However, the results for albendazole have been superior, probably because of its pharmacokinetic profile, which favors intestinal absorption and penetration into the cyst. An intermittent treatment schedule with cycles of 28 days with 14-day periods of rest has been recommended in the past, but evidence suggests that continuous treatment with no monthly interruptions may be equally effective [13]. Administration of albendazole with fat-rich meals facilitates absorption and bioavailability. Adverse reactions (neutropenia, liver toxicity, alopecia and others), reversible upon cessation of treatment, have been noted in a few patients. Examination for adverse reactions (aminotransferases and blood-count) should be performed regularly: every 2 weeks during the first 3 months and then monthly for 1 year. Contraindications to chemotherapy include pregnancy, chronic hepatic diseases and bone marrow depression. The combination of praziquantel and albendazole has been used successfully in the treatment of hydatid disease. Nitazoxanide does not appear to be effective.

PERCUTANEOUS ASPIRATION OF HEPATIC CYSTS UNDER ULTRASONOGRAPHIC GUIDANCE (PAIR)

PAIR is a technique for the treatment of cysts in the liver and other abdominal locations. PAIR consists of: (i) percutaneous puncture using sonographic guidance; (ii) aspiration of substantial amounts of the liquid contents; (iii) injection of a protoscolicidal agent (e.g. 95% ethanol or hypertonic saline) for at least 15 minutes; and (iv) re-aspiration. PAIR is usually indicated for patients who cannot undergo surgery, for those who refuse surgery or for cases of relapse after surgery, or failure to respond to benzimidazoles. PAIR is contraindicated for inaccessible or superficially located liver cysts, for CE2 and CE3b cysts, for inactive or calcified cystic lesions (CE4, CE5) and for lung cysts. The presence of biliary fistulae is also a contraindication for protoscolicide use.

Recent application of PAIR in conjunction with albendazole has been used with good results and offers an alternative to surgery. Some studies have shown that PAIR has a lower rate of complications, shorter (or no) hospitalization and lower costs than does surgical removal, and is the method of choice for the treatment of hepatic cysts in centers having experience with this technique. PAIR should be performed with monitoring so that potential complications of anaphylaxis, asthma or laryngeal edema can be adequately treated. Combined use of albendazole (10 mg/kg/day for 8 weeks) and PAIR has been shown to be more effective than either treatment alone [18–20].

SURGERY

Surgery remains the treatment of choice when cysts are large (>10 cm diameter), secondarily infected or located in certain organs (i.e. brain, heart). The main objective of surgery is total removal of the cyst while avoiding the adverse consequences of spilling its contents. Pericystectomy, is the usual procedure, but simple drainage, capitonage, marsupialization and resection of the involved organ may be used depending on the location and condition of the cyst(s). Preoperative albendazole or mebendazole is indicated to prevent secondary recurrences following leakage or rupture of cyst and spillage of its contents [21].

PREVENTION

Periodic mass treatment of dogs with praziquantel, prohibition of giving raw infected viscera to dogs and adequate inspection of abattoirs, as well as educational measures to change human practices that facilitate hydatid disease transmission, have been effective in controlling echinococcosis [22, 23].

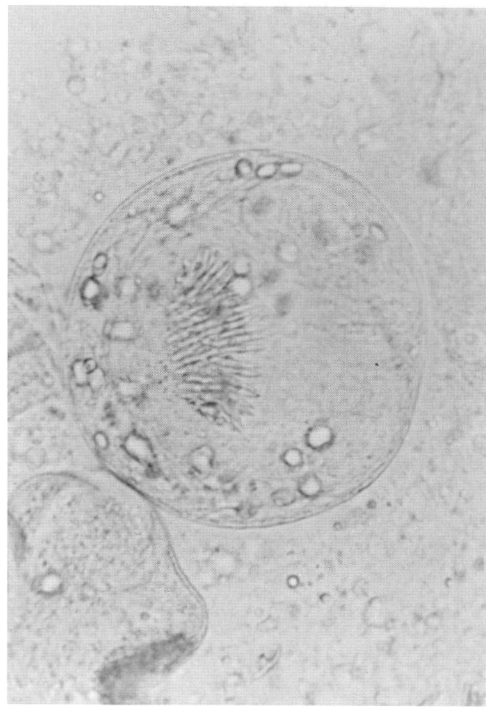
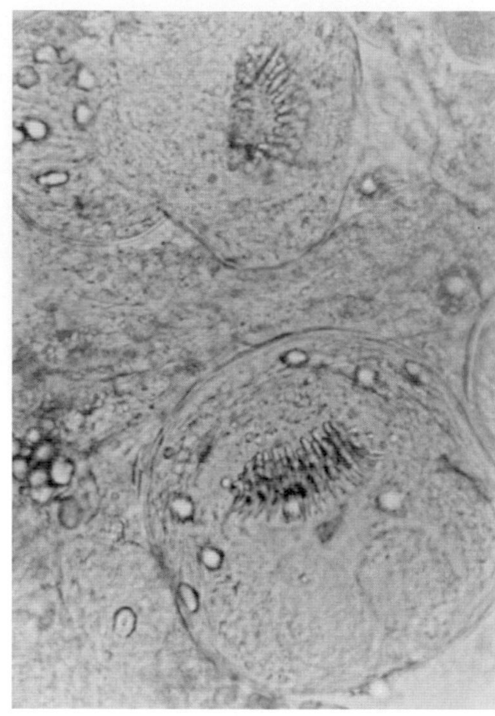

FIGURE 128.5 Hydatid scoleces in fresh unstained smear (left) and iodine-stained smear (right) from a hepatic cyst (×400) *(reproduced from Strickland GT. Diagnosis and treatment of hepatic hydatid cysts with the aid of echo-guided percutaneous cyst puncture. Clin Infect Dis 1995;21:1372.).*

REFERENCES

1. Eckert J, Deplazes P. Biological, epidemiological, and clinical aspects of echinococcosis, a zoonosis of increasing concern. Clin Microbiol Rev 2004;17:107–35.
2. Moro PL, McDonald J, Gilman RH, et al. Epidemiology of *Echinococcus granulosus* in the central Peruvian Andes. Bull WHO 1997;75:553–61.
3. MacPherson CN, Romig T, Zeyhle E, et al. Portable ultrasound scanner versus serology in screening for hydatid cysts in a nomadic population. Lancet 1987;2:259–61.
4. Moro P, Schantz PM. Cystic echinococcosis in the Americas. Parasitol Int 2006;55:S181–6.
5. Gavidia CM, Gonzalez AE, Zhang W, et al. Diagnosis of cystic echinococcosis, central Peruvian Highlands. Emerg Infect Dis 2008;14:260–6.
6. Macpherson CN, Spoerry A, Zeyhle E, et al. Pastoralists and hydatid disease: An ultrasound scanning prevalence survey in East Africa. Trans R Soc Trop Med Hyg 1989;83:243–7.
7. Schantz PM, von Reyn CF, Welty T, et al. Epidemiologic investigation of echinococcosis in American Indians living in Arizona and New Mexico. Am J Trop Med Hyg 1977;26:121–6.
8. Eckert J, Conraths FJ, Tackmann K. Echinococcosis: an emerging or re-emerging zoonosis? Int J Parasitol 2000;30:1283–94.
9. Pawlowski Z, Eckert J, Vuitton DA, et al. Echinococcosis in humans: Clinical aspects, diagnosis and treatment. In: Eckert J, Gemmell MA, Meslin F-X, eds. WHO/OIE Manual on Echinococcosis in Humans and Animals, Paris, Office International des Épizooties. Geneva: World Health Organization; 2001:20–71.
10. Santibanez S, Garcia HH. Pulmonary cystic echinococcosis. Curr Opin Pulm Med 2010;16:257–61.
11. MacPherson CNL, Bartholomot B, Frider B. Application of ultrasound in diagnosis, treatment, epidemiology, public health and control of *Echinococcus granulosus* and *Echinococcus multilocularis*. Parasitology 2003;127(suppl.):S21–35.
12. Verastegui M, Moro P, Guevara A, et al. Enzyme-linked immunoelectrotransfer blot test for diagnosis of human hydatid disease. J Clin Microbiol 1992;30:1557–61.
13. Brunetti E, Kern P, Vuitton DA. Writing Panel for the WHO-IWGE. Expert consensus for the diagnosis and treatment of cystic and alveolar echinococcosis in humans. Acta Trop 2010;114:1–16.
14. Davis A, Pawloski ZS, Dixon H. Multicentre clinical trials of benzimidazole-carbonates in human echinococcosis. Bull WHO 1986;64:383–8.
15. Gil-Grande LA, Rodriguez-Caabeiro F, Prieto JG, et al. Randomized controlled trial of efficacy of albendazole in intraabdominal hydatid disease. Lancet 1993;342:1269–72.
16. Vuitton DA. Benzimidazoles for the treatment of cystic and alveolar echinococcosis: what is the consensus? Expert Rev Anti Infect Ther 2009;7:145–49.
17. Junghanss T, da Silva AM, Horton J, et al. Clinical management of cystic echinococcosis: state of the art, problems, and perspectives. Am J Trop Med Hyg 2008;79:301–11.
18. Khuroo MS, Dar MY, Yatton GN, et al. Percutaneous drainage versus albendazole therapy in hepatic hydatidosis: A prospective, randomized study. Gastroenterology 1993;104:1452–9.
19. Khuroo MS, Wani NA, Javid G, et al. Percutaneous drainage compared with surgery for hepatic hydatid cysts. N Engl J Med 1997;337:881–7.
20. Smego RA, Bhatti S, Khalij AA, Asim Beg M. Percutaneous Aspiration-Injection-Reaspiration-Drainage plus albendazole or mebendazole for hepatic cystic echinococcosis: A meta-analysis. Clin Infect Dis 2003;27:1073–83.
21. Perdomo R, Alvarez C, Monti J, et al. Principles of the surgical approach in human liver cystic echinococcosis. Acta Trop 1997;64:109–22.
22. Heath DD, Jensen O, Lightowlers MW. Progress in control of echinococcosis using vaccination—a review of formulation and delivery of the vaccine and recommendations for practical use in control programs. Acta Trop 2003;85:133–43.
23. Moro PL, Schantz PM. Echinococcosis: historical landmarks and progress in research and control. Ann Trop Med Parasitol 2006;100:703–14.

Alveolar Echinococcosis (Alveolar Hydatid Disease) 129

Pedro L Moro, Peter M Schantz

Key features

- Zoonotic parasitic disease principally transmitted between wild canids (e.g. foxes) and small mammals, mainly rodents. Domestic dogs ands cats can also become infected
- Human alveolar echinococcosis occurs in central Europe, much of Russia, the Central Asian republics and western China, the north-western portion of Canada and western Alaska
- The liver is the primary organ affected by the larval form of *Echinococcosis multilocularis*, but local extension may occur followed by metastases to lungs and brain
- Computed tomography (CT) can identify liver lesions caused by *E. multilocularis*; purified *E. multilocularis* antigens are highly specific and allow discrimination between infections of *E. multilocularis* and *Echinococcosis granulosus*
- Treatment options include surgery, chemotherapy with anthelminthic agents and liver transplantation for advanced cases
- Contact with dogs and foxes in areas where the infection is endemic should be avoided. Infection in dogs and cats prone to eat infected rodents can be prevented by monthly treatments with praziquantel

INTRODUCTION

Alveolar echinococcosis is infection by the larval (metacestode) form of *Echinococcus multilocularis*. It is also known as alveolar hydatid disease.

EPIDEMIOLOGY

Alveolar echinococcosis has been reported in parts of central Europe; much of Russia; the Central Asian republics; north-eastern, north-western and western China; the north-western portion of Canada; and western Alaska [1]. Foxes may play an important role in the zoonotic transmission of alveolar echinococcosis as demonstrated by increased incidence of human alveolar echinococcosis in certain endemic areas of Europe from a mean of 0.10 per 100,000 during 1993–2000 to a mean of 0.26 per 100,000 during 2001–2005 following an increase in the population of foxes [1–3]. It also appears that the parasite has spread from endemic to non-endemic areas in North America and North Island, Hokkaido, Japan, owing primarily to the movement, or relocation, of foxes. Certain occupation groups such as hunters, trappers, and persons who work with fox fur are often exposed to alveolar hydatid disease. Hyperendemic areas are in parts of China with prevalences as high as 15% in some villages.

High rates of infection (hyperendemic foci) have also been reported in some Eskimo villages of the North American tundra, where local dogs develop tapeworm infection as a result of regular feeding on infected rodents that live as commensals around dwellings [4]. Humans become infected with *E. multilocularis* by their association with the dogs. In central Europe, infected foxes expel eggs which are eaten by rodents inhabiting cultivated fields and gardens and these, in turn, may be a source of infection for dogs. Individuals who own dogs that kill game, or dogs that roam outdoors unattended, have a higher risk of alveolar echinococcosis than those who do not [5]. A higher risk of alveolar echinococcosis has been observed in farmers. Foxes and rodents of the genera *Microtus* and *Peromyscus* are involved in the cycle in rural regions of central North America [6].

NATURAL HISTORY, PATHOGENESIS, AND PATHOLOGY

Small mammals, mainly rodents, act as natural intermediate hosts. Humans are accidental, dead-end hosts who acquire infection by ingesting eggs shed in feces by the definitive host—typically foxes that are infected with the adult tapeworm [1]. The embryo or oncosphere hatches from the egg in the small intestine of humans and is transported to the liver where it forms multilocular hydatid cysts. In humans, the larval mass resembles a malignancy in appearance and behavior, because it proliferates indefinitely by exogenous budding and invades the surrounding tissues. Unlike cystic echinococcosis, protoscolices are rarely observed in human infections. Fox and coyote populations have increasingly encroached upon suburban and urban areas of many regions and, as a result, domestic dogs or cats may become infected, developing the tapeworm when they eat infected wild rodents [1].

Alveolar echinococcosis is a serious disease; however, improvements in treatment in the last 30 years have had a positive impact on the life expectancy of patients. A recent study found that the life expectancy of an average 50-year-old patient with alveolar echinococcosis, was reduced by 18.2 and 21.3 years for males and females in 1970 respectively. By 2005, the life expectancy reduction was 3.5 and 2.6 years, for males and females, respectively [7].

CLINICAL FEATURES

In both humans and natural intermediate hosts, the liver is the primary organ affected by the metacestode of *E. multilocularis*, but local extension can occur followed by metastases to lungs and brain [1]. In chronic infections, the lesion consists of a central necrotic cavity filled with a white amorphous material that is covered with a thin peripheral layer of dense fibrous tissue. Areas of calcification may exist, as does extensive infiltration by proliferating vesicles. The initial symptoms of alveolar hydatid disease are usually vague and include upper quadrant and epigastric pain, jaundice, hepatomegaly, sometimes fever and anemia, weight loss, and pleural pain. Mortality in patients can occur from hepatic failure, invasion to adjacent structures, or, less frequently, metastases to the brain. The mortality rate in progressive, clinically manifest cases may be 50–75%. Instances of spontaneous death of the alveolar lesion during its early stage of development have been reported in people with asymptomatic infection [4].

PATIENT EVALUATION, DIAGNOSIS, AND DIFFERENTIAL DIAGNOSIS

Alveolar echinococcosis will generally become symptomatic in older individuals, closely mimicking hepatic carcinoma or cirrhosis. Hepatomegaly and characteristic scattered areas of radiolucency outlined by calcified rings 2–4 mm in diameter can be observed in plain radiographs. CT will typically show indistinct solid tumors with central necrotic areas and perinecrotic, plaque-like calcifications [8].

Serologic tests for *E. multilocularis* are highly sensitive and usually positive at high titers. Discrimination between infections with *E. multilocularis* and *E. granulosus* can be accomplished by using highly specific serological assays that use purified *E. multilocularis* antigens [9,10]. Diagnosis can be confirmed by demonstrating larval elements using needle biopsy. Exploratory laparotomy is often performed for diagnosis, as well as determination of the size and extent of invasion.

TREATMENT

The preferred treatment in alveolar echinococcosis is surgical resection of the entire larval mass, usually by excision of the affected lobe of the liver [1]. Wedge resections of the lesion may be attempted when involvement is extensive. Often the lesion in alveolar echinococcosis is inoperable because disease is advanced when diagnosed. Long-term treatment (over several years) with mebendazole (50 mg/kg/day) or albendazole (15 mg/kg/day) inhibits growth of larval *E. multilocularis,* reduces metastasis and enhances both the quality and length of survival [11, 12]; prolonged therapy can eventually be larvicidal in some patients. Liver transplantation has been employed successfully in otherwise terminal cases. In a Swiss study, therapy for non-resectable alveolar echinococcosis with mebendazole and albendazole resulted in an increased 10-year survival rate of approximately 80% (versus 29% in untreated historical controls) and a 16–20-year survival rate of approximately 70% (versus 0% in historical controls) [13]. Monitoring of patients with alveolar echinococcosis should be done by long-term follow-up with ultrasound at shorter intervals and CT and/or magnetic resonance imaging at 2–3-year intervals. Progression is documented by enlargement of lesions over time. Monitoring of benzimidazole plasma levels after starting treatment is recommended.

Preliminary *in vitro* studies suggest nitazoxanide and albendazole may be parasitocidal against *E. multilocularis* larvae, but further efficacy trials in humans are warranted to assess efficacy [14].

Eliminating *E. multilocularis* from its wild animal hosts is impractical; therefore, contact with dogs and foxes in areas where the infection is endemic should be avoided. Preventing infection in humans depends on education to improve hygiene and sanitation. Tapeworm infection in dogs and cats prone to eat infected rodents can be prevented by monthly treatments with praziquantel. Clearing rubbish from dwellings and preventing rodent access into buildings will help to decrease the rodent population.

REFERENCES

1. Eckert J, Deplazes P. Biological, epidemiological, and clinical aspects of echinococcosis, a zoonosis of increasing concern. Clin Microbiol Rev 2004;17:107–35.
2. Schweiger A. Human alveolar echinococcosis after fox population increase, Switzerland. Emerg Infect Dis 2007;13:878–82.
3. Vuitton DA, Zhou H, Bresson-Hadni S, et al. Epidemiology of alveolar echinococcosis with particular reference to China and Europe. Parasitology 2003;127(suppl.):S87–107.
4. Wilson JF, Rausch RL. Alveolar hydatid disease: a review of clinical features of 33 indigeneous cases of *Echinocccus multilocularis* infection in Alaskan Eskimos. Am J Trop Med Hyg 1980;29:340–9.
5. Kern P, Ammon A, Kron M, et al. Risk factors for alveolar echinococcosis in humans. Emerg Infect Dis 2004;10:2088–93.
6. Kapel CM, Torgerson PR, Thompson RC, Deplazes P. Reproductive potential of *Echinococcus. multilocularis* in experimentally infected foxes, dogs, raccoon dogs and cats. Int J Parasitol 2006;36:79–86.
7. Torgerson PR, Schweiger A, Deplazes P, et al. Alveolar echinococcosis: from a deadly disease to a well-controlled infection. Relative survival and economic analysis in Switzerland over the last 35 years. J Hepatol 2008 49:72–7.
8. Didier D, Weiler S, Rohmer P, et al. Hepatic alveolar echinococcosis: Correlative US and CT study. Radiology 1985;154:179–86.
9. Carmena D, Benito A, Eraso E. The immunodiagnosis of *Echinococcus multilocularis* infection. Clin Microbiol Infect 2007;13:460–75.
10. Ito A, Ma L, Schantz PM, et al. Differential serodiagnosis for cystic and alveolar echinococcosis using fractions of Echinococcus granulosus cyst fluid (antigen B) and E. multilocularis protoscolex (EM18). Am J Trop Med Hyg 1999;60:188–92.
11. Wilson JF, Rausch RL, McMahon BJ, Schantz PM. Parasiticidal effect of chemotherapy in alveolar hydatid disease: Review of experience with mebendazole and albendazole in Alaskan Eskimos. Clin Infect Dis 1992;15:234–49.
12. Brunetti E, Kern P, Vuitton DA; Writing Panel for the WHO-IWGE. Expert consensus for the diagnosis and treatment of cystic and alveolar echinococcosis in humans. Acta Trop 2010;114:1–16.
13. Koch S, Bresson-Hadni S, Miguet JP, et al. Experience of liver transplantation for incurable alveolar echinococcosis: a 45-case European collaborative report. Transplantation 2003;75:856–63.
14 Reuter S, Manfras B, Merkle M, et al. In vitro activities of itraconazole, methiazole, and nitazoxanide versus Echinococcus multilocularis larvae. Antimicrob Agents Chemother 2006;50:2966–70.

Polycystic Echinococcosis (Polycystic Hydatid Disease) 130

Pedro L Moro, Peter M Schantz

Key features

- Zoonotic parasitic disease principally transmitted between the bush dog (host of the adult cestode), *Speothos venaticus*, and the paca (the intermediate host), *Cuniculus paca*. Domestic dogs can become infected with the cestode
- Cestodes that cause polycystic echinococcosis are indigeneous to humid tropical forests in Central America and northern South America
- Nearly all cases of polycystic echinococcosis are caused by *Echinococcus vogeli*; *Echinococcus oligarthus* is a rare cause of disease
- The primary localization of *E. vogeli* infections is the liver, but cysts often invade contiguous sites; the lungs are involved in about 15% of cases
- Treatment options include surgery and chemotherapy with anthelminthic agents

INTRODUCTION

Polycystic echinococcosis is infection by the larval stage of *Echinococcus vogeli* and, less frequently, *Echinococcus oligarthrus*. The cestodes that cause polycystic echinococcosis are indigeneous to humid tropical forests in Central America and northern South America. Humans become infected after accidental ingestion of eggs passed in the feces of definitive hosts—usually domestic dogs or, less likely, bush dogs [1].

EPIDEMIOLOGY

As of 2007, 172 human cases of polycystic echinococcosis have been recorded from Central and South America. Most cases were reported from Brazil (57.6%), Colombia (16.9%) and Ecuador (6.4%) [2]. Polycystic echinococcosis is an emerging disease, as suggested by its increasing frequency. In 1979, there were 12 cases in four countries; by 1997 there were 72 cases; by 1998 there were 86 cases in 11 countries [3, 4]. The natural hosts of *E. vogeli* range throughout neotropical areas of Central and South America, and, as local awareness and availability of diagnostic capability increase, it is probable that more cases will be recorded. A survey of Colombian mammals found that 73 (22.5%) of 325 pacas harbored metacestodes of *E. vogeli* but only three (0.9%) harbored *E. oligarthus* [5]. The known range of *E. oligarthrus* extends from northern Mexico to southern Argentina; the three confirmed cases of human disease caused by this species have been reported from Venezuela and Brazil.

NATURAL HISTORY, PATHOGENESIS, AND PATHOLOGY

The natural hosts of *E. vogeli* are the bush dog, *Speothos venaticus*, and the paca, *Cuniculus paca* [1, 2]. The larval stage occurs occasionally in rodents of other species, including the agouti and spiny rat. Bush dogs are rarely seen animals that are an unlikely source of infection for humans. The intermediate host, the paca, is widely hunted for food in northern South America, and local hunters routinely feed the viscera of pacas to their dogs; thus, dogs may be the primary source of infection for humans.

The definitive hosts of *E. oligarthrus* are felids, including jaguarondi, ocelots, and pumas; the intermediate hosts are the same as for *E. vogeli*. Although the hydatid cysts of both species are similar macroscopically, differentiation of *E. vogeli* and *E. oligarthrus* can be made on the basis of the length and proportions of the rostellar hooks. Human infection with *E. oligarthrus* is extremely rare; only three human cases are documented. The remote behavior of the definitive hosts presumably limits human exposure.

CLINICAL FEATURES

The disease cause by polycystic echinococcosis is also known as polycystic hydatid disease (PHD). Patient ages at diagnosis range from 6 to 78 years (median 44); the most common signs at presentation have been hepatomegaly, palpable peritoneal masses, and jaundice [2, 4]. Polycystic echinococcosis has characteristics intermediate between the cystic and alveolar forms. The primary localization of *E. vogeli* infections is the liver but cysts often invade contiguous sites. Hepatomegaly or tumor-like masses in the liver have been typical findings. The lungs are involved in about 15% of cases. The three known cases of *E. oligarthrus* infection have involved the eyes (two cases) and the heart. The prognosis in polycystic echinococcosis is poor; approximately 14% of patients die of complications of biliary obstruction and portal hypertension.

Five clinical presentations have been described for polycystic echinococcosis [2]: type 1 is most common, occurring in 37% of patients and involving cysts in the liver and abdominal cavity; type II occurs in 26%, involves cysts in the liver and abdominal cavity and is associated with hepatic insufficiency; type III occurs in 14% of patients and cysts occur in the liver and lung/chest; type IV occurs in 16% of patients and the cysts occur in the mesentery of the intestine or of the stomach; and type V occurs in 4% of patients and it involves calcified cysts in the liver and lung.

At laparatomy, polycystic echinococcosis owing to *E. vogeli* appears as a whitish-gray polycystic structure that contains a yellow fluid or gel (Fig. 130.1A). The entire cyst may be only 10 mm in diameter or may form vesicular aggregates that replace most of the liver. The protoscolex with its four circular suckers and rostellum with hooks can be seen in wet mount preparations and tissue sections. The large hooks are 38–46 μm long and the small hooks are 30–37 μm.

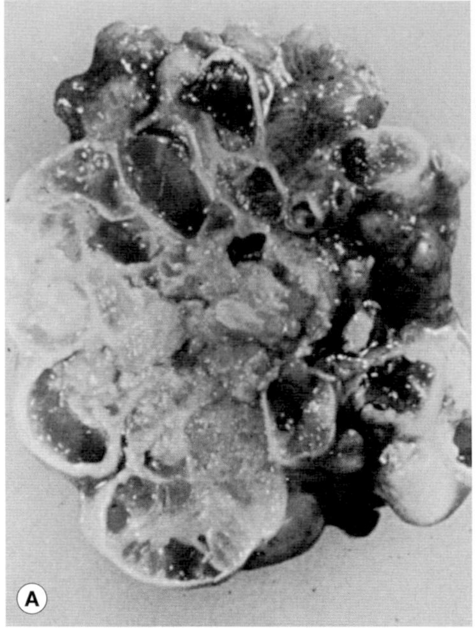

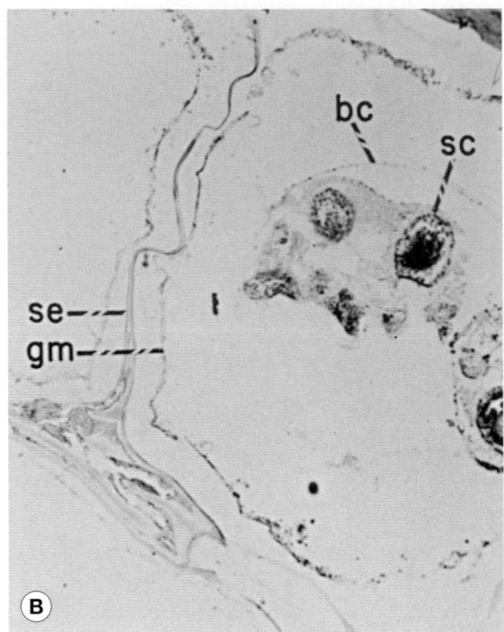

FIGURE 130.1 Polycystic hydatid disease. **(A)** Frontal section of a human heart showing a polycystic hydatid cyst of *Echinococcus vogeli*. **(B)** Histologic section of a portion of a cyst showing internal septa (se), germinal membrane (gm), brood capsules (bc), and necrotic scoleces (sc) *(Reproduced with permission from Alessandro A, Rausch RL, Cuello C, Aristizabal N. Echinococcus vogeli in man, with a review of polycystic hydatid disease in Colombia and neighboring countries. Am J Trop Med Hyg 1979;28:303–17.).*

Numerous vesicles are often seen microscopically and vary in size from a few millimeters to centimeters (Fig. 130.1B). The vesicles are partitioned by septa formed from the hyaline laminated membrane, which is 8–65 µm thick and stains intensely by the periodic acid-Schiff technique. The internal surface of the septa is lined with a germinal membrane that is 3–13 µm thick and contains calcareous corpuscles. The brood capsules bud internally from the germinal epithelium. Externally, the cyst is surrounded by fibrous tissue, with only slight cellular infiltration. Portions of these cysts are frequently necrotic and mineralized, and the only remains of the larval metacestode are the hooks and calcareous corpuscles.

PATIENT EVALUATION, DIAGNOSIS, AND DIFFERENTIAL DIAGNOSIS

The diagnosis of polycystic echinococcosis should be considered in patients who present with abdominal masses and who reside, or previously resided, in rural Central or South American regions. Radiology (x-ray films, ultrasonography, or computed tomography) can demonstrate polycystic structures and diffuse mineralization in the liver or other sites [6]. Serologic tests are helpful for diagnosis but cross-reactivity can occur with *E. granulosus* infection, and with other helminth infections, cancer, and chronic immune disorders [7]. Specific *E. vogeli* antigens may differentiate hydatid disease owing to *E. vogeli* from that caused by *E. granulosus*; however, tests using specific antigens are not widely available. Molecular techniques can be used to distinguish *Echinococcus* species by using PCR followed by sequencing or restriction fragment length polymorphism analysis.

TREATMENT

The principles of management of cystic and alveolar echinococcosis also apply to polycystic echinococcosis [8]. As the lesions are extensive, surgical resection may be difficult and is usually incomplete. A combination of surgery with albendazole is most likely to be successful. In a review of the outcomes of human cases of polycystic echinococcosis, 35 (88%) out of 40 patients who underwent surgery recovered uneventfully and five (12%) died. The number of reported cases treated with albendazole is very small, but of 13 treated with albendazole alone, six improved partially or completely [2].

REFERENCES

1. Eckert J, Deplazes P. Biological, epidemiological, and clinical aspects of echinococcosis, a zoonosis of increasing concern. Clin Microbiol Rev 2004;17:107–35.
2. D'Alessandro A, Rausch RL. New aspects of neotropical polycystic (*Echinococcus vogeli*) and unicystic (*Echinococcus oligarthrus*) echinococcosis. Clin Microbiol Rev 2008;21:380–401.
3. Tappe D, Stich A, Frosch M. Emergence of polycystic neotropical echinococcosis. Emerg Infect Dis 2008;14:292–7.
4. D'Alessandro A. Polycystic echinococcosis in tropical America: *Echinococcus vogeli* and *E. oligarthrus*. Acta Trop 1997;67:43–65.
5. D'Alessandro A, Rausch RL, Morales GA, et al. Echinococcus infections in Colombian animals. Am J Trop Med Hyg 1981;30:1263–76.
6. Pawlowski Z, Eckert J, Vuitton DA, et al. Echinococcosis in humans: Clinical aspects, diagnosis and treatment. In: Eckert J, Gemmell MA, Meslin F-X, eds. WHO/OIE Manual on Echinococcosis in Humans and Animals. Paris: Office International des Épizooties; 2001:20–71.
7. Gottstein B, D'Alessandro A, Rausch RL. Immunodiagnosis of polycystic hydatid disease/polycystic echinococcosis due to Echinococcus vogeli. Am J Trop Med Hyg 1995;53:558–63.
8. Brunetti E, Kern P, Vuitton DA. Writing Panel for the WHO-IWGE. Expert consensus for the diagnosis and treatment of cystic and alveolar echinococcosis in humans. Acta Trop 2010;114:1–16.

Sparganosis 131

Meredith L Holtz, Robert Gilman

Key features

- Sparganosis is a rare parasitic disease caused by infestation by the larvae of tapeworms of the genus *Spirometra*
- It is acquired by ingesting copepods or undercooked meat containing the larvae
- Invasion of tissue by the larvae causes a migratory abscess that is usually subcutaneous, but can appear in any tissue of the body
- CNS infection has the worst prognosis, and presents with seizures, headache, or a slowly evolving paralysis
- The parasite can be distinguished histologically by a head with characteristic deep invagination, body pseudo-segmentation, and the absence of suckers and hooks
- Definitive diagnosis is identification of the worm on extraction, which also can lead to a cure

INTRODUCTION

Sparganosis is a rare parasitic disease of humans caused by invasion of human tissue by plerocercoid tapeworm larvae (spargana) of the genus *Spirometra*. Many species of *Spirometra* have been described. In Southeast Asia the parasite is referred to as *Spirometra mansoni* and in North America as *S. mansonoides*. On other continents it may be called *S. erinacei*, *S. europaei*, *S. theileri* and *S. ranarum* [1]. Adult tapeworms occur in domestic and wild carnivores and are similar to *Diphyllobothrium* (see Chapter 126). The life cycles differ, as *Spirometra* usually use amphibians, reptiles and mammals as second intermediate hosts, and *Diphyllobothrium* use fish (Fig. 131.1).

EPIDEMIOLOGY

Humans are rare incidental hosts. The parasites are prevalent in cats, dogs and wild carnivores in many parts of the world, and are endemic in 48 countries. Human infections are most common in Southeast Asia, but infections have been recorded in East Africa, South America, North America, Australia and parts of Europe [2]. The highest endemicity of infection with *Spirometra* spp. is in Korea and Japan, primarily because of dietary customs [3].

NATURAL HISTORY, PATHOGENESIS AND PATHOLOGY

Humans ingest larvae of *Spirometra* spp. by: 1) drinking contaminated water containing copepods (*Cyclops*) carrying the procercoid larvae; 2) ingesting the plerocercoid larvae while eating undercooked meat from second intermediate hosts such as amphibians, reptiles, rodents or other mammals; or 3) using those meats as a poultice (a traditional self-treatment according to ritual belief) that is applied directly to ulcers, sores, or inflamed eyes. The latter is a more common cause of orbital sparganosis [3].

After ingestion, the spargana migrate to the subcutaneous tissues, where they become encapsulated in inflammatory nodules that can develop into abscesses. These abscesses can occur anywhere in the body, as spargana have the ability to migrate to any tissue, including the brain [1]. The sparganum remains viable inside the nodule, thus the subcutaneous masses may migrate [4]. The parasite can live for up to 30 years inside their host, and their length can vary from a few millimeters to a few centimeters.

CLINICAL FEATURES

The most common clinical presentation is a migrating subcutaneous abscess that may involve localized pain, erythema and pruritus. Other features of the clinical presentation depend on the location and size of the lesion [3]. In the subconjunctival tissues, the larvae provoke acute inflammation with painful conjunctivitis and periorbital edema. If the larvae invade the periorbital tissues, it may result in proptosis and blindness [3]. Sparganosis can infect the central nervous system (CNS), breast, lungs, peritoneal cavity, epididymis, bone, bladder, heart, ear and kidneys. In some locations, such as breast, bone and peritoneal cavity, it could be mistaken for cancer.

CNS infections usually have the worst prognosis. Although CNS involvement is rare, spargana have been reported to cause brain abscesses (that may migrate), intradural spinal canal infection, and extradural spinal cord infection. In these cases, the mass may produce seizures (reported as most common symptom), headache, slowly evolving hemiparesis, paresthesias, memory loss, confusion and radiculalgia, depending on the location [3]. There is no evidence to suggest that immunosuppression influences the risk of CNS infection.

On biopsy, the parasites can usually be extracted alive, and they may be several centimeters in length. They are glistening white, opaque ribbon-like worms with a typical undulating cestode movement (Fig. 131.2A,C). Grossly, the inflammation is nodular and locally fibrotic. Histologically, the inflammation consists of lymphocytes, histiocytes, plasma cells, neutrophils, and multinucleated giant cells; eosinophils may be abundant or absent (Fig. 131.2B).

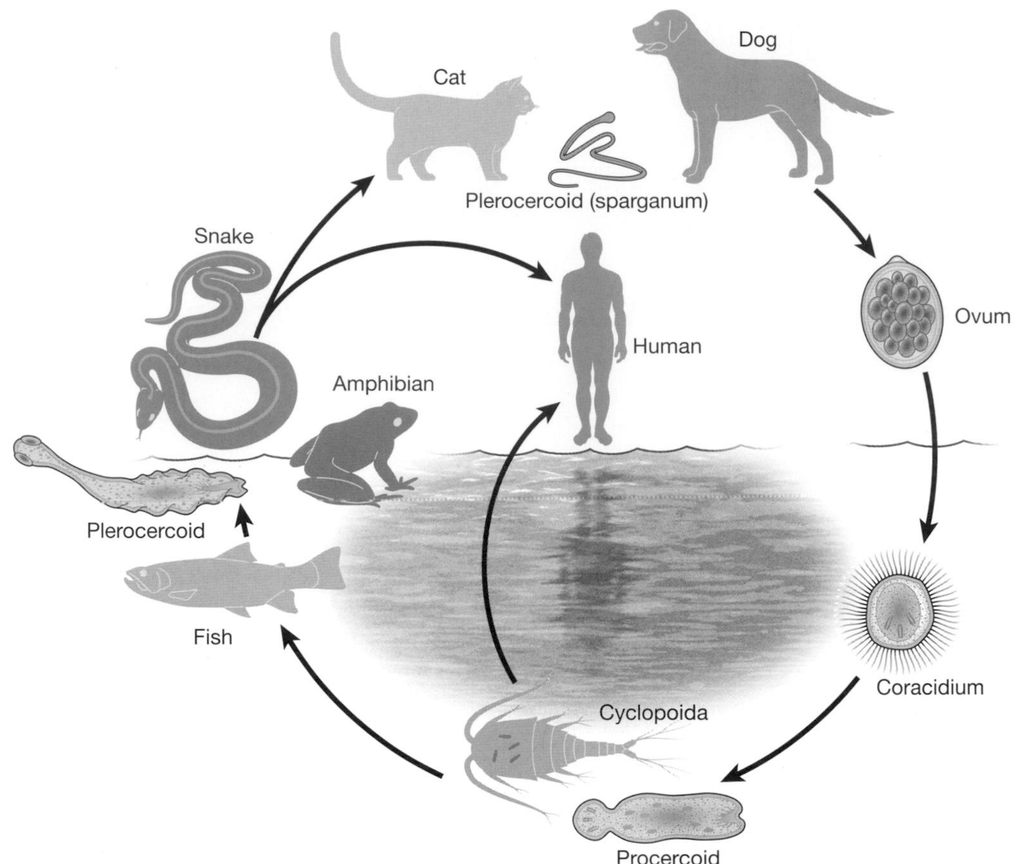

FIGURE 131.1 Lifecycle of *Spirometra* spp. Ova from the adult worm are shed in the feces of the definitive hosts, cats and dogs. The eggs hatch in fresh water into coracidia, which are ingested by the first intermediate host, copepods of the genus *Cyclops,* and grow into the first larval stage, procercoid. Water containing the copepods is ingested by the second intermediate hosts, which include reptiles, amphibians and mammals, where they grow into the plerocercoid larvae. Sparganum develops into an adult worm in the intestines of the definitive hosts.

PATIENT EVALUATION, DIAGNOSIS AND DIFFERENTIAL DIAGNOSIS

In a patient with a subcutaneous infection suspected to be sparganosis, peripheral eosinophilia does not occur, and blood work will provide little help. However, peripheral eosinophilia can be pronounced in CNS infection. Enzyme-linked immunosorbent assay (ELISA) has shown high sensitivity and specificity, but is only available in a research setting [5].

Imaging can be helpful in some cases, especially in CNS infection. Ultrasonographic findings in subcutaneous and musculoskeletal cases include serpiginous, cystic, tubular tracts with an echogenicity. These are not specific to sparganosis [6].

In CNS infection, computed tomography (CT) scan can reveal multifocal areas of low density within white matter, adjacent ventricular dilation, or irregular enhancing lesions. The most distinct features of sparganosis on CT scan are the small punctuate calcifications caused by the calcareous corpuscles the worm leaves in its tract (seen more clearly on CT scan than on magnetic resonance imaging [MRI]) (Fig. 131.3).

Further investigation with MRI in CNS infection has three characteristic features. The first is the tunnel sign, created by the undulating movement of the worm (Fig. 131.4A–C). It is a column-shaped or fusiform-shaped tunnel with a hollow appearance and a smooth, well-defined margin [7]. A second characteristic finding is ring or bead-shaped enhancement, representing inflammatory granuloma. A third sign is a change in the location and shape of the lesion on serial images, due to migration [8]. It is important to look for lesions of multiple ages in the same image, due to the long course of the disease.

Definitive diagnosis is provided by identification of the parasite in a tissue specimen. If the intact parasite is extracted, it can be recognized by its head with a characteristic deep invagination (Fig. 131.2C,D). Histologic sections of the worm show features of cestode larvae (Fig. 131.2D). The surface tegument has multiple infoldings, or pseudosegmentation. The worm-like appearance and the solid body of the spargana along with the absence of suckers and hooks usually distinguish them from the cystic stages of other cestodes that occur in subcutaneous tissues. Within the body of the worm, there are longitudinal muscle fibers, excretory channels and calcareous corpuscles (Fig. 131.3) [9].

Differential diagnosis of parasite-induced cerebral mass lesions includes *Toxoplasma,* infection with various larval forms of other cestodes such as *Coenurus, Echinococcus, Multiceps,* cysticercosis, and paragonimiasis, and can be distinguished microscopically. Gnathostomiasis, paragonimiasis and infection from the filarial nematode *Loa loa* can each cause migratory subcutaneous masses.

TREATMENT

The only effective treatment is complete surgical removal of the intact worm and the surrounding granuloma. In patients with many infections, supplementary treatment with praziquantel may be advisable, but there is little evidence to suggest its effectiveness (see Chapter 128). ELISA after removal can help to determine whether the worm was removed completely.

Coenuriasis 132

Rachel B Webman, Robert H Gilman

Key features

- Coenuriasis is a common zoonosis with rare human infections
- In humans, infection is caused by the larval stage of the cestode *Taenia* (*Multiceps*) species
- Generally a single space-occupying lesion is found subcutaneously, ocularly, or in the CNS
- The coenurus is a thin-walled cyst filled with clear fluid with small scoleces attached to the cyst wall
- Treatment is usually surgical excision combined with antiparasitic medication

INTRODUCTION

Coenuriasis is a zoonotic disease of humans caused by infection with the larval stage of the cestode parasite, *Taenia* (*Multiceps*) species, including *T. multiceps*, *T. serialis*, *T. brauni*, and *T. glomerata*.

EPIDEMIOLOGY

Taenia (*Multiceps*) *multiceps* has a wide distribution in temperate areas, where it usually circulates in a cycle between dogs and herbivorous mammals, including sheep, goats, cattle, and horses. Coenuri infect the brain and spinal cord of the intermediate host and cause a disease of sheep known as *gid* or *staggers*. Human neurocoenuriasis is rare but has been reported from the US, England, France, Africa, the Middle East, and Brazil [1,2].

Taenia (*Multiceps*) *serialis*is also a parasite of temperate areas with wide distribution. Coenuri are usually found in intermuscular connective tissue of lagomorphs and rodents, including the rabbit, squirrel, and nutria. *T. serialis* is rare in humans and has been found in Canada, the US, France, the Middle East, and Africa.

Taenia (*Multiceps*) *brauni* is a tropical tapeworm of eastern Africa with a sylvatic life cycle, including the dog, fox, jackal, and genet as definitive hosts and rodents such as the swamp rat, porcupine, and gerbil as intermediate hosts. The coenuri infect subcutaneous tissue of the intermediate hosts. There are fewer than 100 reports of *T. brauni* in humans.

Taenia (*Multiceps*) *glomeratus* has been found in subcutaneous tissue of humans in Nigeria.

NATURAL HISTORY, PATHOGENESIS, AND PATHOLOGY

Adult tapeworms are found in the small intestines of canids, usually dogs. These definitive hosts pass gravid proglottids at defecation. The proglottids eventually disintegrate to free the eggs, which disperse throughout the environment. When ingested by intermediate hosts, susceptible herbivores or humans, the oncospheres penetrate the wall of the small intestine and travel through the bloodstream to solid organs. There they develop into coenuri in the subcutaneous tissues, muscles, and central nervous system [3].

The coenurus has a thin wall surrounding a single cavity that contains a clear fluid. Numerous scoleces 3 mm in diameter attach to the cyst wall, and unlike the unilocular hydatid cyst of *E. granulosus*, no brood capsules are found (Fig. 132.1). Each scolex has four circular suckers and two rows of hooks on a rostellum. There are large and small hooks. The hook lengths for *T. multiceps* are 150 to 170 μm and 90 to 130 μm; those for *T. serialis* are 135 to 175 μm and 68 to 120 μm; those for *T. brauni* are 95 to 140 μm and 70 to 90 μm; and those for *T. glomeratus* are 90 to 100 μm and 65 to 70 μm (Fig. 132.2) [2].

CLINICAL FEATURES

Patients with coenuriasis usually have a space-occupying lesion caused by a single cyst 2 to 6 cm in diameter. However, cysts up to 10 cm in diameter have been reported [4]. Neural coenuri have been found in the cerebrum, leptomeninges, ventricles, posterior horn of the lateral ventricle, brainstem, and spinal cord and among the cranial nerves. The clinical manifestations of neurocoenuriasis are similar to those of neurocysticercosis. In cerebral cases these include headache, vomiting, papilledema, meningeal symptoms, and seizures, as well as focal neurologic deficits [1].

Subcutaneous coenuri are found in the intercostal region and anterior abdominal wall. They have also been reported in the breast, axilla, lumbar spine, peritoneal cavity, and extremities. These cysts resemble a lipoma, ganglion, or neurofibroma. Ocular coenuri have been recorded in the vitreous, anterior chamber, and conjunctiva [5].

PATIENT EVALUATION, DIAGNOSIS, AND DIFFERENTIAL DIAGNOSIS

Space-occupying lesions in the deep organs are visualized with x-ray, radioisotopic scans, ultrasonography, or more commonly with computed tomography (CT) scans and magnetic resonance imaging (MRI). On CT scans, cysts are seen as a lucent area surrounded by a contrast-enhancing rim (Fig. 132.3). Older, sterile lesions appear calcified on CT. On MRI, cyst fluid resembles cerebrospinal fluid, appearing dark in T1-weighted images and bright in T2-weighted images [3].

Subcutaneous coenuri can be palpated, and ocular coenuri can be observed by ophthalmologic examination.

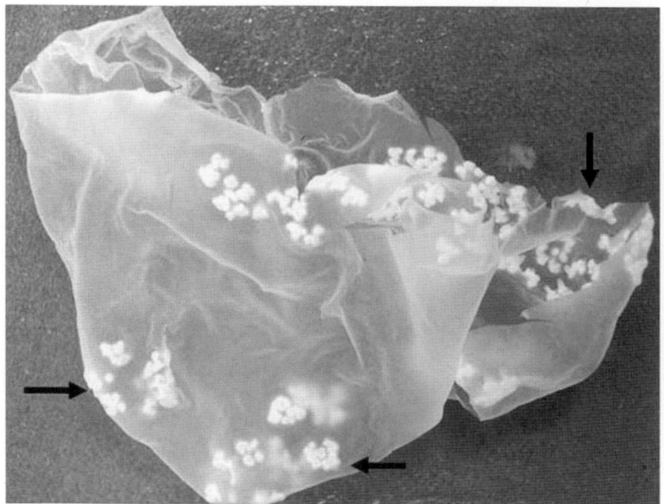

FIGURE 132.1 Macroscopic view of the inner cyst. The arrows show the clusters of protoscolices attached to the inner surface. *Reproduced with permission from Benifla M, Barrelly R, Shelef I, et al. Huge hemispheric intraparenchymal cystcaused by Taenia multiceps in a child. J Neurosurg 2007;107: 511–14.*

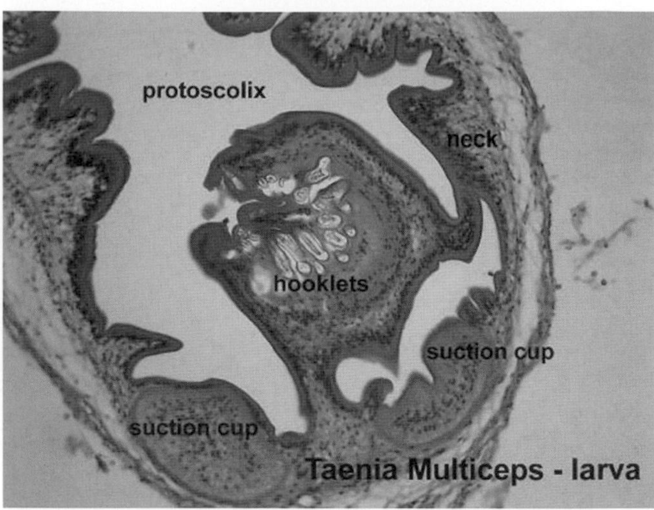

FIGURE 132.2 Photomicrograph of a coenuris protoscolix. Main anatomical details shown and labeled are the neck, hooklets, and two of the four suction cups. *Reproduced with permission from Benifla M, Barrelly R, Shelef I, et al. Huge hemispheric intraparenchymal cystcaused by Taenia multiceps in a child. J Neurosurg 2007;107:511–14.*

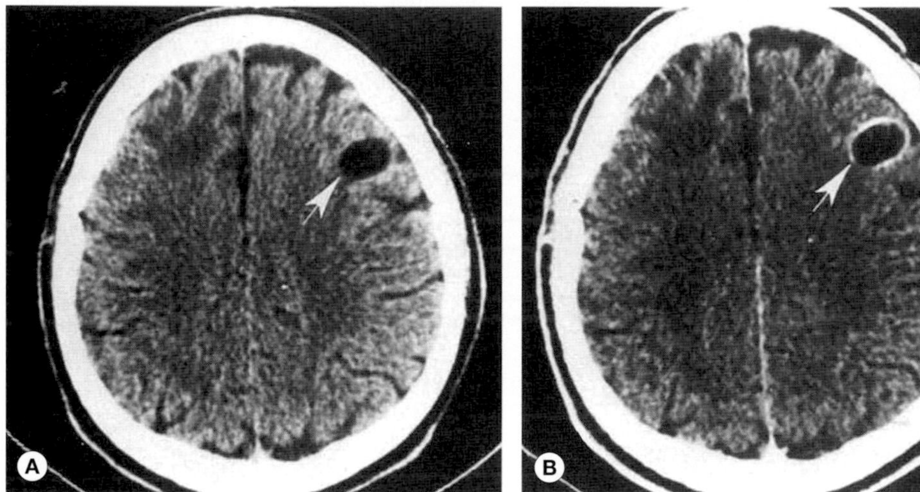

FIGURE 132.3 CT scans of the head before **(A)** and after **(B)** contrast, showing a cyst in the right frontal lobe. Note enhanced cyst rim in post-contrast figure. *Reproduced with permission from Pau A, Turtas S, Brambilla M, et al. Computed tomography and magnetic resonance imaging of cerebral coenurosis. Surg Neurol 1987;27:548–52.*

Definitive diagnosis generally rests on surgical excision followed by microscopic identification, as described in the pathology section. Diagnosis has also been made after fine needle aspiration followed by microscopy. Serology has been used to rule out the more common, *Taenia solium* and *Echinococcus granulosus* infections; however, false-positive results for *T. solium* or *E. granulosus* can occur. PCR has also been used in research settings to identify and differentiate between *T. muliceps* and *T. serialis* [1].

TREATMENT

Surgical excision is the usual treatment, although both praziquantel and albendazole are likely to be effective, as in the treatment of cysticercosis. Patients are treated with a combination of surgical intervention and antiparasitics [1, 4]. Praziquantel can lead to toxic endophthalmitis and loss of vision in intraocular coenurosis and inflammation in other parts of the body.

The best treatment of an intravitreal cestode cystic larva is its removal through a closed vitrectomy [5].

Preventive measures include hygienic practices to reduce contact with dogs and to break the transmission of eggs from dog feces to humans. Elimination of adult worms with praziquantel or niclosamide reduces environmental contamination with eggs. Experimental vaccination of sheep has proven successful and could lead to a halt in the life cycle of *T. multiceps* [6].

REFERENCES

1. Ing M, Schantz P, Turner J. Human coenurosis in North America: case reports and review. Clin Infect Dis 1998;27:519–23.
2. Templeton AC. Anatomical and geographical location of human coenurus infection. Trop Geogr Med 1971;23:105–8.
3. Pau A, Turtas S, Brambilla M, et al. Computed tomography and magnetic resonance imaging of cerebral coenurosis. Surg Neurol 1987;27:548–52.
4. Benifla M, Barrelly R, Shelef I, et al. Huge hemispheric intraparenchymal cyst caused by *Taenia multiceps* in a child. J Neurosurg 2007;107:511–14.
5. Ibechukwu BI, Onwukeme KB. Intraocular coenurosis: a case report. Br J Ophthalmol 1991;75:430–1.
6. Varcasia A, Tosciri G, Sanna Coccone GN, et al. Preliminary field trial of a vaccine against coenurosis caused by *Taenia multiceps*. Vet Parasit 2009;162:285–9.

PART

7

POISONOUS AND TOXIC PLANTS AND ANIMALS

133 Poisonous Plants and Aquatic Animals

133.1 Poisonous Aquatic Animals

David A Warrell

INTRODUCTION: SEAFOOD POISONING [1]

Inhabitants of oceanic islands and sea coasts who are largely dependent on marine animals for their protein intake are particularly at risk from acute gastrointestinal symptoms ("food poisoning") after eating seafood. In some communities, almost 2% of the population is affected each year. Infectious causes include viruses: hepatitis A virus (mollusks, especially clams and oysters), Norwalk virus (clams and oysters) and astro- and caliciviruses (cockles and other molluscs); bacteria: *Vibrio parahaemolyticus* (crustaceans, especially shrimps), *Vibrio cholerae* (crabs and mollusks), non-O group 1 *V. cholerae* (oysters), *Vibrio vulnificus* (oysters), *Aeromonas hydrophila* (frozen oysters), *Plesiomonas shigelloides* (oysters, mussels, mackerel, cuttlefish), *Shigella* spp. (mollusks), *Campylobacter jejuni* (clams), and *Salmonella typhi* (mollusks). Microbial toxins have been responsible for botulism after ingestion of smoked fish and canned salmon. Since 1953, approximately 100,000 Japanese are thought to have been affected by methyl mercury poisoning (Minamata disease) after eating fish and mollusks contaminated with methyl mercury derived from industrial waste dumped in Minamata Bay and at the mouth of the Agano River in Japan. The victims developed severe CNS damage, with a mortality of 33% in the initial outbreak. Pregnant women exposed to methyl mercury gave birth to infants who were mentally retarded and had cerebral palsy and convulsions.

The origins of natural toxins in seafood that give rise to gastrointestinal, neurotoxic and other symptoms can usually be traced down the food chain to algae (dinoflagellates and diatoms) and bacteria, while histamine-like symptoms are attributable to bacterial decomposition of dead fish. Globalization of the seafood industry and expanding appetites for novel gustatory experiences, or use as traditional medicines, now ensures that exotic tropical fish, crustaceans and mollusks are widely available in Western fish markets. As a result, toxic seafood poisoning is becoming more common and geographically widespread.

PREVENTION OF SEAFOOD POISONING

As most marine toxins, such as ciguatera toxin, tetrodotoxin and scombrotoxins, are heat-stable, cooking does not prevent poisoning. However, some toxins are fairly water-soluble and may be leached out by soaking—as such, the water in which exotic fish are cooked should not be drunk. In tropical areas, the flesh of fish should be separated as soon as possible from the head, skin, intestines, gonads and other viscera that may contain high concentrations of toxin. All scale-less fish should be regarded as potentially tetrodotoxic. Fish may accumulate toxins from the food chain throughout their lives and so very large reef fish carry the highest risk of being ciguatera-toxic. Certain species are especially dangerous, such as Moray eels and parrot fish (Scaridae), which should never be eaten because of the high risk of unusually rapid and severe ciguatera and scaritoxic fish poisoning. Scombroid poisoning can be prevented by eating fresh fish or by freezing fish as soon as possible after they are caught. Shellfish should never be eaten during the dangerous seasons, when red tides declare the blooming of toxic dinoflagellates and when there are numbers of dead sea birds, seals, and other marine animals on the beaches.

REFERENCE

1. Sobel J, Painter J. Illnesses caused by marine toxins. Clin Infect Dis 2005; 41:1290–6.

133.2 Fish Poisoning: Gastrointestinal and Neurotoxic Syndromes

David A Warrell

Key features

- Food poisoning from toxins in fish, shellfish, and crustaceans, rather than pathogenic organisms, is prevalent in many ocean communities and is increasingly recognized in travelers and those who eat exotic fish. Toxins are ultimately derived from dinoflagellates, diatoms, and bacteria (Table 133.2.1)
- As most seafood toxins are thermostable, cooking does not remove the risk of poisoning. Very large reef fish (e.g. Moray eels), scale-less fish, and fish viscera should be avoided and shellfish should not be eaten at times of red tide or when marine birds and mammals are dying off
- Diarrheal, neurotoxic, paralytic and amnesic syndromes of shellfish poisoning are recognized. Acute gastrointestinal symptoms are associated variously with paraesthesiae and more serious paralytic and central nervous system (CNS) symptoms that can be fatal. Treatment is symptomatic
- Ciguatera and tetrodotoxic fish poisonings cause acute gastrointestinal symptoms followed by paraesthesiae and neurotoxic or paralytic symptoms
- Scombroid fish poisoning produces anaphylactic, histamine-like symptoms caused by eating fish spoiled by bacterial decomposition
- Palytoxin, carps' gall bladder and *Pfeisteria*-associated poisoning are also discussed

NEUROTOXIC FISH POISONING

Nausea, vomiting, abdominal colic, tenesmus and watery diarrhea may precede neurotoxic symptoms of paraesthesia of the lips, buccal cavity and extremities, distorted temperature perception (so that cold objects impart a burning sensation like dry ice), myalgia, progressive flaccid paralysis, dizziness, ataxia, cardiovascular disturbances, bradycardia and rashes. Two important causes of this syndrome are ciguatera fish poisoning and tetrodotoxin poisoning (Table 133.2-1).

CIGUATERA FISH POISONING [1, 2]

Symptoms develop between 1 and 6 hours (extreme range: minutes to 30 h) after eating fish such as groupers, snappers, parrot fish, mackerel, moray eels (Fig. 133.2.1), barracudas, and jacks. These are warm-water shore or reef fish. The global incidence is thought to exceed 50,000 cases per year. Up to 2% of the population may be affected each year (e.g. in Kiribati, Tokelau, and Tuvalu in the Pacific region) with a case fatality of 0.1%. The toxins responsible are polyethers, such as ciguatoxin (activates Na^+ channels), maitotoxin (activates Ca^{2+} channels) and scaritoxin, ultimately derived along the food chain from benthic dinoflagellates such as *Gambierdiscus toxicus*. They are concentrated in the liver, viscera and gonads, especially of large, carnivorous fish. The increasing market for exotic fish from the Caribbean and elsewhere has led to cases of ciguatera in Britain and other European countries. Geographically-distinct clinical patterns have emerged in the Caribbean (predominantly gastrointestinal), Pacific (more neurotoxic), and Indian Ocean (hallucinations, incoordination, dysequilibration, depression and nightmares), reflecting variation in the prevailing toxins.

Gastrointestinal symptoms of nausea, vomiting, diarrhea and abdominal pain and cramps and, on occasion, a metallic taste in the mouth are followed by neurologic symptoms of paresthesia around the mouth and extremities, reversed hot-cold sensation (dysesthesia), increased salivation, dilatation of the pupils, strabismus, ptosis, weakness and ataxia, usually resolve within a few hours, but paraesthesiae and myalgia may persist for a week, or even months. Pruritus of the soles and palms and a sensation that one's teeth are loose are distinctive symptoms but occur irregularly. Cardiovascular features include braycardia, hypotension and hypovolemia. Rashes are also described. Similar symptoms (chelonitoxication) may follow ingestion of marine turtles in the Indo-Pacific area, but the case fatality is much higher.

TETRODOTOXIN POISONING

Scale-less fish, such as puffer, porcupine (Fig. 133.2.2), toad and sun fish (order: Tetraodonitiformes) may become highly poisonous at certain seasons, such as May to June—the spawning season in Japan. Eating these fish is proscribed in the Old Testament (e.g. Leviticus 11:9–12). Tetrodotoxin, an aminoperhydroquinazoline, is one of the most potent non-protein toxins known. It produces neurotoxic and cardiotoxic effects by blocking voltage-gated sodium ion channels. It is concentrated in the ovaries, viscera, and skin of tetraodontiform fish; in the skin of newts (genus *Taricha*), frogs and toads (genera *Colostethus, Atelopus, Bracycephalus*), and salamanders; in the saliva of octopuses; in the digestive glands of several species of gastropod

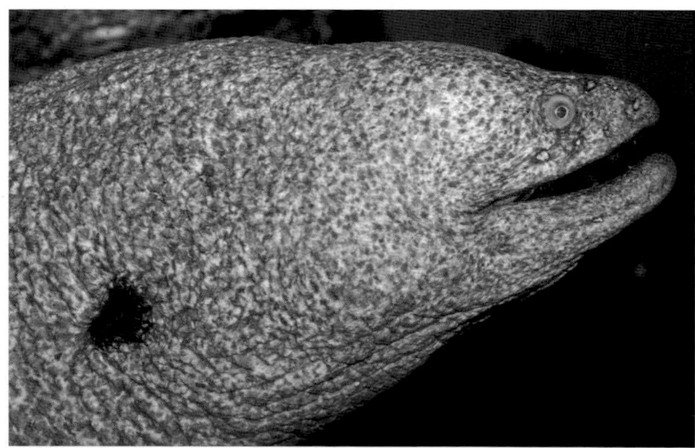

FIGURE 133.2.1 Californian moray eel (*Gymnothorax morda*) (*© David A. Warrell*).

TABLE 133.2-1 Summary of Characteristics of Different Types of Seafood Poisoning All of Which Cause Acute Gastrointestinal Symptoms

Type of poisoning	**Ciguatera**	**Tetrodotoxic**	**Scombroid**
Incubation	1–6 hours	10–45 minutes	5–60 minutes
Duration of symptoms	Days–months	Days	Few hrs
Characteristic symptoms	Paraesthesiae, myalgias	Rapidly developing paralysis, areflexia, erythematous rash	Immediate lip tingling, anaphylactic-like pruritus, urticaria, shock, angioedema, brochospasm, diarrhoea, headache
Seafood affected	Tropical reef fish: red snapper, red bass, coral trout, sea bass, grouper, parrot fish, moray eels, mackerel, tuna, jacks, barracuda	Scale-less fish: puffer ("fugu"), porcupine, sun, toad fish and freshwater puffer fish (Tetraodontiformes) also amphibians, crabs, octopus, molluscs, nermertines, flat worms etc.	Dark-fleshed fish: tuna, skipjack, bonito, mackerel, mahi-mahi; anchovies, sardines, pilchards
Geographical range	Tropical Pacific, Indian and Caribbean oceans	Tropical oceans, Japan, China, SE Asia, also farmed	Global
Toxin and origin	Ciguatoxins and maitotoxins from dinoflagellate *Gambierdiscus toxicus*	Tetrodotoxins (aminoperhydroquinazoline) from bacteria e.g. *Pseudomonas* sp. Saxitoxin in freshwater puffer fish	Histamine, saurine from bacterial (*Proteus, Klebsiella*) decomposition of fish muscle histidine

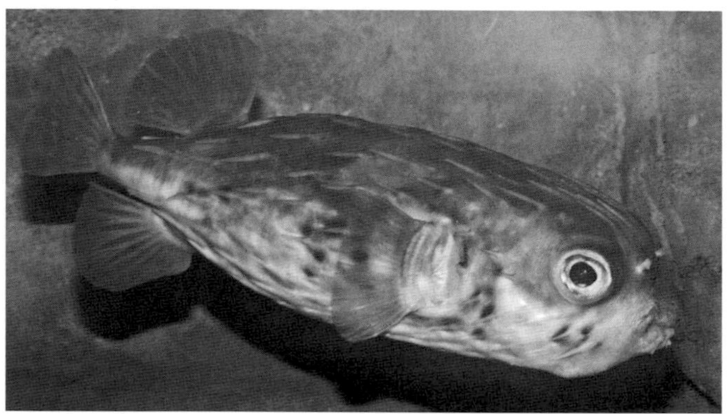

FIGURE 133.2.2 Slender-spined porcupine fish, South Australia (*Diodon nicthemerus*) (© David A. Warrell).

mollusks; and in a starfish, flat worm (*Planorbis* spp.), and nemertine worms in Japan. It is produced by various bacteria (*Pseudomonas, Pseudoalteromonas, Vibrio* spp. etc.). Puffer fish ("fugu") is particularly popular in Japan where, despite stringent regulations, there are still cases of tetrodotoxin poisoning, with about four deaths each year.

Nausea and abdominal pain occur but usually no vomiting or diarrhea, or there may be no gastrointestinal symptoms. Neurotoxic symptoms characterized by rapid onset, within 10–45 minutes, of weakness, dizziness, paresthesiae of the lips, tongue, throat and, later, the limbs. Pallor, sweating and increased salivation may be present. Tachycardia, hypotension, difficulty breathing and flaccid ascending paralysis may lead to respiratory paralysis; death usually occurs 2–6 hours after eating the fish. Usually, consciousness is retained throughout, although they may appear comatose. Patients have developed fixed dilated pupils and brain stem areflexia, so appearing brain dead, but have made a complete recovery after being mechanically ventilated.

Erythema, petechiae, blistering and desquamation may appear. Freshwater puffer fish poisoning in northern Thailand has been attributed to saxitoxin.

HISTAMINE-LIKE SYNDROME (SCOMBROTOXIC POISONING)

The dark red flesh of scombroid fish (tuna, mackerel, bonito, and skipjack) and of canned non-scombroid fish, such as sardines and pilchards, may be decomposed by the action of bacteria such as *Proteus morgani* and *Klebsiella pneumoniae*, which decarboxylate muscle histidine into saurine, histamine, cadaverine and other unidentified toxins: 100 g of spoiled fish may contain almost 1 g of histamine. Histamine absorbed from the gut is normally broken down by *N*-methyl-transferase and diamine oxidase (histaminase), but if the histamine concentration is very high, or the patient is taking a diamine oxidase inhibitor such as isoniazid (as anti-tuberculosis chemotherapy), scombrotoxic poisoning may result. Toxic fish may produce a tingling or smarting sensation in the mouth or a peppery flavor when eaten. Within minutes or up to a few hours after ingestion, flushing, burning, sweating, urticaria and pruritis may develop with headache, abdominal colic, nausea, vomiting, diarrhoea, bronchial asthma, giddiness and hypotension. Full recovery is expected over a few hours but symptoms may persist for up to 24 hours.

PALYTOXIN POISONING [3]

Palytoxin and similar toxins are highly potent Na^+-K^+ ATPase inhibitors occurring in zoanthid corals (*Palythoa toxica*), red alga, a sea anemone and in dinoflagellates such as *Ostrepsis siamensis*. It affects humans lethally when ingested in reef fish, crabs and shellfish (sometimes associated with ciguatoxins, saxitoxins and tetrodotoxin), and non-lethally after dermal and ocular exposure, especially in aquarium keepers. Clinical effects include acute gastrointestinal symptoms followed by paraesthesiae, hypertension, distorted sense of taste (dysguesia), rhabdomyolysis, cardiac dysrhythmias, respiratory failure, and coma, rapidly progressing to death. There is no specific treatment.

POISONING BY INGESTING CARP'S GALLBLADDER [4]

In parts of the Far East, the raw bile and gallbladder of various species of freshwater carp (e.g. grass carp *Ctenopharyngodon idellus* and Jullien's golden carp *Probarbus jullieni*) are believed to have medicinal properties. Patients in China, Taiwan, Hong Kong, Japan, Thailand and elsewhere have developed acute abdominal pain, vomiting and watery diarrhea 2–18 hours after drinking the raw bile or eating the raw gallbladder of these fish. One patient developed flushing and dizziness. Hepatic and renal damage may develop, progressing to oliguric or non-oliguric acute renal failure (acute tubular necrosis). The hepatonephrotoxin has not been identified, but is heat-stable and may be derived from the carp's diet.

PFIESTERIA-ASSOCIATED POSSIBLE ESTUARY ASSOCIATED SYNDROME (PEAS)

Although the toxic dinoflagellate *Pfiesteria piscicida* is commonly associated with fish kills and can be concentrated in shellfish, toxic exposure in humans is thought to be by direct contact with the toxin, absorbed through the skin or from aerosols. It became a major environmental concern in coastal waters of North Carolina, Virginia and Maryland (USA) in the late 1990s. Pfiesteria-associated Possible Estuary Associated Syndrome (PEAS) was characterized by impaired cognitive function and rapid and severe decrements in visual contrast sensitivity. PEAS signs and symptoms responded to cholestyramine treatment supporting the hypothesis that PEAS was a biotoxin-associated illness.

DIFFERENTIAL DIAGNOSIS OF SEAFOOD POISONING

The differential diagnosis of gastrointestinal symptoms of seafood poisoning includes bacterial and viral food poisoning and allergic reactions.

Viral and bacterial food poisoning has a longer incubation period (hours or days), unless it is caused by a preformed toxin, as in the case of staphylococcal, clostridial and *Bacillus cereus* poisoning. However, neurologic symptoms are distinctive, suggesting some kind of neurotoxic seafood poisoning. Allergic reactions produce anaphylactic symptoms (pruritus, urticaria, erythema, angioedema, bronchospasm, and shock), sometimes within minutes of ingestion. Unless there is a past history of specific seafood allergy (e.g. to prawns, tuna) or an epidemiologic clue (several diners affected), it can be very difficult to distinguish allergy from scombroid poisoning, but the emergency treatment is the same for both etiologies.

TREATMENT OF SEAFOOD POISONING [5]

No specific treatments or antidotes are available. Gastric lavage is controversial but elimination of gastrointestinal contents should be attempted if this can be achieved within 1–2 hours of ingestion and without jeopardizing the airway. Activated charcoal adsorbs saxitoxin and other shellfish toxins. Atropine is said to improve gastrointestinal symptoms and sinus bradycardia in patients with gastrointestinal and neurotoxic poisoning. Calcium gluconate may relieve mild neuromuscular symptoms. Oximes and anticholinesterases are ineffective in ciguatera and tetrodotoxin poisoning respectively. Mannitol, once promoted for ciguatera poisoning, has proved useless. In cases of paralytic poisoning, endotracheal intubation and mechanical ventilation and cardiac resuscitation have proved life saving. In Malaysia, a patient with tetrodotoxin poisoning developed fixed dilated pupils and brain stem areflexia, so appearing brain dead, but made a complete recovery after being mechanically ventilated. Symptoms of scrombrotoxic poisoning can be alleviated with epinephrine, anti-H1 histamine blockers and adrenergic β-2 agonist bronchodilators.

REFERENCES

1. Bagnis RA, Kuberski T, Laugier S. Clinical observations on 3009 cases of Ciguatera (fish poisoning) in the Southern Pacific. Am J Trop Med Hyg 1979; 28:1067–73.
2. Halstead BW. Poisonous and Venomous Marine Animals of the World, 2nd edn. Princeton: Darwin Press; 1988.
3. Deeds JR, Schwartz MD. Human risk associated with palytoxin exposure. Toxicon 2009;56:150–62.
4. Lin YF, Lin SH (1999). Simultaneous acute renal and hepatic failure after ingesting raw carp gall bladder. Nephrol Dialysis Transplant 1999;14: 2011–12.
5. Williamson JA, Fenner PJ, Burnett JW, eds. Venomous and Poisonous Marine Animals: A Medical and Biological Handbook. Sydney: University of New South Wales Press; 1996.

133.3 Mushroom Poisoning

Hans Persson

Key features

- Most fungi are nontoxic and most fungal poisonings are not severe, but in other parts of the world, morbidity and mortality may be high
- Mushrooms cannot be considered as essential nutrients but self-harvested mushrooms, intended as a delicacy, still kill people in the 21st century
- The priority in fungal poisoning is prevention
- Amatoxins occur in some *Amanita* species, in *Galerina marginata* and in certain *Lepiota* species. They inhibit protein synthesis, damaging intestinal mucosa, liver and kidneys
- Gastrointestinal symptoms are typically delayed for about 12 hours. On the second day, signs of liver damage may ensue. Silibinin or high-dose benzyl penicillin may reduce the toxic effects

ILLNESS AFTER MUSHROOM INGESTION

Discomfort after ingestion of mushrooms has a number of possible causes aside from exposure to primary fungal toxins. Mushrooms are susceptible to bacteria and parasites, explaining why even nontoxic mushrooms may cause gastrointestinal discomfort, especially if they have been stored for a few days. Mushrooms contain proteins that may induce allergic reactions in hypersensitized individuals. Ingestion of a surfeit of tasty, nontoxic mushrooms may also cause indigestion that raises the suspicion of poisoning.

This chapter is confined to poisonings resulting from the effects of intrinsic mushroom toxins.

FUNGAL POISONING—CAUSES AND CIRCUMSTANCES

The most common cause of true mushroom poisoning is confusion of toxic mushrooms with edible ones; some potentially treacherous confusions are possible. Careless mushroom harvesting because of a

TABLE 133.3-1 Summary of Characteristics of Different Types of Seafood Poisoning All of Which Cause Acute Gastrointestinal Symptoms

Type of poisoning	Ciguatera	Tetrodotoxic	Scombroid
Incubation	1–6 hours	10–45 minutes	5–60 minutes
Duration of symptoms	Days to months	Days	Hours
Characteristic symptoms	Paraesthesiae, myalgias	Rapidly developing paralysis, areflexia, erythematous rash	Immediatelip-tingling,anaphylactic-like pruritus, urticaria, shock, angioedema, brochospasm, diarrhea, headache
Seafood affected	Tropical reef fish: red snapper, red bass, coral trout, sea bass, grouper, parrot fish, moray eels, mackerel, tuna, jacks, barracuda	Scaleless fish: puffer ("fugu"), porcupine, sun, toad fish and freshwater puffer fish (Tetraodontiformes), also amphibians, crabs, octopus, mollusks, nermertines, flat worms, etc.	Dark-fleshed fish: tuna, skipjack, bonito, mackerel, mahi-mahi; anchovies, sardines, pilchards
Geographic range	Tropical Pacific, Indian and Caribbean oceans	Tropical oceans Japan, China, Southeast Asia, also farmed	Global
Toxin and origin	Ciguatoxins and maitotoxins from the dinoflagellate *Gambierdiscus toxicus*	Tetrodotoxins (aminoperhydroquinazoline) from bactéria, e.g. *Pseudomonas* spp.; axitoxin in freshwater puffer fish	Histamine, saurine from bacterial (*Proteus*, *Klebsiella*) decomposition of fish muscle histidine

lack of knowledge and awareness of potential risks may also result in serious mushrooms poisoning. Toddlers, who are happy to put anything into their mouth, may accidentally try mushrooms, but only small amounts are usually ingested, making serious poisoning rare in this situation. Deliberate ingestion of toxic mushrooms occurs as a result of, and is almost exclusively related to, ingestion of psychotropic fungi and, hence, this is looked upon as a variation of abuse.

DIAGNOSIS [1, 2]

Circumstances are often unclear. The history is of fundamental importance. Any information about the mushrooms harvested is essential: supposed species, appearance, site of growth, etc. Some fungal toxins cause typical clinical features, for example the dreaded amatoxins and those causing distinctive neurologic symptoms. Information about specific symptoms and the time for their onset is crucial. The possibility of a cause for the symptoms other than poisoning must also be considered.

Identification of the actual mushrooms by macro- or microscopic examination often requires the assistance of a mycologist. Currently, amatoxin is the only fungal toxin that can be detected (in urine) in clinical practice.

FUNGAL TOXINS

From a clinical point of view, the most relevant and practical way of classifying mushroom poisonings is to group them according to their toxic effects and related symptoms. Applying this pragmatic approach, the following main groups of fungal toxins can be distinguished: cytotoxic agents, neurotoxins and gastrointestinal irritants (Table 133.3-1).

CYTOTOXIC FUNGI [3]

AMATOXINS

Species

Amatoxins are cyclic octapeptides occurring mainly in certain *Amanita* species, for example *Amanita phalloides* (death cap) (Fig. 133.3.1),

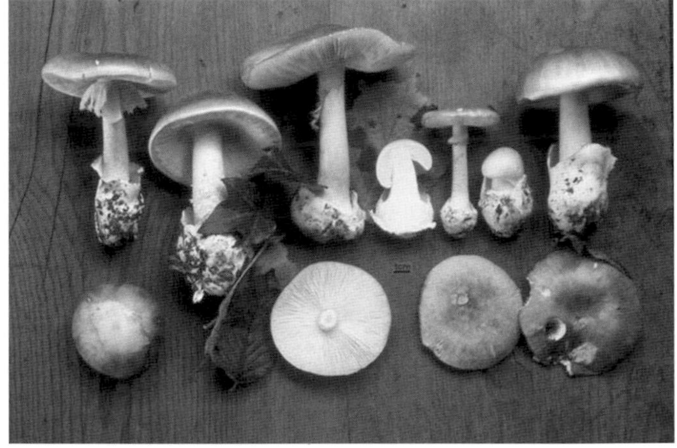

FIGURE 133.3.1 Death cap *(Amanita phalloides)* *(courtesy of Hans Marklund).*

Amanita virosa (destroying angel) and *Amanita verna* (fool's mushroom), in *Galerina marginata* and in certain *Lepiota* species.

Mechanisms of Toxicity

Amatoxins inhibit protein synthesis by blocking nuclear RNA polymerase II, resulting in cell necrosis. There is also some evidence that the toxins may induce apoptosis and glutathione depletion. Target organs are intestinal mucosa, liver and kidneys. The most critical clinical effect is hepatic damage—the degree of which is decisive for the prognosis.

Symptoms

Entirely typical, and of great diagnostic importance, is a delayed onset of gastrointestinal symptoms. The latency period after ingestion may vary from 8 hours to 24 hours (mean: 12 hours). Symptoms are violent with vomiting and intense, watery diarrhea (mimicking cholera). This results in dehydration and metabolic disturbances. On the second day, signs of liver damage may ensue and, in severe cases,

Treatment

Treatment is symptomatic and supportive. Admission to hospital is rarely required. The age and general condition of the patient and the intensity of symptoms will determine whether medical intervention is necessary or not. Children and the elderly may be more at risk. The only medical treatment that may occasionally be indicated is correction of fluid and electrolyte disturbances.

CHLOROPHYLLUM MOLYBDITES

Chlorophyllum molybdites or *Lepiota moybdites* ("false parasol" or "green-spored parasol") and *Lepiota morganii* or *Macrolepiota morganii* ("Morgan's mushroom") contain a gastrointestinal irritant with additional, possible α-receptor-blocking and cholinergic effects.

Symptoms

Intense gastrointestinal symptoms will follow ingestion within 30 min to a few hours. Diarrhea may sometimes become bloody. Fluid and electrolyte imbalance may follow and, in severe cases, renal dysfunction might ensue. Occasionally, cholinergic symptoms are observed.

Treatment

Treatment is symptomatic and supportive, with adequate fluid and electrolyte replacement. Any cholinergic symptoms are reversed by atropine.

OTHER TOXIC EVENTS CAUSED BY FUNGI

ANTABUSE SYNDROME

Species and Mechanisms of Toxicity

An antabuse reaction may be provoked by *Coprinus atramentarius* and possibly other *Coprinus* spp., *Clitocybe clavipes*, and *Boletus luridus*. The toxic principle is the presence of coprin that blocks aldehyde dehydrogenase, explaining why ingestion of these mushrooms in combination with ethanol may result in a typical antabuse syndrome. This risk will last for almost a week post-ingestion.

Symptoms

Symptoms mimic those of an ethanol—disulfiram reaction ("antabuse syndrome"): flushing, sweating, nausea, headache, tachycardia, anxiety, and circulatory disturbances.

Treatment

If the patient is admitted early, activated charcoal and gastric lavage may be useful. Otherwise, treatment is symptomatic and supportive.

Paxillus Syndrome

This syndrome is caused by ingestion of the "roll-rim cap", *Paxillus involutus*. This mushroom can cause problems in two ways. First, it contains thermo-labile, strongly irritating toxins that may cause severe gastroenteritis if the mushroom is not cooked properly. Second, there are antigenic agents in this mushroom that are not denatured by cooking, explaining why people may become sensitized if the fungus is eaten repeatedly. These people may react violently to subsequent meals containing this mushroom. Symptoms are severe gastroenteritis, dehydration, hemolysis and associated kidney failure. Treatment is symptomatic.

REFERENCES

1. Bresinsky A, Besl H. A Colour Atlas of Poisonous Fungi. A Handbook for Pharmacists, Doctors, and Biologists. London: Wolfe Publishing Ltd; 1990.
2. Cooper MR, Johnson AW. Poisonous plants and fungi in Britain. Animal and human poisoning, 2nd edn. London: The Stationary Office; 1998.
3. Karlson-Stiber C, Persson H. Cytotoxic fungi—an overview. Toxicon 2003; 42:339–49.
4. Enjalbert F, Rapior S, Nougier-Soulé J, et al. Treatment of amatoxin poisoning: 20-year retrospective analysis. J Toxicol Clin Toxicol 2002;40:715–57.
5. Holmdahl J. Mushroom poisoning: *Cortinarius speciosissimus* nephrotoxicity. Thesis. Gothenburg: Göteborg University; 2001.
6. Holmdahl J, Blohmé I. Renal transplantation after *Cortinarius speciosissimus* poisoning. Nephrol Dialysis Transplant 1995;10:1920–2.
7. Saviuc P, Danel V. New syndromes in mushroom poisoning. Toxicol Rev 2006; 25:199–209.
8. De Haro L, Prost N, David JM, et al. Syndrome sudorien et muscarinien. Expérience de Centre Antipoisons de Marseille. La Presse Médicale 1999;28: 1069–70.

133.4 Poisoning by Plants

Hans Persson

Key features

- Ingestion of, or contact with, poisonous plants is common, but serious plant poisoning is rare worldwide because most plant exposures are accidental, occurring in small children who eat only a small amount and require no treatment
- Intentional exposures may be with suicidal intent (*Thevetia, Aconitum* and *Colchicum* spp.), or involve psychotropic and hallucinogenic plants that are abused as recreational drugs (*Datura* and *Cannabis* spp.)
- Use of herbal medicines or foods containing plant toxins, for example aconitine in China and cyanide (cassava) in Africa may cause severe poisoning
- Treatment involves cautious decontamination and symptomatic and supportive care
- Specific antidotes are available only for poisoning by plants containing belladonna alkaloids, cardiac glycosides, cyanogenic agents, and colchicine

CIRCUMSTANCES

Accidental exposure to plants is common in small children, related to their curiosity and habit of testing things by putting them into the mouth. However, the amount swallowed is usually trivial and so serious plant poisoning is uncommon in small children. More commonly, toxic plants may be mistaken for edible ones and prepared as

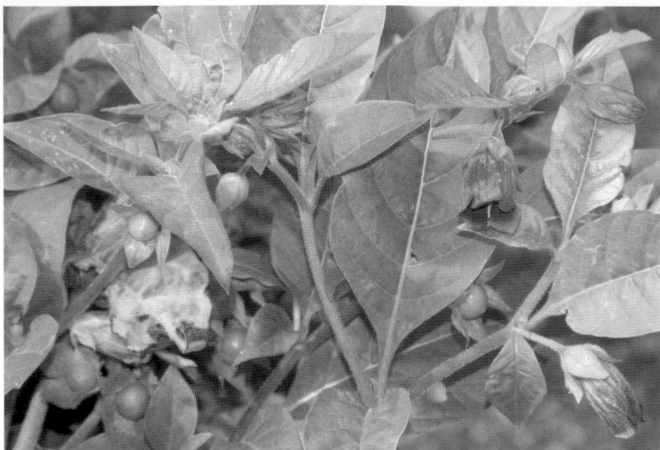

FIGURE 133.4.1 Deadly night shade (*Datura belladonna*) (© David A. Warrell).

food that causes poisoning in both in adults and children. Another cause of significant plant poisoning is deliberate ingestion of plants whose toxins have psychotropic and hallucinogenic properties, such as belladonna alkaloids (e.g. in *Datura* spp.) (Fig. 133.4.1), tetrahydrocannabinols (*Cannabis sativa*) or mescaline (*Lophophora williamsii*). Toxic plants are also used as suicidal agents. In South India and Sri Lanka, yellow oleander (*Thevetia peruviana*) is commonly chosen as an agent for self harm (see below).

Treatment of plant poisoning involves decontamination, symptomatic care and administration of antidotes, such as physostigmine for belladonna alkaloids, digitalis-specific antibodies for cardiac glycosides, hydroxocobalamine or sodium thiosulphate for cyanogenic plant toxins and specific antibodies for colchicine.

BOX 133.4.1 Classification of Plant Toxins—Overview

Gastrointestinal irritants
- Oxalic acid
- Calcium oxalate
- Diterpene esters
- Others

Dermatotoxins
- Calcium oxalate
- Oxalic acid
- Phototoxic psoralens

Neurotoxins
- Belladonna alkaloids
- Hallucinogenic toxins
- Convulsants
- Agents with nicotine-like effects

Cardiotoxins
- Aconitine
- Cardiac glycosides
- Taxin, veratrin, andromedotoxins, phoratoxin

Cytotoxic agents
- Colchicine
- Toxalbumins – ricin, abrin
- Lectins
- Cyanogenic glycosides (bitter cassava root)

Hepatotoxins
- Pyrrolizidine alkaloids

Nephrotoxins
- Terpenes
- Antraquinone glycosides

SPECIFIC PLANT POISONINGS

(Box 133.4.1) [1–5]

GASTROINTESTINAL IRRITANTS

Ingestion of many plants may cause gastroenteritic symptoms (abdominal colic, vomiting, and diarrhea) as the sole toxic manifestation.

Oxalic acid and calcium oxalate crystals occur in a number of popular decorative plants, such as "dumb cane" (*Dieffenbachia* spp.), "elephant's ear" (*Philodenron* spp.) and "cuckoo pint" (*Arum maculatum*). The crystals cause intense irritation of mucous membranes in the mouth, esophagus, stomach and intestine. Increased salivation, reddening, blistering, and dysphagia may ensue. Other decorative plants, for example *Euphorbia* and *Daphne* spp. contain highly irritating diterpene esters that cause burning sensations and pain in the mucous membranes of the gastrointestinal tract and are, in general, most pronounced in mouth and pharynx. Other symptoms are increased salivation, reddening and blisters.

Some of these toxins may also cause skin lesions and minor renal damage (see below).

Treatment is with oral fluids to rinse and dilute the irritant material, together with symptomatic care as required.

SKIN LESIONS

Dieffenbachia and *Euphorbia* spp. are irritating to skin and dermatitis can develop in people who handle these plants frequently. Hypersensitivity reactions may follow exposure to certain plants, for example "poison ivy" (*Rhus radicans*), "western poison oak" (*Toxicodendron diversilobum*) and *Primula obconica*. Treatment is by rinsing the skin with water and symptomatic care.

More dramatic reactions may occur after exposure to plants containing phototoxic psoralens. Examples are "giant hogweed" and other *Heracleum* spp., "rue" (*Ruta graveolens*) and the "gas plant" (*Dictamnus albus*). Skin that is contaminated with sap from these plants and subsequently exposed to sun light may develop a nasty phototoxic reaction involving eczematous skin lesions and extensive, painful bullae. To prevent this unpleasant reaction, exposed skin should be irrigated immediately and sunlight avoided. Established injuries are treated as chemical burns.

NEUROTOXIC PLANTS

BELLADONNA ALKALOIDS

Belladonna alkaloids have long been used in clinical medicine to reduce gastric acid secretion, as spasmolytics, and to treat bradycardia and cholinergic overstimulation. In excess, however, they can prove toxic.

Belladonna alkaloids occur in a number of plants, for example deadly nightshade (*Atropa belladonna*), henbane (*Hyoscyamus niger*), thorn apple/Jimsonweed (*Datura stramonium*) and angels' trumpet (*Brugmansia suaveolens*) (Fig. 133.4.2). The alkaloids inhibit acetylcholine activity at muscarine receptors, resulting in both peripheral and central anticholinergic effects. Exposed patients may present with central nervous system (CNS) symptoms, such as anxiety and excitation – sometimes extreme, hallucinations, mydriasis and fever.

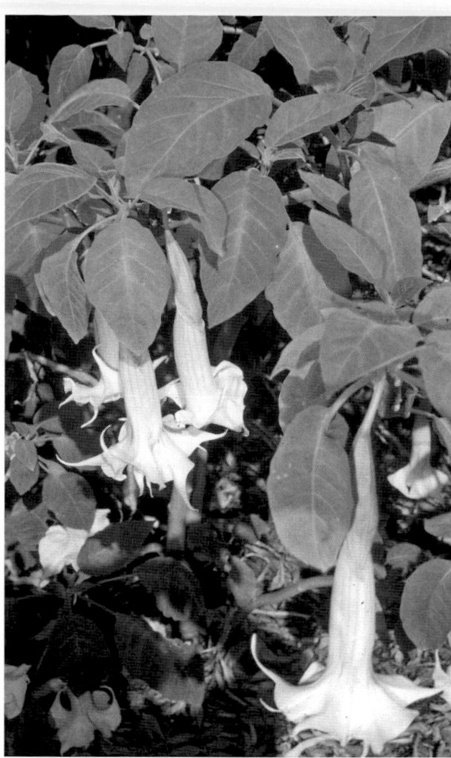

FIGURE 133.4.2 Angels' trumpet (*Brugmansia suaveolens*) (© David A. Warrell).

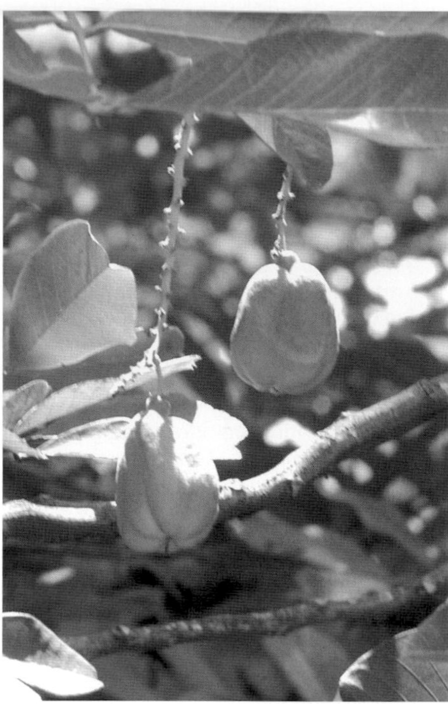

FIGURE 133.4.3 Ackee fruit (*Blighia sapida*) (© David A. Warrell).

Peripheral symptoms include tachycardia, urinary retention, dry mouth, warm skin and flushing. Rarely, and in severe exposure, seizures and unconsciousness may ensue. Differential diagnoses include poisoning by amphetamines and other CNS stimulants, acute organic psychosis and CNS infections.

Treatment is both specific and symptomatic. Sedation, preferably with benzodiazepines, is often effective, but large doses may be required. Physostigmine in a dose of 1–2 mg slowly intravenously (IV) in adults (0.02–0.04 mg/kg slowly IV in children) will more specifically antagonize both central and peripheral anticholinergic symptoms. However, physostigmine should be withheld if cardiotoxic agents have been co-ingested, if the patient is bradycardic and if a diagnostic electrocardiogram (ECG) reveals any conduction abnormalities.

Unilateral mydriasis may be an alarming clinical sign; however, it happens when people who handle anticholinergic plants rub their eye. This has sometimes caused diagnostic confusion, resulting in expensive, but unnecessary, investigations. "Gardener's eye" should be considered in such situations.

HALLUCINOGENIC PLANTS

These plants are popular because of the strong hallucinogenic effects. Most important are tetrahydrocannabinols from cannabis (*Cannabis sativa*) and alkaloids of khat (*Catha edulis*), mescaline in "peyote" (*Lophophora williamsii*) and myristicin in "nutmeg" (*Myristica fragrans*). Ingestion of the plant itself usually causes only moderate toxic exposure. Treatment is symptomatic.

PLANTS CAUSING CONVULSIONS

Cicutoxin occurs in *Cicuta virosa* ("cowbane"), *Cicuta maculata* ("water hemlock") and *Cicuta douglasii* ("western water hemlock"). Oenanthotoxin in *Oenanthe crocata* ("hemlock water dropwort") has the same toxic properties as cicutoxin, one of the most potent convulsants known. Cicutoxin is a potent gamma-aminobutyric acid (GABA) antagonist that induces recurrent seizures and exerts cholinergic effects.

Severe poisoning has occurred in adults who have mistaken these plants for edible ones. The onset of symptoms is dramatic, with initial cholinergic symptoms, such as gastrointestinal upset, hypersalivation and sweating. The most prominent symptoms are recurrent, long-lasting tonic-clonic convulsions. On arrival in hospital, patients may have hypoxia, severe metabolic acidosis, circulatory instability, joint dislocations and rhabdomyolysis.

Treatment requires maximum symptomatic and supportive care in an intensive care unit. Emphasis should be put on eliminating the convulsions which, in the few cases observed so far, have necessitated complete muscle relaxation and ventilator support.

A number of other plants have been associated with seizures. Examples are the "ackee fruit" (*Blighia sapida*) (Fig. 133.4.3), the "chinaberry" (*Melia azedarach*), "moonseed" (*Menispermum canadense*), "May apple" (*Podophyllum pelatum*) and "nux vomica" (*Stychnos nux-vomica*). Treatment is symptomatic and supportive.

PLANTS WITH NICOTINIC EFFECTS

Examples of plants exerting nicotine effects are hemlock (*Conium maculatum*) and the tobacco plant (*Nicotina tabacum*). The unpleasant taste of hemlock does stop people from ingesting it although it has been confused with parsley. Symptoms are variable and not characteristic: salivation, nausea, vomiting, thirst, vision disturbances, sweating, and vertigo. More severe symptoms may follow, such as hypertension and tachycardia, followed by bradycardia and hypotension, muscle fasciculation and seizures. At a later stage, muscular weakness, paralysis and coma may ensue. Treatment is symptomatic and supportive.

Nicotine-like effects may also follow ingestion of "Jessamine" (*Gelsemium sempervirens*)—poisonings are reported from China. Cyticine, the toxic principle of *Laburnum* spp. (e.g. "golden chain") may cause mild nicotine effects, but symptoms observed in children after ingestion of golden chain seeds are mostly just vomiting and diarrhea. Occasionally, and after heavy exposure, typical nicotine symptoms may occur (see above). Ingestion of *Lobelia* spp. may cause similar symptoms.

CARDIOTOXIC PLANTS

CARDIAC GLYCOSIDES (SEE BELOW)

Aconitine

Aconitum spp., such as *Aconitum napellus* ("aconite", "monkshood") and *Aconitum septentrionale* (a northern variant) contain aconitine, one of the most potent plant toxins. Severe poisoning may occur through ingestion of herbal medicines containing aconitine and from deliberate ingestion of the plant to cause self-harm. These dreaded intoxications are not uncommon and numerous fatalities have occurred.

Typically, burning and tingling sensations on lips, in the mouth and in the pharynx develop rapidly. Gastrointestinal and neurotoxic symptoms may develop. numbness and paraesthesia in the extremities and sialorrhea. The most life-threatening features are cardiac arrythmias. Ventricular extrasystoles often precede ventricular tachycardia and fibrillation. Heart failure and shock develop concurrently. These arrythmias are difficult to control and the prognosis is poor. CNS depression and seizures are uncommon symptoms.

Gastrointestinal decontamination should be attempted, energetically and even at a late stage. Treatment is symptomatic and supportive. Advanced methods of cardiopulmonary support are indispensable in severe cases.

Cardiotoxic Plants—Miscellaneous

Yew (*Taxus baccata*) and some other *Taxus* spp. contain toxic alkaloids that may exert significant cardiotoxicity; QRS-widening, AV-block and other arrythmias have been observed. Fatalities have occurred. Veratrine (*Veratrum* and *Zigadenus* spp.) (Fig. 133.4.4) is associated with digitalis-like effects. Cardiotoxic effects have also been associated with exposure to "mountain laurel" (*Kalmia latifolia*), *Menziesia* spp., *Rhododendron* spp. and "American mistletoes" (*Phoradendron* spp.).

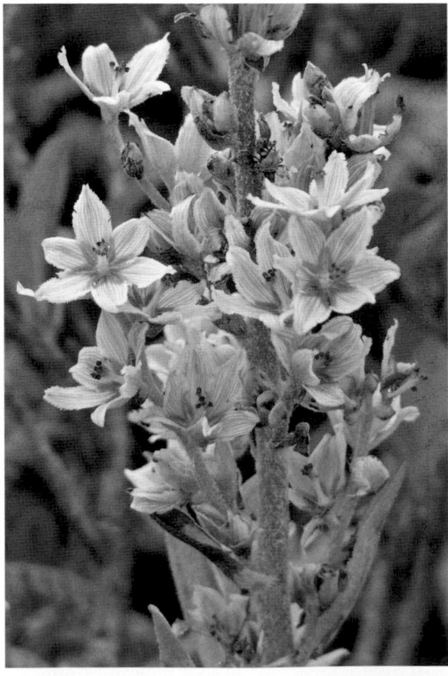

FIGURE 133.4.4 White helleborine (*Veratrum album*) (© *David A. Warrell*).

CYTOTOXIC PLANTS

These plant toxins disturb cell metabolism, affecting mitosis and intracellular protein synthesis.

COLCHICINE

Colchicine is used as a pharmaceutical, for example against gout. It is the toxic principle of *Colchicum autumnale* ("autumn crocus", "meadow saffron") and the magnificent *Gloriosa superba* ("glory lily", "ornamental lily"). Colchicine has antimitotic effects, in particular on cells with rapid turnover, for example intestinal mucosa and bone marrow. However, colchicine is also toxic to heart, liver and kidneys.

Classical colchicine poisoning presents with different phases. There is an initial period with mainly gastrointestinal symptoms that are often intense. Thereafter, serious systemic symptoms may follow with cardiac arrhythmias, CNS depression and seizures, liver and kidney damage and delayed bone marrow depression. Intentional, massive exposures may result in severe, and even fatal, poisoning.

Apart from attempts to reduce absorption, treatment aims to enhance elimination by multiple-dose activated charcoal and, in particular, to provide proper rehydration and other supportive care. In cases of impaired bone marrow function, administration of granulocyte colony-stimulating factor (G-CSF) has proven useful. Colchicine-specific antibodies have been developed but are not yet commercially availability.

TOXALBUMINS

The so called toxalbumins ricin and abrin are water soluble proteins that block protein synthesis and cause cell death. Particularly vulnerable are mucous membranes in the mouth, esophagus and gastrointestinal tract. They occur in *Ricinus communis* ("castor oil plant" or "castor bean") (Fig. 133.4.5) and *Abrus precatorius* ("jequirity bean", "rosary bean" or" rosary pea") (Fig. 133.4.6). Ricin is listed as a chemical weapon. The primary target is the gut. Severe gastroenteritis with extensive fluid and electrolyte loss is the major toxic manifestation. Secondary renal and hepatic damage may ensue.

Treatment is symptomatic and supportive with initial emphasis on fluid and electrolyte replacement, correction of metabolic disturbances, kidney and liver support.

CYANOGENIC GLYCOSIDES

Kernels and fruits of certain plants may contain cyanogenic glycosides. Kernels must be chewed to release their cyanide and large amounts are required to cause poisoning. Glycosides of this type occur in *Prunus* spp., such as almonds, apricots, cherries, and peaches.

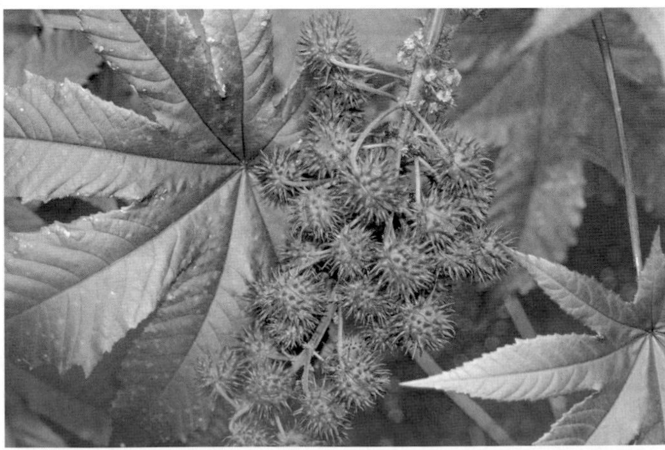

FIGURE 133.4.5 Castor oil plant or castor bean (*Ricinus communis*) (© *David A. Warrell*).

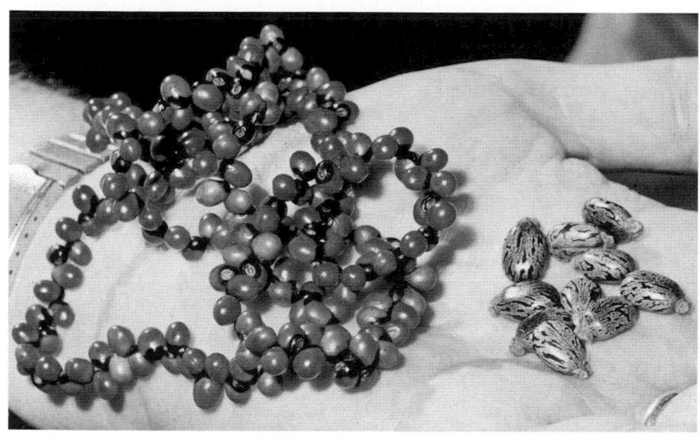

FIGURE 133.4.6 Jequirity bean, rosary bean or rosary pea (*Abrus precatorius*) (© David A. Warrell).

"Loquat" (*Eriobotrya*), "cherry laurel" (*Prunus laurocerasus*) and even apple pips (*Malus* spp.) are claimed to have caused poisoning.

Chewing and swallowing kernels or fruits of this type may result in cyanide release in the stomach. This is a relatively slow process and onset of symptoms is much delayed in comparison with ingestion of cyanide salts or inhalation of hydrogen cyanide, where symptoms are either immediate (inhalation) or start in a few minutes (ingestion). Acute cyanide poisoning induced by plants is rare. Treatment is as for cyanide poisoning of any origin.

"Cassava" (*Manihot esculenta*), an important food crop in arid tropical countries, contains cyanide. Unless it is thoroughly cooked, ingestion of bitter cassava roots can cause acute cyanide poisoning (gastrointestinal symptoms after 30 minutes to hours) or, over a longer period, chronic cyanide poisoning aggravating iodine-deficiency cretinism and causing acute spastic paraparesis ("Konzo") in Tanzania and other East African countries, and tropical ataxic neuropathy in Nigeria and some other countries.

HEPATOTOXIC PLANTS

In contrast to fungi, plant poisoning rarely affects the liver. There is, however, one exception. Plants containing pyrrolizidine alkaloids may cause chronic veno-occlusive disease that gradually impairs liver function. Long-term exposure may result in cirrhosis These alkaloids occur in certain *Senecio, Crotalaria, Heliotropium* and *Symphytum* spp. Clinical cases have been reported from Jamaica, India and Afghanistan, for example. There is no specific treatment available. In recent years, a number of widely distributed herbal medicines have been associated with hepatic toxicity.

NEPHROTOXIC PLANTS

Damage to the kidneys with a temporary decline in renal function is usually secondary to other symptoms such as heavy fluid loss. Direct nephrotoxic effects may be observed after exposure to the anthraquinon glycosides and oxalic acid in rhubarb (*Rheum rhabarbum*). Ingestion of large amounts of stems or leaves may cause irritation in the mouth and intestine, transient renal dysfunction and moderate metabolic acidosis. *Rumex* spp. (docks and sorrels) that also contain oxalates may cause similar effects.

"Spurge laurel" (*Daphne laureda*), "mezereon" (*Daphne mezereum*) and "savin" (*Juniperus savina*) contain terpenes that are irritating and may cause blisters in mouth and gastrointestinal tract, but also nephritis with hematuria and proteinuria.

REFERENCES

1. Audi J, Belson M, Patel M, et al. Ricin poisoning: a comprehensive review. JAMA 2005;294:2342–51.
2. Cooper MR, Johnson AW. Poisonous Plants and Fungi in Britain. Animal and Human poisoning, 2nd edn. London: The Stationary Office; 1998.
3. Chan TY. Aconite poisoning. Clin Toxicol 2009;47:279–85.
4. Froberg B, Ibrahim D, Furbee RB. Plant poisoning. Emerg Med Clin North Am 2007;25:375–433.
5. Schep LJ, Slaughter RJ, Beasley DM. Nicotinic plant poisoning. Clin Toxicol 2009;47:771–81.

133.5 Plant Cardiac Glycoside Poisoning

Michael Eddleston

Key features

- Cardiac glycosides inhibit the Na^+/K^+ ATPase on cardiomyocyte membranes, increasing intracellular sodium and calcium concentrations, cardiac excitability and risk of dysrhythmias
- Most poisoning is suicidal, although unintentional poisoning in children or from medicinal use is recognized
- Acute poisoning results in vomiting, diarrhea, abdominal pain, hyperkalemia, sinus and atrio-ventricular (AV) node block, severe bradycardia and ventricular tachydysrhythmias
- Antidigoxin antibodies effectively reverse poisoning but are rarely available because of cost; symptomatic care involves treating bradycardia and hyperkalemia
- Case fatality from yellow oleander poisoning is 5–10%; cardiac glycoside poisoning kills several thousand people every year—the majority in South Asia

INTRODUCTION

Cardiac glycosides occur in many plant families, including Scrophulariaceae (foxgloves), Apocynaceae (oleanders) and Liliaceae (lilies, sea onion). Each plant species synthesizes several glycosides, for example yellow oleander (*Cascabela thevetia* (L.)) (Fig. 133.5.1) contains thevetins A and B, thevetoxin and neriifolin, while sea mango (odollam tree; *Cerbera manghas* Linn) (Fig. 133.5.2) contains cerberin, neriifolin and cerberoside [1].

The glycosides are made up of a sugar moiety and a non-sugar or aglycone moiety; classification into cardenolides or bufadienolides is based up on the aglycone having a five- or a six-membered lactone ring in the C17 position of the steroid nucleus respectively. The glycosides are not destroyed by either drying or heating of plant material.

EPIDEMIOLOGY

It seems likely that plants containing cardiac glycosides are responsible for more acute deaths each year than any other plant family. Self-poisoning with seeds of the yellow oleander or sea mango causes thousands of deaths every year in South Asia [2, 3]. Unintentional

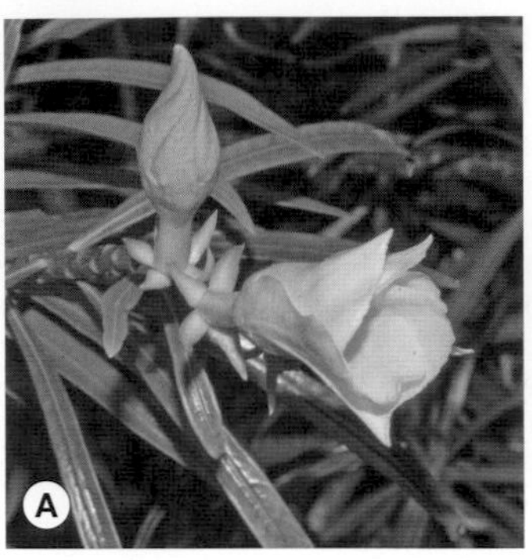
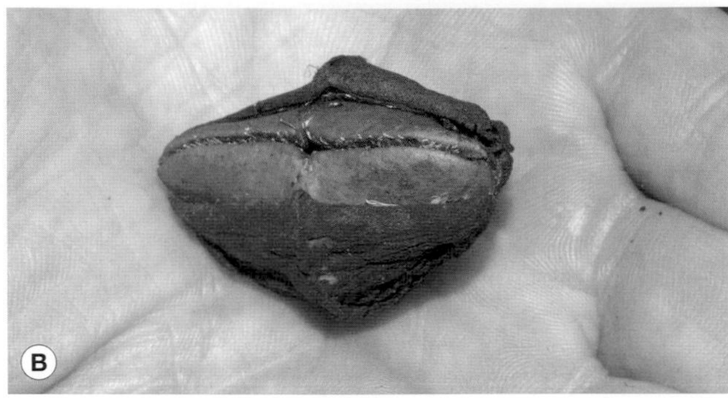

FIGURE 133.5.1 Yellow oleander (*Thevetia peruviana*). **(A)** flower and **(B)** the seed that has been extracted from the fruit.

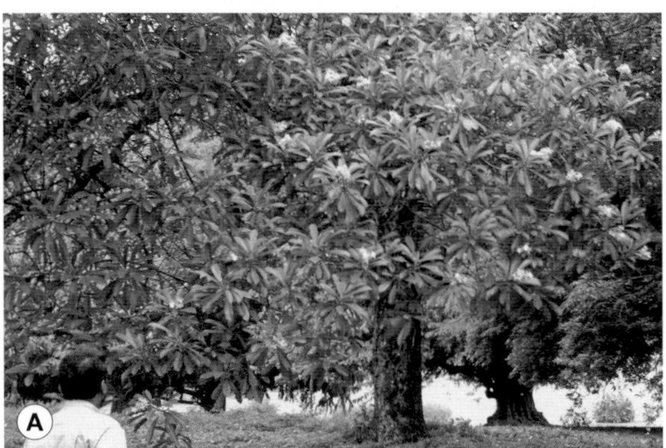
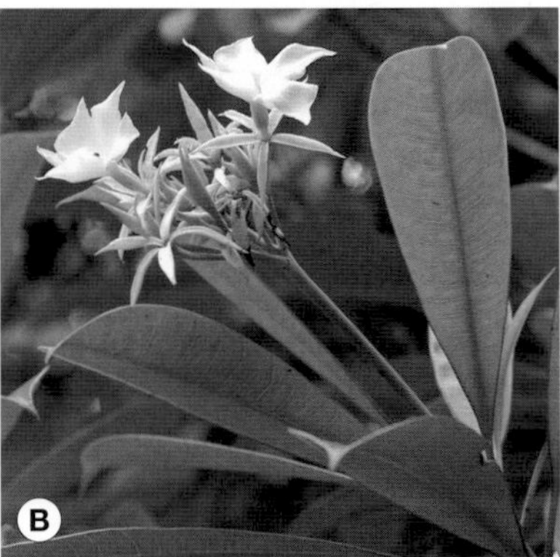
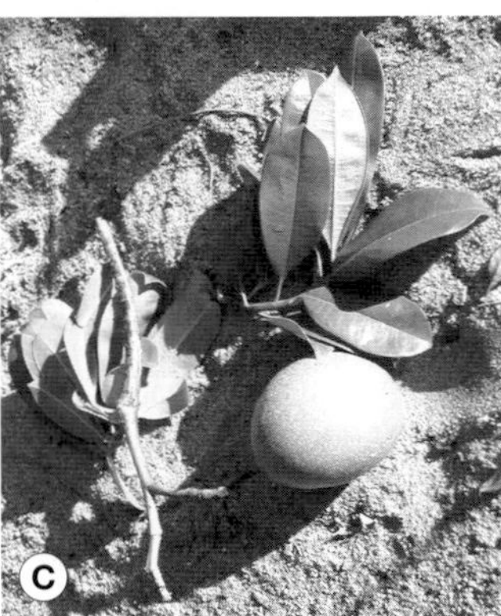

FIGURE 133.5.2 Sea mango, odollam tree or Kerala suicide nut (*Cerbera manghas*). **(A)** tree, **(B)** flower and **(C)** fruit.

pediatric poisoning occurs with yellow oleander in the tropics and subtropics; ingestion of therapeutic teas made from common oleander (*Nerium oleander*) leaves is an occasional cause of severe poisoning [4]. In southern Africa, medicinal use of plants containing cardiac glycosides (such as *Urginea sanguinea*) commonly results in unintentional poisoning [5].

NATURAL HISTORY, PATHOGENESIS, AND PATHOLOGY

Cardiac glycosides inhibit the Na^+/K^+ ATPase on cardiomyocyte membranes, causing a fall in intracellular potassium concentration and rise in sodium [6]. This causes an increase in intracellular calcium owing to loss of Na^+/Ca^{2+} exchange activity which in turn increases calcium release from the sarcoplasmic reticulum, alters membrane resting polarity and increases excitability with risk of dysrhythmias. Cardiac glycosides also increase vagal efferent activity to the heart, reducing sinuatrial firing rate (causing bradycardia) and conduction velocity of electrical impulses through the AV node.

PATIENT EVALUATION, DIAGNOSIS AND DIFFERENTIAL DIAGNOSIS

Diagnosis is made from the history plus typical toxidrome. Symptomatic patients present with gastrointestinal signs (nausea, vomiting, diarrhea, abdominal pain) and with cardiac dysrhythmias, commonly bradycardia and/or sinus or AV node block [3, 7]. Blood tests show hyperkalemia that correlates with severity of poisoning. Cardiac glycosides can be detected using standard laboratory assays for digitalis glycosides. However, these assays are not quantitative and apparent cardiac glycoside concentrations should not be used to determine whether to give treatment.

TREATMENT

Pharmaceutical digitalis poisoning is treated with antidigoxin or digitoxin Fab antibody fragments. The cardiac glycosides in yellow oleander are similar enough to digitalis glycosides for the Fab fragments to be highly effective in reversing gastrointestinal and cardiac toxicity [8, 9]. The indications for administration include complete heart block, Mobitz type-II second-degree block, sinus bradycardia with a heart rate of less than 40 beats per minute (bpm) unresponsive to atropine, sinus arrest or block with sinus pauses longer than two seconds, serum potassium >5.5 mmol/l, or ventricular tachycardias [8]. The best regimen is currently unclear. Consider giving 400 mg over 20 min followed by 400–800 mg over 4–8 hours by infusion to provide a therapeutic concentration for longer. There is less evidence for use of Fab fragments for poisoning with other plant cardiac glycosides but case reports suggest benefit. Unfortunately, the cost of these antibodies precludes their use in many places where cases are common.

Two randomized, controlled trials have tested the effectiveness of multiple doses of activated charcoal (MDAC) in yellow oleander poisoning [6]. The first found a marked reduction in death in patients receiving MDAC compared with a single dose of charcoal (SDAC): case fatality 5/201 (2·5%) patients receiving MDAC versus 16/200 (8%) patients receiving SDAC ($p = 0 \cdot 025$, relative risk [RR] 0·31, 95% confidence interval [CI] 0·12–0·83) [10]. The second, larger trial found no effect on mortality of giving MDAC versus SDAC (23/540 (4·3%) vs. 26/549 [4.7%]; RR 0·90, 0·52–1·56) [11]. The reason for this difference in trial results in unclear and precludes a clear conclusion on the effectiveness of MDAC. However, charcoal was found to be safe in these studies and a single dose is recommended.

The evidence for benefit from other interventions is weak (Table 133.5-1). Gastric lavage is not recommended. Atropine and intravenous fluids are used to keep the heart rate above 60 bpm and systolic

TABLE 133.5-1 Grade of Evidence for Treatments (both recommended and non-recommended) for Plant Cardiac Glycoside Poisoning

Treatment	Efficacy*
Digoxin-specific Fab antibodies	1b Individual RCT (with narrow confidence interval)
Activated charcoal	1a SR of RCTs "-"
Intravenous atropine	Case-series and low quality cohort and case-control studies
Insulin dextrose	Expert opinion
Temporary cardiac pacing	Expert opinion
Gastric lavage or emesis	Expert opinion
Low energy DC cardioversion	Expert opinion

Grade of Recommendation (Oxford Centre for Evidence Based Medicine) http://www.cebm.net/index.aspx?o=1025.
RCT, randomized, controlled trial.

blood pressure above 80 mmHg. Insulin dextrose is given for serum potassium concentrations above 5.5 mmol/L; hypokalemia and hypomagnesemia should be treated until both are back in the high normal range. In the absence of antidigoxin Fab, consider treating severe bradycardia owing to AV block with temporary pacing and ventricular fibrillation with low-energy direct current (DC) defibrillation.

REFERENCES

1. Radford DJ, Gillies AD, Hinds JA, Duffy P. Naturally occurring cardiac glycosides. Med J Aust 1986;144:540–4.
2. Gaillard Y, Krishnamoorthy A, Bevalot F. *Cerbera odollam*: a 'suicide tree' and cause of death in the state of Kerala, India. J Ethnopharmacol 2004;95:123–6.
3. Eddleston M, Ariaratnam CA, Meyer PW, et al. Epidemic of self-poisoning with seeds of the yellow oleander tree (Thevetia peruviana) in northern Sri Lanka. Trop Med Int Health 1999;4:266–73.
4. Bandara V, Weinstein SA, White J, Eddleston M. A review of the natural history, toxinology, diagnosis and clinical management of Nerium oleander (common oleander) and Thevetia peruviana (yellow oleander) poisoning. Toxicon 2010;56(3):273–81.
5. McVann A, Havlik I, Joubert PH, Monteagudo FSE. Cardiac glycoside poisoning involved in deaths from traditional medicines. S Afr Med J 1992;81:139–41.
6. Rajapakse S. Management of yellow oleander poisoning. Clin Toxicol 2009;47:206–12.
7. Eddleston M, Ariaratnam CA, Sjostrom L, et al. Acute yellow oleander (Thevetia peruviana) poisoning – cardiac arrhythmias, electrolyte disturbances, and serum cardiac glycoside levels on presentation to hospital. Heart 2000;83:301–6.
8. Eddleston M, Rajapakse S, Rajakanthan K, et al. Anti-digoxin Fab fragments in cardiotoxicity induced by ingestion of yellow oleander: a randomised controlled trial. Lancet 2000;355:967–72.
9. Roberts DM, Buckley N. Antidotes for acute cardenolide (cardiac glycoside) poisoning. Cochrane Database Syst Rev 2006;4:CD005490.
10. de Silva HA, Fonseka MMD, Pathmeswaran A, et al. Multiple-dose activated charcoal for treatment of yellow oleander poisoning: a single-blind, randomised, placebo-controlled trial. Lancet 2003;361:1935–8.
11. Eddleston M, Juszczak E, Buckley NA, et al. Multiple-dose activated charcoal in acute self-poisoning: a randomised controlled trial. Lancet 2008;371:579–86.

134 Animals Hazardous to Humans

David A Warrell

INTRODUCTION

Animals may prove hazardous to humans through traumatic attacks (e.g. by large felines, bears, crocodiles, sharks, etc.), through poisoning after their flesh has been ingested (see Chapters 133.1, 133.2), through envenoming and allergic hypersensitization (this chapter and Chapter 136) and through transmission of zoonotic infections—see "Bats" (Chapter 134.6 and elsewhere in this book).

VENOMOUS BITES AND STINGS, AND ENVENOMING

Envenoming (American/Australian: "envenomation"), as distinct from poisoning, occurs when venoms secreted by specialized glands are injected through the victim's skin or applied to absorbent mucous membranes. To inject their venoms, venomous snakes and lizards have grooved or cannulated fangs or solid teeth; spiders have venom jaws (chelicerae); vampire bats, insectivorous mammals and leeches have solid teeth; male monotreme mammals (platypus and echidna) have venomous spurs; centipedes have modified legs (maxillipeds, forcipules or prehensors); insects, scorpions, ticks, fish and echinoderms (sea urchins etc.) have rigid, sharpened, barbed stings, spines, or hypostomes; echinoderms have venomous grapples (pedicellariae); cnidarians (jellyfish, coelenterates) have stinging hairs (cnidocytes, nematocysts); octopuses (cephalopods mollusks) have venomous beaks; and cone shells (gastropod mollusks) impale their prey with a venom-filled radular tooth mounted on a harpoon-like proboscis. Some elapid snakes, scorpions, "blister" beetles, millipedes and other arthropods can "spit" or squirt their venoms—a largely defensive ploy.

Venoms are noxious substances secreted by specialized glands. They vary in their complexity from simple organic acids and phenols in some arthropod venoms, to complex mixtures of hundreds of different proteins (polypeptide toxins, enzymes, etc.) and smaller, pharmacologically-active molecules in snake venoms. Evolution has selected venoms and venom-administering organs to immobilize and digest animals' prey, to prevent blood clotting in the case of leeches, vampire bats and other "blood sucking" species, and for defense. A few venom toxins are modified salivary gland secretions, but most venom genes originated from other organs through repeated episodes of gene duplication and gene recruitment.

Here, the venomous animals of greatest medical importance in human and veterinary medicine are selected for discussion: snakes, lizards, fish, arthropods, leeches and the aquatic cnidarians, mollusks and echinoderms.

134.1 Venomous Marine Animals

Key features

- The many species of venomous fish that inhabit tropical and temperate oceans and rivers have stinging apparatus in their fins, gill covers or, in sting rays, at the base of the tail. Common causes of fish stings are weevers (Europe), sting rays (Americas and Amazon tributaries) and scorpion fish that are popular aquarium pets. Stone fish (*Synanceja*) are the most dangerous
- Cnidarians (coelenterates)—including jellyfish, cubomedusoids, sea wasps, Portuguese-men-o'-war or bluebottles, stinging corals and sea anemones—envenom by firing numerous stinging hairs into the dermis, causing pain, weals and sometimes cardiovascular collapse
- Echinoderms (starfish and sea urchins) have sharp venomous spines that can impale waders' feet
- Mollusks capable of causing fatal envenoming are cone shells and blue-ringed octopuses
- The pain of marine stings is relieved by hot (45°C) water. Antivenoms are manufactured for envenoming by scorpion fish and box jellyfish

VENOMOUS FISH [1–3]

Although more than 1200 species of fish are thought to be venomous, only about 200 species can inflict dangerous stings. Rarely, fatal stings are inflicted by cartilagenous fish (class Chondrichthyes), such as sharks and dogfish (order Squaliformes); stingrays and mantas (order Rajiformes); and bony fish (superclass Osteichthyes), such as ray-finned fish (class Actinopterygii) of the orders Siluriformes (catfish), Perciformes [families Trachinidae (weever fish), Uranoscopidae (star-gazers or stone-lifters) and others] and Scorpaeniformes (scorpion fish, stonefish, lion fish—*Synanceja*/*Synanceia* spp.) (Figs 134.1.1 and 134.1.2). Tropical oceans have the richest venomous fish fauna, but dangerous species also occur in temperate northern waters. Large rivers in South America, West Africa and Southeast Asia are inhabited by freshwater stingrays (*Potamotrygon* spp.) (Fig. 134.1.3). Venom glands are embedded in grooves in the spines or, in the case of stingrays, lie beneath a membrane covering the long barbed precaudal spine.

INCIDENCE AND EPIDEMIOLOGY

Some years, hundreds of weever fish stings occur around the British coast and along the Adriatic coast. An estimated 1500 stings by rays and 300 stings by scorpion fish occur in the USA each year. Stings by freshwater rays are common in the Amazon region. Ornate, but aggressive, *Pterois* and *Dendrochirus* spp. (lion, zebra, tiger, turkey or red fire fish) are popular aquarium pets. People wading near the shore

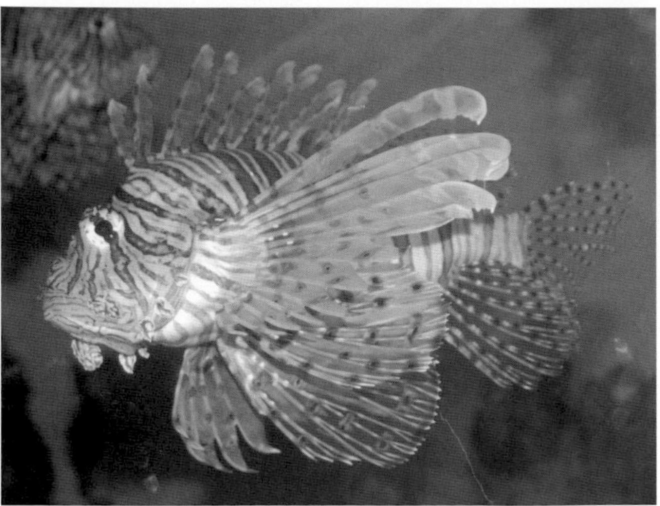

FIGURE 134.1.1 Lion fish (*Pterois volitans*- Scorpaenidae) *(© David A. Warrell).*

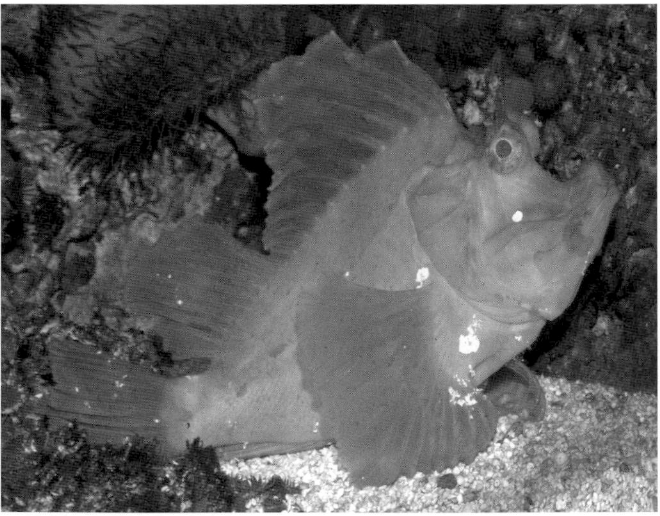

FIGURE 134.1.2 Weedy or pop-eyed scorpionfish *Rhinopias frondosa*—Scorpaenidae) *(© David A. Warrell).*

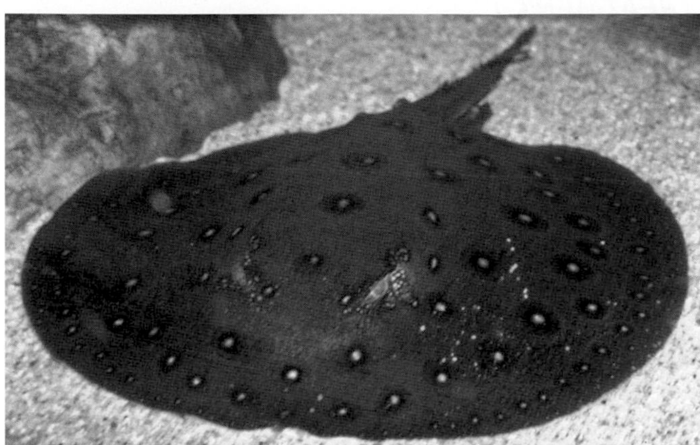

FIGURE 134.1.3 Freshwater stingray (*Potamotrygon* spp.—Potamotrygonidae) *(© David A. Warrell).*

or coral reefs may tread upon well-camouflaged stonefish (*Synanceja* spp.) lying partly covered by sea plants and anemones [1]. Stingrays lash their tails, usually impaling the ankle [2].

PREVENTION

Employing a shuffling gait when wading, avoiding the handling of living or dead fish, and keeping away from fish near tropical reefs all aid in prevention. Footwear protects against most species, except stingrays.

VENOM COMPOSITION

Stingray and weeverfish venoms contain peptides, enzymes, vasoactive kinins, 5-hydroxytryptamine, histamine and catecholamines. Venoms cause local necrosis and target cardiac, skeletal and smooth muscle resulting in electrocardiogram changes, hypotension and paralysis.

CLINICAL FEATURES [3]

Immediate sharp, agonizing pain is typical. Hot, painful, erythematous swelling extends up the stung limb and may persist for days and be complicated by necrosis and secondary infection by marine *Vibrio* spp. (such as *Vibrio vulnificus*) and freshwater *Aeromonas hydrophila,* particularly if the spine is left in the wound. Stingray spines (up to 30 cm long) can cause severe lacerating and penetrating wounds, sometimes with fatal results.

Stings by rays or Scorpaenidae (scorpion and stonefish) may cause nausea, vomiting, diarrhea, sweating and hypersalivation, cardiac arrhythmias, hypotension, respiratory distress, neurologic signs and generalized convulsions. However, fatalities are very rare.

TREATMENT

Treatment is common to all wounds caused by venomous fish and includes: (i) pain relief; (ii) neutralizing effects of venom; (iii) prevention of secondary infection; and (iv) supportive care of systemic symptoms. Immersion of the stung part in uncomfortably hot, but not scalding, water (less than 45 °C) relieves pain and neutralizes venom. Alternatively, inject local anesthetic as a ring block or local nerve block. The barbed venomous spine, its covering membrane and other foreign material should be removed as soon as possible. Systemic effects are treated symptomatically. Cardiopulmonary resuscitation may be required on the beach. In Australia, CSL (Melbourne, Australia) manufacture an antivenom specific for *Synanceja trachynis, Synanceja verrucosa,* and *Synanceja horridus* which has paraspecific activity against venoms of North American scorpion fish (*Scorpaena guttata*) and some other Scorpaenidae. Doxycycline or co-trimoxazole covers *Vibrio* and *Aeromonas* spp.

CNIDARIANS (COELENTERATES)

Cnidarian (Jellyfish, Cubomedusoids, Sea Wasps, Portuguese-Men-O'-War or Bluebottles, Hydroids, Stinging Corals, Sea Anemones, etc.) tentacles are armed with millions of stinging capsules (nematocysts) which, triggered by contact or chemicals, evert stinging hairs that penetrate the skin, producing lines of painful, irritant weals. Venoms contain peptides and other vasoactive compounds provoking pain, inflammation and urticaria.

EPIDEMIOLOGY

The northern Australian box jellyfish or sea wasp (*Chironex fleckeri*) is the most dangerous species, having killed more than 70 people since 1883. The peak season for stings is December through January. Fatal stings in the Indo-Pacific region are attributable to *Chiropsalmus quadrumanus* and *Chiropsalmus quadrigatus* and, elsewhere, Portuguese men-o'-war (*Physalia* spp.) and Chinese *Stomolophus nomurai* have caused a number of fatalities. Irukandji syndrome occurs in northern

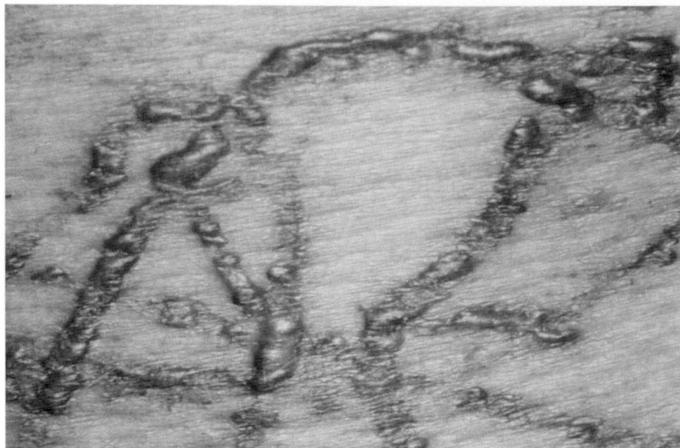

FIGURE 134.1.4 Lines of weals inflicted by a box jellyfish or "sea wasp" (*Chironex fleckeri*—Chirodropidae) sting in Darwin, Australia *(© Bart Currie).*

Queensland and the Florida-Caribbean area, and is caused by stings of tiny cubomedusoids like *Carukia barnesi*. Epidemics of "mauve stinger" *Pelagia noctiluca* stings occur in the northern Adriatic coast where stinging sea anemones (*Anemonia sulcata*) also occur.

PREVENTION

Avoid the sea when warning notices are displayed or bathe only in "stinger-resistant" enclosures. "Lycra" or wetsuits and nylon stockings protect against nematocyst stings.

CLINICAL FEATURES

Stings may produce diagnostic patterns: *C. fleckeri*—striated brownish-purple weals (Fig. 134.1.4); *Carukia barnesi*—a transient erythematous macule; Portuguese man-o'-war (*Physalia* spp.)—chains of oval weals surrounded by erythema. Immediate severe pain is the commonest symptom. Chirodropids (*Chironex* and *Chiropsalmus* spp.) can cause respiratory arrest, generalized convulsions, pulmonary edema, and cardiac arrest within minutes of the sting. Symptoms include cough, nausea, vomiting, abdominal colic, diarrhea, rigors, severe musculoskeletal pains and profuse sweating. Irukandji syndrome comprises severe musculoskeletal pain, anxiety, trembling, headache, piloerection, sweating, tachycardia, hypertension, and pulmonary edema starting about 30 min after a sting by *C. barnesi* and other cubomedusoids) and persisting for hours. Envenoming by *Physalia* species may result in intravascular hemolysis, peripheral gangrene and renal failure.

TREATMENT

To prevent drowning, remove victims from the water as soon as possible. A slurry of baking soda and water [50% (w/v)] is recommended by American authorities for stings by the widely distributed Atlantic genus, *Chrysaora*. For stings by *C. fleckeri* and other cubozoans, including Irukandji, but not for *Chrysaora*, *Physalia* or *Stomalophus* spp., apply vinegar or 3–10% aqueous acetic acid solution, which inhibits nematocyst discharge. Pressure immobilization and verapamil are not recommended. Shave off adherent tentacles with a razor. Hot water treatment (see venomous fish above) relieves the pain of *Physalia* stings [4]. Specific "sea wasp" antivenom for *C. fleckeri* is manufactured in Australia, but its efficacy is questionable.

ECHINODERMATA (STARFISH AND SEA URCHINS) (Fig. 134.1.5)

Echinoderm spines cause penetrating injuries and envenoming. There is severe pain and local swelling, but rarely systemic effects.

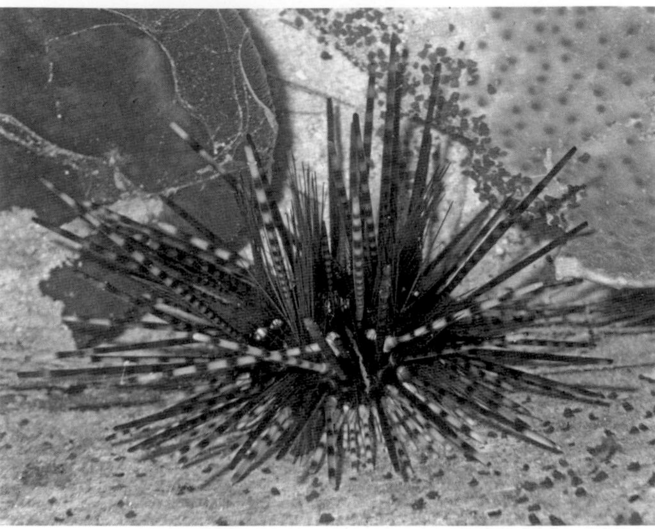

FIGURE 134.1.5 Long-spined sea urchin (*Diadema setosum*—Diadematidae) Papua New Guinea *(© David A. Warrell).*

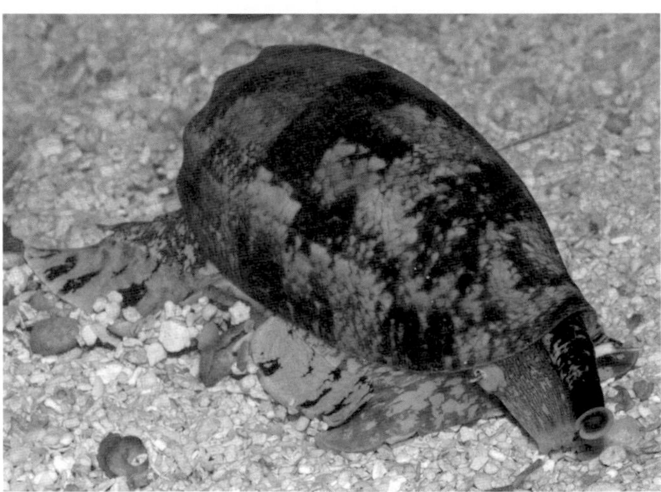

FIGURE 134.1.6 Geography cone (*Conus geographus*—Conidae) *(© David A. Warrell).*

TREATMENT

Hot water (see above) may relieve the pain. Spines should be squeezed out or removed surgically, but this may prove impossible. There is a risk of marine bacterial infections (see above).

MOLLUSCA (CONE SHELLS AND OCTOPUSES)

Cone shells (genus *Conus*) (Fig. 134.1.6) are carnivorous marine snails that harpoon their prey, implanting a radular tooth charged with venom containing a mixture of many small (10–30 amino acid) peptide toxins. Careless handling of these attractive shells may result in a potentially fatal sting. Symptoms of envenoming are nausea, vomiting, paraesthesia and numbness of the lips and site of sting, numbness, dizziness, ptosis, diplopia, dysarthria, dyspnea and loss of consciousness.

Small, blue-ringed octopuses of the Australian and West Pacific region (*Hapalochlaena* spp.) (Fig. 134.1.7) can inject tetrodotoxin when they bite with their powerful beaks. These bites are painful and cause local bleeding, swelling and inflammation. Severe neurotoxic symptoms,

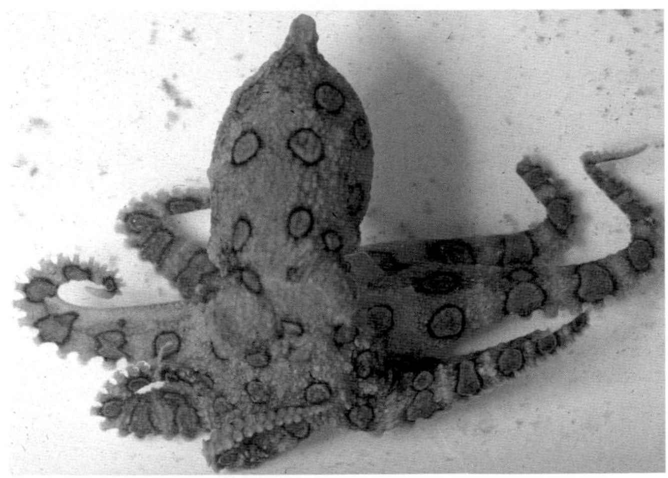

FIGURE 134.1.7 Greater blue-ringed octopus (*Hapalochlaena lunulata*—Octopodidae) Papua New Guinea *(© David A. Warrell)*.

and even fatal generalized paralysis, may develop within 15 minutes of the bite.

TREATMENT

No antivenoms are available. Cardiopulmonary resuscitation and mechanical ventilation may be required.

REFERENCES

1. Bergbauer M, Myers RF, Kirschner M. Dangerous marine animals. London: A&C Black; 2009.
2. Sutherland SK, Tibballs J. Australian animal toxins. The creatures, their toxins and care of the poisoned patient, 2nd edn. Melbourne; Oxford University Press; 2001.
3. Williamson JA, Fenner PJ, Burnett JW, Rifkin JF, eds. Venomous and poisonous marine animals: a medical and biological handbook. Sydney: University of New South Wales Press; 1996.
4. Loten C, Stokes B, Worsley D, et al. A randomised controlled trial of hot water (45 degrees C) immersion versus ice packs for pain relief in bluebottle stings. Med J Aust 2006;184:329–33.

134.2 Leeches (Phylum Annelida, Class Hirudinea)

Key features

- Land and aquatic leeches are blood-sucking annelids, most common in tropical forests, rivers and lakes
- Bleeding continues after the leech has fed and detached because of salivary anticoagulants
- Prevention is by protective clothing and liberal use of diethyl toluamide (DEET) repellent
- Attached leeches should be gently removed. Chemicals may encourage regurgitation into, and infection of, the wound (e.g. with their symbiotic *Aeromonas hydrophila*)

These blood-sucking, hermaphroditic, egg-laying annelids attach their elongated annulated bodies to leaves, rocks or the host by a posterior sucker. By standing on the posterior sucker and waving the anterior sucker, they can sense their prey with amazing efficiency. They drop on to the prey or pursue it with a looping or lashing motion. The anterior sucker contains the mouth, armed with three radially arranged jaws which make a Y-shaped incision and secrete saliva containing a histamine-like vasodilator and anticoagulants, such as hirudin [from the medicinal leech (*Hirudo medicinalis*), which inhibits thrombin and factor IXa]; hementin (from *Haementeria ghilianii*, which is directly fibrinolytic); and hementerin [from *Haementeria depressa* (*Haementeria lutzi*), a plasminogen activator]. Other enzymes include esterases, antitrypsin, antiplasmin and anti-elastase [1].

Land leeches, 1–8 cm long, infest rainforest vegetation and usually attach themselves to the lower legs or ankles after a bite that may be painless. They ingest about a milliliter of blood in one hour and then drop off, but the wound continues to bleed—sometimes for a week.

Aquatic leeches are swallowed when stagnant water is drunk and they invade the mouth, nostrils, eyes, vulva, vagina, urethra or anus of swimmers.

Blood sucking leeches have a global distribution but have the greatest impact in damp forests of the subtropical and tropical regions of the Indo-Pacific region. Pond, lake and stream water is often used for bathing, washing clothes, washing utensils and animals, and human consumption in villages. Leeches are commonly present in ponds, particularly in the rainy season.

PREVENTION

Apply repellents such as dibutyl phthalate and diethyl toluamide to clothing, skin and the inside and outside of footwear. Children should be discouraged from bathing in leech-infested waters and all drinking water should be boiled or filtered.

CLINICAL FEATURES [2]

The main effect is blood loss, but other symptoms include local soreness, secondary infection, residual itching and phobia. Ingested aquatic leeches may penetrate the bronchi or esophagus but usually attach to the pharynx or nasal passages, causing a feeling of movement at the back of the throat with cough, hoarseness, stridor, breathlessness, epistaxis, hemoptysis, hematemesis and fatal upper airway obstruction. Leeches are no longer thought to be a cause of "halzoun" (Lebanon) or "marrara" (Sudan) (Chapter 135). Leeches penetrating the anus may reach the rectosigmoid junction causing perforation and peritonitis. Bleeding may persist for up to a week after the leech has dropped off. Transmission of pathogens has been suggested, but not proved—except in the case of wound infection by *A. hydrophila*, which lives symbiotically in the leeches gut.

TREATMENT [3]

Leeches will detach if salt, alcohol, turpentine or vinegar is applied, but these chemicals may make the leech regurgitate into the wound. Gentle mechanical removal is preferred, but avoid pulling off the leech so roughly that its mouth parts are left in the wound to cause chronic infection. A styptic, such as silver nitrate, or a firm dressing stops the bleeding. Invasive aquatic leeches must be removed by endoscope, aided by 30% cocaine, 10% tartaric acid or dilute (1:10000) adrenaline (epinephrine) in the nasopharynx, larynx, trachea or esophagus, and concentrated salt solution in the genitourinary tract and rectum.

REFERENCES

1. Sawyer RT. Leech Biology and Behaviour. Oxford: Oxford University Press; 1986.
2. Montazeri F, Bedayat A, Jamali L, et al. Leech endoparasitism: report of a case and review of the literature. Eur J Pediatr 2009;168:39–42.
3. Keegan HL. Leeches as pests of man in the Pacific region. In: Keegan HL, McFarlane WR, eds. Venomous and Poisonous Animals and Noxious Plants of the Pacific Region. Oxford: Pergamon Press; 1963:99–104.

134.3 Fish Capable of Inflicting Serious Trauma

Key features

- Shark attacks can be devastating but only 70–100 occur each year with 5–15 fatalities. Florida, Australia and South Africa have the highest risk
- Attacks are best prevented by taking local advice to avoid high risk locations, circumstances and behavior
- Medical problems include extensive trauma, hemorrhagic shock and a high risk of bacterial contamination by unusual marine pathogens
- First aid is securing the victim from drowning, resuscitation, control of bleeding and perforating injuries, intravenous fluid replacement and rapid evacuation to hospital for emergency surgery and treatment of infection
- Other fish capable of causing severe and fatal trauma include barracuda, Moray eels, needle fish, sting rays, piranhas and candiru

SHARKS

Sharks are most common in oceans between latitudes 47° south and 46° north, especially where water temperature is above 20°C. There are about 70–100 shark attacks with 5–15 fatalities each year (case fatality ~8%), mostly in North American (especially Florida), Australian and South African waters [1]. Great white (*Carcharodon carcharias*) (length ~16 m, weight 2250 kg), tiger (*Galeocerdo cuvier*) (5.5 m, 900 kg) (Fig. 134.3.1A–E) and bull (*Carcharhinus leucas*) (3.5 m, 360 kg) sharks are the most dangerous, but attacks have been reported by 32 species; all 70 species exceeding 2 m in length are potentially lethal. Devastating deep wounds, especially of buttocks, thighs or shoulders result in massive bleeding from severed arteries causing shock and the risk of drowning. Shark wounds are characterized by sharp incisions without abrasions, serrated edges, a triangular or rectangular flap of skin, regular spacing corresponding to the shark's teeth, gouge marks on the bones and severing of body parts at the joints without fractures (Fig. 134.3.2A–C) [2]. Bumping or rubbing against shark skin can inflict severe abrasions caused by their placoid scales.

MANAGEMENT

Vascular injury is a major determinant of mortality. Immediate medical care involves resuscitation (control of hemorrhage, fluid replacement and treatment of hypothermia), washout, debridement and follow-up for prevention of infection and closure of more complex wounds [3–5]. A study of shark wounds in Recife, Brazil discovered more than 80 bacterial pathogens, mainly Enterobacteriaceae, all of which were covered by gentamicin, vancomycin and levofloxacin [6]. Isolates include Vibrio spp. such as *Vibrio carchariae, Vibrio parahaemolyticus* and *Photobacterium (Vibrio) damsela* and *Aeromonas* spp.

PREVENTION

Take local advice. Most attacks occur between 06.00 h and 20.00 h, but sharks come closer to the shore and are most active in twilight or darkness. Avoid bathing between sand bars and the ocean, far out to sea, where dead fish or sewage are being discharged and flocks of birds are feeding. Do not bathe if you are injured, bleeding, wearing jewelry or brightly patterned or colored clothes, or with a pet dog. Surfers and surface swimmers are targeted more often than divers. Reduce risk by bathing in groups, close to the shore and only in daylight. If attacked by a shark, fight back—hit it on the nose and claw at its eyes and gills. Chemical and electrical-field repellents and chainmail protective suits have been developed.

OTHER DANGEROUS FISH [4]

Most fish can inflict a painful and damaging bite if handled carelessly on a line or in a net, but the following deserve special mention.

BARRACUDAS

The great barracuda (*Sphyraena barracuda*) of the tropical Atlantic can grow to almost two meters in length. Its powerful jaws and numerous long, razor-sharp, fang-like teeth can sever a digit or even a hand. Hands and ankles may be bitten when a landed fish is thrashing about still on the line or while the hook is being disengaged. Barracudas are attracted by shining objects, such as rings and bracelets on hands dangled in the water and may leap out of the water in pursuit of a fish that is being pulled in on an angler's line.

MORAY EELS (MURAENIDAE)

The giant Moray (*Gymnothorax javanicus*) can reach a length of 3 meters and a weight of 36 kilograms; the Californian Moray (*Gymnothorax mordax*) reaches 1.5 meters in length (Fig. 133.2.1). Moray eels may be encountered by divers exploring coral reefs and wrecks. Attacks are unusual but the eels' multiple rows of long, fang-like, backward-pointing teeth may cause deep puncture wounds with avulsion of tissue if the animal is forcefully removed (Fig. 134.3.3). Despite much speculation, they have no venom apparatus but a major threat is infection of the bite wounds with a variety of marine Vibrio, Aeromonas and Pseudomonas spp. [7].

*NEEDLE FISH (GARFISH) (*TYLOSURUS *SPP. BELONIDAE)* (Fig. 134.3.4A,B)

These Indo-Pacific fish can leap out the sea at speeds of 60 km/h, attracted by light. They have impaled fishermen and, rarely, surfers and divers, sometimes causing fatal injuries (Fig. 134.3.4C–E) [8–10].

STING RAYS (DASYATIDAE)

Sting rays can inflict fatal penetrating trauma with their spines (see below).

PIRANHAS (PIRAÑAS) (CHARACIDAE)

(Fig. 134.3.5A)

These ferocious fish of the Amazon, Orinoco and other South American river systems are alleged to have stripped unwary swimmers to the bone (Fig. 134.3.5B). Such mass attacks on people or animals have rarely been reported, but piranhas sharp teeth can bite out chunks of flesh (Fig. 134.3.5C).

*CANDIRU (VAMPIRE, TOOTH PICK OR PENIS FISH) (*VANDELLIA CIRRHOSA *TRICHOMYCTERIDAE)*

In the Amazon region, these tiny parasitic catfish (Portuguese "candirú", Spanish "canero") (Fig. 134.3.6) are feared more than piranhas. Normally, they attach to the gills of large fish and feed off their blood, but these fish are apparently also attracted to bathers by detecting urine or blood. Once they have burrowed into the urethra, vagina or anus (especially in menstruating women), they erect spines

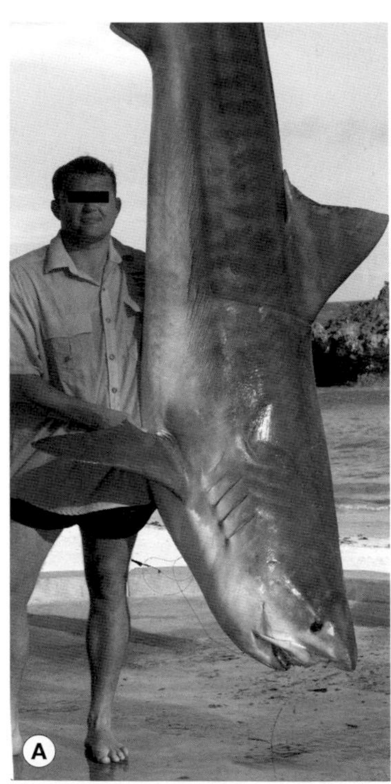

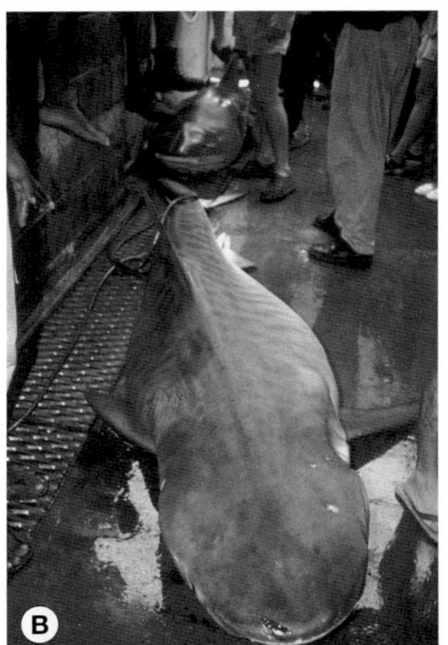

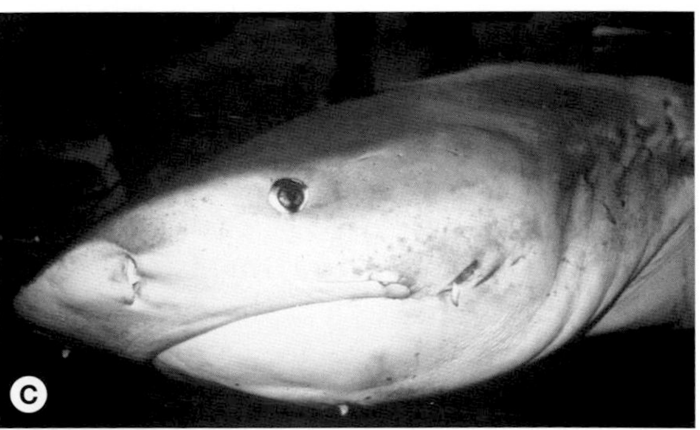

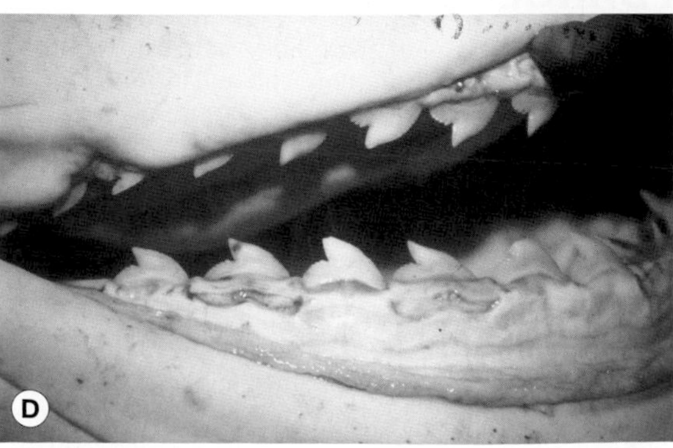

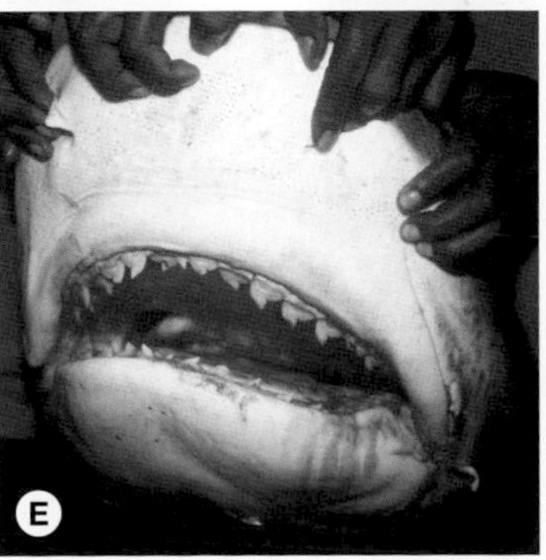

FIGURE 134.3.1 (A) Tiger shark *(Galeocerdo cuvier)*. Specimen weighing 268 kg caught off Watamu, Kenya *(copyright D. A. Warrell)*. **(B–E)** Specimen captured off Madang, Papua New Guinea in 2001 and responsible for the attack illustrated *(© Steve Allen)*.

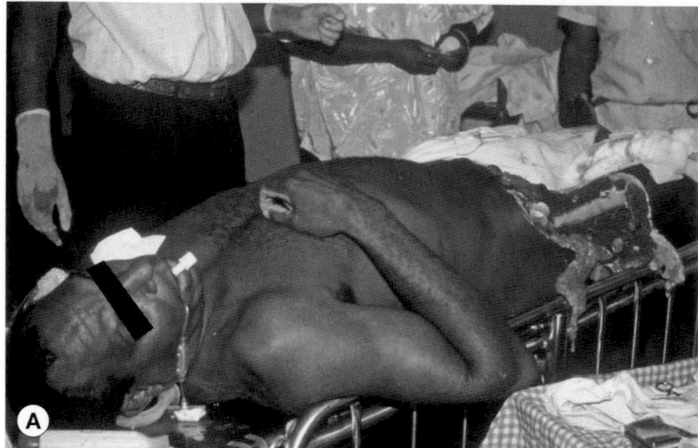

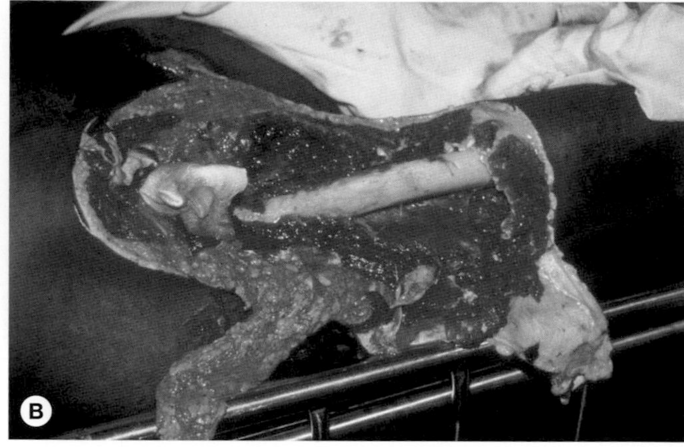

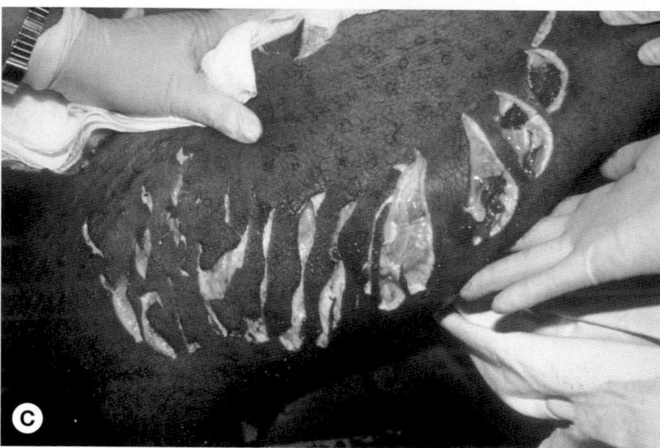

FIGURE 134.3.2 (A–C) Victim of a tiger shark attack off Madang, Papua New Guinea in 2001 *(© Steve Allen).*

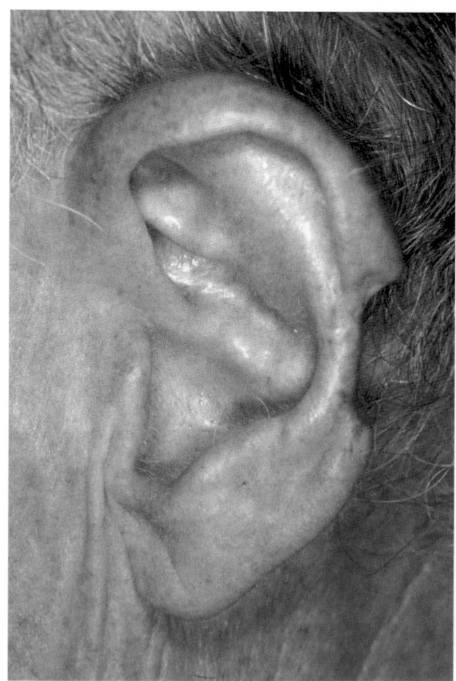

FIGURE 134.3.3 Moray eel injury *(© R. Sautter).*

on their gill covers which prevents removal. One hospital in Puerto Maldonado, Peru, admits more than 10 cases each year. Although several herbal concoctions are said to promote their elimination, surgery or cystoscopy is usually necessary [11, 12].

MANAGEMENT OF INJURIES BY OTHER DANGEROUS FISH

The same principles apply as with shark bites, although trauma is usually on a much smaller scale. Infection with aquatic microorganisms is a serous problem, especially in immunocompromised people; in salt water: *Fusarium solani, Vibrio vulnificus, V. parahaemolyticus, Vibrio alginolyticus, Erysipelothrix rhusiopathiae* (causing erysipeloid, "seal finger" and "whale finger"), *Plesiomonas shigelloides, Acinetobacter* spp., *Chromobacterium violaceum, Flavobacterium* spp., *Pseudomonas aeruginosa, Mycobacterium marinum, Prototheca* spp. and *Staphylococcus aureus* (off populous beeches such as Waikiki, Honolulu); and in freshwater, *Aeromonas hydrophila* and free-living amoebae.

In cases of severe, extensive injuries, especially if there has been delay in presentation, blind antibiotic treatment is appropriate with oral doxycycline or co-trimoxazole or parenteral tetracycline and an aminoglycoside combined with either cefotaxime or a fluoroquinolone. Results of cultures will direct specific therapy.

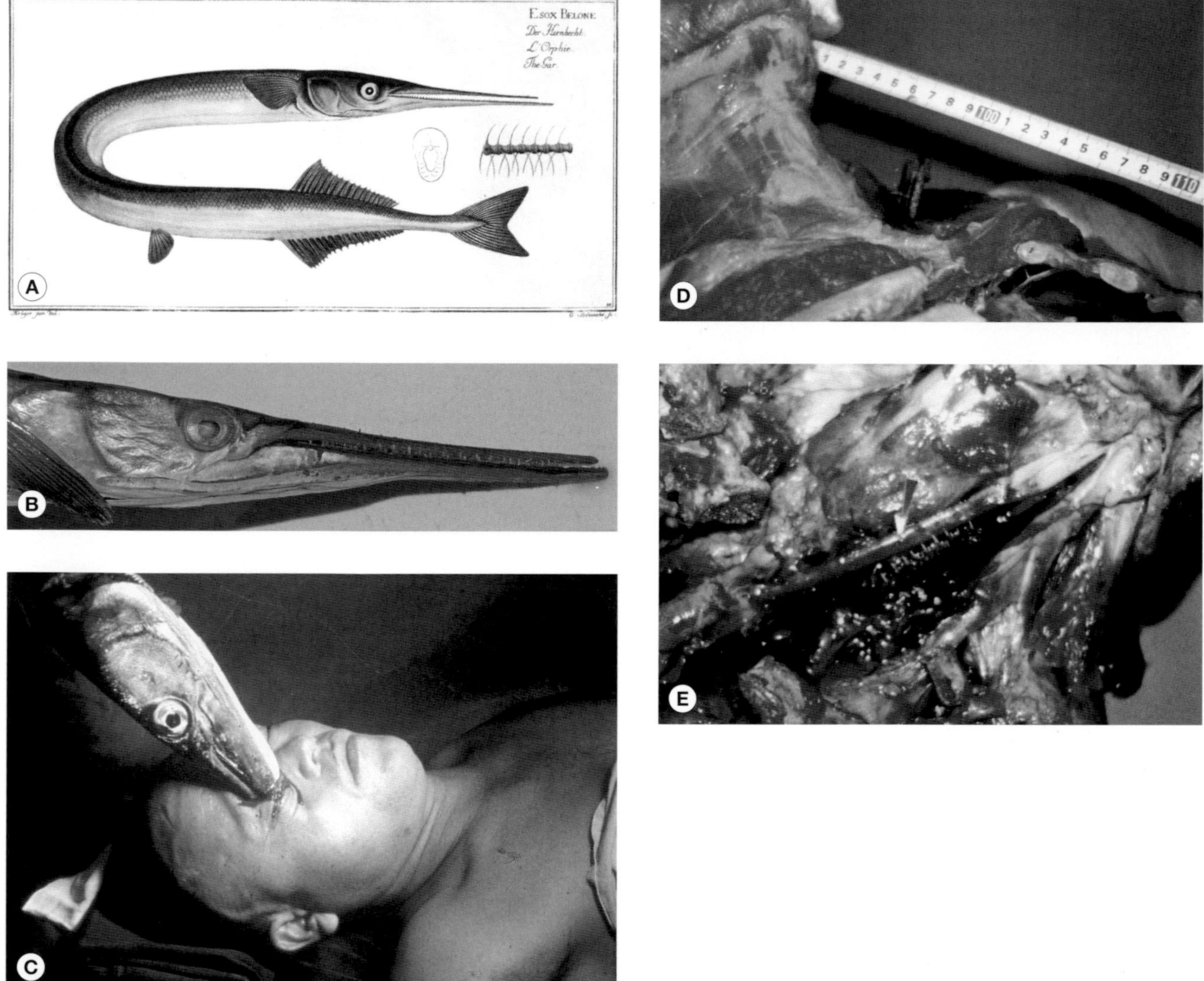

FIGURE 134.3.4 Needle fish (gar fish). **(A)** Illustration from Marcus Elieser Bloch's "Ichthyologie ou histoire naturelle generale et particuliere poisons" Berlin, 1785–1797 *(© David A. Warrell)*. **(B)** *Tylosurus graviloides* *(© David A. Warrell)*. **(C)** Japanese victims of attacks by crocodile needlefish *(Tylosurus crocodilus)*: victim impaled in the orbit *(courtesy of Dr Mashiro Kohama, Okinawa)*. **(D–E)** Victim fatally impaled in the supraclavicular region, rupturing the left subclavian artery and showing the needle like lower jaw with teeth *in situ*.

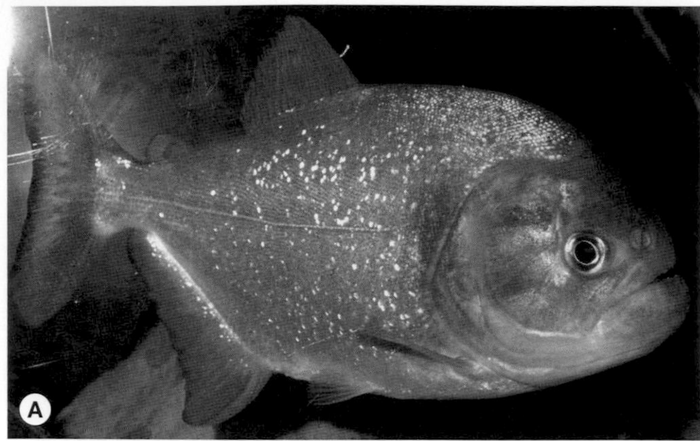

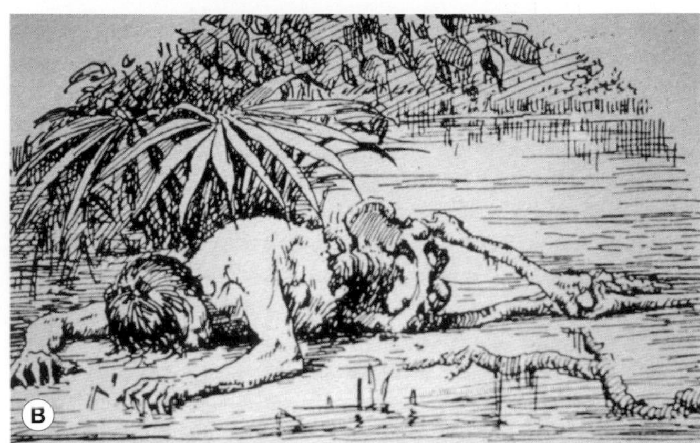

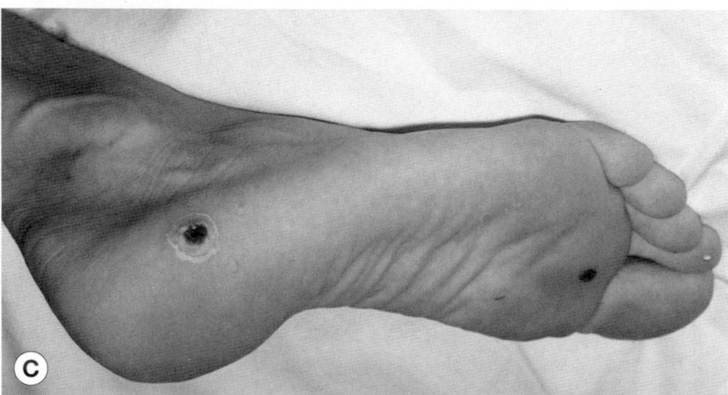

FIGURE 134.3.5 Piranha attack. **(A)** Red-bellied piranha (*Pygocentrus-Serrasalmus-nattereri*) *(© David A. Warrell)*. **(B)** Mythical representation of a mass attack in the Amazon *(© David A. Warrell)*. **(C)** Piranha bite Brazil *(© David A. Warrell)*.

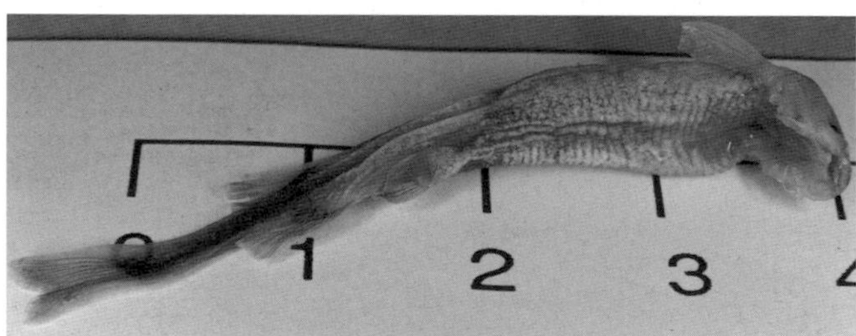

FIGURE 134.3.6 Candiru (*Vandellia cirrhosa*) Brazil *(© David A. Warrell)*.

REFERENCES

1. International Shark Attack File. Available at: http://www.flmnh.ufl.edu/fish/sharks/statistics/2005attacksummary.htm (last accessed 28 December 2011).
2. Ihama Y, Ninomiya K, Noguchi M, et al. Characteristic features of injuries due to shark attacks: a review of 12 cases. Leg Med (Tokyo) 2009;11:219–25.
3. Caldicott DGE, Mahajani R, Kuhn M. The anatomy of shark attack: a case report and review of the literature. Injury Int J Care Injured 2001;32:445–53.
4. Auerbach PS, Burgess GH. Injuries from nonvenomous aquatic animals. In: Auerbach PS, ed. Wilderness Medicine, 5th edn. Philadelphia: Mosby Elsevier, Philadelphia; 2007:1654–91.
5. Lentz AK, Burgess GH, Perrin K, et al. Mortality and management of 96 shark attacks and development of a shark bite severity scoring system. Am Surg 2010;76:101–6.
6. Interaminense JA, Nascimento DC, Ventura RF, et al. Recovery and screening for antibiotic susceptibility of potential bacterial pathogens from the oral cavity of shark species involved in attacks on humans in Recife, Brazil. J Med Microbiol 2010;59:941–7.
7. Erickson T, Vanden Hoek TL, Kuritza A, Leiken JB. The emergency management of Moray eel bites. Annals Emergency Med 1992;21:212–16.
8. Barss PG. Penetrating wounds caused by needle-fish in Oceania. Med J Aust 1985;143:617–18, 621–2.
9. McCabe MJ, Hammon MW, Halstead BW, Newton TH. A fatal brain injury caused by a needlefish. Neuroradiology 1978;15:137–9.
10. Kerkhoffs GMMJ, op den Akker JW, Hammacher ER. Surfer wipe out by predator fish. Br J Sports Med 2003;37:537–9.
11. Gudger EW. Bookshelf browsing on the alleged penetration of the human urethra by an Amazonian catfish called candiru. Am J Surgery 1930;8:170–188, 443–57.
12. Spotte S. Candiru: Life and Legend of the Bloodsucking Catfish. Berkeley: Creative Arts Book Company; 2002.

134.4 Lizards

Key features

- Bites by venomous helodermid lizards (Gila monsters and Mexican beaded lizards of Middle America) are rare: envenoming causes severe pain, swelling, hypotension, nausea, vomiting, sweating and sometimes angioedema and evidence of myocardial effects
- First aid involves urgent disengagement of the animal's jaws. As no antivenom is available, treatment is supportive and symptomatic
- Varanid, iguanid and agamid lizards may be capable of envenoming—notably the Komodo dragon

INTRODUCTION: VENOMOUS LIZARDS

Venomous salivary secretion have been demonstrated in Iguanas (Iguanidae), glass/alligator lizards (Anguidae) and monitors (Varanidae)—notably the Komodo dragon (*Varanus komodoensis*) which has been responsible for human fatalities that were attributed to trauma or infection of the bite wounds [1]. However, the only two lizards of proven medical importance are members of the family Helodermatidae that inhabit dry forests and deserts in western Middle America [2–4]. The Mexican beaded lizard or escorpión (*Heloderma horridum*) (Fig. 134.4.1A, B) is the larger (up to 1 m in total length and 2 kg in weight) with a relatively longer tail and a more arboreal habit. It is found in western Mexico, south to Guatemala. The Gila monster (*Heloderma suspectum*) (Fig. 134.4.1B–D), which reaches a total length of 55 cm and a weight of 1 kg, occurs in the south-western USA (south-east Nevada, south-west Utah, south-east California, south-west New Mexico, Arizona) and adjacent areas of Mexico

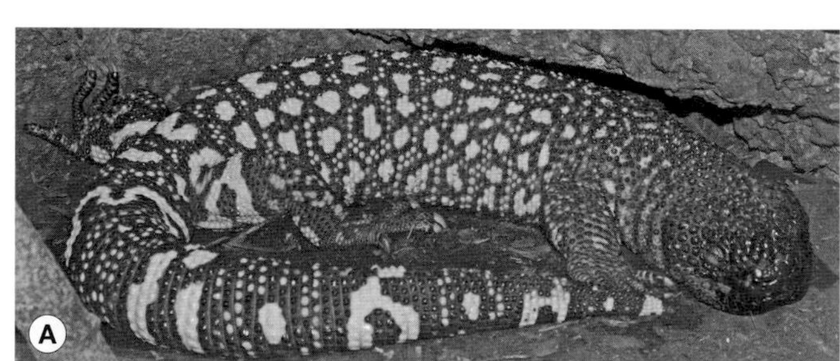

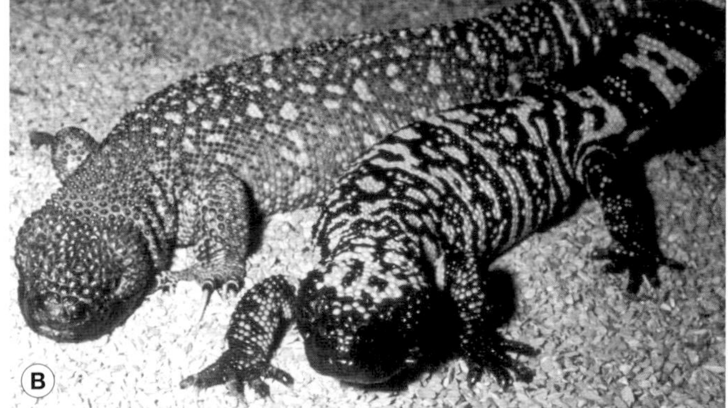

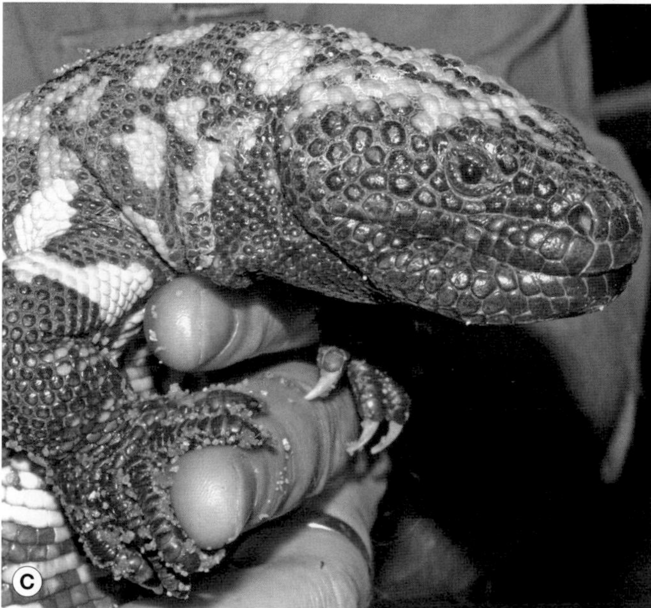

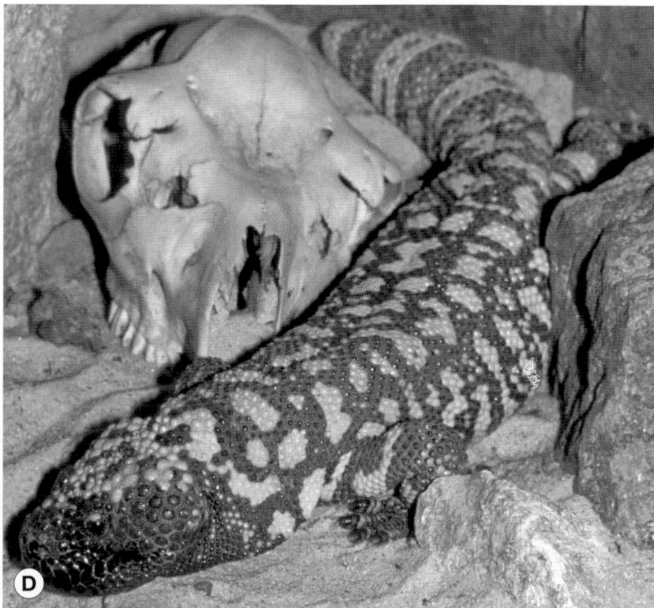

FIGURE 134.4.1 (A) Mexican beaded lizard (*Heloderma horridum exasperatum*) (© David A. Warrell). **(B)** Mexican beaded lizard (*Heloderma horridum horridum*) (left) compared with Gila monster (*Heloderma suspectum*) (right) (courtesy of D. Ball and Zoological Society of London). **(C)** Gila monster (*H. suspectum*) (© David A. Warrell). **(D)** Gila monster (*H. suspectum*) (© David A. Warrell).

(Sonora and northern Sonaloa). The two species overlap in Mexico (southern Sonora and northern Sinaloa).

VENOM APPARATUS

Venom from bulging multi-lobed anterior submandibular glands pools in labial gutters in the lower jaw. When threatened, the lizards open and shut their mouths to promote drooling of venom-enriched saliva. When they bite and chew, venom is inoculated by the mandibular (dentary) teeth of which the fourth to the seventh are most prominently grooved, and the maxillary teeth, which are less grooved.

VENOM COMPOSITION [4, 5]

Heloderma venoms contain toxic proteases, hyaluronidase, phospholipase A_2, horridum toxin (a glycoprotein tissue kallikrein-like enzyme that releases bradykinin and is probably responsible for hypotension in human victims of envenoming), bioactive peptides of great scientific interest, including helospectin (a vasoactive intestinal peptide analogue) and exendins -3 and -4, which are glucagon-like peptide-1 (GLP-1) homologues that stimulate insulin secretion and inhibit glucagon secretion. A synthetic homologue of exendin-4, exenatide, is a high affinity GLP-1 receptor agonist which has been developed for treatment of type 2 diabetes mellitus.

HELODERMA BITES

These are virtually never accidental because helodermids are reclusive and non-aggressive animals that inhabit thinly-populated rural areas. Almost exclusively, bites are inflicted on the fingers, hands and forearms of young men who are handling or trying to catch the lizards. Alcohol consumption seems to have contributed on many occasions, as is the case with bites by pet exotic snakes. Bites may be "slashing" in type, in which the anterior maxillary teeth strike and can envenom but do not engage, and "gripping", when the animal clings on and chews for up to 15 minutes before it can be removed [6]. Not all bites result in envenoming.

SYMPTOMS OF ENVENOMING [6–9]

Envenoming by *H. suspectum* and *H. horridum* causes identical clinical syndromes. Pain may start immediately and is described as throbbing or burning. It may radiate up the bitten limb to the shoulder, chest and epigastrium, and is often excruciating in intensity, persisting for 24 hours or more. Swelling also develops rapidly, extending, in some cases, to involve the whole limb, but although it may be tense, compartment syndrome has never been described. The bite site is erythematous or cyanosed with traumatic ecchymoses and persistent bleeding, but tissue necrosis does not develop. Red lymphangitic lines extend up the limb and regional lymph glands may become tender and enlarged. Local paresthesia, hyperesthesia and even paralysis have been described. The earliest systemic symptoms start within five minutes of the bite: dizziness, weakness, nausea, vomiting, profuse generalized sweating, breathlessness and weakness. Hypotension and tachycardia are commonly recorded. These symptoms may be transient or recurrent. Less commonly, there is angioedema (swelling of lips, tongue, throat and upper airway) [10], increased secretions, chills, fever and tinnitus.

INVESTIGATIONS

Neutrophil leukocytosis is common. In exceptional cases, thrombocytopenia and mild coagulopathy have been described. Electrocardiographic changes include T-wave abnormalities, conduction defects and, in one case, myocardial infarction and acute kidney injury were documented in a previously fit 23-year-old man [11, 12]. Clearly, envenoming may be life-threatening but the few alleged fatalities, all reported before 1930, are difficult to attribute.

TREATMENT: FIRST-AID

The longer the lizard is allowed to retain its grip and to chew, the more venomous saliva will be inoculated into the wound. The priority is to disengage, but the powerful jaws make this difficult. Rejected dangerous and barbaric methods include application of a flame under the animal's jaw, instilling gasoline or chloroform into its mouth or severing its jaw muscles with a knife. Pulling the animal off by its tail is quick but risks extending the bite wounds and detaching teeth. Expert opinion currently favors levering the jaws apart with a screw driver, putting the attached lizard under the tap, placing its four feet on the ground or introducing some alcohol into its mouth.

TREATMENT: MEDICAL

Severe pain is relieved by local anesthetic or systemic analgesia. Opiates may be required. The wound should be explored for shed teeth which are not detectable by radiography. The risk of infection has not been studied, but prophylactic antibiotics are not justified. However, tetanus toxoid is recommended and the wound should be observed for evidence of sepsis. Specific antivenoms have been raised experimentally in rabbits but they are not generally available. Hypotension can be treated with intravenous fluids and, if necessary, with epinephrine or dopamine. Angioedema responds to epinephrine, antihistamine and hydrocortisone. Otherwise, treatment is symptomatic and supportive and the patient may be expected to recover completely in less than 1 week.

REFERENCES

1. Fry BG, Vidal N, Norman JA, et al. Early evolution of the venom system in lizards and snakes. Nature 2006;439:584–8.
2. Bogert CM, Martín del Campo R. The Gila Monster and its Allies. Ohio: Society for the Study of Amphibians and Reptiles; 1993.
3. Brown DE, Carmony NB. Gila Monster. Facts and Folklore of America's Aztec lizard. Silver City: High-Lonesome Books; 1991.
4. Beck DD. Biology of Gila Monster and Beaded lLizards. Berkeley: University of California Press; 2005.
5. Russell FE, Bogert CM. Gila monster, venom and bite—a review. Toxicon 1981;19:341–59.
6. Strimple PD, Tomassoni AJ, Otten EJ, Bahner D. Report on envenomation by a Gila monster (*Heloderma suspectum*) with a discussion of venom apparatus, clinical findings, and treatment. Wilderness Environ Med 1997;8:111–16.
7. Albritton DC, Parrish HM, Allen ER. Venenation by the Mexican beaded lizard (*Heloderma horridum*): report of a case. S D J Med 1970;23:9–11.
8. Ariano-Sánchez D. Envenomation by a wild Guatemalan Beaded Lizard *Heloderma horridum charlesbogerti*. Clin Toxicol (Phila) 2008;46:897–9.
9. Hooker KR, Caravati EM, Hartsell SC. Gila monster envenomation. Ann Emerg Med 1994;24:731–5.
10. Piacentine J, Curry SC, Ryan PJ. Life-threatening anaphylaxis following gila monster bite. Ann Emerg Med 1986;15:959–61.
11. Bou-Abboud CF, Kardassakis DG. Acute myocardial infarction following a gila monster (*Heloderma suspectum cinctum*) bite. West J Med 1988;148:577–9.
12. Preston CA. Hypotension, myocardial infarction, and coagulopathy following gila monster bite. J Emerg Med 1989;7:37–40.

134.5 Snakes

Key features

- Venomous snake bites are largely an occupational/environmental hazard of agricultural workers and their children in rural areas of the tropics. Most bites could be prevented by wearing protective footwear, by using lights while walking at night and by sleeping off the ground or under a well-tucked-in mosquito net
- Snake venoms are rich in toxic proteins that cause necrosis, shock, hemostatic disturbances, paralysis, rhabdomyolysis and acute kidney injury
- Bites by Elapidae (cobras, kraits, mambas, coral snakes, Australasian snakes, and sea snakes) may cause descending flaccid paralysis. Some elapid venoms cause local necrosis, rhabdomyolysis and hemostatic disturbances
- Bites by Viperidae (vipers, adders and pit vipers: rattlesnakes, moccasins, lanceheads) can cause severe local swelling, bruising, blistering and necrosis together with shock, consumptive coagulopathy, spontaneous systemic bleeding, acute kidney injury and, with some species, neurotoxicity
- First aid involves reassurance, immobilization of the whole patient, especially the bitten limb, rapid evacuation to the nearest hospital and avoidance of dangerous traditional methods
- Specific antivenom is given if there is evidence of systemic or severe local envenoming. Assisted ventilation, renal dialysis or cardiovascular support may be required

INTRODUCTION

The three families of venomous snakes—Atractaspididae, Elapidae and Viperidae—contain some 500 species, whereas the fourth—the Colubridae, once considered nonvenomous—contains at least 40 species venomous to humans. Less than 200 species have caused clinically severe envenoming ending in death or permanent disability.

DISTRIBUTION OF VENOMOUS SNAKES [1]

Venomous species are widely distributed, except at altitudes above 5000 meters, in polar regions and in most islands of the western Mediterranean, Atlantic, Caribbean and Pacific. There are no venomous snakes in Madagascar, New Zealand, Ireland, Iceland and Chile. The range of *Vipera berus* extends into the Arctic Circle. Sea snakes exist in the Indian and Pacific oceans and in estuaries, rivers (New Guinea) and lakes (Philippines, Cambodia, Solomon Islands).

SNAKE CLASSIFICATION

Medically-important snakes always possess one or more pairs of enlarged teeth in the upper jaw—the fangs—which penetrate the skin of their victim and conduct venom into the tissues along a groove or through a lumen.

COLUBRIDAE

The fangs of colubrids are relatively short, are situated at the posterior end of the maxilla and are capable of only restricted movement (Fig. 134.5.1). African species, the boomslang *(Dispholidus typus)* and the vine, twig or bird snakes (*Thelotornis* spp.) have killed a few people. The Japanese yamakagashi *(Rhabdophis tigrinus)* has caused coagulopathy and at least two deaths, whereas the related Southeast Asian red-necked keelback *(Rhabdophis subminiatus)* has been responsible for cases of severe envenoming.

ATRACTASPIDINAE

The African and Middle Eastern burrowing asps, also known as burrowing or mole vipers, or adders and stiletto snakes, have long front fangs and strike sideways. Three species are known to have caused fatal envenoming.

ELAPIDAE

This family includes African and Asian cobras, Asian kraits, African mambas, American coral snakes, Australasian terrestrial venomous snakes and sea snakes. The relatively short anterior fangs of these snakes are permanently erect and capable of little movement (Fig. 134.5.2). In the ringhals and African and Asian spitting cobras, the venom channel opens forward before it reaches the tip of the fang, allowing venom to be ejected as a fine spray for a distance of several meters into the eyes of an aggressor.

VIPERIDAE

The fangs are situated anteriorly, are up to 2.5 cm in length, curved and are capable of a wide range of movement (Fig. 134.5.3). Pit vipers (subfamily Crotalinae) comprise rattlesnakes, moccasins, South American lance-headed vipers and Asian pit vipers. They possess a heat-sensitive pit organ behind the nostril (Fig. 134.5.4). The Old World vipers, subfamily Viperinae include the European, African and Asian vipers and adders.

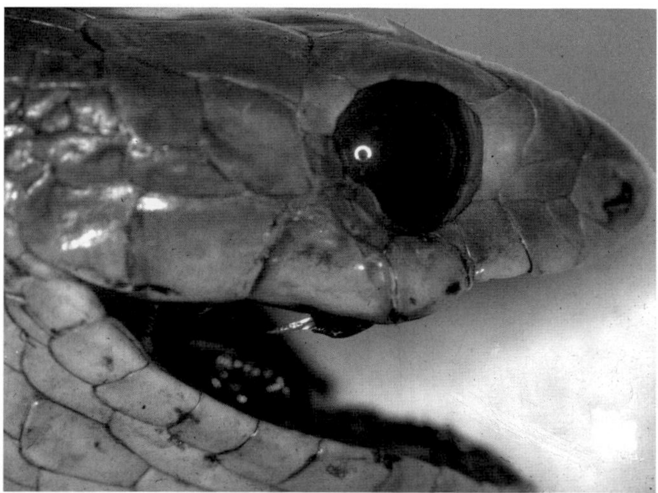

FIGURE 134.5.1 Short posterior maxillary fang of the African Boomslang (*Dispholidus typus*—Colubridae) specimen from Nigeria *(© David A. Warrell)*.

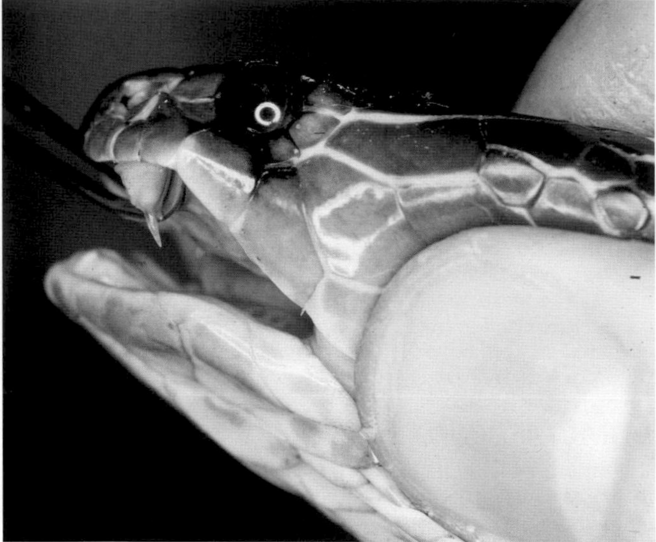

FIGURE 134.5.2 Short fixed front fang in a Sri Lankan cobra (*Naja naja*—Elapidae) *(© David A. Warrell).*

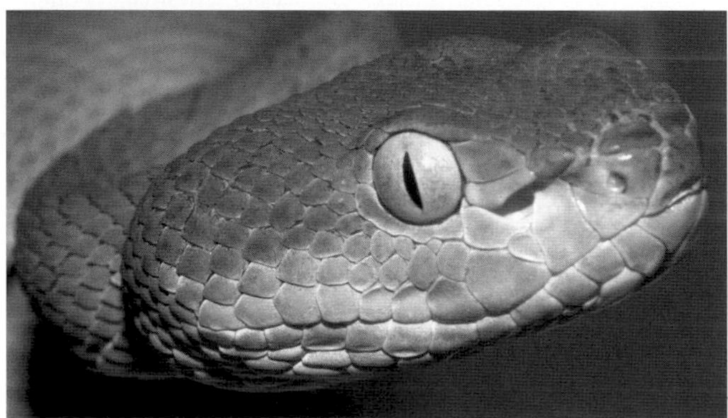

FIGURE 134.5.4 Heat-sensitive pit organ of dark green pit viper [*Cryptelytrops* (*Trimeresurus*) *macrops*—Viperidae, Crotalinae] Thailand *(© David A. Warrell).*

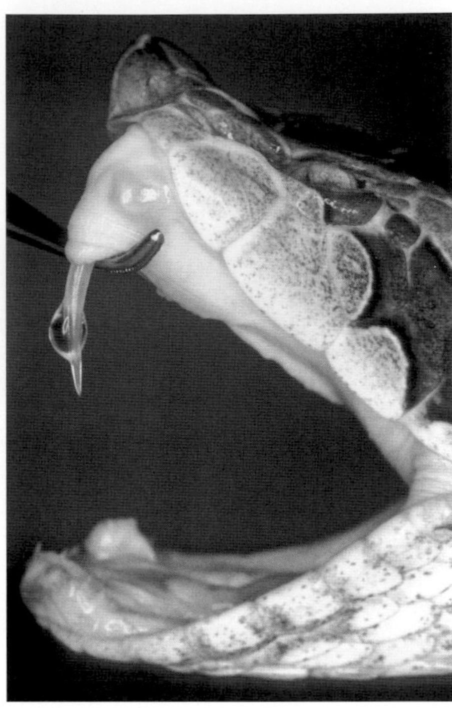

FIGURE 134.5.3 Long hinged front fang of Malayan pit viper (*Calloselasma rhodostoma*—Viperidae, Crotalinae) Thailand *(© David A. Warrell).*

MEDICALLY IMPORTANT SNAKES [1]

Table 134.5.1 lists some of the species commonly responsible for human deaths and serious disability, usually resulting from local necrosis. Scientific and common English names are given.

INCIDENCE AND IMPORTANCE OF SNAKEBITE [2]

Snake bite is an important medical emergency in some parts of the rural tropics but its incidence is usually underestimated because most victims seek the help of traditional healers rather than practitioners of Western-style medicine. In coastal Kenya, where snake bites cause 6.7 deaths per 100,000 per year (0.7% of all deaths), 68% of bitten people had sought treatment from traditional healers. In the Benue Valley of north-east Nigeria, *Echis ocellatus* causes some 500 bites per 100,000 population per year, with a 12% mortality. Recently, a study of snake bite mortality in India, based on verbal autopsy, estimated 46,000 deaths each year. In Burma, Russell's viper bite is a common cause of acute kidney injury and is responsible for most of the estimated 1000 snake-bite deaths each year. In the USA, there are about 45,000 bites and a few deaths each year. Rattlesnakes, especially (*Crotalus adamanteus, Crotalus atrox, Crotalus horridus, Crotalus oreganus, Crotalus scutulatus, Crotalus viridis* and *Sistrurus miliaris*), are the most dangerous species. In Britain, the adder or viper (*Vipera berus*) is the only venomous species, biting more than 200 people each year. Only 14 deaths have been reported since 1876—the last in 1975. This species is important in Scandinavian countries. *Vipera aspis* causes most bites in France, while *Vipera ammodytes* is important in eastern Europe.

Some hunter-gatherer tribes, such as the Yanomamo of Venezuela, the Waorani of Ecuador, the Kaxinawa of Brazil, the Hadza of Tanzania and some tribal groups in Papua New Guinea, suffer high mortality from snake bites. Global estimates of annual snake bite mortality vary from 20,000 to 125,000. Many survivors are left with permanent physical disability.

EPIDEMIOLOGY [3]

Most snake bites are inflicted on the lower limbs of farmers, plantation workers, herdsmen and hunters in rural areas of tropical developing countries. The incidence of bites by a particular species in a particular geographic area depends on the densities of human and snake populations, the snake's irritability (its inclination to bite when trodden on or disturbed) and diurnal rhythm, and the extent to which human activities encroach on its chosen habitat. The snake is usually trodden on at night or in undergrowth. Some species, such as the Asian kraits (*Bungarus* spp.) and African spitting cobras (*Naja nigricollis, Naja mossambica*, etc.), enter human dwellings at night and may bite people who roll over onto them while sleeping on the floor. Snakes do not bite without provocation, but may strike if inadvertently trodden upon or touched. In Europe, North America, and Australia, exotic snakes are increasingly popular pets. In these countries, bites are inflicted on the hands of (usually) males who are picking up their pets, often late at night while drunk. In the USA, 25% of bites result from snakes being attacked or handled. Serious bites by back-fanged (colubrid) snakes usually occur only under these circumstances. Seasonal peaks in the incidence of snake bite are associated with agricultural activities, such as ploughing before the annual rains in the West African Sahel and the rice harvest in Southeast Asia, or to fluctuations in the activity or population of venomous snakes. Severe flooding, by concentrating the human and snake populations, has

TABLE 134.5.1 Species responsible for most deaths and morbidity resulting from snakebite. Specific antivenoms are manufactured for the treatment of envenoming by all these species (see Table 134.5.2 and reference [11])

Area of distribution	Latin name*	English name
North America	*Crotalus adamanteus*	Eastern diamondback rattlesnake
	Crotalus atrox	Western diamondback rattlesnake
	Crotalus oreganus	Pacific rattlesnake
Central America	*Crotalus simus*	Central American rattlesnake
	Bothrops asper	Terciopelo
South America	*Bothrops atrox*	Common lancehead, fer-de-lance, barba amarilla
	Bothrops asper	Terciopelo
	Bothrops jararaca	Jararaca
	Crotalus durissus	South American rattlesnake
Europe	*Vipera berus*	Viper, adder
	Vipera ammodytes	Long-nosed viper
Africa	*Echis* spp.	Saw-scaled or carpet viper
	Bitis arietans	Puff adder
	Naja nigricollis, *Naja mossambica*, etc.	African spitting cobras
	Naja haje	Egyptian cobra
	Dendroaspis spp.	Mambas
Middle East	*Echis* spp.	Saw-scaled or carpet vipers
	Daboia palaestinae	Palestine viper
	Macrovipera lebetina	Levantine viper
Southeast Asia and India	*Naja* spp.	Asian cobras
	Bungarus caeruleus	Common krait
	Daboia russelii	Western Russell's viper
	Daboia siamensis	Eastern Russell's viper
	Echis carinatus	Saw-scaled or carpet viper
	Calloselasma (Agkistrodon) rhodostoma	Malayan pit viper
	Cryptelytrops (*Trimeresurus*) spp.	Green pit vipers
Far East	*Naja atra*	Chinese cobra
	Bungarus multicinctus	Chinese krait
	Gloydius spp.	Mamushis
	Protobothrops flavoviridis	Habu
	Protobothrops mucrosquamatus	Chinese habu
Australasia	*Acanthophis* species	Death adders
	Notechis scutatus	Tiger snake
	Oxyuranus scutellatus	Taipan
	Pseudonaja textilis	Eastern brown snake

*Scientific (Latin) names are important because they are used internationally to describe the range of specificity of antivenoms.

given rise to epidemics of snake bite, notably in Colombia, Pakistan, India, Bangladesh, Nepal, Burma and Vietnam. Invasion of virgin jungle during construction of new highways and irrigation and hydroelectric schemes has led to an increased incidence of snake bite in Brazil and Sri Lanka. On rare occasions, snakebite or injection of snake venom has been used for suicide or murder.

PREVENTION OF SNAKE BITE

To reduce the risk of bites, snakes should never be disturbed, attacked, cornered or handled—even if they are thought to be a harmless species or appear to be dead. Venomous species should not be kept as pets or as performing animals. In snake-infested areas, boots, socks and long trousers should be worn for walks in undergrowth or deep sand, and a light should always be carried at night. Collecting firewood, dislodging logs and boulders with bare hands, pushing sticks or fingers into burrows, holes and crevices, climbing rocks and trees covered with dense foliage, and swimming in overgrown lakes and rivers are particularly hazardous activities. Unlit paths and gutters are especially dangerous after heavy rains. Sleeping on the ground carries a risk of nocturnal krait bites in South Asia and of spitting cobra bites in Africa, but mosquito nets are protective. It is futile and ecologically

TABLE 134.5.2 Guide to initial dosage of some important antivenoms

Species		Manufacturer, antivenom	Approximate initial dose
Latin name	*English name*		
Acanthophis spp.	Death adder	CSL*, monospecific	3000–6000 units
Bitis arietans	Puff adder	Sanofi-Pasteur, Fav Afrique and Favi Rept, SAVP†; polyspecific	80 ml
Bothrops asper	Terciopelo	Instituto Clodomiro Picado	50–100 ml
Bothrops atrox	Common lance head	Suero Antiofidico (Instituto Nacional de Higiene y Medicina Tropical "Leopoldo Izquieta Perez" Guayaquil, Ecuador); Soro Antibotropico (Instituto Butantan, San Paulo, Brazil)	20 ml
Bothrops (*Bothriopsis*) *bilineatus*		As above	20 ml
Bothrops jararaca	Jararaca	Instituto Butantan and other Brazilian manufacturers, Bothrops polyspecific	20 ml
Bungarus caeruleus *Bungarus candidus*	Common krait Malayan krait	Indian manufacturers§, polyspecific Thai Red Cross, Bangkok monospecific	100 ml 100 ml
Calloselasma (*Agkistrodon*) *rhodostoma*	Malayan pit viper	Thai Red Cross, Bangkok, monospecific or hemato-polyvalent	100 ml
Crotalus adamanteus	Eastern diamondback rattlesnakes	Protherics "CroFab"	7–15 vials
Crotalus atrox	Western diamondback rattlesnakes	Protherics "CroFab"	7–15 vials
Crotalus oreganus and *Crotalus viridis* subspp.	Western rattlesnakes	Protherics "CroFab"	7–15 vials
Cryptelytrops (*Trimeresurus*) *albolabris*	Green pit viper	Thai Red Cross, monospecific or hemato-polyvalent	100 ml
Daboia (*Vipera*) *palaestinae*	Palestine viper	Rogoff Medical Research Institute, Tel Aviv, Palestine, viper-monospecific	50–80 ml
Daboia (*Vipera*) *russelii*	Western Russell's viper	Indian manufacturers,§ polyspecific	100 ml
Daboia siamensis	Eastern Russell's viper	Thai Red Cross, monospecific or hemato-polyvalent Myanmar Pharmaceutical Factory monospecific	100 ml 50 ml
Echis ocellatus, *Echis leucogaster*, *Echis pyramidum* (Africa)	African saw-scaled or carpet vipers	SAIMR†, Echis, monospecific; Aventis-Pasteur "Fav Afrique"	20 ml
Elapidae (Hydrophiinae)	Sea snakes	CSL*, sea snake	1000 units
Naja kaouthia	Monocellate Thai cobra	Thai Red Cross, monospecific or neuro-polyvalent	100 ml
Naja naja	Indian cobra	Indian manufacturers,§ polyspecific	100 ml
Notechis scutatus	Tiger snake	CSL*, monospecific	3000–6000 units
Oxyuranus scutellatus	Taipan	CSL*, polyspecific	12,000 units
Pseudonaja textilis	Eastern brown snake	CSL*, monospecific	3000–6000 units
Vipera berus	European adder	Immunoloski Zavod-Zagreb Vipera, polyspecific Protherics Fab. Monospecific "ViperaTAb"	10–20 ml 100–200 mg

*Commonwealth Serum Laboratories, Melbourne, Australia.
†South African Vaccine Producers [formerly SAIMR (South African Institute for Medical Research)].
§Haffkine, Kasauli, Serum Institute of India, Vins, Bharat, Biological Evans, King Institute, etc.
Contacts for procurement of antivenoms: http://www.who.int/bloodproducts/snake_antivenoms/snakeantivenomguide/en/; http://www.searo.who.int/EN/Section10/Section17.htm; http://www.toxinfo.org/antivenoms/ (all websites last accessed 28 December 2011).

undesirable to attempt to exterminate venomous snakes. Various substances toxic to snakes, such as insecticides and methylbromide, have been used to keep human dwellings free of these animals. However, no effective yet harmless snake repellent has been discovered.

VENOM APPARATUS

The venom glands are surrounded by compressor muscles and are situated behind or below the eye. The venom duct opens within a sheath at the base of the fang and venom is conducted toward the tip in a partially or completely closed groove or fang canal. Venomous snakes can inject doses of venom lethal to their natural prey at each of 10 or more consecutive strikes. Whether the dose can be adjusted according to the size of the prey or the intention of the snake is controversial. The high proportion of bites without envenoming ("dry bites") reported for species such as *Calloselasma rhodostoma* (>50%) or *Pseudonaja* spp. (>80%) is more likely to reflect mechanical inefficiency than to voluntary control by the snake, and the concept of a defensive bite may not be valid. There is no support for the popular belief that snakes are less dangerous after they have eaten. The snake uses only a small fraction of the content of its venom gland at each strike.

VENOM COMPOSITION

More than 90% of the dry weight of venom is protein and each venom may contain more than 100 different proteins: enzymes (80–90% of viperid; 25–70% of elapid venoms), non-enzymatic polypeptide toxins and non-toxic proteins such as nerve growth factor. These include digestive hydrolases, hyaluronidase and activators or inactivators of many physiologic processes. Viperid venoms have metalloproteinases, endopeptidase, arginine ester hydrolase, kininogenase, as well as thrombin-like factor X, and prothrombin-activating enzymes responsible for the anti-hemostatic effects of envenoming. Phospholipases A_2 (lecithinase) are found in many venoms. They damage mitochondria, red blood cells, leukocytes, platelets, peripheral nerve endings, skeletal muscle, vascular endothelium and other membranes, and produce presynaptic neurotoxic activity, opiate-like sedative effects and the autopharmacologic release of histamine. Some are anti-coagulant. Hyaluronidase promotes the spread of venom through tissues.

Necrotoxins

A variety of venom myotoxic and cytolytic factors may contribute to local tissue necrosis at the site of the bite. Studies of terciopelo (*Bothrops asper*) venom induced necrosis implicate zinc-dependent metalloproteinases and myotoxic phospholipases A_2. In other cases, other digestive hydrolases, hyaluronidase, polypeptide cytotoxins (Elapidae) and, perhaps, secondary effects of inflammation are involved.

Neurotoxins

Postsynaptic (α-)neurotoxins, such as α-bungarotoxin and cobrotoxin, are three-finger fold polypeptides that bind to acetylcholine receptors on the motor end-plate, like curare, competitively inhibiting acetylcholine. Presynaptic (β-)neurotoxins, such as β-bungarotoxin, crotoxin, taipoxin and notexin, are phospholipases A_2 that prevent release of acetylcholine at the neuromuscular junction and damage the nerve endings irreparably. Myotoxic phospholipases A_2 in venoms of Elapidae, notably sea snakes and some Australasian, American and Asian terrestrial elapids an Viperidae can cause generalized rhabdomyolysis.

Cardiovascular and autopharmacologic toxins

Some venoms release vasodilating autacoids such as histamine and kinins. Venom of the Brazilian jararaca (*Bothrops jararaca*) and other vipers contain bradykinin potentiating and angiotensin converting enzyme (ACE) inhibiting peptides that cause hypotension. Sarafotoxins from the venom of the Israeli burrowing asp (*Atractaspis engaddensis*) are similar to physiologic endothelins. They are potent vasoconstrictors of the coronary arteries and delay atrioventricular conduction.

Variation in Venom Composition

Venom composition varies enormously from species to species but also within a single species throughout its geographic range, at different seasons of the year and as the snake matures.

Pharmacology

When snakes bite humans, venom is usually introduced subcutaneously or intramuscularly. Intravenous injection is a rare possibility. Smaller M_w elapid neurotoxins are rapidly absorbed into the bloodstream, whereas larger M_w phospholipase A_2 presynaptic toxins and viperid enzymes are taken up more slowly through the lymphatics, sometimes causing visible lymphangitis and enlarged, painful lymph nodes. Continuing absorption of venom from the depot at the site of bite may explain delayed or recurrent envenoming after an initial therapeutic response to antivenom. Redistribution of venom toxins into the vascular compartment may occur as a result of antivenom treatment. Envenoming after ingestion of snake venom has not been reported in humans. Most venoms are concentrated and bound in the kidney and some components are eliminated in the urine. Crotaline venoms are selectively bound in the lungs, concentrated in the liver and excreted in bile, while polypeptide neurotoxins, such as α-bungarotoxin, are tightly bound at neuromuscular junctions. Most venom components do not cross the intact blood brain barrier. Central nervous system effects of venoms remain controversial.

CLINICAL EFFECTS [4]

The patient who has been bitten by a snake may present with symptoms resulting from fear, from prehospital treatment and from effects of the venom itself. Snake bite is usually a terrifying experience, especially for those who believe that all bites are rapidly fatal. Physiologic manifestations of anxiety, and even frank hysteria, may confuse the clinical picture. Thus, patients who are bitten, but not envenomed, may feel flushed and breathless, with constriction of the chest, and a thumping pulse, palpitations, sweating and effects of hyperventilation, such as faintness, acroparesthesia and even tetany, may be noticed. Such symptoms dominate many accounts of snake bites written by the victims and are falsely attributed to neurotoxicity. Misguided traditional prehospital treatments can result in swelling and ischemia of limbs whose circulation is occluded by tourniquets, bleeding or sensory loss resulting from local incisions, vomiting and other side effects caused by ingested herbal remedies, smarting eyes and conjunctivitis from instillation of plant juices, and bronchospasm from insufflation of oils. Rarely, snake bite may precipitate vaso-vagal collapse, angina pectoris, myocardial infarction or cardiac arrhythmia.

General symptoms and signs

The evolution of symptoms and signs of envenoming depends on the nature of the venom, the dose and the site of injection. The earliest symptom is usually pain—felt immediately. Local swelling may start within minutes and consumption coagulopathy with undetectable plasma concentrations of fibrinogen and other clotting factors can develop in half an hour (*C. rhodostoma* and *Echis* species). Rarely, death may occur as soon as 15 minutes after an elapid (e.g. *Naja naja* or *Dendroaspis* species) or viper (e.g. *Daboia russelii, Daboia siamensis*) bite. Usually, however, death comes hours after an elapid or sea snake bite and days after a viper bite.

Local effects

This is characteristic of bites by the Viperidae, including the pit vipers of the subfamily Crotalinae, African spitting cobras (e.g. *N. mossambica, N. nigricollis*) and Asian cobras (e.g., *N. naja, Naja kaouthia* and *Naja siamensis*). Tender swelling spreads from the site of the bite and there is early tender enlargement of lymph nodes draining the bitten area. Within a few hours, blood or fluid-filled bullae may appear under the epidermis (Fig. 134.5.5). With elapid bites, blistering is nearly always followed by tissue necrosis, usually superficial, which may extend up the fascial planes of the limb, sometimes as skip

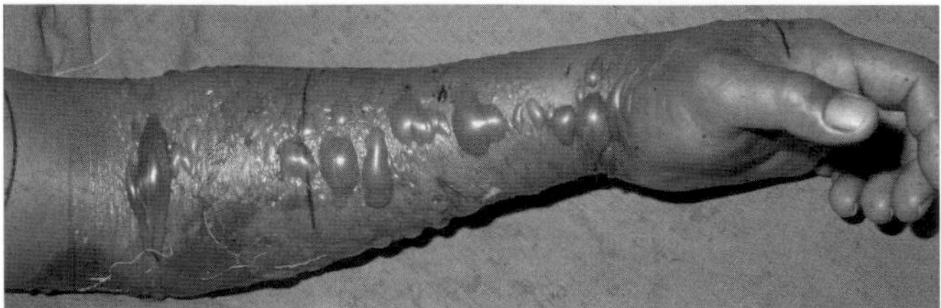

FIGURE 134.5.5 Intense edema, bruising and formation of bullae 25 hours after a bite on the forearm by a Malayan pit viper (*Calloselasma rhodostoma*) in Thailand *(© David A. Warrell).*

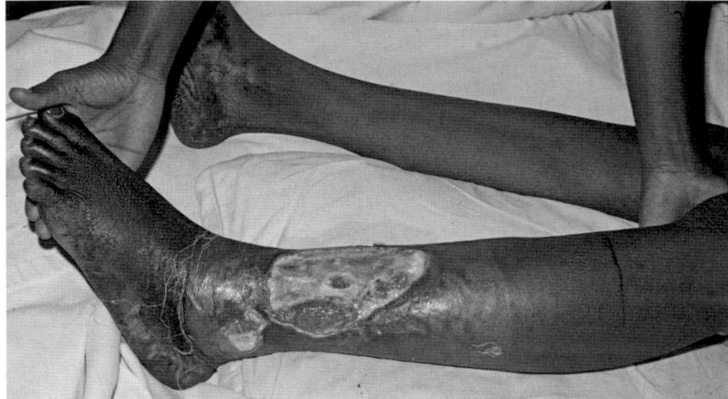

FIGURE 134.5.6 Blistering with necrosis of skin and subcutaneous tissue one week after a bite on the ankle by a black-necked spitting cobra (*Naja nigricollis*) in Nigeria *(© David A. Warrell).*

lesions separated by areas of unaffected skin (Fig. 134.5.6). Bullae caused by Viperidae bites frequently dry up and slough without the development of necrosis. A pale, anesthetic, demarcated area of skin with a characteristic odor of putrefaction signals the appearance of necrosis. This is an effect of the venom, but the necrotic tissue is vulnerable to secondary infection by bacteria, including anaerobes.

Massive swelling of the bitten limb indicates increased permeability leading to extravasation of circulating volume; a swollen limb can accommodate several liters of blood. The result may be hypovolemia and hypotension. Envenoming by rattlesnakes (*Crotalus*) produces local pain with swelling that appears within 15 minutes of the bite and may spread rapidly. Bruising along the path of lymphatics and bullae, and local necrosis may develop. Paresthesias of the tongue and lips and an abnormal metallic taste are common early symptoms following bites by Pacific (*C. oreganus*), eastern diamondback (*C. adamanteus*), western diamondback (*C. atrox*) and timber (*C. horridus*) rattlesnakes. Other symptoms include weakness, rigors, sweating, fasciculation, spontaneous bleeding, neurotoxic effects (*C. adamanteus*, *C. scutulatus*) and gastrointestinal symptoms. Bites by the Mohave rattlesnake (*C. scutulatus*) and *Crotalus durissus terrificus* may produce little, or no, local swelling but severe systemic signs.

Bleeding and clotting disturbances [5]

This combination is characteristic of vipers, pit vipers and some Australasian elapids. Spontaneous bleeding is most frequently detected in the gingival sulci (Fig. 134.5.7). The most common sites of hemorrhage are intracerebral, gastrointestinal and retroperitoneal. Incoagulable blood is suggested by oozing from venipuncture sites or sites of recent trauma.

Hypotension and shock

Early syncope can occur as part of the autopharmacologic syndrome after bites by vipers, Australasian elapids and burrowing asps. Shock is most commonly the result of hypovolemia (Fig. 134.5.8), vasodilatation or direct action of venom on the myocardium.

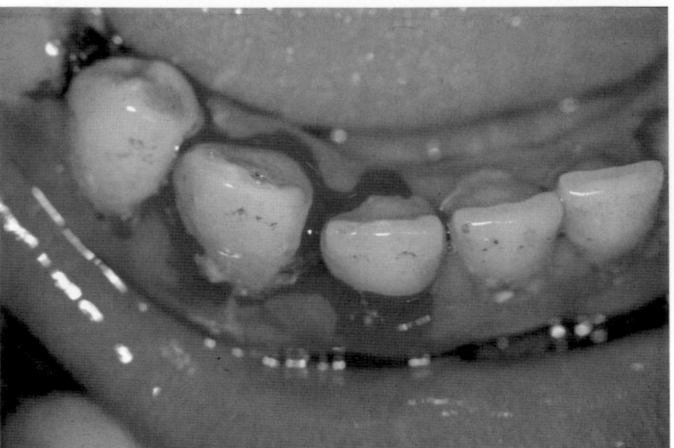

FIGURE 134.5.7 Spontaneous bleeding from gingival sulci after a bite by a West African saw-scaled viper (*Echis ocellatus*) in Nigeria *(© David A. Warrell).*

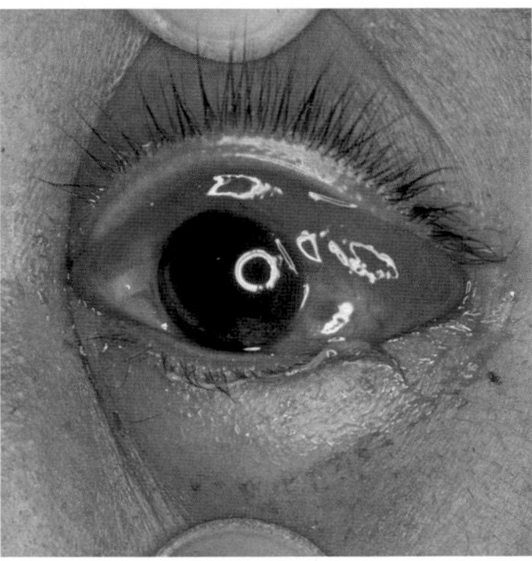

FIGURE 134.5.8 Clinical evidence of increased systemic vascular permeability: chemosis (edema of the conjunctiva) 48 hours after a bite by Russell's viper *(Daboia siamensis)* in Burma *(© David A. Warrell).*

Neurotoxicity

This is a feature of envenoming by elapids. A few species of vipers also produce neurotoxic effects, for example *C. durissus terrificus*, *Gloydius brevicaudus*, *Bitis atropos* and *D. russelii* (especially in Sri Lanka). Typically, neurotoxic symptoms develop early, but after krait bite there may be a delay of 10 or more hours. Symptoms include vomiting, headache, paresthesia, drowsiness, apathy or euphoria, hyperacusis, diplopia, blurred vision, heaviness of the eyelids and difficulty in speaking. The levator palpebrae superioris and extraocular muscles are the most sensitive to neuromuscular blockade and, in some patients, the only feature of envenoming is ptosis and ophthalmoplegia. More serious effects are paralysis of the palate, jaws, tongue, vocal cords, neck muscles and muscles of deglutition and respiration (Fig. 134.5.9). The intercostal muscles are affected before the diaphragm and limbs. Paralyzed patients are fully conscious unless they are hypoxemic (respiratory failure) or hypotensive (circulatory failure). Neurotoxicity is usually completely reversible; in some cases there is a rapid response to specific antivenom or anticholinesterase, and in others there is slow, spontaneous resolution. With no specific

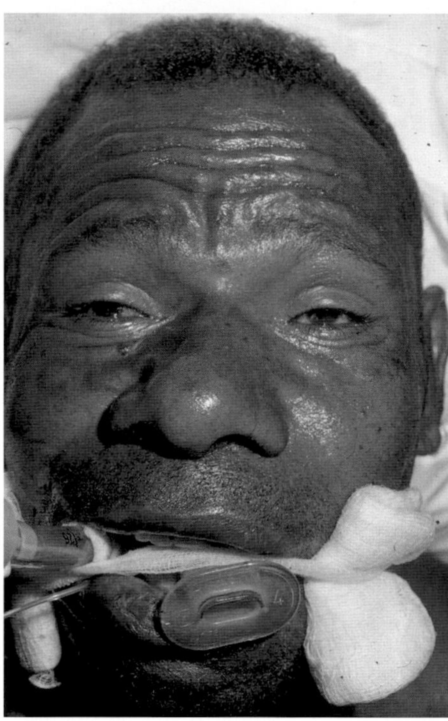

FIGURE 134.5.9 Neurotoxic envenoming after a bite by a Papuan taipan (*Oxyuranus scutellatus canni*). Note bilateral ptosis (the patient is attempting to open his eyes by contracting the frontalis muscle) and inability to breathe spontaneously (mechanical intubation via endotracheal tube) *(© David A. Warrell).*

antivenom, patients supported by artificial ventilation recover sufficient diaphragmatic movement to breathe adequately in 1–4 days. The ocular muscles recover in 2–4 days and there is usually full recovery of motor function in 3–7 days. Upper airway obstruction by the tongue or inhaled vomitus may precipitate respiratory arrest.

Generalized rhabdomyolysis

Envenoming by sea snakes [6], some Australasian elapids, *D. russelii* in Sri Lanka and *C. durissus terrificus* can cause systemic rhabdomyolysis. The symptoms are muscle pain and stiffness with trismus and respiratory muscle paralysis. Myoglobinemia, myoglobinuria, hyperkalemia and renal failure may result.

Acute kidney injury

Renal failure can complicate almost any severe case of snakebite, but it is the major cause of death in victims of sea snakes, some Australasian elapids, Russell's vipers and *C. durissus terrificus*. Mechanisms of renal damage include ischemia (from hypotension, renal vasoconstriction or disseminated intravascular coagulation) (Fig. 134.5.10), hemorrhage, direct nephrotoxicity or pigment nephropathy associated with massive intravascular hemolysis, microangiopathic hemolysis, generalized rhabdomyolysis and associated electrolyte disturbances.

Venom ophthalmia caused by spitting cobras [7]

The ringhals *(Hemachatus haemachatus)* and African and Asian spitting cobras can eject venom in a fine stream from the tips of their fangs for a distance of a few meters. If venom enters the eye, there is intense local pain, leukorrhea, blepharospasm and palpebral edema. Because most patients make an uneventful recovery, these injuries used to be thought trivial, but slit lamp examination reveals corneal erosions in more than half of the cases. There is the same risk of secondary infection as with other corneal injuries (Fig. 134.5.11), leading to

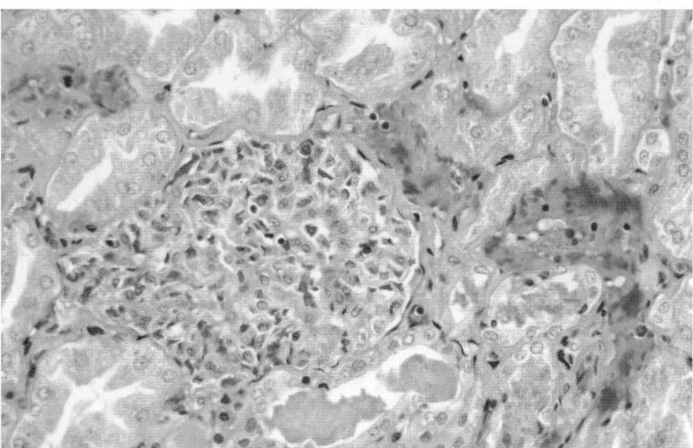

FIGURE 134.5.10 Kidney of a patient who died 15 hours after being bitten by Russell's viper (*Daboia siamensis*) in Burma, showing fibrin thrombi (staining red) in glomerular and peritubular vessels *(© Dr Nicholas Francis).*

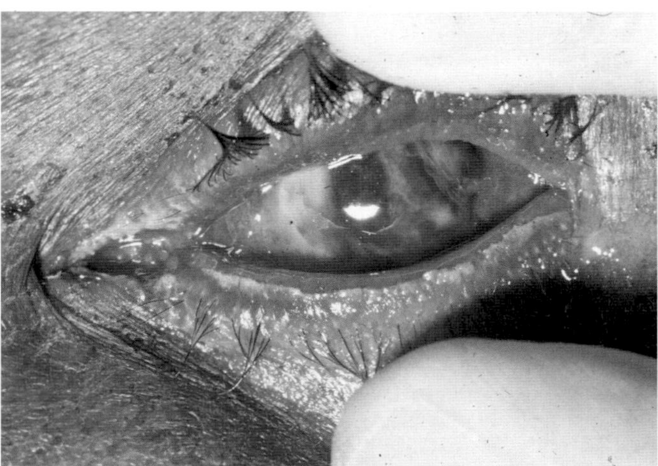

FIGURE 134.5.11 Severe venom ophthalmia that led to blindness in a patient "spat at" by a black-necked spitting cobra *Naja nigricollis* in Nigeria. Failure to treat with a local antimicrobial agent may allow secondary infection of corneal abrasions with these disastrous results (panophthalmitis requiring enucleation) *(© David A. Warrell).*

permanent blindness in some cases. The venom may be absorbed also into the anterior chamber, resulting in anterior uveitis with hypopyon.

LABORATORY INVESTIGATIONS

The peripheral white blood cell count is raised in patients severely envenomed by many species of snakes. Anemia is the result of bleeding or, much more rarely, intravascular and microangiopathic hemolysis. Thrombocytopenia occurs with disseminated intravascular coagulation, together with a hemolytic uremic-like syndrome in victims of some viper and Australian elapid envenomings. Important simple tests for venom-induced defibrination are the 20-minute whole blood clotting test A few milliliters of blood are placed in a new, clean, dry glass test tube, left undisturbed for 20 minutes and then tipped once to check for clotting (Fig. 134.5.12). Serum potassium is elevated by the generalized rhabdomyolysis of sea snake envenoming. Serum enzymes, such as aspartate and alanine aminotransferases and creatine kinase, are mildly elevated in patients with local tissue damage but are grossly raised if there is generalized rhabdomyolysis. Electrocardiographic changes, such as inverted T waves, raised ST segments, prolonged Q-Tc intervals and arrhythmias, have been reported. The urine of snakebite victims commonly

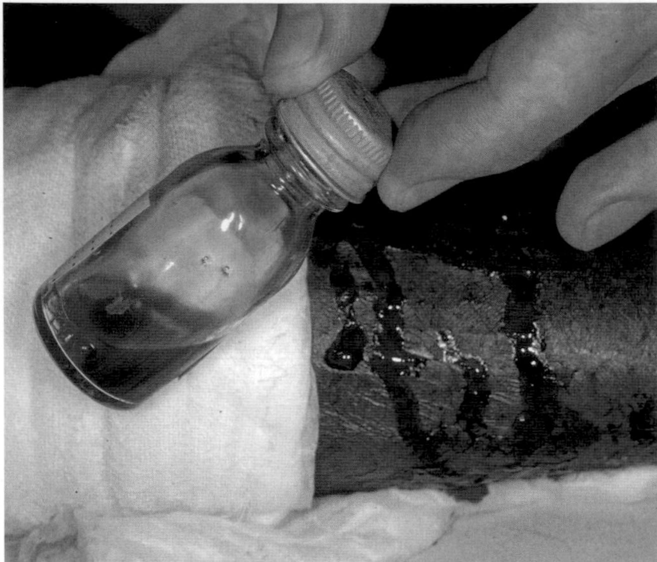

FIGURE 134.5.12 Twenty-minute whole blood clotting test. Blood taken from a patient envenomed by a Papuan taipan (*Oxyuranus scutellatus*) remains incoagulable after standing undisturbed in a glass tube for 20 minutes. The patient with venom-induced consumption coagulopathy continues to bleed from razor cuts made inadvisedly at the site of the bite *(© David A. Warrell).*

contains red and white blood cells and granular casts. Dark urine should be tested for hemoglobin and myoglobin.

VENOM IMMUNODIAGNOSIS

Specific snake venom antigens have been detected in wound swabs, aspirates or biopsies, serum, urine, cerebrospinal fluid and other body fluids. Enzyme immunoassay (EIA) has been the most widely used. Under ideal conditions, relatively high venom antigen concentrations (wound swabs or aspirates) may be detected quickly enough (15–30 min) to allow the selection of the appropriate monospecific antivenom. A commercial venom detection kit for Australian elapids is produced by CSL (Melbourne, Australia). For retrospective diagnosis, including forensic cases, tissue around the fang punctures, wound and blister aspirate, serum and urine should be stored for EIA immunodiagnosis.

TREATMENT OF SNAKE BITE [3, 4, 8–10]

Snakebite is a rare emergency in most parts of the world and because its management is thought to require specialized knowledge, many clinicians close their minds to the simple therapeutic principles that could prevent morbidity and mortality. Management starts with first aid by relatives, friends or fellow workers of the snakebite victim who happen to be present where and when the bite occurs. Therefore, first aid principles should be a priority subject for community health education in schools, at clinics and via the media.

FIRST-AID TREATMENT

Most snakebite victims are terrified and require reassurance. The bitten limb should be immobilized, if possible, with a splint or sling and the patient quickly moved to the nearest treatment facility. Pain can be treated with oral acetaminophen or codeine phosphate. Aspirin and nonsteroidal anti-inflammatory agents should be avoided, if possible, as they may lead to persistent gastric bleeding in patients with incoagulable blood. Local incisions and suction are more likely to introduce infection and cause persistent bleeding than to remove significant amounts of venom from the wound. In one study of viper bites in Jammu, India, 94% of patients who had received incisions developed local infection, compared with none in the group without incisions. Vacuum extractors, potassium permanganate instillation and ice packs can increase local necrosis. Electric shock treatment is potentially dangerous and of unproven value.

Tourniquets

Tight (arterial-occlusive) tourniquets must never be recommended for snake bite first-aid because they have been responsible for gangrenous limbs, peripheral nerve damage and other harmful effects.

Pressure-Immobilization (P-I) and Pressure Pad

These are the only two acceptably safe and promising first-aid methods currently available, but both require further clinical testing. In animal studies, compressing superficial veins and lymphatics in the bitten limb at about 55 mmHg reduced the spread of larger M_w toxins such as the presynaptic phospholipase A_2 toxins of Australian elapid venoms. In practice, the entire bitten limb is bound firmly, using a 10-cm wide elasticated bandage, starting at the toes or fingers and finishing at the groin or axilla. A splint is incorporated to aid immobilization. Anecdotal experience supports the use of the method but it has proved difficult to train people to apply it correctly. However, it is the only known method for delaying the onset of potentially fatal respiratory paralysis after a neurotoxic elapid bite before the patient reaches medical care without incurring the dangers of a tight arterial tourniquet. If the necessary skills and equipment are available immediately, pressure-immobilization (P-I) should be applied, unless it is possible to eliminate the possibility of a neurotoxic elapid bite (e.g. by confident identification of the snake or exclusion on geographical grounds). A local pressure pad applied over the bite wound has been advocated for Russell's viper bites in Burma.

Transport to medical care

Patients should be transported to hospital as quickly, but as passively, as possible. They should be placed on their left side in the recovery position to prevent aspiration of vomit. Persistent vomiting can be treated with chlorpromazine by intramuscular injection (25–50 mg in adults, 1 mg/kg in children) [intravenous (IV) injection risks hypotension] or chlorpromazine or prochlorperazine by intrarectal suppository. Syncope, shock, angio-oedema and other anaphylactic symptoms can be treated with 0.1% adrenaline (epinephrine) by intramuscular injection (0.5 ml for adults, 0.01 ml/kg for children) and an antihistamine such as chlorphenamine maleate, by IV injection (10 mg for adults, 0.2 mg/kg for children). Respiratory distress and cyanosis should be treated by clearing the airway, preventing obstruction by the tongue by jaw-lifting, inserting an oropharyngeal airway and by positioning, giving oxygen and, if necessary, assisted ventilation. If the patient is unconscious and no femoral or carotid pulses can be detected, cardiopulmonary resuscitation must be started immediately.

If the snake has been killed it should be brought to the hospital for identification, but it must be handled cautiously as even snakes that appear dead and severed heads can cause envenoming. They should be carried on a stick or maneuvered into a container.

TREATMENT BY MEDICALLY-TRAINED PERSONNEL IN HOSPITAL OR DISPENSARY

Because of the uncertainties about the type, quantity and quality of venom injected and the variable time course for development of signs of envenoming, all victims of snakebite should be hospitalized and observed for at least 24 hours. Frequent observations of the level of consciousness, blood pressure, and pulse and respiratory rate, and new signs, such as ptosis, should be made. Any ligatures should be released, preferably after starting administration of antivenom (see "*Antivenom Treatment*" below). Physical examination should include assessment of local swelling, tender enlargement of regional lymph nodes draining the bitten area, spontaneous bleeding [most often detected in the gingival sulci (Fig. 134.5.1), nose and gastrointestinal and genitourinary tracts, blood pressure, ptosis [the earliest sign of neurotoxic envenoming (Fig. 134.5.3)] and assessment of respiratory muscle power. If a coagulopathic venom is suspected, hemostasis should be checked at the bedside by the 20-minute whole blood clotting test or by rapid laboratory tests of hemostasis.

ANTIVENOM TREATMENT

Antivenom (also known as antivenin, antivenene and anti-snakebite serum) is the only specific antidote to envenoming. It is the partially purified immunoglobulin (whole IgG, $F(ab')_2$, or Fab fragments) of horses or sheep that have been hyperimmunized with venoms of one species of snake (monovalent) or several species (polyvalent) of greatest medical importance in a particular region [11].

Indications

Because of their high cost and the inherent danger of reactions, antivenoms should not be used indiscriminately. Antivenom is indicated if there is systemic envenoming evidenced by hypotension or other signs of cardiovascular toxicity, signs of neurotoxicity or generalized myotoxicity, impaired consciousness, spontaneous systemic bleeding and incoagulable blood. Supporting evidence of severe envenoming is provided by a peripheral leukocytosis of more than 20×10^9/l, elevated serum enzymes, hemoglobinuria, myoglobinuria, severe anemia or hemoconcentration, uremia and oliguria. In the absence of systemic envenoming, massive local swelling (involving more than half of the bitten limb), bites on fingers or toes and rapidly progressive swelling following bites by species known to cause necrosis are indications for antivenom.

Contraindications

There is no absolute contraindication to antivenom; however, because of the increased danger of severe reactions, atopic individuals and those known to be hypersensitive to equine serum should be pretreated with epinephrine, hydrocortisone and antihistamine (doses above) and watched carefully for at least two hours after completion of antivenom administration.

Administration

Antivenom should be given as soon as indicated, but it may be effective as long as signs of systemic envenoming persist (seven days or more after the bite in the case of patients with viperid bite coagulopathy). To prevent local envenoming, antivenom must be given early, within a few hours of envenoming. Only specific antivenom—one whose range of specificity includes the biting species—should be used. Some antivenoms raised against the venom of one or two species have paraspecific activity against venoms of related species. Antivenom should be diluted in an appropriate volume of fluid and given by "push" injection over 10–15 minutes or by IV infusion over 30–60 minutes. Epinephrine 0.1% solution, 0.5 ml for adults or 0.01 ml/kg for children, must be ready to be given, by intramuscular injection, in case of early anaphylactic reactions during the infusion. The patient must be watched carefully while antivenom is being given and for at least two hours afterward. At the first sign of a reaction, administration of antivenom should be stopped and epinephrine given. Once the symptoms of the reaction have subsided, antivenom infusion can be completed. IV chlorphenamine maleate (10 mg in adults, 0.2 mg/kg in children) and hydrocortisone (100 mg in adults, 2 mg/kg in children) are given to combat released mediators and to calm the patient. Antivenom reactions are not predicted by conjunctival or intradermal "hypersensitivity tests" which can only detect specific IgE. Anti-H1 histamines blockers and corticosteroids have proved ineffective, singly or in combination, in preventing early anaphylactic antivenom reactions, but in a recent, powerful study, epinephrine (adult dose 0.25 ml of 0.1% solution) administered subcutaneously before antivenom was given reduced the frequency of severe early anaphylactic reactions [12]. Appropriate initial doses of antivenom have been established for some antivenoms (Table 134.5.2). Assessment of the antivenom dose will remain a matter of clinical judgment. The dose of antivenom for children and adults should be the same.

Response to antivenom

Spontaneous systemic bleeding usually stops within about 30 minutes of initiating antivenom therapy and blood clotting is usually restored within 6 hours if an adequate neutralizing dose of antivenom has been given. Improvement in neurotoxic symptoms attributable to postsynaptic toxins [e.g. Australian and Papuan death adder (genus *Acanthophis*) and Asian cobras (genus *Naja*)] may be observed within 30–60 minutes. However, severe, local envenoming nephrotoxicity following Russell's viper bites, and presynaptic neurotoxicity, are not reversed by antivenom. Further antivenom should be given if severe signs of envenoming persist after 1–2 hours or if blood coagulability is not restored within about six hours..

ANTIVENOM REACTIONS

Early anaphylactic reactions usually develop within 10–60 minutes of starting IV administration of antivenom. Premonitory symptoms include restlessness, cough, itching of the scalp, nausea, vomiting, a feeling of heat or an increase in pulse rate followed by generalized pruritus and appearance of urticaria, fever, tachycardia, autonomic manifestations and, in a few patients, severe hypotension, airflow obstruction and angioedema. The incidence of early reactions is dose-dependent and also depends on the quality of manufacture. The cause of most reactions is complement activation by IgG aggregates, residual Fc fragments or osmotic effects rather than IgE-mediated type I hypersensitivity to equine serum, which is rare.

Pyrogenic reactions occur within 1–2 hours of antivenom treatment and can precipitate febrile convulsions in children. They are attributable to endotoxin-contamination during manufacture [11].

Late reactions of serum sickness type may develop 5–10 days after antivenom treatment. They are dose-related. Clinical features include fever, pruritus, urticaria, subcutaneous and periarticular swellings, polyarthritis, lymphadenopathy, mononeuritis multiplex and other neurologic symptoms, and proteinuria.

SUPPORTIVE TREATMENT

Neurotoxic Envenoming

Patients unable to cough up or swallow their secretions aspirate and may develop fatal airway obstruction or pneumonia. Others die of respiratory paralysis. Endotracheal intubation should be performed at an early stage, when pooling of secretions in the pharynx becomes evident—before obstruction or respiratory arrest has developed. If respiratory muscle power is inadequate, ventilation must be assisted. Patients have recovered from respiratory paralysis after being manually ventilated by relays of relatives or nurses for up to 30 days and after mechanical ventilation for up to 10 weeks. Most effects of neurotoxic envenoming are fully reversible; therefore, artificial ventilation should always be attempted.

Anticholinesterases have a variable, but potentially useful, effect in patients with neurotoxic envenoming, especially when postsynaptic neurotoxins are involved. The "Tensilon test" can be performed, as with suspected myasthenia gravis. Atropine sulphate (0.6 mg for adults; 50 µg/kg for children) or glycopyrronium is given by IV injection followed by edrophonium chloride (Tensilon) by slow IV injection in an adult dose of 10 mg (0.25 mg/kg for children) or neostigmine bromide or methylsulphate (Prostigmin) by intramuscular injection 0.02 mg/kg for adults (0.04 mg/kg for children). Patients who respond convincingly can be maintained on neostigmine methylsulphate, 0.5–2.5 mg every 1–3 hours up to 10 mg/24 hours maximum for adults or 0.01–0.04 mg/kg every 2–4 hours for children by intramuscular, IV or subcutaneous injection.

Circulatory collapse

Antivenom should be given, as well as plasma expanders. Clinical observation of jugular venous pressure or measurement of central venous pressure or pulmonary wedge pressure (via a Swan-Ganz catheter) helps to prevent fluid overload and precipitation of pulmonary edema. If hypotension persists despite restoration of central venous pressure to +10 to 15 cm H_2O, an infusion of dopamine should be started at an initial dose of 2 μg/kg/minute through the central catheter.

Local necrosis

Once definite signs of necrosis have appeared, surgical debridement is required, with antibiotic prophylaxis to cover anaerobic organisms.

Intracompartmental syndrome and fasciotomy

Increased pressure within tight fascial compartments, such as the digital pulp spaces and anterior tibial compartment, may cause ischemia. Necrosis of digits is especially common. The signs are excessive pain, weakness and tenderness of the compartmental muscles and pain when they are passively stretched, hypoesthesia of skin supplied by nerves running through the compartment, and obvious tenseness of the compartment. Detection of arterial pulses by palpation or Doppler does not exclude intracompartmental ischemia. Intracompartmental pressures exceeding 45 mmHg carry a high risk of ischemic necrosis. In these circumstances, fasciotomy may be justified, but it did not prove effective in saving envenomed muscle in experimental animals. Fasciotomy is contraindicated until blood coagulability has been restored (by adequate doses of antivenom followed by clotting factors) and must be justified by demonstration that the intracompartmental pressure is consistently raised (to less than 30 mmHg below mean arterial pressure). Early adequate antivenom treatment will prevent the development of intracompartmental syndromes in most cases.

LOCAL INFECTION AT THE SITE OF THE BITE

Local infections may result from unusual bacteria derived from the snake's venom or fangs or contamination of the wound from asterile incisions. A booster dose of tetanus toxoid should be given, but prophylactic antibiotics are not indicated unless the wound has been incised or tampered with in any way. If the wound is necrotic, *Clostridium tetani* should be eliminated with a large dose of benzyl penicillin or metronidazole and an aminoglycoside, such as gentamicin, given for 48 h. If a local abscess develops, it should be drained and the patient given a course of antibiotics, such as penicillin, chloramphenicol or erythromycin, which are usually available and affordable.

Acute kidney injury

Some snake bite victims admitted with oliguria and elevated blood urea nitrogen and creatinine levels are simply hypovolemic. Urine output, serum creatinine, urea and electrolytes should be measured each day in patients with severe envenoming and in those bitten by species known to cause acute kidney injury. If urine output drops below 400 ml in 24 h, urethral and central venous catheters should be inserted. If urine flow fails to increase after cautious rehydration, diuretics should be tried (e.g. furosemide by slow intravenous injection, 100 mg followed by 200 mg) and then mannitol. Dopamine (2.5 μg/kg per min by IV infusion) has proved effective in some cases. If these measures are ineffective, the patient should be placed on strict fluid balance. Peritoneal or hemodialysis will usually be required.

Other drugs

Heparin, antifibrinolytic agents (aprotinin, ε-aminocaproic acid), corticosteroids, antihistamines and a variety of herbal and other remedies have been advocated for treatment of snakebite. None has proved effective and many are harmful.

Treatment of snake venom ophthalmia [7]

When cobra venom is "spat" into the eyes, first-aid consists of irrigation with generous volumes of water or any other bland liquid, such as milk—or even urine, which may be available. Unless a corneal abrasion can be excluded by fluorescein staining or slit-lamp examination, treatment should be the same as for any corneal injury; a topical antimicrobial such as tetracycline or chloramphenicol should be applied. Instillation of antivenom is not recommended. Epinephrine (0.1%) or local anesthetic eye drops relieve the pain.

REFERENCES

1. World Health Organization. WHO guidelines for the production, control and regulation of snake antivenom immunoglobulins. Available at: http://apps.who.int/bloodproducts/snakeantivenoms/database/ (last accessed 28 December 2011).
2. Warrell DA. Snake bite. Lancet 2010;376:77–88.
3. Warrell DA. Epidemiology, clinical features and management of snakebites in Central and South America. In: Campbell J, Lamar WW, Greene H, eds. Venomous Reptiles of the Americas. Ithaca: Cornell University Press; 2004;709–61.
4. Meier J, White J, eds. Handbook of Clinical Toxicology of Animal Venoms and Poisons. Boca Raton: CRC Press; 1995.
5. Reid HA, Thean PC, Chan KE, Baharou AR. Clinical effects of bites by Malayan viper (Ancistrodon rhodostoma). Lancet 1963;i:617–21.
6. Gopalakrishnakone P, ed. Sea snake Toxinology. Singapore: Singapore University Press; 1994:1–36.
7. Chu ER, Weinstein SA, White J, Warrell DA. Venom ophthalmia caused by venoms of spitting elapid and other snakes: report of nine cases with review of epidemiology, clinical features, pathophysiology and management. Toxicon 2010;56:259–72.
8. Sutherland SK, Tibballs J. Australian Animal Toxins. The Creatures, Their Toxins and Care of The Poisoned Patient, 2nd edn. Melbourne: Oxford University Press; 2001.
9. Warrell DA. Treatment of bites by adders and exotic venomous snakes. BMJ 2005;331:1244–7.
10. Warrell DA. Bites by venomous snakes outside The Americas. In: Auerbach PA, ed. Wilderness Medicine, 5th edn. Philadelphia: Elsevier; 2007:1086–123.
11. World Health Organization. WHO Guidelines for the Production, Control and Regulation of Snake Antivenom Immunoglobulins. Available at: http://www.who.int/bloodproducts/snake_antivenoms/snakeantivenomguide/en/ (last accessed 28 December 2011).
12. de Silva HA, Pathmeswaran A, Ranasinha CD, et al. Low-dose adrenaline, promethazine, and hydrocortisone in the prevention of acute adverse reactions to antivenom following snakebite: a randomised, double-blind, placebo-controlled trial. PLoS Med 2011;8:e1000435.

USEFUL WEBSITES

Snake bites in South and Southeast Asia: http://www.searo.who.int/EN/Section10/Section17.htm (last accessed 28 December 2011)
Snake bites in Africa: http://www.afro.who.int/en/clusters-a-programmes/hss/essential-medicines/highlights/2731-guidelines-for-the-prevention-and-clinical-management-of-snakebite-in-africa.html (last accessed 02-03-2012)
Envenoming worldwide: http://www.toxinology.com/ (last accessed 28 December 2011)
Antivenoms: http://www.toxinfo.org/antivenoms/ (last accessed 28 December 2011)

134.6 Bats

Key features

- Bats are increasingly recognized vectors and reservoirs of zoonotic infections
- Lyssavirus infections transmissible to humans by bats include Genotypes 1 (classic rabies), 4 (Duvenhage), 5 and 6 (European bat lyssaviruses), and 7 (Australian bat lyssavirus)
- Vampire bats (Desmodontinae) transmit classic rabies to humans and domestic animals in Latin America
- Insectivorous and frugivorous bats are vectors or reservoirs of Lyssaviruses Genotypes 1, 4, 5, 6 and 7, Filoviruses (Ebola and Marburg), Henipaviruses (Hendra and Nipah) and some other viruses, bacteria and fungi
- Bat-transmitted rabies infections can be prevented by vaccination
- Vampire bat rabies can be controlled by vaccinating the bats or killing them with anticoagulants

INTRODUCTION [1, 2]

The medical importance of bats (Order Chiroptera) to human health is increasingly recognized. They are proven, or potential, reservoirs of zoonotic human pathogens and vectors. Transmission may be direct, by bat bites, scratches or more subtle contact; or indirect by infecting other mammalian hosts or by creating in their accumulated feces (bat guano)—a culture medium for pathogenic fungi whose spores may be inhaled by people entering bat caves. Bats may damage fruit crops, and cattle and other domestic animals are vulnerable to bat-transmitted infections. In Latin America, vampire bat-transmitted bovine rabies ("derriengue") and trypanosomiasis (*Trypanosoma evansi* infection causing "surra") threatens meat production. Nipah virus causes fatal disease in pigs in Southeast Asia where epidemics have led to the culling of more than 1 million of these animals. Hendra, Menangle and Tioman viruses have been responsible for fatal diseases in horses and pigs in Australia and Malaysia. However, bats are much less important, medically and economically, than rodents. Rats, mice and voles are vectors and reservoirs of many prevalent zoonotic pathogens, such as Hanta- and Arena- viruses, plague bacillus, leptospires, rickettsiae and parastrongyloids. Rodents also consume crops and food stores and damage human dwellings and installations. In their favor, bats are fascinating and beautiful animals which are protected and conserved in many Western countries and which benefit the environment by controlling insects, pollinating fruit trees and distributing seeds. Bats are eaten medicinally in China and elsewhere and as a delicacy and valuable source of protein in West Africa, Southeast Asia, Indonesia, New Guinea and Australia (by native Australians). Catching and butchering bats and consuming inadequately cooked bats incurs the risk of infection.

BAT BIOLOGY

Bats have a number of special characteristics, some of which are unique. They show extreme diversity, constituting 20% of all mammalian species, and they are widely distributed in all continents except Antarctica and some oceanic islands. Some species breed within the Arctic circle. Bats are enormously abundant, sometimes occuring in colonies, flocks or clouds composed of as many as 20–30 million individual animals. In caves inhabited by Mexican free-tailed bats (*Tadarida brasiliensis*), there may be more than 3000 bats/m^3 in their cave roosts. Bats are the only mammals capable of flying, as opposed to gliding. Some species migrate more than 1500 kilometers and North American hoary bats (*Lasiurus cinereus*—Vespertilionidae) have reached Iceland and the Orkney Islands (UK). The wing membrane is formed by the skin of the back and belly, supported by elongated fingers, externally rotated and adducted legs and, in some cases, the tail. Some bats, such as true vampires, are also capable of quadrupedal gait. Most bats are nocturnal. They are the only vertebrates capable of catching insects in complete darkness, achieved by the use of sophisticated echolocation. Bats are variously insectivorous, frugivorous, flower-feeding, hematophagous or carnivorous. Their weight ranges from 2 g (one of the tiniest vertebrates) to 1.2 kg. Metabolic flexibility allows them to be heterothermic (extreme variation in body core temperature 2–41 °C) and to hibernate. They are the longest-living of tiny mammals (e.g. *Myotis lucifugus*, weighing only 7 g, has lived to 35 years). Bats roost, hanging upside down from their feet or clinging onto surfaces, in human constructions such as roof spaces, eaves and attics of dwellings (bringing them into close contact with people), tombs, temples, mines, pipes, irrigation tunnels and bridges and in caves, rock crevices, foliage, tree cavities, trees and bird and termite nests. Some species can fashion tent-like shelters out of leaves. Recently, an epidemic of white-nosed syndrome has killed more than a million bats in the north-east USA. A cold-growing fungus, *Geomyces destructans*, has been implicated ("WNS fungus"), but this may not be the primary cause. Bats are infested with numerous ectoparasites, including bat flies, fleas, mites, ticks and *Chimex* bugs.

Medically importance species are members of both suborders: Megachiroptera [flying foxes, fruit bats and rousettes (Pteropodidae)] (Figs 134.6.1 and 134.6.2) and Microchiroptera, which include sheath-tailed bats (Emballonuridae), free-tailed bats (Molossidae, e.g. the Mexican free-tailed bat *Tadarida brasileinsis mexicana*) (Fig. 134.6.3), moustache bats (Mormoopidae), slit-faced bats (Nycteridae), New World leaf-nosed bats (Phyllostomidae) (Fig. 134.6.4)—containing the true vampire bats (sub-family Desmodontinae) (Figs 134.6.5, 134.6.6, 134.6.7)—horseshoe bats (Rhinolophidae) and evening bats (Vespertilionidae).

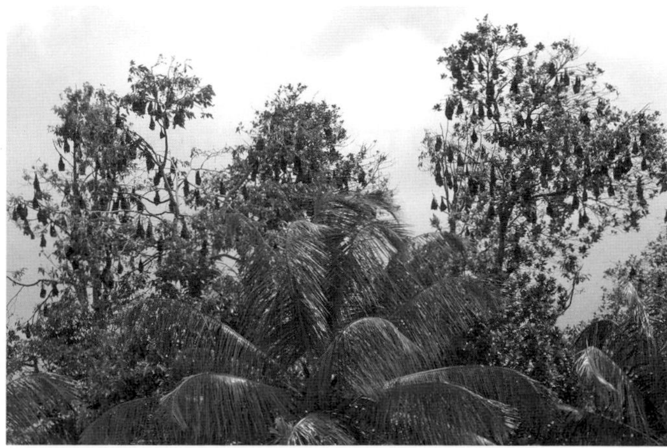

FIGURE 134.6.1 Indian fruit bats (*Pteropus giganteus*—Pteropodidae) roosting at Mawanella, Sri Lanka *(© David A. Warrell)*.

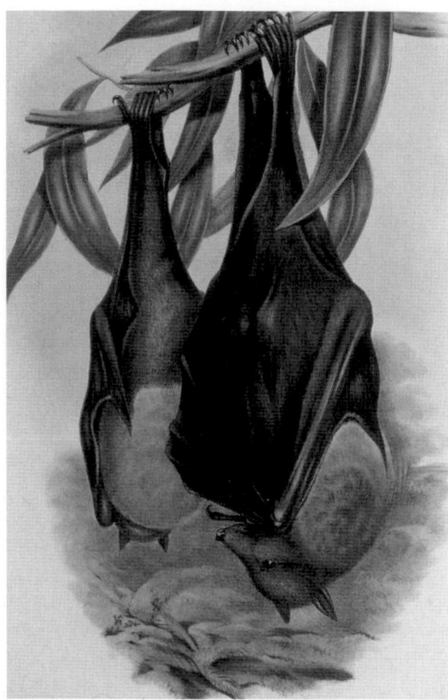

FIGURE 134.6.2 Grey headed fruit bat/flying fox (*Pteropus poliocephalus*—Pteropodidae), as depicted by John Gould.

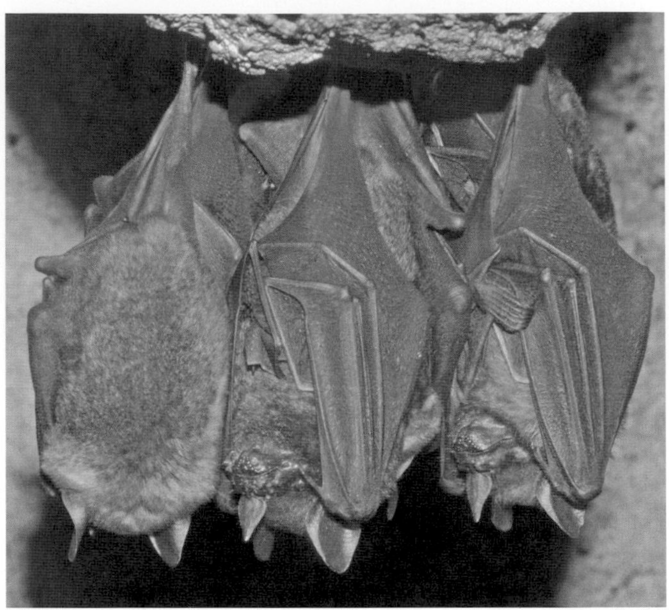

FIGURE 134.6.4 Seba'a short-tailed bat (*Carollia perspicillata*—Phyllostomidae) *(© David A. Warrell).*

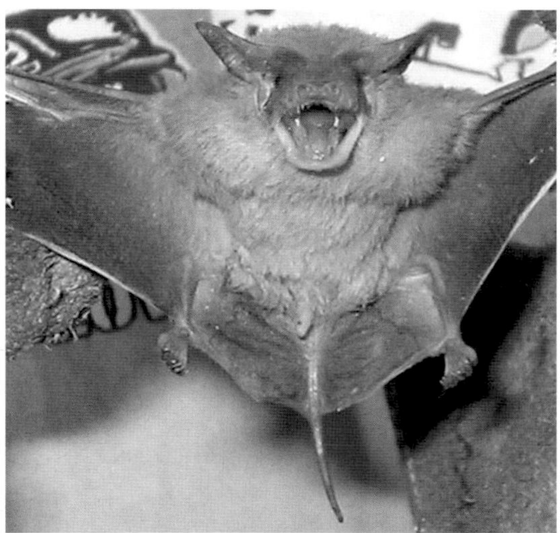

FIGURE 134.6.3 Mexican free-tailed bat (*Tadarida brasiliensis*—Molossidea) in Peru *(© Dr Ivan Vargas Meneses).*

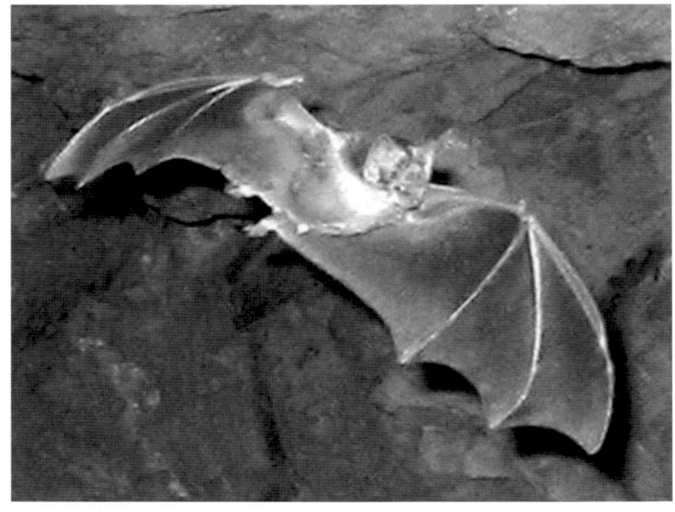

FIGURE 134.6.5 Common vampire bat (*Desmodus robustus*—Desmodontina) flying in a cave roost in Peru *(© Dr Ivan Vargas Meneses).*

BAT-TRANSMITTED INFECTIONS (Table 134.6-1)

RABIES AND RABIES-RELATED LYSSAVIRUSES

See Chapter 34.1 (Rabies) [3, 4]

Genotype 1 (classic) rabies

In the Americas, this virus has been found in bats of the families Molossidae, Phyllostomidae (both in true vampire bats Desmodontinae and in non-vampire bats, such as Seba's short-tailed leaf-nosed bat (*Carollia perspicillata*; Fig. 134.6.4)] and Vespertilionidae. It has been transmitted to humans by members of these families. In India, Genotype 1 was found in Pteropodidae, but transmission to humans has not yet been documented; in China, a patient died of bat-transmitted rabies in Jilin Province in 2002 (bat species and virus type unknown).

Vampire bat rabies (Latin America) [5, 6]

Vampire biology

The three species of true vampire bats (Desmodontinae) must be distinguished from non-hematophagous species that have been named "vampires", such as the spectral vampire bat (*Vampyrum spectrum*—Phyllostomidae)—the largest bat of the New World—and the false vampire bats (Megadermatidae) of Africa, Asia and Australia. The common vampire (*Desmodus rotundus*) (Figs 134.6.5, 134.6.6, 134.6.7), hairy-legged vampire (*Diphylla ecaudata*) and white-winged vampire (*Diaemus youngi*) are confined to Central and South America

TABLE 134.6-1 Viruses, bacteria, fungi and parasites that have been isolated from bats and are capable of causing human disease.

Human pathogen	Bat vector/reservoir	Geographical area
Viruses		
Orthoreoviruses		
Melaka* Pulau, Kampar	Pteropodidae	Malaysia
Orthobunyaviruses		
Kaeng Khoi	Molossidae	Thailand, Cambodia
Phleboviruses		
Toscana	Vespertilionidae	Mediterranean
Coronaviruses	Pteropodidae, Rhinolophidae, Phyllostomidae, Vespertilionidae	China, Brazil
Filoviruses		
Marburg, Ebola*	Pteropodidae, Rhinopholidae	Uganda, Gabon, Democratic Republic of Congo
Flaviviruses		
Dengue	Pteropodidae, Phyllostomidae	Costa Rica, Ecuador, south China
Ilheus	Mormoopidae, Phyllostomidae	Latin America
Japanese encephalitis	Rhinolophidae, Vespertilionidae	Japan, Taiwan
Kyasanur Forest	Pteropodidae, Rhinolophidae	India
Rio Bravo virus	Molossidae	USA, Mexico, Trinidad, Guatemala, Brazil
St Louis encephalitis	Molossidae, Mormoopidae, Phyllostomidae, Natalidae	USA, Guatemala, Trinidad
West Nile	Pteropodidae, Vepertilionidae	India, USA
Yellow fever	Molossidae, Mormoopidae	Ethiopia
Influenza viruses	Pteropodidae, Megadermatidae, Vespertilionidae	Kazakhstan
Paramyxoviruses	Pteropodidae	
Hendra*		Australia
Nipah*		Southeast Asia
Menangle*		Australia
Lyssaviruses		
Genotype I Classic rabies*	Ptropodidae, Molossidae, Phyllostomidae, Vespertilionidae	India, Americas
Genotype 4 Duvenhage virus*	Vespertilionidae	South Africa, Kenya
Genotype 5 European bat lyssavirus-1*	Pteropodidae, Molossidae, Rhinolophidae	Europe
Genotype 6 European bat lyssavirus-2*	Vestpertilionidae	Europe
Genotype 7 Australian bat lyssavirus*	Pteropodidae, Emballonuridae	Australia
Alphaviruses		
Chikungunya	Vespertilionidae	Senegal
Eastern equine encephalitis	Emballonuridae, Phyllostomidae	Latin America
Venezuelan equine encephalomyelitis	Phyllostomidae	Mexico, Guatemala, Ecuador, Panama, USA,
Western equine encephalitis	Phyllostomidae, Vespertilionidae	Panama, USA, Colombia
Bacteria		
Borrelia johnsonii	Vespertilionidae (Eptesicus fuscus)	Iowa, USA (in *Carios kelleyi* bat ticks)
Leptospira	Phyllostomidae, Pteropodidae	Brazil, Peru, Trinidad, Australia
Brucella	*Desmodus rotundus*	Brazil
Fungi		
Histoplasma capsulatum	*Mormoopidae, Vespertilionidae, Natilidae Phyllostomidae*	Panama, Mexico, Colombia, Trinidad, USA
Scopulariopsis, Geomyces, Trichophyton, Aphanoascus, Myceliophthora, Chrysosporium spp.	Rhinolophidae, Vespertilionidae	Mexico, Colombia, France

Evidence of direct or indirect bat to human transmission is documented in cases marked *, but varies with the other pathogens

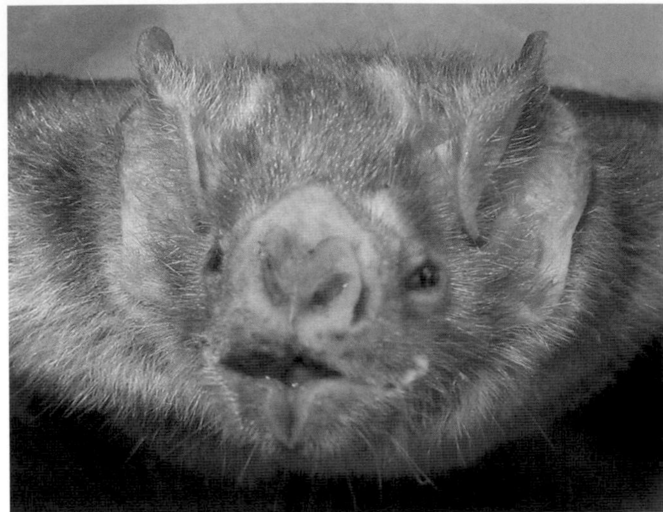

FIGURE 134.6.6 Common vampire bat (*Desmodus robustus*—Desmodontina) showing cleft in lower lip for sucking up the blood meal *(© Dr Ivan Vargas Meneses).*

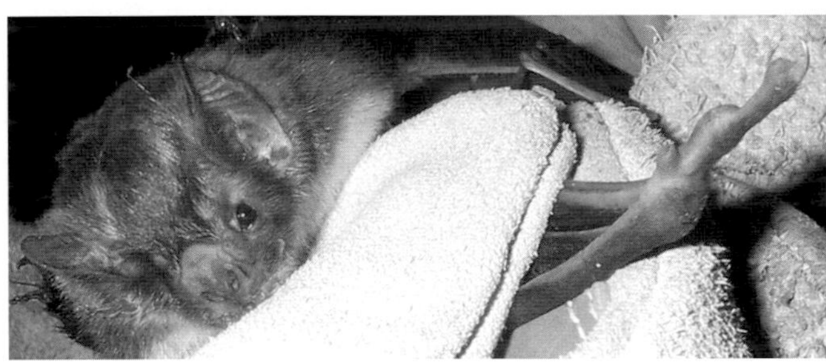

FIGURE 134.6.7 Common vampire bat (*Desmodus robustus*—Desmodontina) showing the enlarged thumb enabling quadrupedal gait *(© Dr Ivan Vargas Meneses).*

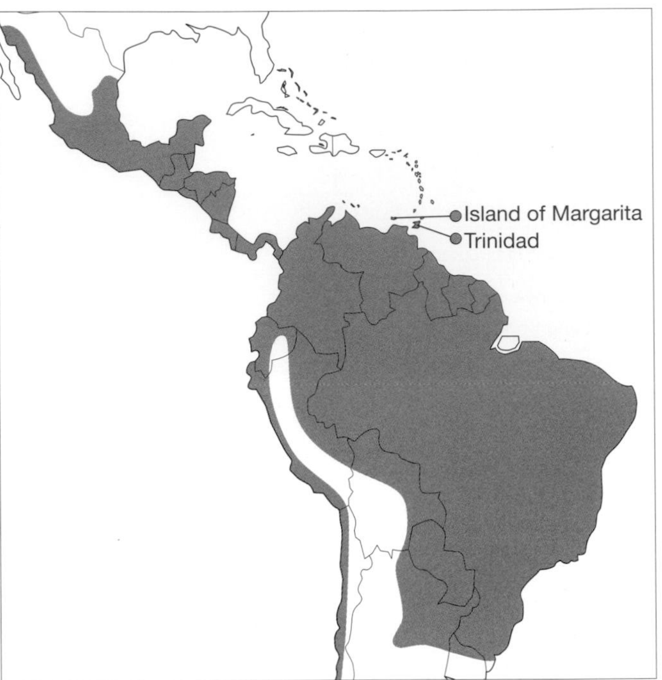

FIGURE 134.6.8 World distribution of vampire bats *(© David A. Warrell).*

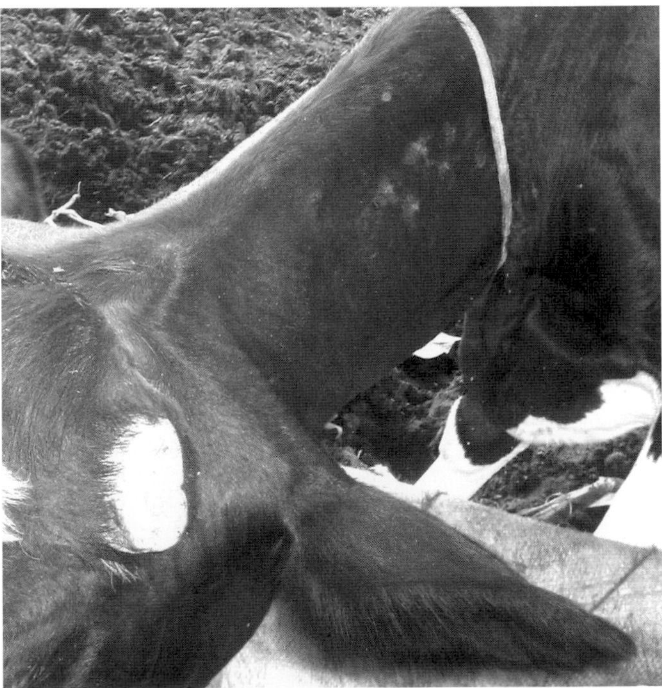

FIGURE 134.6.9 Bite sites of vampire bats on a cow in Peru *(© Dr Ivan Vargas Meneses).*

(Fig. 134.6.8). Vampire bats feed at night on the blood of vertebrates (Figs 134.6.9, 134.6.10): mammals, birds and reptiles. *Diaemus* and *Diphylla* feed largely on birds, while *Desmodus* prefers mammals, especially large domestic herbivores. Self-sharpening incisor and canine teeth are modified to allow painless venesection. The vampire's saliva flows down a groove on the dorsal surface of its tongue into the wound. Salivary toxins increase capillary permeability, inhibit platelet aggregation, inhibit activated factors X and IX ("draculin") and activate plasminogen ("desmoteplase"—currently being developed as a thrombolytic drug, DSPA-alpha-1).

These anti-hemostatic factors ensure blood flow from the wound that the bat sucks up through a cleft in its protruded lower lip (Fig. 134.6.6), underneath its tongue along paired ventral grooves. Predation is facilitated by vampires' ability to clamber, hop and spring using their hind legs and enlarged thumb (Fig. 134.6.7). Vampires can regurgitate blood when they return to the roost, feeding not only their young and relatives, but also other members of the colony—altruistic behavior that is unique among animals. Vampires roost in jungle caves (Fig. 134.6.11), hollow trees and in man-made tunnels and drains (Fig. 134.6.12).

Rabies epizootics

Rabies (classic genotype 1) is enzootic in many, but not all, vampire bat populations. Since the late 14th century, European explorers of the Caribbean and South America reported the association between vampire bat attacks and fatal human illness. Ecologic changes, such as destruction of forest and introduction of cattle ranching, construction of trans-Amazonian highways, the invasion of newly-accessible jungle by gold miners and electric power failures, have led to small epidemics of human rabies transmitted by vampires. These have accounted for more than 500 deaths since 1975, usually affecting rural communities of indigenous Amerindians, such as the Warao

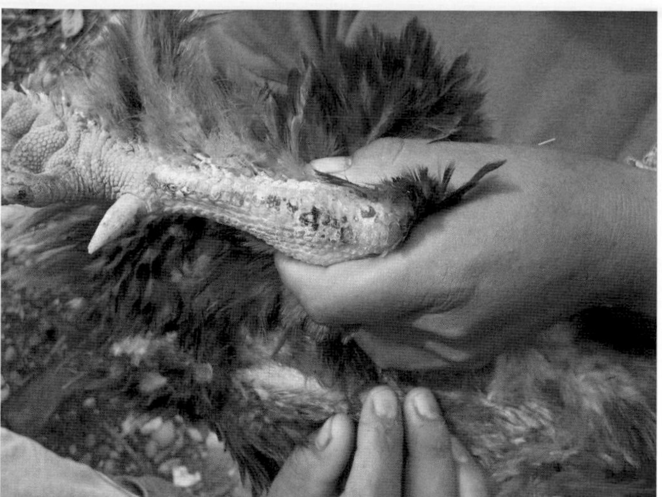

FIGURE 134.6.10 Bite sites of vampire bats on a chicken in Peru *(© Dr Ivan Vargas Meneses).*

in north-east Venezuela. There have been recent outbreaks in Colombia (Chocó, Santander), Peru (Condorcanqui, Bagna, Puerto Maldanado, Ayacucho), Brazil (Para, Maranhão) and Venezuela (Delta Amacuro). Humans are bitten at night on their extremities, ears and faces. Children appear particularly vulnerable. They may not wake up but discover bleeding wounds showing a double puncture made by the incisors (Fig. 134.6.12) or a depressed lesion with raised edge (Figs 134.6.13 and 134.6.14) in the morning. Mosquito nets are normally protective but accessible body parts may be attacked and the vampire's melena stool may be found staining the net (Fig. 134.6.15). Historical epidemics of vampire bat rabies, such as occurred in Trinidad from 1929, were characterized by predominantly paralytic disease, but a minority of patients develop hydrophobia and other features of furious rabies. Vampire bat-related strains of classic Genotype 1 rabies virus have been found in many South American wild and domestic mammals and have been transmitted to humans, for example by pet marmosets in Brazil.

Annually, bovine rabies of vampire bat origin ("derriengue") kills 30,000 cattle in Brazil and 100,000 cattle in the whole of South America, with considerable economic loss. "Derriengue" means limping illness, emphasizing its paralytic nature.

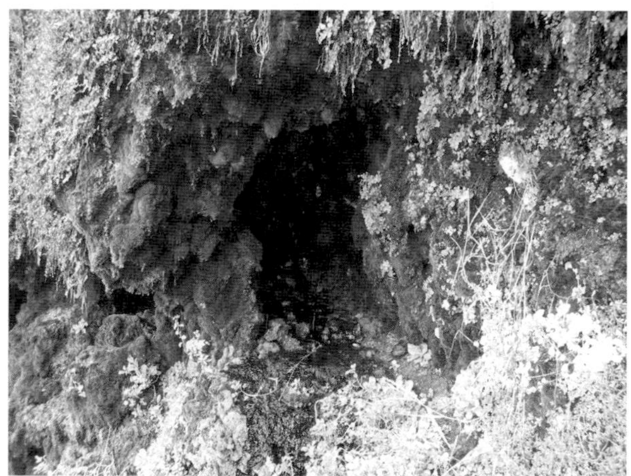

FIGURE 134.6.11 Natural cave roost for vampire bats in Peru *(© Dr Ivan Vargas Meneses).*

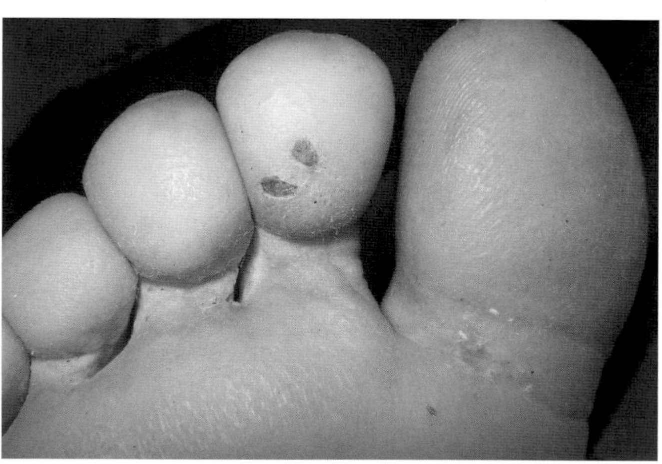

FIGURE 134.6.13 Bite inflicted by a vampire bat in Puerto Maldonado, Peru *(© Dr Ivan Vargas Meneses).*

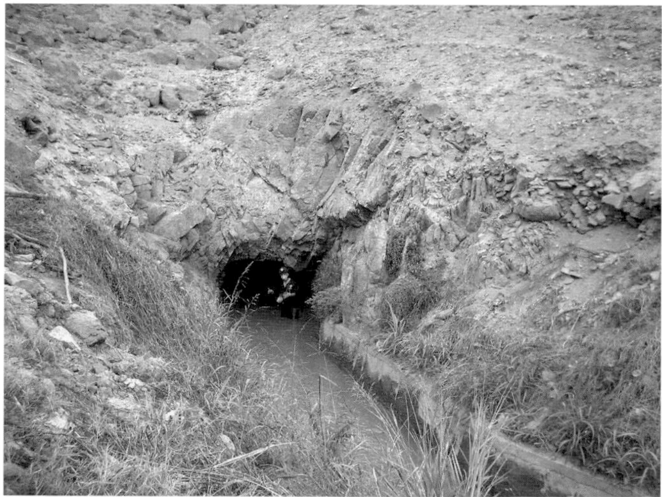

FIGURE 134.6.12 Irrigation drain used as a roost for vampire bats in Peru *(© Dr Ivan Vargas Meneses).*

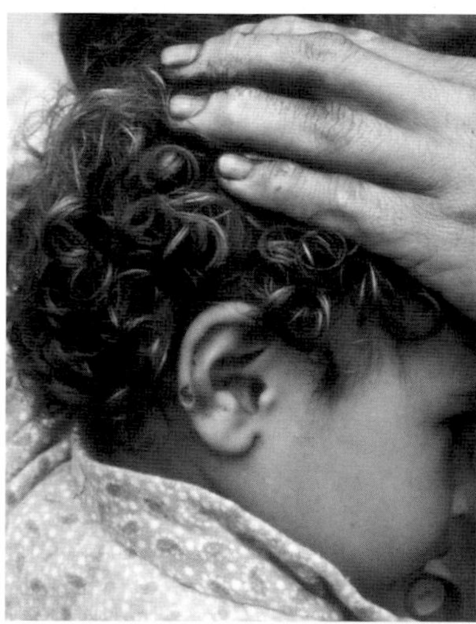

FIGURE 134.6.14 Bite inflicted by a vampire bat in Tapirai, São Paulo State, Brazil *(© João Luiz Costa Cardoso).*

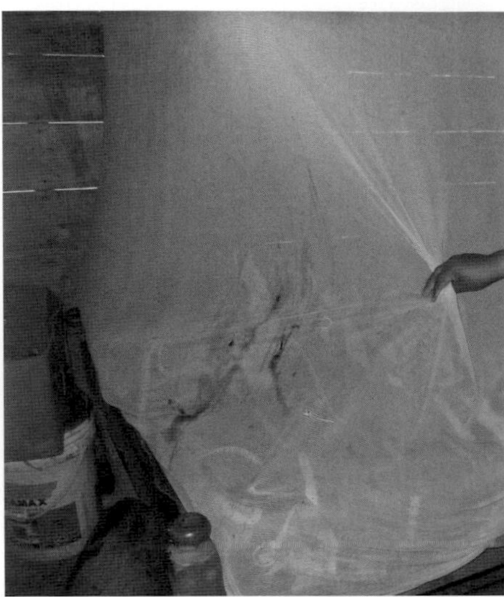

FIGURE 134.6.15 Mosquito net through which a man was bitten by a vampire in Puerto Maldonado, Peru. Note the bat's melena stool staining the net *(© Dr Ivan Vargas Meneses).*

Prevention and control of vampire bat rabies [6]

People, especially children, living in areas where vampire bat bites are common should, ideally, be protected by rabies pre-exposure immunization, but this is rarely practicable. However, the high risk of fatal rabies in affected communities (e.g. 16 of 57 people bitten by vampires in one village in north-east Brazil) reflects the inaccessibility of post-exposure prophylaxis. Bat proofing of dwellings and sleeping under mosquito nets affords some protection and electric house lighting may deter vampires. Vampires are highly susceptible to anticoagulants, such as warfarin, which can be distributed to vampire colonies by capturing the bats and releasing them after plastering them with warfarin paste. Treatment of cattle with controlled doses of warfarin will kill vampires feeding on them. Cattle can be vaccinated using adjuvanted Pasteur Virus strain (PV) vaccine and vampires themselves with recombinant vaccinia-vaccine.

Non-vampire bat rabies

In the USA, 30 of the 40 cases of human rabies reported between 1995 and 2008 were attributed to bat strains of Genotype 1 rabies virus. Fifteen were associated with *Lasionycteris noctivagans* or *Pipistrellus subflavus,* 11 with *Tadarida brasiliensis,* and 1 each with *Myotis* spp. and *Eptesicus fuscus.* However, there was a clear history of a bat bite in only a few of these cases, although some had been in direct contact with bats and others had bats in their homes. This suggests the possibility of subtle contact such as the bat's licking an open wound or intact mucous membranes of a sleeping person [7, 8]. Bat strains of Genotype 1 appear more tolerant of low temperatures and are more able to replicate in endothelial cells than canine strains of Genotype 1. The survival of three American children from bat-transmitted rabies may also suggest decreased virulence of bat strains. Aerosol transmission of rabies was claimed to explain infection of two visitors to Frio Caves in Texas inhabited by 20–30 million *T. brasilensis,* but it is far more likely that they were infected transdermally.

In Asia, evidence of serotype 1 infection was found in insectivorous and frugivorous bats in Cambodia and China.

Genotype 2 Lagos Bat Virus (LGV)

Lyssavirus Genotype 2 is grouped together with Genotype 3 Mokola virus (not found in bats) in Phylogroup II. Although human disease has not been reported, direct or serologic evidence of Lagos bat virus (LGV) infection has been found in several species of fruit bats (Pteropodidae) in Africa: the very widely distributed straw-coloured fruit bat (*Eidolon helvum*) that is often eaten as "bush meat", epauletted fruit bats (*Epomophorsu, Epomops* and *Micropteropus* spp.), Egyptian rousettes (*Rousettus aegyptiacus*); and in vespertilionid species: long-winged bats (*Miniopterus* spp.) and Gambian slit-faced bats (*Nycteris gambiensis*). A new LGV-like lyssavirus (Shomoni virus) has been described in a Commerson's leaf-nosed bat (*Hipposideros commersoni*) in coastal Kenya. Seroprevalence of LGV is 30–70% in *R. aegyptiacus* and *E. helvum.* Serologic evidence of LGV-like infection was found in insectivorous and frugivorous bats in Cambodia.

Genotype 4 Duvenhage virus

Lyssavirus Genotype 4 has been found in insectivorous and frugivorous bats, such as the Egyptian slit-faced bat (*Nycteris thebaica*—Nycteridae), the common bent-wing bat (*Miniopterus schreibersii*) and other vespertilionid species in east and southern Africa. The three identified human cases in South Africa and Kenya showed clinical features indistinguishable from classic rabies encephalomyelitis.

Genotype 5 and 6 European Bat Lyssavirus (EBLV)

This genotype is the only zoonotic virus in European bats. European bat lyssaviurs (EBLV)-1 infection has been found in sorentine bats (*Eptesicus sorentinus*) and *R. aegyptiacus* and EBLV-2 in Daubenton's bats (*Myotis daubentonii*), pond bats (*Myotis dasycneme*) and other *Myotis* spp. and greater horseshoe bats (*Rhinolophus ferrumequinum*).

Genotype 7 Australian Bat Lyssavirus (ABLV)

Genotype 7 Australian bat lyssavirus (ABLV) was first isolated from a black flying fox (*Pteropus alecto*) in New South Wales in 1996 and subsequently from three other species of flying fox (*Pteropus poliocephalus, Pteropus scapulatus, Pteropus conspicillatus*) and one species of insectivorous bat, the yellow-bellied sheath tailed bat (*Saccolaimus flaviventris*—Emballonuridae). Two Queensland women died of diseases indistinguishable from classic rabies, one five weeks after scratches by a *S. flaviventris* and the other more than two years after bites by a flying fox. In the Philippines, ABLV has been found in Lyle's flying foxes (*Pteropis lylei*) obtained from restaurants, and in *Miniopterus schreibersii* and great round-leafed bats (*Hipposideros armiger*) in Cambodia and Thailand.

Other rabies-related viruses

Aravan (Kyrghistan), Khujand (Tajikistan), Irkut (Siberia) and West Caucasian bat lyssaviruses (Phylogroup I) have not yet been classified. They have been isolated in one African and one Eurasian bat. Serologic evidence of West Caucasian bat virus was found in long-winged bats (*Miniopterus* spp.—Vespertilionidae) in Kenya and of Aravan and Khujand bat viruses in Indian fruit bats (*Pteropus giganteus*—Pteropodidae) in Bangladesh, Irkut and in Thailand (*Pteropus lylei*). No transmission to humans has been described.

FILOVIRUSES: MARBURG VIRUS AND EBOLA VIRUS [9, 10]

The environmental reservoirs and vectors of these deadly hemorrhagic fevers have long been debated, but, in Uganda, serologic and PCR evidence of Ebola and Marburg virus infections has been found in Egyptian fruit bats or rousettes (*R. aegyptiacus*), suggesting that this species may be a natural host of both viruses. Evidence of Lake Victoria Marburg virus has been found in *R. aegyptiacus* in Kitum Cave, Mount Elgon, Kenya, and Python and Kitaka Caves in Uganda—sites where humans have been infected. Touching bat feces or being hit by low-flying bats were identified as possible risk factors for acquisition of the infection. Insectivorous bats, such as greater long-fingered bats *Miniopterus inflatus* (Vespertilionidae), and horseshoe bats (*Rhinolophus elocuens*) and round leaf bats (*Hipposideros* spp. Rhinolophidae) have also been implicated in Gabon, Democratic Republic of Congo and Uganda. In Democratic Republic of Congo, hunting of bats, such as migratory hammer-headed or big-lipped bats (*Hypsignathus monstrosus* Pteropodidae) for human consumption was linked to the 2007 outbreak of Ebola virus. In the Philippines, Ebola virus Reston has been found in domestic pigs. Several asymptomatic human infections were reported.

PARAMYXOVIRUSES (NIPAH, HENDRA, MENANGLE) [11]

Three emerging paramyxovirus infections have been described for which bats are the likely natural reservoirs and domestic horses and pigs have proved to be the amplifying vectors for human infection. Hendra and Nipah viruses are Henipaviruses; Menangle is a rubulavirus.

Hendra virus [12]

In 1994, there was an outbreak of fatal respiratory disease in horses and humans in Australia, attributed to a new pathogen, Hendra virus, whose natural reservoir is *Pteropus* spp. (*P. alecto, P. poliocephalus, P. scapulatus, P. conspicillatus*). There have been 13 subsequent outbreaks. In 2008, 2009 and 2011, equine and human victims showed primarily encephalitic features. Among six human cases, three died.

Nipah virus [11]

In 1998, there was an epidemic of encephalitis in Malaysia and Singapore affecting pigs and pig-handlers in whom the case fatality was more than 40%. The causative virus, named Nipah after an affected village, is closely related to Hendra virus. *Pteropus vampyrus* and *Pteropus hypomelanus* are the natural reservoirs. There were outbreaks in Bangladesh in 2001, 2003 and 2004 (case fatality >74%) and in adjacent West Bengal in 2001. So far, more than 440 human cases of Nipah virus encephalitis have been diagnosed. The epidemics have been attributed to disruption of Pteropus ecology by deforestation (e.g. building the new Kuala Lumpur airport), which displaced the bats from their traditional roosts to agricultural areas where they have contact with domestic animals and humans. In Bangladesh, where there have been 130 deaths, human-to-human transmission within families has been inferred.

Menangle and Tioman viruses have been isolated from *Pteropus* spp. in Australia and Malaysia, and from sick pigs. Influenza-like illness in pig farmers with Menangle sero-conversion has been reported.

OTHER VIRUSES

Many of the other viruses that have been isolated from bats have not been proved to be either transmissible to humans, directly or indirectly, or to cause human disease. These include severe acute respiratory syndrome (SARS) viruses [13], the Arenavirus Tacaribe virus, Orthoreoviruse Nelson Bay virus [14], Mojuí dos Campos, Bimiti, Catu, Guama, Manzanilla, Nepuyo, Oriboca, Montana myotis leukoencephalitis, Tamana bat, Nepuyo, Catu, Mount Elgon bat, Entebbe and Astroviruses.

BACTERIAL INFECTIONS

Leptospira and *Brucella* have both been reported to occur naturally in bats. Leptospira-infected bats are found in Asia and Europe, as well as the Americas. *Brucella* infection has been found in vampire bats in Brazil. Bats can be infected with enteric bacteria such as *Samonella* spp. and *Escherichia coli*, but transmission to humans has not been reported. Transmission of Hansen's disease (*Mycobacterium leprosum*) by vampire bats has been suspected but not proven.

Histoplasmosis

Bat guano provides a rich medium for the growth of *Histoplasma capsulatum*; environment in the bat roost fosters this growth. Humans exposed to dried guano have suffered massive infection and death by inhalation.

OTHER FUNGI

Many other fungi have been found in association with bat roosts, including *Candida* and *Scopulariopsis* and *Geomyces* spp. (including White-Nosed Syndrome (WNS) fungus of bats see above), which can infect humans. The involvement of bats seems limited to the provision of a rich environment in the roost as a culture medium for these organisms.

PROTOZOA

Trypanosoma evansi, the causative agent of surra in domestic animals, has been demonstrated in vampire bats. These bats can mechanically transmit the trypanosome from host to host. *Trypanosoma cruzi* has been reported also, but evidence for transmission to humans is lacking.

PREVENTION OF BAT-TRANSMITTED INFECTIONS

For measures against vampire bat rabies see above. Ideally, bats and humans should not share the same microenvironment, but bats are rightly protected in many countries and so expert advice should be sought if they are found roosting in attics. An aggressive bat is likely to be unwell, perhaps rabid. All case of scratches, bites and possible mucosal contact should be reviewed for possible post-exposure rabies prophylaxis. Even the handling of a dead bat has been associated with transmission. Grounded, trapped or sick bats should, ideally, be handled only by experts and never without gloves. The risk of inhaling aerosolized fungal spores and acquiring other bat-related diseases must be recognized by cave explorers (spelunkers) and prevented by wearing appropriate clothing and masks.

REFERENCES

1. Calisher CH, Childs JE, Field HE, et al. Bats: important reservoir hosts of emerging viruses. Clin Microbiol Rev 2006;19:531–45.
2. Wong S, Lau S, Woo P, Yuen KY. Bats as a continuing source of emerging infections in humans. Rev Med Virol 2007;17:67–91.
3. McElhinney LM, Marston DA, Stankov S, et al. Molecular epidemiology of lyssaviruses in Eurasia. Dev Biol (Basel) 2008;131:125–31.
4. Banyard AC, Hayman D, Johnson N, et al. Bats and lyssaviruses. Adv Virus Res 2011;79:239–89.
5. Greenhall AM, Schmidt U, eds. Natural History of Vampire Bats. Boca Raton: CRC Press; 1988.
6. Schneider MC, Romijn PC, Uieda W, et al. Rabies transmitted by vampire bats to humans: an emerging zoonotic disease in Latin America? Rev Panam Salud Publica 2009;25:260–9.
7. Warrell MJ. Human deaths from cryptic bat rabies in the USA. Lancet 1995;346:65.
8. Gibbons RV. Cryptogenic rabies, bats, and the question of aerosol transmission. Ann Emerg Med 2002;39:528–36.
9. Pourrut X, Souris M, Towner JS, et al. Large serological survey showing cocirculation of Ebola and Marburg viruses in Gabonese bat populations, and a high seroprevalence of both viruses in *Rousettus aegyptiacus*. BMC Infect Dis 2009;9:159.
10. Kuzmin IV, Niezgoda M, Franka R, et al. Marburg virus in fruit bat, Kenya. Emerg Infect Dis 2010;16:352–4.
11. Wild TF. Henipaviruses: a new family of emerging Paramyxoviruses. Pathol Biol (Paris) 2009;57:188–96.
12. Field H, Schaaf K, Kung N, et al. Hendra virus outbreak with novel clinical features, Australia. Emerg Infect Dis 2010;16:338–40.
13. Wang LF, Shi Z, Zhang S, et al. Review of bats and SARS. Emerg Infect Dis 2006;12:1834–40.
14. Chua KB, Voon K, Crameri G, et al. Identification and characterization of a new orthoreovirus from patients with acute respiratory infections. PLoS One 2008;3:e3803.

135 Pentastomiasis

David A Warrell

Key features

- Pentastomiasis (synonyms: porocephalosis, linguatulosis, or linguatuliasis) is caused by maxillopod crustaceans known as pentastomids or pentastomes
- *Linguatula* infection is acquired by eating raw offal. In humans, migrating larvae cause obstructive symptoms in various organs or acute nasopharyngeal pentastomiasis (Halzoun or Marrara syndrome)
- *Armillifer* infection is acquired by eating raw snake meat or drinking water contaminated by snakes. Unless infection is massive, it is asymptomatic but revealed by appearance of calcified larvae on abdominal radiographs
- There is no proven chemotherapy, but ivermectin, praziquantel, or mebendazole could be tried in severe symptomatic cases; surgery may be needed to relieve obstructive symptoms
- Prevention is by avoiding eating raw meat and boiling drinking water

INTRODUCTION

Pentastomiasis, also termed porocephalosis, linguatulosis, or linguatuliasis, is a zoonosis caused by pentastomids or pentastomes, now considered a subclass of maxillopod crustaceans [1]. The name pentastome derives from the appearance of two pairs of hooks above the mouth giving "five mouths", while "lingua" refers to the resemblance of some pentastomes to an animal's tongue, hence an alternative name "tongue worm". Adults inhabit the respiratory tracts of their definitive vertebrate hosts – dogs and other carnivorous mammals in the case of *Linguatula* spp., and snakes and other reptiles in the case of *Armillifer* spp. They attach to respiratory tract epithelium by their peri-oral hooks and suck up blood and other tissues, tissue fluids, and secretions [2]. The more than 100 species belong to orders Cephalobaenida (e.g. genus *Raillietiella*) and Porocephalida (e.g. genera *Linguatula, Armillifer, Porocephalus, Leiperia* and *Sebekia*). More than ten species are recognized zoonotic parasites of humans [3, 4]. Visceral pentastomiasis is most often caused by *Linguatula serrata* or *Armillifer armillatus.* Nasopharyngeal pentastomiasis ("Halzoun" or "Marrara syndrome") is caused by *L. serrata*. Subcutaneous pentastomiasis is caused by *Raillietella* and *Sebekia* spp. [3].

LINGUATULA *SPECIES*

Linguatula serrata occurs in Europe, the Middle East, Africa, and North, Central and South America, where canids are the definitive hosts. In some parts of the Middle East, more than 50% of stray dogs are infected with *L. serrata*. These animals harbor adults and larvae in their upper respiratory tracts and shed ova in their nasal secretions, saliva, and feces onto wet vegetation or into water. Ova are ingested by herbivorous intermediate hosts and by humans who can be infected directly by contact with dogs' nasal secretions or contaminated food, developing visceral pentastomiasis and becoming intermediate hosts. Humans can also be infected by ingesting infected offal from ruminants; in which case, they develop nasopharyngeal pentastomiasis ("Halzoun"), becoming temporary definitive hosts. *Linguatula* ova hatch in the gut lumen releasing larvae which burrow into the tissues and encyst. When the intermediate hosts are eaten by carnivores, third-stage larvae hatch from the cysts and migrate to the lungs and nasopharynx where they mature.

CLINICAL FEATURES (LINGUATULOSIS) [5]

VISCERAL PENTASTOMIASIS

When humans ingest *Linguatula* ova, larvae hatch in the gut, burrow through its wall, migrate through the tissues and encyst mainly in the liver. Later larval stages can obstruct or compress biliary, gastrointestinal or respiratory tracts, meninges, brain, or the anterior chamber of the eye, causing iritis and secondary glaucoma.

NASOPHARYNGEAL PENTOSTOMIASIS ("HALZOUN" IN LEBANON, "MARRARA SYNDROME" IN THE SUDAN)

This follows ingestion of raw liver or lymph nodes from sheep, goats, cattle, buffalo, camels, and lagomorphs, containing encysted or migrating third-stage larvae. Larvae migrate from the stomach up the esophagus to the nasopharynx mucosa [6, 7]. Within minutes to a few hours of eating the infected viscera, there is intense irritation of the upper respiratory and gastrointestinal tracts causing coughing, sneezing, rhinorrhea, retching, vomiting, lacrimation, hemoptysis, epistaxis, cervical lymphadenopathy, transient deafness, difficulty in speaking, dysphagia, wheezing, dyspnea, edema of the face and oropharynx, and urticaria. These clinical features suggest a hypersensitivity reaction. Wriggling larvae 5–10 mm long are found in sputum and vomitus. Patients who survive the acute upper airway obstruction usually recover in 1–2 weeks. Persistent infections are rare.

ARMILLIFER *(POROCEPHALUS) SPECIES*

These annulated, non-segmented parasites of up to 20 cm long inhabit the respiratory and digestive tracts of snakes, lizards, crocodilians, and other vertebrates (Fig. 135.1). Human infections have been reported from Africa (especially West Africa), Southeast Asia, the Far East, and America. Ova shed in the snake's nasal secretions and picked up by rodents and other mammals hatch, releasing larvae that encyst in the tissues but will develop into nymphs if ingested by the definitive host. Humans may ingest ova by drinking water contaminated by snakes or by handling pet snakes (including pythons kept as revered peri-domestic totems in West Africa) and then licking their fingers.

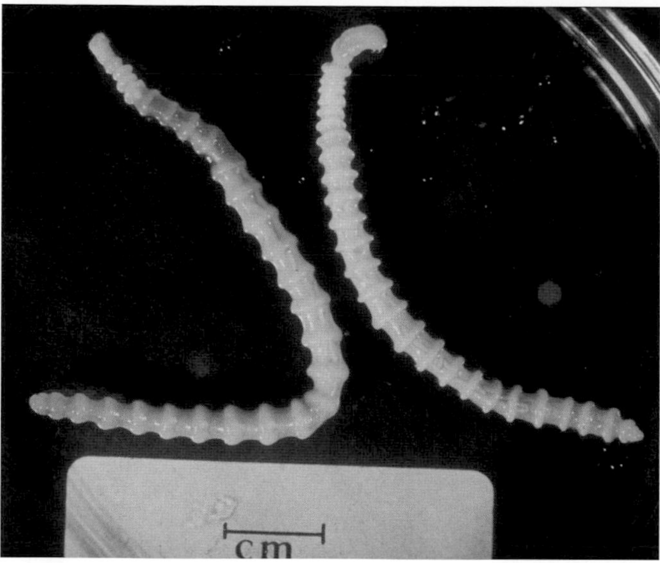

FIGURE 135.1 Pentastomes from the respiratory tract of an Egyptian cobra (*Naja haje*).

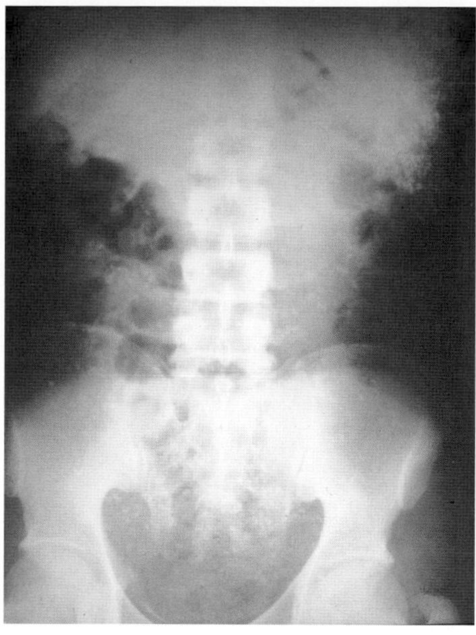

FIGURE 135.2 Straight abdominal radiograph showing characteristic crescentic calcified pentastome larvae, especially dense over the liver.

Ova, larvae, and adult pentastomids may be ingested by eating raw snake as part of widespread *ju ju* rituals in west and central Africa and Southeast Asia, and for medicinal reasons in the Far East. In humans, ingested eggs hatch in the gut, releasing larvae that burrow into the tissues where they encyst, die and calcify or mature, excyst and migrate. Various species infect humans, including *A. armillatus* (Africa and Arabia), *Armillifer grandis* (Africa), *Armillifer moniliformis* (Southeast Asia), *Armillifer agkistrodonti* [8] and *Porocephalus taiwani* (China) [9], *Porocephalus crotali* (USA) [10], and *Leiperia cincinnalis* (Africa).

EPIDEMIOLOGY

Judged by the discovery of calcified larvae in thoracic and abdominal radiographs, these infections can be prevalent in some parts of the world. In south-west Nigeria, they were seen in 7% of men aged 50–59 years, appearing as discrete, crescent-shaped, soft tissue calcifications, 4–8 mm in size, especially in the right upper quadrant because they are situated beneath the peritoneum covering the liver (Fig. 135.2). At autopsy, the prevalence exceeded 20% in some parts of Africa [11].

CLINICAL FEATURES (POROCEPHALOSIS)

Infection is usually asymptomatic – the diagnosis being incidental by radiography or laparaotomy for other purposes or as a chance finding at autopsy. Mass migration of larvae from the gut into the tissue following ingestion of many ova or adult female pentastomes may produce a variety of symptoms and signs, including fever, abdominal pain, diarrhea, hepatosplenomegaly, and obstructive jaundice prompting laparotomy at which hundreds of wriggling nymphs may be discovered beneath the visceral peritoneum. Hemorrhagic enterocolitis and intestinal obstruction, secondary bacterial septicemia and pneumonia are described in the rare fatal cases [11, 12]. The peritoneum, liver and biliary tract, lungs, pleura, pericardium, central nervous system, and anterior chamber of the eye may be affected by the migrating larvae, leading to inflammatory and obstructive symptoms [13].

SUBCUTANEOUS PENTASTOMIASIS

Subcutaneous creeping eruptions, resembling cutaneous larva migrans or larva currens have been associated with *Raillietella hemidactyli* infections in Vietnam, resulting from ingestion of living lizards and with *Sebekia* spp. in Costa Rica [3].

INVESTIGATIONS

Severe infections are associated with neutrophil leukocytosis, sometimes with eosinophila and other features of an inflammatory response and anemia, but results of other routine investigations, including hepatic enzymes, are normal. The crescentic calcified pentastomid larvae produce a distinctive radiographic appearance. Unlike cysticerci, they are not found in muscle, but they must be distinguished from calcified mesenteric lymph glands and calculi [14]. They are usually numerous and most dense in the lower lung fields and abdomen (especially the right upper quadrant) reflecting their subperitoneal disposition. Ultrasound and imaging may detect hyperechoic/dense lesions in the peritoneum, liver, and other viscera, resembling tumors [15].

DIAGNOSIS

Pentastomes may be discovered accidentally in the liver, intestinal wall and other tissues at surgery or autopsy [11]. Their macroscopic and histologic appearances are well-described [12, 16]. Pentastomids have also been identified by consensus PCR [10] and immunologic tests are being developed.

TREATMENT

There is no proven effective chemotherapy for pentostomiasis, but ivermectin, praziquantel, and mebendazole have been used with apparent success in individual cases. This should be reserved for severe and symptomatic cases. Obstruction and compression should be relieved surgically. Hypersensitivity phenomena (halzoun) should be treated with adrenaline (epinephrine), antihistamines, and corticosteroids.

PREVENTION

Pentostomiasis can be prevented by thoroughly cooking all meat of any origin, but especially of the key host species and boiling and/or filtering of drinking water. Eating sheep's lymph nodes is proscribed by the Shiite Moslems of Lebanon.

REFERENCES

1. Haugerud RE. Evolution in the pentastomids. Parasitol Today 1989;5:126–32.
2. Riley J. The biology of pentastomids. Adv Parasitol 1986;25:45–128.
3. Drabick JJ. Pentastomiasis. Rev Infect Dis 1987;9:1087–94.
4. Fain A. The Pentastomida parasitic in man. Annales de la Societé Belge de Medecine Tropicale 1975;55:59–64.
5. Self JT, Hopps HC, Williams AO. Review. Pentastomiasis in Africans. Trop Geogr Med 1975;27:1–13.
6. Schacher JF, Khalil GM, Salman S. A field study of Halzoun (parasitic pharyngitis) in Lebanon. J Trop Med Hyg 1965;68:226–30.
7. Yagi H, el Bahari S, Mohamed HA, et al. The Marrara syndrome: a hypersensitivity reaction of the upper respiratory tract and buccopharyngeal mucosa to nymphs of *Linguatula serrata*. Acta Trop 1996;16:127–34.
8. Chen SH, Liu Q, Zhang YN, et al. Multi-host model-based identification of *Armillifer agkistrodontis* (Pentastomida), a new zoonotic parasite from China. PLoS Negl Trop Dis 2010;4(4):e647.
9. Yao MH, Wu F, Tang LF. Human pentastomiasis in China: case report and literature review. J Parasitol 2008;94(6):1295–8.
10. Brookins MD, Wellehan JF, Roberts JF, et al. Massive visceral pentastomiasis caused by *Porocephalus crotali* in a dog. Vet Pathol 2009;46:460–3.
11. Yapo Ette H, Fanton L, Adou Bryn KD, et al. Human pentastomiasis discovered postmortem. Forensic Sci Int 2003;137:52–4.
12. Tappe D, Büttner DW. Diagnosis of human visceral pentastomiasis. PLoS Negl Trop Dis 2009;3:e320.
13. Lang Y, Garzozi H, Epstein Z, et al. Intraocular pentastomiasis causing unilateral glaucoma. Br J Ophthalmol 1987;71:391–5.
14. Palmer PES, Reeder MM, eds. Pentastomida. In: The Imaging of Tropical Diseases with Epidemiological, Pathological and Clinical Correlation. Berlin: Springer; 2001:389–95. Available at: http://tmcr.usuhs.mil/tmcr/chapter28/intro.htm (last accessed 1 March 2012).
15. Lai C, Wang XQ, Lin L, et al. Imaging features of pediatric pentastomiasis infection: a case report. Korean J Radiol 2010;11:480–4.
16. Ma KC, Qiu MH, Rong YL. Pathological differentiation of suspected cases of pentastomiasis in China. Trop Med Int Health 2002;7:166–77.

Injurious Arthropods 136

David A Warrell

Key features

- Hymenoptera venom anaphylaxis: stings by bees, vespids, and ants may lead to hypersensitization and anaphylaxis, preventable by desensitization with purified venoms and treatable with epinephrine (adrenaline)
- Bites by mosquitoes, midges, flies and other arthropods, and superficial infestations by fleas, lice, bedbugs, etc. are very common nuisances. They cause pruritus, papular urticaria and secondary bacterial infections and may result in hypersensitization
- Scabies remains prevalent in most parts of the world. It causes distressing symptoms and may be complicated by streptococcal infection leading to glomerulonephritis and rheumatic fever
- Skin, wounds and body cavities may be invaded by fly larvae (myiasis) and adult fleas (tungiasis), causing discomfort, infection and tissue destruction
- Spider bites are common in the Americas, Mediterranean, South Africa and Australia but there are few fatalities. Only recluse spiders (*Loxosceles*) are reliably associated with necrotic araneism. Bites by cosmopolitan black and brown widow spiders (*Latrodectus*), Latin American banana spiders (*Phoneutria*) and Sydney funnel web spiders (*Atrax*) cause neurotoxic araneism
- Scorpion stings still cause numerous fatalities in North and South Africa, the Middle East, Mexico, Latin America, and India. Severe local pain and systemic autonomic effects may be fatal, especially in children
- Mass attacks by bees or vespids are uncommon, except during the Africanized killer bee epidemic in the Americas, during which many fatalities occurred
- Lepidopterism and erucism: stinging hairs of many species of moths and their larvae (caterpillars) can excite cutaneous irritation, allergy and, in the case of caterpillars of the genus *Lonomia*, systemic envenoming

Bites and stings by arthropods may have a variety of pathologic consequences:

- allergic reactions – cutaneous or systemic;
- auto-immune reactions, such as endemic pemphigus foliaceus ("fogo selvagem") by *Simulium pruinosum* bites in Brazil (Fig. 136.1) [1];
- infection of the bite site by bacteria and other microorganisms;
- acquisition of systemic infections transmitted by the arthropod vector;
- envenoming.

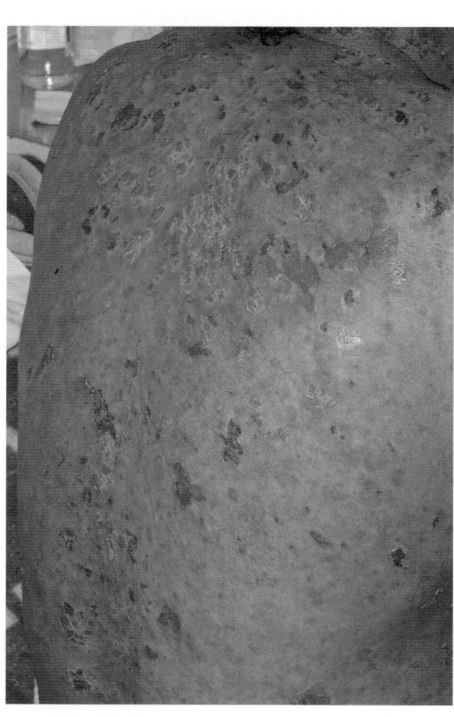

FIGURE 136.1 Fogo salvagem – endemic pemphigus foliaceus, an autoimmune disease associated with bites by black flies (*Simulium pruinosum*) in some parts of South America *(© David A. Warrell).*

ALLERGIC REACTIONS TO ARTHROPODS

Cutaneous, respiratory and systemic hypersensitivity reactions may be caused by a large variety of arthropods. Sensitization results from inoculation of salivary protein allergens during a blood meal in the case of mosquitoes, sandflies, midges, fleas, bed bugs and lice; contact with urticating hairs of Lepidoptera larvae; inhalation of aerosolized arthropod allergens, such as those of non-biting chironomid midges (*Cladotanytarsus lewisi* "green nimmiti" in North and East Africa) [2], or injection of venoms, most commonly by Heminoptera stings. Allergic effects of arthropod proteins must be distinguished from (i) direct toxic effects of their venoms which, by releasing histamine and other mediators, may produce identical clinical effects, (ii) from infections transmitted by these vectors and (iii) secondary infection of the bite wounds.

REFERENCES

1. Culton DA, Qian Y, Li N, et al. Advances in pemphigus and its endemic pemphigus foliaceus (Fogo Selvagem) phenotype: a paradigm of human autoimmunity. J Autoimmun 2008;31:311–24.
2. Tee RD, Cranston PS, Kay AB. Further characterisation of allergens associated with hypersensitivity to the "green nimitti" midge (*Cladotanytarsus lewisi*, Diptera: Chironomidae). Allergy 1987;42:12–9.

136.1 Hypersensitization and Anaphylaxis Caused by Stings of Hymenopteran Insects (Bees, Wasps, Yellow Jackets, Hornets, Ants)

These include members of the families Apidae (e.g. honey bees – *Apis mellifera, Apis cerania, Apis dorsata*, etc. – and bumble bees, *Bombus* spp.), Vespidae [e.g. European wasps (*Vespula germanica, Vespula vulgaris*) American wasps, yellow-jackets and white-faced hornets (*Vespula* and *Dolichovespula* spp.) paper wasps (*Polistes* spp.) and European and Asian true hornets (*Vespa* spp.)], and Formicidae [e.g. American fire ants, genus *Solenopsis* (Fig. 136.1.1) and Australian bull or bulldog ants (*Myrmecia* spp.)]. Venom allergens include phospholipases A, hyaluronidase, acid phosphomonoesterases and polypeptide neurotoxins, such as apamin and melittin (*A. mellifera*). Non-allergenic compounds include vasoactive amines such as histamine, 5-hydroxytryptamine, catecholamines and kinins, cholinesterase (in the venom of *V. germanica*), pheromones, 2-methylpiperidine alkaloids (in venoms of fire ants, *Solenopsis* spp.) and anti-inflammatory peptides from honey bee venom, such as peptide 401 (mast cell degranulating peptide) [1].

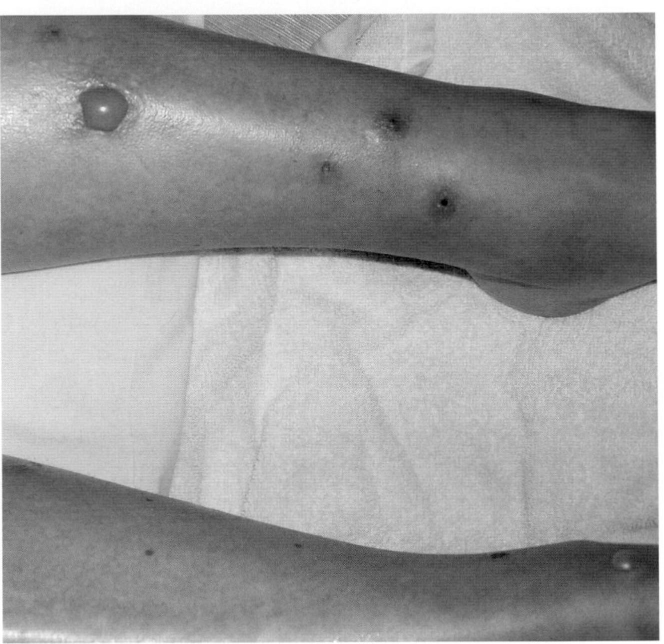

FIGURE 136.1.1 Multiple fire ant (*Solenopsis*) stings in Mexico *(Courtesy of Ms Jean Dickinson).*

EPIDEMIOLOGY

In the USA, 40–50 deaths per year are attributed to hymenoptera sting anaphylaxis; in England and Wales, fewer than 5; and in Australia, 2–3. In children, the annual incidence of systemic reactions to stings by hymenoptera has been reported to be 0.4–0.8% and in an adult population in the USA, the prevalence of systemic allergic sting reactions was found to be 4%, while 20 % of this population showed evidence of venom hypersensitivity by skin testing or radioallergosorbent testing (RAST). Most patients allergic to bee venom are beekeepers or their relatives [2, 3]. Two species of fire ants, *Solenopsis richteri* and *Solenopsis invicta*, were imported into the USA from South America in 1918 and have now spread to 13 southern states, where an estimated 2.5 million people are stung each month. The incidence of systemic allergic reactions is about 4 per 100,000 population per year, and there have been fatalities. In Tasmania and southern Australia, the jack jumper ant (*Myrmecia pilosula*) causes 90% of all ant stings. About 2–3% of the population are hypersensitive and fatal anaphylaxis has occurred [4].

PREVENTION

Patients who with a history of systemic anaphylaxis provoked by a sting and detectable venom-specific IgE should be considered for desensitization with purified venoms. This treatment proved significantly more effective than placebo or whole body extracts of hymenoptera in preventing anaphylactic reactions to sting challenge [5]. Desensitization involves a series of visits to the clinic for administration of gradually increasing doses of venom followed by years of maintenance therapy. Systemic reactions (anaphylaxis) occur in 5–15% of courses and local reactions in 50%.

Wasps are attracted by sweet things and meat in homes, greengrocers, orchards and vineyard. At night, hornets are attracted by light. Some species, such as the Asian *Vespa mandarina*, are so aggressively territorial that their nests must be eradicated before the area can be farmed. Vespid nests may be destroyed by fumigation with insecticides. In aggressive bee colonies, the queens should be replaced.

Death from anaphylaxis can be prevented by self-administered first-aid with epinephrine (adrenaline).

CLINICAL FEATURES

Symptoms of anaphylaxis may start within minutes of the sting. They include itching, which may start in the scalp, palms, soles, axillae and perineum, and then become generalized; flushing; dizziness; syncope; wheezing; epigastric pain, abdominal colic (uterine colic in women), diarrhea, incontinence of urine and feces; tachycardia and visual disturbances – all developing within a few minutes of the sting. Urticaria, angioedema of the lips, gums and tongue, generalized cutaneous erythema and swelling, edema of the glottis, profound hypotension and coma may develop over the next 15–20 minutes. The median time to first cardiac arrest is 10–20 minutes after the sting, but deaths have occurred after only two minutes. A few patients develop serum sickness a week or more after the sting. Reactions are enhanced by β-blockers.

DIAGNOSIS OF ANAPHYLAXIS AND VENOM HYPERSENSITIVITY

Detection of a raised plasma/serum mast-cell tryptase concentration confirms anaphylaxis, excluding panic attacks and other causes of collapse. The peak is 0.5–1.5 hours after the attack but levels persist for 6–8 hours. Type I hypersensitivity is confirmed by detecting venom-specific (Vespidae, Apidae, Formicidae) IgE in the serum using RAST or prick skin tests. Bumble bee and honey bee venoms cross react, as do wasp, yellow-jacket and true hornet venoms. However, venoms of Apidae and Vespidae do not cross react. Patients who have suffered a systemic reaction, have a 50–60% risk of a reaction to their next sting. In the absence of systemic symptoms, even massive and persistent local reactions do not predict a systemic reaction following subsequent stings. Children who have generalized urticaria after a sting have only a 10% chance of a systemic reaction when re-stung. Hypersensitivity to venom may be lost spontaneously in some children and young adults, but this is unpredictable and unreliable. In some countries, live insect sting challenge is used to assess hypersensitivity and response to immunotherapy. The RAST test can be used for a post-mortem diagnosis of hymenoptera sting anaphylaxis.

TREATMENT

The barbed stings of Apidae remain embedded at the site of the sting and continue to inject venom, so they should be removed immediately by any possible means. Vespids can withdraw their stings and sting repeatedly. Wasp stings may become infected because some species feed on rotting meat. Diluted domestic meat tenderizer (papain), ice packs and aspirin relieve local pain in some cases. Systemic antihistamines can be used for more severe local reactions. Severe local reactions may require treatment with antihistamines, nonsteroidal anti-inflammatory agents or even corticosteroids.

TREATMENT OF ANAPHYLAXIS [6]

The patient is laid down in the recovery position. Cardiopulmonary resuscitation may be needed. Epinephrine (adrenaline) should be given immediately by intramuscular injection into the antero-lateral thigh: 0.1% (1:1000) (0.5–1 ml for adults; 0.01 mg/kg for children). If the patient is unconscious or pulseless, epinephrine diluted 1:100,000 is given by slow intravenous (IV) injection. In rare cases, blood pressure fails to respond to even large doses of adrenaline and plasma expanders and requires pressor agents, such as dopamine. Use of IV histamine H_1 blockers such as chlorphenamine maleate (10 mg for adults; 0.2 mg/kg for children) and steroids are of unproven benefit, but may prevent relapses. People with known hypersensitivity should wear an identifying tag in case they are found unconscious after being stung. They should be trained to give themselves adrenaline using an "EpiPen" or "Ana-Pen", but many of those who are prescribed these kits are unable to use them effectively because they have not been trained. Shock and airway obstruction are the main causes of death following insect sting anaphylaxis.

REFERENCES

1. Piek T. Venoms of the Hymenoptera. Biochemical, Pharmacologicaland Behavioural Aspects. London: Academic Press; 1986.
2. Mueller UR. Insect Sting Allergy. Clinical Picture, Diagnosis and Treatment. Stuttgart: Gustav Fischer; 1990.
3. Novartis Foundation. Anaphylaxis. Novartis Foundation Symposium 257. Chichester: Wiley; 2004.
4. Brown SG, Wiese MD, Blackman KE, Heddle RJ. Ant venom immunotherapy: a double-blind, placebo-controlled, crossover trial. Lancet 2003;361:1001–6.
5. Hunt KJ, Valentine MD, Sobotka AK, et al. A controlled trial of immunotherapy in insect hypersensitivity. N Engl J Med 1978;2991:157–61.
6. Soar J, Pumphrey R, Cant A, et al. Working Group of the Resuscitation Council (UK) Statement Paper. Emergency treatment of anaphylactic Reactions – guidelines for healthcare providers. Resuscitation 2008;77:157–69.

136.2 Bites by Other Insects Resulting in Irritation, Allergy and Transmission of Infections [1]

Blood-feeding insects such as mosquitoes, midges, black flies, sand flies, tabanid flies (horse, deer, and stable flies), tsetse flies and triatomine "kissing" bugs (Fig. 136.2.1) carry out brief, blood-feeding attacks on humans and animals, which have a variety of medical consequences.

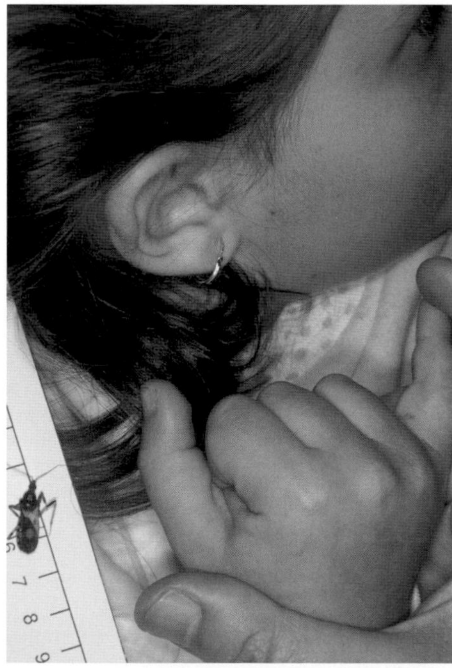

FIGURE 136.2.1 Bug bite, São Paulo, Brazil *(© David A. Warrell)*.

CLINICAL FEATURES

Bites, for example by the large aggressive flies variously known as horse flies, gadflies or cleggs (Tabanidae), may be immediately painful and traumatic but the commonest problem is delayed local swelling and itching from exposure to insects' salivary allergens incurred by previous bites. A small, intensely itchy, reddish lump with a central (hemorrhagic) punctum develops immediately or after a delay of 24–48 hours. A papule, urticarial weal, blister or bulla may develop (e.g. after "Blandford fly" *Simulium posticatum* bites in Oxfordshire, UK), or bites may provoke a more generalized erythema multiforme or, especially in children, papular urticaria, and sometimes even systemic anaphylaxis may be provoked. Triatomine bug bites are usually multiple – often near the eye or angle of the mouth. They are painful, swollen, ooze blood and may be surrounded by black staining from the bug's feces (see Chapter 98, "Chagas' Disease"). Scratching may lead to secondary infection, an inflamed, painful pustule or carbuncle, or a demarcated, hot, bright red, raised area of erysipelas or cellulitis. Causative bacteria include *Staphylococcus aureus* and *Streptococcus pyogenes*. The risk of secondary infection seems to be higher under humid tropical conditions. It may be difficult to distinguish between envenoming or allergy, resulting in early symptoms after minutes or a few hours, and infection, resulting in late symptoms after many hours or even days.

Papular urticaria is a chronic or recurrent rash of numerous very itchy weals and papules with skin edema usually seen on the legs, buttocks, neck and arms of young children. It erupts as weals with visible puncta and progresses to papules surmounted by vesicles or bullae that may become excoriated and infected. It is associated with chronic superficial infestations by fleas (e.g. cat fleas *Ctenocephalides felis*) and bedbugs (see below), and with bites by mosquitoes, mites and other arthropods [2, 3].

SPECIFIC INFECTIONS TRANSMITTED BY BITING FLIES (DIPTERA) AND BUGS (HEMIPTERA)

- Mosquitoes (family Culicidae) transmit many viral infections, malaria, lymphatic filariasis and myiasis.
- Sandflies (subfamily Phlebotominae) transmit Phlebovirus (Pappataci) fever, Oroya fever (*Bartonella bacilliformis*) and leishmaniasis.
- Tsetse flies (family Glossinidae) transmit African trypanosomiasis.
- Chrysops or deer flies (family Tabanidae) transmit *Loa loa*.
- Black flies (family Simuliidae) transmit onchocerciasis.
- Reduviid bugs (family Reduviidae) transmit American trypanosomiasis.
- Giant water bugs (family Belastomatidae) may transmit Buruli ulcer.

TREATMENT

- Apply a cooling antiseptic solution, cream or ointment (e.g. triclosan, hydrogen peroxide, "Savlon") to sooth irritation and prevent secondary infection.
- Reduce itch with counter irritants such as crotamiton ("Eurax") cream/lotion with or without hydrocortisone. Calamine is as useless as it is for prickly heat.
- Topical corticosteroids (e.g. hydrocortisone 0.5% cream or ointment) can be tried but topical antihistamines are not recommended as they may be light-sensitizing.
- For severe pruritus, use oral antihistamines. Try full dose, non-sedating anti-H_1 drugs such as cetirizine (adult dose up to 10 mg twice a day) during the day and chlorphenamine ("Piriton") 4 mg at night.
- Early systemic symptoms of anaphylaxis should be treated with adrenaline (epinephrine) 0.1% (1:1000) by intramuscular injection.
- If inflamed pustules develop, apply a topical antibacterial such as mupirocin ("Bactroban"). They may need to be lanced under aseptic conditions. Multiple infected bites may warrant a course of oral antibiotic, such as flucloxacillin, erythromycin or clindamycin.

PREVENTION

Be prepared for insect bites, not only in tropical rain forests and beaches, but also in the arctic and in cool mountainous terrain such as the Californian Sierra Nevada, Italian Dolomites and Scottish Highlands. The risk of getting bitten varies geographically, seasonally and diurnally. Seek specific advice.

- Sensible clothing should be as ample and protective as comfort (but not vanity) demands. Long sleeves and long trousers should be worn after dusk. Light colors are less attractive to mosquitoes than dark ones. Blue color attracts African tsetse flies (see Chapter 97, "Sleeping Sickness"). Hats and face veils may be necessary to protect against mass attacks on face and scalp by swarms of Scottish midges (Culicoides), or tropical blackflies (Simulium). This protection is recommended in places where there is a high risk of acquiring muco-cutaneous leishmaniasis by bites of tiny sandflies (Phlebotomus, Lutzomyia), for example Manu National Park in Peru.
- Effective repellents include diethyl-toluamide (DEET) and p-methane-diol. These can be applied to exposed skin or impregnated into cotton clothing and socks, and ankle, wrist and head bands.
- Clothes can be impregnated with pyrethroid insecticides but this may impair waterproofing.
- Protect sleeping quarters. Night bites by mosquitoes that transmit malaria, cone-nosed (triatomine) "kissing" bugs (Central and South America) that transmit Chagas' disease, bed bugs, soft ticks that transmit tick-borne encephalitis and tick-borne relapsing fever, and even vampire bats that transmit rabies (see Chapters 34.1 and 134.6), can be prevented by sleeping under a a well tucked-in pyrethroid-impregnated mosquito net. Mosquito proofing of sleeping quarters and insecticide spraying at dusk reduces the risk. Pyrethroid-releasing mosquito coils can be burned or, if there is electricity, plug-in insecticide vaporizers can be used. Fans may deter mosquitoes from biting.

Although not related to insect bites, beware of Chagas' disease acquired through drinking raw jungle fruit and sugar cane juices (e.g. in Brazil and Venezuela) contaminated with infected triatomine bugs (see "American trypanosomiasis").

REFERENCES

1. Shatin H, Canizares O. Dermatoses caused by arthropods. In: Canizares O, Harman RMR, eds. Clinical Tropical Dermatology. Oxford: Blackwell; 1992:372–403.
2. Stibich AS, Schwartz RA. Papular urticaria. Cutis 2001;68:89–91.
3. Naimer SA, Cohen AD, Mumcuoglu KY, Vardy DA. Household papular urticaria. Isr Med Assoc J 2002;4(suppl. 11):911–3.

136.3 Invasive Larvae of Flies (Myiasis) and Fleas (Tungiasis) [1, 2]

MYIASIS

Infestation of living animals by larval flies (Insecta, Diptera) is known as myiasis. In humans, larvae of three families of flies have been associated with myiasis: Oestridae (botflies), Calliphoridae (blowflies) and Sarcophagidae (fleshflies). Myiasis is classified by its location as cutaneous, wound, nasopharyngeal, orbital, ophthalmic, aural, urogenital, pulmonary and intestinal.

Primary or specific myiasis is caused by flies whose larvae are obligate parasites of living tissues.

Opportunistic or secondary myiasis is caused by saprophagous larvae that feed on decaying tissue.

Accidental myiasis is caused by coprophagous larvae that enter the gastrointestinal tract by chance or by inhalation of the gravid female fly to cause pulmonary myiasis.

Aural, nasopharyngeal and malignant wound myiasis are potentially lethal, demanding removal of the larvae, debridement and reconstructive surgery.

Diagnosis is by discovering and expertly identifying larvae in infested patients.

CUTANEOUS MYIASIS [3, 4]

Human bot flies, also known as ver macaque, berne, el torsalo or beefworm (*Dermatobia hominis* Oestridae), are a common cause of dermal myiasis in Central and South America. Their eggs are deposited on biting arthropods, such as mosquitoes, which carry them to the skin of the host. Here, the eggs hatch and the larvae burrow into the skin. As the larva grows over a period of 10 weeks, a boil develops with a small aperture. Larvae may grow to more than 1 cm in length (Fig. 136.3.1A, B). An early symptom is sporadic pain caused by the spiny larva. Unless the eye is involved, infestation is generally harmless. Secondary infection of the wound is the most common complication.

Tumbu flies, also known as putsi fly or ver du cayor (*Cordylobia anthropophaga* Calliphoridae), occur throughout sub-Saharan Africa and southern Spain. Females lay their eggs, usually on urine- or feces-contaminated sand or moist soil, and on clothes hung outside to dry. Skin contact with viable ova on clothing results in infestation. Larvae penetrate the skin and grow rapidly to mature in about 10 days. A painful inflamed boil develops which seems to wriggle, exudes blood-stained pus and has a definite head, through which the larval spiracles may protrude (Fig. 136.3.2). There may be associated fever and lymphadenopathy.

Larvae of warble flies (*Hypoderma* spp.) and horse bot flies, *Gasterophilus* spp. (Oestridae), can invade human skin causing intense itching and a creeping eruption.

PREVENTION AND TREATMENT

Ironing the washing before it is worn destroys the eggs and prevents tumbu fly infestation. Larvae are best excised under local anesthesia. Folk remedies such as the application of raw meat, glue or petroleum jelly to the lesion usually fail. Squeezing may rupture the larva, causing inflammation or a granulomatous reaction.

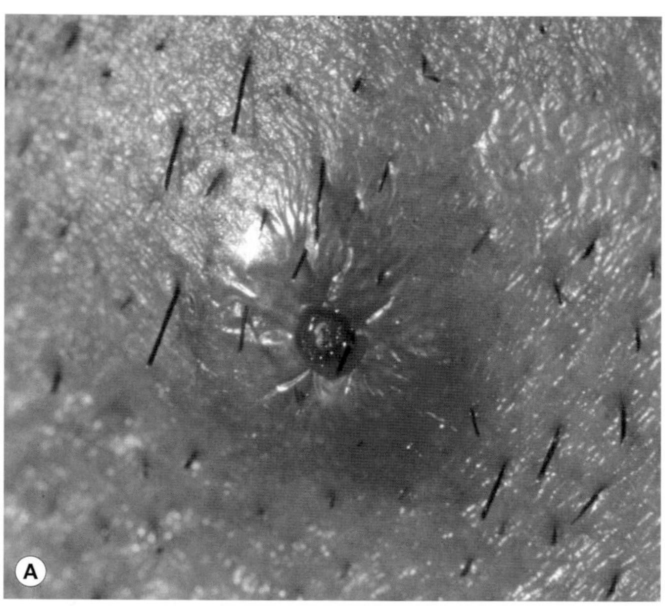

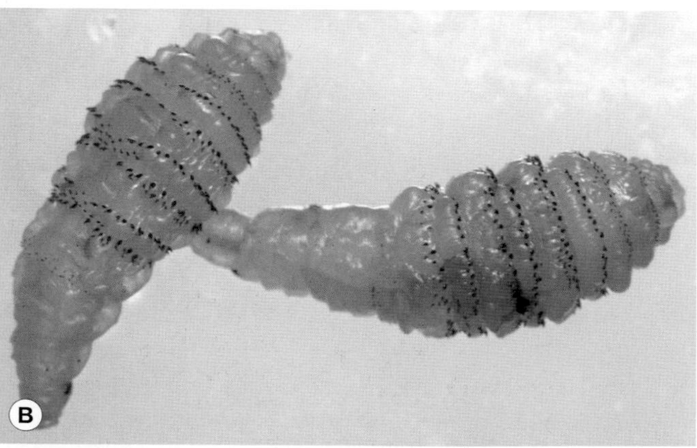

FIGURE 136.3.1 Human bot fly (*Dermatobia hominis*) infestation of the cheek acquired in Costa Rica. **(A)** Boil-like lesion with punctum. **(B)** Extracted larvae.

WOUND MYIASIS

Larvae of many species of flies invade open wounds and feed on necrotic tissue – a habit that has been employed therapeutically to debride wounds and promote healing.

However, New World screw-worms *Cochliomyia hominivorax* (Calliphoridae) in the Americas and North Africa, and the Old World screw-worms, *Chrysomya bezziana* (Calliphoridae) and Wohlfahrt's wound myiasis fly *Wohlfahrtia magnifica* (Sarcophagidae) in the Old World are obligate parasites of living tissue. Larvae hatch from eggs laid on wounds, in ears, in the nasal cavity orbit and on mucous membranes and genitalia. They burrow *en masse* into healthy tissue, causing destruction, and even death, from secondary bacterial infection.

CONTROL, PREVENTION AND TREATMENT

A massive epidemic of *C. hominivorax* myiasis, mainly in sheep, in Northern Africa, started in 1989. It was controlled by releasing 1260 million sterile male *C. hominivorax* flies in the 15,000 km^2 infested area (Fig. 136.3.3).

Wounds should be protected from flies. Treatment involves surgical removal of the larvae, debridement of affected tissue and treatment of secondary infection. Reconstructive surgery may be required.

OPHTHALMOMYIASIS (OCULAR MYIASIS) [5, 6]

Fewer than 5% of cases of human myiasis affect the eye. Usually, only external structures, such as the lids and conjunctivae, are infested but some fly larvae can penetrate the conjunctiva or sclera, causing corneal ulceration and damage to anterior and posterior internal structures that may result in blindness. The usual cause of ophthalmomyiasis externa is *Oestrus ovis*, the cosmopolitan sheep and goat nasal botfly, whose natural host is herbivorous mammals. Although most common in tropical developing countries (especially North Africa, the Middle East and the Caribbean), it still occurs rarely in Western cities. Female flies eject their larvae into the nostrils of the host, where they mature.

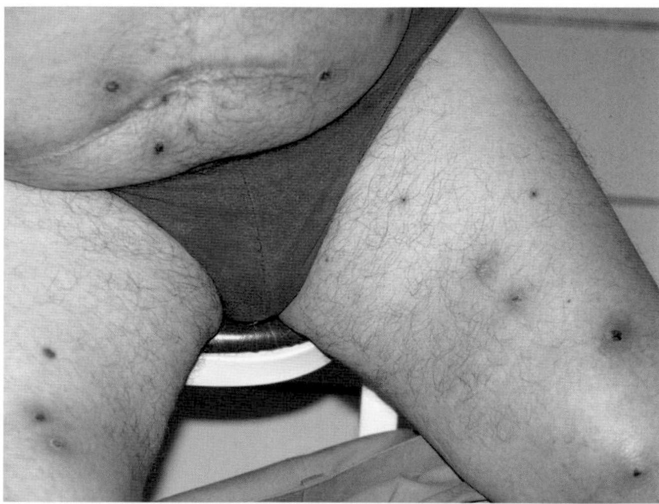

FIGURE 136.3.2 Tumbu fly (*Cordylobia anthropophaga*): multiple lesions in a Peruvain man at Instituto de Medicina Tropical "Alexander von Humboldt" Universidad Peruana Cayetano Heredia, Lima, Peru, who had been working in Zambia *(© David A. Warrell)*.

اللجنة المركزية لمكافحة ذبابة الدودة اللولبية
للوقاية من الإصابة بيرقات ذبابة الدودة اللولبية
اتبع الخطوات التالية :-
- عدم تعرض الحيوان لأي نوع من الجروح.
- ازالة الأشياء الحادة من حظائر وأماكن تربية الحيوان.
- المراقبة والكشف اليومي بواقع مرتين أسبوعيا على الأقل.
- العناية الفائقة بالولادات الحديثة وتطهير الحبل السري ومتابعة علاجه.
- تغطيس الحيوانات أو رشها بالأدوية الوقائية حسب ارشادات الطبيب البيطري.
- التنظيف المستمر لحظائر الحيوانات ورشها بالمبيدات الحشرية.
- الاهتمام بتنظيف الجروح والخدوش فور حدوثها.
- التبليغ الفوري عن ظهور أي حالات إصابة بالدودة في الحيوانات.

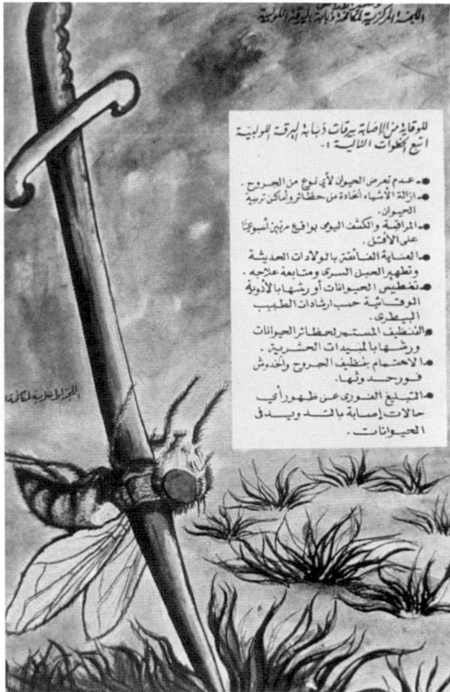

FIGURE 136.3.3 Poster advertising the screw worm control program in North Africa.

Human victims may give a history of having been buzzed in the face or struck on the eye by an insect and later of developing irritation and redness of the eye, foreign body sensation, pain, lacrimation, palpebral edema and signs of purulent conjunctivitis or a stye (hordeolum). *Oestrus ovis* larvae rarely develop beyond the first instar in humans and so symptoms are self-limiting, but they may be more rapidly relieved by slit lamp examination and removal of larvae which cling to the conjunctivae and may cause follicular conjunctival reaction and pseudomembrane formation. Other causes of human ophthalmomyiasis include *Rhinoestrus purpureum, Dermatobia hominis, Hypoderma* spp., (Oestridae), and *Cochlyomyia hominis, Lucilia* spp. and *Phormia* spp. (Calliphoridae). Larvae of *Hypoderma, Cochlyomyia* and *Dermatobia* are more dangerous as they may burrow into the eye, resulting in pain, nausea and destruction. They must be surgically removed.

Congo floor maggots, larvae of the fly *Auchmeromyia luteola* live in earthen floors of huts throughout tropical Africa between latitudes 18°N and 26°S. They suck blood from those sleeping on the ground, causing local swelling and itching.

PREVENTION AND TREATMENT

If possible, avoid sleeping on the ground. Fumigate the hut. Treat bites symptomatically, making sure that no secondary infection is introduced. If there are signs of infection, wipe the skin with tincture of iodine and give systemic antimicrobials.

TUNGIASIS

Tungiasis, also known as "nigua", "pio/bicho de pie" and "pique" is caused by the "chigger", "jigger" or "chigoe" flea (*Tunga penetrans* family Hectopsyllidae) which must not to be confused with trombiculid mites, also known as "chiggers" or harvest mites (see below) Adult female fleas are acquired while walking barefoot in the sand. They burrow into the epidermis of the toes and foot, causing itching or painful lesions.

After fertilization, the female flea jumps (feebly) and burrows alongside the nailfold or into the skin of the groin, loses her legs and produces eggs each night. A painful swelling develops, typically under a toe nail, with the risk of secondary infection and even fatal tetanus. The encapsulated flea must be curetted out and iodine applied. Complete enucleation is required.

PREVENTION

Wear proper shoes; do not walk around bare-footed.

DISTINCTION FROM OTHER CREEPING ERUPTIONS

Arthropod infestations must be distinguished from "Creeping eruption" (cutaneous larva migrans) caused by larvae of cat and dog hook worms, such as *Ancylostoma braziliense, Uncinaria stenocephala* and *Ancylostoma caninum* that are acquired by lying on a beach in Central/Southern America. The larva moves day-by-day producing an itchy or painful tortuous serpiginous track.

REFERENCES

1. Zumpt F. Myiasis in Man and Animals in the Old World. London: Butterworth; 1965.
2. Hall M, Wall R. Myiasis of humans and domestic animals. Adv Parasitol 1995;35:257–334.
3. McGraw TA, Turiansky GW. Cutaneous myiasis. J Am Acad Dermatol 2008;58:907–26.
4. Caissie R, Beaulieu F, Giroux M, et al. Cutaneous myiasis: diagnosis, treatment, and prevention. J Oral Maxillofac Surg 2008;66:560–8.
5. Dunbar J, Cooper B, Hodgetts T, et al. An outbreak of human external ophthalmomyiasis due to *Oestrus ovis* in southern Afghanistan. Clin Infect Dis 2008;46:e124–6.
6. Chodosh J, Clarridge J. Ophthalmomyiasis: a review with special reference to Cochliomyia hominivorax. Clin Infect Dis 1992;14:444–9.

136.4 Superficial Infestations by Ectoparasitic Arthropods: Fleas, Lice, Mites and Ticks

Some blood-feeding invertebrates infest the skin and hair of human bodies and clothing for long periods. Tropical climate, poverty and lack of personal hygiene increase the risk of acquiring ectoparasites from other humans or from the environment and harboring them. These infestations are irritating, distressing, embarrassing and antisocial but it is only in the past century that Westerners have grown less accustomed to being flea-ridden and lousy. The biting and burrowing of these ectoparasites causes pain and irritation and may lead to hypersensitivity, secondary local infection or transmission of systemic infectious diseases.

SPECIFIC INFECTIONS TRANSMITTED BY INFESTING ARTHROPODS

- Fleas transmit rickettsioses and plague.
- Tcks transmit viral encephalitides, viral hemorrhagic fevers, Colorado, Oklahoma and Kemerovo tick fevers, louping ill, spirochaetoses, rickettsioses, bartonelloses, ehrlichiosis, anaplasmosis and protozoal infections (babesiosis).
- Lice transmit spirochaetoses and rickettsioses.
- Trombiculid mites transmit scrub typhus.
- Scabies mites encourage local streptococcal infection leading to acute glomerulonephritis.

FLEAS (INSECTA FAMILY PULICIDAE)

Humans can be infested and bitten by human fleas (*Pulex irritans*) and by dog, cat, rat, pigeon and other animal fleas. Direct contact with an infested person or animal is not necessary. Tropical rodent fleas (Xenopsylla species) transmit plague and murine typhus. The first evidence of fleas is the appearance of small groups of intensely itchy bites producing red macules with a central puncta often in a line a few centimeters apart, especially on the trunk or buttocks. Fleas may not remain on the body after feeding, but retreat to bedding or crevices and cracks in the bed or room. Examination of underclothing or turning back the bedclothes may reveal the jumping fleas.

TREATMENT

Itching bites are treated with counter-irritants, topical corticosteroid or systemic antihistamines (see Chapter 136.2). Domestic animals and the infested environment should be kept as clean as is practicable and treated with pyrethroid or other pesticides.

LICE (INSECTA FAMILY PEDICULIDAE) [1]

Human head lice, body (clothing) lice and pubic lice are obligate human parasitic insects that spread through close physical contact. Nymphs and adults require blood for survival and feed daily.

HEAD LICE (PEDICULUS *CAPITIS*)

Head lice flourish on the human scalp, even in hygienic, affluent conditions (e.g. in English teenage schoolgirls). Eggs ("nits") stuck to head hairs are recovered using a fine comb. Itching and scratching may cause secondary infection with occipital lymphadenopathy.

Treatment

Repeated application of insecticide lotion (pyrethroid, organophosphate or carbamate) and combing.

Prevention

Avoid head-to-head contact and sharing of combs and hair adornments.

BODY LICE (PEDICULUS *HUMANUS*)

Body lice infestation is promoted by poor hygiene (unwashed clothes and bodies) and crowding. Such conditions are common accompaniments of disasters, wars, forced immigration and cold, wet seasons (e.g. highlands of Ethiopia). Lice and their eggs may be discovered on skin, body hair or in clothing, especially in the seams. More than 21,500 lice have been found on one person. Individual bites look like flea bites but lack their linearity. There is only mild local irritation.

Treatment

Clothing is burned or heat-sterilized and impregnated with pyrethroids. Infested people are bathed with soap and 1% lysol.

PUBIC (CRAB) LICE (PTHIRUS PUBIS *FAMILY* PHTHIRIDAE)

Pubic lice cause sexually-transmitted infestation of the pubic hair, body hair, eyebrows and eyelashes, where they provoke itching, scratching, secondary infection and a curious bluish staining (maculae caeruliae). Eggs are stuck to the hairs.

Treatment

Insecticides (see above) are applied to affected areas, left on for 1–2 days and then re-applied after a week. Sexual contacts should also be treated.

MITES (ARACHNIDA) [1]

SCABIES MITES (ASTIGMATA FAMILY SARCOPTIDAE) [2]

The human scabies mite *Sarcoptes scabiei* var. *hominis* causes a chronic infestation. Scabies mites adapted to other mammalian hosts, such as *Sarcoptes scabiei* var. *canis*, cause only self-limiting pruritus in humans. Avian mites *Dermanyssus gallinae* and *Ornithonyssus* spp. occasionally bite humans, causing lesions which resemble scabies.

Prevalence rates increase when there is overcrowding and following social disruption in wartime. For example, prevalence among dermatology patients in Edinburgh rose from 5–30% during the world wars. Outbreaks may occur in nursing homes and hospitals. Most cases are acquired by close contact rather than fomites, as the mites do not survive long away from the body. Symptoms of scabies are caused only by the 3-mm long adult female mites, which burrow through the epidermis within the stratum granulosum and deposit 2–3 eggs daily during their month of life. Six-legged larvae hatch after a few days, migrate to the skin surface and moult to become eight-legged nymphs and later adults, maturing in about 10–14 days. The smaller males die after mating on the epidermis and do not burrow. Females feed on cells of the stratum corneum and its secretions. Mite excretions, saliva and eggs incite a delayed type-IV hypersenstitivity reaction in the host, responsible for the familiar irritation and itching which begins up to three weeks after initial infestation but soon after re-infestation. In an immunocompetent host, a typical infestation involves fewer than 20 mites. Scabies is transmitted by close physical contact often involving whole families.

Clinical features

Burrows most commonly occur in the interdigital clefts between the fingers and on the wrists, but may be widespread (Fig. 136.4.1). Tracks are serpiginous, extending for a few millimeters up to one centimeter, creating linear papulovescular lesions with excoriation, secondary infection, eczematization, lichenification and erythematous papules. Lesions are intensely itchy, especially at night and after a hot bath or shower, provoking scratching – excoriation that promotes secondary infection. In about 7% of cases, very itchy reddish brown nodules occur on the genitalia, groin, buttocks and axillae (nodular scabies). In infants, vesicular, pustular and nodular lesions are found on the axillae, head, face, diaper region, palms and soles. An exuberantly crusting form, Norwegian scabies, occurs in patients immunosuppressed by HIV, human T-lymphotropic virus (HTLV)-1 or by drugs employed in organ transplantation, and in people with trisomy-21. Demarcated, hyperkeratotic, scaly plaques involve, in particular, the extremities, scalp, face, neck and buttocks. The scales contain thousands of mites and the load per patient may exceed 1 million mites. This type of scabies is very infectious and a single case can give rise to nosocomial outbreaks.

Complications

In developing countries, scabetic lesions often become secondarily infected with *Staphylococcus aureus* and *Streptococcus pyogenes*. Strains of the latter organism may cause rheumatic fever, rheumatic heart disease and post-streptococcal glomerulonephritis.

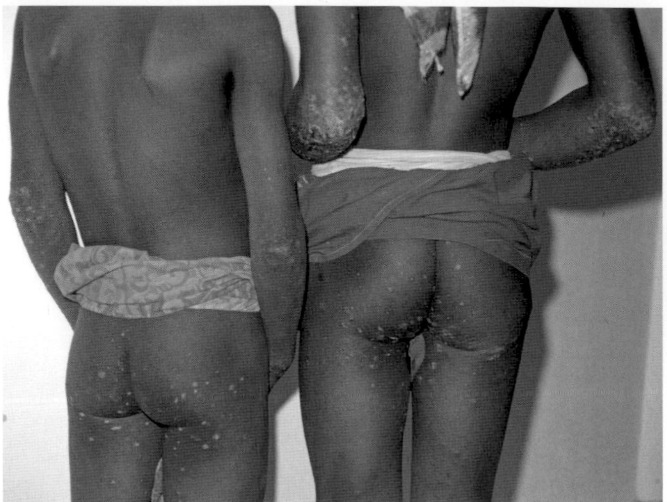

FIGURE 136.4.1 Extensive scabies in two Koranic students in Zaria, Nigeria. In this region, scabies infestation may be associated with streptococcal glomerulonephritis *(© David A. Warrell).*

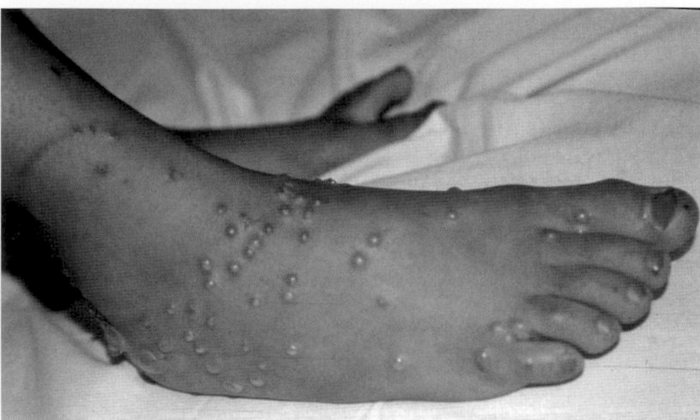

FIGURE 136.4.2 Multiple blistering lesions from bites by Cayenne ticks (*Amblyomma cajennense*) in Brazil. This species can transmit Rocky Mountain Spotted Fever *(Courtesy of Dr João Luiz Costa Cardoso).*

Diagnosis

This is confirmed by microscopy of scrapings from affected areas, especially interdigital spaces, but many cases are atypical and a dermatologic opinion may be required to exclude other causes.

Treatment

Topical aqueous lotions of 0.5% malathion or 5% permethrin are applied to the whole body surface of all affected people and close contacts on two occasions one week apart. Itching may persist and requires topical counter irritants, a corticosteroid (e.g. crotamiton and hydrocortisone) and a sedating antihistamine (chlorphenamine at night). Resistance to permethrin is resulting in treatment failures. Lindane is no longer used in Western countries on the grounds of safety. Nodular scabies may require additional corticosteroid treatment. Patients cured of scabies may be left with persistent post-scabies eczematous rashes. Systemic ivermectin (200 μg/kg, in multiple doses) has proved effective for Norwegian scabies when combined with topical treatment and keratolytics. Ivermectin is being used increasingly to treat and control ordinary scabies in a dose of 200 μg/kg repeated after 1–2 weeks. Successful combined mass treatment campaigns against scabies and intestinal helminthes have been carried out, and elimination of human scabies is envisaged by some optimists.

TROMBICULID (HARVEST) MITES (ACARANI LEPTOTROMBIDIUM *SPP. FAMILY TROMBICULIDAE) [3]*

Sometimes known misleadingly as "chiggers", trombiculid mites can infest in large numbers, especially under tight underpants, causing multiple, persisting, painful, itchy, blistering bites. They occur particularly in grassy, rodent-infested "mite islands" in jungle clearings throughout Asia and the Pacific region, where they are responsible for transmitting scrub typhus.

Prevention

Use diethyl-toluamide (DEET)-containing repellents, tuck trousers into boots and avoid notorious "mite islands", which are densely infested with these trombiculids.

BEDBUGS (INSECTA CIMEX *SPP. FAMILY CIMICIDAE)*

The common bedbug, *Cimex lectularius* is cosmopolitan and, in recent years, infestations have increased in developed countries, such as the UK. In tropical countries, it is replaced by *Cimex hemipterus.* There is no convincing evidence that bedbugs transmit infections such as hepatitis B. Adults reach a length of about 5 mm. Nymphs pass through five instars to reach adulthood after about four months. Nymphs and adults take about 5–10 minutes to obtain a full blood meal. Adults may take several blood meals over several weeks but can survive six months' starvation.

At night, bedbugs emerge from cracks and crevices in the bedroom to bite sleeping humans. Sometimes, bites go unnoticed but bedbugs may cause sleeplessness through pain and allergic reactions to their bites. Swellings, red papules and even disseminated bullous eruptions may appear. Rooms that are heavily infested may acquire an unpleasant odor. Bites are discouraged by keeping the light on all night, by sleeping under a permethrin-impregnated mosquito net and by putting newspaper beneath the under-sheet. Eradication is by thorough cleaning of the environment (heavily-infested furniture may have to be burned), steam cleaning sheets or exposing them to the sun and application of the usual residual insecticides. However, insecticide-resistance has developed and bedbugs are becoming more abundant.

TICKS (ACARINA) [3, 4]

Soft (argasid) ticks (family Argasidae) [5] live in animal burrows and human dwellings. They attach briefly at night, engorge rapidly with blood and then drop off and hide in cracks and crevices. Ticks of the genus *Ornithodorus* transmit relapsing fevers (*Borrelia* spp.).

Hard (ixodid) ticks (family Ixodidae) or their tiny nymphs may be picked up from vegetation or brought into gardens by deer or indoors by dogs. They find a secluded area (groin, perineum, waist, umbilicus, axilla, scalp and even external auditory meatus) and feed for days until they are spherical and engorged. The bite of hard ticks is not usually detected during feeding. Multiple bites may cause local vesicular lesions (Fig. 136.4.2). Some species transmit Lyme disease, Rocky Mountain spotted fever, African tick fevers, European tick-borne encephalitis, Crimean-Congo hemorrhagic fever, Colorado tick fever, louping ill, babesiosis, ehrlichiosis, anaplasmosis and other human infections. Some ticks in North America and Australia can inject a paralyzing neurotoxin (see below).

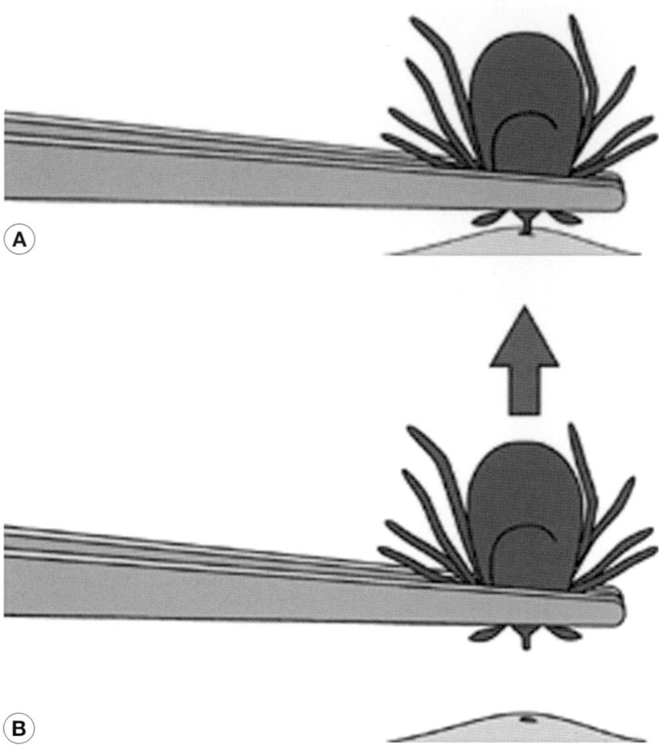

FIGURE 136.4.3 (A, B) Technique for removing ticks *(Courtesy of US Centers for Disease Control and Prevention, Atlanta).*

Prevention of tick-transmitted infections

- Common sites for tick attachment should be examined when undressing at night after being in the field.
- Contact with tick-infested domestic animals should be avoided.
- Light-coloured trousers (pants) allow ticks to be seen more easily.
- Trouser (pant) bottoms should be tucked into boots.
- DEET-containing repellents should be applied.
- Specific antibiotic chemoprophylaxis against tick-transmitted infections is not justified.

Removing ticks

The tick is grasped as close as possible to the skin surface using fine curved (iris) forceps. Squeezing the tick's engorged body should be avoided. The tick should be pulled out gently without twisting (Fig. 136.4.3A, B). If the mouth parts break off, they should be removed separately. The aim is not to leave the barbed hypostome in the wound as it may provoke inflammation and granuloma formation. The tick should be kept for later expert examination in case symptoms develop.

REFERENCES

1. Roberts DT, ed. Lice and Scabies: A Health Professional's Guide to Epidemiology and Treatment. London: Public Health Laboratory Service; 2000.
2. Hengge UR, Currie BJ, Jäger G, et al. Scabies: an ubiquitous neglected skin disease. Lancet Infect Dis 2006;6:769–79.
3. Baker AS. Mites and Ticks of Domestic Animals: An Identification Guide and Information Source. London: The Stationery Office; 1999.
4. Hoogstraal H. Changing patterns of tickborne diseases in modern society. Annu Rev Entomol 1981;26:75–99.
5. Hoogstraal H. Argasid and nuttalliellid ticks as parasites and vectors. Adv Parasitol 1985;24:135–238.

136.5 Envenoming by Arthropods

TICKS (ACARINA OR ACARI)

TAXONOMY AND EPIDEMIOLOGY

Ticks, with mites, form the order Acarana of the class Arachnida. Adult females of about 34 species of hard tick (family *Ixodidae*) and immature specimens of 9 species of soft ticks (family *Argasidae*) have been implicated in human tick paralysis. The tick's saliva contains a neurotoxin which causes presynaptic neuromuscular block and decreased nerve-conduction velocity. The tick embeds itself in the skin with its barbed hypostome introducing the salivary toxin while it engorges with blood [1].

Although tick paralysis has been reported from all continents, most cases occur in western North America (*Dermacentor andersoni*), eastern USA (*Dermacentor variabilis*) and eastern Australia from north Queensland to Victoria (*Ixodes holocyclus*, known as the bush, scrub, paralysis-, or dog- tick). In British Columbia, Canada, there were 305 cases with a 10% case fatality between 1900 and 1968. About 120 cases have been reported in the USA and in New South Wales (Australia), there were at least 20 deaths between 1900 and 1945 [2, 3].

CLINICAL FEATURES [4]

Ticks are picked up in the countryside or from domestic animals, particularly dogs, in the home. The majority of patients and almost all fatal cases are children. After the tick has been attached for 5–6 days, a progressive ascending, lower motor neuron paralysis develops with paraesthesiae. Often, a child, who may have been irritable for the previous 24 h, falls on getting out of bed first thing in the morning and is found to be weak or ataxic. Paralysis increases over the next few days: death results from bulbar and respiratory paralysis and aspiration of stomach contents. Vomiting is a feature of the more acute course of *I. holocyclus* envenoming.

This clinical picture is often misinterpreted as poliomyelitis. Other neurologic conditions, including Guillain–Barré syndrome, paralytic rabies, Eaton-Lambert syndrome, myasthenia gravis or botulism, may also be suspected. Diagnosis depends on finding the tick, which is likely to be concealed in a crevice, orifice or hairy area of the body. The scalp is the commonest place. Fatal tick paralysis has been caused by a tick attached to the tympanic membrane.

TREATMENT

The tick must be discovered and detached without being squeezed (Fig. 136.4.3A, B). It can be painted with ether, chloroform, paraffin, petrol or turpentine, or prized out between the partially separated tips of a pair of small, curved forceps. Following removal of the tick there is usually a rapid and complete recovery; however, in Australia, patients have died even after the tick had been detached. The antivenoms, raised in dogs and rabbits in Australia, are no longer produced.

ARACHNIDA

SPIDERS (ORDER ARANEAE)

All but one family of this enormous order are venomous, but few species have proved dangerous to humans. Spiders bite with a pair of fangs, the chelicerae, to which the venom glands are connected.

Necrotic araneism is caused by recluse spiders, *Loxosceles* (family Sicariidae) (Fig. 136.5.1)

Neurotoxic araneism is caused by:

- black and brown widows *Latrodectus* (family Theriidae) (Fig. 136.5.2);
- wandering, armed or banana spiders *Phoneutria* (family Ctenidae) (Fig. 136.5.3A, B);
- Sydney and other Australian funnel-web spiders *Atrax, Hadronyche* and *Missulena* spp. (Mygalomorphae family Hexathelidae) (Fig. 136.5.4).

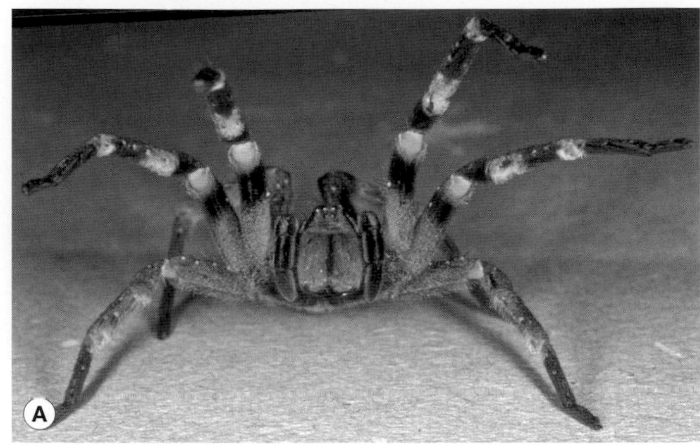

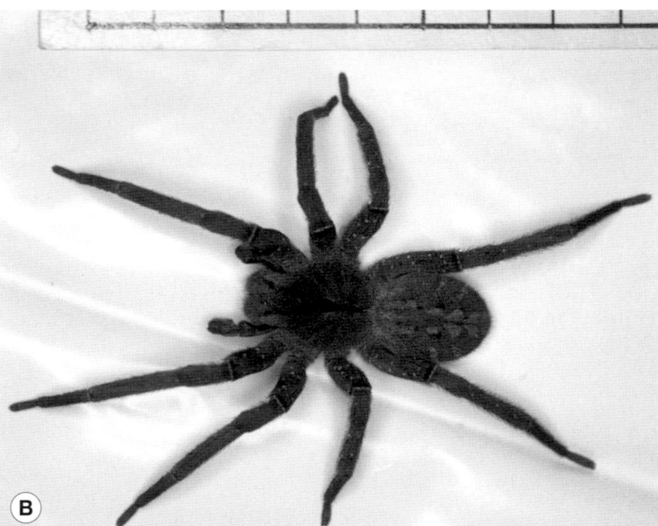

FIGURE 136.5.3 Brazilian armed, wandering or banana spider (*Phoneutria nigriventer*). **(A)** Defensive posture with raised "arms" *(copyright D. A. Warrell).* **(B)** Dorsal view (scale in cm).

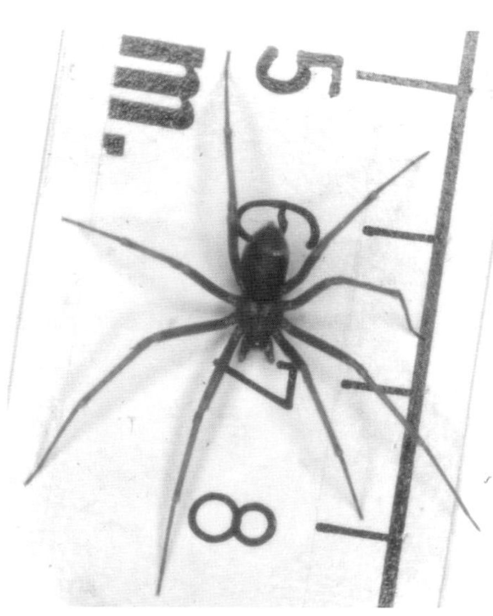

FIGURE 136.5.1 Female Brazilian recluse spider (*Loxosceles gaucho*), Brazil *(© David A. Warrell).*

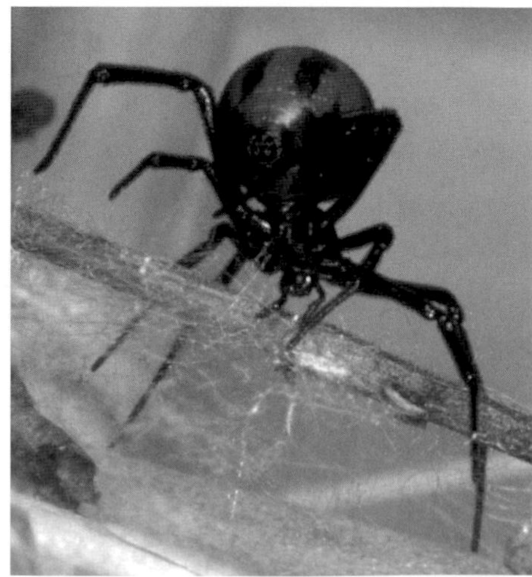

FIGURE 136.5.2 Black widow spider (*Latrodectus curacaviensis*), Brazil *(© David A. Warrell).*

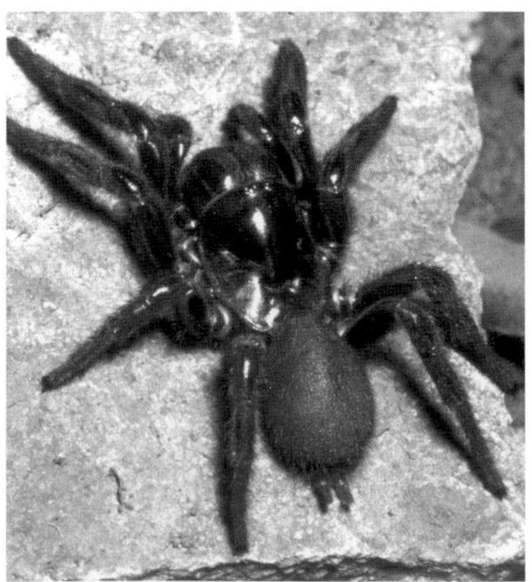

FIGURE 136.5.4 Sydney funnel-web spider (*Atrax robustus*) *(Courtesy of South Australian Museum).*

Epidemiology

Spider bites are common in some parts of the world but there are now few fatalities. Brazil reported 19,634 bites (10/100,000 population) in 2005 with only 9 deaths (0.05%). In Central and Southern America, *Loxosceles* spp. such as *Loxosceles laeta and Loxosceles gaucho* are widely distributed and cause many bites. In Chile, the case fatality of loxoscelism ranges from 1% to 17%. In the south and south-central USA, the brown recluse spider, *Loxosceles reclusa*, caused at least 200 bites and 6 deaths in the USA during the last century. More than 60 cases were reported from Texas between 1959 and 1962. In the Mediterranean region, North Africa, and Israel bites by *Loxosceles rufescens* have been reported. Most bites from *Loxosceles* spp. occur in bedrooms while people are asleep or dressing. In the USA, a number of men were bitten on the genitalia while they sat on outdoor privies in which the spiders had spun their webs.

Black and brown widow spiders are cosmopolitan in distribution. *Latrodectus tredecemguttatus* (sometimes referred to, loosely, as "tarantula") lives in fields in Mediterranean countries and was responsible for a series of epidemics of bites. In Italy, 946 cases were reported between 1946 and 1951 [5]. *Latrodectus hasselti*, the Australian redback spider causes up to 340 bites each year in Australia and 20 deaths have been reported [6, 7]. The black widow spider (*Latrodectus mactans*) was responsible for 63 deaths in the USA between 1950 and 1959. Several species of *Latrodectus* occur in Latin America

Wandering, armed or banana spiders (*Phoneutria* spp.) cause bites and a few deaths in Latin American countries. They have been imported into temperate countries in bunches of bananas, causing a few bites and deaths.

Highly dangerous funnel-web spiders (*Atrax* spp.) are restricted to south-eastern Australia and Tasmania. The Sydney funnel web spider (*Atrax robustus*) is found only within a 160-mile (256 km) radius of Sydney. The aggressive males caused at least 13 deaths between 1927 and 1980. Members of the related genera *Hadronyche* and *Missulena* may be equally dangerous [8].

In England, mild neurotoxic araneism has been described after bites by *Steatoda nobilis* and *Steatoda grossa* (family Theridiidae) [9] and woodlouse spider (*Dysdera crocata* family Dysderidae).

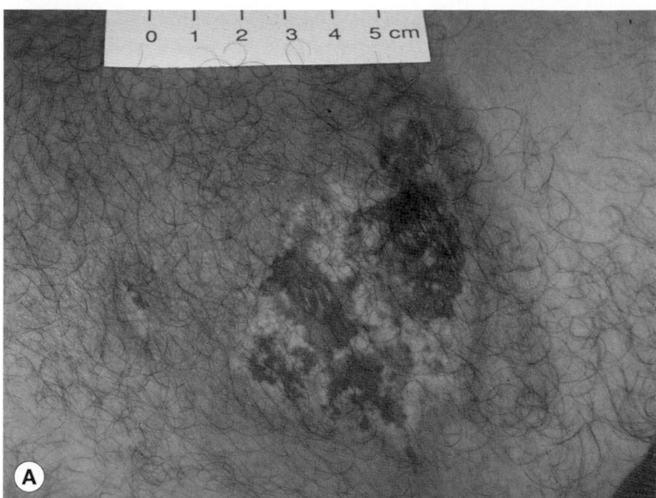

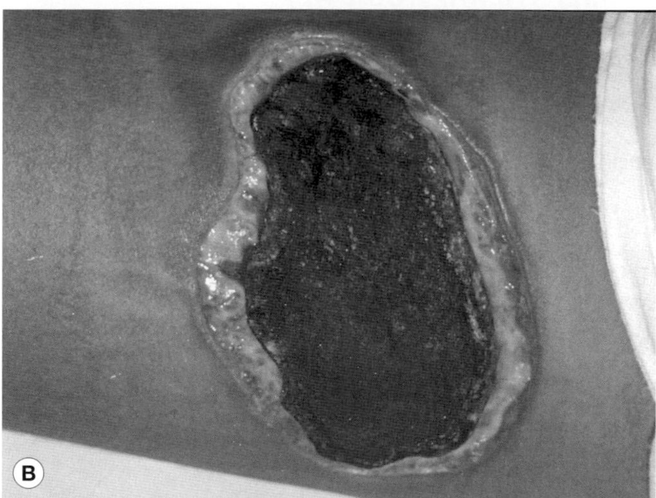

FIGURE 136.5.5 Necrotic araneism. **(A)** "Red-white-and-blue" sign developing 18 hours after a bite by the Brazilian recluse spider (*Loxosceles gaucho*), São Paulo, Brazil *(© David A. Warrell)*. **(B)** Eschar after *Loxosceles amazonica* bite, Belém, Brazil *(Courtesy of Dr Pedro Pardal)*.

Necrotic araneism

Skin lesions varying in severity from mild, localized erythema and blistering to extensive granulomas and tissue necrosis have been falsely attributed to a large variety of familiar peri-domestic species, such as the Australian white-tailed spider (*Lampona cylindrata*), North American hobo spider (*Tegenaria agrestis*), European and South American wolf spiders (*Lycosa*, including the Italian "tarantula" *Lycosa terentula*) and cosmopolitan sac spiders (*Cheiracanthium*) [10]. However, only members of the genus *Loxosceles* have proved capable of causing "necrotic arachnidism/araneism". Venom sphingomyelinase D is implicated in the pathogenesis of dermonecrosis. Neutrophils adhere to the endothelium of cutaneous capillaries and degranulate. The bite itself is usually painless and unnoticed. Burning develops over several hours at the site of the bite, with swelling and development of a characteristic macular lesion – the red-white-and-blue sign (Fig. 136.5.5A) showing areas of red vasodilatation, white vasoconstriction and central blue prenecrotic cyanosis. A blackened eschar develops (Fig. 136.5.5B), which sloughs in a few weeks leaving a full thickness necrotic ulcer. Sometimes, an entire limb or area of the face is involved. Facial bites cause much swelling. Some 13% of cases have systemic symptoms, such as fever, headaches, scarlatiniform rash, jaundice, methaemoglobinemia, and hemoglobinuria resulting from intravascular hemolysis. Acute kidney injury may ensue. The average case fatality is about 5%.

Neurotoxic araneism

The bite is immediately very painful but local signs are minimal (*L. mactans*) or moderate (*L. hasselti*). After about 30 minutes there is painful regional lymphadenopathy, then headache, nausea, vomiting and local sweating with piloerection ("gooseflesh") – a sign highly suggestive of neurotoxic araneism. In cases of bites by *L. mactans* and *L. tredecemguttatus*, there is profuse generalized sweating and fever with painful muscle spasms, tremors and rigidity. This may be sufficiently severe to embarrass respiration. The classic "facies latrodectismica" is an agonized grimace caused by facial spasm and trismus, associated with swollen eyelids, congested conjunctivae, flushing and sweating. Abdominal rigidity may simulate an acute abdomen and prompt laparotomy. Other features include tachycardia, hypertension, restlessness, irritability, psychosis, priapism and rhabdomyolysis. A localized or diffuse rash may appear several days later. Envenoming by *Phoneutria* and *Atrax* spp. produces similar features.

First-aid treatment

In Australia, pressure-immobilization (see Chapter 134.5) is recommended for bites by *A. robustus* and *Hadronyche* species.

Specific treatment

Antivenoms for envenoming by *Latrodectus* spp. are made in Australia, Mexico, South Africa, Brazil and some other South American countries for *Atrax* spp. in Australia [11], for *Loxosceles* spp. in Peru, Brazil, Mexico, and Argentina, and for *Phoneutria* spp. in Brazil. Despite decades of use, there is no decisive evidence for the efficacy of *Loxosceles* antivenoms [12]. Neurotoxic araneism may be more obviously responsive to antivenom [8], but the effectiveness of antivenom for *L. hasselti* bites in Australia has been questioned [13].

Supportive treatment

Oral dapsone (100 mg twice daily) is said to reduce the extent of necrotic lesions by inhibiting neutrophil degranulation and calcium gluconate (10 ml of a 10% solution, given by slow intravenous injection) is said to relieve the pain of muscle spasms caused by the venom of *Latrodectus* spp. rapidly and more effectively than muscle relaxants, such as diazepam or methocarbamol. Unfortunately, evidence for efficacy is lacking. Antihistamines, corticosteroids, α-blockers and atropine have also been advocated. For necrotic araneism caused by *Loxosceles* spp., early surgical debridement, corticosteroids, antihistamines and hyperbaric oxygen all have their advocates, but there is no basis for recommending their use.

TARANTULA SPIDERS (MYGALOMORPHAE, FAMILY THERAPHOSIDAE)

Tarantula spiders are becoming increasingly popular pets, kept and bred by both children and adults in Western countries. The largest of these giant spiders, the goliath birdeater (*Theraphosa blondi*) of Venezuela and Brazil weighs up to 150 g with a leg-span of up to 30 cm. In human victims, a strike by the large vertically-orientated fangs (Fig. 136.5.6) is powerful enough to penetrate a finger nail. However, despite their size, tarantulas are generally perceived to be harmless pets. Bites are uncommon but are under-reported.

New World tarantulas, such as the popular Mexican pink/orange/red-kneed tarantula (*Brachypelma smithi*), can eject urticating abdominal setae, causing kerato-uveal injuries ("ophthalmia nodosa") and irritation of skin, nasopharynx and respiratory tract. Bites may cause allergic reaction, but envenoming appears to be clinically trivial, with the possible exception of a few genera, such as Sericopelma (Theraphosinae).

Old World tarantulas which lack protective urticating hairs, seem more ready to bite. In birds, and mammals (as large as dogs), bites may be lethal [14]. In humans, their bites are increasingly recognized as being potentially dangerous. Apart from intense local pain, inflammation and swelling, severe systemic symptoms may ensue. Episodic, generalized, painful muscle cramps have been reported after bites by Ornithoctoninae spp. Orange-fringed (*Haplopelma doriae*) (Ornithoctoninae) from Borneo, African baboon tarantula (*Pterinochilus murinus*) (Harpactirinae), Indian ornamental tarantula (*Poecilotheria regalis*) (Poecilotheriinae) and Southeast Asian and Australasian *Lampropelma* (Ornithoctoninae), *Eumenophorus* (Eumenophorinae), *Selenocosmia* (Selenocosmiinae) and African *Stromatopelma* and *Heteroscodra* (Stromatopelminae) [15].

Treatment

In the absence of any antivenom, muscle spasms can only be palliated with large doses of benzodiazepines and other muscle relaxants. Dantrolene might be considered.

Prevention

The dangers of tarantula hairs and bites must be recognized and tarantula keepers should be warned of the danger of handling these animals incautiously, especially after drinking alcohol.

SCORPIONS (SCORPIONES: BUTHIDAE, HEMISCORPIIDAE)

Species capable of inflicting fatal stings occur in North Africa and the Middle East (*Androctonus, Buthus, Hemiscorpius* and *Leiurus* spp.) (Fig. 136.5.7), South Africa (*Parabuthus* spp.), India and Nepal (*Hottentota tamulus*), North, Central and Southern America, and Trinidad, and Tobago (*Centruroides* and *Tityus* spp.) (Fig. 136.5.8) [16, 17]. Scorpion toxins target Na^+, K^+, Ca^{2+} and Cl^- channels, causing direct effects and the release of neurotransmitters, such as acetylcholine and catecholamines [18, 19]. Scorpions are nocturnally-active arachnids. Discovery of scorpions during the daytime is usually made by removing their protective shelter in the field (e.g. loose bark, debris, rocks), in the house (e.g. footwear, storage boxes, clothing on the floor) and in other places protected from light.

EPIDEMIOLOGY

In Mexico, there are 250,000 stings with less than 50 deaths/year attributed to *Centruroides limpidus, Centruroides noxius* and *Centruroides suffusus*. In Khuzestan Province, Iran, 25,000 stings (*Hemiscorpius lepturus, Androctonus* and *Buthus* spp.) are treated each year. They are the

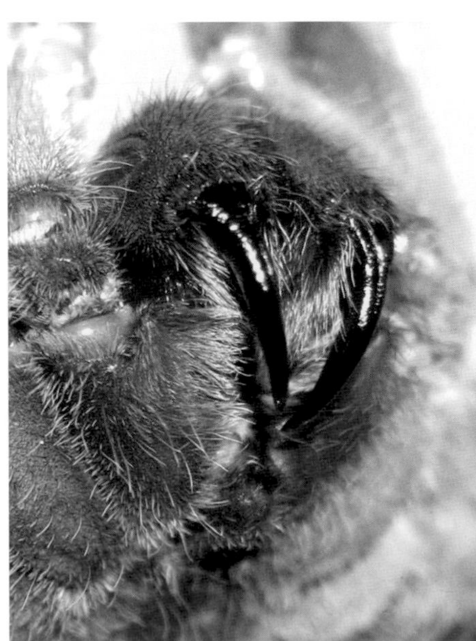

FIGURE 136.5.6 Vertically placed venom jaws (25-mm long) of the East African king baboon tarantula (*Citharischius crawshayi* Eumenophorinae Theraphosidae) *(Courtesy of Peter Kirk).*

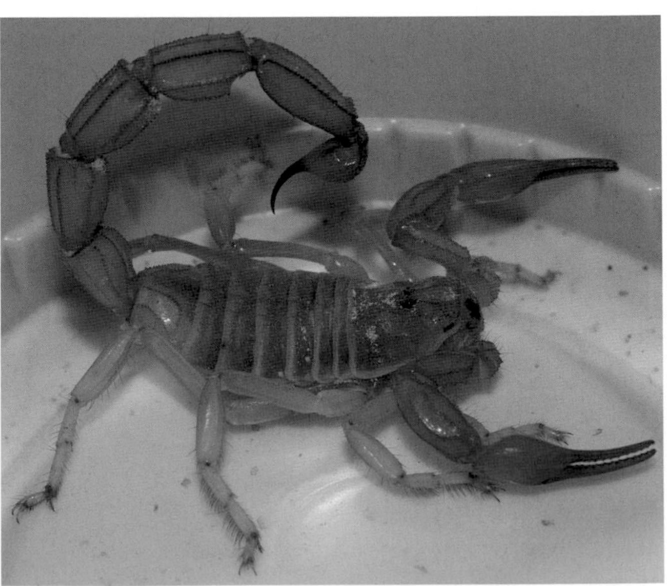

FIGURE 136.5.7 "Death stalker" scorpion (*Leiurus quinquestriatus*), Egypt *(© David A. Warrell).*

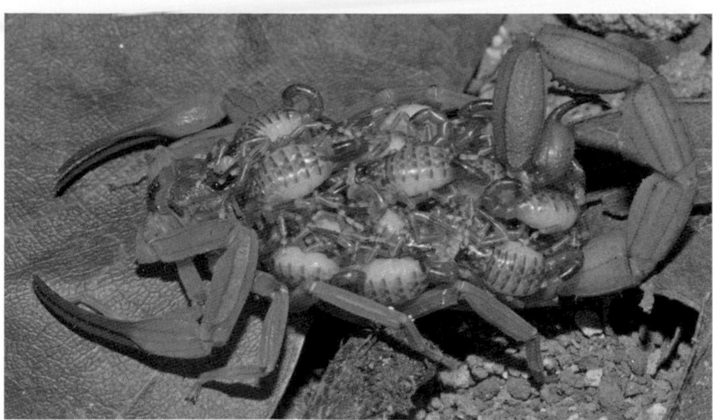

FIGURE 136.5.8 South American scorpion (*Tityus serrulatus*), female with young, São Paulo, Brazil *(© David A. Warrell).*

fourth major cause of death. In Algeria, there were 150 deaths in 1998 and 74 in 2005. In Tunisia, there are about 40,000 stings per year, 1000 hospital admissions and 100 deaths. In Arizona, 15,000 stings, mainly by *Centruroides exilicauda*, are reported each year but there have been no deaths in the USA since 1968. In Brazil, where important species are *Tityus serrulatus* (Fig. 136.5.8) and other *Tityus* spp., there were 36,558 reported stings with only 50 deaths (case fatality 0.14%) in 2005. In India, many people are stung by the red scorpion (*M. tamulus*), with fatalities in adults and children.

PREVENTION

Scorpions can be excluded from houses by incorporating a row of ceramic tiles into the base of the outside wall, making the doorsteps at least 20 cm high, and using residual insecticides, such as 1% lindane or dieldrin powders, indoors.

CLINICAL FEATURES

Buthid scorpion stings cause intense local pain with minimal local edema and tender enlargement of regional lymph nodes. However, stings by *H. lepturus* (Iran, Iraq, Pakistan and Yemen) are relatively painless, but macular erythema, pupura and bullae develops at the site, with induration in 39% of cases, and swelling and necrosis that requires surgery in 20% of cases [20]. Systemic symptoms may develop within minutes or be delayed for as long as 24 hours. Many scorpion venoms stimulate the release of acetylcholine and catecholamines, often resulting in initial transient cholinergic and, later, prolonged adrenergic symptoms [21]. Early symptoms include vomiting, profuse sweating, piloerection, alternating brady- and tachycardia, abdominal colic, diarrhea, loss of sphincter control and priapism. Later, severe life-threatening cardiorespiratory effects may appear: hypertension, shock, tachy- and bradyarrhythmias, electrocardiogram (ECG) changes and pulmonary edema with, or without, evidence of myocardial dysfunction. Severe cardiovascular complications are particularly associated with stings by *Androctonus* spp., *Leiurus quinquestriatus, Hottentota tamulus* and *Tityus* spp. In Arizona, *C. (sculpturatus) exilicauda* stings cause neurotoxic effects, such as erratic eye movements, fasciculation and muscle spasms, that can be misinterpreted as tonic-clonic convulsive movements, and respiratory distress. In southern Africa, *Parabuthus transvaalicus* envenoming is more likely to cause ptosis and dysphagia. Hemiplegia and other neurologic lesions have been attributed to fibrin deposition resulting from disseminated intravascular coagulation, for example after stings by *Nebo hierichonticus* in the Middle East. Hypercatecholaminemia could explain hyperglycemia and glycosuria but, in the case of stings by the black scorpion of Trinidad (*Tityus trinitatis*), there is severe abdominal pain with nausea, vomiting and hematemesis, hyperglycemia and biochemical evidence of acute pancreatitis attributable to simultaneous spasm of the shincter of Oddi and pancreatic exocrine hypersecretion [22]. In Iran and Iraq, stings by *H. lepturus* (Hemiscorpiidae) produce a unique clinical syndrome. Systemic symptoms include dry mouth, thirst, dizziness, nausea, vomiting, fever, cardiac arrhythmias, ECG ST-depression, hypoglycemia, confusion and convulsions, leukocytosis, thrombocytopenia, coagulopathy, hemolytic anemia with hemoglobinuria, proteinuria and renal failure. Twenty percent of pediatric cases require dialysis. Early treatment with Rhazi Institute antivenom proved effective.

TREATMENT

Pain responds temporarily to local infiltration or ring block with local anesthetic. Although they are said to relieve pain, local injection of emetine or dehydroemetine may cause necrosis and systemic myotoxic effects and are not recommended. Parenteral opiate analgesics, such as meperidine (pethidine) or morphine, may be required.

Antivenom is manufactured in several countries. Its use is strongly advocated in Africa and the Americas, but vasodilators have been preferred in Israel and India [23]. If specific antivenom is available, it should be administered intravenously (IV) as soon as possible in patients with systemic envenoming and in young children stung by dangerous species, even before the development of these symptoms. Patients with cardiovascular symptoms benefit from ancillary vasodilator treatment with α-blockers (e.g. prazosin), calcium-channel blockers (e.g. nifedipine), or angiotensin converting enzyme (ACE) inhibitors (e.g. captopril). Atropine should not be used except in cases of sinus bradycardia with hypotension. The use of cardiac glycosides and β-blockers is controversial [24]. Benzodiazepines may be useful in patients with muscle spasms.

WIND SCORPIONS, CAMEL SPIDERS OR SUN SPIDERS (SOLIFUGAE)

These arthropods are neither scorpions nor spiders, but non-venomous solifugids. They may exceed 15 cm in length and have terrified foreign troops in Iraq and Afghanistan. In Turkana (northern Kenya), the local people believe that their bite can cause coma and hypersalivation. However, solifugids lack venom and venom apparatus although they possess formidable jaws. They are mainly nocturnal and seek shade during the day. This has led to the impression that they chase people when they are merely seeking the refuge of the person's shadow.

INSECTA

COLEOPTERA (BEETLES)

The most notorious vesicating beetle is "Spanish fly" – *Lytta vesicatoria* (Meloidae – blister beetles). Its venom contains cantharidin, which causes blistering 2–3 h after application to the skin, and priapism (hence its reputation as an aphrodisiac) and renal failure when given systemically or absorbed after eating the legs of frogs which have fed on meloid beetles [25].

"Nairobi eye" and similar blistering conditions in Australia and Southeast Asia are caused by species of the genus *Paederus* (Staphylinidae), which are 5–10 mm in length [26, 27]. The typical skin lesions (dermatitis linearis) (Fig. 136.5.9), whose appearance may be delayed 12–96 h after contact, consist of erythema, itching and blistering caused by inadvertently crushing and smearing the beetle. Systemic symptoms, such as fever, arthralgia and vomiting, may arise in severe cases. The active principle pederin is the most complex non-proteinaceous insect toxin known. Treatment is palliative. The toxin is easily spread to other sites, such as the eye, by fingers.

HEMIPTERA (BUGS)

Giant water bugs or water beetles (family Belastomatidae) (Fig. 136.5.10) are found in freshwater, especially in the Americas, and may swarm in large numbers in some urban areas. They may exceed 15 cm in length and have powerful mouth parts. Their bites can inject saliva that proved lethal to mice experimentally and can cause severe pain

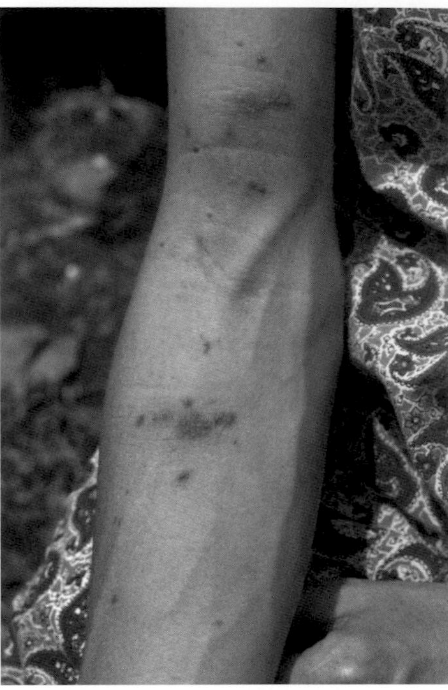

FIGURE 136.5.9 Dermatitis linearis caused by contact with a blister beetle (*Paederus* spp.) in Nigeria *(© David A. Warrell).*

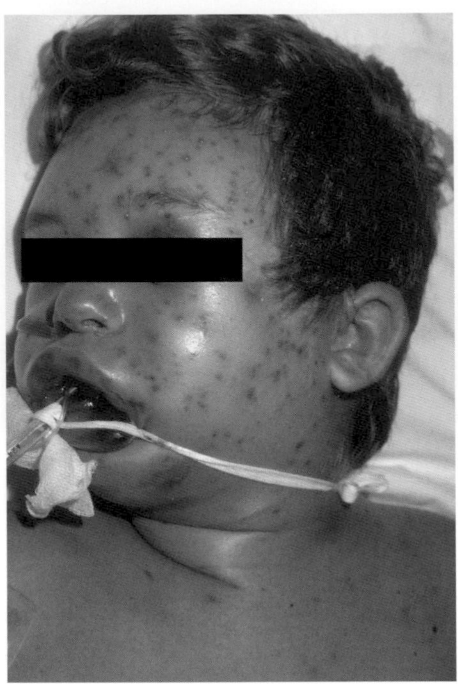

FIGURE 136.5.11 Multiple stings from Africanized bees (*Apis mellifera scutellata*), Brazil *(© David A. Warrell).*

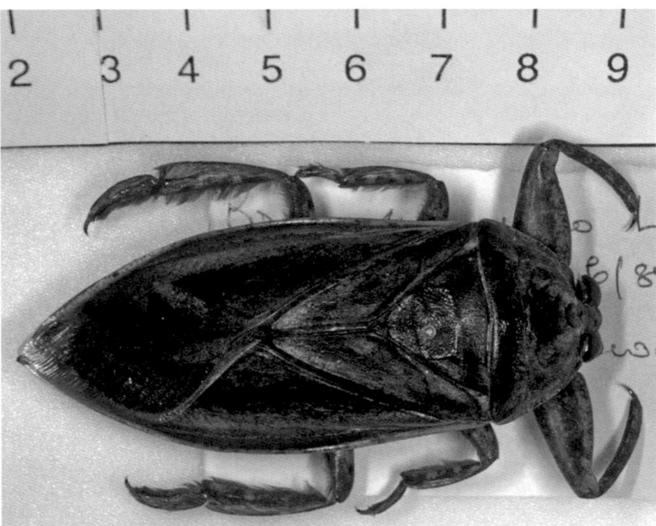

FIGURE 136.5.10 Giant water bug (*Lethocerus* spp.), Darwin, Australia *(© David A. Warrell).*

and swelling in human victims [28, 29]. In North America, *Lethocerus americanus* is known as "toe biter" from its habit of attacking swimmers. Whether or not these bugs have a true venom is unknown.

HYMENOPTERA (see also Chapter 136.1)

In non-sensitized people, a single sting, which, in the case of Vespidae and Apidae, introduces about 50 μg of venom, will rapidly produce a hot, red, painful swelling and weal a few centimeters in diameter, which persists for not more than a few hours. These effects are dangerous only if the airway is obstructed, for example following stings on the tongue. However, as few as 30 bee or wasp stings can cause fatal systemic envenoming in children, but children and adults have survived more than 1000 stings by *Apis mellifera*.

Epidemiology

Accidental release of African queen bees (*Apis mellifera scutellata*) in Brazil in 1957 resulted in the spread of this aggressive genotype throughout Latin America and as far north as Las Vegas, NV, USA [30]. An average of 30 deaths from mass attacks by these insects were reported each year at the height of the epidemic (Fig. 136.5.11). Fatal mass attacks by bees or wasps have been reported as uncommon events in Europe, Africa, Asia and Australia.

Clinical features [31]

Some patients have symptoms suggesting histamine toxicity: vasodilatation, hypotension, vomiting, diarrhea, throbbing headache, coma and bronchoconstriction. In Latin America, victims of attacks by *A. m. scutellata* have shown evidence of generalized rhabdomyolysis (grossly elevated serum creatine kinase, aminotransferases and myoglobin), intravascular hemolysis, hypercatecholaminemia (hypertension, pulmonary edema with hyaline membrane, myocardial damage), bleeding, hepatic dysfunction and acute renal failure. Mass vespid attacks can result in hepatic damage. In non-sensitized people, stings from *Solenopsis* and *Myrmecia* spp. produce pain, itching, swelling and erythema around a central weal which last a few hours, and later vesicles or pustules. In an un-sensitized patient, an estimated 10,000 *Solenopsis invicta* stings caused no systemic envenoming. Multiple traumatic bites by soldiers of army, driver, safari ants or siafu (genus *Dorylus*, Ecitoninae) may ulcerate and become secondarily infected.

Treatment

Severe envenoming from multiple stings by hymenoptera should be treated with epinephrine (adrenaline), IV antihistamines and corticosteroids (doses as above). Intensive care is essential. IV mannitol and bicarbonate may protect the kidneys from the damaging effects of myoglobinuria and hemoglobinaemia ("pigment nephropathy"), as in patients with the crush syndrome. Experimental antivenoms have been produced for bee envenoming, but are not yet commercially available. Exchange transfusion or plasmapheresis might be considered to remove venom in severe cases. Renal dialysis is often needed.

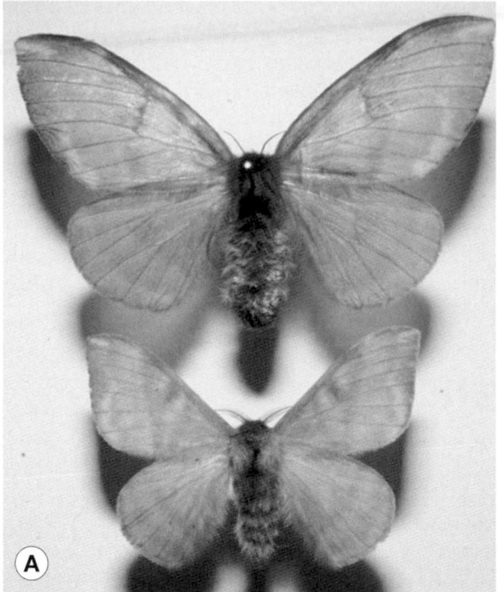

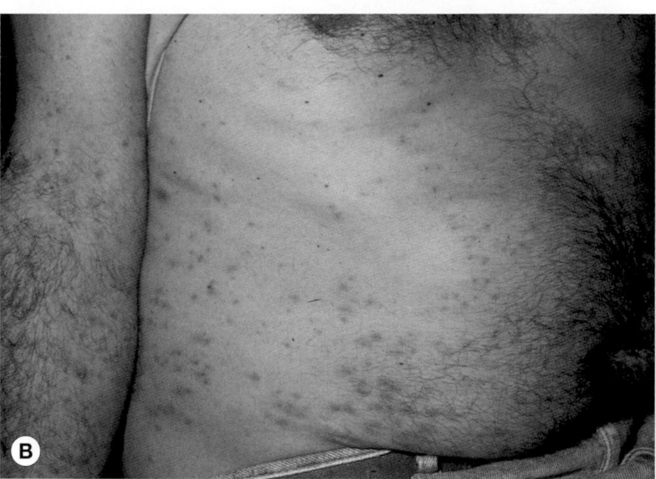

FIGURE 136.5.12 Lepidoperism caused by yellowtail or ashen moths (*Hylesia metabus*). **(A)** *Hylesia metabus* adult moths, Cayenne, French Guiana. **(B)** Vesiculo-papular lesions caused by setae from *Hylesia metabus* moths, Peruibe, São Paulo State, Brazil *(© David A. Warrell).*

LEPIDOPTERA

The stinging abdominal hairs (barbed setae or "flechettes") of some species of adult female moths [genus *Hylesia*, (Fig. 136.5.12A) family Saturniidae] which they use to protect their eggs can cause contact dermatitis and urticaria ("lepidopterism"), while caterpillars of many species of moths can produce local, or even systemic, effects ("erucism") [32]. Venomous lepidoptera are found in all parts of the world, but most cases of lepidopterism are reported from Middle and Southern America.

Common causes of cutaneous urticating vesiculo-papular eruptions and upper respiratory and gastrointestinal tract irritation with a risk of hypersensitization and anaphylaxis are:

- caterpillars of oak processionary moths (*Thaumetopoea processionea* – family Thaumetopoeidae) in central/southern Europe [33];
- caterpillars of moths of the genus *Megalopyge* (Megalopygidae, called "puss caterpillars" in the southern USA) [32];
- adult female yellowtail or ashen moths of the genus *Hylesia* (Saturniidae). Epidemics of stings by these moths have been described, especially from coastal areas of Brazil, (Fig. 136.5.12B), Peru, Venezuela and Mexico, including sailors and travelers [34, 35].

Systemic envenoming:

- caterpillars of the genus *Lonomia* – Saturniidae (*Lonomia obliqua, Lonomia achelous*) (Saturniid moths) (Fig. 136.5.13A) cause thousands of stings each year in Venezuela, Colombia, Brazil, Peru, Paraguay and French Guiana [36]. Venom injected through their bristles contains fibrinolytic (Factor XIII-activator); anticoagulant; procoagulant (prothrombin-, Factor X-, Factor V- activators); kallikrein-like metalloproteinase and phospholipase A_2 activities that cause defibrinogenation and spontaneous bleeding. Symptoms include local burning, erythema, swelling, inflammation, headache, nausea, vomiting, malaise, extensive ecchymoses (Fig. 136.5.13B); bleeding from nose, gums, gut, genito-urinary tract tract and partly-healed scars; polyarthralgia and acute kidney injury [37]. The case fatality of about 2% is usually attributable to cerebral hemorrhage. Laboratory findings in envenomed patients are decreased plasma fibrinogen, Factor V, Factor XIII, and plasminogen concentrations, as well as increased fibrin/fibrinogen degradation products and fibrinolytic activity, but a normal platelet count. A fatal imported case from Peru was reported in Canada [38]. An effective antivenom ("Soro antilonômico") is produced by Instituto Butantan, São Paulo, Brazil [39];

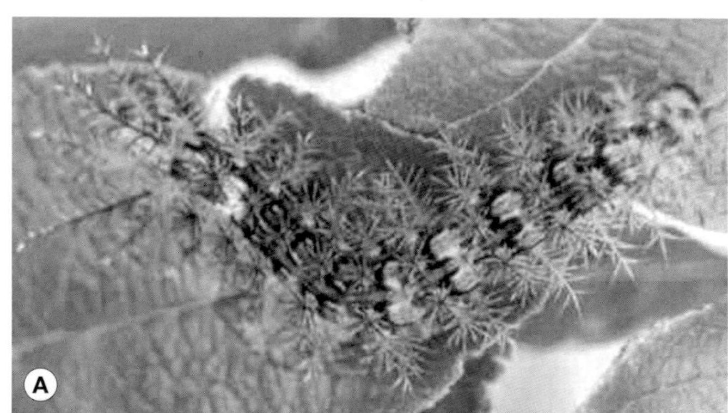

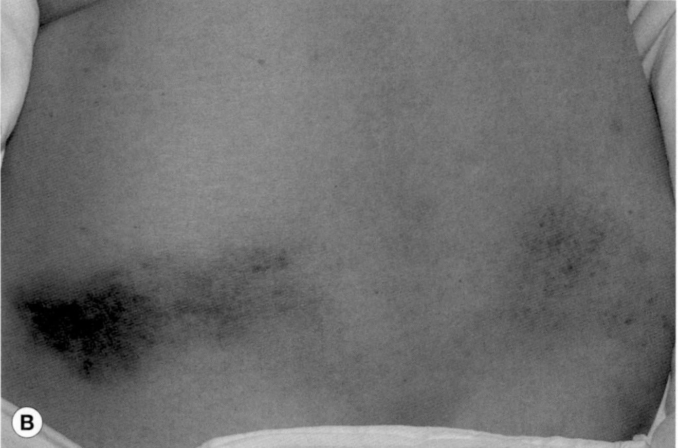

FIGURE 136.5.13 Erucism caused by Saturniid moth caterpillars (*Lonomia obliqua*). **(A)** *Lonomia achelous achelous* caterpillar, Leticia, Colombia. **(B)** Extensive bruising in a 58-year-old woman after contact with *Lonomia obliqua* caterpillars, Boissucanga, São Paulo State, Brazil *(© David A. Warrell).*

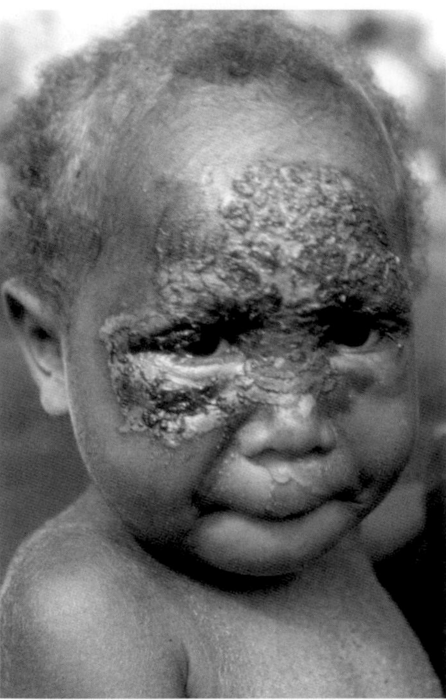

FIGURE 136.5.14 Local reaction to contact with millipedes in Madang, Papua New Guinea *(Courtesy of Dr Bernie Hudson).*

- stinging hairs of caterpillars (*Premolis semirufa*) can cause a disabling arthritis of the hands ("pararama") in rubber tappers in Pará State, Brazil, who are frequently in contact with them [40].

MYRIAPODA (CENTIPEDES AND MILLIPEDES)

CENTIPEDES (CLASS CHILOPODA)

Epimorph centipedes have 15–191 pairs of legs and move rapidly and distractedly. They occur in most parts of the world, including the Arctic Circle. The largest, *Scolopendra gigantea* of South America, can grow to more than 30 cm in length. Many species can inflict painful stings through a pair of modified claws (forcipules) on the post-cephalic segment. More than 3000 stings are reported each year in Brazil. Venoms contain serotonin, histamine, lipids, polysaccharides, proteases and peptides that are neurotoxic to insects. Stings cause intense radiating pain, swelling, inflammation, erythema and lymphangitis, and, sometimes, local necrosis. Systemic effects, such as vomiting, sweating, headache, cardiac arrhythmias, myocardial ischemia, rhabdomyolysis, proteinuria, acute renal failure and convulsions, are extremely rare. The risk of mortality was probably greatly exaggerated in older literature. Hypersensitivity may have played a role in these reactions. Reports of documented fatalities remain elusive but are said to occur on some Indian Ocean islands. The most important genus is *Scolopendra*, which is distributed throughout tropical countries. Local treatment is the same as for scorpion stings. No antivenom is available [41].

MILLIPEDES (CLASS DIPLOPIDA) [42, 43]

Millipedes are widely distributed. They may exceed 35 cm in length, have hundreds (not thousands) of legs, move sluggishly and tend to coil into a ball. Most species possess glands in each of their body segments which secrete, and in some cases squirt out, irritant liquids for defensive purposes. These contain hydrogen cyanide and a variety of aldehydes, esters, phenols and quinonoids. Members of at least eight genera of millipedes have proved injurious to humans. Important genera are *Rhinocricus* (Caribbean), *Spirobolus* (Tanzania and Papua New Guinea), *Spirostreptus* and *Iulus* (Indonesia), and *Polyceroconas* (*Salpidobolus*) (Papua New Guinea). Children are particularly at risk when they handle or try to eat these large arthropods. When venom is squirted into the eye, intense conjunctivitis results and there may be corneal ulceration and, allegedly, blindness. Skin lesions initially stain brown ("mahogany stains") or purple, blister after a few days and then peel (Fig. 136.5.14). They have been mistaken for signs of child abuse. First aid is generous irrigation with water. Eye injuries should be treated as for snake venom ophthalmia (see Chapter 134.5).

REFERENCES

1. Gothe R, Kunze K, Hoogstraal H. The mechanism of pathogenicity in the tick paralyses. J Med Entomol 1979;16:357–69.
2. Murnaghan MF, O'Rourke FJ. Tick paralysis. In: Bettini S, ed. Arthropod Venoms. Handbook of Experimental Pharmacology, Vol. 48. Berlin: Springer-Verlag; 1979:419.
3. Stone BF. Toxicoses induced by ticks and reptiles in domestic animals. In. Harris JB, ed. Natural Toxins: Animal, Plant and Microbial. Oxford: Oxford University Press; 1987:56–71.
4. Pearn J. The clinical features of tick bite. Med J Aust 1977;2:313.
5. Mareti Z, Lebez D. Araneism with Special Reference to Europe. Pula-Ljubjan: Novit; 1979.
6. Clark RF, Wethern-Kestner S, Vance MV, Gerkin R. Clinical presentation and treatment of black widow spider envenomation: a review of 163 cases. Ann Emerg Med 1992;21:782–7.
7. Southcott RV. Arachnidism and allied syndromes in the Australian region. Records of the Adelaide Children's Hospital 1976;1:97–186.
8. Isbister GK Fray MR, Balit CR, et al. Funnel-web spider bite: a systematic review of recorded clinical cases. Med J Aust 2005;182:407–11.
9. Warrell DA, Shaheen J, Hillyard PD, Jones D. Neurotoxic envenoming by an immigrant spider (*Steatoda nobilis*) in southern England. Toxicon 1991;29: 1263–5.
10. Isbister GK, White J, Currie BJ, et al. Spider bites: addressing mythology and poor evidence. Am J Trop Med Hyg 2005;72:361–4.
11. Sutherland SK, Tibballs J. Australian Animal Toxins. The Creatures, Their Toxins and Care of the Poisoned Patient, 2nd edn. Melbourne: Oxford University Press; 2001.
12. Pauli I, PUka J Gubert IC, Minozzo JC. The efficacy of antivenom in loxoscelism treatment. Toxicon 2006;48:123–37.
13. Isbister GK. Antivenom efficacy or effectiveness: the Australian experience. Toxicology 2010;268:148–54.
14. Isbister GK, Seymour JE, Gray MR, Raven RJ. Bites by spiders of the family Theraphosidae in humans and canines. Toxicon 2003;41:519–24.
15. Ahmed N, Pinkham M, Warrell DA. Symptom in search of a toxin: muscle spasms following bites by Old World tarantula spiders (*Lampropelma nigerrimum, Pterinochilus murinus, Poecilotheria regalis*) with review. Q J Med 2009;102:851–7.
16. Fet V, Selden PA, eds. Catalog of the Scorpions of the World. (1758–998). New York: New York Entomological Society; 2000.
17. Polis GA, ed The Biology of Scorpions. Stanford: Stanford University Press; 1990.
18. Bettini S, ed. Athropod Venoms. Handbook of Experimental Pharmacology, Vol. 48. Berlin: Springer-Verlag; 1978:977.
19. Brownell P, Polis G, eds. Scorpion Biology and Research. New York: Oxford University Press; 2001.
20. Pipelzadeh MH, Jalali A, Taraz M, et al. An epidemiological and a clinical study on scorpionism by the Iranian scorpion *Hemiscorpius lepturus*. Toxicon 2007;50:984–92.
21. Ismail M. The scorpion envenoming syndrome. Toxicon 1995;33:825–58.
22. Waterman JA. Some notes on scorpion poisoning in Trinidad. Trans Soc Trop Med Hyg 1938;31:607–24.
23. Bawaskar HS, Bawaskar PH. Management of the cardiovascular manifestations of poisoning by the Indian red scorpion (Mesobuthus tamulus). Br Heart J 1992;68:478–80.
24. Freire-Maia L, Campos JA, Amaral CFS. Treatment of scorpion envenoming in Brazil. In: Bon C, Goyffon M, eds. Envenomings and Their Treatments. Lyon: Edition Fondation Marcel Mérieux; 1996:301–10.
25. Eisner T, Conner J, Carrel JE, et al. Systemic retention of ingested cantharidin by frogs. Chemoecology 1990;1:57–62.
26. Southcott RV. Injuries from Coleoptera. Med J Aust 1989;151:654–9.

27. Frank JH, Kanamitsu K. *Paederus sensu lato* (Coleoptera: Staphylinidae): natural history and medical importance. J Med Entomol 1987;24:1555–91.
28. Vigors Earle K. Injuries produced by tropical "water-beetles". Trans R Soc Trop Med Hyg 1948;42:101–4.
29. Haddad V, Jr, Schwartz EF, Schwartz CA, Carvalho LN. Bites caused by giant water bugs belonging to Belostomatidae family (Hemiptera, Heteroptera) in humans: A report of seven cases. Wilderness Environ Med 2010;21:130–3.
30. Winston ML. Killer Bees. The Africanized Honey Bee in the Americas. Cambridge, MA: Harvard University Press; 1992.
31. França FOS, Benvenuti LA, Fan HW, et al. Severe and fatal mass attacks by 'killer' bees (Africanised honey bees – Apis melliferascutellata in Brazil: clinicopathological studies with measurement of serum venom concentrations. Q J Med 1994;87269–82.
32. Hossler EW. Caterpillars and moths: Dermatologic manifestations of encounters with Lepidoptera. J Am Acad Dermatol 2010;62:1–10, 13–28.
33. Maier H, Spiegel W, Kinaciyan T, et al. The oak processionary caterpillar as the cause of an epidemic airborne disease: survey and analysis. Br J Dermatol 2003;149:990–7.
34. Rodriquez J, et al. External morphology of abdominal setae from male and female Hylesia metabus adults (Lepidoptera: Saturniidae) and their function. Florida Entomologist 2004;87:30–6.
35. Rodriguez-Morales AJ, Arria M, Rojas-Mirabal J, et al. Lepidopterism due to exposure to the moth *Hylesia metabus* in northeastern Venezuela. Am J Trop Med Hyg 2005;73:991–3.
36. Kelen EMA, Picarelli ZP, Duarte AC. Hemorrhagic syndrome induced by contact with caterpillars of the genus Lonomia (Saturniidae, Hamileucinae). J Toxicol: Toxin Rev 1995;14:283–308.
37. Carrijo-Carvalho LC, Chudzinski-Tavassi AM. The venom of the Lonomia caterpillar: an overview. Toxicon 2007;49:741–57.
38. Chan K, Lee A. Onell R, et al. Caterpillar-induced bleeding syndrome in a returning traveller. CMAJ 2008;179:158–61.
39. Da Silva WD, Campos CM, Gonçalves LR, et al. Development of an antivenom against toxins of *Lonomia obliqua* caterpillars. Toxicon 1996;34:1045–9.
40. Costa RM, Atra E, Ferraz MB. "Pararamose": an occupational arthritis caused by lepidoptera (*Premolis semirufa*). An epidemiological study. Rev Paul Med 1993;111:462–5.
41. Bettini S, ed. Arthropod Venoms. Handbook of Experimental Pharmacology, Vol. 48. Berlin: Springer-Verlag; 1978: 977.
42. Radford AJ. Millipede burns in man. Trop Geogr Med 1975;27:279–87.
43. Radford AJ. Giant millipede burns in Papua New Guinea. PNG Med J 1976;18:138–41.

USEFUL WEBSITE

http://www.ntnu.no/ub/scorpion-files/links.php (last accessed 03-03-2012)

PART

8

NUTRITIONAL PROBLEMS AND DEFICIENCY DISEASES

137 General Principles

Benjamin Caballero, Wafaie Fawzi

Nutritional problems in tropical areas are almost always associated with deficiency states, with protein-energy malnutrition, hypovitaminosis A and iron and iodine deficiencies being the most prevalent. Other micronutrient deficiencies, including deficiencies in B vitamins tend to co-exist in the same communities. Emerging evidence indicates that vitamin D deficiency is also highly prevalent in many regions of thes world. Over 20% of the world population consumes amounts of foods insufficient to sustain health and an active and productive life; malnutrition contributes to more than one third of all child deaths.

Insufficient dietary intake of protein, energy, and/or micro-nutrients is only one factor leading to nutritional diseases in the tropics. The unsanitary environment leads to frequent infections of the gastrointestinal tract, which, even if relatively minor, cause malabsorption of essential nutrients, reduced intake resulting from loss of appetite and altered metabolic processes associated with infection, collectively leading to worsening of nutritional status. A child living in an unsanitary environment can have as many as ten or more episodes of acute gastroenteritis in a year. Each episode leads to a negative balance between intake and losses, with consequent weight loss and delay in longitudinal growth. In addition, many children living in a highly contaminated environment exhibit a state of chronic immune stimulation; this constant stimulation may also contribute to a significant nutritional cost. Children who survive recurring illnesses early in life may never recover from their growth delay, becoming permanently stunted adults. Conversely, an impaired nutritional status increases the risk of infection by affecting cellular and humoral immune systems, facilitating microorganism colonization, and increasing the frequency and severity of infectious illnesses. This vicious cycle of malnutrition leading to more frequent and severe forms of infections, which, in turn, contributes to further deterioration of nutritional status, contributes to higher mortality rates observed among children in tropical developing countries. This cycle can be interrupted through nutritional interventions, as well as other measures that reduce the risk of infections, such as enhanced water quality and sanitation in these settings.

Although nutritional deficiencies are by far the most common in developing countries, there is an increasing trend, particularly in urban areas, toward diseases, commonly associated with nutritional excess, such as obesity, diabetes, and cardiovascular disease. The majority of humans now live in cities and the rapid migration to the cities has produced drastic changes in lifestyle and food choices in children and adults. Energy expenditure for physical activity is reduced owing to a more sedentary way of life, and more "empty" calories and processed foods are consumed; although the diet may still be marginal in certain nutrients, it is likely to contain more calories from fat, including more saturated fats. As a consequence, stunting in linear growth and excess body fat can be observed in many children in the poor slums of large urban areas in developing countries. The increasing prevalence of these conditions will continue to pose a challenge to health care systems, which have historically focused on the management of nutritional deficiencies in resource-limited settings. As such, strengthening of health systems is critical to addressing both under- and over-nutrition in resource-limited settings, including enhancing quality of care through expanded and improved training of health workers for the prevention and management of nutritional disorders. Scaling-up these services in community-based settings to reach women and children who have difficulty accessing health facilities is also urgently needed. Quite simply, a greater investment of resources in nutritional services could play a very significant role in preventing the major causes of disease and death globally.

Protein-energy Malnutrition in Children

138

Tahmeed Ahmed, M Iqbal Hossain, Munirul Islam, AM Shamsir Ahmed, M Jobayer Chisti

Key features

- Protein-energy malnutrition (PEM) is the most common childhood ailment in the world and is primarily caused by deficiency of energy, protein and micronutrients
- PEM manifests as underweight (low body weight compared with healthy peers), stunting (poor linear growth), wasting (acute weight loss) or edematous malnutrition (kwashiorkor)
- Case fatality rates among children hospitalized with severe wasting or edema (also known as severe acute malnutrition [SAM]) range from 5% to 30%
- All forms of PEM are associated with increased risk of infectious illnesses and cognitive deficit
- Management of most forms of PEM can be done in the community setting by improving household food security, promoting appropriate complementary food, providing micronutrients, providing anti-helminthic treatment and preventing (e.g. by vaccines) and treating infectious illnesses
- Children with SAM and associated acute illnesses should be treated in a hospital setting using World Health Organization (WHO) guidelines. Children with SAM who are not acutely ill and have an appetite can be managed in the community using ready-to-use-therapeutic foods, preferably made locally

INTRODUCTION

Protein-energy malnutrition (PEM) includes a number of distinct disorders of growth in children primarily caused by deficiency of nutrients, notably protein and energy. Micronutrient deficiencies are also common in these disorders. PEM includes the following conditions:

- Underweight: a child with a body weight less than that of normal children of same age and sex (more than two standard deviations [SD] below the median weight of World Health Organization [WHO] growth standards). Severe underweight is defined as a body weight less than -3SD.
- Stunting: a child with a height or length less than that of normal children of same age and sex (more than two SD below the median height or length of WHO growth standards). Severe stunting is defined as a height or length less than -3SD.
- Wasting: a child has wasting if the body weight is more than two SDs below the median weight of normal children of same height or length of WHO growth standards. A child has severe wasting if the weight-for-height (WHZ)/length is less than -3SD.
- Severe acute malnutrition (SAM): a serious condition characterized by the presence of any of the following features – severe wasting, bilateral pedal edema and a mid-upper arm circumference (MUAC) of less than 11.5 cm. It includes marasmus, kwashiorkor and marasmic kwashiorkor.

Chronic deprivation of nutrients usually results in stunting, while wasting occurs when there is an acute deprivation of nutrients over a short interval. An underweight child may also have wasting and stunting. Wasting and stunting are commonly seen in children between the ages of 1 and 2 years, but by 3–4 years of age, children in developing countries are more stunted than wasted. This indicates that these children have stopped growing in height, but may have a normal WHZ. The earliest account of kwashiorkor – a severe form of PEM characterized by edema – was published in 1865 by Hinajosa in Mexico. The acuteness of kwashiorkor has been the focus of attention of nutritionists and as many as 70 names have been given to this condition in different parts of the world. Cicely Williams first introduced the name kwashiorkor in 1935, which in the Ga language of West Africa means "the disease of the deposed child". This literally refers to the child who develops edema after being weaned with starchy gruels following the birth of a sibling who is breastfed.

EPIDEMIOLOGY AND CONSEQUENCES

About one-third of all children under the age of five years in developing countries are stunted, while 20% are underweight. An estimated 178 million children are stunted and, of them, 74 million live in south-central Asia (Fig. 138.1). A total of 36 countries account for 90% of all stunted children worldwide; India alone has more than 61 million stunted children. Most of these children are from the poorest segments of the population. Wasting, which is also known as moderate acute malnutrition (MAM), has a global prevalence of 10% (55 million children affected).

Underweight, stunting and wasting contribute to 19%, 14.5% and 14.6% of deaths respectively, among children under the age of five years in the developing world. Case fatality rates among children admitted to a hospital with severe acute malnutrition are very high and range from 5% to 30%. Among survivors, comorbidities are common. Because of reduced immunocompetence (impaired delayed hypersensitivity to antigens, selective B cell and complement malfunction), prevalence and severity of infections, notably the infectious diarrheas, are greater compared with well nourished peers. Impairment of cognitive function commonly occurs in malnourished children and this may be irreversible. For every 10% increase in stunting, the proportion of children reaching the final grade of primary school drops by 7.9%.

CAUSES OF PROTEIN-ENERGY MALNUTRITION (PEM)

Malnutrition because of lack of food and the interplay of infections is known as primary malnutrition, which is responsible for most malnutrition seen in the developing world. However, there is a host of basic and underlying causes of malnutrition that operate at national and societal levels (Fig. 138.2). The root causes of malnutrition are

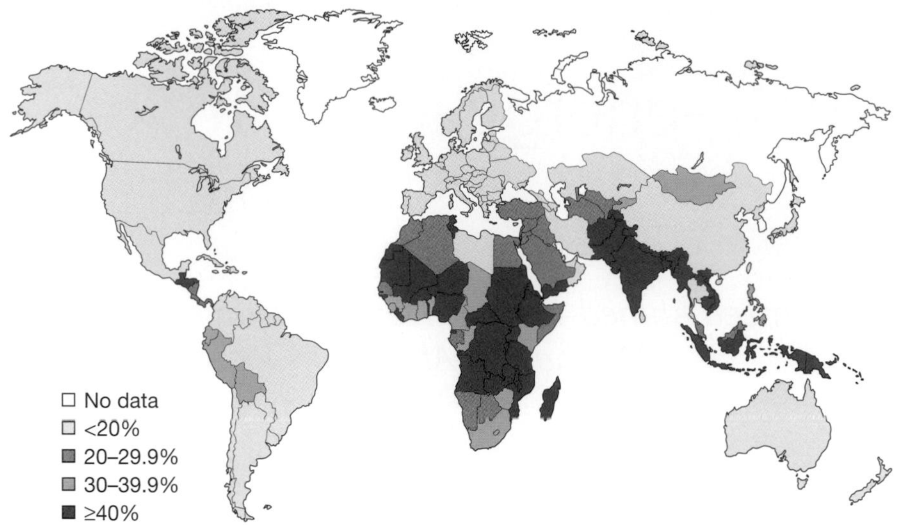

FIGURE 138.1 Global prevalence of stunting in children under 5 years of age. Most of the burden of stunting is in South Asia and sub-Saharan Africa. *(From [1]).*

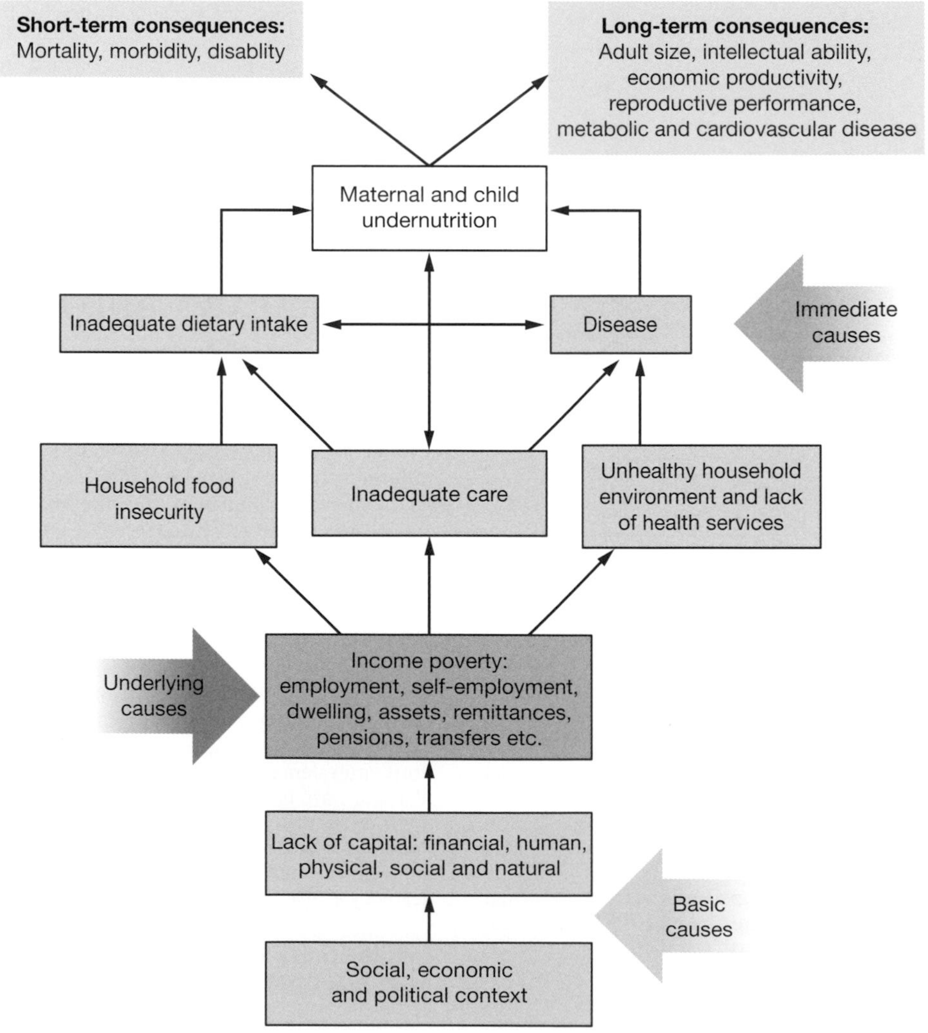

FIGURE 138.2 Framework of causes of maternal and child malnutrition. *(From [1]).*

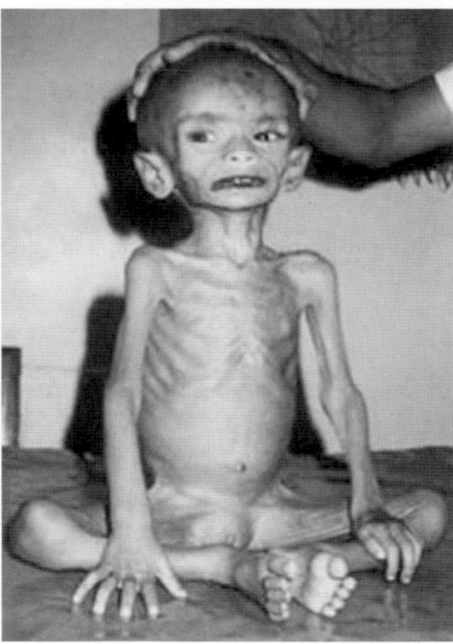

FIGURE 138.3 Severe wasting occurs when there is loss of body fat, subcutaneous tissues and muscles.

political in nature interlaced with issues of social and gender inequity, particularly of income and education. Civil conflicts and social inequalities are important precipitating factors. Malnutrition occurring as a result of chronic diseases, such as chronic kidney, liver or heart disease, is known as secondary malnutrition.

CLINICAL FEATURES

Thinness and short stature may be the only features of moderate underweight, stunting and wasting. The manifestation of severe acute malnutrition can be quite dramatic and the major signs include severe wasting, edema, skin changes or dermatosis, and eye signs. Severe wasting occurs when there is loss of body fat, subcutaneous tissues and muscles. In a severe case, the body appears to have only skin and bones with wrinkling of the skin, the head looks disproportionately large and the ribs are markedly visible (Fig. 138.3). The skin becomes redundant on the severely wasted buttocks, giving a "baggy pants" appearance (Fig. 138.4). A WHZ of less than -3SD and a MUAC less than 11.5 cm indicate severe wasting.

In the absence of other causes of edema, such as nephrotic syndrome, the presence of bilateral pedal edema is a sign of SAM. A decrease in serum albumin level is partly responsible for development of edema. Other factors that contribute to the development of edema in SAM include decreased body potassium and reduced inactivation of antidiuretic hormone. Edema is detected by pressing on the dorsum of the foot for 3–5 seconds; an indentation on release of pressure indicates pedal edema (Fig. 138.5).

Based on severity, there are three categories of edema:

Mild: both feet (can include ankles), grade +;
Moderate: both feet, lower legs, hands or lower arms, grade + +;
Severe: generalized bilateral pitting edema including both feet, legs, hands, arms and face, grade + + +.

Dermatosis is a skin condition that is common in severe acute malnutrition. A child with dermatosis may have patches of skin that are abnormally light or dark in color, shedding of skin in scales or sheets, and ulceration of the skin of the perineum, groin, limbs, behind the ears and in the armpits. There may be weeping lesions. There may be severe rash in the distribution of a diaper. Secondary infection can occur.

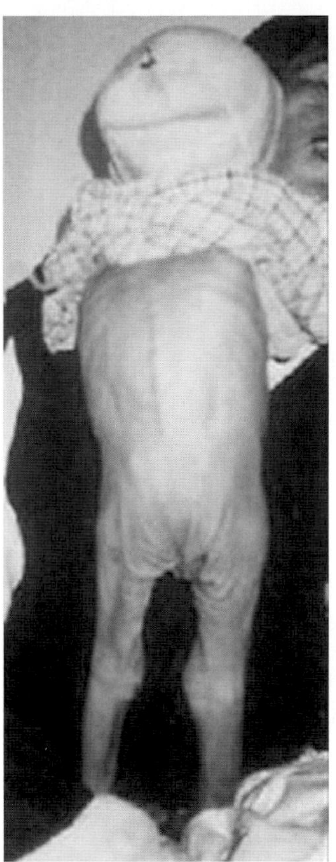

FIGURE 138.4 "Baggy pants" appearance in severe wasting or severe acute malnutrition.

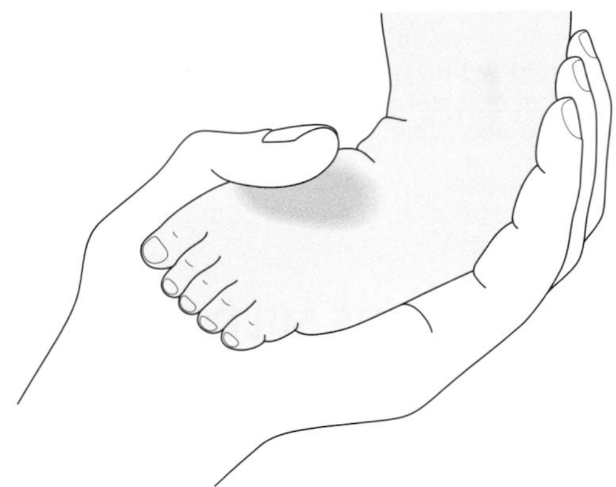

FIGURE 138.5 Detection of pedal edema.

The extent of dermatosis is described in the following way:

Mild: discoloration or a few rough patches of skin, grade +;
Moderate: multiple patches on arms and/or legs, grade ++;
Severe: flaking skin, raw skin, fissures (openings in the skin), grade +++.

Clinical terms describing severe PEM are used mostly in hospital settings. A child with a weight-for-age of less than -3SD and no edema is said to have "marasmus", while a child with a weight-for-age of more than -3SD and bilateral pedal edema has "kwashiorkor". "Marasmic kwashiorkor" is the condition where weight-for-age is less than -3SD and edema is present.

Marasmus has been recognized for centuries. It is usually seen in infancy and is characterized by severe weight reduction, gross wasting of muscle and tissue beneath the skin, stunting and no edema.

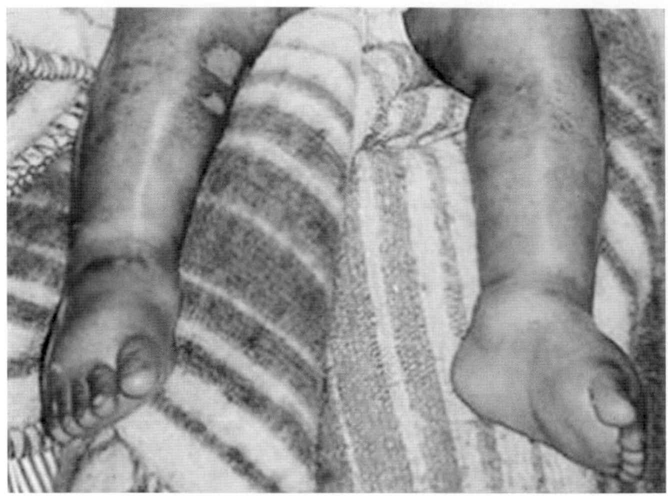

FIGURE 138.6 Bilateral pedal edema in a child with kwashiorkor.

Usually, the child is irritable. Marasmus occurs as a result of severe deficiency of energy, protein, vitamins and minerals, although the primary cause is inadequate energy intake. This deficiency often results when there is a decrease or absence of breastfeeding, feeding on diluted milk formula or a delay in introducing solid foods in the diet. In marasmus, the body generally adapts itself to the deficiency of energy and protein. The muscles provide amino acids leading to the production of proteins including albumin and β-lipoprotein. Adequate amounts of albumin and β-lipoprotein prevent the development of edema and fatty enlargement of the liver in marasmus.

Kwashiorkor, which occurs mostly in children 1–3 years of age, results from a deficiency of dietary protein and is usually associated with an infection. Typically, there are skin lesions (pigmented or de-pigmented areas with or without ulceration), scanty lustre-less hair, loss of interest in the surroundings and loss of appetite (Fig. 138.6). The edema is usually noticed in the feet, but can also occur in other parts of the body. β-lipoprotein is not produced in adequate amounts, resulting in impaired transport of fat and an enlarged fatty liver.

A child with marasmic kwashiorkor has clinical findings of both marasmus and kwashiorkor. There may be mild hair and skin changes, and an enlarged, fatty liver.

MANAGEMENT OF MILD OR MODERATE MALNUTRITION

Mildly- or moderately-malnourished children account for the major burden of malnutrition in any developing country. These children have an increased susceptibility to infections and have impaired intellectual capabilities. They can progress to severe malnutrition so management of these children is, therefore, important from a public health perspective. Management of these children takes place at household and community levels. The focus should be on the counseling of parents on health and nutrition education so that the diet of the child is improved through breastfeeding and appropriate complementary feeding; that proper care is taken during common illnesses, including diarrhea; that micronutrients are provided, either through food or by supplementation; that routine vaccines are administered; and, in many countries, that periodic deworming is done. This is commonly done in developing countries by a strategy called growth monitoring and promotion (GMP) where children under the age of five years are weighed at regular intervals and a package of interventions provided at the visits for promoting growth. Potential strengths of GMP are that it provides frequent contact with health workers and a platform for child health interventions. However, the success of GMP depends on how sincerely the promotion part, particularly counseling for changing behavior, is carried out by community health workers.

There is now an increased interest in improving water quality, sanitation and hygiene as a means of reducing malnutrition. This is based on the premise that children in developing countries are continuously exposed to pathogenic bacteria. These bacteria may not result in enteric disease, but colonize the small intestine causing atrophy of the intestinal villi. As a result, there is malabsorption and malnutrition. This condition is called environmental enteropathy and is believed to be responsible for 40% of childhood malnutrition in some countries. Food supplementation through large scale programs has also been tried with limited success in reducing moderate acute malnutrition. However, the ultimate goal in the management of moderate malnutrition is to reduce food insecurity through increased availability and access to food and its utilization.

PHASES OF MANAGEMENT OF SEVERE ACUTE MALNUTRITION (SAM)

The management of children with SAM can be divided into three phases.

1. Acute phase: problems that endanger life, such as hypoglycemia or an infection, are identified and treated. Feeding and correction of micronutrient deficiencies are initiated during this phase. Small, frequent feeds are given (about 100 kcal/kg and 1–1.5 g protein/kg per day). Broad-spectrum antibiotics are started. The main objective of this phase is to stabilize the child. Case fatality is highest during this phase of management, the principal causes of death being hypoglycemia, hypothermia, infection and water-electrolyte imbalance. Most deaths occur within the first 1–2 days of admission. This treatment phase usually takes about 3–5 days.
2. Nutritional rehabilitation: the aim of this phase is to recover lost weight by intensive feeding. The child is stimulated emotionally and physically, and the mother is trained to continue care at home. Around 150–250 kcal/kg and 3–5 g protein/kg are provided daily during this phase. Micronutrients, including iron, are continued. The mothers are counseled on health and nutrition. This phase takes 2–4 weeks if the criterion of discharge is WHZ -2 without edema. It can take longer if the child is managed on an outpatient basis.
3. Follow-up: follow-up is done to prevent relapse of severe malnutrition and to ensure proper physical growth and mental development of the child. The likelihood of relapse into SAM is highest within one month of discharge. Follow-up visits should be fortnightly initially and then monthly until the child has achieved WHZ >-1. Nutritional status and general condition are assessed and the care givers counseled. Common illnesses are treated.

STEP 1: TREAT/PREVENT HYPOGLYCEMIA

Hypoglycemia and hypothermia usually occur together and are signs of infection. The child should be tested for hypoglycemia on admission or whenever lethargy, convulsions or hypothermia are found. If blood glucose cannot be measured, all children with SAM suspected to have hypoglycemia should be treated accordingly.

If the child is conscious and blood glucose is <3mmol/l or 54mg/dl:

> 50 ml bolus of 10% glucose or 10% sucrose solution (1 rounded teaspoon of sugar in 3.5 tablespoons water) is given orally or by nasogastric (NG) tube. The starter diet F-75 (see Step 7) is given every 30 min for two hours (giving one quarter of the two-hourly feed each time). Thereafter, two-hourly feeds are continued for first 24–48 hours.

If the child is unconscious, lethargic or convulsing:

> sterile 10% glucose (5 ml/kg) is given intravenously (IV), followed by 50 ml of 10% glucose or sucrose by NG tube. Then the starter diet F-75 is given as above (Box 138.1).

BOX 138.1 Recipes for F-75 and F-100

If you have cereal flour and cooking facilities, use one of the top three recipes for F-75:

Alternatives	Ingredients	Amount for F-75
If you have dried skimmed milk	Dried skimmed milk	25 g
	Sugar	70 g
	Cereal flour	35 g
	Vegetable oil	30 g
	Mineral mix*	20 ml
	Water to make 1000 ml	*1000 ml***
If you have dried whole milk	Dried whole milk	35 g
	Sugar	70 g
	Cereal flour	35 g
	Vegetable oil	20 g
	Mineral mix*	20 ml
	Water to make 1000 ml	*1000 ml***
If you have fresh cow's milk, or full-cream (whole) long life milk	Fresh cow's milk, or full-cream (whole) long life milk	300 ml
	Sugar	70 g
	Cereal flour	35 g
	Vegetable oil	20 g
	Mineral mix*	20 ml
	Water to make 1000 ml	*1000 ml***

If you do not have cereal flour, or there are no cooking facilities, use one of the following recipes for F-75: / **No cooking is required for F-100:**

Alternatives	Ingredients	Amount for F-75	Amount for F-100
If you have dried skimmed milk	Dried skimmed milk	25 g	80 g
	Sugar	100 g	50 g
	Vegetable oil	30 g	60 g
	Mineral mix*	20 ml	20 ml
	Water to make 1000 ml	*1000 ml***	*1000 ml***
If you have dried whole milk	Dried whole milk	35 g	110 g
	Sugar	100 g	50 g
	Vegetable oil	20 g	30 g
	Mineral mix*	20 ml	20 ml
	Water to make 1000 ml	*1000 ml***	*1000 ml***
If you have fresh cow's milk, or full-cream (whole) long life milk	Fresh cow's milk, or full-cream (whole) long life milk	300 ml	880 ml
	Sugar	100 g	75 g
	Vegetable oil	20 g	20 g
	Mineral mix*	20 ml	20 ml
	Water to make 1000 ml	*1000 ml***	*1000 ml***

*Contents of mineral mix are given in Appendix 4 of the manual. Alternatively, a commercial product called *Combined Mineral Vitamin Mix (CMV)* may be used.
(From World Health Organization. Management of Severe Malnutrition: A Manual for Physicians and Other Senior Health Workers. Geneva: World Health Organization; 1999).

**Important note about adding water: Add just the amount of water needed to make 1000 ml of formula. (This amount will vary from recipe to recipe, depending on the other ingredients.) Do not simply add 1000 ml of water, as this will make the formula too dilute. A mark for 1000 ml should be made on the mixing container for the formula, so that water can be added to the other ingredients up to this mark.

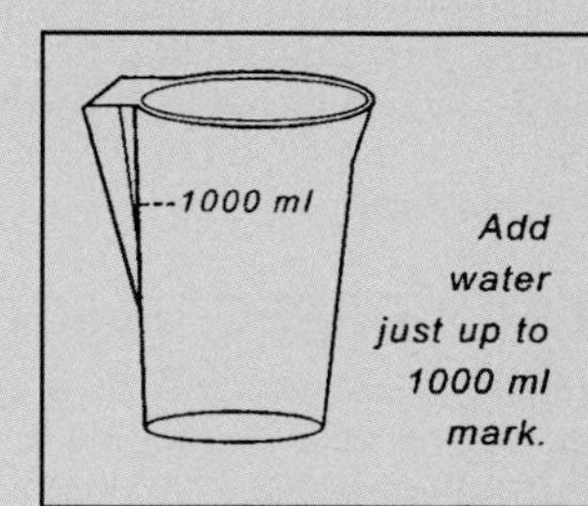

BOX 138.2 Recipe for ReSoMal

Ingredients	Amount
Water (boiled and cooled)	1.7 liters
WHO-ORS (hypo-osmolar)	One 1 liter sachet
Sugar	40 g
Electrolyte/mineral solution*	33 ml

ReSoMal contains approximately <45 mmol/l sodium, 40 mmol/l potassium and 3 mmol/l magnesium.

- Every 30 minutes for first 2 hours, ReSoMal 5 ml/kg body weight is given orally or by NG tube.
- Then, in alternate hours for up to 10 hours, ReSoMal is given 5–10 ml/kg/h (the amount to be given should be determined by how much the child wants, and stool loss and vomiting). F-75 is given in alternate hours during this period until the child is rehydrated.

*See Box 138.3.

NG, nasogastric; WHO-ORS, World Health Organization-Oral Rehydration Solution.

STEP 2: TREAT/PREVENT HYPOTHERMIA

If the axillary temperature is <35.0°C or the rectal temperature is <35.5°C, the child is given feeds and re-warmed by covering with a warm blanket or placing the child on the mother's bare chest (skin-to-skin) and covering them with a blanket. A heater or lamp may be placed nearby. The child must be kept dry and away from drafts.

STEP 3: TREAT/PREVENT DEHYDRATION

Assessment of dehydration can be difficult in a severely malnourished child. All children with watery diarrhea should be assumed to have dehydration and given ReSoMal, a special rehydration solution for children with SAM. It contains less sodium and more potassium and glucose than the standard oral rehydration solution (ORS) (Box 138.2).

If diarrhea is severe, then the standard hypo-osmolar WHO-ORS (75 mmol sodium/l) may be used as loss of sodium in stool is high and symptomatic hyponatremia can occur with ReSoMal. Severe diarrhea can be caused by cholera or rotavirus infection, and is usually defined as stool output >5 ml/kg/hr.

Return of tears, moist mouth, eyes and fontanelle appearing less sunken, and improved skin turgor are signs that rehydration is proceeding. It should be noted that many severely malnourished children will not show these changes, even when fully rehydrated. Signs of over-hydration are increasing respiratory rate and pulse rate, increasing edema and puffy eyelids. If these signs occur, fluids are stopped immediately and the child reassessed after one hour. IV rehydration should be used only in case of shock, infusing slowly to avoid overloading the heart.

STEP 4: CORRECT ELECTROLYTE IMBALANCE

All severely malnourished children have excess body sodium, even though serum sodium may be low. Deficiencies of potassium and magnesium are also present and may take at least two weeks to correct. Edema is partly caused by these imbalances and must never be treated with a diuretic. The following are given to a child with SAM:

- extra potassium 3–4 mmol/kg/day;
- extra magnesium 0.4–0.6 mmol/kg/day.

BOX 138.3 Recipe for Electrolyte/Mineral Solution

	Amount (g)	Molar content of 20 ml
Potassium chloride	224	24 mmol
Tripotassium citrate	81	2 mmol
Magnesium chloride	76	3 mmol
Zinc acetate	8.2	300 μmol
Copper sulphate	1.4	45 μmol
Water up to	2500 ml	

The extra potassium and magnesium are not required if electrolyte/mineral solution is used in preparing ReSoMal and the feeds (Box 138.3).

STEP 5: TREAT INFECTION

In severe malnutrition, the usual signs of infection, such as fever, are often absent. Therefore, broad-spectrum antibiotics based on local antimicrobial resistance patterns are given routinely on admission.

If the child appears to have no complications:

- oral amoxicillin 15 mg/kg eight-hourly for five days

If the child appears sick or lethargic, or has complications (hypoglycemia, hypothermia, skin lesions, respiratory tract or urinary tract infection):

- ampicillin 50 mg/kg intramuscularly (IM)/IV six-hourly for two days, then oral amoxicillin 15 mg/kg eight-hourly for five days;
- gentamicin 7.5 mg/kg IM/IV once daily for seven days.

If the child fails to improve clinically by 48 hours or deteriorates after 24 hours, a third-generation cephalosporin (e.g. ceftriaxone 50–75 mg/kg/day IV or IM once daily may be started with gentamicin). Ceftriaxone, if available, should be the preferred antibiotic in cases of septic shock or meningitis. Anti-malarial treatment is provided if the child has a peripheral blood film positive for malaria parasites.

STEP 6: CORRECT MICRONUTRIENT DEFICIENCIES

All severely malnourished children have vitamin and mineral deficiencies. Although anemia is common, iron is not given until the child has a good appetite and starts gaining weight (usually by the second week). Vitamin A should be given orally on day 1 (for age >12 months, 200,000 IU; for age 6–12 months, 100,000 IU; for age 0–5 months, 50,000 IU) unless there is definite evidence that a dose has been given in the last month. If the child has xerophthalmia, the same doses of vitamin A are repeated on days 2 and 14, or on day of discharge.

The following micronutrients are provided daily for the entire period of nutritional rehabilitation (at least four weeks):

- multivitamin supplements;
- folic acid 1 mg/day (5 mg on day 1);
- zinc 2 mg/kg/day;
- copper 0.3 mg/kg/day;
- iron 3 mg/kg/day, but only when gaining weight.

A combined electrolyte/mineral/vitamin mix for severe malnutrition is available commercially. This can replace the electrolyte/mineral solution and multivitamin and folic acid supplements mentioned in

TABLE 138-1 Frequency and Volume of F-75 During Acute Phase of Treatment

Days	Frequency	Vol/kg/feed	Vol/kg/day
1–2	2-hourly	11 ml	130 ml
3–5	3-hourly	16 ml	130 ml
6–7+	4-hourly	22 ml	130 ml

Steps 4 and 6. However, the large single dose of vitamin A and folic acid on day 1 are still given.

STEP 7: START CAUTIOUS FEEDING

During the stabilization phase, a cautious approach is required because of the child's fragile physiologic state and reduced capacity to handle large feeds. Feeding should be started as soon as possible after admission. The WHO-recommended starter formula, F-75, contains 75 kcal/100 ml and 0.9 g protein/100 ml. Very weak children may be fed by spoon, dropper or syringe. Breastfeeding is encouraged between the feeds of F-75. A recommended schedule in which volume is gradually increased and feeding frequency gradually decreased is shown in Table 138-1. If intake does not reach 80 kcal/kg/day despite frequent feeds, coaxing and re-offering, give the remaining feed by nasogastric tube.

Criteria for Increasing Volume/Decreasing Frequency of F-75 Feeds

1. If vomiting, lots of diarrhea or poor appetite, continue two-hourly feeds.
2. If little, or no vomiting, modest diarrhea (less than five watery stools per day) and finishing most feeds, change to three-hourly feeds.
3. After a day on three-hourly feeds (if no vomiting, less diarrhea and finishing most feeds), change to four-hourly feeds.

In case of SAM infants less than 6 months old, feeding should be initiated with F-75. During the nutritional rehabilitation phase, F-75 can be continued and, if possible, re-lactation should be done.

STEP 8: ACHIEVE CATCH-UP GROWTH

During the nutritional rehabilitation phase, feeding is gradually increased to achieve a rapid weight gain of >10 g gain/kg/day. The recommended milk-based F-100 contains 100 kcal and 2.9 g protein/100 ml. Modified porridges or modified family foods can be used provided they have comparable energy and protein concentrations. Readiness to enter the rehabilitation phase is signaled by a return of appetite – usually about one week after admission. A gradual transition is recommended to avoid the risk of heart failure, which can occur if children suddenly consume huge amounts.

To change from starter to catch-up formula:

1. replace F-75 with the same amount of catch-up formula F-100 every 4 hours for 48 hours;
2. then, increase each successive feed by 10 ml until some feed remains uneaten. The point when some remains unconsumed after most feeds is likely to occur when intakes reach about 30 ml/kg/feed (200 ml/kg/day).

If weight gain is:

- poor (<5 g/kg/day): the child requires full reassessment for other underlying illnesses, for example tuberculosis (TB);
- moderate (5–10 g/kg/day): check whether intake targets are being met or if infection has been overlooked;
- good (>10 g/kg/day): continue to praise staff and mothers.

STEP 9: PROVIDE SENSORY STIMULATION AND EMOTIONAL SUPPORT

In severe malnutrition there is delayed mental and behavioral development. Just giving diets will improve physical growth, but mental development will remain impaired. This is improved by providing tender loving care and a cheerful, stimulating environment. The play sessions should make use of toys made of discarded material.

STEP 10: PREPARE FOR FOLLOW-UP AFTER RECOVERY

A child who has achieved WHZ -2SD can be considered to have improved. At this point, the child is still likely to have a low weight-for-age because of stunting. Good feeding practices and sensory stimulation should be continued at home. Parents or care givers should be counseled on:

- feeding energy- and nutrient-dense foods;
- providing structured playtimes for the children;
- bringing the child back for regular follow-up checks;
- ensuring that booster immunizations are given;
- ensuring that vitamin A and anti-helminthic drugs are given every six months.

TREATMENT OF COMPLICATIONS

Children with SAM may experience a number of severe complications; supportive treatment for shock, very severe anemia, vitamin deficiencies, dermatoses, parasitic infection, TB and lactose intolerance are often required.

COMMUNITY-BASED MANAGEMENT OF SAM

In countries with a heavy burden of SAM, facilities and resources for taking care of such children are far from being adequate. It is now agreed that children with SAM who have good appetites but no complications can be treated at the community level. Because the number of facilities is always sub-optimal in developing countries, facility-based treatment cannot cater to the huge numbers of severely malnourished children living in the community. In addition, feeding therapeutic diets including F-75 and F-100 at home is not recommended because of the propensity of these liquid diets to become contaminated in the home environment. To overcome this problem, ready-to-use-therapeutic food (RUTF) has been developed and used in field situations. If prepared as per prescription, RUTF has the nutrient composition of F-100 but is more energy dense and does not contain any water. Bacterial contamination, therefore, does not occur and the food is also safe for use in home conditions. The prototype RUTF is made of peanut paste, milk powder, vegetable oil, mineral and vitamin mix as per WHO recommendations. It is available as a paste in a sachet, does not require any cooking and children can eat directly from the sachet.

RUTF seems to play an important role in the management of severe malnutrition in disaster and emergency settings. A supplementary feeding program providing food rations to families of affected children should be in place. A stabilization center for taking care of acutely ill, severely malnourished children who need inpatient care based on WHO guidelines should also be provided. For countries in Asia, including India, Bangladesh and Pakistan, which have the highest burden of child malnutrition, there is a need for research on cost-effectiveness and sustainability of management of severe malnutrition using RUTF. To make a program cost-effective and sustainable, RUTF made of locally-available food ingredients and pertaining to the characteristics of an ideal RUTF is always preferable.

Children with SAM being considered for outpatient nutritional rehabilitation must fulfill the following attributes:

- free of any acute illness;
- have a good appetite;

TABLE 138-2 Minimum Amount of RUTF a Child Should Consume to Pass the Appetite Test

Weight of the child (kg)	Minimum amount of 1 RUTF sachet the child should consume willingly within 30 min (92 g sachet giving 500 kcal)
<4	⅛
4–9.9	¼
10–14.9	½
15 kg and above	¾

RUTF, ready-to-use-therapeutic food.

- have a care giver at home;
- live within a reasonable distance from the outpatient facility.

Testing for a good appetite is done by offering RUTF to the child in a quiet room. If the child consumes a certain amount of RUTF within 30 minutes, it is assumed that the child has a good appetite (Table 138-2).

DOSE OF READY-TO-USE-THERAPEUTIC FOOD (RUTF)

A child should be given RUTF to provide 200 kcal/kg/day. The care giver is counseled to offer the daily ration of RUTF in 5–6 divided doses and to provide potable water during feeding. Rations of RUTF should be provided weekly or fortnightly, depending on staff availability as well as the distance of the child's residence. At the start of treatment, oral amoxicillin should be provided, as well as vitamin A and folic acid. There should be adequate facilities in the out-patient department for counseling regarding preparation and offering of homemade nutritious foods, as well as recognition of danger signs of acute illnesses.

REFERENCE

1. Black R, Allen LH, Bhutta ZA, et al, for the Maternal and Child Undernutrition Study Group. Maternal and child undernutrition: global and regional exposures and health consequences. Lancet 2008;371:243–60.

FURTHER READING

Ahmed T, Ali M, Ullah M, et al. Mortality in severely malnourished children with diarrhoea and use of a standardised management protocol. Lancet 1999;353:1919–22.

Ahmed T, Begum B, Badiuzzaman, et al. Management of severe malnutrition and diarrhea. Ind J Pediatr 2001;68:45–51.

Collins S. Treating severe acute malnutrition seriously. Arch Dis Child 2007;92:453–61.

Sattar S, Ahmed T, Rasul CH, et al. Efficacy of a high-dose in addition to daily low-dose vitamin A in children suffering from severe acute malnutrition with other illnesses. PLoS ONE 2012;7(3):e33112. doi:10.1371/journal.pone.0033112.

World Health Organization. Management of Severe Malnutrition: A Manual for Physicians and Other Senior Health Workers. Geneva: World Health Organization; 1999.

World Health Organization. Management of the Child with a Serious Infection or Severe Malnutrition: Guidelines for Care at the First-Referral Level in Developing Countries (WHO/FCH/CAH/00.1). Geneva: World Health Organization; 2000.

Vitamin Deficiencies 139

Jeffrey K Griffiths

Key features

- Vitamin deficiencies remain common globally
- Vitamin deficiencies affect all ages, and frequently co-exist with mineral (zinc, iron, iodine) deficiencies
- Vitamin A deficiency leads to xerophthalmia and night blindness, deficient formation and function of epithelial surfaces, impaired growth and bone formation, adverse reproductive capacity, and diminished immunity. The World Health Organization has estimated that providing vitamin A to deficient children could decrease global death rates in children under 5 years of age by 23%
- Vitamin B_1 (thiamine) deficiency can lead to beriberi: dry beriberi – peripheral neuropathy with burning/tingling sensations, limb weakness, ataxia and paraesthesias; or wet beriberi – cardiac failure and edema (of the limbs, trunk and face with ascites or pleural effusions). Thiamine deficiency is also associated with Wernicke's encephalopathy that includes confusion, ophthalmoplegia, nystagmus, diplopia and ataxia
- Vitamin B_2 deficiency (ariboflavinosis) is associated with cheilitis, angular stomatitis, glossitis, oral ulcers, sore throat, watery itchy bloodshot eyes and seborrheic dermatitis
- Vitamin B_3 (niacin) deficiency can lead to pellagra that includes dermatitis, diarrhea, dementia and death (the "four Ds")
- Vitamin B_9 (folate) and vitamin B_{12} (cobalamin) deficiency can lead to megaloblastic anemia. Folate deficiency in pregnant women is also associated with neural tube defects in offspring. Vitamin B_{12} deficiency can also lead to ataxia and dementia, memory loss and, in infants, movement disorders
- Vitamin C (ascorbic acid) deficiency can lead to scurvy that predominantly relates to impaired connective tissue synthesis (weakness, ecchymoses, bleeding from gums, an inability of wounds to heal, the loss of teeth, death)
- Vitamin D deficiency can lead to osteomalacia, rickets, disorders of calcium homeostasis and immune dysregulation

INTRODUCTION AND SIGNIFICANCE

Vitamin deficiencies remain common globally. Unless severe, they are often clinically unrecognized, yet even mild deficiency may have significant adverse consequences. Vitamin deficiencies affect all ages and frequently co-exist with mineral (zinc, iron, iodine) deficiencies. The groups most susceptible to vitamin deficiencies are pregnant and lactating women, and young children, because of their relatively high needs for these compounds and susceptibilities to their absence. These include death from infectious diseases, anemia, death during pregnancy or childbirth and impaired cognition and physical development. The effects of vitamin deficiencies are related to the biochemical roles they play. Some of the most common deficiencies relate to vitamin A, various B vitamins, folate and vitamin D. Supplementation programs have made diseases such as scurvy (vitamin C deficiency) or pellagra (niacin deficiency) rare. New information suggests that vitamin D deficiency, which causes osteomalacia and rickets, is associated with abnormal immunoregulation and infectious diseases. Table 139-1 lists the most important consequences of deficiency and the recommended dietary intakes for the vitamins discussed in this chapter.

VITAMIN A

Vitamin A is lipid-soluble and essential to cellular differentiation. It is ingested either as the preformed retinyl ester or carotenoid provitamins (including beta-carotene) from plant sources and stored in the liver. It is transported from the liver to the rest of the body by retinol binding protein (RBP) and gains entry into cells via a specific receptor. Once intracellular, it is transformed to retinoic acid and modulates gene regulation and transcription. Overt deficiency occurs when hepatic retinol stores are exhausted. Its aldehyde—retinal—helps form visual pigments (rhodopsins). Thus, vitamin A deficiency (VAD) leads to xerophthalmia and night blindness, and is the leading cause of preventable childhood blindness worldwide [1]. VAD also leads to the deficient formation and function of epithelial surfaces, impaired growth and bone formation, adverse reproductive capacity and diminished immunity. Hematopoesis is dependent upon vitamin A, as well as iron and folate; anemia remediation requires adequate vitamin A.

Through poorly understood mechanisms, VAD children suffer more severe episodes of infectious diseases. Furthermore, children with infections excrete both vitamin A and its serum carrier protein, worsening VAD. Overt VAD can be precipitated during acute infections (such as measles, pneumonia, diarrhea, varicella) leading to acute severe xerophthalmia [2]. Mortality can approach 50% in VAD children with measles and giving vitamin A to them can decrease mortality rates by half. The World Health Organization (WHO) has estimated that providing vitamin A to deficient children could decrease global death rates in children under 5 years of age by 23%.

Young children and women of childbearing age are at particular risk of VAD. It is most common in Southeast Asia and Africa. The WHO Global Database on Vitamin A Deficiency (2009) [3] estimates that 5.2 million preschool-age children and 9.8 million pregnant women have night blindness. As judged by low serum retinol concentrations (<0.70 μmol/l), 190 million preschool children and 19.1 million pregnant women have subclinical VAD which predisposes them to increased morbidity and mortality from infectious diseases. Serum retinol levels are an insensitive indicator of VAD as serum retinol is homeostatically maintained within a narrow range until body stores are nearly depleted. Other assays, such as the modified relative dose

TABLE 139-1 Common Vitamin Deficiencies and Recommended Intakes

	Vitamin A	**Thiamine Vitamin B_1**	**Riboflavin Vitamin B_2**	**Niacin Vitamin B_3**	**Folate Vitamin B_9**	**Cobalamin Vitamin B_{12}**	**Ascorbic Acid Vitamin C**	**Vitamin D**
Deficiency:	Xerophthalmia, anemia, high moribidity from infectious diseases	Beriberi: neurologic dysfunction and cardiac failure	Ariboflavinosis – oral, ocular, genital syndrome: angular cheilitis, photophobia, dermatitis	Pellagra: dermatitis, dementia, diarrhea, death	Anemia, neural tube defects	Anemia, neurologic dysfunction	Scurvy	Rickets Osteomalacia Probable linkage to increased infectious diseases
Recommended Dietary Allowances & Adequate Intakes (Food and Nutrition Board, Institute of Medicine, US National Academies, 2011).* Recommended Dietary Allowances (>12 months of age) are based upon meeting the needs of 97–98% of normal persons. Adequate Intakes (0–12 months of age) are mean intakes observed in normal breastfed children.								
Intake units	**μg/day retinol**[†] **(retinol activity equivalents [RAE])**	**mg/day**	**mg/day**	**mg/day**	**μg/day**	**μg/day**	**mg/day**	**μg/day, IU/ day (1 μg = 40 IU units)**
Infants 0–6 months	400	0.2	0.3	2	65	0.4	40	10 (400)
Infants 6–12 months	500	0.3	0.4	4	80	0.5	50	10 (400)
1–3 years	300	0.5	0.5	6	150	0.9	15	15 (600)
4–8 years	400	0.6	0.6	8	200	1.2	25	15 (600)
9–13 years	600	0.9	0.9	12	300	1.8	45	15 (600)
14–18 years, male/female	900/700	1.2/1.0	1.3/1.0	16/14	400/400	2.4/2.4	75/65	15/15 (600/600)
19–70 years, male/female	900/700	1.2/1.1	1.3/1.1	16/14	400/400	2.4/2.4	90/75	15/15 (600/600)
>70 years, male/female	900/700	1.2/1.1	1.3/1.1	16/14	400/400	2.4/2.4	90/75	20/20 (800/800)
Pregnancy	770	1.4	1.4	18	600	2.6	85	15 (600)
Lactation	1300	1.4	1.6	17	500	2.8	120	15 (600)

*Reference documents for these vitamins and other vitamins and minerals can be found at www.nap.edu.

[†]One μg retinol has the same bioavailability as 2 μg of β-carotene in oil, 12 μg of dietary β-carotenoids or 24 μg of other dietary provitamin-A carotenoids. International units (IU) are no longer recommended for use. One IU of vitamin A was equivalent to 0.3 μg retinol. Thus, the World Health Organization recommendation to give children 0–6 months of age 100,000 IU of vitamin A twice-yearly is equivalent to the administration of 30,000 μg (30 mg) of preformed retinol twice-yearly.

response (MRDR) test, better assess total body stores, but remain research tools at this time [4].

Liver, milk, cheese and eggs are rich in vitamin A esters, and green and orange-yellow vegetables are rich in carotenoid precursors. Although breast milk provides adequate vitamin A for nursing infants, young children after weaning may be given a diet of monotonously starchy foods deficient in vitamin A precursors and little, or no, animal protein. Because the conversion of intestinal carotenoids to retinol is not efficient, VAD may occur where the sole dietary sources of vitamin A or carotenoids are vegetables and fruits. Pregnancy and lactation greatly increase maternal vitamin A requirements and overt xerophthalmia may be precipitated during pregnancy.

CLINICAL MANIFESTATIONS, DIAGNOSIS AND PREVENTION OF VITAMIN A DEFICIENCY (VAD)

Xerophthalmia

The ocular manifestations of VAD include reversible and non-reversible changes. They are the only clear clinical signs of VAD available to the clinician. Moderate VAD may escape diagnosis if ocular changes are absent. Night-blindness ("XN") results from inadequate formation of rhodopsin. Bitot spots ("X1B") are corneal lesions which represent worsening keratinizing conjunctival metaplasia ("X1A"). The entire cornea may keratinize, leading to xerosis ("X2"). These changes are reversible with vitamin A ingestion. Further progression, associated with profoundly low serum retinol levels, includes corneal necrosis and localized ("X3A") or complete ulceration ("X3B"). Vitamin A should be given to children with irreversible X3A or X3B changes, as it may prevent death from infections or the loss of sight in the other eye. Unfortunately, the infectious, hematological and other manifestations of VAD are indirect and no clinical VAD indicators other than xerophthalmia exist.

Diagnosis of vitamin A deficiency (VAD)

Xerophthalmia, as described above, indicates severe VAD. Serum retinol testing, when available, will identify only some individuals with moderate deficiency as retinol levels may be normal, despite nearly-depleted body stores. Research tests, such as the MRDR, examine the biochemical avidity of VA uptake as measured by comparing serum levels of VA with those of synthetic vitamin A_2 and provide a better measure of total body VA stores. Xerophthalmia prevalence is used as a population-wide indicator for severe VAD.

Prevention of vitamin A deficiency (VAD)

Consumption of adequate amounts of vitamin A or carotenoid precursors prevents VAD. Exclusively breastfed children are at risk of VAD if their mothers have VAD, as the infant's sole source of vitamin A is breast milk. Household gardening and consumption of green, leafy vegetables rich in carotenoids is widely promoted. VAD can be prevented in non-exclusively breastfed children if their diet includes such vegetables and/or animal proteins (eggs, milk or fish). In developed and newly industrialized countries, vitamin A food biofortification is common. When vitamin A enriched staples, such as sweet potatoes (yams), are adopted by a population, VAD rates decrease dramatically. The WHO recommends that infants and children be given large doses of vitamin A (30 mg retinol activity equivalents [RAE], formerly known as 100,000 IU, in children <12 months of age, and 60 mg RAE, formerly 200,000 IU, if older) twice-yearly where VAD is common. Women of childbearing age, particularly pregnant and lactating women with high vitamin A needs, also benefit from vitamin A supplementation (Table 139-1).

CLINICALLY IMPORANT B VITAMIN DEFICIENCIES

BERIBERI AND THIAMINE (VITAMIN B_1)

Thiamine is a water soluble, labile vitamin which lacks natural body storage and has high turnover and excretion rates. Thiamine deficiency (also known as beriberi) can appear within weeks of a deficient diet. Its current global prevalence is not known and is most frequently recognized in populations who consume thiamine-deficient cassava, sago, de-germinated maize, polished rice or wheat. Removal of the bran from rice or the germ and aleuron layer from wheat effectively removes thiamine (and niacin). Thiamine deficiency is often reported in refugees, confined populations (prisoners) or migrants fed thiamine-deficient foods, and from populations (e.g. Ghana) where a diverse, thiamine-rich diet has been replaced by one high in polished rice. Exercise, diabetes, pregnancy, fever, dysentery and alcoholism are risk factors [5, 6]. Thiamine deficiency has been described in socially-isolated youths who consume refined carbohydrates (dried noodles and soft drinks), as well as the elderly in Europe [7].

Thiamine deficiency has nonspecific symptoms, such as anorexia, weakness and peripheral paraesthesias, as well as (in more severe forms) cardiac involvement and peripheral neuropathy [8]. Peripheral neuropathy with burning/tingling sensations, limb weakness, ataxia and paraesthesias were termed "dry" beriberi. Cardiac failure and edema (of the limbs, trunk, face, with ascites or pleural effusions) were termed "wet" beriberi – characteristically a "collapsing" pulse with an increased systolic and decreased diastolic pressure, and a visibly exaggerated venous jugular pulse wave are seen. Thiamine deficiency can also co-exist, or be confused, with severe thyrotoxicosis, severe anemia, pregnancy, the edema of nephritis, nephrotic syndrome or kwashiorkor. Thiamine deficiency is the only major form of malnutrition which occurs in adequately breastfed infants owing to maternal thiamine deficiency. Acute heart failure with edema leading to death is seen in thiamine-deficient breastfed babies aged 1–3 months. It can be confused with sepsis, malaria, pneumonia and typhoid. Aphonic beriberi is typically seen in infants aged 4–6 months who develop hoarseness progressing to aphonia. Somewhat older infants (7–9 months old) may develop nystagmus, twitching, convulsions and unconsciousness, which mimics encephalitis and meningitis, or malaria.

Thiamine deficiency can manifest as the Wernicke-Korsakoff syndrome in people with genetic abnormalities of transketolase, a thiamine dependent enzyme. Wernicke's encephalopathy is caused by lesions of the brainstem, hypothalamus and mamillary bodies which lead to confusion, ophthalmoplegia, nystagmus, diplopia and ataxia. Memory loss (Korakov's psychosis) appears after recovery [9].

Mild thiamine deficiency can be treated with 10 mg/day orally for a week and then 3–5 mg/day thereafter for at least six weeks. In the presence of heart failure, convulsions or coma in infants, 25–50 mgs of intravenous (IV) thiamine can be given followed by 10 mg/day intramuscularly (IM). This dose should be doubled in critically-ill adults. In infants and adults with cardiac failure, symptomatic relief is dramatic and can occur within hours. Peripheral neuropathy may take weeks to improve. Wernicke's encephalopathy responds within hours to IV thiamine, but Korsakov's psychosis may never resolve.

Grains are the most common source of thiamine; 0.5 mg per 1000 kilocalories of food should be consumed daily, or about 1.0–1.5 mgs in adults (Table 139-1). Thiamine deficiency can be prevented by the ingestion of whole grains, fortified polished rice or de-germinated wheat, or milk. Meats, vegetables and almost all foodstuffs also contain some thiamine.

ARIBOFLAVINOSIS AND RIBOFLAVIN (VITAMIN B_2)

Riboflavin is a precursor for the essential enzymatic cofactors flavin-adenine-dinucleotide (FAD) and riboflavin-5′-phosphate. Flavoproteins have a wide range of redox potentials and are intermediates in many critical biochemical reactions, such as ATP synthesis. Dietary sources are primarily of animal origin. Vegetables such as spinach, broccoli and asparagus also contain riboflavin, as do mushrooms, yeast, tomatoes, whole grains and almonds. Cereals and rice, when milled or polished, become riboflavin-poor, as with thiamine. Cereals and milk are often riboflavin-fortified. Riboflavin degrades when exposed to light, but not heat. Riboflavin deficiency (ariboflavinosis) usually occurs in populations with little fish, eggs, meat or dairy dietary protein, and in combination with other deficiencies. Isolated riboflavin deficiency is extremely rare. Infants are at high risk if, during weaning, they are fed non-fortified cereals and little animal protein. Other groups at risk include: alcoholics, through poor nutritional intake; individuals taking antipsychotic medications (imipramine, amitryptiline, chlorpromazine, others) or antiparasitics (quinacrine) which impair riboflavin metabolism; and those with adrenal or thyroid deficiency, which precipitates clinical aribinoflavinosis. Subclinical deficiency has been documented in women on oral contraceptives, persons with eating disorders (e.g. anorexia nervosa), HIV/AIDS, inflammatory bowel disease, the elderly and in the general population of children in sub-Saharan Africa [10].

Cheilitis, angular stomatitis, glossitis, oral ulcers, sore throat, watery itchy bloodshot eyes and seborrheic dermatitis are common manifestations. Ariboflavinosis is linked to the classic oral-ocular-genital syndrome of angular cheilitis, photophobia and scrotal or labial dermatitis [11]. Normochromic normocytic anemia, photophobia, corneal vascularization and dementia with personality changes are seen in severe deficiency. In contrast to niacin deficiency (pellagra), riboflavinosis dermatitis usually is facial (eyes, nasolabial folds), in the flexures of the extremities and in the genital region. Zinc deficiency dermatitis differs from ariboflavinosis as it usually involves the trunk and extremities and is perioral.

Ariboflavinosis may be suspected on clinical grounds and confirmed with measurement of erythrocyte glutathione reductase (which requires FAD) *in vitro* with and without added FAD. An enzymatic difference of >30% after addition (ratio 1.30 : 1) is confirmatory. Urinary excretion of <19 μg/g creatinine or <40 μg/day, also indicates deficiency. Adults should consume ~ 1.2 mg/day or 2 mg/day during pregnancy. The recommended dietary allowance is 0.3–0.4 mg/day for infants and 0.6–0.9 mg/day for older children. Deficiency can be treated with 5 mg daily until clinical signs resolve and blood testing is normal. Ingestion of 400 mg/day for three months has not led to reported side effects.

PELLAGRA AND NIACIN (VITAMIN B_3)

Niacin deficiency leads to pellagra (from "rough skin" in Italian), which is manifested by a dermatitis especially of areas exposed to sunlight or to pressure (elbows and knees). Niacin is required for the synthesis of nicotinamide adenosine dinucleotide (NAD) and its phosphate (NADP) – cofactors for many enzymatic processes. Niacin can be ingested or endogenously synthesized from the essential amino acid tryptophan in the presence of vitamin B_6 and riboflavin. Isoniazid and azathioprine are known to impair the conversion of tryptophan to niacin and can precipitate pellagra. Pellagra occurs when diets are poor in niacin and animal proteins (which are rich in tryptophan). When unfortified maize (corn) is the major dietary staple it is common. In Central and South America, maize flour is usually treated with lime, unlike in Africa or other parts of the world, and so pellagra remains endemic outside of the Americas [12, 13].

Dermatitis, diarrhea, dementia and eventual death (the "four Ds") are characteristic of pellagra [14]. The diarrhea is secondary to protein deficiency-related atrophic intestinal mucosa. The dementia ranges from hallucinations to seizures and overt dementia, and is related to decreased serotonin (5-hydroxytryptamine) neurotransmitter synthesis. Diagnosis can be made from the characteristic dermatitis and symptoms or by measuring urinary metabolite excretion, which is superior to measurement of erythrocyte NAD or whole blood NAD/NADP concentrations [15]. The skin findings may be mistaken for ariboflavinosis but, with the latter, the lesions are in flexure regions and skin folds. Kwashiorkor may also have similar skin findings, but they are not localized to areas exposed to sun, and pure pellagra is not marked by edema. Pellagra can be prevented by ingestion of 15–20 mgs per day in an adult (Table 139-1) and symptomatic improvement can be seen within two days of treatment.

FOLATE (VITAMIN B_9)

Folate, vitamin B_9, is present in fruits, legumes such as beans and peas, dairy products and green leafy vegetables. Along with vitamin B_{12} deficiency, folate deficiency leads to megaloblastic anemia. Folate deficiency is extremely common globally, including in newly industrialized countries [16, 17]. If low maternal dietary intake occurs during pregnancy, fetuses are at elevated risk of being born with neural tube defects such as spina bifida or anencephaly. Women of child-bearing age should ingest 400 µg/day or more of folate, as its prevention of neural tube defects is most effective during the first month of conception. Other than anemia, the symptoms of folate deficiency are subtle. They include diarrhea, depression, impaired cognition, elevated risks of heart disease and stroke, all of which may occur for other reasons. Because folate deficiency is widespread, it should be co-administered with iron supplements for the prevention or treatment of anemia. After widespread folate biofortification began in the late 1990s, rates of congenital neural tube defects dropped dramatically in many countries [18]. Recent recommendations are that adults ingest 400 µg/day of folate, and 600 µg/day during pregnancy. Infants up to the age of 6 months should receive 65 µg, those aged 7–12 months should receive 80 µg and children aged 1–3 years, 150 µg/day. Alcoholics, others with liver disease, persons on dialysis and those who take dilantin may also develop folate deficiency.

VITAMIN B_{12} (THE COBALAMINS)

Vitamin B_{12} deficiency is associated with macrocytic anemia [19]. Found in animal, but not plant, foods, it is required for erythrocyte formation, DNA synthesis and normal neurologic function. Intestinal absorption of dietary vitamin B_{12} requires gastric acid to separate it from animal protein and intrinsic factor – a glycoprotein secreted by parietal cells of the gastric mucosa. The vitamin B_{12}-intrinsic factor complex is taken up in the distal ileum by receptor-mediated endocytosis. Vegetarians, persons with decreased gastric acid (such as the elderly with atrophic gastritis) or intrinsic factor production, inflammatory bowel disease or who have had surgery to remove the stomach or ileum are at substantial risk of deficiency. Pernicious anemia is an autoimmune disorder which leads to gastric atrophy and a lack of intrinsic factor and, thus, to anemia from vitamin B_{12} deficiency. Neurologic signs of deficiency include ataxia and dementia, memory loss and, in infants, movement disorders. Severe, irreversible neurologic damage can occur in infants of vegan or lacto-ovo vegetarian mothers, as breast milk is the sole source of vitamin B_{12} for infants and deficiency is common in these mothers. Persons taking drugs to reduce gastric acid (proton-pump inhibitors or H_2-blockers) or metformin for diabetes may also be at risk for deficiency. Oral supplements can prevent deficiency so long as intrinsic factor is present [20]; in its absence, IM injections are widely used.

The fish tapeworm, *Diphyllobothrium latum* and related species, is acquired by eating raw fish. These human parasites are found in South America, Uganda and northern Asia, Europe and the Americas. The parasite itself is usually asymptomatic but can cause severe vitamin B_{12} deficiency through uptake of most of the dietary intake [21].

SCURVY AND VITAMIN C (ASCORBIC ACID)

Scurvy is caused by vitamin C deficiency [22]. Humans, unlike most animals, cannot synthesize vitamin C and it is an essential vitamin obtained primarily from fresh fruit and vegetables, such as watercress. Scurvy can develop a month after vitamin C is removed from the diet, although three months or more is more typical. Ascorbate (the active form) promotes hydroxylation of proline and lysine after their incorporation into collagen, and the manifestations of scurvy are primarily related to impaired connective tissue synthesis. Nondescript weakness and fatigue are followed by follicular hyperkeratosis and cutaneous petechial or ecchymotic bleeding after minor trauma. Bleeding from the oral mucosa and spongy enlargement of the gums are common; classically, the gingival interdental papillae between the teeth are bright red. Disease progression leads to depression, profound weakness, an inability of wounds to heal, the loss of all teeth, jaundice and neuropathy, before death. In infants and children, scurvy is manifested by tenderness of the bones, linked to subperiosteal hemorrhage, such that they cry when their bones are touched. Crawling and standing are avoided because of the pain. Bleeding at the osteochondral rib junctions may mimic the ricketic "rosary" of vitamin D or calcium deficiency [23]. Anemia can also be seen because of blood loss and because ascorbate promotes intestinal iron absorption.

Endemic scurvy no longer exists in high-income countries but persists elsewhere [24]. Scurvy occurs in those who ingest grains but not fruit [25]; in socially isolated persons, prisoners [26] or alcoholics with poor diets; and in persons with inflammatory bowel disease. Breast milk contains vitamin C and scurvy may occur in the infants of vitamin C-deficient mothers. Infants and children fed grains, but not fruit, vegetables or fresh animal protein, are also at risk. Because heat destroys vitamin C, it is added to milk after pasteurization. Curing and drying fresh meat destroys the vitamin C it contains. This, and the lack of fresh vegetables or fruit, accounted for the high incidence of scurvy in sailors whom, historically, often lived solely on dried grains, dried vegetables, such as beans, and dried meat.

The diagnosis should be suspected when these characteristic signs and symptoms are present [27]. Capillary fragility may be a manifestation of many other diseases, as may petechial bleeding. Vitamin C can be measured in plasma (reflecting recent intake) and in leukocytes (reflecting tissue content and total body reserves). Individuals with scurvy typically have undetectable plasma levels of vitamin C.

Treatment with up to a gram a day of vitamin C has been advocated for scurvy, although clinical studies have shown that as little as 10 mg/day is curative. Scurvy can be prevented in infants by ensuring maternal intake of vitamin C and by feeding them vitamin C-rich or fortified foods.

RICKETS, OSTEOMALACIA AND VITAMIN D

Vitamin D promotes calcium absorption from the proximal intestine and bone mineralization. Along with parathyroid hormone and calcitonin, it tightly regulates serum calcium and phosphate levels via control of bone, kidney, parathyroid gland and intestinal physiology.

Its primary action on bone is to mobilize calcium and phosphorus via bone resorption to maintain serum calcium levels [28]. At the cell nucleus it regulates the transcription of hundreds of genes and affects signal transduction and voltage-gated calcium flux at the cell membrane. Vitamin D has potent immunoregulatory properties and there is an inverse association between vitamin D and infectious diseases [29]. In addition, vitamin D modulates the renin-angiotensin system and vitamin D deficiency (VDD) has been linked to hypertension and adverse cardiac status [30].

Vitmain D is unlike other vitamins in that endogenous synthesis occurs, as ultraviolet B sunlight converts cutaneous 7-dehydrocholesterol into previtamin D_3. After isomerization into cholecalciferol (vitamin D_3) it is then transported throughout the body by vitamin D-binding protein. Two subsequent hydroxylations (to 25-hydroxyvitamin D_3 and then to 1α,25 dihydroxyvitamin D_3) in the kidney render it an active compound. Sunlight-related synthesis of D_3 is predictably decreased as skin melanin increases, by clothing, during the temperate zone winter and by air pollution at the equator. High concentrations of vitamin D are found in fatty fishes, fish liver oils and egg yolks. Small amounts of vitamin D_2 (ergocalciferol) are found in some plants. In tropical regions, sunlight exposure is the major source of vitamin D, whereas in temperate or circumpolar regions, ingestion is a more significant source.

With vitamin D absent, intestinal calcium uptake is negligible. This leads, in growing children, to inadequate bone mineralization and, clinically, to rickets [31]. In adults, VDD results in bone resorption and osteomalacia. Rickets (also seen with calcium deficiency) develops during bone growth, while osteomalacia develops after epiphyseal fusion. Children with rickets have "knobby" enlargements at bone growth sites, such as the epiphyseal and costochondral junctions of the long bones and the ribs, and bossing of the skull. "Beaded" (enlarged) rib costochondral junctions are called a "rachitic rosary". Radiographs of bone epiphyses reveal ragged, irregular and poorly mineralized growth zones. Legs may become bowed after weight-bearing begins in children. Adults with osteomalacia develop pseudofractures of the ribs and pelvis, and frequently suffer true bone fractures. They complain of bone and muscle pain, and weakness, consistent with both pseudofractures and hypocalcemia-induced muscle dysfunction. Radiographs may show pseudofractures at right angles to the bone shaft, poor bone calcification and loss of trebeculae, and concave vertebrae. Pregnant and lactating women require substantial calcium for the developing fetus and for breast milk; VDD during this period can lead to severe maternal bone damage. Maternal pre-eclampsia and eclampsia is treated with calcium; however, the relationship between VDD, eclampsia and hypocalcemia is not well defined. VDD in tropical countries occurs when people with high melanin levels have inadequate sunlight exposure, when clothing blocks sunlight exposure and from dietary deficiency. Breast fed, swaddled infants born to VDD mothers are at particular risk of VDD. Vegetarians who do not eat fish or eggs and who do not have much direct light exposure, or institutionalized persons, are also "classic" risk groups.

DIAGNOSIS OF VITAMIN D DEFICIENCY (VDD)

Overt VDD can be diagnosed clinically when characteristic rickets are seen in children, or via radiographs or serum testing. Because of vitamin D's tight regulation, serum 1α,25 dihydroxyvitamin D_3 is usually normal in VDD, whereas the precursor 25-hydroxyvitamin D_3 levels are low. Serum calcium and phosphorus levels are decreased depending upon the stage of the illness, while parathyroid hormone and alkaline phosphate levels are elevated. In children with severe rickets and hypocalcemia, hypotonia, muscle weakness and tetany develop. This may be so severe that abdominal muscle protrusion, umbilical herniation and respiratory compromise and death may occur. Dental enamel hypoplasia and poor formation of permanent teeth are also observed. Like moderate VAD, moderate VDD may be related to increased risks of infectious diseases, hypertension and maternal mortality, but the magnitude and degree of causality remain undefined [29–30].

TREATMENT OF VITMAIN D DEFICIENCY (VDD)

Both vitamin D and calcium should be given to children or adults with VDD. Four hundred IU of vitamin D given daily over prolonged periods is efficacious; however, this amount is now less than the recommended dietary allowance for adults (Table 139-1). Larger doses (5000 IU per day for two months, or 50,000 IU per week in adults) are often utilized. Children should receive 800 mgs (adults 1000 mgs) of calcium daily with vitamin D therapy.

PREVENTION OF VITAMIN D DEFICIENCY (VDD)

An adequate diet containing vitamin D and sunlight exposure prevent VDD. Institutionalized persons may require either increased dietary vitamin D or specific actions to ensure sunlight exposure. In developed and newly industrialized countries, milk is often fortified with vitamin D. There is active controversy over what the "correct" levels for biofortification of foods and daily intake should be, with a strong bias towards increasing current recommendations [29, 31].

REFERENCES

1. World Health Organization. Micronutrient deficiencies. Available at: www.who.int/nutrition/topics (last accessed 31st May 2012).
2. Sommer A. Vitamin A deficiency and clinical disease. J Nutr 2009;139:1835–9.
3. World Health Organization. Global Prevalence of vitamin A deficiency in populations at risk 19955–2005. Geneva: World Health Organization; 2009. Available at: http://www.who.int/nutrition/publications/micronutrients/vitamin_a_deficiency/9789241598019/en/index.html (last accessed 31st May 2012).
4. Tanumihardjo SA. Vitamin A: biomarkers of nutrition for development. Am J Clin Nutr 2011;94:6585–655.
5. Padilha EM, Fujimori E, Borges ALV, et al. Epidemiological profile of reported beriberi cases in Maranhao State, Brazil, 20065–2008. Cadernos de Saude Publica 2011;27:449–59.
6. Cerroni MP, Barrado JCS, Nobrega AA, et al. Outbreak of beriberi in an Indian population of the upper Amazon Region, Roraima State, Brazil 2008. Am J Trop Med Hyg 2010;83:1093–7.
7. Toffanello ED, Inelmen EM, Minicuci N, et al. Ten-year trends in vitamin intake in free-living healthy elderly people: the risk of subclinical nutrition. J Nutr Health Aging 2011;15:99–103.
8. Carpenter KJ. Beriberi, White Rice, and Vitamin B: A Disease, a Cause, and a Cure. Berkeley, Los Angeles: University of California Press; 2000:282.
9. Kumar N. Acute and subacute encephalopathies: deficiency states (nutritional). Sem Neurol 2011;31:169–83.
10. Rohner F, Zimmermann MB, Wegmueller R, et al. Mild riboflavin deficiency is highly prevalent in school-age children but does not increase risk for anaemia in Cote d'Ivoire. Br J Nutr 2007;97:970–6.
11. Karthikeyan K, Jaisankar TJ, Thappa DM. Non-venereal dematoses in male genital region – prevalence and patterns in a referral centre in south India. Ind J Dermatol 2001;46:185–22.
12. Scrimshaw NS. Fifty five-year personal experience with human nutrition worldwide. Ann Rev Nutr 2007;27:1–18.
13. Seal AJ, Creeke PI, Dibari F, et al. Low and deficient niacin status and pellagra are endemic in postwar Angola. Am J Clin Nutr 2007;85:2185–24.
14. Hegyi J, Schwartz RA, Hegyi V. Pellagra: dermatitis, dementia, and diarrhea. Int J Dermatol 2004;43:1–5.
15. Creeke PI, Dibari F, Cheung E, et al. Whole blood NAD and NADP concentrations are not depressed in subjects with clinical pellagra. J Nutr 2007;137:2013–17.
16. Cordero JF, Do A, Berry RJ. Review of interventions for the prevention and control of folate and vitamin B12 deficiencies. Food Nutr Bull 2008;29:2(suppl.):S188–95.
17. Borwankar R, Sanghvi T, Houston R. What is the extent of vitamin and mineral deficiencies? Magnitude of the problem. Food Nutr Bull 2007;28:1(suppl. 2):S174–81.
18. Oakley GP, Jr. The scientific basis for eliminating folic acid-preventable spina bifida: a modern miracle from epidemiology. Ann Epidemiol 2009;19:226–30.
19. Milman N. Anemia – still a major health problem in many parts of the world. Ann Hematol 2011;90:369–77.
20. Andres E, Fothergill H, Mecili M. Efficacy of oral cobalamin (vitamin B12) therapy. Exp Opin Pharmacother 2010;11:249–56.

21. Von Bonsdorff B, Gordin R. Castle's test (with vitamin B12 and normal gastric juice) in the ileum in patients with genuine and patients with tapeworm pernicious anemia. Acta Med Scand 1980;208:193–7.
22. Magiorkinis E, Beloukas A, Diamantis A. Scurvy: past, present, and future. European J Int Med 2011;22:147–52.
23. Ratanachu-Ek S, Sukswai P, Jeerathanyasakun Y, Wongtapradit L. Scurvy in pediatric patients: a review of 28 cases. J Med Assoc Thailand 2003;86(suppl. 3):S734–40.
24. Loewenberg S. Afghanistan's hidden health issue. Lancet 2009;374:9700, 1487–8.
25. Cheung E, Roya Mutahar Fitsum Ververs MT, Nasiri SM, et al. An epidemic of scurvy in Afghanistan: assessment and response. Food Nutr Bull 2003;24: 247–55.
26. Bennett M, Coninx R. The mystery of the wooden leg: vitamin C deficiency in East African prisons. Tropical Doctor 2005;35:81–4.
27. Raynaud-Simon A, Cohen-Bittan J, Gouronnec A, et al. Scurvy in hospitalized elderly patients. J Nutr Health Aging. 2010;14:407–10.
28. Feldman D, Malloy PJ. Vitamin D deficiency, rickets, and osteomalacia. In: Martini L, ed. Encyclopedia of Endocrine Diseases, Vol. 4. Elsevier Inc., San Diego; 2004: 666–73.
29. Taylor CE, Camargo CA, Jr. Impact of micronutrients on respiratory infections. Nutr Rev 2011;69:259–69.
30. Anderson JL, May HT, Horne BD, et al. Relation of vitamin D deficiency to cardiovascular risk factors, disease status, and incident events in the general healthcare population. 2010. Am J Cardiol 2010;106:963–68.
31. Holick MF. Vitamin D deficiency. N Engl J Med 2007;357:266–81.

Mineral Deficiencies 140

Anuraj H Shankar

Key features

- Minerals are not manufactured by the human body and must be obtained through diet or supplementation
- The human body requires 17 minerals for biological function and health
- Deficiencies are widespread, with the greatest burden affecting young children and women of childbearing age
- From a public health perspective, the most important deficiencies are of iron, zinc, and iodine
- Iron: deficiency affects about 2 billion people globally and is associated with anemia, decreased work capacity, decreased cognition and increased susceptibility to infection. Treatment of deficiency involves improved intake and decreased losses due to infections such as hookworm, malaria and others
- Zinc: deficiency affects about 1 billion people globally, with another 1 billion at risk of zinc deficiency, and is associated with reduced growth, impaired immunity, and decreased resistance to infection. It is especially important for rapidly dividing cells, including immune cells and those within epithelial surfaces. The human body does not store zinc at appreciable quantities, and sufficient daily intake is needed. Supplementation reduces the severity and duration of diarrhea, and may improve outcome of other conditions including pneumonia and tuberculosis, and possibly malaria. Deficiency is best addressed by supplementation, fortification, and dietary diversification
- Iodine: deficiency affects about 2 billion people globally and is associated with infant mortality, miscarriages, mental deficiency and brain damage, as well as thyroid hormone-related abnormalities. Iodine deficiency is the leading preventable cause of brain damage in infancy. The most effective control mechanism for addressing iodine deficiency is salt iodization
- Other minerals of significant public health importance include selenium, calcium, magnesium and fluoride

INTRODUCTION

Minerals are essential elements required for human life, and typically exclude the organic building blocks of carbon, hydrogen, nitrogen and oxygen [1]. They cannot be made by the body and must therefore be obtained in the diet in adequate amounts required for proper health. Minerals are distinct from vitamins in that they are not organic molecules comprised of multiple atoms. The human body requires 17 different minerals, as indicated in Table 140-1, and these comprise 4% of the total body mass [2, 3]. They are classified as major minerals (daily requirement of at least 100 mg), trace minerals (daily requirement of less than 100 mg), and ultra trace minerals (typically 1 μg or less per day) [4]. Minerals are naturally present in food or may be added through food fortification or dietary supplements.

Minerals play a variety of crucial biologic roles, including maintenance of proper electrolyte balance and conductivity functions for muscle and nerve excitation, acid-base balance, as cofactors in enzymes required for metabolism, in forming and stabilizing proteins, and in the crystalline structure of bones and teeth, as well as other functions [5]. It is crucial to note that many minerals interact with each other and with vitamins; for example, healthy bones require a balance between vitamin D, calcium, phosphorus, magnesium, zinc, fluoride, chloride, manganese, copper and sulfur. Deficiency in any of these would influence skeletal health. Interactions in absorption may also be important; for example, high intakes of iron may decrease zinc absorption, or high intake of zinc may result in copper deficiency. A balanced diet provides all required minerals and in the proper quantities and ratios.

Unfortunately, mineral deficiencies are widespread, particularly for persons residing in low-income countries, and have a large impact on global health and tropical medicine. For some minerals, requirements are sufficiently low that even poor diets provide the needed amounts, or reserves or nutrient recycling may mitigate the effects of chronically low intakes, and in some cases, loss of mineral-dependent functions may be partially compensated by alternative biologic pathways. Under these scenarios, clinical manifestations of mineral deficiency may be absent or mild, and only recognized in rare cases of severe chronic deficiency. However, for some minerals, reserves are limited and the physiologic roles are such that even mild deficiencies may adversely affect health. From a public health perspective, based on the prevalence and impact on morbidity, mortality and quality of life, deficiencies of the trace minerals iron, zinc and iodine have the greatest burden on health and are reviewed in detail below. The roles of other minerals are briefly discussed thereafter.

IRON

GLOBAL BURDEN OF IRON DEFICIENCY

Iron deficiency is widespread and affects more than two billion persons worldwide [6]. Chronic anemia associated with iron deficiency results in impaired work capacity, reduced cognitive performance and increased susceptibility to infection [7–10]. Globally, iron deficiency is associated with 841,000 annual deaths and 35 million disability-adjusted live years (DALYs) [6].

OVERVIEW OF IRON BIOLOGY

Iron has multiple physiologic roles; among the most crucial being the primary functional element of hemoglobin [7, 8]. The ferrous ion (Fe^{+2}) combined with the protoporphyrin IX ring structure forms heme, the oxygen-carrying component of hemoglobin and myoglobin. Iron deficiency leads to lower heme levels and reduced erythropoiesis, resulting in hypochromic microcytic anemia. Iron also has a crucial role in the electron transport chain in mitochondria through the

TABLE 140-1 Essential Minerals in Descending Order by Recommended Daily Intake Levels, and Key Biological Functions and Dietary Sources

Dietary mineral	RDA/AI	Functional significance	Dietary sources
Potassium	4700 mg	Systemic electrolyte needed to maintain membrane action potentials; essential for ATP regulation	Legumes, potato skin, tomatoes and bananas
Chlorine	2300 mg	Production of hydrochloric acid in the stomach and in cellular pump functions	Table salt (sodium chloride) is the main dietary source
Sodium	1500 mg	Systemic electrolyte needed to maintain membrane potential and action potentials; essential in co-regulating ATP with potassium	Table salt (sodium chloride, the main source), sea vegetables, milk and spinach
Calcium	1000 mg	Needed for muscle contractility, heart and digestive system health, builds bone, supports synthesis and function of blood cells	Dairy products, canned fish with bones (e.g. salmon or sardines), green leafy vegetables, nuts and seeds
Sulfur	850 mg	Critical in tertiary protein structure including connective tissue and skin, for example collagen and keratin. A component of bile acids for fat absorption and in B vitamins thereby facilitating energy production. Needed for several enzymes and antioxidant molecules, including glutathione and coenzyme A	Mustard, egg, seafood, beans, milk, milk products, nuts and meat. Sulfur in proteins are the main dietary source, followed by sulfates in water, fruits and vegetables
Phosphorus	700 mg	Key component of bones and energy processing via ATP and related molecules	Meat, yeast, wheat germ, soybean flour, meat, poultry, cheese, milk, canned fish, nuts and cereals
Magnesium	420 mg	Required for processing ATP and for bones	Nuts, soybeans and cocoa mass
Zinc	11 mg	Required for production of immune cells and their function, is an antioxidant, is cofactor in nearly 300 enzymes including carboxypeptidase, alcohol dehydrogenase and carbonic anhydrase	Liver, shellfish, oysters, meat, canned fish, hard cheese, whole grains, nuts, eggs and pulses. Vegetables and cereals may also contain phytates and oxalates which reduce zinc absorption
Iron	8 mg	Required for oxygen carrying capacity of hemoglobin and myoglobin, and as cofactor for several other enzymes	Red meat, leafy green vegetables, fish (tuna, salmon), eggs, dried fruits, beans, whole and enriched grains
Fluorine	3.8 mg	Forms compounds with calcium and phosphorus that are stronger and less soluble than other calcium salts, leading to stronger teeth and bones	Tea, meat, fish, cereals and fruit
Manganese	2.3 mg	Required cofactor for enzymes of energy production and synthesis of DNA and RNA. Key component of potent antioxidant enzyme superoxide dismutase	Cereals, spinach, wholemeal bread, nuts, pulses, fruit, dark green leafy vegetables, root vegetables, tea and liver
Copper	900 µg	Needed for connective tissue formation and release of iron from storage sites and maturation of red blood cells. Crucial for function of antioxidant enzyme superoxide dismutase. Needed for T cell function and maturation	Liver, shellfish, brewer's yeast, olives, nuts, whole grains, beans and chocolate
Chromium	200µg	Needed for normal sugar metabolism via GTF that enhances glucose utilization. Roles in fat and protein metabolism, and maintaining healthy cholesterol levels	Meat and whole-grain products, as well as some fruits, vegetables and spices
Iodine	150 µg	Required for synthesis of thyroid hormones, thyroxine and triiodothyronine to prevent goiter, may function as an antioxidant for organs, such as mammary and salivary glands, gastric mucosa and the thymus	Sodium or potassium iodide added to table salt, vegetables grown in iodine-rich soil, kelp, onions, milk, milk products, salt water fish and seafood
Selenium	55 µg	A cofactor essential to activity of antioxidant enzymes such as glutathione peroxidase	Organ meats, fish and shellfish, muscle meats, whole grains, cereals, dairy products and vegetables such as broccoli, mushrooms, cabbage and celery
Molybdenum	45 µg	Key component of oxidases including xanthine oxidase, aldehyde oxidase and sulfite oxidase	Milk, beans, bread, liver and cereals
Cobalt	1 µg	Critical component of vitamin B_{12} and thereby influences DNA synthesis, production of red blood cells and nerve function	Green leafy vegetables, some fish, liver, kidney and milk

Some sources further consider the trace minerals boron, nickel, silicon, strontium, tin, and vanadium to be essential, but consensus is pending.
AI, adequate intake; GTF, glucose tolerance factor; RDA, recommended daily allowance.
From NHS Direct Online (2012): Vitamins and Minerals. Available from: www.nhs.uk/Conditions/vitamins-minerals/Pages/vitamins-minerals.aspx. (Accessed 04/19/2012).

family of cytochromes, with the iron-porphyrin ring functioning to reduce ferrous to ferric iron. The iron sulfur family of enzymes also acts as electron carriers in the respiratory chain involving NADH and oxygen [7]. Iron is a critical component of peroxide and nitrous oxide generating enzymes and microbicidal reactions critical for immune function and may be involved in regulation of cytokine production and second-messenger cascade systems [7]. Fetal and infant neurologic development and brain function are also affected by iron deficiency as a result of changes in neurotransmitter regulation, myelin formation and energy metabolism [8].

CAUSES OF IRON DEFICIENCY

Iron deficiency results when iron loss outstrips intake to the degree that iron reserves are depleted. This can occur because of chronically low intake levels of iron rich foods, or result from increased demand owing to blood loss from parasitic helminth infections, such as hookworm and schistosomiasis, disrupted iron metabolism from malaria and other infections, or impaired absorption owing to gut inflammation from infectious diseases [11, 12]. Prevention and treatment of iron deficiency and its consequences typically requires actions to both improve intake and reduce losses. Iron absorption from the intestine and mobilization from iron stores in macrophages and hepatocytes are tightly controlled processes regulated by hepcidin, a small polypeptide hormone, and its receptor, known as ferroportin—an iron export protein [13].

ASSESSMENT OF IRON STATUS

As stated above, anemia is the clinical condition most commonly associated with iron deficiency. It is assessed by measuring hemoglobin levels, hematocrit, mean red blood cell volume or blood reticulocyte counts. In some cases palm, nail bed or conjunctival pallor have been used. Because anemia may have other etiologies, confirmation of iron deficiency as a cause requires an indictor of iron status; these include ferritin, transferrin saturation, soluble transferrin receptor, erythrocyte zinc protoporphyrin levels and bone marrow biopsy [14–17].

PERSONS AFFECTED AND CONSEQUENCES OF IRON DEFICIENCY

Women and children are most adversely affected by iron deficiency and related anemia as the demands of rapid growth and pregnancy leave them more vulnerable. For women of reproductive age, menstrual iron loss accounts for approximately 0.5 mg/day [18]. During pregnancy, the iron demands for maternal and fetal growth increase from 0.8 mg/day in the first trimester, to 7.5 mg/day in the third trimester [19, 20]. Blood loss at delivery further depletes iron stores. These factors are exacerbated by early onset of childbearing, greater number of births, limited birth spacing and poor access to antenatal care, including dietary iron supplements [21]. Currently, the World Health Organization (WHO) recommends iron supplementation of 60 mg/day for six months for pregnant women as part of the standard package of prenatal care, along with anti-malaria prophylaxis as appropriate.

Infants are at risk for developing iron deficiency, especially low birth weight and preterm infants who are born with reduced iron stores. For all neonates, delayed cord clamping at delivery is important to optimize transfer of as much iron-rich blood from the placenta. The iron content of breast milk is low but highly bioavailable, and exclusive breastfeeding for the first six months of life is advocated [22], followed by use of iron-fortified complementary foods for weaning, along with prevention and rapid detection and treatment of infectious disease [23, 24]. In addition to anemia and associated effects, iron deficiency in young children compromises early childhood cognitive development [7, 9].

CONTROL OF IRON DEFICIENCY

Current control measures include periodic deworming of pregnant women and children for hookworm, schistosomiasis and trichuris. Reduction of malaria transmission in malaria endemic areas has also resulted in reduction of iron deficiency. Improved iron intake through counseling and promotion of consumption of iron-rich foods has met with limited success [25]. However, supplementation and food fortification has been successful in reducing iron deficiency in some areas [14]. Currently, control of iron deficiency remains a global priority with the primary focus being on infants and pregnant women, and renewed attention to adolescents.

Over the last 40 years, some, but not all, studies reported that iron supplementation increased the risk of developing, or reactivating, malarial illness. An initial systematic review and meta-analysis of controlled trials concluded that oral iron supplementation at WHO-recommended doses resulted in a non-significant 9% increased risk of a clinical malaria episode, a significant (17%) greater risk of infection and tendency toward higher levels parasitemia. In these same studies, the risk of anemia in children was reduced by 50% [26]. A subsequent large-scale trial in Tanzanian children indicated that daily oral iron supplementation led to a 12% increased risk of mortality and a significant (11%) increased risk of all-cause hospitalization [27]. This led to the current WHO/United Nations Children's Fund (UNICEF) recommendation to restrict iron supplementation to iron-deficient children in *Plasmodium falciparum* endemic areas. Issues have been raised with regard to the practicality of this recommendation for programs. Moreover, the current recommendation has been challenged by a recent meta-analysis of 68 trials indicating limited adverse effects of iron supplementation in malaria endemic areas [28]. The role of iron-fortified foods or food additives for improving iron status are not yet evaluated for potential adverse effects on malaria. Co-implementation of malaria control activities in conjunction with programs that increase iron intake would be prudent.

CONCLUSION

Iron deficiency remains a serious public health problem, especially for pregnant women and children, and there is urgent need to scale-up effective prevention and treatment. This will require coordinated efforts and improved implementation.

ZINC

GLOBAL BURDEN OF ZINC DEFICIENCY

Zinc is the second most abundant trace mineral in the body following iron. Because zinc and iron share similar dietary sources, deficiencies tend to coexist and zinc deficiency is similarly widespread. In contrast to iron, the body does not generally retain zinc reserves and when daily intake falls below requirements, the onset of the adverse effects is relatively rapid. Currently, it is estimated that 1 billion persons worldwide suffer from zinc deficiency, and it is associated with 780,000 annual deaths and 29 million disability-adjusted live years (DALYs) [29]. Similar to iron, this burden falls predominantly on children and pregnant women in low income countries because of their growth needs and exposure to poor diets and diseases [29].

OVERVIEW OF ZINC BIOLOGY

Zinc is a cofactor in more than 200 enzymes with myriad roles in basic cellular functions, such as division, programmed cell death, DNA replication and RNA transcription [30, 31], and also functions as an antioxidant and can stabilize membranes [32]. Multiple body functions are therefore affected by zinc deficiency, including growth, sexual maturation, neuro-behavioural development and resistance to infectious diseases. Zinc status is particularly important for tissues with rapid cell turnover, such as epithelial linings of the gut and respiratory tract [33], and the immune system. Zinc affects multiple aspects of immunity, from the barrier of the skin to gene regulation within lymphocytes. While zinc deficiency impairs the normal function of cells mediating nonspecific immunity, such as neutrophils and macrophages, specific immunity mediated by T and B lymphocytes is more strongly affected, as growth and maturation of these cells is impaired, and basic functions, such as cytokine and antibody production are dysregulated [32].

Clinically, even moderate zinc deficiency results in reduced physical growth, impaired immunity and decreased resistance to infection. Moderate-to-severe zinc deficiency can cause hair loss, skin lesions, diarrhea and wasting of body tissues. Sensory functions may also be affected, including eyesight, taste and smell. In severe zinc deficiency, a wide range of disturbances occur, including severe growth retardation and impaired bone development, along with delayed sexual maturation, frequent dermatitis, impaired taste acuity and behavioral changes [34]. As indicated above, defects in the immune system result in increased susceptibility to, and severity of, diarrhea, pneumonia and malaria.

Several clinical trials have demonstrated the importance of zinc supplements given during acute or persistent diarrhea to reduce the severity and duration of diarrhea [35, 36]. Supplemental zinc is currently recommended as an adjunct therapy during the treatment of diarrhea in children at a recommended dosage equivalent to two times the age specific recommended daily amount (RDA) per day for 10–14 days. Studies strongly indicate that zinc treatment with oral rehydration therapy (ORT) is significantly more effective than ORT alone in reducing the duration and severity of diarrheal episodes, decreasing stool output and lessening the need for hospitalization. In addition, zinc may also prevent future diarrhea episodes for up to three months [37]. Further research is required for therapeutic supplementation for other infectious diseases, such as pneumonia and tuberculosis and viral infections (including HIV).

CAUSES OF ZINC DEFICIENCY

As described above, zinc deficiency is generally caused by low dietary intake. Persons in low-income countries tend to consume diets that are predominantly plant-based, which tend to be low in both total zinc and bioavailable zinc owing to high levels of tannins and phytates that reduce absorption [38]. Deficiency can also be precipitated and/or exacerbated by infectious diseases, such as acute or chronic diarrhea, that may affect absorption and/or loss of zinc in the feces. Viral, bacterial and protozoan pathogens, including rotavirus, *Shigella* and cryptosporidium have been linked to fecal zinc loss, and subsequent deficiency [34, 38]. Non-infectious chronic diseases, including diabetes and liver and kidney diseases of multiple etiologies, also compromise zinc status [39, 40]. Lastly, certain genetic conditions can perturb zinc metabolism or limit absorption, such as sickle-cell disease, and acrodermatitis enteropathica.

ASSESSMENT OF ZINC STATUS

Diagnosis of zinc deficiency is not as straightforward as for iron [41]. For individual persons, this has generally relied on depressed levels of plasma zinc (typically <70 μg/dL but with age, pregnancy and sex-specific cut-offs) and the presence of clinical signs of deficiency, such as loss of taste or repeated bouts of infectious disease, and low intake based on dietary assessment. However, these measures are not considered definitive because of homeostatic control mechanisms and the influence of infection that tends to depress plasma zinc levels as part of the acute phase response. As such, documented changes in plasma zinc and related clinical signs of deficiency following supplementation are recommended to confirm the diagnosis.

Similarly, at the population level, determining zinc deficiency relies on several criteria as indicated by WHO/UNICEF/International Atomic Energy Agency (IAEA)/International Zinc Nutrition Consultative Group (IZINCG) recommendations. These include population-based prevalence of 25% or more of zinc intakes below the estimated average requirement (EAR), 20% or more of the population with low serum zinc concentrations (based on age- and sex-specific cut-offs) or 20% or more of children less than 5 years of age with height-for-age less than -2 standard deviations (SD) below the age-specific median of the reference population. Moreover, changes in the prevalence of low plasma zinc and mean population plasma zinc levels following intervention further confirm widespread zinc deficiency. However, it is notable that because mean plasma zinc concentration usually increases following enhanced zinc intake, clinical improvement in population-based health, such as reduced incidence or severity of diarrhea, provides the best evidence for the improvement of zinc deficiency and status.

PERSONS AFFECTED AND CONSEQUENCES OF ZINC DEFICIENCY

Women and children are at the greatest risk for zinc deficiency. Maternal zinc deficiency can affect the zinc nutrition of exclusively breastfed infants [42]. Mothers without zinc deficiency can satisfy a newborn's zinc requirement through the first six months of life [43]. After this age, infants must consume complementary foods containing sufficient absorbable zinc. In many low-income countries, neither of these requisites is satisfied.

The increased nutritional demands during pregnancy and lactation predispose women to developing zinc deficiency. Physiologic adjustments in zinc absorption among lactating women have been found to help meet lactation needs [44], although these compensatory adaptations are limited. Another factor of concern is iron intake, as several studies have demonstrated that supplemental iron (greater than 25 mg) might decrease zinc absorption [1, 45–47].

Infants and young children are at greater risk of zinc deficiency because of the increased requirements during growth. Low birth weight (<2500 g) infants have poor hepatic stores of zinc [48] placing them at increased risk. Likewise, in premature infants, zinc status is further compromised because most of the zinc from the mother is transferred to the fetus during the last trimester of pregnancy; premature infants also have reduced zinc absorption from their immature gastrointestinal tract. Infants in low income countries may also experience suboptimal complementary feeding practices, such as delayed introduction of foods and use of foods with low total and absorbable zinc. Moreover, complementary foods which have high phytate content can interfere with zinc absorption [49].

Adolescence and old age are additional life stages affected by zinc deficiency. In adolescence, zinc deficiency occurs because of increased physiologic requirements at the time of the pubertal growth spurt [50]. For the elderly, in addition to poor zinc intakes, there is some evidence that the efficiency of zinc absorption my decrease with age [51, 52].

CONTROL OF ZINC DEFICIENCY

The three major intervention strategies to address zinc deficiency are supplementation, fortification and dietary diversification. Supplementation is further divided into preventive supplementation and therapeutic supplementation. The choice of intervention depends upon the available resources and technical feasibility. While the health benefits of zinc supplementation are well established [53], health programs specifically targeted at high-risk populations are in need of expansion.

Preventive supplementation of zinc in programs already delivering daily or weekly nutrient supplements for prevention of iron deficiency anemia and other micronutrient deficiencies appears most feasible. Consideration of the specific form of zinc used is important as it may affect its bioavailability. In addition, supplementation programs must take into account the prevailing diet, as bioavailability of zinc in the diet is influenced by the food source, as well as other components of the diet that inhibit or promote absorption of zinc. Continued research is required on the best forms of zinc that are both readily absorbed and do not have antagonistic interactions with other minerals.

Dietary diversification and modification represent a sustainable long-term approach to improving the intakes of several nutrients simultaneously, including zinc. Home gardening and education interventions have been effective food-based strategies to address dietary inclusion of multiple micronutrients, and supplementation programs are useful for targeting at-risk population subgroups. Information on locally-available, low-cost, culturally-acceptable zinc-rich foods is needed. Likewise, information is required on the best ways of implementing both large-scale and home-based food processing interventions to enhance zinc absorption from the usual diet.

In populations where zinc deficiency is widely distributed and food distribution channels are established, food fortification is generally the more cost-effective and sustainable strategy [54]. Success has been seen in fortification programs targeted to specific high-risk groups, such as infants and young children, in the form of infant formulas and complementary foods. Further research on improved agricultural practices including plant cultivation to enhance dietary zinc content is required.

CONCLUSION

It is estimated that nearly one billion people in the developing world are deficient in zinc, with another one billion at risk for deficiency [55]. In children, zinc deficiency causes an increase in infection and diarrhea, contributing to the death of about 780,000 children worldwide per year [56]. Zinc supplements are critical in treating diarrheal disease and helping to prevent diarrheal and respiratory disease (and possibly malaria), and to reduce mortality, especially among children with low birth weight or stunted growth. Numerous strategies to address zinc deficiency exist; however, careful examination is required on the zinc absorption, acceptability and cost of fortified products.

IODINE

GLOBAL BURDEN OF IODINE DEFICIENCY

As with iron and zinc, it is estimated that two billion individuals have an insufficient iodine intake, with South Asia and sub-Saharan Africa being most affected. However, about 50% of Europe remains mildly iodine deficient, and iodine intakes in other industrialized countries, including the USA and Australia, have fallen in recent years [57]. Iodine deficiency has multiple adverse effects, termed iodine deficiency disorders (IDD), owing to inadequate thyroid hormone production. Iodine deficiency and associated disorders increase infant mortality, miscarriage and stillbirth. IDD is the main cause of preventable mental retardation and brain damage owing, primarily, to effects on the fetus and children in the first few years of life. Globally, the annual burden of IDD includes two million DALYs [58].

OVERVIEW OF IODINE BIOLOGY

Iodine is an essential component of thyroxine (T3) and triiodothyronine (T4) produced by the thyroid gland. These are required for normal neuronal migration and myelination of the brain during fetal and early postnatal life. Hypothyroxinemia during these critical periods causes irreversible brain damage, with mental retardation and neurologic abnormalities [59]. Gestational iodine deficiency may impair fetal growth and neurodevelopment and increase mortality. Deficiency during infancy and childhood reduces growth and motor functions, and impairs cognitive development. Absorption of iodide, the most readily absorbed dietary form of iodine, involves a specialized sodium/iodine symporter (NIS) expressed on enterocytes and cells of the thyroid [60]. A healthy adult maintains approximately 20 mg of iodine reserves, with 70% in the thyroid [61]. Adaptations to low intake include elevated thyroid-stimulating hormone (TSH) levels, reduced thyroid T3 and T4 production, and enhanced NIS expression for greater uptake of iodine. This leads to the characteristic pattern onset during deficiency of elevated TSH, a low serum T4 and a normal or high T3 [62]. Thyroid failure and cretinism is seen in areas of chronic and severe iodine deficiency with low T4 and T3 levels and highly elevated TSH [63, 64]. The effects of iodine deficiency on development of goiter vary considerably between populations and individuals as a result of environmental, genetic and other poorly-understood factors.

CAUSES OF IODINE DEFICIENCY

The iodine content of most foods is low, with typical servings containing less than 5% of daily needs [65, 66]. The content in foods is strongly influenced by iodine in the soil and/or in fertilizers in irrigation and livestock feeds. Marine plants, particularly seaweed, and animals concentrate iodine from seawater and tend to be good dietary sources. Other primary sources include bread and dairy products, and, particularly, iodized table and cooking salt. Certain dietary substances, termed goitrogens can interfere with thyroid metabolism and exacerbate iodine deficiency [67]. These include cruciferous vegetables, such as cabbage, cauliflower or broccoli, and rapeseed oil – all of which contain glucosinolates; and cassava, sorghum and sweet potatoes, which contain cyanogenic glucosides. In such cases, their metabolites can compete with iodine for uptake by the thyroid. In many low-income countries, particularly in sub-Saharan Africa, cassava is widely consumed and, if not properly prepared, can exacerbate IDD [68]. Cigarette smoking is also associated with higher serum levels of thiocyanate that may limit iodine uptake by the thyroid [69]. Deficiencies of selenium, iron and vitamin A exacerbate the effects of iodine deficiency.

ASSESSMENT OF IODINE STATUS

Four methods are generally recommended for assessment of iodine nutrition in populations: urinary iodine concentration (UI), the goiter rate, serum TSH and serum thyroglobulin (Tg). These indicators are complementary in that UI is a sensitive indicator of recent iodine intake (days) and Tg shows an intermediate response (weeks-to-months), whereas changes in the goiter rate reflect long-term iodine nutrition (months-to-years) [70]. However, assessment of iodine status in pregnancy is difficult and it remains unclear whether iodine intakes are sufficient in this group, leading to calls for iodine supplementation during pregnancy in several industrialized countries [71].

PERSONS AFFECTED AND CONSEQUENCES OF IODINE DEFICIENCY

Iodine deficiency affects nearly two billion individuals worldwide in all segments of society, with the greatest impacts on pregnant women and children. Based on a recent WHO global review [72] more than a third of school-age children are iodine deficient, the majority of whom live in Southeast Asia, Africa and the Western Pacific.

The most devastating outcomes of IDD are increased perinatal mortality, mental retardation and cretinism. Iodine deficiency is the greatest cause of preventable brain damage in childhood and goiter is the most visible manifestation of IDD. If iodine deficiency occurs during the fetal stage up to the third month after birth, when much of the brain development occurs, the resulting thyroid failure will lead to irreversible alterations in brain function [73, 74]. In severely endemic areas, cretinism may affect up to 5–15% of the population.

CONTROL OF IODINE DEFICIENCY

The most effective means of controlling iodine deficiency in populations is universal salt iodization. It is among the most cost-effective interventions to promote economic and social development in areas of iodine deficiency and has resulted in declining prevalence of IDD worldwide [75]. Efforts are required to identify alternative dietary vehicles for supplementation, such as circumstances where predisposing factors may limit the consumption of iodized salt (e.g. risks of hypertension) or to increase the bioavailability for high-risk groups, such as infants and pregnant women.

CONCLUSION

Iodine is crucial for health, and deficiency during pregnancy is especially harmful. Salt iodization remains the most cost-effective way of delivering iodine and of improving health and cognition in iodine-deficient populations. Worldwide, the annual costs of salt iodization are estimated at US $0.02–0.05 per child covered; the costs per child death averted are US $1000, and per DALY gained are US $34–36 [76]. However, this intervention must be sustained and continued advocacy and investments must be made to continue these successes.

OTHER MINERALS OF CLINICAL AND PUBLIC HEALTH IMPORTANCE

SELENIUM

Selenium is an essential nutrient for growth and reproduction. Biochemically, selenium is a component of the enzyme glutathione peroxidase, which, along with other nutrients, protects against damage to cellular components by preventing the accumulation of peroxides in the tissue (S7). Severe deficiency of selenium is associated with cardiomyopathy, especially in children and women of childbearing age [77].

Selenium is critical for the proper functioning of the immune system [78]. Selenium deficiency is associated with decreased immune cell counts, increased disease progression and high risk of death in the HIV/AIDS population [79–81]. Moreover, HIV/AIDS malabsorption can deplete levels of many nutrients, including selenium. Selenium has antioxidant properties that help protect cells from oxidative stress, thus potentially slowing progression of the disease [82].

Researchers continue to investigate the relationship between selenium and HIV/AIDS, including the effect of selenium levels on disease progression and mortality. Current laboratory experiments have shown that selenium has an inhibitory effect on HIV *in vitro* through antioxidant effects of glutathione peroxidase and other selenoproteins. Moreover, in several randomized controlled trials, selenium supplementation has reduced hospitalizations and diarrheal morbidity, and improved $CD4^+$ cell counts; however, the evidence remains equivocal [83]. Continued research is needed to study the effect of selenium supplementation on HIV disease-related comorbidities in the context of anti-retroviral therapy in both developing and developed countries [83].

CALCIUM AND MAGNESIUM

There are significant health impacts of calcium and magnesium deficiencies. Both calcium and magnesium play important roles in bone structure, muscle contraction, nerve impulse transmission, blood clotting and cell signaling [84]. Inadequate intake of calcium results in rickets and a risk of osteoporosis, as well as hypertension and stroke. Magnesium deficiency affects neurologic and neuromuscular function, resulting in anorexia, muscular weakness and lethargy. Calcium and magnesium deficiencies for both adults and children are widespread, especially in developing countries [85].

For women, both calcium and magnesium are known to play an important role in the prevention and treatment of pre-eclampsia and eclampsia during pregnancy [86]. Pre-eclampsia is one of the most common causes of maternal and fetal morbidities and mortalities worldwide, with incidence rates in the range of 4–8% of all pregnancies [87, 88]. Calcium plays an important role in muscle contraction and regulation of water balance in cells, as modification of plasma calcium concentration can lead to the alteration of blood pressure [89]. Magnesium is an essential cofactor for many enzyme systems and plays an important role in neurochemical transmission and peripheral vasodilatation [88]. It is well documented that lowering of serum calcium and the increase of intracellular calcium can cause an elevation of blood pressure in pre-eclamptic mothers. In addition, serum magnesium also decreases in women with preeclampsia [89].

Recent Cochrane reviews have examined the effects of calcium and magnesium supplementation on pre-eclampsia and eclampsia during pregnancy [90, 91]. In the case of calcium, supplementation appears to approximately halve the risk of pre-eclampsia and thus reduces the risk of preterm birth [91]. Magnesium sulfate remains the drug of choice for the management of pre-eclampsia and has also been shown to reduce the risk of preterm birth [90, 92]. Moreover, magnesium sulfate given to women with eclampsia considerably reduces the risk ratio of maternal death and of recurrence of seizures, even compared with seizure-reducing drugs such as diazepam [93]. The success of supplementation programs such as these described requires continued efforts to enhance implementation and expand coverage.

FLUORIDE

The role of fluoride in preventing tooth decay is well established [94, 95]. Despite significant successes with community-based programs, a recent review of global epidemiologic data indicates a marked increase in the prevalence of dental caries, especially in developing countries [96, 97]. Researchers emphasize the need for focused efforts to promote water fluoridation, topical fluoride application and rinses and a renewed effort to include oral health within educational programs. Tooth decay is widespread and is known to disproportionately affect lower socio economic groups. Water and salt fluoridation should be implemented where deemed feasible and the use of affordable fluoride toothpastes should be encouraged.

SUMMARY

Mineral deficiencies negatively affect billions of individuals worldwide, imposing a heavy burden on wellbeing and economic productivity. Most prominently, deficiencies in iron, zinc and iodine have the largest negative impact on public health; however, other minerals, including calcium, magnesium, selenium and fluoride, contribute significantly to the health burden. While the causes of mineral malnutrition are complex, the primary determinant is insufficient dietary intakes. Efforts aimed at fortifying foods or providing supplements to reduce mineral deficiencies have had some success, but substantial efforts are still needed to get effective programming at scale [98]. To ensure sufficient impact, several mutually-reinforcing strategies need to be put in place to increase access and consumption to those in need. As most nutrient deficiencies do not occur in isolation, measures for prevention and control will need to rely on dietary diversification, as well as education to promote optimum dietary intakes.

REFERENCES

1. Institute of Medicine, Food and Nutrition Board. Dietary Reference Intakes for Vitamin A, Vitamin K, Arsenic, Boron, Chromium, Copper, Iodine, Iron, Manganese, Molybdenum, Nickel, Silicon, Vanadium, and Zinc. Washington: National Academy Press; 2001.
2. McDowell LR. Minerals in Animal and Human Nutrition, 2nd edn. Elsevier, Philadelphia; 2003.
3. Gropper SS, Smith JL, Groff JL. Advanced Nutrition and Human Metabolism, 5th edn. Wadsworth: Cengage Learning; 2009.
4. Offenbacher EG, Pi-Sunyer FX, Stoecker BJ. Chromium. In: O'Dell BL, Sunde RA, eds. Handbook of Nutritionally Essential Mineral Elements. New York: Marcel Dekker; 1997:389.
5. O'Dell BL, Sunde RA. Handbook of Nutritionally Essential Mineral Elements. New York: Marcel Dekker, Inc.; 1997.
6. Ezzati M, Lopez AD, Rodgers A, Murray CJL. Comparative quantification of health risks: global and regional burden of disease attributable to selected major risk factors. Geneva: World Health Organization; 2004.
7. McLean E, Cogswell M, Egli I, et al. Worldwide prevalence of anaemia, WHO Vitamin and Mineral Nutrition Information System, 1993–2005. Public Health Nutr 2009;12:444–54.
8. Beard JL. Iron biology in immune function, muscle metabolism and neuronal functioning. J Nutr 2001;131:568–80.
9. Beard JL. Iron deficiency alters brain development and functioning. J Nutr 2003;133:1468–72.
10. Haas JD, Brownlie TT. Iron deficiency and reduced work capacity: a critical review of the research to determine a causal relationship. J Nutr 2001; 131(suppl.):676–88.
11. Brooker S, Akhwale W, Pullan R, et al. Epidemiology of plasmodium-helminth co-infection in Africa: populations at risk, potential impact on anemia, and prospects for combining control. Am J Trop Med Hyg 2007; 77(suppl. 6):88–98.
12. Prentice AM, Ghattas H, Doherty C, Cox SE. Iron metabolism and malaria. Food Nutr Bull 2007;28(suppl. 4):S524–39.
13. Ganz T, Nemeth E. Regulation of iron acquisition and iron distribution in mammals. Biochim Biophys Acta 2006;1763:690–9.
14. Zimmermann MB, Hurrell RF. Nutritional iron deficiency. Lancet 2007; 370:511–20.
15. Zimmermann MB. Methods to assess iron and iodine status. Br J Nutr 2008;99(suppl. S3):S2–9.
16. Ramakrishnan U. Nutritional Anemias. CRC Series in Modern Nutrition. Boca Raton: CRC Press; 2001:260.

17. Prevention. WHOCfDCa. Assessing the iron status of populations: a report of a joint World Health Organization/Centers for Disease Control technical consultation on the assessment of iron status at the population level. Geneva: World Health Organization; 2004.
18. Guillebaud J, Bonnar J, Morehead J, Matthews A. Menstrual blood-loss with intrauterine devices. Lancet 1976;307:387–90.
19. Milman N. Iron and pregnancy – a delicate balance. Ann Hematol 2006; 85:559–65.
20. Bothwell TH. Iron requirements in pregnancy and strategies to meet them. Am J Clin Nutr 2000;72:257–64.
21. Kalaivani K. Prevalence and consequences of anaemia in pregnancy. Ind J Med Res 2009;130:627–33.
22. Allen LH. Multiple micronutrients in pregnancy and lactation: an overview. Am J Clin Nutr 2005;81:1206–12.
23. Chaparro CM. Setting the stage for child health and eevelopment: Prevention of iron deficiency in early infancy. J Nutr 2008;138:2529–33.
24. Chaparro CM, Neufeld LM, Tena Alavez G, et al. Effect of timing of umbilical cord clamping on iron status in Mexican infants: a randomised controlled trial. Lancet 2006;367:1997–2004.
25. Dewey KG. Increasing iron intake of children through complementary foods. Food Nutr Bull 2007;28(suppl. 4):S595–609.
26. Shankar AH. Malaria and nutrition. In: Semba RD, Bloem MW, eds. Nutrition and Health in Developing Countries, 2nd edn. New York: Springer Publishing Company; 2008.
27. Sazawal S, Black RE, Ramsan M, et al. Effects of routine prophylactic supplementation with iron and folic acid on admission to hospital and mortality in preschool children in a high malaria transmission setting: community-based, randomised, placebo-controlled trial. Lancet 2006;367:133–43.
28. Ojukwu JU, Okebe JU, Yahav D, Paul M. Oral iron supplementation for preventing or treating anaemia among children in malaria-endemic areas. Cochrane Database Syst Rev 2009;3:CD006589.
29. Caulfield L, Black RE. Zinc deficiency. In: Ezzati M, Lopez AD, Rodgers A, Murray CJL, eds. Comparative Quantification of Health Risks: Global and Regional Burden of Disease Attributable to Selected Major Risk Factors. Geneva: World Health Organization; 2004.
30. Haase H, Rink L. Functional significance of zinc-related signaling pathways in immune cells. Annu Rev Nutr 2009;29:133–52.
31. Hotz C, Brown KM. Assessment of the risk of zinc deficiency in populations and options for its control. Food Nutr Bull 2004;25:99–199.
32. Shankar AH, Prasad AA. Zinc and immune function: the biological basis of altered resistance to infection. Am J Clin Nutr 1998;68:447S.
33. Tuerk MJ, Fazel N. Zinc deficiency. Curr Opin Gastroenterol 2009;25: 136–43.
34. Prasad AS. Impact of the discovery of human zinc deficiency on health. J Am Coll Nutr 2009;28:257–65.
35. Bhutta ZA, Bird SM, Black RE, et al. Therapeutic effects of oral zinc in acute and persistent diarrhea in children in developing countries: Pooled analysis of randomized controlled trials. Am J Clin Nutr 2000;72:1516–22.
36. Baqui AH, Black RE, El Arifeen S, et al. Effect of zinc supplementation started during diarrhoea on morbidity and mortality in Bangladeshi children: community randomised trial. BMJ 2002;325:1059.
37. Bhutta ZA, Black RE, Brown KH, et al. Prevention of diarrhea and pneumonia by zinc supplementation in children in developing countries: pooled analysis of randomized controlled trials. Zinc Investigators' Collaborative Group. J Pediatr 1999;135:689–97.
38. Solomons NW. Dietary Sources of zinc and factors affecting its bioavailability. Food Nutr Bull 2001;22:138–54.
39. Tudor R, Zalewski PD, Ratnaike RN. Zinc in health and chronic disease. J Nutr Health Aging 2005;9:45–51.
40. DiSilvestro RA. Zinc in relation to diabetes and oxidative disease. J Nutr 2000;130:1509–11.
41. Gibson R. Principles of Nutritional Assessment. Oxford: Oxford University Press; 2005.
42. Dórea JG. Zinc deficiency in nursing infants. J Am Coll Nutr 2002; 21:84–7.
43. Krebs NF, Hambidge KM. Zinc requirements and zinc intakes of breast fed infants. Am J Clin Nutr 1986;43:288–92.
44. King JC. Determinants of maternal zinc status during pregnancy. Am J Clin Nutr 2000;71:1334.
45 Whittaker P. Iron and zinc interactions in humans. Am J Clin Nutr 1998;68:442–6.
46. Hambidge KM, Krebs NF, Sibley L, English J. Acute effects of iron therapy on zinc status in pregnancy. Obstet Gynecol 1987;70:593–6.
47. O'Brien KO, Zavaleta N, Caulfield LN, et al. Prenatal iron supplements impair zinc absorption in pregnant Peruvian women. J Nutr 2000;130: 2251–5.
48. Zlotkin SH, Cherian MG. Hepatic metallothionein as a source of zinc and cystein during the first year of life. Pediatr Res 1988;24:326–9.
49. Bell JG, Keen CL, Lönnerdal B. Effect of infant cereals on zinc and copper absorption during weaning. Am J Did Child 1987;141:1128–32.
50. King JC. Does poor zinc nutriture retard skeletal growth and mineralization in adolescents? Am J Clin Nutr 1996;64:375–6.
51. Mares-Perlman JA, Subar AF, Block G, et al. Zinc intake and sources in the US adult population: 1976–1980. J Am Coll Nutr 1995;14:349–57.
52. August D, Janghorbani M, Young VR. Determination of zinc and copper absorption at three dietary Zn-Cu ratios by using stable isotope methods in young adult and elderly subjects. Am J Clin Nutr 1989; 50: 1457–63.
53. The WHO/UNICEF Joint Statement May 2004 on the Clinical Management of Acute Diarrhoea. New York: The World Health Organization and United Nations Children's Fund.
54. Edejer TT, Aikins M, Black R, et al. Cost effectiveness analysis of strategies for child health in developing countries. BMJ 2005;331:1177.
55. Prasad AS. Zinc deficiency. BMJ 2003;326:409.
56. Hambidge KM, Krebs NF. Zinc deficiency: a special challenge. J Nutr 2007; 137:1101.
57. de Benoist B, McLean E, Andersson M, Rogers L. Iodine deficiency in 2007: global progress since 2003. Food Nutr Bull 2008;29:195–202.
58. Caulfield LE, Richard SA, Rivera JA, et al. Stunting, wasting, and micronutrient deficiency disorders 2006. In: Dean T, Jamison DT, Breman JG, et al, eds. Disease control priorities in developing countries, 2nd edn. New York: Oxford University Press; 2006:551–68.
59. Morreale de Escobar G, Obregon MJ, Escobar del Rey F. Role of thyroid hormone during early brain development. Eur J Endocrinol 2004;151(suppl. 3):U25–37.
60. Nicola JP, Basquin C, Portulano C, et al. The Na+/I-symporter mediates active iodide uptake in the intestine. Am J Physiol Cell Physiol 2009;296:C654–62.
61. Fisher DA, Oddie TH. Thyroid iodine content and turnover in euthyroid subjects: validity of estimation of thyroid iodine accumulation from short-term clearance studies. J Clin Endocrinol Metab 1969;29:721–7.
62. Delange F, Camus M, Ermans AM. Circulating thyroid hormones in endemic goiter. J Clin Endocrinol Metab 1972;34:891–5.
63. Dumont JE, Ermans AM, Bastenie PA. Thyroid function in a goiter endemic. V. Mechanism of thyroid failure in the Uele endemic cretins. J Clin Endocrinol Metab 1963;23:847–60.
64. Morreale de Escobar G, Obregon MJ, Escobar del Rey F. Role of thyroid hormone during early brain development. Eur J Endocrinol 2004;151(suppl. 3):U25–37.
65. Pennington JAT, Schoen SA, Salmon GD, et al. Composition of core foods in the U.S. food supply, 1982–1991. J Food Comp Anal 1995;8:171–217.
66. Haldimann M, Alt A, Blanc A, Blondeau K. Iodine content of food groups. J Food Comp Anal 2005;18:461–71.
67. Gaitan E. Environmental goitrogenesis. Boca Raton: CRC Press; 1989.
68. Ermans AM, Delange F, Van der Velden M, Kinthaert J. Possible role of cyanide and thiocyanate in the etiology of endemic cretinism. Adv Exp Med Biol 1972;30:455–86.
69. Laurberg P, Nøhr SB, Pedersen KM, Fuglsang E. Iodine nutrition in breast-fed infants is impaired by maternal smoking. J Clin Endocrinol Metab 2004;89: 181–7.
70. Delange F, de Benoist B, Pretell E, Dunn JT. Iodine deficiency in the world: where do we stand at the turn of the century? Thyroid 2001;11:437–47.
71. Zimmerman MB. Iodine Deficiency. Endocrine Reviews 2009;30:376–408.
72. De Benoist B, Andersson M, Egli I, et al., eds. Iodine status worldwide: WHO Global Database on Iodine Deficiency. Geneva: World Health Organization; 2004.
73. Bleichrodt N, Born MP. A meta-analysis of research on iodine and its relationship to cognitive development. In: Stanbury JB, ed. The damaged brain of iodine deficiency. New York: Cognizant Communication; 1994:195–200.
74. Zimmermann MB. The adverse effects of mild-to-moderate iodine deficiency during pregnancy and childhood: a review. Thyroid 2007;17:829–35.
75. World Health Organization, United Nations Children's Fund, International Council for the Control of Iodine Deficiency Disorders. Assessment of Iodine Deficiency Disorders and Monitoring Their Elimination. A Guide for Programme Managers. (WHO/NHD/01.1), 2nd edn. Geneva: World Health Organization; 2001.
76. Caulfield LE, Richard SA, Rivera JA, et al. Stunting, wasting, and micronutrient deficiency disorders 2006. In: Dean T, Jamison DT, Breman JG, eds. Disease control priorities in developing countries, 2nd edn. New York: Oxford University Press;2006:551–68.
77. Levander OA. A global view of human selenium nutrition. Ann Rev Nutr 1987;7:227–50.
78. Rayman MP. The importance of selenium to human health. Lancet 2000; 356:233–41.

79. Look MP, Rockstroh JK, Rao GS, et al. Serum selenium versus lymphocyte subsets and markers of disease progression and inflammatory response in human immunodeficiency virus-1 infection. Biol Trace Elem Res 1997; 56:31–41.
80. Singhal N, Austin J. A clinical review of micronutrients in HIV infection. J Int Assoc Physicians AIDS Care 2002;1:63–75.
81. Baum MK, Shor-Posner G. Micronutrient status in relationship to mortality in HIV-1 disease. Nutr Rev 1998;56:S135–9.
82. Patrick L. Nutrients and HIV; Part One – Beta carotene and selenium. Altern Med Rev 1999;4:403–13.
83. Stone CA, Kawai K, Kupka R, Fawzi WW. Role of selenium in HIV infection. Nutr Rev 2010;68:671–81.
84. Food and Agriculture Organization/World Health Organization Expert Consultation. Magnesium. In: Human Vitamin and Mineral Requirements. Rome and Geneva: Food and Agriculture Organization of the United Nations and World Health Organization; 2002.
85. Combs GF, Nielsen FH. Health significance of calcium and magnesium: Examples from human studies. In: Cotruvo J, Bartram J, eds. Calcium and magnesium in drinking-water: public health significance. Geneva: World Health Organization; 2009.
86. American Congress of Obstetricians and Gynecologists practice bulletin. Diagnosis and management of preeclampsia and eclampsia. Number 33, January 2002. Obstet Gynecol 2002;99:159–67.
87. Walker JJ. Pre-eclampsia. Lancet 2000;356:1260–5.
88. Norwitz ER, Robinson JN, Repke JT. Prevention of preeclampsia: is it possible? Clin Obstet Gynecol 1999;42:436–54.
89. Hofmeyr GJ, Duley L, Atallah A. Dietary calcium supplementation for prevention of pre-eclampsia and related problems: a systematic review and commentary. BJOG 2007;114:933–43.
90. Duley L, Matar HE, Almerie MQ, Hall DR. Alternative magnesium sulphate regimens for women with pre-eclampsia and eclampsia. Cochrane Database Syst Rev 2010;8:CD007388.
91. Hofmeyr GJ, Lawrie TA, Atallah AN, Duley L. Calcium supplementation during pregnancy for preventing hypertensive disorders and related problems. Cochrane Database Syst Rev 2010;8:CD001059.
92. Doyle LW, Crowther CA, Middleton P, et al. Magnesium sulphate for women at risk of preterm birth for neuroprotection of the fetus. Cochrane Database Syst Rev 2009;1:CD004661.
93. Duley L, Henderson-Smart DJ, Walker GJ, Chou D. Magnesium sulphate versus diazepam for eclampsia. Cochrane Database Syst Rev 2010;12: CD000127.
94. Truman BI, Gooch BF, Sulemana I, et al. Reviews of evidence on interventions to prevent dental caries, oral and pharyngeal cancers, and sports-related craniofacial injuries. Am J Prev Med 2002;23(suppl. 1):21–54.
95. Hausen HW. Fluoridation, fractures, and teeth. BMJ 2000;321:844–5.
96. Bagramian RA, Garcia-Godoy F, Volpe AR. The global increase in dental caries. A pending public health crisis. Am J Dent 2009;22:3–8.
97. Blinkhorn AS, Davies RM. Caries prevention. A continued need worldwide. Int Dent J 1996;46:119–25.
98. Allen L, de Benoist B, Dary O, Hurrell R. World Health Organization and Food and Agriculture Organization. Guidelines on the food fortification with micronutrients. 2006.

PART

9

VECTOR TRANSMISSION OF DISEASES AND ZOONOSES

141 Arthropods in Disease Transmission

Duane J Gubler

Key features

- Vector-borne diseases are among the most important global public health problems
- These diseases occur primarily in the tropics, but expand to affect human and animal populations in temperate areas
- Vector-borne diseases are transmitted by hematophagous arthropods, the most important of which are mosquitoes
- Globally, the most important vector-borne diseases are caused by viruses; however, in Africa, malaria is the most important
- Most vector-borne diseases exist in complex zoonotic cycles involving a variety of birds, rodents, and other vertebrate hosts
- The emergence/re-emergence of vector-borne diseases in the past 40 years has been driven by population growth, urbanization, globalization and lack of public health infrastructure

HISTORY

Although early scholars recognized a relationship between arthropods and illness in humans and animals, the concept of disease transmission by insects is relatively new. The first demonstration that a parasite of humans required a developmental phase in an insect to complete its life cycle occurred about 135 years ago. Sir Patrick Manson, working in China in 1877, showed that the human filarial parasite *Wuchereria bancrofti* required an obligatory period of development in the mosquito *Culex pipiens fatigans* (*Cx. pipiens quinquefasciatus*). This discovery was followed over the next 30 years by a series of observations that demonstrated transmission of protozoa, helminths, viruses and bacteria by ticks, flies, mosquitoes, fleas and lice (Table 141-1) [1]. Since that time, many important disease pathogens of humans and animals have been shown to depend on arthropods to complete their transmission cycles.

The pathogens transmitted to humans by arthropods fall into four categories: nematodes or roundworms, protozoa, bacteria (including rickettsiae and spirochetes), and viruses. Some are true parasites of humans (e.g. *W. bancrofti*), but most are zoonotic, with other primary vertebrate hosts (reservoirs). In these cases, humans become an incidental host, and although they may contribute to the transmission cycle on a temporary basis, they are not required for survival of the pathogen in nature.

DISEASE TRANSMISSION

An arthropod can transmit a disease agent from one person or animal to another in one of two basic ways.

MECHANICAL TRANSMISSION

This consists of transfer of the organism on contaminated mouthparts or other body parts. There is no multiplication or developmental change of the pathogen on or in the insect. Examples include some enteroviruses, bacteria, and protozoa of humans that have a direct fecal–oral transmission cycle. Insects, such as houseflies, can become contaminated with these pathogens while feeding on feces and can transport them directly to the food of humans.

BIOLOGIC TRANSMISSION

The second and most important type of disease transmission by arthropods is biologic. The pathogen must undergo development in the insect vector in order to complete its life cycle. There are four types of biologic transmission.

Propagative

This occurs when the organism is ingested with a blood meal and undergoes simple multiplication in the body of the arthropod. Examples are the arboviruses, which replicate extensively in the tissues of the arthropod, and are transmitted to a new host in the saliva when another blood meal is taken.

Cyclopropagative

The pathogen undergoes a developmental cycle (changes from one stage to another) as well as multiplication in the body of the arthropod. The best example of cyclopropagative transmission is malaria, in which a single zygote may give rise to >200,000 sporozoites.

Cyclodevelopmental

The pathogen undergoes developmental changes from one stage to another, but does not multiply. With the filariae, for example, a single microfilaria ingested by a mosquito can result in only one infective larva. In most instances, however, the number of infective larvae is lower than the number of microfilariae ingested with the blood meal.

Transovarial or Vertical

Some viral and rickettsial disease agents are transmitted from the female parent arthropod through the eggs to the offspring. If the pathogen can infect the developing egg germ cells, it is termed transovarial transmission. With some arboviruses, only the ovarial sheath and oviduct are infected; the egg is infected as it passes down the

TABLE 141-1 Early History of the Discovery of the Arthropod Transmission of Human and Animal Disease

Year	Scientist	Disease	Vector	Host
1877	Manson	Filariasis	*Culex* mosquitoes	Human
1891	Smith & Kilborne	Piroplasmosis	*Boophilus* ticks	Cattle
1896	Bruce	Nagana	*Glossina* flies	Cattle
1895	Ross	Malaria	*Culex* mosquitoes	Birds
1900	Manson	Malaria	*Anopheles* mosquitoes	Human
1900	Reed	Yellow fever	*Aedes aegypti*	Human
1902	Graham	Dengue	*Aedes* mosquitoes	Human
1903	Bruce	African sleeping sickness	*Glossina* flies	Human
1904	Dutton	African tick fever	Soft ticks	Human
1905	Liston	Plague	Rat fleas	Human
1906	Ricketts	Rocky Mountain spotted fever	Hard ticks	Human
1907	Mackie	Relapsing fever	Lice	Human
1908	Chagas	Chagas disease	Reduviid bugs	Human

Adapted from Philip CB, Rozeboom LE. Medico-veterinary entomology: a generation of progress. In: Smith RF, Mittler TE, Smith CN, eds. History of Entomology. Palo Alto, CA: Annual Reviews; 1973:333–59.

oviduct and is inseminated. This is distinguished from transovarial transmission and is called vertical transmission. In either case, the newly hatched larval stages are infected with the pathogen, which is then transmitted to subsequent developmental stages of the arthropod (transstadial transmission). Finally, venereal transmission of certain viruses has also been documented. Thus, male mosquitoes that become infected transovarially or vertically, can transfer the infective virus to female mosquitoes in the seminal fluid during copulation. These latter types have epidemiologic importance in the infection of humans or other animals and in the maintenance of the pathogen in nature.

Extrinsic Incubation Period

In all types of biologic transmission, a period of time is required for the pathogen to develop the arthropod vector to an infective stage that can be transmitted. With arboviruses, transmission requires replication in the salivary glands; for the malaria parasite, there is invasion of the salivary glands by the infectious sporozoites; and with filariae, there is development of the juvenile worms to the infective stage III larvae. This period of time between infection of the arthropod vector and transmission is called the extrinsic incubation period. The extrinsic incubation period is generally 7 to 14 days but can be longer, depending on the pathogen, the vector, and various environmental factors, especially temperature.

FACTORS INFLUENCING TRANSMISSION

The ability of insects to transmit an agent depends on the interaction of complex intrinsic and extrinsic factors. Successful mechanical transmission depends on the degree of contact insects have with humans, and on the arthropod feeding behavior. For example, the domestic housefly has been incriminated as a mechanical vector of various intestinal pathogens, primarily because this insect breeds in large numbers, lives in intimate contact with humans, and has the habit of feeding on feces and food. Tabanid flies are efficient mechanical vectors of viruses and protozoa because of frequent interrupted blood feeding. Certain flies can mechanically transmit the bacteria that cause yaws and other tropical diseases from open sores.

The ability to transmit a pathogen biologically varies greatly among species of arthropods and even among geographic strains within a species. There can be variation in the susceptibility to becoming infected and subsequently to transmitting a pathogen. Most work has been done with mosquitoes, and variation in vector competence has been documented with all of the major disease agents they transmit (i.e. malaria, filarial parasites, and arboviruses). Thus, within a single mosquito species it is common to find geographic strains that are good and poor vectors. Because vector competence (susceptibility to infection, growth of the pathogen, and transmission) is genetically controlled, it may be expected to change as a result of selective pressures on either the pathogen or the arthropod over time.

In addition to innate susceptibility to infection, the overall vectorial capacity is influenced by other biologic and behavioral characteristics of the arthropod. The degree of contact the species has with humans is influenced by the blood meal host preference, the intrinsic blood-feeding and resting behavior of the arthropod, and the population density of the vector, animal and human hosts. Longevity, resting behavior, flight behavior and oviposition (breeding) behaviors are important intrinsic factors which are influenced by extrinsic environmental factors, such as temperature, humidity, wind and rainfall.

Other extrinsic factors may influence whether an individual insect becomes infected with a pathogen. For example, it has been shown that mosquitoes ingesting blood containing both microfilariae and Rift Valley fever virus have a higher viral infection rate because disseminated virus infection is facilitated by microfilariae escaping from the midgut into the hemocoel. Other factors can also influence this "leaky gut" phenomenon. Finally, infection of the arthropod and subsequent transmission is influenced by the strain of pathogen. This is especially important with the arboviruses, where certain strains or subtypes of virus have greater infectivity and more rapid replication in the vectors [2].

Because arthropods are cold-blooded, transmission of diseases in temperate regions is seasonal, usually only occurring during warm months. Cessation of transmission in these regions is usually determined by temperature and day length. In the tropics and subtropics, transmission generally occurs year-round. In these areas, increased seasonal transmission is most frequently correlated with the rainy season.

SYSTEMATICS

The order Diptera is by far the most important, primarily because of the family Culicidae (mosquitoes). Most vector-borne pathogens are zoonoses (pathogens of animals), and have a primary vertebrate reservoir host and a primary arthropod vector that maintains the transmission cycle in nature; this is usually via horizontal transmission, but is sometimes facilitated by transovarial or vertical transmission. This primary cycle is usually silent to humans and domestic animals. On occasion, the pathogen may be introduced into the peri-domestic or urban environment by secondary vectors or by the vertebrate host, which often establish a secondary transmission cycle involving other vertebrate hosts and arthropod vectors. Humans and domestic animals are usually infected by bridge vectors from these secondary cycles, and are often dead-end or incidental hosts, not contributing to the transmission cycle by infecting the arthropod vectors. A basic vector-borne pathogen transmission cycle is shown in Figure 141.1.

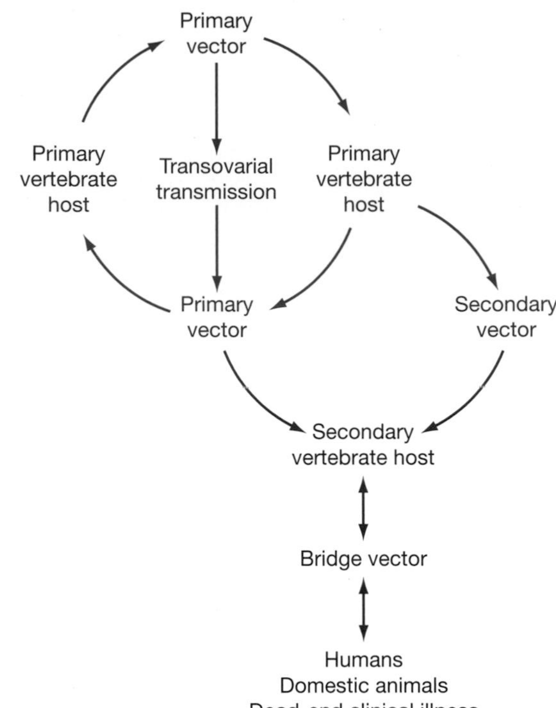

FIGURE 141.1 Transmission cycles for arthropod-borne infections.

TABLE 141-2 Vector-Borne Infections of Man and Animals

Pathogens	Disease	Animal reservoirs	Geographic distribution	Vector
Viruses				
Togaviridae				
	Chikungunya	Primates, humans	Africa, Asia	Mosquitoes
	Ross River	Marsupials, humans	Australia, South Pacific	Mosquitoes
	Mayaro	Birds	South America	Mosquitoes
	Onyong-nyong fever	Not known	Africa	Mosquitoes
	Sindbis fever	Birds	Asia, Africa, Australia, Europe, Americas	Mosquitoes
	Eastern equine encephalomyelitis	Birds	Americas	Mosquitoes
	Western equine encephalomyelitis	Birds, rabbits	Americas	Mosquitoes
	Venezuelan equine encephalomyelitis	Rodents	Americas	Mosquitoes
	Barmah Forest	Not known	Americas	Mosquitoes
Flaviviridae				
	Dengue (serotypes 1–4)	Primates, humans	Worldwide in tropics	Mosquitoes
	Yellow fever	Primates, humans	Africa, South America	Mosquitoes
	Kyasanur Forest disease	Primates, rodents, camels	India, Saudi Arabia	Ticks
	Omsk hemorrhagic fever	Rodents	Asia	Ticks
	Japanese encephalitis	Birds	Asia	Mosquitoes
	Murray Valley encephalitis	Birds	Australia	Mosquitoes
	Rocio	Birds	South America	Mosquitoes
	St Louis encephalitis	Birds	Americas	Mosquitoes
	West Nile encephalitis	Birds	Asia, Africa, Americas, Europe	Mosquitoes
	Tick-borne encephalitis	Rodents	Europe, Asia, North America	Ticks
Bunyaviridae				
	Sandfly fever	Not known	Europe, Africa, Asia	Sandflies

TABLE 141-2 Vector-Borne Infections of Man and Animals—cont'd

Pathogens	Disease	Animal reservoirs	Geographic distribution	Vector
	Rift Valley fever	Cattle, sheep, camels	Africa	Mosquitoes
	La Crosse encephalitis	Rodents	North America	Mosquitoes
	California encephalitis	Rodents	North America, Europe, Asia	Mosquitoes
	Crimean-Congo hemorrhagic fever	Rodents, sheep	Europe, Asia, Africa	Ticks
	Oropouche fever	Not known	Central and South America	Midges, mosquitoes
Rhabdoviridae				
Vesicular stomatitis virus	Vesicular stomatitis	Cattle, horses, pigs	Global	Phlebotomus flies, mosquitoes
Orbiviridae				
Bluetongue virus	Bluetongue	Cattle, sheep, goats	Global	Culicoides flies
Bacteria				
Yersinia pestis	Plague	Rodents	Global	Fleas
Francisella tularensis	Tularemia	Rabbits, rodents	North America, Europe, Asia	Ticks, tabanid flies
Coxiella	Q fever	Ungulates	Global	Ticks
Rickettsia rickettsii	Rocky Mountain spotted fever	Rabbits, rodents, dogs	Western hemisphere	Ticks
Rickettsia typhi	Murine typhus	Rats	Global	Ticks
Rickettsia conorii	Boutonneuse fever	Dogs, rodents	Europe, Africa	Ticks
Rickettsia australis	Queensland tick typhus	Rodents	Australia	Ticks
Rickettsia sibirica	Siberian tick typhus	Rodents	Asia	Ticks
Rickettsia africae	African tick fever	Rodents	Sub-Saharan Africa, Caribbean	Ticks
Orientia tsutsugamushi	Scrub typhus	Rodents	Asia, Australia	Mites
Borrelia species	Relapsing fever	Rodents	Global	Ticks and lice
Borrelia burgdorferi	Lyme disease	Rodents	Americas, Europe	Ticks
Protozoa				
Plasmodium spp	Malaria	Primate, humans	Global	Anopheline mosquitoes
Trypanosoma rhodesiense	African trypanosomiasis (sleeping sickness)	Ungulates	Eastern Africa	Glossina flies
Trypanosoma qambiense	African trypanosomiasis (sleeping sickness)	Pig, ungulates	Africa	Glossina flies
Trypanosoma cruzi	Chagas disease	Dogs, cats, opossum	Western hemisphere	Triatomid bugs
Leishmania spp	Leishmaniasis	Dogs, rodents	Asia, Africa, Europe, Central and South America	Phlebotomus flies
Babesia spp	Babesiosis	Ungulates, rodents	Global	Ticks
Filaria				
Wuchereria bancrofti	Bancroftian filariasis	Humans	Global	Mosquitoes
Brugia malayi	Brugian filariasis	Humans, primates	Asia	Mosquitoes

Adapted from Gubler DI. Vector-borne diseases. Rev Sci Tech Off Int Epiz 2009;28;583–8.

IMPORTANCE

Collectively, arthropods are responsible for hundreds of millions of cases of disease each year. The most important vector-borne diseases of man and domestic animals are presented in Table 141-2. In the past 40 years, the world has experienced a dramatic global re-emergence of epidemic infectious disease in general and vector-borne diseases in particular, e.g. malaria, leishmaniasis, dengue hemorrhagic fever, yellow fever, Japanese encephalitis, West Nile encephalitis, chikungunya, epidemic polyarthritis, and many more [3]. In addition, several new vector-borne diseases have emerged, e.g. Barmah Forest in Australia, Alkhurma virus, a flavivirus that causes hemorrhagic disease in Saudi Arabia, and Lyme disease and ehrlichiosis in the US. The arboviruses have been the most important emergent and re-emergent vector-borne pathogens, with expanding distribution of epidemics of severe diseases [3].

The shrinking world, with highly increased human mobility due to air travel and commerce using containerized shipping (globalization), has made vector-borne diseases not just problems of the tropics; they present the world community with one of its greatest health problems, and are a threat to regional and global economic security [3]. For example, over 1000 cases of malaria are imported into the US each year, and there are several fatalities, mainly because of late diagnosis. With anopheline vectors in many areas of the US, there has been sporadic transmission documented in some coastal states, including California, New Jersey, Georgia and Florida. Similarly, many cases of dengue fever are imported into the US each year. The principal vector, *Aedes aegypti*, occurs in most Gulf Coast states, and in 1985, another important vector, *Ae. albopictus*, was found in Texas. This species subsequently spread throughout the eastern US. The first indigenous dengue transmission since 1945, secondary to imported disease, was documented in Texas in 1980. and since then there has been sporadic autochthonous transmission in Texas, initiated by introduced viruses. In 2001, a small outbreak occurred in Hawaii, caused by dengue viruses from Tahiti, and in 2009–2010, a small outbreak recurred in Florida as a result of introduced viruses [4]. In 2007, chikungunya virus was introduced to Italy from India, causing the first outbreak in Italy [5]. The transmission episodes underscore the need for physicians in non-endemic areas to be aware of vector-borne diseases and to be knowledgeable about how to diagnose and treat them.

In tropical regions, the incidence of dengue has increased dramatically, occurring not only as larger and more frequent epidemics but also newly occurring in some countries. Moreover, severe and fatal dengue, dengue hemorrhagic fever, has also spread geographically and is now a major public health problem in Asia, the Pacific and the Americas. Other viruses such as yellow fever, Japanese encephalitis, Ross River, West Nile, Venezuelan equine encephalitis, chikungunya, Rift Valley fever and O'nyong-nyong have expanded their geographic distribution and caused major epidemics. The re-infestation of the American tropics by *Ae. aegypti* has put that region at the highest risk for urban epidemics of yellow fever in more than 60 years.

The factors responsible for this dramatic twentieth-century re-emergence of epidemic vector-borne disease are several [3]. The successes in controlling malaria, leishmaniasis, African trypanosomiasis, yellow fever, dengue, Japanese encephalitis, and plague in the years following World War II, which led to complacency, a redirection of resources, and deterioration in public health infrastructure, were contributing factors, as were changing lifestyles and environment. Although vector-borne diseases are climate-sensitive, there is no good evidence that global warming has contributed to the re-emergence. Other drivers of this re-emergence have been demographic and societal. Population growth has been a principal driver of environmental change, as well as animal husbandry practices. Population growth combined with economic development have led to unprecedented urbanization in developing countries over the past 50 years, which has driven globalization. Annually, there is an unprecedented movement of people, animals, commodities and pathogens into new geographic areas where there is a lack of effective vector control. The result has been the dramatic re-emergence of epidemic vector-borne disease in the past 40 years.

REFERENCES

1. Philip CB, Rozeboom LE. Medico-veterinary entomology: a generation of progress. In: Smith RF, Mittler TE, Smith CN, eds. History of Entomology. Palo Alto, CA: Annual Reviews; 1973:333–59.
2. Gubler DI. Vector-borne diseases. Rev Sci Tech Off Int Epiz 2009;28;583–8.
3. Gubler DJ. The global threat of emergent/reemergent vector-borne diseases. In: Vector-Borne Diseases: Understanding the Environmental, Human Health, and Ecological Connections. Washington, DC: National Academies Press; 2008:43–64.
4. Centers for Disease Control and Prevention. Locally acquired Dengue – Key West, Florida, 2009–2010. MMWR Morb Mortal Wkly Rep 2010;59:577–81.
5. Rezza G, Nicoletti L, Angelini R, et al. Infection with chikungunya virus in Italy: an outbreak in a temperate region. Lancet 2007;370:1840–6.

PART

10

THE SICK RETURNING TRAVELER

142 General Principles

David R Hill

Key features

- Returned travelers should be evaluated with a history that identifies the itinerary, exposure risks, and predominant symptoms
- Clinicians need a knowledge of the geographic distribution and incubation periods of potential diseases generated in the differential diagnosis
- Common syndromes in returned travelers are fever, diarrheal disease, skin rash, and respiratory conditions
- After a physical exam, targeted laboratory testing can help to confirm or rule out diagnostic considerations, leading to appropriate treatments
- Implementation by health professionals of pre-travel guidance and recommendations, and compliance by travelers of prevention measures, will help to decrease illness in travelers

In 2010 there were 940 million international tourist arrivals throughout the world (Fig. 142.1). While the majority of trips were taken to Europe, an increasing number are to low-income, more tropical countries. These numbers do not include the many thousands who are internally displaced or who cross international borders without documentation to flee famine or violence, or to seek employment.

Widespread international travel has the well-recognized ability to carry a pathogen from one part of the world to a distant destination in the span of less than a day. This was best illustrated by the global spread of pandemic influenza A (H1N1) in the spring and summer of 2009. The World Health Organization (WHO) remarked during the early phases of the pandemic, "During previous pandemics, influenza viruses took >6 months to spread as widely as the new influenza A (H1N1) pandemic virus has taken to spread in <6 weeks."[1]

Over the last two decades, a partnership between the United States Centers for Disease Control and Prevention (CDC) and the International Society of Travel Medicine established the GeoSentinel surveillance network (http://www.istm.org/geosentinel/main.html) [2]. This is a global network of travel and tropical medicine clinics that contribute information about ill returned travelers that have been seen at their centers [3]. The network has published numerous articles on ill returned travelers that help define the epidemiology of syndromes such as fever [4], skin conditions [5], and diarrhea [6], as well as the types of illness that occur in defined groups of travelers, for example those who are visiting friends and relatives (VFR travellers) [7] and child travelers [8]. Although the database suffers from not being able to define the actual risk of acquisition of a pathogen or syndrome, as the total number of travelers to each destination is not known, it does add important information on the geographic risk of common and uncommon travel-related conditions.

In addition to defining the predominant symptoms, returned travelers should also be asked about their destinations, activities, exposure risks and duration at each location (Box 142.1). Understanding the geographic risk of infectious diseases and modes of transmission (e.g. fecal–oral, vector, person-to-person via respiratory secretions) is key to being able to develop a differential diagnosis of illness in returned travelers. If a traveler has not had freshwater exposure in Africa, the likelihood of schistosomiasis is greatly reduced. The incubation period of illness is also helpful. Enteric bacterial infections usually have a short incubation (<7–10 days), *Plasmodium falciparum* malaria has an intermediate incubation (1 week to 1 month) and helminths and viral hepatitis a long incubation (≥1 month) (Table 142-1) [9].

The frequency of illness can help to narrow the differential. The most common syndromes in returned travellers are fever (Chapter 143), acute and chronic diarrhea (Chapter 146), skin rash (Chapter 147), and respiratory conditions [3]. All clinicians, whether they are experts in tropical medicine or nurses who triage ill returned travelers, should be able to evaluate severity in each of these syndromes and either manage them directly or refer them for appropriate investigation and care. No traveler should return with *P. falciparum* malaria that is missed by an unsuspecting clinician. Helpful algorithms

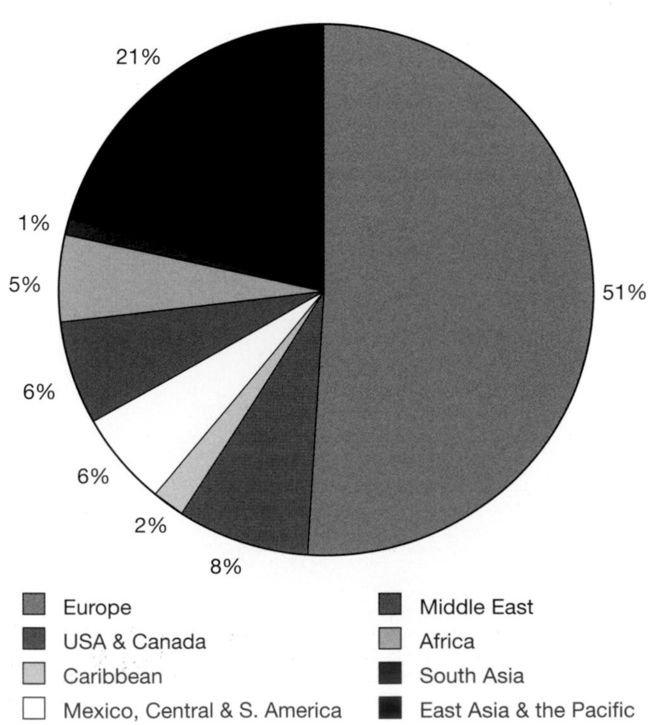

FIGURE 142. 1 Global international tourist arrivals of 940 million travellers for 2010. *Data from the United Nations World Tourism Organization: www.unwto.org/index.php.*

BOX 142.1 Key features to apply to an illness in returned travelers

Itinerary and exposure risks

Geographic distribution of infectious diseases

Incubation periods

Frequency of illness in returned travelers

Pre-travel prevention measures

TABLE 142-1 Typical incubation periods for infectious diseases in returned travelers*

Short (<7–10 days)	Intermediate (1 week to 1 month)	Long (>1 month)
Diarrhea: bacterial and viral	Malaria: *Plasmodium falciparum*	Malaria: *Plasmodium vivax*
Pneumonia: bacterial and viral	Diarrhea: protozoal	Tuberculosis
Influenza	Enteric fever: *Salmonella* Typhi and Paratyphi	Viral hepatitis
Arboviruses: dengue, chikungunya	Brucellosis	Rabies
Rickettsial infection, e.g. African tick fever	Leptospirosis	Amebic liver abscess
STIs: gonorrhea, chancroid, chlamydia, herpes simplex	Lassa fever	Leishmaniasis: visceral
Hemorrhagic fevers: Ebola, Marburg	STIs: chlamydia, syphilis, LGV, genital warts	Trypanosomiasis: west African
Meningitis, bacterial	Lyme borreliosis	Onchocerciasis
Japanese encephalitis	Trypanosomiasis: east African; acute Chagas disease	Schistosomiasis
	Strongyloidiasis	Filariasis
	Acute HIV infection	

*Incubation periods are a useful guide, but many diseases have a wide range of incubation periods
LGV, lymphogranuloma venereum; STIs, sexually transmitted infections.

for evaluating returned travelers can be found in Health Information for Overseas Travellers [10].

The pre-travel preparations undertaken by an individual traveler can rule out certain illnesses. The high efficacy of some vaccines, for example those against hepatitis A and B, and yellow fever, makes these diseases unlikely in a returned traveler who has received them. In contrast, the limited efficacy of typhoid vaccine does not preclude enteric fever in a VFR traveler returned from Bangladesh. And, while most cases of malaria occur in persons who have not taken any chemoprophylaxis or who have been incompletely compliant, a history of malaria chemoprophylaxis does not eliminate malaria as a consideration in a febrile returned traveler.

TABLE 142-2 Laboratory testing in the returned traveler

Screening tests
Complete blood count, with eosinophil count Malaria blood smear or RDT Liver enzymes BUN, creatinine and electrolytes Urine analysis Stool culture, ova and parasite exam, antigen detection Acute phase serum for possible analysis*
Secondary tests
Tuberculin skin testing or interferon gamma release assay Sputum exam and culture Chest x-ray Blood cultures Hepatitis serology Syphilis and HIV testing Lumbar puncture Upper and lower endoscopy Ultrasound, MRI, CT scanning Tissue biopsy

*Paired acute and convalescent serum for arboviral infection; single test for schistosomiasis, *Strongyloides* and filaria.
BUN, blood urea nitrogen; CT, computed tomography; MRI, magnetic resonance imaging; RDT, rapid diagnostic test for malaria.

Investigations are directed by the predominant syndrome. Some long-term or expatriate travelers will be asymptomatic and screened for infectious disease to reassure them or to provide an exit evaluation for their company or non-governmental organization (see Chapter 145). Other times, investigations will be directed toward a single laboratory finding, such as eosinophilia (Chapter 148).

All travelers should have a careful physical exam with vital signs taken, including their weight. Particular attention can be paid to the skin (rash, eschar), lymphatic system (lymphadenopathy), conjunctiva (injection, icterus), chest (dullness, rales), and abdomen (pain, organomegaly). Suggested laboratory testing is outlined in Table 142-2.

The following chapters detail the evaluation and management of the major syndromes in returned travelers, as well as present other emerging topics in travel medicine: immigrant medicine, international adoptions, medical tourism, and the effect of transplantation on the acquisition and expression of tropical disease. Lastly, some travelers think they have a parasitic or other tropical illness when actually they have a fixed delusion about being infected. This is a challenging clinical condition that requires patience, expertise, and collaboration with other health providers.

Most of the syndromes and infectious agents described can be prevented if the travel medicine clinician is informed and the traveler takes the proper preventive measures. There are excellent resources for health professionals to use in the pre-travel consultation: the WHO (http://www.who.int/ith/en/), the CDC (http://wwwnc.cdc.gov/travel/default.aspx) and many national organizations (e.g. Public Health Agency of Canada [http://www.phac-aspc.gc.ca/tmp-pmv/prof-eng.php], the United Kingdom National Travel Health Network and Centre [www.nathnac.org], and Switzerland [http://www.safetravel.ch]). If physicians and nurses accessed this information and travelers understood and complied with the recommended preventive measures, there should be less illness in returned travelers.

REFERENCES

1. World Health Organization. New influenza A (H1N1) virus: global epidemiological situation, June 2009. Wkly Epidemiol Rec 2009;84:249–57.
2. Marano C, Freedman DO. Global health surveillance and travelers' health. Curr Opin Infect Dis 2009;22:423–9.
3. Freedman DO, Weld LH, Kozarsky PE, et al. Spectrum of disease and relation to place of exposure among ill returned travelers. N Engl J Med 2006;354: 119–30.
4. Wilson ME, Weld LH, Boggild A, et al. Fever in returned travelers: results from the GeoSentinel Surveillance Network. Clin Infect Dis 2007;44:1560–8.
5. Lederman ER, Weld LH, Elyazar IR, et al. Dermatologic conditions of the ill returned traveler: an analysis from the GeoSentinel Surveillance Network. Int J Infect Dis 2008;12:593–602.
6. Greenwood Z, Black J, Weld L, et al. Gastrointestinal infection among international travelers globally. J Travel Med 2008;15:195–202.
7. Leder K, Tong S, Weld L, et al. Illness in travelers visiting friends and relatives: a review of the GeoSentinel Surveillance Network. Clin Infect Dis 2006; 43:1185–93.
8. Hagmann S, Neugebauer R, Schwartz E, et al. Illness in children after international travel: analysis from the GeoSentinel Surveillance Network. Pediatrics 2010;125:e1072–80.
9. Johnston V, Stockley JM, Dockrell D, et al. Fever in returned travellers presenting in the United Kingdom: recommendations for investigation and initial management. J Infect 2009;59:1–18.
10. Field VK, Ford L, Hill DR, ed. Health Information for Overseas Travel. Prevention of Illness in Travellers from the UK. London: National Travel Health Network and Centre; 2010.

Fever in the Returned Traveler 143

Victoria Johnston, Michael Brown

Key features

- Travel, especially to developing countries, is associated with an increased risk of infections not usually seen in high-income countries, e.g. malaria, enteric fever, dengue, and schistosomiasis
- While gastroenteritis, respiratory tract infections, and self-limiting viral infections are common, an important minority of patients will have a potentially life-threatening tropical infection
- The evaluation of an ill returned traveler therefore requires a detailed travel history together with an understanding of the geographic distribution of infections, risk factors for acquisition, incubation periods, clinical presentations and appropriate laboratory investigations
- A syndromic approach to specific investigations, and to presumptive therapy pending laboratory confirmation of the diagnosis, is appropriate
- As a rule, malaria should be excluded in all travelers presenting with a fever who have visited the tropics

INTRODUCTION

Up to 70% of travelers to developing countries report health problems, the majority of which are self-limiting; however 8–15% of travelers are ill enough to seek medical attention while abroad or on return home, with fever as a common presenting complaint [1–4]. While for many the underlying cause is a self-limiting globally endemic infection, such as gastroenteritis, physicians are increasingly encountering conditions not normally seen in the patient's country of origin. In some cases these are potentially life-threatening, such as malaria, and others have potential public health consequences, such as enteric fever.

To evaluate returned travelers presenting with fever, an understanding of the geographic distribution of infections, risk factors for acquisition, incubation periods and clinical presentations is required. With this understanding, a risk assessment can be undertaken, initial investigations instigated, and, when appropriate, presumptive therapy started.

EPIDEMIOLOGY

Fever in returned travelers is a syndrome with an epidemiology that reflects factors relating to the individual traveler and to the wide spectrum of etiologic pathogens. Organ-specific infections – for example, gastroenteritis or respiratory tract infections, particularly upper respiratory tract infections – are common. Amongst patients with undifferentiated fever, malaria, dengue and enteric fever are the most common diagnoses (see Fig. 143.1) [3].

The following factors influence an individual's risk of acquiring infection (see Table 143-1) [5]:

Individual Factors

- *Purpose and duration of travel:* individuals visiting friends and relations (VFR) and long-stay travelers (e.g. aid-workers) are at greatest risk of acquiring malaria, enteric fever, hepatitis A, tuberculosis, and sexually transmitted infections, including HIV. This is in part due to longer duration of travel and closer proximity to the local population.
- *Immune status:* migrants returning to their home countries may be immune to certain infections, such as hepatitis A and acute schistosomiasis; however, they may incorrectly consider themselves immune to others, such as malaria. Consequently, VFR travelers are less likely to seek pre-travel advice, take malaria prophylaxis or receive vaccines [6]. Travelers with HIV, malignancy or on immunosuppressant drugs are at increased risk of opportunistic infections, including nontyphoidal *Salmonella* and penicilliosis.
- *Risk activities:* certain risk activities expose individuals to infection, e.g. freshwater exposure and schistosomiasis, unprotected sexual intercourse and HIV.

Pathogen Factors

- *Geographic distribution:* the risk of acquiring a specific infection varies with country and environment, e.g. urban or rural, mountains or coastal plains. While malaria is the most common infection diagnosed in travelers returned from sub-Saharan Africa, dengue is more prevalent among travelers returning from South-east Asia and enteric fever from south central Asia (see Table 143-1 and Fig. 143.1).
- *Incubation period:* most travelers become symptomatic within 21 days of exposure, with the majority presenting within 1 month of return. However, some pathogens have a much longer incubation period (e.g. *Plasmodium vivax* and tuberculosis); patients may present months or rarely years later (see Table 143-2).

CLINICAL FEATURES

Patients can present with undifferentiated fever or with organ-specific symptoms, such as gastroenteritis or respiratory infection. The most common causes are discussed below, with the focus on returned travelers. For more detailed descriptions, relevant chapters on specific infections should be consulted.

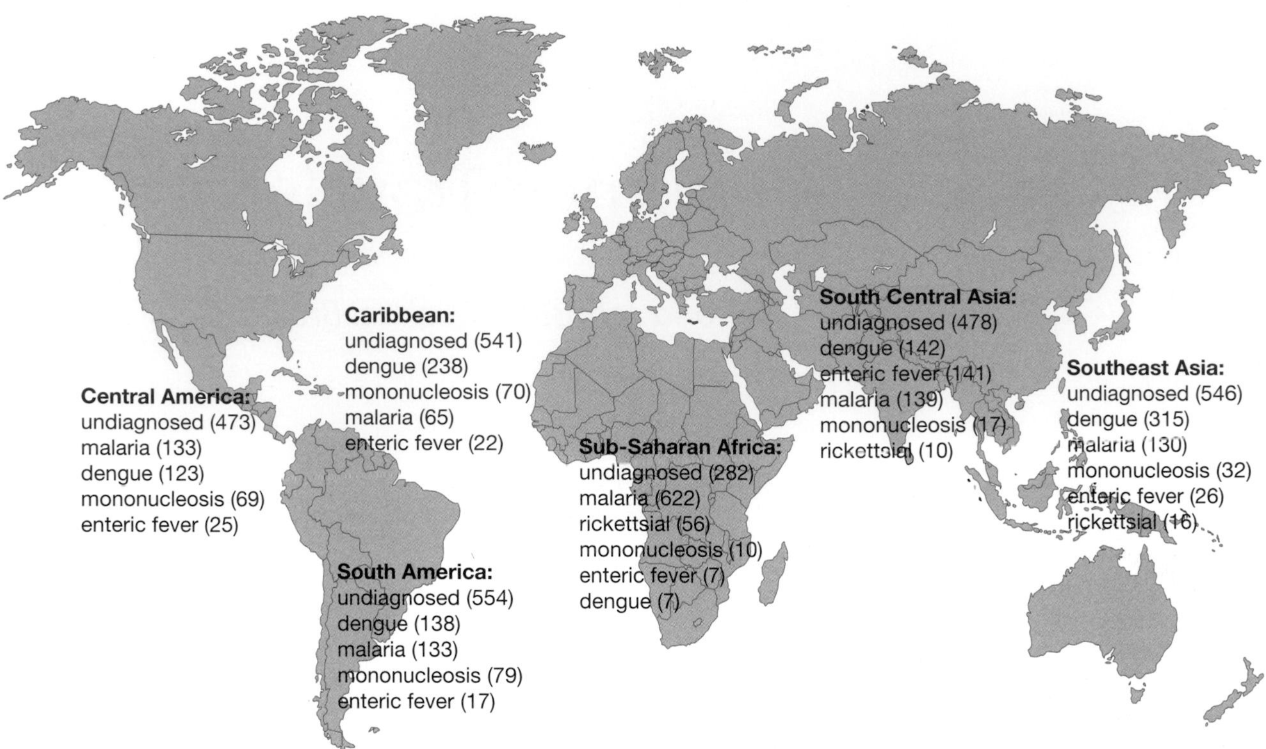

FIGURE 143.1 Spectrum of disease in relation to place of exposure amongst travelers with systemic febrile illness (per 1000 patients with systemic febrile illness; N = 3907). *(Frequency data from Freedman DO, Weld LH, Kozarsky PE, et al. Spectrum of disease and relation to place of exposure among ill returned travelers. N Engl J Med 2006;354: 119–30.)*

UNDIFFERENTIATED FEVER

Malaria [7]

Malaria is an important, potentially fatal infection in travelers returning from the tropics, particularly from sub-Saharan Africa. It should be excluded in all returned travelers with a history of fever. Most short-term travelers present within 1 month of return, however *P. falciparum* occasionally presents up to 6 months later and *P. vivax*, *P. ovale* and *P. malariae* can present a year or more following return [8]. Many travelers do not take chemoprophylaxis, or take it inadequately [6]. When malaria is acquired despite chemoprophylaxis, the onset of symptoms is often delayed, severity of illness reduced, and microbiologic diagnosis may be obscured [9]. Because chemoprophylaxis may obscure the diagnosis, in cases where malaria is thought likely, chemoprophylaxis should be stopped while patients are investigated [7].

Nearly all patients with malaria give a history of fever; however, up to half are afebrile on presentation and specific fever patterns are uncommon [10]. Headache, myalgia, arthralgia, and malaise are frequently described, with some patients reporting diarrhea or cough. Complications occur mainly with *P. falciparum* infection. In patients with confusion, seizures or reduced conscious level, cerebral malaria or hypoglycemia should be considered; hypoxia, tachypnea, and signs of pulmonary edema indicate respiratory involvement.

Enteric Fever (*Salmonella typhi, S. paratyphi*)

Enteric fever is a potentially life-threatening infection which requires early diagnosis and management. It is a cause of fever, particularly in VFR travelers returning from Asia [3]. With an incubation period of 7–18 days (range up to 60 days) most patients will present within a month of return; however, later presentations are possible. A history of vaccination pre-travel has little predictive value; it provides incomplete protection against *S. typhi* and no protection against *S. paratyphi*.

In addition to fever, symptoms include headache, constipation/diarrhea, and dry cough. Complications, in particular encephalopathy and gastrointestinal bleeding and intestinal perforation, occur infrequently; they are more likely if the duration of illness is >2 weeks.

Rickettsiae

The most common traveler-associated rickettsial infections are due to *R. africae* (African tick typhus). Endemic throughout sub-Saharan Africa, it is a common diagnosis in travelers who have visited game parks in southern African. *R. conorii* (Mediterranean spotted fever or tick bite fever), endemic throughout sub-Saharan Africa, the Mediterranean, Caspian littoral, Indian subcontinent and Middle East, is also well described. Travelers infected with *R. typhi* (murine typhus) and *Orientia tsutsugamushi* (scrub typhus) are rarely encountered.

Rickettsiae have a short incubation period (5–7 days; up to 10 days) and similar presentations. More than 80% of patients infected with *R. africae* or *R. conorii* describe fever, headache and myalgia. The classic signs of inoculation eschar, rash and lymphadenitis are seen in <50%; however, retrospective cohorts report higher rates (Fig. 143.2) [11]. Complications, for example. reactive arthritis, are rarely encountered in African tick typhus; mortality rates of up to 32% have been reported for Mediterranean tick bite fever, 17% for scrub typhus and 4% for murine typhus [12–14].

Arbovirus

There are over 500 arthropod-borne viruses worldwide; not all cause disease in humans. The majority are restricted to specific geographic locations; for example, Ross River virus in Australia. They have short incubation periods (<1 week) and result in self-limiting illnesses. Four clinical presentations predominate:

- systemic febrile illness, e.g. all arboviruses
- hemorrhagic fever, e.g. dengue, yellow fever, Rift Valley fever, Congo-Crimean hemorrhagic fever
- acute encephalitis, e.g. Japanese encephalitis, Rift Valley fever, West Nile virus, Eastern and Western equine encephalitis viruses
- polyarthralgia or arthritis, e.g. chikungunya, Ross River.

TABLE 143-1 Common or Important Causes of Fever Associated With Geographic Areas and Specific Risk Factors

Risk factor	Common	Occasional	Rare but important
Geographic area			
Sub-Saharan Africa	HIV-associated infections (inc seroconversion) Malaria Rickettsiae	Acute schistosomiasis (Katayama) Amebic liver abscess Brucellosis Dengue Enteric fever Meningococcus	Histoplasmosis Other arbovirus, e.g. Rift Valley, West Nile fever, yellow fever Trypanosomiasis Viral hemorrhagic fever (Lassa, Ebola, Marburg, CCHF) Visceral leishmaniasis
North Africa, Middle East and Mediterranean		Brucellosis Q fever Toscana (sandfly fever)	Visceral leishmaniasis
Eastern Europe and Scandinavia		Lyme disease	Hantavirus Tick-borne encephalitis Tularemia
South and Central Asia	Dengue Enteric fever Malaria	Chikungunya Visceral leishmaniasis	CCHF Japanese encephalitis Other arbovirus (Nipah virus) Rickettsiae
Southeast Asia	Chikungunya Dengue Enteric fever Malaria	Leptospirosis Melioidosis	Hantavirus Japanese encephalitis Other arbovirus (Nipah virus) Paragonimiasis Penicilliosis Scrub typhus
North Australia		Dengue Murray Valley Q fever Rickettsiae Ross River fever	Barmah Forest Melioidosis
Latin America and Caribbean	Dengue Enteric fever Malaria	Brucellosis Coccidioidomycosis Histoplasmosis Leptospirosis	Acute trypanosomiasis (Chagas) Hanta virus Yellow fever
North America		Coccidioidomycosis Histoplasmosis Lyme disease Rocky Mountain spotted fever	Babesiosis Anaplasmosis Ehrlichiosis West Nile fever
Specific risk factors			
Game parks	Tick typhus		Anthrax Trypanosomiasis
Freshwater exposure		Acute schistosomiasis Leptospirosis	
Caves		Histoplasmosis	Marburg Rabies
HIV	Amebiasis Nontyphoidal salmonella Tuberculosis	STI, e.g. syphilis Visceral leishmaniasis	*Blastomycosis* Coccidioidomycosis Histoplasmosis Penicilliosis

Abbreviations: CCHF, Congo-Crimean hemorrhagic fever; STI, sexually transmitted infection.
Table adapted with permission from British Infection Society. Fever in returned travellers presenting in the United Kingdom: recommendations for investigation and initial management [5].

TABLE 143-2 Incubation Periods

Incubation period	Infection
Short (<10 days)	Arboviral infections, e.g. dengue, chikungunya Gastroenteritis, acute (bacterial, viral) Melioidosis Meningitis (bacterial, viral) Relapsing fever (*Borrelia* spp.) Respiratory tract infection (bacterial, viral including H1N1 and avian influenza) Rickettsial infection, e.g. tick typhus, scrub typhus
Medium (10–21 days)	Bacterial • Brucellosis • Enteric fever (typhoid and paratyphoid fever) • Leptospirosis • Melioidosis • Q fever (*Coxiella burnetii*) Fungal • Coccidioidomycosis • Histoplasmosis (can be as short as 3 days) Protozoal • Chagas disease, acute • Malaria (*Plasmodium falciparum*) • *Trypanosoma rhodesiense* Viral • CMV, EBV, HIV, viral hemorrhagic fevers
Long (>21 days)	Bacterial • Brucellosis • Tuberculosis Fluke • Schistosomiasis, acute Protozoal • Amebic liver abscess • Malaria (including *Plasmodium falciparum*) • *Trypanosomiasis gambiense* • Visceral leishmaniasis Viral • HIV • Viral hepatitis (AE)

Table adapted with permission from British Infection Society. Fever in returned travellers presenting in the United Kingdom: recommendations for investigation and initial management [5].

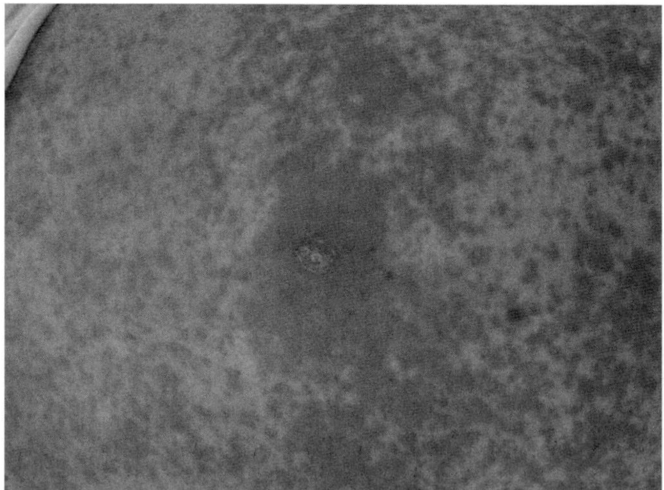

FIGURE 143.2 Patient returned 2 days previously from a safari holiday in Botswana. On further examination, an eschar was found. Diagnosis: tick typhus.

Dengue is the most prevalent arbovirus in travelers. Although widespread, it is a common cause of fever only in those returning from Asia, the Caribbean and South America [15]. Most travelers present with a febrile illness associated with headache, retro-orbital pain, myalgia, arthralgia (especially back pain) and rash [15]. The rash is initially erythrodermic, and becomes petechial with disease progression (Fig. 143.3). Hepatitis, myocarditis, encephalitis and neuropathy can occur. Bleeding gums, epistaxis and gastrointestinal bleeding occur but are not necessarily indicative of dengue hemorrhagic fever, which like dengue shock syndrome is rare in travelers. Chikungunya is increasingly reported in returning travelers from the islands of the Indian Ocean, South and Southeast Asia [16]. The clinical presentation is similar to classic dengue fever; however, arthralgia is more prominent. In the majority of cases, the arthralgia settles; 5–30% develop chronic arthropathy with pain, stiffness and swelling lasting months to years [17,18].

Acute Schistosomiasis (Katayama Fever)

This should be considered in febrile travelers returning from Africa. Travelers give a history of freshwater exposure 4–6 (up to 9) weeks prior to symptom onset. Some describe a self-resolving itchy rash immediately following exposure (swimmer's itch). Symptoms and signs include fever, lethargy, myalgia, arthralgia, cough, wheeze, headache, urticarial rash, diarrhea and hepatosplenomegaly [19]. The

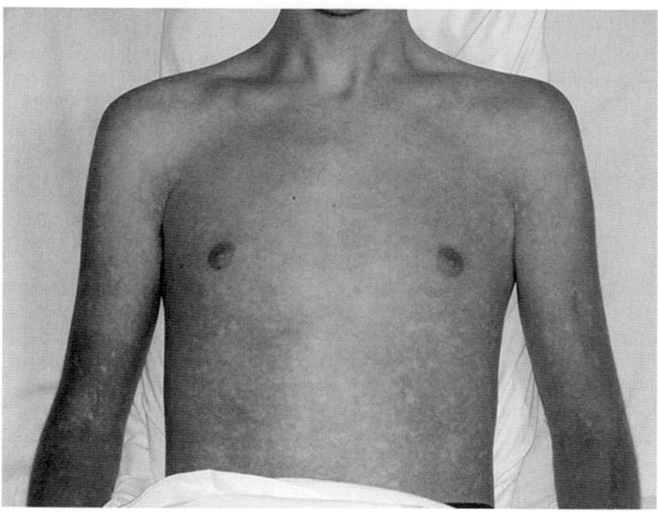

FIGURE 143.3 Patient returned 4 days previously from a beach holiday in Thailand. He describes developing "sunstroke" on the last day of his holiday (sunburn, headache, feverish). Symptoms have not settled. Diagnosis: dengue.

eosinophil count is usually elevated at presentation of acute schistosomiasis and provides supportive evidence for the diagnosis, but it may only appear a few days after symptom onset. Acute symptoms are self-limiting in most cases.

Leptospirosis

Leptospirosis has a global distribution. Infection occurs through exposure to rodent or dog urine-contaminated fresh water; for example, through recreational water-sports, flooding, or occupational exposure. Following an incubation period of 7–12 days, patients classically present with a biphasic illness comprising a bacteremic phase with flu-like symptoms lasting 4–7 days, followed 1–3 days later by an immune phase characterized by fever, myalgia, hepatorenal syndrome and hemorrhage [20]. This severe end of the spectrum, Weil's disease, occurs infrequently but has a high case-fatality rate of 10–15%. Gastrointestinal and respiratory presentations and meningitis, myocarditis and pancreatitis are occasionally described.

Amebic Liver Abscess [21]

This should be considered in all patients with fever and a raised right hemi-diaphragm on chest radiography. It has a global distribution, with a higher prevalence in developing countries. Travelers, exposed through faecal–oral transmission, will often present weeks to months following return (incubation period: 8–20 weeks). Most patients report fever and (often localized) abdominal pain; hepatomegaly is common. Only 20% give a history of dysentery and only 10% have diarrhea at presentation.

Brucellosis [22]

Brucellosis is acquired through ingestion of unpasteurized milk, although transmission may also occur through direct contact with animal parts or, in laboratories, through inhalation of aerosolized particles. It has a global distribution, with a higher prevalence found in the Middle East, Balkan Peninsula, former USSR, Mediterranean and South America. Symptoms develop 2–4 weeks following exposure (up to 6 months described) and vary from an acute febrile illness to a chronic low-grade relapsing fever; signs include lymphadenopathy, hepatomegaly and splenomegaly. Complications of brucellosis are common – in particular, large-joint septic arthritis, sacroiliitis, and, less commonly, spondylitis of the lumbar spine. Other complications include epididymo-orchitis, septic abortion, neurologic involvement (meningitis, encephalitis and abscess) and endocarditis.

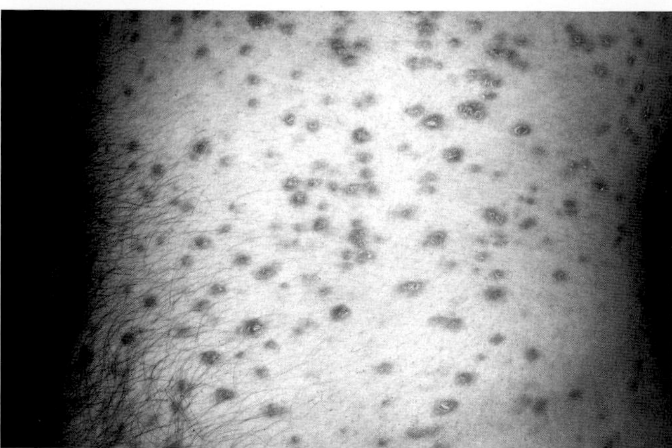

FIGURE 143.4 Patient returned 1 month previously from a 2-week holiday in Thailand. Two days ago, he developed fever, headache and rash. On further questioning, he reported having unprotected sexual intercourse during his holiday. Diagnosis: secondary syphilis.

Q Fever (*Coxiella burnetii*) [23]

Although rarer than brucellosis, Q fever has a similar epidemiologic and clinical history. It has a global distribution, with most cases related to occupational exposure, predominantly through inhalation of aerosolized particles. Community outbreaks, as reported in the Netherlands in 2008, occur [24] The majority of cases are asymptomatic; however, the diagnosis should be considered in patients presenting with fever, pneumonia or hepatitis following exposure to farms or animals. Complications, including chronic infection, are well described, particularly endocarditis.

HIV and Other STIs

Between 5% and 51% of short-term travelers take part in casual sex while abroad, with higher rates reported in long-term travelers [25]. The prevalence of HIV in many tropical countries is high and often not restricted to certain risk groups. Many STIs can present as a febrile illness, including HIV seroconversion, secondary syphilis (Fig. 143.4) and gonorrhea. People living with HIV who travel to the tropics are also at increased risk of opportunistic infections (see Table 143-1) [26].

RESPIRATORY TRACT INFECTIONS

Respiratory tract infections are diagnosed as the underlying cause of febrile illness in 7–24% of returning travelers [5]. These include sinusitis, pharyngitis, tonsillitis, bronchitis, influenza, pneumonia and pulmonary eosinophilia. Influenza is the commonest vaccine-preventable infection acquired by travelers.

Upper Respiratory Tract Infections

- Diphtheria: patients with severe pharyngitis on return from Indian subcontinent, Southeast Asia, Haiti or South America

Lower Respiratory Tract Infections

- Histoplasmosis or coccidioidomycosis: exposure to damp conditions, e.g. bat-occupied caves or dusty conditions, respectively. Coccidioidomycosis is restricted to certain areas in the Americas
- Legionella: exposure to air-conditioning or other aerosolized water sources in cruise ships or hotels
- Melioidosis (*Burkholderia pseudomallei*): febrile patients from Southeast Asia with upper lung zone infiltrates or cavitation on chest radiography, or septicemia
- Q fever: fever, pneumonia or hepatitis following exposure to farms or animals

- Tuberculosis: travel to areas of high endemicity, particularly amongst VFRs, long-stay travelers, healthcare workers and the immune-compromised; active disease is uncommon [27]
- Fever, respiratory symptoms and peripheral eosinophilia: consider Loeffler's syndrome (*Ascaris*, hookworm, *Strongyloides*), acute schistosomiasis, tropical pulmonary eosinophilia (filaria), leaking hydatid cyst, visceral larva migrans, and paragonimiasis [28].

GASTROINTESTINAL INFECTIONS

Diarrhea

Travelers' diarrhea has a reported incidence of at least 200 cases/1000 ill returned travelers [3]. Fever is self-reported in one-third of these patients, making it an important underlying etiology in febrile travelers. Specific pathogens vary according to destination, setting and season; however, enteric bacteria including *Escherichia coli*, *Campylobacter*, *Salmonella*, and *Shigella* are the most common. In up to 50%, no pathogen is identified. The combination of fever and bloody diarrhea is suggestive of bacterial or amebic dysentery, with the latter (uncommon in the returning traveler) often having a more indolent onset. In both cases, empiric antibiotics should be considered (see below). It should be noted that any systemic febrile infection may have diarrhea at presentation; for example, severe sepsis, malaria, pneumococcal pneumonia.

Abdominal Pain

Enteric fever, amebic liver abscess, viral hepatitis, and, rarely, leaking or secondarily infected hydatid cysts may all cause fever and abdominal pain.

Jaundice

Infections presenting with fever and jaundice are listed in Table 143-3.

NEUROLOGIC INFECTIONS

Neurologic presentations, including meningitis and encephalitis, are reported in 15/1000 ill returned travelers [3]. Cerebral malaria, which may present with encephalopathy, meningismus, seizures or focal signs, should always be excluded.

TABLE 143-3 Infectious Causes of Fever and Jaundice

Hepatic	EBV, CMV Enteric fever (typhoid and paratyphoid) Hepatitis A–E* Leptospirosis (Weil's disease) Nontyphoidal *Salmonella plus* HIV *P. falciparum* malaria, severe Relapsing fevers (*Borrelia* spp) Septicemia, including pneumococcal sepsis Typhus Viral hemorrhagic fever
Post-hepatic	Ascending cholangitis (including occasionally helminths)
Hemolytic	Bartonellosis Hemolytic-uremic syndrome (*Shigella* spp., *E. coli*) Malaria *Mycoplasma pneumoniae* Sickle cell crisis with infective trigger

*Fever and jaundice rarely present concurrently.
Table adapted with permission from British Infection Society. Fever in returned travellers presenting in the United Kingdom: recommendations for investigation and initial management [5].

Meningitis

Typical bacterial and viral causes should be considered. In addition, causes of predominantly lymphocytic meningitis include: arboviruses, brucellosis, leptospirosis, Lyme disease, Q fever, relapsing fevers, syphilis, tuberculosis, HIV seroconversion, and HIV-related opportunistic infections, for example cryptococcal meningitis. Some infections, such as enteric fever, can rarely present with meningismus but the CSF is normal.

Encephalitis

In addition to typical causes of encephalitis, travel-related causes to be considered include: arboviruses (e.g. Japanese encephalitis, tick-borne encephalitis), brucellosis, rabies, rickettsial infections, African trypanosomiasis, and tuberculosis. African trypanosomiasis (sleeping sickness) has been described in travelers returning from game parks in East and Central Africa, including Tanzania, Malawi, and Zambia.

PATIENT EVALUATION, DIAGNOSIS, AND DIFFERENTIAL DIAGNOSIS [5]

The evaluation of fever in returned travelers requires an understanding of the epidemiologic factors which influence exposure to specific pathogens. These factors are reflected in the travel history and include geographic destinations visited, dates of particular risk exposures, time of onset and duration of symptoms. The first two determine which infections the traveler may have been exposed to and the last two allow for an estimation of the incubation period (see Tables 143.1 & 143.2).

As can be seen from Figure 143.1, the travel history is vital for determining the likely diagnosis, as many infections can have similar clinical presentations. Certain symptoms and signs may give further clues; relevant examination findings include rash, eschar, hepatosplenomegaly and jaundice (see Tables 143-3, 143-4 & 143-5). Table 143-6 lists the differential diagnosis in patients with chronic fever (>2 weeks), and is a reminder that noninfectious causes of fever are seen in this group.

Travelers presenting with undifferentiated fever should have a number of initial recommended investigations performed (see Table 143-7). Following this, specific investigations may be appropriate, depending on the differential diagnosis (see Table 143-8). Where tuberculosis is considered, it is essential that adequate samples of sputum or tissue for mycobacteria culture are obtained. Tuberculin skin tests and interferon-gamma release assays have a limited role in evaluation of patients with chronic fever.

Rarely, fever in the returned traveler may be due to a viral hemorrhagic fever such as Lassa, Ebola, Marburg or Congo-Crimean hemorrhagic fever. The diagnosis should be considered in travelers who have visited endemic regions within 21 days of symptom onset [29,30], in particular, travel to rural areas of sub-Saharan Africa (particularly West Africa); contact with suspected cases, healthcare facilities, rats or wild animals raises the index of suspicion. Symptoms and signs vary according to pathogen, with bleeding in advanced cases. Although rare, these infections can be severe and have implications for nosocomial transmission. Malaria must be excluded; however, PCR of blood may be required, before further investigations (which might result in exposure of healthcare staff) are performed. A high index of suspicion and close liaison with specialists are necessary to manage such patients appropriately.

TREATMENT

The relevant chapters should be consulted for detailed advice on the treatment of individual infections. In particular situations, presumptive treatment may be instigated, before the cause of the febrile illness is known (see Table 143-8) [5].

TABLE 143-4 Acute Fever and Rash or Ulcer

Rash	Infection
Maculopapular	Arboviral infection, e.g. dengue, chikungunya "Childhood viral illness", e.g. measles, rubella, parvovirus Drug hypersensitivity reaction Fungal infection (papule/nodules), e.g. histoplasmosis, penicilliosis Infectious mononucleosis group, e.g. EBV, CMV, HIV seroconversion Leprosy (reaction) Rickettsial infection, e.g. tick typhus Syphilis Viral hemorrhagic fever, e.g. Ebola
Vesicular	Herpes simplex virus, disseminated Herpes zoster virus (chickenpox or disseminated zoster) Monkey pox Rickettsial infection
Erythroderma	Dengue Kawasaki's disease Staphylococcal or streptococcal toxin related syndromes, e.g. toxic shock syndrome, scarlet fever Sunburn *Vibrio vulnificus*
Purpuric	Dengue hemorrhagic syndrome Gonococcal infection Herpes zoster virus, hemorrhagic Meningococcal infection Plague Rickettsial infection, severe Severe sepsis ± disseminated intravascular coagulation Viral hemorrhagic fever, e.g. Lassa, Ebola, CCHF, Rift Valley fever
Ulcer	Chancre: *Trypanosoma rhodesiense, Yersinia pestis* (Bubonic plague) Eschar: African tick typhus, anthrax Genital ulcer: syphilis, herpes simplex virus Skin ulcer: anthrax, diphtheria, fungal infection, superinfected bacterial ulcer, tropical ulcer, Buruli ulcer

Table adapted with permission from British Infection Society. Fever in returned travellers presenting in the United Kingdom: recommendations for investigation and initial management [5].

Malaria

Parasitic confirmation (smears, RDTs, or PCR) of suspected malaria is preferred and empiric treatment is not recommended in clinical settings with good diagnostic facilities. However, diagnostic results must be accurate, timely, and available to the treating physician. Accuracy will depend upon the skills of the microscopist; RDT and PCR results reflect the performance characteristics of the assay. When accurate results will not be available for more than 6 hours, presumptive treatment is encouraged, as delay in treatment has been associated with poor clinical outcomes, especially in patients with severe malaria [7].

Amebic Liver Abscess

Metronidazole 500 mg three times daily for 7–10 days or tinidazole 2 g daily for 3 days should be commenced empirically in patients with an appropriate travel history, clinical presentation, imaging, and,

TABLE 143-5 Fever and Hepatomegaly, Splenomegaly or Hepatosplenomegaly

Bacterial	Brucellosis Enteric fever (typhoid and paratyphoid) Leptospirosis Q fever (*Coxiella burnetii*) Relapsing fever (borreliosis) Rickettsial infection, e.g. tick typhus
Flukes	Fascioliasis Schistosomiasis, acute (Katayama syndrome)
Protozoal	Amebic liver abscess Malaria (acute)* Trypanosomiasis Visceral leishmaniasis*
Viral	Dengue Hepatitis, acute (A, B, E) HIV, CMV or EBV seroconversion
Non-infectious	Chronic myeloid leukemia* Hemoglobinopathy Lymphoma* Myelofibrosis*

*May cause massive splenomegaly.
Table adapted with permission from British Infection Society. Fever in returned travellers presenting in the United Kingdom: recommendations for investigation and initial management [5].

TABLE 143-6 Chronic Fever (>14 Days)

Bacterial	Brucellosis Infective endocarditis Enteric fever (typhoid and paratyphoid) Pyogenic deep-seated abscess Q fever (*Coxiella burnetii*) Tuberculosis
Fungal	Coccidioidomycosis Cryptococcosis Histoplasmosis Paracoccidioidomycosis Penicilliosis
Helminth	Schistosomiasis, acute (Katayama syndrome) Strongyloides hyperinfestation syndrome
Protozoal	Amebic liver abscess Toxoplasmosis Visceral leishmaniasis
Viral	HIV *plus* opportunistic infection
Noninfectious	Autoimmune disorders Drugs Malignancy Pulmonary embolus Vasculitis

Table adapted with permission from British Infection Society. Fever in returned travellers presenting in the United Kingdom: recommendations for investigation and initial management [5].

TABLE 143-7 Recommended Initial Investigations in Returning Travelers Presenting With (Undifferentiated) Fever*

Investigation	Interpretation
Malaria film and dipstick antigen test (RDT)	• Perform in all patients who have visited a tropical country within 1 year of presentation • The sensitivity of a thick film read by an expert is equivalent to that of an RDT, however blood films are necessary for speciation and parasite count • Three thick films/RDTs over 72 hours (as an outpatient if appropriate) should be performed to exclude malaria with confidence • Positive blood films (thick and thin) should be sent to the reference lab for confirmation • Patients, returned from Asia (particularly Malaysia) with a high *P. malariae* parasite count should have the potentially lethal *P. knowlesi* excluded by PCR.
FBC	• Lymphopenia: common in viral infection (dengue, HIV) and typhoid • Eosinophilia (>0.45 × 10^9/L): incidental or indicative of infectious (e.g. parasitic, fungal) or noninfectious cause – see Table 143-8 • Thromobocytopenia: malaria, dengue, acute HIV, typhoid, also seen in severe sepsis
Blood cultures	• Two sets should be taken prior to any antibiotic therapy • Sensitivity of up to 80% in typhoid • Notify the laboratory if the diagnosis of enteric fever or brucellosis is being considered
U&E, LFTs	See Table 143.5
Serum save†	• HIV should be offered to all patients with pneumonia, aseptic meningitis/encephalitis, diarrhea, viral hepatitis, mononucleosis-like syndrome, unexplained lymphadenopathy, fever or blood dyscrasia • Other e.g. arboviral, brucella, Q fever serology if indicated
EDTA sample for PCR†	• Consider if other features suggestive of arboviral infection, VHF
Urinalysis	• Proteinuria and hematuria in leptospirosis • Hemoglobinuria in malaria (rare)
CXR ± liver U/S	

*As an infection control precaution, the diagnosis of VHF should be considered and excluded before performing blood tests.
†To ensure that the correct tests are done, an adequate travel history MUST be documented on request forms. This includes locations visited, dates of travel, dates of symptom onset and risk activities undertaken. Pathogen-specific request forms may be required by reference laboratory for some infections, e.g. dengue and other arbovirus.

where available, serology (which may be falsely negative in early disease). Most patients demonstrate clinical improvement, with resolution of fever within 48–72 hours. The main differential diagnosis is a pyogenic liver abscess; therefore, patients with evidence of sepsis require broad-spectrum antibiotics until the diagnosis is confirmed. Surgical or percutaneous drainage is rarely required and should only be considered if there is diagnostic uncertainty, symptoms persist after 4 days of treatment, or if there is imminent risk of rupture into critical sites (e.g. left-lobe abscess rupturing into pericardium) [31]. After completion of treatment, all patients should be given 10 days of a luminal amebicide to prevent relapse: diloxanide furoate (500 mg orally three times daily), or paromomycin (30 mg/kg orally in three divided doses).

Enteric Fever

When there is a strong suspicion a parenteral third-generation cephalosporin (e.g. ceftriaxone) can be commenced pending blood culture results. Fluoroquinolone-resistant isolates are reported in patients returning from Asia, but rarely reported in those returning from Africa [32]. Ciprofloxacin 750 mg twice daily remains the treatment of choice for fully sensitive isolates. Azithromycin 1 g followed by 500 mg daily should be used as follow-on therapy where fluoroquinolone resistance is suspected or confirmed. Regardless of which antibiotic is used, fever takes some time to resolve; failure to defervesce is not a reason to change antibiotics where the isolate is confirmed as sensitive.

Leptospirosis

Due to the potential severity of the illness, the nonspecific nature of initial investigations, and a minimum period of 6–10 days before confirmatory serology becomes available, a 5–7-day course of penicillin (benzylpenicillin 1.5 million units four times daily) or doxycycline (100 mg twice daily) should be considered in patients with a flu-like illness within 7–12 days of freshwater exposure.

Rickettsiae

Fever and headache, with or without rash, developing within 10 days of exposure to ticks in southern African game parks should prompt treatment with doxycycline 100 mg twice daily while other infections are excluded. A response is expected within 24–48 hours.

Acute Schistosomiasis

Empiric treatment should be offered to travelers presenting with fever, urticarial rash, and eosinophilia (>0.45 × 10^9/L) within 4–8 weeks of freshwater exposure [28]. Praziquantel, 40 mg/kg, in a divided dose 4 hours apart, will kill mature but not immature schistosomes (***Schistosoma japonicum:*** 60 mg/kg in three divided doses). Treatment should therefore be given at the time of diagnosis, but repeated 6–8 weeks later. Corticosteroids are generally advocated to help alleviate acute symptoms.

Bacterial Sepsis

International travel, particularly to India, Middle East, and Africa, is associated with an increased risk of acquiring extended-spectrum β-lactamase (ESBL)-producing Gram-negative pathogens [33]. Fluoroquinolone-resistant Campylobacter isolates are increasingly reported in travelers returning from Asia. This should be taken into account when empiric antibiotics are indicated.

TABLE 143-8 Summary of Diagnostic Tools and Presumptive Therapy by Geographic Area of Travel and Clinical Presentation

1. This table applies to patients in whom **malaria has been excluded**

2. Diseases that present commonly in non-travelers with fever are omitted – respiratory tract infections, diarrhea, EBV, lymphoma, etc.

Undifferentiated fever

	SSA	SEA	SCA	ME/NA	SA	Diagnostics	Comments/empiric Rx
Amebic liver abscess						Serology (>92% sensitive at presentation); U/S abdomen	Empiric tinidazole/metronidazole if suggestive clinical and travel history with abscess on U/S. Serology is positive in 25% of healthy individuals in endemic areas
Brucellosis						Extended BC, serology	Suspect if contact with livestock/unpasteurized milk
Chikungunya						PCR (1–4 days) or IgM (>5 days)	Manage symptomatically as outpatient
Dengue						Dengue PCR (1–8 days after symptom onset) IgM ELISA (>4 days)	Manage symptomatically as outpatient with daily FBC unless high risk of shock (high hematocrit, falling platelets). Supportive management but avoid aspirin. Vaccination (YF, JE, TBE) history required to interpret results
Enteric fever (typhoid / paratyphoid)						Multiple BC (> 80% sensitive in first week). Stool and urine cultures become positive after the first week	If clinically unstable, Rx empirically with ceftriaxone. If traveled from SSA, ciprofloxacin remains an alternative. If confirmed sensitive, switch to ciprofloxacin. If resistant, use azithromycin empirically as oral follow-on agent
HIV						HIV (RNA or antigen and antibody)	Many serologic tests do not pick up seroconversion illness
Leptospirosis						Acute phase (EIA IgM >5 days) + 3-6 wk serum	Rx on suspicion with doxycycline/penicillin. Serology used for diagnostic confirmation. Culture has limited role; although consider BC/CSF if within 5 days of exposure
Rickettsia						Acute phase + 3–6-week serum	Consider empiric Rx doxycycline if exposure to ticks in game park, headache, fever ± rash/eschar
Schistosomiasis, acute						Not helpful	Empiric Rx praziquantel if appropriate presentation and exposure 4–8 weeks previous. Consider steroids

Fever with rash

	SSA	SEA	SCA	ME/NA	SA	Diagnostics	Comments/empiric Rx
Dengue						Dengue PCR (1–8 days after symptom onset) IgM ELISA (>4 days)	Manage symptomatically as outpatient with daily FBC unless high risk of shock (high hematocrit, falling platelets). Supportive management but avoid aspirin. Vaccination (YF, JE, TBE) history required to interpret results
HIV						HIV (antigen and antibody)	Many rapid tests do not pick up seroconversion illness
Rickettsia						Acute phase + 3–6-week serum	Consider empiric Rx doxycycline if exposure to ticks in game park, headache, fever ± rash/eschar
Schistosomiasis, acute						Not helpful	Empiric Rx praziquantel if appropriate presentation and exposure 4–8 weeks previous. Consider steroids
VHF						PCR to ref lab	**Always** contact regional center. VHF are endemic in South America (arenaviruses) and Europe/Asia (Congo-Crimean hemorrhagic fever), however are rarely encountered in travelers

continued

TABLE 143-8 Summary of Diagnostic Tools and Presumptive Therapy by Geographic Area of Travel and Clinical Presentation—cont'd

	SSA	SEA	SCA	ME/NA	SA	Diagnostics	Comments/empiric Rx
Fever with jaundice							
Leptospirosis						Acute phase (EIA IgM >5 days) + 3–6-week serum	Rx on suspicion with doxycycline/penicillin. Serology used for diagnostic confirmation. Culture has limited role; although consider BC/CSF if within 5 days of exposure
Viral hepatitis						Anti-HAV IgM, Hep B SAg, Hep E IgM	Acute hepatitis C should also be considered in homosexual men
VHF						PCR to ref lab	**Always** contact regional center. VHF are endemic in South America (arenaviruses) and Europe/Asia (Congo-Crimean hemorrhagic fever), however are rarely encountered in travelers
Yellow fever						EDTA (blood) ± CSF for PCR; IgG/IgM serology	Require confirmation of YF vaccine history
Fever with hepato-(and/or) splenomegaly							
	SSA	**SEA**	**SCA**	**ME/NA**	**SA**	**Diagnostics**	**Comments/empiric Rx**
Amebic liver abscess						Serology (>92% sensitive at presentation), U/S abdomen	Empiric tinidazole/metronidazole if suggestive clinical and travel history with abscess on U/S. Serology is positive in 25% of healthy individuals in endemic areas
Brucellosis						Extended BC, serology	Suspect if contact with livestock/unpasteurized milk
Leptospirosis						Acute phase (EIA IgM >5 days) + 3–6-week serum	Rx on suspicion with doxycycline/penicillin. Serology used for diagnostic confirmation. Culture has limited role; although consider BC/CSF if within 5 days of exposure
Trypanosomiasis						Blood film	Travel to game parks in SSA
Visceral leishmaniasis						Leishmaniasis serology, bone marrow aspirate	Travel to Mediterranean, Horn of Africa, Bihar, Nepal, Bangladesh, Brazil

Serious/very common — Common — Rare

SSA, sub-Saharan Africa; SEA, Southeast Asia; SCA, South Central Asia; ME/NA, Middle East, Mediterranean, North Africa; SA, South America, Caribbean.

YF, yellow fever; JE, Japanese encephalitis; TBE, tick-borne encephalitis; VHF, viral hemorrhagic fever; BC, blood culture; CSF, cerebrospinal fluid; Rx, treatment.

Table adapted with permission from British Infection Society. Fever in returned travellers presenting in the United Kingdom: recommendations for investigation and initial management [5].

REFERENCES

1. Hill DR. Health problems in a large cohort of Americans traveling to developing countries. J Travel Med 2000;7:259–66.
2. Rack J, Wichmann O, Kamara B, et al. Risk and spectrum of diseases in travelers to popular tourist destinations. J Travel Med 2005;12:248–53.
3. Freedman DO, Weld LH, Kozarsky PE, et al. Spectrum of disease and relation to place of exposure among ill returned travelers. N Engl J Med 2006;354: 119–30.
   Key reference detailing geographic risk of imported infection, utilizing the GeoSentinel database of more than 17,000 returned travelers.
4. Wilson ME, Weld LH, Boggild A, et al. Fever in returned travelers: results from the GeoSentinel Surveillance Network. Clin Infect Dis 2007;44:1560–8.
   GeoSentinel study examining subset of travelers who returned with fever.
5. Johnston V, Stockley JM, Dockrell D, et al. Fever in returned travellers presenting in the United Kingdom: recommendations for investigation and initial management. J Infect 2009;59:1–18.
   Important UK guidelines for evaluation of febrile returned travelers.
6. Smith AD, Bradley DJ, Smith V, et al. Imported malaria and high risk groups: observational study using UK surveillance data 1987-2006. BMJ 2008;337: a120.
7. Lalloo DG, Shingadia D, Pasvol G, et al. UK malaria treatment guidelines. J Infect 2007;54:111–21.
8. Leder K, Black J, O'Brien D, et al. Malaria in travelers: a review of the GeoSentinel surveillance network. Clin Infect Dis 2004;39:1104–12.
9. Reyburn H, Behrens RH, Warhurst D, Bradley D. The effect of chemoprophylaxis on the timing of onset of falciparum malaria. Trop Med Int Health 1998;3:281–5.
10. Nic Fhogartaigh C, Hughes H, Armstrong M, et al. Falciparum malaria as a cause of fever in adult travellers returning to the United Kingdom: observational study of risk by geographical area. QJM 2008;101:649–56.
11. Jensenius M, Fournier PE, Vene S, et al. African tick bite fever in travelers to rural sub-Equatorial Africa. Clin Infect Dis 2003;36:1411–17.
12. de Sousa R, Nobrega SD, Bacellar F, Torgal J. Mediterranean spotted fever in Portugal: risk factors for fatal outcome in 105 hospitalized patients. Ann N Y Acad Sci 2003;990:285–94.
13. Civen R, Ngo V. Murine typhus: an unrecognized suburban vectorborne disease. Clin Infect Dis 2008;46:913–18.
14. Kumar K, Saxena VK, Thomas TG, Lal S. Outbreak investigation of scrub typhus in Himachal Pradesh (India). J Commun Dis 2004;36:277–83.
15. Jelinek T, Muhlberger N, Harms G, et al. Epidemiology and clinical features of imported dengue fever in Europe: sentinel surveillance data from TropNetEurop. Clin Infect Dis 2002;35:1047–52.
16. [Anonymous]. Outbreak and spread of chikungunya. Wkly Epidemiol Rec 2007;82:409–15.
17. Borgherini G, Poubeau P, Jossaume A, et al. Persistent arthralgia associated with chikungunya virus: a study of 88 adult patients on reunion island. Clin Infect Dis 2008;47:469–75.
18. Brighton SW, Prozesky OW, de la Harpe AL. Chikungunya virus infection. A retrospective study of 107 cases. S Afr Med J 1983;63:313–15.
19. Bottieau E, Clerinx J, de Vega MR, et al. Imported Katayama fever: clinical and biological features at presentation and during treatment. J Infect 2006;52: 339–45.
20. Katz AR, Ansdell VE, Effler PV, et al. Assessment of the clinical presentation and treatment of 353 cases of laboratory-confirmed leptospirosis in Hawaii, 1974-1998. Clin Infect Dis 2001;33:1834–41.
21. Stanley SL Jr. Amoebiasis. Lancet 2003;361:1025–34.
22. Pappas G, Akritidis N, Bosilkovski M, Tsianos E. Brucellosis. N Engl J Med 2005;352:2325–36.
23. Raoult D, Marrie T, Mege J. Natural history and pathophysiology of Q fever. Lancet Infect Dis 2005;5:219–26.
24. Delsing CE, Kullberg BJ. Q fever in the Netherlands: a concise overview and implications of the largest ongoing outbreak. Neth J Med 2008;66:365–7.
25. Matteelli A, Carosi G. Sexually transmitted diseases in travelers. Clin Infect Dis 2001;32:1063–7.
26. Bottieau E, Florence E, Clerinx J, et al. Fever after a stay in the tropics: clinical spectrum and outcome in HIV-infected travelers and migrants. J Acquir Immune Defic Syndr 2008;48:547–52.
27. Cobelens FG, van Deutekom H, Draayer-Jansen IW, et al. Risk of infection with *Mycobacterium tuberculosis* in travellers to areas of high tuberculosis endemicity. Lancet 2000;356:461–5.
   One of the few study quantifying the risk of tuberculosis in long-stay travelers to high tuberculosis incidence countries. Healthcare workers had the highest risk of infection (7.9 cases/1000 person months) and clinical disease.
28. Checkley AM, Chiodini PL, Dockrell DH, et al. Eosinophilia in returning travellers and migrants from the tropics: UK recommendations for investigation and initial management. J Infect 2010;60:1–20.
29. Woodrow CJ, Eziefula AC, Agranoff D, et al. Early risk assessment for viral haemorrhagic fever: experience at the Hospital for Tropical Diseases, London, UK. J Infect 2007;54:6–11.
30. Advisory Committee on Dangerous Pathogens. Management and Control of Viral Haemorrhagic Fevers. London: The Stationary Office; 1996.
31. Khan R, Hamid S, Abid S, et al. Predictive factors for early aspiration in liver abscess. World J Gastroenterol 2008;14:2089–93.
32. Cooke FJ, Day M, Wain J, et al. Cases of typhoid fever imported into England, Scotland and Wales (2000-2003). Trans R Soc Trop Med Hyg 2007;101:398–404.
33. Laupland KB, Church DL, Vidakovich J, et al. Community-onset extended-spectrum beta-lactamase (ESBL) producing *Escherichia coli*: importance of international travel. J Infect 2008;57:441–8.

144 Malaria in the Returned Traveler

David G Lalloo

Key features

- *Plasmodium falciparum* malaria is a potential medical emergency as patients can deteriorate rapidly; patients with suspected malaria should be evaluated immediately
- Symptoms of malaria are often nonspecific
- A careful exposure history is necessary: country and area of travel, including stop-overs, date of return, date of symptoms and details of prophylaxis (if any)
- Falciparum malaria is most likely to occur within the first 1–3 months of return from an endemic area. The incubation period for falciparum malaria is at least 6 days
- Three negative slides over a period of 48–72 hours are necessary to exclude malaria
- Consider other travel-related infections: e.g. typhoid, hepatitis, dengue, influenza, acute HIV, meningitis/encephalitis and viral hemorrhagic fevers (VHF)
- Initiate therapy with rapidly active agents. Artemisinin-containing treatments are the most effective for falciparum

INTRODUCTION

Malaria is one of the most important illnesses in the returned traveller. It accounts for a large proportion of the patients admitted with a fever after foreign travel and has the potential to cause a rapidly fatal illness. Recognition and prompt management of the disease by physicians at all levels of the system is important.

EPIDEMIOLOGY

In the USA, approximately 1300–1600 patients are diagnosed with malaria each year, with up to 7 deaths. Similar numbers of cases are seen in the UK and in France – up to 3000 cases are reported annually. The majority of cases (60–80%) are caused by *Plasmodium falciparum* with a further 10–25% being *Plasmodium vivax*. Those most at risk include recent immigrants or foreign visitors and people visiting friends and relatives (VFR travellers) in their country of origin. Appropriate pre-travel advice and education about recognition of symptoms of malaria on return from endemic countries is particularly important in this latter group. Travellers to sub-Saharan Africa have the highest risk: falciparum malaria is the most common post-travel diagnosis in this group [1]. Most deaths from malaria in Western countries are associated with delays in the recognition of the disease by patients and health personnel. Therefore, the importance of a thorough travel history for all febrile patients needs to be emphasized.

CLINICAL FEATURES

UNCOMPLICATED MALARIA

There are few specific symptoms or signs of malaria. Fever, or a history of fever, may be associated with nonspecific malaise, chills or rigors, respiratory symptoms, or gastrointestinal upset. A classic fever pattern, such as an every other day spike with *P. vivax*, is rarely seen. Practitioners should have a high index of suspicion for malaria in anyone who has returned from an endemic area in the last year: the minimum incubation period is 6 days. Nearly all patients with falciparum malaria will present within 3 months of exposure and usually in the first month after return [2]. Presentation of infection by other species may occur later after exposure and can be delayed for over a year. In patients with a history of fever, the presence of splenomegaly or jaundice makes malaria more likely [3] ; hepatomegaly or splenomegaly are more common in children.

Individuals who may have taken sub-optimal chemoprophylaxis regimens or were not completely adherent to their regimen may have a subacute, or even insidious, onset of clinical symptoms. They may present with atypical symptoms [4–9] to include fatigue, low back pain, nausea and anorexia, and depression. On occasion, these individuals will be afebrile. With long-acting drugs, such as mefloquine, atovaquone and choroquine-proguanil, the clinical presentation may be delayed by weeks after return. They often have very low and intermittent parasitemias, making conformation by microscopy difficult. In addition, patients who present to emergency departments with nonspecific febrile syndromes often get empirically treated with antibiotics such as azithromycin, tetracyclines, sulfa drugs and clindamycin, that have significant anti-malaria activity. This can temporarily result in clinical improvement and lead to delay and confusion over the diagnosis of malaria in the otherwise nonimmune returning traveller.

SEVERE OR COMPLICATED MALARIA

The clinical manifestations of severe malaria in returned travellers are similar to those in endemic regions (Table 144-1). Cerebral malaria and respiratory distress predominate in children; severe anaemia tends to be less common than in endemic populations. In adults, cerebral malaria, respiratory distress syndrome and multi-organ failure, including renal failure predominate. Severe malaria should be considered a medical emergency. Pregnant women, those who have lost their spleen and patients with advanced HIV are at higher risk of severe malaria. Severe or complicated malaria is usually associated with falciparum infection but there is growing evidence that a small proportion of patients with vivax develop severe malaria [10].

PATIENT EVALUATION AND DIFFERENTIAL DIAGNOSIS

Initially, it is most important to suspect the diagnosis and take an appropriate history. Many patients from an endemic area consider themselves to be immune but immunity is lost relatively rapidly after

TABLE 144-1 Features of Severe and Complicated Malaria

Adults
Impaired consciousness or seizures Acidosis (pH <7.3) Hypoglycemia (<2.2 mmol/l) Pulmonary edema **or** acute respiratory distress syndrome (ARDS) Renal impairment (oliguria <0.4 ml/kg bodyweight per hour or creatinine >265 μmol/l) Hemoglobin ≤8 g/dL Spontaneous bleeding/disseminated intravascular coagulation Shock (algid malaria – BP <90/60 mmHg) Hemoglobinuria (without G6PD deficiency) Parasitemia >2% red blood cells parasitized
Children
Impaired consciousness or seizures Respiratory distress or acidosis (pH <7.3) Hypoglycemia (<2.2 mmol/l) Severe anemia (<8 g/dl) Prostration Parasitemia >2% red blood cells parasitized

TABLE 144-2 Options for Management of Uncomplicated Falciparum Malaria in Adults

Drug	Dose	Frequency and duration
Artemether-lumefantrine (Coartem®) in the USA and Canada (Riamet®) in Europe (Tablet contains 20 mg artemether and 120 mg lumefantrine)	If weight >35 kg, 4 tablets	0, 8, 24, 36, 48 and 60 hours
Atovaquone-proguanil (Malarone®) (Adult tablet: 250 mg atovaquone-100 mg proguanil)	4 "adult" tablets	Daily for 3 days
Quinine sulfate	600 mg (salt)	Every 8 hours for 5–7 days
must be combined with:		
doxycycline OR	200 mg	Daily for 7 days
clindamycin	450 mg	Every 8 hours for 7 days
Dihydroartemisinin-piperaquine (licensed in Europe)	36–75 kg: 3 tablets > 75 kg: 4 tablets	Daily for 3 days
In rare areas of chloroquine sensitivity*		
Chloroquine	600 mg (base) 300 mg (base)	Initial dose 6, 24 and 48 hours

*Many clinicians would still advocate an alternative drug because of the difficulty of determining sensitivity.

leaving an endemic area and patients can still develop severe malaria [11]. The most useful investigations are thick and thin blood films, or a rapid diagnostic test. In experienced hands, a thick film is more sensitive but in many Western settings where microscopy experience is limited, rapid diagnostic tests are commonly reported and the diagnosis confirmed by a reference laboratory. If performed correctly, rapid tests are highly sensitive for the detection of falciparum malaria but can miss other species; newer-generation rapid diagnostic tests (RDTs) are better at detecting non-falciparum species. Blood films are still essential for confirming speciation and estimating the parasitemia which has prognostic significance. Repeated blood films may be necessary to detect low parasitemias, particularly if patients have been taking chemoprophylaxis. At least three thick films taken over 24–48 hours should be examined before the diagnosis can be excluded.

A full blood count, urea and electrolytes, liver enzymes and blood glucose should be taken routinely. Mild anemia is common and the presence of thrombocytopenia or hyperbilirubinemia are strongly predictive of malaria [3]. Elevation of hepatic transaminases and abnormalities of renal function can occur in more severe disease. Hypoglycemia commonly occurs in severe malaria because of the disease itself and if the patient has been treated with quinine, quinine-induced hyperinsulinemia, particularly in children or pregnancy. In severe disease, elevated lactate levels are common and clotting function should be evaluated to detect the rare cases who develop disseminated intravascular coagulation (DIC; Table 144-1). Blood cultures should be considered: Gram-negative bacteremia can be a complication of severe malaria, particularly in children. A lumbar puncture should be performed in those with impaired consciousness to exclude meningitis or encephalitis: significantly raised cerebrospinal fluid (CSF) white cell counts are rare in cerebral malaria.

The differential diagnosis of malaria in the returned traveller is wide; it is essentially that of a febrile illness. A detailed travel history, including precise destinations visited, duration of visit and activities whilst abroad and preventive measures taken, can help to determine the likelihood of malaria. The most important differential diagnoses to be considered are typhoid, arboviral diseases, including dengue, and the rare hemorrhagic fevers which are important to consider because of their public health significance (e.g. the need for isolation).

TREATMENT

Most of the evidence for managing malaria comes from the endemic setting. The strength of the evidence for the treatment of malaria in all settings is summarized in World Health Organization (WHO) guidelines [12] and in Chapter 96.

UNCOMPLICATED DISEASE

There are a number of options for the management of uncomplicated malaria (Tables 144-2, 144-3 and 144-4). The choice of antimalarial depends upon the species of malaria and the geographic region where the infection is likely to have been acquired. Malaria should be managed in consultation with someone experienced in managing malaria. In the USA, advice can be obtained from the Centers for Disease Control and Prevention (CDC) [13]. To speak with a malaria clinician, the CDC's Emergency Operations Center can be reached at (770) 488–7100.

Non-Falciparum

Chloroquine has been traditionally used for the treatment of all non-falciparum species and still remains highly effective for treating *Plasmodium ovale, Plasmodium malariae* and *Plasmodium knowlesi* infection (Table 144-4). However, there is increasing evidence of the spread of chloroquine resistance in *P. vivax* acquired in some regions of the Pacific and Southeast Asia. Opinions vary on how best to treat vivax

TABLE 144-3 Options for Management of Uncomplicated Falciparum Malaria in Children

Drug	Dose	Frequency and duration
Co-artem (Riamet®)	>35 kg: 4 tablets 25–35 kg: 3 tablets 15–24 kg: 2 tablets 5–14 kg: 1 tablet	0, 8, 24, 36, 48 and 60 hours
Atovaquone-proguanil (Malarone®): (Adult tablet: 250 mg atovaquone-100 mg proguanil) (Ped tablet: 62.5 mg atovaquone-25 mg proguanil)	> 40 kg: 4 "adult" tablets 31–40 kg: 3 "adult" tablets 21–30 kg : 2 "adult" tablets 11–20 kg: 1 "adult" tablet 9–10 kg:- 3 "pediatric" tablets 5–8 kg :-2 " pediatric" tablets	Daily for 3 days
Quinine sulfate:	10 mg/kg (of quinine salt)	Every 8 hours for 5–7 days
must be combined with	3.5 mg/kg	Daily for 7 days
Doxycycline (not given to children <12 or 8 years depending upon national recommendations) OR	7 mg/kg	Every 8 hours for 7 days
Clindamycin (<12 years or 8 years depending upon national recommendations)		
Dihydroartemisinin-piperaquine (licensed in Europe)	12–23 kg: 1 tablet 24–35 kg: 2 tablets 36–75 kg: 3 tablets Over 75 kg: 4 tablets	Daily for 3 days

infection acquired in this region: one approach is to use chloroquine and re-treat with another drug if there is failure to respond or early recrudescence. The alternative is to use a different drug, particularly for infections from Papua New Guinea and Indonesia, where the risk of chloroquine resistance is highest. There is limited evidence that most antimalarials are effective against chloroquine-resistant vivax including co-artemether, mefloquine, atovaquone-proguanil and quinine-doxycycline [14]. Patients with mixed infections or uncertainty about the infecting species should be treated as though they have falciparum malaria.

Patients with *P. ovale* or *P. vivax* infection also require treatment to eradicate hepatic hypnozoites: relapse may occur in 10–100% of patients with vivax who are treated with chloroquine alone depending on the strain and geographic area where infection was acquired. Primaquine is the only drug that is currently licensed for this purpose; other drugs, such as tafenoquine are currently being evaluated. Higher doses of primaquine [30 mg (base) daily for 14 days] are needed for vivax than for ovale (15 mg daily) and patients should be tested for G6PD deficiency before administration. Anti-relapse therapy with primaquine is more effective if administered simultaneously with

TABLE 144-4 Treatment of Non-Falciparum Malaria

Acute treatment		
Drug	***Dose***	***Duration and frequency***
Chloroquine: Adult	600 mg (base)	Initial dose
	300 mg	6, 24 and 48 hours
Child	10 mg/kg (base)	Initial dose
	5 mg/kg base	6, 24 and 48 hours
Quinine/co-artem/ atovaquone-proguanil	As for uncomplicated falciparum	
Preventing relapse		
Drug	***Dose***	***Duration and frequency***
Primaquine: *ovale* Adult Child	 15 mg 0.25 mg/kg	 Daily for 14 days
Primaquine: *vivax* Adult Child	 30 mg 0.5 mg/kg	 Daily for 14 days
Primaquine: *Mild G6PD deficiency* Adult	 45–60 mg	 Weekly dose for 8 weeks
Child	0.5–0.75 mg/kg (max. 30 mg)	As a single weekly dose for 8 weeks

chloroquine during the treatment of the acute infection [14]. Primaquine should not be given in pregnancy; for those with mild G6PD deficiency, weekly regimens can be safely given to most patients following expert advice.

Falciparum

Malaria caused by *P. falciparum* needs to be treated promptly because of the potential for patients to deteriorate and develop severe disease (Tables 144-2 and 144-3). The choice of drug depends upon the origin of the infection. Chloroquine resistance is widespread and chloroquine is only effective for falciparum malaria acquired in parts of central America, Haiti and the Dominican Republic, and parts of the Middle East. Outside those regions, there are four main choices of oral antimalarials for uncomplicated disease: quinine and doxycline or clindamycin, mefloquine, atovaquone-proguanil and artemether-lumefantrine. Two other oral artemisinin combinations have been submitted for registration in Europe: dihydroartemesinin-piperaquine and pyronaridine-artesunate. There are limited data in returned travellers to assess which drug is best but substantial endemic data show that artemisin combination treatments (ACTs) reduce parasitemia more rapidly and they should now be considered the drugs of choice in a developed setting when available. Atovaquone-proguanil is well tolerated and widely available owing to its use as a prophylactic medication. Mefloquine is least well tolerated in single-dose treatment doses [15] and is not effective for malaria from areas of Southeast Asia where resistance is widespread. If mefloquine is used for treatment, a split dose is recommended as three tablets (750 mg) followed by a second dose of two tablets (500 mg) given 6–12 hours later. Split-dose mefloquine is better tolerated. Oral quinine should be accompanied by either doxycycline or clindamycin to ensure a full therapeutic response: most patients will complain of tinnitus. Patients with uncomplicated falciparum should be observed closely and many physicians suggest that they should be managed as in-patients in the initial stages.

SEVERE DISEASE

Chemotherapy

Parenteral therapy should be given to all those with severe or complicated malaria and to those who cannot tolerate oral therapy (Table 144-5). Many clinicians also advocate parenteral therapy for those with high levels of parasitemia (>2%). Parenteral quinine or quinidine has been the mainstay of treatment of severe malaria for over 50 years; however, two major trials have now clearly demonstrated the superiority of parenteral artesunate over quinine in endemic settings, in both adults and children, with reduction in mortality [16]. Although these studies were not performed in a Western setting, they constitute the best evidence that is ever likely to be available. Parenteral artesunate should now be considered the drug of choice for the management of severe malaria in the returned traveller.

The major difficulty in using artesunate has been the poor availability of a quality-assured parenteral drug. The Chinese product used in the studies did not reach international regulatory standards of good manufacturing and quality control. In the USA, a formulation of intravenous artesunate manufactured in accordance with good manufacturing practices is available as an Investigational New Drug via the CDC; elsewhere, local health authorities have developed mechanisms to quality-assure imported artesunate. Both the Chinese and the USA parenteral artesunate formulations are moving towards registration. Artesunate should be given as a slow, intravenous infusion at 0, 12 and 24 hours and then daily until oral medication can be taken. Each treatment dose is 2.4 mg/kg with no modification for altered renal status. Treatment should be completed with a full course of an oral ACT, atovaquone-proguanil, mefloquine or quinine-doxycycline. Artesunate appears to be well tolerated, although transient reticulocytopenia and neutropenia have been noted with higher doses; full blood counts should be monitored.

If not available, or if administration of artesunate is likely to be delayed, therapy should be started with intravenous quinine or quinidine using a loading dose followed by infusion three times a day (quinine) or continuous infusion (quinidine). The electrocardiography (ECG) should be monitored continuously and if parenteral therapy is continued for more than 48 hours, the dose should be reduced. Once the patient is well enough, oral quinine should be commenced to complete at least 5 days of treatment. Quinine or quinidine should be combined with 7 days of either doxycycline or clindamycin (children or pregnant women) to ensure full cure. A full course of atovaquone-proguanil or an ACT could also be used to complete treatment.

TABLE 144-5 Drug Management of Severe Malaria in Travellers (Adults and Children)

- Quinine: loading dose of 20 mg/kg quinine dihydrochloride in 5% dextrose or dextrose saline over 4 hours. Followed by: 10 mg/kg over 4 hours every 8 hours for first 48 hours (or until patient can swallow). Frequency of dosing should be reduced to 12-hourly if intravenous quinine continues for more than 48 hours.
- Quinidine: loading dose of 10 mg/kg quinidine gluconate IV over 1–2 hours then continuous infusion of 0.02 mg/kg/min for at least 24 hours. Alternatively, 24 mg/kg quinidine gluconate IV over 4 hours, followed by 12 mg/kg over 4 hours every 8 hours.
- Artesunate: 2.4 mg/kg given IV at 0, 12 and 24 hours then daily thereafter.
- If quinine or quinidine given, parenteral therapy is normally followed by oral quinine to complete 5–7 days treatment along with 7 days of doxycycline or clindamycin (pregnancy, children). Atovaquone-proguanil or a full course of an artemisin combination treatment (ACT) can also be used.
- If parenteral artesunate given, treatment can be completed with a full course of an ACT, atovaquone-proguanil, mefloquine, or quinine and doxycycline or clindamycin.

Supportive Therapy

In addition to chemotherapy, supportive treatment of the patient is extremely important. Patients with severe or complicated malaria or with high parasite counts need careful observation in a high dependency or intensive care unit. Blood glucose should be closely monitored and corrected if low. Achieving an optimum fluid balance is also important: under-perfusion may exacerbate hyperlactatemia, whilst fluid overload can contribute to pulmonary edema and respiratory distress syndrome. There is no consensus on the optimum type or volume of fluids to use in severe malaria. Patients with anemia may need transfusion. Broad-spectrum antibiotics may be appropriate in those patients, particularly children, who have sepsis-like syndromes caused by concomitant Gram-negative bacteremia. Patients with renal failure should be treated with hemofiltration which is superior to peritoneal dialysis [17].

Adjunctive Treatment

Although many adjunctive treatments have been studied in severe malaria, none have been proven effective and none are indicated in routine clinical practice. Exchange transfusion has been most extensively studied with anecdotal success but has never been evaluated in a randomized, controlled trial [18]. Prior to the availability of artesunate, many experienced clinicians advocated exchange transfusion for those with hyperparasitemia of more than 20% or in patients with parasitaemia >10% and signs of severe disease. Given the broad stage specificity of artesunate and its rapid effect in reducing parasitemia, it is now uncertain whether there is any role for exchange transfusion if parenteral artesunate is available. If artesunate is not available, or access is significantly delayed, there may still be a role for red blood cell exchange [19].

MONITORING AND PROGNOSIS

There is little value in measuring parasite counts more than daily, as variations in peripheral falciparum parasitemia occur according to the stage of the infection. Most patients who do not have very high initial parasite counts should clear peripheral parasites by 72 hours after the start of treatment. Those with uncomplicated malaria usually recover without sequelae, although fatigue and mild anemia can take a number of weeks to resolve. The case fatality rate in falciparum malaria is around 4–8/1000; approximately 7–15% of those with severe and complicated malaria die, depending upon definitions [20, 21]. Those who are pregnant and who are elderly [22] can have worse outcomes. Individuals over the age of 70 years reported a case fatality rate of over 30%. Subtle neurologic sequelae can follow cerebral malaria in children, diminishing over time, but sequelae are rare in adults.

REFERENCES

1. Freedman DO, Weld LH, Kozarsky PE, et al. Spectrum of disease and relation to place of exposure among ill returned travelers. N Engl J Med 2006;354:119–30.
2. Leder K, Black J, O'Brien D, et al. Malaria in travelers: a review of the GeoSentinel surveillance network. Clin Infect Dis 2004;39:1104–12.
3. Taylor SM, Molyneux ME, Simel DL, et al. Does this patient have malaria? JAMA 2010; 304:2048–56.
4. Stuiver PC, van Rijsunjk JB, Visser LG. Delayed onset of malignant tertian malaria through the inappropriate use of doxycycline: another threat to patients returning from malarious areas. J Travel Med 1996;3:193.

5. Reyburn H, Behrens RH, Warhurst D, Bradley D. The effect of chemoprophylaxis on the timing of onset of falciparum malaria. Trop Med Int Health 1998;3:281–5.
6. Day JH, Behrens RH. Delay in onset of malaria with mefloquine prophylaxis. Lancet 1995;345:398.
7. Wetsteyn JCFM, De Geus A. Chloroquine-resistant falciparum malaria imported into the Netherlands. Bull World Health Org 1985;63:101–8.
8. Lewis SJ, Davidson RN, Ross EJ, Hall AP. Severity of imported falciparum malaria: effect of taking antimalarial prophylaxis. BMJ 1992;305:741–3.
9. Klement E, Chauveheid MP, Thellier M, et al. Subacute clinical forms of *Plasmodium falciparum* malaria in travelers receiving chloroquine-proguanil prophylaxis. Clin Infect Dis 2001;33:e1–2.
10. Kochar DK, Saxena V, Singh N, et al. *Plasmodium vivax* malaria. Emerg Infect Dis 2005;11:132–4.
11. Jennings RM, DE Souza JB, Todd JE, et al. Imported *Plasmodium falciparum* malaria: are patients originating from disease-endemic areas less likely to develop severe disease? A prospective, observational study. Am J Trop Med Hyg 2006;75:1195–9.
12. World Health Organization. Guidelines for the treatment of malaria – 2nd edition. Available at: http://whqlibdoc.who.int/publications/2010/9789241547925_eng.pdf.
13. Centers for Disease Control and Prevention. Treatment of Malaria: Guidelines For Clinicians (United States). Available at: http://www.cdc.gov/malaria/diagnosis_treatment/treatment.html.
14. Baird JK. Resistance to therapies for infection by *Plasmodium vivax*. Clin Microbiol Rev 2009;22:508–34.
15. Ranque S, Marchou B, Malvy D, et al. Treatment of imported malaria in adults: a multicentre study in France. QJM 2005;98:737–43.
16. Sinclair D, Donegan S, Lalloo DG. Artesunate versus quinine for treating severe malaria. Cochrane Database Syst Rev 2011;3:CD005967.
17. Phu NH, Hien TT, Mai NT et al. Hemofiltration and peritoneal dialysis in infection-associated acute renal failure in Vietnam. N Engl J Med 2002;347:895–902.
18. Riddle MS, Jackson JL, Sanders JW, Blazes DL. Exchange transfusion as an adjunct therapy in severe *Plasmodium falciparum* malaria: a meta-analysis. Clin Infect Dis 2002;34:1192–8.
19. Shelat SG, Lott JP, Braga MS. Considerations on the use of adjunct red blood cell exchange transfusion in the treatment of severe *Plasmodium falciparum* malaria. Transfusion 2010;50:875–80.
20. Legros F, Bouchaud O, Ancelle T, et al. Risk factors for imported fatal *Plasmodium falciparum* malaria, France, 1996–2003. Emerg Infect Dis 2007;13:883–8.
21. Smith AD, Bradley DJ, Smith V, et al. Imported malaria and high risk groups: observational study using UK surveillance data 1987–2006. BMJ 2008;337:a120.
22. Greenberg AE, Lobel HO. Mortality from *Plasmodium falciparum* malaria in travelers from the United States, 1959 to 1987. Ann Intern Med 1990;113:326–7.

Screening of the Asymptomatic Long-term Traveler 145

Vanessa Field

Key features

- Screening aims to identify risks that may have implications for the health of an individual
- A sound knowledge of destination-specific risks, mode of acquisition and incubation periods of diseases, and knowledge of the utility of screening tests is necessary
- The clinician must take a detailed history in order to assess the likelihood of exposure to infectious and noninfectious travel-associated risks and assess the magnitude and potential impact of that risk; e.g. exposure to schistosomula, sexually transmitted and blood-borne infections, tuberculosis, and malaria
- A physical examination and targeted testing according to exposure is recommended, with findings of eosinophilia necessitating specific evaluation
- Referral to a specialist center is essential for those clinicians with little or no experience of managing returned travelers

INTRODUCTION

The long-term traveler can be defined as those traveling or residing overseas for more than 6 months and includes those going on extended holidays (gap year/backpackers/visiting friends and relatives) and those residing overseas in order to work or volunteer (expatriates). The type and extent of risk to the health of long-term travelers, and the screening of them on return, varies considerably according to the individual, their destination/s, duration, and purpose of travel.

Screening of travelers is a medical review undertaken to identify risk factors that may have implications for the health of the traveler. Screening can lead to more extensive evaluation or can be diagnostic on its own. There are little data and no uniformly accepted guidelines or extensive cost/benefit analyses for screening of the asymptomatic long-term traveler.

It is accepted that a post-travel consultation is an opportunity to:

1. Discuss exposure to infectious disease risks and assess the necessity for and timing of screening.
2. Target investigations of latent infections that may have deleterious consequences if unrecognized.
3. Counsel the traveler and reduce the risk of secondary transmission of infections, e.g. tuberculosis, salmonellosis, scabies, and HIV.
4. Inform the traveler of potential disease manifestations that can occur at a later stage, e.g. *Plasmodium vivax* malaria, and consider presumptive treatment strategies.
5. Offer reassurance and/or confirm diagnosis or proof of cure following illness, such as febrile systemic illness, diarrheal disease, or rash, that occurred during travel.
6. Provide information about the consequence of any illness during travel in view of future travel, e.g. dengue.
7. Review a traveler's compliance with preventative measures, including their experience of malaria chemoprophylaxis, and review their vaccination status.
8. Provide a lifestyle assessment – diet, exercise, alcohol, smoking, BMI, stress.
9. Review pre-existing medical conditions and medication; provide a cardiovascular, neoplastic (cervical, breast, prostate, colon), and psychological review.
10. Where relevant, determine fitness at the end of a period of work.

There is uncertainty about the ideal timing of conducting a post-travel consultation. Infections with a long incubation may be overlooked. An additional medical visit 3 months after return may be recommended in order to detect infections such as HIV.

Referral to a specialist center for advice and management is essential for those clinicians with little or no experience of managing returned travelers. A sound knowledge of destination-specific risks, mode of acquisition and incubation periods of diseases, and of the sensitivity and specificity of screening tests is necessary.

HOW DOES A CLINICIAN EVALUATE AN ASYMPTOMATIC LONG-TERM TRAVELER ON RETURN?

HISTORY

History is the cornerstone of the post-travel consultation. The clinician must take a detailed history in order to assess the likelihood of exposure to infectious and noninfectious travel-associated risks and assess the magnitude and potential impact of that risk [1].

The clinician should ask, what might this person, from this place, have been exposed to, that may cause them ill health at some time? And so they must consider:

- *Person* – age, gender, socioeconomic status (including immigrant/refugee status), occupation, sexual orientation, travel experience/knowledge, personal risk profile (risk aversion/perception), pre-existing health conditions (including medication), pre-travel preparation (vaccinations, chemoprophylaxis), compliance during travel with pre-travel advice, and any illness.
- *Place* – exact destination, itinerary, season, accommodation, duration, and date of return. Diseases can be destination-specific: e.g. *Loa loa* is confined to equatorial regions of West Africa, tick typhus is a disease of the East and southern African savannah, and gastrointestinal and soil-transmitted infections are ubiquitous.
- *Exposures* – an exposure history should detail:

- Safety risks: threats experienced to personal safety.
- Environmental risks: exposures to altitude, sun, extremes of temperature, and specific environments, including soil-transmitted helminths (strongyloides, hookworm, other intestinal helminths), freshwater contact (schistosomiasis, leptospirosis), caves (histoplasmosis), game parks (trypanosomiasis), safari (African tick typhus) equatorial forest (loiasis, onchocerciasis), and marine environments (stings, coral infections/necrosis).
- Food- and water-borne risks: general hygiene measures, water access, ingestion of raw/undercooked meat/fish, and unpasteurized products (e.g. amebiasis, brucellosis, giardiasis, intestinal helminths).
- Vector-borne risks (including animals): measures taken to prevent insect exposures; bites/skin wounds received (e.g. malaria, filariasis, trypanosomiasis, rabies).
- Airborne risks: close contact with people potentially infected with tuberculosis.
- Sexual health and blood-borne virus risks: unprotected contact and potential exposure to HIV, hepatitis B and C, and other sexually transmitted infections.
- Skin health: skin wounds, UV damage, rash, and any symptoms such as itch.
- Psychological health: positive and negative experiences of travel, readjustment issues, and any ongoing mental health concerns.

EXAMINATION

In asymptomatic travelers, physical examination is often of limited value. However, examination may reveal previously undetected lymphadenopathy, hepatosplenomegaly, hypertension, cardiac/pulmonary dysfunction, and skin disorders. A full examination is therefore necessary.

GENERAL SCREENING TESTS

Laboratory tests are often insensitive, nonspecific and may not be available for conditions in their pre-clinical stage, as is the case for malaria. Minimal laboratory tests comprise a total blood count and differential, liver transaminases, blood urea, and creatinine levels, as well as targeted serologic markers according to exposure (see below). Microscopic examination of stool for ova, cysts, and parasites, a urine dip-stick and, when appropriate a "terminal urine" for schistosomiasis, should be performed. Fasting blood glucose, lipids, thyroid function tests, and neoplastic markers (e.g. PSA) are optional for those wanting a comprehensive health review (Fig. 145.1).

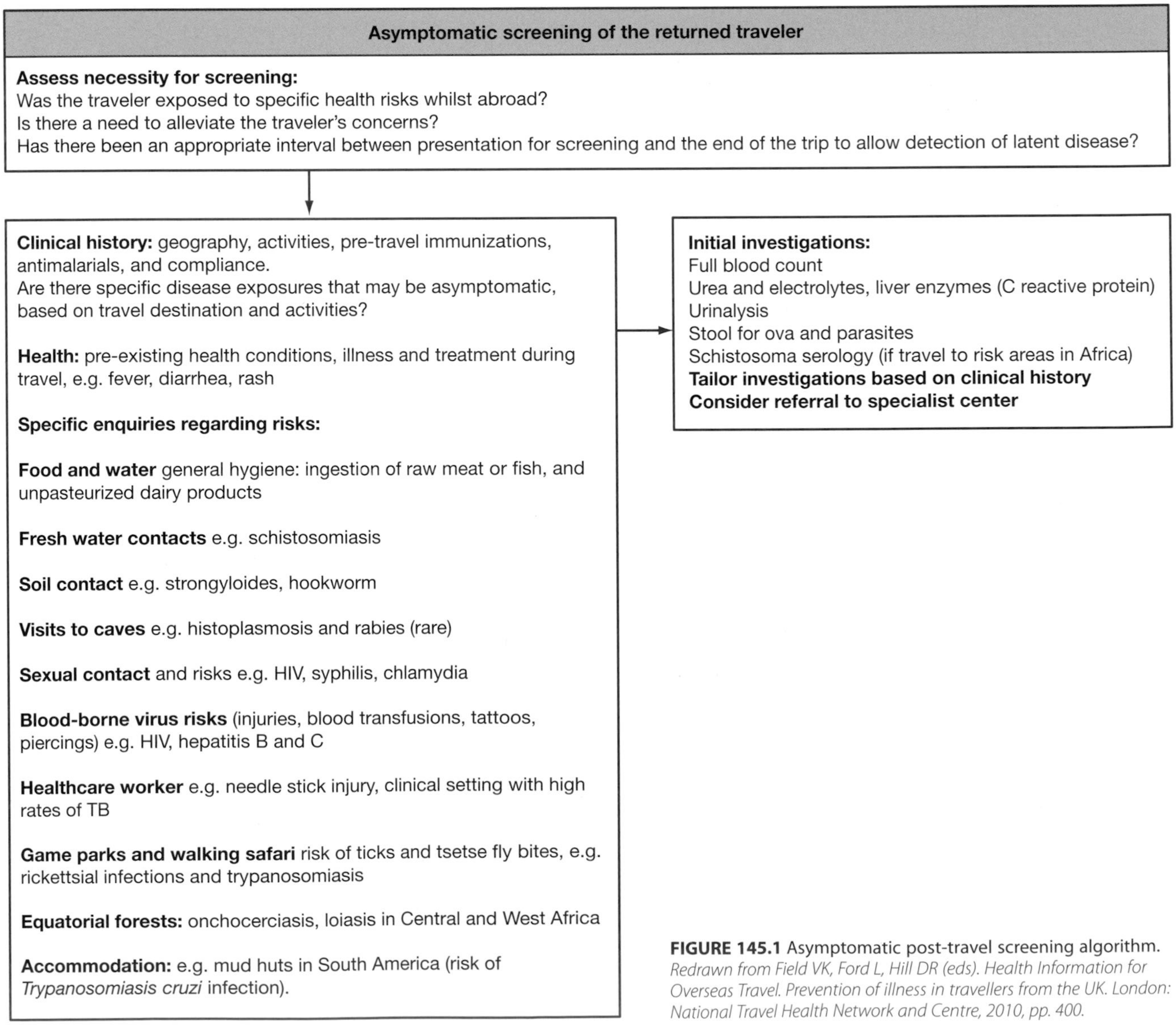

Asymptomatic screening of the returned traveler

Assess necessity for screening:
Was the traveler exposed to specific health risks whilst abroad?
Is there a need to alleviate the traveler's concerns?
Has there been an appropriate interval between presentation for screening and the end of the trip to allow detection of latent disease?

Clinical history: geography, activities, pre-travel immunizations, antimalarials, and compliance.
Are there specific disease exposures that may be asymptomatic, based on travel destination and activities?

Health: pre-existing health conditions, illness and treatment during travel, e.g. fever, diarrhea, rash

Specific enquiries regarding risks:

Food and water general hygiene: ingestion of raw meat or fish, and unpasteurized dairy products

Fresh water contacts e.g. schistosomiasis

Soil contact e.g. strongyloides, hookworm

Visits to caves e.g. histoplasmosis and rabies (rare)

Sexual contact and risks e.g. HIV, syphilis, chlamydia

Blood-borne virus risks (injuries, blood transfusions, tattoos, piercings) e.g. HIV, hepatitis B and C

Healthcare worker e.g. needle stick injury, clinical setting with high rates of TB

Game parks and walking safari risk of ticks and tsetse fly bites, e.g. rickettsial infections and trypanosomiasis

Equatorial forests: onchocerciasis, loiasis in Central and West Africa

Accommodation: e.g. mud huts in South America (risk of *Trypanosomiasis cruzi* infection).

Initial investigations:
Full blood count
Urea and electrolytes, liver enzymes (C reactive protein)
Urinalysis
Stool for ova and parasites
Schistosoma serology (if travel to risk areas in Africa)
Tailor investigations based on clinical history
Consider referral to specialist center

FIGURE 145.1 Asymptomatic post-travel screening algorithm. *Redrawn from Field VK, Ford L, Hill DR (eds). Health Information for Overseas Travel. Prevention of illness in travellers from the UK. London: National Travel Health Network and Centre, 2010, pp. 400.*

TARGETED DISEASE EVALUATION

Eosinophilia

Eosinophilia can indicate parasitic infection with helminths, especially with nematodes, trematodes, or larval cestodes (see also Chapter 143). It is more marked when blood and tissue migration occurs, as in *Strongyloides stercoralis*, schistosomiasis, blood filariasis, and intestinal helminths (ascaris, hookworm), but less so in lymphatic filariasis. Individuals with such infections may also have normal eosinophil counts.

The sensitivity of eosinophilia as a screening tool for helminth infection in asymptomatic long-term travelers can be as low as 27% [2]. Three stool examinations, together with parasite serologies for strongyloidiasis, schistosomiasis and filariasis, are more sensitive (89%) [2]. The predictive value of eosinophilia is higher in travelers with particularly high eosinophil counts (absolute count >1000/mm^3), and further work-up of these individuals is justified [3].

Schistosomiasis

Infection with *Schistosoma* spp. should be suspected in any traveler who has been in contact with potentially infected fresh water in endemic areas. Schistosomiasis has been reported following both short-term [4, 5] and long-term travel [6, 7]. Heavy parasite loads in travelers are rare and so late-stage disease manifestations are also rare. The cost-effectiveness of diagnosing an occult asymptomatic parasitic infection such as schistosomiasis is not known. Specialist referral should be considered.

Testing is recommended 2–4 months after last exposure in those who are asymptomatic (Fig. 145.2). Stool and urine microscopy is an insensitive method of diagnosis. Rectal snip is more sensitive [8] but has been largely superseded by schistosomal antibody testing, which is both sensitive and specific, with seroconversion usually occurring within 3 months (occasionally up to 1 year). A positive test does not necessarily indicate active disease, as titers can remain detectable for many years after successful eradication. Schistosomal antigen tests may provide more reliable measures of active infection in the future.

Sexual Health and HIV Screening

Sexual health screening in returned asymptomatic long-term travelers is an important part of the post-travel consultation, limiting secondary transmission and reassuring the traveler.

HIV serologic testing is reliably specific and sensitive and can be routinely offered to any traveler with a history of sexual contact with a new partner [9]. Individuals should be offered an HIV test (with saliva testing or rapid serum HIV testing) after counseling and informed consent has been gained, at the initial consultation, and again at 12 weeks post-exposure. A repeat test at 6 months may be recommended.

If potentially exposed to HIV within 72 hours of the consultation and depending on the type of exposure (skin penetration, type of bodily fluid exchange, likelihood of donor positivity), HIV post-exposure prophylaxis (PEP) should be considered. Donor testing should be arranged if possible. Safe sexual practices should be encouraged in the period before testing.

Hepatitis B, C and syphilis (*Treponema pallidum)* serology, *Neisseria gonorrhoea* and *Chlamydia trachomatis* (direct urethral/cervical sampling, or indirect urine sampling), should also be considered and an examination performed for warts, ulcers, and discharge. Specialist advice should be sought when necessary.

Screening for HIV, hepatitis B surface antigen, and hepatitis C core antibodies, should be performed in those whose exposure history reveals risk factors e.g. needlestick injury, needle shared by intravenous drug users, receipt of blood/blood product, exposure to contaminated needle/syringe during medical/dental treatment, or procedures in which contaminated instruments may have been used, such as during tattooing or body piercing.

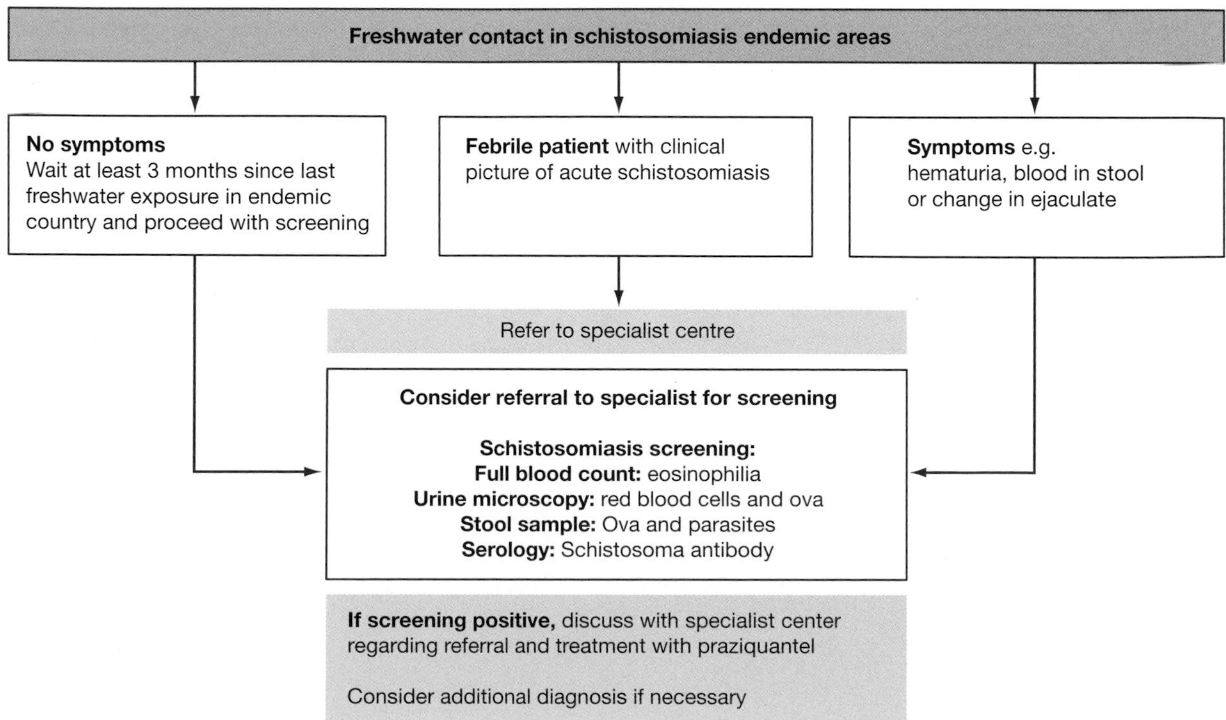

FIGURE 145.2 Schistosomiasis screening algorithm. *Redrawn from Field VK, Ford L, Hill DR (eds). Health Information for Overseas Travel. Prevention of illness in travellers from the UK. London: National Travel Health Network and Centre, 2010, pp. 400.*

Trypanosomiasis

Serologic tests are sensitive for *Trypanosoma cruzi* (Chagas disease) and *Trypanosoma brucei gambiense*, the two forms of trypanosomiasis that may be latent. Screening should be restricted to those travelers whose history suggests significant exposure, e.g. poor housing in an area endemic in South America for triatomid bugs and *T. cruzi*, or exposure to tsetse fly in areas of Central and West Africa known for intense transmission of *T. brucei gambiense*. Guidelines have recently been published for management of latent Chagas disease [10].

Tuberculosis

Incidence rates of TB infection in some long-term travelers are comparable to those of the indigenous populations [11, 12]. Latent TB (positive purified protein derivative [PPD] or interferon-gamma release assay [IGRA]) was diagnosed significantly more commonly in long-term than in short-term travelers [7]. Healthcare workers, those who visit friends and relatives, and children under the age of 5 years, can be at particular risk, some of them to MDR and XDR TB [11, 13].

The American Thoracic Society recommends screening for tuberculosis in people likely to be recently infected, particularly those who have been in close contact with a known infectious case [14]. Screening should be targeted to those at high risk such as healthcare workers with prolonged travel in a country with an annual incidence of ≥40 TB cases/100,000 population. Tuberculin testing (Mantoux, PPD) before and after exposure is recommended in this group. A change from a negative to a positive tuberculin skin test is more sensitive and specific than a chest x-ray and occurs 6 weeks to 4 months after TB exposure. Administration and interpretation of the test require expertise and timing. False-negative reactions are common when not performed correctly [15]. A more recent cost-effectiveness model proposed a single post-travel tuberculin skin test in people originally from countries with a low incidence of TB [16].

Testing is less reliable in those who are immunocompromised and in those previously vaccinated with BCG. IGRA testing can be considered as an alternative test in cases with prior BCG vaccination. A chest x-ray should be taken for those with a positive test. Post-exposure prophylactic treatment averts progression to active disease in most cases.

Rabies PEP

Long-term asymptomatic travelers should be asked of their potential for exposure to rabies as well as their pre-exposure vaccine history. Rabies vaccine and IgG should be considered, depending on the exposure type and time.

Malaria

Malaria may become symptomatic after the initial post-travel period, and so all returned travelers from malaria-endemic areas should be educated about nonspecific symptoms and signs, especially fever, during the first few months after return. They should be advised to seek an early medical opinion and inform health professionals of their travel history, should these symptoms occur.

PSYCHOLOGICAL HEALTH

Psychological diagnoses were reported significantly more frequently in long-term travelers as compared to short-term travelers [7]. Many long-term travelers fail to make a successful transition to their country of posting or to their home country on return. The returnee may be hesitant to voice their concerns because of issues of confidentiality or fear of stigma/embarrassment. Debriefing sessions, time for rest and relaxation, as well as readjustment and re-adaptation should be encouraged.

CONCLUSIONS

All asymptomatic long-term travelers should have a post-travel consultation on their return. This should include a detailed personal, travel and exposure history and physical examination. Little additional testing need be done, except when indicated by risk. The post-travel consultation is also an opportunity to re-emphasize primary prevention messages and perform a general health review.

REFERENCES

1. Field VF, Ford L, Hill DR, eds. The post-travel consultation. In: Health Information for Overseas Travel. London: National Travel Health Network and Centre; 2010:179–91.
   New practical manual for travel medicine providers with comprehensive information of risk assessment and risk management in the pre-travel consultation, guidance on special needs travelers, algorithms for managing returned travelers, and an extensive disease guide.
2. Libman MD, MacLean JD, Gyorkos TW. Screening tests for schistosomiasis, filariasis, and strongyloides among expatriates returning from the tropics. Clin Infect Dis 1993;17:353–9.
3. Schulte C, Krebs B, Jelinek T, et al. Diagnostic significance of blood eosinophilia in returning travelers. Clin Infect Dis 2002;34:407–11.
4. Schwartz E, Kozarsky P, Wilson M, Cetron M. Schistosome infection among river rafters on Omo River, Ethiopia. J Travel Med 2005;12:3–8.
5. Leshem E, Maor Y, Meltzer E, et al. Acute schistosomiasis outbreak: clinical features and economic impact. Clin Infect Dis 2008;47:1499–506.
   Recent analysis of a cluster of schistosomiasis and its impact in short-term travelers to Tanzania.
6. Trachtenberg JD, Jacobson M, Noh JC, et al. Schistosomiasis in expatriates in the Arusha region of Tanzania. J Travel Med 2002;9:233–5.
7. Chen LH, Wilson ME, Davis X, et al. Illness in long-term travelers visiting GeoSentinel clinics. Emerg Infect Dis 2009;15:1773–82.
   Analysis of differences in illness in returned long-term travelers (>6 months) vs. short-term travelers utilizing the GeoSentinel database of travel and tropical medicine clinics throughout the world. Areas of concern for long-term travelers were vector-borne diseases, contact-transmitted diseases, and psychological problems.
8. Strickland GT. Gastrointestinal manifestations of schistosomiasis. Gut 1994;35:1334–7. doi:10.1136/gut.35.10.
9. Bos JM, Fennema JS, Potsma MJ. Cost-effectiveness of HIV screening of patients attending clinics for sexually transmitted diseases in Amsterdam. AIDS 2001;15:2031–6.
10. Bern C, Montgomery SP, Herwaldt BL, et al. Evaluation and treatment of Chagas disease in the United States: a systematic review. JAMA 2007;298:2171–81.
    Excellent review of the complexity of evaluating symptomatic and asymptomatic people with Chagas disease.
11. Cobelens FG, van Deutekom H, Draayer-Jansen IW, et al. Risk of infection with *Mycobacterium tuberculosis* in travelers to areas of high endemicity. Lancet 2000;356:461–5.
12. Jung P, Banks RH. Tuberculosis risk in US Peace Corps Volunteers, 1996 to 2005. J Travel Med 2008;15:87–94.
13. Leder K, Tong S, Weld L, et al. Illness in travelers visiting friends and relatives: a review of the GeoSentinel Surveillance Network. Clin Infect Dis 2006;43:1185–93.
14. Blumberg HM, Burman WJ, Chaisson RE, et al. American Thoracic Society/Centers for Disease Control and Prevention/Infectious Diseases Society of America: treatment of tuberculosis. Am J Respir Crit Care Med 2003;15:603–62.
15. Lifson AR. *Mycobacterium tuberculosis* infection in travelers: tuberculosis comes home (commentary). Lancet 2000;356:461–5.
16. Tan M, Menzies D, Schwartzman K. Tuberculosis screening of travelers to higher-incidence countries: a cost-effectiveness analysis. BMC Public Health 2008;8:201.
    Modelling of the cost-effectiveness of post-travel tuberculosis skin-test screening of travelers from low-incidence countries to countries of varying incidence. For all travelers, a single post-trip tuberculin test was most cost-effective. Screening was more cost-effective with increasing trip duration and infection risk.

Persistent Diarrhea in the Returned Traveler 146

Stephen G Wright

Key Features

- Persistent diarrhea (diarrhea lasting ≥14 days) is one of the most common syndromes in returned travelers
- Etiologies range from infectious causes—often protozoan parasites such as *Giardia* spp. or bacteria—to post-infectious irritable bowel syndrome (IBS) to non-infectious inflammatory bowel syndromes
- Evaluation combines stool examinations and culture with laboratory testing for eosinophilia. A malabsorption work-up and more extensive testing may be warranted if initial studies are negative
- If an infectious etiology is determined, appropriate treatment should be given
- Management of non-infectious etiologies can include dietary change (e.g. for lactose intolerance), symptomatic management of IBS, or interventions for inflammatory bowel disease

INTRODUCTION

Diarrheal disease is common among populations in tropical regions of the world and is a frequent illness in returned travelers. Acute and chronic diarrhea were the most common reasons for individuals seeking post-travel medical care in the GeoSentinel surveillance network of 17 tropical and travel medicine clinics throughout the world [1]. Presentation with acute diarrhea occurred at a rate of 222 visits per 1000 travelers seeking medical care, and chronic diarrhea occurred at a rate of 113 per 1000 visits, with the highest relative rates from South Asia [1, 2]. At the Hospital for Tropical Diseases in London, gastrointestinal complaints were responsible for 39% of attendances at the walk-in clinic over the course of a year in which over 3000 patients used the service. Following an episode of diarrhea during travel, approximately 2% of individuals will go on to chronic illness [3].

ETIOLOGY

Etiologies of diarrhea in returned travelers can be divided into infectious, usually parasitic and bacterial [4–6], post-infectious, for example lactose intolerance and irritable bowel syndrome (IBS) [7], and non-infectious, such as inflammatory bowel disease (Table 146-1). There is a wide range of microbial agents that cause diarrhea. Many episodes of travelers' diarrhea caused by enterotoxigenic *Escherichia coli* will be self-limiting; however, invasive bacterial infections, such as *Shigella* spp., can produce more serious infections that will need antimicrobial treatment. For diarrhea that lasts more than 14 days post-travel, protozoan parasites are more common: *Giardia*, the most frequently identified agent and travel to South Asia, the highest risk [6]. Although parasites are considered more common with chronic disease, bacterial diarrhea can also persist beyond a week [8].

While *Giardia* is the commonest parasitic cause of persisting diarrhea, *Cryptosporidium* spp. and, less commonly, *Cyclospora cayetanensis* are also recognized. Amebiasis is uncommon in short-term travelers, being typically seen in long-term travelers or expatriates. Intestinal helminths usually do not cause diarrheal symptoms with low worm burdens. Acute hookworm infection can occasionally be associated

TABLE 146-1 Causes of Persistent Diarrhea in Returned Travelers*

Clinical category	Possible causes
Diarrhea with weight loss	Giardiasis Cryptosporidosis Cyclospora Hookworm infection (uncommon) Whipworm infection Strongyloidiasis (less common with GI symptoms) Celiac disease (gluten sensitive enteropathy) HIV/AIDS Tropical sprue (rare) Inflammatory bowel disease Colonic cancer Pancreatic disease Anatomical causes (diverticula, strictures, blind loops)
Diarrhea with normal body weight	Post-infective irritable bowel Lactose intolerance (can be post-infectious) Food intolerance
Diarrhea with blood	Amebiasis Invasive bacteria (e.g. *Shigella*, *Campylobacter*) *Clostridium difficile*-associated diarrhea Hemorrhagic *Escherichia coli* (shiga-toxin producing) Schistosomiasis Inflammatory bowel disease (especially ulcerative colitis) Carcinoma of the colon Colonic polyps Diverticulitis Ischemic colitis

*There can be overlap of clinical presentations.
GI, gastrointestinal.

with persistent diarrhea. Colonic schistosomiasis and trichuris infection which can cause diarrhea in indigenous populations are uncommon causes in travelers.

Post-infectious IBS, identified at 6 months following return, is a recognized complication of travelers' diarrhea. Although the incidence has varied, with some studies reporting it as high as 15%, it is likely that it occurs less than 5% of the time [7]. Factors associated with increased risk of developing IBS are multiple episodes of diarrhea during travel, longer duration of illness and increased severity.

Celiac disease is relatively common in temperate parts of the world, occurring in approximately 1 in 200 persons. It should also be considered in migrants with persisting diarrhea. The range of countries where this is recognized is increasing. The first presentation of inflammatory bowel disease (IBD) can occur following an episode of diarrhea during travel.

ASSESSMENT

The goals in assessing patients are to:

- determine if there is a persisting, treatable infection—often giardiasis or another protozoal infection;
- consider the possibility of gastrointestinal disease, such as celiac disease, brought to light as a consequence of intestinal infection, or IBD presenting for the first time;
- consider whether the patient has a disease unrelated to travel.

If, after careful evaluation, an infectious cause is ruled out and there is no underlying non-infectious bowel disease, the patient is likely to have post-infectious IBS. In this case, managing persisting symptoms becomes the main objective.

Weight loss during tropical travels is common, but this is usually regained when the traveler returns to their usual diet. When this does not happen, malabsorption needs to be considered in a patient with continuing diarrhea. Pale, foul-smelling stools are typical of malabsorption. Both foul-smelling flatus and stools are typical of giardiasis. Soreness of tongue or mouth can be associated with folate deficiency, consistent with celiac disease and tropical sprue, but uncommon in giardiasis. Tropical sprue is now uncommon in travellers, perhaps related to the ready use of antibiotics in the treatment of travelers' diarrhea.

Physical examination should assess for abdominal masses, colonic tenderness, and organ enlargement. Signs of advanced nutrient depletion such as glossitis, anemia, and ankle edema suggesting hypoproteinemia, are unusual. It is essential to record body weight at initial evaluation so that changes over time and after treatment can be monitored.

A history of blood in the stools needs careful evaluation. The cause may be as simple as an anal fissure from frequent bowel movements and irritation at the mucocutaneous junction, or bleeding from hemorrhoids. In these cases, small amounts of fresh blood are seen on the outside of the stool or left on the toilet paper after a bowel movement. Blood can be associated with invasive organisms, shiga-toxin producing *E. coli* [9], and non-infectious etiologies (Table 146-1). Colonoscopy may be is often needed to investigate non-local causes.

In older travelers, conditions unrelated to travel need consideration, for example diverticulitis, ischemic colitis and colonic cancer. IBD can affect any age and an intestinal infection has been associated with the first presentation of disease.

INVESTIGATIONS (Table 146-2)

Stool culture and microscopy should be routine in persons with prolonged diarrhea. Although microscopy has been the mainstay of diagnosis for parasites, antigen detection assays for *Giardia* and *Cryptosporidium* are more sensitive and specific than visual detection [10]. When there is a broad differential, it remains important to carry out microscopy, or etiologies other than those identified by antigen detection will be missed. When amebiasis is suspected, a freshly passed stool should be examined promptly under direct microscopy and evaulated by antigen detection assay. Concentration methods for parasite diagnosis can improve the yield and are discussed in Chapter 154.1. Examination of formed or semi-formed stools for polymorphonuclear cells indicates inflammation in the colonic wall, often from invasive bacteria or amebiasis. It is likely that molecular methods for fecal parasite diagnosis will become increasingly used in the next few years.

Fecal cultures for bacteria should be obtained. If the patient has taken antibiotics, a toxin assay for *Clostridium difficile* should be assessed [11]. *Clostridium difficile*-associated diarrhea can occur, even after short-course antibiotic treatment of travelers' diarrhea. While helminths are uncommon causes of persisting diarrhea in the traveler, eosinophilia raises the possibility of hookworm, strongyloidiasis and schistosomiasis. *Strongyloides* hyperinfection syndrome in the immunocompromised patient is not associated with eosinophilia.

TABLE 146-2 Investigations of Persistent Diarrhea

First-line investigations	
Stool	Microscopy of saline wet mount, iodine stained and concentrated stool specimens for parasites (usually × 3) Fecal leukocytes Antigen detection* for *Giardia*, *Cryptosporidium* and *Entamoeba histolytica* Modified acid fast staining for *Cryptosporidium* and *Cyclospora* Bacterial cultures
Blood	Complete blood count with an eosinophil count Sedimentation rate, C-reactive protein Liver enzymes, albumin, creatinine and BUN and electrolytes
Urine	Urine analysis
Serology	Amebiasis, strongyloidiasis, schistosomiasis (depending on geographic risk)
Second-line investigations	
	Hydrogen breath studies Lactose tolerance test Fecal elastase (pancreatic insufficiency) Fecal calprotectin (indicator of colonic inflammation) Celiac disease screening Folate & vitamin B12 Thyroid function tests Serum immunoglobulin levels HIV serology SeHCAT scan (bile salt malabasorption) CT/MRI scanning Upper and lower gastrointestinal endoscopy with biopsies

*Antigen detection is available for *Entamoeba* spp. but will usually not distinguish between *E. histolytica* and the non-pathogen, *Entamoeba dispar*. *E. histolytica* adhesin ELISA assay distinguishes *E. histolytica*.
BUN, blood urea nitrogen; CT, computed tomography; MRI, magnetic resonance imaging.

Serum folic acid and vitamin B12 levels should be requested when malabsorption is suspected. Based on the geographic risk and the clinical scenario, serology for amebiasis and schistosomiasis can be useful. A serologic screen for celiac disease is needed as part of testing for non-dysenteric diarrhea when infectious etiologies have been eliminated. Upper and lower gastrointestinal endoscopy with appropriate biopsies are needed for patients with diarrhea and weight loss in whom no cause is found from initial investigations. Small bowel biopsies can be useful to identify pathogens such as *Cyclospora*, as well as define the histology in complex cases, such as HIV-associated enteropathies.

MANAGEMENT

Routine testing as outlined in Table 146-2 will usually reveal a diagnosis. If an infectious agent is discovered through culture or microscopy, this should be treated as described in the specific pathogen chapters of this textbook. If studies are negative, including those for non-infectious etiologies, some advocate empirical treatment for giardiasis using a single dose of a nitroimidazole, usually tinidazole at 2 g for adults. However, with current antigen-detection tests, it is less likely that the patient will have giardiasis in the face of negative testing.

If first-line investigations are negative, a more extensive work-up for malabsorption may be appropriate that includes upper and lower endoscopy with biopsy, and imaging tests. These tests should be able to rule out IBD.

For those without malabsorption and in whom no other cause is identified, or who have recurrent diarrhea after treatment of an infection, post-infectious lactose intolerance is possible and a dietary change (avoiding dairy products) can be made to see if there is improvement. Cholestyramine sequestration of unabsorbed bile salts can control symptoms in patients in whom there is bile salt malabsorption.

For patients with long-term symptoms (months) and no etiology, post-infectious IBS becomes most likely and symptom management is the main consideration. The Rome criteria for IBS include recurrent abdominal discomfort for at least three days per month for three months, plus a change in stool frequency and form with relief by defecation. Many measures have been tried without consistent benefit. Dietary changes, including an increase in fiber intake, antispasmodics, and antimotility agents, probiotics, serotonin-receptor agonists and antidepressants given in low dose for their anti-parasympathetic side effects, have each had variable success [12]. A recent study of rifaximin in diarrhea-predominant IBS showed marginal improvement compared with placebo for three months after treatment [13].

As the differential diagnosis of persistent diarrhea in returned travelers is broad, the clinician should take a careful history to clarify symptoms, pursue a diagnostic work-up based on the differential diagnosis and work closely with the patient to treat and manage symptoms.

REFERENCES

1. Freedman DO, Weld LH, Kozarsky PE, et al. Spectrum of disease and relation to place of exposure among ill returned travelers. N Engl J Med 2006; 354:119–30.
2. Greenwood Z, Black J, Weld L, et al. Gastrointestinal infection among international travelers globally. J Travel Med 2008;15:195–202.
3. Hill DR, Beeching NJ. Travelers' diarrhea. Curr Opin Infect Dis 2010; 23:481–7.
4. Okhuysen PC. Traveler's diarrhea due to intestinal protozoa. Clin Infect Dis 2001;33:110–14.
5. Shah N, DuPont HL, Ramsey DJ. Global etiology of travelers' diarrhea: systematic review from 1973 to the present. Am J Trop Med Hyg 2009;80: 609–14.
6. Swaminathan A, Torresi J, Schlagenhauf P, et al. A global study of pathogens and host risk factors associated with infectious gastrointestinal disease in returned international travellers. J Infect 2009;59:19–27.
7. Pitzurra R, Fried M, Rogler G, et al. Irritable bowel syndrome among a cohort of European travelers to resource-limited destinations. J Travel Med 2011;18: 250–6.
8. Pandey P, Bodhidatta L, Lewis M, et al. Travelers' diarrhea in Nepal: an update on the pathogens and antibiotic resistance. J Travel Med 2011;18:102–8.
9. Frank C, Werber D, Cramer JP, et al. Epidemic profile of shiga-toxin-producing *Escherichia coli* O104:H4 outbreak in Germany—preliminary report. N Engl J Med 2011;365:1771–80.
10. Youn S, Kabir M, Haque R, Petri WA, Jr. Evaluation of a screening test for detection of *Giardia* and *Cryptosporidium*. J Clin Microbiol 2009;47:451–2.
11. Norman FF, Perez-Molina J, Perez de Ayala A, et al. *Clostridium difficile*-associated diarrhea after antibiotic treatment for traveler's diarrhea. Clin Infect Dis 2008;46:1060–3.
12. Brandt LJ, Chey WD, Foxx-Orenstein AE, et al. An evidence-based position statement on the management of irritable bowel syndrome. Am J Gastroenterol 2009;104(suppl. 1):S1–35.
13. Pimentel M, Lembo A, Chey WD, et al. Rifaximin therapy for patients with irritable bowel syndrome without constipation. N Engl J Med 2011;364: 22–32.

147 Skin Lesions in Returning Travelers

Eric Caumes

Key points

- Skin diseases are one of the three most common health problems in returning travelers
- Insect bites, localized cutaneous eruption, and pruritic rashes are the most frequent reasons for consultation
- Travel-related dermatoses include infectious and environmental diseases of exotic or cosmopolitan origin
- Common skin infections include bacterial diseases (pyoderma, cellulitis), dermatophytosis and scabies
- The main exotic dermatoses are hookworm-related cutaneous larva migrans, localized cutaneous leishmaniasis, tungiasis and furuncular myiasis
- Environmental skin diseases include sunburns, arthropod-related reactions, contact dermatitis, marine-life dermatitis, and superficial injuries

INTRODUCTION

Dermatoses are a leading cause of health problems in returning travelers, being reported in approximately 20% of ill patients. The most common dermatologic problems are skin and soft tissue infections (pyoderma, cellulitis), hookworm-related cutaneous larva migrans (HrCLM), and reactions to arthropod bite or sting (with or without secondary infection) [1–3]. Amongst skin disease in returned travelers, imported disease accounts for 24% to 54% of cases. Approximately 10% of the patients are ill enough to be hospitalized [1].

APPROACH TO A TRAVELER WITH A SKIN LESION

The patient's history should systematically evaluate the type of travel, use of preventive measures, risk exposure, and history of similar signs and symptoms in fellow travelers. The dermatologic history will focus on the initial presentation and onset relative to potential exposures, the progression of lesions, and their duration.

Clinical examination will focus on the morphologic characteristics of the lesions (papule, nodule, vesicle, bullous, plaque, ulcer, creeping dermatitis) (Fig. 147.1) together with their anatomic distribution (i.e. localized, generalized or limited to a specific anatomic location) and the presence of pruritus. Any associated local and systemic signs and symptoms will need to be taken into account. Further diagnostic procedures may be warranted according to the findings of the clinical examination.

LOCALIZED SKIN DISEASES

SKIN AND SOFT TISSUE INFECTION

Bacterial skin infections are the most common skin diseases observed in returned travelers [4]. The clinical spectrum ranges from impetigo and abscess to erysipelas and necrotizing cellulitis [1,3,5]. Infections are usually due to *Streptococcus pyogenes* (GAS) and/or *Staphylococcus aureus*. Arthropod bites or stings can become superinfected with the bite acting as a portal of entry (Fig. 147.2) or becoming infected secondary to scratching.

The clinical presentation provides clues toward a specific microbial agent. Impetigo (Fig. 147.3) (presenting as bullae, pustules or post-bullous erosions) is more often due to *S. aureus* than to *Streptococcus* spp. [1,5]. Ecthyma (Fig. 147.4) (presenting as a crusted lesion) is more likely secondary to *S. pyogenes* [5]. Folliculitis, carbuncles, and abscesses (Fig. 147.5) are almost exclusively due to *S. aureus* [5]. Erysipelas and cellulitis (Fig. 147.6) are more likely due to *S. pyogenes* but other bacteria (*S. aureus*, anaerobes, *Aeromonas hydrophila*, *Vibrio vulnificus*, *Pasteurella* spp.) should be considered in the case of dog bite or marine envenomation, for example.

S. aureus may be either methicillin-resistant (MRSA) or methicillin-sensitive (MSSA). Both can carry the gene of the Panton-Valentine leukocidin (PVL), a cytotoxin that confers higher morbidity. PVL-positive *S. aureus* strains acquired abroad can be transmitted after arrival home [4]. *S. pyogenes* remains sensitive to penicillins [5].

CREEPING DERMATITIS

Creeping eruption is defined as a linear or serpiginous cutaneous track that is slightly elevated, erythematous and migrating (Fig. 147.7). The clinical characteristics of the cutaneous trail (length, width, speed of migration, location, duration) help to differentiate between causes. Hookworm-related cutaneous larva migrans (HrCLM) caused by penetration of the skin by nonhuman (cat, dog) hookworm larvae is the most common cause of creeping dermatitis [6]. HrCLM is widely distributed in tropical and subtropical countries worldwide and is usually acquired while lying or walking on the beaches in hot seaside areas, particularly in Southeast Asia or the Caribbean. The striking symptom of HrCLM is pruritus localized at the site of the eruption and the clinical sign is creeping dermatitis. Edema or local swelling and vesiculobullous lesions along the course of the larva are reported in approximately 10% of the patients. Hookworm folliculitis is a particular form of HrCLM (Fig. 147.8).

The most frequent anatomic locations of HrCLM are the feet followed by the buttocks and thighs. Without any treatment, the eruption usually lasts weeks. Creeping eruptions may also be seen in diseases involving non-hookworm larvae (e.g. "larva currens" of strongyloidiasis), maggots, adult nematodes, trematode larvae, and mites (Box 147.1).

Oral ivermectin (200 μg/kg, single dose) and albendazole (400 to 800 mg per day, according to weight, for 3 days) are the first-line

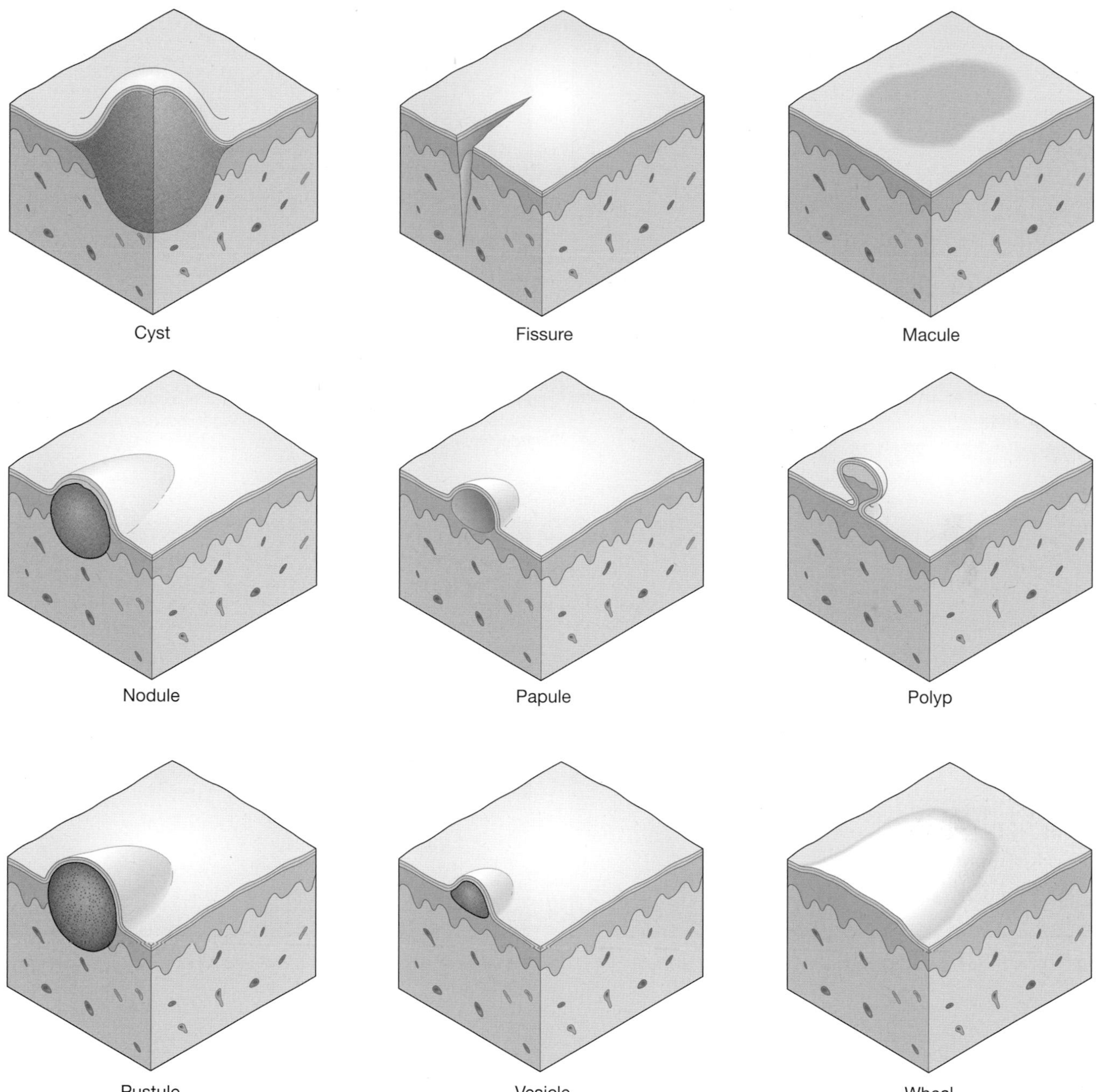

FIGURE 147.1 Skin lesion morphology.

treatments of HrCLM. Taken in a single dose, ivermectin is well tolerated and highly efficacious with cure rates of 94–100% in all but one of the largest series [6].

CUTANEOUS ULCER

Beside pyodermas, the main cause of cutaneous ulcer is cutaneous leishmaniasis (CL) (Fig. 147.9). Old World CL (caused primarily by *Leishmania major* and *L. tropica*) usually occurs in travelers to sub-Saharan and North Africa, the Mediterranean basin, and the Middle East. New World CL (caused primarily by species of *L. braziliensis* and *L. mexicana* complexes) usually occurs in travelers to the forested areas of South and Central America. The clinical forms of CL also include papules, nodules, plaques and nodular lymphangitis [4]. The average number of cutaneous lesions varies from one to three and rarely exceeds ten per patient. Usual features of CL include return from an endemic country in the New or Old World, anatomic location on exposed skin (face, arms, legs), absence of pain, chronicity (more than 1 month duration), and failure of antibiotic treatment (which is often prescribed to treat "pyoderma").

Other causes of cutaneous ulcer in returned travelers include inoculation eschars seen during rickettsioses (e.g. African tick bite fever) (Fig. 147.10), the early stage of African trypanosomiasis (trypanosomal chancre) (Fig. 147.11), and less commonly, cutaneous anthrax. Sporotrichosis and Buruli ulcer (cutaneous manifestation of *Mycobacterium ulcerans* infection) more often present as chronic lesions (Box 147.2).

FIXED LOCALIZED PAPULES AND NODULES

There are several causes of fixed papules and nodules (Box 147.3). Myiasis and tungiasis are among the most common. Myiasis is infestation of human tissue by larvae or maggots of flies (*Diptera*). Furuncular myiasis (caused by *Cordylobia anthropophaga* in sub-Saharan Africa and *Dermatobia hominis* in Central and South America)

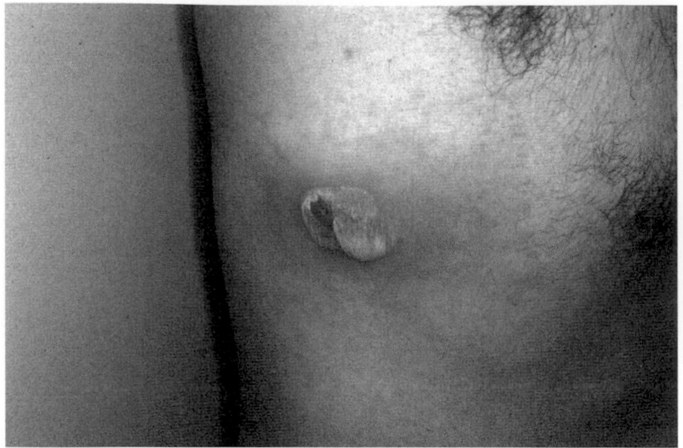

FIGURE 147.2 Bullous bacterial cellulitis complicating an insect bite (return from Central Africa).

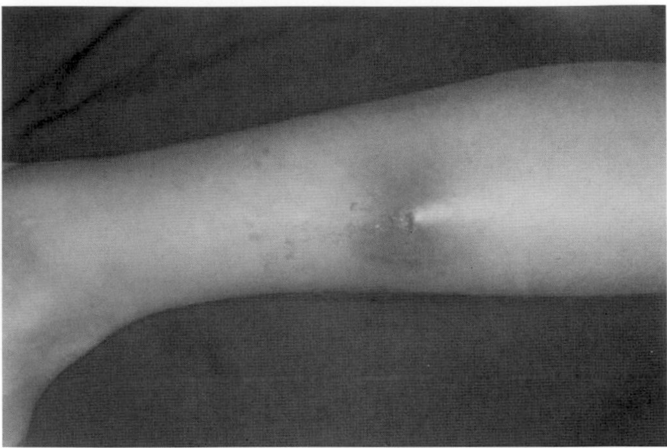

FIGURE 147.5 Abscess of the leg due to a methicillin-susceptible but Panton-Valentine-producing strain of *Staphylococcus aureus* after return from Ivory coast.

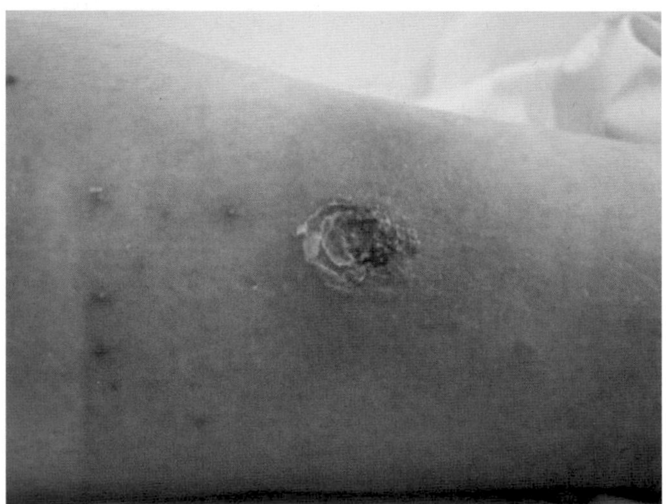

FIGURE 147.3 Limited post-bullous erosion of the leg (impetigo).

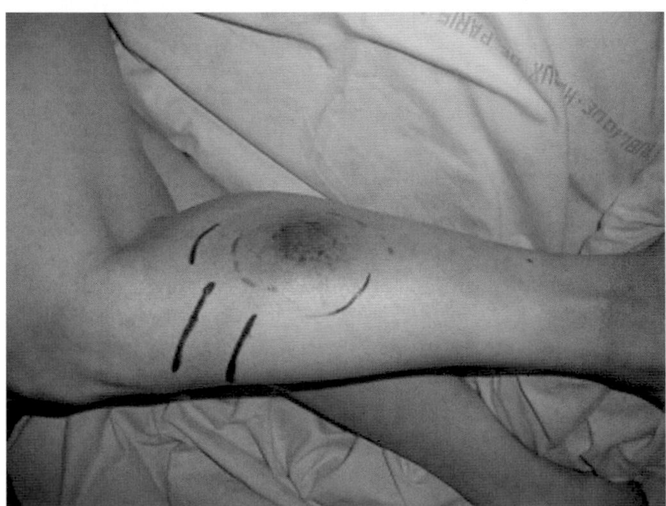

FIGURE 147.6 Cellulitis of the calf associated with a cutaneous trail of lymphangitis.

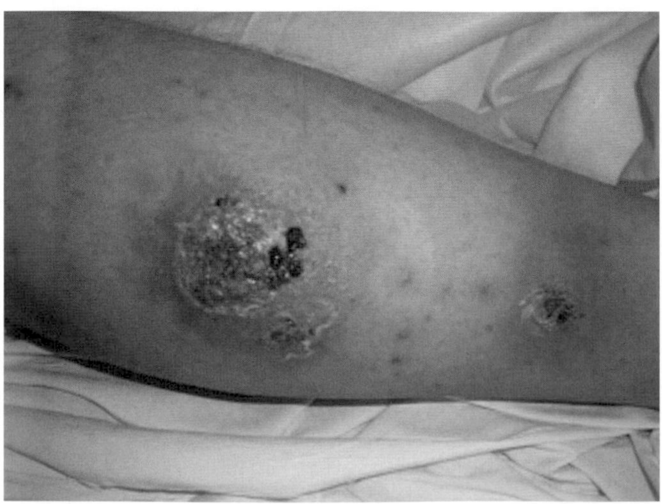

FIGURE 147.4 Large crusted cutaneous lesion of the thigh (ecthyma).

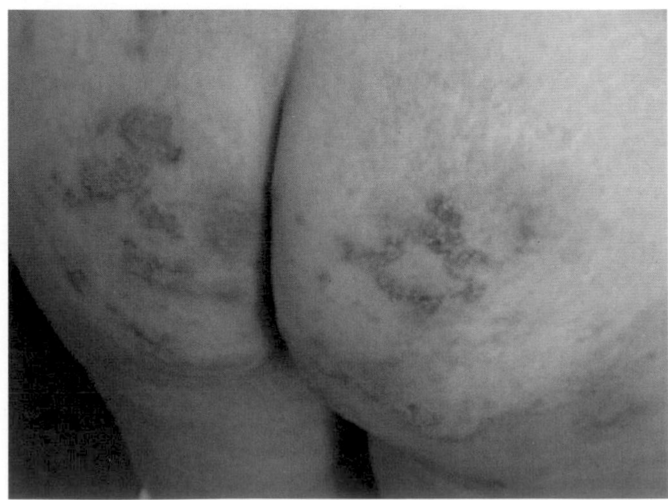

FIGURE 147.7 Creeping dermatitis of the buttocks after return from French West Indies (hookworm-related cutaneous larva migrans).

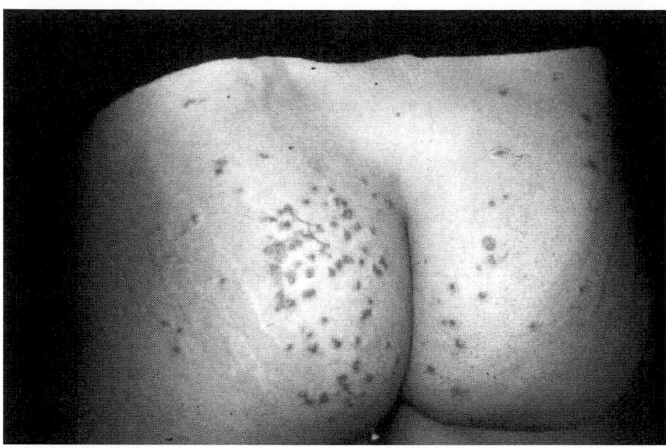

FIGURE 147.8 Creeping dermatitis and folliculitis due to hookworm-related cutaneous larva migrans (return from Thailand).

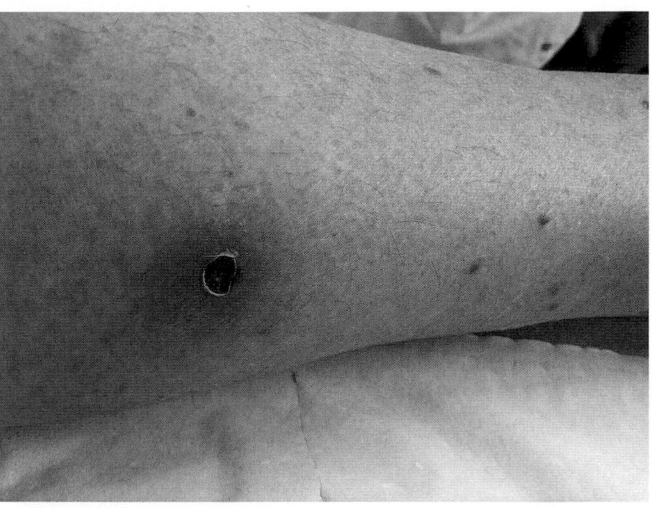

FIGURE 147.10 Eschar of African tick bite fever acquired on walking safari in South Africa.

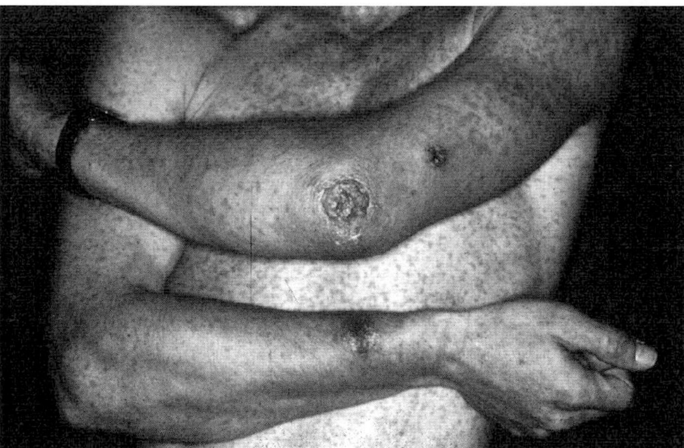

FIGURE 147.9 Chronic cutaneous ulcer due to cutaneous leishmaniasis (return from French Guyana) and febrile exanthem associated with an adverse cutaneous drug reaction secondary to amoxicillin.

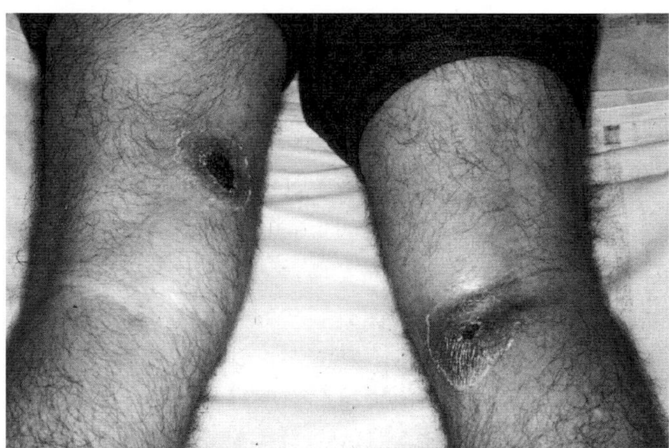

FIGURE 147.11 Acute cutaneous ulcer of West African trypanosomiasis due to *T. brucei gambiense* (trypanosomal chancre) (evacuation from Gabon).

BOX 147.1 Causes of Creeping Eruption in Travelers

- Nematode's larvae
  - Animal hookworms (HrCLM)*, *Pelodera strongyloides*, zoonotic *Strongyloides* spp.
  - Gnathostomiasis (*Gnathostoma* spp.)
  - Larva currens (*Strongyloides stercoralis*)
- Adult nematodes
  - Loiasis (*Loa loa*)
  - Dracunculiasis (*Dracunculus medinensis*)
  - Dirofilariasis (*Dirofilaria immitis*)
- Trematode's larvae
  - Fascioliasis (Fasciola gigantica)
- Fly maggots
  - Migratory myiasis (*Gasterophilus* spp.)
- Mite
  - Scabies (Sarcoptes scabiei)*
  - Pyemotes dermatitis (*Pyemotes ventricosus*)

HrCLM: hookworm-related cutaneous larva migrans.
*Common cause.

BOX 147.2 Causes of Cutaneous Ulcer in Travelers

- Noninfectious causes: spider bite, cupping
- Bacterial infection: ecthyma*, tick eschar* (rickettsiosis), syphilis, anthrax, mycobacterial infection (*M. ulcerans*), melioidosis, glanders, tularemia, cutaneous diphtheria, plague
- Parasitic infection: leishmaniasis*, trypanosomal chancre (African trypanosomiasis), chagoma (American trypanosomiasis), cutaneous amebiasis
- Fungal infection: sporotrichosis, mycetomas, West African histoplasmosis, North American blastomycosis, paracoccidioidomycosis, chromomycosis
- Viral infection: herpes simplex infection

*Common cause.

BOX 147.3 Causes of Fixed Localized Papules and Nodules in Travelers

- Noninfectious: arthropod bites*, sea urchin granuloma, tick granuloma, acne exacerbation
- Bacterial infection: mycobacterial infection (leprosy, tuberculosis)
- Parasitic infection: leishmaniasis*, tungiasis*, myiasis*, scabies*, onchocerciasis, gnathostomiasis, cysticercosis, late cutaneous schistosomiasis, dirofilariasis, paragonimiasis, sparganosis, trypanosomiasis
- Fungal infection: lobomycosis, mycetoma, paracoccidioidomycosis, chromomycosis, sporotrichosis, West African histoplasmosis
- Viral infection: Orf, milker's nodules

*Common cause.

gives rise to a papule then a nodule with a central punctum, and the patient typically complains of a crawling sensation inside the lesion. Cases due to *Cochliomyia hominivorax, Oestrus ovis, C. ruandae* and *C. rodhani* have been seen [4].

Tungiasis is caused by penetration of the gravid female sand flea *Tunga penetrans,* which burrows into the skin of its host, usually on the feet or a toe, where it appears as a slowly growing nodule. The infection is acquired via direct contact (e.g. bare feet) with infested soil or beach sand. Tungiasis (also called chigoe flea, jigger flea) is widely distributed throughout Latin America, the Caribbean, Africa and Asia up to the west coast of India [4].

FIXED AND LOCALIZED PRURITIC ERUPTION

Arthropod-Related Dermatitis

Arthropod-related dermatitis is caused by fleas, sand flies, chiggers, bedbugs, and less commonly mosquitoes, and mites. The bites can result in vesiculobullous lesions, cellulitis-like reactions, papular urticaria and prurigo. Identification of the implicated arthropod can be difficult but is without significant consequence as the treatment is the same. Corticosteroid-based ointments are indicated in mild to moderate cases, whereas systemic corticosteroids can be discussed in more severe cases. Oral antihistamines may improve the symptoms. An antibiotic is usually indicated if secondarily infected.

Contact Dermatitis

Allergic contact dermatitis has been widely reported after contacts with plants such as cashew nut tree, poison ivy/oak (poison ivy dermatitis), mango and pistachio. Irritant contact dermatitis has been described after contacts with moths as well as nocturnal beetles of the genus *Paederus*. Paederus dermatitis, also called blister beetle dermatitis, occurs when nocturnal beetles of the genus *Paederus* (rove beetles) are crushed on the skin. One or 2 days after crushing the insect and release of paederin, linear, erythematous plaques with a "burnt" aspect, and the appearance of vesicles or pustules occurs [7]. The lesions are usually on the neck, face or arms. Contact with the conjunctiva and/or cornea can induce severe eye disease ("Nairobi eye"). In the case of irritant dermatitis, the irritant should be removed by washing.

Phytophotodermatitis is a cutaneous phototoxic reaction that occurs after contact with a variety of plant substances (e.g. limes, lemons) followed by sunlight exposure. The acute presentation is similar to sunburn but with well-delimited and circumcised erythema and vesicles. Secondarily the involved skin has marked hyperpigmentation [8].

Dermatophytosis

Dermatophytes are distributed worldwide but their incidence is higher in the tropics. They rank among the most common skin diseases observed after travel abroad [2–4]. They can present as tinea corporis (infection of the non-hairy glabrous skin), tinea cruris and axillaris (infection of the groin or axillae), tinea of the feet (the most common dermatophytic infection) and tinea capitis (often in children returning from visiting friends and relatives or adopted in Africa) [4].

OTHER LOCALIZED DERMATOLOGIC SYNDROMES

The most frequent cause of nodular lymphangitis (defined by the presence of nodular and/or ulcerative lesions distributed along the line of lymphatic drainage) is leishmaniasis and bacterial lymphangitis. Localized erythematous edema can be due to a cellulitis-like reaction after an insect bite or a bacterial cellulitis [4]. Marine dermatitis or envenomation can be traced to contact with jellyfish, fire coral, stone fish, sea anemones, urchins, or other sea creatures.

DISSEMINATED SKIN DISEASES

FEBRILE EXANTHEM

A febrile exanthem deserves particular attention because it can reveal potentially life-threatening disease (Box 147.4). The main etiologies are arboviruses, usually dengue fever, and rickettsioses, often African tick bite fever [9].

Chikungunya and dengue rashes are difficult to differentiate; both have diffuse (potentially pruritic) macular or maculopapular exanthems in which small islands of skin are spared. Arthralgia is more frequent with chikungunya, and leukopenia and thrombocytopenia is more frequent in dengue [9]. Other less common arboviral diseases presenting with fever and rash (e.g. West Nile and O'Nyong Nyong) could be involved.

African tick bite fever (ATBF) is the most commonly encountered rickettsiosis in travelers, mostly in those returning from rural subequatorial Africa [4]. ATBF can occur in clusters of travelers exposed to *Amblyomma* ticks during game hunting, safaris, adventure races, and military exercises. Clinical presentation includes fever, headache, neck myalgia, one to several inoculation eschars (see Fig. 147.10), maculopapular or vesicular cutaneous rash, and regional adenopathy. It is usually a mild disease. Other rickettsioses that may be observed in travelers are Rocky Mountain spotted fever (in Americas), Mediterranean spotted fever (in Mediterranean Europe, Africa and Asia), scrub typhus (in rural south and southeastern Asia and the western Pacific), and murine typhus (in tropical and subtropical regions).

Other life-threatening infections include meningococcal disease, toxic staphylococcal and streptococcal infection, leptospirosis and other rickettsioses [4,9]. Although rare, viral hemorrhagic fevers (VHFs) such as Lassa, Marburg and Ebola, Rift Valley fever, and Crimean-Congo hemorrhagic fever, have been reported in travelers [4,10]. Yellow fever should also be suspected in non-vaccinated travelers returning from areas of endemicity.

Hypersensitivity reaction to drugs must always be considered in the diagnosis of fever and exanthem (see Fig. 147.9).

URTICARIA

Acute schistosomiasis (Katayama fever) is a leading cause of urticaria in a traveler [4]. Acute urticaria can also be seen during the invasive phase of other helminth infections such as ascariasis, strongyloidiasis or fascioliasis, whereas chronic urticaria is more often related to toxocariasis and trichinosis (Box 147.5). Hypersensitivity reaction to drugs and, less commonly, viral hepatitis A can be considered in the differential diagnosis of acute urticaria.

BOX 147.4 Causes of Febrile Exanthem in Travelers

- Noninfectious causes: adverse drug reaction*
- Viral infection: dengue*, chikungunya*, other arboviral infections, measles, rubella, HIV, EBV and cytomegalovirus primary infection, viral hemorrhagic fever
- Bacterial infection : rickettsial infections*, typhoid, meningococcemia (purpura), syphilis, rat-bite fever, leptospirosis, brucellosis
- Parasitic infection : African trypanosomiasis, trichinellosis, toxoplasmosis

*Common cause.

BOX 147.5 Causes of Urticaria in Travelers

- Noninfectious causes: adverse drug reaction*
- Viral infection: hepatitis A infection
- Parasitic infection: invasive phase of helminthic diseases (ascariasis, hookworm, strongyloidiasis, anisakiasis, gnathostomiasis, schistosomiasis*, fascioliasis), chronic helminthic infections where humans are dead end host (trichinellosis, toxocariasis) and rupture of cyst during hydatid disease

*Common cause.

DISSEMINATED PRURITUS WITH OR WITHOUT RASH

Scabies is the most common cause of diffuse pruritic skin disease [4]. The patient complains of generalized and intense itching, worsening at night, usually sparing the face and head. Specific skin findings include 5- to 10-mm burrows, and papulonodular genital lesions. The classic distribution of lesions are the interdigital web spaces, flexor surfaces of the wrists, the elbows, the axillae, the buttocks and genitalia, and on the breasts of women. Other skin changes are secondary to pruritus and include excoriation and lichenification.

Ciguatera is a cause of localized pruritic neurosensory manifestations (perioral and distal extremity paresthesias) without cutaneous manifestations. There should be a history of fish consumption, other cases among travelers sharing the same meal, a short incubation period (2–30 hours), and the association of gastrointestinal and neurological signs. The latter can last for months after the initial event. This fish poisoning is acquired by the ingestion of fish containing the toxins produced by the dinoflagellate *Gambierdiscus toxicus*, which is found in damaged coral reef systems in tropical and subtropical regions.

Seabather's eruption (also called sea lice) is a highly pruritic maculopapular eruption that occurs after swimming in the ocean and is generally confined to the skin under swimwear. It is caused by larval forms of sea anemones (e.g. *Edwardsiella lineata*) and jellyfish (e.g. *Linuche unguiculata*) that become trapped under swimwear.

Cercarial dermatitis (swimmer's itch) is also a pruritic maculopapular eruption but is predominantly distributed on uncovered body areas. It results from penetration of the skin by cercariae of nonhuman schistosomes while swimming in fresh water. It can last for several days.

From the "skin" point of view, travelers must be instructed to avoid arthropod bites, sun overexposure, walking barefoot, and scratching in the case of pruritus. They should be up-to-date against tetanus. Travel first aid kits should include insect repellents, corticosteroid ointments, and appropriate dressings and bandages. Travelers can consider carrying antibiotics to treat streptococcal and staphylococcal skin infection.

REFERENCES

1. Caumes E, Carriere J, Guermonprez G, et al. Dermatoses associated with travel to tropical countries: a prospective study of the diagnosis and management of 269 patients presenting to a tropical disease unit. Clin Infect Dis 1995;20: 542–8.
2. Ansart S, Perez L, Jaureguiberry S, et al. Spectrum of dermatoses in 165 travelers returning from the tropics with skin diseases. Am J Trop Med Hyg 2007; 76:184–6.
3. Lederman ER, Weld LH, Elyazar IR, et al. Dermatologic conditions of the ill returned traveler: an analysis from the GeoSentinel Surveillance Network. Int J Infect Dis 2008;12:593–602.
   Information form the GeoSentinel global network of travel and tropical medicine clinics. Allows destination-specific comparison of risk.
4. Hochedez P, Caumes E. Common skin infections in travelers. J Travel Med 2008;15:223–33.
   Comprehensive review of skin conditions in returned travelers.
5. Hochedez P, Canestri A, Lecso M, et al. Skin and soft tissue infections in returning travelers. Am J Trop Med Hyg 2009;80:431–4.
6. Hochedez P, Caumes E. Hookworm-related cutaneous larva migrans. J Travel Med 2007;14:339–46.
7. Dursteler BB, Nyquist RA. Outbreak of rove beetle (Staphylinid) pustular contact dermatitis in Pakistan among deployed U.S. personnel. Mil Med 2004;169:57–60.
8. Weber IC, Davis CP, Greeson DM. Phytophotodermatitis: the other "lime" disease. J Emerg Med 1999;17:235–7.
9. Hochedez P, Canestri A, Guihot A, et al. Management of travelers with fever and exanthema, notably dengue and chikungunya infections. Am J Trop Med Hyg 2008;78:710–13.
10. Beeching NJ, Fletcher TE, Hill DR, Thomson GL. Travellers and viral haemorrhagic fevers: what are the risks? Int J Antimicrob Agents 2010;36:S26–35.

148 Eosinophilia in Migrants and Returned Travelers: A Practical Approach

Anna M Checkley, Christopher JM Whitty

Key features

- All individuals returning from tropical areas should be investigated with stool microscopy for ova and parasites and strongyloides serology. An HIV test should be considered
- Individuals returning from Africa should in addition be investigated with schistosomiasis and filariasis serology and microscopy of filtered urine for schistosoma ova
- In those returning from West Africa, day blood microscopy for microfilaria should additionally be performed and night bloods for microfilaria and skin snips for onchocerciasis should be considered

INTRODUCTION

Eosinophilia, defined here as an absolute eosinophil count greater than 0.45×10^9/L, occurs in about 10% of migrants and travelers returning from the tropics who seek post-travel care [1]. In this group, the presence of eosinophilia usually signifies an underlying helminth infection [2], most frequently with a nematode (round worm, e.g. *Ascaris*) or trematode (fluke, e.g. schistosomiasis) [3].

The cause of eosinophilia varies depending on the patient group and regions visited. Eosinophilia is often higher in travelers, most of whom have been recently infected with helminths, than in chronically infected migrants [4]. Certain helminth infections, such as Katayama syndrome, tropical pulmonary eosinophilia and strongyloides infection are also associated with a higher eosinophilia ($>2 \times 10^9$/L), as are multiple helminth infections. The prevalence of imported helminth infections is highly dependent on the geographic area visited, and this is reflected in published case series in migrants and travelers. Studies from North America, where many migrants are from Asia and Latin America, report a higher proportion of strongyloides infection [5]. Those from Europe, where a higher proportion of travelers and migrants are from Africa, report more schistosomiasis [2].

It is important to investigate eosinophilia in returning travelers and migrants; although helminth infections are often self-limiting and cause little harm, they occasionally cause long-term health problems. For example, strongyloides infection can result in a dangerous hyperinfection syndrome [5], and schistosomiasis is occasionally associated with bladder carcinoma.

Eosinophilia has numerous noninfectious causes, most commonly drugs, atopy (asthma and eczema) and allergy. These and uncommon but serious noninfectious causes such as hemopoietic malignancies and connective tissue disorders are summarized in Table 148-1. Long-standing moderate-/high-grade eosinophilia ($>1.5 \times 10^9$/L) can itself result in end-organ damage.

GENERAL PRINCIPLES

HISTORY AND PHYSICAL EXAMINATION

A medical history can establish which parasites the individual may have been exposed to. This is mainly determined by the geographic regions they have visited. This should be noted in detail, including travel within the country (urban or rural), activities undertaken, and the timings of these events. A history of relevant exposures should also be sought, including swimming in fresh water, particularly in Africa (schistosomiasis), barefoot exposure to soil or sand (strongyloidiasis, hookworm), food consumed (parasites of uncooked seafood or meat) and occupation (hydatid disease in sheep farmers). It should be kept in mind, however, that risk factors for exposure to infectious agents are frequently underreported. Eosinophilia can be asymptomatic, but symptoms such as fever, cough, diarrhea, dysuria and rash should be specifically queried. The possibility of a noninfectious cause should be explored by taking a careful drug history, and asking about pre-existing medical conditions such as allergic rhinitis or asthma.

Physical examination is not helpful in reaching a diagnosis in many cases [6], but attention should be paid to the presence of rashes suggestive of skin conditions that can result in eosinophilia; other disease-specific findings are mentioned below.

LABORATORY INVESTIGATIONS

Laboratory investigations, guided by the geographic area of travel, are the key to the effective diagnosis of eosinophilia. The timing at which tests are taken in the course of helminth infection is particularly important in interpreting the results. Eosinophilia is often greatest during the tissue migration phase of the parasite, for example in Katayama syndrome, before eggs can be detected in the stool. The period before eggs can be detected is termed the ***pre-patent period***, and it is important to be aware that during this phase, samples for microscopy for ova or parasites may be negative. Eosinophilia can be transient, or absent from helminth infections without a tissue migration stage of infection, for example the beef tapeworm *Taenia saginata*. Therefore, the absence of eosinophilia does not exclude helminth infection.

Direct Microscopy

Concentrated stool microscopy identifies most soil-transmitted helminths (e.g. *Ascaris lumbricoides, Trichuris trichiura*, hookworm spp.) and is useful in patients from all geographic areas. However, it has a low sensitivity in detecting strongyloides. Microscopy of urine for *Schistosoma haematobium* and of filtered blood for filarial infections is useful in patients from relevant geographic areas.

Serology

Most serologic tests do not become positive until 4–12 weeks after infection, so can be negative when eosinophilia is first detected. It may be worth repeating serologic investigations at 3 months if they were initially negative and eosinophilia persists. Many serologic tests

TABLE 148-1 Noninfectious Causes of Peripheral Eosinophilia

Cause						
Atopy	*Dermatologic*	*Drug*	*Gastrointestinal*	*Hematologic*	*Vasculitis*	*Other*
Asthma	Immunobullous disorders: dermatitis herpetiformis and pemphigoid	NSAIDs	Inflammatory bowel disease	Hodgkin lymphoma	Churg–Strauss syndrome	Allergic bronchopulmonary aspergillosis
Eczema	Atopic dermatitis	Beta-lactam antibiotics	Eosinophilic gastroenteritis	Non-Hodgkin lymphoma	Polyarteritis nodosa	Sarcoidosis
Allergic rhinitis	Eosinophilic cellulitis (Well's syndrome)	Sulfa-containing antibiotics	Chronic pancreatitis	Chronic eosinophilic leukemia	Wegener's granulomatosis	Addison's disease
Seasonal rhinitis		Tetracycline	Eosinophilic cholangitis	Systemic mastocytosis	Other connective tissue diseases and vasculitides	Eosinophilic myocarditis
		Acetylsalicylic acid		Chronic myelomonocytic leukemia	Rheumatoid arthritis	Familial eosinophilic syndromes
		Carbamazepine		Chronic myeloid leukemia		Heavy metal poisoning
		Colchicine		Acute myeloid leukemia		Idiopathic eosinophilic pneumonias
		Nitrofurantoin		Myelodysplastic syndrome		Immunodeficiency syndromes
		Dapsone				Cholesterol embolization
		Minocycline				

NSAIDs, nonsteroidal anti-inflammatory drugs.

for helminths cross-react, so taking expert advice is recommended. Table 148-2 outlines common helminths, their microscopic appearance, diagnostic tests and treatments.

MANAGEMENT

The management of certain important conditions is outlined below, and is covered in greater detail in disease-specific chapters and in Table 148-2. Empiric albendazole (400 mg twice daily for 3 days) is recommended by some experts for those recently returned from the tropics, to cover the possibility of pre-patent geohelminth infection (e.g. *Ascaris* and hookworm) as the cause of a transient eosinophilia with negative stool microscopy.

FOLLOW-UP ISSUES

Eosinophilia should resolve following the treatment of the underlying cause, and it is important to establish that this has happened. Occasionally, a finding such as positive schistosoma serology in a long-term resident of an endemic area can be mistaken to be the cause of eosinophilia, when in fact there is another cause. Serology often remains positive for many years, and is not a good measure of effective treatment.

CLINICAL SYNDROMES

ASYMPTOMATIC EOSINOPHILIA

We suggest investigating this common presentation [3] of helminth infection from the basis of the travel history, and therefore the geographic distribution of helminth infections. The soil-transmitted helminths *Ascaris lumbricoides, Trichuris trichiura* and hookworm have a worldwide distribution. Others, especially those with a life cycle involving an intermediate host or vector, or those associated with certain foods, have defined geographic limits. The most common pathogens causing eosinophilia in all returned travelers and migrants are intestinal helminths, especially strongyloidiasis, and in those returning from Africa, schistosomiasis and filariasis in addition.

All patients presenting with eosinophilia should be investigated with concentrated stool microscopy and strongyloides serology [2]. Strongyloides stool culture and an HIV test should also be considered. Other initial screening investigations are region-specific. Terminal urine microscopy (for ova) and serology for schistosomiasis should be performed in those returning from Africa. The filarial infections *Loa loa, Onchocerca volvulus* and *Wuchereria bancrofti* are more common in patients from West Africa, so filarial serology and filtered blood microscopy for microfilaria should be requested (see "dermatologic presentations").

If initially negative, stool microscopy should be performed on a total of three occasions, and serology should be repeated at 3 months if it was first taken less than 12 weeks after the time of probable exposure. If initial investigations are negative, attention should also be paid to the possibility of noninfectious causes. An empiric course of albendazole can be considered.

Table 148-3 lists common helminth infections by geographic area and summarizes clinical presentations.

FEVER AND/OR RESPIRATORY SYMPTOMS

Katayama Syndrome

This occurs during acute schistosomiasis infection 2–9 weeks following exposure [7]. It presents with fever and high-grade eosinophilia ($>5 \times 10^9$/L), dry cough, urticarial rash and sometimes pulmonary infiltrates on chest radiograph. Serology and stool and terminal urine microscopy are often negative. Empiric treatment can be given when this presentation is accompanied by a history of freshwater exposure in Africa: praziquantel 40 mg/kg single dose and oral prednisolone 20 mg/day for 5 days. Praziquantel is relatively ineffective against immature stages of schistosomiasis, so treatment should be repeated at 6–8 weeks.

Loeffler's Syndrome

The relatively rare Loeffler's syndrome is caused by larvae of helminths such as *Ascaris*, hookworm and *Strongyloides* migrating through the lungs during acute infection. It presents similarly to Katayama syndrome, with fever, urticaria, wheeze and dry cough. Diagnosis is clinical as symptoms occur before eggs can be detected in the stool. Migratory pulmonary infiltrates may be seen on chest radiograph. Albendazole 400 mg/day for 3 days is recommended.

GASTROINTESTINAL/GENITOURINARY SYMPTOMS

Strongyloidiasis

This is widely distributed throughout the tropics. It is transmitted when larvae penetrate the skin of humans walking barefoot. It often presents with larva currens, an itchy, linear, urticarial rash which

TABLE 148-2 Microscopic Appearance, Distribution, Diagnosis and Treatment of the More Common Imported Helminth Infections

Name	Picture	Geographic distribution	Diagnosis	Treatment
Ankylostoma duodenale/ Necator americanus (hookworm)		Worldwide	Concentrated stool microscopy	Albendazole 400 mg single dose
Ascaris lumbricoides (ascariasis, roundworm)		Worldwide	Concentrated stool microscopy	Albendazole 400 mg single dose (mebendazole 500 mg single dose)
Echinococcus granulosus (hydatid)		Worldwide	Serology	Seek specialist advice. Combination of praziquantel 20 mg/kg twice daily for 14 days pre- and post-procedure, prolonged course of albendazole 400 mg twice daily, PAIR, surgery
Loa loa (eye worm)		Africa (Central and West predominantly)	Microscopy of blood taken within 2 h of midday, serology	Seek specialist advice. First exclude coexisting onchocerciasis. DEC 50 mg day 1 increasing by day 4 to 200 mg three times daily which is then given for 3 weeks; pretreat with prednisolone if microfilariae seen on blood film
Onchocerca volvulus (river blindness, onchocerciasis)		Africa (Central and West predominantly)	Skin snips (specialist centers), filarial serology	Ivermectin 200 µg/kg monthly doses for 3 months, repeat every 3–6 months usually for several years; seek ophthalmologic advice; observe first dose
Schistosoma haematobium (schistosomiasis)		Africa (*S. haematobium/S. mansoni*) Southeast Asia (other species)	Microscopy of nitrocellulose-filtered terminal urine (*S. haematobium*), concentrated stool microscopy (*S. mansoni* and other species), serology (all species)	Praziquantel 40 mg single dose
S. mansoni (schistosomiasis)				
Strongyloides stercoralis (strongyloidiasis)*		Worldwide	Concentrated stool microscopy, serology, stool culture (charcoal or agar plate method)	Ivermectin 200 µg/kg (single dose albendazole 400 mg twice daily for 3 days)
Wucheria bancrofti/ Brugia malayi (lymphatic filariasis)		Worldwide, tropical (*W. bancrofti*), South/Southeast Asia (*B. malayi*)	Microscopy of blood taken within 2 h of midnight, serology	Seek specialist advice. First exclude coexisting onchocerciasis. DEC 50 mg day 1 increasing by day 4 to 200 mg three times daily, which is then given for 3 weeks

DEC, diethylcarbamazine; PAIR, puncture, aspiration of cyst contents, injection of a substance toxic to the immature "scolices" and re-aspiration.
Figures are reproduced courtesy of the Centers for Disease Control and Prevention (CDC), apart from *Ascaris lumbricoides* which is courtesy of Kansas State University, *Echinococcus granulosus* which is courtesy of CDC and Dr LLA Moore Jr, *Onchocerca volvulus* which is kindly provided by Eric A T Bienen, Department of Parasitology, Leiden University Medical Centre, and *Wuchereria bancrofti* which is courtesy of CDC and Dr Mae Melvin.

TABLE 148-3 Common Helminth Infections Summarized by Geographic Area and Clinical Presentation

Helminth	Common name/ syndrome	Distribution	Respiratory	Gastrointestinal	Hepatic	Neurological	Cutaneous/ muscular	Other
Ancylostoma duodenale	Hookworm	Worldwide	Wheeze, dry cough (Loeffler's syndrome)	Nausea, vomiting, diarrhea, abdominal pain			Transient itch/ maculopapular rash	Fever (Loeffler's syndrome)
Ancylostoma spp.	Cutaneous larva migrans	Worldwide, tropical only					Serpiginous rash	
Angiostrongylus cantonensis	Eosinophilic meningitis, rat lung worm	SE Asia, Oceania, Caribbean				Severe headache, meningism, focal neurological signs		
Angiostrongylus costaricensis		South America, Caribbean		Severe abdominal pain, diarrhea, constipation				
Anisakis spp.	Fish tapeworm	SE Asia, S America, Europe		Severe abdominal pain, nausea and vomiting				Anaphylaxis
Ascaris lumbricoides	Roundworm	Worldwide	Wheeze, dry cough (Loeffler's syndrome)	Abdominal pain, diarrhea	Biliary obstruction		Urticarial rash (Loeffler's syndrome)	Fever (Loeffler's syndrome)
Brugia malayi	Lymphatic filariasis	SE Asia, S Asia, Oceania	Dry cough, wheeze, breathlessness (tropical pulmonary eosinophilia)				Lymphadenitis, lymphedema	Fever (tropical pulmonary eosinophilia)
Clonorchis sinensis	Clonorchiasis	SE Asia			Hepatomegaly, biliary obstruction, (acute) Abdominal pain (acute), cholangiocarcinoma (chronic)		Urticarial skin rash	Fever
Coccidioides immitis	Coccidioidomycosis	South, Central and North America	Fever, cough, pleuritic chest pain			Chronic meningitis	Rash	
Echinococcus granulosus	Cystic hydatid	Worldwide	Cough, pleuritic pain, breathlessness		Asymptomatic/right upper quadrant pain			Anaphylaxis
Echinococcus multilocularis	Alveolar hydatid	Middle East, SE Asia, Central Asia, Europe			Asymptomatic/right upper quadrant pain			Disseminated infection to any organ late in infection
Enterobius vermicularis	Pinworm/threadworm	Worldwide		Diarrhea, abdominal pain, weight loss			Pruritus ani	Vaginal discharge
Fasciola hepatica	Fascioliasis	Worldwide			Upper abdominal pain (acute), biliary obstruction and hepatic abscesses (chronic)			Fever
Gnathostoma spinigerum	Gnathostomiasis	SE Asia, Central and South America, Caribbean		Abdominal pain		Severe meningoencephalitis and myelitis, focal neurology, subarachnoid and intracerebral hemorrhage	Intermittent subcutaneous swelling, pruritus, edema	
Hymenolepis nana	Dwarf tapeworm	Worldwide, tropical only		Diarrhea, abdominal pain				
Loa loa	Eye worm, Calabar swelling	Africa (Central and West predominantly)					Calabar swelling	Conjunctival worm migration
Necator americanus	Hookworm	Worldwide	Wheeze, dry cough (Loeffler's syndrome)	Nausea, vomiting, diarrhea, abdominal pain			Transient itch/ maculopapular rash	Fever (Loeffler's syndrome)
Onchocerca volvulus	Onchocerciasis/river blindness	Africa (Central and West predominantly), Middle East, Central Asia, Central and South America					Nodules, pruritic dermatitis, limb swelling	Keratitis, anterior uveitis, choroidoretinitis

Opisthorchis spp.	Opisthorchiasis	SE Asia, Europe (Siberia)			Hepatomegaly, biliary obstruction, (acute) Abdominal pain (acute), cholangiocarcinoma (chronic)		Urticarial skin rash	Fever
Paracoccidioides brasiliensis	Paracoccidioidomycosis	South, Central and North America	Cough, night sweats, weight loss, malaise			Chronic meningitis	Ulcerative oral/nasal/ cutaneous lesions	
Paragonimus spp.	Paragonimiasis	Africa (Central and West predominantly), SE Asia, Central and South America	Pleuritic chest pain, pleural effusion, cough, hemoptysis	Abdominal pain, diarrhea		Meningoencephalitis, transverse myelitis, myelopathy	Subcutaneous migratory nodules	
Pseudoterranova decipiens	Fish tapeworm	SE Asia, South America and Europe		Severe abdominal pain, nausea and vomiting				
Schistosoma haematobium	Bilharzia/Katayama fever	Africa (all), Middle East and Central Asia	Dry cough (Katayama fever)			Paraplegia, spinal cord syndromes	Urticarial rash (Katayama fever)	Fever (Katayama fever), hematuria, proteinuria, dysuria, hematospermia
Schistosoma japonicum	Bilharzia/Katayama fever	SE Asia	Dry cough (Katayama fever)	Abdominal pain, diarrhea	Hepatosplenomegaly, portal hypertension	Focal neurological signs/ seizures	Urticarial rash (Katayama fever)	Fever (Katayama fever)
Schistosoma mansoni	Bilharzia/Katayama fever	Africa (all), South America, Caribbean, Middle East and Central Asia	Dry cough (Katayama fever)	Abdominal pain, diarrhea	Hepatosplenomegaly, portal hypertension	Paraplegia, spinal cord syndromes	Urticarial rash (Katayama fever)	Fever (Katayama fever)
Schistosoma spp	Cercarial dermatitis	Worldwide					Itchy maculopapular rash	
Strongyloides stercoralis	Strongyloidiasis	Worldwide	Wheeze, dry cough (Loeffler's syndrome), hyperinfestation syndrome	Diarrhea, abdominal pain, bloating, hyperinfestation syndrome			Itchy urticarial rash (larva currens)	Fever (Loeffler's syndrome)
Taenia saginata	Beef tapeworm	Worldwide		Abdominal pain, diarrhea, segments expelled per rectum				
Taenia solium	Pork tapeworm, cysticercosis	Worldwide, tropical only		Abdominal pain, diarrhea, segments expelled per rectum		Usually space-occupying lesions without eosinophilia. Rarely eosinophilic meningoencephalitis		
Toxocara canis/ cati	Visceral larva migrans	Worldwide	Wheeze, cough	Abdominal pain	Hepatosplenomegaly	Meningoencephalitis		
Trichinella spiralis	Trichinellosis/ trichinosis	Worldwide		Upper abdominal pain, fever, vomiting, diarrhea Dysphagia		Meningoencephalitis	Periorbital edema, urticaria, myalgia, muscle weakness	Myocarditis, cardiac conduction disturbances
Trichuris trichiura	Whipworm	Worldwide		Diarrhea Dysentery			Myalgia, muscle weakness, edema, urticarial rash	
Wuchereria bancrofti	Lymphatic filariasis/ tropical pulmonary eosinophilia	Worldwide, tropical only	Dry cough, wheeze, breathlessness (tropical pulmonary eosinophilia)				Lymphadenitis, lymphedema	Fever (tropical pulmonary eosinophilia)

(dark shading)	More commonly imported condition
(medium shading)	Usual presentation
(light shading)	Uncommon presentation

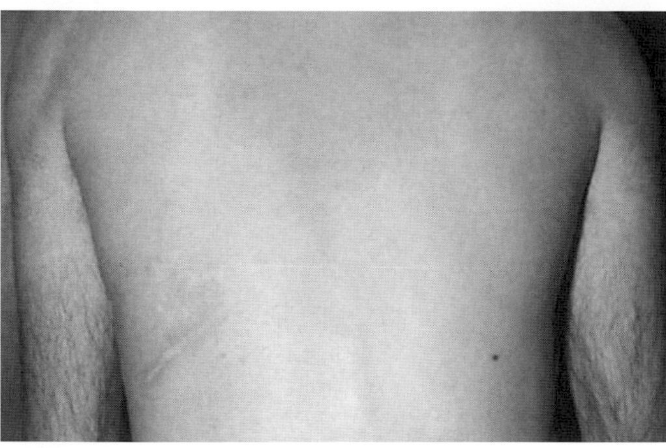

FIGURE 148.1 Linear, urticarial rash of *larva currens*. *(Reproduced courtesy of the Centers for Disease Control and Prevention.)*

typically moves several millimeters per second (Fig. 148.1). Nonspecific gastrointestinal symptoms include diarrhea and abdominal bloating. In immunocompromised individuals, strongyloides can present decades after exposure as *hyperinfection syndrome* [6] with paralytic ileus and Gram-negative sepsis. This condition is due to uncontrolled replication of the parasite and is life-threatening.

Diagnosis of strongyloides infection can be difficult: serology is usually the most sensitive test and stool microscopy is often negative. The reverse applies in the hyperinfection syndrome, where stool samples contain abundant larvae but serology may be negative and eosinophilia absent. Stool culture (performed in specialist laboratories) is recommended. Treatment is with a single dose of ivermectin 200 μg/kg, or (less effective) albendazole 400 mg twice daily for 3 days [8]. Hyperinfection should be treated with a prolonged course. Migrants from all tropical regions should be screened for strongyloides before starting treatment with immunosuppressive drugs.

Soil-Transmitted Helminths (Geohelminths)

These have a worldwide distribution but are most prevalent in the tropics. *Ascaris* and *Trichuris* are transmitted via the fecal–oral route, and hookworm is acquired when larvae penetrate the skin of humans walking barefoot on affected soil. They are often asymptomatic. Hookworm may present with a transient itch and maculopapular rash, followed weeks later by nausea, vomiting, diarrhea and abdominal pain. *Ascaris* may present as Loeffler's syndrome, or weeks later with abdominal pain, diarrhea, and occasionally gastrointestinal or biliary obstruction. Visible worms may be passed in stools. *Trichuris* infection is usually asymptomatic, but heavy infections can cause morbidity in children, including anemia, dysentery and rectal prolapse. All are diagnosed by concentrated stool microscopy. Ascaris and hookworm are treated with a single dose of albendazole 400 mg; trichuriasis requires albendazole 400–800 mg twice daily 3 days.

Schistosomiasis/Bilharzia: *Schistosoma mansoni, S. japonicum* and *S. haematobium*

Schistosomiasis is widely distributed, particularly in Africa (*S. haematobium* and *S. mansoni*) and Southeast Asia (*S. japonicum*) [9]. It is acquired following freshwater exposure, usually swimming. Infection is often asymptomatic. *S. haematobium* affects the genitourinary system and can present with hematuria, proteinuria, dysuria and hematospermia. *S. mansoni* and *S. japonicum* affect the gastrointestinal tract and can present with abdominal pain or diarrhea; portal hypertension and hepatosplenomegaly occur in chronic infection. Schistosomiasis is diagnosed by serology and microscopy of either nitrocellulose-filtered terminal urine (*S. haematobium*) or concentrated stool samples (*S. mansoni* and *S. japonicum*). Treatment is with praziquantel 40mg/kg. *S. haematobium* infection has been linked to squamous cell carcinoma of the bladder, and heavy infections require further investigation.

Hydatid

Hydatid disease is most often seen in individuals returning from sheep-rearing areas, especially the Middle East, although it also occurs in North and East Africa, Asia, Europe and the Americas. Affected individuals are usually asymptomatic; eosinophilia, right upper quadrant pain, and fever can indicate cyst leakage or infection. Diagnosis is by serology with characteristic appearances on ultrasound or computed tomography (CT). Treatment depends on factors such as cyst size, location and stage [10,11]. Options include "PAIR" (puncture, aspiration of cyst contents, injection of a substance toxic to the immature "scolices" and re-aspiration), prolonged albendazole, surgery, or a combination of methods. Surgical and percutaneous intervention carry a risk of anaphylaxis and cyst dissemination, and should be performed in specialist centers.

Liver Flukes

Liver flukes including *Fasciola hepatica, Clonorchis sinensis* and *Opisthorchis* spp. typically present with hepatomegaly and symptoms of bile duct obstruction such as right upper quadrant pain and jaundice. They are diagnosed by stool microscopy (low sensitivity in fasciola infection) and serology, and treated with triclabendazole (*Fasciola*) and praziquantel (*Opisthorchis* and *Clonorchis*).

NEUROLOGICAL SYMPTOMS

Rarely, parasites invade the central nervous system (CNS) and cause an eosinophilic meningitis, encephalitis or myelitis. The commonest cause of eosinophilic meningitis is *Angiostrongylus cantonensis*, the rat lung worm. This occurs in the Caribbean, Hawaii and Southeast Asia, and is acquired following the ingestion of larvae in undercooked snails, prawns, crabs or frogs. It presents with severe acute headache, meningism, visual disturbance, paresthesias and cranial nerve palsies. Gnathostomiasis is less common, occurring in Southeast Asia. It is acquired by consuming inadequately cooked fish, frog, snake or chicken, and presents with a severe meningoencephalitis and myelitis, which can be fatal. Diagnosis of both infections is by serology; treatment is with albendazole and corticosteroids.

Schistosomiasis can rarely present with CNS involvement. Seizures or focal neurologic signs can occur, most commonly in *S. japonicum* infection. Involvement of the spinal cord, usually with paraplegia, is more widely reported with *S. mansoni* and *S. haematobium*. Treatment consists of an extended course of praziquantel and high-dose steroids.

DERMATOLOGIC PRESENTATIONS

Filariasis: Onchocerciasis, Lymphatic Filariasis and *Loa loa*

The major filariases are onchocerciasis, lymphatic filariasis (*Wucheria bancrofti* and *Brugia malayi*) and *Loa loa*.

Onchocerciasis or river blindness occurs around fast-flowing rivers mainly in Africa. It presents with an itchy rash which over a long period can develop into a "leopard skin" pattern of hypopigmented patches and nodules. Migration of microfilariae within the eye results in keratitis, anterior uveitis and choroidoretinitis, with eventual blindness. Lymphatic filariasis has a worldwide tropical distribution, although it is most common in Africa. Presentation is with fever, lymphangitis, and lymphedema that can include the scrotum. Loiasis occurs mainly in Central and West Africa. It causes migratory soft tissue "Calabar" swellings. Sometimes the adult worm is seen migrating across the conjunctiva [4].

Serology is most sensitive for diagnosing lymphatic filariasis, but can be positive in any of the filariases. Microfilariae of *W. bancrofti*, *B. malayi* and *Loa loa* circulate in the bloodstream with a diurnal periodicity, and can be diagnosed by blood taken around midnight (lymphatic filariasis) or midday (*Loa loa*). In routine practice, day bloods (taken around midday) for microscopy of filtered blood are often adequate. They are the investigation of choice for *Loa loa* and should detect *W. bancrofti*. In difficult cases, bloods taken around midnight have higher sensitivity for *W. bancrofti*. *Loa loa* can also be diagnosed clinically when conjunctival migration is seen. Onchocerciasis can be diagnosed by microscopy of skin snips (shallow snips of skin are taken, then incubated in saline prior to microscopy), or if microfilariae are seen on slit lamp examination of an affected eye.

Treatment is associated with significant risks and should be carried out in specialist centers. Lymphatic filariasis and *Loa loa* are treated with diethylcarbamazine (DEC), after onchocerciasis has been excluded, as DEC can cause severe reactions including blindness in individuals infected with onchocerciasis. Encephalopathy can occur following treatment of *Loa loa*, and prednisolone pretreatment is necessary if there are high levels of microfilariae in the blood. Onchocerciasis is treated with ivermectin 200 μg/kg monthly for 3 months, repeated every 3–6 months usually for several years.

REFERENCES

1. Libman MD, MacLean JD, Gyorkos TW. Screening for schistosomiasis, filariasis, and strongyloidiasis among expatriates returning from the tropics. Clin Infect Dis 1993;17:353–9.
   Large North American series of 1605 returning travelers and migrants, reporting high prevalences of imported schistosomiasis and filariasis. The relative lack of cases of strongyloides is probably due to the fact that the study was performed before strongyloides serology was widely available.
2. Whetham J, Day JN, Armstrong M, et al. Investigation of tropical eosinophilia; assessing a strategy based on geographical area. J Infect 2003;46:180–5.
   Series of 261 patients undergoing investigation of eosinophilia in a London tropical medicine clinic, following return from the tropics. 21% of patients were asymptomatic; the suggested approach to investigating this group is used in this chapter.
3. Schulte C, Krebs B, Jelinek T, et al. Diagnostic significance of blood eosinophilia in returning travelers. Clin Infect Dis 2002;34:407–11.
   Large series of 14,298 returning travelers investigated in a German infectious diseases department. Eosinophilia was defined as greater than 7%, a definition which may overestimate the prevalence of the problem. In common with other studies, they observed a greater prevalence of eosinophilia in returnees from Africa, in particular West Africa, compared to other geographic regions. The greater the degree of eosinophilia, the greater its predictive value for an underlying helminth infection. A definite diagnosis was reached in 36% of individuals. Of note, as is the case in many case series published more than 5 years ago, strongyloides serology was not routinely performed.
4. Nutman TB, Miller KD, Mulligan M, Ottesen EA. *Loa loa* infection in temporary residents of endemic regions: recognition of a hyperresponsive syndrome with characteristic clinical manifestations. J Infect Dis 1986;154:10–8.
5. Gill GV, Welch E, Bailey JW, et al. Chronic *Strongyloides stercoralis* infection in former British Far East prisoners of war. QJM 2004;97:789–95.
6. Whitty CJ, Carroll B, Armstrong M, et al. Utility of history, examination and laboratory tests in screening those returning to Europe from the tropics for parasitic infection. Trop Med Int Health 2000;5:818–23.
7. Visser LG, Polderman AM, Stuiver PC. Outbreak of schistosomiasis among travelers returning from Mali, West Africa. Clin Infect Dis 1995;20:280–5.
8. Marti H, Haji HJ, Savioli L, et al. A comparative trial of a single-dose ivermectin versus three days of albendazole for treatment of *Strongyloides stercoralis* and other soil-transmitted helminth infections in children. Am J Trop Med Hyg 1996;55:477–81.
9. Gryseels B, Polman K, Clerinx J, Kestens L. Human schistosomiasis. Lancet 2006;368:1106–18.
10. Junghanss T, da Silva AM, Horton J, et al. Clinical management of cystic echinococcosis: state of the art, problems, and perspectives. Am J Trop Med Hyg 2008;79:301–11.
11. WHO Informal Working Group on Echinococcosis. Guidelines for treatment of cystic and alveolar echinococcosis in humans. Bull World Health Organ 1996;74:231–42.

Immigrant Medicine 149

Sandra K Schumacher, Elizabeth D Barnett

Key features

- Immigration is increasing and health professionals need to be aware of key health concerns of immigrants and refugees
- Health professionals must consider where the immigrant has lived and traveled prior to arriving in the US. Knowing the immigrant's underlying health status, age, and duration of time in the US is also necessary to determine needs for screening and potential illnesses
- Screening for tuberculosis and hepatitis B are important for all migrants
- Standardized screening protocols can help identify common infectious diseases of immigrants
- Noninfectious processes such as depression and stress are common among immigrants

INTRODUCTION

Almost 200 million people live outside their country of birth – about 3% of the world's population. Between 1965 and 1990, the number of international migrants grew by an annual rate of 2.1%; today this rate is 2.9%. The number of foreign-born individuals living in the US increased from just over 9 million in the 1960s to over 37 million in 2008. The proportion of foreign-born individuals from Europe has decreased, while the proportions of those from Latin America, Asia, and Africa have increased more than tenfold during this period. Health providers must be prepared to address the health issues of immigrants [1].

Health status of immigrants reflects circumstances in their birth countries, exposures and experiences during their route of migration, and the situation at their destination. Infections contracted at birth, such as hepatitis B, may not manifest until decades after migration. Infections contracted in adolescence or adulthood, such as human papillomavirus, can lie dormant until years after migration. The route of migration may increase the risk of infections such as tuberculosis (TB), malaria, or schistosomiasis by exposing individuals to more crowded conditions or to vectors and diseases not present in their region of birth. Health providers must now, more than ever before, be prepared to address infectious diseases that may be unfamiliar or have been eliminated by immunization and public health programs in the area in which they trained.

PRE-DEPARTURE AND POST-ARRIVAL HEALTH ASSESSMENT

Some immigrants may have received health screening or assessment before departure from their birth country. Well-defined procedures for health screening pre- and post-migration to some countries exist for refugees and internationally adopted children, but other groups may have received minimal or no health preparation. Access to healthcare following immigration can be highly variable. Any health professional may see an immigrant for their first contact with the health system, whether a dentist, emergency room nurse or physician, primary care provider, or school nurse [2].

There is general agreement that some screening tests should be performed routinely for all immigrants, based upon prevalence of these conditions, availability and accuracy of screening tests, existence of effective interventions once these conditions are identified, and the potential risk that lack of identification of these conditions poses to both the immigrant and potentially to their contacts (Box 149.1). The first such disease is TB. Since early this century, the largest proportion of new TB cases identified in the US is in immigrants. Elimination of TB in the US and many other countries depends on treating and eliminating TB where it is endemic, but also identifying and treating latent TB infection in new arrivals [3].

Hepatitis B is another condition for which there is general agreement about testing. Recent data indicate that the majority of newly identified cases of hepatitis B in the US are in foreign-born individuals. The Centers for Disease Control and Prevention (CDC) recommends routine testing for hepatitis B infection in all immigrants from areas of the world where prevalence of hepatitis B infection is ≥2%, and for US-born children not immunized at birth whose parents were born where prevalence of hepatitis B infection is ≥8% [4,5].

Additional evaluation of new immigrants, or those who have not received a thorough health assessment in the past, should include complete history and physical examination, including vital signs, hearing, vision, and dental screening, and mental health assessment. Some information may not be revealed until development of a trusting and therapeutic relationship with health professionals, particularly when immigrants have experienced traumatic experiences or are unfamiliar with the US health system and its focus on preventive strategies and health promotion.

Helpful laboratory screening tests include complete blood count with differential (identifies anemia, possible hemoglobinopathy, eosinophilia, or other blood abnormality), urinalysis (identifies hematuria, proteinuria, or glucosuria), and lead levels for children. All immigrants should be offered the same age-appropriate screening and immunizations that are given to US-born individuals. Stool for ova and parasites is appropriate for immigrants from most regions, especially South America, Asia, and Africa; additional serologic tests for

BOX 149.1 Suggested Initial Immigrant Evaluation

Complete history and physical including:
- Vital signs
- Hearing
- Vision
- Dental screening
- Mental health assessment

Basic laboratory screening:
- Complete blood count with differential
- Tuberculin skin test
- Hepatitis B screening (HBSAg, HBSAb, and HBcoreAb)
- When appropriate:
  - Stool examination for ova and parasites
  - Urinalysis
  - Lead level
  - Vitamin D level
  - Parasite serologies

Age-appropriate immunizations or titers to prove immunity

specific parasites may be needed in addition to stool tests for individuals with eosinophilia or with signs or symptoms of parasitic diseases not diagnosed through stool examination. Detailed information about screening and assessment of new immigrants is available from other sources [6,7].

INFECTIOUS DISEASES OF IMMIGRANTS

FEBRILE ILLNESSES

Priority should be given to identifying illnesses that can be fatal rapidly or pose a threat to public health. Delayed diagnosis of *Plasmodium falciparum* malaria can be lethal, and undiagnosed TB or measles can lead to secondary cases.

Fever soon after immigration from malarial countries could be malaria; 90% of *P. falciparum* cases occur within 1 month of arrival. Fever with rash suggests dengue, while fever with rash and arthritis may indicate chikungunya virus. Early fevers may also be due to typhoid and paratyphoid fevers, rickettsial infections, and amebic liver abscesses. Fever months after migration may be caused by TB, primary malarial infection, or relapse of *P. vivax* and *P. ovale.* Many less common infections can be associated with fever, though other accompanying signs and symptoms may suggest these diagnoses. Other febrile illness with short incubation periods, such as influenza or meningococcemia, can occur in immigrants exposed after migration, but may be more relevant to returning travelers [8]. This chapter will focus on infectious diseases that can be seen by clinicians at any time following migration and that are likely to be related to the individual's country of origin or migration process.

PULMONARY

TB is undoubtedly the most important pulmonary infection of immigrants and refugees. All immigrants should have a tuberculin skin test (TST), and those with a positive TST evaluated for active TB. If there are no signs or symptoms of disease, a diagnosis of latent TB infection is appropriate, and treatment, usually with INH, is recommended. Of note, prior vaccination with BCG vaccine is not a contraindication to administration of a TST, and interpretation of a TST is made without regard to prior BCG vaccine except in extraordinary circumstances. Interferon-gamma release assays, unlike TSTs, are not affected by prior BCG vaccination and their use may be considered in these circumstances. Susceptibility testing of TB isolates is important in guiding therapy, especially when immigrants are from areas of multidrug-resistant or, less commonly, extensively drug-resistant TB [9].

Cavitary pneumonia, localized extrapulmonary disease, or disseminated infection suggest histoplasmosis, coccidioidomycosis, or blastomycosis. Disease can occur as a result of reactivation of latent infection in the setting of an underlying condition such as AIDS. *Histoplasma capsulatum* is widely distributed in Latin America, the Caribbean, and Southeast Asia. In Africa, a variant strain, *Histoplasma capsulatum* var. duboisii, involves skin and bones rather than the lungs. Parts of Mexico and Central and South America are endemic for *Coccidioides immitis*. Paracoccidioidomycosis is endemic in southern Mexico and Central and South America. *Blastomyces dermatitidis* can be seen in immigrants from Mexico, Central America, and Africa. Melioidosis caused by *Burkholderia pseudomallei* and paragonimiasis, caused by the lung fluke *Paragonimus westermani*, can be found in immigrants most commonly from Southeast Asia. Melioidosis is associated with chest pain but also a nonproductive or productive cough with normal sputum findings. A chronic cough may suggest paragonimiasis.

Cystic lesions in the lung suggest hydatid disease caused by *Echinococcus granulosus* and should be distinguished from cavitary lesions. Immigrants from the Middle East and other sheep-raising parts of the world can harbor hydatid cysts of the lung that can reach a large size without producing symptoms.

Eosinophilia with wheezing may be associated with tropical pulmonary eosinophilia (TPE), a hypersensitivity reaction of lymphatic filarial parasites which usually affects people living in the tropics of India, Southeast Asia, and certain parts of China and Africa. Peripheral eosinophilia >3000 cells/mm^3 is suggestive of TPE. These patients also have high titers of antifilarial antibodies, an absence of microfilariae in the blood, and a raised serum total IgE.

Pulmonary infiltrates in an immigrant receiving corticosteroids or other immunosuppressive medications should raise the question of hyperinfection due to strongyloidiasis, even if there is no peripheral blood eosinophilia. Strongyloides is unique because of its ability to complete the life cycle within the human host; an individual remains infected, often asymptomatically, for years. If an individual becomes immunosuppressed, strongyloides hyperinfection syndrome, a condition where larvae multiply rapidly and disseminate widely, may occur and can lead to death if left untreated [10].

GASTROINTESTINAL

Helicobacter pylori infection is prevalent in the developing world, where it is usually acquired at a young age. *H. pylori* infection may be asymptomatic, but a wide range of symptoms, including abdominal pain, weight loss, nausea, dyspepsia, vomiting, and bloating, have been attributed to this infection. *H. pylori* does cause chronic gastritis and increases the risk of duodenal and gastric ulcers, and persistent infection increases the risk of gastric cancer. Treatment is recommended for those with gastric ulcer disease or malignancy; treatment for other clinical manifestations associated with *H. pylori* infection remains controversial [11].

Infection with intestinal nematodes is common among immigrants from developing countries and may cause abdominal pain, though often is asymptomatic. The hookworms *Ancylostoma duodenale* and *Necator americanus* may be associated with anemia and protein deficiency due to blood loss. *Ascaris lumbricoides* can cause an impaired nutritional status, especially in children. *Trichuris trichiura* can cause pus-filled, bloody stools and rectal prolapse.

Diarrhea in immigrants may be the result of bacterial, viral, or parasitic infection. Time since arrival, recent exposures, and specific clinical symptoms help focus the evaluation appropriately. *Giardia lamblia,* a common cause of diarrhea in children, is more often asymptomatic in immigrants. Chronic diarrhea or epigastric pain, particularly in the immunosuppressed, can suggest a diagnosis of *Strongyloides stercoralis* [12].

Entamoeba histolytica may be asymptomatic, but has the potential to cause invasive disease if not diagnosed and treated. This parasite is associated with a dysentery-like illness, with blood or pus in the stool along with abdominal pain and fever. Liver abscess can present with fever, right upper quadrant pain, weight loss, hepatomegaly, and jaundice. It usually presents within several months of departure from endemic areas and occurs frequently in young men. Most cases of amebic dysentery or liver abscess in the US originate from Mexico, but other Latin American countries, South Africa, India, and Southeast Asia also have high rates of amebic disease.

Prolonged constipation or dysphagia among immigrants from Latin America south of the equator can indicate chronic Chagas disease caused by *Trypanosoma cruzi*. Infected individuals can have symptoms of achalasia, or evidence of megaesophagus or megacolon. Infection can be diagnosed by testing for IgG antibodies. Infection can be transmitted congenitally and through blood donation; the US, Canada, parts of Latin and South America, and parts of Europe routinely test blood donors for infection.

Jaundice may be associated with hepatitis, schistosomiasis, or the liver fluke *Clonorchis sinensis*. Hepatitis A and B can also present with abdominal pain, but may be accompanied by fatigue, nausea, and jaundice. Acute hepatitis A is unusual in older immigrants from developing countries because of prior infection. Hepatitis B and C infection may be asymptomatic and put the individual at risk for late complications of cirrhosis or hepatocellular carcinoma. Hepatitis E is rare in immigrants but is worthy of note because the case fatality rate is high in pregnant women.

NEUROLOGIC AND OPHTHALMOLOGIC

Seizures can be caused by neurocysticercosis, TB, and, less commonly, toxoplasmosis, especially if there is co-infection with HIV, and may occur years after infection. Although rare, Gambian sleeping sickness, which occurs in West Africa and is caused by *Trypanosoma brucei gambiense*, and East African trypanosomiasis, caused by *Trypanosoma brucei rhodesiense*, can present as altered day–night sleeping patterns. East African trypanosomiasis is less common in migrants and presents acutely, whereas West African trypanosomiasis is more common and chronic so should be considered years after infection.

Visual deficits can occur with onchocerciasis caused by *Onchocerca volvulus*. Loiasis can present acutely when an adult *Loa loa* worm migrates across the conjunctiva, though infection may have occurred remotely. Immigrants from Africa, the Middle East, and Asia may show evidence of sequelae of trachoma, the leading cause of blindness worldwide, caused by *Chlamydia trachomatis;* acute disease is not commonly seen in immigrants to the US.

Ocular toxocariasis is associated with eye pain, leukocoria, strabismus, and loss of visual acuity, and may be mistaken for retinoblastoma. Toxoplasmosis can present with blurry vision, floaters, eye pain, conjunctivitis, and photophobia; chorioretinitis is the hallmark of this condition, especially in congenital infection. Syphilis and TB are associated with uveitis, chorioretinitis, and visual loss.

CARDIAC

Symptomatic atrioventricular block or sustained ventricular tachycardia in immigrants from Mexico or Central and South America suggests Chagas disease. Spain is second to the US in having the largest number of immigrants from Latin America [13], and many of these immigrants from Latin America are from *Trypanosoma cruzi*-endemic areas such as Bolivia, which has the highest prevalence of *Trypanosoma cruzi* infection [14]. An estimated 10 million people are infected, and although most are asymptomatic, about 25% develop arrhythmias, heart block, or congestive heart failure years to decades after infection. Reactivation of chronic Chagas disease can occur in people with HIV or other immunosuppressive conditions.

Structural abnormalities of the heart include aortic aneurysms associated with syphilis and aortic or mitral valve abnormalities associated with rheumatic fever. Recurrent rheumatic fever can present with fatigue, fever, chest pain, and a changing or new murmur on the background of previous rheumatic valvular disease. It is sometimes indistinguishable from the clinical manifestations of endocarditis. TB may present with pericarditis and should be included on the differential of an immigrant with chest pain.

GENITOURINARY

Screening urinalysis is helpful in identifying glycosuria associated with diabetes; hematuria, which suggests schistosomiasis [15] and other chronic kidney diseases; and proteinuria, which could be associated with recurrent urinary tract infections, HIV, glomerulonephritis, polycystic kidney disease, or chronic kidney disease.

Painless genital ulcers may appear with syphilis or granuloma inguinale, caused by the bacteria *Klebsiella granulomatis*, seen rarely in the US but not uncommon in developing countries. Rash follows the ulcer of syphilis and is usually what prompts the infected individual to seek medical care. Painful ulcers suggest *herpesvirus* or chancroid, caused by the bacteria *Haemophilus ducreyi*. The incubation period of herpes is usually a few days to a week, whereas chancroid typically presents a few days to 2 weeks after exposure.

Hydroceles, acute episodes of local inflammation of the skin or lymph nodes, or periodic limb swelling, suggests lymphatic filariasis, endemic in Asia, Africa, and Central and South America. Lymphatic dysfunction can also lead to lymphedema of the breast, penis, and scrotum. Buboes or abscesses in the groin can indicate lymphogranuloma venereum, caused by the invasive serovar L1, L2, or L3 of *Chlamydia trachomatis*. Symptoms occur days to a month after exposure. Rectal pain and inflammation after anal sex also can be associated with this infection.

Infections that can present as infertility include schistosomiasis and TB. Prior gonococcal or chlamydia infection can also be associated with an inability to conceive.

DERMATOLOGIC

Erythema nodosum may occur with TB, leprosy, and infections with dimorphic fungi. Erythema can also signify cellulitis; recurrent cellulitis is a complication of the lymphedema of lymphatic filariasis. Areas of depigmentation are seen with onchocerciasis, leprosy, and yaws.

Ulcerative skin lesions can be caused by leishmaniasis in immigrants from the Indian subcontinent, Southwest and Central Asia, Southern Europe, the Middle East, East Africa, Central America, and South America. Less common causes of ulcerations include an ulcer with eschar from the bacteria *Bacillus anthracis* and painless, large Buruli ulcers usually seen on the extremities from *Mycobacterium ulcerans*.

The nematode *Loa loa* can cause erythematous, pruritic, occasionally painful subcutaneous swelling on the extremities. *Paragonimus*, usually non-*westermani*, can cause migratory swellings or firm, mobile, and tender subcutaneous nodes, often in the lower abdominal and inguinal regions. The trematode *Fasciola* is associated with larger, possibly 5 cm, subcutaneous nodules. Onchocerciasis presents with depigmentation, severe itching, and subcutaneous nodules.

Superficial migratory lesions include larva currens, caused by infection with *Strongyloides stercoralis*, and cutaneous larva migrans, usually seen on the feet, buttocks, or abdomen, caused by dog and cat hookworms. Pruritus and excoriations from scratching are typical of onchocerciasis, scabies, and pinworms. Scabies mites burrow into the webs of fingers and toes, the wrists and backs of elbows, the knees, and around the waist and umbilicus, and can cause characteristic linear lesions. An itchy rectal area suggests pinworms [16].

NONINFECTIOUS DISEASES OF IMMIGRANTS

Fatigue, bruising, and nonhealing sores can suggest blood disorders, including anemias and thalassemias, particularly among people from the Mediterranean, Africa, and Asia. Some of these blood disorders are genetic, whereas others are caused by nutritional disorders such as iron, B12 or folate deficiency, or chronic diseases such as hookworm infestation, HIV, lead intoxication, kidney disease, or malignancy. In the future, it is likely that immigrants will bear a disproportionate burden of disease due to infection-associated cancers, such as hepatoma from chronic hepatitis B and C, carcinoma of the cervix caused by human papillomavirus, Epstein-Barr virus-associated Burkitt lymphoma, human herpesvirus-8-associated Kaposi sarcoma, and HIV-associated lymphomas.

Malnutrition and stunting of growth can be especially severe in immigrant children and refugees as a result of food deprivation and infections. Malabsorption can result from intestinal protozoan infections or, rarely, tropical sprue; lactose intolerance is common among African and certain Asian immigrant groups. Immigrants may present with specific nutritional disorders such as bowing of the legs in children or osteomalacia in adults with vitamin D deficiency, xerophthalmia secondary to vitamin A deficiency, endemic goiter associated with iodine deficiency, or acrodermatitis with zinc deficiency.

Depression and stress are common among immigrants who are adapting to a new culture and language. Post-traumatic stress disorder and other psychiatric problems are not uncommon among refugees, especially those who have experienced torture, rape, and other physical trauma in war-torn countries. Those who care for immigrants may find that disclosures of trauma occur only after development of a trusting relationship with the healthcare provider. There are many validated screening instruments available, including the Harvard Trauma Questionnaire to check for post-traumatic stress disorder, the Hopkins Symptom Checklist which screens for anxiety, and the Beck Depression Inventory [17].

CONCLUSION

Diseases seen in immigrants may be the result of exposures in their country of origin, during migration, or exposures occurring after arrival at their destination. Health professionals must take a detailed history about the type and duration of symptoms and think systematically while remembering where an immigrant has lived. It is always necessary to consider noninfectious processes as well, particularly mental health issues, which may not manifest until after arrival in the US.

REFERENCES

1. International Organization for Migration. About migration. http://www.iom.int/jahia/Jahia/about-migration/lang/en (accessed 12 April 2010).
2. US Citizenship and Immigration Services. Immigration medical examinations. http://www.uscis.gov/portal/site/uscis/menuitem.eb1d4c2a3e5b9ac89243c6a7543f6d1a/?vgnextoid=288a0a5659083210VgnVCM100000082ca60aRCRD&vgnextchannel=288a0a5659083210VgnVCM100000082ca60aRCRD (accessed 12 April 2010).
3. Centers for Disease Control and Prevention. CDC immigration requirements: technical instructions for tuberculosis screening and treatment. http://www.cdc.gov/immigrantrefugeehealth/pdf/tuberculosis-ti-2009.pdf (accessed 12 April 2010).
4. Centers for Disease Control and Prevention. A comprehensive immunization strategy to eliminate transmission of hepatitis B virus infection in the United States: recommendations of the Advisory Committee on Immunization Practices (ACIP) Part 1: immunization of infants, children, and adolescents. MMWR Recomm Rep 2005;54:1–23.
5. Centers for Disease Control and Prevention. A comprehensive immunization strategy to eliminate transmission of hepatitis B virus infection in the United States: recommendations of the Advisory Committee on Immunization Practices (ACIP) Part II: immunization of adults. MMWR Recomm Rep 2006;55:1–25.
6. Barnett E. Infectious disease screening for refugees resettled in the United States. Clin Infect Dis 2004;39:833–41.
   This article reviews screening, types of infectious diseases, and immunizations for refugees to the US.
7. Walker PF, Barnett ED. Immigrant Medicine. Philadelphia: Elsevier; 2007.
   This book details immigration medicine. It focuses on infectious and noninfectious diseases of immigrants with information separated by sections and chapters. It is highlighted throughout with tables and charts, including a listing of diseases by geography.
8. Wilson ME, Weld LH, Boggild A, et al. Fever in returned travelers: results from the GeoSentinel Surveillance Network. Clin Infect Dis 2007;44:1560–8.
   Using a large, multicenter database, this article shows the frequency of fever in returned travelers and defines the causes of fever by place of exposure and traveler characteristics.
9. Centers for Disease Control and Prevention. Emergence of Mycobacterium tuberculosis with extensive resistance to second-line drugs – worldwide, 2000–2004. MMWR Morb Mortal Wkly Rep 2006;55:301–5.
10. Newberry AM, Williams DN, Stauffer WM, et al. Strongyloides hyperinfection presenting as acute respiratory failure and gram-negative sepsis. Chest 2005;128:3681–4.
11. Suerbaum S, Michetti P. Helicobacter pylori infection. N Engl J Med 2002;347:1175–86.
12. Thielman NM, Guerrant RL. Acute infectious diarrhea. N Engl J Med 2004:350:38–47.
13. Schmunis GA. Epidemiology of Chagas disease in non-endemic countries: the role of international migration. Mem Inst Oswaldo Cruz 2007;102:75–85.
14. Schmunis GA, Cruz JR. Safety of the blood supply in Latin America. Clin Microbiol Rev 2005;18:12–29.
15. Ross AGP, Bartley PB, Sleigh AC, et al. Schistosomiasis. N Engl J Med 2002;346:1212–20.
16. Lucchina LC, Wilson M, Caumes E, et al. Colour Atlas of Travel Dermatology. WileyBlackwell: Oxford; 2007.
   This book details dermatologic concerns in immigrants and travelers. The book has detailed, colored pictures supplemented by concise, descriptive text. Each chapter includes etiology, prevalence, incubation, clinical features, differential diagnosis, and treatment.
17. Kandula NR, Kersey M, Lurie N. Assuring the health of immigrants: what the leading health indicators tell us. Annu Rev Public Health 2004;25:357–76.

International Adoption 150

Cynthia R Howard

Key features

- The demography of international adoption is in constant flux
- Growth failure is the most common medical problem on arrival
- Tuberculosis infection is the most serious medical diagnosis commonly identified
- Young international adoptees may be acutely infected, asymptomatic and shedding HAV
- Ninety per cent of international adoptees need catch-up immunizations
- International adoptees are at risk for developmental delay

INTRODUCTION

Between 25,000 and 40,000 children are adopted each year by citizens from a country other than the child's country of birth [1]. Underlying reasons for loss of parents remain constant and include extreme poverty, death of one or both parents, abandonment due to gender or disability, armed conflict resulting in separation from parents, maternal substance abuse, or other social or cultural determinants. The HIV epidemic has led to an increase in the number of orphaned children, particularly on the African continent. One hundred and forty-three million children are estimated to have been orphaned by one or both parents [2].

The demography of international adoption is in constant flux. Consequently, the epidemiology of diseases in this population of children shifts from year to year. For example, in 1990, United States citizens adopted children predominantly from South Korea (38%), Colombia (9%), the Philippines (6%) and Peru (6%). In 2009, China (24%), Ethiopia (18%), Russia (12%), South Korea (8.5%) and Guatemala (6%) were the predominant countries of birth [3]. Individual health risks vary depending on intrauterine exposure to infections and toxins, genetic heritage, congenital anomalies, caregiver environment (foster care versus institutional care), food security, exposure to infection, circumstances leading to the loss of parental care, and birth region.

Common medical problems for international adoptees (IA) include chronic malnutrition, anemia, latent tuberculosis infection, and intestinal parasites. Approximately 50% of IA will experience an acute infection within the first month following arrival in the US. Most can be successfully treated as outpatients. Upper respiratory infections and diarrhea are common. Skin conditions such as scabies, impetigo, and molluscum contagiosum are relatively common. Evaluation of the sick IA depends on both the epidemiology of diseases in the country of origin and on the medical and social history of the child. Birth family history and immunization records may be unavailable or unreliable.

Growth failure is the most common medical problem children have on arrival. Psychosocial deprivation, particularly long-term institutionalization, adversely affects growth in height, weight and head circumference [4]. Children may arrive with a low weight-for-height secondary to lack of protein and calories. In a study of 869 children adopted between 1986 and 2001 from 33 different countries, 28% were chronically malnourished, and 5% were acutely malnourished [5]. In Miller's study of 452 IA from China, z-scores of ≤ -2 were found for 39% of children for height, 24% for head circumference and 18% for weight. Although some children arrive from Ethiopia with a history of severe protein–energy malnutrition, they appear to be growing better than their peers who arrive from long-term orphanage care [6]. Micronutrient deficiencies including zinc, vitamin D and iron deficiency have been documented in children from all countries.

Lead toxicity is well documented, particularly among children adopted from Asia, with children from China at highest risk. In one study, 13% of children from China had elevated lead levels ranging from 11.1 to 51 µg/dL [7].

Internationally adopted children come from countries with a high or intermediate prevalence of tuberculosis, hepatitis A, and hepatitis B. They are routinely screened for hepatitis B, tuberculosis, and HIV in their birth countries. However, the reliability of the pre-adoption screens varies from country to country. In one study, 50% of newly arrived children had an undiagnosed medical condition. Of these, more than 50% were diagnosed with an infectious disease [8].

TUBERCULOSIS

Tuberculosis is one of the most serious medical diagnoses identified among IA. In one study of 527 IA, 21% had a positive tuberculin skin test (TST) on arrival. Of those who were negative initially, 46.9% were retested at 3 months or more after arrival, and 20% of these initially negative skin tests had converted to positive. No active cases of tuberculosis were found in this group [9]. Possible explanations for conversion include exposure immediately prior to departure from birth country, and improvement in nutritional status with boosting of the skin test. Interferon-gamma release assays (IGRA), which can distinguish BCG immunity from tuberculosis infection, are being studied in children. QuantiFERON GOLD is currently recommended as an alternative method of diagnosing infection in children ≥ 5 years old.

In a study of 869 IA from 33 different countries between 1986 and 2001, 12% had evidence of *M. tuberculosis* infection (TST ≥ 10 mm) on initial screening and no active disease. The frequency of positive TST screens did not depend on birth region or nutritional status [5]. The continent of Africa was not represented in that study. International adoption in significant numbers of children from African countries, particularly Ethiopia, began in 2004. A 2008 study reported a positive TST for 16% of 54 Ethiopian children [6].

Screening for tuberculosis should be done for all children older than 3 months of age. TSTs may be negative in young infants, if their exposure to tuberculosis was recent, they are malnourished or otherwise immunocompromised, or they recently received a live-virus vaccine. The TST should take place within 2 weeks of arrival and be repeated within 3 to 6 months for those children who had a TST <10 mm on arrival [5,9]. The TST should be placed regardless of BCG vaccination status. QuantiFERON GOLD may be substituted for the TST in children 5 years of age or older. A physical examination and chest radiograph to assess for extrapulmonary and pulmonary tuberculosis are indicated for every child with a positive TST. A child with a positive TST but no evidence of active disease should be treated with isoniazid for latent tuberculosis infection. If positive for active disease, every effort should be made to isolate the organism, particularly if the child is from a region of the world with a high rate of multidrug-resistant TB, such as Eastern Europe, Russia, Asia, or certain countries in Africa, e.g., South Africa.

Children ≥2 years old arriving from countries highly endemic for tuberculosis are required to be evaluated for TB prior to entering the US [10]. However, following natural disasters such as the January 2010 earthquake in Haiti, orphans may not have received routine screening prior to arrival in the adoptive country.

HEPATITIS A

Infants and young children from hepatitis A (HAV)-endemic areas may be acutely infected, asymptomatic and shedding virus with the potential to infect nonimmune adoptive families and others with whom they may come in contact (e.g. day care). Serology has proven useful in identifying these children. In 2009, the Advisory Committee on Immunization Practices (ACIP) recommended that people anticipating close contact with an IA within 60 days after arrival from a country known for intermediate or high rates of hepatitis A should be vaccinated against hepatitis A [11]. Among IA <6 years of age, the prevalence of total HAV antibody ranges from 10% (among Chinese children) to 55–72% (of Ethiopian children) [12].

HEPATITIS B

Hepatitis B (HBV) infection in the IA can be silent or acutely symptomatic. The prevalence of hepatitis B among IA ranges from 1% to 5%. In a study of 1282 IA between 1999 and 2006, 1.1% were identified with acute or chronic infection. An additional 2.9% had evidence of resolved infection. The highest rates were among children from Ethiopia and Bulgaria [13]. Children found to be hepatitis B surface antigen (HBsAg)-positive must be tested again. Persistence of the surface antigen for 6 months or more indicates chronic hepatitis B infection. Children who initially test negative for hepatitis B surface antibody and antigen must be retested within 6 months. All members of the household adopting a child who is HBV-infected should be immunized and should have post-immunization antibody titers to determine whether levels are consistent with protection.

HEPATITIS C

Hepatitis C (HCV) seroprevalence among IA is less than 1%. Routine screening is not recommended. The AAP recommends consideration of HCV screening for children from Russia, Eastern Europe, and China. Screening of children from other regions may be indicated depending on the prevalence of HCV in the country of origin, history of blood transfusions, and maternal drug history [14].

SYPHILIS

Screening for *Treponema pallidum* is recommended. Though uncommon among IA, a prevalence of 1.7% or less has been reported [15]. If prior sexual abuse is suspected, a syphilis screen should be repeated 1 month after arrival. Children from tropical regions may have positive tests due to spirochete infections other than syphilis, but differentiation between syphilis and other treponeme infections (yaws, pinta, and bejel) may be impossible unless active lesions are present. Care must be taken in the interpretation of either the treponemal or nontreponemal test result. If syphilis cannot be excluded satisfactorily, a full evaluation for disease must be undertaken and appropriate treatment given.

HIV

Despite the increasing number of children orphaned due to HIV, the prevalence of HIV infection among IA has been low in multiple studies [15]. In the future, increasing numbers of IA will likely be HIV-positive as adoptive parents more favorably consider adopting children who have the infection. All children should be screened on arrival for HIV antibodies. If they are less than 6 months of age they also should have HIV DNA PCR done. Some experts recommend a follow-up antibody screen 6 months post arrival to detect infection that may have occurred immediately prior to departure from the country of origin.

INTESTINAL PATHOGENS

Diarrhea and abdominal distention are common among newly arrived children. In one study, >25% of IA had one or more intestinal parasites [16]. Other common stool pathogens include *Blastocystis hominis*, *Dientamoeba fragilis*, and *Hymenolepis nana*. Stool samples should be cultured for enteric bacteria in any child with diarrhea.

Helicobacter pylori must be considered in the evaluation of abdominal pain, anemia, or growth failure. Risk factors include orphanage residence (versus foster care), older age at adoption, and intestinal parasite infection. Stool for *H. pylori* antigen is a noninvasive screening method [17].

Screening for malaria parasites should be considered for all IA coming from areas where malaria is holoendemic (Haiti or most countries in sub-Saharan Africa). In a small study of Liberian immigrant children in Minnesota, 28 of 43 (65%) were positive for a *Plasmodium* species, but one-third were asymptomatic and one-third had splenomegaly as the only sign of infection [18].

EOSINOPHILIA

An absolute eosinophil count greater than 450 requires etiologic investigation. This should include stool for ova and parasites, although this test alone is insufficient if the eosinophilia is persistent or high. Serologic tests for *Strongyloides stercoralis*, *Schistosomia* spp., lymphatic filariasis, *Toxocara canis*, echinococcosis, *Entamoeba histolytica*, and visceral or cutaneous larval migrans are indicated as guided by history, physical examination and country of birth. Patients with eosinophilia often are asymptomatic. Empiric treatment with albendazole or ivermectin is recommended for the patient who has persistent eosinophilia without a cause [18].

IMMUNIZATIONS

More than 90% of IA need catch-up immunizations to meet standards in the US. Availability and reliability of pre-adoption immunization records are variable. Practitioners can choose from two clinically sound approaches: (a) either screening for quantitative antibody levels to verify immunity in the infant >6 months of age based on vaccine record and/or knowledge of immunizations available in the birth country; or (b) immunization according to age and catch-up schedule [19]. Typically measles vaccine as a single antigen is administered in most birth countries rather than full MMR. MMR is recommended over serologic testing for measles antibody. Varicella testing for children coming from tropical countries is not recommended prior to 12 years of age unless there is a history of disease. In the tropics, varicella is a disease of adolescents and adults.

CONCLUSIONS

IA come from countries with a high prevalence of endemic diseases that are potentially life-threatening. All IA should be screened for

TABLE 150-1 Clinical Screening Protocol Recommended for Newly Arrived International Adoptees (IA)

			Notes
INITIAL VISIT	STOOL	Ova and parasites	Three early-morning stools separated by 24 h
		Giardia-specific antigen	One early-morning stool; note: if child has watery diarrhea, add stool studies for *Cryptosporidium*, routine stool culture, and stool culture for *Yersinia*. Recheck stool 2–3 weeks after completion of treatment
	URINE	*Helicobacter pylori* antigen	Consider for IA with persistent abdominal pain and/or refractory iron deficiency anemia
		CCU or bag urine for urinalysis	Urinalysis is a simple screen for renal and systemic disease. *Schistosoma haematobium* should be considered in the older IA who has asymptomatic hematuria if the country of origin is located in Africa
	BLOOD	Hemogram	Include red blood cell indices and white blood cell differential
		Ferritin, serum iron, iron saturation, transferrin	
		Vitamin D	25 OH Total
		Calcium	
		Phosphorous	
		Hgb electrophoresis	If sickle cell disease is prevalent in country of birth or RBC indices indicate thalassemia
		Thyroid-stimulating hormone, free thyroxine	
		G6PD	If G6PD deficiency is common in country of birth or if prescribing primaquine
		Hepatitis A IgG antibody	If positive, then hepatitis A core IgM antibody
		Hepatitis B testing	HBsAg, HBcAb (if positive IgM), HBsAb
		Hepatitis C antibody	Perform if history suggests possible exposure. If positive, then hepatitis C RNA by PCR
		HIV types 1 and 2 antibodies	HIV DNA PCR if <6 months old
		RPR, ART or VDRL	Treponemal test to confirm (MHA-TP or FTA-ABS)
		Newborn metabolic screen	For infants (0–12 months)
		Malaria PCR or thin and thick smears for malaria parasites	If country is endemic for malaria
		Lead	
		Diphtheria anti-toxoid antibody	If ≥6 months old
		Tetanus anti-toxoid antibody	If ≥6 months old
		Poliovirus types I, II, and III neutralizing antibody	If ≥6 months old; note that neutralizing antibodies must be ordered unless acute infection is suspected. Titer to type III often not predictive of protective level, and repeating vaccine is not recommended
		Varicella	For children >12 years old or with history of infection
		Measles, mumps and rubella antibodies	If MMR is documented
		Tuberculin skin test	CXR and treat if ≥10 mm (see Box 150.1)
	TST	Hepatitis B panel	Only if child did not have immunity at initial visit Repeat at 6 months after initial testing if initial serology results are negative (no anti-HBs IgG) or if child is <12 months of age at initial testing
		Hepatitis C antibody	Repeat if history suggests exposure
6 MONTHS POST INITIAL VISIT	BLOOD	HIV types 1 and 2 antibody	Some experts recommend repeating at 6 months post arrival
		Iron studies	
		Tuberculin skin test	Only if first test was negative
	TST		

ART, automated reagin test; FTA-ABS, fluorescent treponemal antibody absorption; HBcAb, hepatitis B core antibody; HBsAb, hepatitis B surface antibody; HBsAg, hepatitis B surface antigen; MHA-TP, microhemagglutination test for *Treponema pallidum*; RPR, rapid plasma regain; VDRL, Venereal Disease Research Laboratories.

BOX 150.1 Definition of a Positive Tuberculin Skin Test (TST) in Internationally Adopted Children

Induration ≥5 mm if:

- evidence of immunosuppression
- history of contact with active tuberculosis
- signs and symptoms of tuberculosis
- abnormal chest radiograph

Induration ≥10 mm in all other internationally adopted children

Reprinted from Brunette GW, ed. *The Yellow Book, Health Information for International Travel.* Atlanta: Mosby Elsevier; 2009.

TABLE 150-2 Growth and Development Risk Factors and Potential Outcomes in Internationally Adopted Children*

Risk factor	Potential outcome
Prenatal alcohol exposure	Fetal alcohol spectrum disorders
Low birthweight (<2500 g)	Behavioral and academic problems
Small head circumference ≤–2.8 SD	Mental retardation
Vision and hearing issues	Fine motor and speech delay; hearing and vision screens are recommended for all new arrivals
Social neglect	Sensory processing delay, global delay
Malnutrition	Underweight, stunting, gross motor delay
Micronutrient deficiency: iron	Cognitive delay
Long-term institutional care	Cognitive delay, attachment disorder
Lack of play/sensory experiences	Global delay
Multiple transitions	Attachment delay, behavioral problems, sleep disturbance
Transition to a second language	Language delay
History of physical and/or sexual abuse	Depression, personality disorders
Early deprivation of physical/social needs	Early puberty in girls
Previously undiagnosed medical conditions	Complex neurobehavioral problems

*Most newly arrived international adoptees (IA) are underweight and will catch up within 6 months of arrival. The majority of IA have developmental delays, and most will catch up quickly. To mitigate long-term effects, developmental screening is recommended at arrival and 6 months post arrival. Vision and hearing screening is recommended within 3 months of arrival.

acute and infectious diseases as noted above. Likewise, family members, including the extended family and childcare providers, should be current on their routine immunizations. Protection against hepatitis A, hepatitis B, and measles should be ensured.

Children with previously unidentified chronic medical conditions may appear healthy. Therefore, specialized laboratory screening and examination by a professional skilled in caring for this population are needed to identify and treat potential long-term issues. IA are at risk for developmental delays, fetal alcohol spectrum disorders, and failure to thrive. Orphans are at increased risk for neglect of physical and social needs and physical abuse, placing them at increased risk for mental illness. In addition, congenital anomalies and genetic disorders must be considered on examination. The initial examination is recommended within 2 weeks of arrival, or sooner if the child is acutely ill with fever or diarrhea. A thorough history and physical examination should be performed with particular attention to specific details (Table 150-1 & Box 150.1).

A detailed developmental examination that includes sensory evaluation by an occupational therapist is necessary. Consultation with a child psychologist experienced in international adoption issues is recommended if there is a history of multiple transitions, physical signs of fetal alcohol syndrome, long-term institutional care, known mental health issues, acute attachment issues, birth parent depression, physical or sexual abuse, or if the child is older than 4 years at the time of adoption (Table 150-2).

REFERENCES

1. Department of Economic and Social Affairs, Population Division. Child adoption: trends and policies. United Nations Population Newsletter 2008; 85:1–2.
2. UNICEF/UNAIDS/USAID. Children on the brink 2004. A joint report of new orphan estimates and a framework for action. http://www.unicef.org/publications/files/cob_layout6-013.pdf (accessed 25 March 2010).
3. U.S. Department of State. IR3 - IH3 - IR4 - IH4 Visa Issuances for FY-2009. http://adoption.state.gov/pdf/adoption_visa_issuance_2009.pdf (accessed 25 March 2010).
4. Johnson DE. Long-term medical issues in international adoptees. Pediatr Ann 2000;29:234–41.
The author has extensive experience in international adoption, having founded the first international adoption clinic in the United States in 1986 that offered both pre- and post-adoption services. The concise, descriptive review of major medical problems is an excellent follow-up to articles written by the same author 10 years earlier. However, the data reviewed were collected prior to the arrival of significant numbers of international adoptees from Africa.
5. Mandalakas AM, Kirchner HL, Iverson S, et al. Predictors of *Mycobacterium tuberculosis* infection in international adoptees. Pediatrics 2007;120:e610–16.
The lead author is an expert in pediatric tuberculosis. The retrospective chart review examines risk factors, including the impact of malnutrition, region of birth, and age, among a large number of internationally adopted children. One must keep in mind that children from Africa are not represented in this review.
6. Miller LC, Tseng B, Tirella LG, et al. Health of children adopted from Ethiopia. Matern Child Health J 2008;12:599–605.
This descriptive article, the only one of its kind published to date, examines the medical findings of 54 children adopted from Ethiopia. The risk of active hepatitis A virus shedding, potentially infecting non-immune adoptive family members, is not addressed. Dr Miller has also authored a comprehensive, practical manual intended for the practicing clinician, The Handbook of International Adoption Medicine (Oxford University Press, 2005).
7. Miller LC, Hendrie NW. Health of children adopted from China. Pediatrics 2000;105:e76.
8. Hostetter MK, Iverson SI, Dole K, Johnson DE. Unsuspected infectious diseases and other medical diagnoses in the evaluation of internationally adopted children. Pediatrics 1989;83:559–64.
9. Trehan I, Meinzen-Derr JK, Jamison L, Staat MA. Tuberculosis screening in internationally adopted children: the need for initial and repeat testing. Pediatrics 2008;122:e7–14.
10. Centers for Disease Control. CDC immigration requirements: technical instructions for tuberculosis screening and treatment: using cultures and directly observed therapy. 2009:1-1-35.
11. Centers for Disease Control. Updated recommendations from the Advisory Committee on Immunization Practices (ACIP) for use of hepatitis A vaccine

in close contacts of newly arriving international adoptees. http://www.cdc.gov/mmwr/preview/mmwrhtml/mm5836a4.htm (accessed 8 June 2010).
12. Sharapov UM, Teshale E. Viral hepatitis A among international adoptees. Presented at: Adoption Stakeholders Meeting, Center for Disease Control and Prevention October 5, 2009.
13. Stadler LP, Mezoff AG, Staat MA. Hepatitis B virus screening for internationally adopted children. Pediatrics 2008;122:1223–8.
14. American Academy of Pediatrics. Medical evaluation of internationally adopted children for infectious diseases. In: Pickering LK, Baker CJ, Kimberlin DW, Long SS, eds. Red Book: 2009 Report of the Committee on Infectious Diseases, 28th ed. 2009:183.
15. Murray TS, Groth ME, Weitzman C, Cappello M. Epidemiology and management of infectious diseases in international adoptees. Clin Microbiol Rev 2005;18:510–20.
16. Staat MA. Infectious disease issues in internationally adopted children. Pediatr Infect Dis J 2002;21:257–8.
17. Miller LC, Kelly N, Tannemaat M, Grand RJ. Serologic prevalence of antibodies to *Helicobacter pylori* in internationally adopted children. Helicobacter 2003;8:173–8.
18. Stauffer WM, Kamat D, Walker PF. Screening of international immigrants, refugees, and adoptees. Prim Care 2002;29:879–905.
19. Barnett ED. Immunizations for internationally adopted children. Vaccine Quarterly 2009;3:3–4.

151 Medical Tourism

Stephen T Green

Key features

- Medical tourism is the practice of traveling outside of a patient's local area for the purpose of accessing medical services; this often includes international travel
- Associated risks include risks known within travel medicine, such as the risk of acquiring tropical diseases and the additional risks related to the medical or surgical treatment
- Quality control, risk, and safety of treatment facilities in the destination country are key issues but difficult to control, especially if the provider is not engaged in independent accreditation or a robust external review process
- Patients can return to their home country with ongoing needs related to their treatment and problems resulting from having traveled overseas
- Medical tourism raises ethical and legal issues that merit further clarification

INTRODUCTION

Throughout history people have traveled for reasons of accessing healthcare. The Ancient Greeks were possibly the first to lay the foundations of a medical tourism network when, in honour of Aesculapius, the God of medicine, they erected the Asculepia Temples. These became organized health centers to which people traveled from all over the ancient world. In 1248 AD, the Mansuri Hospital was built in Egypt and it became the largest and most advanced hospital in the world, with a capacity of 8000 people; it was a magnet for foreigners seeking healthcare, regardless of race or religion. During the 16th century, Europe's wealthy elite rediscovered Roman baths and flocked to spa towns such as Bath, St Moritz, Ville d'Eaux, Aachen, and Baden Baden to "take the waters" on the promise that it would prove beneficial for a vast variety of conditions.

From the end of the 20th century there has been increasing growth in the movement of patients, medical technology, capital funding and healthcare professionals across national borders. This has internationalized the delivery of medical services. The phenomenon known as "medical tourism" (or sometimes medical travel) has arisen for several reasons. Patients travel because of high costs of healthcare in their home country, excessive delays in accessing a medical or surgical intervention, and to seek treatments that may be considered inadequate, unsafe or unavailable in their home countries [1].

Medical tourism has given rise to new risks emerging from the medical/surgical treatment and from the international travel. Therefore, it represents a means by which:

- persons will travel to potentially unfamiliar places where they may come into contact with unfamiliar diseases, including tropical diseases;
- microorganisms can be transported across international borders, some of which may be antibiotic resistant or unfamiliar to medical staff in the country of origin;
- new challenges are generated for domestic healthcare provider systems as they see returned travelers with post-treatment complications;
- new ethical and quality assurance dilemmas are generated.

WHAT SERVICES ARE AVAILABLE VIA MEDICAL TOURISM?

Marketing material, both print and internet-based, indicate that the range of investigations and treatments available around the world for medical tourists vary widely. Examples include:

- health check-ups and diagnostics;
- cosmetic surgery, for example liposuction, dermabrasion, and breast, face, and botox injections;
- cardiology/cardiac surgery, for example coronary revascularization, percutaneous transluminal septal myocardial ablation;
- dentistry, for example cosmetic, reconstruction and implants;
- orthopedic surgery, for example hip replacement and resurfacing, knee replacement;
- bariatric surgery, for example gastric bypass, gastric banding;
- fertility/reproductive system, for example *in vitro* fertilization, preconception sex selection, transgender reassignment;
- organ, cell and tissue transplantation, for example renal and hemi-liver transplantation;
- eye surgery, for example refractive surgery such as laser-assisted in-situ keratomileusis (LASIK), cataract surgery;
- opiate and alcohol detoxification services;
- spa services;
- Complementary and traditional medicine services, for example Ayurvedic medicine, Chinese traditional medicine.

Some of these procedures may not be legal or acceptable in all regions of the world.

HOW MANY MEDICAL TOURISTS ARE THERE AND WHERE DO THEY COME FROM?

There are no reliable estimates of the number of medical tourists and their origin.

A report from 2007 authored by the international consultancy Deloitte, estimated that the number of US citizens seeking treatment outside of the USA was 750,000 [2]. US-origin medical tourists are thought to represent 9% of the worldwide number of medical tourists [3]. This indicates that annually there could be between 30 and 50 million traveling abroad for reasons of medical tourism. Support for these numbers comes from a report that a single hospital in Bangkok admitted about 430,000 patients in 2003, with that hospital admitting 93,000 Arab patients. Conservative estimates of medical tourism to India place the annual number at 150,000 and the equivalent figure for Singapore is around 400,000 [4]. In contrast, a US-based study in 2008 surveyed 45 companies promoting medical tourism (representing an estimated 70% of companies promoting such services) found that only 13,500 US patients traveled for healthcare overseas [5].

WHERE ARE MEDICAL TOURISM SERVICES PROVIDED?

The cost of accessing healthcare is much less in Asia [6], South and Central America, and Africa, and is one of the important drivers for the growth of medical tourism. However, the procedure or treatment cost does not include the potential increased costs related to poor standards of care and quality. Increasingly, facilities in Asia and South America are seeking international accreditation as an important stamp of approval for their services.

Medical tourism destinations include:

- Asia: India, Malaysia, Singapore, Korea, and Thailand;
- the Middle East: Dubai;
- South Africa;
- South and Central America: Brazil, Costa Rica, and Mexico;
- eastern Europe: Hungary, Poland, and Ukraine;
- southern Europe and the Mediterranean: Cyprus and Malta.

Estimates of the number of country-specific medical tourists that are based on industry sources may be biased and inaccurate.

INFECTION-RELATED RISKS

Some procedures carry the risk of hemorrhage and the need for blood product transfusions, with attendant risks of blood-borne viruses, such as HIV and hepatitis B [7]. Other pathogens, such as *Trypanosoma cruzi*, may be a risk in Latin America [8]. The cross-border transmission of antimicrobial resistance as a consequence of undergoing surgery overseas has been well-described [9].

Rabies [10] and West Nile Virus have been transmitted at the time of transplantation [11].

If such events are to be avoided, it is necessary that hospitals and clinics providing medical tourism services maintain the highest standards of clinical governance. Ensuring that this is the case is a challenge.

A second area of relevance is the need for pre-travel preventative medicine. Some countries (e.g. India, Thailand, Brazil) where medical tourism services are advertised are also countries where people travel for holiday, business, or to visit friends and relatives. For these travelers, as well as medical tourists, there is the need to seek pre-travel advice and prevention measures for malaria and other tropical diseases. As examples, non-vaccine-preventable diseases, such as dengue and chikungunya, can be a risk in South Asia; food- and water-transmitted enteric infection are widely distributed; and personal safety and the prevention of sexually transmitted infections are all important.

Medical tourists may also need advice regarding the prevention of deep venous thrombosis during long-distance air flights, particularly on the return journey. This could involve fitted lower-extremity compression stockings or the use of low molecular weight heparin.

QUALITY CONTROL, SAFETY, AND RISK

Provision of healthcare is a complex and challenging process with medical, dental, social, political, ethical, business, and financial ramifications. For example, there cannot be effective infection control in a hospital ward, outpatient clinic, kitchen, mortuary, laboratory, or blood bank without good governance in place throughout the organization.

Medical tourism compounds these difficulties; only through independent and transparent scrutiny is it possible to establish if a hospital, clinic or staff member is fit for purpose and functioning in a safe way. Worldwide, independent external assessment is increasingly being used to regulate, improve and market healthcare providers in the medical tourism field. The most common models are accreditation, peer review, statutory inspection, International Organization for Standardization (ISO) certification and evaluation (usually internal) against the "business excellence" framework [12].

The most robust model, from a clinical perspective, is accreditation.

"Accreditation is usually a voluntary program, sponsored by a non-governmental agency (NGO), in which trained external peer reviewers evaluate a health care organization's compliance with pre-established performance standards. Accreditation addresses organizational, rather than individual practitioner, capability or performance. Unlike licensure, accreditation focuses on continuous improvement strategies and achievement of optimal quality standards, rather than adherence to minimal standards intended to assure public safety" [13].

Accreditation systems are structured to provide objective measures for evaluation of quality management in a hospital or clinic; the results can be used by the general public, governments, and third-party payers, as examples. Independent accreditation schemes include the Joint Commission International (JCI) from the USA, QHA Trent Accreditation from the UK and Accreditation Canada International. Currently, it is not compulsory for private sector providers, such as hospitals and clinics, to go through independent accreditation anywhere in the world. However, without accreditation, it may not be possible for persons with private health insurance to seek reimbursement. Additionally, without reputable external scrutiny, it is challenging to see how interested parties can have a clear idea whether a hospital or clinic will safely deliver excellence in care.

When complaints arise concerning the delivery of healthcare, for example an incident of medical negligence or a medical accident affecting a medical tourist, it may be difficult, or impossible, to obtain a satisfactory resolution of the problem within a foreign legal jurisdiction. In some countries, for example Malaysia and Singapore, doctors routinely carry medical indemnity from organizations such as the Medical Protection Society (UK), which will help protect patients and providers if successful legal action is taken. However, in other countries, such as Thailand or India, it is not routine for doctors to subscribe to a medical indemnity organisation [4] and hence medical tourists might not enjoy the same level of protection in the event of an iatrogenic injury.

The lack of legal safeguards is occasionally taken advantage of by patients, such as when they seek stem cell injections to treat conditions where there is no scientific evidence to justify their usage [14], or pre-conception sex selection [15].

Deaths are also well documented among medical tourists. In 2005, the wife of a prominent African politician died after undergoing liposuction in Spain [16]. In another instance, a UK resident went to the USA to receive cosmetic silicone injections and died of complications [17].

THE RETURNED MEDICAL TOURIST

Upon returning home, patients may require routine follow-up after undergoing gastric band surgery, for example. Sometimes, the overseas medical tourism provider will make arrangements for this to happen in the patient's home country.

For medical tourists who return ill, it should be established if they are:

- ill from the surgery or treatment itself;
- ill because of a complication of the surgery, for example a wound infection, possibly with a multidrug resistant organism;
- ill because of an intervention associated with the surgery or treatment, for example a blood transfusion;

- ill secondary to the journey, for example deep venous thrombosis, with or without pulmonary embolus;
- ill as a result of acquiring a tropical disease, for example malaria or typhoid.

When complications have occurred as a result of treatment overseas as a medical tourist, the patient's medical insurance in their home country may not always cover this care. This should be clarified before undergoing an overseas procedure. In addition, consular services may not always be available to medical tourists. As an example, UK travelers will not be contacted nor visited in the overseas country by Foreign and Commonwealth personnel if a complication occurs from treatment specifically arising from medical tourism.

CONCLUSION

If an individual plans to become a medical tourist, the details of the procedure and the destination should be conveyed to the travel health provider so that proper prevention measures can be taken, for example hepatitis B vaccination and malaria chemoprophylaxis. Likewise, if a hemodialysis patient plans to have a kidney transplant overseas that might otherwise have been impossible for them to obtain in their home country, steps can be taken prospectively by the home medical team to improve the outcome, such as outlining measures that should be taken to assure the survival of the transplanted kidney.

There remain ethical issues around medical tourism, such as concern about how organs for transplantation are obtained. These have yet to be adequately resolved, although there are international guidelines addressing the issue [18].

Primum non nocere can be a challenging maxim to apply to medical tourism, but as its prevalence increases it is increasingly something that healthcare workers and healthcare provider systems are going to have to confront. For some patients and healthcare systems, it has the power to provide answers for problems that might otherwise seem intractable.

REFERENCES

1. Crooks VA, Snyder J. Medical tourism: What Canadian family physicians need to know. Can Fam Physician 2011;57:527–9.
2. Deloitte's report reduction in US medical tourism due to the recession. Int Med Tourism J 2009. Available at: http://www.imtj.com/news/?EntryId82=166602 (last accessed 31 December 2011).
3. Ehrbeck T. Guervara C. Margo PD. McKinsey Quarterly. Mapping the market for medical travel. 2008. Available at: http://www.medretreat.com/templates/UserFiles/Documents/McKinsey%20Report%20Medical%20Travel.pdf (last accessed: 25th April 2012).
4. Mortensen J. International trade in health services: assessing the trade and the trade-offs. 2008. Available at: http://www.arengufond.ee/upload/Editor/teenused/Tervise%20lugemine/International_Trade_in_Health%20Services_DK_Mortensen%202008.pdf (last accessed 25th April 2012).
5. Alleman BW, et al. Medical tourism services available to residents of the United States. J Gen Intern Med 2011;26:492–7.
6. Shetty P. Medical tourism booms in India, but at what cost? Lancet 2010;376:671–2.
7. Ounibi W. High HIV and HbsAg infection rate in recipients of commercial transplants. J Am Soc Nephrol 1993;4:957.
8. Trivedi M, Sanghavi D. Knowledge deficits regarding Chagas' disease may place Mexico's blood supply at risk. Transfus Apher Sci 2010;43:193–6.
9. Kumarasamy KK, Toleman MA, Walsh TR, et al. Emergence of a new antibiotic resistance mechanism in India, Pakistan, and the UK: a molecular, biological, and epidemiological study. Lancet Infect Dis 2010;10:597–602.
10. Bronnert J, Wilde H, Tepsumethanon V, et al. Organ transplantations and rabies transmission. J Trav Med 2007;14:177–80.
11. Iwamoto M, Jernigan DB, Guasch A, et al. Transmission of West Nile virus from an organ donor to four transplant recipients. N Engl J Med 2003; 348:2196–203.
12. Shaw C. The external assessmentof health services. World Hospitals and Health Services 2003:40(1), Available at: http://www.who.int/management/External%20Assessment%20of%20Health%20Services.pdf (last accessed 25th April 2012).
13. Rooney AL, van Ostenberg PR. Licensure, Accreditation, and Certification: Approaches to Health. Bethesda: Quality Assurance Project; 1999. Available at: www.qaproject.org/indexl.html (last accessed 25th April 2012).
14. Henderson M. Patients warned over dangers of untested stem-cell wonder cures. 29 August 2006. http://www.timesonline.co.uk/tol/news/uk/health/article621777.ece (last accessed 25th April 2012).
15. Sex selection: Getting the baby you want. April 2010. Available at: http://www.guardian.co.uk/lifeandstyle/2010/apr/03/sex-selection-babies (last accessed 25th April 2012).
16. Stella Obasanjo's doctor jailed for negligence. September 2006. Available at: http://thenationonlineng.net/web2/articles/19341/1/Stella-Obasanjos-doctor-jailed-for-negligence/Page1.html (last accessed 25th April 2012).
17. 'Buttocks injection' death: Police quiz woman in US. February 2011. Available at: http://www.bbc.co.uk/news/world-us-canada-12410546 (last accessed 25th April 2012).
18. Delmonico FL. The implications of Istanbul Declaration on organ trafficking and transplant tourism. Curr Opin Organ Transpl 2009;141:116–9.

Transplant Patients and Tropical Diseases 152

Neha Nanda, Frank J Bia

Key features

- "Travel for transplantation" differs from "transplant tourism", which is driven by commercialism, involves organ trafficking, diversion of resources, and is associated with greater risks of infection and lower graft survival rates
- Solid organ transplant (SOT) recipients are less immunocompromised than stem cell transplant (SCT) recipients. The resulting disparities in quality of life and medical problems following transplantation can lead to acquisition of tropical infections during travel
- Exposure to tropical pathogens depends upon the geography of travel; presenting clinical syndromes are often atypical, since immunosuppression can alter the usual pathogenesis
- Malaria predominates among tropical pathogens acquired abroad by travelers who have received SCT or SOT
- Few cases of visceral leishmaniasis have been reported in SCT recipients. Visceral leishmaniasis is well described in SOT recipients and is generally not acquired during travel; infections reflect the endemicity of leishmaniasis in the recipient's country of origin
- Acute Chagas disease in the SCT population causes severe illness, while in the immunocompetent host the course is often benign. Most SOT-related cases of Chagas disease have been described in Latin America. Acquisition during transplantation, particularly cardiac transplantation, is well documented
- *Campylobacter* infections can result in Guillain–Barré syndrome (GBS) in transplant recipients; immunosuppressive regimens do not prevent this from occurring

INTRODUCTION

International travel and transplantation present many opportunities for acquisition of tropical diseases. These include infections related to trafficked organs, those acquired during transplantation, and infections among post-transplant recipients who are immunocompromised by drugs used to prevent transplant rejection.

The Istanbul Declaration on Organ Trafficking and Transplant Tourism (2008) provides useful guidance and information. The Declaration distinguishes between "travel for transplantation" and "transplant tourism". When organs, donors, recipients, or professionals move across jurisdictional borders, it is designated as travel for transplantation, which may be justified. When organ trafficking, commercialism, and diversion of resources undermine the ability of a host country to provide transplant services for its own population, it becomes unethical transplant tourism (Table 152-1) [1,2].

TRANSPLANT TOURISM

The Istanbul Declaration is curtailing such practices, but risks for donors and recipients persist, particularly for recipient acquisition of serious tropical diseases under conditions of immunosuppression.

Stem cell transplants occurring among medical tourists have resulted in a recipient brain tumor from unproven neural stem cell therapy performed in Moscow, and meningitis from stem cell transplants in China for spinal cord injuries [3]. Graft survival rates are lower and infection rates are generally higher among transplant tourists. Kidney is the most common organ procured through transplant tourism. At UCLA, 17 of 33 (52%) recipients who received the organ from another country experienced post-transplant infections requiring hospitalization [2]. One recipient acquired hepatitis B and died of multi-organ failure [4]. Given the long waiting list for organ transplantation in the US, and challenges involved in regulating the practice of transplant tourism, it is reasonable to expect a rise in tropical infections occurring in transplant recipients.

In 2008, a total of 27,966 solid organ transplants were performed in the US, of which two-thirds were from deceased donors. There were approximately 16,000 kidney transplants and 6000 liver transplants. In Europe during the same year, about 4000 liver transplants were done. The median wait time for liver transplantation in the US varies from 76 days to 459 days. In 2008, about 400 patients with acute myelogenous leukemia (AML) underwent transplantation and 3500 patients with multiple myeloma [5–7]. Worldwide, organ trafficking and transplant tourism account for about 10% of annual organ transplants, providing ample opportunity for the acquisition of unrecognized tropical diseases and reactivation of latent infections from the donated organ [1].

This chapter focuses upon travelers who have undergone transplantation under ideal circumstances, who then visit areas where tropical diseases remain endemic. How do such travelers fare when they receive pharmaceutical agents designed to prevent organ rejection and are exposed to tropical agents whose pathogenesis may be altered by immunosuppression? Infections may become more pathogenic, and clinically unrecognizable, even to experienced clinicians.

DEGREES OF IMMUNOSUPPRESSION

In the last 20 years, new immunomodulating agents have been introduced for induction and maintenance of immunosuppression in a transplant recipient (Table 152-2) [8–13]. These include tacrolimus and cyclosporine, which are calcineurin inhibitors; corticosteroids that inhibit multiple cytokines; sirolimus, an (mTOR) inhibitor of mammalian rapamycin affecting cellular protein synthesis; mycophenolate mofetil, an antimetabolite; daclizumab and basiliximab, antibodies directed against interleukin-2; and alemtuzumab or thymoglobulin, with antibodies directed against T and B lymphocytes. As a result of potent therapies, the rate of graft survival and quality of life after transplantation have improved. In kidney transplant recipients, 1-year graft survival now approaches 95% and incidence of rejection at 1 year is only 15%. The quality of life for organ recipients 10 years after liver transplantation is generally good. Multiple studies have shown long-term improvement in quality of life after allogeneic stem cell transplantation [14–16].

Immunosuppressive therapy started immediately after transplant is more potent and is referred to as induction therapy. This regimen generally consists of thymoglobulin, alemtuzumab, daclizumab, or basiliximab. Lifetime maintenance immunotherapy is less potent and consists of calcineurin inhibitors, mTOR inhibitors, and steroids. In the setting of acute rejection, more potent agents like rituximab, an anti-CD20 antibody, and intravenous corticosteroids are employed. Most of these agents are associated with increased susceptibility to infection (Table 152-2). In stem cell transplantation (SCT), conditioning with total body irradiation eradicates disease and reduces the likelihood of early rejection.

TABLE 152-1 Differences Between "Travel for Transplant" and "Transplant Tourism"

Travel for transplant	Transplant tourism
Movement of organs, donors, recipients, or transplant professionals across jurisdictional borders for transplantation, which may be justified	Practice of transplantation during which transplant resources are diverted to a recipient from another country. The interests of the residents of the host country are therefore undermined
Patients' interests are first priority	Driven largely by commercialism and monetary gain
Ethical practices in organ acquisition	Unethical practices such as organ trafficking

SCT recipients are the most immunosuppressed. As a result of conditioning therapy and graft-versus-host disease (GVHD), cutaneous and mucosal breakdown, neutropenia, lymphopenia, hypogammaglobinemia, and loss of immune memory occur. Following engraftment, SCT recipients inherit their donor's hematopoietic profile. Solid organ transplant (SOT) recipients are less immunocompromised. Among SOT recipients, kidney transplant recipients require relatively minimal immunosuppression, liver and heart require moderate amounts, and small bowel and lung require higher levels.

IMMUNOSUPPRESSION AND TROPICAL DISEASES

There are very few case reports or series on tropical infections in the SCT recipient: tuberculosis in endemic areas, asymptomatic Chagas disease, and toxoplasmosis. In contrast, there are numerous reports, case series, and reviews of tropical infections in the SOT recipient. This disparity is partially a result of variations in the quality of life (QOL), including opportunities for travel, within each subgroup. In SOT, there is improvement in QOL [14,17]. However, in SCT, there is a reduction in QOL until year 1 post-transplant; 60% reported improvement in QOL by year 1, but 25% reported ongoing medical problems.

DISEASE DISTRIBUTION IN RETURNING TRAVELERS

In a cross-sectional survey of 2554 SOT recipients at the Mayo Clinic, 27% of the recipients reported travel outside of the US and Canada after their transplant. Ninety-six percent of the travelers did not seek medical care prior to travel; 8% required medical attention due to illness [18]. Pre-travel counseling and vaccination can help in reducing morbidity in this population. Generally, SOT recipients are urged to delay travel until 3–6 months following transplant. Detailed information about pre-travel advice has been published [19,20].

Relevant data on all traveler types are available from approximately 30 GeoSentinel sites on six continents. However no database similar to that of the GeoSentinel network exists for transplant recipients. The

TABLE 152-2 Immunosuppressive Agents Used in Transplantation

Name	Trade name	Mechanism	Use	Impact on infections
Alemtuzumab [8,9]	Campath, MabCampath	Humanized monoclonal antibody directed against CD52, a glycoprotein expressed on B and T lymphocytes, monocytes, and natural killer cells	1. B-cell lymphoid leukemia 2. For induction and maintenance of acute rejection after SOT	Increases risk of CMV infection and BK virus nephropathy
Mycophenolate mofetil (MMF) [10,11]	Cellcept	Inhibitor of IMPDH enzyme, resulting in inhibition of both T and B cells	Maintenance immunosuppression after SOT and SCT	Increases risk of bacterial infections compared to calcineurin inhibitors and increases risk of CMV infection
Calcineurin inhibitors – cyclosporine (CsA) and tacrolimus (TAC) [12]	CsA – Gengraf, Neoral, Restasis, Sandimmune TAC – Prograf	Blocks transcription of cytokines responsible for T-cell activation by inhibiting calcineurin	Same as MMF	Increases risk of BK virus nephropathy when TAC used with MMF
Sirolimus [13]	Rapamune	Inhibits T-cell activation and proliferation	Same as MMF and also used in drug-eluting coronary stents	Reduces risk of CMV reactivation compared to TAC

IMDPH, inosine-5′-monophosphate dehydrogenase.

reader is referred to a review article by Franco-Paredes et al. detailing three categories of tropical infections in transplant patients: those related to donor, to the recipient, and to de novo acquisition [20].

Approximately 8% of all travelers need medical care during or following travel, regardless of their immunologic status. Diagnoses that contributed to death in travelers included severe and complicated malaria, pulmonary embolism, pneumonia, and pyogenic abscesses. Among the more than 17,000 patients reported via the GeoSentinel network from June 1996 through August 2004, most were seen for illness within a month of travel [21]. Diagnoses for 67% of these travelers fell into four major syndrome categories: systemic febrile illnesses, acute diarrhea, dermatologic disorders, and chronic diarrhea. This classification is of epidemiologic value in predicting disease in transplant patients.

MALARIA

Malaria is the most likely tropical disease acquired abroad by travelers who previously received SCT or SOT, as it is for all travelers.

MALARIA IN STEM CELL AND SOLID ORGAN TRANSPLANT RECIPIENTS

There are few case reports of malaria in stem cell recipients. A 20-year-old Bangladeshi woman successfully underwent autologous SCT for acute myelogenous leukemia. She received the transplant in Italy. Within a week after her transplant, she developed fevers in the setting of neutropenia. Despite recovery of her neutrophil counts, and treatment with broad-spectrum antimicrobials, fevers continued. A peripheral blood smear showed 4% *Plasmodium vivax* parasitemia. Within 48 hours of initiation of antimalarial therapy, fevers resolved. Infection was presumed to be a recrudescence of a primary *vivax* malaria [22].

A 20-year-old Indian man who underwent an allogeneic SCT for chronic myeloid leukemia in India, had a subtle presentation of malaria. Although the patient engrafted, he had continued pancytopenia, and 70 days following transplant he developed splenomegaly and persistent pancytopenia despite a bone marrow examination showing good cellularity. He had *P. vivax* on peripheral blood smear. Following malaria treatment, his blood counts normalized and the spleen reduced in size. In retrospect, he gave a history of malaria 5 years prior to transplant [23]. Based on limited reports, *vivax* appears to be the most common species in SCT recipients. The prolonged latency of *vivax* hypnozoites make recrudescence feasible.

Literature and data on SOT recipients who have acquired malaria *de novo* are minimal. Rather, acquisition of malaria infection during SOT appears to occur through infected blood products or transplanted organs. Most of the nearly 50 cases of malaria in SOT recipients have involved renal transplant patients [24], likely reflecting their larger numbers; a majority were caused by *P. falciparum*. Most had favorable outcomes; however, some deaths have occurred with *P. falciparum*. Case data are insufficient to allow description of pathogenesis, levels of parasitemia and response to antimalarial therapy in SOT recipients who acquired malaria independent of transplantation.

LEISHMANIASIS IN STEM CELL AND SOLID ORGAN TRANSPLANT RECIPIENTS

Among SCT recipients, at least two individuals have developed visceral leishmaniasis as a result of *de novo* infection. One report describes a 57-year-old man who developed fevers 66 weeks after he had received a peripheral blood SCT in France [25]. It was complicated by GVHD, and treated with antithymoglobulin, anti-CD25 monoclonal antibody, and mycophenolate mofetil. One year following successful treatment of nodular pulmonary aspergillosis, fevers recurred and serum antibodies to *Leishmania* were detected. Amastigotes were seen in bone marrow; blood and bone marrow cultures showed *L. infantum* promastigotes. Retrospective analysis revealed that during the first febrile episode, asymptomatic circulation of *Leishmania* occurred. Prior to the second episode of fever, there was active infection. Pretransplant donor and recipient blood did not show *Leishmania* organisms or antibodies. Acquisition of visceral leishmaniasis was attributed to a sandfly bite a few weeks before his initial presentation. Fever abated after restarting therapy with amphotericin B, followed by an uneventful course at 1 year [25].

A 59-year-old male in the Netherlands presented with cytomegalovirus (CMV) and Epstein-Barr virus (EBV) reactivation 3 months after receiving an HLA-matched SCT. He had no constitutional symptoms and his physical examination was unremarkable, but he was pancytopenic. Amastigotes of *L. infantum* were observed on bone marrow biopsy and in peripheral blood. No antibodies against *Leishmania* were detected in peripheral blood. Pre-transplant donor and recipient sera were antibody-negative. The patient had traveled to southern France, where leishmaniasis is endemic, 4 weeks before the transplant. He received liposomal amphotericin B, resulting in negative blood smears and bone marrow [26].

More than 60 cases of visceral leishmaniasis have been described in SOT recipients; the vast majority had received renal transplants [24]. Most were *not* acquired during travel, but reflected endemicity of leishmaniasis in the recipients' country of origin. Clues to the development of visceral leishmaniasis in this population include fever, hepatomegaly, and splenomegaly. Approximately 50% can show pancytopenia. Symptoms may be atypical due to immunosuppression, and diagnosis can be delayed.

Antibody detection tests such as the rk39-based immunochromatographic test have shown promise in the diagnosis of visceral leishmaniasis in endemic areas and can assist in the early diagnosis in a returning transplant recipient as well. However, these diagnostic modalities have yet to be studied in this group of individuals [27].

CHAGAS DISEASE (AMERICAN TRYPANOSOMIASIS) IN STEM CELL AND SOLID ORGAN TRANSPLANT RECIPIENTS

Presentations of Chagas disease in SCT recipients range from asymptomatic parasitemia to fulminant fatal disease. Asymptomatic parasitemia can occur with reactivation of latent infection in individuals from endemic areas. A patient from northern Argentina developed parasitemia 3 months after allogeneic SCT. During a presentation with pneumococcal bacteremia, asymptomatic *Trypanosoma cruzi* infection was detected in blood cultures. Treatment achieved a favorable outcome [28].

A 31-year-old male with chronic Chagas disease was found to have asymptomatic circulating trypomastigotes and neutropenia following conditioning therapy 4 days prior to SCT. He underwent successful transplantation and treatment for Chagas, with no evidence of reactivation of *T. cruzi* at 4 years [29].

Acute disseminated Chagas disease acquired *de novo* can present during episodes of severe immunosuppression. A 25-year-old male developed fever and neuropsychiatric symptoms approximately 10 days after an unrelated cord blood transplant. One month after transplantation, *T. cruzi* was observed in peripheral blood and bone marrow. Despite antiparasitic therapy, his decline was rapid. Autopsy showed *T. cruzi* myocarditis and encephalitis. In retrospect, his pretransplant evaluation had shown pancytopenia with diffuse ST-T wave changes and abnormal Q waves on the electrocardiogram [30].

A 20-year-old man developed acute Chagas disease after allogeneic SCT, possibly via infected blood products. Three months following his transplant, fever, weakness, and generalized edema occurred with a normal neurologic examination. Hypogammaglobinemia was present and trypomastigotes were observed in peripheral blood and cerebrospinal fluid (CSF) with an otherwise normal CSF analysis. Therapy was initiated, but he developed bacteremia and shock and died [31].

Most SOT-related cases of Chagas disease have been described in Latin America; reactivation does not occur in all patients who undergo immunosuppression [24,32]. Acquisition during transplantation, particularly cardiac transplantation is well documented, and travel for transplantation represents the most likely source of Chagas disease. Donors from areas of high endemicity such as Latin America require careful screening to prevent transmission and subsequent reactivation in the immunosuppressed recipient. Cardiac transplantation utilizing the heart of a patient with chronic infection is considered an absolute contraindication since chagasic myocarditis can readily evolve during periods of immunosuppression.

STRONGYLOIDIASIS IN STEM CELL AND SOLID ORGAN TRANSPLANT RECIPIENTS

Strongyloidiasis in SCT presents as a hyperinfection syndrome that is often fatal. Frequently a result of a subclinical *S. stercoralis* infection prior to transplantation in SOT recipients, the disease usually occurs within the first 3 months after transplantation. In SCT, it can have an earlier presentation [33].

Two people with SCT developed hyperinfection syndrome with alveolar hemorrhage. A 52-year-old man from Puerto Rico, who had undergone an autologous SCT in the US for advanced follicular lymphoma, presented 24 days after SCT with acute-onset abdominal pain, nausea, and vomiting. Duodenal biopsy showed acute inflammation with *S. stercoralis* larvae and rare CMV inclusions. Stools were negative for larvae. Eosinophilia had been observed 3 months prior to the transplant. Initial improvement occurred following administration of ivermectin, thiabendazole, phosphonoformate (Foscarnet®), and ganciclovir. However, his course was complicated by pneumonia and bacteremia. On bronchoalveolar lavage, *S. stercoralis* larvae were detected. He died in septic shock with alveolar hemorrhage [34].

A 44-year-old woman residing in Florida with acute myelomonocytic leukemia had intermittent eosinophilia. Two days following myeloablative conditioning and allogeneic SCT, she developed fever, hypotension, bilateral pulmonary infiltrates, and bacteremia. Bronchoalveolar lavage showed *S. stercoralis* larvae and she received ivermectin and immunosuppression reduction. Stools were negative for larvae before and after transplantation. Eleven days into her illness, she died despite therapy [35].

For SOT recipients, travel for transplantation again represents the most likely scenario for acquisition of infection [24]. This may be particularly true for pancreatic transplantation where a portion of the infected duodenum can carry larvae. Patients who are immunosuppressed following SOT and acquire a new infection are at similar risk.

CAMPYLOBACTER INFECTIONS IN STEM CELL AND SOLID ORGAN TRANSPLANT RECIPIENTS

Campylobacter jejuni is the agent most frequently associated with Guillain–Barré syndrome (GBS). Reports of *C. jejuni* in SCT recipients are sparse. Campylobacteriosis varies from asymptomatic bacteremia to symptomatic enteritis with or without bacteremia. None of the reported cases of *C. jejuni* infection were attributed to either recent or remote history of travel in this group [36].

Among SOT recipients there are few reports of *C. jejuni* infection or associated GBS; it is far more likely to occur following CMV infection. In 1998, Maccario et al. reported a case of high-grade bacteremia in a renal transplant recipient nearly 200 days following transplantation [37]. Immunosuppression did not prevent detection of IgM antibody production directed against GM1 ganglioside and subsequent GBS. In 2002, Colle et al. reported *Campylobacter fetus* infection and subsequent GBS 70 days following liver transplantation [38]. They suggested that GBS and subsequent clinical recovery were largely mediated by autoimmune antibody production that was largely unaffected by transplant immunosuppression directed at T cells. In 2005, Toussaint et al. reported a severe case of CMV-associated colitis and vasculitis [39]. In this case *Campylobacter*-induced inflammatory cytokine production could have led to CMV reactivation.

In summary, travel to endemic regions can place transplant recipients at risk of tropical infections during their chronic immunosuppression (Tables 152-3 & 152-4). However, transplant tourism within facilities

TABLE 152-3 Tropical Infections Occurring in Stem Cell Transplant Recipients*

Syndrome	Outcome
Systemic febrile illness	
Malaria	Cured
Leishmaniasis	Cured
Chagas disease	Some cases are fatal
Disseminated infection	
Strongyloidiasis	Often fatal
Toxoplasmosis	Often fatal
Asymptomatic infection	
Chagas disease	Cured

*Data obtained from case reports only; estimates for the frequency of each disease in this population are not available.

TABLE 152-4 Tropical Infections Occurring in Solid Organ Transplant Recipients

Syndrome	Frequency	Outcomes
Systemic febrile illness		
Malaria	At least 45 cases have been reported [24]; most have occurred in renal transplant recipients	Majority were cured
Leishmaniasis	At least 60 cases have been reported; most have occurred in renal transplant recipients	Cured
Disseminated infection		
Strongyloidiasis	At least 63 cases have been reported	Often fatal
Histoplasmosis	1 case per 1000 transplant person years in endemic areas	Cured
Asymptomatic infection		
Chagas disease	Varies, depending on the endemic area	Cured

located in endemic regions for tropical diseases, where either blood transfusions or organs may already be infected with tropical pathogens, is of equal or greater importance. Atypical presentations, widespread systemic illness and delayed diagnoses are likely to occur under both circumstances.

REFERENCES

1. Delmonico FL. The implications of Istanbul Declaration on organ trafficking and transplant tourism. Current Opin Organ Transplant 2009;14:116–19.
2. Delmonico FL. The hazards of transplant tourism. Clin J Am Soc Nephrol 2009;4:249–50.
3. Barclay E. Stem-cell experts raise concerns about medical tourism. Lancet 2009;373:883–4.
4. Gill J, Madhira BR, Gjertson D, et al. Transplant tourism in the United States: a single-center experience. Clin J Am Soc Nephrol 2008;3:1820–8.
5. OPTN. http://optn.transplant.hrsa.gov/latestData/rptData.asp
6. European Liver Transplant Registry. http://www.eltr.org/spip.php?article146
7. Bone Marrow and Cord Blood Donation and Transplantation. http://bloodcell.transplant.hrsa.gov/RESEARCH/Transplant_Data/US_Tx_Data/Data_by_Disease/national.aspx
8. Peleg AY, Husain S, Kwak EJ, et al. Opportunistic infections in 547 organ transplant recipients receiving alemtuzumab, a humanized monoclonal CD-52 antibody. Clin Infect Dis 2007;44:204–12.
9. Park SH, Choi SM, Lee DG, et al. Infectious complications associated with alemtuzumab use for allogeneic hematopoietic stem cell transplantation: comparison with anti-thymocyte globulin. Transpl Infect Dis 2009;11:413–23.
10. Hanvesakul R, Kubal C, Jham S, et al. Increased incidence of infections following the late introduction of mycophenolate mofetil in renal transplant recipients. Nephrol Dial Transplant 2008;23:4049–53.
11. Ritter ML, Pirofski L. Mycophenolate mofetil: effects on cellular immune subsets, infectious complications, and antimicrobial activity. Transpl Infect Dis 2009;11:290–7.
12. Binet I, Nickeleit V, Hirsch HH, et al. Polyomavirus disease under new immunosuppressive drugs: a cause of renal graft dysfunction and graft loss. Transplantation 1999;67:918–22.
13. Haririan A, Morawski K, West MS, et al. Sirolimus exposure during the early post-transplant period reduces the risk of CMV infection relative to tacrolimus in renal allograft recipients. Clin Transplantat 2007;21:466–71.
14. Zand MS. Immunosuppression and immune monitoring after renal transplantation. Semin Dial 2005;18:511–19.
15. Desai R, Jamieson NV, Gimson AE, et al. Quality of life up to 30 years following liver transplantation. Liver Transpl 2008;14:1473–9.
16. Pidala J, Anasetti C, Jim H. Quality of life after allogeneic hematopoietic cell transplantation. Blood 2009;114:7–19.
17. Kawagishi N, Takeda I, Miyagi S, et al. Quality of life and problems affecting recipients more than 10 years after living donor liver transplantation. Transplant Proc 2009;41:236–7.
18. Uslan DZ, Patel R, Virk A. International travel and exposure risks in solid-organ transplant recipients. Transplantation 2008;86:407–12.
19. Kotton CN, Ryan ET, Fishman JA. Prevention of infection in adult travelers after solid organ transplantation. Am J Transplant 2005;5:8–14.
20. Franco-Paredes C, Jacob JT, Hidron A, et al. Transplantation and tropical infectious diseases. Int J Infect Dis 2010;14:e189–96.
21. Freedman DO, Weld LH, Kozarsky PE, et al. Spectrum of disease and relation to place of exposure among ill returned travelers. N Engl J Med 2006;354:119–30.
   This is an important summary of the epidemiology of travel-related infections based upon clinical surveillance data obtained in over 17,000 ill returning travelers reported through 30 GeoSentinel sites on six continents.
22. Salutari P, Sica S, Chiusolo P, et al. *Plasmodium vivax* malaria after autologous bone marrow transplantation: an unusual complication. Bone Marrow Transplant 1996;18:805–6.
23. Raina V, Sharma A, Gujral S, Kumar R. *Plasmodium vivax* causing pancytopenia after allogeneic blood stem cell transplantation in CML. Bone Marrow Transplant 1998;22:205–6.
24. Martin-Davila P, Fortun J, Lopez-Velez R, et al. Transmission of tropical and geographically restricted infections during solid-organ transplantation. Clin Microbiol Rev 2008;21:60–96.
   This article represents an important comprehensive summary of tropical disease acquisition and presentations in the population of patients who have received solid organ transplants. The issues of diseases acquired during transplantation versus those encountered during travel following transplantation are well discussed.
25. Sirvent-von Bueltzingsloewen A, Marty P, Rosenthal E, et al. Visceral leishmaniasis: a new opportunistic infection in hematopoietic stem-cell-transplanted patients. Bone Marrow Transplant 2004;33:667–8.
26. Agteresch HJ, van 't Veer MB, Cornelissen JJ, Sluiters JF. Visceral leishmaniasis after allogeneic hematopoietic stem cell transplantation. Bone Marrow Transplant 2007;40:391–3.
27. Chappuis F, Sundar S, Hailu A, et al. Visceral leishmaniasis: what are the needs for diagnosis, treatment and control? Nature Rev 2007;5:873–82.
28. Altclas J, Sinagra A, Jaimovich G, et al. Reactivation of chronic Chagas' disease following allogeneic bone marrow transplantation and successful pre-emptive therapy with benznidazole. Transpl Infect Dis 1999;1:135–7.
29. Dictar M, Sinagra A, Veron MT, et al. Recipients and donors of bone marrow transplants suffering from Chagas' disease: management and preemptive therapy of parasitemia. Bone Marrow Transplant 1998;21:391–3.
30. Fores R, Sanjuan I, Portero F, et al. Chagas disease in a recipient of cord blood transplantation. Bone Marrow Transplant 2007;39:127–8.
31. Villalba R, Fornes G, Alvarez MA, et al. Acute Chagas' disease in a recipient of a bone marrow transplant in Spain: case report. Clin Infect Dis 1992;14:594–5.
   This represents a very well-written and -documented clinical presentation of acute Chagas disease after an allogeneic bone marrow transplantation.
32. Centers for Disease Control and Prevention (CDC). Chagas disease after organ transplantation – United States, 2001. MMRW Morb Mortal Wkly Rep 2002;51:210–12.
33. Roxby AC, Gottlieb GS, Limaye AP. Strongyloidiasis in transplant patients. Clin Infect Dis 2009;49:1411–23.
   The authors have compiled all strongyloidiasis cases in SCT and SOT recipients. They provide an excellent summary of clinical presentations, timing of appearance, and outcomes, along with prevention strategies in this population.
34. Gupta S, Jain A, Fanning TV, et al. An unusual cause of alveolar hemorrhage post hematopoietic stem cell transplantation: a case report. BMC Cancer 2006;6:87.
35. Wirk B, Wingard JR. *Strongyloides stercoralis* hyperinfection in hematopoietic stem cell transplantation. Transpl Infect Dis 2009;11:143–8.
36. Lau SK, Woo PC, Leung KW, Yuen KY. Emergence of cotrimoxazole- and quinolone-resistant *Campylobacter* infections in bone marrow transplant recipients. Eur J Clin Microbiol Infect Dis 2002;21:127–9.
37. Maccario M, Tarantino A, Nobile-Orazio E, Ponticelli C. *Campylobacter jejuni* bacteremia and Guillain-Barre syndrome in a renal transplant recipient. Transpl Int 1998;11:439–42.
38. Colle I, Van Vlierberghe H, Troisi R, et al. *Campylobacter*-associated Guillain-Barre syndrome after orthotopic liver transplantation for hepatitis C cirrhosis: a case report. Hepatol Res 2002;24:205.
39. Toussaint N, Goodman D, Langham R, et al. Haemorrhagic *Campylobacter jejuni* and CMV colitis in a renal transplant recipient. Nephrol Dial Transplant 2005;20:823–6.

153 Delusional Parasitosis

Kathryn N Suh, Jay S Keystone

Key features

- An uncommon, unfounded, irrational belief of infestation that cannot be corrected by reasoning, persuasion, or logic
- More common in women and in older age groups (>50 years)
- Patients may be otherwise highly functional
- Rarely, may be associated with underlying medical or psychiatric disease, substance abuse, or medications
- Longstanding history of cutaneous complaints and dermatologic findings, often for months to years before diagnosis
- Skin lesions are common and often asymmetric, reflecting the range of the dominant upper limb
- Effective therapies (neuroleptics) are available but often difficult for patients to accept
- **Synonyms**: delusional (or delusions of) infestation; delusions of parasitosis
  - *less commonly*: chronic tactile hallucinosis, cocaine bugs, delusional ectoparasitosis, delusory parasitosis, Ekbom's syndrome, formication, praeseniler dermatozoenwahn (presenile dermatozoic delusion), psychogenic parasitosis
  - *others*: acaraphobia, dermatophobia, entomophobia, parasitophobia (technically these are not correct since they indicate a phobia rather than belief)

INTRODUCTION

Delusional parasitosis (DP), first described in 1894, is a disorder in which affected individuals have a delusion – an unshakeable belief – that they are infected by "bugs": parasites, worms, bacteria, mites, or other living organisms, associated with abnormal cutaneous sensations. While the disease remains rare, there is increasing awareness of and advancement in the pharmacologic therapy of DP. However, recognition and management of this problem continues to be challenging.

EPIDEMIOLOGY

Delusional disorders are rare, being slightly more common among women. Their incidence and prevalence were previously estimated to be 0.7–3.0 and 24–30 cases per 100,000 population, respectively [1]. More recent data suggest that these may be underestimates; in one Swedish cohort, the lifetime prevalence of delusional disorders was estimated at 0.30 per 100 population [2].

Rates of DP are difficult to determine. Since patients with DP generally refuse psychiatric help, the true incidence and prevalence of this disorder may be greatly underestimated in the psychiatric literature. In southwest Germany, the incidence and prevalence of DP were estimated to be 16.6 and 83.2 cases per million population per year, respectively [3]. In his 1995 review, Trabert [4] had identified a total of 1223 cases in the literature; as of 2008, reports of over 1400 cases were published [5]. Most have been reported from North America and Europe, and recently from most other areas of the world except Africa.

While DP affects adults of all ages, it is much more common in older age groups (> 50 years). In Trabert's review, the mean age of onset was 57 years and 84% of patients were over age 50, with men presenting at a slightly younger age than women [4]. Overall, women outnumber men by a 2–3 : 1 ratio [4,6]. Although the sex distribution is almost equal in early adulthood, the female : male ratio exceeds 3 : 1 in individuals over 50 years of age [4,6].

Patients can be from any socioeconomic background. Many are single and may be considered "loners". A higher than expected prevalence of personality disorders has been observed in some case series [6,7]. However, many affected individuals are both educated and highly functional; in Lyell's survey [6], several of the 282 patients described were professionals, including physicians and psychologists.

NATURAL HISTORY, PATHOGENESIS, AND PATHOLOGY

In its truest form, DP is a delusional disorder of the somatic type: "delusions that the person has some physical defect of general medical condition" [8]. Munro [9] first suggested that DP was a form of monosymptomatic hypochondriasis or monosymptomatic hypochondriacal psychosis (MHP), a fixed, single hypochondriacal belief that exists when no other thought disorder is present. Delusions of parasitosis are the most common form of MHP.

The pathophysiology of somatic delusional disorders is unknown. Some have theorized that abnormal sensations experienced by patients (*as if* something was crawling on the skin) lead to the conviction that parasites are present (that something really *is* crawling on the skin). An incident during which exposure to parasites might have occurred, such as sleeping in unclean bedsheets, borrowing another's clothing, or travel to an exotic destination, may be a trigger for DP. In some, newly acquired knowledge or awareness of a disease (through heightened public health or media interest, or the internet, for example) can amplify and perpetuate new or pre-existing symptoms; reasons for this symptom amplification are unclear. Stress can also exacerbate somatic complaints, and the stress induced by the severity of the perceived illness may augment symptoms further.

It has also been suggested that DP may be due to central nervous system abnormalities. Response of many patients to the dopamine

BOX 153.1 Diagnostic Criteria for Delusional Disorder

1. Non-bizarre delusions involving situations that occur in real life, lasting >1 month
2. Does not meet all criteria for diagnosis of schizophrenia (see text)
3. Function is otherwise not markedly impaired
4. Mood episodes, if concurrent, are of brief duration compared with duration of delusions
5. Substance abuse, medication side effects, and general medications must be ruled out

Adapted from American Psychiatric Association. DSM-IV-TR. Diagnostic and Statistical Manual of Mental Disorders, 4th edn, Text Revision. Washington, DC: American Psychiatric Association, 2000;323–9.

antagonist pimozide supports the theory that DP results from excess extracellular dopamine within the striatum of the brain [10]. In some patients, structural abnormalities in the basal ganglia, in particular the putamen and caudate nucleus, have been documented [11,12]; most of these patients also responded favorably to dopamine antagonists. Such findings must be interpreted with caution, however, given the small number of patients studied and the lack of comparison with age-matched normal controls.

CLASSIFICATION OF DELUSIONAL PARASITOSIS

No definite classification of DP exists. Broadly speaking, three different forms can be described.

PRIMARY DELUSIONAL PARASITOSIS

Primary DP is a somatic delusional disorder (Box 153.1). Patients with delusional disorders do not meet the diagnostic criteria for schizophrenia or other psychiatric disorders. Specifically, hallucinations, disorganized speech, schizophrenic behavior, and other "negative" symptoms are absent, although hallucinations that are *secondary* to the delusional theme (i.e. tactile hallucinations) may be present. Similarly, anxiety or depression *secondary* to the delusional disorder may be present.

SECONDARY DELUSIONAL PARASITOSIS ASSOCIATED WITH UNDERLYING PSYCHIATRIC DISEASE

Delusions of parasitosis may be a manifestation of an underlying psychiatric illness, such as schizophrenia, anxiety, depression, obsessive compulsive disorder, schizophreniform disorder, bipolar disorder, or post-traumatic stress disorder. It is essential to distinguish this form of DP from primary DP as the management differs, but this may be challenging, particularly for the non-psychiatrist physician who is most likely to encounter such patients.

SECONDARY DELUSIONAL PARASITOSIS ASSOCIATED WITH UNDERLYING MEDICAL CONDITIONS

Although up to 25% of cases of DP have been attributed to underlying medical conditions [4,7], in our experience this is remarkably rare. Delusional parasitosis has been attributed to diseases of most organ systems, most commonly the central nervous system (Table 153-1). Substance abuse should be considered, especially when DP presents in younger age groups. Numerous prescription medications have been implicated in DP; in such cases, symptoms generally resolve

TABLE 153-1 Some Medical Conditions and Medications Associated With Delusions of Parasitosis

Neurologic disorders	Dementia Head trauma Infarction Infection Multiple sclerosis Multiple system atrophy Postoperative complication of neurosurgery Tumors of the central nervous system
Endocrine disorders	Diabetes mellitus Hyperthyroidism
Hematologic disorders	Severe anemia Leukemia Polycythemia vera
Infectious diseases	HIV infection Leprosy Tuberculosis Prior infestation
Malignancy	Lymphoma Solid organ: breast, colon, lung
Nutritional deficiency	B12, folate, thiamine deficiency Pellagra
Drugs or toxins	Alcohol Amphetamines, including methylphenidate Cocaine Heroin
Prescription medications	Amantadine Ciprofloxacin Corticosteroids Ketoconazole Pargyline Pegylated interferon-alpha Phenelzine Topiramate

Adapted from Slaughter JR, Zanol K, Rezvani H, et al.: Psychogenic parasitosis: a case series and literature review. Psychosomatics 1998;39:491–500; and Johnson GC, Anton RF: Delusions of parasitosis: differential diagnosis and treatment. South Med J 1985;78:914–18.

once the offending drug is discontinued. Documented parasitic infection rarely (2% of all cases) precedes the development of DP [6].

CLINICAL FEATURES

Patients with DP have unfounded, irrational beliefs of infestation that cannot be corrected by reasoning, persuasion or logic. Symptoms and beliefs are variable, ranging from a non-disruptive feeling of infestation to delusions that may interfere with daily activities. Patients with primary DP generally have intact mental function, lack other manifestations of psychiatric disease, and have otherwise normal behavior. Their delusions are limited in scope and usually do not interfere with personal and professional aspects of their lives. Although they initially cannot appreciate their delusional state, it may subsequently become evident to them during therapy. Patients with secondary DP may have signs and symptoms of underlying disease. Younger patients are more likely to have DP associated with head injuries, substance abuse and schizophrenia, and are more likely to be involved in shared delusions [6,13]. Delusions due to substance abuse are usually transient and of inadequate duration to meet the criteria for delusional disorder.

Longstanding dermatologic complaints are common, including rashes, pruritus, and sensations of stinging, biting and formication.

Most patients have chronic symptoms, at least 6 months in duration and often longer, before the diagnosis is established. The median and average duration of symptoms before diagnosis in Trabert's study was 1 year and 3 years, respectively [4]. Patients may have received repeated courses of dermatologic and antiparasitic therapies despite the lack of an objective diagnosis. They frequently bring in specimens for examination which they have picked from their skin – the "matchbox" or "Ziploc® bag" sign [14,15] – and which typically contain normal skin flakes or dust, hair, or occasionally parts of non-pathogenic insects. Patients may produce bizarre and exhaustive descriptions and diagrams of the parasites and their reproductive cycles. Patients who attribute their disease to household pets may have visited veterinarians repeatedly, seeking treatment for their pets. Consultation with pest-control services and exterminators, and use of potentially toxic pesticides (on themselves and their belongings), may be attempted. Those driven to extremes may move, or rid themselves of their belongings. For some, fear of transmission of their "infection" to others may cause them to be socially isolated, even from family members. Recently, as a result of web searches, some believe that they have "Morgellons disease", an unexplained condition characterized by diverse cutaneous symptoms, foreign material (e.g. fibers) on the skin, and skin lesions.

Others, particularly family members, may occasionally be drawn into the patient's delusional system, usually by a woman [16]. Between 8% and 25% of delusions of parasitosis are shared [6,7,16], most often with one other person (folie à deux), usually a partner or spouse (less commonly offspring). On occasion, trios (folie à trois), or even larger groups, may be involved.

BOX 153.2 Suggested Initial Investigations in Patients with Delusional Parasitosis

In all patients:

- Complete blood count and differential
- Electrolytes, urea, creatinine
- Liver function tests and enzymes
- Fasting blood sugar
- Thyroid-stimulating hormone level
- B_{12} and folate levels
- Calcium and magnesium
- Erythrocyte sedimentation rate and C-reactive protein
- Chest radiograph

Based on the individual's risk factors and symptoms:

- Drug and toxin screen
- Serology for HIV infection and syphilis
- Tuberculin skin test
- Additional radiologic imaging (e.g. computerized tomography or magnetic resonance imaging of the brain)

PATIENT EVALUATION, DIAGNOSIS, AND DIFFERENTIAL DIAGNOSIS

Delusional parasitosis should be suspected when an individual presents with an irrational, fixed belief that he or she is infected with internal or external parasites in spite of reassurance and ample evidence to the contrary. It is important to determine the following: 1) is the belief founded in reality, and the patient truly infected; 2) if infection can be excluded, is the patient truly delusional, or is the patient hypochondriacal and the belief "shakeable"; and 3) if the patient is delusional, what form of DP is present? The optimal therapy differs depending on the answers to these questions. If an organic cause can be ruled out, the major challenge is then to determine whether the patient is suffering from a primary delusional disorder or has an underlying psychiatric illness. A psychiatric opinion is invaluable in such instances, but most patients with DP will refuse a psychiatric assessment.

The initial assessment(s) should focus on the patient's primary complaints, eliminating both true infection and an organic disease(s) as causes of their symptoms. A thorough history to elicit symptoms of underlying disease, and use of prescription and illicit drugs, should be obtained; important clues about underlying medical or psychiatric illness can be discovered by thorough careful questioning and listening. A complete physical examination is essential, looking for findings of underlying conditions and paying particular attention to the skin, since most patients have cutaneous symptoms. Ulcers, scratches, denuded skin and scars may be present from attempts to remove the organisms from the skin by using fingernails, knives, pins, duct-tape or other objects. Lesions are often absent in the upper back where the patient cannot reach. Contact or irritant dermatitis may be present from excessive cleaning or the use of abrasive soaps or chemicals.

Evaluation by a dermatologist can be beneficial and may reassure the patient that his/her symptoms are being taken seriously. If the patient has brought his/her own specimens, reassure the patient that these will be sent to a proper laboratory and/or entomologist for examination. The patient should be provided with specimen bottles containing preservative to collect additional specimens, thereby reducing the chance that parasites will be missed because of improper collection and reassuring the patient that you "believe" him/her. Skin biopsies are rarely required. Negative results, especially from repeated examinations of submitted specimens, can eliminate the possibility of a real parasitic infection. Appropriate initial investigations should be obtained (Box 153.2).

Follow-up visits fulfill multiple needs. In addition to providing more opportunity for the patient to develop trust in the physician, serial examination of skin lesions during repeat visits can be performed and additional specimens (or other investigations) obtained as required. Repeated assessments may also be helpful in determining whether the patient has a shakeable belief (hypochondriasis) rather than true delusions, if this remains unclear. Since most patients will not agree to psychiatric care, long-term follow-up with the primary care physician may be most appropriate.

PSYCHIATRIC ASSESSMENT

Secondary DP associated with underlying psychiatric disorders is best managed by a psychiatrist. Some suggest that most patients with DP should be managed by primary care physicians, dermatologists, or infectious disease consultants for fear of losing them to medical care altogether by suggesting they see a psychiatrist, while others recommend that a psychiatrist be at least consulted at some point in the patient's care. However, many healthcare practitioners are not trained or prepared to provide the pharmacotherapy that can benefit the patient with DP.

Convincing patients with DP of the need for and importance of a psychiatric referral is extremely difficult. The treating physician's credibility often dissipates and trust is lost at the mere mention of the need for psychiatric consultation or therapy; there is a significant risk of losing the patient altogether. Gradual introduction of the topic over the course of several visits, emphasizing the need for expert guidance to *manage the effects that DP has had on the patient's life* (such as stress or depression) may result in greater success. In some situations it may be helpful to discuss the case with a psychiatrist prior to commencing therapy.

TREATMENT

Psychotherapy, psychosurgery, and electroconvulsive therapy have met with little success in the treatment of DP, with low cure rates comparable to the rate of spontaneous resolution (17). Antidepressant and anxiolytic medications may improve secondary mood disorders but generally have no role in the treatment of primary DP.

A strong therapeutic relationship with the patient is critical. A sympathetic, non-judgmental approach, acknowledgment that patients' symptoms are real (and, if necessary that they are *not* mentally ill), and empathetic exploration into the effects their symptoms have had on their daily lives can instill a sense of trust into the relationship. A conservative, non-confrontational approach is recommended [17–19]. Use of phrases such as "I cannot see any parasites today" rather than "There are no parasites" [6], and acknowledgment that their problem *may* have resulted from a previous infection may accomplish this, while further gaining the patient's trust. It is important not to dismiss patients' complaints as trivial, even when they are clearly delusional, but equally important not to openly support their beliefs and feed into their delusional system. Reassurance that they can be helped is also valuable.

In spite of the limited evidence of their efficacy, with few clinical trials and no substantial randomized controlled trials conducted, antipsychotic medications have become the mainstay of therapy for DP [20]. The goal of therapy should be improvement in the patient's symptoms, and not necessarily cure. Convincing patients to take antipsychotic agents poses another significant obstacle, however. Even if patients do agree to start medication, adherence may be an issue. How does one convince psychotic patients who steadfastly believe that they are not psychotic to take antipsychotics? One strategy that we have used with considerable success is the approach that *"the parasitic infection" is no longer present, but symptoms continue as a result of a "biochemical imbalance" resulting from the initial infestation*. Introducing the need for an antipsychotic is accomplished by indicating that although the drug was originally designed for schizophrenia (*"but of course, you are not schizophrenic"*), it is being used for another purpose, i.e. to rebalance body chemistry. This statement should be followed by examples of other medications that have more than one use, such as aspirin for pyrexia and coronary artery disease, or amitriptyline for depression and neuritis. Patients are much more likely to agree to take medication for treatment of a "chemical imbalance" than for a psychiatric problem. Some patients may be persuaded if they are told that patients with a similar condition have experienced great relief in their symptoms using similar medications. Bargaining with a patient is fraught with potential problems; however, the physician may agree to a patient's request (for example, treatment with an antiparasitic agent) on the condition that the patient also begin an antipsychotic medication.

Efficacy comparisons of different agents are hindered by publication bias, the paucity of controlled trials, the inclusion of patients with both primary and secondary DP in many studies, and the lack of standardized criteria for assessing response to therapy.

First-Generation Antipsychotic Agents

While many first-generation antipsychotics have been used successfully for treatment of DP, pimozide has been the most extensively studied, with the highest reported success rate. Case series from the late 1990s reported response rates of up to 87% (33% to 52% complete, 28% to 35% partial) [21,22], and two small double-blind trials both demonstrated efficacy of greater than 90% [23,24].

Pimozide selectively blocks dopamine type 2 receptors. It has minimal effect on other central nervous system neurotransmitters, although its antagonistic effects on opiate receptors may also reduce sensations of pruritus and formication [23]. The most common adverse effects are extrapyramidal reactions (tremor, bradykinesia, shuffling gait), which occur in up to 15% of patients [13].

Doses between 1 and 12 mg daily are usually effective for treatment of DP. An initial dose of 0.5 to 1 mg daily can be increased gradually (e.g. by 1 mg weekly) either to the maximum daily dose of 20 mg, or until the desired clinical effect has been achieved, which may take several weeks. Most patients respond to doses much lower than 10 mg per day. Once a satisfactory response has been obtained, the patient should be maintained on the same dose for several months, and the dose can then be tapered gradually (by 1 mg every 1 to 2 weeks) until the drug is discontinued [13,25]. If relapses occur, they often respond to re-institution of the drug. Some patients will require prolonged or indefinite therapy in order to control their symptoms.

Second-Generation Antipsychotic (SGA) Agents

Many psychiatrists today would choose a newer atypical antipsychotic over pimozide, particularly in the elderly and those with known cardiac disease, because of the better safety profile, greater tolerability, and more specific actions. In a recent retrospective case series of patients with primary and secondary DP treated with various SGAs, partial or full remission was achieved in 37% and 38% of 63 cases, respectively, and overall, SGAs were felt to be as effective as traditional first-generation drugs, albeit with a lower rate of complete remission [26].

Risperidone is considered by some to be the first-line therapy for DP. Risperidone has been effective for some patients who have failed therapy with pimozide [26,27]. Risperidone preferentially blocks serotonin receptors while still maintaining some activity against dopamine receptors. Between 0.25 and 8 mg daily, administered in one or two doses, are required for clinical response, although most patients require 2–4 mg [26]. Adverse effects, including extrapyramidal reactions, can occur. A possible increased risk of cerebrovascular accidents in dementia patients receiving risperidone [28] has not been reported in patients with delusional disorders.

Olanzapine at doses of 2.5 to 20 mg daily also appears to be effective, but its use has been reported less frequently [26]. Success has also been reported with many other SGAs.

OUTCOME AND PROGNOSIS

Delusional parasitosis was previously considered a progressive disorder with only a 10% to 30% chance of spontaneous remission [11,17]. Antipsychotic therapy has resulted in markedly improved outcomes.

Prognostic factors include the type of DP (primary versus secondary), duration of illness prior to therapy, and the duration of therapy. In patients treated with SGAs, the time to onset of any effect and to maximal effect was shorter, and response rates higher (80% versus 68%) in secondary DP compared with primary DP, but these differences were not statistically significant [26]. Maximum effects of therapy were generally noted by 10 weeks in responders, suggesting that a lack of response by this time should prompt a change in treatment. The duration of symptoms may also affect outcome. In Trabert's study [4], the likelihood of a full remission was inversely correlated with the duration of symptoms, although this was not observed in patients treated with SGAs [26]. Sustained therapy of at least 8 weeks' duration and treatment supervision by a psychiatrist may also be associated with improved response rates [26]. Relapse rates are difficult to determine; they appear to be common and tend to respond well to re-institution of therapy, regardless of the antipsychotic agent used [6,15].

REFERENCES

1. Kendler KS. Demography of paranoid psychosis (delusional disorder): a review and comparison with schizophrenia and affective illness. Arch Gen Psychiatry 1982;39:890–902.
2. Bogren M, Mattisson C, Isberg PE, Nettelbladt P. How common are psychotic and bipolar disorders? A 50-year follow-up of the Lundby population. Nord J Psychiatry 2009;63:336–46.
3. Trabert W. Zur Epidemiologie des Dermatozoenwahns. Nervenarzt 1991; 62:165–9.
4. Trabert W. 100 years of delusional parasitosis: meta-analysis of 1,223 case reports. Psychopathology 1995;28:238–46.
   The earliest and largest case series in the literature which provides many observations about many features of DP.
5. Freudenmann RW, Lepping P. Delusional infestation. Clin Microbiol Rev 2009;22:690–732.
   A recent, very thorough review of all aspects of DP as they are currently understood.
6. Lyell A. Delusions of parasitosis. Br J Dermatol 1983;108:485–99.

7. Skott A. Delusions of infestation. Reports from the Psychiatric Research Center. No. 13. Göteborg, Sweden: St. Jörgen's Hospital, University of Göteborg, 1978.
8. American Psychiatric Association. DSM-IV-TR. Diagnostic and Statistical Manual of Mental Disorders, 4th edn, Text Revision. Washington, DC: American Psychiatric Association, 2000;323–9.
9. Munro A. Monosymptomatic hypochondriacal psychosis manifesting as delusions of parasitosis. A description of four cases successfully treated with pimozide. Arch Dermatol 1978;114:940–3.
10. Huber M, Kirchler E, Karner M, Pycha R. Delusional parasitosis and the dopamine transporter. A new insight of etiology? Med Hypotheses 2007; 68:1351.
11. Huber M, Karner M, Kirchler E, et al. Striatal lesions in delusional parasitosis revealed by magnetic resonance imaging. Prog Neuropsychopharmacol Biol Psychiatry 2008;32:1967–71.
12. Narumoto J, Ueda H, Tsuchida H, et al. Regional cerebral blood flow changes in a patient with delusional parasitosis before and after successful treatment with risperidone: a case report. Prog Neuropsychopharmacol Biol Psychiatry 2006;30:737–40.
13. Driscoll MS, Rothe MJ, Grant-Kels JM, Hale MS. Delusional parasitosis: a dermatologic, psychiatric, and pharmacologic approach. J Am Acad Dermatol 1993;29:1023–33.
14. [Anonymous]. The matchbox sign [letter]. Lancet 1983;2:261.
15. Zanol K, Slaughter J, Hall R. An approach to the treatment of psychogenic parasitosis. Int J Dermatol 1998;37:56–63.
16. Musalek M, Kutzer E. The frequency of shared delusions in delusions of infestation. Eur Arch Psychiatr Neurol Sci 1990;239:263–6.
17. Wykoff RF. Delusions of parasitosis: a review. Rev Infect Dis 1987;9:433–7.
18. Lynch PJ. Delusions of parasitosis. Semin Dermatol 1993;12:39–45.
19. Winsten M. Delusional parasitosis: a practical guide for the family practitioner in evaluation and treatment strategies. J Am Osteopath Assoc 1997;97:95–9.
20. Lepping P, Russell I, Freudenmann RW. Antipsychotic treatment of primary delusional parasitosis: systematic review. Br J Psychiatry 2007;191:198–205.
A review of the literature focusing on therapy with both traditional and atypical antipsychotic agents. Publications included here are limited non-randomized studies (crossover studies and case series) as no randomized clinical trials have been performed.
21. Bhatia MS, Jagawat T, Choudhary S. Delusional parasitosis: a clinical profile. Int J Psych Med 2000;30:83–91.
22. Zomer SF, de Wit FRE, van Bronswijk JEH, et al. Delusions of parasitosis: a psychiatric disorder to be treated by dermatologists? An analysis of 33 patients. Br J Dermatol 1998;138:1030–2.
23. Ungvari G, Vladar K. Pimozide treatment for delusions of infestation. Act Nerv Super (Praha) 1986;28:103–7.
24. Hamann K, Avnstorp C. Delusions of infestation treated by pimozide: a double-blind crossover clinical study. Acta Derm Venereol 1982;62:55–8.
25. Koo J, Gambla C. Delusions of parasitosis and other forms of monosymptomatic hypochondriacal psychosis: general discussion and case illustrations. Dermatol Clin 1996;14:429–38.
26. Freudenmann RW, Lepping P. Second-generation antipsychotics in primary and secondary delusional parasitosis: outcome and efficacy. J Clin Psychopharmacol 2008;28:500–8.
The largest case series of patients with DP treated with second-generation (atypical) antipsychotic agents.
27. Wenning MT, Davy LE, Catalano G, Catalano MC. Atypical antipsychotics in the treatment of delusional parasitosis. Ann Clin Psychiatry 2003;15: 233–9.
28. Mazzucco S, Cipriani A, Barbui C, Monaco S. Antipsychotic drugs and cerebrovascular events in elderly patients with dementia: a systematic review. Mini Rev Med Chem 2008;8:776–83.

PART

11

LABORATORY DIAGNOSIS OF PARASITIC DISEASES

154 General Principles

John H Cross[†], Brett E Swierczewski

A detailed travel history combined with the clinical presentation can help the clinician form a differential diagnosis and choose the most appropriate diagnostic testing. Confirmation of a clinical diagnosis will depend on the results of laboratory studies.

The techniques in the following chapters (Chapters 154.1 and 154.2) primarily describe tests for morphologic identification of parasites in stool, urine, blood, sputum, and tissue. Many of the tests can be performed by a clinician in the field and most should be available in basic laboratories throughout the world.

Increasingly, the diagnosis of parasitic infections relies upon immunologic tests that are highly sensitive and specific. Some serologic tests can be performed successfully in the field or clinical laboratory, whereas others require specialized laboratories not available in low-income settings. Similarly, molecular techniques such as PCR are useful in diagnosis, but are not widely available. However, antigen detection methods, such as rapid diagnostic tests for malaria (RDTs) are being rolled-out worldwide in the global effort to diagnose and treat malaria. Each of the individual pathogen chapters will discuss the immunologic and molecular diagnostic tests that are available.

154.1 Preparation of Samples for Morphologic Diagnosis of Parasites in Stool and Urine Specimens

John H Cross[†], Brett E Swierczewski

It is difficult to identify a parasite unless the correct method of examination is used. As feces and urine may also be infected with nonparasitic agents, universal precautions such as gloves, laboratory coats, safety glasses and, on some occasions, biologic safety cabinets may be needed.

PHYSICAL CHARACTERISTICS OF THE SPECIMEN

The consistency of a stool specimen is important. Trophozoites of intestinal protozoa are usually found in liquid or soft stools, but almost never in fully formed ones. Cysts of protozoa will usually be found in formed stools. Helminth eggs may be present in either liquid or formed stool.

Stools should first be examined for macroscopic parasites: pinworm, *Ascaris*, and tapeworm proglottids may be found. If blood is seen on the surface of stools, it is usually a sign of hemorrhoids; bloody mucus is suggestive of amebiasis, although it can be as a result of other conditions that cause inflammation of the colon. Blood-tinged mucus should always be examined for amebic trophozoites. Occult blood can be caused by parasites, but may also indicate other gastrointestinal disorders.

The age of an unpreserved specimen can determine whether or not parasites are found. Freshly passed specimens are essential for the detection of trophozoites. Liquid or soft stools are best examined *within one-half hour of the time of passage*. If this is not possible, part of the specimen should be preserved for subsequent examination. The immediate examination of fully formed specimens is not as critical, but when they cannot be examined on the day of collection they should be preserved if possible.

Most laboratories rely on specimens preserved in various fixative solutions available in commercial kits. The specimens can then be submitted to the laboratory for examination at a convenient time.

TECHNIQUES OF STOOL EXAMINATION

For detection of all types of parasites, trophozoites, cysts, and helminth eggs, a combination of two or more methods is desirable.

DIRECT WET FILM

This method should be reserved for examination of freshly passed liquid or soft stools or the mucoid portion of formed specimens. It also allows study of the motility of protozoa. Cysts and helminth eggs can be seen on wet film; however, concentration methods are more efficient for their detection.

In the preparation of a wet film, a small portion of feces is mixed with a drop of normal saline on a slide; a coverslip is placed on the preparation and examined unstained. The film should be thin enough so that newsprint can easily be read. After the wet film has been checked for trophozoites of amoeba and flagellates, an iodine stain can be used. Iodine stains cysts and reveals details that cannot be seen in an

[†]Deceased

unstained preparation. D'Antoni iodine solution is preferable. Organisms present in small numbers may not be seen on direct examination, but can be detected after concentration of the specimen.

MODIFIED D'ANTONI IODINE SOLUTION

Distilled water: 100 mL
Potassium iodide: 1 g
Powdered iodine crystals: 1.5 g

The potassium iodide solution should be saturated with iodine, with some excess remaining in the bottle. It is best to store it in brown, glass-stoppered bottles in the dark. The solution is ready for use after 4 days; sufficient quantity for daily use is decanted into a brown glass dropping bottle and discarded after 1 day. The stock solution remains good as long as an excess of iodine remains in the bottle.

PERMANENT STAINING OF FIXED SPECIMENS

The trichrome stain is used in most laboratories especially for amebae. A modified, acid-fast stain, such as the Kinyoun carbol-fuchin stain, is used for *Crypotosporidium, Cyclospora,* and *Isospora*. See [1] for staining methods; kits are commercially available.

Frequently, it is difficult to make an identification of protozoa—the cytologic detail revealed by one of the permanent stains is essential.

When fresh stool specimens are used, a small quantity of feces is transferred to a slide with an applicator stick. The material is then streaked out in a thin uniform film. When using fresh specimens, it is essential that the film be placed in fixative immediately to prevent drying out.

When polyvinyl alcohol (PVA) fixed material is used, the slides are allowed to dry for about 2 hours at room temperature. Gomori trichrome stain is the method frequently used. Helminth eggs can be difficult to identify in a trichrome stain.

CONCENTRATION METHODS

Concentration of stool specimens should be routinely done. Special techniques have been devised for the concentration of nematode eggs and larvae. These are simple to perform and should be used whenever the presence of parasites is suspected if they cannot be demonstrated by more direct examination.

The formalin-ethyl-acetate sedimentation technique is excellent for the concentration of both cysts and eggs. Concentration methods and reagent preparations are described in [1] and [2].

After concentration, two drops of the concentrated material are examined the same way for direct wet mounts using drops of iodine and saline.

EXAMINATION OF URINE AND VAGINAL SECRETIONS

Eggs of *Schistosoma haematobium*, microfilariae of *Wuchereria* and *Onchocerca*, and trophozoites of *Trichomonas vaginalis* can be found in urine and in prostatic and vaginal secretions. Organisms are best recovered by examination of centrifuged or membrane-filtered urine specimens. *Trichomonas vaginalis* in a fresh specimen of urine or in vaginal or prostatic exudate can be identified by its jerky motility.

SPECIAL DETECTION METHODS

AGAR PLATE CULTURE FOR STRONGYLOIDES LARVAE [3]

Agar medium is poured in a thin layer into a Petri dish, covered and allowed to harden overnight. A few grams of feces are placed into the center of the agar and incubated for 2–5 days at 28 °C. Tracks made in the agar by the larvae of *Strongyloides* can be seen and recovered by a Pasteur pipette. The collected material is placed onto a slide and examined microscopically for specific identification.

CELLOPHANE TAPE SWAB FOR ENTEROBIUS AND TAENIA EGGS

The test is easily performed with cellophane tape everted on an applicator stick and applied several times to the perianal region. The tape is then placed onto a slide and microscopically examined. Falcon™ Pinworm Paddles (Becton Dickinson, Franklin Lakes, NJ) are commercially available and are more easily used.

DUODENAL SAMPLING AND BIOPSY

Sampling of duodenal contents is a reliable means of recovery of *Strongyloides* larvae and other small intestinal parasites. Specimens can be obtained by intubation or by use of the enteric capsule or string test (Enterotest). Antigen detection tests have largely replaced duodenal sampling for *Giarda* and *Cryptosporidium* [4].

Biopsy of small intestinal mucosa may reveal *Giardia, Cryptosporidium,* and *Microsporidia*, as well as *Strongyloides* larvae.

METHODS FOR ESTIMATION OF WORM BURDEN

Estimates of daily egg output have been made for a number of hepatic and intestinal worms. This makes it possible to follow the results of therapy in a quantitative manner by periodic egg counts, allowing comparison of the efficacy of different medications. See [1] for methods.

KATO-KATZ THICK-SMEAR TECHNIQUE

This technique is particularly used in control programs and to evaluate treatment of intestinal helminths [5]. Kits are commercially available. A new technique—FLOTAC (flotation-translation)—is considered more sensitive than the Kato-Katz. Adaptation of FLOTAC allows the count of the parasites in 1 g of feces [6].

SPECIAL METHODS FOR INTESTINAL HELMINTHS

PLATYHELMINTHS

Gravid proglottids of *Diphyllobothrium* found in the feces can usually be identified by the presence of a uterine rosette in the middle of each segment. If no rosette is seen, the segments are probably those of *Taenia*. To differentiate between the two taenid species, segments should be rinsed in tap water and placed between two microscope slides that are separated at the edges by thin pieces of cardboard. The preparation can be fastened by means of rubber bands at each end of the slides so that the segments become somewhat flattened. The uterine branches should be visible under low-power microscopy. India ink injected into the segments can enhance the uterine branches.

NEMATODES

Nematodes found in the feces can be readily recognized by their internal structure. This may be made visible by clearing in glycerin or lactophenol.

REFERENCES

1. Ash L, Orihel T. Atlas of Human Parasitology, 5th edn. Chicago: ASCP Press; 2007.
2. Garcia LS. Diagnostic Medical Parasitology, 5th edn. Washington: ASM Press; 2007.
3. Arakaki T, Iwanaga M, Kinjo F, et al. Efficacy of agar-plate culture in detection of *Strongyloides stercoralis* infection. J Parasitic 1990;73:425.

4. Aldeen WE, Carroll K, Robison A, et al. Comparison of nine commercially available enzyme-linked immunosorbent assays for the detection of *Giardia lamblia* in fecal specimens. J Clin Microbiol 1998;36:1338–40.
5. Tarafder MR, Carabin N, Joseph L, et al. Estimating the sensitivity and specificity of Kato-Katz stool examination technique for the detection of hookworm, *Ascaris lumbricoides and Trichuris trichura* in human in the absence of a gold standard. Int J Parasitol 2010;40:399–404.
6. Knoop S, Speich B, Hattendorf J, et al. Diagnostic accuracy of Kato-Katz and FLOTAC for assessing anthelminthic drug efficacy. PLoS Negl Trop Dis 2011;5(4):e1036.doi: 10/1371/journal.pntd.0001036.

154.2 Examination of Blood, Other Body Fluids, Tissues, and Sputum

Brett E Swierczewski, John H Cross[†]

EXAMINATION OF FRESH BLOOD

Microscopic examination of fresh blood is useful for detection of trypanosomes and microfilariae. A small drop of blood is placed on a slide and covered with a coverglass. The high-dry objective with reduced illumination is suitable for trypanosomes, while low-power is used for detection of microfilariae.

THE THIN FILM

Thin and thick blood films are used for species identification of malarial parasites (Chapter 96), trypanosomes (Chapters 97 and 98), and microfilariae (Chapters 110–113). To prepare a thin film, place a small drop of blood from the fingertip, earlobe, or vial of blood near one end of a microscope slide. Raise the end of the slide farthest from the drop of blood and take a second slide as a spreader, making an angle of approximately 30 degrees with the first. Allow the blood to touch the spreader slide and begin to run out toward the edges. Before the blood has a chance to reach the edges, pull the spreader slide in an even, quick motion so that the drop is drawn out into a thin film. This will form a "comet's tail" toward the end of the slide.

Thin films must be fixed in absolute methyl alcohol for 1 minute and air-dried before being placed in diluted Giemsa (1 part Giemsa to 9 parts buffered water) and stained. After 45 minutes, slides are washed in buffered water and allowed to dry. If the slide contains a thick film and a thin film, fix only the thin portion then stain both parts of the film simultaneously.

THICK BLOOD FILMS

When a thick layer of blood is used, many more parasites will be present in each field; however, increased distortion of the parasites is common. To prepare a thick film, place three drops of blood close together near one end of the slide. With a corner of another slide, stir the blood, mingling the three drops over an area 2 cm in diameter. After the films are thoroughly dry, immerse the slide in buffer solution prior to staining or in Giemsa's stain itself. When Giemsa's stain is used for thick films, the procedure is the same as for thin films except that the fixation step is omitted. Thick and thin films can be made on the same slide.

ESTIMATING NUMBERS OF MALARIA PARASITES IN BLOOD

Determine the patient's white blood cell count. On a thick blood smear, count the number of parasites seen per 100 white blood cells; the total number per cubic millimeter of blood can then be determined. Parasites can also be quantified as a percent of the number of red blood cells infected, for example 2%.

[†]Deceased

BLOOD CONCENTRATION PROCEDURES

Buffy coat films serve to concentrate white cells (in which *Leishmania* may be found) and are useful for detection of trypanosomes and microfilariae. A centrifugation technique is used to check for trypanosomes when they are too sparse to be seen in thick blood films. Small numbers of microfilariae in the blood can be detected by a membrane filtration technique.

QUANTITATIVE BUFFY COAT

The QBC Malaria Test is a rapid diagnostic method used for malaria parasites.

RAPID DIAGNOSTIC TESTS FOR MALARIA

Histidine-rich protein (PF HRP-2) is released by *Plasmodium falciparum* and can be detected on a nitrocellulose and glass fiber dipstick pretreated with a monoclonal antibody against HRP-2. The dipstick is placed in hemolyzed blood followed by a drop of reagent and read visually. There are several other malaria rapid diagnostic tests (RDTs) on the market and the World Health Organization has reviewed these (www.wpro.who.int/sites/rdt/home.htm).

EXAMINATION OF CEREBROSPINAL FLUID

Trophozoites of *Naegleria* (Chapter 102) and trypanosomes (Chapter 97) can be found in the cerebrospinal fluid (CSF). Detection of helminths in the CSF may also be possible in patients with severe infections. The CSF must be examined promptly, as trypanosomes will survive for only about 20 minutes, and *Naegleria* may become rounded and non-motile. The CSF is centrifuged (7000 × *g* for 10 minutes), the supernatant removed and the sediment examined under reduced illumination.

TISSUE IMPRESSIONS

Tissue impression smears stained with Giemsa's stain can be used for detection of *Leishmania* and *Toxoplasma*. Fresh lymph nodes, liver biopsy material, or bone marrow is lightly impressed on a slide, allowed to dry at room temperature and stained like a thin blood film. When dealing with lymph nodes or other tissue, it is best to prepare the smear from a freshly cut surface.

BIOPSY AND ASPIRATION

Spleen, liver, and bone marrow biopsies are used in the diagnosis of visceral leishmaniasis. Aspiration of enlarged posterior cervical or other involved lymph nodes will at times reveal African trypanosomes when the blood is apparently free of them. The lymph nodes are less often involved in Rhodesian (East African) sleeping sickness than in the Gambian (West African) form, or in Chagas' disease (American trypanosomiasis).

Aspiration of fluid from a hydatid cyst (done under ultrasonographic guidance) may reveal hydatid sand, but it must be remembered that certain hydatid cysts are sterile so the absence of scoleces or hooklets from the sediment is not necessarily evidence against the parasitic nature of the cyst. Aspiration of an amebic abscess will yield few parasites as they tend to occur in the tissue surrounding the abscess cavity.

Eggs of *Schistosoma mansoni* and *Schistosoma japonicum* can be found in tissue from the rectal mucosa when they cannot be recovered from the stool. Mucosa from the bladder wall, taken at cystoscopy or a rectal snip biopsy, may likewise reveal eggs of *Schistosoma haematobium* (Chapter 122). Larvae of *Trichinella spiralis* may be abundant in muscle. Microfilariae of *Onchocerca volvulus, Mansonella ozzardi*, and *Mansonella streptocerca* can be demonstrated in skin snips.

EXAMINATION OF SPUTUM

Examination of the sputum is indicated when there is a question of pulmonary paragonimiasis; eggs can also found in the feces. *Entamoeba histolytica* can be detected in the sputum of patients with pulmonary abscesses. *Pneumocystis jirovecii* (now designated a fungus) can be found in sputum, but is more readily seen in bronchial aspirates or in impression smears of lung biopsy material (Chapter 86). *Cryptosporidium* has occasionally been found in sputum and lung biopsy. Ruptured hydatid cysts can be recognized by the presence of hooklets in the sputum. *Strongyloides* larvae may also be found in sputum in disseminated infections.

Sputum specimens should be induced, if possible. Specimens should be examined by wet mount while fresh or preserved in polyvinyl alcohol (PVA) fixative for protozoa.

RAPID METHENAMINE SILVER STAIN FOR PNEUMOCYSTIS JIROVECII

The best results for detection of *Pneumocystis* are obtained with a methenamine silver impregnation technique [1]. *Pneumocystis jirovecii* will have a delicately stained wall, usually brownish or grayish, and rather transparent. Mucin will be taupe to dark gray.

CULTURE METHODS

Acanthamoeba and *Naegleria*, the leishmanias (Chapter 99), *Trypanosoma cruzi*, and *Toxoplasma* (Chapter 101) can be cultured with specific media.

OTHER CULTURE METHODS

Acanthamoebaa, Naegleria, and *Balamuthia* can be established in axenic cultures, as well as in cell culture. Novy–Mac Neal–Nicolle (NNN) medium is used for *Leishmania* and *Trypanosoma cruzi*, and Culbertson's medium for *Acanthamoeba*. Culture of *Toxoplasma* has been described [2] and is applicable to blood, CSF, placental and other tissues.

ANIMAL INOCULATION

Trypanosoma brucei gambiense and *Trypanosoma brucei rhodesiense* infections can be established in a number of laboratory animals. White rats, white mice, and guinea pigs are most useful for diagnosis and the maintenance of laboratory strains. Young animals are most easily infected. Rats infected with *T. brucei gambiense* will survive for several months with a low-grade parasitemia; if infected with *T. brucei rhodesiense*, they die within a short time with an overwhelming parasitemia. *Trypanosoma rangeli* multiplies in common laboratory animals but does not cause apparent disease. Young white rats and white mice can be infected with *T. cruzi*; the white mouse is best for diagnostic inoculation. Intraperitoneal or subcutaneous inoculation should be used; amounts of up to 2 ml of blood are injected, depending on the size of the animal. It is important to check rats for the presence of their common parasite, *Trypanosoma lewisi*, before inoculation.

For isolation of *Leishmania*, the hamster is most satisfactory. Following intraperitoneal or intratesticular inoculation, hamsters will develop a generalized infection with any form of *Leishmania*, and the organisms can be demonstrated in spleen impression smears or in testicular aspirates. This infection develops slowly, and culture methods are generally regarded as being superior for diagnostic use.

Toxoplasma gondii shows little host specificity and will infect all common laboratory animals. White rats and mice are generally used; rats develop a chronic infection and are good for maintenance of the strain, whereas intraperitoneal infection of mice results in proliferation of the organisms in the ascitic fluid and death of the mice within a few days. Mouse peritoneal fluid, rich in organisms, is used as a source of *Toxoplasma* for the Sabin-Feldman dye test and other diagnostic procedures.

Xenodiagnosis can be considered a special case of animal inoculation; the term was originally applied to the diagnosis of Chagas disease by feeding uninfected reduviid bugs on a patient suspected of having the disease. Subsequent examination of the bugs will reveal developmental stages of the parasites if the test result is positive.

REFERENCES

1. Yu PKW, Uhl JR, Anhalt JP. Rapid methenamine silver stain. Arch Pathol Lab Med 1989;113:111.
2. Shepp DH, Mackman RC, Conley FK, et al. *Toxoplasma gondii* reactivation identified by detection of parasitemia in tissue culture. Ann Intern Med 1985;103:218–21.

PART

12

DRUGS USED IN TROPICAL MEDICINE

Mebendazole

Allyson K Bloom, Edward T Ryan

DESCRIPTION

Methyl 5-benzoylbenzimidazole-2-carbamate.

AVAILABLE PRODUCTS

1. Mebendazole chewable tablets (generic mebendazole, Teva Pharmaceuticals) are available in 100 mg.
2. Mebendazole oral tablets can also be found under other names in other countries, including Anelmin®, Pantelmin® and Wormin®.
3. The manufacturer has discontinued production of mebendazole in the US.

INDICATIONS

1. Treatment of infections caused by nematodes, including *Ascaris* spp., hookworm, *Enterobius* spp., *Trichuris* spp., *Trichinella* spp., visceral and cutaneous larva migrans and *Capillaria* spp.
2. Mebendazole has also been reported to shorten the course of *Angiostrongylus* infection (unlabeled).
3. Mebendazole has been used for treatment of echinococcal disease as second-line therapy behind albendazole (unlabeled).

MODE OF ACTION

Benzimidazoles bind to, and inhibit the polymerization of, beta-tubulin. This inhibits cytoplasmic microtubule formation and glucose uptake within the parasite. This leads to immobilization and death of adult worms.

PHARMACOKINETICS

Bioavailability of mebendazole is poor, but is increased when ingested with food. As a result of poor absorption it can be used to target luminal-dwelling adult worms. Higher doses and longer courses are required for treatment of systemic disease. Absorbed drug undergoes rapid, first pass hepatic metabolism into inactive metabolites and excretion of absorbed drug is half renal and half biliary. There is significant intra- and inter-individual variability.

DOSE ADJUSTMENTS IN RENAL FAILURE

Adjustments for short courses are likely unnecessary. Close monitoring of long-term therapy is recommended.

DOSE ADJUSTMENTS IN LIVER FAILURE

Close monitoring of long-term therapy is recommended if biliary obstruction is present.

DOSE

For adults and children >2 years of age unless otherwise indicated.

- Treatment of ascariasis and trichuriasis:
  100 mg twice daily for three days or 500 mg once
  (drug of choice, but some studies report low cure rates for triuchuriasis).
- Treatment of capillariasis:
  200 mg twice daily for 21 days
  (second-line therapy behind albendazole).
- Treatment of enterobiasis:
  100 mg once, repeat at two weeks.
- Treatment of hookworm:
  100 mg twice daily for three days
  (less effective than albendazole for *Necator* spp.).
- Treatment of trichinellosis:
  200–400 mg three times daily for three days then 400–500 mg three times daily for 10 days
  (with steroids; second-line therapy behind albendazole).
- Treatment of visceral larva migrans:
  100–200 mg twice daily for five days.
- Treatment of strongyloidiasis:
  100 mg twice daily for three days
  (longer therapy may be required for cure; second-line therapy behind ivermectin).
- Treatment of mansonellosis:
  100 mg twice daily for 21 days
  (second-line therapy, but may be alternate to diethylcarbamazine [DEC] in onchocerca-endemic areas).
- Treatment of echinococcal hydatid disease:
  20–50 mg/kg daily for 3–6 months
  (second-line therapy behind albendazole).
- Treatment of alveolar echinococcosis:
  20–50 mg/kg daily for prolonged course
  (second-line therapy behind albendazole).

ROUTE OF ADMINISTRATION

Oral.

ADVERSE EVENTS AND SERIOUS ADVERSE EVENTS

Generally very well tolerated, especially for courses of three days or less. Abdominal pain, diarrhea and elevated liver function tests have been reported. With prolonged therapy and higher-than-recommended doses, neutropenia and hepatitis have rarely occurred. Rare hypersensitivity reactions include rash, urticaria and angioedema.

KEY DRUG INTERACTIONS

Decreased mebendazole levels have been reported when mebendazole has been co-administered with phenytoin or carbamazepine, and dose increases may be warranted in treatment of systemic infections.

CONTRAINDICATIONS

Avoid if previous serious adverse effect or hypersensitivity.

USE IN SPECIAL POPULATIONS

PREGNANCY

Category C. Mebendazole is teratogenic in animals, but has not been well studied in humans. No increased morbidity reported in case reports of women inadvertently treated during pregnancy. However, there was a trend towards increased congenital defects with exposure in the first trimester.

LACTATION

Mebendazole is excreted in animal milk; not well studied in humans.

PEDIATRICS

Studies in children <2 years old are limited, but the few available suggest that it is well tolerated.

ELDERLY (AGE > 60 YEARS)

No recommendations for dose adjustments are available for patients >60 years of age.

RESISTANCE

In livestock, decreased binding to tubulin has led to resistance to benzimidazoles; this has not yet been demonstrated in humans, although some studies suggest decreasing efficacy.

STORAGE

Store at room temperature.

FURTHER READING

Dayan AD. Albendazole, mebendazole and praziquantel. Review of non-clinical toxicity and pharmacokinetics. Acta Tropica 2003;86:141–59.

Drugs for Parasitic Infections. Med Lett Drugs Ther 2004;46:e1–12.

Horton J. Mebendazole. In: Grayson ML, ed. Kucer's Antibiotics, 6th ed. London: Hodder; 2010;2240–4.

Lexi-Comp Online. Available at: http://online.lexi.com (last accessed 1st March 2012).

Liu LX, Weller PF. Antiparasitic Drugs. New Engl J Med 1996;334:1178–84.

Luder PJ, Siffert B, Witassek F, et al. Treatment of hydatid disease with high oral doses of mebendazole: Long term follow up of plasma mebendazole levels and drug interactions. Eur J Clin Pharm 1986;31:443–8.

Albendazole

Allyson K Bloom, Edward T Ryan

DESCRIPTION

Methyl 5-(propylthio)-2-benzimidazole carbamate.

AVAILABLE PRODUCTS

1. Albendazole tablets (Albenza®, GlaxoSmithKline) are available in 200 mg.
2. Albendazole oral tablets can also be found under other names in other countries including Albex®, Alzental®, Eskazole®, Helmidazole®, Parhel® and Zentel®.
3. Albendazole suspension (Zentel®, GlaxoSmithKline) is available in some countries in 100 mg per 5 ml.

INDICATIONS

1. Treatment of neurocysticercosis caused by *Taenia solium*.
2. Treatment of hydatid disease caused by *Echinococcus* spp.
3. Treatment of nematode infection, including those caused by *Ascaris* spp., hookworm, *Enterobius* spp., *Trichuris* spp., *Strongyloides* spp., cutaneous and visceral larva migrans, trichinella, *Gnathostoma* spp., *Capillaria* spp. and *Gongylonema* spp. (unlabeled).
4. Treatment of giardiasis (unlabeled).
5. Treatment of AIDS-related microsporidiosis (unlabeled).
6. Treatment of infection caused by *Clonorchis sinensis* (unlabeled).
7. Albendazole has also been used for treatment of anisakiasis, prevention of clinical disease in patients who may have been exposed to *Baylisascaris procyonis* and as second-line or adjunctive therapy in filariasis (unlabeled).

MODE OF ACTION

The active metabolite of albendazole – albendazole sulfoxide – binds to, and inhibits, the polymerization of beta-tubulin. This inhibits cytoplasmic microtubule formation and glucose uptake within the parasite. This leads to immobilization and death of adult worms and prevents hatching of eggs.

PHARMACOKINETICS

Bioavailability of albendazole is poor, but is increased when ingested with food. Absorption can be increased five-fold when albendazole is ingested with high-fat foods. Albendazole is rapidly converted to albendazole sulfoxide via first pass hepatic metabolism, reaching peak levels 2–5 hours after ingestion. Albendazole sulfoxide is 70% protein bound in plasma and is distributed throughout tissue, including cerebrospinal fluid. Concentrations in hydatid cyst fluid are higher than those seen for mebendazole. The mean half-life is 8–12 hours, with excretion probably through the biliary system. Conversion to albendazole sulfoxide also occurs in the gut epithelium, where the metabolite is then excreted directly into the lumen. There is significant intra- and inter-individual variability.

DOSE ADJUSTMENTS IN RENAL FAILURE

Dose adjustments are likely unnecessary, as urinary excretion of albendazole and its metabolites are negligible.

DOSE ADJUSTMENTS IN LIVER FAILURE

Close monitoring is recommended if biliary obstruction is present.

DOSE

All doses are for adults. For children: 15 mg/kg/day up to maximum daily dose of 800mg.

- Treatment of echinococcal hydatid disease:
  400 mg twice daily with fatty food
  (often in conjunction with surgical resection/aspiration, as clinically indicated).
  Duration of therapy ranging from few weeks to prolonged, depending on clinical course and indication.
- Treatment of alveolar echinococcosis:
  400 mg twice daily with fatty food over prolonged course.
- Treatment of neurocysticercosis caused by *Taenia solium*:
  400 mg twice daily for 8–28 days, repeated as necessary
  (in setting of viable cysts, with steroids and anti-seizure therapy).
- Treatment of ascariasis and hookworm infection:
  400 mg once
  children <2 years: 200 mg once
  (more effective for *Ancylostoma* than *Necator*; increased duration to three days may improve efficacy).
- Treatment of enterobiasis:
  400 mg once, repeated at two weeks.
- Treatment of chronic strongyloidiasis:
  400 mg twice daily for three days
  (second-line therapy behind ivermectin).
- Treatment of trichuriasis:
  400 mg daily for three days.
- Treatment of trichinellosis:
  400 mg twice daily for 8–14 days
  (with steroids).
- Treatment of capillariasis:
  400 mg daily for ten days.
- Treatment of cutaneous larva migrans:
  400 mg daily for three days.
- Treatment of visceral larva migrans:
  400 mg daily for five days.
- Treatment of giardiasis:
  400 mg daily for five days.
- Treatment of AIDS-related microsporidiosis:
  400 mg twice daily for ≥2–3 weeks.

- Treatment of clonorchiasis:
  10 mg/kg daily for seven days.
- Treatment of gnathostomiasis:
  400 mg twice daily for 21 days
  (with surgical resection if possible).
- Treatment of gongylonemiasis:
  10 mg/kg daily for three days
  (with surgical resection).
- Treatment of mansonellosis:
  400 mg twice daily for 7–10 days
  (not effective against microfilariae).
- Treatment of onchocerciasis:
  400 mg daily for 3–7 days
  (second-line therapy, may be synergistic with ivermectin).
- Treatment of loiasis:
  400 mg twice daily for 3–7 days
  (second line therapy).
- Treatment of lymphatic filariasis:
  400 mg once in combination with antifilarial agents.

ROUTE OF ADMINISTRATION

Oral.

ADVERSE EVENTS AND SERIOUS ADVERSE EVENTS

Generally very well tolerated. Adverse events are rarely reported with courses less than seven days and when they do occur tend to be mild and transient. Symptoms from dying parasites may also contribute to the incidence of adverse effects.

- Gastrointestinal: elevations in liver enzymes can occur, usually mild, with rarer cases of hepatitis and liver failure. Abdominal pain, nausea and vomiting have been reported.
- Hematologic: bone marrow suppression can rarely occur and is more common in patients with underlying hepatic dysfunction. Usually resolves with discontinuation of treatment.
- Neurologic: headaches and dizziness. Use with caution in individuals with retinal cysticercosis owing to inflammation and risk of detachment.
- Dermatologic: alopecia and more rarely hypersensitivity reactions, erythema multiforme and Stevens-Johnson syndrome.

KEY DRUG INTERACTIONS

Albendazole is a minor substrate of the CYP1A2 and CYP3A4 isoenzymes and a weak inhibitor of the CYP1A2 isoenzyme. Steroids and praziquantel have been reported to increase plasma levels of albendazole sulfoxide, which may be clinically desirable. Chloroquine and other anti-malarials may decrease the level of anthelminthics, but this has not been demonstrated specifically for albendazole. Ritonavir use may decrease plasma levels of albendazole. Conivaptan strongly inhibits CYP3A4 and should be discontinued at least seven days prior to initiation of CYP3A4 substrates.

CONTRAINDICATIONS

Avoid if previous serious adverse effect or hypersensitivity.

USE IN SPECIAL POPULATIONS

PREGNANCY

Category C. Albendazole is teratogenic in animals, but has not been well studied in humans. No increased morbidity reported in case reports of women inadvertently treated during pregnancy. The World Health Organization (WHO) endorses treatment of pregnant women in the second and third trimesters (but not the first) for intestinal helminthiasis/anemia, if clinically indicated.

LACTATION

Albendazole is excreted in animal milk; not well studied in humans.

PEDIATRICS

Studies in children younger than 6 years are limited, but several studies have shown albendazole to be safe in children as young as 1 year of age. For children 1–2 years old, a dose of 200 mg is recommended. Use of albendazole in children <1 year old is not recommended.

ELDERLY (AGE >60 YEARS)

No recommendations for dose adjustments are available for patients >60 years of age.

RESISTANCE

In livestock, decreased binding to tubulin has led to resistance to benzimidazoles; this has not yet been demonstrated in humans, although some studies suggest decreasing efficacy.

STORAGE

Store at room temperature. Shield suspension form from light.

FURTHER READING

Abba K, Ramaratnam S, Ranganathan LN. Anthelmintics for people with neurocysticercosis (Review). Cochrane Database System Rev 2010;3:CD000215.

Bethony J, Brooker S, Albonico M, et al. Soil-transmitted helminth infections: ascariasis, trichuriasis, and hookworm. Lancet 2006;367:1521–32.

Corti N, Heck A, Rentsch K, et al. Effect of ritonavir on the pharmacokinetics of the benzimidazoles albendazole and mebendazole: an interaction study in healthy volunteers. Eur J Clin Pharm 2009;65:999–1006.

Drugs for Parasitic Infections. Med Lett Drugs Ther 2004;46:e1–12.

Lexi-Comp Online. Available at: http://online.lexi.com (last accessed 1st March 2012).

Liu LX, Weller PF. Antiparasitic Drugs. New Engl J Med 1996;334:1178–84.

Horton J. Mebendazole. In: Grayson ML, ed. Kucer's Antibiotics, 6th edn. London: Hodder; 2010:2227–39.

Ndyomugyenyi R, Kabatereine N, Olsen A, Magnussen P. Efficacy of Ivermectin and Albendazole alone and in combination for treatment of soil-transmitted helminths in pregnancy and adverse effects: A randomized open label controlled intervention in Masindi District, Western Uganda. Am J Trop Med Hyg 2008;79:856–63.

Solaymani-Mohammadi S, Genkinger JM, Loffredo CA, Singer SM. A meta-analysis of the effectiveness of albendazole compared with metronidazole as treatments for infection with *Giardia duodenalis*. PLOS Neg Trop Dis 2010;3:e682.

Anti-Tuberculosis Drugs

Sonya S Shin, Kwonjune J Seung

Anti-tuberculosis drugs, dosing (including pediatric dosing), interactions, adverse events and monitoring requirements, including interactions with anti-retroviral treatment regimens (see Chapter 27.1 for discussion of tuberculosis and Chapter 27 for discussion of HIV)

Appendix 1A Anti-Tuberculous Medications and Their Side Effects, from the "*PIH Guide To the Medical Management of Multidrug-Resistant Tuberculosis*"

Drug name (abbreviation)	Description and adult dose	Side effects	Monitoring requirements and comments
Isoniazid (H)	Bactericidal; inhibits mycolic acid synthesis most effectively in dividing cells; hepatically metabolized. Dose: 300 mg/day or 900 mg/day twice or thrice weekly	Common: hepatitis (10–20% have elevated transaminases), peripheral neuropathy (dose-related; increased risk with malnutrition, alcoholism, diabetes, concurrent use of aminoglycoside (AG) or ETO). Less common: gynecomastia, rash, psychosis, seizure	Monitoring: consider baseline and monthly aspartate aminotransferase (SGOT), especially if age greater than 50 years. Comments: give with pyridoxine 50 mg/day if using large dose or if patient is at risk for peripheral neuropathy (diabetes, alcoholism, HIV, etc.)
Rifamycins Rifampin (R) Rifabutin (RFB)	Bactericidal; inhibits protein synthesis by blocking mRNA transcription and synthesis; hepatically metabolized. Dose: R, 600 mg/day; RFB, 300 mg/day	Common: orange-colored bodily secretions, transient transaminitis, hepatitis, GI distress. Less common: cholestatic jaundice	Monitoring: baseline SGOT and bilirubin, repeat if symptoms (jaundice, fatigue, anorexia, weakness, or nausea and vomiting) for more than three days
Pyrazinamide (Z)	Bactericidal; mechanism unclear; effective in acidic milieu (e.g. cavitary disease, intracellular organisms); hepatically metabolized, renally excreted. Dose: 15–30 mg/kg/day	Common: arthritis/arthralgias, hepatotoxicity, hyperuricemia, adominal distress. Less common: impaired diabetic control, rash	Monitoring: baseline and monthly SGOT; uric acid can be measured if arthalgias, arthritis or symptoms of gout are present. Comments: usually given once daily, but can split dose initially to improve tolerance
Ethambutol (E)	Bacteriostatic at conventional dosing (15mg/kg); inhibits lipid and cell wall metabolism; renally excreted. Dose: 15–25 mg/kg	Common: generally well tolerated. Less common: optic neuritis, GI distress, arthritis/arthralgia	Monitoring: baseline and monthly visual acuity and red/green color vision test when dosed at greater than 15 mg/kg/day (more than 10% loss is considered significant); regularly question patient about visual symptoms

Appendix 1A Anti-Tuberculous Medications and Their Side Effects—cont'd

Drug name (abbreviation)	Description and adult dose	Side effects	Monitoring requirements and comments
Aminoglycosides (AG) Amikacin (AMK) Kanamycin (K) Streptomycin (S) **Polypeptides** Capreomycin (CM) Viomycin (VM)	Bactericidal; aminoglycosides inhibit protein synthesis through disruption of ribosomal function; less effective in acidic, intracellular environments; polypeptides appear to inhibit translocation of the peptidyl-tRNA and the initiation of protein synthesis; renally excreted. Dose: 15–20 mg/kg/day	Common: pain at injection site, proteinuria, serum electrolyte disturbances. Electrolyte disturbances are more common in patients receiving CM. Less common: cochlear ototoxicity (hearing loss, dose-related to cumulative and peak concentrations, increased risk with renal insufficiency, may be irreversible), nephrotoxicity (dose-related to cumulative and peak concentrations, increased risk with renal insufficiency, often irreversible), peripheral neuropathy, rash, vestibular toxicity (nausea, vomiting, vertigo, ataxia, nystagmus), eosinophilia. Otoxocity potentiated by certain diuretics, especially loop diuretics	Monitoring: baseline and then biweekly creatinine, urea, and serum potassium; more frequently in high risk patients. If potassium is low, check magnesium and calcium. Baseline audiometry and monthly monitoring in high risk patients (elderly, diabetic, or HIV-positive patients, or patients with renal insufficiency). Comments: observe for problems with balance; increase dosing interval or reduce dose and monitor serum drug concentrations as needed to control side effects.
Fluoroquinolones Ofloxacin (OFX) Levofloxacin (LFX) Moxifloxacin (MFX)	Bactericidal; DNA-gyrase inhibitor; renally excreted. Dose: OFX 800 mg/day; LFX 750–1000 mg/day; MFX 400 mg/day	Common: Generally well tolerated, well absorbed. Less common: diarrhea, dizziness, GI distress, headache, insomnia, photosensitivity, rash, vaginitis, psychosis, seizure (CNS effects seen almost exclusively in elderly)	Monitoring: no laboratory monitoring requirements. Comments: do not administer with antacids, sucralfate, iron, zinc, calcium or oral potassium and magnesium replacements; LFX and MFX have the most activity against *M. tuberculosis*
Cycloserine (CS)	Bacteriostatic; alanine analogue; interferes with cell-wall proteoglycan synthesis; renally excreted. Dose: 500–1000 mg/ day, initiate at 500 mg/day for 2–3 days, then gradually increase to full dose	Common: neurologic and psychiatric disturbances, including headaches, irritability, sleep disturbances, aggression and tremors. Less common: psychosis, peripheral neuropathy, seizures (increased risk of CNS effects with concurrent use of ethanol, H, ETO or other centrally acting medications), hypersensitivity	Monitoring: consider serum drug monitoring to establish optimal dosing. Comments: give 50 mg for every 250 mg of CS (to lessen neurologic adverse effects)
Thiamides Ethionamide (ETO) Prothionamide (PTO)	May be bactericidal or bacteriostatic depending on susceptibility and concentrations attained at the infection site; the carbotionamide group, also found on thiacetazone, and the pyridine ring, also found on H, appear essential for activity; hepatically metabolized, renally excreted. Dose: 500–1000 mg/day, initiate at 500 mg/day for 2–3 days, then gradually increase to full dose	Common: GI distress (nausea, vomiting, diarrhea, abdominal pain, loss of appetite), dysgeusia (metallic taste), hypothyroidism (especially when taken with PAS). Less common: arthralgias, dermatitis, gynecomastia, hepatitis, impotence, peripheral neuropathy, photosensitivity	Monitoring: consider baseline and monthly SGOT. Comments: may split dose or give at bedtime to improve tolerability; ETO and PTO efficacies are considered similar; PTO may cause fewer GI side-effects
Para-aminosalicylic acid (PAS)	Bacteriostatic; disrupts folic acid metabolism (thought to inhibit the biosynthesis of co-enzyme F in the folic acid pathway); hepatic acetylation, renally excreted. Dose: 12 g/day divided into 3 doses	Common: GI distress (nausea, vomiting, diarrhea), hypersensitivity, hypothyroidism (especially when taken with ETO). Less common: hepatitis, electrolyte abnormalities. Drug interactions: decreased H acetylation, decreased R absorption in non-granular preparation, decreased B12 uptake	Monitoring: no laboratory monitoring requirements. Comments: some formulas of enteric coated granules need to be administered with an acidic food or beverage (i.e. yogurt or acidic juice)

CNS, central nervous system; GI, gastrointestinal.
Available at: http://ftp.pih.org/inforesources/pihguide-mdrtb.html.

Appendix 1B Pediatric Dosing of Tuberculosis Drugs, from "*World Health Organization Guidelines for the Programmatic Management of Drug-Resistant Tuberculosis*"

Medication (abbreviation)	Dose	Maximum daily dose
Isoniazid (H)	10–15 mg/kg daily	300 mg
Rifampicin (R)	10–20 mg/kg daily	600 mg
Ethambutol (E)	15–25 mg/kg daily	1200 mg
Pyrazinamide (Z)	30–40 mg/kg daily	1500 mg
Streptomycin (S)	20–40 mg/kg daily	1000 mg
Kanamycin (K)	15–30 mg/kg daily	1000 mg
Capreomycin (CM)	15–30 mg/kg daily	1000 mg
Ofloxacin (OFX)	15–20 mg/kg daily	800 mg
Levofloxacin (LFX)	15–25 mg/kg daily	1000 mg
Moxifloxacin (MFX)	7.5–10 mg/kg daily	400 mg
Ethionamide (ETO)	15–20 mg/kg daily	1000 mg
Cycloserine (CS)	10–20 mg/kg daily	1000 mg
Para-aminosalicylic acid (PAS)	150 mg/kg daily	8 g (PASER™)

PASER, brand-name formulation of enteric-coated PAS.
Available at: whqlibdoc.who.int/publications/2011/9789241501583_eng.pdf.

Appendix 1C World Health Organization (WHO)-Recommended Use of Fixed-Dose Combinations for First-Line Treatment for Adults, from "*Who Tuberculosis Care With TB-HIV Co-Management*"

Weight	Initial phase (two months)	Continuation phase (four months)
	2 (HRZE)	4 (HR)
	Daily 56 total doses	Daily 112 total doses
	(Isoniazid 75 mg + rifampin 150 mg + pyrazinamide 400 mg + ethambutol 275 mg)	(Isoniazid 75 mg + rifampin 150 mg)
30–39 kg	2	2
40–54 kg	3	3
55–70 kg	4	4
Over 70 kg	5	5

HR, isoniazid + rifampin; HRZE, isoniazid, rifampin, ethambutol + pyrazinamide.

Appendix 2A Recommendations for Concomitant Treatment of Tuberculosis and HIV Infection, from the United States Centers for Disease Control and Prevention's (CDC) *"Managing Drug Interactions in the Treatment of HIV-related Tuberculosis"*

Combined regimen for treatment of HIV and tuberculosis	Pharmacokinetic effect of the rifamycin	Tolerability/toxicity	Antiviral activity when used with rifampin	Recommendation (comments)
Efavirenz-based ART* with rifampin-based TB treatment	Well-characterized, modest effect	Low rates of discontinuation	Excellent	Preferred (efavirenz should not be used during the first trimester of pregnancy)
PI-based ART* with rifabutin-based TB treatment	Little effect of rifabutin on PI concentrations, but marked increases in rifabutin concentrations	Low rates of discontinuation (if rifabutin is appropriately dose-reduced)	Favorable, though published clinical experience is not extensive	Preferred for patients unable to take efavirenz[†]
Nevirapine-based ART with rifampin-based TB treatment	Moderate effect	Concern about hepatotoxicity when used with isoniazid, rifampin and pyrazinamide	Favorable	Alternative for patients who cannot take efavirenz and if rifabutin not available
Zidovudine/lamivudine/abacavir/tenofovir with rifampin-based TB treatment	50% decrease in zidovudine, possible effect on abacavir not evaluated	Anemia	No published clinical experience	Alternative for patients who cannot take efavirenz and if rifabutin not available
Zidovudine/lamivudine/tenofovir with rifampin-based TB treatment	50% decrease in zidovudine, no other effects predicted	Anemia	Favorable, but not evaluated in a randomized trial	Alternative for patients who cannot take efavirenz and if rifabutin not available
Zidovudine/lamivudine/abacavir with rifampin-based TB treatment	50% decrease in zidovudine, possible effect on abacavir not evaluated	Anemia	Early favorable experiences, but this combination is less effective than efavirenz-based regimens in persons not taking rifampin	Alternative for patients who cannot take efavirenz and if rifabutin not available
Super-boosted lopinavir-based ART with rifampin-based TB treatment	Little effect	Hepatitis among healthy adults, but favorable experience among young children (<3 years)	Good among young children (<3 years)	Alternative if rifabutin not available; preferred for young children when rifabutin not available

ART: *antiretroviral therapy.*
**With 2 nucleoside analogues.*
[†]*Includes patients with non-nucleoside reverse transcriptase inhibitor (NNRTI)-resistant HIV, those unable to tolerate efavirenz and women during the first 1–2 trimesters of pregnancy.*

Appendix 2B Recommendations for Co-Administration of Anti-Retroviral Drugs with Rifampin, from the United States Centers for Disease Control and Prevention's (CDC) *"Managing Drug Interactions in the Treatment of HIV-related Tuberculosis"*

Non-nucleoside reverse transcriptase inhibitors			
	Recommended change in dose of antiretroviral drug	*Recommended change in dose of rifampin*	*Comments*
Efavirenz	None (some experts recommend 800 mg for patients > 60 kg)	No change (600 mg/day)	Efavirenz AUC ↓ by 22%; no change in rifampin concentration. Efavirenz should not be used during the 1st trimester of pregnancy
Nevirapine	No change	No change (600 mg/day)	Nevirapine AUC ↓ 37–58% and Cmin ↓ 68% with 200 mg twice/day dose
Delavirdine	Rifampin and delavirdine should not be used together		Delavirdine AUC ↓ by 95%
Etravirine	Etravirine and rifampin should not be used together		Marked decrease in etravirine predicted, based on data on the interaction with rifabutin
Single protease inhibitors			
	Recommended change in dose of antiretroviral drug	*Recommended change in dose of rifampin*	*Comments*
Ritonavir	No change	No change (600 mg/day)	Use with caution. Ritonavir AUC ↓ by 35%; no change in rifampin concentration. Monitor for antiretroviral activity of ritonavir
fos-Amprenavir	Rifampin and fos-amprenavir should not be used together		
Atazanavir	Rifampin and atazanavir should not be used together		Atazanavir AUC ↓ by >95%
Indinavir	Rifampin and indinavir should not be used together		Indinavir AUC ↓ by 89%
Nelfinavir	Rifampin and nelfinavir should not be used together		Nelfinavir AUC ↓ 82%
Saquinavir	Rifampin and saquinavir should not be used together		Saquinavir AUC ↓ by 84%
Dual protease-inhibitor combinations			
	Recommended change in dose of antiretroviral drug	*Recommended change in dose of rifampin*	*Comments*
Saquinavir/ritonavir	Saquinavir 400 mg + ritonavir 400 mg twice-daily	No change (600 mg/day)	Use with caution; the combination of saquinavir (1000 mg twice-daily), ritonavir (100 mg twice-daily), and rifampin caused unacceptable rates of hepatitis among healthy volunteers
Lopinavir/ritonavir (Kaletra™)	Increase the dose of lopinavir/ ritonavir (Kaletra™) – 4 tablets (200 mg of lopinavir with 50 mg of ritonavir) twice-daily	No change (600 mg/day)	Use with caution; this combination resulted in hepatitis in all adult healthy volunteers in an initial study
"Super-boosted" lopinavir/ritonavir (Kaletra™)	Lopinavir/ritonavir (Kaletra™) – 2 tablets (200 mg of lopinavir with 50 mg of ritonavir) + 300 mg of ritonavir twice-daily	No change (600 mg/day)	Use with caution; this combination resulted in hepatitis among adult healthy volunteers. However, there are favorable pharmacokinetic and clinical data among young children
CCR-5 receptor antagonists			
	Recommended change in dose of antiretroviral drug	*Recommended change in dose of rifampin*	*Comments*
Maraviroc	Increase maraviroc to 600 mg twice-daily	No change (600 mg/day)	Maraviroc Cmin ↓ by 78%. No reported clinical experience with increased dose of maraviroc with rifampin
Integrase inhibitors			
	Recommended change in dose of antiretroviral drug	*Recommended change in dose of rifampin*	*Comments*
Raltegravir	No change	No change (600 mg/day)	No clinical experience; raltegravir concentrations ↓ by 40–61%

Appendix 2C Recommendations for Co-Administration of Anti-Retroviral Drugs with Rifabutin, from the United States Centers for Disease Control and Prevention's (CDC) *"Managing Drug Interactions in the Treatment of HIV-related Tuberculosis"*

	Antiretroviral dose change	*Rifabutin dose change*	*Comments*
Non-nucleoside reverse-transcriptase inhibitors			
Efavirenz	No change	↑ to 450–600 mg (daily or intermittent)	Rifabutin AUC ↓ by 38%. Effect of efavirenz + protease inhibitor(s) on rifabutin concentration has not been studied. Efavirenz should not be used during the 1st trimester of pregnancy
Nevirapine	No change	No change (300 mg daily or thrice-weekly)	Rifabutin and nevirapine AUC not significantly changed
Delavirdine	Rifabutin and delavirdine should not be used together		Delavirdine AUC ↓ by 80%; rifabutin AUC ↑ by 100%
Etravirine	No change	No change (300 mg daily or thrice-weekly)	No clinical experience; etravirine Cmin ↓ by 45%, but this was not thought to warrant a change in dose
Single protease inhibitors	*Antiretroviral dose change*	*Rifabutin dose change*	*Comments*
fos-Amprenavir	No change	↓ to 150 mg/day or 300 mg 3 times/week	No published clinical experience
Atazanavir	No change	↓ to 150 mg every other day or 3 times/week	No published clinical experience. Rifabutin AUC ↑ by 250%
Indinavir	1000 mg every 8 hours	↓ to 150 mg/day or 300 mg 3 times/week	Rifabutin AUC ↑ by 170%; indinavir concentrations ↓ by 34%
Nelfinavir	No change	↓ to 150 mg/day or 300 mg 3 times/week	Rifabutin AUC ↑ by 207%; insignificant change in nelfinavir concentration
Dual protease inhibitor combinations	*Antiretroviral dose change*	*Rifabutin dose change*	*Comments*
Lopinavir/ritonavir (Kaletra™)	No change	↓ to 150 mg every other day of 3 times/week	Rifabutin AUC ↑ by 303%; 25-O-des-acetyl rifabutin AUC ↑ by 47.5-fold
Ritonavir (any dose) with saquinavir, indinavir, amprenavir, fos-amprenavir, atazanavir, tipranavir or darunavir	No change	↓ to 150 mg every other day of 3 times/week	Rifabutin AUC ↑ and 25-O-des-acetyl rifabutin AUC ↑, by varying degrees
CCR-5 receptor antagonists			
Maraviroc	No change	No change	No clinical experience; a significant interaction is unlikely, but this has not yet been studied
Integrase inhibitors			
Raltegravir	No change	No change	No clinical experience; a significant interaction is unlikely, but this has not yet been studied

Appendix 2D Overlapping Toxicities of Anti-Retroviral and Tuberculosis Drugs, from the "*PIH Guide to the Medical Management of Multidrug-Resistant Tuberculosis*"

Toxicity	Antiretroviral agent	Antituberculosis agent	Comments
Peripheral neuropathy	**Stavudine (D4T), didanosine (ddI), zalcitabine (ddC)**	**Linezolid (LZD), CS, H,** Aminoglycosides, ETO/PTO, E	Avoid use of D4T, ddI and ddC in combination with CS or LZD because of theoretically increased peripheral neuropathy. If these agents must be used and peripheral neuropathy develops, replace the anti-retroviral agent with a less neurotoxic agent
Central nervous system (CNS) toxicity	**Efavirenz (EFV)**	**CS**, H, ETO/PTO, Fluoroquinolones	Efavirenz has a high rate of CNS side-effects (confusion, impaired concentration, depersonalization, abnormal dreams, insomnia and dizziness) in the first 2–3 weeks, which typically resolve on their own. If the CNS side-effects do not resolve on their own consider substitution of the agent. At present, there are limited data on the use of EFV with CS; concurrent use is accepted practice with frequent monitoring for CNS toxicity. Frank psychosis is rare with EFV alone
Depression	**EFV**	**CS**, Fluoroquinolones, H, ETO/PTO	Severe depression can be seen in 2.4% of patients receiving EFV.* Consider substituting EFV if severe depression develops. The severe socioeconomic circumstances of many patients with chronic disease can also contribute to depression
Headache	**Zidovudine (AZT), EFV**	**CS**	Rule out more serious causes of headache such as bacterial meningitis, cryptococcal meningitis, CNS toxoplasmosis, etc. Use of analgesics (ibuprofen, paracetamol) and hydration may help. Headache secondary to AZT, EFV and CS is usually self-limited
Nausea and vomiting	**Ritonavir (RTV), D4T**, nelvirapine (NVP) and most others	**ETO/PTO, PAS, H, E, Z** and others	Nausea and vomiting are common adverse effects and can be managed. Persistent vomiting and abdominal pain may be a result of developing lactic acidosis and/or hepatitis secondary to medications
Abdominal pain	**All anti-retroviral treatment has been associated with abdominal pain**	**ETO/PTO, PAS**	Abdominal pain is a common adverse effect and often benign; however, abdominal pain may be an early symptom of severe adverse effects, such as pancreatitis, hepatitis, or lactic acidosis
Pancreatitis	**D4T, ddI, ddC**	**LZD**	Avoid use of these agents together. If an agent causes pancreatitis suspend it permanently and do not use any of the pancreatitis-producing anti-HIV medications (D4T, ddI, or ddC) in the future. Also consider gallstones or alcohol as a potential cause of pancreatitis
Diarrhea	**All protease inhibitors, ddI (buffered formula)**	**ETO/PTO, PAS,** Fluoroquinolones	Diarrhea is a common adverse effect. Also consider opportunistic infections as a cause of diarrhea or *Clostridium difficile* (a cause of pseudomembranous colitis)
Hepatotoxicity	**NVP, EFV, all protease inhibitors (RTV > other protease inhibitors), all nucleoside reverse transcriptase inhibitors (NRTIs)**	**H, R, E, Z,** PAS, ETO/ PTO, Fluoroquinolones	Also consider TMP/SMX as a cause of hepatotoxicity if the patient is receiving this medication. Also rule out viral etiologies as cause of hepatitis (Hepatitis A, B, C and cytomegalovirus), as well as other AIDS-related complications (*Mycobacterium avium* complex, lymphoma, etc.)
Skin rash	**Abacavir (ABC), NVP, EFV, D4T** and others	**H,R, Z, PAS,** Fluoroquinolones, and others	Do not re-challenge with ABC (can result in life-threatening anaphylaxis). Do not re-challenge with an agent that caused Stevens-Johnson syndrome. Also consider TMP/SMX as a cause of skin rash if the patient is receiving this medication. Thioacetazone is contraindicated in HIV because of life-threatening rash
Lactic acidosis	**D4T, ddI, AZT, lamivudine (3TC)**	**LZD**	If an agent causes lactic acidosis replace it with an agent less likely to cause lactic acidosis

Continued

Appendix 2D Overlapping Toxicities of Anti-Retroviral and Tuberculosis Drugs, from the "*PIH Guide to the Medical Management of Multidrug-Resistant Tuberculosis*"—cont'd

Toxicity	Antiretroviral agent	Antituberculosis agent	Comments
Renal toxicity	Tenofovir (TDF)	**Aminoglycosides, CM**	TDF may cause renal injury with the characteristic features of Fanconi syndrome, hypophosphatemia, hypouricemia, proteinuria, normoglycemic glycosuria and, in some cases, acute renal failure. There are no data on the concurrent use of TDF with aminoglycosides or CM. Use TDF with caution in patients receiving aminoglycosides or CM. Even without the concurrent use of TDF, HIV-infected patients have an increased risk of renal toxicity secondary to aminoglycosides and CM. Frequent creatinine and electrolyte monitoring every 1–3 weeks is recommended. Many anti-retroviral and anti-tuberculosis medications need to be dose adjusted for renal insufficiency
Nephrolithiasis	**Indinavir (IDV)**	None	No overlapping toxicities regarding nephrolithiasis have been documented between ART and anti-tuberculosis medications. Adequate hydration prevents nephrolithiasis in patients taking IDV. If nephrolithiasis develops while on IDV, substitute with another protease inhibitor if possible
Electrolyte disturbances	TDF (rare)	**CM, Aminoglycosides**	Diarrhea and/or vomiting can contribute to electrolyte disturbances. Even without the concurrent use of TDF, HIV-infected patients have an increased risk of both renal toxicity and electrolyte disturbances secondary to aminoglycosides and CM
Bone marrow suppression	AZT	**LZD**, R, RFB, H	Monitor blood counts regularly. Replace AZT if bone marrow suppression develops. Consider suspension of LZD. Also consider TMP/SMX as a cause if the patient is receiving this medication. Consider adding folinic acid supplements, especially if receiving TMP/SMX
Optic neuritis	ddI	**E**, ETO/PTO (rare)	Suspend agent responsible for optic neuritis permanently and replace with an agent that does not cause optic neuritis
Hyperlipidemia	**Protease inhibitors, EFV**	None	No overlapping toxicities regarding hyperlipidemia have been documented between ART and anti-tuberculosis medications. Follow WHO ART guidelines for management of hyperlipidemia
Lipodystrophy	**NRTIs (especially D4T and ddI)**	None	No overlapping toxicities regarding lipodystrophy have been documented between ART and anti-tuberculosis medications. Follow WHO ART guidelines for management of lipodystrophy
Dysglycemia (disturbed blood sugar regulation)	**Protease inhibitors**	ETO/PTO	Protease inhibitors tend to cause insulin resistance and hyperglycemia. ETO/PTO tend to make insulin control in diabetic patients more difficult and can result in hypoglycemia and poor glucose regulation. Gatifloxacin is no longer recommended for use in treatment of tuberculosis as a result of this side-effect
Hypothyroidism	D4T	**ETO/PTO, PAS**	There is potential for overlying toxicity; however, evidence is mixed. Several studies show subclinical hypothyroidism associated with HAART, particularly stavudine. PAS and ETO/PTO, especially in combination, can commonly cause hypothyroidism

*Bristol-Myers Squibb, letter to providers, March 2005.
TMP/SMX, trimethoprim-sulfamethoxazole.
Available at: http://ftp.pih.org/inforesources/pihguide-mdrtb.html.

Diethylcarbamazine (DEC)

LeAnne M Fox, Amy D Klion

DESCRIPTION

N,N-Diethyl-4-methylpiperazine-1-carboxamide dihydrogen citrate.

AVAILABLE PRODUCTS

1. DEC tablets (available from US Centers for Disease Control and Prevention): 50 mg.
2. DEC tablets can be found under other names in other countries, including Hetrazan®, Banocide® and Notézine®.

INDICATIONS

1. Treatment of *Loa loa*.
2. Prophylaxis for *L. loa*.
3. Treatment of lymphatic filariasis (*Wuchereria bancrofti, Brugia malayi, Brugia timori*).
4. Treatment of tropical pulmonary eosinophilia (TPE).
5. Treatment of *Mansonella streptocerca* infection (streptocerciasis).

MODE OF ACTION

The mechanism of action of DEC is poorly understood. It has no filaricidal effect *in vitro*, but appears to render microfilariae more susceptible to destruction by host defense mechanisms through effects on the surface membrane [1] and parasite motility [2]. The mechanism of action against adult worms is unknown [1], although some studies have suggested that DEC compromises intracellular processing and transport of certain macromolecules to the plasma membrane [3].

PHARMACOKINETICS

Peak serum levels are achieved in 1–2 hours after a single oral dose and plasma half-life varies from 2–10 hours, depending on the urinary pH. DEC is excreted by both urinary and extra-urinary routes; more than 50% of the oral dose appears in acidic urine as the unchanged drug. Alkalinizing the urine can elevate plasma levels, prolong half-life and increase the therapeutic effect and toxicity of DEC.

DOSE ADJUSTMENTS IN RENAL FAILURE

Consider dose adjustment in severe renal impairment [4].

DOSE ADJUSTMENTS IN LIVER FAILURE

None.

DOSE

- Treatment of *L. loa*:
  Adults and children >18 months of age: 3 mg/kg three times daily for 21 days.
- Prophylaxis against *L. loa*:
  Adults and children >18 months of age: 6 mg/kg up to 300 mg dose once weekly.
- Treatment of lymphatic filariasis*:
  Adults and children >18 months of age: 6 mg/kg/day divided in 3 doses for 12 consecutive days OR 6 mg/kg/day as a single dose.
- Treatment of TPE:
  Adults and children >18 months of age: 6 mg/kg/day divided in 3 doses for 14–21 days.

ROUTE OF ADMINISTRATION

Oral.

HOW TO GIVE THE DRUG

Administering with food can lessen intestinal upset.

ADVERSE EVENTS AND SERIOUS ADVERSE EVENTS

DUE TO THE DRUG ITSELF

- Gastrointestinal: nausea, gastrointestinal upset.
- Systemic: drowsiness.
- Other (rarely reported): rash.

DUE TO THE EFFECT ON THE PARASITE

- Hematologic: eosinophilia.
- Renal: hematuria, proteinuria.
- Gastrointestinal: abdominal pain, nausea.
- Neurologic *(L. loa)*: headache and, rarely, neuropsychiatric problems, entrapment neuropathy or encephalopathy.
- Skin and soft tissue: rash, subcutaneous nodules, angioedema, urticaria.
- Lymphatic *(W. bancrofti* and *Brugia spp)*: adenitis, lymphangitis and, rarely, acute lymphedema or hydrocele, scrotal nodules, epididymitis.
- Systemic: fever, headache, malaise, myalgia, arthralgia, orthostatic hypotension.

*For patients with microfilariae in the blood, some experts recommend starting with a lower dosage and scaling up: day 1: 50 mg, day 2: 50 mg three times/day, day 3: 100 mg three times/day, day 4–12: 6 mg/kg divided in three doses.

KEY DRUG INTERACTIONS

None.

CONTRAINDICATIONS

Onchocerciasis should be excluded in all patients with a consistent exposure history owing to the possibility of severe exacerbations of skin and eye involvement (Mazzotti reaction). DEC should be used with extreme caution in patients with circulating *L. loa* microfilarial levels >2500/mm^3 owing to the potential for life-threatening side effects, including encephalopathy and renal failure. Neither steroids pretreatment nor slow dose escalation prevents these complications.

USE IN SPECIAL POPULATIONS

PREGNANCY

Category C.

LACTATION

There is no information on DEC and breastfeeding.

PEDIATRICS

Safe and effective in children at least 18 months of age.

ELDERLY (AGE > 60)

No adjustment.

RESISTANCE

Not reported to date.

STORAGE

Room temperature, protected from light.

AVAILABILITY IN THE USA

DEC is not currently licensed for commercial use in the USA, but is available to US-licensed physicians from the CDC under an Investigational New Drug (IND) protocol for treatment of loiasis and lymphatic filariasis and chemoprophylaxis of loiasis.

COMMENTS ON USE

Dosing recommendations are empiric as no formal studies have been conducted. Consequently, lower doses may be prudent depending on the initial microfilarial load, patient age, weight and/or medical status (e.g. renal disease).

REFERENCES

1. Hawking F. Diethylcarbamazine and new compounds for the treatment of filariasis. Adv Pharmacol Chemother 1979;16:129–94.
2. Langham ME, Kramer TR. The "in vitro" effect of diethylcarbamazine on the motility and survival of *Onchocerca volvulus* microfilariae. Tropenmed Parasitol 1980;31:59–66.
3. Spiro RC, Parsons WG, Pery SK, et al. Inhibition of post-translational modification and surface expression of a melanoma-associated chondroitin sulfate proteoglycan by diethylcarbamazine or ammonium chloride. J Biol Chem 1986;261:1521–9.
4. Adjepon-Yamoah KK, Edwards G, Breckenridge AM, et al. The effect of renal disease on the pharmacokinetics of diethylcarbamazine in man. Br J Clin Pharm 1982;13:829–34.

Ivermectin

Philip J Cooper, Thomas B Nutman

DESCRIPTION

22,23-dihydroderivative of avermectin B_1.

AVAILABLE PRODUCT

Stromectol®/Mectizan® tablets (Merck Sharpe & Dohme): 3 mg and 6 mg.

INDICATIONS

1. Treatment of onchocerciasis (*Onchocerca volvulus*).
2. Treatment of lymphatic filariasis (*Wuchereria bancrofti, Brugia malayi*) in combination with albendazole or diethylcarbamazine.
3. Treatment of strongyloidiasis (*Strongyloides stercoralis*).
4. Treatment of scabies (*Sarcoptes scabies*).
5. Treatment of intestinal helminth infections:
   a. *Ascaris lumbricoides* – highly effective;
   b. *Trichuris trichiura* – more effective in combination with albendazole;
   c. hookworm – possible benefits by adding ivermectin to albendazole.
6. Ivermectin is effective for the treatment of other ectoparasitic infections, including human body lice and head lice.
7. Ivermectin appears to be effective for the treatment of cutaneous larva migrans caused by animal hookworms.

MODE OF ACTION

Ivermectin blocks transmission across nerve synapses that use glutamate-gated anion channels or γ–aminobutyric acid (GABA)-gated chloride channels through stimulation of GABA by presynaptic nerve endings and enhancement of binding to postsynaptic nerve endings. This effect prevents nerve impulse conduction causing parasite paralysis and death.

PHARMACOKINETICS

Peak serum levels are reached 4–5 hours after oral ingestion [1]; highly lipid soluble with highest concentrations observed in liver and fat [2] and extremely low levels in brain; plasma half-life is approximately 18 hours: liver metabolism and almost all ivermectin and/or its metabolites are excreted in feces and just 1% in the urine.

DOSE ADJUSTMENTS IN RENAL FAILURE

None.

DOSE ADJUSTMENTS IN LIVER FAILURE

None.

DOSE

- Treatment of onchocerciasis:
  Children/adults >15 kg weight: 150 μg/kg for one dose annually for ~5 years.
- Treatment of lymphatic filariasis [3]
  :Children/adults >15 kg weight: single dose of 150 μg/kg.
- Treatment of strongyloidiasis and other intestinal helminth infections [3, 4]:
  Children/adults >15 kg weight: single dose of 200 μg/kg.
- Treatment of scabies [5]:
  Children/adults >15 kg weight: single dose of 200 μg/kg. Repeat dose after 1–2 weeks.
- Treatment of human body lice and head lice [5]:
  Children/adults >15 kg weight: single dose of 200 μg/kg. Repeat dose after 1–2 weeks.
- Treatment of cutaneous larva migrans [5]:
  Children/adults >15 kg weight: single dose of 200 μg/kg.

ROUTE OF ADMINISTRATION

Oral.

HOW TO GIVE THE DRUG

On an empty stomach.

ADVERSE EVENTS AND SERIOUS ADVERSE EVENTS

Dermatologic: a Mazzotti-type reaction may follow 2–4 days after the administration of ivermectin in individuals with *O. volvulus* infection [6]. Such reactions are associated with localized pruritus and edema accompanied by papular or urticarial rashes. Occasionally, the patient may have systemic features, such as fever, postural hypotension, arthralgia, myalgia and headache. Pruritus and maculopapular rashes have been reported 2–4 days after treatment of scabies [5].

- Gastrointestinal: nausea and vomiting.
- Hematologic: single oral doses of ivermectin have been associated with prolongation of prothrombin times and occasional hematomas [7], but concern about hematologic effects in mass drug distribution does not appear to be justified [1].
- Hepatic: a temporary mild-to-moderate elevation of alanine amino transferase has been reported in some patients [8].
- Ocular: mild ocular irritation associated with death of *O. volvulus* microfilariae in the cornea and anterior chamber of the eye.

KEY DRUG INTERACTIONS

Rare post-marketing reports of increased International Normalized Ratio when co-administered with warfarin; may enhance some of the pharmacologic actions of diazepam.

CONTRAINDICATIONS

Possible concurrent infection with *Loa loa*. The death of *L. loa* microflariae may cause a severe, or even fatal, encephalopathy – individuals with heavy microfilaremia are particularly at risk. Individuals who may have an exposure history to *L. loa* should have heavy infections excluded by examination of thin blood films obtained at midday.

USE IN SPECIAL POPULATIONS

PREGNANCY

Category C.

LACTATION

Small quantities of ivermectin (2%) enter breast milk [2]. Treatment is not recommended in lactating women with infants less than one week of age.

PEDIATRICS

Recommended for use only in children >15 kg weight.

ELDERLY (AGE > 60)

No adjustment.

RESISTANCE

Resistance to ivermectin is widespread among veterinary parasites but still no proven resistance among parasites of human populations. Some evidence of reduced responsiveness of *O. volvulus* to ivermectin among a few individuals [9].

STORAGE

Room temperature, protect from light.

AVAILABILITY IN THE USA

Oral tablets (Stromectol®) available.

COMMENTS ON USE

None.

REFERENCES

1. Canga AG, Prieto AHS, Liebana MJD, et al. The pharmacokinetics and interactions of ivermectin in humans – a mini-review. AAPS J 2008;10:42–6.
2. Reynolds JEF, ed. Martindale. The Extra Pharmacopoeia, 30th edn. London: Pharamceutical Press; 1993.
3. Olsen A. Efficacy and safety of drug combinations in the treatment of schistosomiasis, soil-transmitted helminthiasis, lymphatic filariasis, and onchocerciasis. Trans R Soc Trop Med Hyg 2007;101:747–58.
4. Reddy M, Gill SS, Kalkar SR, et al. Oral drug therapy for multiple neglected tropical diseases. JAMA 2007;298:1911–24.
5. Dourmishev AL, Lyubmoir LA, Schwartz RA. Ivermectin: pharmacology and application in dermatology. Int J Dermatol 2005;44:981–8.
6. World Health Organization. Drug information. Geneva: World Health Organization; 1990: 48–9.
7. Homeida MM, Bagi IS, Gahlib HW, et al. Prolongation of prothrombin time with ivermectin. Lancet 1988;1:1346–7.
8. Ali BH, Bashir AA. Ivermectin in human filariasis: a mini-review. Vet Hum Toxicol 1990;32:110–13.
9. Osei-Atweneboana MY, Eng JK, Boakye DA, et al. Prevalence and intensity of *Onchocerca volvulus* infection and efficacy of ivermectin in endemic communities in Ghana: a two-phase epidemiological study. Lancet 2007;369: 2021–9.

Pentavalent Antimony

Alan J Magill

DESCRIPTION

Pentavalent antimony (SbV) is usually given as sodium stibogluconate (SSG) or meglumine antimoniate (MA).

AVAILABLE PRODUCTS

1. SSG (Pentostam®, GlaxoSmithKline) is available in a 100-ml amber glass bottle sealed with synthetic butyl rubber closures and aluminum collars. There are 100 mg of SbV per ml. Pentostam® also contains chlorocresol BP, glucono-delta-lactone HSE and sterile water for injections.
2. MA (Glucantime®, Sanofi-Aventis) is available in 5-ml glass ampoules each containing 85 mg per ml.
3. Generic SSG manufactured by Albert David Ltd (Calcutta, India) is available in multi-dose vials. Thirty ml contains SSG equivalent to 100 mg SbV in each ml.
4. There are many other manufacturers of SbV products around the world. The manufacturing consistency and quality of these products are not known.

INDICATIONS

Treatment of visceral leishmaniasis, cutaneous leishmaniasis and mucosal leishmaniasis. SbV is of less utility for the treatment of leishmaniasis recidivans, diffuse cutaneous leishmaniasis and post-kala azar dermal leishmaniasis as rhese syndromes require extended dose regimens.

MODE OF ACTION

Not known.

PHARMACOKINETICS

Following intravenous (IV) or intramuscular (IM) administration of sodium stibogluconate, antimony is excreted rapidly via the kidneys, the majority of the dose being detected in the first 12-hour urine collection. This rapid excretion is reflected by a marked fall in serum or whole blood antimony levels to approximately 1–4% of the peak level by eight hours after an IV dose. During daily administration, there is a slow accumulation of sodium stibogluconate into the central compartment so that tissue concentrations reach a theoretical maximum level after at least seven days.

DOSE ADJUSTMENTS IN RENAL FAILURE

There are no studies although most authorities recommend very careful monitoring if given to individuals with significant renal compromise.

DOSE ADJUSTMENTS IN LIVER FAILURE

There are no data in humans. High concentrations of antimony are found in the livers of animals after repeated dosage with SbV. Pentostam® should therefore be used with caution in patients with hepatic disease.

DOSE

Twenty mg/kg/day for 10–28 days depending on the clinical syndrome and parasite being treated. Older literature and current drug labels may still reference an upper limit of 850 mg given daily; however, the current recommendation is for 20 mg/kg without reference to an upper limit. [1,2]

ROUTE OF ADMINISTRATION

SbV is given intravenously (IV) and intramuscularly (IM) or intralesional (IL) injection. There are no oral forms of the drug.

Owing to the presence of particulates (size range: 20–300 μm) Pentostam® solution should be drawn up through a filter immediately prior to administration. These particulates are insoluble complexes formed by an interaction between product preservative and the antioxidant in the rubber stopper. Filters of pore size ≤5 μm and membrane types polyvinylidene difluoride, polyethersulphone, polysulphone, nylon, surfactant-free cellulose acetate and mixed cellulose esters have been shown to be suitable. Where sterile filters are not available, the risks and benefits of administering unfiltered Pentostam® therapy should be assessed by the clinician on an individual basis.

HOW TO GIVE THE DRUG

IV: the appropriate weight-determined dose can be added to 250 ml of dextrose and water and infused slowly over 20–30 minutes via a peripheral antecubital vein. Access can be obtained with a "butterfly" steel needle placed daily. Patients do not require an indwelling plastic catheter.

ADVERSE EVENTS AND SERIOUS ADVERSE EVENTS

- Immediate reactions: in the unlikely event of coughing, vomiting or substernal pain, administration should be discontinued immediately. In such cases, extreme care should be taken if Pentostam® is re-administered by this route.
- Gastrointestinal: some degree of anorexia, nausea, vomiting, diarrhea and/or abdominal pain is very common. Transient rises in serum lipase and amylase usually occur during treatment with

SSG. Symptomatic pancreatitis and deaths caused by pancreatitis have been reported. SbV commonly causes mild elevation (2–5-fold increase) of hepatic enzymes in serum which later return to normal.

- Systemic: malaise, headache and lethargy.
- Musculoskeletal: myalgias and arthralgias are quite common. Large joint (shoulders, hips) arthralgias can be quite severe, are dose-dependent and tend to become apparent by day 7–10 of treatment. Nonsteroidal anti-inflammatory drugs (NSAIDs) do not seem to offer much relief.
- Cardiac: electrocardiogram (ECG) changes, including reduction in T-wave amplitude, T-wave inversion and QT prolongation, are commonly observed. Prolongation of the QTc interval has been observed in some patients taking SSG and appears to be dose-related. There have also been reports of fatal cardiac arrhythmias in patients receiving higher dose antimonial therapy for visceral leishmaniasis. Therefore, ECG monitoring is recommended before and during (at least weekly) therapy with SSG. Where ECG monitoring is not available, the risks and benefits of SSG therapy should be assessed on an individual basis. If clinically significant prolongation of QTc interval occurs, SSG should be discontinued. ECG changes, notably alterations in T wave amplitude, may be expected in the majority of patients given SSG. These appear to be reversible on cessation of therapy and are not of serious significance. SSG should be used with caution in patients with cardiovascular disease, a history of ventricular arrhythmias or other risk factors known to predispose towards QT prolongation, for example those with congenital QTc prolongation or taking concomitant drugs known to significantly prolong the QT interval (e.g. class III anti-arrhythmics such as sotalol and amiodarone).
- Respiratory: transient coughing immediately following injection was reported with varying frequency during several trials.
- Hematologic: transient reductions in platelets, white blood cells and hemoglobin are not uncommon.
- Other (rarely reported) side-effects include fever, rigor, sweating, vertigo, facial flushing, worsening of lesions on the cheek, bleeding from the nose or gums, substernal pain, jaundice and rash. IV injection of Pentostam® may cause transient pain along the course of the vein and eventually thrombosis of that vein.

KEY DRUG INTERACTIONS

There are no known drug interactions. Past reports of sudden cardiac death have been reported when patients were treated with amphotericin B after they failed treatment with SbV.

CONTRAINDICATIONS

Pentostam® should not be given to any patient who has experienced a serious adverse reaction to a previous dose. Pentostam® should not be given to any patient with significantly impaired renal function as kidneys are the route of excretion.

USE IN SPECIAL POPULATIONS

PREGNANCY

SbV is contraindicated in pregnancy [3].

LACTATION

SbV is found in breast milk after IV dosing [4]. Children should not be breast-fed by mothers receiving Pentostam.

PEDIATRICS

SbV is used in infants, children and adolescents.

ELDERLY (AGE >60 YEARS)

There is little information on the effects of Pentostam on elderly individuals.

RESISTANCE

Therapeutic failures occur worldwide in all forms of leishmaniasis. Therapeutic failures likely due to resistance are especially high in Bihar, India for visceral leishmaniasis.

STORAGE

All products are light sensitive and should be stored in the dark. Do not freeze and do not store at temperatures >25 °C.

PRODUCT INSERT

1. Pentostam®: http://www.medicines.org.uk/EMC/medicine/2182/SPC/Pentostam+Injection/.
2. Glucantime.

AVAILABILITY IN THE USA

No SbV products are approved by the Unites States Food and Drug Administration (FDA) for any indication. Pentostam® is available under an Investigational New Drug (IND) application for civilians from the US Centers for Disease Control and Prevention (CDC) [http://www.cdc.gov/laboratory/drugservice/release-information.html] and for military personnel from the Walter Reed Army Medical Center in Washington, DC, USA.

COMMENTS ON USE

When serious or bothersome adverse events such as epigastric pain, marked chemical pancreatitis and pancytopenias occur, briefly stopping SbV (a "drug holiday") for 2–4 days until symptoms are resolving and laboratory abnormalities are returning to baseline is recommended. Interestingly, these symptoms and laboratory abnormalities do not recur when re-starting the drug at previous dose levels.

REFERENCES

1. Herwaldt BL, Berman JD. Recommendations for treating leishmaniasis with sodium stibogluconate (Pentostam) and review of pertinent clinical studies. Am J Trop Med Hyg 1992 Mar;46(3):296–306.
2. Control of the leishmaniasis: report of a meeting of the WHO Expert Committee on the Control of Leishmaniases, Geneva, 22-26 March 2010. (WHO technical report series; no. 949)
3. Mueller M, Balasegaram M, Koummuki Y, et al. A comparison of liposomal amphotericin B with sodium stibogluconate for the treatment of visceral leishmaniasis in pregnancy in Sudan. J Antimicrob Chemother 2006;58:811–15.
4. Berman JD, Melby PC, Neva FA. Concentration of Pentostam in human breast milk. Trans R Soc Trop Med Hyg 1989;83:784–5.

Pentamidine

Allyson K Bloom, Edward T Ryan

DESCRIPTION

4,4-[1,5-pentanediylbis(oxy)]bis-benzenecarboximidamid.

AVAILABLE PRODUCTS

1. Pentamidine isethionate for injection (Pentam-300®, APP Pharmaceuticals); available in 15-ml vials as 300 mg of lyophilized powder for reconstitution.
2. Pentamidine isethionate for aerosolization (Nebu-Pent®, APP Pharmaceuticals); available in 15-ml vials as 300 mg of lyophilized powder.
3. Dosing recommendations are usually based on the pentamidine isethionate formulation, which is labeled according to the weight of the isethionate salt compound. A mesylate salt compound is also available; dosing of the mesylate salt is based on the weight of pentamidine alone; 1.74 mg of pentamidine isethionate is equivalent to 1 mg of pentamidine alone.
4. Inhaled and injectable pentamidine can also be found under other names in other countries, including Pentacarinat®.

INDICATIONS

1. Treatment and prophylaxis of *Pneumocystic jiroveci* pneumonia (PCP).
2. Treatment and prophylaxis of *Trypanosoma brucei gambiense* (unlabeled):
   a. early stage without central nervous system (CNS) involvement.
3. Possible treatment of visceral leishmaniasis (unlabeled):
   a. in relapse after pentavalent antimony;
   b. some clinical trials report efficacy in cutaneous leishmaniasis.

MODE OF ACTION

Unclear *in vivo* mechanism.

PHARMACOKINETICS

Peak levels achieved at end of intravenous (IV) infusion or 40 minutes following intramuscular (IM) administration. Half-life: 6–9 hours. Distributes to kidneys, liver, spleen, lungs. Unknown metabolism. Excreted unchanged in the urine. Aerosol administration results in low systemic absorption.

DOSE ADJUSTMENTS IN RENAL FAILURE

- CrCl 10–50 ml/min: administer dose every 24–36 hours.
- CrCl <10: administer dose every 48 hours.

Not removed by renal replacement therapy, including dialysis.

DOSE ADJUSTMENTS IN LIVER FAILURE

None.

DOSE

INJECTABLE

- Treatment of PCP:
  3–4 mg/kg IV or IM daily × 14–21 days.
- Prevention of PCP:
  4 mg/kg IV or IM once every month.
- Treatment of blood-stage trypanosomiasis caused by *T. b. gambiense*:
  4 mg/kg IV or IM daily × 7–10 days.
- Prophylaxis of trypanosomiasis caused by *T. b. gambiense*:
  4 mg/kg IV or IM once every 3–6 months.
- Treatment of leishmaniasis (alternative agent for certain types of cutaneous leishmaniasis):
  2–3 mg/kg IV or IM daily or every other day for 4–7 doses.

INHALED

- Prevention of PCP:
  300 mg inhaled via Respirgard II nebulizer once every four weeks.

ROUTE OF ADMINISTRATION

IV, IM or inhaled. No oral preparation.

HOW TO GIVE THE DRUG

Do not reconstitute with sodium chloride (precipitation will occur).

- IM: dissolve the 300 mg contents of the vial in 3 ml sterile water. Administer the calculated dose via deep IM injection.
- IV: dissolve the 300 mg contents of the vial in 3 ml sterile water. Further dilute the calculated dose in 250 ml 5% dextrose in water. Infuse the calculated dose over 1–2 hours to a supine patient; monitor blood pressure.
- Inhaled: dissolve the 300 mg contents of the vial in 6 ml sterile water. Transfer into Respirgard II nebulizer reservoir. Using a 40–50 pounds per square inch (PSI) air or oxygen source, set the flow rate at 5–7 liters per minute.

ADVERSE EVENTS AND SERIOUS ADVERSE EVENTS

Administration of parenteral pentamidine has been associated with severe hypotension, hypoglycemia, pancreatitis, cardiac arhythmias and death. Extravasation of IV preparation can lead to necrosis. Sterile abscesses can occur at IM administration site.

- Renal: nephrotoxicity common. Hyperkalemia, hypocalcemia, hypomagnesemia.
- Endocrine: damages pancreatic islet cells; can lead to insulin release, hypoglycemia and eventual diabetes.
- Gastrointestinal: anorexia, nausea, vomiting common. Pancreatitis and hepatitis.
- Cardiac: prolonged QT prolongation and torsades de pointes.
- Respiratory: inhalational administration induces cough and bronchospasm.
- Hematologic: leukopenia, anemia, thrombocytopenia.

KEY DRUG INTERACTIONS

Do not administer with other drugs associated with QT prolongation (particularly arthemether, lumefantrine, nilotinib, quinine, chloroquine, ciprofloxacin, tetrabenazine, thioridazine, ziprasidone). As a substrate of CYP2C19, levels may be decreased by strong CYP2C9 inducers, such as carbamazepine, phenytoin, ritonavir and rifampin. Avoid concurrent use with other nephrotoxins, including amphotericin B, aminoglycosides and foscarnet.

CONTRAINDICATIONS

As above.

USE IN SPECIAL POPULATIONS

PREGNANCY

Category C.

LACTATION

Unknown.

PEDIATRICS

Dosing and safety in children >4 months old comparable to use in adults.

ELDERLY (AGE >60 YEARS)

No specific recommendations.

RESISTANCE

Leishmania resistance reported. Resistance may relate to decreased transport across protozoal membranes (for *Trypanosoma*) and into mitochrondria (for *Leishmania*).

STORAGE

Room temperature; protect from light.

AVAILABILITY IN THE USA

Available in the USA.

COMMENTS ON USE

Monitor glucose, electrolytes, renal function, hepatic function, blood pressure and EKG-QTc.

FURTHER READING

Bray PG, Barrett MP, Ward SA, Koning HP. Pentamidine uptake and resistance in pathogenic protozoa: past, present, and future. Trends Parasitol 2003;19: 232–9.

Ena J, Amador C, Pasqau F, et al. Once-a-month administration of intravenous pentamidine to patients infected with Human Immunodeficiency Virus as prophylaxis for *Pneumocystis carinii* pneumonia. Clin Inf Dis 1994;18:901–4.

Lexi-Comp Online. Available at: http://online.lexi.com (last accessed 1st March 2012).

O'Brien JG, Dong BJ, Coleman RL, et al. A 5-year retrospective review of adverse drug reactions and their risk factors in Human Immunodeficiency Virus-infected patients who were receiving intravenous pentamidine therapy for *Pneumocystic carinii* pneumonia. Clin Inf Dis 1997;24:854–9.

Soto-Mancipe J, Grogl M, Berman JD. Evaluation of pentamidine for the treatment of cutaneous leishmaniasis in Colombia. Clin Inf Dis 1993;16:417–25.

Nitazoxanide

Allyson K Bloom, Edward T Ryan

DESCRIPTION

2-acetyloxy-N-(5-nitro-2-thiazolyl)benzamide.

AVAILABLE PRODUCTS

1. Nitazoxanide tablets (Alinia®, Romark Laboratories); 500 mg.
2. Nitazoxanide oral suspension (Alinia®, Romark Laboratories); 100 mg/5ml; reconstituted form available in bottles of 60 ml.
3. Nitazoxanide tablets and oral suspension under other names in other countries, including Heliton® (Argentina), Annita® (Brazil), Celectan® (Colombia, Ecuador, Venezuela), Repinox® (Costa Rica, Dominican Republic, Guatemala, Honduras, Nicaragua, Panama, El Salvador), Nodik® (Guatemala), Daxon® (Mexico), Dexidex® (Mexico), Kidonax® (Mexico), Pacovanton® (Mexico), Paramix® (Mexico), Anelmin® (Paraguay) and Colufase® (Peru).

INDICATIONS

1. Treatment of giardiasis.
2. Treatment of cryptosporidiosis:
   a. in children aged 1–11 years;
   b. in immunocompetent adults;
   c. in patients with HIV/AIDS (unlabeled).
2. Clinical trials demonstrate efficacy in treating diarrhea associated with (unlabeled):
   a. protozoa: *Entamoeba histolyticum, Isospora belli, Balantidium coli;*
   b. helminths: *Ascaris lumbricoides, Trichuris trichiura, Hymenolepsis nana, Taenia saginata, Enterobius vermicularis, Ancylostsoma duodenale, Strongyloides stercoralis, Fasciola hepatica;*
   c. bacteria: *Clostridium difficile;*
   d. viruses: rotavirus.

MODE OF ACTION

Blockage of electron transport and anerobic metabolism through inhibition of pyruvate-ferredoxin oxidoreductase. Through an unknown mechanism, nitazoxanide also demonstrates activity against several organisms that do not contain pyruvate-ferredoxin oxidoreductase.

PHARMACOKINETICS

Food increases bioavailability. Metabolized in blood to active metabolite tizoxanide (desacetyl-bitazoxabide) which is glucuronidated in liver. Highly plasma protein-bound (99%). Excreted in urine, bile, and feces.

DOSE ADJUSTMENTS IN RENAL FAILURE

Use with caution.

DOSE ADJUSTMENTS IN LIVER FAILURE

None.

DOSE

- Treatment of infectious diarrhea:
  Adults/adolescents >12 years of age: 500 mg every 12 hours for three days.
  Children aged 4–11 years: 200 mg every 12 hours for three days.
  Children aged 1–3 years: 100 mg every 12 hours for three days.
- Treatment of cryptosporidiosis in adults with HIV:
  1000 mg every 12 hours for two weeks.

ROUTE OF ADMINISTRATION

Oral.

HOW TO GIVE THE DRUG

Give orally with food.

ADVERSE EVENTS AND SERIOUS ADVERSE EVENTS

Well tolerated.

- Gastrointestinal: nausea, vomiting, diarrhea, abdominal pain; events generally mild and self-limited when reported.

KEY DRUG INTERACTIONS

No major.

CONTRAINDICATIONS

Avoid in individuals with previous nitazoxanide serious adverse effect.

USE IN SPECIAL POPULATIONS

PREGNANCY

Category B.

LACTATION

Unknown.

PEDIATRICS

Not evaluated in children <1 year of age. Safe and efficacious in children >1 year of age.

ELDERLY (AGE >60 YEARS)

No adjustment.

RESISTANCE

None reported to date.

STORAGE

Room temperature. Reconstituted formula can be stored for up to seven days.

AVAILABILITY IN THE USA

Tablet and suspension available in the USA.

COMMENTS ON USE

No specific recommendations.

FURTHER READING

Fox KM, Saravolatz LD. Nitazoxanide: A new thiazolide antiparasitic agent. Clin Inf Dis 2005;40:1173–80.

Hoffman PS, Sisson G, Croxen MA, et al. Antiparasitic drug nitazoxanide inhibits the pyruvate oxidoreductases of *Helicobacter pylori*, selected anaerobic bacteria and parasites, and *Campylobacter jejuni*. Antimicrob Agents Chemother 2007;51:868–76.

Lexi-Comp Online. Available at: http://online.lexi.com (last accessed 1st March 2012).

Musher DM, Logan N, Bressler AM, et al. Nitazoxanide versus vancomycin in *Clostridium difficile* infection: A randomized, double-blind study. Clin Inf Dis 2009;48:e41–6.

Dapsone

Allyson K Bloom, Edward T Ryan

DESCRIPTION

4,4-diaminodiphenyl sulfone.

AVAILABLE PRODUCTS

1. Dapsone tablets (Jacobus Pharmaceuticals): 25 mg and 100 mg.
2. Topical formulation (Aczone® 5% topical gel, Allergan); packaged in 30 g tubes.
3. Dapsone oral tablets can also be found under other names in other countries, including: Dapsone® (Australia), Daps® (Argentina), Avlosulfon® (Canada), Disulone® (Czech Republic), Dapson®, (Denmark, Egypt, the Netherlands, Norway), Dapson-Fatol® (Germany), Dapsoderm-X® (Mexico), Dapsona® (Paraguay), Lepravir® (Phillipines), Sulfona® (Portugal), Dopsan® (Thailand) and Lennon-Dapsone® (South Africa).

INDICATIONS

1. Treatment of leprosy (in combination with other anti-leprosy agents).
2. Prophylaxis of *Pneumocystis jiroveci* pneumonia (PCP) (unlabeled).
3. Treatment of PCP (in combination with trimethorprim) (unlabeled).
4. Prophylaxis against toxoplasmosis in HIV (in combination with pyrimethamine) (unlabeled).
5. Treatment of acne vulgaris (topical formulation).

Dapsone has been demonstrated to be effective in the treatment of various autoimmune and inflammatory conditions, including recluse spider bites, dermatitis herpetiformis, bullous pemphigoid, relapsing polychondritis, leukocytoclastic vasculitis and rheumatoid arthritis.

MODE OF ACTION

Dapsone inhibits the synthesis of dihydrofolic acid by competing with para-aminobenzoate for the active site of dihydropteroate synthetase. Detailed mechanism unknown; however, dapsone may inhibit neutrophil function through prevention of the respiratory burst and inhibition of adherence to vascular endothelium.

PHARMACOKINETICS

Peak serum levels are achieved in 2–8 hours; 70–90% protein bound; widely distributed in the body, concentrating in liver, kidney, skin, muscle. Metabolized in the liver through acetylation. Metabolites are eliminated in the urine as glucuronide conjugates.

DOSE ADJUSTMENTS IN RENAL FAILURE

Decreasing dose in severe renal compromise may be indicated.

DOSE ADJUSTMENTS IN LIVER FAILURE

None.

DOSE

- Treatment of leprosy:
  Adults/adolescents >15 years: 100 mg once daily for months–years.
  Children: 2 mg/kg once daily for months–years
  (with one or more other anti-leprosy agent).
- Prophylaxis against PCP:
  Adults: 100 mg once daily or 50 mg twice daily.
  Children: 2 mg/kg once daily or 4 mg/kg (max 200 mg) once weekly.
- Treatment of PCP:
  Adults: 100 mg once daily for 21 days.
  Children: 2mg/kg once daily for 21 days
  (with trimethoprim).
- Prophylaxis against toxoplasmosis in HIV:
  Adults: 50 mg–100 mg once daily or 200 mg once weekly.
  Children: 2 mg/kg daily
  (with pyrimethamine and leucovorin).

ROUTE OF ADMINISTRATION

Usually oral. Topical formulation available for treatment of acne vulgaris.

HOW TO GIVE THE DRUG

Administering with food can lessen intestinal upset.

ADVERSE EVENTS AND SERIOUS ADVERSE EVENTS

- Gastrointestinal: nausea, vomiting, diarrhea, abdominal pain, hepatitis, pancreatitis can occur.
- Hematologic: hemolysis occurs in majority of patients on doses of 200 mg or greater a day resulting in a 1–2g/dl decrease in hemoglobin, may be life-threatening if G6PD deficiency. Dapsone

also associated with methemoglobinemia. Agranulocytosis can occur.

- Systemic: a hypersensitivity reaction can occur, and may include fever, lymphadenopathy, rash, anemia, hepatitis. Erythema nodosum leprosum and reversal reactions can occur in patients with leprosy.
- Other (rarely reported): peripheral neuropathy, pneumonitis, nephrotic syndrome, renal papillary necrosis, rashes, photosensitivity, erythema multiforme, exfoliative dermatitis and toxic epidermal necrolysis.

KEY DRUG INTERACTIONS

Dapsone is a substrate of the CYP3A4 and CYP2C9 isoenzymes; dapsone levels decreased by rifampin and rifabutin; increased with saquinavir, amprenavir, bosentan, conivaptan, imatinib. Non-enteric coated didanosine preparations may decrease absorption of dapsone, leading to clinical failure; dose staggering may attenuate this effect. Concomitant trimethoprim and dapsone therapy may increase the levels of each drug, and should be closely monitored. Concomitant use with anti-malarials may increase the incidence of hemolysis, especially in patients with G6PD deficiency. Avoid concurrent use with probenicid.

CONTRAINDICATIONS

G6PD deficiency. Hypersensitivity to sulfones; cross-sensitivity of sulfonamides and sulfones 0–55%.

USE IN SPECIAL POPULATIONS

PREGNANCY

Category C.

LACTATION

Dapsone enters breast milk in large quantities. Avoid breastfeeding during use.

PEDIATRICS

Safe and effective in children of at least four weeks of age.

ELDERLY (AGE > 60)

No adjustment.

RESISTANCE

Mycobacterium leprae can develop resistance to dapsone, especially during monotherapy.

STORAGE

Room temperature; protect from light.

AVAILABILITY IN THE USA

Oral and topical dapsone is available in the USA.

COMMENTS ON USE

G6PD levels should be checked prior to use. A complete blood count should be monitored regularly throughout treatment: weekly for the first month, monthly for six months, every six months subsequently.

FURTHER READING

Beumont MG, Graziani A, Ubel PA, MacGregor RR. Safety of dapsone as *Pneumocystis carinii* pneumonia prophylaxis in Human Immunodeficiency Virus-infected patients with allergy to trimethoprim/sulfamethoxazole. Am J Med 1996;100:611–16.

Coleman MD. Dapsone: Modes of action, toxicity, and possible strategies for increasing patient tolerance. Br J Derm 1993;129:507–13.

Lexi-Comp Online. Available at: http://online.lexi.com (last accessed 1st March 2012).

Mills J, Leoung G, Medina I, et al. Dapsone Treatment of *Pneumocystis carinii* pneumonia in the Acquired Immunodeficiency Syndrome. Antimicrob Agents and Chemo 1988;32:1057–60.

Mohle-Boetani J, Akula SK, Holodniy M, et al. The sulfone syndrome in a patient receiving dapsone prophylaxis for *Pneumocystis carinii* pneumonia. West J Med 1992;156:303–6.

Safrin S, Finkelstein DM, Feinberg J, et al. Comparison of three regimens for treatment of mild to moderate *Pneumocystis carinii* pneumonia in patients with AIDS: A double-blind, randomized trial of oral trimethoprim-sulfamethoxazole, dapsone-trimethoprim, and clindamycin-primaquine. Ann Intern Med 1996;124:792–802.

Subject Index

Page numbers followed by "f" indicate figures, "t" indicate tables, and "b" indicate boxes.

A

B

C

E

F

J

K

M

O

S

T

U

V

W

X